Anatomy of Breast

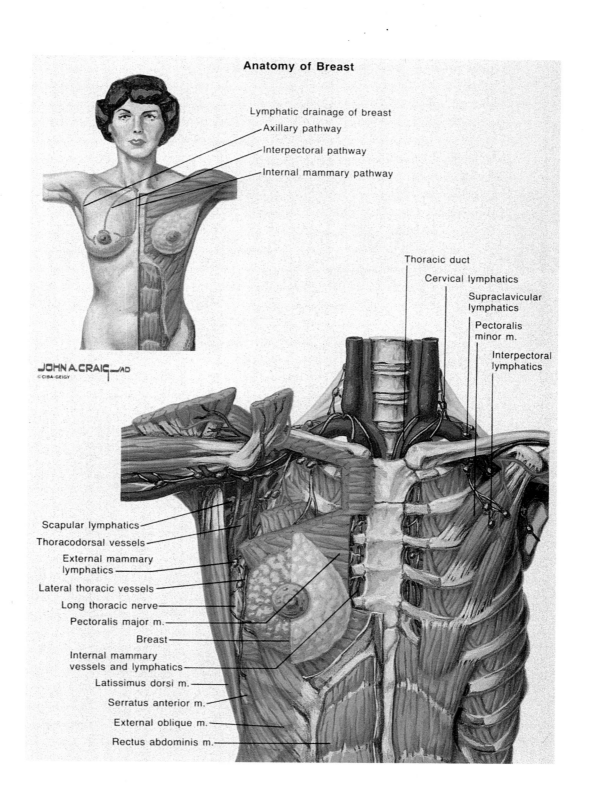

Lymphatic drainage of breast
Axillary pathway
Interpectoral pathway
Internal mammary pathway

Thoracic duct
Cervical lymphatics
Supraclavicular lymphatics
Pectoralis minor m.
Interpectoral lymphatics

JOHN A. CRAIG AD
©CIBA-GEIGY

Scapular lymphatics
Thoracodorsal vessels
External mammary lymphatics
Lateral thoracic vessels
Long thoracic nerve
Pectoralis major m.
Breast
Internal mammary vessels and lymphatics
Latissimus dorsi m.
Serratus anterior m.
External oblique m.
Rectus abdominis m.

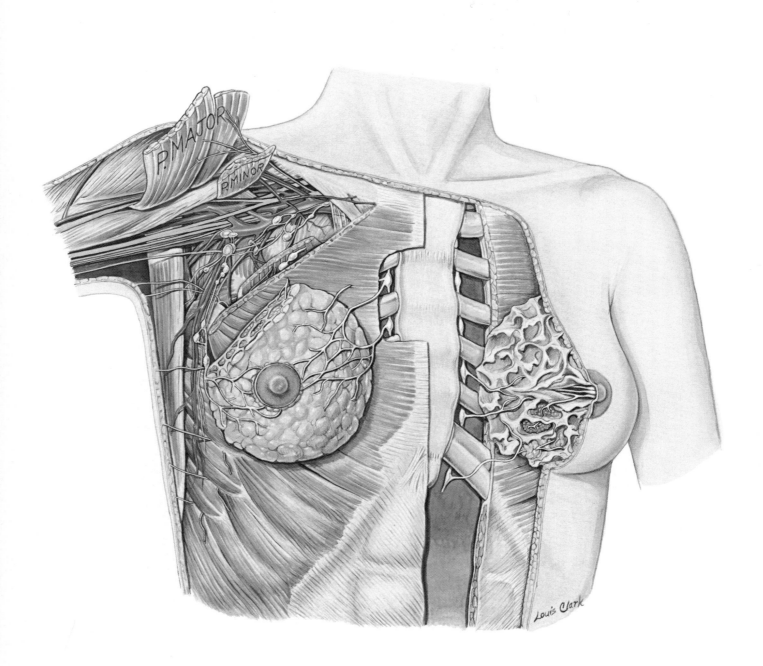

P. MAJOR

P. MINOR

Louis Clark

THE
BREAST

COMPREHENSIVE MANAGEMENT OF BENIGN AND MALIGNANT DISEASES

Edited by

KIRBY I. BLAND, M.D.

Professor and Associate Chairman
Department of Surgery
University of Florida College of Medicine
Gainesville, Florida

EDWARD M. COPELAND III, M.D.

Edward R. Woodward Professor and Chairman
Department of Surgery
University of Florida College of Medicine
Gainesville, Florida

W.B. SAUNDERS COMPANY
Harcourt Brace Jovanovich, Inc.
Philadelphia London Toronto Montreal Sydney Tokyo

W. B. SAUNDERS COMPANY
Harcourt Brace Jovanovich, Inc.

The Curtis Center
Independence Square West
Philadelphia, PA 19106

Library of Congress Cataloging-in-Publication Data

The Breast: comprehensive management of benign and malignant diseases. Edited by Kirby I. Bland and Edward M. Copeland III.

p.   cm.

1. Breast—Cancer—Treatment.   2. Breast—Diseases—
Treatment.   I. Bland, K. I.   II. Copeland, Edward M.
[DNLM: 1. Breast Diseases—therapy.
WP 900 B828]
RC280.B8B674 1991   618.1'9—dc20   DNLM/DLC
ISBN 0–7216–2234–8   90–8927
                                                               CIP

Editor: Edward H. Wickland, Jr.
Developmental Editor: Kathleen McCullough
Designer: Joan Wendt
Production Manager: Bill Preston
Manuscript Editors: Constance Burton and Kendall Sterling
Illustration Coordinator: Peg Shaw
Indexer: Linda Van Pelt

Art by Louis Clark and Jonathan Bland, copyright 1987. Reproduced with permission from the Clincal Symposia, John Craig, M.D. All rights reserved.

The Breast: Comprehensive Management of Benign
              and Malignant Diseases   ISBN 0–7216–2234–8

Last digit is the print number: 9   8   7   6   5   4   3   2

To our wives,
Lynn and Martha,
in appreciation for the generous support they provided to our careers
which allowed the development of this book,
and to our mentors,
Edward R. Woodward, Jonathan E. Rhoads, and Richard G. Martin, Sr.

Associate Editors

David L. Page, M.D.
Professor of Pathology
Director of Anatomic Pathology
Vanderbilt University Medical School
Vanderbilt University Medical Center
Nashville, Tennessee

Nancy Price Mendenhall, M.D.
Associate Professor
Department of Radiation Oncology
University of Florida College of Medicine
Gainesville, Florida

Warren E. Ross, M.D.
Executive Associate Dean
Professor of Medicine
University of Florida College of Medicine
Gainesville, Florida

Edward J. Wilkinson, M.D.
Professor of Pathology
Department of Pathology and Laboratory Medicine
University of Florida College of Medicine
Director of the Section of Surgical Pathology and Cytopathology
Shands Hospital at the University of Florida
Gainesville, Florida

Contributors

JOSEPH C. ALLEGRA, M.D.
Professor and Chairman, Department of Medicine, University of Louisville School of Medicine, Louisville, Kentucky.

FREDERICK C. AMES, M.D.
Associate Professor of Surgery, University of Texas Medical School at Houston; Chief, Breast Surgical Section, Robert F. Fly Chair in Surgery, M.D. Anderson Cancer Center, Houston, Texas.

MICHAEL J. ANDERSON, M.D.
Assistant Professor of Medicine, Uniformed Services University of the Health Sciences; Commander, Medical Corps, U.S. Navy; Head, Medical Oncology Division, National Naval Medical Center, Bethesda, Maryland.

RODRIGO ARRIAGADA, M.D.
Universite Paris-Sud; Radiation Oncologist, Institut Gustave-Roussy, Villejuif Cedex, France.

CHARLES M. BALCH, M.D.
Professor and Head, Division of Surgery, and Chairman, Department of General Surgery, M.D. Anderson Cancer Center; Associate Chairman, Department of Surgery, University of Texas Medical School at Houston, Houston, Texas.

ALFRED A. BARTOLUCCI, Ph.D.
Professor and Chairman, Department of Biostatistics and Biomathematics, University of Alabama at Birmingham, Birmingham, Alabama.

MICHAEL BAUM, Ch.M.
Professor of Surgery, The Institute of Cancer Research and The Royal Marsden Hospital; Honorary Director, Cancer Research Campaign Clinical Trials Centre, King's College School of Medicine and Dentistry, London, England.

ELLEN BENHAMOU, M.D.
Departement de Biostatistique et D'épidémiologie, Institut Gustave-Roussy, Villejuif Cedex, France.

SIMONE BENHAMOU, M.Sc.
Institut National de la Santé et de la Reserche Médicale; Institut Gustave-Roussy, Villejuif Cedex, France.

ROBERT BIRCH, Ph.D.
Assistant Professor, Department of Biostatistics and Biomathematics, University of Alabama at Birmingham, Birmingham, Alabama.

KIRBY I. BLAND, M.D.
Professor and Associate Chairman, Department of Surgery, University of Florida College of Medicine, Gainesville, Florida.

MARILYN BROWN, R.N., B.S.N.
Registered Nurse Specialist, Data Coordinator, Department of Surgery, University of Florida College of Medicine, Gainesville, Florida.

BLAKE CADY, M.D.
Associate Professor of Surgery, Harvard Medical School; Chief of Surgical Oncology, New England Deaconess Hospital, Boston, Massachusetts.

JEAN CHAVAUDRA, D.Sc.
Associate Professor, Faculty of Medicine, Universite Paris-Sud; Head, Medical Physics Department, Institut Gustave-Roussy, Villejuif Cedex, France.

JANE McGEE COLBURN, M.A.
Coordinator of Infant Care for Occupational and Physical Therapy in the Neonatal Intensive Care Unit and Special Care Nurseries, The Children's Hospital of Alabama, Birmingham, Alabama.

GENEVIÈVE CONTESSO, M.D.
Chief, Department of Anatomy and Pathology, Institut Gustave-Roussy, Villejuif Cedex, France.

EDWARD M. COPELAND III, M.D.
Edward R. Woodward Professor and Chairman, Department of Surgery, University of Florida College of Medicine, Gainesville, Florida.

ANNE R. CRAMER, M.D.
Breast Reconstruction Fellow, Eastern Virginia Medical Center, Norfolk, Virginia.

JEFFREY M. CRANE, M.D.
Clinical Instructor, University of North Carolina at Chapel Hill; Staff Physician, Rex Cancer Center, Raleigh, North Carolina.

WILLIAM S. DALTON, M.D., Ph.D.
Associate Professor of Internal Medicine and Pharmacology, University of Arizona College of Medicine; Arizona Cancer Center, University Medical Center, Tucson, Arizona.

JOHN M. DALY, M.D.
Jonathan E. Rhoads Professor and Chief, Division of Surgical Oncology, University of Pennsylvania School of Medicine, Philadelphia, Pennsylvania.

JOHN A. DEWAR, M.D.
Honorary Senior Lecturer, Ninewells Hospital and Medical School, Dundee; Consultant, Radiotherapy and Oncology, Ninewells Hospital, Dundee, Scotland.

ROBERT B. DICKSON, Ph.D.
Associate Professor of Anatomy and Cell Biology, Lombardi Cancer Research Center, Georgetown University School of Medicine, Washington, D.C.

ARTHUR J. DONOVAN, M.D.
Professor and Chairman, Department of Surgery, University of Southern California School of Medicine; Active Staff, Kenneth Norris Jr. Cancer Hospital, Los Angeles County (LAC)-USC Medical Center, Los Angeles, California.

MARILYN C. DOSS, M.A.
Special Assistant to the Vice President for Health Affairs, University of Alabama at Birmingham; University of Alabama Hospitals, Birmingham, Alabama.

WILLIAM D. DUPONT, Ph.D.
Associate Professor and Director, Division of Biostatistics, Vanderbilt University Medical School, Nashville, Tennessee.

PHILIP L. DUTT, M.D., J.D.
Fellow in Surgical Pathology, Department of Pathology, Vanderbilt University Medical School, Nashville, Tennessee.

LEE M. ELLIS, M.D.
Junior Faculty Associate, Department of Surgery, Clinical Surgical Oncology Fellow, M.D. Anderson Cancer Center, University of Texas Medical School at Houston, Houston, Texas.

JOSEPH T. ENNIS, M.D.
Director, Institute of Radiological Sciences, Mater Misercordine Hospital, Dublin, Ireland.

HOLLY EYLES, R.N., O.C.N.
Medical Oncology Specialist, Division of Medical Oncology, Shands Hospital at the University of Florida, Gainesville, Florida.

LESLEY J. FALLOWFIELD, D.Phil.
Senior Lecturer in Health Psychology, The London Hospital Medical College; Honorary Lecturer, Department of Surgery, Kings College Hospital, London, England.

ISAIAH J. FIDLER, D.V.M., Ph.D.
Professor of Pathology and Cell Biology, Graduate School of Biomedical Sciences, University of Texas Health Science Center; Chairman, Department of Cell Biology, M.D. Anderson Cancer Center, University of Texas Medical School at Houston, Houston, Texas.

BERNARD FISHER, M.D.
Distinguished Service Professor, University of Pittsburgh School of Medicine; Surgeon, Presbyterian-University Hospital, Pittsburgh, Pennsylvania.

GILBERT H. FLETCHER, M.D.
Professor of Radiotherapy, M.D. Anderson Cancer Center, University of Texas Medical School at Houston, Houston, Texas.

FRANÇOISE FONTAINE, M.D.
Department of Radiotherapy, Institut Gustave-Roussy, Villejuif Cedex, France.

DAISY A. FRANZINI, M.D.
Associate Professor, Department of Pathology, University of Florida College of Medicine; Attending Pathologist, Shands Hospital at the University of Florida; Chief, Anatomic Pathology Service, Veterans Administration Medical Center, Gainesville, Florida.

ERIC R. FRYKBERG, M.D.
Assistant Professor of Surgery, University of Florida Health Science Center; Chief, Divisions of General Surgery and Oncology, University Medical Center, Jacksonville, Florida.

THOMAS A. GASKIN, M.D.
Chief of Surgery, Baptist Medical Center-Princeton; Clinical Assistant Professor, University of Alabama School of Medicine, Birmingham, Alabama.

EDWARD P. GELMANN, M.D.
Professor of Medicine and Anatomy and Cell Biology, Georgetown University School of Medicine; Director, Division of Medical Oncology, Department of Medicine, Georgetown University Hospital, Washington, D.C.

WILLIAM H. GOODSON, III, M.D.
Associate Professor in Residence, Department of Surgery, University of California San Francisco, San Francisco, California.

JOHN T. HAMM, M.D.
Assistant Professor of Medicine, Division of Medical Oncology, University of Louisville School of Medicine, Louisville, Kentucky.

HERBERT C. HOOVER, Jr., M.D.
Associate Professor of Surgery, Harvard Medical School; Chief, Surgical Oncology Research, Associate Visiting Surgeon, Massachusetts General Hospital, Boston, Massachusetts.

J. SHELTON HORSLEY, III, M.D.
Professor of Surgery, Virginia Commonwealth University Medical College of Virgina; Medical College of Virginia Hospitals, Richmond, Virginia.

CHARLES E. HORTON, M.D.
Professor of Plastic Surgery, Eastern Virginia Medical School; Plastic Surgeon, Norfolk General Hospital; Children's Hospital of the King's Daughters; Leigh Memorial Hospital; DePaul Hospital, Norfolk, Virginia.

SCOTT A. HUNDAHL, M.D.
Associate Professor of Surgery, University of Hawaii John A. Burns School of Medicine; Queen's Medical Center; Kuakini Medical Center; Honolulu, Hawaii.

HUGO JAPAZE, M.D.
Chairman, Department of Pathology, University of Tucuman; Director of Pathology, University of Tucuman Hospital, Tucuman, Argentina.

MAUREEN KELLER-WOOD, Ph.D.
Assistant Professor, Department of Pharmacodynamics, College of Pharmacy, University of Florida College of Medicine, Gainesville, Florida.

PATRICIA ANN KELLY, P.T.
Assistant Director of Physical Therapy, Spain Rehabilitation Center, University of Alabama at Birmingham, Birmingham, Alabama.

EILEEN B. KING, M.D.
Clinical Professor of Pathology, Department of Pathology, Department of Epidemiology and Biostatistics, University of California San Francisco, San Francisco, California.

BARNETT S. KRAMER, M.D.
Professor of Medicine, Uniformed Services University of the Health Sciences; Senior Investigator, National Cancer Institute—Navy Medical Oncology Branch and National Naval Medical Center, Bethesda, Maryland.

STEPHEN S. KROLL, M.D.
Associate Professor of Surgery, M.D. Anderson Cancer Center, University of Texas Medical School at Houston; Clinical Associate Professor of Plastic Surgery, Baylor College of

Medicine; Assistant Surgeon, M.D. Anderson Cancer Center, Houston, Texas.

JEAN LaCOUR, M.D.
Head of the Department of Oncological Surgery, Institut Gustave-Roussy, Villejuif Cedex, France.

PHILLIPE LASSER, M.D.
Institut Gustave-Roussy, Villejuif Cedex, France.

MONIQUE G. LÊ, M.D.
Institut National de la Santé et de la Recherche Médicale; Institut Gustave-Roussy, Villejuif Cedex, France.

THIERRY LE CHEVALIER, M.D.
Universite Paris-Sud; Institut Gustave-Roussy, Villejuif Cedex, France.

HENRY PATRICK LEIS, JR., M.D.
Clinical Professor of Surgery in Breast Surgical Oncology and Honorary Director of Breast Center, University of South Carolina School of Medicine, Columbia, South Carolina. Professor Emeritus of Surgery, Emeritus Chief of the Breast Service and Emeritus Co-Director of the Institute of Breast Diseases, New York Medical College, Valhalla, New York.

MARC E. LIPPMAN, M.D.
Professor of Medicine and Pharmacology, Georgetown University School of Medicine, Washington, D.C. Clinical Professor of Medicine and Pharmacology, Uniformed Services University of the Health Sciences, Bethesda, Maryland. Director, Lombardi Cancer Research Center, Georgetown University Hospital, Washington, D.C.

HENRY T. LYNCH, M.D.
Professor and Chairman, Department of Preventive Medicine and Public Health, Creighton University School of Medicine, Omaha, Nebraska.

JANE LYNCH, B.S.N., R.N.
Instructor, Department of Preventive Medicine, Creighton University School of Medicine, Omaha, Nebraska.

DAVID MANT, M.B., M.F.C.M.
Clinical Lecturer, in General Practice, and Senior Clinical Scientist, Imperial Cancer Research Fund General Practice Research Group; Specialist, Community Medicine, Oxford District Health Authority, Oxford, England.

JOSEPH N. MARCUS, M.D.
Associate Professor of Pathology, Creighton University School of Medicine; Director, Flow Cytometry Laboratory, and Director, Immunopathology Laboratory, AMI Saint Joseph Hospital, Omaha, Nebraska.

SHAHLA MASOOD, M.D.
Associate Professor, Department of Pathology, University of Florida; Assistant Chairman, Department of Pathology, University Medical Center; Jacksonville, Florida.

JOHN B. McCRAW, M.D.
Professor, Plastic and Reconstructive Surgery, Eastern Virginia Medical School; Plastic Surgeon, Norfolk General Hospital, Leigh Memorial Hospital, Children's Hospital of the King's Daughters, and DePaul Hospital, Norfolk, Virginia.

MARSHA D. McNEESE, M.D.
Associate Professor, Department of Radiotherapy, M.D. Anderson Cancer Center, University of Texas Medical School at Houston, Houston, Texas.

NANCY PRICE MENDENHALL, M.D.
Associate Professor, Department of Radiation Oncology, University of Florida College of Medicine, Gainesville, Florida.

CAROLYN MIES, M.D.
Assistant Professor, Department of Pathology, University of Miami School of Medicine, Miami, Florida.

ANTHONY B. MILLER, M.B.
Professor, Department of Preventive Medicine and Biostatistics, University of Toronto Faculty of Medicine; Associate Member, Department of Surgery, Mount Sinai Hospital, Toronto, Ontario, Canada.

RODNEY R. MILLION, M.D.
Professor and Chairman, Department of Radiation Oncology, University of Florida College of Medicine; Medical

Director, Radiation Oncology Department, Shands Hospital at the University of Florida, Gainesville, Florida.

ELEANOR D. MONTAGUE, M.D.
Professor Emeritus, Department of Radiotherapy, M.D. Anderson Cancer Center, University of Texas Medical School at Houston, Houston, Texas.

GARTH L. NICOLSON, Ph.D.
Professor of Tumor Biology, Graduate School of Biomedical Sciences, University of Texas Health Science Center, Houston; Chairman, Department of Tumor Biology, M.D. Anderson Cancer Center, University of Texas Medical School at Houston, Houston, Texas.

JOHN E. NIEDERHUBER, M.D.
Professor of Surgery, Oncology, and Molecular Biology and Genetics, Johns Hopkins University School of Medicine; Division of Surgical Oncology, Johns Hopkins Hospital, Baltimore, Maryland.

MICHAEL P. OSBORNE, M.D., M.S.
Associate Professor of Surgery, Cornell University Medical College; Associate Member, Memorial Sloan-Kettering Cancer Center; Associate Attending Surgeon, Memorial Hospital for Cancer and Allied Diseases, New York, New York.

MARY JANE OSWALD, B.S.
Data Base Coordinator, Department of Radiotherapy, M.D. Anderson Cancer Center, University of Texas Medical School at Houston, Houston, Texas.

DAVID L. PAGE, M.D.
Professor of Pathology, Director of Anatomic Pathology, Vanderbilt University Medical School; Vanderbilt University Medical Center, Nashville, Tennessee.

RESAD PASIC, M.D., Ph.D.
Assistant Professor, Department of Obstetrics and Gynecology, University of Sarajevo; Women's Hospital, University of Sarajevo, Sarajevo, Yugoslavia.

K KENDALL PIERSON, M.D.
Professor and Chief of Anatomic Pathology, University of Florida College of Medicine; Attending Pathologist,

Shands Hospital at the University of Florida, Gainesville, Florida.

RAPHAEL E. POLLOCK, M.D., Ph.D.
Associate Professor of Surgery, M.D. Anderson Cancer Center, University of Texas Medical School at Houston; Associate Surgeon, M.D. Anderson Cancer Center, Houston, Texas.

MARILYN RANEY, M.A.
Statistician/Instructor, Department of Biostatistics and Biomathematics, University of Alabama at Birmingham, Birmingham, Alabama.

JOHN REYNOLDS, M.D.
Senior Registrar, St. Vincent's Hospital, Dublin, Ireland.

FRANCE ROCHARD, M.D.
Assistant Chirurgien, Institut Gustave-Roussy, Villejuif Cedex, France.

LYNN J. ROMRELL, Ph.D.
Professor of Anatomy and Cell Biology and Associate Dean for Education, University of Florida College of Medicine, Gainesville, Florida.

FRANCIS E. ROSATO, M.D.
Professor and Chairman, Department of Surgery, Jefferson Medical College of Thomas Jefferson University; Thomas Jefferson University Hospital, Philadelphia, Pennsylvania.

ANNE L. ROSENBERG, M.D.
Assistant Professor of Surgery, Jefferson Medical College of Thomas Jefferson University; Thomas Jefferson University Hospital, Philadelphia, Pennsylvania.

WARREN E. ROSS, M.D.
Executive Associate Dean, Professor of Medicine, University of Florida College of Medicine, Gainesville, Florida.

DANIÈLE SARRAZIN, M.D.
Chief, Radiotherapy Service, Institut Gustave-Roussy, Villejuif Cedex, France.

LORI J. SHEHI, M.D.
Assistant Professor, Department of Pathology, University of Florida College of Medicine, Gainesville, Florida.

S. P. SHETH, M.D.
Assistant Professor of Medical Oncology, Department of Medicine, University of Louisville School of Medicine, Louisville, Kentucky.

JEAN F. SIMPSON, M.D.
Assistant Professor, Vanderbilt University Medical School; Director, Immunocytochemistry Laboratory, Vanderbilt University Medical Center, Nashville, Tennessee.

WILEY W. SOUBA, M.D., Sc.D.
Assistant Professor of Surgery and Biochemistry, University of Florida College of Medicine, Gainesville, Florida.

MARC SPIELMANN, M.D.
Institut Gustave-Roussy, Villejuif Cedex, France.

DEMPSEY S. SPRINGFIELD, M.D.
Associate Professor in Orthopedics, Harvard Medical School; Visiting Orthopedic Surgeon, Massachusetts General Hospital, Boston, Massachusetts.

ANNE T. STOTTER, Ph.D.
Acting Assistant Director, Academic Surgical Unit, St. Mary's Hospital, London, England.

TONCRED STYBLO, M.D.
Assistant Professor, Department of Surgery, Emory University School of Medicine, Atlanta, Georgia.

SANDRA M. SWAIN, M.D.
Assistant Professor of Medicine, Director, Comprehensive Breast Center, Georgetown University School of Medicine, Lombardi Cancer Center, Washington, D.C.

NITIN T. TELANG, Ph.D.
Assistant Laboratory Member, Memorial Sloan-Kettering Cancer Center; Assistant Attending Biochemist, Department of Surgery Breast Service, Memorial Hospital for Cancer and Allied Diseases, New York, New York.

DANIEL W. TENCH, M.D.
Assistant Professor of Pathology, Mercer University School of Medicine, Macon, Georgia.

JEAN-PAUL TRAVAGLI, M.D.
Institut Gustave-Roussy, Villejuif Cedex, France.

JEROME A. URBAN, M.D.
Clinical Professor Emeritus of Surgery, Cornell University Medical Center; Memorial Sloan-Kettering Cancer Center, Memorial Hospital for Cancer and Allied Diseases, New York, New York.

UMBERTO VERONESI, M.D.
Director General, Istituto Nazionale per lo Studio e la Cura dei Tumori, Milan, Italy.

MARTIN P. VESSEY, M.D.
Professor of Social and Community Medicine, University of Oxford; Specialist in Community Medicine, Oxford District Health Authority, and Oxfordshire Regional Health Authority, Oxford, England.

FREDERICK B. WAGNER, JR., M.D.
Grace Revere Osler Professor Emeritus of Surgery and University Historian, Jefferson Medical College of Thomas Jefferson University; Honorary Attending Surgeon, Thomas Jefferson University Hospital, Philadelphia, Pennsylvania.

HAROLD J. WANEBO, M.D.
Professor of Surgery, Director, Surgical Oncology, Brown University Program in Medicine; Chief of Surgery, Roger Williams General Hospital, Providence, Rhode Island.

PATRICE WATSON, Ph.D.
Assistant Professor, Department of Preventive Medicine, Creighton University School of Medicine, Omaha, Nebraska.

MORTON C. WILHELM, M.D.
Joseph Farrow Professor of Surgical Oncology, University of Virginia School of Medicine; Attending Staff, University of Virginia Hospital; Consulting Surgeon, Veterans Administration Hospital (Salem); Charlottesville, Virginia.

EDWARD J. WILKINSON, M.D.
Professor, Department of Pathology and Laboratory Medicine, University of

Florida College of Medicine; Director of the Section of Surgical Pathology and Cytopathology, Department of Pathology, Shands Hospital at the University of Florida, Gainesville, Florida.

JAMES L. WITTLIFF, Ph.D.
Professor of Biochemistry, Director of Hormone Receptor Laboratory, University of Louisville School of Medicine; James Graham Brown Cancer Center, University of Louisville School of Medicine, Louisville, Kentucky.

TIMOTHY J. YEATMAN, M.D.
Junior Faculty Associate, Department of Surgery, Clinical Surgical Oncology Fellow, M.D. Anderson Cancer Center, University of Texas Medical School at Houston, Houston, Texas.

Preface

For some time, we have been urged to develop a comprehensive textbook that bridges multiple disciplines for the treatment of diseases of the breast. One readily recognizes the impact of breast disease in westernized societies, as carcinoma of this organ continues to increase exponentially in industrialized nations. In the United States, breast carcinoma remains one of the most common and, perhaps, feared health problems for women. Current estimates note that one of every ten American women will develop some variant of breast cancer, one of every three women will consult her physician for breast disease, and approximately one of every five women will undergo breast biopsy.

During the past two decades we have witnessed unparalleled advances in the treatment of neoplastic diseases of the breast. The integration of multidisciplinary approaches, including surgery, radiation oncology, medical oncology, pathology, radiology, pharmacology, genetics, and biostatistics, represents only a portion of the diagnostic and therapy team members implemented in treating cancer of the breast.

The purpose of the first edition of *The Breast: Comprehensive Management of Benign and Malignant Diseases* is to organize in a comprehensive, readable text the basic principles necessary for the diagnosis and treatment of various benign and malignant breast diseases. The ambitious task of organizing this volume has brought together many recognized authorities in the treatment of physiological, metabolic, and neoplastic derangements of the mammary gland. Although we consider this text to be comprehensive, it is neither intended to replace standard books of surgery and medicine nor thought to be a fundamentally encyclopedic recitation of the myriad of pathological permutations that may exist with the various diseases of this organ site. Rather, our purpose is to familiarize the reader with the various surgical and medical illnesses that exist in derangements of normal breast physiology, growth, and neoplastic transformation encountered in diagnostic clinics throughout the world. This text is therefore intended to coexist with other major medical and surgical reference books. Each chapter makes a notation of carefully selected monographs, journal articles, or chapters within major reference texts that the contributors of the individual chapters consider valuable resources. In essence, this tome represents a distillation of the fundamental and heralded contributions of innumerable physicians, physiologists, anatomists, geneticists, and other health-related workers who have devoted their lives to the management of diseases of the breast.

To comprehensively review the fundamental information included in this text, the book has been organized into 20 sections and 55 chapters. The first section deals with the history of breast diseases, including the major contributions of the twentieth century. Sequential sections are organized to review anatomy, physiology, pathology, genetics, surgery, pharmacokinetics, radiation biology, and biostatistics, as well as the special problems encountered in management of benign and malignant diseases of this organ site. Although some overlap invariably exists among multiple chapters, we have made every effort to minimize repetition, except when used to reiterate controversial or "state-of-the-art" issues for management. We also recognize that in the past several decades many have continued to emphasize the increasingly symbiotic relationship between the basic sciences of medicine and their clinical counterparts to provide an integration of these disciplines that allows for the successful approach to the diagnosis and management of breast disease.

To publish a comprehensive treatise for the diseases of this organ demanded the cooperation of the associate editors and the multiple contributors of this volume, many of whom are busy clinicians. We are most appreciative of the efforts of our associate editors and the respective authors of the individual sections.

In summary, we have prepared *The Breast* with the specific goal of assembling and collating basic and clinical scientific data essential to the multidisciplinary principles and practices in the treatment of breast diseases. We gratefully acknowledge the opportunity provided by the immense challenge entrusted to us by the publisher, and we are hopeful that this goal has been attained.

KIRBY I. BLAND
EDWARD M. COPELAND III

Acknowledgments

We are indebted to the Associate Editors and each contributor for the first edition of *The Breast: Comprehensive Management of Benign and Malignant Diseases*. The untold hours necessary to prepare this treatise represent time taken from busy clinical practices, laboratories, and families. The diligent efforts of the contributors to provide a comprehensive, insightful, state-of-the-art presentation while adhering to a standard format to achieve a uniform style is gratefully acknowledged. The updating of respective contributions is praiseworthy, and the choice of selective illustrations, tables, and references brings the text to a focused, readable state of completeness.

We pay tribute to the staff members of the W. B. Saunders Company, who have made the publication of this first edition possible. Edward Wickland has provided strong support for the initiation and completion of this edition and has supervised all phases of organization and preparation of *The Breast*. In addition, Kathleen McCullough, Mary Anne Folcher, and Bill Preston have provided incalculable assistance to the planning, preparation, and editorial review of the contributions of all the authors. Special appreciation goes to our program assistant, Ervene Katz, and senior word processor, Marge McGarva, who have contributed numerous hours to diligent review, typing, and editing of the manuscripts submitted by authors of the various sections. We also express gratitude to Louis Clark and Jonathan Bland, who skillfully prepared the illustrations and line drawings for multiple chapters of the text.

We are indebted to our residents and research fellows in surgery and medicine for their intellectual stimulation and their encouragement to proceed with the development of this textbook. To the faculty and residents who have read and reviewed manuscripts and provided opinions and suggestions for the various presentations of clinical data in this text, we gratefully acknowledge their interest, enlightening commentary, and critique.

Finally, to the many friends and colleagues who have expressed interest and encouragement in the development of this textbook, we are hopeful that the goals set forth by the editorial staff have been achieved.

KIRBY I. BLAND
EDWARD M. COPELAND III

Contents

Section I

Historical Perspectives of Breast Disease and Its Treatment

Chapter 1

HISTORY OF BREAST DISEASE AND ITS TREATMENT

Frederick B. Wagner, Jr., M.D.

Diseases of the breast, with their uncertain causes and confusion of treatments, have intrigued the attention of physicians and medical historians throughout the ages. Despite centuries of theoretical meanderings and scientific inquiry, cancer of the breast remains one of the most dreaded of human ills. While primarily thought of as a disease of women, it may occasionally afflict men with results just as lethal. The breast as a paired organ further increases its exposure to disease. As an appendage of the skin it usually reveals its disorders to touch or sight. The story of efforts to cope with these problems is complex. In breast cancer there is no happy ending as in diseases for which cause and cure have been found. Progress has been made, nevertheless, in humanizing the horrors that formerly devastated the body and psyche. In highlighting the mainstream of this history, the names of countless important contributors must be omitted.

ANCIENT CIVILIZATIONS

Egyptian. The oldest of recorded medical history comes from ancient Egypt. In addition to engraving or painting hieroglyphics on stone, the Egyptians etched their cursive script on thin sheets of papyrus leaf. Among six principal papyri, the most informative one with respect to diseases of the breast is that acquired by Edwin Smith (1822–1906) at Thebes (now Luxor and Karnak) in 1862. Dating to about 1600 B.C., it is a roll about 15 feet long, with writing on both sides. The front contains 17 columns with 48 cases devoted to clinical surgery.[9] References are made to diseases of the breast such as abscess, trauma, and infected wounds. Case 45 is perhaps the earliest recording of breast cancer with the title of *Instructions Concerning Tumors on His Breast*

(Fig. 1–1). The examiner is told that a breast with bulging tumors, very cool to the touch, is an ailment for which there is no treatment.

The Egyptian physicians limited themselves to the treatment of single types of disease, such as for the eyes, head, or intestines, or internal disorders. There was a rule that a surgeon had to declare a stand when solicited. He had to contract that he could cure the ailment; that he could not cure the ailment and thus refuse treatment; or that he required a longer period of observation to determine whether he could produce a cure. There were no concessions for therapeutic failure. Surgical treatment was limited to burning with fire or removal with sharpened instruments.

Medical practice declined in Egypt as the centuries passed, until by the Alexandrian period many of their physicians went to Greece for study.

Babylonian. Babylon around the beginning of the second millenium B.C. under King Hammurabi produced the famous Code with 282 clauses. This city of wealth, luxury, and vice in Mesopotamia has been considered

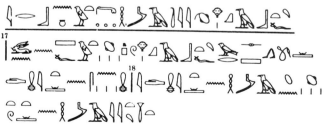

Figure 1–1. Recording of the earliest known case of breast cancer (ca. 1600 B.C.). (From *The Edwin Smith Papyrus*. Published in facsimile and hieroglyphic transliteration with translation and commentary by James Henry Breasted. Birmingham, AL, The Classics of Medicine Library, 1984, p 405. Reprinted by permission.)

the founding site of Oriental civilization with respect to mathematics, astronomy, and art. Initially there were no identifiable physicians, because failure in treatment would cause their hands to be cut off. This led to the practice of the sick to collect in the marketplace and solicit the advice of passers-by who had suffered from and possibly been cured of the same affliction. Through this custom "the whole people was the physician." The term "curb stone consultation" in modern use is an historic carryover of this practice.

Later on the Code of Hammurabi (ca. 1950 B.C.) disclosed that physicians regained public esteem sufficiently to obtain a fee and practice was regulated by law. Internal medicine consisted mainly of a recitation of litanies and incantations against the demons that concentrated in the earth, air, and water. Surgery consisted of opening an abscess with a bronze lancet. The custom persisted, however, that if the patient lost his life or eye, the physician would lose his hands.

Classical Greek Period (460–136 B.C.). European medicine had its origins in ancient Greece. Its scientific advancement was due to Hippocrates (460–370 B.C.), who also inculcated its ethical ideals. His basic philosophy was the linkage of the four cardinal humors of the body (blood, phlegm, yellow bile, and black bile) with the four universal elements (earth, air, water, and fire). Perfect health depended upon proper balance in the dynamic qualities of the humors. Throughout the centuries to follow, the humoral theory would persist but with subsequent writers holding vague and conflicting notions as to the composition, origin, and role of these body humors. It was generally believed that blood was in the arteries and veins, phlegm in the brain, yellow bile in the liver, and black bile in the spleen. Hippocrates rescued medicine from the realm of the supernatural to realistic observation of the patient within his own environment. He divided diseases into three general categories: those curable by medicine as the most favorable; those not curable by medicine, but by the knife; and those not curable by the knife that would be curable by fire.

One case history of Hippocrates described a woman with carcinoma of the breast associated with bloody discharge from the nipple. She died when the discharge became arrested. He associated breast cancer with cessation of menstruation leading to mammary engorgement and indurated nodules. He clearly stated that in cases of deep-seated cancer it was better to give no treatment, because treatment hastened death. The omission of treatment might prolong life. There is no record that he recommended surgery for breast cancer.

Alexandria on the Nile, founded by Alexander the Great in 332 B.C., became the world focal point of Greek science during its peak period of the third and second centuries B.C. As many as 14,000 students studied there at one time in the various branches of Hellenistic knowledge contained in 700,000 scrolls of the largest library in antiquity. Anatomical studies, although rudimentary, were conducted and led to progress in the tools and techniques of surgery. Surgery was further advanced by introduction of the vascular ligature.

Greco-Roman Period (150 B.C.–500 A.D.). With the destruction of Corinth in 146 B.C., Greek medicine migrated to Rome. The Romans during the preceding six centuries had lived without physicians. They employed medicinal herbs, assorted concoctions, votive objects placed in the temples, religious rites, and superstitions (Fig. 1–2). The Roman citizen had a household god for most known diseases and his own herbal medicines. Archagathus, who came to Rome in 220 B.C. as the first Greek physician to practice there, was known for his cruelty in surgery.

Leonides, a Greek physician in the first century A.D., is credited with the first recorded operative treatment for breast cancer. His method consisted of an initial incision into the uninvolved portion of the breast, followed by applications of the cautery to stop bleeding. Repeated incisions and applications of cautery were continued until the entire breast and tumor had been removed and the underlying tissues were covered with an eschar. The aftercare consisted of poultices and a diet avoiding cold beverages and withholding food difficult to digest.

Aurelius Cornelius Celsus, a Roman who lived in the first century A.D. as an encyclopedist and not a physician, wrote about contemporary Greek medicine in polished

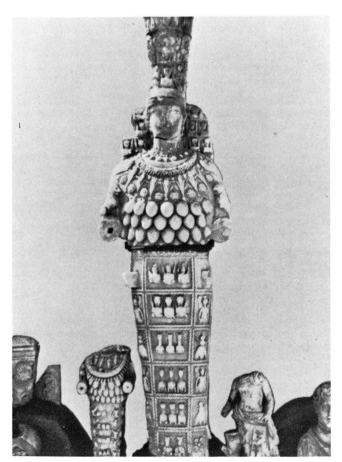

Figure 1–2. Statue of Diana of Ephesus, a fertility deity invoked by Roman women, displaying 20 accessory pectoral breasts. (From Haagensen CD: Diseases of the Breast. 2nd ed. Philadelphia, WB Saunders, 1971, p 5. Reprinted by permission.)

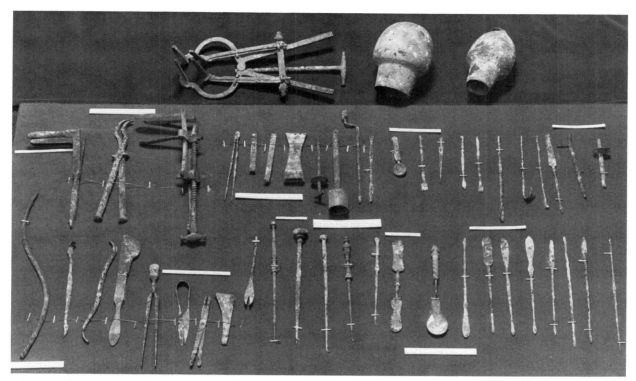

Figure 1–3. Surgical instruments (79 A.D.) from excavations of Pompei and Herculaneum. (Courtesy of Archives of Thomas Jefferson University, Philadelphia, PA.)

Latin. In his treatise there is the first clinical description of cancer. He mentions the breasts of women as one of the sites with description of a fixed irregular swelling with hardness or softness, dilated tortuous veins, and with or without ulceration. He also delineated four clinical stages, namely malignancy (apparently simple or early), carcinoma without ulcer, ulcerated cancer, and ulcerated cancer with flower-like excrescences that bled easily. Celsus opposed treatment of the last three stages by any method, since aggressive measures would irritate the condition or lead to inevitable recurrence. Furthermore, if surgery were considered in a favorable case, he did not give any details.

Under the Romans, surgery, including obstetrics and

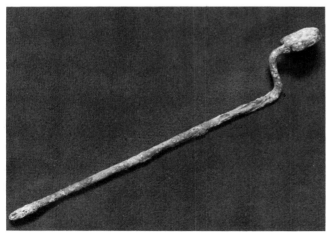

Figure 1–4. Roman cautery (79 A.D.) depicted from Figure 1–3.

ophthalmology, reached a stage of technology that it would not attain again until the time of the Renaissance. Surgical instruments became highly specialized, as witnessed by the finding of over 200 different instruments in the excavations of Pompei and Herculaneum (Fig. 1–3 and 1–4).

The greatest Greek physician after Hippocrates was Galen (131–201 A.D.). He was born on the Mediterranean coast of Asia Minor, studied in Alexandria, and practiced for the rest of his life in Rome. He studied anatomy from apes, dogs, cows, and pigs rather than humans, with speculation on function that credited him as the founder of experimental physiology. His system of pathology again combined the humoral ideas of Hippocrates and the theory of the four universal elements within his own concept of a spirit controlling the whole. Until the time of Vesalius (1514–1564), European medicine respected his authority in anatomy, physiology, and disease. Following his death there was no significant progress until well into the sixteenth century.

In his humoral theory, Galen considered black bile, especially when extremely dark or thick, to be the most harmful of the four constituents and the ultimate cause of cancer. Congestion of black bile could cause scirrhus, a hard and heavy tumor, or cancer that was very hard and malignant and could ulcerate. The vague relationship of scirrhus to carcinoma would await the nineteenth century for its ultimate elucidation.

Galen described mammary cancer as a swelling with distended veins resembling the shape of a crab's legs. He made no mention of metastasis or the process by which death occurred. To prevent accumulation of black bile the patient should be purged and bled. Menstruation in women under 50 should be encouraged by hot baths, exercise, and massage. Emmenagogues and dietary measures were employed. He claimed to have cured the disease in its early stage by surgery when the tumor was on the surface of the body and all the roots could be extirpated. The "roots" were not derived from the tumor but were the dilated veins filled with morbid black bile. In removing the tumor in a circle the surgeon had to be aware of the danger of profuse hemorrhage from large blood vessels. On the other hand, the surgeon should allow the blood to flow freely for a while to allow the escape of black blood and also squeeze out the vessels to evacuate the thick part of the blood.

Late antiquity produced only medical compendia and collections of recipes without any further original contributions. The ancient period is considered to have ended with the writings of Galen.

MEDIEVAL PERIOD

When the Middle Ages began and ended is a matter of opinion, but in European history it may be considered the period between the downfall of Rome and the beginning of the Renaissance.[72] The doctrine of the four humors, which formed the basis of Hippocratic medicine and was endowed with authority by Galen, governed all aspects of medical thinking throughout and beyond the Middle Ages. This may be traced through Christian, Jewish, and Arabic tradition.

Christian. From the Christian standpoint, medicine throughout the Middle Ages was maintained by monks and clerics who constituted the educated class. Almost from the beginning of Christian monastic life, certain monks would undertake the care of sick brethren, but with the founding of the Monastery on Monte Cassino in central Italy by Saint Benedict in 529 there arose an interest in medicine in the scattered cloisters of the Roman Church. Monte Cassino fostered the teaching and practice of medicine, along with copying and preserving ancient manuscripts. It developed many satellites throughout Christendom in which the monks, under the example of their sainted founder, treated the sick and copied medical manuscripts. Monastic schools spread under the Benedictines to England, Scotland, Ireland, France, Switzerland, and most of the European continent. Unfortunately, their libraries contained only a few texts, mainly with parts of Hippocrates, Galen, Celsus, and Dioscorides. The last-named was a Greek army surgeon in the service of Nero around 60 A.D. and who originated materia medica. Furthermore, reliance on the texts was secondary to prayer, relics of saints, amulets, and miracles. The Church invoked one or more saints for nearly every disease. The patron saint for breast disease was Saint Agatha. She had been a martyr in Sicily in the middle of the third century when her two breasts were torn off with iron shears because of resistance to the advances of the governor Quintiamus (Fig. 1–5). On Saint Agatha's day, two loaves of bread representing her breasts are carried on a tray.

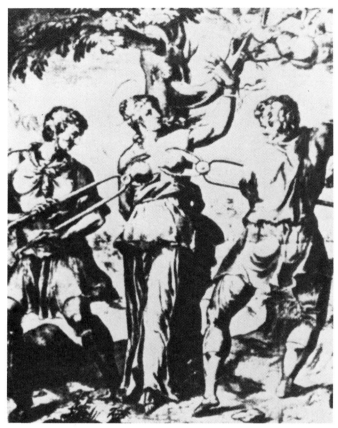

Figure 1–5. Martyrdom of St. Agatha. (Robinson JO: Treatment of breast cancer through the ages. Am J Surg 151:318, 1986. Reprinted by permission.)

One product of the cloister was the *Physica* of Saint Hildegarde of Bingen (1098–1180). She was the first female writer upon medicine in the German countries. Partly in Latin and partly in German she described medicinal plants with prescriptions for various diseases. Her work revealed remarkable learning but added nothing of significance to medical advancement.

The Council of Rheims (1131) prohibited monks and the clergy to practice medicine. From that time on medical teaching and practice were increasingly carried on by laymen. Even earlier, sometime in the ninth century, a lay medical school developed in Salerno in southern Italy. It became famous not only for its teaching but also for its visits to the bedsides of the sick. Cathedral schools, although in clerical hands, profited from a greater freedom than the monasteries and enjoyed the intellectual contacts of the large cities. Further growth of cities in the eleventh and twelfth centuries led to the rise of universities, which became the final force in wresting medicine from monastic influence.

Jewish. Jewish physicians were active at Salerno from its beginning in the ninth century. They achieved great distinction not only in the art of healing but also in their literary efforts. Despite recurrent persecutions by Church and State, their services were sought by popes, kings, and noblemen. In a time when poisoning of enemies and rivals was common, the Jews were considered the safest medical advisers. The Arabian rulers and Egyptian caliphs also preferred them to their Mohammedan doctors, who practiced magic and astrology in treating disease.

Under the tolerant Moors of Spain and the early Christian rulers of Spain and Portugal, the Jews became leaders in the medical profession. The foremost among them was Moses Maimonides (1135–1204). Born in Cordova, Spain, he studied medicine at Cairo and became the physician to Saladin, the Sultan of Egypt. In addition to his own principal medical treatise, *Book of Counsel*, he translated from Arabic into Hebrew the *Canon* of Avicenna (980–1037), the authoritative storehouse of medicine during the Middle Ages. Maimonides also made a collection of the aphorisms of Hippocrates and Galen. He was cautious to prescribe drugs only when needed and to allow nature a chance to cure trivial illness. His death was mourned by Arabs, Jews, and Christians alike.

Jewish physicians remained prominent in Spain under the Western Caliphate until they were banished from the country in 1492. The Salerno School exploited them as teachers until it had enough indigenous talent to proceed without them. Even at Montpellier in southern France the Jews became excluded in 1301. It would not be until the onset of the modern industrial movement that they would again be admitted to citizenship throughout Europe and given university freedom, which once more liberated their brilliant medical talent.

Arabic. The western world owes its main debt to Arabic medicine in that it preserved some of the Greek writings that might otherwise have been lost. Arabian medicine of the Middle Ages exists principally in the sense that the Arabic language was used, but the true Arabs contributed little to medicine beyond their name. Those classed as Arabian medical writers were of such diverse origins as Persian, Syrian, Saracen, and Jewish because of their use of the Arabic language. The Mohammedans made translations of the Greek authors with great zeal, and Bagdad, the capital of the Islamic Empire in Iraq, became the center of such learning. In Western Islam the library at Cordova had 600,000 manuscripts and the one at Cairo had 18 rooms of books. The Tartars raided the library in Bagdad in 1260 and threw the books into the river.

Rhazes (860–932), one of the great Arabic physicians, condoned excision of the breast for cancer only if it could be completely removed and the underlying portion cauterized. From what had been written before and evidently from his own experience, he warned that incising a breast cancer would only produce an ulceration.

Haly ben Abbas, a Persian who died in 994, authored an encyclopedic work, *Royal Book*, in medicine and surgery based on Rhazes and the Greek sources. He endorsed the removal of breast cancers with allowance of bleeding to evacuate melancholic humors. It was widely believed for many centuries that various forms of melancholy predisposed to cancer. He did not tie the arteries and made no mention of cautery.

Avicenna (980–1037) was the successor to Haly ben Abbas and known as "the Prince of Physicians." He was chief physician to the hospital at Bagdad and was the author of the *Canon*, which remained authoritative for four centuries. For external cancer he recommended a milk diet and excision with the cautery.

Albucassis (1013–1106), born in Spain, wrote a large treatise of three books, the *Collection*, which became a leading textbook on surgery during the next two centuries. He agreed that small tumors in which the entire breast could be removed was advisable, but that he had never cured such a case.

The great Arab hospitals were at Bagdad, Damascus, and Cairo. Medical instruction was given at these hospitals or at academies in the cities. The emphasis was on clinical medicine, with neglect of anatomy and surgery. In all the cultures of the Middle Ages the surgery, when employed, used the knife and cautery alone or in combination. Ignorance, the horror, and the poor results of surgery for breast and other diseases could well put a label of "Dark Ages" upon this period. Except for a few erudite surgeons such as those mentioned, surgery was practiced by barbers and men of low intellect with virtually no education. This situation would continue until the dawn of the Renaissance.

THE RENAISSANCE

The transition from the medieval to the modern era occurred in the latter part of the fifteenth century, with the introduction of gunpowder into warfare, the discovery of America, and the invention of the printing press. The boundaries of the Renaissance are ill defined but may well be included within the sixteenth and seventeenth centuries. Medical teaching began to flourish in the universities previously founded in Montpellier, Bologna, Padua, Paris, Oxford, and Cambridge.

Andreas Vesalius (1514–1564), the Flemish surgeon-anatomist, was a pivotal figure of paramount importance in his dissections of the human body at Padua. In his *De Fabrica Humani Corporis* (1543) he broke through the tradition of Galen by the rejection of animal anatomy. This provided surgery with a new practical basis. For breast tumors he advised wide excision and the use of ligatures instead of cautery.

Ambrose Paré (1510–1590) studied medicine in Paris and through his experience in wars became the greatest surgeon of his time. His books on anatomy and surgery, *Oeuvres complètes* (1575), were written in his native French and read throughout Europe. He encouraged compassion in surgery by use of the vascular ligature and avoidance of cautery and boiling oil. He condoned the excision of superficial cancers but attempted to treat breast cancers by application of lead plates, which were intended by compression of the blood supply to arrest the growth. He made the important observation that breast cancer often caused swelling of the axillary glands.

Michael Servetus (1509–1553), a Spaniard who studied in Paris, was later burned at the stake for "the crime of honest thought." His heretical discovery was that blood in the pulmonary circulation passes into the heart after having been mixed with air in the lungs. In cancer of the breast he felt that the underlying muscle should be removed and also the glands described by Paré. This constituted a forerunner concept of radical mastectomy.

Wilhelm Fabry (1560–1624) is regarded as the "Father of German Surgery." His name was honored by the placement of a wreath at his statue in Hilden near Düsseldorf by members of the International Society of the History of Medicine in 1986 (Fig. 1–6). He devised an instrument that compressed and fixed the base of the breast so that a knife could amputate it more swiftly and less painfully (Fig. 1–7).[28] He stipulated that the tumor should be mobile and that no remnants should be left behind. It is claimed that he also removed the axillary nodes, but by what approach is not clear.

The other famous German surgeon of this period was Johann Schultes (1595–1645), known as Scultetus, who was an illustrator of surgery and inventor of surgical instruments. His book, *Armamentarium chirurgicum*, published posthumously in 1653, contained plates of surgical procedures, one of which represented amputation of the breast.[74] He used heavy ligatures on large needles, which transfixed the breast so that traction would facilitate its removal by the knife. Hemostasis was secured by cauterization of the base (Fig. 1–8).

In Rouen, France, Guillaume de Houppeville in 1693 reported mastectomy with the surrounding healthy tissue and a portion of the underlying pectoral muscle. In this he was ahead of other surgeons of his time.

With only a few outstanding surgeons in each of the

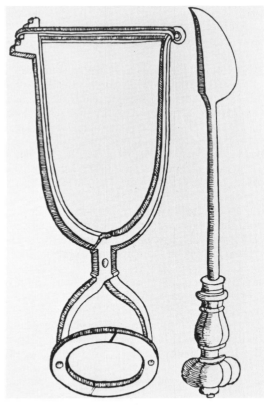

Figure 1–7. Mastectomy instruments of Fabry von Hilden in late sixteenth century. (From Robinson JO: Treatment of breast cancer through the ages. Am J Surg 151:319, 1986. Reprinted by permission.)

important countries of Europe, coupled with the pain, bleeding, infection, and mortality that accompanied breast surgery, it must be realized that few amputations for cancer could actually be performed. Women in the many small towns had no access to anything resembling proper care, and the average life expectancy was only 35 years. Scientific journals as a method of medical communication other than by textbooks made a rudimentary beginning only toward the end of the seventeenth century. A few books with home remedies for common ailments, including those of the breast, were in print (Fig. 1–9).[53]

EIGHTEENTH CENTURY

The eighteenth century has been termed the "Age of Enlightenment" (de Moulin) and the "Age of Theories and Systems" (Garrison).[30, 31] Despite these optimistic designations, this century was slow to develop significant changes in pathological and physiological concepts. Textbooks described preternatural tumors which included scrofula, aneurysms, skin diseases, varicose veins, scirrhus, and cancer. The separation of scirrhus and cancer in the arbitrary doctrine of Galen was still held and argued as to etiology and differentiation. Scirrhus was considered by some to be a benign growth that under adverse circumstances could undergo malignant degeneration, whereas others regarded it as an

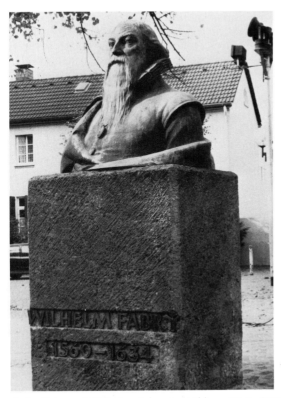

Figure 1–6. Statue of Wilhelm Fabry in Hilden, West Germany. (Courtesy of Dr. Ellen Wiederhold, Burgermeister of Hilden.)

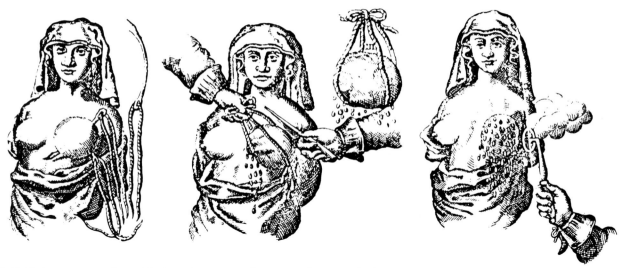

Figure 1–8. Mastectomy procedure of Scultetus in seventeenth century. (Courtesy of Robinson JO: Treatment of breast cancer through the ages. Am J Surg 151:320, 1986. Reprinted by permission.)

existing stage of cancer. The majority believed that scirrhus originated in stagnation and coagulation of body fluids within the mammary gland (local cause). Others believed it to occur by a general internal derangement of the body juices (systemic cause). In accepting both causes, authors conceded that the local cause could be a precipitating factor in a predisposed patient. Hermann Boerhaave (1668–1738) taught that Galen's yellow bile was blood serum rather than bile itself, that phlegm was altered serum into which yellow bile had changed by standing, and that black bile was a part of the clot which separated off and became a darker color.[49] Thus, the four humors in this concept were only different components of the blood.

Pieter Camper (1722–1789) described and illustrated the internal mammary lymph nodes, and Paolo Mascagni (1752–1815) did the same for the pectoral lymph drainage. Death by metastasis from cancer was not yet understood. At best, in the French *Encyclopedie* this condition meant the spreading of disease from the skin to some internal organ or vice versa, a mysterious sympathy existing between different parts of the body. Death, if not due to hemorrhage, was ascribed to a general decomposition of the humors with prolonged fever and pain. Toward the end of the century there were a few reports of remarkable cases related to duration. One such was an 80-year-old patient who had

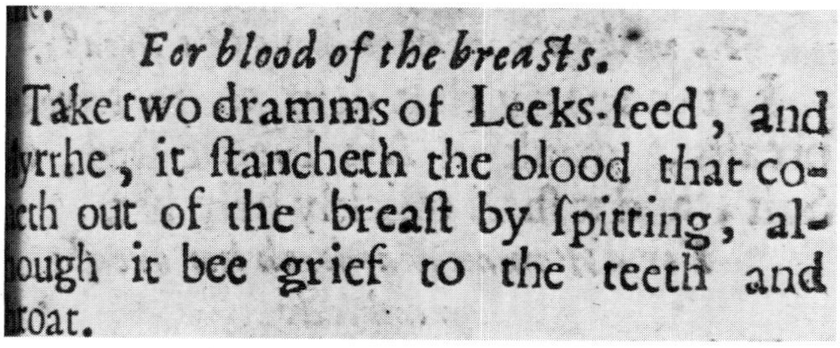

> For blood of the breasts.
> Take two dramms of Leeks-feed, and
> yrrhe, it stancheth the blood that co-
> eth out of the breast by spitting, al-
> ough it bee grief to the teeth and
> roat.

Figure 1–9. Home remedy "for blood of the breasts" (1664).

suffered for more than 30 years with an open breast cancer that destroyed the entire breast and denuded the ribs.

In Edinburgh, strongly oriented to university teaching, the separation of surgeons from barbers was accomplished by 1718. In London, where Barber-Surgeon Guilds had existed, the separation occurred in 1745. A new era of British surgery was instituted when William Cheselden (1688–1752), surgeon to St. Thomas' and St. George's Hospitals, first established private courses in anatomy and surgery. The Hunter brothers, John (1728–1793) and William (1718–1783), likewise in London, followed suit. These courses attracted students from all over the country, the continent, and America. John Hunter remains credited as the founder of experimental surgery and surgical pathology.

In France, Henri Francois le Dran (1685–1770) (Fig. 1–10) concluded that cancer was a local disease in its early stages, and that spread to the lymphatic system signaled a worsened prognosis.[52] This was a courageous contradiction to the humoral theory of Galen, which had persisted for a thousand years and was still to be upheld by many for two centuries to come. A colleague of le Dran, Jean Louis Petit (1674–1750), first Director of the French Academy of Surgery, supported these principles. He advocated removal of the breast, the underlying pectoral muscle, and the axillary lymph nodes. Petit thus recommended what could be considered the first radical mastectomy.[70] It differed from the modern operation in that he failed to remove an extensive area of skin. In leaving the greater portion of skin, he included the nipple unless it was actually involved. Also, he did not mention whether the axillary nodes were removed in continuity.

In Germany, Lorenz Heister (1683–1758) was one of the great surgeons during the first half of the eighteenth century. He favored the use of a guillotine machine, using the traction strings of Scultetus. This not only was rapid but also removed all the skin of the breast. In

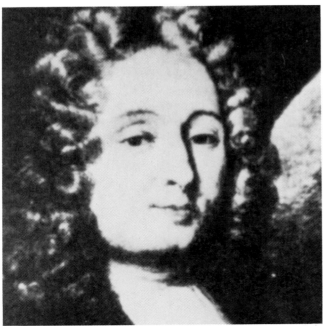

Figure 1–10. Henri François le Dran (1685–1770) noted that lymphatic spread worsened the prognosis of breast cancer. (From Robinson JO: Treatment of breast cancer through the ages. Am J Surg 151:321, 1986. Reprinted by permission.)

addition, he advised removal of the underlying pectoral muscle and the axillary lymph nodes. It is likely that only large and superficial nodes were removed because of danger of bleeding from the great vessels. For Heister, anesthesia for surgery was a century away. He described the patient-surgeon relationship as follows: "Many females can stand the operation with the greatest courage and without hardly moaning at all. Others, however, make such a clamour that they may dishearten even the most undaunted surgeon and hinder the operation. To perform the operation, the surgeon should therefore be steadfast and not allow himself to become disconcerted by the cries of the patient."[17]

Mastectomies were performed in larger numbers during the beginning of the eighteenth century. They decreased during the second half of the century because of the poor results and indiscriminate mutilation. Camper reported in 1757 that in a densely populated town such as Amsterdam with 200,000 inhabitants "not six times a year a breast was amputated with reasonable chance of a cure."[16]

NINETEENTH CENTURY

Two monumental contributions to surgery of the breast were to highlight the nineteenth century. The first was the introduction of anesthesia by William T.G. Morton in the United States in 1846, and the other was the principle of antisepsis by Joseph Lister in Great Britain in 1867. The greatest horrors of surgery, namely pain and sepsis, thus became alleviated. The latter part of the century also witnessed the perfection of the modern radical mastectomy and statistics on various

aspects of breast cancer. It is proper to trace what was happening on both sides of the Atlantic.

European Surgery

At the beginning of the nineteenth century the treatment for breast cancer remained in confusion and may have regressed. In 1811, Samuel Young in England revived the outmoded and disproved method of Paré, in which compression was used to cut off the blood supply of the tumor.[84] Nooth, another English surgeon, sprayed the breast with carbolic acid, which was a modified form of the ancient practice of cauterization.

In 1822, James Elliott reported the first case of a tumor examined under the microscope. It was an axillary node removed during breast surgery and diagnosed as a sarcoma.[26]

James Syme (1799–1870) was the famous surgeon of Edinburgh whose daughter married Lord Lister. Much of his breast surgery was performed during the era before the advent of anesthesia.[76] His third surgical apprentice, Dr. John Brown (1810–1882), became a successful clinician as well as a writer. The latter's book, *Rab and His Friends* (1858), contains a classic vivid description of breast surgery as performed by the 28-year-old Dr. Syme in the Minto House Hospital of Edinburgh. Brown, who was acting as a clerk, gives the account as follows: "The operating theater is crowded; much talk and fun and all the cordiality and stir of youth. The surgeon with his staff of assistants is there. In comes Allie (the patient): one look at her quiets and abates the eager students. Allie stepped upon a seat, and laid herself on the table, as her friend the surgeon told her; arranged herself, gave a rapid look at James (her husband), shut her eyes, rested herself on me (Brown), and took my hand. The operation was at once begun; it was necessarily slow; and chloroform—one of God's best gifts to his suffering children—was then unknown. The surgeon did his work. The pale face showed its pain, but was still and silent. Rab's (a mastiff) soul was working within him; he saw that something strange was going on—blood flowing from his mistress, and she suffering; his ragged ear was up, and importunate; he growled and gave now and then a sharp impatient yelp; he would have liked to have done something to that man. But James had him firm, and gave him a glower from time to time, and an intimation of a possible kick—all the better for James, it kept his eye and his mind off Allie. It is over: she is dressed, steps gently and decently down from the table, looks for James; then turning to the surgeon and the students, she curtsies—and in a low, clear voice, begs their pardon if she has behaved ill. The students—all of us—wept like children; the surgeon helped her up carefully—and resting on James and me, Allie went to her room, Rab following. Four days after the operation what might have been expected happened. The patient had a chill, the wound was septic, and she died."[10, 75]

Later in life, Syme was able to operate with the blessing of anesthesia. He felt it incumbent upon the surgeon to search very carefully for axillary glands in the course of the operation, but stated that the results were almost always unsatisfactory no matter how perfectly they seemed to have been removed.

Sir James Paget (1814–1899) questioned in 1856 whether operation added length of life or comfort to justify the risk. He reported an operative mortality of 10 percent in 235 patients and always a recurrence within eight years. In 139 patients with scirrhous carcinoma, those without operation lived longer than those with surgery.[65] In 1874 he published the paper stamping his name in surgical history, *On Disease of the Mammary Areola Preceding Cancer of the Mammary Gland.*[64]

Robert Liston (1794–1874), an influential surgeon from the University College Hospital, London, in the preanesthesia era, could advocate operation only under the most favorable circumstances. He considered it rash and cruel to attempt removal of the axillary glands.[55]

Charles Moore (1821–1879) of the Middlesex Hospital in London championed the belief that the only hope of cure for breast cancer was by wider and more extensive surgery, despite the frequent disastrous results (Fig. 1–11). His famous paper, *On the Influence of Inadequate Operation on the Theory of Cancer* (1867), was widely accepted.[61] He stressed that the tumor should not be cut into and that recurrences originated by dispersion from the primary growth and not by independent organic origin. His operation called for removal of the entire breast with special attention to including the sternal edge, and removal of the skin in continuity with the main mass of the tumor. He did not remove the pectoralis major muscle.

Joseph Lister (1827–1912), one of England's most respected surgeons, agreed with Moore's principles and advocated division of the origins of both pectoral muscles to gain better exposure of the axilla for the nodal dissection. His epoch-making contribution of the carbolic acid spray was not widely accepted before a lapse of 15 to 20 years.[54]

In 1877, Mitchell Banks of Liverpool advocated removal of the axillary nodes in all cases of breast surgery

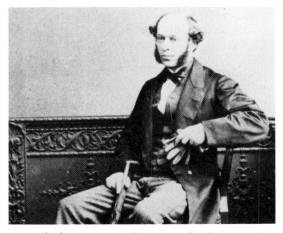

Figure 1–11. Charles Moore, British surgeon of mid-nineteenth century, advocated wider and more extensive breast surgery. (From Robinson JO: Treatment of breast cancer through the ages. Am J Surg 151:323, 1986. Reprinted by permission.)

for cancer. He washed the wound with carbolic acid solution but avoided the spray because of its cooling effect on the patient.[3]

In France, Alfred-Armand-Louis-Marie Velpeau (1795–1867), originally apprenticed to the blacksmith trade, rose to become Professor of Clinical Surgery at the Paris Faculty (1834–1867). In 1854 in his *Treatise on Diseases of the Breast* he claimed to have seen more than 1,000 breast tumors, benign or malignant, during a practice of 40 years.[80] In those times, once the tumor had been excised the patient and surgeon usually parted company. Follow-up until death was unusual. Despite this, Velpeau felt he had cured a good many cases. Statistical studies in France in the middle of the century failed to support Velpeau's optimism, based on anecdotal impressions. In 1844, Jean-Jacques-Joseph Leroy d'Etiolles (1798–1860) conducted an inquiry with 174 answers on 1192 patients. The conclusion was that operation was more harmful than beneficial.[18] The 1854 Congress of the Academie de Medicine discussed the question of whether cancer should be treated at all.

New practices started in Germany in 1875, when Richard von Volkmann (1830–1889) removed the entire breast, no matter how small the primary tumor, as well as the pectoral fascia with occasionally a thick layer of the underlying muscle, and extirpated the axillary nodes.[81] Theodor Billroth (1829–1894) also removed the whole breast, but was not certain that in small tumors a local excision with a surrounding zone of normal tissue would not do just as well. In fixed tumors, however, he included the pectoral fascia along with a thick layer of the underlying muscle. Ernst Georg Ferdinand Kuster (1839–1922) of Berlin recommended in 1883 that the axillary fat be removed in all cases along with the nodes. Lothar Heidenhain (1860–1940), a pupil of Volkmann, recommended removal of the superficial portion of the pectoralis major muscle even if the tumor was freely mobile, but the entire muscle with its underlying connective tissue if the tumor was fixed.[46]

By the turn of the century there was still a high mortality due to gross infection in spite of Lister's carbolic spray. Voices were still heard which claimed that patients with breast cancer lived longer if not operated upon.

American Surgery

Throughout most of the nineteenth century, Philadelphia was the undisputed medical center of the United States. It harbored the country's oldest medical college (University of Pennsylvania, founded in 1765), the Jefferson Medical College, founded in 1824, and more than 50 other medical schools that became extinct. It established a permanent medical college for women, and one in homeopathy as well as osteopathy. Contributions of Philadelphia surgeons who dominated this period will be discussed first.

Joseph Pancoast (1805–1882) was a dextrous surgeon-anatomist who in the flowery language of his era was said "to have an eye as quick as a flashing sunbeam and a hand as light as floating perfume." His *Treatise on Operative Surgery,* published in 1844 in the preanesthetic and preantiseptic era, illustrates a mastectomy.[67] The patient is awake with eyes open and is semireclining. An assistant compresses the subclavian artery above the clavicle with the thumb of one hand. Larger vessels in the wound are compressed with the thumb and index finger of the assistant's other hand. Ligatures are left long and brought through the lower pole of the wound, where they act as a drain and can be pulled out later as they slough off. In the smaller left lower sketch the axillary glands are shown in continuity with the breast through the single incision that has extended into the axilla. This was the first description of an en bloc removal of the breast with its axillary lymphatic drainage. Skin removal, however, was scanty with easy approximation of the wound with five wide adhesive strips (Fig. 1–12).

Samuel D. Gross (1805–1884) was designated by Fielding Garrison as "The Greatest American Surgeon of his Time."[31] His approach to cancer of the breast, however, was more conservative than that of Pancoast, his colleague. He described extirpation of the breast as "generally a very easy and simple affair."[35] Using a small elliptical incision, he attempted in all cases to save enough skin for easy reunion of the edges of the wound. He aimed for healing by first intention, which was less

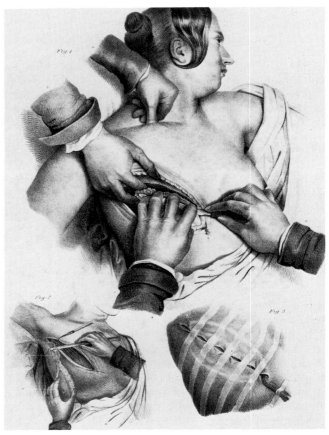

Figure 1–12. Mastectomy (1844) of Dr. Joseph Pancoast in preanesthetic and preantiseptic era. En bloc removal with axillary lymphatic drainage.

likely if the wound were permitted to gape. In dealing with inordinately vascular tumors he ligated each vessel upon its division, but generally considered this as awkward and unnecessary. Lymph nodes in the axilla were removed only if grossly involved, and in that case through the outer angle of the incision or through a separate one, with enucleation of the glands with the finger or handle of the scalpel. It was his rule not to approximate the skin until four or five hours after the operation, "lest secondary hemorrhage should occur, and thus necessitate the removal of the dressings." In the sixth edition of his *System of Surgery* (1882) he devoted 30 pages to diseases of the mammary gland.

Samuel W. Gross (1837–1889) took a much more aggressive approach than that of his eminent father. He stated in 1887 that "no matter what the situation of the tumor may be, or whether glands can or cannot be detected in the armpit, the entire breast, with all the skin covering it, the paramammary fat, and the fascia of the pectoral muscle are cleanly dissected away, and the axillary contents are extirpated. It need scarcely be added that aseptic precautions are strictly observed."[36] Removal of all the skin of the breast led to its designation as the "dinner plate operation." Against the criticism that an open large wound resulted in granulations from which cancer would again develop he said, "When fireplugs produce whales, and oak trees polar bears, then will granulations produce cancer, and not until then."[14]

The younger Gross personally examined under the microscope all the tumors he removed. He was the histologist to the Philadelphia Academy of Surgery, the oldest surgical society in the United States, which he helped his father to found in 1879. Following his premature death in 1889, his widow married William Osler. In her will of 1928, Lady Osler bequeathed an endowment for a lectureship at the Jefferson Medical College in honor of her first husband for his special interest in tumors.

D. Hayes Agnew (1818–1892) at the University of Pennsylvania also held a leadership position in American surgery as author of *Principles and Practice of Surgery* (1878) in three volumes, which endorsed Listerian antisepsis.[1] He shared the pessimistic view of many eminent surgeons of his era that few cases were ever cured by surgery. *The Agnew Clinic* by Thomas Eakins is a masterpiece of American art depicting mastectomy in 1889 under conditions that would have been considered ideal for the time (Fig. 1–13).

Toward the end of the nineteenth century, Philadelphia had to share the limelight with an increasing number of cities throughout the country, and especially with Baltimore, where the Johns Hopkins Hospital Medical School produced a revolution in medical education and research. At that institution, William Steward Halsted (1852–1922) was to provide a landmark in the history of the treatment of breast cancer. He recommended that "the suspected tissues should be removed in one piece lest the wound become infected by the division of tissue invaded by the disease, or by division of the lymphatic vessels containing cancer cells, and

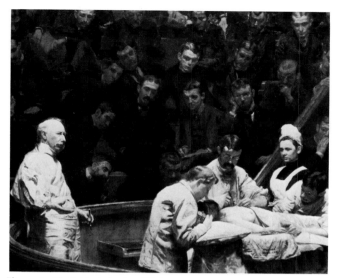

Figure 1–13. Eakins' *Agnew Clinic* (1889) depicting mastectomy under ideal conditions of the time. (Courtesy of University of Pennsylvania School of Medicine, Philadelphia, PA.)

because shreds or pieces of cancerous tissue might be readily overlooked in a piecemeal extirpation." He advocated such wide removal of the skin that a graft would be required and recommended that the pectoralis major muscle be part of the en bloc specimen regardless of the size of the tumor.[41] Later, he went on to favor removal of the sheaths of the upper portion of the rectus abdominis, serratus anterior, subscapularis, latissimus dorsi, and teres major muscles.[40] Although there was nothing dramatically new in Halsted's operation, he placed it on a logical and scientific basis, spelled out the exact technique, and dispersed his principles widely throughout the profession (Fig. 1–14).

As so often happens, Willie Meyer (1854–1932), of the New York Graduate School of Medicine, described a similar technique only ten days after Halsted's published paper.[59] He advocated removal of the pectoralis minor muscle in addition to the major. His operation has frequently been referred to as the Willie Meyer modification of the Halsted procedure.

Cullen in 1895 credited William Welch, the pathologist at Hopkins, as being the first to employ frozen section in the diagnosis of breast lesions.[12] Welch is stated to have employed this procedure in 1891 on one of Halsted's patients who was determined to have a benign breast tumor.

By the end of the century, the Halsted radical mastectomy had basically been established as the ideal method for surgical treatment of operable breast cancer. It would prevail as the standard procedure for the next 70 years or more.

TWENTIETH CENTURY

As the twentieth century commenced it seemed that if the causes of breast diseases were still not understood, at least the surgery for their various manifestations had

been widely exploited. It became evident, however, in the instance of breast cancer that significantly higher rates of cure were not to be anticipated by surgery alone. This damper on surgical expectations stimulated scientific inquiry through epidemiological studies, laboratory research, and statistical analysis of practical experiences with surgery in the various pathological stages. The search for other modalities to enhance or replace surgery included radiation, hormones, chemicals, and immune responses. The developments in these areas during this century will be traced briefly.

Surgery

The classic radical mastectomy of Halsted and Meyer, although extensive, did not include the supraclavicular and internal mammary nodes. Halsted himself in 1907 reported the removal of supraclavicular nodes in 119 patients.[42] In 44 with metastatic deposits, only two were alive and well after five years. In 1910, Westerman reported a patient with local recurrence in whom he disarticulated the arm and resected three ribs.[83] The thoracic wall defect was repaired with a pedicled flap. In two other cases he carried out a partial excision of the thoracic wall and closed the defect with tissue from the contralateral healthy breast. These last two patients died within weeks, and the follow-up on the first was only for one and a half years. These supraradical operations were discontinued within a few years, because of increased operative mortality and unimproved survival rate.

The importance of the internal mammary nodes was

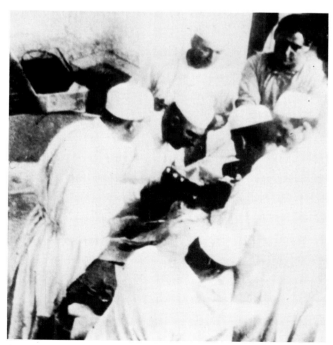

Figure 1–14. Dr. William S. Halsted performing radical mastectomy. Note absence of masks. (Courtesy of College of Physicians of Philadelphia, Philadelphia, PA.)

neglected until the third decade of the century. In 1927, William S. Handley (1872–1962) of the Middlesex Hospital directed attention to the frequency of internal mammary node involvement, especially by the time the axillary nodes were enlarged.[43] He reported removal of internal mammary nodes as an extension of radical mastectomy. After World War II, Jerome A. Urban and Owen H. Wangensteen, among others, advocated "supraradical mastectomy," in which the dissection was carried into the mediastinum and the neck.[79, 82]

For approximately 70 years the Halsted radical mastectomy remained the generally accepted surgical treatment for carcinoma of the breast. Cushman D. Haagensen (Fig. 1–15) of Columbia-Presbyterian Medical Center in New York dedicated his life to the surgical and pathological study of breast diseases over the period of a half century, in which he classified breast cancers according to size, clinical findings, and nodal status while establishing a breast unit where statistics and data were maintained and analyzed from his private patients.[38] Throughout this time he remained a loyal advocate of radical mastectomy. He was the first to propose self-examination of the breast and to suggest that lobular neoplasia (in situ) was not actual carcinoma. The fact that survival statistics for breast cancer, which were increased from three to ten years and beyond, did not change over 75 years has led to more limited types of surgery augmented with adjunctive modalities.

At the end of World War II, radical mastectomy was the standard operation for breast cancer, but divergence of opinions and reports began to produce confusion. In

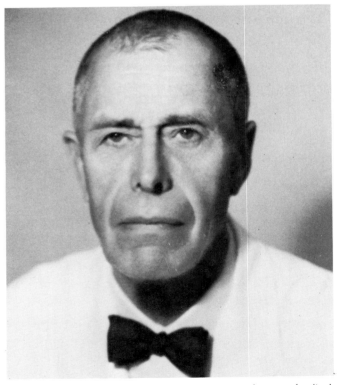

Figure 1–15. Dr. Cushman D. Haagensen, a strong advocate of radical mastectomy, who classified and analyzed breast cancer for half a century. (Courtesy of Dr. Gordon Schwartz.)

1948 two reports appeared that were destined to change the management and become accepted as general principles in the management of localized disease. The first was the concept of modified radical mastectomy by Patey and Dyson from the Middlesex Hospital in London, and the second was the method of treatment by simple mastectomy and radiotherapy by McWhirter of the University of Edinburgh.[58, 68] Subsequent studies of patients treated by simple, radical, and modified radical mastectomies with or without radiotherapy revealed a striking similarity in survival rates.

Since 1970 the surgical trend for cancer has been more and more to limited procedures such as wedge resection or tylectomy with inclusion of a wide zone (2 to 3 cm) of normal surrounding breast tissue. Axillary dissection in many instances became confined to sampling of the Level I nodes. Limited surgery with improved radiotherapy became increasingly employed to control local disease, with chemotherapy and hormonal manipulation for systemic manifestations.

To the alleviation of the horrors of pain and infection by the advent of anesthesia and aseptic technique was added the relief from sexual disfigurement by breast reconstruction. Although considered a recent innovation, breast reconstruction dates back to 1895, when Vincenz Czerny transplanted a large lipoma to replace a breast that had been removed for benign disease.[13] The following year, Tansini of Padua University reported the first radical mastectomy with reconstructive surgery by a latissimus dorsi musculocutaneous flap.[77] Serious consideration of this procedure had to await the era of antibiotics. In 1954 the Ivalon sponge was introduced by Pagman and Wallace, followed by the use of silicone advocated by Cronin and Gerow in 1963.[11, 66] This was an improvement but tended to displace upward and was associated with capsular contraction and occasional skin necrosis. Better results were achieved in the 1970s with implantation of the prosthesis beneath the pectoral muscle.

Concern for patients at high risk for cancer because of strong family history led to prophylactic subcutaneous bilateral mastectomy. This was mainly replaced by the more effective total mastectomy with subpectoral prosthesis implant and reconstruction of the nipple.

Surgery, in whatever form and aided by other modalities, does not appear to have increased the cure rate, but has definitely extended the survival with lessened local recurrence. The zeal to achieve the ideal of prevention or cure remains unabated in the profession and remains an ongoing challenge.

Radiation

Emile Grubbe (1875–1960), a second-year medical student in Chicago, within two months after the discovery of x-rays in 1895 by Wilhelm Conrad Roentgen (1845–1923), irradiated a patient with cancer of the breast. He protected the skin surrounding the lesion with tinfoil. Survival was only one month. This interest led to his becoming the world's first Professor of Roentgenology at the Hahnemann Medical College of Philadelphia.[37] In 1896, Hermann Gocht (1869–1938) at Hamburg treated two late cases with protection of the adjacent skin with flexible lead. Some palliation was achieved. Survival was for 17 days and for 3 months, respectively.[33]

Georg Clemens Perthes (1869–1927), Professor of Surgery in Leipzig, in 1903 ascribed the "curative effect" of x-rays to inhibition of cell division.[69]

Early difficulties related to the measurement of dosage and to the amount required. The effects could produce erythema, epilation, vesication, or necrosis. Nevertheless, radiotherapy became the treatment of choice for inoperable cases.

In 1902, Guido Holzknecht (1872–1931) of Vienna introduced a practical dosimeter. He became one of the early pioneers who died as a result of working with these rays. By 1919, 169 physicians of the world were listed as victims for their work in this field, and by 1954 there were 190 additional names.[19]

Radiology as a specialty became recognized in the 1920s. Its use was then extended from inoperable cases to the anticipation that residual cancer cells after surgery would be killed by the rays. Postoperative irradiation was initiated in many hospitals of America and Europe. The equipment until World War I permitted a maximum voltage of only 150 kV but after the war the voltages ranged from 170 to 200 kV. Radical mastectomy became enhanced with radiotherapy as standard treatment in many centers.

In 1927, Robert Monod of Paris reported a case considered inoperable that lent itself to surgery by preoperative irradiation.[19] The patient was still in good condition three years later.

Harrington of the Mayo Clinic reported in 1929 the follow-up of 1859 cases treated from 1910 to 1923, with expressed doubts as to the value of ancillary radiotherapy.[44] Controversy continued between enthusiasts and opponents, even with improved apparatus.

George Edward Pfahler (1874–1957) of Philadelphia advised postoperative irradiation in all cases, starting two weeks after surgery. In his report of 1022 cases he found no significant improvements in Stage I disease but a definitely improved five-year survival for patients in Stage II.[71]

Irradiation alone had been used for inoperable cases from about the beginning, but it was not until 1922 that a claim was made for its sole use in operable cases. William Stephen Stone (1867–1946) of New York City claimed the superiority of radiotherapy over radical surgery for treatment of operable mammary cancer.[20] He based his conclusions on experience with 10,000 cases of breast malignancy. Surgeons remained skeptical, although local recurrences and Stage II cases presumably fared better than if not treated by irradiation.

Geoffrey Langdon Keynes (b. 1887) of St. Bartholomew's Hospital in London reported in 1932 on the use of radium as a source of radiation.[50] After experience with this modality as an adjunct to surgery, he extended its use to being the sole treatment. He claimed a five-year survival of 77.1 percent in the absence of enlarged

axillary nodes and 36.3 percent with axillary involvement.

Supervoltage x-rays became available in the 1930s, capable of generating voltages beyond 1 million volts. This led to increased reliance on the palliative and curative powers of the ionizing rays with development of new methods of patient management.

François Baclesse (1896–1967) of Paris championed local excision of breast cancer followed by adequate radiotherapy.[21] From the Curie Foundation he reported cases studied between 1937 and 1953, with the conclusion that for Stage I and Stage II the results were equal to those of the orthodox radical mastectomy.

In 1948, Robert McWhirter (b. 1904), previously alluded to, proposed simple mastectomy followed by radiotherapy.[58] He argued that radical mastectomy for Stage I disease was an overkill but that often it was inadequate for Stage II, when the disease frequently spreads beyond the axillary nodes. His method gained more adherents in Britain at the time than in America.

In the 1960s, even higher voltage x-rays were developed along with the radioactive cobalt beam. Further improvement in technology has allowed 6000 to 7000 rads, including implantation of Ir^{192} in the breast, with good cosmesis, low incidence of radiation pneumonitis, and less than 7 to 10 percent rate of recurrence in clinical Stages I and II patients.

At present it is still difficult to assess scientifically the contributions of local therapy to the cure of breast cancer. No single type has emerged as distinctly superior to all others. It is not certain that more intensive surgical procedures or the addition of more advanced radiation improves the welfare of most patients.

Mammography

Before and even after World War I the early diagnosis of breast cancer was most difficult. Patients sought advice only when they easily felt a hard lump, usually by accident, which was gradually increasing in size. Surgeons looked for skin retraction and inversion of the nipple and palpated the breast and axilla for masses. Roentgen rays were about to make another significant contribution in the form of mammography for early diagnosis.

In 1913, Salomon in Germany studied 3000 amputated breasts radiographically and was able to differentiate scirrhous forms of cancer from the nodular types.[73] He noted the microcalcifications in intraductal carcinomas but failed to appreciate their significance. In 1927, Kleinschmidt wrote a book in which he described mammography as an aid in diagnosis.[51] These studies were extended in other parts of the world, but the method was slow to be accepted. Baraldi in 1933 in Buenos Aires injected carbon dioxide into the retromammary and premammary spaces for finer delineation of breast structure.[4] Benzadon, his colleague, pursued this method, which failed to be accepted.[6]

Jacob Gershon-Cohen of Philadelphia studied roentgen mammary patterns from 1937 to 1948 and made notable progress in accurate diagnosis of malignant tumors. He tirelessly advocated the use of roentgenograms as an aid to clinical diagnosis and in 1948 was the first to demonstrate the feasibility of detecting occult carcinomas.[32] Progress was hampered by unsatisfactory technique and lack of pathological knowledge.

Egan in 1962 at the M.D. Anderson Hospital in Texas reported a classic study of 2522 mammograms in which the differentiation of benign and malignant tumors was made without the aid of clinical findings.[24] The fear of inducing breast cancer by repeated mammographic studies was alleviated by improved technology with much smaller doses and the use of xerography. The accuracy of this study has progressed to beyond 90 percent and led to the finding of nonpalpable carcinomas. These minute lesions may now be biopsied under radiological control with careful needle insertion.

In 1978 there was a consensus report of the National Institutes of Health/National Cancer Institute with respect to breast screening by mammography.[63] It emphasized the distinction between mammography used for diagnosis, the value of which was unquestioned, versus its use for screening to detect possible disease in women below 40 years of age. The recommendation was limited to women who have no symptoms or clinical signs whatsoever. The panel found no convincing justification for routine mammographic screening for women under 50 years of age, but did not question the importance of physical examination and breast self-examination for women of any age. The panel further recommended routine mammography for women who are 40 to 49 years of age with a personal history of breast cancer or with a mother or sister(s) having a breast cancer history. In women below 40 years of age, the recommendation was limited to women with a personal history of breast cancer.

Hormonal Therapy

Hormonal treatment for breast cancer was considered even before the beginning of the twentieth century. In 1889, Albert Schinzinger (1827–1911) of Freiburg, Germany, proposed oophorectomy in menstruating women prior to mastectomy in order to cause what he thought would be early aging.[21] This was based on his experience and belief that the prognosis of breast cancer was worse in younger patients. George Thomas Beatson (1848–1933) of Glasgow reported in 1896 and again in 1901 on three cases of advanced breast cancer that had responded favorably to oophorectomy.[5] He based his reasoning on the effect of castration in cows after calving in prolonging lactation and thus a relationship of ovaries to cellular activity in the breast. During the first decade of the century, surgical castration was performed in cases of advanced cancer in young women by some surgeons, but with varying success. It was estimated that perhaps one third of such patients were benefited.

The term "hormone" was first coined by Starling in 1905. In that same year the modality of radiation-castration was introduced, in which, according to MacMahon and Cahill, interest waned after about 1914 because of unfavorable results.[56] Although oophorectomy faded from the clinical armamentarium, research in the field continued in the laboratory in the twenties and thirties.

The modern era of endocrine surgery started around 1940 with the work of Huggins on the beneficial effects of castration in the male for cancer of the prostate.[8] In 1953 he advocated the renewal of surgical oophorectomy to remove the major source of estrogens in the body.[48] The adrenals, which also produce steroid hormones, were also deemed indicated for removal once corticosteroids had become available for substitution. Some cases responded with dramatic remissions while others remained unaffected. In the early fifties, hypophysectomy for advanced breast cancer was recommended, with results similar to those of adrenalectomy.

Clinical administration of hormones started in 1939 when P. Ulrich reported the beneficial effect of testosterone in two cases of breast cancer.[78] Alexander John Haddow (b. 1912) of Edinburgh with his collaborators in 1944 observed a favorable effect of synthetic estrogen in advanced breast cancer.[39] Stilbestrol was synthesized by Edward Dodds of London in 1938.[23] Its effect on advanced breast cancer was reported by Nathanson in 1946.[62] In the fifties and sixties, estrogens and androgens remained in active use.

During the last three decades much investigation has been devoted to the regulation of breast tumor growth. In 1973 the properties of estrogen receptors were demonstrated in human breast tumors by McGuire.[57] In 1975, Horowitz identified progesterone receptors in hormone-dependent breast cancer.[47] The identification of receptors for estrogen, progesterone, and prolactin became useful markers in hormone dependence and their associated susceptibility to manipulation. Although cure by hormones is not likely, their improved aid in management of breast cancer may be anticipated with new advances.

Chemotherapy

The use of chemical compounds, especially arsenic, in the treatment of breast cancer dates to ancient times. In modern terms, however, Paul Ehrlich (1854–1915) may be credited as the "Father of Chemotherapy." He coined the designation "chemotherapy" and by 1898 had isolated the first alkylating agent. In a series of historic experiments he methodically studied a group of compounds that led by 1910 to the discovery of salvarsan, which successfully treated syphilis in rabbits.[25] It was not until just after World War II that his work was revived to be applied to the treatment of tumors.

During World War II the United States Office of Scientific Research had produced nitrogen mustard, an alkylating agent. A ship containing this substance blew up in Naples harbor, and the sailors who were exposed developed marrow and lymphoid hypoplasia.[22] Experimental work with such alkylating agents had begun at Memorial Hospital in New York in the treatment of lymphosarcoma, but the results were withheld until the war secrecy ban was lifted in 1946. Analogues of these compounds such as cyclophosphamide, busulfan, phenylalanine, and chlorambucil appeared for experimental and clinical use.

Engell in 1955 reported the presence of circulating malignant cells in the blood stream, which stimulated much interest in their destruction by systemic administration of chemicals.[27] Actually, malignant cells within the blood stream of a patient with a malignant tumor of the skin had been reported by Ashworth in Australia as far back as 1869.[2]

Other antineoplastic drugs that were investigated and brought into clinical use were the purine and pyrimidine antagonists. Heidelberger and collaborators in 1957 reported the action of 5-fluorouracil against solid tumors, which has remained particularly useful in cancer of the breast.[45] A proliferation of antineoplastic agents resulted in many protocols to study their action in the various clinical stages, pathological types, and age groups of patients with breast cancer. The National Institutes of Health in 1957 organized a cancer and chemotherapy national service in which the first patient was entered in 1958 in a randomized, double-blind study using thiotriethylenephosporamide, an alkylating agent. Prospective trials with single agents were extended into combination chemotherapeutic regimens. Greenspan and his group in New York in 1963 was one of the first to engage in combination trials, using the antimetabolite methotrexate and the alkylating agent thiotepa.[34]

Multiple clinical trials were carried out throughout the world, such as the National Surgical Adjuvant Breast Project (1956), combination trials in Great Britain, and the Milan project of Bonadonna and Valagussa (1981).[7] These multidrug trials indicated that it was possible to increase survival in women with operable breast cancer and constituted the most active modern treatment of the disease.[29] While no marked increase in cure rate has resulted, the five-year survival rates have increased, particularly in premenopausal women with metastases.

Immunotherapy

At present there is no accepted form of immunotherapy for practical clinical use in cancer of the breast. Nevertheless, exploration of the potential for this modality, either alone or in combination with other forms of therapy, is being conducted in prospectively randomized studies, especially by the National Cancer Institute of the United States National Institutes of Health.

The agents under investigation are high-dose recombinant interleukin 2 (IL-2), lymphokine-activated killer cells (LAK), and bacillus Calmette-Guérin (BCG). In varying combinations with cyclophosphamide/methotrexate/5-fluorouracil (CMF) and radiotherapy, the protocols are aimed at advancing the frontier for improvement of patients with histologically proven involvement of the axillary nodes or disseminated disease.

The ultimate utopian dream for breast cancer would be an effective immunization against its onset.

References

1. Agnew DH: The Principles and Practice of Surgery, Vol III. Philadelphia, JB Lippincott, 1883, p 710.
2. Ashworth TR: A case of cancer in which cells similar to those in the tumours were seen in the blood after death. Med J Aust 14:146–148, 1869.
3. Banks MD: A plea for the more free of cancerous growths. Liverpool & Manchester Surg Rep, 1898, pp 192–206.
4. Baraldi A: Roentgeno-neumo-mastia. Bol Soc Cir Buenos Aires 18:1254–1267, 1934.
5. Beatson GT: The treatment of cancer of the breast by oophorectomy and thyroid extract. Br Med J II:1145–1148, 1901.
6. Benzadon J: Contribucion al estudio de la roentgen-neumo-mastia. Semna Med 2:1085–1091, 1935.
7. Bonadonna G, Valagussa P: Dose-response effect of adjunct chemotherapy in breast cancer. N Engl J Med 304:1–15, 1981.
8. Bordley J III, Harvey AM: Two Centuries of American Medicine, 1776–1976. Philadelphia, WB Saunders, 1976, p 679.
9. Breasted JH: The Edwin Smith Surgical Papyrus. Classics of Med Lib, Vol III. Chicago, University of Chicago Press, 1930, p 405.
10. Brown J: Horae Subsecivae. 2nd Ser. London, Adam & Charles Black, 1910, pp 277–278.
11. Cronin TD, Gerow FJ: Augmentation mammoplasty, a new "natural feel" prosthesis. Trans Third Internat Cong Plastic Surg. Amsterdam, Excerpta Medica Foundation, 1964, pp 41–49.
12. Cullen IS: A rapid method of making permanent specimens from frozen sections by the use of formalin. Bull J Hopkins Hosp 6:67–73, 1895.
13. Czerny V: Plasticher Ersatz der Brustdruse durch ein Lipom. Verh Dtsch Ges Chir 24:216–217, 1895.
14. DaCosta JC: Speeches and Papers of John Chalmers DaCosta, M.D., LL.D. Philadelphia, WB Saunders, 1931, p 225.
15. de Moulin D: A Short History of Breast Cancer. The Hague, Martinus Nijhoff, 1983, p 31.
16. de Moulin D: A Short History of Breast Cancer. The Hague, Martinus Nijhoff, 1983, p 47.
17. de Moulin D: A Short History of Breast Cancer. The Hague, Martinus Nijhoff, 1983, p 49.
18. de Moulin D: A Short History of Breast Cancer. The Hague, Martinus Nijhoff, 1983, p 80.
19. de Moulin D: A Short History of Breast Cancer. The Hague, Martinus Nijhoff, 1983, p 99.
20. de Moulin D: A Short History of Breast Cancer. The Hague, Martinus Nijhoff, 1983, p 100.
21. de Moulin D: A Short History of Breast Cancer. The Hague, Martinus Nijhoff, 1983, p 102.
22. Devita VT: Cancer principles: Practice of Oncology. Philadelphia JB Lippincott, 1982, p 133.
23. Dodds EC: Significance of synthetic estrogens. Acta Med Scand 90(Suppl):141–145, 1938.
24. Egan RL: Experience with mammography in a tumor institution. Radiology 25:894–900, 1960.
25. Ehrlich P: Closing Notes on Experimental Chemotherapy of Spirillosco. Berlin, J Springer, 1910.
26. Elliott J: Sarcomatous tumour of the breast successfully removed. Lond Med Phys J 48:305–308, 1822.
27. Engell HC: Cancer cells in the circulating blood. Acta Chir Scand 207(Suppl):1–70, 1955.
28. Fabry W: Observationum et curationum chirurgicarum centuriae, cent II: I.A. Huguetan, 1641, pp 267–269.
29. Fisher B, Redmons C, Fisher ER: The contribution of recent clinical trials of primary breast cancer therapy to an understanding of tumor biology. Cancer 46:1009–1025, 1980.
30. Garrison FH: An Introduction to the History of Medicine. Philadelphia, WB Saunders, 1929, p 310.
31. Garrison FH: An Introduction to the History of Medicine. Philadelphia, WB Saunders, 1929, p 599.
32. Gershon-Cohen J: Atlas of Mammography. New York, Springer-Verlag, 1970.
33. Gocht H: Therapeutische Verwendung der Rontgenstrahlen. Fortschr Geb Roentgenstr 1:14–22, 1897.
34. Greenspan EM, Fisher M, Lesnick G, Edelman S: Response of

advanced breast carcinoma to the combination of the antimetabolic methotrexate and the alkylating agent thio-TEPA. Mt Sinai J Med 33:1–26, 1963.

35. Gross SD: System of Surgery, Vol II, 5th ed. Henry C. Lea's Son & Co., 1872, p 1003.

36. Gross SW: An analysis of two hundred and seven cases of carcinoma of the breast. Med News 51:613–616, 1887.

37. Grubbe EH: X-ray Treatment: Its Origin, Birth and Early History. St. Paul, Bruce Pub., 1949.

38. Haagensen CD: Diseases of the Breast. 3rd ed. Philadelphia, WB Saunders, 1986.

39. Haddow A, Watkinson JM, Patterson D: Influence of synthetic estrogen upon advanced malignant disease. Br Med J II:393–398, 1944.

40. Halsted WS: A clinical and histological study of certain adenocarcinomata of the breast. Ann Surg 28:557–576, 1898.

41. Halsted WS: The results of operations for the cure of cancer of the breast performed at the Johns Hopkins Hospital from June 1889 to January 1894. Johns Hopkins Hosp Rep 4:297–350, 1894–1895.

42. Halsted WS: The results of radical operations for cure of cancer of the breast. Ann Surg 46:1–19, 1907.

43. Handley WS: Parasternal invasion of the thorax in breast cancer and its suppression by the use of radium tubes as an operative precaution. Surg Gynecol Obstet 45:721–782, 1927.

44. Harrington SW: Carcinoma of the breast; surgical treatment and results. JAMA 92:280, 1929.

45. Heidelberger C, Chaudhuri NK, Danneberg P, et al: Fluorinated pyrimidines, a new class of tumor inhibitory compounds. Nature 179:663–666, 1957.

46. Heidenhain L: Ueber die Ursachen der localen Krebsrecidive nach Amputation Mammae. Arch Klin Chir 39:97–166, 1889.

47. Horowitz KB: Progesterone receptors and hormone dependent breast cancer. Doctoral Dissertation, University of Texas Southwestern Medical School, Dallas, 1975.

48. Huggins C, Doa TLY: Adrenalectomy and oophorectomy in the treatment of advanced carcinoma of the breast. JAMA 151:1388–1394, 1953.

49. King LS: The Medical World of the Eighteenth Century. Huntington, NY, RE Krieger, 1971, pp 59–121.

50. Keynes GL: The radium treatment of carcinoma of the breast. Br J Surg 19:415–480, 1932.

51. Kleinschmidt O: In Zweife P, Payr E, Hurzel S (eds) Brustdruse in die Klinik der Bosartigsten Geschwulste. Leipzig, 1927.

52. le Dran F: Memoire avec une precis de plusiers observations sur le cancer. Mem Acad Roy Chir Paris 3:1–56, 1757.

53. Levens P: The Pathway to Health. London, 1664, p 109. In special collections of Thomas Jefferson University Library, Philadelphia, PA.

54. Lister J: On the antiseptic principle in the practice of surgery. Lancet II:95, 353, 668, 1867.

55. Liston R: Practical Surgery. 3rd ed. London, Churchill, 1840, p 336.

56. MacMahon CE, Cahill JL: The evolution of the concept of the use of surgical castration in the palliation of breast cancer in premenopausal females. Ann Surg 184:713–716, 1976.

57. McGuire WL, De La Garza M: Similarity of estrogen receptors in human and rat mammary carcinoma. J Clin Endocrinol Metab 36:548–552, 1973.

58. McWhirter R: The value of simple mastectomy and radiotherapy in the treatment of cancer of the breast. Br J Radiol 21:599–610, 1948.

59. Meyer W: An improved method of the radical operation for carcinoma of the breast. Med Rec 46:746–749, 1894.

60. Monod R: Cancer du sein rendu operable par la radiotherapie, Guerison se maintenant depuis trois ans et trois mois. Bull Med Soc Natl Chir 54:92–94, 1927.

61. Moore C: On the influence of inadequate operations on the theory of cancer. R Med Chir Soc Lond 1:244–280, 1867.

62. Nathanson IT: The effect of stilboestrol in advanced cancer of the breast. Cancer Res 6:484, 1946.

63. National Institutes of Health/National Cancer Institute Consensus Development Meeting on Breast Cancer: Issues and Recommendations. J Natl Cancer Inst 60:6, 1978.

64. Paget J: On disease of the mammary areola preceding cancer of the mammary gland. St Bart Hosp Rep 10:87–89, 1874.

65. Paget J: On the average duration of life in patients with scirrhous cancer of the breast. Lancet 1:62–63, 1856.

66. Pagman WJ, Wallace RM: The use of a plastic prosthesis in breast and other soft tissue injury. Presented at 60th Congress of Pan-Pacific Surgery Association, October 7, 1954.

67. Pancoast J: Treatise on Operative Surgery. Philadelphia, Carey & Hart, 1844, p 268.

68. Patey DH, Dyson WH: The prognosis of carcinoma of the breast in relation to the type of operation performed. Br J Cancer 2:7–13, 1948.

69. Perthes GC: Ueber den Einfluss der Roentgenstrahlen auf epitheliale Gewebe, insbesondere auf das Carcinom. Langenbecks Arch Klin Chir 7:955–1000, 1903.

70. Petit JL: Oeuvres completes, section VII. Limoges, R. Chapoulard, 1837, pp 438–445.

71. Pfahler GE: Results of radiation therapy in 1,022 private cases of carcinoma of the breast from 1902 to 1928. Am J Roentgenol 27:497, 1932.

72. Riesman D: Medicine in the Middle Ages. New York, Paul B Hoeber, 1935.

73. Salomon A: Beitrage zur Pathologic und Klinik der Mammar-Carcinom. Arch Klin Chir 105:573–668, 1913.

74. Scultetus J: Armamentarium chirurgicum. Ulm, B Kuhnen, 1653, pp 50–51.

75. Sugarman J: Striking memories of medical education; A glimpse of three physician writers. Pharos 50:30–35, 1987.

76. Syme J: Principles of Surgery. London, H Balliere, 1842.

77. Tansini I: Sopra il mio nuovo processo per l'amputazzione della mammella per cancere. Reforma Medica 12:3, 1896.

78. Ulrich P: Testosterone (hormone male) et son role possible dans le traitement de certains cancers du sein. Int Union Against Cancer 4:377, 1939.

79. Urban JA, Baker HW: Radical mastectomy in continuity with en bloc resection of the internal mammary lymph chain. Cancer 5:992–1008, 1952.

80. Velpeau AALM: Traite des Maladies du Sein et de la Region Mammaire. Paris, V Masson, 1854.

81. Volkmann R: Beitrage zur Chirurgie. Leipzig, Breitkopf & Hartel, 1875, pp 320–338.

82. Wangensteen OH: Discussion to Taylor and Wallace: Carcinoma of the breast, fifty years' experience at the Massachusetts General Hospital. Ann Surg 132:839–841, 1950.

83. Westerman CWG: Thoraxexcisie bij recidief van carcinoma mammae. Geneesk Med Lydschr 54:1681–1690, 1910.

84. Young S: Minutes of cases of cancer and cancerous tendency successfully treated, with a preparatory letter addressed to the Governors of the Middlesex Hospital by Samuel Whitbread. London, E Coxe & Son, 1815.

Section II

Anatomy and Physiology of the Normal and Lactating Breast

Chapter 2

ANATOMY OF THE BREAST, AXILLA, CHEST WALL, AND RELATED METASTATIC SITES

Lynn J. Romrell, Ph.D. and Kirby I. Bland, M.D.

Mammary glands, or breasts, are a distinguishing feature of mammals. They have evolved as milk-producing organs to provide nourishment to the offspring, which are born in a relatively immature and dependent state. The act of nursing the young provides physiological benefit to the mother by aiding in postpartum uterine involution and to the young in transferring passive immunity. The nursing of the young is also of significance in the bonding between the mother and her offspring.

During embryological development there is growth and differentiation of the breasts in both sexes (for a review see Morehead[25]). Paired glands develop along paired lines, the *milk lines,* extending between the limb buds from the future axilla to the future inguinal region. Among the various mammalian species the number of paired glands varies greatly and is related to the number of young in each litter. In the human and most other primates, normally only one gland develops on each side in the pectoral region. An extra breast (polymastia) or nipple (polythelia) may occur as a heritable condition in about 1 percent of the female population. These relatively rare conditions also may occur in the male. When present, the supernumerary breast or nipple usually forms along the milk lines; about one third of the affected individuals have multiple extra breasts or nipples.

In postnatal life, in the male, there is normally little additional development and the gland remains rudimentary. In the female, the breasts undergo extensive further development, which is correlated with age and is regulated by hormones that influence reproductive function. By about 20 years of age the breast has reached its greatest development, and by the age of 40 it begins atrophic changes. During each menstrual cycle, structural changes occur in the breast under the influence of changes in ovarian hormone levels. Striking changes occur not only in the functional activity of the breast but also in the amount of glandular tissue during pregnancy and lactation. The actual secretion and production of milk is induced by prolactin from the pituitary and somatomammotropin from the placenta. With the changes in the hormonal environment that occur at menopause, the glandular component of the breast regresses, or involutes, and is replaced by fat and connective tissue.[17]

GROSS ANATOMICAL STRUCTURE—SURFACE ANATOMY

Form and Size

The breast is located within the superficial fascia of the anterior thoracic wall. It consists of 15 to 20 lobes of glandular tissue of the tubuloalveolar type, fibrous connective tissue connecting its lobes, and adipose tissue in the intervals between the lobes.[7] Subcutaneous connective tissue surrounds the gland and extends as septa between the lobes and lobules, providing support for the glandular elements, but it does not form a distinctive capsule around the components of the breast. The deep

17

layer of the superficial fascia, which lies on the deep, or posterior, surface of the breast, rests upon and fuses with the deep (pectoral) fascia of the thoracic wall. A distinct space, the *retromammary bursa,* can be identified surgically on the posterior aspect of the breast between the deep layer of the superficial fascia and the deep investing fascia of the pectoralis major and contiguous muscles of the thoracic wall (Fig. 2–1). The retromammary bursa contributes to the mobility of the breast on the thoracic wall. Fibrous thickenings of the connective tissue interdigitate between the parenchymal tissue of the breast extending from the deep layer of the superficial fascia (hypodermis) and attaching to the dermis of the skin. These suspensory structures, called *Cooper's ligaments,* insert perpendicular to the delicate superficial fascial layers of the dermis, or corium, permitting remarkable mobility of the breast while providing support.

At maturity, the glandular portion of the breast has a unique and distinctive protuberant conical form. The base of the cone is roughly circular, measuring 10 to 12 cm in diameter and 5 to 7 cm in thickness. Commonly, breast tissue extends into the axilla as the axillary tail of Spence. There is tremendous variation in the size of the breast. A typical nonlactating breasts weighs between 150 to 225 gm, whereas the lactating breast may exceed 500 gm.[33] In a recent study of breast volume in 55 women, Smith et al.[30] reported that the mean volume of the right breast was 275.46 ml (SD = 172.65, median = 217.7, minimum = 94.6, maximum = 889.3) and the left breast was 291.69 ml (SE = 168.23, median = 224.0, minimum = 106.9, maximum = 893.9).

The breast of the nulliparous female has a typical hemispheric configuration with distinct flattening above the nipple. The multiparous breast, which has experienced the hormonal stimulation associated with pregnancy and lactation, is usually larger and more pendulous. As has been noted, during pregnancy and lactation the breast increases dramatically in size and becomes more pendulous. With increasing age the breast usually decreases in volume, becomes somewhat flattened and pendulous, and is less firm.

Extent and Location

The mature female breast extends inferiorly from the level of the second or third rib to the inframammary

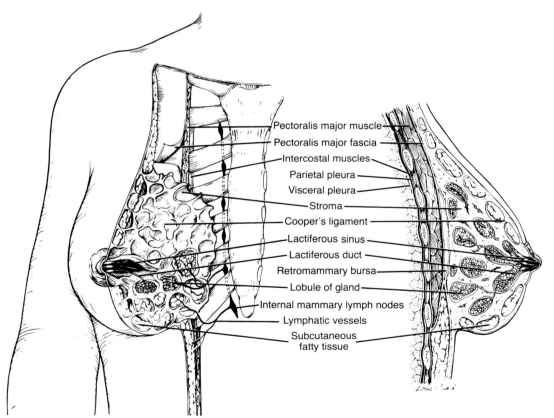

Figure 2–1. A tangential view of the breast on the chest wall and a cross-sectional (sagittal) view of the breast and associated chest wall. The breast lies in the superficial fascia just deep to the dermis. It is attached to the skin by the suspensory ligaments of Cooper and is separated from the investing fascia of the pectoralis major muscle by the retromammary bursa. Cooper's ligaments form fibrosepta in the stroma that provide support for the breast parenchyma. Fifteen to 20 lactiferous ducts extend from lobules composed of glandular epithelium to openings located on the nipple. A dilation of the duct, the lactiferous sinus, is present near the opening of the duct in the subareolar tissue. Subcutaneous fat and adipose tissue distributed around the lobules of the gland give the breast its smooth contour and, in the nonlactating breast, account for most of its mass. Lymphatic vessels pass through the stroma surrounding the lobules of the gland and convey lymph to collecting ducts. Lymphatic channels ending in the internal mammary (or parasternal) lymph nodes are shown. The pectoralis major muscle lies adjacent to the ribs and intercostal muscles. The parietal pleura, attached to the endothoracic fascia, and the visceral pleura, covering the surface of the lung, are shown.

fold, which is at about the level of the sixth or seventh rib, and laterally from the lateral border of the sternum to the anterior or midaxillary line. The deep or posterior surface of the breast rests upon portions of the deep investing fasciae of the pectoralis major, serratus anterior, and external abdominal oblique muscles and the upper extent of the rectus sheath. The axillary tail (of Spence) of the breast extends into the anterior axillary fold. The upper half of the breast, and particularly the upper outer quadrant, contains more glandular tissue than does the remainder of the breast.

MICROSCOPIC ANATOMICAL STRUCTURE

Nipple and Areola

The epidermis of the nipple and areola is highly pigmented and somewhat wrinkled. It is covered by keratinized, stratified squamous epithelium. The deep surface of the epidermis is invaded by unusually long dermal papillae that allow capillaries to bring blood close to the surface, giving the region a pinkish color in immature and blond individuals. At puberty this skin becomes pigmented, and the nipple becomes more prominent. During pregnancy the areola becomes larger and the degree of pigmentation increases. Deep to the areola and nipple, bundles of smooth muscle fibers are arranged radially and circumferentially in the dense connective tissue and longitudinally along the lactiferous ducts that extend up into the nipple. These muscle fibers are responsible for the erection of nipple that occurs in response to various stimuli (for a review of the anatomy of the nipple and areola see Giacometti and Montagna[9]).

The areola contains sebaceous glands, sweat glands, and accessory areolar glands (of Montgomery), which are intermediate in their structure between true mammary glands and sweat glands. The accessory areolar glands produce small elevations on the surface of the areola. The sebaceous glands (which usually lack associated hairs) and sweat glands are located along the margin of the areola. Whereas the tip of the nipple contains numerous free sensory nerve cell endings and Meissner's corpuscles in the dermal papillae, the areola contains fewer of these structures.[35] In a review of the innervation of the nipple and areola, Montagna and Macpherson reported observing fewer nerve endings than described by other investigators.[23] They reported that most of the endings were at the apex of the nipple. Neuronal plexuses are also present around hair follicles in the skin peripheral to the areola, and pacinian corpuscles may be present in the dermis and in the glandular tissue. The rich sensory innervation of the breast, particularly the nipple and areola,[5] is of great functional significance because the suckling infant initiates a chain of neural and neurohumoral events resulting in the release of milk and maintenance of glandular differentiation that is essential for continued lactation.

Inactive Mammary Gland

The adult mammary gland is composed of 15 to 20 irregular lobes of branched tubuloalveolar glands. The lobes, separated by fibrous bands of connective tissue, radiate from the *mammary papilla,* or *nipple,* and are further subdivided into numerous lobules. Those fibrous bands that connect with the dermis are the *suspensory ligaments of Cooper.* Abundant adipose tissue is present in the dense connective tissue of the interlobular spaces. The intralobular connective tissue is much less dense and contains little fat.

The tubuloalveolar glands, derived from modified sweat glands in the epidermis, lie in the subcutaneous tissue. Each lobe of the mammary gland ends in a *lactiferous duct* (2 to 4 mm in diameter), that opens through a constricted orifice (0.4 to 0.7 mm in diameter) onto the nipple (Fig. 2–1). Beneath the areola each duct has a dilated portion, the *lactiferous sinus.* Near their openings, the lactiferous ducts are lined with stratified squamous epithelium. The epithelial lining of the duct shows a gradual transition to two layers of cuboidal cells in the lactiferous sinus and then becomes a single layer of columnar or cuboidal cells through the remainder of the duct system. Myoepithelial cells of ectodermal origin lie within the epithelium between the surface epithelial cells and the basal lamina.[28] These cells, arranged in a basket-like network, are present in the secretory portion of the gland but are more apparent in the larger ducts. They contain myofibrils and are strikingly similar to smooth muscle cells in their cytology.

The morphology of the secretory portion of the mammary gland varies greatly with age and during pregnancy and lactation (Fig. 2–2). In the inactive gland the glandular component is sparse and consists chiefly of duct elements (Fig. 2–3). Most investigators believe that the secretory units in the inactive breast are not organized as alveoli and consist only of ductules. During the menstrual cycle the inactive breast undergoes slight cyclical changes. Early in the cycle the ductules appear as cords with little or no lumen. Under estrogen stimulation, at about the time of ovulation, secretory cells increase in height, lumens appear as small amounts of secretions accumulate, and fluids and lipid accumulate in the connective tissue. Then, in the absence of continued hormonal stimulation, the gland regresses to a more inactive state through the remainder of the cycle.

Active Mammary Glands—Pregnancy and Lactation

During pregnancy, in preparation for lactation, the mammary glands undergo dramatic proliferation and development. These changes in the glandular tissue are accompanied by relative decreases in the amount of connective and adipose tissue. Plasma cells, lymphocytes, and eosinophils infiltrate the fibrous component of the connective tissue as the breast develops in response to hormonal stimulation. The development of the glandular tissue is not uniform, and variation in the

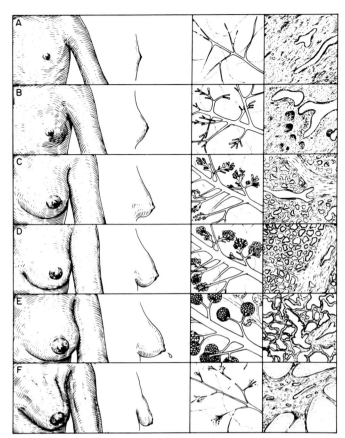

Figure 2–2. Schematic drawing illustrating mammary gland development. Anterior and lateral views of the breast are shown in columns 1 and 2. The microscopic appearances of the ducts and lobules are illustrated in columns 3 and 4, respectively. Panels: A, prepubertal (childhood); B, puberty; C, mature (reproductive); D, pregnancy; E, lactation; F, postmenopausal (senescent) state. (From Copeland EM III, Bland KI: The breast. *In* Sabiston DC Jr. (ed): Essentials of Surgery. Philadelphia, WB Saunders, 1987. Reprinted by permission.)

degree of development may occur within a single lobule. The cells vary in shape from low columnar to flattened. As the cells proliferate by mitotic division, the ductules branch and alveoli begin to develop. In the later stages of pregnancy, alveolar development becomes more prominent (Fig. 2–4). Near the end of pregnancy the actual proliferation of cells declines, and subsequent enlargement of the breast occurs through hypertrophy of the alveolar cells and accumulation of their secretory product in the lumens of the ductules.

The secretory cells contain abundant endoplasmic reticulum, a moderate number of large mitochondria, a supranuclear Golgi complex, and a number of dense lysosomes.[36, 38] Depending on the secretory state of the cell, large lipid droplets and secretory granules may be present in the apical cytoplasm. Two distinct products that are released by different mechanisms are produced by the cells.[39] The protein component of the milk is synthesized in the granular endoplasmic reticulum, packaged in membrane-limited secretory granules for transport in the Golgi apparatus, and released from the cell by fusion of the granule's limiting membrane with the plasma membrane. This type of secretion is known as

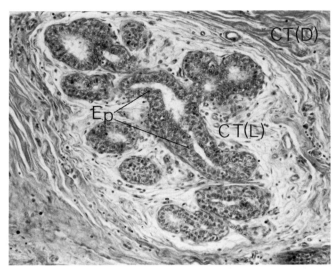

Figure 2–3. Inactive or resting human mammary gland. The epithelial (Ep) or glandular elements are imbedded in loose connective tissue [CT(L)]. Within the lobule the epithelial cells are primarily duct elements. Dense connective tissue [CT(D)] surrounds the lobule. × 160. (Courtesy of Michael H. Ross, Ph.D., University of Florida College of Medicine, Gainesville, FL.)

merocrine secretion. The lipid, or fatty, component of the milk arises as free lipid droplets in the cytoplasm. The lipid coalesces into large droplets that pass to the apical region of the cell and project into the lumen of the acinus prior to their release. As they are released from the cell, the droplets are invested with an envelope of plasma membrane. A thin layer of cytoplasm is trapped between the lipid droplet and plasma membrane as lipid is being released. It should be emphasized that only a very small amount of cytoplasm is lost during this

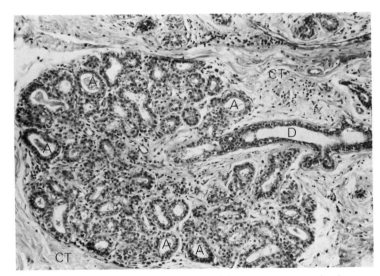

Figure 2–4. Proliferative or active (pregnant) human mammary gland. The alveolar elements of the gland become conspicuous during the early proliferative period (compare with Figure 2–3). Within the lobule of the breast, distinct alveoli (A) are present. The alveoli are continuous with a duct (D). The alveoli are surrounded by highly cellular connective tissue (CT). The individual lobules are separated by dense connective tissue septa. × 160. (Courtesy of Michael H. Ross, Ph.D., University of Florida College of Medicine, Gainesville, FL.)

secretory process that is classically known as *apocrine secretion.*

The milk released during the first few days following childbirth is known as *colostrum.* It has a low lipid content but is believed to contain considerable quantities of antibodies that may provide the newborn with some degree of passive immunity. The lymphocytes and plasma cells that infiltrate the stroma of the breast during its proliferation and development are believed to be, in part, the source of the components of the colostrum. As the plasma cells and lymphocytes decrease in number, the production of colostrum stops and lipid-rich milk is produced.

Hormonal Regulation of the Mammary Gland

Production of estrogens and progesterone by the ovary at puberty stimulates and influences the initial growth of the mammary gland (see Chapter 3, pp 36–38). Subsequent to this initial development, slight changes occur in the morphology of the glandular tissue with each ovarian, or menstrual, cycle. During pregnancy the corpus luteum and placenta continuously produce estrogens and progesterone, which stimulate proliferation and development of the mammary gland. The growth of the glands is also dependent on the presence of prolactin, produced by the adenohypophysis; somatomammotropin (lactogenic hormone), produced by the placenta; and adrenal corticoids.

The level of circulating estrogens and progesterone drops abruptly at parturition with the degeneration of the corpus luteum and loss of the placenta. The secretion of milk is then brought about by increased production of prolactin and adrenal cortical steroids. A neurohormonal reflex regulates the high level of prolactin production and release. The act of suckling by the infant initiates impulses from receptors in the nipple that regulate cells in the hypothalamus. The impulses also cause the release of oxytocin in the neurohypophysis. The oxytocin stimulates the myoepithelial cells of the mammary glands, causing them to contract and eject milk from the glands.[19] In the absence of suckling, secretion of milk ceases and the glands regress and return to an inactive state.

After menopause the gland atrophies, or involutes. As the release of ovarian hormones is diminished, the secretory cells of the alveoli degenerate and disappear, but some of the ducts remain. The connective tissue also demonstrates degenerative changes, marked by a decrease in the number of stromal cells and collagen fibers.

THORACIC WALL

The thoracic wall is composed of both skeletal and muscular components. The skeletal components include the 12 thoracic vertebrae, the 12 ribs and their costal cartilages, and the sternum. The spaces between the ribs, the *intercostal spaces,* are filled with the *external, internal,* and *innermost intercostal muscles* and the associated *intercostal vessels and nerves* (Fig. 2–5). Some anatomists refer to the innermost layer as the *intima* of the *internal intercostal muscle.* The terminology chosen is of no particular consequence; the relationship that should be appreciated is that the intercostal veins, arteries, and nerves pass in the plane that separates the internal intercostal muscle from the innermost (or intimal) layer. The *endothoracic fascia,* a thin fibrous layer of connective tissue forming a fascial plane continuous with the most internal component of the investing fascia of the intercostal muscles and the adjacent layer of the periosteum, marks the internal limit of the thoracic wall. The parietal pleura rests upon the endothoracic fascia.

It is important to recognize that the muscles and skeletal girdles of the upper extremities almost completely cover the thoracic wall anteriorly, laterally, and posteriorly. For the surgeon concerned with the breast, a knowledge of the anatomy of the axilla and pectoral region is essential. The anatomy of the axilla is presented in a separate section; this section will emphasize the anatomy of the pectoral region.

The 11 pairs of *external intercostal muscles* whose fibers run downward and forward form the most superficial layer (see section on the innervation of the breast and Fig. 2–11). The muscle begins posteriorly at the tubercles of the ribs and extends anteriorly to the costochondral junction. Between the costal cartilages the muscle is replaced by the *external intercostal membrane.* The fibers of the 11 pairs of *internal intercostal muscles* run downward and posteriorly. The muscle fibers of this layer reach the sternum anteriorly. Posteriorly, the muscle ends at the angle of the ribs and then the layer continues as the *internal intercostal membrane.* The *innermost intercostal muscles (intercostales intimi)* form the most internal layer and have fibers that are oriented vertically but almost in parallel with the internal intercostal muscle fibers. The muscle fibers of this layer occupy approximately the middle half of the intercostal space. This is the least well developed of the three layers. It can best be distinguished by the fact that its fibers are separated from the internal intercostals by the intercostal vessels and nerves.

The *subcostalis* and *transversus thoracis muscles* are located on the internal surface of the thoracic wall. They occur in the same plane as the innermost internal costal muscles and are considered by many anatomists to be anterior and posterior extensions of this layer. The subcostal muscles are located posteriorly and have the same orientation as the innermost intercostal muscles. They are distinct because they pass to the second or third rib below (that is, they pass over at least two intercostal spaces). Anteriorly, the *transversus thoracis muscles* form a layer that arises from the lower internal surface of the sternum and extends upward and laterally to insert on the costal cartilages of the second to sixth ribs (Fig. 2–6). These fibers pass deep to the internal thoracic artery and accompanying veins.

All these muscles are innervated by the intercostal nerves that are associated with them. These nerves also

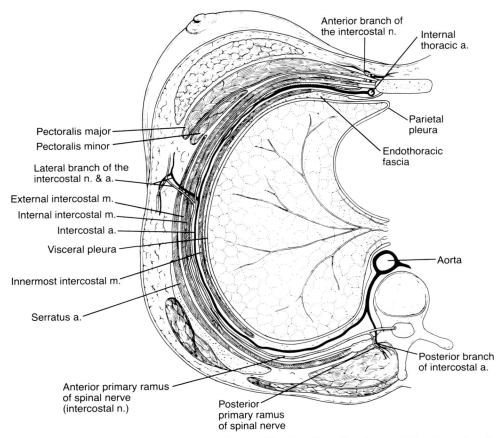

Figure 2–5. Cross section of the breast and chest wall illustrating the layers of the thoracic wall and paths of blood vessels and nerves. The intercostal muscles occur in three layers—external, internal, and innermost. The intercostal vessels and nerves pass between the internal and innermost layers. The posterior intercostal arteries arise from the aorta and pass anterior to anastomose with the anterior intercostal arteries that are branches of the internal thoracic artery. The veins are not shown but basically follow the course of the arteries. The intercostal nerves are direct continuations of the anterior primary rami. They supply the intercostal muscles and give anterior and lateral branches that supply the overlying skin, including that of the breast. The breast lies superficial to the pectoralis major muscle and the underlying pectoralis minor muscle. The serratus anterior muscle originates from eight or nine fleshy digitations on the outer lateral surface of the ribs and inserts on the ventral surface of the medial (vertebral) border of the scapula. Parietal pleura attaches to the endothoracic fascia that lines the thoracic cavity. Visceral pleura covers the surface of the lungs. The thin channels in the substance of the lung represent lymphatic channels that convey lymph to pulmonary lymph nodes located in the hilum of the lung. Lymphatic channels draining the thoracic wall and overlying skin and superficial fascia are not illustrated but follow the path of the blood vessels that supply the region (see text).

give branches to the overlying skin. In a similar fashion the intercostal vessels supply intercostal muscles and give branches to the overlying tissues. The intercostal nerves are direct continuations of the ventral primary rami of the upper 11 thoracic spinal nerves. The twelfth thoracic spinal nerve is called the *subcostal nerve.* As the nerves pass anteriorly they give branches to supply the intercostal muscles. Additionally, each nerve gives a relatively large lateral cutaneous branch, which exits the intercostal space along the midaxillary line near the attachment sites of the serratus anterior muscle on the ribs. The lateral cutaneous nerves then give branches that extend anteriorly and posteriorly. As the intercostal nerve continues anteriorly, it gives additional branches to the intercostal muscles. Just lateral to the border of the sternum the upper five intercostal nerves pierce the internal intercostal muscle and the external intercostal membrane to end superficially as the *anterior cutaneous nerve* of the chest. These nerves give rise to medial and lateral branches that supply the overlying skin. The

lower six intercostal nerves continue past the costal margin into the anterior abdominal wall and are therefore identified as *thoracoabdominal nerves.*

The *intercostal arteries* originate in two groups, the anterior and posterior intercostal arteries. The *posterior intercostal arteries,* except for the first two spaces, arise from the thoracic aorta. The posterior intercostals for the first two spaces arise from the superior (or supreme) intercostal artery, which is a branch of the costocervical trunk. The anterior intercostals are usually small paired arteries that extend laterally to the region of the costochondral junction. The anterior intercostal arteries of the upper five intercostal spaces arise from the internal thoracic (or mammary) artery; those of the lower six intercostal spaces arise from the musculophrenic artery. The anterior and posterior intercostal veins demonstrate a similar distribution. Anteriorly, they drain into the musculophrenic and internal thoracic veins. Posteriorly, the intercostal veins drain into the azygos system of veins.

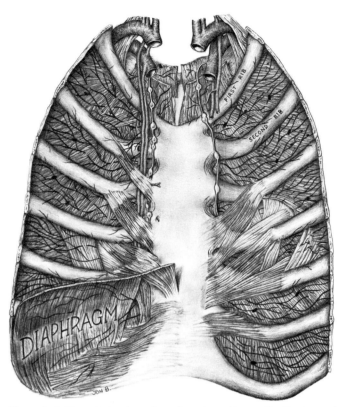

Figure 2–6. The anterior thoracic wall as viewed internally. The internal thoracic arteries and veins can be seen as they pass parallel to and about 1 cm from the sternal margin. Except in the upper two or three intercostal spaces the transversus thoracis muscle lies deep to these vessels. The internal thoracic lymphatic trunks and associated parasternal lymph nodes accompany these vessels. Lymphatic channels located in the intercostal spaces convey lymph from the thoracic wall anteriorly to the parasternal nodes or posteriorly to the intercostal nodes.

The superficial muscles of the pectoral region and their innervation and blood supply are described in the section on the axilla. The *pectoralis major* is a fan-shaped muscle with two divisions. The clavicular division (or head) originates from the clavicle and is easily distinguished from the larger costosternal division that originates from the sternum and costal cartilages of the second through sixth ribs. The fibers of the two divisions converge laterally and insert into the crest of the greater tubercle of the humerus along the lateral lip of the bicipital groove. The *cephalic vein* serves as a convenient landmark defining the separation of the upper lateral border of the pectoralis major muscle from the deltoid muscle. The cephalic vein can be followed to the deltopectoral triangle, where it pierces the *clavipectoral fascia* and joins the axillary vein. The pectoralis major muscle acts primarily in flexion, adduction, and medial rotation of the arm at the shoulder joint. This action brings the arm across the chest. In climbing, the pectoralis major muscles along with the latissimus dorsi muscles function to elevate the trunk when the arms are fixed. The pectoralis major muscle is innervated by both the medial and the lateral pectoral nerves, which arise from the medial and lateral cords of the brachial plexus.

Located deep to the pectoralis major muscle, the *pectoralis minor muscle* arises from the external surface of the second to the fifth ribs and inserts on the coracoid process of the scapula. Although its main action is to lower the shoulder, it may serve as an accessory muscle of respiration. It is innervated by the medial pectoral nerve.

The *subclavius muscle* arises from the first rib near its costochondral junction and extends laterally to insert into the inferior surface of the clavicle. It functions to lower the clavicle and stabilize it during movements of the shoulder girdle. It is innervated by a nerve arising from the upper trunk of the brachial plexus, the *nerve to the subclavius.*

AXILLA

A knowledge of the anatomy of the axilla and its contents is of paramount importance to the clinician. It is also essential that the surgeon be thoroughly familiar with the organization of the deep fascia and neurovascular relationships of the axilla.

Boundaries of the Axilla

The axilla is a pyramidal compartment between the upper extremity and the thoracic walls (Fig. 2–7). It is described as having four walls, an apex, and a base.

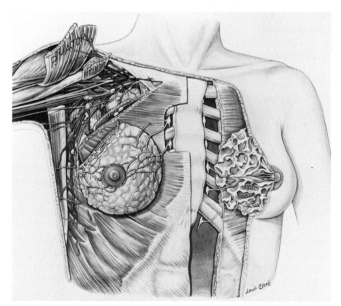

Figure 2–7. The anterior chest illustrating the structure of the chest wall, breast, and axilla. See text for details of the structure of the axilla and a description of its contents. On the right side, the pectoralis major has been cut lateral to the breast and reflected laterally to its insertion into the crest of the greater tubercle of the humerus. This exposes the underlying pectoralis minor and the other muscles forming the walls of the axilla. The contents of the axilla, including the axillary artery and vein, components of the brachial plexus, and axillary lymph node groups and lymphatic channels, are exposed. On the left side, the organ is cut to expose the structure of the breast in sagittal view. The lactiferous ducts and sinuses can be seen. Lymphatic channels passing to parasternal lymph nodes are also shown.

The curved *base* is made of axillary fascia. Externally, this region, the *armpit*, appears dome-shaped (and covered with hair after puberty). The *apex* is not a roof but an aperture that extends into the posterior triangle of the neck through the *cervicoaxillary canal*. The cervicoaxillary canal is bounded anteriorly by the clavicle, posteriorly by the scapula, and medially by the first rib. Most structures pass through the cervical axillary canal as they course between the neck and upper extremity. The *anterior wall* is made up of the pectoralis major and minor muscles and their associated fasciae. The *posterior wall* is composed primarily of the subscapularis muscle, located on the anterior surface of the scapula, and to a lesser extent by the teres major and latissimus dorsi muscles. The *lateral wall* is a thin strip of the arm, the bicipital groove, between the insertions of the muscles of the anterior and posterior walls. The *medial wall* is made up of serratus anterior muscle that covers the thoracic wall (in this region over the upper four or five ribs and their associated intercostal muscles).

Contents of the Axilla

The axilla contains the great vessels and nerves of the upper extremity. These, along with the other contents, are surrounded by loose connective tissue. Figure 2–7 illustrates many of the key relationships of structures within the axilla. The vessels and nerves are closely associated with each other and are enclosed within a layer of fascia, the *axillary sheath*. This layer of dense connective tissue extends from the neck and gradually disappears as the nerves and vessels branch. The *axillary artery* may be divided into three parts within the axilla: (1) The first segment, located medial to the pectoralis minor muscle, gives one branch—the supreme thoracic that supplies the thoracic wall over the first and second intercostal spaces. (2) The second part, located posterior to the pectoralis minor, gives two branches—the thoracoacromial trunk and the lateral thoracic artery. The thoracoacromial trunk divides into the acromial, clavicular, deltoid, and pectoral branches. The lateral thoracic passes along the lateral border of the pectoralis minor on the superficial surface of the serratus anterior muscle. Pectoral branches of the thoracoacromial and lateral thoracic supply both the pectoralis major and minor muscles and must be identified during surgical dissection of the axilla. The lateral thoracic is of particular importance in surgery of the breast because it supplies the *lateral mammary branches*. (3) The third part, located lateral to the pectoralis minor, gives off three branches—the anterior and posterior humeral circumflex arteries which supply the upper arm and contribute to the collateral circulation around the shoulder, and the subscapular artery. Although the latter artery does not supply the breast, it is of particular importance in the surgical dissection of the axilla. It is the largest branch within the axilla, giving rise after a short distance to its terminal branches, the subscapular circumflex and the thoracodorsal, and it is closely associated with the central and subscapular lymph node groups. In the axilla the thoracodorsal artery crosses the subscapularis and gives branches to it and to the serratus anterior and the latissimus dorsi. A surgeon must use care in approaching this vessel and its branches so as to avoid undue bleeding that obscures the surgical field.

The *axillary vein* has tributaries that follow the course of the arteries just described. They are usually in the form of venae comitantes, paired veins that follow an artery. The *cephalic vein* passes in the groove between the deltoid and pectoralis major muscles and then joins the axillary vein after piercing the clavipectoral fascia.

Throughout its course in the axilla, the axillary artery is associated with various parts of the *brachial plexus* (Fig. 2–8). The cords of the brachial plexus—medial, lateral, and posterior—are named according to their relationship with the axillary artery. A majority of the branches of the brachial plexus arise in the axilla. The *lateral cord* gives three branches, namely, the *lateral pectoral nerve* (supplying the pectoralis major and often giving a branch that communicates with the medial pectoral nerve) and two terminal branches—the *musculocutaneous nerve* and the *lateral root of the median nerve*. The *medial cord* usually gives five branches, the *medial pectoral nerve* (which supplies both the pectoralis major and minor), the *median brachial cutaneous*, the *medial antebrachial cutaneous*, and two terminal branches—the *ulnar and the lateral root of the median nerve*. The *posterior cord* usually has five branches. Three of these nerves arise from the posterior cord in rapid succession—the *upper subscapular*, the *thoracodorsal*, and the *lower subscapular*; the cord then divides into its two terminal branches—the *axillary* and *radial nerve*.

Two additional nerves that are of particular interest to surgeons are found in the axilla. The *long thoracic nerve* is located on the medial wall of the axilla. It arises in the neck from the fifth, sixth, and seventh roots of the brachial and then enters the axilla through the cervicoaxillary canal. It lies on the surface of the serratus anterior muscle, which it supplies. The long thoracic nerve is covered by the serratus fascia and is sometimes accidentally removed with the fascia during surgery.

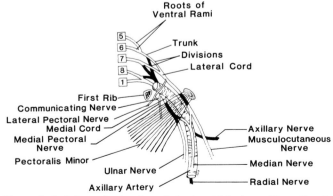

Figure 2–8. Schematic drawing of the brachial plexus illustrating its basic components. The cords are associated with the axillary artery and lie behind the pectoralis minor muscle. The names of the cords reflect their relationship to the artery. Compare with Figure 2–7 to identify the course of these structures in more detail.

This results in paralysis of part or all of the serratus anterior muscle. The functional deficit is inability to raise the arm above the level of the shoulder (or extreme weakness when one attempts this movement). A second nerve, the *intercostobrachial*, is formed by the joining of a lateral cutaneous branch of the second intercostal nerve with the medial cutaneous nerve of the arm. This nerve supplies the skin of the floor of the axilla and the upper medial aspect of the arm. Sometimes a second intercostobrachial nerve may form an anterior branch of the third lateral cutaneous nerve.

Lymph nodes are also present in the axilla. They are found in close association with the blood vessels. The lymph node groups and their location are described in the section on the lymphatic drainage of the breast.

Axillary Fasciae

The anterior wall of the axilla is composed of the pectoralis major and minor muscles and the fascia that covers them. The associated fascia occurs in two layers: (1) a superficial layer investing the pectoralis major muscle, called the *pectoral fascia*, and (2) a deep layer that extends from the clavicle to the axillary fascia in the floor of the axilla, called the *clavipectoral (or costocoracoid) fascia*. The clavipectoral fascia encloses the subclavius muscle located below the clavicle and the pectoralis minor muscle (Fig. 2–9).

The upper portion of the clavipectoral fascia, the *costocoracoid membrane*, is pierced by the cephalic vein, the lateral pectoral nerve, and branches of the thoracoacromial trunk. The medial pectoral nerve does not pierce the costocoracoid membrane, but enters the deep surface of the pectoralis minor supplying it and passes through the anterior investing layer of the pectoralis minor to innervate the pectoralis minor. The lower portion of the clavipectoral fascia, located below the pectoralis minor, is sometimes called the *suspensory ligament of the axilla* or the *coracoaxillary fascia*.

As the costocoracoid membrane is cut, the axillary artery and vein are exposed. *Halsted's ligament,* a dense condensation of the clavipectoral fascia, extends from the medial end of the clavicle and attaches to the first rib (Figs. 2–7 and 2–9A). The ligament covers the subclavian artery and vein as they cross the first rib.

FASCIAL RELATIONSHIPS OF THE BREAST

The breast is located in the superficial fascia in the layer just deep to the dermis, the *hypodermis*. In approaching the breast a surgeon may dissect in a bloodless plane just deep to the dermis. This dissection leaves a layer 2 to 3 mm in thickness in thin individuals in association with the skin flap. The layer may be several millimeters thick in obese individuals. The blood vessels and lymphatics passing in the deeper layer of the superficial fascia are left undisturbed.

Anterior fibrous processes, the *suspensory ligaments of Cooper,* pass from the septa that divide the lobules

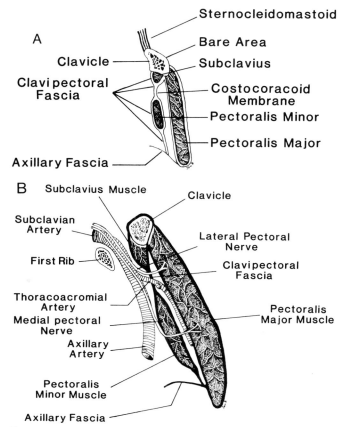

Figure 2–9. Sagittal sections of the chest wall in the axillary region. *A,* The anterior wall of the axilla. The clavicle and three muscles inferior to it are shown. *B,* Section through the chest wall illustrating the relationship of the axillary artery and medial and lateral pectoral nerves to the clavipectoral fascia. The clavipectoral fascia is a strong sheet of connective tissue that is attached superiorly to the clavicle and envelops the subclavius and pectoralis minor muscles. The fascia extends from the lower border of the pectoralis minor to become continuous with the axillary fascia in the floor of the axilla.

of the breast to insert into the skin. The posterior aspect of the breast is separated from the deep, or investing, fascia of the pectoralis major muscle by a space filled with loose areolar tissue, the *retromammary space or bursa* (see Fig. 2–1). The existence of the retromammary space and the suspensory ligaments of Cooper allows the breast to move freely against the thoracic wall. The space between the well-defined fascial planes of the breast and pectoralis major is easily identified by the surgeon removing a breast. Connective tissue thickenings, called *posterior suspensory ligaments*, extend from the deep surface of the breast to the deep pectoral fascia. Since breast parenchyma may follow these fibrous processes, it has been common practice to remove the adjacent portion of the pectoralis major muscle with the breast.

It is important to recognize, particularly with movements and variation in the size of the breast, that its deep surface contacts the investing fascia of other muscles in addition to the pectoralis major. (The external investing fascial layer of all of the superficial muscles of the body wall contributes to the layer known as the deep fascia.) Only about two thirds of the breast overlies the pectoralis major muscle. The lateral portion of the breast may contact the fourth through seventh slips of the serratus anterior muscle at the attachment to the thoracic wall. Just medial to this the breast contacts the upper portion of the abdominal oblique muscle where it interdigitates with the attachments of the serratus anterior muscle. As the breast extends to the axilla it has contact with deep fascia present in this region.

BLOOD SUPPLY OF THE BREAST

The breast receives its blood supply from (1) perforating branches of the internal mammary artery, (2) lateral branches of the posterior intercostal arteries, and (3) several branches from the axillary artery, including highest thoracic, lateral thoracic, and pectoral branches of the thoracoacromial (Fig. 2–10). For reviews of the blood supply of the breast, see Cunningham,[8] Marliniac,[20] and Sakki.[29]

Branches from the second, third, and fourth anterior perforating arteries (Figs. 2–10 and 12–11) pass to the breast as *medial mammary arteries.* These vessels enlarge considerably during lactation. The lateral thoracic artery is an important vessel in the axilla. It gives branches to the serratus anterior muscle, both pectoralis muscles, and the subscapularis muscle and also supplies axillary lymph nodes. In the female the lateral thoracic artery is relatively large and gives rise to *lateral mam-*

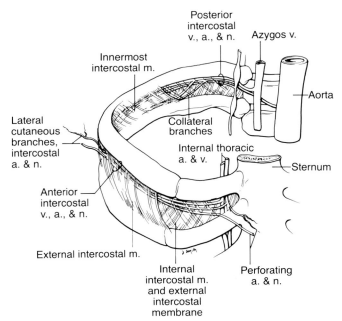

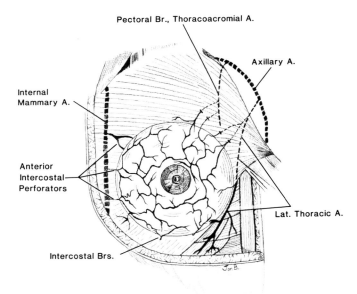

Figure 2–10. Arterial distribution of blood to the breast, axilla, and chest wall. The breast receives its blood supply via three major arterial routes: (1) medially from anterior perforating intercostal branches arising from the internal thoracic artery; (2) laterally from either pectoral branches of the thoracoacromial trunk or branches of the lateral thoracic artery (the thoracoacromial trunk and the lateral thoracic arteries are branches of the axillary artery); and (3) from lateral cutaneous branches of the intercostal arteries that are associated with the overlying breast. The arteries indicated with a dashed line lie deep to the muscles of the thoracic wall and axilla. Many of the arteries must pass through these muscles before reaching the breast.

Figure 2–11. A segment of the body wall illustrating the relationship of structures to the ribs. Two ribs are shown as they extend from the vertebrae to attach to the sternum. The orientation of the muscle and connective tissue fibers is shown. The external intercostal muscle extends downward and forward. The muscle layer extends forward from the rib tubercle to the costochondral junction, where the muscle is replaced by the aponeurosis, called the external intercostal membrane. The internal intercostal muscle fibers with the opposite orientation can be seen through this layer. The innermost intercostal muscle fibers are present along the lateral half of the intercostal space. The intercostal nerve and vessels pass through the intercostal space in the plane between the internal and innermost (or intima of the internal) intercostal muscle layers. Anterior intercostal arteries arise from the internal thoracic artery; anterior intercostal veins join the internal thoracic vein. Posterior intercostal arteries arise from the aorta; posterior intercostal veins join the azygos system on the right and the hemiazygos system on the left. Lymphatics follow the path of the blood vessels. Anteriorly, lymphatics pass to parasternal (or internal mammary) nodes that are located along the internal mammary vessels; posteriorly, they pass to intercostal nodes located in the intercostal space near the vertebral bodies.

mary branches that wrap around the lateral border of the pectoralis major to reach the breast. In the second, third, and fourth intercostal spaces, the posterior intercostal arteries give off *mammary branches;* these vessels increase in size during lactation.

The thoracodorsal branch of the subscapular artery is not involved in the supply of blood to the breast, but it is important to the surgeon who must deal with this artery during the dissection of the axilla. The central and scapular lymph node groups are intimately associated with this vessel. Bleeding that is difficult to control may result from cutting of branches of these vessels.

A fundamental knowledge of the pattern of venous drainage is important because carcinoma of the breast may metastasize through the veins and because lymphatic vessels often follow the course of the blood vessels. The veins of the breast basically follow the path of the arteries, with the chief venous drainage toward the axilla. The superficial veins demonstrate extensive anastomoses, and that may be apparent through the skin overlying the breast. The distribution of these veins has been studied by Massopust and Gardner[21] and Haagensen[13] using photographs taken in infrared light. Around the nipple the veins form an anastomotic circle, the *circulus venosus.* Veins from this circle and from the substance of the gland transmit blood to the periphery of the breast and then into vessels joining the internal thoracic, axillary, and internal jugular veins.

Three principal groups of veins are involved in the venous drainage of the thoracic wall and the breast: (1) perforating branches of the internal thoracic vein, (2) tributaries of the axillary vein, and (3) perforating branches of posterior intercostal veins. Metastatic emboli traveling through any of these venous routes will pass through the venous return to the heart and then be stopped as they reach the capillary bed of the lungs, providing a direct venous route for metastasis of breast carcinoma to the lungs.

The *vertebral plexus of veins (Batson's plexus)* may provide a second route for metastasis of breast carcinoma via veins.[3, 4, 18] This venous plexus surrounds the vertebrae and extends from the base of the skull to the sacrum. Venous channels exist between this plexus and veins associated with thoracic, abdominal, and pelvic organs. In general, these veins do not have valves, making it possible for blood to flow through them in either direction. Furthermore, it is known that increases in intra-abdominal pressure may force blood to enter these channels. These vessels provide a route for metastatic emboli to reach the vertebral bodies, ribs, and central nervous system. (The spread of carcinoma of the prostate to the vertebral bodies and central nervous system occurs through these venous communications.) These venous communications are of particular significance in the breast, where the posterior intercostal arteries are in direct continuity with the vertebral plexus. The potential pathway explains the metastasis of breast carcinoma to the vertebrae, skull, pelvic bones, and central nervous system when there is no pulmonary metastasis.

INNERVATION OF THE BREAST

Miller and Kasahara[22] have described the microscopic anatomic features of the innervation of the skin over the breast. They suggest that the specialization of the innervation of the breast, areola, and nipple is associated with the erection of the nipple and flow of milk mediated through a neurohormonal reflex. As was explained previously, the act of suckling initiates impulses from receptors in the nipple that regulate cells in the hypothalamus. In response to the impulses, oxytocin is released in the neurohypophysis. The oxytocin stimulates the myoepithelial cells of the mammary glands, causing them to contract and eject milk from the glands. In the dermis of the nipple, Miller and Kasahara found large numbers of multibranched free nerve endings; in the dermis of the areola and peripheral, Ruffini-like endings and Krause end-bulbs. The latter two receptor types are associated with tactile reception of stretch and pressure.

Sensory innervation of the breast is supplied primarily by the *lateral and anterior cutaneous branches of the second through sixth intercostal nerves* (Fig. 2–11). Although the second and third intercostal nerves may give rise to cutaneous branches to the superior aspect of the breast, the nerves of the breast are derived primarily from the fourth, fifth, and sixth intercostal nerves. A limited region of the skin over the upper portion of the breast is supplied by nerves arising from the cervical plexus, specifically the anterior, or medial, branches of the *supraclavicular nerve.* All these nerves convey sympathetic fibers to the breast and overlying skin and therefore influence flow of blood through vessels accompanying the nerves and secretory function of the sweat glands of the skin. However, the secretory activity of the breast is chiefly under the control of ovarian and hypophyseal (pituitary) hormones.

The lateral branches of the intercostal nerves exit the intercostal space at the attachment sites of the slips of serratus anterior muscle. The nerves divide into anterior and posterior branches as they exit the muscle. As the anterior branches pass in the superficial fascia, they supply the anterolateral thoracic wall; the third through sixth branches, also known as *lateral mammary branches,* supply the breast. The lateral branch of the second intercostal nerve is of special significance because a large nerve, the *intercostal brachial,* arises from it. This nerve, which can be seen during surgical dissection of the axilla, passes through the fascia of the floor of the axilla and usually joins the medial cutaneous nerve of the arm. However, it is of little functional significance. If this nerve is injured during surgery, the patient will have some loss of cutaneous sensation from the upper medial aspect of the arm.

The anterior branches of the intercostal nerves exit the intercostal space near the lateral border of the sternum. These nerves send branches medially and laterally over the thoracic wall. The branches that pass laterally reach the medial aspect of the breast and are sometimes called *medial mammary branches.*

LYMPHATIC DRAINAGE OF THE BREAST

Lymph Nodes of the Axilla

The primary route of lymphatic drainage of the breast is through the axillary lymph node groups (Figs. 2–7 and 2–12). Therefore, it is essential that the clinician understand the anatomy of the grouping of lymph nodes within the axilla. Unfortunately, the boundaries of groups of lymph nodes found in the axilla are not well demarcated. Thus, there has been considerable variation in the names given to the lymph node groups. Anatomists usually define five groups of *axillary lymph nodes*[11, 26]; surgeons usually identify six primary groups.[13] The most common terms used to identify the lymph nodes are indicated as follows:

1. The *axillary vein group,* usually identified by anatomists as the *lateral group,* consists of four to six lymph nodes that lie medial or posterior to the axillary vein.

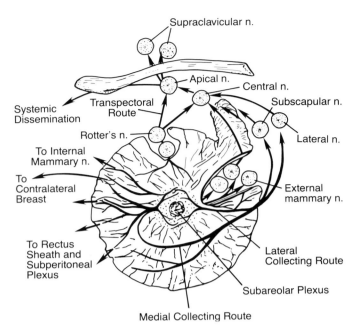

Figure 2–12. Schematic drawing of the breast identifying the position of lymph nodes relative to the breast and illustrating routes of lymphatic drainage. The clavicle is indicated as a reference point. See the text and Figure 2–14 to identify the group or level to which the lymph nodes belong. Level I lymph nodes include the external mammary (or anterior), axillary vein (or lateral), and scapular (or posterior) groups; Level II, the central group; and Level III, the subclavicular (or apical). The arrows indicate the routes of lymphatic drainage (see text).

These lymph nodes receive most of the lymph draining from the upper extremity (Fig. 2–13). The exception is lymph that drains into the *deltopectoral lymph nodes,* a lymph node group sometimes called *infraclavicular.* The deltopectoral lymph nodes are not considered to be part of the axillary lymph node group, but are outlying lymph nodes that drain into the subclavicular (or apical) lymph node group (see below).

2. The *external mammary group,* usually identified by anatomists as the *anterior or pectoral group,* consists of four or five lymph nodes that lie along the lower border of the pectoralis minor in association with the lateral thoracic vessels. These lymph nodes receive the major portion of the lymph draining from the breast. Lymph drains primarily from these lymph nodes into the central lymph nodes. However, lymph may pass directly from the external mammary nodes into the subclavicular lymph nodes.

3. The *scapular group,* usually identified by anatomists as the *posterior or subscapular group,* consists of six or seven lymph nodes that lie along the posterior wall of the axilla at the lateral border of the scapula in association with the subscapular vessels. These lymph nodes receive lymph primarily from the lower back of the neck, the posterior aspect of the trunk as low as the iliac crest, and the posterior part of the shoulder region. Lymph from the scapular nodes passes to the central and subclavicular nodes.

4. The *central group* (both anatomists and surgeons use the same terminology for this group) consists of three of four large lymph nodes that are embedded in

the fat of the axilla, usually behind the pectoralis minor muscle. They receive lymph from the three preceding groups and may receive afferent lymphatic vessels directly from the breast. Lymph from the central nodes passes directly to the subclavicular (apical) nodes. This group is often superficially placed beneath the skin and fascia of the midaxilla and is centrally located between the posterior and anterior axillary fold. This nodal

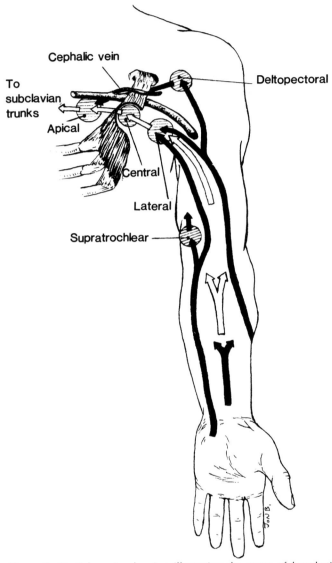

Figure 2–13. Schematic drawing illustrating the route of lymphatic drainage in the upper extremity. The relationship of this drainage to the major axillary lymph node groups is indicated by the arrows. All the lymph vessels of the upper extremity drain directly or indirectly through outlying lymph node groups into the axillary lymph nodes. The outlying lymph nodes are few in number and are organized into three groups: (1) supratrochlear lymph nodes (one or two, located above the medial epicondyle of the humerus adjacent to the basilic vein); (2) deltopectoral lymph nodes (one or two, located beside the cephalic vein where it lies between the pectoralis major and deltoid muscle just below the clavicle); and (3) variable small isolated lymph nodes (few and variable in number; may be located in the cubital fossa or along the medial side of the brachial vessels). Note that the deltopectoral lymph node group drains directly into the subclavicular, or apical, lymph nodes of the axillary group.

group is commonly palpable, owing to its superficial position, and allows the clinical estimation of metastatic disease.[1, 13]

5. The *subclavicular group,* usually identified by anatomists as the *apical group,* consists of 6 to 12 lymph nodes located partly posterior to the upper border of the pectoralis minor and partly above it. The lymph nodes extend into the apex of the axilla along the medial side of the axillary vein. They receive lymph from all the other groups of axillary lymph nodes. The efferent lymphatic vessels from the subclavicular lymph nodes unite to form the *subclavian trunk.* The course of the subclavian trunk is highly variable. It may directly join the internal jugular vein, the subclavian vein, or the junction of these two; likewise, on the right side of the trunk it may join the right lymphatic duct, and on the left side it may join the thoracic duct. Efferent vessels from the subclavicular lymph nodes may also pass to deep cervical lymph nodes.

6. The *interpectoral or Rotter's group,*[12] a group of nodes identified by surgeons[13] but usually not by anatomists, consists of one to four small lymph nodes that are located between the pectoralis major and minor associated with the pectoral branches of the thoraco-acromial vessels. Lymph from these nodes passes into central and subclavicular nodes.

Surgeons also define the axillary lymph nodes with respect to their relationship with the pectoralis minor (Fig. 2–14).[1, 6] These relationships are illustrated schematically in Figure 2–15. Lymph nodes that are located lateral to or below the lower border of the pectoralis minor are called *Level I* and include the external mammary, axillary vein, and scapular lymph node groups. Those lymph nodes located deep to, or behind, the pectoralis minor are called *Level II* and include the central lymph node group and possibly some of the subclavicular lymph node group. Those lymph nodes located medial to or above the upper border of the pectoralis minor are called *Level III* and include the subclavicular lymph node group.

Surgeons use the term *prepectoral* to identify a single lymph node that is only rarely found in the subcutaneous tissue associated with the breast or in the breast itself in its upper outer sector.[13] Haagensen reports finding only one or two prepectoral nodes each year among the several hundred mammary lesions studied.

Lymph Flow

A conceptualization of lymphatic drainage of the breast is essential to the student of this organ's pathophysiology. Metastatic dissemination occurs predominantly by lymphatic routes, which are rich and extensive and arborize in multiple directions through skin and mesenchymal (intraparenchymal) lymphatics. The delicate lymphatics of the corium are valveless; flow encompasses the lobular parenchyma and thereafter parallels major venous tributaries to enter the regional lymph nodes. This unidirectional lymphatic flow is pulsatile as a consequence of the wavelike contractions of the lym-

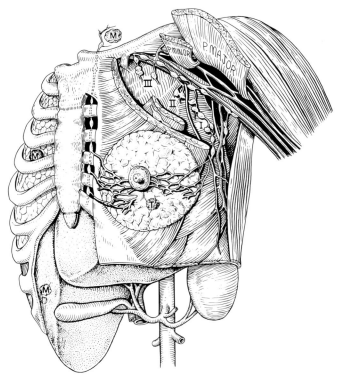

Figure 2–14. Lymphatic drainage of the breast. The pectoralis major and minor muscles, which contribute to the anterior wall of the axilla, have been cut and reflected. This exposes the medial and posterior walls of the axilla as well as the basic contents of the axilla. The lymph node groups of the axilla and the internal mammary nodes are depicted. Also shown is the location of the long thoracic nerve on the surface of the serratus anterior muscle (on the medial wall of the axilla). The scapular lymph node group is closely associated with the thoracodorsal nerve and vessels.

phatics to allow rapid transit and emptying of the lymphatic vascular spaces that interdigitate the extensive periductal and perilobular network. As a consequence of obstruction to lymph flow by inflammatory or neoplastic diseases, a reversal in lymphatic flow is evident and can be appreciated microscopically as endolymphatic metastases of the dermis or breast parenchyma. This obstruction of lymphatic flow accounts for the neoplastic growth in local and regional sites remote from the primary neoplasm.

In contradistinction to blood circulation, lymphatic flow is unidirectional, except in the pathological state, and has preferential flow from the periphery toward the right side of the heart. Lymphatic capillaries end blindly in tissues from which the lymph is collected; throughout their course these capillaries anastomose and fuse to form fewer lymphatic channels that terminate in the large left thoracic duct or the smaller right lymphatic duct. The thoracic duct empties into the left subclavian vein, whereas the right lymphatic duct drains preferentially into the right subclavian vein at the point of entry for the internal jugular vein.

Haagensen emphasized that lymphatics of the dermis are intimately associated with deeper lymphatics of the underlying fascial plains, which explains the multidirectional potential for drainage of superficial breast neoplasms. Preferential lymphatic flow toward the axilla is observed in lesions of the upper anterolateral chest. In contrast, at the level of the umbilicus, tributaries diverge such that chest and upper anterior and lateral abdominal wall lymph will enter channels of the axilla. Thus, carcinomatous involvement of skin, even of the inframammary region, has preferential flow to the axilla rather than to the groin.[13]

Anson and McVay and Haagensen acknowledged two accessory directions for lymphatic flow from breast parenchyma to nodes of the apex of the axilla: the *transpectoral* and *retropectoral routes* (see Fig. 2–12). Lymphatics of the transpectoral route, i.e., interpectoral nodes, lie between the pectoralis major and minor muscles and are referred to as *Rotter's nodes*. The transpectoral route begins in the loose areolar tissue of the retromammary plexus and interdigitates between the pectoral fascia and breast to perforate the pectoralis major muscle and follow the course of the thoracoacromial artery and terminate in the subclavicular (Level III) group of nodes.

The second accessory lymphatic drainage group, the retropectoral pathway, drains the superior and internal aspects of the breast. Lymphatic vessels from this region of the breast join lymphatics from the posterior and lateral surface of the pectoralis major and the pectoralis minor muscles. These lymphatic channels terminate at the apex of the axilla in the subclavicular (Level III) group. This route of lymphatic drainage is found in approximately one third of individuals and is a more direct mechanism of lymphatic flow to the subclavicular group. This accessory pathway is also the major lymphatic drainage by way of the external mammary and central axillary nodal groups (Levels I and II, respectively).[1, 13]

The recognition of metastatic spread of breast carcinoma into internal mammary nodes as a primary route of systemic dissemination is credited to the British surgeon W.S. Handley. Extensive investigation confirmed that central and medial lymphatics of the breast will pass medially and parallel the course of major blood vessels to perforate the pectoralis major muscle and thereafter terminate in the internal mammary nodal chain.

The internal mammary nodal group (see Figs. 2–6 and 2–14) is anatomically situated in the retrosternal interspaces between the costal cartilages approximately 2 to 3 cm within the sternal margin. These nodal groups also traverse and parallel the internal mammary vasculature and are invested by endothoracic fascia. The internal mammary lymphatic trunks eventually terminate in subclavicular nodal groups (Figs. 2–6, 2–12, and 2–15). The right internal mammary nodal group enters the right lymphatic duct, and the left enters the main thoracic duct (see Fig. 2–16A, B). The presence of supraclavicular nodes (Stage IV disease) results from lymphatic permeation and subsequent obstruction of the inferior, deep cervical group of nodes of the jugular-subclavian confluence. In effect, the supraclavicular nodal group represents the termination of efferent trunks from subclavian nodes of the internal mammary nodal

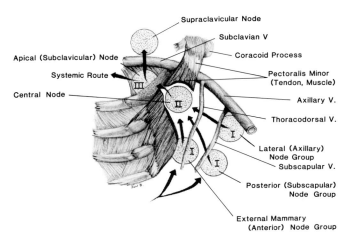

Figure 2–15. Schematic drawing illustrating the major lymph node groups associated with the lymphatic drainage of the breast. The Roman numerals indicate three levels or groups of lymph nodes that are defined by their location relative to the pectoralis minor. Level I includes lymph nodes located lateral to the pectoralis minor; Level II, lymph nodes located deep to the muscle; and Level III, lymph nodes located medial to the muscle. The arrows indicate the general direction of lymph flow. The axillary vein and its major tributaries associated with the pectoralis minor are included.

group. These nodes are situated beneath the lateral margin of the inferior aspect of the sternocleidomastoid muscle beneath the clavicle and represent common sites of distant metastases from mammary carcinoma.

Cross-communication from the interstices of connecting lymphatic channels from each breast provides ready access of lymphatic flow to the opposite axilla. This observation of communicating dermal lymphatics to the contralateral breast explains occasional metastatic involvement of the opposite breast and axilla. Structures of the chest wall, including the internal and external intercostal musculature (see Fig. 2–11), have extensive lymphatic drainage that parallels the course of their major intercostal blood supply. As expected, invasive neoplasms of the lateral breast that involve deep musculature of the thoracic cavity will have preferential flow toward the axilla. Invasion of medial musculature of the chest wall will allow preferential drainage toward the internal mammary nodal groups, whereas bidirectional metastases may be evident with invasive central or subareolar cancers.

The lymphatic vessels that drain the breast occur in three interconnecting groups:[37] (1) A primary set of vessels originate as channels within the gland in the interlobular spaces and along the lactiferous ducts; (2) vessels draining the glandular tissue and overlying skin of the central part of the gland pass to an interconnecting network of vessels located beneath the areola, called the *subareolar plexus;* and (3) a plexus on the deep surface of the breast communicates with minute vessels in the deep fascia underlying the breast. Along the medial border of the breast, lymphatic vessels within the substance of the gland anastomose with vessels passing to parasternal nodes.

Using autoradiographs of surgical specimens, Turner-Warwick demonstrated that the main lymphatic drainage of the breast is through the system of lymphatic vessels occurring within the substance of the gland and not through the vessels on the superficial or deep surface.[37] The main collecting trunks run laterally as they pass through the axillary fascia in the substance of the axillary tail. The subareolar plexus plays no essential part in the lymphatic drainage of the breast.[10] Using vital dyes, Halsell and coworkers[14] demonstrated that this plexus receives lymph primarily from the nipple and the areola and conveys it toward the axilla. The lymphatics communicating with minute vessels in the deep fascia play no part in the normal lymphatic drainage of the breast and only provide an alternative route when the normal pathways are obstructed. More than 75 percent of the lymph from the breast passes to the axillary lymph nodes (see Fig. 2–12). Most of the remainder of the lymph passes to parasternal nodes. Some authorities have suggested that the parasternal nodes receive lymph primarily from the medial part of the breast. However, Turner-Warwick reported that both the axillary and the parasternal lymph node groups receive lymph from all quadrants of the breast, with no striking tendency for any quadrant to drain in a particular direction.

Other routes for the flow of lymph from the breast have been identified. Occasionally, lymph from the breast reaches intercostal lymph nodes, located near the heads of the ribs (see below). Lymphatic vessels reach this location by following lateral cutaneous branches of the posterior intercostal arteries. Lymph may pass to lymphatics within the rectus sheath or subperitoneal plexus by following branches of the intercostal and musculophrenic vessels. Lymph may pass directly to subclavicular, or apical, nodes from the upper portion of the breast. Haagensen[13] has recently reported treating a patient who had apparently demonstrated direct metastasis from the breast to the supraclavicular nodes.

The skin over the breast has lymphatic drainage via the *superficial lymphatic vessels,* which ramify subcutaneously and converge on the axillary lymph nodes. The anterolateral chest and the upper abdominal wall above the umbilicus demonstrate striking directional flow of lymph toward the axilla. Below the umbilicus (the umbilicus establishing a "watershed"), superficial lymphatics carry lymph to the inguinal lymph node groups. It is important to recognize that the skin of the inframammary region drains into the axillary lymph nodes and not into the inguinal nodes. Lymphatic vessels near the lateral margin of the sternum pass through the intercostal space to the *parasternal lymph nodes,* which are associated with the internal thoracic vessels. Some of the lymphatic vessels located on adjacent sides of the sternum may anastomose in front of the sternum. In the upper pectoral region, a few of the lymphatic vessels may pass over the clavicle to *inferior deep cervical lymph nodes.*

The lymphatic vessels from the deeper structures of the thoracic wall drain primarily into parasternal, intercostal, or diaphragmatic lymph nodes (see below).

Lymph Nodes of the Thoracic Wall

The lymphatic drainage of the skin and superficial tissues of thoracic and anterior abdominal walls is described in the section on the lymphatic drainage of the breast. Three sets of lymph nodes and associated vessels—*parasternal, intercostal,* and *diaphragmatic*—are involved in the lymphatic drainage of the deeper tissues of the thoracic wall:

1. The *parasternal, or internal thoracic, lymph nodes* consist of small lymph nodes that are located about 1 cm lateral to the sternal border in the intercostal spaces along the internal thoracic, or mammary, vessels (see Figs. 2–1 and 2–6). The parasternal nodes lie in the areolar tissue underlying the endothoracic fascia bordering the space between the adjacent costal cartilages. The distribution of the nodes in the upper six intercostal spaces has been the subject of several studies since Stibbe's report in 1918 of an average total of 8.5 internal mammary nodes per subject, including both sides.[34] Stibbe reported that they usually occurred in the pattern of four on one side and five on the other. Each of the three upper spaces usually contained one lymph node, as did the sixth space. Frequently, there were no lymph nodes in the fourth or fifth space; an extra node usually was found in one of the upper three spaces on one of the sides. Soerensen[31] reported finding an average of seven nodes of minute size per subject in 39 autopsies, with an average of 3.5 on each side. Ju (as reported by Haagensen[13]) studied 100 autopsy subjects and found an average of 6.2 parasternal nodes per subject, with an average of 3.1 per side. A majority were found in the upper three spaces. However, in contradiction to Stibbe's findings, a lower but similar frequency of nodes was seen in all three of the lower intercostal spaces. Putti[27] studied 47 cadavers and found an average of 7.7 nodes per subject—again, with a majority of the nodes in the upper three spaces and many fewer in the lower spaces. Arão and Abrão[2] studied 100 autopsy specimens and found a much higher frequency of lymph nodes than previously reported. They found an average total of 16.2 per subject, with an average of 8.9 on the right side and 7.3 on the left. In 56.6 percent of the subjects they found retromandibular nodes between the right and left lymphatic trunks at the level of the first intercostal space. An average of 6.6 nodes were seen when the retromandibular nodes were present.

2. The *intercostal lymph nodes* consist of small lymph nodes located in the posterior part of the thoracic cavity within the intercostal spaces near the head of the ribs (see Fig. 2–11). One or more may be found in each intercostal space in relationship with the intercostal vessels. These lymph nodes receive the deep lymphatics from the posterolateral thoracic wall, including lymphatic channels from the breast. Occasionally small lymph nodes occur in the intercostal spaces along the lateral thoracic wall. Efferent lymphatics from the lower four or five intercostal spaces, on both the right and the left sides, join to form a trunk that descends to open into either the cisterna chyli or the initial portion of the thoracic duct. The upper efferent lymphatics from the intercostal nodes on the left side terminate in the thoracic duct; the efferent lymphatics from the corresponding nodes on the right side end in the right lymphatic duct.

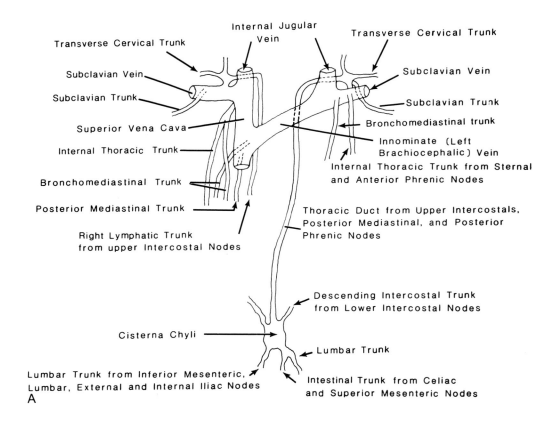

Figure 2–16. *A*, Schematic of the major lymphatic vessels of the thorax and the root of the neck. The thoracic duct begins at the cisterna chyli, a dilated sac that receives drainage from the lower extremities and the abdominal and pelvic cavities via the lumbar and intestinal trunks. Lymph enters the systemic circulation via channels that join the great veins of the neck and superior mediastinum. The lymphatic vessels demonstrate considerable variation as to their number and pattern of branching. A typical pattern is illustrated here. Most of the major trunks, including the thoracic and right lymphatic ducts, end at or near the confluence of the internal jugular with the subclavian.

3. The *diaphragmatic lymph nodes* consist of three sets of small lymph nodes (anterior, lateral, and posterior) located on the thoracic surface of the diaphragm.

The *anterior set of diaphragmatic lymph nodes* includes two or three small lymph nodes (also known as *prepericardial lymph nodes*) located behind the sternum at the base of the xiphoid process, which receive afferent lymphatics from the convex surface of the liver, and one or two nodes located on each side near the junction of the seventh rib with its costal cartilage, which receive afferents from the anterior aspect of the diaphragm. Afferent lymphatics also reach the prepericardial nodes by accompanying the branches of the superior epigastric blood vessels that pass from the rectus abdominis muscle and through the rectus sheath. Efferent lymphatics from the anterior diaphragmatic nodes pass to the *parasternal nodes*. In 1927, Handley identified this lymphatic channel as a potential route by which metastases from the breast may invade the parasternal region, with the potential for spread to the liver. As Haagensen[13] suggests, metastasis via this (rectus muscle) route most likely occurs only when the internal mammary lymphatic trunk is blocked higher in the upper intercostal spaces. When blockage occurs, the flow of lymph may be reversed and carcinoma emboli from the breast may reach the liver. It is significant to note that the autopsy subjects studied by Handley[16] who demonstrated this route of metastasis had locally advanced breast carcinoma. Handley and Thackray[15] described the importance of the parasternal lymph nodes in carcinoma of the breast. Clearly, as Haagensen[13] and others have suggested, this route is not of importance in early cancer

of the breast unless the primary tumor is located in the extreme lower inner portion of the breast where it overlies the sixth costal cartilage.

The *lateral set of diaphragmatic lymph nodes* consists of two or three small lymph nodes on each side of the diaphragm adjacent to the pericardial sac where the phrenic nerves enter the diaphragm. On the right side they are located near the vena cava; on the left, near the esophageal hiatus. Afferent lymphatic vessels reach these nodes from the middle region of the diaphragm; on the right side, afferent lymphatics from the convex surface of the liver also reach these nodes. Efferent lymphatics from the lateral diaphragmatic nodes may pass to the parasternal nodes via the anterior diaphragmatic nodes, to posterior mediastinal nodes, or to anterior nodes via vessels that follow the course of the phrenic nerve.

The *posterior set of diaphragmatic lymph nodes* consists of a few lymph nodes located adjacent to the crura of the diaphragm. They receive lymph from the posterior aspect of the diaphragm and convey it to posterior mediastinal and lateral aortic nodes.

Lymph Nodes of the Thoracic Cavity

Three sets of nodes are involved in the lymphatic drainage of the thoracic viscera—*anterior mediastinal (brachiocephalic)*, *posterior mediastinal*, and *tracheobronchial* (Fig. 2–16). Although a knowledge of the lymphatic drainage of the thoracic viscera may not be particularly significant in treating carcinoma of the

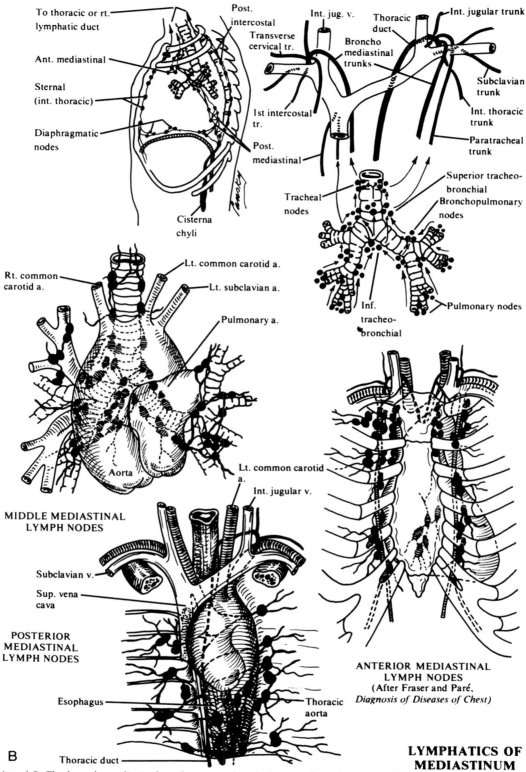

Figure 2–16 *Continued B,* The bronchomediastinal trunks receive lymph drainage from the organs of the thoracic cavity. Lymph from the breast usually passes through the internal thoracic trunk and the right lymphatic or the thoracic duct. See text for details. (From Pansky B: *In* Review of Gross Anatomy. Ed. 5. New York, Macmillan, 1984. Reprinted by permission.)

breast, it is important that one understand the system of collecting lymphatic trunks in this region, which all empty into the confluence of the internal jugular and subclavian veins.

For better comprehension of the pattern of lymphatic drainage in this region, a brief description of the regions and organs drained by the three thoracic lymph node groups is provided. The *anterior mediastinal group* (Fig. 2–16) consists of six to eight lymph nodes located in the upper anterior part of the mediastinum in front of the brachiocephalic veins and the large arterial trunks arising from the aorta. These correspond to the *retromanubrial nodes* as identified by Arão and Abrão.[2] The anterior mediastinal nodes receive afferent lymphatics from the thymus, thyroid, pericardium, and the lateral diaphragmatic lymph nodes. Their efferent lymphatic vessels join with those from the tracheobronchial nodes to form the *bronchomediastinal trunks*.

The *posterior mediastinal group* (Fig. 2–16B) consists of eight to ten nodes located posterior to the pericardium in association with the esophagus and descending thoracic aorta. They receive afferent lymphatics from the esophagus, the posterior portion of the pericardium, the diaphragm, and the convex surface of the liver. Most of their efferent lymphatic vessels join the thoracic duct, but some pass to *tracheobronchial nodes*.

The *tracheobronchial group* (Fig. 2–16B) consists of a chain of five subgroups of lymph nodes—tracheal, superior tracheobronchial, inferior tracheobronchial, bronchopulmonary, and pulmonary—located adjacent to the trachea and bronchi, as is indicated by the descriptive names. The bronchopulmonary nodes are found in the hilus of each lung; the pulmonary nodes, within the substance of the lung in association with the segmental bronchi. The tracheal nodes receive afferent lymphatics from the trachea and upper esophagus. The remaining nodes within this group form a continuous chain with boundaries of lymphatic drainage that are not well defined. The pulmonary and bronchopulmonary nodes receive afferent lymphatic vessels from the lungs and bronchial trees. The inferior and superior tracheobronchial nodes receive afferent lymphatic vessels from the bronchopulmonary nodes; the inferior tracheobronchial nodes also receive some afferent lymphatic vessels from the heart and posterior mediastinal organs. Efferent vessels from the subgroups of tracheobronchial group pass sequentially to the level of the tracheal nodes. Efferents from the latter unite with efferents from parasternal and anterior mediastinal nodes to form the *right* and *left bronchomediastinal trunks*. The left trunk may terminate by joining the thoracic duct, and the right trunk may join the right lymphatic duct. However, it is more common for the right and left trunks to open independently into the junction of the internal jugular and subclavian veins, each on their own side. Figure 2–16 illustrates the major lymphatic channels conveying lymph from the lymph nodes of the thoracic wall and cavity.

VENOUS DRAINAGE OF THE MAMMARY GLAND

Lymphatic drainage of the epithelial and mesenchymal components of the breast is the primary route for metastatic dissemination of adenocarcinoma of this organ. However, the vascular route for tumor embolization via venous drainage systems has a major role for dissemination of neoplasms to the lung, bone, brain, liver, and so forth. The three groups of deep veins that drain the breast (Fig. 2–17) and serve as vascular routes include:

1. The *intercostal veins,* which traverse the posterior aspect of the breast from the second to the sixth intercostal spaces and arborize to enter the vertebral veins posteriorly and the azygos vein centrally to terminate in the superior vena cava.

2. The *axillary vein,* which may have variable tributaries that provide segmental drainage of the chest wall, pectoral muscles, and the breast.

3. The *internal mammary vein perforators,* which represent the largest venous plexus to allow drainage of the mammary gland. This venous network traverses the rib interspaces to enter the innominate vein. Thus, perforators that drain the parenchyma and epithelial components of the breast allow direct embolization to the pulmonary capillary spaces to establish metastatic disease.[1, 13]

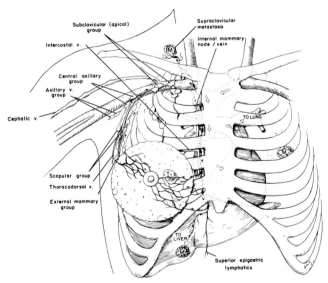

Figure 2–17. Venous drainage of the breast and its relationship to the lymphatics. Lymphatic vessels parallel the course of the three major groups of veins serving the breast and provide routes for metastasis: intercostal, axillary, and internal mammary veins. Visceral metastases to the liver or lungs are possible via vessels providing venous or lymphatic drainage of the breast as these structures communicate with the major venous trunks. (From Copeland EM III, Bland KI: The breast. *In* Sabiston DC Jr (ed): Essentials of Surgery, Philadelphia, WB Saunders, 1987. Reprinted by permission.)

References

1. Anson BJ, McVay CB: Thoracic walls: Breast or mammary region. *In* Anson, BJ, McVay CB (eds): Surgical Anatomy, Vol I. Philadelphia, WB Saunders, 1971, pp 330–369.

2. Arão A, Abrão A: Estudo anatomico da cadeia ganglionar mamaria interna em 100 casos. Rev Paul Med 45:317, 1954.
3. Batson OV: The function of the vertebral veins and their role in the spread of metastases. Ann Surg 112:138–149, 1940.
4. Batson OV: The role of the vertebral veins and metastatic processes. Ann Int Med 16:38–45, 1942.
5. Cathcart EP, Gairns FW, Garven HSD: The innervation of the human quiescent nipple, with notes on pigmentation, erection, and hyperneury. Trans R Soc Edinb 61:699, 1948.
6. Copeland EM III, Bland KI: The breast. In Sabiston DC Jr (ed): Essentials of Surgery, Philadelphia, WB Saunders, 1987, pp 288–326.
7. Cowie AT: Overview of mammary gland. J Invest Dermatol 63:2–9, 1974.
8. Cunningham L: The anatomy of the arteries and veins of the breast. J Surg Oncol 9:71–85, 1977.
9. Giacometti L, Montagna W: The nipple and areola of the human female breast. Anat Rec 144:191–197, 1962.
10. Grant RN, Tabah EJ, Adair FF: The surgical significance of subareolar lymph plexus in cancer of the breast. Surgery 33:71–78, 1953.
11. Gray H: The lymphatic system. In Clemente CD (ed): Anatomy of the Human Body. 30th American ed. Philadelphia, Lea & Febiger, 1985, p 866.
12. Grossman F: Ueber dic axillaren Lymphdrusen. Inaug. Dissert., Berlin, C. Vogt, 1896.
13. Haagensen CD: Anatomy of the mammary glands. In Haagensen CD (ed): Diseases of the Breast, 3rd ed. Philadelphia, WB Saunders, 1986, p 1.
14. Halsell JT, et al: Lymphatic drainage of the breast demonstrated by vital dye staining and radiography. Ann Surg 162:221–226, 1965.
15. Handley RS, Thackray AC: The internal mammary lymph chain in carcinoma of the breast. Lancet 2:276–278, 1949.
16. Handley WS: The radium treatment of sternal recurrences in cancer of the breast. Clin J 56:73, 1927.
17. Helminen HJ, Ericsson JLE: Studies on mammary gland involution. I. On the ultrastructure of the lactating mammary gland. J Ultrastruct Res 25:193–213, 1968.
18. Henriques C: The veins of the vertebral column and their role in the spread of cancer. Ann R Coll Surg Engl 31:1–22, 1962.
19. Linzell JL: The silver staining of myoepithelial cells particularly in the mammary gland, and their relation to ejection of milk. J Anat (Lond) 86:49–57, 1952.
20. Maliniac JW: Arterial blood supply of the breast. Arch Surg 47:329–343, 1943.
21. Massopust LC, Gardner WD: Infrared photographic studies of the superficial thoracic veins in the female. Surg Gynecol Obstet 91:717–27, 1950.
22. Miller MR, Kasahara M: Cutaneous innervation of the human breast. Anat Rec 135:153–167, 1959.
23. Montagna W, Macpherson EA: Some neglected aspects of the anatomy of the human breasts. J Invest Dermatol 63:10–16, 1974.
24. Montagu A: Natural selection in the form of the breast in the female. JAMA 180:826–827, 1962.
25. Morehead JR: Anatomy and embryology of the breast. Clin Obstet Gynecol 25:353–357, 1982.
26. Mornard P: Sur deux cas de tumeurs malignes des mammelles axillaires aberrantes. Bull Mnem Soc Natl Shir Paris 21:487, 1929.
27. Putti F: Richerche Anatomiche sui linfonodi mammari interni. Chir Ital 7:161, 1953.
28. Radnor CJP: Myoepithelium in the prelactating and lactating mammary glands of the rat. J Anat (Lond) 112:337–353, 1972.
29. Sakki S: Angiography of the female breast. Ann Clin Res 6:(Suppl 12) 1–47, 1974.
30. Smith DJ, Jr, Palin WE, Jr, Katch WL, Bennett JE: Breast volume and anthropomorphic measurements: Normal values. Plast Reconstr Surg 78:331–335, 1986.
31. Soerensen B: Recherches sur la localisation des ganglions lymphatiques parasternaux par rapport aux espaces intercostaux. Int J Chir 11:501, 1951.
32. Spratt JS: Anatomy of the breast. Major Probl Clin Surg 5:1–13, 1979.
33. Spratt JS Jr, Donegan WL: Anatomy of the breast. In Donegan WL, Spratt JS Jr (eds): Cancer of the Breast. 3rd ed. Philadelphia, WB Saunders, 1979, p 2.
34. Stibbe EP: The internal mammary lymphatic glands. J Anat 52:527, 1918.
35. Sykes PA: The nerve supply of the human nipple. J Anat (Lond) 105:201, 1969.
36. Tobon H, Salazar H: Ultrastructure of the human mammary gland. I. Development of the fetal gland throughout gestation. J Clin Endocrinol Metab 39:443–456, 1974.
37. Turner-Warwick RT: The lymphatics of the breast. Br J Surg 46:574–582, 1959.
38. Waugh D, Van Der Hoeven E: Fine structure of the human adult female breast. Lab Invest 11:220–228, 1962.
39. Wellings SR, Grunbaum BW, DeOme KB: Electron microscopy of milk secretion in the mammary gland of the C3H/Crgl mouse. J Natl Cancer Inst 25:423–437, 1960.

Chapter 3

BREAST PHYSIOLOGY

Breast Physiology in Normal, Lactating, and Diseased States

Maureen Keller-Wood, Ph.D. and Kirby I. Bland, M.D.

The development and function of the mammary gland are stimulated by a variety of hormones, including the sex steroids, prolactin, oxytocin, cortisol, thyroid hormone, and growth hormone. The trophic and tropic effects of the reproductive hormones estrogen, progesterone, and prolactin are most important in normal breast development and function. Estrogen has potential mitotic (carcinogenic) effects on the mammary epithelium and initiates ductal development. Estrogen also increases the number of estrogen and progesterone receptors on epithelial cells.[12] Progesterone is responsible for the differentiation of the epithelial cells and causes lobular development. Additionally, progesterone may reduce estrogen binding in mammary epithelium and limit proliferation of the tubular system.[12] Prolactin contributes to the development of adipose tissue and is required, with the presence of growth hormone and cortisol, for the growth and development of the mammary epithelium. Prolactin increases the number of estrogen receptors and epithelial cells[13] and acts synergistically with estrogen in ductal development and progesterone in lobuloalveolar development.[5] Prolactin is also the primary hormonal stimulus for lactogenesis during late pregnancy and the postpartum period; prolactin stimulates differentiation of the milk-producing cells of the breast and synthesis of the components of milk. The precise roles of growth hormone (GH), cortisol, and thyroid hormone are less clear; effects of these hormones have been demonstrated in vitro and in vivo in a variety of animal models.[5] However, their relative importance in the human female is unclear.

Secretion of the mammogenic hormones is regulated by the neurohormones of the hypothalamus and the tropic hormones of the pituitary (Fig. 3–1). Ovarian secretion of estrogen and progesterone is regulated by the secretion of the gonadotropins, luteinizing hormone (LH), and follicle-stimulating hormone (FSH) from the basophilic cells of the anterior pituitary. These, in turn, are regulated by secretion of gonadotropin-releasing hormone (GnRH) from the hypothalamus. Secretion of GnRH, LH, and FSH are all altered by positive and negative feedback effects of estrogen and progesterone.

The secretion of mammogenic hormones varies throughout the life of normal females, and these changes in the hormonal milieu are responsible for the normal pattern of breast development. In the female fetus, plasma estrogen and progesterone concentrations are low, because there is minimal secretion of sex steroids by the fetal ovaries. However, placental production of estrogen and progesterone contributes significantly to the estrogen and progesterone concentrations present in fetal blood. In the human female neonate, plasma estrogen and progesterone decrease on the day following birth. Throughout childhood, plasma estrogen and progesterone remain low as a result of the high sensitivity of the hypothalamopituitary axis to the negative feedback effects of the sex steroids. With the onset of puberty there is an increase in central drive to the hypothalamus, a decrease in sensitivity to negative feedback by estrogen and progesterone, and an increase in sensitivity to positive feedback by estrogen. These physiological events initiate an increase in GnRH secretion, increases of LH and FSH secretion, and ultimately increases in ovarian estrogen and progesterone secretion. With the development of positive feedback by estrogen, the menstrual cycle begins.[18]

The human menstrual cycle is characterized by changing patterns of gonadotropin and sex steroid concentrations in plasma. In the *early follicular phase* of the menstrual cycle, increasing FSH and LH concentrations stimulate ovarian follicular growth and secretion of estrogen. The increasing plasma estrogen concentration limits further increases in LH and FSH by negative feedback inhibitory effects. With onset of the *late follicular phase* of the cycle, the very high plasma estrogen concentration stimulates the midcycle surge in LH and FSH via a positive feedback effect. Ovulation follows the midcycle surge in LH, and the follicular epithelium and stroma form the corpus luteum. During the *luteal phase* of the menstrual cycle, plasma progesterone and estrogen concentrations increase.

In early *pregnancy*, progesterone and estrogen are secreted by the ovarian corpus luteum under the influence of chorionic gonadotropin (hCG). Following the twelfth week of gestation, the placenta remains the primary source of plasma progesterone and estrogen.

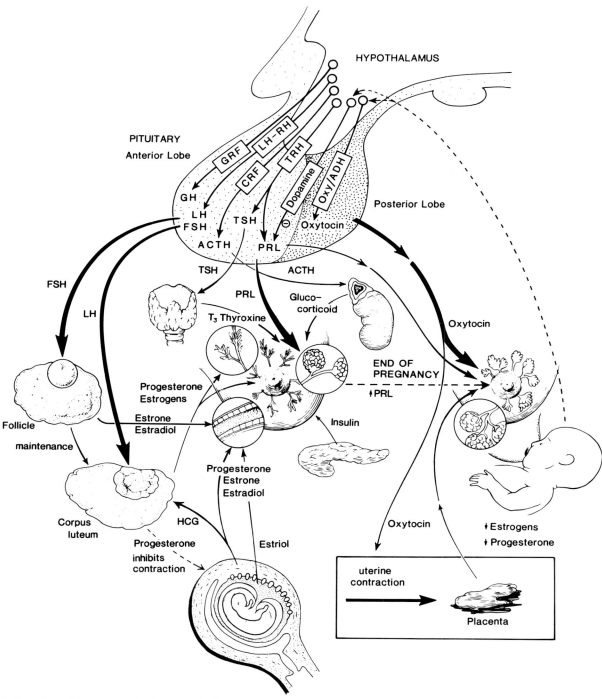

Figure 3–1. Overview of the neuroendocrine control of breast development and function with relationship to gonadotropic hormones of the anterior pituitary and ovary. Basophil secretion of LH and FSH is responsible for ovarian synthesis and release of progesterone and estrogen, respectively. The mammotropic effects of estrogen and progestin initiate myoepithelial and alveolar development. Ductal and stromal enlargement with pregnancy occur as a result of progestin and estrogen secretions in excess from the corpus luteum (first 12 weeks) and thereafter from the placenta. Acidophil cell secretion of prolactin (PRL) is initiated following evacuation of the gravid uterus and is mammotropic to the lobular alveoli. The suckling reflex initiates oxytocin release from the posterior pituitary and is stimulatory to alveolar myoepithelial cells to initiate milk release. Neuroendocrine organs other than the pituitary and ovary secrete hormones (glucocorticoid, GH, insulin, thyroxine) that are tropic to ductal and glandular maintenance and growth.

Placental production of estrogen is dependent upon precursors produced by the maternal and fetal adrenals. Plasma progesterone and estrogen concentrations are maintained in the mother and progressively increase with pregnancy.

During pregnancy, maternal plasma prolactin concentrations also increase. By *late gestation,* plasma prolactin levels are increased tenfold above those of the nonpregnant state. The primary control for prolactin secretion by the anterior pituitary in the nonpregnant female is the hypothalamic inhibitory factor, dopamine. Prolactin secretion may also be stimulated by a hypothalamic releasing hormone whose identity is not yet known; thyrotropin-releasing hormone, the hypothalamic releasing hormone for thyrotropin (TSH), may act as a prolactin-releasing hormone under some circumstances. However, during pregnancy, the high circulating concentrations of prolactin are thought to be a consequence of the high plasma estrogen concentrations, which cause hypertrophy and hyperplasia of the lactotrophs and increase prolactin synthesis and release.[14]

In the following sections the changes in the physiology of the human breast will be described in terms of its relationship to these changes in hormone secretion.

FETAL AND NEONATAL MAMMARY DEVELOPMENT

In the human fetus, the development of rudimentary breast structures is evident. This early development of the mamma may be controlled by the secretion of placental estrogen and progesterone and fetal prolactin.[8] In the human fetus, measurable levels of plasma prolactin are present in the pituitary by midgestation, and in the terminal weeks of pregnancy, fetal prolactin concentrations are similar to maternal prolactin concentrations.[18] Because the ovaries are relatively inactive in steroid biosynthesis, the circulating estradiol and progesterone concentrations are determined by placental production in both female and male fetuses, and there seems to be no sexual dimorphism of breast development in humans before puberty. At birth, the mammary gland consists of a branching system of ducts that converge as an ampulla on the nipples, and there is early evidence of secretory activity in the budding alveoli.[5, 8, 17]

Within the first weeks after birth, there is frequently a measurable, but slight, secretion from the breasts of both male and female neonates. This secretion, often referred to as "witch's milk," is a clear fluid similar to colostrum, with a composition predominantly of water, fat, and cellular debris. The increased secretion after birth parallels that in the maternal mammary gland and is presumably related to the decrease in placental steroids in the presence of relatively high prolactin concentrations secreted by the neonatal pituitary.[1, 5]

During childhood, plasma estrogen levels are quite low, and the mammary gland remains inactive and nonsecretory. Growth of the breast is isometric with proliferation of the stromal tissue and elongation of the ducts in proportion to overall body growth. There is absence of lobular development before puberty (see Fig. 2–2A).[4, 17]

PUBERTAL DEVELOPMENT

Allometric growth of the breast in human females begins with the increase in ovarian secretion of estrogen and progesterone during adolescence. Breast bud development is usually the first configurational change of puberty and correlates most closely with the change in plasma estradiol concentration; there is also a positive, but weaker, correlation with insulin-like growth factor I (IGF-I or somatomedin-C) levels.[1, 4, 8]

In primates, pubertal development of the breast is dependent upon the normal increase in circulating estrogen but also requires normal (active) pituitary function. Treatment of normal prepubertal females with estrogen initiates induction and premature growth of the mammary gland. Normal development is apparent in patients with gonadal dysgenesis and normal pituitary function if they are treated with estrogen replacement. However, in the absence of active pituitary function, normal pubertal breast development does not occur following therapy with supplemental replacement of estrogen alone. The pituitary effect does not appear to be prolactin mediated, as normal breast development occurs in primates that are treated with drugs known to inhibit prolactin secretion. This effect may be mediated, in part, by growth hormone, although estrogen and growth hormone used concomitantly do not restore normal development in hypopituitary primates, and normal breast development occurs in ateliotic dwarfs in the absence of growth hormone. The pituitary effect is possibly mediated by ACTH and TSH release from the pituitary; in rodents, normal adrenal and thyroid function appears to be essential for normal development of the breast ductal epithelium.[11]

Estrogen stimulates proliferation of the ductal epithelial and myoepithelial cells and the surrounding stromal cells of the breast parenchyma. Progesterone, together with estrogen, initiates the formation of the secretory acinar components at the distalmost aspect of the ductules. With *menarche,* the cyclical increases in estrogen and progesterone cause further ductal development and formation of lobules (see Fig. 2–2B). Progesterone and estrogen stimulate the proliferation of connective tissue that subsequently replaces adipose tissue and provide support for the developing ducts. The ovarian steroids also stimulate proliferation of adipose tissue and enhance proportional enlargement and pigmentation of the nipple and areola. Usually, within the first one to two years following menarche, the breast has acquired the structure of a mature breast (see Fig. 2–2C) and has changed from a conical to hemispherical configuration. The ultimate size, density, and inherent shape of the mature breast varies remarkably and is determined by genetic, nutritional, and conditioning factors. In the adult female, the size of the nonpregnant breast parallels proportional alterations in body size and body fat content.[4, 17, 18]

The changes in the human breast with the onset of puberty can best be described as proceeding through a series of morphological development stages described by Tanner (Table 3–1).[19] In initial stages of development, the breast is maintained in the prepubertal phase without development or elevation of the papilla. The next phase (Stage II) is characterized as the "breast bud" stage, with elevation of the breast and papilla as a small mound beneath an enlarged areola. Subsequently, with continual mammotrophic stimuli, there is further enlargement of the breast and areola, although there is absence of separation of the contour of the areola from the remainder of the breast. The papilla and areola enlarge *isometrically* (Stage IV) to form a secondary projection above the level of the breast parenchyma. The final phase of breast development is evident in the fully mature adult breast with projection of the papilla above the areola, which morphologically becomes contiguous with the contour of the breast.

CHANGES IN THE BREAST DURING THE MENSTRUAL CYCLE

Changes in breast volume occur in the mature human breast with establishment of the menstrual cycle. Breast volume is greatest in the second half of the cycle, following a premenstrual increase in size, density, nodularity, and sensitivity. There is some evidence that progesterone may stimulate glandular growth in the luteal phase, as one researcher[16] found an increase in the sprouting and budding of ducts in premenstrual samples collected at autopsy. Changes in the mitotic rate of glandular components have been found to be greater in the luteal phase than in the follicular phase.[4] Additional data suggest that the premenstrual increase in breast volume occurs as a consequence of an increase in size of the lobule without any evidence of epithelial proliferation.[4, 8] Subsequently, there is engorgement of the stroma, lobules, and ducts with an increase in the size of ducts and acini as the lumens dilate. Thereafter, the epithelium becomes vacuolated, and the stroma becomes loose and infiltrated with protein-free fluid and lymphoid and plasma cells. This progressive parenchymal engorgement and edema subside with the onset of menses. This effect may be mediated, in part, by the preceding increase in plasma estrogen during the follicular phase of the menstrual cycle, as estrogens enhance stromal volume during puberty.[21]

PREGNANCY

With pregnancy, there is dramatic secretion and release of circulating ovarian placental estrogen and progestin and, as a consequence of these physiological steroids, the breast undergoes a similarly dramatic alteration in form and substance. The breast enlarges, the areolar skin darkens and the areolar glands become more prominent, the nipple enlarges and becomes erect, the ducts and lobules proliferate, and alveolar development proceeds. Finally, the gland has ductal and lobular preparation for active secretion (see Fig. 2–2D).[8, 17]

The ductular structures of the mammary gland begin to sprout, enlarge, and branch by the third week of pregnancy. During the *first trimester,* lobuloalveolar formation begins as the ductal tree branches to form multiple alveoli. With the increase in lobular size, the proliferating glandular epithelium begins to replace the connective tissue and adipose tissue components of the breast. These early changes are presumably initiated by estrogen and progesterone secreted by the corpus luteum.[3, 14, 17]

The proliferation of the ductular elements increases during the *second trimester* following stimulation of estrogens and progestins secreted by the placenta. Estrogens are responsible for the proliferation and differentiation of the alveolar epithelium. Progesterone and estrogen, together with prolactin, cause the arborization of the glandular structures to form alveoli. A true lobuloalveolar system develops and the secretory epithelium becomes more active, as is evident with the accumulation of colloid within the alveoli.[3, 17]

In the *third trimester* there is further evidence of secretory activity as fat droplets accumulate in the alveolar cells and colostrum fills the alveolar and ductular space. In addition, mammary blood flow increases and the myoepithelial cells hypertrophy.[3, 17, 21]

As pregnancy progresses, the increase in prolactin secretion induces proliferation and differentiation of stem cells to form presecretory alveolar cells and myoepithelial cells. The lactotropic or mammogenic action of prolactin requires the presence of cortisol, insulin, growth hormone, and epidermal growth factor. Placental lactogen (hPL) or somatomammotropin may also participate in this lactotropic action and is structurally related to prolactin. The secretion of hPL increases during gestation in parallel with the increase in placental weight. Further, hPL is less potent than prolactin but clearly has lactogenic activity. In primates treated with estrogen and progesterone, hPL stimulates milk production. However, during normal human pregnancy this placental lactogenic hormone is considered of minor importance relative to that of pituitary prolactin, and it

---

Table 3–1. THE DEVELOPMENTAL STAGES OF BREAST GROWTH

Stage I	Preadolescent: elevation of papilla only.
Stage II	Breast bud stage: elevation of breast and papilla as small mound. Enlargement of areolar diameter.
Stage III	Further enlargement and elevation of breast and areola with no separation of their contours.
Stage IV	Projection of areola and papilla to form a secondary mound above the level of the breast.
Stage V	Mature stage: projection of papilla only, due to recession of the areola to the general contour of the breast.

Tanner JM: Growth at Adolescence. Oxford, Blackwell Scientific Publications, 1961. Reprinted by permission.

may actually inhibit the effect of prolactin by binding to mammary prolactin receptors.[2, 5, 14, 20-22]

In the last weeks of pregnancy, limited synthesis of milk fats and proteins is initiated. This synthetic process is stimulated by the lactogenic effect of prolactin on breast lobules. Other pituitary hormones also may have trophic effects on the mammary gland during pregnancy. Experimentation in rats suggests that normal plasma concentrations of growth hormones and cortisol are required in addition to maintenance of estrogen, progesterone, and prolactin activity for normal lobulo-alveolar growth and development. Following hypophysectomy of humans during pregnancy, neither mammary development nor postpartum initiation of milk secretion is inhibited, suggesting that placental steroids, and perhaps other placental peptides, can induce mammary gland growth and function in the hypopituitary state.[3, 5, 14]

POSTPARTUM LACTATION

Following delivery of the placenta, circulating progesterone and estrogen concentrations are observed to decrease over the next several days. The quantitative decrease in the plasma estradiol and progesterone concentration allows the full expression of the lactogenic actions of prolactin (see Fig. 2-2E). In contrast, during pregnancy the plasma estrogens are observed to inhibit prolactin effects on the breast by decreasing the relative number of prolactin receptors, while progesterone inhibits the biosynthesis of milk products. In the postpartum state, prolactin induces the differentiation of presecretory cells into secretory cells, stimulates synthesis of RNA for production of the specific milk proteins casein and α-lactalbumin, and allows induction of the enzymes galactosyl transferase and lactose synthetase. In addition, prolactin stimulates production of ribosomal proteins and mitochondrial and endoplasmic reticulum lipids. Prolactin is probably responsible for the increase in prolactin receptors in the mammary gland. To physiologically achieve the lactogenic effects of this hormone, the presence of insulin, cortisol, GH, and thyroxine is required. In animals, milk yield is reduced with pituitary stalk transection despite the presence of high circulating plasma values of prolactin. Replacement of growth hormone, thyroxine, insulin, and cortisol are observed to restore milk yield.[2, 3, 15, 20]

The maintenance of lactation requires regular removal of milk and stimulation ("milk let-down") of the neural reflex to prolactin secretion. Basal plasma prolactin levels are high in the first few weeks postpartum and increase further with the suckling reflex. By week six postpartum, basal prolactin concentrations in blood decrease to concentrations within the normal range; however, there is still an increase in prolactin levels with suckling. The magnitude of the suckling-induced surge of prolactin tends to decrease over time, probably as a consequence of the decreased duration and frequency of nursing. In rodents, an increase in duration of the nonsuckling interval will increase the time required for prolactin to reaccumulate in the pituitary; as the non-suckling interval approaches 12 hours, the release of prolactin with suckling is inhibited. For lactating women, the frequency of nursing is observed to effect the return of basal prolactin levels to normal. While high prolactin levels in the initial postpartum period are required for lactogenesis, reduced prolactin values of the late postpartum period are sufficient for galactopoiesis.[2, 5, 6]

Milk production and ejection in nursing women is controlled by neural reflex arcs originating in free nerve endings of the nipple-areolar complex. Stimulation of afferent nerves in the nipple stimulates release of oxytocin from the posterior pituitary and prolactin from the anterior pituitary. Oxytocin initiates contraction of the smooth muscle components of the myoepithelial cells surrounding the alveoli; thereafter, compression of the alveoli occurs and expulsion of milk under pressure into the lactiferous sinuses is evident. Oxytocin release can also be produced by auditory, visual, olfactory, or other stimuli associated with nursing or with vaginal stimulation and can be inhibited by pain or embarrassment. Oxytocic effects on myoepithelial cells are also influenced by the sympathetic system, which controls the tone of myoepithelial smooth muscle. Thus, the maintenance of lactation in women requires an intact hypothalamic-pituitary axis, adequate diet and nutrition, the regular release (suckling) of secreted milk, and the absence of psychological stresses that interfere with normal control of oxytocin or prolactin.[2, 3, 5, 6, 22]

POSTWEANING INVOLUTION

Following weaning of the infant from breast feeding, the gland returns to an inactive state. Because milk is no longer synthesized and removed, prolactin and oxytocin release is not stimulated. Thereafter, the secretory activity of the lactogenic epithelium decreases. The unremoved dormant milk subsequently increases intramammary pressure, and alveolar rupture can be appreciated morphologically and clinically. The retained secretory products are phagocytosed, the lobular structure atrophies, and the secretory cells degenerate.[2, 17]

POST MENOPAUSE

After the menopause, the decrease in ovarian secretion of estrogen and progesterone causes progressive involution of the ductular and glandular components of the breast (see Fig. 2-2F). There is a quantitative decrease in the number and size of the glandular elements of the breast, with the epithelium of the lobules and ducts becoming hypoplastic or atrophic. The surrounding fibrous tissue matrix increases in density and the parenchyma of the breast is replaced, to a variable degree, with adipose and stromal tissue rather than glandular structures. As fat content and supporting stroma are progressively lost with the aging process, the breast shrinks and loses its lobular structure, density, and contour.[2, 8]

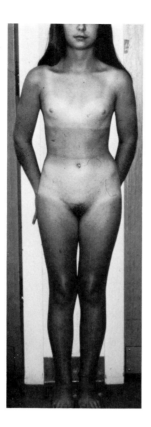

Figure 3–2. Turner syndrome of gonadal agenesis or dysgenesis with the absence of functional ovaries in a 19-year-old phenotypic female (45,XO) with evidence of sexual infantilism and absence of breast development at puberty. (Courtesy of Dr. A. Rosenbloom, Division of Pediatric Endocrinology, University of Florida, Gainesville, FL.)

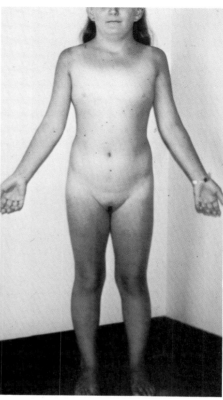

Figure 3–3. Anteroposterior view of a 15-year-old patient with Turner syndrome (XO/XX) emphasizing the short webbed neck, widely separated nipples, short bilateral metacarpals, and congenital lymphedema of the distal extremities. These patients often have renal abnormalities and a variety of skeletal malformations. Note the typical shield-like chest configuration, hypoplastic nipples, and lack of breast development. (Courtesy of Dr. A. Rosenbloom, Division of Pediatric Endocrinology, University of Florida, Gainesville, FL.)

DISEASE STATES

Because the mammary gland is sensitive to the changes in circulating concentrations of the ovarian steroids and a number of pituitary hormones, alterations in the breast can be detected in a variety of endocrine disturbances.

Disturbances in Sexual Differentiation

Disorders of sexual development frequently affect maturation of the secondary sex characteristics, including breast growth at puberty. The degree to which breast morphology is affected will subsequently depend upon the extent to which the normal pattern of increased estrogen secretion at puberty is altered. In the syndrome of *gonadal agenesis* or *dysgenesis (Turner syndrome),* the absence of functional ovaries in phenotypic females (45, XO) is evident as sexual infantilism and absence of breast development at puberty.[7, 10] Some girls, particularly with mosaicism (XO/XX), may have enough ovarian function to have spontaneous breast development.

The typical patient with Turner syndrome is short of stature, with a short webbed neck, widely separated nipples, bilateral short metacarpals, puffiness of the dorsa of the fingers, congenital lymphedema of the feet and hands, renal abnormalities, and a variety of skeletal abnormalities (Fig. 3–2). These patients typically have a shield-like chest configuration, maldevelopment of the breasts and hypoplasia of the nipples (Fig. 3–3). Most

characteristic, perhaps, is the distinctive facies: micrognathia, epicanthal folds, prominent low-set and frequently deformed ears, a fishlike mouth, and ptosis. The gonads in these patients are vestigial (with streaks), and consequently, plasma estrogen levels are low. The genital ducts and external genitalia are female, because of the absence of testicular androgens, but are immature. There is no development of the oogonia or oocytes. These patients undergo adrenarche, and the normal increase in production of adrenal androgens causes development of sparse pubic and axillary hair. The absence of normal production of ovarian estrogen results in failure of development of secondary sex characteristics. Cyclical estrogen therapy may be used, beginning after 15 years of age, to induce development of secondary sex characteristics and to prevent osteopenia.[7, 10, 18]

In *seminiferous tubule dysgenesis* (47, XXY), or typical *Klinefelter syndrome,* the patients are phenotypic males with small atrophic testes, hyalinization of the seminiferous tubules, and interstitial cell hyperplasia. Plasma testosterone concentrations are variable but are generally lower than normal, and postpubertal gynecomastia is frequent (about 90 percent), as are other signs of androgen deficiency: reduced facial and body hair, female escutcheon, small phallus, poor muscular devel-

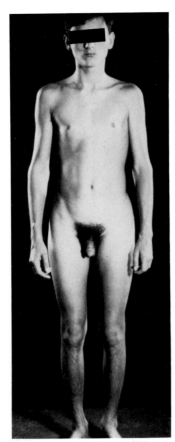

Figure 3–4. Klinefelter syndrome with seminiferous tubular dysgenesis (47,XXY) in a pubertal male. Patients are phenotypic males with small atrophic testes. Postpubertal gynecomastia is frequent, and patients have evidence of androgen deficiency with reduced facial and body hair, small phallus, poor muscular development, and disproportionately long legs compared with total body length. (Courtesy of Dr. A. Rosenbloom, Division of Pediatric Endocrinology, University of Florida, Gainesville, FL.)

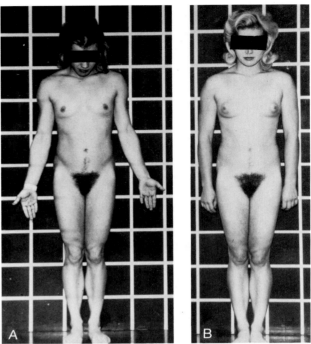

Figure 3–5. A, 21β-Hydroxylase deficiency with sexual infantilism in a 16-year-old female. These patients have normal ovarian estrogen production with increased androgen production; thus, these patients have the disorder of phallic enlargement, precocious pubic and axillary hair development, amenorrhea, and breast hypoplasia. The patient is quite muscular with minimal subcutaneous fat, male-type hairline, and sharp masculine features. B, Same patient at age 17 years following therapy for ten months with hydrocortisone, resulting in cessation of androgen production. This treatment allowed physiologic stimulation of her ovarian function with excellent breast development and other estrogenic effects on the subcutaneous fat and skin. (Courtesy of Dr. A. Rosenbloom, Division of Pediatric Endocrinology, University of Florida, Gainesville, FL.)

opment, and disproportionately long legs compared with total body length (Fig. 3–4). These patients with gynecomastia also have an increased predisposition to breast cancer.[7, 10]

In other variants of gonadal dysgenesis or mosaicism, the degree of breast development in phenotypic females or typical gynecomastia (Chapter 7) in phenotypic males results from the production of circulating plasma estrogen or androgen and thus depends upon the extent of gonadal development.[7]

Sexual infantilism also occurs in cases in which estrogen synthesis is profoundly reduced following deficiencies in the activity of the 17α-hydroxylase or 17,20-desmolase enzymes in the ovary. With *11β-hydroxylase* or *21β-hydroxylase deficiency*, ovarian estrogen production is normal; however, adrenal androgen production is increased. Females with this disorder have phallic enlargement, precocious pubic and axillary hair development, amenorrhea, and breast hypoplasia (Fig. 3–5). In disorders of impairment of testosterone biosynthesis *(17β-hydroxysteroid dehydrogenase deficiency)*, androgen insensitivity in males occurs to produce *testicular feminization*, and genetic males (XY) are phenotypic

females until puberty. Breast development, as evidenced by gynecomastia and areolar pigmentation and virilism, generally occurs at the onset of puberty. These clinical events result from increased testosterone production with rising plasma LH concentrations in the presence of an incomplete enzyme deficiency and a low androgen-to-estrogen ratio. In patients with testicular feminization, target tissue resistance to androgens results in an absence of virilization, and the lack of androgen action to oppose endogenous estrogen effects initiates growth of the breast. The breasts of these prepubertal male patients are generally large, but the nipple and areola are pale and immature.[7]

Pubertal Disorders

The breast may be affected by physiological disorders that occur concurrent with puberty. Premature breast development, with enlargement of the labia minora and majora and dulling of the vaginal mucosa, occurs following prolonged exposure of these premature tissues to estrogen. Clinical presentation of *premature puberty* (precocious development) is frequently caused by iatrogenic exposure to estrogens. Excessive estrogen secretion can also occur as a consequence of true or *central precocious puberty, estrogen-secreting neoplasms,* or *ovarian cysts.* True precocious puberty (Fig. 3–6) may originate from CNS tumors or other CNS disorders, but in females, true precocious puberty is usually idiopathic in origin. In true precocious puberty, the amplitude of LH pulses, and the LH response to GnRH are in the pubertal range. Low plasma LH and FSH concentrations, as the result of negative feedback inhibition, are associated with estrogen-secreting neoplasms or cysts.[18]

In cases of sexual precocity with premature breast development, *galactorrhea* may be observed. Sexual precocity may occur consequent to *primary hypothyroidism* (Figure 3–7) with *Hashimoto's thyroiditis.* In postpubertal females, an increased prolactin secretion may physiologically initiate galactorrhea. Further, HCG and hPL are occasionally secreted by estrogen-secreting *teratomas* or *teratocarcinomas;* for such cases in which hPL is secreted, galactorrhea may occur.[18]

Precocious development of the breast *(premature thelarche)* can occur in the absence of sexual or phenotypic precocity. In premature thelarche, unilateral or bilateral breast enlargement is evident without maturation of other secondary sex characteristics (Figure 3–8). There is generally an absence of nipple development, and breast enlargement commonly regresses in a few months, although this enlargement may persist for several years. Premature thelarche is most often observed in the first two years of life and rarely occurs after age four.[18] The premature breast enlargement of this syndrome occurs as a consequence of the transient increase in estrogen secretion, possibly by ovarian cysts, in response to transient increases in FSH concentrations or ovarian sensitivity to FSH.

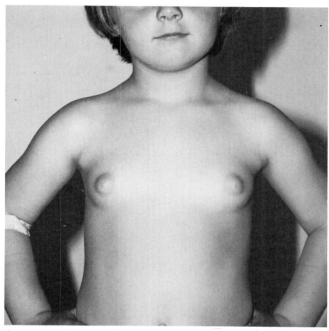

Figure 3–6. A 19-month-old female with central precocious puberty characterized by adolescent levels of gonadotropins and estrogens. This patient has adolescent-type breast development, including nipple maturation. (Courtesy of Dr. A. Rosenbloom, Division of Pediatric Endocrinology, University of Florida, Gainesville, FL.)

Lactational Disorders

In adult women, endocrine disorders can produce both *galactorrhea* and *lactational deficiency.* Galactorrhea is defined as a persistent discharge of milk or milklike secretions from the breast in the absence of parturition, or discharge in the non-nursing mother

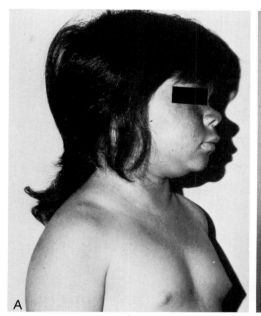
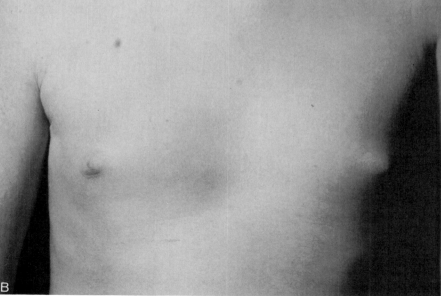

Figure 3–7. *A,* Acquired primary hypothyroidism in a 13-year-old female resulting in central precocity due to stimulation of gonadotropin-releasing hormone. This physiologic effect is related to the high output of thyrotropin-releasing hormone (TRH) from the hypothalamus. *B,* Note the true breast development despite a markedly delayed bone age and short stature. Regression of breast development occurred following therapy with thyroid hormone and conversion to a euthyroid state. (Courtesy of Dr. A. Rosenbloom, Division of Pediatric Endocrinology, University of Florida, Gainesville, FL.)

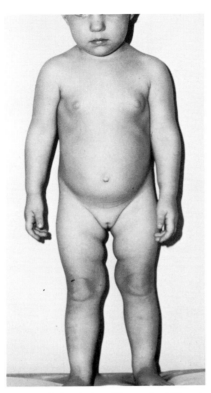

Figure 3–8. Premature thelarche in a 19-month-old female with bilateral precocious breast development and absence of sexual or phenotypic precocity. (Courtesy of Dr. A. Rosenbloom, Division of Pediatric Endocrinology, University of Florida, Gainesville, FL.)

beyond six months postpartum. This condition is often associated with increased plasma prolactin concentrations. In many cases, however, plasma prolactin levels are not elevated at the time the patient presents, although previous physiological mammary stimulation by prolactin may be important in the etiology of galactorrhea.[5]

Galactorrhea with hyperprolactinemia frequently results from a *prolactin-secreting adenoma* of the pituitary gland. These tumors are generally microadenomas of chromophobe cell origin (Fig. 3–9), with increased lactotrophs demonstrable by special strains. A small percentage of these patients also have elevated serum growth hormone concentrations and *acromegaly* as well as hyperprolactinemia. These patients are best treated by surgical removal of the microadenoma or with suppression of prolactin secretion following administration of the dopamine agonist bromocriptine mesylate (Parlodel). Amenorrhea is common in these cases. Galactorrhea may also be the predominant clinical symptom when prolactin levels are augmented following the administration of antipsychotic drugs (pimozide, chlorpromazine, haloperidol) that antagonize the physiological effects of dopamine.[5, 9, 21, 22]

Some women have galactorrhea and amenorrhea in the absence of pituitary microadenomas or a history of drug ingestion. In the rare presentation of the *Chiari-Frommel syndrome*, galactorrhea and amenorrhea persist for greater than six months postpartum in the clinical and radiological absence of a pituitary tumor. Circulating prolactin values are elevated in some patients with this syndrome, suggesting that it etiologically results following stimulation of the mammotrope by estrogens during pregnancy to produce *occult microadenomas*. Similarly, some patients have galactorrhea with usage of *oral contraceptives*. Milk production in these women is probably initiated as a result of the withdrawal of estrogen and progesterone. A small number of these individuals will develop microadenomas of the pituitary.[5]

Other conditions that may infrequently produce galactorrhea include primary hypothyroidism, chest surgery or pulmonary disease, chronic renal failure, and a variety of hypothalamic and pituitary diseases. These conditions physiologically produce galactorrhea by enhancing prolactin secretion.[5]

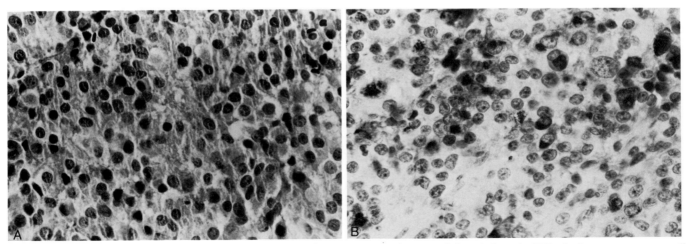

Figure 3–9. *A,* Hematoxylin and eosin photomicrograph of prolactin-secreting adenoma of the pituitary (×250). Such tumors are generally microadenomas of chromophobe cell origin that have evidence of increased lactotrophs demonstrable by special stains. This patient had galactorrhea with hyperprolactinemia as a consequence of the pituitary adenoma. Surgical removal of the microadenoma was curative. *B,* Immunoperoxidase stain for prolactin in the same prolactin-secreting adenoma with demonstration of positive cytoplasmic stain. Cytoplasm of tumor cells is composed of black granules, and clumping is evident near the nuclei. In the central area of the photomicrograph, one can see several tumor cells (×250). (Courtesy of Dr. W.E. Ballinger, Jr., Department of Pathology, University of Florida, Gainesville, FL.)

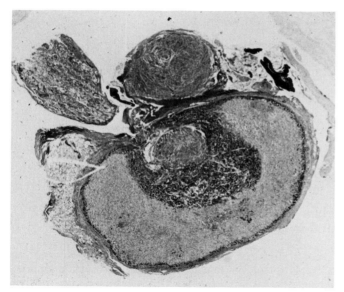

Figure 3–10. Hematoxylin and eosin–stained section of pituitary gland with infarction and necrosis as a consequence of Sheehan's syndrome (×20). The majority of the gland reveals necrosis with preservation of some tissue in the center of the gland and the outer rim. Hypopituitarism resulted with hypoprolactinemia that initiated mammary involution and failure to lactate. (Courtesy of Dr. W.E. Ballinger, Jr., Department of Pathology, University of Florida, Gainesville, FL.)

The largest population of patients with galactorrhea, however, occurs in individuals with the clinical presentation of *idiopathic galactorrhea* and *normal menses.* The majority of these women have persistent postpartum lactation despite prolactin levels in the normal range.[5] The abnormality in these cases may result from increased responsiveness of the target breast tissue to physiological serum concentrations of circulating prolactin.

A *lactational deficiency* of endocrine origin is expressed as *Sheehan's syndrome.* This disorder occurs as a result of damage to the pituitary vascular supply secondary to postpartum hemorrhage and shock. Acute pituitary necrosis generally follows from the damage to this highly vascular organ (Fig. 3–10). The pituitary gland is particularly vulnerable to decreased blood flow at the end of gestation because of its increased size and thus is more sensitive to hypoperfusion and necrosis. The degree of *hypopituitarism* that emanates from hypoperfusion is variable; however, *hypoprolactinemia* generally results, causing mammary involution and the failure of lactation. Other signs of pituitary hormone deficiency (diabetes insipidus, amenorrhea, hypothyroidism, loss of axillary hair, sparse regrowth of pubic hair) may become evident. Spontaneous recovery may occur and generally depends upon the extent of infarction and/or the rate of pituitary cellular regeneration.[5, 23]

References

1. Anderson RR: Endocrinological control in the development of the mammary gland. *In* Larson BL, Smith VR (eds): Lactation, A Comprehensive Treatise, Vol 1. New York, Academic Press, 1974, pp 97–140.
2. Cowie AT, Forsyth IA, Hart IC: Hormonal Control of Lactation. Berlin, Springer-Verlag, 1980, pp 1–263.
3. Cowie AT, Tindal JS: The physiology of lactation. Monogr Physiol Soc 22:1–282, 1971.
4. Drife JO: Breast development in pregnancy. Ann NY Acad Sci, 464:58–65, 1986.
5. Frantz AG, Wilson JD: Endocrine disorders of the breasts. *In* Wilson JD, Foster DW (eds): Williams Textbook of Endocrinology. 7th ed. Philadelphia, WB Saunders, 1985, pp 402–421.
6. Grosvenor CE, Mena F: Neural and hormonal control of milk secretion and milk ejection. *In* Larson BL, Smith VR (eds): Lactation, A Comprehensive Treatise, Vol 1. New York, Academic Press, 1974, pp 272–276.
7. Grumbach MM, Conte FA: Disorders of sexual differentiation. *In* Wilson JD, Foster DW (eds): Williams Textbook of Endocrinology. 7th ed. Philadelphia, WB Saunders, 1985, pp 312–401.
8. Haagensen CD: The normal physiology of the breasts. *In* Haagensen CD (ed): Diseases of the Breast. Philadelphia, WB Saunders, 1986, pp 47–55.
9. Jacobs LS, Daughaday WM: Physologic regulation of prolactin secretion in man. *In* Josimovich JB (ed): Lactogenic Hormones, Fetal Nutrition and Lactation. New York, John Wiley & Sons, 1974, pp 351–377.
10. Jaffe RB: Disorders of sexual development. *In* Jaffe R, Yen SC (eds): Reproductive Endocrinology. Philadelphia, WB Saunders, 1986, pp 183–312.
11. Kleinberg DL, Newman CB: The pituitary gland in primate mammary development: evidence that prolactin is not essential. Ann NY Acad Sci 464:37–43, 1986.
12. Mauvais-Jarvis P, Kuttenn F, Gompel A: Estradiol/progesterone interaction in normal and pathologic breast cells. Ann NY Acad Sci 464:152–167, 1986.
13. Muldoon TG: Steroid hormone receptor regulation by various hormonal factors during mammary development and growth in the normal mouse. Ann NY Acad Sci 464:27–36, 1986.
14. Robyn C: Endocrinological aspects of breast physiology. *In* Angeli A, Bradlow HL, Dogliotti L (eds): Endocrinology of Cystic Breast Disease. New York, Raven Press, 1983, pp 25–34.
15. Roby C, Brandts N, Rozenberg S, Meuris S: Advances in physiology of human lactation. Ann NY Acad Sci 464:66–74, 1986.
16. Rosenberg A: Uber menstruelle, dursch das Corpus Luteum bedingte Mammaveränderungen. Frankfurt Ztsch Path 27:466, 1922.
17. Salazar H, Robon H: Morphologic changes of the mammary gland during development, pregnancy and lactation. *In* Josimovich JB (ed): Lactogenic Hormones, Fetal Nutrition and Lactation. New York, John Wiley & Sons, 1974, pp 221–278.
18. Styne DM, Grombach MM: Puberty in the male and female. *In* Jaffe R, Yen SC (eds): Reproductive Endocrinology. Philadelphia, WB Saunders, 1986, pp 313–384.
19. Tanner JM: Growth at adolescence. Oxford, Blackwell Scientific Publications, 1962, p 35.
20. Tucker HA: General endocrinological control of lactation. *In* Larson BL, Smith VR (eds): Lactation, A Comprehensive Treatise, Vol I. New York, Academic Press, 1974, pp 277–318.
21. Vorherr H: Human lactation and breast feeding. *In* Larson BL, Smith VR (eds): Lactation, A Comprehensive Treatise, Vol IV. New York, Academic Press, 1978, pp 182–280.
22. Yen SSC: Prolactin in human reproduction. *In* Yen SSC, Jaffe R (eds): Reproductive Endocrinology. Philadelphia, WB Saunders, 1986, pp 237–263. 1986.
23. Yen SSC: Chronic anovulation due to CNS-hypothalamic pituitary dysfunction. *In* Yen SSC, Jaffe R (eds): Reproductive Endocrinology. Philadelphia, WB Saunders, 1986, pp 434–435.

Discharges and Secretions of the Nipple*

Eileen B. King, M.D. and William H. Goodson III, M.D.

The frequency of discharges and secretions of the nipple necessitates a comprehensive discussion in the management of breast diseases. The purpose of this chapter is threefold. First, it will inform the reader about nipple aspirate fluid (NAF) findings related to breast physiology, pathology, and risk of cancer. Second, it will discuss nipple discharge in diagnosis and management of breast disease, especially cancer and its precursors. Third, it will describe methods for sample collection and preparation to assure optimum quality for the best diagnostic results.

The terms *discharges* and *secretions* of the nipple are defined as follows: *Discharge* is fluid that escapes spontaneously from the nipple. *Secretion* is fluid present in the ducts that must be collected by nipple aspiration (NAF) or by other means such as conventional breast pump or gentle massage and expression from the ducts (nonspontaneous secretion).

SECRETION IN THE NONLACTATING BREAST

The secretory activity of the female breast is manifested at varying levels throughout life—at birth, after puberty, and well into menopause. Secretion of this modified apocrine gland exhibits milk-like characteristics, and lactation represents the ultimate secretory product. Nipple secretion is usually not clinically appreciated in nonlactating women because dense keratotic material plugs the openings of the lactiferous sinuses (Fig. 3–11). Such secretion is observed, however, in duct lumens displayed in histological sections of breast tissue (Fig. 3–12). By removing the keratotic plugs and using a simple nipple aspirator device, fluid can easily be obtained in a large proportion of women (Fig. 3–13).[10, 59, 64, 72] Researchers have also obtained secretions by using a breast pump or with gentle manual expression.[25, 26, 52, 53, 62]

Both secretory and absorptive activities appear to be inevitable components of breast physiology. Reabsorption has been studied in rabbits by injecting breast ducts with various substances and observing their distribution in tissue, lymphatics, and blood.[9, 29] Suspensions of India ink could be traced to these sites, and diphtheria antitoxin injected into ducts was subsequently measured in blood. Sartorius and coworkers performed ductography using a water-soluble contrast medium in humans and noted that reabsorption occurred at different rates depending upon the presence of lesions.[64]

Fluid Availability Related to Age, Race, and Other Factors

In a study of 606 normal nonlactating women, the availability of NAF was examined by race, age, menstrual history, menopausal status, and use of oral contraceptives or estrogen replacement therapy.[59] Samples of NAF were collected by a modified Sartorius technique. This procedure is noninvasive, simple, and well tolerated by the patient. Fluid availability was defined as a drop or more. On the average, from 20 to 30 μl was obtained. Fluid was most often obtained from Caucasian and Filipino women (70 percent) and was less frequently available from black, Mexican-American, Japanese, and Chinese women (Table 3–2). Age was a significant factor, regardless of race, and women over age 50 were less likely to yield fluid (Table 3–3). Phase of the menstrual cycle and history of pregnancy did not significantly affect the availability of NAF. Similarly, oral contraceptives and estrogen replacement therapy had little effect, although in postmenopausal women there was some increase in the amount of NAF obtained from those receiving estrogen replacement therapy. A comparison of secretory and menopausal status in Caucasian and Chinese women showed that significantly more premenopausal than postmenopausal women yielded fluid and that the difference was most striking in Chinese women (Table 3–4). The mammary and ceruminous glands are both apocrine in type. A relatively high frequency of fluid availability in Caucasian women corresponded to a high incidence of the genetically determined wet earwax in these women.[55, 56] This is particularly interesting because the international mortality and frequency rates for breast cancer seem to be associated with the frequency of the alleles for wet earwax.

In an additional study of 103 women with suspicious breast lesions, a higher frequency of NAF (88.4 percent) was obtained than from normal women, suggesting an association of NAF availability with breast disease.[59] Of 22 women in this study later found to have carcinoma, 16 (72 percent) had yielded NAF. Theoretically, breast epithelium, if displaying more secretory activity, would be more likely to be exposed to endogenous and exogenous carcinogens than would epithelium displaying less evidence of secretory activity.

Wynder and colleagues have evaluated NAF in rela-

*Supported by research grant CA 13556-17 from the National Cancer Institute, Bethesda, MD.

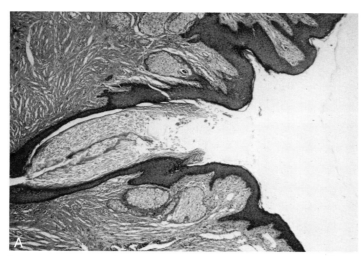
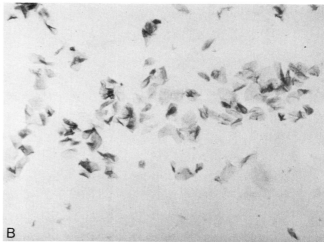

Figure 3–11. *A,* Sagittal section of nipple duct opening demonstrates the usual plug of keratotic plaques obstructing the duct (H and E stain; original magnification ×25).

B, NAF sample contains abundant anucleate keratotic plaques from duct opening (Papanicolaou stain; original magnification ×25).

tion to age, menarchal age, and parity as well as other epidemiological factors in breast disease. Their findings are very similar to those described in the other studies using the Sartorius technique.[10, 59, 64, 72] These studies show that the availability of breast fluid among nonlactating women depends on a number of factors, age, race, menopausal status, and breast disease status being among the most important.

Biochemical and Cytological Composition

NAF has many of the characteristics of colostrum or milk. Chemical analyses show that it is a secretion of both endogenous and exogenous substances. The fluid varies in color and appearance related to its composition. Like colostrum and milk, it contains exfoliated epithelial cells and nonepithelial cells of hematogenous and immune system origin. These components may vary in relationship to the functional aspects of the breast, its pathology, and risk factors for breast cancer.

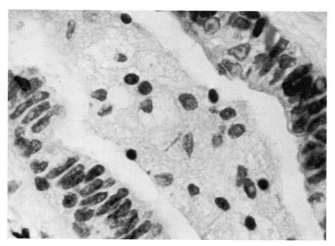

Figure 3–12. Breast duct with lumen containing secretory material and exfoliated lining cells (H and E stain; original magnification ×250).

Biochemical Composition

The biochemical composition of NAF has been studied using micromethods to analyze the small volumes of available ductal secretion. The NAF contains lactose, α-lactalbumin, immunoglobulin, cholesterol, fatty acids, a number of steroids, and other endogenous substances.[57] Substances from exogenous sources are also secreted into the fluid. Examples are technetium, barbiturate, fatty acid, caffeine, pesticides, and nicotine and cotinine related to cigarette smoking. Approximately 10 percent of NAF samples demonstrate mutagenic activity with the Ames salmonella test. These findings demonstrate that breast fluid is a true secretory product. Detailed analysis has been made of many of these components, and their concentrations in breast secretion has been compared with those in plasma. Other studies have considered differences in composition of secretions among women with different risk factors for breast cancer. Among compounds of particular interest, because of their possible role in the pathogenesis of benign and malignant breast disease, are the estrogens and cholesterol with its epoxides and triol.

In a study of estrogen (estrone and estradiol) levels in serum and NAF, Petrakis and colleagues evaluated samples from one or both breasts in 104 women and found estrogen levels to be 5 to 45 times higher in NAF than in serum.[61] They also found that NAF estrogen

Table 3–2. NIPPLE ASPIRATE FLUID (NAF) AVAILABILITY AMONG VARIOUS RACIAL GROUPS

Group	Number with NAF	Number Attempted (%)
Caucasian	158/225	(70.2)
Filipino	7/10	(70.0)
Black	23/37	(62.2)
Mexican-American	37/71	(52.1)
Asian	65/263	(24.7)

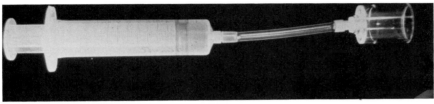

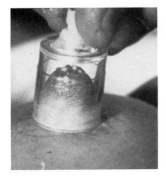 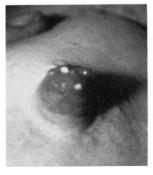 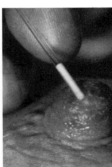

Figure 3–13. Nipple aspirator is a cup-shaped plastic device fitted with tubing to connect with a syringe. The negative pressure created by the syringe causes drops of fluid to appear at each duct opening. The drops are then collected in a capillary tube.

levels were lower in parous than in nulliparous women. This finding suggests that prolonged levels of estrogen in breast fluid after full-term delivery and lactation may in part explain the relative reduction in breast cancer risk in parous compared with nulliparous women. In contrast, the serum estrogen levels were unrelated to parity.

Cholesterol and its oxidation products, 5,6 α and β epoxides and their common hydrolysis product cholestane triol, were measured in NAF by Gruenke and associates.[22] Both these epoxides have been implicated in oncogenic behavior in a number of different studies demonstrating induction of sarcomas, in vitro transforming of embryo hamster cell lines, chromosome damage and inhibition of DNA repair, and mutagenic activity.[6, 27, 28, 54] In a study of 105 women without breast disease, levels of cholesterol and its β epoxide were found to increase with age but were reduced in parous women. The lower levels persisted for a minimum of two years following delivery or lactation. As a result, parous women have less cumulative exposure to these biochemical substances with carcinogenic potential.[22]

That the color of NAF varies greatly is easily observed clinically. Excluding bloody fluids, the colors range from clear to black, with gradations classified as white, pale yellow, dark yellow, brown, and green. In a retrospective study of NAF from 2343 women, the colors of the samples were compared with their biochemical compositions.[58] Each sample had been coded at the time of collection in one of the seven color categories before biochemical analysis. Cholesterol, cholesterol 5,6 α and β epoxides, cholestane triol, lipid peroxide, estradiol and estrone, and immunoglobulin levels were measured. The results were transformed into natural logarithms, and the means and standard deviations were determined for each breast fluid color group. Statistical significance was tested with a one-way analysis of variance. The mean concentrations of cholesterol, its epoxides, and triol were strongly related to darker colorations. Higher concentrations of these substances were also associated with the darker colorations. Similar relationships were obtained for lipid peroxides, estrone, and estradiol. However, the immunoglobulin concentrations showed no relation to color. Although the exact mechanism of color production is unknown, the association with biochemical properties of the NAF is of clinical interest and will be discussed further (see Secretions Associated with Breast Disease).

Cytological Composition

The cytology of breast fluid was first reported by Donne, who in 1838 described the presence of foam

Table 3–3. NIPPLE ASPIRATE FLUID (NAF) AVAILABILITY AND AGE

Age Group (yr)	Number with NAF/Number Attempted (%)	
	All Races	*Caucasian*
≤20	9/18 (50.0)	4/6 (66.6)
21–30	66/121 (54.5)	36/48 (75.0)
31–40	77/145 (53.1)	44/57 (77.2)
41–50	70/125 (56.0)	37/47 (78.7)
51–60	30/78 (38.5)	21/35 (60.0)
≥60	23/86 (26.7)	16/32 (50.0)
Total	266/555 (47.9)	158/225 (70.2)

Table 3–4. NIPPLE ASPIRATE FLUID (NAF) AVAILABILITY AND MENOPAUSAL STATUS IN CAUCASIAN AND CHINESE WOMEN

Group	Number with NAF/Number Attempted (%)	
	Caucasian*	*Chinese†*
Premenopausal	112/138 (81.2)	47/156 (30.1)
Postmenopausal	46/77 (59.7)	3/80 (3.8)

*$X^2 = 24.7$, $P<0.001$
†$X^2 = 20.4$, $P<0.001$

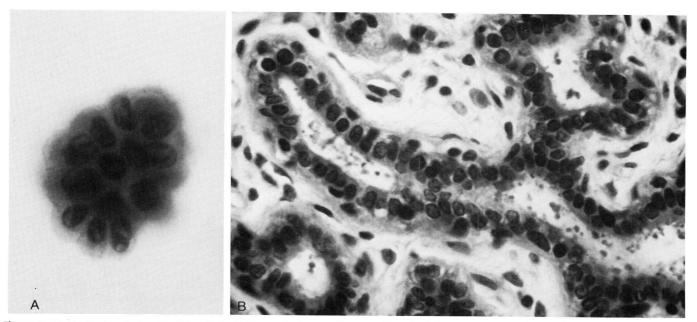

Figure 3–14. *A,* Benign duct epithelial cells in NAF sample have uniform small oval nuclei and columnar shape (Papanicolaou stain; original magnification ×250). *B,* These cells correspond with the normal ductal lobular epithelium depicted in this section of benign breast tissue (H and E stain; original magnification ×250).

cells in colostrum.[18] The main attention remained focused on studies of colostrum, milk, and spontaneous nipple discharge. In an early study of nonspontaneous secretion, Jackson and Severance routinely attempted to express fluid from both breasts during the course of breast examination.[25, 26] They described the presence of red blood cells, vacuolated epithelial cells, and dark-staining epithelial cells, usually in clusters in air-dried smears on Wright's stain. Papanicolaou and colleagues made a thorough and systematic study of the cytology of nonspontaneous breast secretions using a hand breast pump to obtain the specimen.[53] Over 50 percent of the 1600 patients they examined yielded fluid by this method. These investigators emphasized that cytology of abnormal breast conditions could not be properly evaluated without adequate knowledge of what was normal, and they provided a description of the benign cellular findings. They noted that the two cell types most often encountered were foam cells and duct epithelial cells. A few small histiocytes and lymphocytes were also frequently present. Ringrose achieved similar results and noted the same type of cytological findings in fluid from asymptomatic women.[62]

The cytological findings in NAF from women without breast disease are primarily of interest in providing a knowledge of "normal." Such knowledge is essential for comparisons of findings related to benign and malignant breast lesions and to ensure accurate interpretation of clinically significant disease. Benign findings have been evaluated microscopically by determining total cellularity and identifying cell types and the percentage of each type.[31] The samples from women without breast symptoms contain an average of 16,200 ± 6500 cells of all types. The cellularity varies with age and is increased in samples from women in the fourth decade compared with those of younger and older women. It must be emphasized, however, that there is a wide range in cellularity among individuals regardless of age. The timing of greater average cellularity in NAF samples can be considered fortuitous for the study of breast cancer precursors developing in women from ages 30 to 50.

Benign epithelial cells, when present, consist of a few ductal cells; only rarely are apocrine metaplastic cells found in the absence of breast symptoms (Figs. 3–14 and 3–15). Occasionally, one finds the squamous epithelial cells and transitional cell forms from the ampullary and distal portions of the duct within the nipple (Fig. 3–16). Duct openings frequently yield anucleate keratotic plaques that may be abundant when preparation before nipple aspiration has been inadequate (see Fig. 3–11).

Foam cells are most often present and may be abundant. They show predominantly histiocytic characteristics when evaluated cytochemically with monoclonal antibodies or by other conventional means. However, they are a distinct category and remain controversial as to origin (Fig. 3–17). The abundant, finely vacuolated cytoplasm of foam cells may contain yellow-brown pigment granules. Some granules have morphological, electron microscopic, and staining features of lipofuscin and ceroid contained in lysosomes (Fig. 3–18). Other pigmented granules represent hemoglobin and its products staining positively for iron (Fig. 3–18). Other cells are of hematogenous and immune system origin and consist of neutrophils, lymphocytes, and small histiocytes.

The mean percentage of various cell types in NAF from asymptomatic women and those with benign cytology and pathology is illustrated in Figure 3–19. In summary, "normal" cellular findings consist of few or

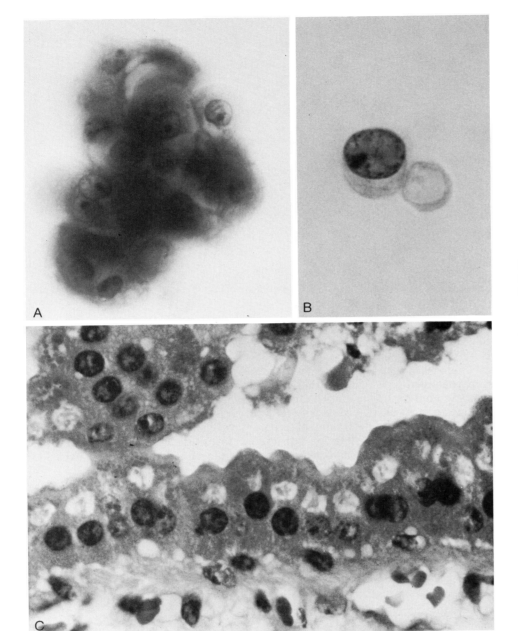

Figure 3–15. *A,* A group of apocrine metaplastic cells in NAF have abundant granular and sometimes vacuolated cytoplasm. *B,* An apocrine bleb containing a large vacuole with a thin cytoplasmic envelope is separating from the border of this single cell (A & B Papanicolaou stain; original magnification ×250). *C,* Multilayered apocrine metaplastic epithelium with tufts of cells separating into the duct lumen are depicted in this tissue section (H and E stain; original magnification ×250).

no duct epithelial cells, a preponderance of foam cells, and moderate numbers of cells of hematogenous origin in samples of modest cellularity.

Menstrual Cycle Changes

Menstrual cycle effects on breast could potentially change the availability and composition of NAF. If there were cyclical changes in breast secretory activity, these changes would be reflected by the presence or absence of fluid at different times in the cycle. Particularly essential would be a knowledge of any ductal lobular epithelial proliferative activity related to the cycle. Cyclical changes would affect the accuracy of diagnosis and interpretation of the cytological findings in both NAF and nipple discharge. Much is already known about the histological changes during the menstrual cycle that would lead one to expect cyclical variations in NAF.

Breast tissue studies have shown cyclical changes related to follicular and luteal phases. Similar observations on changes in histological pattern, cellular morphology, mitoses, and DNA content have been made.[20, 43, 45, 47] Ductal lobular proliferative activity is demonstrated by increased numbers of mitoses and DNA synthesis in the luteal phase corresponding to the combination of estrogen and progesterone influences. Vogel and associates found similar histological changes except that mitoses were observed early in the follicular phase.[69] Some disagreement among such studies may be a result

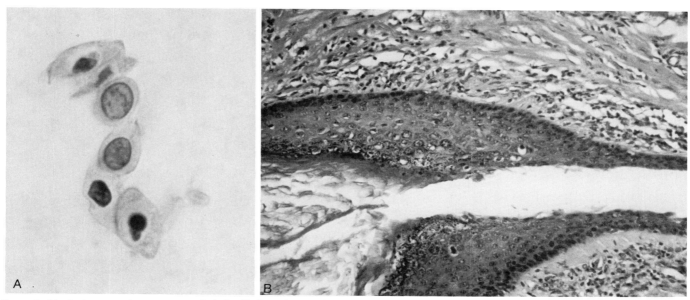

Figure 3–16. *A,* A group of squamous epithelial cells from ducts within the nipple have nuclei of variable size and staining with pyknosis in one (Papanicolaou stain; original magnification ×250). *B,* Note the parabasal squamous maturation of epithelium in the duct lining from which these cells are derived (H and E stain; original magnification ×25).

of inherent problems: heterogeneity of lobular development within the individual breast, variability between subjects, and inaccuracy in cycle data. Some of these problems have been addressed in more recent studies that have given special attention to sample selection and size and to statistical methods. Longacre and Bartlow found excessive lymphocytes, duct epithelial degenerative changes, and sloughing into duct lumens in the late secretory and early menstrual phases.[41] Ferguson and Anderson also found cell depletion through a process of apoptosis in this time interval and peaking on day 28.[20]

Some of the reports indicate that both breasts were examined and that no significant differences were found in morphological changes.

Objective measures of breast epithelial cyclical changes are provided by DNA quantitative cytochemistry previously described in tissue sections and by image cytometry of fine needle aspirate (FNA) samples. In fine needle aspirate biopsies, image cytometry using five nuclear features (area, circumference, boundary fluctuation, chromatin granularity, and stain intensity) successfully discriminated samples from women in follicular

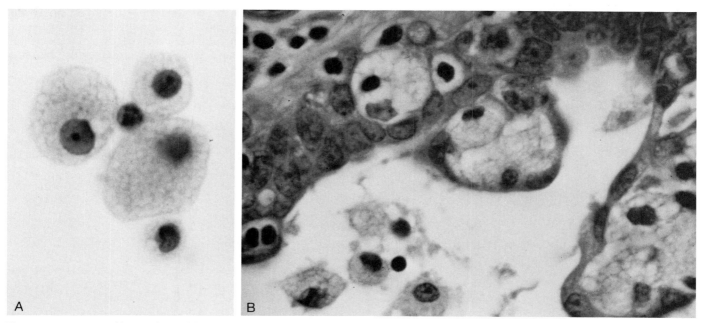

Figure 3–17. *A,* Typical large spherical foam cells with abundant finely vacuolated cytoplasm in NAF. Nuclei are isodiametric and have prominent nucleolei (Papanicolaou stain; original magnification ×250). *B,* In the tissue section, the duct foam cells appear intraepithelial and also within the duct lumen (H and E stain; original magnification ×250).

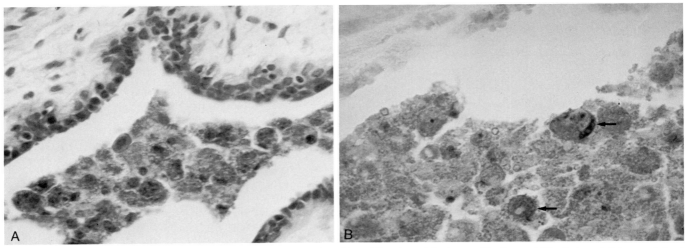

Figure 3–18. *A,* Foam cell containing golden brown pigment granules. (H and E stain; original magnification ×160); *B,* Iron-staining particles in foam cells (Prussian blue stain at arrows; original magnification ×250).

phase and those in luteal phase.[42] This approach, applied to the individual woman, was 100 percent correct in identifying the phase of the cycle. Concerned by the proliferative changes that mimic atypia or malignancy in the postovulatory phase, the authors recommended that fine needle aspiration be done only in the preovulatory phase.

The first report of the cytology of nonspontaneous secretion related to the menstrual cycle was of Papanicolaou and associates.[52] In 1958 they reported on fluid availability with a technique of gentle massage and breast pump application on the breasts of nonlactating women. From 46 of 129 women, aged 20 to 39 years, who yielded breast fluid, the fluid was most often obtained in the fourth (55 percent) or the first (40 percent) week of the cycle. Duct epithelial cells were scant or absent, and foam cells were the most common constituent. These workers noted some cell enlargement and clusters of cells with cytoplasmic vacuolization that appeared different from small undifferentiated duct ep-

ithelial cells. They proposed that these differences are related to the endocrine status of the individual. However, the findings were not analyzed with respect to the day or week of the menstrual cycle.

In our studies of NAF, there are some differences in fluid availability and cellularity associated with the phase of the menstrual cycle. However, these differences do not appear to be significant. In a study of 117 Caucasian women, 70.8 percent yielded fluid in the first week, 83.9 percent in the second week, 75.8 percent in the third week, and 82.8 percent in the fourth week of the menstrual cycle.[59] No significant differences were noted in cellularity or types of cells present. A group of 38 NAF samples from different women were selected for approximately equal distribution among the four weeks of a 28-day cycle. They were analyzed for total cellularity and cell types. Duct epithelial cells occurred singly and in groups, accompanied occasionally by apocrine metaplastic cells; foam cells were almost always present and abundant; and there were a few histiocytes, lympho-

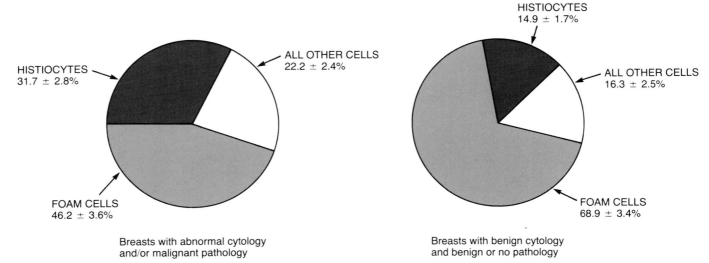

Breasts with abnormal cytology and/or malignant pathology

Breasts with benign cytology and benign or no pathology

Figure 3–19. Comparison of percentage of foam cells in two clinical groups.

cytes, and neutrophils. Although the measure of total cellularity, percentage of single duct cells, histiocytes, and lymphocytes have demonstrated trends toward elevation in the fourth week in the menstrual cycle, the results were not significant on discriminant analysis.

Complete cycles sampled at weekly intervals were evaluated in 14 women. Serum and NAF estrone and estradiol were determined at each examination and serum hormonal levels compared with the menstrual history. In women having serum hormonal patterns consistent with a normal ovulatory cycle, no cytological changes suggesting proliferation or degeneration were noted and there were no significant variations in cellularity or cell types. However, some increase in total cellularity and in percentage of lymphocytes did occur in the late postovulatory and early preovulatory phases.

Our studies of menstrual cycle changes in NAF cytology have revealed no significant differences that might affect the accuracy or diagnostic value of these findings. The sample size is small and more data are needed before definitive conclusions can be drawn.

PREGNANCY AND LACTATION ASSOCIATED SECRETIONS

Responding to a variety of hormonal influences during pregnancy and lactation, the breast becomes fully developed anatomically and functionally. Development of the terminal ductal lobular unit involves proliferation of ductal and lobular epithelium and the manufacture of secretory products, colostrum, and milk. The anatomical and physiological features of the breast and its secretory products have been widely studied and amply discussed elsewhere (see Chapter 2). However, histological studies in humans are limited by the availability of tissue from biopsies.[16, 19] In lieu of human tissue, animal studies have provided some insights into breast changes during pregnancy and lactation.[14]

During pregnancy, the ductal lobular system undergoes extensive hyperplasia with rapid proliferation of epithelial linings as they form new ductules. These are arranged in close proximity with scant supporting stroma. This process is most marked in the first half of the pregnancy and is followed by some development of the stromal component and infiltration of lymphocytes, plasma cells, and eosinophils. Evidence of secretory activity appears in the later months of pregnancy with the presence of protein-rich fluid in dilated duct lumens. The epithelial lining varies from flat to low columnar and exhibits merocrine secretory activity typical of glandular epithelium in other organs. The so-called apocrine secretion consists of lipid droplets that are free within the cytoplasm, become oriented at the free margin of the cell, and separate from the cell bounded by a thin envelope of cytoplasm.[8]

The "normal" cytology of breast secretions during pregnancy is characterized by increased cellularity compared with the resting breast. This is especially true in the later months of pregnancy. Cell types are the same as those found in the absence of pregnancy but show some differences in the proportions of various cells. Epithelial cell clusters are numerous and sometimes have a configuration suggesting papillary structure. In the late third trimester and following delivery, neutrophils are abundant. Postpartum cellular patterns vary depending upon the presence or suppression of lactation.[23, 31]

An interesting point of view about the importance of breast cytology during pregnancy and lactation was expressed by Holmquist and Papanicolaou and by Papanicolaou and colleagues.[23, 53] They propose that cytological studies of breast secretion offer a noninvasive method for studying the effects of altered hormonal stimuli on breast epithelium during pregnancy and lactation. Such studies may also be relevant in demonstrating epithelial changes that might predate development of neoplastic disease of the breast. In their study of 20 antepartum and 39 postpartum women with clinically normal breasts, all the subjects had full-term deliveries and the mean age was 27.2 (17 to 43) years. The cytological samples were generally more cellular than those from nonpregnant women. The cell appearance and predominant cell type varied among individuals, sometimes between the right and left breast of the same individual, and among trimesters. Cell types were the same as those found in the absence of pregnancy or lactation; however, definite alterations in structure were noted. The cell types listed were foam cells, leukocytes, histiocytes, and gland epithelial cells consisting of single cells and cell clusters. *Foam cells* were found to have the same appearance as cells referred to as colostrum bodies, which have been described in "normal" breast fluid samples from nonpregnant women. Among the pregnant patients, Holmquist and Papanicolaou noted that the foam cells exhibited nuclear enlargement, binucleation, multinucleation, and increased cytoplasmic vacuolization compared with those from nonpregnant women.[23] They found an unexpectedly large number of *ductal epithelial cells* during pregnancy and lactation. The groups of cells were papillary in structure and similar to papillary fronds from intraductal papilloma. Differences were also noted in the cytology of postpartum smears from lactating patients compared with those of secretion following estrogen suppression of lactation. The former became virtually acellular at the end of the first week post partum, whereas the latter exhibited cellularity and various types of cell clusters characteristic of those found during pregnancy.

Kline and Lash studied the cytology of breast secretions obtained during the third trimester from 50 pregnant women aged 16 to 39 years.[36] This study was stimulated by the erroneous interpretation of cytological findings during pregnancy based on the papillary groupings and changes similar to those described by Holmquist and Papanicolaou. In the Kline and Lash study, 43 of the 50 women had papillary groupings, whereas the remaining seven had only foam cells and leukocytes. Tissue from four biopsies obtained in the third trimester revealed tufts of cells forming "spurs" or invaginations into duct and alveolar lumens and similar structures that were desquamated into lumens and were suggestive of groups of cells found in the breast secretions. These investigators noted that the "spurs" were closely associated with the formation of new alveoli, and this offered a mechanism for their origin. Delicate capillary networks within these tufts of cells could be easily traumatized and result in blood escaping into the breast secretion. Bloody secretion without significant breast pathology occurs in pregnant and postpartum patients. In a later study, these authors reported persistence of the antepartum cellular findings in 31 of 72 postpartum women; however, no information was provided on lactation or estrogen suppression of lactation.[37] Changes persisted beyond two months post partum in only five women. Additional histological studies of eight breast biopsies demonstrated findings similar to those described during pregnancy and lasting up to two months post partum.

King et al. also found increased cellularity associated with pregnancy.[31] The occurrence of duct epithelial cells was compared in 136 samples, 68 from 34 pregnant women and 68 from 48 nonpregnant women. From 1 to 80 groups of duct cells were found in 82 of the 136 individual samples. The total number of cells per group tended to be greater in pregnant and premenopausal nonpregnant women than in postmenopausal women. However, in comparing all the data from the three groups (using the Kolmogorov-Smirnov test) the only significant difference was between pregnant and postmenopausal patients. Recent studies of pregnancy effects were made on NAF from 27 women selected for equal distribution according to trimester and age. In this analysis, the cellularity was quite variable among women and trimester; the mean cellularity was moderately increased compared with that of nonpregnant normal women (Table 3–5).

Breast fluid cytology during pregnancy and lactation reveals increased cellularity that is most marked in the later months of pregnancy and varies in the postpartum period. Increased numbers of duct epithelial cells in groups were reported by some to have changes like those associated with intraductal papilloma or papillary hyperplasia.[23, 36, 37] In addition, blood may be found in secretions from pregnant and lactating patients in the absence of clinically evident lesions.[36, 37] These findings justify caution in the interpretation of secretions from pregnant or lactating women.

SECRETIONS ASSOCIATED WITH BREAST DISEASE

Nonspontaneous secretions or NAF display cellular patterns related to a variety of disease processes in the

Table 3–6. TERMINOLOGY AND CRITERIA FOR HISTOLOGICAL CLASSIFICATION OF BREAST DISEASE IN TISSUE SECTIONS

Nonproliferative lesions: Lesions such as adenosis, apocrine metaplasia, cysts, duct ectasia, fibroadenoma, inflammation, and squamous metaplasia.
Hyperplasia (mild): Increase in layers of duct lining cells to three or four without cytologic atypia.
Moderate hyperplasia: Multilayering of duct linings, sometimes papillary; bridging of duct lumen forming new irregular lumens; cellular and nuclear variability and minimal atypia.
Atypical hyperplasia (ductal or lobular): *Ductal* changes appear more advanced than those in moderate hyperplasia. Increasing monotony of the cell population suggestive of modal distribution. Some, but not all, the features of carcinoma in situ. *Lobular* changes are increased in number of cells expanding the ductule diameter but not completely filling the lumen.
Carcinoma in situ (ductal or lobular): *Ductal* lesions may be subclassified as solid large cell, comedo, papillary, or cribriform. Nuclear and cellular features of malignancy range from low to high grade. *Lobular* lesions composed of monotonous population of small discohesive cells that completely fill and expand the ductules.

breast. Evaluation of duct fluid for screening or diagnostic purposes has met with varying degrees of success. Significant problems are caused by the limitations in sample availability and cellularity. Despite these considerations, cytological abnormalities in NAF and nonspontaneous secretion have significant association with breast lesions of clinical and prognostic importance. The following discussions summarize the NAF patterns and histological correlates for benign breast disease with and without increased risk of cancer and those associated with malignancy.

Benign Disease Without Increased Risk of Breast Cancer

Cytological findings in NAF previously described as "normal" and those referred to as "hyperplasia" of minimal degree have no apparent association with increased risk of breast cancer. The histological correlates are those defined in a Consensus Meeting, "Is Fibrocystic Disease Precancerous?"[15] Lesions not associated with increased risk of cancer were apocrine metaplasia, cyst, duct ectasia, fibroadenoma, fibrosis, mastitis, periductal mastitis, squamous metaplasia, and mild hyperplasia. Cytological patterns in NAF are nonspecific and inadequate for definitive diagnosis of most benign lesions in this category. The histological lesion referred to as mild hyperplasia is in concordance with changes of Welling's Type ALA 1 or 2 and Black and Chabon's Grade 2 lesions. It is described by the Consensus Meeting as a lesion with three to four layers of cells without significant atypia lining breast ducts.[7, 15, 32, 63, 70] King et al. noted cytological findings in NAF that correlate with this mild degree of hyperplasia (Tables 3–6 and 3–7; Fig. 3–20).[32]

Significant differences between cytologic findings in NAF from "normal" breasts and those with benign breast disease include increased average total cellularity

Table 3–5. NAF AVAILABILITY IN PREGNANT COMPARED WITH NONPREGNANT WOMEN

Group	No.	Cellularity X 10³ (mean)	Range	Age (mean)	Range
First trimester	8	79.4	5.7–304	31	23–41
Second trimester	9	52.7	16.6–104	29	23–35
Third trimester	9	90.4	40.9–218	29	23–35
Nonpregnant	6	21.8	0.9–64	30	23–45

Table 3–7. TERMINOLOGY AND CRITERIA FOR CYTOLOGICAL CLASSIFICATION OF NAF, SECRETION, OR DISCHARGE SAMPLES

Benign, nonproliferative changes: Duct epithelial or apocrine metaplastic cells within normal limits.
Hyperplasia (mild): Minimal cellular changes, slight cellular and nuclear enlargement. Cell distribution predominantly in groups; papillary or apocrine metaplastic changes are subcategorized.
Moderate hyperplasia: Moderate cellular changes; cell and nuclear enlargement disproportionate with N:C ratio increase; chromatin granularity becomes distinctive.
Atypical hyperplasia: Cellular abnormalities are similar but more marked than in moderate hyperplasia. Increased coarseness of chromatin. Tendency for more single cells as well as groups of cells.
Malignant cells: Single cells and groups of cells with unequivocal nuclear features of malignancy.

and slightly greater prevalence of duct epithelial cells and groups of duct cells (Table 3–8). Apocrine metaplastic cells are also more likely to be seen in these samples. Proportionately fewer foam cells are found in samples from women with cytologic abnormality and/or breast lesions (see Fig. 3–19). While there are distinct differences between "normal" samples and those associated with benign breast disease, the only cytological features that correlate with specific lesions are those associated with hyperplasia and papilloma.

Benign Disease Associated with Increased Risk of Cancer

Cytological findings in NAF referred to as moderate hyperplasia or atypical hyperplasia, and in some studies grouped in one category called atypical hyperplasia, have shown a close association with histological changes in these same categories and with an increased risk of breast cancer.[7,15,32,60,63,70] When compared with similar women with no biopsy, those with moderate hyperplasia had 1.5 to 2 times, and those with atypical hyperplasia 5 times, the risk of breast cancer.[15] The histological changes are defined in Table 3–6 and illustrated in Figures 3–21 and 3–22. Also included in those with 1.5 to 2 times increased risk are women having papilloma with a fibrovascular core.

The significance of NAF cytology was evaluated by Petrakis and associates in a preliminary follow-up study of women examined between 1972 and 1980.[60] Among 5206 women without known breast cancer, there were 3194 (61 percent) with adequately cellular NAF. Atypical hyperplasia (moderate and atypical hyperplasia combined) was found in samples from 420 women (13 percent). Matching for age and race, follow-up data from 335 of these women were compared with findings from an equal number of women having samples without atypical hyperplasia. Records of the San Francisco Bay Area Cancer Registry were used for the follow-up 8 to 15 years after the original NAF examination. Nineteen of the women with atypical hyperplasia and six of those without this cytological abnormality had developed breast cancer during this period (P<0.01, chi-squared). The increased risk of subsequent breast cancer associated with the cytological abnormality referred to as atypical hyperplasia appears similar to that found by Page and associates (see Section III, Chapter 6; Section V, Chapter 14) in breast tissue lesions defined as moderate and atypical hyperplasia.[60]

NAF samples from moderate and atypical hyperplasia exhibit duct epithelial cells in cohesive groupings of nonpapillary or papillary pattern as well as isolated duct epithelial cells; however, they make up a very small

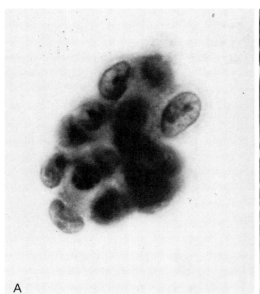
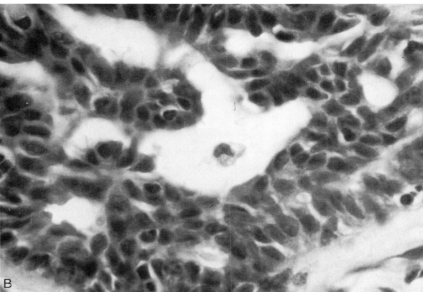

Figure 3–20. *A*, Hyperplasia in NAF represented here by a multilayered ball-like epithelial cell cluster with some nuclear enlargement and variability in size and staining (Papanicolaou stain; original magnification ×250). *B*, In mild hyperplasia, the duct lining cells are three or four layers in thickness and show some luminal bridging (H and E stain; original magnification ×250).

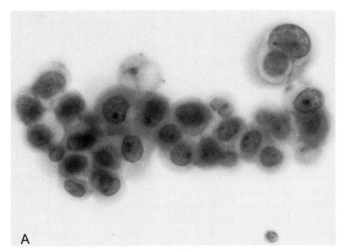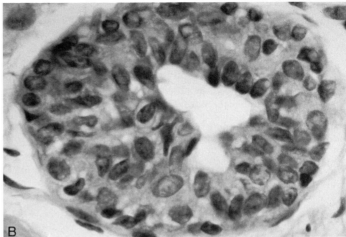

Figure 3–21. *A,* Moderate hyperplasia depicted in a group of cells that have some enlargement of nuclei as well as variability in nuclear and cell sizes. The granularity is both fine and coarse, and nucleoli are evident in some (Papanicolaou stain; original magnification ×250). *B,* The tissue section has similar cytologic changes evident in the moderately hyperplastic ductal lining (H and E stain; original magnification ×250).

proportion of all cells in a sample. The individual cells within groups and isolated cells also show increasing degrees of nuclear enlargement, altered N:C ratio, and nuclear hyperchromasia. Nucleoli may be obscured or distinct and sometimes are enlarged. As the cytological features become more monotonous and present a modal pattern there also tends to be a loss of cohesiveness and an increase in single cells and smaller, loosely arranged groups. Calcific material or typical psammoma bodies have been found in central portions of cell clusters or within the cell cytoplasm.[73] The most significant changes that determine classification of moderate and atypical hyperplasia are in the nuclear and chromatin structure. In correlating the NAF cytology findings with *benign breast biopsies,* 54 percent of those biopsies having histological lesions of atypical hyperplasia also had cytological findings of atypical hyperplasia (Table 3–8).[32]

Although there is a significant relationship of atypical hyperplasia with NAF and the subsequent changes in tissue, it is apparent that NAF cytology does not have sufficient predictive value to make it useful for screening or diagnostic purposes. However, the NAF collection technique is simple and noninvasive and the results do warrant consideration of its use as an adjunct to other procedures for evaluation of the breast and in the context of risk factor assessment.

Biochemical as well as cytological findings in NAF are associated with atypical hyperplasia and increased risk of breast cancer. In a study of 135 control women and 68 women with benign breast disease, Wrensch and associates found the cholesterol and its beta epoxide in NAF increased in women with a first-degree relative with breast cancer.[71] In that study, benign breast disease was classified histologically by the most marked ductal lobular epithelial abnormality. Increased cholesterol and beta epoxide levels were significantly associated with proliferative breast disease. Progressively increasing concentrations of these substances were found with increasing degrees of histological abnormalities. As already noted, the color of breast fluid is a good indicator of biochemical composition. Dark colors such as green and brown are associated with high cholesterol, cholesterol epoxides, and estrone and estradiol. Observations of dark breast fluid can be considered in combination with other factors in assessing the risk of atypical hyperplasia and breast cancer.

A different approach to classification of breast disease and risk of cancer with NAF cytology is being tested. It involves image analysis of foam cells.[33] These ubiquitous cells have been of major interest in studies of NAF cytology and continue to challenge investigators as to their origin and function. They are found in nearly 100 percent of samples from women with benign breast disease and 70 percent of women with breast cancer. Conventional microscopic examination has shown no distinctive diagnostic features that discriminate among the foam cells in the presence of breast lesions. Using digital imaging microscopy of foam cell nuclei, several nuclear shape and chromatic textural parameters were sufficient to discriminate among four categories of benign and malignant breast disease as determined by subsequent breast tissue biopsy: nonproliferative lesions, mild hyperplasia, atypical hyperplasia, and carcinoma. In preliminary studies, 100 percent of proliferative lesions could be distinguished from nonproliferative

Table 3–8. NAF CELLULARITY IN BENIGN BREAST DISEASE

	"Normal"*	Benign Breast Disease
Average cellularity	$6.2 \pm 6.5 \times 10^3$	$24.9 \pm 13.1 \times 10^3$
Average number of duct cell groups per sample	4.2 ± 1.5	10.8 ± 3.2
Single duct cells (%)	3.1 ± 1.7	10.5 ± 7.5

*Asymptomatic

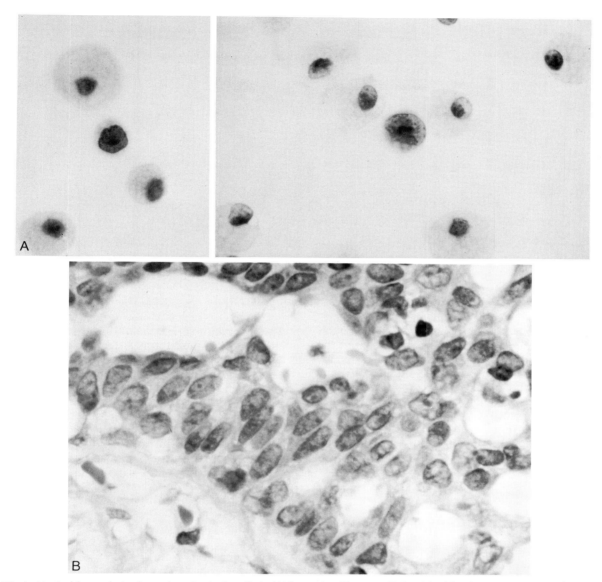

Figure 3–22. *A,* Atypical hyperplasia shown here in single cells in NAF samples. They are distinguished by disproportionate nuclear enlargement, irregular chromatinic membranes, and distinct granularity or hyperchromasia of chromatin (Papanicolaou stain; original magnification ×250). *B,* Atypical hyperplasia in tissue section with similar disproportionate nuclear to cytoplasmic ratio and somewhat monotonous cell population (H and E stain; original magnification ×250).

ones by foam cell classification using the digital imaging method. This type of analysis has the advantage of being both objective and reproducible.

Benign Disease with Unknown Risk of Cancer

Referring again to histological risk categories for benign breast disease as described by the Consensus Meeting, there were two benign lesions not included in risk categories because of insufficient data.[15] These were radial scar and lactiferous sinus solitary papilloma. Papilloma with a fibrovascular core was associated with a slightly increased risk of carcinoma in comparison with women with no breast biopsy.

Radial scar may have varying degrees of atypical proliferative change in the ductal epithelium. NAF cytological findings in association with this lesion have not yet been evaluated.

The NAF cytology of papillary lesions is sufficiently distinctive to warrant further comment. In a study of 1309 asymptomatic women, Jackson and associates obtained breast secretions that were diagnostic of a papillary lesion in 160.[26] Intraductal or intracystic papilloma was confirmed in breast tissue examinations. It was noted that 46 percent were detected by cytological examination as the initial finding. A complete description of cytological findings associated with papilloma is provided by Papanicolaou et al.[53] It is based upon a study of 73 cases with histological diagnosis of papilloma or papillomatosis. Only two of the papillomas were

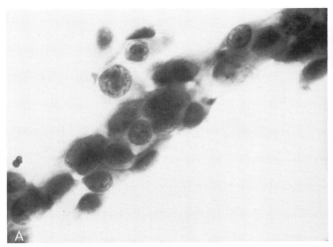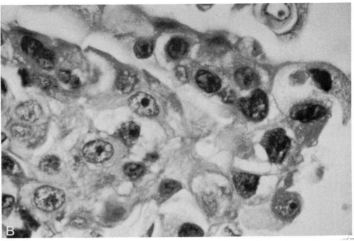

Figure 3–23. *A,* Malignant cells in a group from a NAF sample exhibit nuclear hyperchromasia, coarse granularity, and irregularity in configuration (Papanicolaou stain; original magnification ×250). *B,* Cytological features of ductal carcinoma are similar to those in the NAF sample (H and E stain; original magnification ×250).

found in asymptomatic women from whom breast secretion was obtained with a breast pump. The remainder had a mass and/or nipple discharge. In 48 percent of the 73 cases, the diagnosis of papilloma was suggested by cytology. Most characteristic was the finding of many large groups of epithelial cells. The groups were long and branching and occasionally had a fibrovascular core. Borders of the groups tended to be scalloped, and cells sometimes cupped around each other. Although cytoplasm was homogeneous, vacuolization was not uncommon. Nuclei were small and hyperchromatic—rarely "active" and undergoing mitosis. Occasionally the cells were binucleate or multinucleate. A background of blood, macrophages, and foam cells was typical. The authors emphasized that similar findings in secretions during pregnancy and post partum did not have the same diagnostic significance and should not be relied upon for diagnosis of papilloma.

In our study of women with papilloma, the cytological findings in NAF were correlated with histology and clinical findings in 110 cases. The diagnosis of papilloma was suggested on cytology in 60 percent of these cases. In 32 percent there was bloody discharge and/or an impression of papilloma based on the clinical findings. Distinctive papillary groupings were noted in 91 percent and heavy or moderate cellularity in 89 percent. Blood was present in 64 percent. Papillary groupings of duct epithelial cells with an identifiable fibrous or hyaline stalk were the most distinctive diagnostic finding. Other papillary groups of cells, apocrine metaplastic cells, foam cells along with hemosiderin-laden macrophages, and red blood cells form a frequent cellular accompaniment. Often, the cytological findings represent only a few of these components, and although not entirely diagnostic of the lesion, can be correlated with the clinical presentation.

Carcinoma, In Situ and Invasive

The cytological patterns of malignancy in breast secretions are interpreted in terms of the anticipated

histological patterns to the extent that this is possible. The two major categories of breast carcinoma are ductal and lobular. These terms are applied to histological and cytological patterns and not necessarily to the anatomical site of origin. The tumors may be in situ or invasive. Subclassification of these main categories depends on variations in histological pattern and cytological differentiation. Terms applied to the subclassifications include tubular, alveolar, signet-ring cell, medullary, mucoid, and papillary (cribriform). Paget's disease of the nipple is readily accessible for cytological sampling and presents with or without clinical carcinoma of the breast. The reader is referred to Chapters 8, 9, and 10 for complete descriptions of the histological patterns of breast carcinoma.

Papanicolaou and associates described and analyzed in detail the cytological findings and their significance in breast secretions from 171 (18.5 percent) of 917 asymptomatic women.[53] They concluded that despite its limitations, cytology of breast secretions was valuable in differential diagnosis of mammary diseases and carcinoma. The sensitivity and specificity of the cytological findings in benign breast disease was not mentioned; however, a cytological diagnosis of malignancy was highly reliable. The criteria for diagnosis of malignant cells were based primarily on nuclear abnormalities. In secretions from 613 breasts of 438 asymptomatic women, one unsuspected carcinoma in situ was found. In 510 symptomatic women, 27 (60 percent) of 45 subsequently proven carcinomas were diagnosed on cytology and there were no false positive diagnoses. The differences in cytological pattern associated with various types of mammary carcinoma are clearly described and illustrated. The generally recognized criteria of malignancy characterized the cells, and they were found either isolated or in small clusters. In groups of cells, the nuclei were often crowded and overlapped. Difficulty in identifying the malignant cells was sometimes associated with a background of predominantly inflammatory cells or of red blood cells and blood pigment.

The introduction of a more effective method for breast fluid collection from asymptomatic women led to recent reports on the cytology of NAF.[10, 32, 64] Cytological patterns of carcinoma in NAF are described in limited terms by Sartorius et al.[64] They reported seven carcinomas detected in cytology of NAF samples from asymptomatic women. An additional 11 women had cytological evidence of carcinoma in the NAF; however, their results were also positive by palpation or mammography.

Cytological diagnosis of malignancy in NAF samples examined by King et al. was positive in only 20.6 percent of cases.[32] The distribution of cellular findings associated with benign and malignant breasts is shown in Figure 5–19.[34] When malignant cells are present, they are associated with a highly cellular sample compared with samples from breasts with benign diseases and with those from normal breasts. Cells are distributed in small, loosely cohesive clusters, and there are increased numbers of isolated cells. The size of the cells and nuclei depends upon the histological lesion from which they are derived. However, diagnostic features representative of specific histological patterns have not been identified owing to the limited number of cases available for evaluation in this material. Nuclei show the chromatin changes generally considered representative of malignancy: hyperchromasia, coarse granularity, and condensation at the chromatinic membrane. A nucleolus is usually present and may be large, or there may be more than one. Cytoplasm varies in amount, is usually blue-green, and may contain vacuoles. N:C ratio is often altered because of disproportionate nuclear enlargement. The background findings are a disproportionate increase in histiocytes compared with foam cells; lymphocytes, neutrophils, red blood cells, and protein precipitate are also part of the diathesis (Fig. 3–23).

The low yield of positive cytological diagnoses in NAF samples appears to be related to the unusual histopathology in this consecutive series of breast carcinomas. The selection was based upon NAF sample availability and adequacy defined as ten or more duct epithelial cells. In this series, 26.6 percent of the lesions were carcinoma in situ. Nipple duct involvement within 1 cm of the surface of the nipple is infrequent (8 percent) in such tumors with an extent of less than 2.5 cm.[38] The

better results in other series, some including symptomatic women, correspond with a higher frequency (50 percent) of nipple duct involvement within 1 cm of the surface associated with invasive lesions.[1]

NAF samples are of value in identifying the cytological patterns associated with atypical hyperplasia in the presence of breast cancer. Atypical hyperplasia is much more prevalent in association with breast carcinoma and is infrequent in the absence of carcinoma. The results of NAF cytology related to the presence and absence of atypical hyperplasia associated with carcinoma are seen in Table 3–9.

NAF does not have a role in screening or diagnosis of breast carcinoma because of the limitation of fluid availability and sample adequacy. In the future, it may prove valuable in assessing women for risk of breast carcinoma and in planning appropriate patient follow-up and management.

SPONTANEOUS NIPPLE DISCHARGE ASSOCIATED WITH BREAST DISEASE

Nipple discharge has been reported in 10 to 15 percent of women with benign breast disease and in 2.5 to 3 percent of those with carcinoma.[39, 68] The discharge is often classified according to its appearance as milky, green, brown, bloody, serous, cloudy, or purulent. The significance of bloody discharge is its association with intraductal papilloma and other papillary lesions or carcinoma; however, it is also frequently found in the absence of such lesions. In a review of 386 nipple discharges without associated mass, 177 (46 percent) were bloody. Of patients with benign disease, 38 percent had bloody discharge compared with 69 percent among women with carcinoma. Kilgore and associates classify serous or bloody discharge as pathological and discharge with evidence of secretory products as physiological.[30] Funderburk found serous or bloody fluid in 63 percent (106 of 167) and milky, colored, or clear fluid in 37 percent (61 of 167).[21] The serous or bloody fluids were associated with carcinoma, papilloma, or other papillary lesions in 74 percent (78 of 106); fibrocystic change in 22 percent; and duct ectasia, drugs, and other conditions in 4 percent. The majority (94 percent) of fluids with secretory components were associated with fibrocystic change and other nonproliferative breast lesions; only 6 percent (4 of 61) were associated with papilloma. These findings are similar to those of other investigators.

The clinical significance of nipple discharge and appropriate management choices become most important when there is no palpable mass. Kilgore[30] found 35 percent of carcinoma associated with nipple discharge that had no palpable mass, whereas Funderburk[21] noted 82 percent of nipple discharge without palpable mass.

The cytological diagnosis of nipple discharge samples has been most successful in association with breast cancer, Paget's disease of the nipple, and benign papilloma or papillary disease. Some examples of diagnostic results with nipple discharge appear in Table 3–10.[21, 35, 43, 53, 67] Uei and associates[67] analyzed the cytomorphology

Table 3–9. NAF CYTOLOGY RELATED TO HISTOLOGICAL DIAGNOSIS IN BREASTS IN PRESENCE AND ABSENCE OF APD*

| Cytological Classification | Histological Classification | | | |
| | Benign (%) | | Malignant (%) | |
	APD n = 39	No. APD n = 61	APD n = 27	No. APD n = 7
Benign	20.5	59.0	22.2	28.6
Hyperplasia	25.6	16.4	7.4	14.3
Atypical hyperplasia*	53.9	24.6	70.4	57.1

*APD and atypical hyperplasia refer to moderate hyperplasia and atypical hyperplasia classification combined.

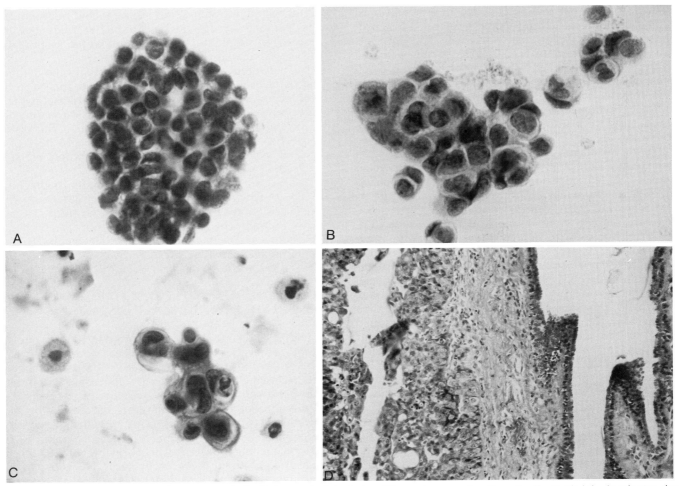

Figure 3–24. Cellular features of malignancy in nipple discharge. *A,* Spherical multilayered group of malignant cells. *B,* Slightly discohesive sheet of malignant cells with prominent nuclear molding. *C,* Cluster of malignant cells with cellular detritus in the background. (*A–C,* Papanicolaou stain; original magnification ×250). *D,* Major duct involvement by tumor at base of nipple and adjacent uninvolved duct (H and E stain; original magnification ×40).

in NAF from both benign and malignant lesions. They noted some distinctive features in the structure of cell groups that improved the accuracy in diagnosis of breast cancer (41 to 66.3 percent) but also increased the false positive interpretations from 0.9 to 3.6 percent (Fig. 3–23). The cellular characteristics associated with breast carcinoma are the same as those described for cytology of nonspontaneous nipple secretions. Of interest is the

finding of a disproportionate number of cases of ductal carcinoma in situ and the unusual papillary carcinoma in the presence of malignant nipple discharge.[21, 32, 53]

Papilloma was diagnosed cytologically by Papanicolaou and associates in 79 percent (34 of 43) and confirmed on tissue biopsy.[53] Others have reported similar success with the cytological diagnosis of intraductal papilloma.[30]

In a consecutive series of 212 nipple discharge samples, we encountered 3 (1.4 percent) with malignant cells (Fig. 3–24). Follow-up of these three revealed infiltrating ductal carcinoma. In one of the three, the discharge occurring on a single occasion was the only clinical finding and the mammogram was unremarkable. Ductography was not performed; however, intraductal carcinoma was located by obtaining a biopsy at a depth of 1.0 to 1.5 cm below the nipple. The initial biopsy was borderline atypical hyperplasia and ductal carcinoma in situ. Node sampling revealed metastatic disease, and subsequent mastectomy provided evidence of microinvasive ductal carcinoma. A second case was similar in that the patient had no palpable mass and the lesion

Table 3–10. REPORTED RESULTS WITH CYTOLOGY OF NIPPLE DISCHARGE

Author	Year	No.	With CA	Positive Cytology No.	Positive Cytology %	False Positive Cytology No.	False Positive Cytology %
Papanicolaou[53]	1958	495	45	45	(60)	3	(1)
Kjellgren[35]	1964	216	25	21	(89)	15	(8)
Masukawa[45]	1966	94	16	6	(43)	1	(1)
Funderburk[21]	1969	182	7	6	(86)	—	
Uei[67]	1980	190	80	53	(66)	4	(4)

was located within 1 cm of the nipple surface. Thus in two of the three with carcinoma, there was neoplastic involvement of a major duct at the nipple base and in the remaining case, malignant cells were found free floating in a duct within routine sections of the nipple (Fig. 3–24).

These cases illustrate the clinical usefulness of cytology for evaluation of spontaneous nipple discharge in the absence of a palpable mass or significant mammographic findings. Cytology is indicated when the discharge is bloody or serous and there is no clinically evident mass.

CLINICAL EVALUATION AND MANAGEMENT OF THE PATIENT WITH NIPPLE DISCHARGE

Spontaneous nipple discharge is the chief complaint in 3 to 6 percent of women coming to breast specialty services. Nipple discharge is, however, often ignored. Newman et al. found spontaneous discharge in 270 (10 percent) of 2685 women on routine examination at a union health service.[50] It is rare for cancer to present as an isolated discharge. Chaudary et al. reported that only 16 (<1 percent) of 2476 cancers presented with discharge and no other finding.[12] Devitt reported, however, that 2 percent of all breast cancers did have a discharge.[17]

Etiology

The majority of nipple discharges are caused by benign conditions. Among women with nipple discharge, malignancy is found in only a small percentage. The majority of discharges are caused by either duct ectasia or benign papillomatosis. Papilloma and duct ectasia are more frequent in young women (Fig. 3–25).[49]

Duct ectasia is a dilatation with loss of elastin in the duct walls and presence of chronic inflammatory cells, especially plasma cells, around the walls. The etiology

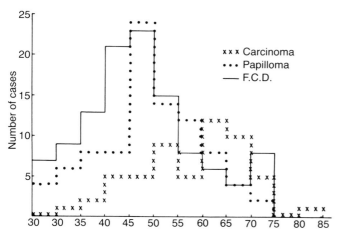

Figure 3–25. Age distribution of patients with nipple discharge. Cancer is much more common in women over the age of 50 years. F.C.D. = fibrocystic disease. (From Murad TM, et al: Ann Surg 195:259, 1982. Reprinted by permission.)

is uncertain, and theories range from collection and then transudation of secretions in ducts dilated from previous pregnancy to primary periductal inflammation. It has been noted that up to 62 percent of nipple discharges in duct ectasia contain bacteria (*Enterococcus*, anaerobic *Streptococcus*, *Staphylococcus aureus*, and *Bacteroides*), but whether this infection is the primary cause or a secondary supercontamination is not known.[11] Duct ectasia is benign, with no known relationship to subsequent cancer.

Papilloma is a benign lesion of epithelium, usually with supporting stroma, growing within ducts independently of the walls. Most common is solitary intraductal papilloma located in the major ducts near the nipple. It is almost always benign and only rarely associated with cancer.

Much less common are peripheral papillomas. Ohuchi et al. reported that 6 of 25 patients with multiple peripheral papillomas had associated ductal carcinoma in situ.[51] It has been suggested that these peripheral papillary lesions are uncommon because in reality they are an intermediate step in the formation of invasive cancer and often progress to cancer before they are diagnosed.[49] Papillary type lesions are also seen at the confluence of major ducts late in normal pregnancy and the early postpartum period and probably account for the bloody secretions sometimes seen during pregnancy.[37] The latter have no association with cancer.

Nipple discharge may also be associated with cancer, although if that is the case, there is most often an associated mass in physical examination or mammography. Occult carcinoma presenting with discharge is usually ductal carcinoma in situ or papillary carcinoma. Fourteen to 34 percent of occult carcinomas and 25 percent of ductal carcinomas present with discharge. In the presence of microinvasion, discharge is less frequent.[65] Drugs and pituitary and other hormonal disorders are rare causes of discharge, but should be considered (see under History).

Evaluation

Not all discharges require biopsy for diagnosis. A careful history and examination can be used to guide biopsy. Special studies other than mammography usually are not helpful. Careful biopsy provides both definitive therapy and diagnosis.

History

History should cover the circumstances in which a discharge occurs, a complete reproductive and endocrine review of systems, and inquiry about trauma or stimulation and drug use.

The single most important point in the history is whether the discharge is spontaneous or elicited. Literature from various cancer societies stresses the point that discharge may be a sign of cancer, when in fact one or more drops of liquid can be expressed in about half of women during the reproductive years.

Breast discharge can be a response to a variety of stimuli other than underlying breast pathology. Disordered hormone production may induce pathophysiological responses in the breast. Spontaneous discharges have been reported with a variety of anovulatory syndromes.[2]

Prolactinemia from pituitary adenoma is a potential cause of nipple discharge and has been reported in up to 47 percent of cases in some series. In general, however, the 2.2 percent reported by Newman et al. is probably more representative of the frequency of prolactin tumors in patients with discharge.[50] Normal serum prolactin levels are 20 mg per ml. If values are repeatedly elevated, plain films and, often, thin-section computer tomography of the sella turcica are indicated. Patients with only moderate elevation frequently have normal radiological studies, but they should be followed closely. With advanced prolactin tumors, patients may show visual field loss or optic nerve compression and often have a history of infertility.

Because the breast is "a gland without feedback mechanisms, prolonged secretory response may follow short, often unrecognized surges in circulating prolactin."[51] These transient rises in prolactin may explain the nipple discharge seen in other situations such as breast stimulation (especially sucking at the nipple), chest trauma, or following thoracotomy.

High doses of such tranquilizers as phenothiazines, reserpine, and methyldopa can induce lactation. Hooper et al. noted galactorrhea in 24 of 100 inpatients; 23 of the 24 were on major tranquilizers.[24] Lactation ceases after the drug is discontinued and many times will not return if lower doses are reinstituted.[2] One should also inquire about possible industrial or agricultural exposure to estrogens.[48]

Examination

Examination should seek the duct or ducts producing the discharge, its color and nature, and other signs of breast pathology. The number of ducts producing discharge is almost as useful a guide as spontaneous discharge. Discharges from multiple ducts are rarely malignant, whereas single-duct discharge can represent a genuine risk of malignancy. Ciatto et al. reported that single-duct discharge has a relative risk of 4.07 (confidence interval 2.7–6) of malignancy compared with an asymptomatic population, whereas multicentric or bilateral discharges have risks similar to those of the general population.[13] Murad et al. report that none of their patients with cancer had bilateral discharges.[49]

The consistency of breast discharges has been evaluated by Leis et al.[40] They found that four types of discharge—serous, serosanguineous, sanguineous, and watery—were associated with cancer in ascending frequency (6.3, 11.9, 24.0, and 45.5 percent, respectively).

Chaudary et al. focused on the presence or absence of heme, as detected by laboratory test sticks (as used for urine dip testing).[12] The stick test detects as few as 5 to 15 red blood cells per ml, which would not be visible as bloody fluid. In their series, 16 of 16 patients with cancer had hemoglobin in nipple secretions. However, the tests have limited specificity, since 107 of 132 intraductal papillomas and 67 of 94 duct ectasias also had hemoglobin in the discharge. Normal pregnancy can also cause blood in nipple discharge. Kline and Lash found intact blood cells in 20 percent of nipple discharges from pregnant women.[36]

Single-duct discharges often have a trigger point on the breast, where pressure induces a discharge. This is important when planning surgical excision of a specific duct (see below). The patient should be examined in a standard position, preferably supine with the ipsilateral hand behind her head. Direct pressure is then applied at various points around the areola until the point producing the maximum discharge is found. It is my preference to check this on the initial visit and on the repeat visit before planning surgical duct excision.

An associated mass should always be sought, since it is a strong indication of possible cancer. Devitt found in his series of patients with discharge that eight of ten women with cancer had palpable masses; one patient had nipple distortion but no mass.[17] Leis et al. reported palpable masses in 88.1 percent of 67 patients with nipple discharge and cancer.[40]

Special Studies

Patients with spontaneous discharge and no mass should have mammograms. Others advocate galactography and routine cytological studies.

Mammography is a way to expand upon physical examination to seek a specific lesion associated with the discharge. It should be considered in all cases of single-duct discharge unless a specific lump or lesion has already been identified.

Galactography is "the only known method for preoperative determination of the nature, location and extent of the lesions" causing nipple discharge.[66] Various techniques are used, but all involve cannulation of the single, previously identified duct with a small nylon catheter or needle (often with a 90 degree bend a few millimeters from the tip) and injection of a water-soluble contrast agent. Water-solubility is important, since oil-based contact can be damaging or cause a serious systemic reaction; 0.10 to 1.5 ml is injected. Pain or discomfort marks the absolute time to cease injection. Tabar et al. reported that 18 of 18 women with cancer were identified by galactography but that only half of them had a mass lesion on routine mammograms.[66] They, therefore, recommend this method to evaluate spontaneous discharge without a palpable mass. Burni and de Guili, however, report only a 79 percent accuracy, based on patients who went on to surgical biopsy after galactography.[5]

A single procedure is always more desirable, and since histological confirmation will be needed, galactography may be omitted. Routinely injecting the duct in

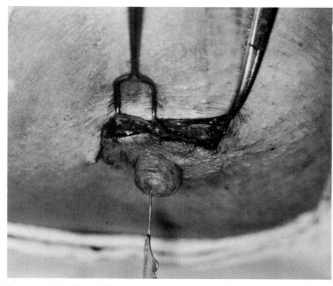

Figure 3–26. Use of lacrimal duct probe to identify duct producing discharge. This procedure was carried out using local anesthesia (see text). A small carcinoma was identified adjacent to the duct producing the discharge in this patient.

question with methylene blue as a purported guide to surgery also seems dubious, since simple duct excision is not the radical operation that Tabar et al. suggest, and there are other techniques for identifying the duct (see below).[66]

Diagnosis

Diagnosis is based on microscopic study of material from the duct. Exfoliative cytology is useful when positive, but a very high false negative rate with current techniques precludes its use for routine diagnostic purposes.

Initial evaluation of a single duct's spontaneous discharge should use examination to localize the pressure point described above and physical examination or mammography to look for a specific lesion. If the latter two are positive, biopsy should be directed to that area. If no specific lesion is identified, duct excision should be undertaken.

The patient is brought to the outpatient operating room. No sedation is needed; most patients can be made quite comfortable with conversation. The skin is disinfected and the patient draped appropriately. The circumareolar incision is marked to encompass approximately 50 percent of the circumference of the areola, but not more. The midportion of the incision should be as close as possible to the trigger point.

One percent Lidocaine (Xylocaine) with epinephrine (or other long-acting anesthetic) is infiltrated into the skin at the site of the proposed incision. Lidocaine is then infiltrated into the tissue under the areola and around the nipple. Direct infiltration into the nipple is quite painful and unnecessary, since within a few minutes the area will be blocked by diffusion of the surrounding anesthetic.

The incision is made, and meticulous hemostasis is maintained in the dermis with judicious use of electrocoagulation. Dissection is then carried out with blunt tenotomy scissors to elevate the skin of the areola into the area directly behind the nipple, where the ducts are identified. Using small blunt scissors allows gentle dissection and precludes large cuts. The edge of the areola is usually elevated with a skin hook. The skin hook is held with the thumb and two fingers of the nondominant hand, and the ring finger of the same hand is used to evert the skin and areola so that the dissection can be carried out with gentle tension. Dissection is continued until the duct in question is found.

There are two ways to find the duct. The simplest way is to pass a small (No. 3-0) lacrimal duct probe through the skin opening (Fig. 3–26). If this is not possible, the duct is identified by gentle dissection behind the nipple (Fig. 3–27). Once the duct is identified, it is dissected free from other ducts in the nipple. By continuing gentle eversion of the nipple, the duct is followed into the nipple and dissected into the dermis, where it is removed, usually with a tiny fragment of skin from the nipple. It is often useful to divide the duct under the nipple by placing two small hemostats on it. This facilitates complete excision from the nipple; on occasion, small papillomas have been found in this location.

After removal of the duct from the nipple, the duct leading deeper into the breast is grasped gently and with gentle traction dissected free from the surrounding tissue (Fig. 3–28). In general, very little local anesthesia is required for this part of the dissection so long as the surgeon uses small instruments, which force slow progress. Judicious application of anesthesia to blood vessels prevents most discomfort.

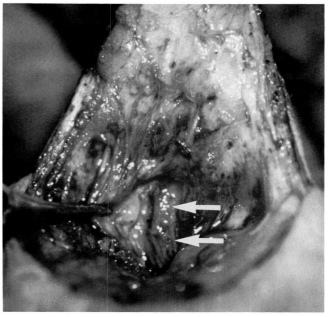

Figure 3–27. Dilated duct is identified behind the nipple. This procedure is performed under local anesthesia, without premedication (see text).

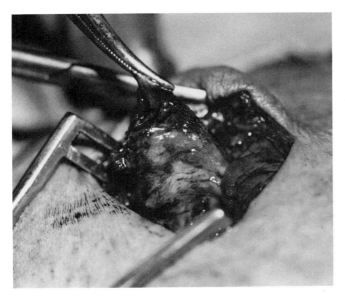

Figure 3–28. Following separation of the duct from the nipple, gentle traction is maintained to identify the segment of breast to be removed. This procedure is done under local anesthesia (see text).

The procedure usually removes a cone of tissue of a diameter that increases as it extends deeper into the breast. The tissue is easily identified as an independent segment of the breast, since it is denser than the immediately adjacent tissue and often surrounded by either loose connective tissue or fatty tissue. If a duct containing discharge is transected in the course of the dissection, it should be secured with a hemostat for later identification; after completion of the main portion of dissection, it should be excised entirely.

Hemostasis must be maintained meticulously. The outer edge of the adjacent breast tissue is approximated with small, interrupted, absorbable sutures. A purse-string of absorbable suture is usually placed loosely to evert the nipple in order to prevent inversion. A few interrupted sutures are used to draw the areola across to its normal position. The skin is then closed with subcuticular, absorbable suture and tape skin closures.

The patient is given a simple dressing, advised to wear her brassiere for support for 72 hours, and asked to avoid vigorous activity during that time. To preserve platelet function, she is directed to use no aspirin for approximately seven days before and after surgery. Acetaminophen should be used for pain; narcotics are not usually prescribed.

Prognosis

The prognosis after the diagnosis of nipple discharge has not been studied extensively but seems good if cancer is not found in the initial evaluation. McPherson and Mackenzie found recurrence of discharge in 5 of 72 patients between two weeks and nine years following surgery.[46] Three of the 72 subsequently developed cancer, but two of the three lesions were in the contralateral breast and none of the three patients had recurrent discharge.

SAMPLE COLLECTION, PREPARATION, AND EXAMINATION

An adequate sample for breast cytology will help assure good results with this method. The preparatory methods for breast cytology include direct smears from spontaneous nipple discharge and membrane filtration of NAF samples. Cytological examination needs to be systematic and thorough, and a classification system should utilize terminology related to the anticipated histopathology.

Sample Collection

Spontaneous nipple discharge is expressed directly onto the glass slide, which is held at the opening of the duct and moved across the drop of fluid and the surface of the nipple to make a thin spread. A specimen bottle of 95 percent ethanol should be held close to the breast so that the slide can be immediately placed in the fixative. It is suggested that from four to six smears be prepared from each discharge, since the material is often more cellular in the last drops of fluid. If blood-tinged fluid is observed to be coming from one duct, its location should be noted and an attempt made to keep the sample from that duct separate from the remaining discharge. This can be accomplished by utilizing a capillary pipette to collect the sample directly from the duct opening.[44]

NAF samples are collected using a suction-cup device placed over the nipple and attached to a 10 ml syringe with a short length of plastic tubing (see Fig. 3–13). Negative pressure to the cup over the nipple is achieved by withdrawing the plunger 5 to 6 ml and maintaining the pressure until fluid appears at the nipple, or for 15 seconds. The amount of negative pressure achieved is 100 to 175 mm of mercury and similar to the negative pressures developed by suckling infants.[57]

The steps in the NAF collection procedure are summarized as follows:

1. To remove any accumulated secretory material and exfoliated squamous cells from the nipple surface and duct openings, the nipple is first cleaned using a moist gauze or plastic sponge.

2. Then the nipple is soaked with Cerumenex (3 percent) to loosen plugs.

3. Subsequent gentle squeezing expresses the plugs, and the nipple is wiped dry.

4. Using suction combined with gentle hand pressure, the nipple aspirate specimen is obtained. The suction device is placed over the nipple, and negative pressure is applied by withdrawing the plunger of the attached syringe. During aspiration, gentle hand pressure is applied to the breast starting at the base and extending toward the nipple.

5. Generally, one or more beads of fluid appear on the surface of the nipple.

6. The specimen is then removed from the nipple into capillary tubes, suspended in 2 ml physiological salt

solution and transported at once to the laboratory, or refrigerated when this is not possible.

or

7. If direct smears are to be prepared from the nipple, have the patient hold a bottle of fixative to one side of her breast. Smear the fluid lengthwise on a microscope slide and immerse *immediately* in the fixative.

Sample Preparation

Two important aspects of specimen preparation are concentration of cells and recovery of cells. Cell concentration refers to increasing the number of cells per unit volume or area. Cell recovery is the efficiency in collecting cells per unit volume of sample or the percentage of total cells in a sample. In NAF samples, the cell recovery is especially important because of the scant cellularity. If concentration techniques lead to a differential loss of cells, the preparatory method may interfere with the diagnostic value of the sample.

Direct smears require no special laboratory preparation other than appropriate staining with Papanicolaou stain or other stains preferred by the laboratory.

NAF samples are concentrated and recovered on membrane filters. Millipore filters are preferred because of the high rate of cell recovery (approximately 80 percent of cells per sample) and because of good quality of cytomorphology.[3] The following steps in membrane filtration are recommended to produce a filter of optimum quality with well-preserved cellular morphology:

1. Label the edge of a 46 mm Millipore filter (5 μ pore size) with a laundry ink pen and pre-expand the filter for 10 seconds in 95 percent ethanol.

2. Assemble Millipore filtration apparatus using the glass base and a stainless steel screen.

3. Moisten screen and glass base with physiological saline, allowing it to pool on the surface.

4. Place the pre-expanded filter on the pooled saline.

5. Clamp on glass funnel and add 25 to 30 ml physiological salt solution.

6. Adjust suction to a gentle drip.

7. Pour the entire well-mixed sample into the funnel. Allow filtration to proceed until the solution just covers the surface of the filter; never allow the filter to dry.

8. When the last saline has been suctioned through the filter and a small amount of solution still covers the filter, add 95 percent ethanol. This ethanol should be added without disrupting the filter surface.

9. Discontinue suction and, adding more ethanol above the filter, allow the cells to fix for 2 minutes before completing the suctioning. Never let the filter dry.

10. Remove the filter and store in 95 percent ethanol until staining is done.

Precautions

1. Do not overload the filter. If filtration stops, immediately stop the vacuum and aspirate the remaining unfiltered specimen out of the funnel. Add 95 percent ethanol to the funnel, just covering the filter.

2. Never allow the filter to dry.

3. Bloody specimens can be treated with 50 percent ethanol after washing with physiological salt solution and before fixation with 95 percent ethanol.

Staining of Millipore filter preparations can be accomplished by carrying the filter through the solutions on a clamp-style paper clip of a plastic filter holder. This method allows uniform diffusion of stains and solutions providing consistently even staining. Filters should not be clipped to glass slides, because uneven staining occurs.

Mounting Millipore filters requires special attention because of the thickness of the filter (130 ± 10 μm). Excess clearing solvent (xylene or toluene) should be removed before mounting by placing the filter, cell side up, on an absorbent paper towel. The filter must not be allowed to dry. Sufficient mounting medium (Permount, Eukitt, or Kleermount) should be spread evenly across a glass slide and the filter floated, cell side up, on the mounting medium. An additional drop of mounting fluid should be dropped on the filter surface before applying a No. 1 thickness coverslip.

Cytological Examination

Slides are first examined by a cytotechnologist with special training and experience in evaluation of NAF and breast discharge cytology. Every microscopic field on the slide is viewed, and fields are overlapped so as not to overlook any of the cells with abnormalities. A complete and systematic examination is required because epithelial cells are few and tend to be small; significant cells or groups of cells can easily be missed. Abnormal cells are marked with an ink dot, and a qualitative assessment is made of the cellular composition, including types of cells and degree of cellularity. A preliminary evaluation by the cytotechnologist is based upon the changes in epithelial cells and the accompanying cellular findings.[4]

The pathologist who makes the final diagnosis reviews the entire slide, paying particular attention to marked areas. An interpretation is based on the cytological findings considered in the light of clinical information. The pathologist must also be experienced in this specialized area of cytopathology.

The appropriate diagnostic terminology used for the cellular findings in NAF and nipple discharge is that which conforms with the expected pathology in subsequent biopsy. Morphological terminology that is universally understood and consistent with standard nomenclature is to be preferred over systems that use numbers or nonspecific terms that are subject to a variety of interpretations.

Examples of diagnostic cytology terminology for NAF, spontaneous secretion, or nipple discharge are given here.

Benign: No significant cellular abnormalities.

Apocrine metaplasia: May be associated with fibrocystic change and may have varying degrees of atypia that require qualifying remarks.

Calcific deposits within cell groups (with or without atypia): Mammograms should be reviewed for presence of significant calcification.

Changes of a type seen with intraductal papilloma
Papillary groups and changes suggestive of intraductal papilloma

Hyperplasia: Minimal cellular abnormality associated with benign duct epithelial changes. "Papillary" may be used as a qualifying description; such cell groups have been related to papillomatosis (epitheliosis).

Moderate hyperplasia: Moderate cellular abnormality associated with benign duct epithelial changes.* "Papillary" may be used as a qualifying description as in the preceding category. These changes may be seen with papillomatosis (epitheliosis). The breast having these cytological findings should be examined for evidence of benign lesions such as fibrocystic change, fibroadenoma, adenosis, and so forth. Coexistent breast cancer is rarely encountered in patients with these cytological findings.

Atypical hyperplasia: Severe cellular abnormality associated with marked duct epithelial changes.* This degree of cellular abnormality is expected to be associated with more advanced forms of benign breast disease. These changes are not diagnostic of malignancy but have been found more often with coexistent breast cancer than have any of the lesser degrees of cellular abnormality. The breast having these cellular changes should be examined clinically for any findings that would indicate a need for biopsy. Review of previous mammograms may be of interest.

Malignant cells consistent with mammary carcinoma
Malignant cells of the type seen in Paget's disease of the nipple

References

1. Anderson JA, Pallesen RM: Spread to the nipple and areola in carcinoma of the breast. Ann Surg 189:367–372, 1979.
2. Barnes AB: Diagnosis and treatment of abnormal breast secretions. N Engl J Med 275:1184–1187, 1966.
3. Barrett DL, King EB: Comparison of cellular recovery rates and morphological detail obtained using membrane filter and cytocentrifuge techniques. Acta Cytol 20:174–180, 1976.
4. Barrett DL, King EB, Hasson PL: Collection and cytopreparatory techniques for serous effusions and cerebrospinal fluids; Part I. Lab Med 9:9–22, 1978.
5. Berni D, de Guili E: The value of ductogalactography in the diagnosis of intraductal papilloma. Tumori 69:539–544, 1983.
6. Bischoff F: Carcinogenic effects of steroids. Adv Lipid Res 7:165–244, 1969.
7. Black MM, Chabon AB: In situ carcinoma of the breast. Pathol Annu 4:185–210, 1969.
8. Bloom W, Fawcett DW: A Textbook of Histology. 9th ed. Philadelphia, WB Saunders, 1968, pp 767–775.
9. Bonser GM, Dossett SA, Jull SW: Human and Experimental Breast Cancer. Springfield, IL, CC Thomas, 1961.
10. Buehring GC: Screening for breast atypias using exfoliative cytology. Cancer 43:1788–1799, 1979.
11. Bundred NJ, Dixon JMJ, Lumsden AB, Radford D, Hood J, Miles RS, Chetty U, Forrest APM: Are the lesions of duct ectasia sterile? Br J Surg 72:844, 1985.
12. Chaudary MA, Millis RR, Davies GC, Hayward JL: Nipple discharge; the diagnostic value of testing for occult blood. Ann Surg 196:651–655, 1982.
13. Ciatto S, Bravetti P, Cariaggi P: Significance of nipple discharge; clinical patterns in selection of cases for cytologic examination. Acta Cytol 30:17–20, 1986.
14. Cole HA: The mammary gland of the mouse during the oestrous cycle, pregnancy and lactation. Proc R Soc Lond B 114:136–160, 1933.
15. Consensus Meeting: Is "fibrocystic disease" of the breast precancerous? Arch Pathol Lab Med 110:171–173, 1986.
16. Dawson EK: A histological study of the normal mamma in relation to tumor growth. II, The mature gland in pregnancy and lactation. Edinb Med J 42:569–598, 633–660, 1935.
17. Devitt JE: Management of nipple discharge by clinical findings. Am J Surg 149:789–792, 1985.
18. Donne A: Die Milch und insbesondere die Milch der Ammen. Weimar, Landes Industrie Komptoir, 1838.
19. Engels S: An investigation of the origin of the colostrum cells. J Anat 87:362–372, 1953.
20. Ferguson DJP, Anderson TJ: Morphological evaluation of cell turnover in relation to the menstrual cycle in the "resting" human breast. Br J Cancer 44:177–181, 1981.
21. Funderburk WW, Syphax B: Evaluation of nipple discharge in benign and malignant diseases. Cancer 24:1290–1296, 1969.
22. Gruenke LD, Wrensch MR, Petrakis NL, Miike R, Ernster VL, Craig JC: Breast fluid cholesterol and cholesterol epoxides: Relationship to breast cancer risk factors and other characteristics. Cancer Res 47:5483–5487, 1987.
23. Holmquist DG, Papanicolaou GN: The exfoliative cytology of the mammary gland during pregnancy and lactation. Ann NY Acad Sci 63:1422–1435, 1956.
24. Hooper JH, Welch VC, Shackelford RT: Abnormal lactation associated with tranquilizing drug therapy. JAMA 178:506–507, 1961.
25. Jackson D, Severance AO: Cytological study of nipple secretions; an aid in the diagnosis of breast lesions. Tex State J Med 41:512–514, 1946.
26. Jackson D, Todd DA, Gorsuch PL: Study of breast secretion for detection of intramammary pathologic change and of silent papilloma. J Int Coll Surg 15:552–568, 1951.
27. Kelsey MI, Pienta RJ: Transformation of hamster embryo cells by neutral sterols and bile acids. Toxicol Lett 9:177–182, 1981.
28. Kelsey MI, Pienta RJ: Transformation of hamster embryo cells by cholesterol-alpha-epoxide and lithocholic acid. Cancer Lett 6:143–149, 1979.
29. Keynes G: Chronic mastitis. Br J Surg 11:89–121, 1923.
30. Kilgore AR, Fleming R, Ramos MM: The incidence of cancer with nipple discharge and the risk of cancer in the presence of papillary disease of the breast. Surg Gynecol Obstet 96:649–660, 1953.
31. King EB, Kromhout LK, Chew KL, Mayall BH, Petrakis NL, Jensen RH, Young IT: Cellular composition of the nipple aspirate specimen of breast fluid: The benign cells. Am J Clin Pathol 64:728, 1975.
32. King EB, Chew KL, Petrakis NL, Ernster VL: Nipple aspirate cytology for the study of breast cancer precursors. J Natl Cancer Inst 71:1115–1121, 1983.
33. King EB, et al: Analytic studies of foam cells from breast cancer precursors. Cytometry 5:124–130, 1984.
34. King EB, et al: Cytopathology of abnormal mammary duct epithelium. *In* Nieburgs HE (ed): Prevention and Detection of Cancer. Part II, Detection, Vol 2, Cancer Detection in Specific Sites. New York, Marcel Dekker, 1976.
35. Kjellgren O: The cytologic diagnosis of cancer of the breast. Acta Cytol 8:216–217, 1964.
36. Kline TS, Lash SR: Nipple secretion in pregnancy; a cytologic and histologic study. Am J Clin Pathol 37:626–632, 1962.
37. Kline TS, Lash SR: The bleeding nipple of pregnancy and postpartum period; a cytologic and histologic study. Acta Cytol 8:336, 1964.
38. Lagios MD, Westdahl PR, Rose MR: The concept and implications of multicentricity in breast carcinoma. Pathol Annu 16:83–102, 1981.
39. Leis HP Jr, Dursi MD, Mersheimer WL: Nipple discharge:

---

*There is an increased risk of subsequent breast cancer associated with these changes.[61]

Significance and treatment. NY State J Med 67:3105–3110, 1967.

40. Leis HP, Cammarata A, LaRaja RD, Higgins H: Breast biopsy and guidance for occult lesions. Int Surg 70(2):115–118, 1985.

41. Longacre TA, Bartlow SA: A correlative morphologic study of human breast and endometrium in the menstrual cycle. Am J Surg Pathol 10:382–393, 1986.

42. Malberger E, Gutterman E, Bartfeld E, Zajicek G: Cellular changes in the mammary gland epithelium during the menstrual cycle; a computer image analysis study. Acta Cytol 31:305–308, 1987.

43. Masters JRW, Drife JO, Scarisbreck JJ: Cyclical variations of DNA synthesis in human breast epithelium. J Natl Cancer Inst 58:1263–1265, 1977.

44. Masukawa T: Improved cell collection technique in breast cytology. Cytotech Bull 7:4, 1970.

45. Masukawa T, Lewison EF, Frost JK: The cytologic examination of breast secretions. Acta Cytol 10:261–265, 1966.

46. McPherson VA, Mackenzie WC: Lesions of the breast associated with nipple discharge; prognosis after local excision of benign lesions. Can J Surg 5:6–11, 1962.

47. Meyer JS: Cell proliferation in normal human breast ducts, fibroadenomas, and other duct hyperplasias, measured by nuclear labelling with tritiated thymidine; Effects of menstrual phase, age, and oral contraceptive hormones. Hum Pathol 8:67–81, 1977.

48. Mills JL, Jeffreys JL, Stolley PD: Effects of occupational exposure to estrogen and progestogens and how to detect them. J Occup Med 26:269–272, 1984.

49. Murad TM, Contesso G, Mouriesse H: Nipple discharge from the breast. Ann Surg 195:259–264, 1982.

50. Newman HF, Klein M, Northrup JD, Ray BF, Drucker M: Nipple discharge; Frequency and pathogenesis in an ambulatory population. NY State J Med (83):928–933, 1983.

51. Ohuchi N, Abe R, Kasai M: Possible cancerous change of intraductal papillomas of the breast. Cancer 54:605–611, 1984.

52. Papanicolaou GN, Bader GM, Holmquist DG, Falk EA: Cytologic evaluation of breast secretions. Ann NY Acad Sci 63:1409–1421, 1956.

53. Papanicolaou GN, Holmquist DG, Bader GM, Falk EA: Exfoliative cytology of the human mammary gland and its value in the diagnosis of cancer and other diseases of the breast. Cancer 11:377–409, 1958.

54. Parsons PG, Goss P: Chromosome damage and DNA repair induced in human fibroblasts by UV and cholesterol oxide. Aust J Exp Biol Med Sci 56:287–296, 1978.

55. Petrakis NL: Cerumen genetics and human breast cancer. Science 173:347–349, 1971.

56. Petrakis NL: Genetic cerumen type, breast secretory activity and breast cancer epidemiology. In Mulvihill JJ, Miller RW, Fraumeni JF Jr (eds): Genetics of Human Cancer. New York, Raven Press, 1977.

57. Petrakis NL: Physiologic, biochemical, and cytologic aspects of nipple aspirate fluid. Breast Cancer Res Treat 8:7–19, 1986.

58. Petrakis NL, Lee RE, Miike R, DuPuy ME, Morris M: Coloration of breast fluid related to concentration of cholesterol, cholesterol epoxides, estrogen and lipid peroxides. Am J Clin Pathol 89:117–120, 1988.

59. Petrakis NL, Mason L, Lee R: Association of race, age, menopausal status, and cerumen type with breast fluid secretion in nonlactating women, as determined by nipple aspiration. J Natl Cancer Inst 54:829–834, 1975.

60. Petrakis NL, Wrensch MR, Ernster VL, Miike R, King EB, Goodson WH: Prognostic significance of atypical epithelial hyperplasia in nipple aspirates of breast fluid. Lancet 2:505, 1987.

61. Petrakis NL, Wrensch MR, Ernster VL, Miike R, Murai J, Simberg N, Siiteri PK: Influence of pregnancy and lactation on serum and breast fluid estrogen levels: Implications for breast cancer risk. Int J Cancer 40:587–591, 1987.

62. Ringrose CA: The role of cytology in early detection of breast disease. Acta Cytol 10:373–375, 1966.

63. Rogers LW, Page DL: Epithelial proliferative disease of the breast; A marker of increased cancer risk in certain age groups. Breast 5:2–7, 1979.

64. Sartorius OW, Smith HS, Morris P, Benedict P, Friesen L: Cytologic evaluation of breast fluid in the detection of breast disease. J Natl Cancer Inst 59:1073–1078, 1977.

65. Schuh ME, Takuma N, Penetrante RB, Rosner D, Dao TL: Intraductal carcinoma; analysis of presentation, pathologic findings, and outcome of disease. Arch Surg 121:1303–1307, 1986.

66. Tabar L, Dean PB, Penetek Z: Galactography; the diagnostic procedure of choice for nipple discharge. Radiology 149:31–38, 1983.

67. Uei Y, Watanabe Y, Hirota T, Yamamoto H, Watanabe H: Cytologic diagnosis of breast carcinoma with nipple discharge; special significance of the spherical cell cluster. Acta Cytol 24:522–528, 1980.

68. Urban JA, Egeli RA: Non-lactational nipple discharge. CA 28:130–140, 1978.

69. Vogel PM, Georgiade NG, Fetter BF, Vogel FS, McCarty KS Jr.: The correlation of histologic changes in the human breast with the menstrual cycle. Am J Pathol 104:23–34, 1981.

70. Wellings SR, Jensen HM, Marcum RG: An atlas of subgross pathology of the human breast with special reference to possible precancerous lesions. J Natl Cancer Inst 55:231–273, 1975.

71. Wrensch MR, et al: Breast fluid cholesterol and cholesterol beta-epoxide concentrations in women with benign breast disease. Cancer Res 49:2168–2174, 1989.

72. Wynder EL, Lahti H, Laakso K, Cheng S, DeBevoise S, Rose DP: Nipple aspirates of breast fluid and the epidemiology of breast disease. Cancer 56:1473–1478, 1985.

73. Zimmerman AL, Barrett DL, Petrakis NL: The incidence and significance of intracytoplasmic calcifications in nipple aspirate specimens. Acta Cytol 21:685–692, 1977.

Section III

Pathology of Benign and Premalignant Lesions

Chapter 4

CONGENITAL AND ACQUIRED DISTURBANCES OF BREAST DEVELOPMENT AND GROWTH

Kirby I. Bland, M.D. and Lynn J. Romrell, Ph.D.

DEVELOPMENT OF THE BREAST

The mammary glands, or breasts, are considered to be highly modified sudoriferous glands. Basically, the glands develop as ingrowths from the ectoderm, which form the ducts and alveoli. The supporting vascularized connective tissue is derived from mesenchyme. At about the fifth or sixth week of development, two ventral bands of somewhat thickened ectoderm, called the mammary ridges (or "milk lines"), are present in the embryo (Fig. 4–1). In many mammals, paired mammary glands develop along these ridges, which extend from the base of the forelimb (future axilla) to the region of the hindlimb (inguinal region). The ridges are not prominent in the human embryo and disappear shortly after their formation except for a small portion that persists in the pectoral region, where a single pair of glands usually develop. Accessory nipples (polythelia) or accessory mammary glands (polymastia) may occur along the original mammary ridges or milk lines (Fig. 4–2) if the structure fails to undergo its normal regression.

Each gland develops as the ingrowth of the ectoderm forms a primary bud of tissue in the underlying mesenchyme (Fig. 4–3A). Each primary bud gives rise to 15 to 20 secondary buds, or outgrowths (Fig. 4–3B). During the fetal period, epithelial cords develop from the secondary buds and extend into the surrounding connective tissue. By the end of prenatal life, lumens have developed in the outgrowths, forming the lactiferous ducts and their branches (Fig. 4–3C). At birth the lactiferous ducts open into a shallow epithelial depression, known as the mammary pit. The pit becomes elevated and transformed into the nipple, shortly after birth, as a result of proliferation of the mesenchyme underlying the presumptive nipple and areola (Fig. 4–3D). Failure of the elevation of the pit to occur results in a congenital malformation known as inverted nipple.

In newborn infants of both sexes, the breasts often show a transient enlargement and may produce some secretion, often called witch's milk. These transitory changes occur in response to maternal hormones that

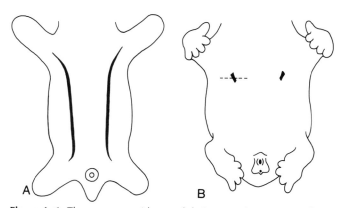

Figure 4–1. The mammary ridges and their regression. *A,* Ventral view of an embryo at the beginning of the fifth week of development (about 28 days), showing the mammary ridges that extend from the forelimb to the hindlimb. *B,* A similar view of the ventral embryo at the end of the sixth week, showing the remains of the ridges located in the pectoral region.

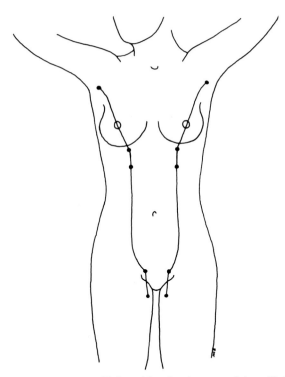

Figure 4–2. Mammary milk line. After development of the milk bud in the pectoral area of ectodermal thickening, the "milk streak" extends from the axilla to the inguinal areas. At week nine of intrauterine development, atrophy of the bud has occurred except for the presence of the supernumerary nipples or breast.

cross the placenta during fetal development. At birth the breasts appear similar in both sexes, demonstrating only the presence of the main lactiferous ducts. The glands remain underdeveloped until puberty, when in the female the breasts enlarge rapidly in response to estrogen and progesterone secretion by the ovaries. The hormonal stimulation causes proliferation of the glandular tissue as well as fat and other connective tissue elements associated with the breast. The glandular tissue remains incompletely developed until pregnancy occurs. At this time the intralobular ducts undergo rapid development and form buds that become alveoli.

AMASTIA

The congenital absence of one or both breasts (amastia) is a rare clinical anomaly. The first recorded reference to amastia is found in The Song of Solomon (8:viii): "We have a little sister, and she hath no breast: What shall we do for our sister in the day when she shall be spoken for?" Froriep first described true absence of the breast in 1839.[34] The association of bilateral amastia with other congenital anomalies was described in 1882 by Gilly,[36] with the description of a 30-year-old woman who presented with absence of the ulna and the ulnar aspect of the right hand. Approximately 50 case reports of amastia were recorded by Deaver and McFarland[24] in their treatise of the breast in 1917. Reports in the literature prior to the 1960s rarely gave details of amastia

or its less severe manifestations. There have been only a few reports of bilateral amastia, defined as complete absence of both breasts and nipples. An extensive review of the literature by Trier[107] documented 43 cases for which data were available. Three presentations were observed: (1) bilateral absence of breasts with congenital ectodermal defects (seven cases); (2) unilateral absence of the breasts (20 cases); and (3) bilateral absence of the breast (16 cases) with variable associated anomalies (Table 4–1).

Subsequently, Tawil and Najjar[104] reported an additional case of congenital bilateral absence of breasts and nipples in a 12-year-old Arab girl with abnormal ears, macrostomia, and chronic glomerulonephritis. Previously, Goldenring and Crelin[40] described a mother and daughter with similar phenotypes. More recently, Nelson and Cooper[83] documented a family in which the father and two of three daughters were found to have bilateral absence or hypoplasia of the nipples/breast tissue with associated minor defects. The mode of inheritance of this combination of defects is autosomal dominant.

Unilateral absence of the breast (Fig. 4–4) is more common than bilateral amastia, and such subjects are most commonly female. This rare physical defect occurs as a result of complete failure of the development of the mammary ridge at about the sixth week in utero. Most often, abnormalities are not associated with bilateral absence of nipple and breast tissue. However, Trier[107] has observed amastia in association with cleft palate, hypertelorism and saddle nose, and anomalies of the pectoral muscle, ulna, hand, foot, palate, ears, genitourinary tract, and habitus. Occasionally, several members of a family have been affected. At least four reports[32, 40, 107, 114] document the transmission of this anomaly with pedigree penetrance consistent with dominant inheritance.

Rich and associates[99] recently described a case of ureteral triplication as a component of an autosomal dominant syndrome comprising bilateral amastia, pectus excavatum, umbilical hernia, patent ductus arteriosus, dysmorphic low-set ears, ptosis, epicanthic folds with an antimongoloid slant of the eyes, ocular hypertelorism, high-arched palate, flat broad nasal bridge, tapered digits, cubitus valgus, and syndactyly. Nelson and Cooper[83] have also reported the autosomal dominant transmission of breast hypoplasia or absence of the nipples in association with webbing of the fingers. Rich et al.[99] are the only investigators to report genetically transmitted ureteral triplication, alone or in association with bilateral amastia.

UNILATERAL CONGENITAL DEFECTS OF THE BREAST WITH ASSOCIATED DEFECTS OF THE CHEST WALL, IPSILATERAL MUSCULATURE, SUBCUTANEOUS TISSUES, AND BRACHYSYNDACTYLY (POLAND'S SYNDROME)

In 1841, Alfred Poland[92] published in *Guy's Hospital Report* the description of a patient who presented with

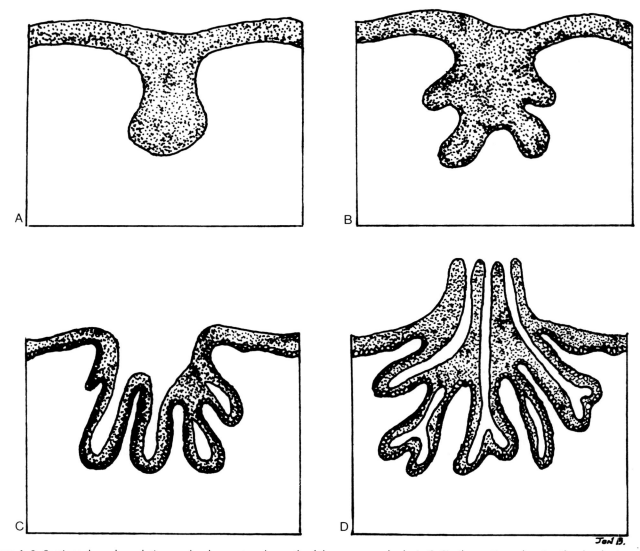

Figure 4–3. Sections through evolutionary development and growth of the mammary bud. *A–C,* Similar sections showing the developing gland at successive stages between the twelfth week and birth. The mammary pit develops, and major lactiferous ducts are present at the end of gestation. *D,* A similar section showing the elevation of the mammary pit by proliferation of the underlying connective tissue forming the nipple soon after birth.

absence of musculature (pectoralis major and minor) of the shoulder girdle and malformations of the ipsilateral upper limb. In this original report of unilateral congenital absence of the pectoralis major and minor muscles, there was associated absence of the external oblique and partial absence of the serratus anterior. Thereafter, numerous authors have reported similar findings with the additional observation of hypoplasia or complete absence of the breast or nipple, costal cartilage and rib defects (ribs 2, 3, and 4 or 3, 4, and 5), hypoplasia of subcutaneous tissues of the chest wall, and brachysyndactyly. This constellation of clinical findings, whether all or partially present, is currently known as *Poland's syndrome.* Clinical manifestations of this disorder are extremely variable, and rarely can all features be recognized in a single individual.[63, 65, 109]

Poland's syndrome is invariably unilateral, with a higher incidence in female than in male patients. When the chest wall defect (ribs, cartilage, or both) is evident, there is usually a deep concavity on expiration and lung herniation with inspiration (Fig. 4–5). The right side is more commonly affected than the left.[23] The most common defect, breast hypoplasia, is readily recognized, and the rudimentary breast tissue is usually higher on the involved side and medially displaced from its normal anatomical position.

While the etiology is unclear, this syndrome is seldom familial. Leukemia has been associated with the syndrome, as have other rare congenital anomalies. Similar defects have been noted with exposure to drugs, such as thalidomide.

Treatment of patients with Poland's syndrome varies with the number of anomalies and their physical expression. With the presentation of one or two typical characteristics of Poland's syndrome, the patients usually complain only about their appearance. These patients

Table 4–1. CONGENITAL ANOMALIES ASSOCIATED WITH BILATERAL ABSENCE OF THE NIPPLES AND BREAST TISSUES

No. of Patients	Reported Anomalies
1	Atrophy of the right pectoral muscle; absence of the ulna and ulnar side of the hand
1	Absence of finger on the right hand; deformity of the right foot
1	Bilateral lobster-claw deformity of the hands and feet; cleft palate
2	Sparse axillary and pubic hair; saddle nose; hypertelorism; high-arched palate
1	Short status; short small nose; a broad nasal root; protrusion of the external ear; high-arched palate
10	No anomalies

From Trier WC: Complete breast absence. Case report and review of the literature. Plast Reconstruct Surg 36:431, 1965. Reprinted by permission.

are not functionally embarrassed by their lack of anterior chest wall muscle mass or the small size of their breast. Only in extreme cases, as with total absence of the costal cartilage or segments of the anterior ribs, are patients physically impaired and emotionally disturbed by their deformity. Surgical procedures to correct the deformities of the chest wall have been documented[109] and include (1) subperiosteal grafts from adjacent ribs with free flaps of latissimus dorsi or external oblique[5]; (2) autologous split-rib grafts[97]; (3) split-rib grafts with periosteum that has been detached posteriorly and rotated from the anterior aspect of the defective rib to the sternum[95]; (4) heterologous bone grafts[46]; and (5) metallic mesh implants followed by rib grafts from the opposite chest wall.[30] Ravitch[96] popularized the use of split-rib grafts from the opposite chest wall that are placed across the defect and reinforced with Teflon felt. The technique described by Amoroso and Angelats[2] utilizes autologous tissue of the latissimus dorsi myocutaneous flap for augmenting the hypoplastic breast and to contour the anterior chest wall while simultaneously augmenting the involved hypoplastic breast. This procedure, initially attempted by Asp and Sulamaa[5] of Finland, was unsuccessful using a free latissimus dorsi flap. Thus, the procedure was abandoned because of transplanted muscle atrophied as a result of the omission of the neurovascular pedicle from the transplant, emphasizing the value of preservation of the pedicle when employing this technique. In 1950, Campbell[14] described the use of a latissimus dorsi muscle flap transferred through the axilla for anterior chest wall reconstruction with preservation of the neurovascular bundle. He, too, abandoned this technique as the flap was associated with a cutaneous component and/or applied over a breast prosthesis unsuccessfully.

Schneider et al.[101] emphasized the value of a single-stage reconstruction. The high success rate and the reliability of this technique, which uses the latissimus dorsi myocutaneous flap, represents remarkable advance over the aforementioned methods. The cosmetic and functional results of this technique appear superior to those obtained with standard multiple-stage procedures.

At least two recent reports confirm a variant of Poland's syndrome associated with large melanotic spots. As breasts and melanocytes both have origin from the ectoderm, abnormalities of breast hypoplasia and hyperpigmentation probably develop from within this germinal layer. Moore and Schosser[78] reported on Becker's melanosis associated with hypoplasia of the breast

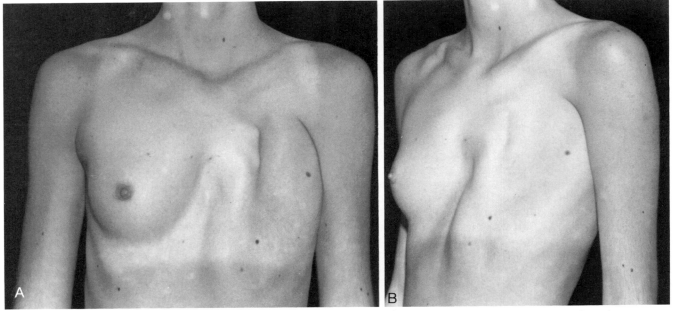

Figure 4–4. A and B, Unilateral amastia in 20-year-old female with concomitant chest wall deformity of ipsilateral ribs 3–6 and cartilage. In contrast to those with Poland's syndrome, this patient has accessory musculature of the shoulder, including pectoralis major and minor, latissimus dorsi, and serratus anterior muscles. (Courtesy of Dr. John McGraw, Norfolk, VA.)

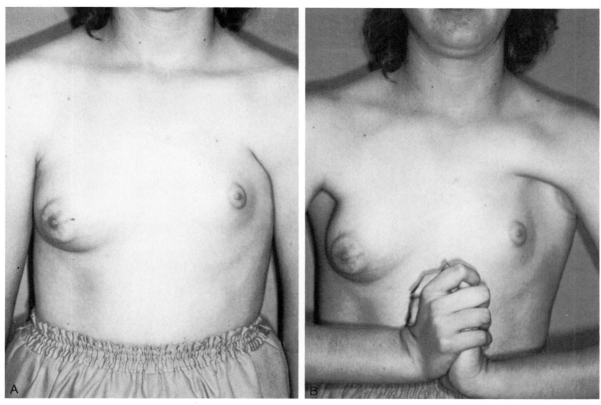

Figure 4–5. Poland's syndrome: A 15-year-old girl with Poland's syndrome of left breast (A) with shoulder girdle musculature actively contracted. B, There is accentuation of the left hypoplastic breast. There is absence of the sternal head of the pectoralis major although the clavicular head is present. (Courtesy of Dr. Hollis H. Caffee, Division of Plastic and Reconstructive Surgery, University of Florida College of Medicine, Gainesville, FL.)

and pectoralis major muscle. Zubowicz and Bostwick[116] also confirmed two patients with areas of diffuse hyperpigmentation overlying a unilaterally hypoplastic breast. Treatment was directed toward reconstructing the breast mound and symmetrically sizing the two areolae. Patients often do not request treatment of the pigmented abnormalities, and standard methods utilized in the therapy of hyperpigmentation frequently yield unsatisfactory results. Such hyperpigmented areas appear to have no neoplastic risk.

IATROGENIC FACTORS THAT INITIATE BREAST HYPOPLASIA

The failure of complete development of the vestigial male or female breast may occur as a consequence of developmental hypomastia (Fig. 4–6) or may be initiated by therapeutic manipulation and/or injury of the mammary anlage in infancy or in the prepubertal interval. Rudimentary breast tissue in the male or female infant lies beneath the primitive nipple-areola complex at approximately the fourth intercostal space. Thus, *trauma, incisions, abscess, infectious lesions, or radiation therapy* to the breast bud in the infantile or prepubertal era can initiate maldevelopment with hypoplasia of the vestigial breast. The surgeon must be especially aware of the necessity and technique of any incision for drainage of

lesions of the areolar complex or masses within the breast bud to avoid subsequent maldevelopment. Further, unilateral development of breast tissue in the adolescent female may represent nonisometric growth of breast tissue in precocious or early pubertal states. With this presentation, cautious observation of the contralateral breast is in order. The surgeon should not biopsy by incisional or excisional techniques the rudimentary breast structure or the nipple-areola complex. The risk of neoplastic lesions is infinitesimally small in this younger age group, whereas the travesty of irreversible damage to the breast bud with subsequent hypoplasia of the breast or amastia is a distinct possibility. The bilaterally symmetrical nipple-areola and breast complexes overlie the fourth intercostal space of the infant. In the fully developed breasts of the sexually mature female, the complex may extend to the seventh and eighth intercostal spaces. Thus, excisional biopsies of any chest wall lesions that are initiated prior to full maturation of the mammae, must be approached cautiously.

Cherup and associates[18] documented breast and pectoral muscle maldevelopment after *anterolateral and posterolateral thoracotomies* in children. Incisions placed through the third and fourth intercostal spaces for repair of congenital heart lesions were evaluated in 28 patients by these authors. In this series, standard anterolateral thoracotomies resulted in a high frequency of breast or

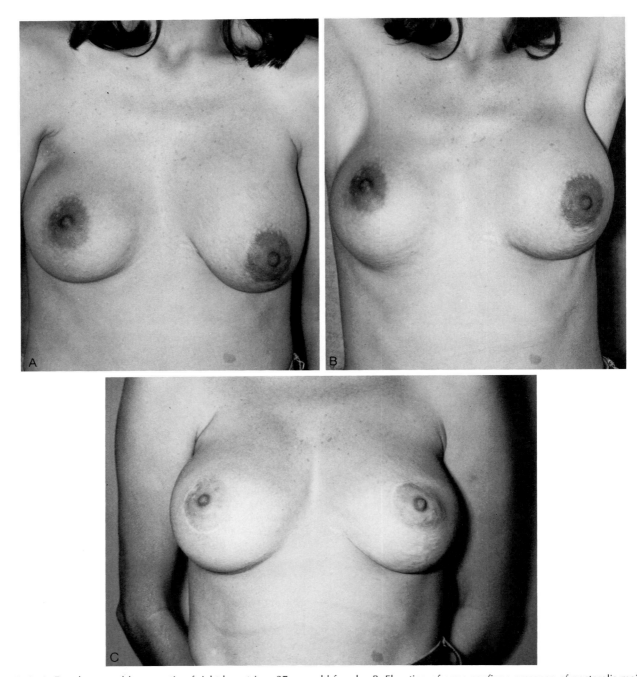

Figure 4–6. *A,* Developmental hypomastia of right breast in a 27-year-old female. *B,* Elevation of arms confirms presence of pectoralis major and shoulder girdle musculature on side of hypomastia. *C,* Final cosmetic appearance of breasts following augmentation mammaplasty of right breast and reduction mammaplasty with mastopexy of left breast. (Courtesy of Dr. Hal G. Bingham, Division of Plastic and Reconstructive Surgery, University of Florida, College of Medicine, Gainesville, FL.)

pectoral muscular maldevelopment. Using measurements of volumes of the breast and pectoral muscles with plaster molds and linear dimensions of each chest side, the authors concluded that 60 percent of patients with these incisions had greater than a 20 percent difference in volume between the two sides. To avoid these maldevelopment syndromes, when the anterolateral or posterolateral thoracotomy must be used, it should be started anteriorly in the seventh or eighth interspace, below the level to which the breast will extend by adulthood, and the incision should be carried no higher than the sixth interspace to avoid the extension of the breast to the axilla. Further, the pectoralis muscles should not be divided, but elevated superiorly as a unit from the inferior edge and retracted, to avoid subsequent injury to this organ as well. This technique avoids injury to the neurovascular pedicles of the pectoralis muscles and the breast bud itself.

Moss[80] in 1959 reported that in the prepubertal interval, when the human breast consists mainly of an expanding ductular system, 1500 to 2000 rad of *radiation* delivered through a single portal over an eight-day period will initiate striking maldevelopment of this organ. Further, 3000 to 4000 rad administered over 30 days not only permanently arrests growth of glandular epithelium but also concomitantly produces severe fibrosis and hypoplasia of the breast. Following 3000 rad, the end result was essentially complete loss of lobules and shrinkage of ductules of breast tissue. Williams and Cunningham,[114] in evaluating the histological changes of irradiated breasts of women, state that irradiated areas show intense obliterative endarteritis and in the end stages, marked fragmentation of elastic tissue.

Underwood and Gaul[108] documented severe breast hypoplasia as a consequence of *radium therapy implants* for a cavernous hemangioma in the region of the left breast of an infant. Subsequently, the contralateral breast matured normally while the ipsilateral involved breast failed to develop. Similar reports of hypoplasia have been recorded by Mathews[68] with the use of radium needles applied to the surface of the hemangioma, close to the nipple, when the patient was in her infancy. The report by Weidman et al.[111] addresses the necessity of observation of breast hemangiomas and the cautious application of radiotherapy in the treatment of hemangiomas or other lesions of the breast with ionizing radiation. Further, contemporary approaches to the therapy of intrathoracic or chest wall neoplasms dictate modification of irradiation portals that traverse the nipple-areola complex or the breast bud in infantile or prepubertal patients.

PREMATURE THELARCHE

The term premature thelarche refers to isolated breast development in the *absence* of additional signs of sexual maturation. This clinical presentation is represented by precocious development (Fig. 4–7) without other signs of puberty in girls younger than eight years of age. Wilkins and colleagues[113] postulate an increased sensitiv-

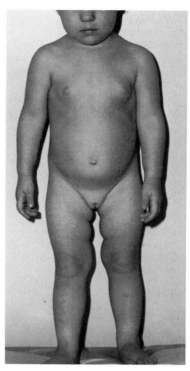

Figure 4–7. Premature thelarche in a 19-month-old female with isolated breast development in the absence of additional signs of sexual maturation. (Courtesy of Dr. Arlan L. Rosenbloom, Department of Pediatrics, University of Florida College of Medicine, Gainesville, FL.)

ity of breast tissue to low circulating levels of estrogens (estrone, estradiol) secreted during early childhood as the etiology of this premature breast development. Several authors have suggested normal or slightly increased plasma estradiol and basal gonadotropin (LH and FSH) levels with the presentation. Conflicting results with regard to gonadotropin responsiveness by synthetic gonadotropin-releasing hormone (LH-RH) have been observed. In premature thelarche, the basal LH and FSH concentrations have been reported as normal or slightly elevated.[55, 76] In a series of 15 patients reported by Caufriez et al.,[17] all patients with premature thelarche had normal basal LH and FSH levels for their age and normal responses to LH-RH. The observations of these investigators are in agreement with those of Reiter and associates.[98] These reports suggest that patients with premature thelarche do have normal regulation of the hypothalamo-pituitary-gonadal axis.

Caufriez et al.[17] confirmed a normal prolactin secretion in basal conditions and in response to thyrotropin-releasing hormone (TRH) for girls with premature thelarche. Prolactin does not convincingly appear to have a role in the genesis of isolated breast development in prepubertal girls. The endocrinological relationship of this clinical presentation has been further investigated by Pasquino et al.[89] in nine young girls with premature thelarche who were compared with nine healthy girls and six girls with true precocious puberty. The gonadotropin stimulation test with LH-RH was used. Girls with premature thelarche were observed to have LH responses that resemble those of normal girls, and FSH responses were similar to those of patients with precocious puberty. This study suggests that in premature thelarche there is partial activation of the diencephalic-hypophyseal-gonadal axis, which affects FSH alone. The authors conclude that premature thelarche should be considered as one of the disorders that results from altered sensitivity of the hypothalamic receptors that regulate sexual maturation. From a practical point of view, this study emphasizes the utility of the *gonadotropin stimulation test* with LH-RH in girls with premature breast development as a test to distinguish between *premature thelarche* and true *precocious puberty*.

Data by Ilicki et al.[48] in the long-term follow-up of 68 girls with premature thelarche confirmed that 85 percent of patients with the disorder had onset before the age of two years. In 30.8 percent, this clinical finding was recognized at birth; in 44 percent there was a regression after 3 2/12 ± 2 8/12 years (SD). In this study, basal levels of plasma FSH and response to LH-RH were significantly higher (p<0.001) than in prepubertal controls. Twenty-seven of 52 patients evaluated had increased plasma estradiol, and in 27 of 40 patients tested, urocystograms or vaginal smears confirmed estrogenization. Basal levels of LH and responses to LH-RH were prepubertal. In this study, girls with premature thelarche were significantly taller than normal controls of the same age (p<0.001). These investigators suggest that premature thelarche is an incomplete form of precocious sexual development, probably occurring secondary to a derangement in the maturation of the hypothalamo-pituitary-gonadal axis that results in a higher than normal secretion of FSH. The authors conclude that the end result appears to be a defect in the peripheral sensitivity to the sexual hormones.

In follow-up of the natural history and endocrine findings of premature thelarche, a longitudinal study from the Institute of Paediatrics, University of Rome, Italy, was completed by Pasquino et al.[90] This study of 40 girls with premature thelarche confirmed that when the disorder occurred *prior* to the age of two years, it usually regressed completely, thus representing an isolated and transient phenomenon. However, this disorder occurring *after* two years of age persisted more frequently and may represent the first sign of sexual development, generally leading to early simple puberty. These observations were confirmed by Mills et al.,[76] who likewise conducted longitudinal studies of the natural history of the disorder by contacting 46 patients with previously diagnosed cases. These authors observed palpable breast tissue that persisted for three to five years in 57 percent of the subjects. Only 11 percent reported that their breast had continued to enlarge. Patients in whom breast tissue had been present at birth and had persisted were significantly more likely to have progressive enlargement. Comparison of these patients with matched-control subjects showed no relationship between premature thelarche and maternal obstetrical problems, exposure to medications, diet, or prenatal infections. Further, girls with premature thelarche were no more likely than control subjects to have other medical or sexual problems develop during the interval of follow-up.

Escobar and coworkers[29] evaluated the plasma concentration of extradiol-17β in premature thelarche and in varying types of sexual precocity. All patients with idiopathic precocious puberty had elevated plasma estradiol concentrations for their ages that showed wide variations. No correlation between the grade of sexual development and the level of estradiol was observed. The plasma estradiol concentrations confirmed good correlation with clinical signs of estrogenic effects in prepubertal and adolescent normal girls (Fig. 4–8). Seven of their 10 patients with premature thelarche had prepubertal levels of estradiol. Girls with higher estradiol levels were seven years older and had urocystograms with moderate estrogenic activity. The findings in these younger girls confirmed the hypothesis that premature thelarche specifically resulted from higher sensitivity of breast tissue to prepubertal estrogen levels, since other estrogen target tissues did not show this stimulatory effect.

JUVENILE (ADOLESCENT, VIRGINAL) HYPERTROPHY OF THE FEMALE BREAST

Juvenile or adolescent hypertrophy of the breast is a commonly observed occurrence in the young adolescent female following a normal puberty. This clinical presentation denotes the adolescent breast that does not cease its rapid pubertal growth and continues to enlarge even into mature years. The majority of patients with juvenile hypertrophy of the breast have symmetrical, *bilateral* involvement (Fig. 4–9), although *unilateral* juvenile hypertrophy has been described. There have been a few reported cases of massive breast hypertrophy during pregnancy,[62, 79, 85] in which rapid enlargement is evident soon after conception with predominant growth occurring during the second trimester.

Several conditions may initiate breast asymmetry,

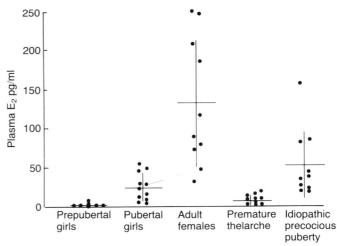

Figure 4–8. Estradiol-17β plasma values in normal females, premature thelarche, and idiopathic precocious puberty. Mean values are indicated by horizontal lines and standard deviations by vertical lines. (From Escobar ME, et al: Acta Endocrinol. 81:351, 1976. Reprinted by permission.)

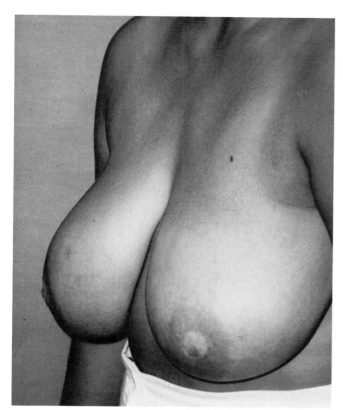

Figure 4–9. Bilateral juvenile hypertrophy in a 17-year-old nulliparous Hispanic female. The patient presented with mastodynia related to her large breast size. She was on no medications known to induce breast gigantism. Therapy consisted of reduction mammaplasty. (Courtesy of Dr. Hollis H. Caffee, Division of Plastic and Reconstructive Surgery, University of Florida College of Medicine, Gainesville, FL.)

including maldevelopment, neoplasms, incisional or excisional biopsies, trauma, and radiotherapy. As noted earlier, developmental abnormalities account for the majority of these lesions. Mayl, Vasconez, and Jurkiewicz[69] suggested that juvenile hypertrophy, also referred to as *macromastia,* may occur secondary to a primary defect of the breast or an endocrinological disorder. The general tenet has been that an augmented plasma level of estrone or estradiol may induce hypertrophy of the mamma. However, the measurement of various mammotropic hormones as etiological for the disorder has not yielded precise clinical correlates with breast enlargement. Nonetheless, substantial *decreases* in plasma *progesterone* levels have been documented for juvenile hypertrophy in the presence of *normal* plasma *estrogen* and *growth hormone* values. These substantial decreases of progesterone may be etiological for the abnormality. One could also postulate that target organ tissues (ductal epithelium, collagen and stroma of the adolescent female breast) may have estrogen receptors that are highly responsive to minimal concentrations of the mammotropic steroid hormones (e.g., estrogens, progesterone) that regulate breast growth and development.[7]

Sperling and Gold[103] and Mayl et al.[69] have recommended the use of the antiestrogen drugs, dydrogesterone (Gynorest) and medroxyprogesterone acetate (Pro-

vera) in the treatment of virginal hypertrophy. Ryan and Pernoll[100] were successful in preventing regrowth of breast parenchyma following reduction mammaplasty in several patients with adolescent hypertrophy by the use of the drug dydrogesterone. However, a subsequent follow-up report by these investigators suggested its ineffectiveness. Thereafter, partial success for prevention of regrowth was achieved with tamoxifen citrate (Nolvadex). Treatment with tamoxifen may be of value following reduction mammaplasty (subcutaneous mastectomy) in patients with strongly positive estrogen receptor profiles in the removed breast tissue. Using an escalating dose of 10 to 40 mg of tamoxifen citrate per day, these authors were able to achieve reduction of breast bulk with the drug. Theoretically, with the use of this compound, estrogen receptors can be converted to a negative profile status. The infrequent usage of tamoxifen in the treatment of juvenile hypertrophy of the breast suggests that a prospective controlled clinical trial may be of value to determine its efficacy for this condition.

The most commonly applied technique for the treatment of adolescent (juvenile) hypertrophy continues to be the *subcutaneous mastectomy* described by Furnas[35] as a reduction mammaplasty. However, the technique, as reported by Cardoso de Castro,[15] does not represent a panacea for this disorder. Modifications of the subcutaneous mastectomy have subsequently been described by Courtiss and Goldwyn,[22] employing an inferior pedicle technique as an alternative to free nipple and areola grafting for severe *macromastia* or *extreme ptosis.* For recurrent adolescent hypertrophy following previously successful reduction mammaplasty, the *total glandular mastectomy* with *subpectoral augmentation* may be considered. This aggressive technique, as previously described by Bland and coworkers,[8] should only rarely be necessary in the premenopausal female (Fig. 4–10). The success of this more radical approach is dependent upon the extirpation from the chest wall of all breast tissue that has estrogen hypersensitivity and, thus, the potential for regrowth.

DRUG INDUCTION OF GIGANTISM

Drug-related induction of *breast gigantism* has previously been described. This disorder may occur in the adolescent or in the fully mature adult breast (Fig. 4–11). D-Penicillamine as an etiological factor in breast enlargement is poorly understood but is a well-recognized cause of sudden gigantism. Desai[27] postulates an effect on sex hormone binding globulin by D-penicillamine to increase the amount of circulating free estrogen. Taylor and associates[105] suggest that it is likely that D-penicillamine produces a local effect on the breast, as patients do not show changes in menstrual function while receiving the drug or during the time of maximal breast growth. These authors confirm the effect of danazol (17-α-pregna-2,4-dien-20-ynol(2,3-d) isoxazol-17β-0; Danocrine) to act by interfering with the sensitivity of the breast parenchymal estrogen receptor,

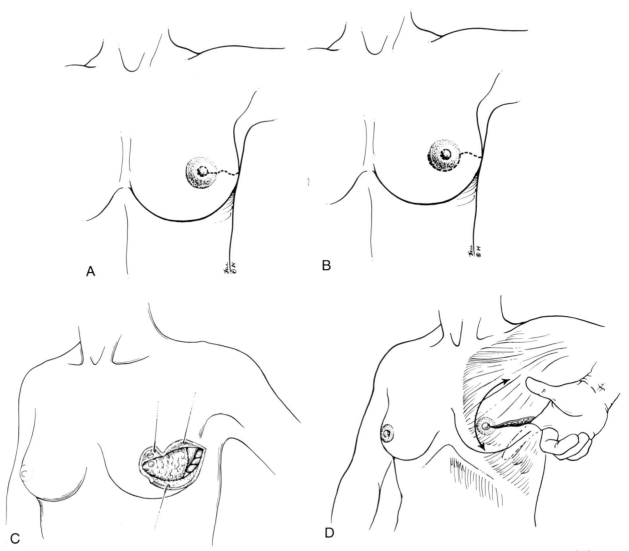

Figure 4–10. Technique for one-stage simple mastectomy with immediate reconstruction *(A).* Circumferential nipple incision extended transareolarly and in "lazy S" pattern over lateral portion of breast. Nipple and ductal system remain with breast specimen. *B,* When pre-existing para-areolar scar is present, or inferior skin envelope must be reduced, circumareolar incision is used. Nipple is circumscribed as in *A. C,* Flap elevation via circumareolar incision with development of skin thickness and extent of dissection identical to modified radical mastectomy technique. *D,* Entering submuscular plane via muscle-splitting incision of serratus anterior at fifth rib level, serratus anterior muscle origins are avulsed from their ribs to beyond sixth rib, and blunt dissection of subpectoralis major plane is continued superiorly to clavicle and medially to sternum. (From Bland KI, et al: Arch Surg 121(2):221, 1986. Reprinted by permission.)

thereby diminishing growth. These studies confirmed both dimunition in breast size during the first courses of danazol administration and that these reductions occurred simultaneously with a reduction in plasma circulating estradiol concentrations. Further, the cessation of danazol administration with an increase in breast volume indicated that a reduction in breast size was not simply a coincidental spontaneous remission. This clinical trial did not determine whether the breast shrinkage that resulted with the drug was produced by a reduction in circulating estrogen concentrations or by a local effect. The blocking of estrogen receptors by danazol may mimic the postmenopausal condition and has been successfully applied by Buckle[12] for the treatment of gynecomastia in males.

BREAST HYPERTROPHY WITH PREGNANCY (GIGANTOMASTIA)

Massive hypertrophy of the breast with pregnancy is a rare condition of unknown etiology that is often referred to as *gigantomastia of pregnancy*. The first recorded report of this condition was made by Palmuth in 1648.[87] In the exhaustive review of 55 cases in the world literature by Moss,[79] 33 patients with this condition had previously been reported by Deaver and McFarland in 1917.[24] These reviews reveal that this condition may affect women of all races during the child-bearing years. The disorder is less common than juvenile (virginal) hypertrophy of the breast, which classically progresses independent of pregnancy and occurs usually between

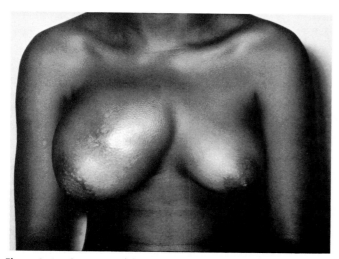

Figure 4–11. Gigantism of drug induction. An 18-year-old black female with painful unilateral gigantism of the right breast following treatment with D-penicillamine.

the ages of 11 and 19 years. In distinction, gigantomastia of pregnancy usually occurs during the first few months of pregnancy and may progress to necrosis, incapacity, and possibly death.[79]

The typical history is that of a healthy pregnant woman who observed gradual bilateral massive enlargement of her breasts within the first few months of pregnancy. The breasts may enlarge to several times their normal weight and size to become grotesque, huge, and incapacitating. The skin and parenchyma become firm, edematous, and tense and may have prominent subcutaneous veins with a diffuse peau d'orange appearance. As a consequence of rapid breast enlargement and skin pressure, insufficient vascularity of the skin may initiate ulceration, necrosis, infection, and/or hemorrhage.

In the immediate postpartum period, the hypertrophied breasts recede to approximately their previous volume. When the woman delivers, the breasts regress in size but almost always hypertrophy again with succeeding pregnancies. Most authors agree that this condition is hormonal in etiology, but its precise mechanism is unclear. Whether there is an overproduction of mammotropic hormone from the pituitary or an enhanced sensitivity of breast parenchyma to the hormones of pregnancy (e.g., estriol, estradiol, HCG, progestins) has not been established. Parham[88] determined that estrogen and testosterone were of no value in the treatment of gigantism of pregnancy; however, norethindrone may be of value. Hydrocortisone therapy has been attempted without success by Nolan[85]; testosterone has been used with divided results. Moss[79] used fluoxymesterone without results, while diuretics were successfully used with moderate temporary effect.

Luchsinger[62] was one of the first to suggest that this condition may occur as a consequence of specific individual reactivity of the breast to hormonal stimuli. This author questioned whether, in addition to possible hormonal dysfunction, estrogenic placental hormones were

sufficiently metabolized in the presence of insufficient liver function. Lewison et al.[58] postulated that gigantism of pregnancy may be due to the depression of all steroid hormones and decreased liver function as measured by the salicylate conjugation test. These investigators advocated the use of the progestational agent norethindrone to reduce breast size; however, it was used with mestranol and had to be discontinued when thrombophlebitis occurred. While liver dysfunction and the inability to decompose estrogenic hormones have been postulated to be etiological for the disorder, it must be noted that many normal pregnancies are accompanied by severe liver failure without the development of gigantomastia.

In most instances, gigantomastia is self-limiting and does not progress to pyogenic abscesses, skin ulcerations, necrosis, or systemic illness. For the majority of patients, breast size will spontaneously regress to its approximate nonpregnant configuration. The patient should be advised of proper brassiere support, good skin hygiene, and adequate nutrition. On occasion, diuretics are of value. Operative intervention may be necessary to relieve severe pain, massive infection, necrosis, slough, and ulceration or hemorrhage if delivery is not imminent. Post delivery, the patient should be advised that gigantism will almost certainly recur with subsequent pregnancies, and *reduction mammaplasty* may be considered.

SYMMASTIA: MEDIAL CONFLUENCE OF THE BREAST

Symmastia (Greek, *syn* "together" and *mastos* "breast") is the newly coined terminology for medial confluence of the breast. This rare clinical anomaly represents a webbing across the midline in breasts that are usually symmetrical (Fig. 4–12). More common, however, is the presternal blending (confluence) of the breast tissue that is associated with macromastia. These conditions are most often recognized in individuals who seek reduction mammaplasty.[102]

Like many anomalies of ectodermal origin, a broad spectrum of defects may be observed with this congenital lesion. Cases may range from an empty skin web to those with an apparent confluence of major portions of symmetrical breast tissue within the midline. The common denominator is the need for resection of presternal skin to varying degrees. Spence et al.[102] recommend correction of the web defect using three methods: (1) elevation of an *inferiorly based triangular skin flap* that is advanced superiorly in an inverted Y-V manner following division of excessive medial soft tissue. Thereafter, the divided medial soft tissue is sutured superiorly to the medial pectoralis fascia to create a brassiere-band sling effect. (2) These authors have also used a *superiorly based medial flap* that contains both skin and soft tissue. Excess skin and soft tissue were excised, and the remaining flap was tailored to fit into a V-shaped defect in the inferior incision. (3) A third option suggested by the authors consists of the vertical division and superior

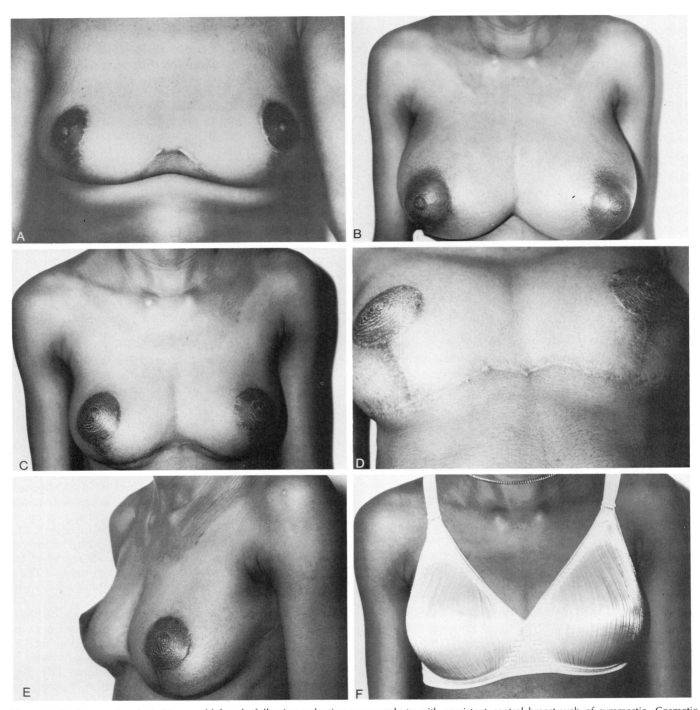

Figure 4–12. Symmastia. *A,* A 24-year-old female following reduction mammaplasty with persistent central breast web of symmastia. Cosmetic congenital defect was corrected with inserted Y-V advancement flap. *B,* A 19-year-old female with large, painful breasts and prominent central webbing reportedly present since the beginning of breast development. *C–F,* Postoperative appearance of breasts after correction of symmastia with reduction mammaplasty using the inferior pedicle technique. (From Spence RJ, et al: Plast Reconstruct Surg 73:2, 1984. Reprinted by permission.)

rotation of the excess subcutaneous tissue flaps with elevation of a *superiorly based skin flap* inserted into a V-shaped defect in the inferior incision. No reports currently exist on the application of the new *liposuction* techniques for this disorder; however, it seems predictable, as reported by McKissock,[71] that the same limitations will apply to the breast as advocates of liposuction have professed exist elsewhere in the body. Thus, the amount of skin involved in the web medially, and its resiliency, will determine the applicability of liposuction techniques for this anomaly.

SUPERNUMERARY NIPPLES (POLYTHELIA)

The presence of supernumerary or accessory nipples (Fig. 4–13) is a relatively common minor congenital

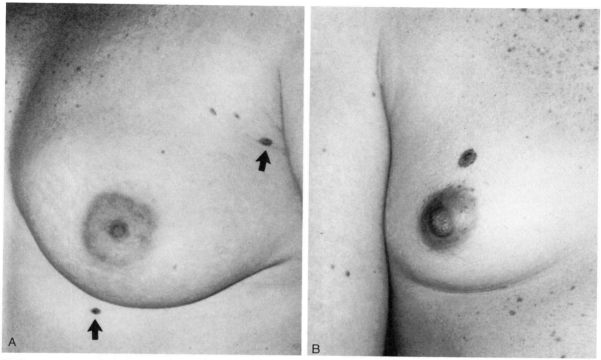

Figure 4–13. Supernumerary nipple. *A,* A 38-year-old female with supernumerary nipples above (in axilla) and below the normal left breast in the mammary milk line. *B,* Supernumerary nipple and areolar complex (rudimentary) in upper right breast of a 22-year-old woman. Excisional biopsy was the preferred treatment.

anomaly that occurs in both sexes with an estimated frequency of 1 in 100 to 1 in 500 persons.[20] Méhes[72–74] reported the frequency of supernumerary nipples as 0.22 percent in a white European population, significantly lower than the incidence of 1.63 percent found by Rahbar[93] in black American neonates. This represents a 7.4-fold increase for the anomaly in blacks. In the newborn Jewish population reported by Mimouni et al.,[77] the higher incidence of 2.5 percent for polythelia was observed. This high frequency of supernumerary nipples could possibly be due to ethnic differences, but as acknowledged by some authors, may be related to a systematic technique for examination of the newborn.

Polythelia should be searched for in the routine physical examination of every newborn, and the presence of the condition should be reported to the parents. This is important for the following reasons as reported by Mimouni[77]: (1) Supernumerary breasts in females may respond to fluctuations in hormones in a physiological manner such that pubertal enlargement, premenstrual swelling, tenderness, and lactation during pregnancy and parturition may occur; (2) patients with polythelia may be subject to the same spectrum of pathological diseases observed in normal breasts (e.g., neoplasms, fibroadenoma, papillary adenoma, cysts, or carcinoma); and (3) the supernumerary nipples may be associated with other congenital diseases such as vertebral anomalies, cardiac arrhythmias, or renal anomalies. Table 4–2 summarizes the associated abnormal conditions that may occur with polythelia.

Moore and Schosser[78] observed that supernumerary

nipples usually develop just below the normal breast in the white population, with less common occurrence in abdominal or inguinal sites. Abramson[1] observed bilateral supernumerary nipples in approximately one half of patients with polythelia. In the ectopic sites, polythelia takes origin from the extra mammary buds that are present along the ventral embryonic mammary ridges (see Fig. 4–3*A*). Only a minority of persons with this clinical anomaly have greater than two extra nipples.[78]

While various malformations have been associated with polythelia (Table 4–2), recently attention has been drawn to the high incidence of *renal anomalies* and *malignancies in children* with supernumerary nipples.

Table 4–2. POLYTHELIA AND ASSOCIATED CONDITIONS

Urinary Tract Abnormalities	Cardiac Abnormalities	Miscellaneous Abnormalities
Renal agenesis Renal cell carcinoma	Cardiac conduction disturbances, especially left bundle branch block	Pyloric stenosis Epilepsy
Obstructive disease Supernumerary kidney(s)	Hypertension Congenital heart anomalies	Ear abnormalities Arthrogryposis multiplex congenita

From Pellegrini JR, Wagner RF Jr.: Polythelia and associated conditions. Am Fam Physician 28:129–132, 1983. Reprinted by permission.

The association between supernumerary nipples and occult anomalies of the urogenital system, has been reported in at least two non–United States pediatric populations. These studies from Hungary[72] and Israel[110] report that 23 and 40 percent, respectively, of children with polythelia had obstructive renal abnormalities or duplications of the excretory system. In embryogenesis, polythelia occurs during the third month of gestation when the embryonic mammary ridge fails to regress normally—an event coincident with the development of the urogenital and other organ systems. Therefore, it is not surprising that various congenital anomalies, particularly of the genitourinary tract, appear to occur excessively with polythelia. The studies by Goedert et al.[37, 38] and Méhes et al.[74] suggest that polythelia is also associated with cancers of the testis and kidney. *Familial occurrence* has been reported by the authors, including the association of polythelia with renal cancer and in three families, the combination of urogenital anomalies, germ cell tumors, and renal cancer.

Goedert et al.[38] evaluated 299 medical students, of whom 8 (2.7 percent) had polythelia. This frequency of the anomaly yielded an estimated relative risk of testicular cancer for men with polythelia of 4.5 (95 percent confidence interval, 1.6–12.4). In the first Health and Nutrition Examination Survey (HANES) dermatological examination, polythelia was observed in 108 (0.5 percent) of the total series of 20,749 persons and in 27 (0.4 percent) of the 7004 white males. Using the HANES white males as controls, these authors estimate the relative risk of testicular cancer associated with polythelia to be 31.8 (95 percent confidence interval, 13.9–72.6). Obviously, the estimated magnitude for risk of testicular cancer in men with polythelia is expected to vary according to the nature of the comparison group and the methods for determination of the disorder. The prevalence of polythelia of 2.5 percent as reported by Mimouni et al.[77] suggests that this rate closely resembles the 2.7 percent prevalence evident in the medical student population determined by Goedert et al.[38] Thus, an intensive evaluation and search for the anomaly would expectantly change the frequency when compared with the HANES dermatological examination. Overall, it would appear that the estimated 4.5-fold relative risk of testicular cancer in men with polythelia is a more accurate determination than the relative risk of 31.8 based on the HANES survey. Although the association between the disorder and testicular cancer is statistically highly significant, the estimated incidence of testicular cancer in men with polythelia appears to be less than five cases per 10,000 per year. Despite this low frequency of testicular carcinoma, the association with renal anomalies must be sought. It was also suggested that children with polythelia, especially male children, should be evaluated to exclude urinary tract anomalies. For these children, kidney ultrasonography is indicated. Radiological examinations of the urogenital tract are indicated in every patient in whom there is suspicion of pathology in this organ system. As noted above, Rahbar[93] acknowledged the high frequency of accessory nipples in black Americans to be almost 7.4-fold greater than in white

Europeans. However, the association of the wide range of anomalies reported in whites with polythelia has thus far not been experienced in black Americans.

Only a few cases of bilateral *intra-areolar polythelia* have been recorded. Multiplicity of nipples is not uncommon, and they are bilateral in approximately one half of patients so affected. As many as ten nipples have been recorded in a single patient.[25] Atypical locations have been noted secondary to the displaced embryonal primordium. Intra-areolar polythelia represents a nipple-areola unit within the mammary ridge such that a dichotomy of the vestigial breast and nipple-areola complex exists.

The presence of supernumerary nipples may necessitate operative therapy in instances in which discharge, tumor, or cyst formation is evident. Simple excision elliptically placed in lines of cleavage or skin folds is preferred in order to achieve maximum cosmesis. Primary closure is usually possible and allows the surgeon to achieve a superior cosmetic result.

SUPERNUMERARY BREAST (POLYMASTIA)

While congenital supernumerary nipples or breasts may occur in any size or configuration along the mammary milk line, the most common site to observe the abnormally placed mamillae is a line extending from the nipple to the symphysis pubis. As noted above, the supernumerary nipple anomaly may be easily overlooked in young infants, in whom these ectopic lesions often appear only as a small spot with a diameter of 2 to 3 mm. The importance of recognition of this anomaly, clearly, is the potential need for investigation of other associated anomalies. In contradistinction, polymastia results when the embryonic mammary ridge (see Fig. 4–1A) fails to undergo normal regression (see Fig. 4–1B). Causal factors are as yet unknown.

A familial occurrence of the polymastia anomaly has been observed.[86] DeGrouchy and Turleau[26] document the association of polymastia with *congenital cytogenetic syndromes,* especially those involved with chromosomes 3 and 8. The prevalence of polymastia was 0.1 percent in the Collaborative Perinatal Project reported by Chung and Myrianthopoulos,[19] although Orti and Qazi[86] suggest a frequency approaching 1 percent. In a longitudinal survey of minor congenital defects, Méhes[72-74] observed that supernumerary breasts were present in 0.2 percent of children; 8 of the 20 affected children in the study also had *major renal anomalies.* Further, other congenital anomalies, notably *Turner syndrome* (ovarian agenesis and dysgenesis with chromosomal karyotypes of 45,X, but mosaic patterns (45,X/46,XX or 45,X/46,XX/47,XXX) are seen) and *Fleischer's syndrome* (lateral displacement of the nipples to the midclavicular lines with bilateral renal hypoplasia[31]), may have polymastia as a component of the syndrome (Fig. 4–14).

Goeminne[39] documented that renal anomalies often occur together with an abnormal number and/or location of nipples. Previous reports suggest the association between renal adenocarcinoma and renal malformations,

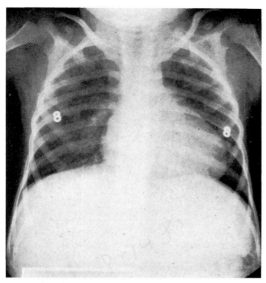

Figure 4–14. Fleischer's syndrome. Posteroanterior chest roentgenogram of a 5-year-old with bilateral renal hypoplasia. Although the clavicles are not horizontal, the lateral displacement of the nipples (designated by the lead markers 8) is apparent. (From Fleischer DS: J Pediatr 69:5(1)806, 1966. Reprinted by permission.)

and one half of the patients with polymastia and kidney cancer in the study by Goedert and coworkers[37] had duplicate renal arteries. The aforementioned reports suggest the association between polymastia, renal anomalies, and renal adenocarcinoma. The observations of Cohen et al.[20] and Fraumeni[33] of renal cancer in young patients with polymastia in comparison with those without this breast anomaly are consistent with earlier onset of several hereditary neoplasms.

ACCESSORY (ECTOPIC) AXILLARY BREAST TISSUE

Ectopic axillary breast tissue is a relatively uncommon occurrence but is a relatively common variant of supernumerary breast tissue. In the human embryo, the mammary ridge first becomes apparent in the 7 to 8 mm long embryo with atrophy prior to birth. It is the persistence of mammalian tissue along the milk line that results in ectopically displaced or accessory breast tissue (see Figs. 4–1 and 4–2). This congenital anomaly is commonly bilateral and is often unaccompanied by the areola or the nipple (Fig. 4–15). Greer[41] noted the presence of accessory axillary breast tissue to be apparent only at or after puberty, with the most rapid growth observed during pregnancy. Kajava[53] classified accessory axillary breast tissue into eight categories as follows: (1) the presence of a complete breast with mammary gland tissue and the nipple-areola complex; (2) the presence of gland tissue and nipple; (3) gland tissue and areola; (4) solitary gland tissue; (5) nipple-areola with fat replacement of the mammary gland tissue *(pseudomamma)*; (6) the nipple alone *(polythelia)*; (7) the areola alone *(polythelia areolaris)*; and (8) the presence of a small patch of hair-bearing tissue *(polythelia pilosa)*.

Clearly, polythelia represents the most common variant of supernumerary breast components and occurs predominantly between the breast and the umbilicus.[41] However, glandular tissue compatible with complete or variable components of breast parenchyma, can occur within the mammary ridge at sites between the axilla and the groin. Jeffcoate[49] suggests that axillary breast tissue may represent true ectopic tissue not contiguous with the breast, but more commonly represents an enlargement of the axillary tail of Spence. Thus, to determine the presence or absence of accessory axillary breast tissue, one must distinguish between an enlargement of the axillary tail and ectopically displaced mammary tissues of the milk line.

The discovery of accessory axillary breast tissue usually occurs during the first pregnancy as a consequence of the secondary changes initiated with hormonal stimulation by ovarian estradiol and placental estriol. The symptomatic axillary breast tissue becomes painfully enlarged and, on rare occasion, may develop galactoceles with milk secretion via contiguous skin pores.[94] While these anomalies may not become evident until the first pregnancy, once the lesions are recognized, they continue to recur with subsequent pregnancies and may undergo cyclical changes during menstruation. DeCholnoky[25] noted pathological findings in 26 cases of axillary breast tissue that included normal breast tissue (nine), cystic disease (ten), fibroadenoma (three), mastitis (four), and atypical ductal hyperplasia (one) or carcinoma (two). Frequently, the clinician will identify the lesion as excess axillary fat, although lymphadenitis, lymphoma, metastatic carcinoma, and hidradenitis suppurativa are frequent misdiagnoses. Following identification of the hormonal dependency with pregnancy or menstruation, the clinician can often establish the diagnosis, especially if a history of lactation during the puerperium is confirmed.

Management consists of reassuring the patient of its common benignity and its embryological origin. However, accessory axillary tissue may be misdiagnosed for

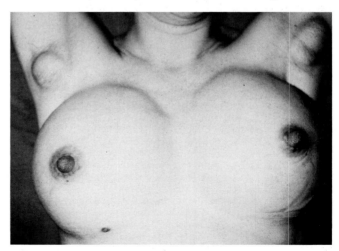

Figure 4–15. Supernumerary breasts presenting as accessory (ectopic) breast tissue bilaterally in the axilla and a right supernumerary inframammary nipple presenting in the mammary milk line. (From Greer KE: Arch Dermatol 109:88, 1974. Reprinted by permission.)

the symptomatic alterations inherent with pathological changes of breast tissue (e.g., carcinoma and the benign breast tissue spectrum). Treatment of symptomatic accessory breast tissue during the puerperium and pregnancy involves conservative management for the majority of clinical presentations. The presence of dense, nodular masses suggestive of malignant transformation necessitates aggressive approaches to rule out carcinoma. As this hormonally dependent accessory breast tissue rapidly regresses when lactation ceases, the patient can be reassured but should be admonished that enlargement and painful, lactating, accessory tissue may recur with subsequent pregnancy. Elliptically placed incisions in skin folds of the axilla allow complete dissection and removal of the breast tissue beneath the skin and over the underlying fascia. The cosmetically oriented resections of the accessory tissue are usually curative, although the lesion may recur if excision is incomplete.

ACKNOWLEDGMENT

The authors gratefully acknowledge the technical assistance and photograms supplied by Dr. Arlan L. Rosenbloom, Department of Pediatrics, and Dr. Hal G. Bingham and Dr. H. Hollis Caffee, Division of Plastic Surgery, University of Florida.

References

1. Abramson DJ: Bilateral intra-areolar polythelia. Arch Surg 110:1255, 1975.
2. Amoroso PJ, Angelats J: Latissimus dorsi myocutaneous flap in Poland syndrome. Ann Plast Surg 6(4):287–290, 1981.
3. Anderson KC, Li FP, Marchetto DJ: Dizygotic twinning, cryptorchism, and seminoma in a sibship. Cancer 53:374–376, 1984.
4. Argenta LC, VanderKolk C, Friedman RJ, Marks M: Refinements in reconstruction of congenital breast deformities. Plast Reconstr Surg 73–80, 1985.
5. Asp K, Sulamaa M: On rare congenital deformities of the thoracic wall. Acta Chir Scand 118:392, 1959.
6. Blackard CE, Mellinger GT: Cancer in a horseshoe kidney: A report of two cases. Arch Surg 97:616–627, 1968.
7. Bland KI, Copeland EM III: Breast disease: Physiologic considerations. In Miller T, Rowlands B (eds): The Physiological Basis of Modern Surgical Care. St Louis, CV Mosby, 1988, pp 1019–1056.
8. Bland KI, O'Neal B, Weiner LJ, Tobin GR II: One-stage simple mastectomy with immediate reconstruction for high-risk patients: An improved technique. The biologic basis for ductal-glandular mastectomy. Arch Surg 121(2):221–225, 1986.
9. Blaydes RM, Kinnebrew CA: Massive breast hyperplasia complicating pregnancy. Obstet Gynecol 12:601–602, 1958.
10. Boenhein F: Uber das Vorkommen uberzahlinger Mamillen und Kombination derselben mit anderen Degenerations-Zeichen. Anat Hefte Arb Anat Inst 57:583–609, 1919.
11. Brightmore TG: Cystic lesion of a dorsal supernumerary breast in a male. Proc R Soc Med 64:662–663, 1971.
12. Buckle R: Studies on the treatment of gynecomastia with danazol/danol. J Int Med Res 5(Suppl 3):114–123, 1977.
13. Camisa C: Accessory breast on the posterior thigh of a man. J Am Acad Dermatol 3:467–469, 1980.
14. Campbell DA: Reconstruction of the anterior thoracic wall. J Thorac Surg 19:456, 1950.
15. Cardoso de Castro C: Subcutaneous mastectomy for gigantomastia in an adolescent girl: Case report. Plast Reconstr Surg 59:575, 1977.
16. Carella A: Supernumerary breast associated with multiple vertebral malformation: Case report. Acta Neurol 26:136–138, 1971.
17. Caufriez A, Wolter R, Govaerts M, L'Hermite M, Robyn C: Gonadotropins and prolactin pituitary reserve in premature thelarche. J Pediatr 91(5):751–753, 1977.
18. Cherup LL, Siewers RD, Futrell JW: Breast and pectoral muscle maldevelopment after anterolateral and posterolateral thoracotomies in children. Ann Thorac Surg 41:492–497, 1986.
19. Chung CS, Myrianthopoulos NC: Factors affecting risks of congenital malformations. I. Epidemiologic analysis. Birth Defects 11(10):1–22, 1975.
20. Cohen AF, Li FP, Berg S, Marchetto DJ, Tsai S, Jacobs SC, Brown RS: Hereditary renal-cell carcinoma associated with a chromosomal translocation. N Engl J Med 301:592–595, 1979.
21. Copeland EM III, Bland KI: The breast. In Sabiston DC Jr (ed): Essentials of Surgery. Philadelphia, WB Saunders, 1987, pp 288–326.
22. Courtiss EH, Goldwyn RM: Reduction mammaplasty by the inferior pedicle technique: An alternative to free nipple and areola grafting for severe macromastia or extreme ptosis. Plast Reconstr Surg 59:500, 1977.
23. David TJ: Nature and etiology of the Poland anomaly. N Engl J Med 287:487, 1972.
24. Deaver JB, McFarland J: The Breast: Anomalies, Diseases and Treatment. Philadelphia, P Blakiston's & Sons, 1917.
25. DeCholnoky T: Accessory breast tissue in the axilla. NY State J Med 51:2245–2248, 1951.
26. DeGrouchy J, Turleau C: Clinical Atlas of Human Chromosomes. New York, John Wiley & Sons, 1977.
27. Desai SN: Sudden gigantism of the breasts. Drug induced? Br J Plast Surg 26:371–372, 1973.
28. Echert M, Hammann HF: Mammaektopic an Rücken. Dtsch Med Wochenschr 100:1395, 1975.
29. Escobar ME, Rivarola MA, Bergadá C: Plasma concentration of oestradiol-17β in premature thelarche and in different types of sexual precocity. Acta Endocrinol 81:351–361, 1976.
30. Fevre M, Hannouche D: Les bréches thoraciques par aplasie ou par anomalies costales. Ann Chir Infant 9:153, 1968.
31. Fleisher DS: Lateral displacement of the nipples, a sign of bilateral renal hypoplasia. J Pediatr 69:5(1):806–809, 1966.
32. Fraser FC: Dominant inheritance of absent nipples and breasts. Novanta anni delle leggi mendeliane. Roma, Istituto Gregorio Mendel, 1956, pp 360–362.
33. Fraumeni JF Jr.: Clinical patterns of familial cancer. In Mulvihill JJ, Miller RW, Fraumeni JF, Jr. (eds): Genetics of Human Cancer. New York, Raven Press, 1977, pp 223–233.
34. Froriep L: Beobachtung eines Falles von Mangel der Brustdruse. Notizen aus dem Gebiete der Natur and Heilkunst 1:9–16, 1839.
35. Furnas DW: Subcutaneous mastectomy for juvenile hypertrophy of the breast. Report of case. Br J Plastic Surg 35:367–370, 1982.
36. Gilly E: Absence complete de mamelles chez une femme mère: Atrophie de membre supérieur droit. Courrier Med 32:27, 1882.
37. Goedert JJ, McKeen EA, Fraumeni JF Jr.: Polymastia and renal adenocarcinoma. Ann Intern Med 95:182–184, 1981.
38. Goedert JJ, McKeen EA, Javadpour N, Ozols RF, Pottern LM, Fraumeni JF Jr.: Polythelia and testicular cancer. Ann Intern Med 101(5):646–647, 1984.
39. Goeminne L: Synopsis of mammorenal syndromes. Humangenetik 14:170–171, 1972.
40. Goldenring J, Crelin ES: Mother and daughter with bilateral congenital amastia. Yale J Biol Med 33:466–467, 1961.
41. Greer KE: Accessory axillary breast tissue. Arch Dermatol 109:88–89, 1974.
42. Guerry RL, Pratt-Thomas HR: Carcinoma of supernumerary breast of vulva with bilateral mammary cancer. Cancer 38:2570–2574, 1976.
43. Guillebaud J, Fraser IS, Thorburn GD, Jenkin G: Endocrine effects of danazol in menstruating women. J Int Med Res 5(Suppl 3):57–66, 1977.
44. Guyda HF, Johanson AJ, Migeon CJ, Blizzard RM: Determination of serum luteinizing hormone (SLH) by radioimmuno-

assay in disorders of adolescent sexual development. Pediatr Res 3:538, 1969.

45. Hassim AM: Bilateral fibroadenoma in supernumerary breasts of the vulva. Br J Obstet Gynaecol 76:275–277, 1969.
46. Hecker WC, Daum R: Chirurgisches vorgehen bei kongenitalen brustwanddefekten. Chirurg 11:482, 1964.
47. Hubert C: Etude sur l'amastie. Thesis. Paris, A Michalon, 1907.
48. Ilicki A, Lewin RP, Kauli R, Kaufman H, Schachter A, Laron Z: Premature thelarche—natural history and sex hormone secretion in 68 girls. Acta Paediatr Scand 73:756–762, 1984.
49. Jeffcoate TNA: Principles of Gynecology. London, Butterworth & Co, 1967, pp 158–159.
50. Jessing A: Excessive mammary hypertrophy in pregnancy treated with androgenic hormones. Nord Med 63:237–239, 1960.
51. Job JC, Guilhaume B, Chaussain JL, Garnier PE: Le développement prématuré isolé des seins chez les fillettes. Arch Fr Pédiatr 32:39, 1975.
52. John C: Uber akzessorische Milchdrüsenaand Warzen, insbesondere über milchdrüsenähnliche Bildungen in der Achselhöe. Arch Gynakol 126:689, 1925.
53. Kajava Y, quoted by Brightmore T: Bilateral double nipples. Br J Surg 59:55–57, 1972.
54. Kenny RD, Flippo JL, Black EB: Supernumerary nipples and renal anomalies in neonates. Am J Dis Child 141:987–988, 1987.
55. Kenny FM, Midgley AR, Jaffe RB, Garces LY, Vasquez A, Taylor FH: Radioimmunoassayable serum LH and FSH in girls with sexual precocity, premature thelarche and adrenarche. J Clin Endocrinol Metab 29:2372, 1969.
56. Kumar S, Cederbaum AI, Pletka PG: Renal cell carcinoma in polycystic kidneys: Case report and review of literature. J Urol 124:708–709, 1980.
57. Lau FT, Henline RB: Ureteral anomalies: Report of a case manifesting three ureters on one side with one ending blindly in an aplastic kidney and a bifid pelvis with a single ureter on the other side. JAMA 96:587, 1931.
58. Lewison EF, Jones GS, Trimble FH, Lima L da C: Gigantomastia complicating pregnancy. Surg Gynecol Obstet 110:215–223, 1960.
59. Li Z, Tong Z, Luo B, Cai H: Congenital hypertrichosis universalis associated with gingival hyperplasia and macromastia. Chin Med J 99(11):916–918, 1986.
60. Lorbek W: Ein Fall von Ureter trifidus. Wien Med Wochenschr 102:222, 1952.
61. Lorino CO, Finn M: Unilateral juvenile hypertrophy of the breast. Br J Radiol 60:193–195, 1987.
62. Luchsinger J: Bilateral mammary hypertrophy during pregnancy. Rev Obstet Ginec Venez 20:707–710, 1960.
63. Mace JW, Kaplan JM, Schanberger JE, Gotlin RW: Poland's syndrome: Report of seven cases and review of the literature. Clin Pediatr 11:98, 1972.
64. Martin JA: Treatment of cystic hygromas. Tex J Med 50:217–222, 1954.
65. Martin LW, Helmsworth JA: The management of congenital deformities of the sternum. JAMA 179:82, 1962.
66. Máte K: Association of polythelia and aberrant ventricular conduction. Orv Hetil 117:1863–1865, 1976.
67. Máte K, Horváth K, Schmidt J, et al: Polythelia associated with disturbances of cardiac conduction. Cor Vasa 21:112–116, 1979.
68. Mathews DN: Treatment of hemangiomata. Br J Plast Surg 6:83–93, 1953.
69. Mayl N, Vasconez LO, Jurkiewicz M: Treatment of macromastia in the actively enlarging breast. Plast Reconstr Surg 54:6, 1974.
70. McFarland WL, Wallace S, Johnson DE: Renal carcinoma and polycystic kidney disease. J Urol 107:530–532, 1972.
71. McKissock PK: Discussion of: Symmastia: The problem of medial confluence of the breast. Plast Reconstr Surg 73:267–269, 1984.
72. Méhes K: Association of supernumerary nipples with other anomalies. J Pediatr 94:274–275, 1979.
73. Méhes K: Association of supernumerary nipples with other anomalies. J Pediatr 102:161, 1983.
74. Méhes K, Szüle E, Törzsök F, Meggyessy V: Supernumerary nipples and urologic malignancies. Cancer Genet Cytogenet 24:185–188, 1987.

75. Miller G, Bernir L: Adenomatose erosive du mamelon. Can J Surg 8:261–266, 1965.
76. Mills JL, Stolley PD, Davies J, Moshang T Jr: Premature thelarche. Am J Dis Child 135:743–745, 1981.
77. Mimouni F, Merlob P, Salomon H, Reisner BM: Occurrence of supernumerary nipples in newborns. Am J Dis Child 137:952–953, 1983.
78. Moore JA, Schosser RH: Becker's melanosis and hypoplasia of the breast and pectoralis major muscle. Pediatr Dermatol 3(1):34–37, 1985.
79. Moss TW: Gigantomastia with pregnancy. Arch Surg 96:27–32, 1968.
80. Moss TW: Therapeutic Radiology. St Louis, CV Mosby, 1959.
81. Mulvihill JJ: Genetic repertory of human neoplasia. In Mulvihill JJ, Miller RW, Fraumeni JF Jr. (eds): Genetics of Human Cancer. New York, Raven Press, 1977, pp 137–143.
82. Nelson KG: Premature thelarche in children born prematurely. J Pediatr 103:756–758, 1983.
83. Nelson MM, Cooper CKN: Congenital defects of the breast—an autosomal dominant trait. S Afr Med J 61(12):434–436, 1982.
84. Ng RCK, Suki WN: Renal cell carcinoma occurring in a polycystic kidney of a transplant recipient. J Urol 124:710–712, 1980.
85. Nolan JJ: Gigantomastia: Report of case. Obstet Gynecol 19:526–529, 1962.
86. Orti E, Qazi QH: Polymastia. In Bergsma D (ed): Birth Defects Compendium. New York, Alan R Liss, 1979, p 874.
87. Palmuth P: Observationem medicarum centuriae tres poshumae, Braunschweig. Cent ii, OBS p. 89, 1648.
88. Parham KJ: Gigantomastia: Report of a case. Obstet Gynecol 18:375–379, 1961.
89. Pasquino AM, Piccolo F, Scalamandre A, Malvaso M, Ortolani R, Boscherini B: Hypothalamic-pituitary-gonadotrophic function in girls with premature thelarche. Arch Dis Child 55:941–944, 1980.
90. Pasquino AM, Tebaldi L, Cioschi L, Cives C, Finocchi G, Maciocci M, Mancuso G, Boscherini B: Premature thelarche: A follow up study of 40 girls. Arch Dis Child 60:1180–1192, 1985.
91. Pers M: Aplasias of the anterior thoracic wall, the pectoral muscles, and the breast. Scand J Plast Surg 2(2):125–135, 1968.
92. Poland A: Deficiency of the pectoral muscles. Guys Hosp Rep 6:191, 1841.
93. Rahbar F: Clinical significance of supernumerary nipples in black neonates. Clin Pediatr 21:46–47, 1982.
94. Raux JP: Lactation from axillary tail of breast. Br Med J 1:28, 1955.
95. Ravitch MM: Congenital Deformities of the Chest Wall and Their Operative Correction. Philadelphia, WB Saunders, 1977, p 233.
96. Ravitch MM: Disorders of the sternum and the thoracic wall. In Sabiston DC Jr, Spencer FC (eds): Gibbon's Surgery of the Chest. 3rd ed. Philadelphia, WB Saunders, 1976, pp 324–369.
97. Ravitch MM: Operative treatment of congenital deformities of the chest. Am J Surg 101:588, 1961.
98. Reiter EO, Kaplan SL, Conte FA, Grumbach MM: Responsivity of pituitary gonadotrophins to luteinizing hormone–releasing factor in idiopathic precocious puberty, precocious thelarche, precocious adrenarche and in patients treated with medroxy-progesterone acetate. Pediatr Res 9:111, 1975.
99. Rich MA, Heimler A, Waber L, Brock WA: Autosomal dominant transmission of ureteral triplication and bilateral amastia. J Urol 137:102–105, 1987.
100. Ryan RF, Pernoll ML: Virginal hypertrophy. Plast Reconstr Surg 75(5):737–742, 1985.
101. Schneider WJ, Hill HL Jr, Brown RG: Latissimus dorsi myocutaneous flap for breast reconstruction. Br J Plast Surg 30:277, 1977.
102. Spence RJ, Feldman JJ, Ryan JJ: Symmastia: The problem of medial confluence of the breasts. Plast Reconstr Surg 73:261–269, 1984.
103. Sperling RL, Gold JJ: Use of an antiestrogen after a reduction mammaplasty to prevent recurrence of virginal hypertrophy of breasts: Case report. Plast Reconstr Surg 52:439, 1973.

104. Tawil MH and Najjar SS: Congenital absence of the breasts. J Pediatr 73(5):751, 1968.
105. Taylor PJ, Cumming DC, Corenblum B: Successful treatment of D-penicillamine–induced breast gigantism with danazol. Br Med J 282:362–363, 1981.
106. Tollerud DJ, Blattner WA, Fraser MC, Brown LM, Pottern L, Shapiro E, Kirkemo A, Shawker TH, Javadpour N, O'Connell K, Stutzman RE, Fraumeni JR, Jr.: Familial testicular cancer and urogenital developmental anomalies. Cancer 55:1849–1954, 1985.
107. Trier WC: Complete breast absence. Case report and review of the literature. Plast Reconstr Surg 36:430–439, 1965.
108. Underwood GB, Gaul LB: Disfiguring sequelae from radium therapy: Results of treatment of a birthmark adjacent to the breast of a female infant. Arch Dermatol 57:918–919, 1948.
109. Urschel HC, Byrd HS, Sethi SM, Razzuk MA: Poland's syndrome: Improved surgical management. Ann Thorac Surg 37:204–211, 1984.
110. Varsano IB, Jaber L, Garty BZ, Mukamel MM, Grunebaum M: Urinary tract abnormalities in children with supernumerary nipples. Pediatrics 73(1):103–105, 1984.
111. Weidman AI, Zimany A, Kopf AW: Underdevelopment of the human breast after radiotherapy. Arch Dermatol 93:708–710, 1966.
112. Weinberg W: Zur vererbung des zwergwuchses. Arch Rass Ges Biol 9:710, 1912.
113. Wilkins L, Blizzard RM, Migeon CJ: The Diagnosis and Treatment of Endocrine Disorders in Childhood and Adolescence. 3rd ed. Springfield, IL, Charles C Thomas, 1965, pp 106–107.
114. Williams IG, Cunningham GJ: Histological changes in irradiated cancer of the breast. Br J Radiol 24:123–133, 1951.
115. Wilson MG, Hall EB, Ebbin AJ: Dominant inheritance of absence of the breast. Humangenetik 15:268–270, 1972.
116. Zubowicz V, Boswick J III: Congenital unilateral hypoplasia of the female breast associated with a large melanotic spot: Report of two cases. Ann Plast Surg 12:204–206, 1984.

Chapter 5

INFLAMMATORY, INFECTIOUS, AND METABOLIC DISORDERS OF THE MAMMA

Kirby I. Bland, M.D.

BREAST DUCTS AND PARENCHYMA

Inflammatory states of the breast are most often recognized following retrograde bacterial infections that result from disruption of the epithelial interface of the nipple-areola complex. *Staphylococcus aureus* and streptococcal bacteria are the organisms evident on Gram stain and culture that are most frequently recovered from nipple discharge in an active inflammatory condition of the breast. Abscess is often related to *lactation in the puerperium* and typically occurs within the first few weeks of breast feeding. Progression of the inflammatory process can result in diffuse breast *cellulitis* with *loculated subcutaneous, subareolar, interlobular (periductal), retromammary, or central unicentric and multicentric abscesses* (Fig. 5–1). Through the diffuse network of the lactiferous duct system, multilocular abscesses may be seen with the presentation of diffuse cellulitis in the systemically ill patient.

In classic streptococcal infections of the breast, there is evidence of diffuse cellulitis with no localization (pointing) until a more advanced stage of disease, when the patient presents with systemic manifestations and bacteremia. In contradistinction, *S. aureus* abscesses tend to have a more localized, deeply invasive, and suppurative presentation with acute and chronic abscess formation. The multilocular abscess, as evidenced in Figure 5–1, is typically seen in staphylococcal infections that initiate loculated suppuration interspersed within interlobular (periductal) sites of the fibrosepta of Cooper's ligaments.

The presentation of an advanced abscess of the breast (Fig. 5–2) necessitates immediate surgical intervention. The diffuse cellulitis of streptococcal lymphatic permeation is often adequately treated with local wound care, including the application of focal heat compresses and the administration of appropriate antibiotics (e.g., penicillin or cephalosporin derivatives). A superficial or deep abscess with overgrowth of any bacterial organism usually presents with point tenderness, erythema, and hyperthermia of the breast. The identification of this clinical disorder necessitates immediate and adequate operative drainage of fluctuant areas to abrogate bacteremia and subsequent sepsis. Thorough debridement of the abscess via a circumareolar incision or multiple nonradial incisions placed in the direction of Langer's lines is recommended. The surgeon must ensure full egress of debris and purulence of the abscess with attention to hygienic evacuation of the cavity. Design of appropriate incisions is essential to avoid necrosis of

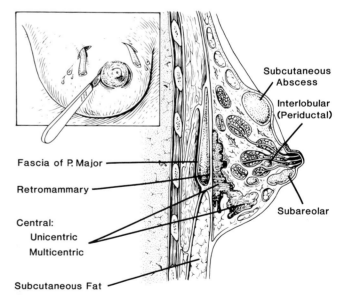

Subcutaneous Abscess

Interlobular (Periductal)

Fascia of P. Major

Retromammary

Central:
 Unicentric
 Multicentric

Subcutaneous Fat

Subareolar

Figure 5–1. Sagittal view of the breast with sites of potential abscess formation that include subcutaneous, subareolar, interlobular (periductal), retromammary, and central areas. Central abscesses may be focal or multicentric. Retromammary abscesses may be seen in chronic infectious or neoplastic processes (e.g., tuberculosis, carcinoma). Deep abscesses may be multilocular and may communicate with subcutaneous or subareolar sites. Painful, diffuse cellulitis is often apparent with deeper abscesses in subcutaneous, interlobular, or subareolar planes. *Insert* above depicts the necessity of thorough drainage and complete evacuation of the abscess via incisions that parallel Langer's lines.

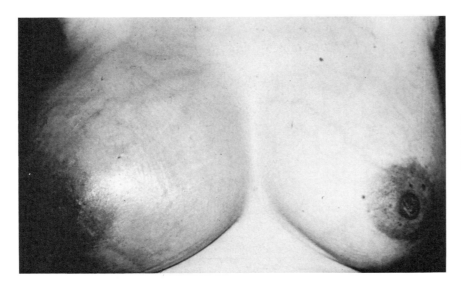

Figure 5–2. Acute, superficial, and deep suppurative abscess of the right breast in a nulligravid 30-year-old female. Following incision and drainage via a periareolar incision, *Staphylococcus aureus* was cultured from the abscess.

skin and subcutaneous tissues. Excision of deep or extensive abscesses with contiguous breast tissue and skin is to be condemned, as postoperative nipple-areola retraction and breast atrophy may result.

Chronic inflammatory states of the breast with abscess formation is unusual, and the clinician must include in the differential diagnosis chronic infectious disorders and neoplastic processes (e.g., tuberculosis, sarcoidosis, carcinoma). Further, one must be aware of the *subacute inflammatory state* of puerperal mastitis observed in the lactating female.

Puerperal (Lactational) Mastitis

Epidemic mastitis has been observed by Colbeck,[41] Sherman,[174] and Ravenholt et al.[155] as a hospital-acquired puerperal infection of the breast that occurs in nursing women who suffer from *milk stasis, noninfectious inflammation, or infectious mastitis.* Thomsen et al.[191] note that recent studies suggest that nursing women with the aforementioned inflammatory symptoms of the puerpera may have these diagnoses based upon leukocyte counts of the milk and quantitative cultures for bacteria. Most commonly, epidemic mastitis is caused by highly virulent strains of penicillin-resistant *S. aureus* transmitted via the suckling neonate.[41, 155, 174] This variant of mastitis is associated with other neonatal staphylococcal infections and may result in substantial morbidity, although rare mortality, in the untreated patient. Often, pus may be expressed from the nipple in epidemic mastitis, as it has been proposed by Gibbard[74] that the inflammatory disorder primarily involves the glandular component of the breast parenchyma.

The presentation of epidemic mastitis makes it incumbent upon the gynecologist to wean the infant from breast feeding, since prolongation of the inflammatory-infectious process will inevitably lead to abscess formation.[95, 174, 178] If weaning and the suckling reflex is not discontinued, the infection may persist or recur, as the

infant may harbor and continue to transmit highly pathogenic strains of staphylococcus.

Nonepidemic (sporadic) puerperal mastitis typically involves the interlobular connective tissue of the breast parenchyma.[74] Gibbard[74] and Newton and Newton[141] observed nipple fissuring and milk stasis as primary pathological mechanisms that initiate this secondary invasive retrograde bacterial infection (Fig. 5–3). Marshall et al.[123] identified similar primary etiological factors, but the causes of the fissuring and stasis were not identified. Leary[111] documented the incidence of sporadic mastitis associated with the puerperal period to be 1.04 percent; Fulton[71] identified the incidence to be 8.9 percent with abscess formation in 4.8[111] to 11 percent.[53] Thomsen et al.[192] noted that for nursing women with inflammatory symptoms, it is possible on the basis of

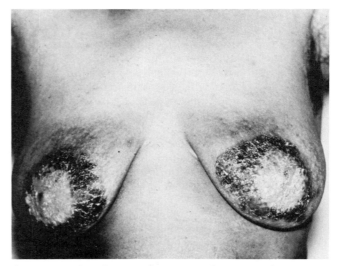

Figure 5–3. Bilateral, nonepidemic (sporadic) puerperal mastitis in a 28-year-old multigravid female that persisted into the sixth week postpartum with breast suckling. Discontinuance of breast feeding, administration of antibiotics, and emptying of the breast allowed rapid resolution of the inflammatory process, which presented with nipple-areolar fissuring and milk stasis.

the leukocyte count of milk and quantitative cultivation of bacteria to classify these cases into (1) milk stasis (counts $< 10^6$ leukocytes and $< 10^3$ bacteria per ml of milk); (2) noninfectious inflammation (counts $> 10^6$ leukocytes and $< 10^3$ bacteria); and (3) infectious mastitis (counts $> 10^6$ leukocytes and $> 10^3$ bacteria). These authors compared the duration and outcome of cases without intervention with those treated by systematic and intensive emptying of the breasts. In many cases this was supplemented by antibiotic therapy as directed by susceptibility tests and culture. The course of milk stasis was of short duration, and the authors confirmed that outcome was excellent and independent of therapy. For cases of untreated noninfectious inflammation, symptoms persisted for several days, and one half the patients developed infectious mastitis. Emptying of the ductal and lobular systems of the breast resulted in a significant decrease in duration of symptoms and a significantly improved outcome. Infectious mastitis *without* treatment was followed by a good result in only 15 percent of cases; 11 percent subsequently developed abscesses. In contrast, emptying of the breast increased the rate of good outcome to 50 percent and significantly decreased duration of symptoms (Table 5–1). Further, the addition of antibiotic therapy was shown by Thomsen et al.[191] to result in a good outcome in 96 percent of cases treated synchronously with emptying of the breast. This combination therapy allows a significant reduction of persistence of symptoms related to the infectious puerperal state. Emptying of the breast has previously been shown by Marshall et al.[123] and Niebyl and coworkers[143] to shorten the duration of symptoms and significantly improve the outcome, with a remarkable reduction in recurrence of the infectious mastitis. Soltau and Hatcher[178] suggest that weaning is important to prevent recurrence of infections from pathogenic bacteria that exist in the infant's nostrils. Erno[66] and Thomsen[190] previously demonstrated that for cases of

infectious mastitis, antibodies develop within a few days in the mammary glands and may protect against recurrence.

Bacteriological assessment of human milk is often difficult because of contamination with the normal flora of skin bacteria. Moon and Gilbert[136] determined that a jet of milk taken from the normal mother and cultured on blood agar will be sterile in over one half the samples. Further, Wright[217] confirmed that colony counts of the bacterial growths vary from 10 to 4500 colonies per ml. Marshall et al.[123] determined that nonepidemic (sporadic) acute puerperal mastitis was evident in 2.5 percent of mothers who elected to nurse their infants. Interestingly, *S. aureus* was cultured from the milk in 23 of 48 (47.9 percent) infected breasts and was identified bacteriologically from only one breast of 19 normal mothers. Further, 41 of 48 (85.4 percent) women with mastitis continued to nurse without difficulty for an average of 13 weeks, although mastitis recurred in 8.3 percent. Breast abscesses that resulted from mastitis and that required therapy were evident in only 4.6 percent of these patients with acute, puerperal, nonepidemic mastitis. Marshall et al.[123] state that, considering the limitations of their culture technique, it is possible that the skin of the nipple and areola of women with mastitis is more likely to be colonized with *S. aureus* than is the skin of the noninfected mother. However, despite the presence of *S. aureus* within the cultured milk, the continuation of nursing during therapy for mastitis caused no apparent illness in any infant in this reported series. Duncan and Walker[59] have previously noted that bacteria in maternal milk does not appear pathogenic to the infant. Further, maintenance of lactation during mastitis has been shown by Applebaum[8] to enhance resolution of the inflammatory process by the reduction in congestion of the breast parenchyma. In this series, continuation of lactation allowed greater than two thirds of 61 women with mastitis to continue breast feeding for an average of 13 weeks.

With breast feeding in the postpartum state and evidence of progressive stasis, mastalgia, and persistent growth of bacteria in the lactiferous ducts, discontinuance of lactation is essential to enable resolution of the inflammatory process. The use of a breast suction pump may, on occasion, be advantageous to empty stagnant milk ducts and central abscess collections. The continuance of lactation following removal of the suckling reflex may necessitate the use of intramuscular injections of stilbestrol or testosterone enanthate/estradiol valerate (Deladumone). Usually, the addition of these antilactational drugs is not necessary, as discontinuance of suckling and provision of adequate breast support are sufficient to initiate cessation of lactation.

We agree with Thomsen et al.[191] that the treatment of infectious mastitis requires emptying of the breast and the administration of appropriate antibacterial coverage. Patients with signs and symptoms of florid mastitis should immediately be treated by penicillinase-resistant penicillins, regardless of the bacterial or leukocytes counts of expressed milk.

Patients who present with nonpuerperal infectious

Table 5–1. COURSE OF INFECTIOUS MASTITIS WITH AND WITHOUT TREATMENT THAT CONSISTS OF EMPTYING OF THE DUCT AND LOBULAR SYSTEMS OF THE BREAST ALONE OR IN COMBINATION WITH SYSTEMIC ANTIBIOTIC THERAPY

Treatment	No. of Cases	Duration of Symptoms (days, mean)	Result (No. of Cases)	
			Normal Lactation	*Poor**
None	55	6.7	8	47
Emptying of the breast	55	4.2	28	27
Antibiotics and emptying of the breast	55	2.1	53	2

*Breast abscess, 6 cases; symptoms of sepsis, 12 cases; recurrence of symptoms, 32 cases; duration of > 14 days, 20 cases; impaired lactation only, 27 cases.

From Thomsen AC, Espersen T, Maigaard S: Am J Obstet Gynecol 149:492, 1984. Reprinted by permission.

mastitis or noninfectious inflammations of the breast should have mammography followed by prompt drainage of the abscess with biopsy of any viable tissue near or within the abscess cavity. Differential diagnosis of an inflammatory breast mass presenting in the nonlactating female includes chronic recurring subcutaneous or subareolar infections, carcinoma, tuberculosis, inflammatory cysts, and duct ectasia. Finally, the reader is reminded that suppurative mastitis may occur in *infants* and is most often related to *S. aureus* or gram-negative organisms.[30, 181] Prompt expression of the nipple with Gram staining and culture of the discharge is important prior to incision and drainage of the offending bacterial infection. The surgeon should not resect local breast tissues with inflammatory lesions of the nipple, areola, or breast parenchyma in the infant or child, as such practices may cause maldevelopment or agenesis of rudimentary structures of the organ.

Mamillary Fistula

The entity mamillary fistula was initially proposed in 1953 by Hedley Atkins[10] to describe a fistulous opening from the periareolar or areolar skin into a lactiferous duct. The process had been described by Zuska and colleagues[219] some four years earlier, but it was Atkins who described in detail its presentation and therapy. This fistulous process establishes itself as a chronically discharging lesion in or near the region of the areola and is often predated by a history of subcutaneous breast abscess that discharges and then recurs. Atkins acknowledges that many patients have undergone repeated operations and that the process appears refractory to incision and drainage.[10]

Initial recommendations by Atkins included passage of a probe into the discharging sinus with entry into the fistulous tract and an exit via the nipple-areolar duct mechanism. Thereafter, the tract was saucerized and allowed to heal by granulation. In 1958, Patey and Thackeray[149] suggested that complete excision of the tract is appropriate, while Hadfield[85] recommended excision of the major duct system for this benign process.

Pathology. Often the fundamental pathological process cannot be determined at operation. Confusion about the etiology and pathology of the mamillary fistulas includes that in the original descriptions by Zuska et al.,[219] who noted that squamous epithelium lined the fistula and considered same to be a dilated lactiferous duct. Thereafter, Patey and Thackeray[149] observed the fistula to be lined by granulation tissue that communicated with one of the major mammary ducts. Lambert et al.[109] observed nonspecific chronic inflammation to be common, whereas communication between the fistulous tract and a lactiferous duct was clearly demonstrated in only 4 of 38 cases (10.5 percent). Several authors repeatedly failed to identify communication between the areola and the lactiferous duct either macroscopically or microscopically and suggest that the fistula originates and remains in the subepidermal glands.[35, 36, 120] Further, Abramson,[1] Tedeschi et al.,[186] and Sandison and

Walker[169] suggest the fundamental abnormality is stasis with dilatation of the major ducts. This pathological observation was not confirmed by Lambert et al.,[109] although communication with the duct system may be demonstrated in some patients.

Therapy. Mamillary fistulas should be suspected and sought in any patient who presents with periareolar or subcutaneous abscesses juxtaposed to the nipple and/or areolar complex. The lesions are painful and may be associated with toxic shock syndrome (which will be discussed subsequently). Therapy is similar to that described in the following section on periareolar abscess in the nonlactating breast. With presentation as a discharging abscess, a fine lacrimal probe may be inserted within the fistula tract under local anesthesia and manipulated to emerge via the nipple. When a subareolar abscess is present, pressure on the abscess may initiate discharge of pus via the nipple or the site of probe placement. Many cases can be adequately managed by simply laying open the tract along the course of the lacrimal duct probe. Larger fistulas with well-established epithelialized tracts are optimally treated with excision of the fistulous tract in its entirety and packing of the wound abscess. The defect is allowed to granulate, or it may be loosely approximated with fine monofilament nylon suture. All suppurative wounds should be cultured, as bacterial flora that exist antecedent to toxic shock syndrome should have established sensitivities to cultures prior to recognition of the clinical syndrome.

Caswell and Maier[36] and Maier et al.[120] stress that reconstruction of an inverted nipple (Fig. 5–4) is an important surgical concept for treatment of this process. Lambert et al.[109] made no attempt to evert the nipple in the majority of their cases, and no recurrence ensued. These authors caution that attempts to cosmetically correct and restore contour of the nipple may lead to incomplete excision of the fistulous tract and the possibility of recurrence.

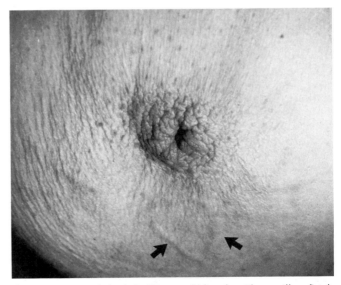

Figure 5–4 Inverted nipple in 35-year-old female with mamillary fistula. Dilated venous plexus (*arrows*) can be seen circumscribing the periareolar abscess.

Periareolar Abscess in the Nonlactating Breast

The nipple-areola complex is a highly sensitive end-organ in which neurosensory stimuli are easily recognized. Moreover, inflammatory states of this component of the breast can result in early and sometimes disabling symptoms. Retrograde bacterial infections commonly induce *periareolar abscesses* as a consequence of disruption of the epithelial interface, with subsequent entry of normal flora of skin bacteria. As noted with lactational mastitis, streptococcal bacteria and *S. aureus* are the organisms most commonly identified on Gram stain and culture that initiate periareolar abscess in the nonlactating female. Because the abscess is superficial and has associated cellulitis, simple drainage is often insufficient (Fig. 5–5). While various operative procedures for this condition have been introduced in several clinics, uniformly successful therapy has not been established. Further, Watt-Boolsen et al.[210] identified few reports that have explicitly dealt with primary therapy of *central abscesses* of the breast since these lesions are often the cause of relapse. These authors attempted to identify therapeutic failures requiring additional therapy and proposed a treatment policy. The estimated recurrence rate for periareolar abscesses of the nonlactating breast in this Danish series was 38 percent at eight years following simple incision of the abscess. Similar relapse rates have been identified by Leach et al.[110] In contradistinction, Rosenthal and associates[164] reported superior results following repeated needle aspiration of pus from the abscess and concomitant administration of systemic antibiotics. The recurrence rate for this series was 10 percent at an average follow-up time of 18 months. Further, only those patients treated initially with incisions in the Rosenthal series had development

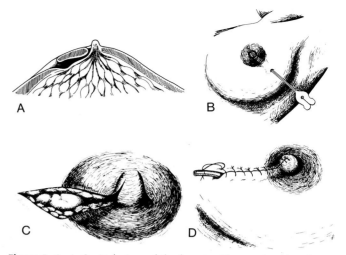

Figure 5–6. *A,* Sagittal view of the breast with a periareolar abscess and nipple sinus. *B,* A probe is passed through the sinus tract between the abscess and the nipple. *C,* Extent of excision required to remove the infected sinus tract and correct the nipple inversion when present. *D,* Primary closure over a Penrose drain or small Robinson catheter. (From Maier WP: Am J Surg 144:359, 1982. Reprinted by permission.)

of a fistula. Watt-Boolsen et al.[210] note that 10 of 11 recurrences represented fistulas within the line of surgical incision. This concept was originally proposed by Deaver et al.[51] in 1918 in their classic treatise on the breast. Moreover, Patey and Thackeray,[149] Hadfield,[85] and Urban[200] independently concluded that *excisional therapy* for the small periareolar abscess is associated with a lower recurrence rate than is *incisional therapy.* Excisional therapy has also been supported by other investigators.[84, 106, 120] We concur with Ekland and Zeigler[64] that the higher recurrence rate observed in the aforementioned series utilizing incisional techniques is expectant and that this approach, predictably, is unlikely to result in resolution of the primary abscess. Further, the inability of these authors to identify recurrences early in the natural history of the disease, and the tendency for some abscesses to recur, suggest that etiologically the origin of these periareolar abscesses is multifactorial. Investigators suggest that primary bacterial invasion is the cause for the ductal inflammatory state[28] or that the cause is related to primary ductal disease with secondary bacterial invasion from normal skin flora.[1, 84, 92, 94, 169, 186, 189, 196, 219] Kilgore and Fleming[106] and Maier et al.[120] postulate that a primary inflammatory process of the periareolar and areolar components (sweat and sebaceous glands) and the accessory mammary glands may be involved in the process.

We agree with the therapeutic strategy proposed by Maier and associates[120] in that treatment of the primary abscess is optimal with use of a small, periareolar, nonradial incision. Following incision, the breast abscess cavity is evacuated and the wound is dressed and maintained over the next few days with scrupulous hygienic care (Fig. 5–6). Two to three days after resolution of the acute inflammatory process, a fine probe is inserted into the cavity in an attempt to identify the sinus tract

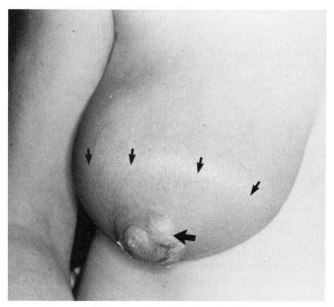

Figure 5–5. Superficial subareolar and periareolar abscess (*large arrow*) in the lactating breast of a 35-year-old multigravid female. Small arrows denote advancing margins of cellulitis.

(Fig. 5–6B). When the tract is discovered, a small radial incision (Fig. 5–6C) is created with excision of a small amount of the overlying skin and areola. The excision of this portion of the skin should be inclusive of all infected tissue but should not include uninvolved quadrants of the breast. When the tract communicates with the nipple, a V-shaped incision of this segment of the nipple is appropriate (Fig. 5–6C). Thereafter, the wound is saucerized and allowed to granulate with strict attention to hygienic wound care. The application of topical antibacterial agents is optional. In the experience of the author and others,[120, 149, 210] healing usually occurs within six to eight weeks with superior cosmetic results. Using the aforementioned techniques allows a remarkable decrease in recurrence of the periareolar abscess.

Atkins[10] identified the coexistence of *carcinoma of the breast with periareolar abscesses*. This infrequent occurrence is coincidental, and the periareolar abscess does not represent a premalignant lesion. The presentation of a periareolar abscess in the pre- or postmenopausal era should prompt the physician to search for an inflammatory carcinoma. The presence of a subareolar mass with overlying cellulitis is suggestive of, but not to be confused with, this ominous neoplastic process (see Chapter 9). Xeromammography is appropriate following identification of a subareolar mass and *prior* to drainage of the abscess. In selected patients, incision of a fluctuant abscess associated with a carcinoma may be necessary prior to initiating therapy of the neoplasm. Sufficient biopsy material to establish the diagnosis of the neoplastic process should be obtained at the time of drainage of the periareolar abscess.

Toxic Shock Syndrome Following Breast Surgery

In 1978, Todd and associates[195] described toxic shock syndrome (TSS) associated with phage group 1 staphylococci. The majority of the initial reports related to menstruating women and the use of intravaginal tampons. More recently, however, TSS has been recognized following various surgical procedures, the majority of which involve some variant of foreign body placement (prostheses, tampons) or packing of a wound or body cavity.[194] Barnett et al.,[16] Uretsky et al.,[201] and Bresler[26] document varying time intervals in which TSS occurred from occult postoperative wound infections related to augmentation mammaplasty. The criteria of the toxic shock syndrome are given in Table 5–2. The typical patient is premenopausal and has had remote operations on the breast, typically, with recent biopsy or augmentation mammaplasty. The onset of symptoms is temporarily related to a biopsy two to three days earlier, or in some reports, to the insertion of a tampon. Often, within 72 hours, the patient becomes lethargic, tachypneic, hyperthermic, and tachycardic with precipitous changes in the systolic blood pressure.[198] Wannemaker[208] and Jacobson et al.[97] suggest involvement of at least three organ systems to meet the classic criteria of TSS. Organ system involvement may include gastrointestinal,

Table 5–2. CRITERIA FOR TOXIC SHOCK SYNDROME

Fever—temperature ≤ 38.9°C (102°F)
Rash—diffuse macular erythroderma
Desquamation—one to two weeks after onset of illness, particularly of palms and soles
Hypotension—systolic blood pressure ≤ 5th percentile by age for children 16 years or younger; orthostatic fall in diastolic blood pressure ≥ 15 mm Hg from lying to sitting; orthostatic syncope or orthostatic dizziness
Involvement of at least three of the following organ systems:
  Gastrointestinal—vomiting or diarrhea at onset of illness
  Mucous membranes—vaginal, oropharyngeal, or conjunctival hyperemia
  Renal—blood urea nitrogen or creatinine levels ≥ 2 X ULN, or ≥ 5 leukocytes per high-power field, in the absence of urinary tract infection
  Hepatic—total bilirubin, serum aspartate aminotransferase or serum alanine aminotransferase levels > 2 X ULN
  Hematologic—platelets ≤100,000 per μl
  Central nervous system—disorientation or alteration in consciousness without focal neurological signs when fever and hypotension are absent
Negative results on the following tests if obtained:
  Blood, throat or cerebrospinal fluid cultures, although blood cultures positive for *Staphylococcus aureus* are accepted by some authors
  Serological tests for Rocky Mountain spotted fever, leptospirosis, or rubeola

ULN = upper limit of normal.
Bresler MJ: Toxic shock syndrome due to occult postoperative wound infection. Case Report. West J Med 139(5):710–713, 1983.
Wannemaker L: Toxic shock: Problems in definition and diagnosis of a new syndrome. Ann Intern Med 96:775–777, 1982.
Ganem D: Toxic Shock Syndrome—Medical Staff Conference, University of California, San Francisco. West J Med (Nov); 135:383–388, 1981.
From Follow-up on toxic-shock syndrome. MMWR 29:441–445, 1980.

musculoskeletal, mucous membranes, kidneys, liver, hematopoietic, or central nervous systems. Postoperative wound infection was a rare cause of TSS, accounting for less than 1 percent of all cases reported to the Centers for Disease Control between January 1, 1980 and July 31, 1981.[18] The TSS cases identified in our institution are typically associated with an occult wound infection with absence of physical signs of a local infectious process. Such innocuous, occult presentations have also been documented by Reingold et al.[157] Typically, the wound abscess is not discovered or appears to be innocuous at the time of attempted drainage with removal of the augmentation implant. A majority of the cases have been associated with postoperative staphylococcal wound infections, and the bacterium is commonly coagulase-positive.

Infections related to insertion of breast implants are relatively uncommon. In the series reported by Courtiss et al.,[46] *S. aureus* is by far the most prevalent organism and may be a component of a mixed infection with *Pseudomonas aeruginosa* or *Staphylococcus epidermidis*. These infections occur in the postoperative period and have a higher incidence if associated with postoperative hematoma formation. In cases without toxic shock syndrome, treatment by conservative drainage and intravenous antibiotics may allow salvage of the implants.

Clegg and associates[40] noted paraprosthetic infections secondary to the mycobacterium bacilli *(M. fortuitum and M. chelonei)* over a 3.5-year period following implantation of prostheses for breast augmentation. These wounds may initially appear innocuous or occult but are often chronic and refractory to therapy with various antimicrobial agents. In a survey of plastic surgeons by Clegg and associates,[39] there was no evidence of epidemic mycobacterial wound infections following 39,455 augmentation mammaplasties. This survey determined that the estimated rate of wound infection by all organisms following this procedure was 0.64 percent, with only five cases of mycobacterial wound infections documented. Further, this species of bacteria was not implicated in the toxic shock syndrome. Although *S. epidermidis* represents a potentially common cause of subclinical infections in breast prostheses, which is perhaps related to capsular contracture around silicone implants,[173] no data exist that implicate *S. epidermidis* in the causation of TSS.

A clinical study conducted by Ransjö et al.[154] concluded that subclinical infections play a role in capsular formation around silicone breast implants. In evaluating the role of antibiotic prophylaxis in preventing capsular formation, these authors acknowledged that bacterial cultures of breast wounds are essential to identify potential agents causing capsular contraction. Samples taken from 25 patients (49 breasts) perioperatively at the time of reduction mammaplasty were cultured on agar plates and incubated both aerobically and anaerobically. In over 90 percent of the samples, bacteria grew abundantly. The species of bacteria most commonly identified were *S. epidermidis* and propionibacteria. Both organisms were sensitive to penicillin G and/or isoxapenicillin. The authors were unable to conclusively demonstrate that prophylactic antibiotics will decrease capsular formation during augmentation mammaplasty.

More recently, Thornton and associates[193] studied endogenous microbiological flora of the human breast and its role in breast infections following subglandular augmentation or reduction mammaplasty. A total of 231 cultures were obtained from 59 breasts of 30 patients who were followed over 12 months. Thornton et al.[193] identified no fungi cultured from any specimen; 53 percent were positive for coagulase-negative staphylococcus. Common aerobic flora included lactobacillus, D-enterococcus, diphtheroids, micrococcus, and Á-hemolytic streptococcus. The most frequently cultured anaerobic bacterium was *Propionibacterium acnes.* Other anaerobes included *Clostridium sporogenes* and peptococcus. These authors found no correlation between the type of bacterial flora and the depth within the breast from which the culture was obtained. Postoperative wound infections were identified in 2 of 19 patients (10.5 percent) undergoing reduction mammaplasty. Importantly, a 25 percent capsular rate at one year was identified in 20 subglandular augmentation mammaplasties. No bacteria were identified at the time of mammaplasty surgery in two capsules, whereas three were associated with coagulase-negative staphylococcus, diphtheroids, and *P. acnes.* The authors established that

breast tissue in areas remote from the nipple contains a flora that is similar to that of normal skin. Further, cases of infection were identified in which endogenous bacteria were correlated with later infection.

Therapy. The low-grade, innocuous-appearing wound infection may be misleading in the early phases of TSS. Presentation with progressive *rash formation* (diffuse macular erythroderma), *fever* ($\geq$ 38.9°C), and continual *deterioration of hemodynamic parameters* necessitates rapid resuscitation and identification of the occult infectious source. Progressive involvement of the aforementioned organ systems is indicative of an overwhelming bacteremia related to the *S. aureus,* which is often coagulase-positive. Rapid fluid administration and initiation of systemic intravenous antibiotics (e.g., synthetic penicillins specific for coagulase-positive staphylococci) have important roles in resuscitation. Intravenous β-lactamase–resistant antibiotics, such as the synthetic penicillins or cephalosporins, should be administered prophylactically when the potential for TSS exists. Crucial to therapy, however, is operative drainage of the infected site, which may require opening of the breast operative site or re-excision of infected, necrotic tissues. TSS related to augmentation mammaplasty should be suspected, even weeks to months following placement of the prosthesis. With the emergence of new staphylococcal strains of bacteria that are capable of inducing severe septicemia with consequent hemodynamic and multisystem organ failure, a high index of suspicion is necessary to abort this potentially lethal clinical syndrome.

Mammary Tuberculosis

Tuberculous mastitis is a rare entity. Gottschalk et al.[78] and Haagensen[83] estimate that approximately 700 cases have been reported in the medical literature. The first description of tuberculous mastitis is credited in 1829 to Sir Astley Cooper, who stated, "In young women who have enlargement of the cervical absorbent glands, I have sometimes, though rarely, seen tumors of a scrofulous nature form in their bosoms."[43, 88, 142, 211] However, in the 40 years following Cooper's original description, only two cases, both in men, were reported.[211] Azzopardi[11] and Hamit and Ragsdale[87] note the incidence of the disease to vary from 0.025 to 4.5 percent of all surgically treated breast diseases. In India, the documented incidence of breast tuberculosis has been reported to be between 1 and 4.5 percent.[54, 57, 139] It is estimated that between 9 million and 10 million people suffer from pulmonary tuberculosis in India.[148] However, few cases of tuberculous mastitis have been documented, perhaps because of lack of patient awareness with manifestation of the disease and the lack of adequate (available) medical care in Third World countries. The disease is extraordinarily rare in Western countries and is confined mainly to the immigrant population.[77] Despite the frequency with which tuberculosis was reported in the era that preceded antimicrobial chemotherapy, recognition and documentation of tuberculous mastitis were unusual.

The majority of reported cases of tuberculosis of the breast have appeared from Western countries; the infrequency of the disease is related to the present rarity of pulmonary and other variants of tuberculosis. Schaefer[171] documented two cases in 2141 breast specimens received for histopathological examination, while Wilson and MacGregor[214] identified only five cases of tuberculous mastitis in a population of 500,000 over a 15-year period.

Clinical Presentation. The disease is seen almost exclusively in females. In the series of 439 patients reported by Morgan,[137] 4 percent were males. For females, tuberculous mastitis has been reported from the age of 6 months to 84 years.[54, 77] Epidemiological data confirm that women in the reproductive age group, and especially during the lactational period, are more vulnerable to the infection.[137, 139, 214] Thus, growth of the tuberculous bacilli is augmented by the vascularity and stasis of the lactating breast. In the review by Banerjee et al.,[14] 82.5 percent of patients were in the reproductive age group and 33 percent were lactating at the time of clinical presentation. Although both breasts are equally vulnerable to the disease, bilateral disease is rare and was observed by Wilson and MacGregor[214] in only 3 percent of patients with tuberculous mastitis. Duration of symptoms varies from a few months to several years, but the majority have symptoms for less than 12 months.[57, 137, 139]

The most frequent symptom is a single nodule of the breast;[5, 54] multiple masses are rare.[54] The presentation of tuberculous mastitis is that of mastalgia more often than is seen with carcinoma. Banerjee et al.[14] noted infrequent involvement of the nipple-areola complex. Fixation to skin is frequent;[214] however, the breast remains mobile unless the mastitis is secondary to extension from tuberculosis of the underlying ribs and/or chest wall. The lump is often irregular, firm, and ill defined. As regional lymph nodes are often involved, evidence of fixation and an ill-defined mass on examination make the clinical distinction of tuberculous mastitis from carcinoma difficult.[14] In the series reported by other authors,[79, 130] there may be associated nipple retraction and peau d'orange with *coexisting tuberculosis and carcinoma of the breast.* Careful review of the literature and critical analysis of reported cases by these authors indicate that this unique pathological combination was originally described in 1899 by Warthin.[209] Four additional cases[117, 134, 177, 207] were reported between 1902 and 1933. The report by Miller and associates[130] suggests that of reported cases of breast tuberculosis, approximately 5 percent were associated with cancer. As this frequency approximates the lifetime probability of a woman in the United States developing breast cancer, it would appear that the coexistence of cancer and tuberculosis is coincidental. No evidence has been presented that establishes a causal relationship of the two diseases.

Mode of Infection. Wilson and MacGregor[214] initially determined that as much as 60 percent of breast tuberculosis was *primary.* However, it is now accepted that mammary tuberculosis is almost invariably *secondary* to a tuberculous process of contiguous or remote sites.[54] Gupta et al.[82] suggested that coincidental tuberculosis of the faucial tonsils of suckling infants is the most common route of infection for the primary variant of tuberculous mastitis in the Indian population. Retrograde extension of the acid-fast *Mycobacterium tuberculosis* bacilli may occur in a way physiologically similar to that described previously for breast infections with inoculation through the nipple and into the duct system. Abrasions of the skin may also be portals of entry for bacteria, although this is a less frequent route of infection. Dharkar et al.[54] note that tuberculous mastitis is most commonly initiated via retrograde lymphatic spread from cervical or axillary lymphatics, and less commonly from the primary pulmonary site to the paratracheal and internal mammary lymphatics. Hematogenous dissemination and direct spread from contiguous structures are additional routes for extension of the primary infection.

McKeown and Wilkinson[127] in their classic description of tuberculous mastitis note five histological types:

1. *Acute miliary tubercular mastitis,* in which the disease is established from blood-borne infection as part of a generalized miliary spread. It is recognized primarily in an autopsy series of patients who died of acute fulminant tuberculosis.

2. *Nodular tuberculous mastitis,* the most common variant, exhibiting caseation and chronic abscess formation with and without sinuses in a single quadrant of the breast.[139]

3. *Disseminated tuberculous mastitis,* the second most common variant, in which tubercles are found throughout the breast with multiple sinuses.

4. *Sclerosing tuberculous mastitis,* in which there is minimal caseation, characterized by shrinkage of breast parenchyma with early skin retraction and late sinus formation. Clinically, this variant is often indistinguishable from carcinoma.

5. *Tuberculous mastitis obliterans,* the rarest form, in which there is intraductal infection with obliteration of the ductal system and fibrosis. Sinus tract formation is rare in this variant.

Diagnosis and Treatment. Hale et al.[86] note this entity to be a disease of women between the ages of 20 and 40 years; it is rare in men, the elderly, and prepubescent girls. Evidence to support the diagnosis of tuberculous mastitis includes local pain, purulent discharge, and the presence of tuberculosis in a remote site of the body. However, the most reliable diagnostic studies comprise bacteriological cultures of the acid-fast bacilli aspirate, histological examination of tissue, and guinea pig inoculation.[87] D'Orsi et al.[56] note the microscopic appearance of biopsy material to typically consist of granulomatous inflammatory infiltrates with central caseation.

Following wedge or excisional biopsy with appropriate bacteriological cultures to confirm the diagnosis, patients should be started on active systemic chemotherapy. Dharkar has used local streptomycin successfully.[54] The therapy of tuberculous mastitis requires a combination of antituberculous drugs (*streptomycin, INH* [isonicotine hydrazine], and *thiacetazone* or *PAS [para-amino salicylic acid])* *with surgery.* In 1963 Wilson and MacGregor[214] recommended simple mastectomy, since local recurrence developed in the majority when lesser procedures were applied. Today most authorities agree that antimicrobial therapy with the aforementioned triple therapy or rifampin substituted for streptomycin combined with excision of necrotic tissue and drainage is adequate.

Mukerjee et al.[139] attempted repeated needle aspiration of a tuberculous breast in an elderly woman who had intercurrent medical disease and was considered inoperable. The success of this conservative method prompted recommendation of antituberculous drugs in conjunction with repeated needle aspiration for six months. In Western countries, conservative approaches are dictated by the presence of intercurrent residual disease, patient noncompliance, the potential for unreliability of patient therapy, and therapeutic responses. The consensus is that optimal results are achieved following *excisional therapy* and a course of *antituberculous drugs.*

Although mammary tuberculosis is rare in industrialized and Western societies, widespread travel is changing the epidemiological characteristics of many diseases. Despite the rarity of tuberculous mastitis, this primary or secondary infection should be considered in the differential diagnosis for inflammatory disorders of the mamma.

Mammary Sarcoidosis

Sarcoidosis is a multisystem, idiopathic disorder with a diverse clinical spectrum that is characterized morphologically by the presence of granulomas that classically involve lymph nodes, lungs, spleen, liver, eyes, bone marrow, and the parotids. Despite its multiorgan involvement, sarcoidosis of the breast is rare, as evidenced by the paucity of reported cases. Gansler and Wheeler[24, 72, 73, 153, 170, 172, 179] document 19 cases of mammary sarcoidosis up to 1984. Until the 1940s, the rarity of mammary sarcoidosis was accounted for by the inability to distinguish sarcoidoisis from tuberculosis on a morphological and bacteriological basis. Indeed, early reports of mammary sarcoidosis include a patient with positive tuberculin skin tests,[49] while another patient described by Rubin and Penner[165] had acid-fast bacilli that were subsequently identified in autopsy tissues.

Clinical Presentation and Diagnosis. Mammary sarcoidosis may present clinically in variable forms (Fig. 5–7). The patient may have a solitary, mobile, nontender breast mass that is indistinguishable from and suspect for carcinoma. Wedge or excisional biopsy of the lesion confirms *noncaseating granulomas* at microscopic examination. This diagnosis should not be confirmed until other potential causes of granulomatous mastitis have been excluded.[175] In rare cases, granulomatous mastitis may be the clinical manifestation of typhoid, brucellosis, leprosy, cryptococcosis, phycomycosis, North or South American blastomycosis, sporotrichosis, histoplasmosis,

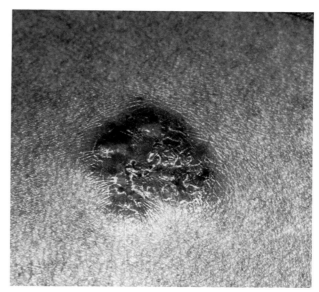

Figure 5–7. Cutaneous extension of mammary sarcoidosis with an encrusted, draining peripheral lesion of upper outer quadrant of breast. This nontender breast mass was thought to be a carcinoma. The patient had noncaseating granulomas in the breast. Thereafter the patient was confirmed to have pulmonary sarcoidosis.

coccidioidomycosis, hydatid disease, cysticercosis, filariasis, or *Oxyuris* infestation.[11, 33, 72, 83, 116, 127, 156, 158, 160, 168, 185, 212, 218] Gram stain and cultures for specific organisms are appropriate and are usually more sensitive than histological stains. Sections prepared with stains should not contain acid-fast bacteria, metazoa, foreign bodies, or fungi.

The patient with this variant of granulomatous mastitis often has a documented history of lymphatic or pulmonary sarcoidosis. The parenchymal breast lesions of nonspecific granulomatous mastitis and mammary sarcoidosis contain granulomas, giant cells, and chronic inflammatory cell populations. However, necrosis of ductal epithelium, microabscess formation, and fat necrosis are rarely seen histopathologically in mammary sarcoidosis. In contradistinction, granulomas that are noncaseous are pathognomonic of sarcoidosis, especially in the patient with pre-existing lymph node or pulmonary sarcoidosis and anergy to a battery of skin tests. Diagnosis is commonly established on the radiographic evidence of bilateral hilar lymphadenopathy and elevated serum concentrations of *angiotensin converting enzyme (ACE)* and the serum *lysozyme.*[163, 183] In addition to anergy of skin tests, the *Kveim test* is usually strongly positive with multiple epithelioid granulomas.[15]

Therapy. Ablative surgery is not necessary unless there is histopathological confusion with carcinoma, in which case total mastectomy for a diffuse infectious process may be appropriate. Bodo et al.[22] were able to establish the diagnosis with fine needle aspiration cytology, thereby avoiding ablative surgery. Following excision or wedge biopsy of infectious tissue, the diagnosis may be established histopathologically and may be confirmed with supporting adjunctive tests (ACE, lysozyme, Kveim test). As mammary sarcoidosis may be clinically mistaken for malignant or benign neoplasms of the breast, biopsy must be performed on clinically suspicious lesions whether or not disseminated sarcoidosis is evident. Therapy is directed at systemic manifestations of the disease.

Oleogranulomatous Mastitis

This rare variant of mastitis is an illness that appears to be exclusively endemic to Hong Kong women who wish to improve the size and form of their breast. Etiologically, oleogranulomatous mastitis occurs from a relatively inexpensive form of mammaplasty that involves the injection of liquefied paraffin wax or beeswax into the breast parenchyma. While the results of the mammaplasty are immediately gratifying, the long-term effects of injections present the surgeon with serious dilemmas that include the differentiation from carcinoma, breast abscesses, skin and tissue sloughing, and breast necrosis.

Oleogranulomas are easily confused with carcinoma of the breast, as it is often possible for these patients to present initially with an advanced ulcerating mass of the breast and/or chest wall.[4] In nonsuppurative oleogranulomatous mastitis, bilateral presentation; the absence of nipple retraction, peau d'orange, or enlarged lymphatics; and the lack of skin involvement despite the extensive presentation of the process suggests a benign etiology. Despite this presentation, biopsy is essential to differentiate oleogranulomas from carcinoma. Pathologically, the histological features include (1) chronic granulomas with foreign body giant cells that contain lipid vacuoles, foam histiocytes, and an inflammatory cell population; and (2) the total absence of caseating granulomas indicative of tuberculous mastitis. The history of liquefied paraffin or beeswax injection is confirmatory. In the series reported by Alagaratnam,[4] uninfected paraffinomas were successfully treated by simple excision, whereas infected ulcerating lesions required extensive wide excision and drainage and, on occasion, simple mastectomy. Preservation of uninvolved skin is essential, and in appropriate cases, subcutaneous mastectomy followed by placement of a subpectoral mammary prosthesis is possible.

Parasitic Infestations

Parasitic infections of the breast are infrequent and are primarily confined to isolated cases in nonindustrialized societies. The majority of case reports describe *hydatid disease, filariasis,* and infestation with the *guinea worm.*

In 1924, Mills[131] documented the mechanism of infection by *hydatid cysts* of the *Echinococcus.* Ingestion of food contaminated by eggs of the echinococcus allows the protective membrane of the eggs to be dissolved by gastric and duodenal secretory enzymes. This digestive process frees the hexacanth embryos, which burrow into the mucosal capillaries and then infest the liver via the portal venous blood. Venous filtration of embryos by the liver and pulmonary microcirculation occurs in approximately 85 percent of infestations; thus, 15 percent are left to develop into cysts within other organs of the body. The *Casoni test* is positive in the majority of patients with hydatid echinococcosis. Hydatid disease occurs throughout the world and especially, in countries where sheep raising is a primary occupation. Despite the possibility of infestation of any organ, the breast is perhaps the organ least often involved by hydatid disease. Herrera-Vegas[90] collected reports of 970 cases of the disease in his 1909 treatise of hydatid disease; only two patients had documented involvement of the breast. Mirza and associates[133] noted that the presenting symptom is a mass in the infected breast, which may be confused with carcinoma. Makki[121] reported three cases of hydatid cysts of the breast that were successfully treated by surgical excision via a radial incision. Axillary lymph node dissection in one patient confirmed nonspecific lymphadenitis. Makki suggested that hydatid disease may be confused with fibroadenomas, chronic cystic mastitis, or carcinoma.[121]

Chandrasoma and Mendis[37] and Cooray[44] previously identified *filarial infections* of the breast; many of these parasitic infestations occurred in women from Sri Lanka. The presenting feature of the infection is a firm mass that appears in less than three months within a segment or quadrant of the breast. In many instances, the presentation of peau d'orange, skin fixation, and a hard, dense mass is suggestive of a malignant process. Excision of the involved inflammatory process is curative. Histologically, an inflammatory process encapsulates the filarial worms.

Dracunculiasis, or *guinea worm infestation,* was observed by Stelling[180] to be endemic to the Middle East, Pakistan, India, and areas of Africa. Infestation with the guinea worm occurs by ingestion of water contaminated with the parasite. Frequently, the patient presents clinically with a skin vesicle overlying a site of calcified intramammary parenchymal dracunculus. Stelling observed mammagraphically calcified and retained worms of the adult female in breast parenchyma that is surrounded with fatty replacement. This author points out that other parasitic diseases may likewise calcify. Hydatid disease produces a fine, ringlike calcification, while filariasis presents as calcified worms shorter than 4 mm in total length.

Actinomycosis of the Breast

Few cases of documented actinomycosis of the mamma have been reported since the 1893 documentation of this bacterial infection by Ammentrop.[7] Actinomycosis is a chronic granulomatous bacterial infection that clinically resembles a deep fungal process, initiated in man by the etiological agent *Actinomyces israelii*. This microaerophilic or anaerobic bacterium grows only in tissues where the oxygen tension is reduced or in devitalized subcutaneous spaces. Pathognomic of the disease is the formation of granulomatous draining sinus tracts from which the clinician can identify sulfur "granules." Skin and sinus tract involvement occurs secondary to extension from the underlying focus as it burrows to the skin surface.

While cervicofacial actinomycosis ("lumpy jaw") is the most common clinical manifestation and is expressed as a nodular enlargement beneath the mandible, one may also see abdominal and thoracic variants. The cervicofacial form accounts for essentially two thirds of all cases. Breast actinomycosis may occur either primarily or secondarily by extension of the infection from the lungs into and through the parietal pleura of the thoracic cage.[96] Only rarely will the physician be suspicious of this rare diagnosis, owing to the variety of clinical presentations that more commonly affect the mamma. The thoracic variant of actinomycosis may not be a primary process but rather may occur as a complication of lung abscess, lung cancer, bronchiectasis, or other pulmonary infections favorable to the growth of this anaerobic bacterium.

Minsker of Russia reported on a complement fixation test that utilizes an antigen-like substance called actinolysat.[132] This test was positive in the majority of cases in which the actinomyces or characteristic filaments were identified. The differential diagnosis from cancer must be established, as the infection may mimic an inflammatory variant of carcinoma. Further, Gogas et al.[76] suggested that when sinus tract formation from actinomycosis occurs, the disease must be differentiated from chronic suppurative mastitis, syphilis, tuberculosis, and chronic osteomyelitis of the ribs.

Therapy. The therapy of this rare but aggressive mammary infection is primarily medical. Penicillin remains the most effective antibiotic for the therapy of *A. israelii*. For severe actinomycotic infections, penicillin should be initially administered intravenously in large quantities (4 million to 6 million units per day). For patients with documented allergies to penicillin, tetracycline or erythromycin may be substituted. The sulfonamides are less effective antibacterials for this organism.

Mammary actinomycosis that is refractory to prolonged antibacterial therapy with penicillins or a penicillin substitute (tetracyline, erythromycin) requires operative management and debridement. This more radical form of therapy usually necessitates abscess drainage, extensive debridement, or in rare cases, simple mastectomy or radical mastectomy. Pemberton[150] documented the rare necessity of radical mastectomy to operatively manage extensive actinomycosis that involves breast skin, parenchyma, and/or musculature of the chest wall. All operative debridement or extirpation procedures should be covered perioperatively and postoperatively with antimicrobials active against the organism.

Subcutaneous Fungal Infections of the Breast (Superficial and Deep Mycoses)

Fungal infestations of the breast parenchyma are rare. Köhlmeier and Kreitner[107] reported on mammary *blastomycosis*, and Jung[100] reported on *sporotrichosis*. Israel[96] notes that the breast parenchyma may be involved either primarily or secondarily by extension of fungal infections from the lung through the thoracic cage. Preoperative diagnosis of mammary fungal infections is rarely established by clinical examination or xeromammography owing to the various clinical presentations that must be distinguished from more common breast lesions of primary and secondary origin.

Lloyd-Davies[115] considered the nipple to be the site of entry for mammary infections. In support of this observation, the majority of patients have lesions that are located in the region of the areola, while sinus tracts and abscess cavities are in proximity to the lesions. Further, Cope[45] and Lloyd-Davies[115] considered the infection to be caused by intraoral fungi that were inoculated into the breast parenchyma by the suckling infant or with kissing. Such fungal infections may present as recurrent mammary abscesses juxtaposed to the nipple or the areola; advanced cases confirm distortion of the nipple-areola complex with fibrosis, scarring, and sinus tract formation. Thin pus may be expressed from the sinus tracts near the nipple, and the discharge may be admixed with blood. With radial spread of the infection, the gland adheres to underlying tissue of the chest wall. Progression of the fungal process allows extension into the thoracic or abdominal cavity. Gogas and associates[76] noted that lymph nodes are not involved by the disease. However, secondary infection of sinus tracts with lymphangitic extension of the fungal infection will lead to inflammatory enlargement of regional lymphatic glands, making the distinction from carcinoma difficult.

Diagnosis. The diagnosis of fungal infections is established by histological examination of fluids and tissues infected with the organisms. Characteristic filaments of the various fungal classes are evident. With expression of thin pus from the abscess or sinus tract, diagnosis can be established by culture of the causative organism or by staining of smears containing fluid or tissue obtained from the abscess or tract. Because fungi are fastidious with respect to culture and isolation, more than one examination and culture is often necessary. The diagnosis of cutaneous *mammmary blastomycosis* is confirmed by collecting material from the miliary abscess and demonstrating round budding organisms in potassium hydroxide mount or a McMannus-stained smear. Cultures are essential, and biopsies from the border of the lesions may be necessary for diagnosis. As the organism is weakly antigenic, complement-fixing antibodies are ordinarily not detectable. Aspiration of unruptured subcutaneous breast nodules in disseminated cases may be excellent sources of culture material.

For the diagnosis of *mammary sporotrichosis*, cultures from unopened lesions permit definitive diagnosis; the fungi, which exhibit thermal dimorphism, are readily grown. Staining of biopsy smears with periodic acid–

Schiff reaction after digestion with diastase often identifies the fungal elements. Serological and sensitivity reactions are adjunctive techniques that may assist the clinician in diagnosis. Circulating antibodies (agglutinins, complement-fixing antibodies, and precipitins) are often present in cases with systemic involvement. Essentially all patients with sporotrichosis have cutaneous reactivity to a heat-killed vaccine or to a polysaccharide prepared from fungal medium.

Therapy. The treatment of fungal infections of the breast skin and parenchyma is both medical and surgical. The medical therapy of fungi in the preantibiotic area consisted primarily of application of thymol and potassium iodide. Appropriate cultures and sensitivity tests from the purulent discharge are essential to select the antibiotic that represents the most effective antifungal agent. Amphotericin B and stilbamidine derivatives are the most effective antifungal agents active against *blastomycosis*. After a test dose of a few milligrams, the initial dose of stilbamidine is 0.25 mg per kg body weight; this may be increased to 0.6 mg per kg to a total of 3 gm. Dihydroxystilbamidine may be effective for breast blastomycosis associated with pulmonary disease. The daily dose is 225 mg in 500 ml of saline given to a total dose of 8 gm.

Iodides continue to be specific chemotherapy for the typical cutaneous variant of *sporotrichosis* but are ineffectual for systemic, disseminated, or internal forms of the fungal disease. In fact, this is the only mycosis in which curative administration of iodides is beyond dispute.[6] The mode of action of iodides as antifungal agents is unknown, but they apparently increase the resistance of the host nonspecifically. Potassium iodide is administered in increasing doses to tolerance (e.g., 5 drops three times daily over one month to 40 drops three times per day). With rising agglutination titers or complement fixation tests, amphotericin B is considered necessary treatment. For disseminated and extracutaneous sporotrichosis, amphotericin B is indicated, especially in the presence of a rising titer with complement fixation tests or agglutination. This drug is given in doses similar to those used in the therapy of blastomycosis. The dosages must be individualized because of the well-known toxicity of amphotericin B. Amphotericin must be given by slow intravenous infusion, and therapy must be individualized to reduce hepatotoxicity, nephrotoxicity, hypokalemia, and anemia; it can be gradually escalated to a maximal daily dose of 0.6 mg per kg. A total dosage of 3 gm is usually sufficient. Dihydroxystilbamidine is quite effective in patients with minor pulmonary symptoms and few or single cutaneous lesions. It is of particular value in patients with pre-existing renal disease. This drug is administered as a daily dose of 225 mg in 500 ml of saline to a total dose of 8 gm.

Antifungal therapy may be necessary for months, and in many cases may eliminate the necessity of surgical intervention. When indicated, however, drainage of the abscess, quadrantectomy, or simple mastectomy may be essential to eradicate the refractory infection.

Candidal Intertrigo of the Breast

This seemingly innocuous variant of *Candida albicans* is classified as a systemic mycosis. Patients so infected have the demonstration of large quantities of *C. albicans* in scrapings from the lesion, thus providing the primary criterion for diagnosis of candidal intertrigo. Characteristically, the inframammary area is involved with a weeping, eroded lesion that has scalloped borders with a definable margin of sodden scales and an intensely red surrounding skin margin (Fig. 5–8). The presence of satellite flaccid vesicopustules supports the diagnosis. Other common sites of involvement include the groin, the axilla, and the intergluteal fold. The lesions are

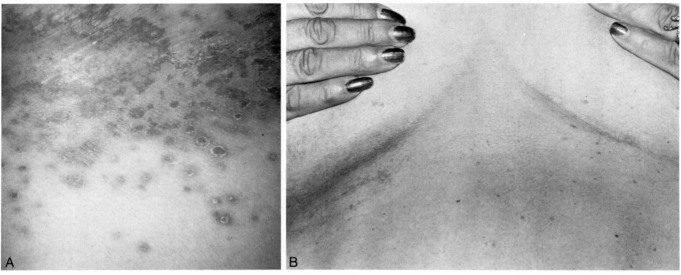

Figure 5–8. *A,* Close-up view of advancing cutaneous *Candida albicans* intertrigo involving the inframammary folds of 64-year-old diabetic female. *B,* Resolution of candidal inframammary infection following control of the hyperglycemic diabetic state and treatment of the intertriginous infection with topical nystatin.

commonly confused with seborrheic dermatoses, and the two lesions may exist concurrently.

Diagnosis. The diagnosis is established with identification of abundant quantities of filaments and budding cells in material obtained from the vesicopustules. Isolation by culture technique is essential to confirmation. Serological reactions offer little evidence of *C. albicans,* and skin tests have no value in diagnosis. Blood of many patients with systemic candidiasis contains anticandidal agglutinins in low titer. These agglutinins may become escalated in extensive systemic variants of the disease. The recently introduced immunodiffusion test has proved to be of diagnostic value in chronic disseminated forms.

Therapy. Therapy of candidal intertrigo necessitates the removal of predisposing factors of inframammary skin maceration. Water-miscible preparations of clotrimazole or nystatin should be used, as ointment vehicles serve to perpetuate the maceration. The combination of nystatin with antibacterial antibiotics or steroids is to be condemned if the diagnosis is established. Clotrimazole is the most widely used preparation, as it has antifungal and bactericidal activity.

Superficial Fungal Infections of the Breast

Tinea (Pityriasis) Versicolor

This common superficial fungal infection is known solely through its habitation of the skin surface of living persons. Easily diagnosed, tinea versicolor is noninflammatory, chronic, and asymptomatic. It is considered noncontagious and is seen in greater frequency in patients who are geographically exposed to excessive humidity and heat. Sweating plays a major role in exacerbation and recurrence of the organism *Pityrosporum,* which is responsible for this superficial mycosis.

Lesions of tinea versicolor may develop a curious confluent pattern that is easily visualized with a Wood's lamp. Typical lesions are macular patches of varying sizes, shapes, and color that vary from white to fawn to brown—thus the designation "versicolor" (Fig. 5–9). The skin most frequented and subsequently colonized by the varying strains of *Pityrosporum* is the upper torso; other common sites include the neck, face, lower abdomen, and proximal extremities. The pruritus associated with the lesions and the subsequent scratching initiate a fine scaling that contains numerous organisms of *P. orbiculare* or *P. ovale.*

Diagnosis and Treatment. Diagnosis is established by direct microscopic examination of scrapings with staining of strains of the fungi using the Hotchkiss-McMannus stain. Almost any of the active fungicidals have activity against tinea versicolor, including clotrimazole, miconazole, sodium thiosulfate, and haloprogin. The daily application of these solutions or creams initiates prompt disappearance of the patches, decreasing of the pruritic response, and eventual clearing of involved skin. Enhancement of the response may be achieved with a suspension of selenium sulfide. Adequate therapy requires that all involved areas be treated with antifungal agents, which include shampoos with selenium sulfide. As recurrence is common, the patient should be advised to promptly re-treat specific sites if necessary.

Common Viral Infections of the Breast

Molluscum Contagiosum

This common poxvirus infection of the skin occurs predominantly in children and young adults. Lesions of childhood molluscum appear predominantly on the trunk, face, and limbs as a consequence of skin-to-skin, and possibly, fomite-to-skin transmission. Becker et al.[19] note the infection to be one of several sexually transmitted diseases of viral etiology that occur worldwide.

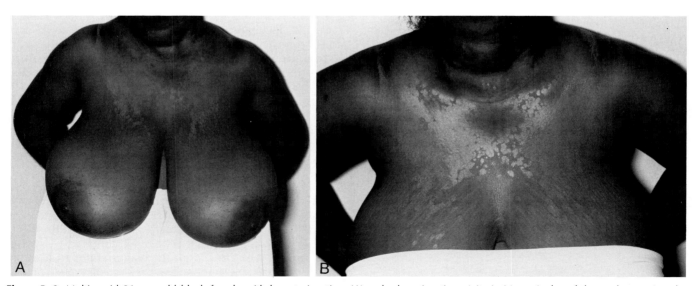

Figure 5–9. Multigravid 31-year-old black female with breast gigantism *(A)* and advancing tinea (pityriasis) versicolor of the neck, anterior chest wall, and breasts *(B).* The superficial fungal infection rapidly resolved following clotrimazole therapy.

Lesions that appear on the breast or upper torso are characteristically discrete, slightly umbilicated, pink to gray, dome-shaped papules. The papules range in size from 2 to 5 mm but may be as large as 1 to 2 cm.

On pathological examination, the epidermis is observed to grow into the dermis to form the saccules that harbor clusters of the molluscum contagiosum virus (Fig. 5–10). As intracytoplasmic inclusions move into the upper stratum of the epidermis, they will stain eosinophilic. These characteristic intracytoplasmic inclusion bodies harbor mature, immature, and incomplete forms of the virus that are referred to as the molluscum body.

Diagnosis. On light microscopic examination of the central portion of the lesions, Giemsa or Wright stain reveals the brick-shaped inclusions that are readily identified. Recently, Penneys and coworkers[151] used tissue obtained from formalin-fixed, paraffin-embedded blocks containing the virus as a source of antigen to generate a polyclonal antibody against the virus. This antibody was capable of recognizing an antigen in molluscum bodies that was preserved during routine fixation and embedding.

Therapy. The treatment of molluscum contagiosum cutaneous involvement of the breast and thorax is surgical. The lesions can be merely shelled-out with a curette. Low-voltage electrocautery, light cryosurgical freezing, or laser therapy is often effective as well. Every effort should be made to preserve breast contour and skin cosmesis following excision of these benign lesions.

Herpes Simplex and Herpes Zoster

The *herpes simplex virus* is one of the most ubiquitous infections of man. Involvement of the breast alone by herpes simplex is extraordinarily rare. Infections with the virus usually become manifest by two mechanisms: (1) primary infection, in which the susceptible individual has no neutralizing antibodies to the H. simplex virus;

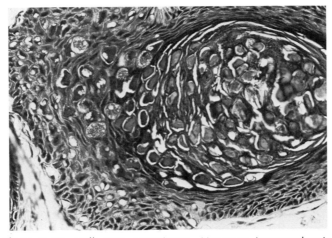

Figure 5–10. Molluscum contagiosum. Numerous intracytoplasmic viral inclusions, called molluscum bodies, appear in the lower epidermis, increase in size as they move toward the surface, and eventually compress and displace the nucleus. (Courtesy of Dr. Lori Shehi, Department of Pathology, University of Florida, Gainesville, FL.)

and with (2) recurrent infections in individuals who have previously been inoculated with the virus and possess specific H. simplex antibody. The latter infection is extraordinarily common; primary infections infrequently produce recognizable clinical symptoms in patients.

In contradistinction, *herpes zoster (shingles)* and *varicella (chickenpox)* are morphologically and etiologically indistinguishable, encapsulated herpetic viral infections that produce similar cytopathological changes, complement-fixation reactions, and cross-reacting antibodies (IgM and IgG).[29] It is postulated that epidemics of chickenpox frequently follow exposure to the H. zoster viral infection, and varicella is regarded as the primary manifestation of the varicella-zoster viral exposure. These viruses lie dormant in dorsal root ganglia to recur in the form of the zoster infection that follows the sensory nerve root to the cutaneous surface distribution, where the vesicles become evident. Recurrence of the H. zoster infection is observed when antibodies, either complement-fixing or neutralizing, fall below an infectious level. These infections may occur in any season but have a predilection for winter months. The most contagious phase is in the prodromal and vesicular stages, in which the transmission is airborne or by contact. Neonatal passive immunity is minimal for the H. zoster infection in comparison with the immunity for H. simplex.

Distribution. The lesions of recurrent H. simplex infection are observed primarily on the perioral and lip area or the genital region. However, herpes simplex lesions may occur on any cutaneous area and are a serious form of conjunctivitis and associated keratitis. These recurrent herpes simplex lesions may occur in a distribution similar to that of H. zoster, and differentiation may be difficult. Vesicles of the typical lesion occur invariably in a herpetiform fashion with an erythematous base. They may appear as eight to ten grouped lesions or as single vesicles, 2 to 3 mm in size, that do not coalesce.

In contrast, varicella infections that involve the dermatomal segments of the skin of the breast have a natural incubation of 10 to 20 days and a 24-hour prodrome characterized by malaise, fever, and exanthem. Soon after, there are eruptions of scarlatiniform pink to red papules, typically 2 to 4 mm in diameter, that coalesce to form a central 3 to 4 mm vesicle surrounded by a red halo. Thereafter, the vesicular lesions become turbid with leukocyte infiltration; the lesion becomes umbilicated and then dries and crusts to form a thick scale and scar. The distribution is typically central, with predominant involvement of the scalp, face, and trunk, often with involvement of one or both breasts (Fig. 5–11).

Treatment. No established or consistent therapy is possible for the latent herpes simplex viral infection. Type I variant, which is usually associated with nongenital lesions, is the strain that most commonly involves the breast. The prevention of bacterial superinfections is of considerable importance. Should the neck or face be involved concomitantly, an ophthalmological antibiotic solution may be used. When multiple sites have

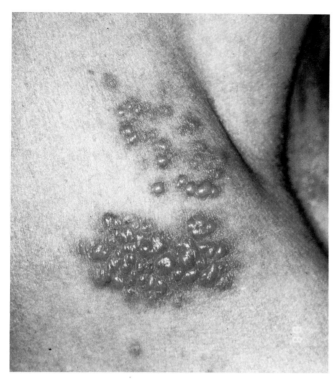

Figure 5–11. The typical appearance of vesicular eruptions of herpes zoster (shingles) in dermatomal distribution of the torso, axilla, and left breast. These painful lesions subsequently became umbilicated, dried, and encrusted to form a scale and scar in the axilla and upper outer quadrant of the breast. (Courtesy of Dr. Frank Flowers, Division of Dermatology, Department of Medicine, University of Florida, Gainesville, FL.)

serious diffuse involvement that is unresponsive to topical steroid instillation, the administration of systemic steroids may be appropriate. For associated keratitis or keratoiritis, the hourly instillation of idoxuridine arabinoside, acyclovir, or trifluorothymidine may be necessary. The possibility of recrudescence of the infection in similar areas of the breast, face, or neck is possible, as the virus is often harbored in the epithelial cells or contiguous neurons. Activation of these latent "phases" will reactivate the virus.

Currently, no specific chemotherapy for varicella exists. Fortunately, this self-limited childhood infection requires no active therapy. In the childhood variant, lesions of the breast and chest wall should be kept dry, and pruritic sites should be treated with a shake solution and oral antihistamines. The administration of prophylactic antibiotics, particularly in a child, is to be discouraged, as such therapy may initiate antibiotic-resistant infections. As the primary infection induces immunity, recrudescence is uncommon. In the immunosuppressed patient, hyperimmune gamma globulin should be administered. Further, adenine arabinoside may be administered for five to seven days in the severely ill patient, as may acyclovir.

Shingles that appear in the dermatomal distribution of the torso, breast, and neck often initiate severe pain as a long-lasting postherpetic neuralgia that should be treated with dry compresses and appropriate analgesics.

In the prodromal phases of pain with shingles, the administration of corticosteroids may be attempted but is rarely of value. Eaglestein and associates[62] recommend the administration of steroid equivalents of 40 mg of prednisone a day for three to six weeks unless contraindicated. Unfortunately, postherpetic neuralgia may persist for months or years. Cordotomy and rhizotomy are rarely effective. Little success has been obtained with the subcutaneous administration of analgesics and steroids into the trigger areas of the dermatomal segments involved with the active H. zoster infection. Kernbaum and Hauchecorne[105] observed decrease of H. zoster pain and a decrease in the probability of postherpetic neuralgia following administration of levodopa (100 mg) with benzerazide (25 mg) three times per day for ten days.

Hidradenitis Suppurativa of the Breast Areolae

This chronic inflammatory process of the apocrine glands was originally described in 1839 by Velpeau,[203] who documented the clinical presentation of axillary and perineal abscesses. However, it was Verneuil,[205] in 1844, who correctly stated that the infection had origin within sweat glands.

The presentation of *hidradenitis suppurativa* of the breast areola is infrequent and has been confirmed by Glass and Vecchione.[75] The chronic inflammatory state originates within the large sebaceous glands (apocrine glands of Montgomery) that are located as tubercles on the surface of the areola. The glands of Montgomery secrete a thick, proteinaceous, and lipoid material responsible for lubrication and skin protection of the nipple during nursing and exposure. These glands are most active in the two decades that follow puberty. Dvorak et al.[61] postulated that patients with chronic acne have a greater propensity to develop hidradenitis suppurativa in multiple sites despite an intact host-defense immune system. The nipples are usually spared the inflammatory process that supervenes.

Diagnosis and Therapy. The clinical course is that of chronicity—recurring abscesses about the nipple and areola with associated draining sinuses, vesicles, cellulitis, and furuncles. With progression of a superimposed bacterial infection, deep central or subareolar abscesses are possible. The history often confirms repeated treatment with incisions and drainage, the administration of systemic and topical antibiotics, and possibly the injection of steroids. This chronic inflammatory state may mimic frankly invasive carcinoma, Paget's disease of the nipple-areola, or chronic inflammatory states (e.g., tuberculosis, sarcoidosis, superficial and deep mycoses, and actinomycosis). Usually the breast maintains symmetry and the parenchyma is well preserved without demonstrable abscesses or lesions that are evident on mammography. With compression of sinus tracts, scars, or pustules, the clinician may express purulent discharge from the glands of Montgomery in one or both areolae.

The patient is rarely systemically ill from this superficial cutaneous infection.

Therapy is directed at control of the inflammatory process by elimination of the chronic infection of the apocrine glandular system of the areolae. Excision may be accomplished under local anesthesia and sedation. When areolae are partially involved, the nipples may be preserved. Defects created with partial loss of the areolae may be covered with advancement flaps from the ipsilateral breast or split-thickness skin grafts from noncontiguous sites. Usually, complete excision of the areolae is essential to abrogate the infectious process and donor split-thickness grafts are required to cover the debrided areolae. Options include total resection of the nipple-areola complex and reconstruction with labia or inner thigh skin with free graft of skin to form a neonipple.

Syphilis of the Breast

In this era, the presentation of *primary* or *secondary syphilis* with chancres or secondary gummas of the breast is rare in developed countries. This infectious disease is initiated by *Treponema pallidum*, a motile, spiral organism of the spirochete family. The infection is acquired primarily through sexual exposure; untreated syphilis in pregnancy may result in congenital syphilis in the offspring. Thus, the disease may occur in both acquired and congenital forms.

Both primary and secondary variants of cutaneous involvement of the breast have been reported. Gummas of the breast (Fig. 5–12) have been reported by Adair[3] and by Braunstein and Woolsey.[25] Because the diagnosis of syphilis of the mamma in the early twentieth century was difficult, these cases must be considered dubious as to their authenticity.

Diagnosis. The diagnosis of *primary syphilis* is established with darkfield examination and the finding of *T. pallidum* and with reagin and treponemal blood test results. The blood reagin assay may not be reactive if the chancre has been present for less than one week. The rapid plasma reagin circle-card test (RPR-CT) is a supersensitive assay that can be performed in five to ten minutes, it came into use following the original application of the Venereal Disease Research Laboratory (VDRL) test. The RPR-CT is usually reactive by the seventh day of appearance of the chancre; the VDRL test may not be reactive at this time and may need to be repeated. The fluorescent treponemal antibody-absorption (FTA-ABS) test will also be positive when the reagin test is reactive and is more sensitive than this test. Within two to six weeks, the primary chancre of the breast will heal without treatment and the patient will then progress to *secondary syphilis*. The secondary stage follows the onset of primary syphilis by 9 to 90 days (average, three weeks). Thus, the chancre is frequently in the healing phase or has completely disappeared at the time of recognition. The presentation of secondary syphilis has been grouped into three syndromes: (1) influenza-like presentation with fever,

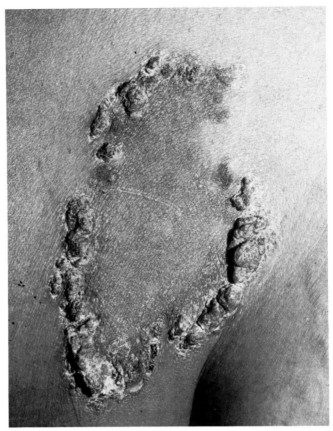

Figure 5–12. Gumma of secondary syphilis in upper outer quadrant of left breast. Syphilis was confirmed by RPR-CT and VDRL. Treatment included benzathine penicillin-G, 2.4 million units, for two consecutive weeks. Thereafter, the gumma healed and the reagin blood test became seronegative.

weight loss, anemia, lymphocytosis; (2) diffuse lymphadenopathy; and (3) a generalized rash that follows the lines of cleavage, especially along the trunk. There is a special predilection for the palms and soles. This generalized rash frequently involves the upper chest and breasts. Lesions are discrete and sharply demarcated and have a coppery hue. The early cutaneous expression of secondary syphilis includes the macular or erythematous eruptions that may appear on the breast six to eight weeks following the infectious exposure.

Therapy. Recognition of *primary syphilis* necessitates rapid administration of benzathine penicillin G, 2.4 million units intramuscularly each week for two consecutive weeks (total, 4.8 million units). For patients allergic to penicillin, tetracycline hydrochloride, 500 mg four times daily for 12 days, or doxycycline or minocycline, 100 mg every 12 hours for 12 days, or erythromycin, 2 gm per day peroral for 12 days, is administered. With this primary presentation the chancre of the breast is expected to heal within two to four weeks following therapy. Patients should be advised that they are sexually infectious for at least the 24 hours following initial administration of the penicillin or for five days following administration of nonpenicillin substitutes.

Therapy of *secondary syphilis* is similar to that for the primary infection. The Jarisch-Herxheimer reaction, or "therapeutic shock," will be experienced by the patient some two to four hours following therapy with penicillin. The treated patient frequently complains of fever, headache, joint pain, and chills. Thereafter, the rash that involves the breast, chest wall, and other sites becomes edematous and more brilliant. Such reactions are not to be confused with penicillin allergies. The therapy of the Jarisch-Herxheimer reaction includes the administration of aspirin or aspirin substitutes, bed rest, and fluids. This reaction does not occur following tetracycline therapy. The patient should be evaluated monthly until the reagin blood test becomes seronegative, an event that is expected within 24 months following the patient's first exposure to syphilis.

Osteoradionecrosis of the Thoracic Wall with Cellulitis

Cellulitis that accompanies osteoradionecrosis of the chest wall may be a formidable presentation in the postmastectomy patient. Frequently, the patient is many years post modified or radical mastectomy and has no evidence of regional or systemic disease. Depending upon the degree of advancing cellulitis and/or associated abscess formation, the process may involve partial- or full-thickness aspects of the chest. The process is usually initiated by radiation therapy for either breast or for pulmonary malignancies.[112]

The biological principles for delivery of radiation suggest that this modality has the inherent potential for tissue necrosis. Older orthovoltage irradiation machines (250 kV) produced considerable cutaneous damage secondary to the progressive vascular intimal sclerosis.[27] As a consequence of this high energy to focal sites of the chest wall, acute and insidiously chronic skin, muscle, and bony injuries were common. Wolbach[216] described radiation dermatitis over 60 years ago and suggested

that the cause has an increased tissue fragility secondary to vasculitis. The advent of state-of-the-art megavoltage radiotherapeutic devices with electron beams has reduced regional tissue damage, which produces osteoradionecrosis in the therapeutic site.

Diagnosis. Clinical presentation of *acute osteoradionecrosis* is that of a second- or third-degree thermal burn with erythema, tenderness, blistering, and edema. There is frequently diffuse concentric dermatitis, often with a central site of full-thickness tissue destruction (Fig. 5–13). The central defect is variable, and its extent is dependent upon the duration of the neglected wound and the presence of superinfection with the bacterial flora. The more frequent presentation is *chronic osteoradionecrosis* that presents as a debilitating, severe ischemia of variable extent of the anterior chest wall. It occurs secondary to irradiation ischemia and fibrosis to induce tissue destruction, ulceration, infection, and even secondary malignancies (e.g., sarcomas).

Characteristic microscopic histology includes atrophy of the dermal appendages, epidermal thinning, endarteritis, proliferative fibrosis, and endophlebitis. As bone and cartilage have a marginal vascular supply, these areas are more susceptible to radiation injury and subsequent transmural extension of the destructive process to include the parietal pleura and the lung. Chest computed tomography and routine x-rays may be helpful in determination of the extent of the destructive process.

Therapy. Frequently, acute radionecrosis with accompanying cellulitis requires the administration of systemic antibiotics. As penetrance of the inflammatory and ischemic process by antimicrobial agents is rarely of value, this form of therapy is to be discouraged except in the case of systemic sepsis or intrathoracic extension of the suppurative process. Vesicles, sinus tracts, and abscesses should be drained externally. Devitalized tissue should be sharply debrided in a controlled, sterile environment; this often necessitates general anesthesia.

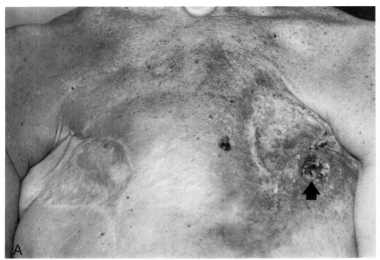
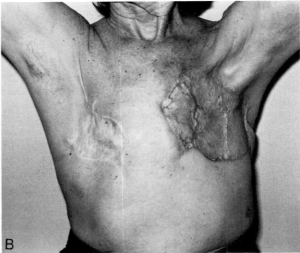

Figure 5–13. *A,* Osteoradionecrosis of left chest wall in a 68-year-old female 18 years status post bilateral radical mastectomies and orthovoltage irradiation to the operative site. Extensive transmural necrosis (*arrow*) of the irradiated site necessitated chest wall resection and reconstruction. *B,* Reconstruction results nine weeks following resection of the osteoradionecrotic chest wall site (ribs 3–7) and transfer of latissimus muscle over defect. No tumor was evident in any of the sections from the necrotic lesion.

Identification of intrathoracic extension of the abscess or sinus tract often requires full-thickness chest wall debridement with rib resection and the possibility of chest wall reconstruction using synthetic mesh and myocutaneous flaps (see Chapters 30 and 45).

SUPERFICIAL AND DEEP VEINS OF THE BREAST AND CHEST WALL

Anticoagulant-Related Necrosis of the Breast

Since the introduction of the anticoagulant dicumarol (bishydroxycoumarin) and related compounds in 1941, numerous hemorrhagic complications have been reported. The severe complication of tissue necrosis associated with hemorrhage as a complication of dicumarol therapy is only rarely observed. One site where hemorrhage and necrosis may present is the female breast.

Flood and associates,[69] in 1943, were the first to report necrosis of the breast following therapy with bishydroxycoumarin. However, it was Verhagen,[204] in 1953, who documented the association between tissue necrosis and therapy with anticoagulants of the coumarin group. The typical patient presenting with necrosis of the breast is a middle-aged or elderly female who develops thrombophlebitis of the lower extremity, for which she is placed on dicumarol therapy.[138, 144] Within three to eight days of therapy, the patient complains of severe pain in the breast. Thereafter, she observes edema, tenderness, and within a short interval, dry, blue-black discoloration of skin and a diffuse erythematous halo (Fig. 5–14). The recognition of anticoagulant-related necrosis and subsequent discontinuance of the drug had no effect on progression of the disease despite coumarin reversal with vitamin K. Initially, blisters often formed containing sterile serosanguineous fluid.

Histology. The histological changes in the mammary parenchyma due to anticoagulant-related complications, reported by Nudelman and Kempson,[144] included extensive interstitial hemorrhage and necrosis. Further, there was degeneration of ducts, venous thrombosis, and acute inflammatory cellular infiltration of the walls of small and medium-sized arteries. These findings are in striking contrast to the hemorrhagic lesions that complicate dicumarol therapy, in which vasculitis and necrosis are absent. Thus, histological changes in the breast that follow anticoagulant therapy resemble the hemorrhagic necrosis one might expect following arterial thrombosis. Hypothetical explanations for the paradoxical changes seen in histological sections include the following: (1) Necrosis may be a manifestation of generalized thrombosis and/or thrombophlebitis that occurs despite anticoagulant therapy; (2) a hypersensitivity reaction to dicumarol may be evident with associated necrotizing vasculitis; and (3) necrosis occurs secondary to diffuse interstitial parenchymal hemorrhage; however, thrombosis and vascular inflammation are not typical components of the pattern of hemorrhage.[144] None of these possibilities is a satisfactory explanation of the extensive soft tissue necrosis found in breasts of these patients.

However, hemorrhagic necrosis may occur secondary to the disruption of the vascular supply of the breast. While venous thrombosis may occur secondary to a generalized hypercoagulable defect, or even secondary to vasculitis, the exact etiology cannot be determined. The most cogent explanation for this rare complication would be the hypersensitivity reaction to dicumarol, with vascular damage initiating thrombosis and spontaneous breast infarction. This explanation is supported by the observations of others[13, 48, 81, 89, 103, 108, 184, 187] that breast necrosis is extraordinarily rare in the absence of anticoagulant therapy with dicumarol. Only the case reported by Boersma and Enler[23] documented the development of gangrene of the breast in the absence of anticoagulant therapy for thrombophlebitis of the leg.

Therapy. Coumarin necrosis has a marked predilection for areas that have abundant subcutaneous fat, such as thighs, buttocks, and less commonly, the abdomen and breast. As the lesion occurs typically before the tenth day of anticoagulant therapy, the temporal relationship of administration of the drug and occurrence of the lesion suggests this diagnosis. Coumarin therapy should be discontinued, with conversion to anticoagulation with intravenous heparin. Immediate anticoagulation with heparin is essential to abrogate exacerbation of the deep venous thrombosis and potential pulmonary embolism. Previous reports[101, 152] suggest the need for debridement of focal sites of tissue necrosis and hemorrhage; others recommend treatment of the extensive necrosis with unilateral or bilateral simple mastectomy.[50, 55] Martin and Phillips[124] and Mason[125] observed the similarities between *purpura fulminans* and coumarin-related tissue necrosis. Quick,[152] in an extensive analysis of anaphylactoid purpura, considers purpura fulminans and Schönlein-Henoch purpura to be manifestations of the Sanarelli-Shwartzman phenomenon. It was the opinion of these authors that radical surgical

Table 5–3. CLASSIFICATION OF CASES OF MAMMARY INFARCTION REPORTED IN THE LITERATURE

Breast Infarcts Mimicking Carcinoma	Breast Infarcts Not Mimicking Carcinoma
Intraductal papilloma[89]	Associated with anticoagulants[140]
Isolated proliferated lobules in sclerosing adenosis[89]	Gangrene complicating postpartum abscess[47, 156]
Adenoma[212]	Postpartum gangrene of breast skin[156]
Fibroadenoma[52]	Hemolytic streptococcal gangrene of breast[122] (not documented by histology)
Hyperplastic breast tissue in pregnancy or lactation[89, 212]	Thrombophlebitis migrans disseminata with gangrene of the breast[69] (anticoagulants also may have played a role)
Syphilitic gumma[215]	Mitral stenosis and congestive heart failure[81] (multiple venous occlusions of the breast)
Wegener's granulomatosis[65, 146]	Mitral stenosis[34] (not documented by histology)

Adapted from Robitaille Y et al: Cancer 33: 1188, 1974.

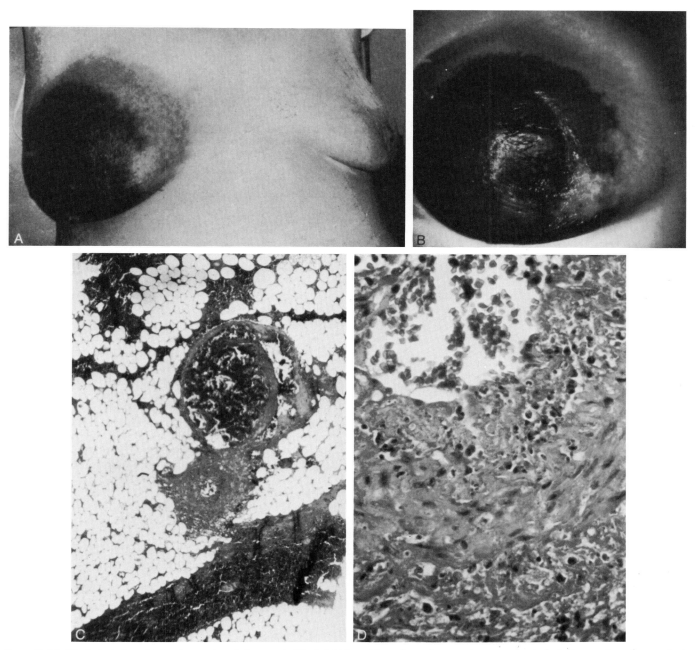

Figure 5–14. Warfarin-induced infarction and partial necrosis *(A)* of right breast four days after symptoms were noted. *B,* Progression of necrosis six days following onset of symptoms. Note the dense eschar evident over the central breast. *C,* Photomicrograph of the histologic vascular lesion in anticoagulant gangrene with evidence of venous thrombosis and necrotizing arteritis (H and E stain, × 70). *D,* Higher power magnification of warfarin-related arterial inflammation with progressive intimal necrosis (H & E stain, × 800). (From Davis, C Jr, Faulconer RJ, Wiley WB: Ann Surg 175(5):647–656, 1972.)

ablation of the necrotic breast should be replaced by medical therapy. A trial with combination heparin, corticosteroids, dextran, and antibiotics may have merit when the diagnosis of coumarin-related tissue necrosis of the breast is established. Prompt resolution without extension of the coumarin-related necrosis is theoretical. In the majority of cases, extensive debridement of the focal necrotic tissue is essential following discontinuance of dicumarol therapy and substitution with heparin anticoagulation.

Spontaneous Infarction of the Breast

Infarction of physiological hyperplastic breast tissue associated with *lactation* or *pregnancy* has been reported, with fewer than 15 cases recorded in the American and British literature.[89, 118, 147, 169, 212] In these cases, vascular lesions were not demonstrable; thus, the pathogenesis of the breast infarction remains speculative. The report by Lucey,[118] described the clinical and pathological features of five cases of spontaneous infarction, with

Table 5–4. MAJOR CLINICOPATHOLOGICAL CHARACTERISTICS OF TWO GROUPS OF PATIENTS WITH MAMMARY INFARCTION

Mimicking Carcinoma	Not Mimicking Carcinoma
Less frequent	More frequent
Predominant in women under 40 years of age	Predominant in obese women over 40 years of age
Low incidence of associated necrosis of the mammary skin	High incidence of associated necrosis of the skin
Usually a pale infarct	Usually a hemorrhagic infarct
When blood vessels are involved, the lesions are predominant in arteries	Blood vessels always involved, predominantly veins
High incidence of underlying hyperplastic breast tissue or benign tumors	No underlying hyperplastic breast tissue or benign tumors
Low incidence of associated diseases with high morbidity	Higher incidence of associated diseases with high morbidity and mortality*

*Thrombophlebitis, pulmonary emboli, cardiovascular diseases.
Adapted from Robitaille Y, et al: Cancer 33: 1189, 1974.

infarcts usually appearing in the third trimester of pregnancy or early in the puerperium.

Diagnosis and Therapy. In the cases reported by Hasson and Pope,[89] in 1961, with infarction of physiological hyperplastic breast tissue, the patients presented clinically with breast neoplasms. As mentioned above, the lesions are typically detected in the third trimester, often in the last month, of pregnancy or in the lactating state. The patients experience diffuse, tender, palpable breast lumps. Multiple nodules are often present; bilateral lesions are rare. As the disease is more commonly unilateral, a pregnancy-related malignancy (see Chapter 50) must be considered.

With infarction of the mammary region in elderly patients, the suspicion of malignancy is greater.[161] Needle core or open biopsy is diagnostic. The features of nonspecific panarteritis, focal endarteritis obliterans, and inflammation of small veins are demonstrative of massive ischemic fat necrosis. In the review by Robitaille and associates,[161] it became apparent that mammary infarction could be divided into two groups: one representing lesions that mimic carcinoma, and the other representing lesions that do not. The clinical and pathological characteristics that are evident in each category are presented in Tables 5–3 and 5–4. Partial mastectomy may be necessary to provide adequate biopsy material that excludes a neoplastic process.

Superficial Migratory Thrombophlebitis (Thrombophlebitis Migrans) with Associated Visceral Carcinoma (Trousseau Syndrome)

Armand Trousseau,[199] in 1860, described the association of carcinoma with thrombophlebitis of large and small veins throughout the body. Sack et al.[167] have more recently implicated carcinoma of the body or tail

of the pancreas as a primary related cause of the syndrome; although malignancies of the lung, stomach, and breast have been reported.

The syndrome may be idiopathic or associated with infections, Behçet's disease, or thromboangiitis obliterans. While visceral carcinomas have been associated with isolated reports of embolism, hemorrhagic episodes, and thrombophlebitis, the most specific sign of underlying carcinoma is superficial migratory thrombophlebitis. Straus and Straus[182] regard this presentation so characteristic as to indicate intensive investigation for an undisclosed malignancy.

Diagnosis. Migratory recurrent thrombophlebitis may involve the superficial veins of the extremities, chest wall, abdominal wall, and flanks and will produce successive crops of tender nodular or linear cords that may clinically resemble nodular vasculitis, erythema nodosum, and many of the panniculitides. Two thirds of patients with the syndrome are men over the age of 35 years.[167] Lesions are erythematous and are located along the course of an involved vein. There may be one or several lesions evident over the large and small veins in the affected site. Fever and leukocytosis often accompany the cutaneous lesions. Edwards[63] and Barron et al.[17] observed nonbacterial thrombotic endocarditis or "marantic" endocarditis to develop in association with superficial migratory thrombophlebitis, probably secondary to the cachexia and debility the patient sustains with the underlying malignancy. Further, the complication usually develops in patients with neoplastic diseases or other debilitating cachectic states. These marantic endocarditis lesions may be detected by the presence of a heart murmur on physical examination and may be confirmed by electrocardiography or cardiac ultrasonography (ECHO).

James[98] documented the association of Trousseau syndrome with disseminated breast carcinoma. This report, with that of Lieberman et al.,[113] suggests that the association with breast cancer is possible and, when recognized, the syndrome serves as a stimulus to investigate the underlying malignancy.

Therapy. In distinction from idiopathic thrombophlebitis, superficial migratory thrombophlebitis associated with carcinoma may show less inflammatory reaction and typically does not respond to anticoagulant therapy. The syndrome may result from a hypercoagulable state. Sack et al.[167] note that warfarin (Coumadin) is not an effective therapeutic modality. Therapy consists of that given for the underlying breast cancer or tumors of other organ sites. As curative extirpation of the malignancy is usually not possible or practical owing to the extensive metastases, heparin has been administered successfully with resolution of the recurrent thrombophlebitis.[98] Phenylbutazone, fibrolysin, aspirin, and nonsteroidal anti-inflammatory drugs are often empirically used for symptomatic relief.

Subclavian and Axillary Vein Thrombosis

Thrombosis of the subclavian and axillary vein may result from injury, venous stasis, and abnormalities of coagulation. Venous thrombosis of the upper extremity that occurs secondary to neoplastic disease is well recognized. Further, subclavian and axillary thrombosis has been reported following direct operative injury in radical mastectomy, from tumor or lymph node compression, and as a manifestation of superficial migratory thrombophlebitis (Trousseau syndrome).[213]

Etiological factors that do not appear to be directly associated with malignancy include strenuous physical exercise (Paget-Schroetter syndrome), central venous cannulization, clotting diatheses, and congestive heart failure. Mavor et al.[126] and Wilson et al.[213] reported thrombosis of the axillary and subclavian veins developing in two patients initially treated by radiotherapy for carcinoma of the breast. Wilson and associates[213] suggest that radiation fibrosis may have been the major etiological factor, but these patients were also treated with the antiestrogen tamoxifen, which may have contributed to venous thrombosis. Other authors[20, 114] claim that tamoxifen may contribute to phlebitis, thrombophlebitis, and thrombosis. Prior to these reports, upper limb venous thrombosis was well documented following combination mastectomy and radiotherapy,[42, 202] but reports did not attribute venous thrombosis to radiotherapy without antecedent major surgery. The infrequency of upper limb venous thrombosis after irradiation suggests that this complication is rare despite clinically detectable fibrosis following ionizing radiotherapy.

Rubin and Casarett[166] confirmed experimentally that radiation produces sclerosis of the vasa vasorum and proliferation of subendothelial and medial elements that leads to vessel luminal narrowing. Controversy exists regarding the effect of radiation on endothelial function and whether direct endothelial damage is a necessary component of vascular thrombogenesis.[188]

Diagnosis. The presentation of axillary or subclavian vein thrombosis following radiotherapy for cancer of the breast is usually delayed several years post treatment; this is a chronic insidious process. Evidence of thrombosis may occur in the presence or absence of recurrent breast carcinoma. The presentation is typically that of an acutely painful swelling of the ipsilateral arm and shoulder several years following the primary therapy. The arm and hand are edematous and often dusky blue.[213] Radiation fibrosis often can be palpated in the involved axilla, although gross evidence of tumor in the axilla or chest wall may be absent. Venography or ultrasound-directed Doppler evaluation of the ipsilateral venous system is confirmatory in most patients. Small collaterals may be visible, and it can be assumed that large vessels are completely occluded by the thrombus.

Therapy. Initial therapy is aimed at dissolution of the thrombus and resolution of the associated inflammatory process and edema. The patient is initially treated with intravenous heparin (5000 units intravenous bolus; 1000 units per hour by continuous infusion) to maintain the partial thromboplastin time (PTT) 2 to 2.5 greater than control values. Primary therapy includes elevation of the involved extremity until regression of the edema and cellulitis occurs; thereafter, the arm may be treated with active and passive range-of-motion exercises until reso-

lution of the venous obstruction occurs. The patient should then have conversion from intravenous heparin to oral anticoagulation with dicumarol (sodium warfarin). Patients taking tamoxifen should have discontinuance of the drug because of its associated thrombogenic activity with depression of antithrombin III activity. Further, patients should have discontinuance of estrogen replacement and oral contraceptives, as both have thrombotic potential.

Mondor Disease (Superficial Thrombophlebitis of the Thoracoabdominal Wall)

Thrombophlebitis of superficial veins of the anterior chest wall and breast was described in 1922 by the French investigators Fiessinger and Mathieu.[99] Kaufman[104] notes that 40 years prior to this report, Faage reported a similar physical finding that he mistakenly attributed to scleroderma. Favre, in 1929, provided yet another report of the disease that was followed in 1931 and 1932 by the first reports in the American literature.[104] However, it was not until 1939 that the classical description was provided by the French surgeon Henry Mondor[12, 135] of four cases of "subcutaneous angiitis" of the chest wall. Thereafter, this investigator reclassified the disease as venous phlebitis. To date, approximately 250 to 300 cases of Mondor disease have been described in the world literature. Owing to its infrequency, most authors acknowledge only a small series of the clinical entity. In 1955, Farrow[67] published the largest series to date, which is inclusive of 43 cases.

The eponymic designation Mondor disease describes a special, rare, benign variant of thrombophlebitis of superficial veins of the anterior thoracoabdominal wall. Typically, it is described in relationship to an area contiguous with the breast and is detected as a thrombosed vein that presents as a tender cordlike structure ("string phlebitis").

Mondor disease classically presents as a single clinical entity; Abramson[2] concluded that the disease should be considered a benign, self-limited lesion and not an indicator of neoplasia. Local or regional inflammatory states and scars of previous surgical procedures may be associated. Skipworth et al.[176] note that cases sporadically have been reported concurrent with lymphoma, lupus erythematosus, appendicitis, and rheumatoid arthritis. Vieta and Heymann[206] described a patient with Mondor disease and simultaneous preoperative carcinoma of the breast. Chiedozi and Aghahowa[38] reported the presence of Mondor disease thought to be initiated by carcinoma of the breast. Association of breast neoplasia with the entity is rare. In the reports by Miller et al.[129] and by Chiedozi and Aghahowa,[38] the presence of pain secondary to thrombophlebitis prompted the investigation and diagnosis of breast cancer. Except for the case reported by Miller and coworkers,[129] palpable axillary nodes have been absent at diagnosis.

Pathophysiology. The precise pathophysiology that initiates Mondor disease is speculative. Hogan[91] postulates that pressure on the lateral thoracic veins leads to

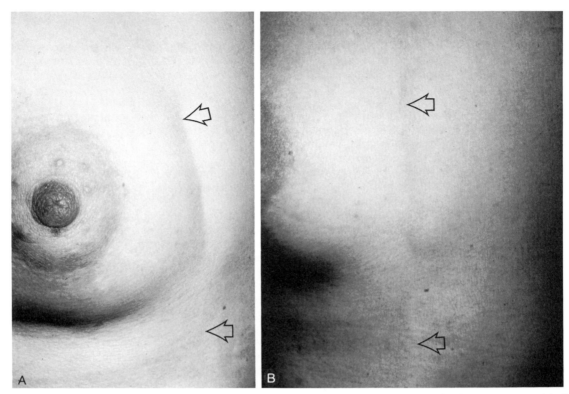

Figure 5–15. Thirty-seven-year-old Hispanic female who presented with acute pain in the left breast in the distribution (*arrows*) of the lateral thoracic vein *(A)*. The tender cord in the anterolateral thorax was treated with warm compresses and aspirin. There was gradual resolution of the inflammatory response with progressive skin retraction over the next eight weeks. *B,* In long-term follow-up, indentations (*arrows*) caused by skin retraction are still evident.

stasis of blood or direct trauma of the vein. Others suggest that previous surgical procedures, infectious processes, and stress-related exercises of the upper extremity, especially with repetitive movements, initiate the syndrome.[67, 162] Superficial veins of the anterior chest wall and abdomen that may be involved include the *lateral thoracic vein,* the *thoracoepigastric vein,* and more rarely, the *superficial epigastric vein.*

In the initial descriptions of Mondor disease, there was disagreement as to whether the affected vessel was an artery,[93] a lymphatic channel,[9] or a vein.[99, 102, 145] Bircher and associates[21] suggested that the fibrous lesion was actually a remnant of the mammary ridge (milk line) (see Chapter 2), and thus the designation "vestigial mastitis" was applied. It is now generally accepted, however, that the disease represents superficial phlebitis of one of the three major veins of the anterior chest or abdominal walls. Johnson and associates[99] delineated four stages of evolution of Mondor disease: (1) The first stage is characterized by thrombus formation within the lumen of the aforementioned veins and the presence of a surrounding inflammatory infiltrate admixed with polymorphonuclear leukocytes. (2) In Stage II, the thrombus becomes better organized, with evidence of early recanalization and the microscopic appearance of solid fibrous cords. (3) With Stage III, multiple sites of recanalization coalesce to form a single lumen of the vein. (4) In the final stage of evolution, the affected vein is completely recanalized with a firm, thickened fibrous wall with

remarkable reduction in the perivascular response. The duration of the entire evolutionary sequence will vary from 2 to 24 weeks.

Diagnosis. The typical patient with Mondor disease has the acute presentation of pain in the lateral one half of the involved breast or the anterior chest wall. Thereafter, the patient notices the appearance of a tender, firm cord that follows the distribution of one of the three major superficial veins of the chest or abdominal wall. When the skin at each end of the involved fibrotic vein is stretched, the cord will assume the configuration of a bowstring. Oldfield termed the actual lesions described by patients to have the appearance of a "goose quill," "drumstick," or "bowstring."[145]

Physical examination discloses a tender, fibrous erythematous cord of variable length and diameter present in the distribution of the affected vein (Fig. 5–15). Although the tender fibrous cord is usually unilateral, bilateral lesions have been described.[2, 67] Only rarely will the process simultaneously involve veins of the chest and abdominal walls. The majority of patients have no evidence of thrombophlebitis in other anatomical sites.[12, 31, 32, 58, 60, 68] Usually, no evidence of axillary adenopathy, breast trauma, infection or nipple discharge will be present at examination.

Therapy. An established diagnosis, usually afforded by the history and physical examination, is essential to appropriate therapy of the disease. Whenever the clinician is uncertain of the diagnosis, or if a contiguous mass is present near the fibrous cord, confirmation must be established by excisional biopsy. No consistent pattern of laboratory or radiological abnormalities has been described in association with Mondor disease.

As this clinical entity is a benign, self-limiting process, the physician must first allay the patient's concern of a breast or chest wall malignancy. The administration of anticoagulants or antibiotics is to be discouraged. The mainstay of therapy includes liberal use of salicylates and heat compresses that provide symptomatic relief of pain along the course of the involved vein. Further, the patient should have restriction of brassiere supports and, on occasion, a sling to limit mobility of the ipsilateral arm and shoulder. Abramson[2] recommended disruption of the fibrous cord by manual traction when pain is unduly severe. Millar[128] suggested an aggressive operative approach for painful cords of the disease. Treatment included division of the "bowstrings" above and below the area of involvement.

The patient should be advised that this benign process will resolve over two to eight weeks; although the inflammatory process in evolution may last 24 weeks. Kaufman[104] and Lunn and Chir[119] noted recurrence of the disease, and these isolated instances have been associated with major disorders[80, 91] (deep venous thrombosis and rheumatic arthritis). For associated systemic illnesses concurrent with Mondor disease, specific treatment of the serious underlying ailment should take precedence over superficial thrombophlebitis of thoracoabdominal veins.

References

1. Abramson DJ: Mammary duct ectasia, mammillary fistula and subareolar sinuses. Ann Surg 169:217–226, 1960.
2. Abramson DJ: Mondor's disease and string phlebitis. JAMA 196:1087–1089, 1966.
3. Adair FE: Gumma of the breast; its differential diagnosis from carcinoma. Ann Surg 79:44–54, 1924.
4. Alagaratnam TT: Uncommon forms of mastitis. Aust NZ J Surg 51(1):45–48, 1981.
5. Algaratnam TT, Ong GB: Tuberculosis of the breast. Br J Surg 67:125–126, 1980.
6. Allen HB, Rippon JW: Superficial and deep mycoses. In Moschella SL, Hurley HJ (eds): Dermatology. Philadelphia, WB Saunders, 1985, pp 774–816.
7. Ammentrop L: Om Aktinomykose. Biblioth. Laeg, Kjùbenh., 7.R., iv, 433–472, 1893.
8. Applebaum RM: The modern management of successful breast feeding. Pediatr Clin North Am 17:203–225, 1970.
9. Ashken MH: String phlebitis. Br J Surg 50:689–693, 1963.
10. Atkins JHB: Mammillary fistula. Br Med J 2:1473–1474, 1955.
11. Azzopardi JF: Problems in Breast Pathology. Philadelphia, WB Saunders, 1979, pp 399–400.
12. Bahal V, Mansel RE: Mondor's disease secondary to breast abscess in a male. Case report. Br J Surg 73:931, 1986.
13. Bamberger R: Total gangran der mamma als teilerscheinung puerperaler sepsis. Munch Med Wochnschr 49:2680, 1912.
14. Banerjee SN, Anathakrishnan N, Mehta RB, Parkash S: Tuberculous mastitis: A continuing problem. World J Surg 11:105–109, 1987.
15. Banik S, Bishop PW, Ormerod LP, O'Brien TEB: Sarcoidosis of the breast. J Clin Pathol 39:446–448, 1986.
16. Barnett A, Lavey E, Pearl RM, Vistnes LM: Toxic shock syndrome: From an infected breast prosthesis. Ann Plast Surg 10:408–410, 1983.
17. Barron KD, Siqueira E, Hirano A: Cerebral embolism caused by a nonbacterial thrombotic endocarditis. Neurology 10:391–397, 1960.
18. Bartlett P, Reingold A, Graham D, et al: Toxic shock syndrome associated with surgical wound infections. JAMA 247:1448–1450, 1982.
19. Becker TM, Blount JH, Douglas J, Judson FN: Trends in molluscum contagiosum in the United States, 1966–1983. Sex Transm Dis 13(2):88–92, 1986.
20. Beex L, Pieters G, Smals A, Kaenders A, Benrand T, Kloppenborg P: Tamoxifen versus ethinyl estradiol in the treatment of postmenopausal women with advanced breast cancer. Cancer Treat Rep 65:179–185, 1981.
21. Bircher J, Schirger A, Clagett OT, Harrison EJ Jr.: Mondor's disease. A vascular rarity. Mayo Clin Proc 37:651–656, 1962.
22. Bodo M, Debrossy L, Sugar J: Boeck's sarcoidosis of the breast: Cytologic findings with aspiration biopsy cytology. Acta Cytol 22:1–2, 1978.
23. Boersma D, Enler H: Gangrenous breast from venous thrombosis. Surgery 54:876–879, 1963.
24. Bonecchi L, Nanni MR: Sarcoide di Boeck della mammella. Radiol Med 67:656–657, 1981.
25. Braunstein AL, Woolsey RD: Gummatous Mastitis. Am J Syph Gonor Vener Dis 24:43–47, 1940.
26. Bresler MJ: Toxic shock syndrome due to occult postoperative wound infection. Case report. West J Med 139(5):710–713, 1983.
27. Brown J, McDowell F, Fryer M: Surgical treatment of radiation burns. Surg Gynecol Obstet 88:609–622, 1949.
28. Bundred NJ, Dixon JM, Lumsden AB, Radford D, Hood J, Miles RS, Chetty U, Forrest AP: Are the lesions of duct ectasia sterile? Br J Surg 72:844–845, 1985.
29. Burnett JW, Crutcher WA: Viral and rickettsial infections. In Moschella SL, Hurley HJ (eds): Dermatology. Philadelphia, WB Saunders, 1985, pp 683–689.
30. Burry VF, Beezley M: Infant mastitis due to gram-negative organisms. Am J Dis Child 124:736–737, 1972.
31. Camiel MR: Mondor's disease in the breast. Am J Obstet Gynecol 152:879–881, 1985.
32. Camiel MR, Benninghoff DL: Mondor's disease in the breast. Superficial thrombophlebitis of the thoracoabdominal wall. J Natl Med Assoc 63(5):352–353, 1971.
33. Campbell FC, Eriksson BL, Angorn IB: Localized granulomatous mastitis: An unusual presentation of typhoid. S Afr Med J 57:793–795, 1980.
34. Canigia A: Un raro disturbo di circolo della ghiandola mammaria. Folia Cardiol 12(1): 3–12, 1953.
35. Caswell HT, Burnett WE: Chronic recurrent breast abscess secondary to inversion of the nipple. Surg Gynecol Obstet 102:439–442, 1956.
36. Caswell HT, Maier WP: Chronic recurrent periareolar abscess secondary to inversion of the nipple. Surg Gynecol Obstet 12:587–598, 1969.
37. Chandrasoma PT, Mendis KN: Filarial infection of the breast. Am J Trop Med Hyg 27:770–773, 1978.
38. Chiedozi LC, Aghahowa JA: Mondor's disease associated with breast cancer. Surgery 103(4):438–439, 1988.
39. Clegg HW, Bertagnoll P, Hightower AW, Baine WB: Mammaplasty-associated mycobacterial infection: A survey of plastic surgeons. Plast Reconstr Surg 72(2):165–169, 1983.
40. Clegg HW, Foster MT, Sanders WE Jr, Baine WB: Infection due to organisms of the *Mycobacterium fortuitum* complex after augmentation mammaplasty: Clinical and epidemiologic features. J Infect Dis 147(3):427–433, 1983.
41. Colbeck JC: An extensive outbreak of staphylococcal infections in maternity units: Use of bacteriophage typing in investigation and control. Can Med Assoc J 61:557–568, 1949.
42. Coon WW, Willis PW: Thrombosis of subclavian and axillary veins. Am Heart J 25:355–371, 1943.
43. Cooper A: Illustration of the Diseases of the Breast, Part I. London, Longman, Rees, Orme, Brown, and Green, 1829, p 73.
44. Cooray GH: Some observations on filarial infection in Ceylon with special reference to its histopathology. Indian J Malariol 14:617–632, 1960.
45. Cope Z: Visceral actinomycosis. Ann R Coll Surg Engl 5:394–410, 1949.

46. Courtiss EH, Goldwyn RM, Caspar WA: The fate of breast implants with infections around them. Plast Reconstr Surg 63(6)812–816, 1979.

47. Creyssul J, Bèraud M: Gangrene massive spontanée du sein—Abcès gangrèneux pulmonaire causècutif. Lyon Chir 4:615–617, 1946.

48. Cutler EC: Apoplexy of the breast. JAMA 82:1763–1764, 1924.

49. Dalmark G: Lymphogranulomatose benigne: Un cas avec des alterations mammaires comme seul symptome. Acta Chir Scand 96:168–178, 1942.

50. Davis CE, Wiley WB, Faulconer RJ: Necrosis of the female breast complicating oral anticoagulant treatment. Ann Surg 173(5):647–656, 1972.

51. Deaver JB, McFarland J, Herman JL: The Breast: Its Anomalies, Its Diseases and Their Treatment. London, William Heinemann 1918, pp 198–199.

52. Delarue J, Redon J: Les infarctus des fibroadènames mammaires. Sem Hop 25:2991–2996, 1949.

53. Devereux WP: Acute puerperal mastitis: Evaluation of its management. Am J Obstet Gynecol 108:78–81, 1970.

54. Dharkar RS, Kanhere MH, Vaishy ND, Bisarya AK: Tuberculosis of the breast. J Indian Med Assoc 50:207–209, 1968.

55. DiCato MA, Ellman L: Coumadin-induced necrosis of breast, disseminated intravascular coagulation, and hemolytic anemia. Ann Intern Med 83(2):233–234, 1975.

56. D'Orsi CJ, Feldhaus L, Sonnenfeld M: Unusual lesions of the breast. Radiol Clin North Am 21:67–80, 1983.

57. Dubey MM, Agarwal S: Tuberculosis of the breast. J Indian Med Assoc 51:358–359, 1968.

58. Duff P: Mondor disease in pregnancy. Case report. Obstet Gynecol 58(1):117–120, 1981.

59. Duncan JT, Walker J: Staphylococcus aureus in the milk of nursing mothers and the alimentary canal of their infants: Report to the Medical Research Council. J Hyg 43:474–484, 1942.

60. Durham RH: Thrombophlebitis migrans and visceral carcinoma. Arch Intern Med 96:380–386, 1955.

61. Dvorak VC, Root RK, MacGregor RR: Host-defense mechanisms in hidradenitis suppurativa. Arch Dermatatol 115:450–455, 1977.

62. Eaglestein WH, Katz R, Brown JA: The effects of early corticosteroid therapy on the skin eruption and pain of herpes zoster. JAMA 211:1681–1683, 1970.

63. Edwards EA: Migrating thrombophlebitis associated with carcinoma. N Engl J Med 240:1031–1035, 1949.

64. Ekland DA, Zeigler MG: Abscess in the nonlactating breast. Arch Surg 107:398–401, 1973.

65. Elsner B, Harper FB: Disseminated Wegener's granulomatosis with breast involvement—Report of a case. Arch Path 87:544–547, 1969.

66. Ernö H: Mycoplasmosis: Experimental mastitis. Demonstration of antibody in milk. Acta Vet Scand 12:451–453, 1971.

67. Farrow JH: Thrombophlebitis of the superficial veins of the breast and anterior chest wall. Surg Gynecol Obstet 101:63–68, 1955.

68. Fischl RA, Kahn S, Simon BE: Mondor's disease. An unusual complication of mammaplasty. Plast Reconstr Surg 56(3):319–322, 1975.

69. Flood EP, Redish MH, Boeick SJ, Shapiro S: Thrombophlebitis migrans disseminata: Report of a case in which gangrene of a breast occurred. NY J Med 43:1121–1124, 1943.

70. Follow-up on toxic-shock syndrome. MMWR 29:441–445, 1980.

71. Fulton AA: Incidence of puerperal and lactational mastitis in an industrial town of some 43,900 inhabitants. Br Med J 1:693–696, 1945.

72. Gansler TS, Wheeler JE: Mammary sarcoidosis. Arch Pathol Lab Med 108:673–675, 1984.

73. Geschicter CF: Diseases of the Breast. Philadelphia, JB Lippincott, 1947, p 164.

74. Gibbard GF: Sporadic and epidemic puerperal breast infections. Am J Obstet Gynecol 65:1038–1041, 1953.

75. Glass LW, Vecchione TR: Hidradenitis suppurativa of the breast areolae. Plast Reconstr Surg 61:449–451, 1978.

76. Gogas J, Sechas M, Diamantis S, Sbokos C: Actinomycosis of the breast. Case report. Int Surg 57(8):664–665, 1972.

77. Goldman KP: Tuberculosis of the breast. Tubercle 59:41–45, 1978.

78. Gottschalk FAB, Decker GAG, Schmaman A: Tuberculosis of the breast. S Afr J Surg 14:19–22, 1976.

79. Grausman RI, Goldman ML: Tuberculosis of the breast. Report of nine cases including two cases of co-existing carcinoma and tuberculosis. Am J Surg 67:48–56, 1945.

80. Grow JL, Lewison EF: Superficial thrombophlebitis of the breast. Surg Gynecol Obstet 116:180–182, 1963.

81. Gruber JB: Infarktbildung in der mamma. Munch Med Wochenschr 44:2328–2330, 1911.

82. Gupta R, Gupta AS, Duggal N: Tubercular mastitis. Int Surg 67:422–424, 1982.

83. Haagensen CD: Diseases of the Breast. Philadelphia, WB Saunders, 1971, pp 339–341.

84. Habif DV, Perzin KH, Lipton R, Lattes R: Subareolar abscess associated with squamous metaplasia of lactiferous ducts. Am J Surg 119:523–526, 1970.

85. Hadfield J: Excision of the major duct system for benign disease of the breast. Br J Surg 47:472–477, 1960.

86. Hale JA, Peters GN, Cheek JH: Tuberculosis of the breast: Rare but still extant. Am J Surg 150:620–624, 1985.

87. Hamit HJ, Ragsdale TH: Mammary tuberculosis. J R Soc Med 75:764–765, 1982.

88. Harrington SW: Tuberculosis of the breast. Surg Gynecol Obstet 63:797–798, 1936.

89. Hasson J, Pope C: Mammary infarcts associated with pregnancy presenting as breast tumors. Surgery 49:313–316, 1961.

90. Herrera-Vegas M, Cranwell DJ: Los quistes hidatìdicos en la Republica Argentina. Buenos Aires, Coni Hermanos, 1909.

91. Hogan GF: Mondor's disease. Arch Intern Med 113:881–885, 1964.

92. Holck S: Subareolar abscess of the breast. Ugeskr Laeger 142:870, 1980.

93. Hughes ESR: Sclerosing peri-angeitis of the lateral thoracic wall. Aust NZ J Surg 22:17–24, 1952.

94. Hughes LE: Bacteroides and breast abscess. Lancet 1:198, 1976.

95. Huntingford PJ: Staphylococcal infection in maternity hospitals. Lancet 2:1179, 1958.

96. Israel J: Gelungene Anlegung liner magenfistel. Berl Klin Wochenschr xvi, 89, 1879.

97. Jacobson JA, Burke JP, Benowitz BA, et al: Varicella zoster and staphylococcal toxic shock syndrome in a young man. JAMA 249:922–923, 1983.

98. James WD: Trousseau's syndrome. Int J Dermatol 23:205–206, 1984.

99. Johnson WC, Wallrich R, Helurg EB: Superficial thrombophlebitis of the chest wall. JAMA 180:103–108, 1962.

100. Jung-Greifswald: Disseminierte Gilchristsche Blastomykose und sporotrichom der mamma mit Bild-und Kulturdemonstration. Arch Dermatol Syph 191:482–484, 1950.

101. Kahn S, Stern HD, Rhodes GA: Cutaneous and subcutaneous necrosis as a complication of coumarin-congener therapy. Plast Reconstr Surg 48(2):160–166, 1971.

102. Karlan M, Traphagen DW: Superficial phlebitis of the breast. Am J Surg 94:981–983, 1957.

103. Katz H: Symmetrische nekrose beider brustwarzen im wochenbett. Zentralbl Gynakol 5:175–178, 1924.

104. Kaufman PA: Subcutaneous phlebitis of the breast and chest wall. Ann Surg 144:847–853, 1956.

105. Kernbaum S, Hauchecorne J: Administration of levodopa for relief of herpes zoster pain. JAMA 246:132–134, 1981.

106. Kilgore AR, Fleming R: Abscesses of the breast: Recurring lesions in the areolar area. Calif Med 77:190–191, 1952.

107. Köhlmeier W, Kreitner H: Blastomykose der Mamma. Wein Klin Wochenschr 65:13–15, 1953.

108. Labry R, Picault H: Epithelioma du sein avec spacèle du mamelon et accidents hemorrhagiques avant d'imposer l'intervention. Lyon Med 87:252, 1955.

109. Lambert ME, Betts CD, Sellwood RA: Mammillary fistula. Br J Surg 73:367–368, 1986.

110. Leach RD, Phillips I, Eykin SJ, Corrin B: Anaerobic subareolar breast abscess. Lancet 2:35–37, 1979.

111. Leary WG Jr: Acute puerperal mastitis—A view. Calif Med 68:147–151, 1948.

112. Lewitt S: Radiation therapy after definitive surgery for breast carcinoma. JAMA 2:237, 1977.
113. Lieberman JS, Borrero J, Urdaneta E, Wright IS: Thrombophlebitis and cancer. JAMA 177:542–545, 1961.
114. Lipton A, Harvey HA, Hamilton RW: Venous thrombosis as a side effect of tamoxifen treatment. Cancer Treat Rep 68(6)887–889, 1984.
115. Lloyd-Davies JA: Primary actinomycosis of the breast. Br J Surg 38:378–381, 1951.
116. Longcope WT, Freiman DG: A study of sarcoidosis. Medicine 31:1–121, 1944.
117. Lucchese G: Tuberculosis e cancro della mammella assosiati. Ann Ital Chir 10:217, 1931.
118. Lucey JJ: Spontaneous infarction of the breast. J Clin Pathol 28:937–943, 1975.
119. Lunn GM, Chir M: Mondor's disease. (Subcutaneous phlebitis of the breast region.) Br Med J 1:1074–1076, 1954.
120. Maier WP, Berger A, Derrick BM: Periareolar abscess in the nonlactating breast. Am J Surg 144:359–361, 1982.
121. Makki H: Some rare cases of hydatid disease. Br J Clin Pract 24(3):125–129, 1970.
122. Marcus R: Haemolytic streptococcal gangrene of breast successfully treated with streptomycin. Br Med J 2:394–395, 1950.
123. Marshall BR, Hepper JK, Zirbel CC: Sporadic puerperal mastitis: An infection that need not interrupt lactation. JAMA, 233(13)1377–1379, 1975.
124. Martin BF, Phillips JD: Gangrene of the female breast with anticoagulant therapy. Am J Clin Pathol 53:622–626, 1970.
125. Mason JR: Haemorrhage-induced breast gangrene. Br J Surg 57(9):700–702, 1970.
126. Mavor GE, Kasenally AT, Harper DR, Woodruff PH: Thrombosis of the subclavian-axillary artery following radiotherapy for carcinoma of the breast. Br J Surg (60)(12):983–985, 1973.
127. McKeown KC, Wilkinson KW: Tuberculous disease of the breast. Br J Surg 39:420–429, 1952.
128. Millar DM: Treatment of Mondor's disease. Case report. Br J Surg 54:(1)76–77, 1967.
129. Miller DR, Cesario TC, Slater LM: Mondor's disease associated with metastatic axillary nodes. Cancer 56:903–904, 1985.
130. Miller RE, Solomon PF, West JP: The co-existence of carcinoma and tuberculosis of the breast and axillary lymph nodes. Am J Surg 121:338–340, 1971.
131. Mills HW: Hydatid cysts of the spleen, with report of four cases. Surg Gynecol Obstet 38:491–505, 1924.
132. Minsker OB: Actinomycosis of the mammary gland. Khirurgiia (Mosk) 39:107–112, 1963.
133. Mirza NB, Pamba HO, O'Leary P: Hydatid cyst of the breast: Case report. East Afr Med J 56:235–236, 1979.
134. Moak H: On the occurrence of carcinoma and tuberculosis in the same organ or tissue. J Med Res 8:128–147, 1902.
135. Mondor H: Tronsculite sous-cutanée subaigue de la paroi thoracique antérioalatèle. Men Acad Chir 65:1271–1278, 1939.
136. Moon AA, Gilbert B: A study of acute mastitis of the puerperium. J Obstet Gynaecol Br Commonw 42:268–282, 1935.
137. Morgan M: Tuberculosis of the breast. Surg Gynecol Obstet 53:593–605, 1931.
138. Moses RG, Warren JR: Coumarin necrosis. Med J Aust 2:76–77, 1973.
139. Mukerjee P, George M, Maheshwasi HB, Rao CP: Tuberculosis of the breast. J Indian Med Assoc 62:410–412, 1974.
140. Nalbandian RM, Maeder IJ, Barrett JL, Pearce FS, Rupp EC: Petechiae, ecchymoses, and necroses of skin induced by coumadin cogeners. JAMA 192:603–608, 1965.
141. Newton M, Newton NR: Breast abscess: Result of lactation failure. Surg Gynecol Obstet 91:651–655, 1950.
142. Nicolson WP, Gillespie CE: Tuberculosis of the breast. South Surg 10:825–846, 1941.
143. Niebyl JR, Spence MR, Pharmley TH: Sporadic (nonepidemic) puerperal mastitis. J Reprod Med 20:97–100, 1978.
144. Nudelman HL, Kempson RL: Necrosis of the breast. A rare complication of anticoagulant therapy. Am J Surg (3):728–733, 1966.
145. Oldfield MC: Mondor's disease: A superficial phlebitis of the breast. Lancet 1:994–996, 1962.
146. Pambakian H, Tighe JR: Breast involvement in Wegener's granulomatosis. J Clin Pathol 24:343–347, 1971.
147. Pambakian H, Tighe JR: Mammary infarction. Br J Surg 58:601–602, 1971.
148. Park JE, Park K: Textbook of Preventative and Social Medicine. 7th ed., Jabalpur, India, Ms. B. Bhanot, 1979, p 344.
149. Patey DH, Thackeray AC: Pathology and treatment of mammary-duct fistula. Lancet 2:871–873, 1958.
150. Pemberton M: A case of primary actinomycosis of the breast. Br J Surg 29:353–354, 1942.
151. Penneys NS, Matsuo S, Mogollon R: The identification of molluscum infection by immunohistochemical means. J Cutan Pathol 13:97–101, 1986.
152. Quick AJ: Secondary non-thrombocytopenic purpura. In Hemorrhagic Diseases and Thrombosis. Philadelphia, Lea & Febiger, 1966, pp 254–269.
153. Ramioul H, Liegeois A, Dejardin R, et al: Un cas de mastite granulomateuse simulant la mastite neoplastique. Gynakol Rundsch 21(Suppl):78–83, 1981.
154. Ransjö U, Asplund OA, Gylbert L, Jurell G: Bacteria in the female breast. Scand J Plast Reconstr Surg 19:87–89, 1985.
155. Ravenholt RT, Wright P, Mulhern M: Epidemiology and prevention of nursery-derived staphylococcal disease. N Engl J Med 257:789–795, 1957.
156. Ravina and Jamain: Les gangrènes du sein pendant la lactation. Gynecol Obstet 48:49–55, 1949.
157. Reingold A, Hargrett N, Dan B, et al: Nonmenstrual toxic shock syndrome: A review of 130 cases. Ann Intern Med 96:871–874, 1982.
158. Reisner D: Boeck's sarcoid and systemic sarcoidosis. Am Rev Tuberc 49:437–462, 1944.
159. Rickert RR, Rajan S: Localized breast infarcts associated with pregnancy. Arch Pathol 97:159–161, 1974.
160. Ridgen B: Sarcoid lesion in breast after probable sarcoidosis in lung. Br Med J 2:1533–1534, 1978.
161. Robitaille Y, Seemayer TA, Thelmo WL, Cumberlidge MC: Infarction of the mammary region mimicking carcinoma of the breast. Cancer 33:1183–1189, 1974.
162. Roscher AA, Weinstein E: The clinico-pathological spectrum of Mondor's disease: An important surgical entity. Int Surg 65:(4):325–329, 1980.
163. Rosen Y, Vuletin JC, Pertschuk LP, Silverstein E: Sarcoidosis: From the pathologist's vantage point. In Sheldon SC, Rosen PP (eds): Pathology Annual. East Norwalk, CT, Appleton Century Crofts, 1979.
164. Rosenthal LJ, Greenfield DS, Lesnick GJ: Breast abscess. Management in subareolar and peripheral disease. NY State J Med 81:182–183, 1981.
165. Rubin EH, Penner M: Sarcoidosis: One case report and review of autopsied cases. Am Rev Tuberc 49:146–169, 1944.
166. Rubin P, Casarett GW: Clinical Radiation Pathology, Vol. I. Philadelphia, WB Saunders, 1968, pp 512–514.
167. Sack GH, Levin J, Bell WR: Trousseau's syndrome and other manifestations of chronic disseminated coagulopathy in patients with neoplasms: Clinical, pathophysiologic and therapeutic features. Medicine 56:1–37, 1977.
168. Salfelder K, Schwarz J: Mycotic 'pseudotumors' of the breast: Report of four cases. Arch Surg 110:751–754, 1975.
169. Sandison AT, Walker JC: Inflammatory mastitis, mammary duct ectasia, and mammillary fistula. Br J Surg 50:57–64, 1962.
170. Scadding JG: Sarcoidosis. London, Eyre & Spottswoode, 1967, pp 335–336.
171. Schaefer G: Tuberculosis of the breast. Am Rev Tuberc 72:810–824, 1955.
172. Scott RB: The sarcoidosis of Boeck. Br Med J 2:777–781, 1938.
173. Shah Z, Lehman JA Jr, Tan J: Does infection play a role in breast capsular contracture? Plast Reconstr Surg 68(1):34–38, 1981.
174. Sherman AJ: Puerperal breast abscess: I. Report of an outbreak at Philadelphia General Hospital. Obstet Gynecol 7:268–273, 1956.
175. Shinoda M, Nomi S, Iwai K, et al: A case of breast sarcoid. Nippon Geka Hokan 48:404–410, 1979.
176. Skipworth GR, Morris JB, Goldstein N: Bilateral Mondor's disease. Arch Dermatol 95:95–97, 1967.
177. Smith LW, Mason RL: The concurrence of tuberculosis and cancer of the breast. Surg Gynecol Obstet 43:70–72, 1926.

178. Soltau DHK, Hatcher GW: Some observations on the aetiology of breast abscess in the puerperium. Br Med J 1:1603–1607, 1970.
179. Stallard HB, Tait CBV: Boeck's sarcoidosis: A case record. Lancet 4:440–442, 1939.
180. Stelling CB: Dracunculiasis presenting as sterile abscess. Am J Roentgenol 138:1159–1161, 1982.
181. Stetler H, et al: Neonatal mastitis due to Escherichia coli. J Pediatr 76:611–613, 1970.
182. Straus B, Straus M: Peripheral manifestations of visceral cancer. NY State J Med 58:3109–3013, 1958.
183. Studdy PR, Lapworth R, Bird R: Angiotensin-converting enzyme and its clinical significance: A review. J Clin Pathol 36:938–947, 1983.
184. Switzer PK: Gangrene of the breast associated with diabetes mellitus. JSC Med Assoc 46:42–44, 1950.
185. Symmers W St C: Systemic Pathology, Vol 4. New York, Churchill Livingstone, 1978, pp 1770–1774.
186. Tedeschi LG, Ahari S, Byrne JJ: Involutional mammary duct ectasia and periductal mastitis. Am J Surg 106:517–521, 1963.
187. Tesar O: Gangrene of breast and gangrene following carbon monoxide poisoning: two rare cases. Rozhl Chir 30:132–139, 1951.
188. Thomas DP, Merton RE, Wood RD, Hockley DJ. The relationship between vessel wall injury and venous thrombosis: An experimental study. Br J Haematol 59:449–457, 1985.
189. Thomas WG, Williamson RCN, Davies JD, Webb AJ: The clinical syndrome of mammary duct ectasia. Br J Surg 69:423–425, 1982.
190. Thomsen AC: Infectious mastitis and occurrence of antibody-coated bacteria in milk. Am J Obstet Gynecol 144:350–351, 1982.
191. Thomsen AC, Espersen T, Maigaard S: Course and treatment of milk stasis, noninfectious inflammation of the breast, and infectious mastitis in nursing women. Am J Obstet Gynecol 149:492–495, 1984.
192. Thomsen AC, Hansen KB, Müller BR: Leukocyte counts and microbiological cultivation in the diagnosis of puerperal mastitis. Am J Obstet Gynecol 146:938–941, 1983.
193. Thornton JW, Argenta LC, McClatchey KD, Marks MW: Studies on the endogenous flora of the human breast. Ann Plast Surg 20:39–42, 1988.
194. Tobin G, Shaw RC, Goodpasture HC: Toxic shock syndrome following breast and nasal surgery. Case report. Plast Reconstr Surg 80(1):111–114, 1987.
195. Todd J, Fishaut M, Kapral F, Welch T: Toxic-shock syndrome associated with phage-group-1 staphylococci. Lancet 2:1116–1121, 1978.
196. Toker C: Lactiferous duct fistula. J Pathol 84:143–146, 1962.
197. Toranto IR, Malow JB: Atypical mycobacteria periprosthetic infections—Diagnosis and treatment. Plast Reconstr Surg 66(2):226–228, 1980.
198. Toxic-shock syndrome—United States. MMWR 29:229–230, 1980.
199. Trousseau A: Clinique médicale de l'hôtel de Dieu de Paris. 5th ed, Vol III. Paris, Paillière et Fils, 1877, pp 105, 700 (Lectures 71 and 96).
200. Urban JA: Excision of the major duct system of the breast. Cancer 16:516–520, 1963.
201. Uretsky BF, O'Brien JJ, Courtiss EH, Becker MD: Augmentation mammaplasty associated with a severe systemic illness. Case report. Ann Plast Surg 3(5):445–447, 1979.
202. Veal JR, Hussey HH: Thrombosis of the subclavian and axillary veins. Am Heart J 25:355–371, 1943.
203. Velpeau A: In Becket Z (ed): Aiselle's Dictionnaire de Medecine, un repertoire general des science medicales son le rapport theorique et pratique. Vol. 11, p 91. Paris, Jeune, 1932.
204. Verhagen H: Local hemorrhage and necrosis of the skin and underlying tissues during anticoagulant therapy with Dicumarol or dicumacyl. Acta Med Scand 148:453–467, 1954.
205. Verneuil A.: Etudes sur les tumeurs de la plan et quelques maladies des glandes sudoripores. Arch Gen Med 4:447, 693, 1844.
206. Vieta JO, Heymann AD: Mondor's disease with carcinoma of the breast. NY State J Med 120–121, 1977.
207. Villard E, Martin JF: Coexistence de cancer et de tuberculose du sein et des ganglions axillaires. Bull Assoc Franc Etude Cancer 22:128–139, 1933.
208. Wannemaker L: Toxic shock: Problems in definition and diagnosis of a new syndrome. Ann Intern Med 96:775–777, 1982.
209. Warthin AS: The coexistence of carcinoma and tuberculosis of the mammary gland. Am J Med Sci 118:25–34, 1899.
210. Watt-Boolsen S, Rasmussen NR, Blichert-Toft M: Primary periareolar abscess in the nonlactating breast: Risk of recurrence. Am J Surg 153:571–573, 1987.
211. Webster CS: Tuberculosis of the breast. Am J Surg 45:557–562, 1939.
212. Wilkinson L, Green WO, Jr.: Infarction of breast lesions during pregnancy and lactation. Cancer 17:1567–1572, 1964.
213. Wilson CB, Lambert HE, Scott RD: Subclavian and axillary vein thrombosis following radiotherapy for carcinoma of the breast. Clin Radiol 38:95–96, 1987.
214. Wilson TS, MacGregor JW: The diagnosis and treatment of tuberculosis of the breast. Can Med Assoc J 89:1118–1124, 1963.
215. Witaker HT, Moore RM: Gumma of the breast. Surg Gynecol Obstet 98:473–477, 1954.
216. Wojtanowski MH, Mandel MD: Osteoradionecrosis of the thoracic wall and its surgical management. Am J Surg 138:434–438, 1979.
217. Wright J: Bacteriology of the collection and preservation of human milk. Lancet 2:121–124, 1947.
218. Yuehan C, Qun X: Filarial granuloma of the female breast: A histopathological study of 131 cases. Am J Trop Med Hyg 30:1206–1210, 1981.
219. Zuska JJ, Crile G, Ayres WW: Fistulas of lactiferous ducts. Am J Surg 81:312–317, 1951.

Chapter 6

BENIGN, HIGH-RISK, AND PREMALIGNANT LESIONS OF THE MAMMA

David L. Page, M.D. and Jean F. Simpson, M.D.

NONPROLIFERATIVE LESIONS
(Benign lesions without cancer risk implications)

Benign breast conditions have a diverse array of clinical presentations; the subjective discomfort of mammary pain and clinical signs of lumpiness have little correlation with histological alterations. Thus, establishment of clear-cut clinicopathological entities is not possible, and the establishment of meaningful categories is accepted as difficult. *Lumpiness* on physical examination is common to many benign and malignant situations. *Pain* is notorious for its seemingly spontaneous appearance and departure, making careful study of dietary and therapeutic interventions precarious.[49] Rigorous quantitative study in this area is in its infancy.[89, 93] In such circumstances one has a choice of two alternatives: grouping everything into a "catch-all phrase," or placing each element into reliable categories to examine interrelationships and correlates with menstrual history, parity, neoplasia, and so forth. The former approach negates an evaluation of individual elements, and the latter makes it difficult to recognize the clustering of elements. Indeed, without fostering this latter reductionist approach, the oversimplified, "lumping" approach will continue to be used without illumination of the situation. During most of this century a flurry of terms has been used.[147] These were largely "lumping" or "catch-all" phrases, most with an emphasis on one or another sign, symptom, or anatomical finding. These terms may be clarified, but not adequately defined in terms of disease entities or completely absolved of controversy. The continued use of such broad or lumping terms of convenience as *fibrocystic disease* (FCD) and *benign breast disease* (BBD) is not only because they are deeply embedded in clinical parlance. Despite the imprecision of applying these terms, they do have utility precisely because of this imprecision, familiarity, and wide reference. Thus, *FCD* has been in use along with *mammary dysplasia* and other synonyms for many decades, referring in a general way to any deviation from perfect symmetry: from vague clinical lumpiness to large cysts and from mild cyclical mammary discomfort to local, constant pain. In surgical pathology or histopathology

these terms had no precise reference and provided no clear understanding of pathogenesis; they essentially denoted that a biopsy had been clinically indicated because some alterations were present microscopically. This statement is true despite the valiant attempt of Foote and Stewart to codify five alterations (Table 6–1) as the defining elements within the notation of fibrocystic disease.[62] The following discussion highlights anatomical pathology, but this is done acknowledging that histopathology is an empty exercise without clinical correlates and predictability. Thus, we will be highlighting those changes that have clinical implications.

The term "benign breast *disease*" may be appropriate in some settings, as it allows for reference to a solitary term (although intrinsically imprecise) avowedly including all elements except carcinoma. However, the use of the analogous term "fibrocystic *disease*" has caused problems despite its intent of giving ready clinicopathological correlation between lumpiness and histological alterations.[15] The difficulty probably arises from the use of the term "disease" without "benign," which has reinforced the widely held belief that cancer risk was elevated in this setting.[33] This belief has been supported by studies of women who have undergone a benign breast biopsy indicating that they have a risk of subsequent carcinoma in the range of two to three times that of the general population.[48, 88] It was the intent of many in the recent past to set this slate right and remove the cancer implications of FCD by changing the term.[44, 81, 96] The need to further stratify this risk indication has been only partially met by histological evaluations of breast biopsies noted below and in Chapter 14.[48] The link between BBD and FCD is made clear

Table 6–1. FIBROCYSTIC DISEASE COMPLEX

Cysts
Sclerosing adenosis
Fibrosis
Papillomatosis (common type of hyperplasia)
Apocrine change

Modified from Foote FW, Stewart FW: Ann Surg 121:6–53, 197–222, 1945.

with the understanding that most benign biopsies have been termed FCD, and studies of cancer risk have held that the performance of a biopsy constituted BBD with its attendant increased risk of cancer. This discussion is dominantly referable to the era preceding mammography. It is evident that the introduction of this powerful diagnostic tool will aid the acceptance of a rigorous reductionist approach in which terms are technique-bound (physical examination, mammogram, and so forth) and must be individually compared. Thus a large cyst may be easily understood to produce a lump, but is it fibrosis when cysts are absent, or a regional variation in fat interposed between breast parenchyma which might be responsible for a palpable abnormality? These questions often are not resolvable.

The view, noted above, that considers *fibrocystic changes* to be largely a term of convenience is not held uniformly. Many would consider that placing some confines of definition on this "condition" would support its acceptance as an entity. Bartow and colleagues[15] have studies in different ethnic groups that support the idea of fibrocystic changes or fibrocystic disease as an entity, because these alterations are quite uncommon in low-risk cancer groups, such as American Indians. It is also true that the commonly grouped histopathological changes that tend to be correlated with lumpy and firm breasts are also correlated with age and menstrual status. All these fibrous and cystic changes increase rapidly in incidence in the 10 or 15 years prior to the menopause.[63, 139] Although it may be very difficult to draw sharp borders of definition for these changes, it is certain that they occur in over 50 percent of the immediately premenopausal population of high-risk North Americans. However, if these broad terms of convenience are of further use to indicate an elevation of breast cancer risk, then they overstate the risk if it is to be used within a high-risk population. The presence of cysts without hyperplasia and other changes noted as proliferative breast disease do not identify a higher risk group of women when compared with others within the same ethnic or geographically defined risk group.[44] It is likely that hyperplastic changes are more common in breasts that are clinically lumpy, but no formal recent analysis of co-occurrence of these conditions is available.

Breast symptoms of pain and/or lumpiness are the dominant presenting complaints of benign breast disease. Often breast pain has no physical or pathologically evident basis. Breast pain may be either cyclical, with premenstrual or midcycle discomfort most common, or noncyclical. Cyclical pain may respond to hormonal therapy and disappears with menopause. Noncyclical pain occurs in a slightly older age group and shows no response to hormonal therapy, making management more difficult. In either case, pain may be focal or diffuse and may or may not be associated with palpable lumps.[117]

Breast lumpiness is most evident in women around the time of menopause. Lumpiness may be quite varied, from diffuse small irregularities to discrete masses. Changes related to menstrual cycle are most evident in the week preceding menses.

Blichert-Toft et al.[20] have designed a diagnostic strategy for the management of patients with vague symptoms and atypical palpatory findings. Included in the system is close collaboration between the primary care physician, radiologist, surgeon, and pathologist, with the result of greater diagnostic accuracy.

In a recent study, Bright et al.[25] identified various risk factors for benign breast disease and made histological and mammographic correlates. Parity, use of oral contraceptives, and use of exogenous estrogen after menopause were protective against breast symptoms of pain and/or signs of lumpiness, termed benign breast disease (BBD). Furthermore, parity was negatively correlated with both the histological changes of intra- or extralobular fibrosis and mammographic changes of homogeneous densities. A summary of clinical findings is presented in Table 6–2.

Histopathology

Considered foremost among all the benign histological changes in the breast are *cysts* and the pink cell *apocrine change* that so commonly accompanies them. They may be recognized in sizes from 1 mm or so to many centimeters. It is remarkable that cysts are usually unilocular within the breast. The reason for this is thought to be that they arise as lobular lesions in which the individual acini or terminal ductules dilate, untwist, and unfold to produce a solitary locule that then enlarges as a cyst (Fig. 6–1).[149] Whether other lobular units and duct structures are recruited in the process of enlargement is unknown. The smaller cysts are often inapparent on gross examination of tissue. Whether associated fibrosis may make smaller cysts palpable is unclear, but possible. Haagensen indicated that clusters of cysts, each cyst being 2 to 3 mm in diameter, were palpable and termed them gross cysts along with larger cysts.[67, 68] In any case, these correlates of palpability have become less important, particularly when many accept the fact that a biopsy may well be appropriate from clinical or mammographic findings even if histology demonstrates no determinate abnormality. Understandably, fibrosis is often reported by pathologists in an attempt to explain clinical palpability or mammographic density. Few large cysts occasion excisional biopsy, as they may be definitely diagnosed by mammography, in company with ultrasound and/or needle aspiration. The gross appearance of large cysts is often blue, a reflection of the slightly cloudy, brown fluid usually found within. These are accorded the eponymous designation "blue-domed cyst of Bloodgood," after Joseph Bloodgood, who studied them and their cancer association in the first part of this century.[22]

Most cysts are lined by cells having a characteristic cytoplasmic pattern. The cells have many mitochondria and secretory granules that appear pink by the usual eosin staining. The nuclei are also quite characteristic, but less defining in that they are regularly round and often have a prominent round and eosinophilic nucleolus as well. Frequently, this epithelium is of columnar

Histopathological Diagnosis	Age	Palpable Mass	Mammographic Abnormality
FCC + PDWA	35–50 (premenopausal)	May be present	May be present
ADH	Increases after menopause	Incidental	Rare*
ALH	Decreases after menopause	Incidental	Rare*
Sclerosing adenosis	25–50 (premenopausal)	Frequent in "aggregate adenosis"	Often, with benign calcification
Fibroadenoma	20–30	More prominent in older patients	More prominent as fat increases with atrophy
CSL/RS	Not established; probably wide age range	Rare	Frequent

Table 6–2. CLINICAL FEATURES OF BENIGN LESIONS OF THE BREAST

*Has favored relation with calcification elsewhere in the breast.
Abbreviations: ADH = atypical ductal hyperplasia; ALH = atypical lobular hyperplasia; CSL/RS = complex sclerosing lesion/radial scar; FCC = fibrocystic change; PDWA = proliferative disease without atypia.

character and has a single protuberance at the apical aspect of the cytoplasm appearing as a bleb or "snout." Often the apocrine cells are grouped in tufted or papillary clusters and sometimes produce prominent papillary prolongations from the basement membrane region, which may or may not contain fibrovascular stalks (Figs. 6–2 and 6–3). The cysts, particularly larger ones, may not have any evidence of an epithelial lining or may have a simple squamous lining with an extremely flattened and undifferentiated epithelialized surface. There have been several studies differentiating these two types of cysts, apocrine and simple, indicating that the former has a high potassium content and is characterized by different steroid hormones.[40] There is some suggestion that there is a cancer risk difference between the kinds of cysts, which is unproved.[39] The apocrine type cysts are probably more commonly associated with multiplicity and recurrence than the nonapocrine cysts.[41, 144, 149] Whether this alteration of mammary epithelium to resemble that of apocrine sweat glands is a true metaplasia seems a point of practical irrelevance. However, much has been written on this point, and many scholars have felt that enzymatic profiles and ultrastructural evidence

support a true metaplasia.[7] Even so, the frequency of a slight to marked protuberance of cell groups (papillary apocrine change) rather than a smooth, single cell layer is quite different in the breast as compared with the apocrine sweat glands. A protein marker, GCDFP-15, is characteristically present and may be a useful marker.[100] Not only the cytoplasm of characteristic apocrine alteration is decorated with this marker. It is found in other settings with eosinophilic cytoplasm, such as nondistended lobular units and, less often, sclerosing adenosis.

There is no proven linkage of cysts alone to breast cancer risk. Recent and intensive studies have not indicated that cysts alone are associated with risk even when larger ones are separately analyzed.[44, 118] It is apparent that cysts are more common in high-risk geographical groups but are not determinants of cancer risk within geographical groups.[16] Other geographical considerations of risk for breast cancer are discussed in Chapter 23. The studies of Dupont and Page[44] did demonstrate a very slight elevation of risk for women with a family history and cysts as opposed to women with a family history of breast cancer alone. This must be considered

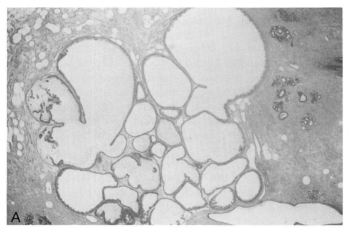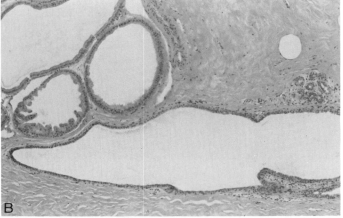

Figure 6–1. *A,* Apocrine cysts. Acini of this lobular unit have dilated and become distorted. Note entering lobular terminal duct at lower right. Low magnification, × 40. *B,* Higher power of *A,* showing apocrine-like epithelium lining dilated terminal duct and cysts. × 80.

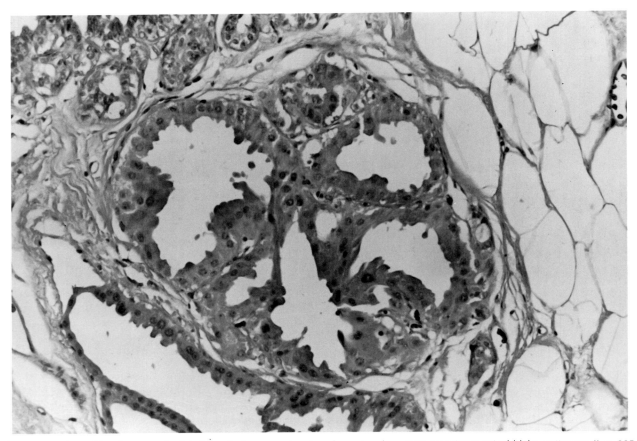

Figure 6–2. These dilated spaces of a lobular unit show prominent coalescent arches. Note prominent apical blebs or "snouts." × 225.

very mild evidence for premalignant indication of cysts, particularly because this interaction was not present with other indicators and remains an isolated observation. Although epithelial hyperplasia (see below), which is related to increased cancer risk, often coexists with cysts, either change may be present without the other in an individual biopsy specimen or entire breast. For this

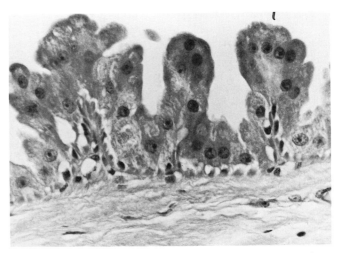

Figure 6–3. Papillary apocrine change. The lining of this cyst shows complex papillary tufts. Note prominent centrally placed nucleoli. × 320.

reason, cysts and hyperplastic epithelial changes should be diagnosed separately. Indeed, the separate consideration of cysts from epithelial changes was well established 50 years ago.[64]

The apocrine cytoplasmic alteration is also of no proven importance with regard to breast cancer risk. Apocrine change was found by Wellings and Alpers to be more commonly present concurrently with breasts associated with cancer than those without.[148] However, it is not an indicator of breast cancer risk in a predictive fashion. The notation of Page et al.[121] that papillary apocrine change was associated with a slight elevation of risk for women over the age of 45 was based on a very small number of patients. In the studies of Black et al.[19] done in the fashion of a case control study, some apocrine lesions were grouped with other hyperplastic lesions, but their separate indication as a risk indicator was not determined. In summary, neither cysts nor apocrine change may be viewed as significantly elevating cancer risk in an individual woman in the absence of other considerations.

Chronic inflammation, edema, and pigment-laden macrophages are often found around cysts. The last are likely the result of cytochromes from dead cells present at some time in the remote past. Occasionally, of course, some of the pigment material may represent hemosiderin. Although duct ectasia and cysts have some similarities histologically, they are usually easily separable because of the general contour of the lesions and the greater degree of inflammation and/or scarring associated with duct ectasia. It is also true that duct ectasia is usually present adjacent to the nipple, although it may extend quite a distance into the breast.

EPITHELIAL HYPERPLASIA AND PROLIFERATIVE BREAST DISEASE

The classification of epithelial hyperplasia in the breast espoused here is based largely upon a large follow-up (cohort) epidemiological study (see also Chaper 14) that sought to link epithelial histological patterns to magnitudes of breast cancer risk.[44] The positive relation of more extensive and complex examples of hyperplasia with carcinoma is supported in many concurrent and prospective studies.[28, 45, 51, 91, 105, 149] While the categories of histological alteration can be readily compared with many classification systems previously proposed, a major consideration marks this approach as different. Rather than supposing a regular stepwise progression or continuum from no change through carcinoma *in situ*, this approach takes as its foundation an absolute separation between carcinoma *in situ* and other hyperplastic appearances.[116] It further recognizes that small examples of lesions with features of carcinoma *in situ* may be reproducibly recognized because of their small size or their lack of some of the features of well-developed carcinoma *in situ*. These less than fully developed examples of carcinoma *in situ* are recognized by the term *atypical hyperplasia*.[120] This term does not, if it is taken to indicate a moderate increased risk of later carcinoma, include all examples of hyperplasia thought to be unusual. The remainder of the hyperplastic lesions of the breast, lacking features of carcinoma *in situ*, are separated by quantitative features only.

Definition and Background

Consistent with its definition elsewhere in the body, hyperplasia of the breast may be understood to mean an increased number of cells relative to a basement membrane. Thus, the increased number of glands without a concomitant increase relative to the basement membrane would not constitute hyperplasia, but rather "adenosis." Hyperplasia may be considered then to represent an increased number of cells above the basement membrane, and because this number is normally two, then three or more cells above the basement membrane constitutes hyperplasia. The discussion that follows is based upon the presentations of Wellings and Jensen[149] as well as those of our own group.[44] These represent a series of concurrent and prospective studies that seek to reproducibly define subgroups of patients and demonstrate their relationship or lack of relationship to carcinoma present at the same time,[149] or developing in the future in a prospective fashion.[44, 120]

One seemingly difficult portion of this discussion is that terminology differing from that presented here is in general usage. However, in most cases, different terms may be analogized and compared if the same definitions for atypical hyperplasia are used. We do not use the term "epitheliosis" because it has indicated both completely benign and worrying changes approaching carcinoma *in situ*.[131] The usefulness of the term as a condition of epithelium as opposed to a condition of increased glands is, of course, still appropriate.[34] The analogous term "papillomatosis" was proposed by Foote and Stewart.[62] This term is still in general usage in North America, where it indicates the common or usual hyperplasias of moderate and florid degree.

Our approach to the stratification of the hyperplasias is to recognize an atypical series of lobular type, a series of apocrine type, and a series of "usual" type that includes the remainder of the hyperplastic lesions found in the breast.[130] The three groups recognize patterns that are regularly found within the breast and do not imply a pathogenetic sequence or a site of origin. The intent of the term "usual" is to relay the idea that these are the common patterns of cytology and cell relationships seen when cell numbers are increased within the basement membrane–bound spaces within the human breast. The usual type or common patterns of hyperplasia have in the past been termed "ductal," largely to contrast them with the lobular series. Because these lesions regularly occur within acini of lobular units, it seems better to avoid the designation of "ductal" as an implication for either site of occurrence or site of origin of these cellular populations. Proliferative lesions in true ducts are unusual and are often truly papillary, that is, having branching, fibrous stalks (see below). It is recognized, however, that the term "ductal hyperplasia" is also in general use largely as a synonym for "papillomatosis."

The stratification of these hyperplastic lesions of usual type depends largely on quantitative changes. When the alterations begin to approximate patterns seen in carcinoma *in situ*, these lesions must be differentiated from those termed *atypical ductal hyperplasia* (ADH). Note that the features at the lesser end of the spectrum between mild and moderate hyperplasia of usual type depend upon quantity and that the separation of the larger lesions from ADH depends upon qualitative features of intercellular patterns and cytology (see atypical hyperplasia, below).

Mild hyperplasia of usual type is characterized by the presence of three or more cells above the basement membrane in a lobular unit or duct. These lesions are commonly of "inflammatory" type because of separation of the epithelial cells by inflammatory cells and their presence around the spaces. Frequently these lesions are associated with greatly attenuated cytoplasmic projections similar to those seen in reactive changes of cervical epithelium. These alterations of mild degree are not associated with any increased cancer risk. When hyperplastic lesions reach five or more cells above the basement membrane and have a tendency to cross and distend the space in which they occur, they are recognized as moderate. The appellation of florid is used when these changes are more pronounced, without any firm definition separating the moderate and the florid categories (Fig. 6–4). The reason for this is not to deny that there are quantitatively lesser and greater phenomena but that the progression of change makes reliable separation difficult. Moderate and florid hyperplasia of the usual type will be found in over 20 percent of biopsies. In follow-up studies, the cancer risk between these two groups was found to be similar (Chapter 14). Risk categories may be stratified into slight, moderate, and marked, with "slight" indicating a risk of 1.5 to 2 times that of the general population and "marked" indicating about a tenfold increased risk (see Chapter 14). The current status of these assignments of histological parameters to risk groups is shown in Table 6–3 and is little changed from that presented by a consensus conference that was supported by the American Cancer Society and the College of American Pathologists.[82] The clinical significance of usual hyperplasia of moderate and florid degree rests in the positive demonstration of a slight increased risk (1.5–2×) of subsequent invasive carcinoma. Clinical features are presented in Table 6–2.

The positive histological features of this group (Figs. 6–5 to 6–7) include (1) a mild variation of size and shape of cells, and more specifically, nuclei. This feature is of great importance in differentiating these lesions from those of atypical hyperplasia and nonco-

medo ductal carcinoma *in situ*. They are most commonly present within lobular units and terminal ducts. (2) The cells are frequently related to each other by a pattern of swirling or streaming. (3) There is a varied shape of secondary lumens, which are often slitlike and are present between the cells within individual spaces. (4) The secondary lumens, particularly in larger, more cellular lesions, may be present peripherally; that is to say, they are present immediately above the cells that surmount the basement membrane of the containing space. (5) The cells appear to be varied, not only in their cytological appearance but also in their placement. Thus, nuclei are not evenly separated one from the other. This may be understood to be a concomitant to the swirling or streaming change noted above.

ATYPICAL HYPERPLASIA

It is the intent of this term, "atypical hyperplasia" (AH), to indicate a group of fairly specific histological patterns that not only are "atypical" or "unusual" but also have been shown to have the implication of an increased risk of later breast cancer development (see Table 6–3 and Chapter 14).[120] This linkage of these histological patterns to a magnitude of breast cancer risk that has been termed moderate is not a universal no-

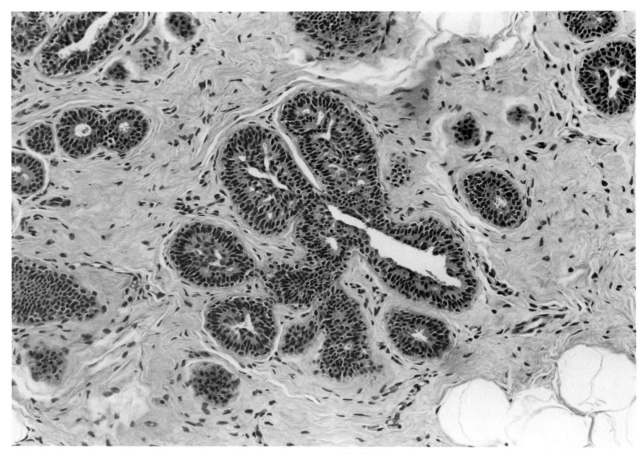

Figure 6–4. Moderate hyperplasia of the usual type. The ductules are partially filled by a heterogeneous population of cells. Note the normally polarized layer of cells just above the basement membrane. × 175.

Table 6–3. RELATIVE RISK FOR INVASIVE BREAST CARCINOMA BASED ON HISTOLOGICAL EXAMINATION OF BREAST TISSUE WITHOUT CARCINOMA*

No increased risk (no proliferative disease)
  Apocrine change
  Duct ectasia
  Mild epithelial hyperplasia of usual type
Slightly increased risk (1.5–2 times)
  Hyperplasia of usual type, moderate or florid
  Sclerosing adenosis†, papilloma
Moderately increased risk (4–5 times) (atypical hyperplasia or
    borderline lesions)
  Atypical ductal hyperplasia and atypical lobular hyperplasia
High risk (8–10 times) (carcinoma *in situ*)
  Lobular carcinoma *in situ* and ductal carcinoma *in situ* (non-
    comedo)

---

*Women in each category are compared to women matched for age who have had no breast biopsy with regard to risk of invasive breast cancer in the ensuing 10 to 20 years. *Note:* These risks are not lifetime risks.

†Jensen et al.[86] have shown sclerosing adenosis to be an independent risk factor for subsequent development of invasive breast carcinoma.

Modified from Hutter RVP, and others: Arch Pathol Lab Med 110:171–173, 1986.

menclature. Rather, it is the result of a group of studies that sought to restrict the term to a small number of histological patterns having some of the same features as the analogous CIS lesions. While many studies have supported the linkage of epithelial hyperplasia to premalignant states in the breast, many also termed any hyperplastic lesion "atypical."[18, 149] In order to separate groups, numbers were assigned, with "five" representing carcinoma *in situ* in both of the best known systems, those of Black and Chabon[18] and Wellings et al.[149] The system of Black and Chabon has a two-character alphanumerical code, in which the first character indicates the histological location of the lesion. The second digit refers to the degree of proliferation within the lesion and may range from 1 through 5: 1 being normal, 2 indicating hyperplasia, 3 and 4 indicating atypia, and 5

indicating carcinoma *in situ*. The system of Wellings et al.[149] includes two different types of atypical lobules (AL), each with a numerical scale of cellular alterations and hyperplasia from mild (I) to CIS (V), based on their advanced forms, either ductal carcinoma *in situ* (ALA) or lobular carcinoma *in situ* (ALB). The ALA lesions are subdivided into five grades (I–V), based on clearly defined histological and cytological patterns. Basically, our cases of AH are most analogous to the categories termed "four" by Black and Chabon as well as Wellings et al. Chapter 14 discusses the predictive utility of this classification system when tested in the forum of an epidemiological study. It is relevant that even when diagnostic terms in general use in the 1970s by hospital pathologists were grouped into analogous categories, a similar but lesser separation of risk groups was accomplished.[28] Atypical hyperplasia has been shown to be more common in the contralateral breast of women who have breast carcinoma.[101]

The atypical hyperplastic lesions have some of the same features as the carcinomas *in situ* (CIS) but either lack a major defining feature of CIS or have the features in less than fully developed form.[120] This general approach has also been used by others.[1, 6, 11, 57] Specific histological features separate each of the atypical hyperplasias from lesser categories as well as from the analogous CIS lesions after which they are named: lobular and ductal CIS. Thus the histological definitions are not viewed as resting within spectra of changes. On the contrary, these histological categories attempt to accept natural pattern groupings within the complex array of mammary alterations reflected in histological preparations. However, when no natural grouping is identified, an arbitrary separation is accepted. This latter approach was used in the separation of atypical lobular hyperplasia from lobular carcinoma *in situ* (see below).

Lobular carcinoma *in situ* (LCIS) (see also Chapter 8) is recognized when there is a well-developed example of filling, distention, and distortion of over half the acini of a lobular unit by a uniform population of characteristic cells. This follows the intent of the original descrip-

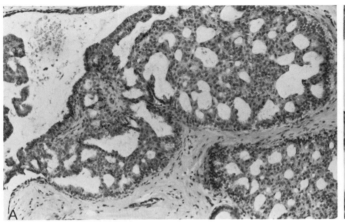
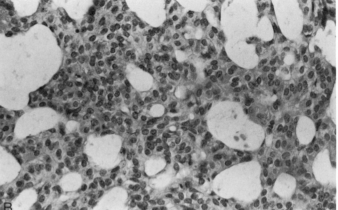

Figure 6–5. *A,* Florid hyperplasia, usual type. Ductules are partially filled with irregular arcade of cells. Note the irregularly shaped secondary lumens. × 150. *B,* Higher power of *A.* There is mild nuclei variability and irregular placement of cells, features supporting the lack of atypia. × 280.

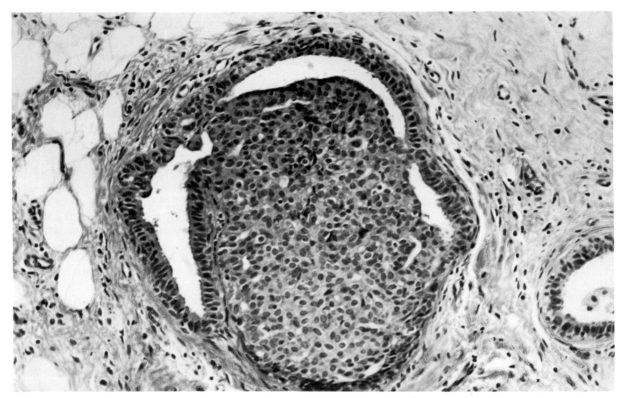

Figure 6–6. Florid hyperplasia of usual type with solid pattern and peripheral placement of secondary spaces. Nuclei are predominantly heterogeneous. × 350.

tion.[62] The analogous AH lesion, atypical lobular hyperplasia (ALH), is recognized when fewer than one half of the acini in a lobular unit are completely so involved, but the appearance is otherwise similar (Fig. 6–8).

This arbitrary recognition of ALH and LCIS in a series of changes from a few cells of appropriate appearance within a lobular unit to extreme examples with uniform cellular populations and extreme distortion and filling of acini imposes a stratification in what is otherwise an undivided continuum. Many pathologists prefer to use one diagnostic term for this range of histological appearances, for example, "lobular neoplasia."[74] This latter approach is espoused by us providing one term

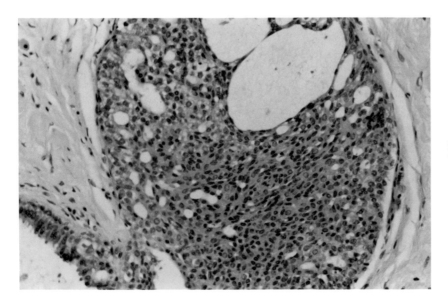

Figure 6–7. Florid hyperplasia of usual type demonstrating prominent nuclear streaming or swirling. × 200.

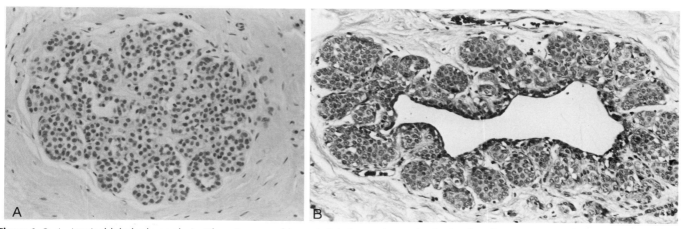

Figure 6–8. *A,* Atypical lobular hyperplasia. There is a resemblance to lobular carcinoma *in situ,* but less than 50 percent of the individual acini are uniformly distended. × 180. *B,* ALH undermining a different luminal cellular population. The same appearance may occur in LCIS; the defining diagnostic features must be present in lobular units to distinguish ALH from LCIS. × 180. (From Page DL, Anderson TJ: Diagnostic Histopathology of the Breast. Edinburgh, Churchill Livingstone, 1987. Reprinted by permission).

that indicates both ALH and LCIS. However, in diagnostic practice, more clinical guidance is given by the use of the separate designations: *LCIS* and *ALH* (see Chapter 14 for risk implications).

A specific feature of lobular neoplasia is the tendency to undermine an otherwise normal and certainly different cell population. As this is the interposition of an abnormal epithelial cell population within another, it has been termed pagetoid spread because of the obvious analogy to Paget's disease of the nipple. This phenomenon has been used by some to indicate diagnostic certainty for LCIS; however, it does occur when the degree of involvement within lobular units only reaches the diagnostic level of ALH. The histological patterns produced are usually more subtle in ALH,[54] and the solid pattern of LCIS ductal involvement is not seen with ALH. This pattern of involvement of ductal spaces outside of lobular units by the cells of lobular neoplasia in the presence of ALH has been termed ductal involvement in ALH and has been shown to be associated with a higher risk of subsequent breast carcinoma than is found with involvement of the lobular units alone. It is a magnitude of risk approaching that experienced after patients or women experience LCIS.[119]

The philosophical underpinnings of the diagnostic phrase "atypical ductal hyperplasia" or "ADH" are the same as those for ALH. Thus, the same features present in the analogous carcinoma *in situ* lesion are evident but not in fully developed form. In practice, the definition for AH in the ductal pattern series was more difficult to attain. When first attempted, this approach did not attain a subsequent risk elevation prediction of higher than double.[121] Rigorous analysis of the patterns accepted in that study revealed that many were pronounced examples of usual pattern hyperplasia. Confinement of ADH to lesions with both the pattern and the cytological features of noncomedo DCIS brought predictability of breast cancer risk to the quadruple level (see Table 6–3 and Chapter 14). This note of only historic interest is made to emphasize the point that

lesions indicating a relatively high risk of cancer not only are unusual but also have features of carcinoma *in situ.*

Because the criteria of atypical ductal hyperplasia are derived from those of ductal carcinoma *in situ,* it is mandatory to understand histological criteria for the latter. Two major criteria required for the diagnosis of ductal carcinoma *in situ* are: First, a uniform population of neoplastic-appearing cells must populate the entire basement membrane–bound space. We further require that this alteration must involve at least two such spaces. Second, an intercellular pattern of rigid arches and even placement of cells must be uniformly present. A helpful secondary criterion is hyperchromatic nuclei, which may not be present in all cases.[85]

Atypical ductal hyperplasia is most often diagnosed when these patterns of carcinoma *in situ* are present, but not completely so, throughout a given membrane-bound space (Figs. 6–9 and 6–10). ADH is also diagnosed when there is a small amount of variation in cell placement or when the intracellular patterns of sharply sculptured geometrical array are not well formed. The pattern of comedo ductal carcinoma *in situ* is not even mentioned here, because its characteristic extreme nuclear atypia is far beyond the patterns seen in atypical ductal hyperplasia.

Some cases of ADH share features with the so-called clinging carcinoma described by Azzopardi.[9] A recently reported study from Northern Italy indicates a considerable overlap of clinging carcinoma with ADH in histological patterns as well as in risk of subsequent cancer development.[51]

LOCALIZED SCLEROSING LESIONS

The classic example of such lesions is *sclerosing adenosis,* long accepted as a gross and histological mimicker of invasive carcinoma. It is in that capacity that it still has its greatest utility as a recognized diagnostic

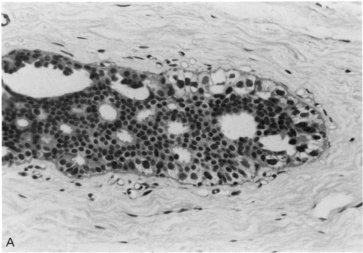

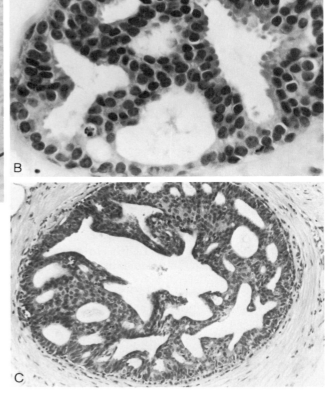

Figure 6–9. *A,* Atypical ductal hyperplasia is evident in this ductule cut longitudinally. Note regular placement of hyperchromatic nuclei and regularity of centrally placed secondary lumens. × 190. *B,* Rigid bar crossing central portion of photograph suggests DCIS; however, the cell pattern is not maintained throughout the remainder of the space. Note the polarity of cells at lower portion of space, a finding that indicated ADH rather than DCIS. × 350. *C,* Although there is some uniformity of some of the intercellular spaces, the cellular prolongations tend to taper and there is a tendency for peripheral placement of secondary spaces. The pattern and cytological criteria for DCIS are not clearly uniformly met, and therefore this is an example of ADH. × 170. (From Page DL, Anderson TJ: Diagnostic Histopathology of the Breast. Edinburgh, Churchill Livingstone, 1987. Reprinted by permission.)

term and histological pattern in the armamentarium of histopathologists.

In its most usual form, sclerosing adenosis is present as a microscopic lesion, probably unrecognized in both clinical and gross examination of tissues. Sclerosing adenosis (SA) is diagnosed only when a clearly lobulo-

centric change gives rise to enlargement and distortion of lobular units with a combination of increased numbers of acinar structures and a coexistent fibrous alteration. (Fig. 6–11). The normal two-cell population is maintained above the basement membrane in most areas, and the glandular units are regularly deformed. The

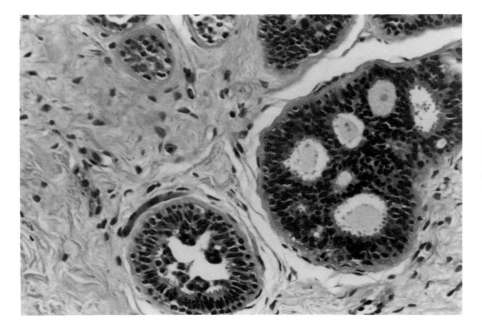

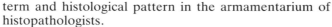

Figure 6–10. Florid hyperplasia of usual type. Although there is hyperchromatism and regularly spaced secondary spaces, there is not a uniform population of evenly spaced cells; this is not diagnostic of ADH. × 225.

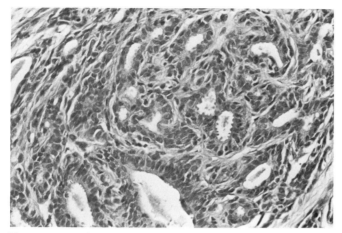

Figure 6–11. Sclerosing adenosis. Glandular elements are deformed and surrounded by stromal fibrous alteration. Two-cell population (basal or myoepithelial and luminal) is focally inapparent. × 240.

term was proposed by Ewing[53] and further described by Dawson[35] in order to clearly separate this increase in glands from lesions involving increased numbers of cells within an enclosure of basement membrane (hyperplasia of usual type, epitheliosis).

Enlarged lobular units appearing otherwise normal, or with slight gland deformity, may not be recognized as sclerosing adenosis but may rather be recognized by the noncommittal and appropriately descriptive term "adenosis." There is a favored association of SA with atypical lobular hyperplasia.[86] Diagnostic patterns of atypical lobular hyperplasia (ALH) are usually present in nonsclerosed lobules elsewhere in the biopsy and are certainly very difficult to recognize when present within a focus of sclerosing adenosis. This may be because of the maintenance of relatively small spaces within readily identifiable lesions of sclerosing adenosis (see under ALH). The cytological features of apocrine change may also be seen in adenosis.[50]

A palpable mass may be created by aggregations of microscopic foci of sclerosing adenosis ("aggregate adenosis"). This situation has been termed "adenosis tumor"[69] in order to indicate that a clinically palpable tumor may be produced. Sclerosing adenosis also frequently contains foci of microcalcification and, when present in this aggregate form, may be detectable by mammography. These features are summarized in Table 6–2.

The differential diagnosis of these lesions has been presented often as a series or listing of criteria. These most often seek to differentiate sclerosing adenosis from infiltrating tubular carcinoma and its variants (Table 6–4). Little thought has been given in these listings as to what is done if, for example, three criteria are consistent and the remaining are not. They must, then, be regarded as guidelines and not hard and fast criteria. Fortunately, most of the time the various criteria are consistent. Such is the variation of the biology of breast disease, or at least the variation of the anatomical expression of breast disease, that occasionally the guidelines will fail or at least be inconsistent. Usually, careful attention to the

fact that sclerosing adenosis is lobulocentric will suffice to correctly identify SA. It is also true in sclerosing adenosis that adjacent tubules tend to take approximately the same or similar shape as their immediate neighbors, although minor variations become marked if one skips to several ductular structures away. Equally true is that occasional ductal structures may be surrounded by a PAS-positive basement membrane in a benign condition, which tends to be lost in carcinoma. However, many carcinomas will have at least an irregular basement membrane and may show immunolocalization of proteins of basement membrane, such as Type 4 collagen or laminin.[32, 140] This is then a helpful but not an absolute criterion. The spaces of a tubular carcinoma tend to be open, occasionally producing an irregular extension of the cluster of cells at one edge, resembling a teardrop. The cells of an infiltrating tubular carcinoma usually are layered singly and when multilayered, the cells appear similar.

A rare condition known as microglandular adenosis (MGA) that may also mimic tubular carcinoma has been well described in the recent past,[31, 132, 142] although it had been noted years before.[102] In this condition, irregular, nonlobulocentric, small glandular spaces are present in increased numbers and appear to dissect and infiltrate through stroma and fat. A clinically palpable mass of several centimeters may be produced, which may be irregularly demarcated from surrounding tissue. The importance of this rare lesion is in its ability to mimic tubular carcinoma. A similar lesion composed of myoepithelial cells has been described and may show multiple recurrences.[90] MGA complicated by hyperplastic foci has been reported in two patients who subsequently developed carcinoma.[132] Additionally, Rosenblum et al.[135] reported seven cases of infiltrative carcinoma in the background of MGA. Because of the rarity of this condition, such associations are not certain. Clinical judgment may suggest various options in this setting, but a conservative stance should be emphasized. In other words, in the differential diagnosis between a benign lesion and "cancer" of little lethality (tubular carcinoma), one should favor benignancy in enigmatic settings.

Radial Scar and Complex Sclerosing Lesions. These entities have some similarities to sclerosing adenosis. These similarities are that carcinoma may be mimicked either clinically or histologically; it is by mammography that the mimicry of carcinoma by the larger complex sclerosing lesions is complete. Similar lesions were first described by Fenoglio and Lattes[56] as mimickers of carcinoma. Indeed, the advent of mammography has made the formal recognition of these lesions mandatory (see Table 6–2). The lesions appear spiculated—hence the term "radial scar." The lesions are not lobulocentric but evidently incorporate several very deformed lobular units within their makeup, having as probable origin the point of terminal duct branching from a more major stem. This is particularly true of the very large lesions. These are all characterized by a central scar from which elements radiate that may vary through the full range of histological appearances of the breast, including cystic

Table 6–4. HISTOPATHOLOGICAL CRITERIA FOR SCLEROSING ADENOSIS AND TUBULAR CARCINOMA

Feature	Sclerosing Adenosis	Tubular Carcinoma
Periphery	Smooth circumscription	Infiltrative
Confinement to lobular units	Yes	No
In situ carcinoma	Absent	Usually present
Double cell layer	Present	Absent, classically
Apical cytoplasmic 'snouts'	Seldom	Often present
Central spaces or lumens	Most often, flattened, or oblong	Uniform, round or angulated
Elastic tissue masses	Insignificant	Common
Relation of glandular element to scar	Not applicable	Infiltrates beyond scar

Modified from Page DL, Anderson TJ: Diagnostic Histopathology of the Breast. Edinburgh, Churchill Livingstone, 1987, p 211.

dilatation as well as units demonstrating hyperplasia and lobulocentric sclerosis like that of sclerosing adenosis. The microscopic features are determined by the degree of maturation, since it is now realized that the classic appearance (Fig. 6–12) represents the well-developed stage.[3] Lesions at an earlier stage show noticeable spindle cells and chronic inflammatory cells around the central parenchymal components, which are less distorted. The association of hyperplasia and cystic and apocrine change becomes more evident as the lesion matures.

The progressive nature of these lesions was further studied ultrastructurally by Battersby and Anderson.[17] A feature associated with "early" lesions was myofibroblasts in close proximity to degenerating parenchymal structures. "Mature" radial scars showed relatively few, sparsely distributed stromal myofibroblasts.

Within the central scar there are "entrapped" epithelial elements that have been appropriately characterized as pseudoinvasive (Fig. 6–13). While these are the elements that most frequently mimic carcinoma histologically, atypical hyperplastic lesions may be found within the preformed epithelial spaces in the outer portions of the lesion. The entrapped epithelial units may closely mimic tubular carcinoma, and this differential diagnosis may be very difficult. However, it should

be recalled that tiny tubular carcinomas pose very little threat to life and a conservative posture in the diagnosis of these lesions will benefit more patients.

Anderson and Battersby[3] analyzed the qualitative and quantitative features of over 100 examples of radial scars from the cases with and without cancer. Their frequency is similar in both groups and is heavily dependent on diligence of search and amount of tissue assessed. Bilaterality and multifocality were present in both groups as was the full range of histological appearance. No premalignant definition of these lesions was supported.

A wide variety of terms have been proposed for these lesions. However, it is likely that "radial scar" will gain and maintain dominance in usage over the next few decades. This is because it is the term favored by radiologists who perform mammography, and the majority of papers written on this subject are found in their literature. The other terms listed here for the fostering of understanding include scleroelastic lesions,[52] nonencapsulated sclerosing lesions,[58] and complex, compound heteromorphic lesions.[149] Except for the term highlighting the usual presence of elastica in the scars, the terms seem to add little to the ones preferred here. We do favor the term "complex sclerosing lesion" for the larger examples in this series. This is because they do tend to have a variety of appearances, and their complexity with

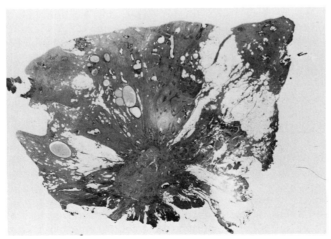

Figure 6–12. Mature radial scar with sclerotic center showing microcystic peripheral parenchyma. × 5.

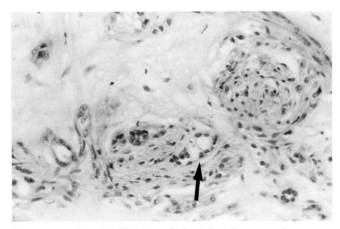

Figure 6–13. Pseudoinfiltration of glandular elements adjacent to a nerve (*arrow*) from a case of radial scar. The entrapped epithelial elements may closely mimic tubular carcinoma. × 300.

regard to mimicry of carcinoma is clearly portrayed by the term "complex." The term "radial" also is useful to indicate the spiculated nature of the lesions mimicking the classic scirrhous or sclerosing infiltrating mammary carcinoma.

DUCT ECTASIA AND FAT NECROSIS

Duct Ectasia

Duct ectasia is an entity or group of entities that still has unclear confines of definition. Some recognize only dilated ducts, as the term would indicate, as representing this condition. When this approach is taken, the condition is very common but is uncommonly associated with clinical pain or scarring.

Most current observers would reserve the diagnostic term for those conditions in which a clinical presentation includes palpable lumpiness in the region of the breast under the areola. Ducts tend to be involved in a segmental fashion; that is, adjacent ducts extending out into the breast from the nipple are involved. Nipple discharge is a common but not invariable accompaniment of this condition, and undoubtedly the periductal scarring attendant to the later stages of this process is responsible for the majority of cases of benign, acquired nipple inversion.[128]

Periductal inflammation is a histological hallmark of this condition.[10] It is now generally believed that the process begins with such a change and proceeds by destruction of the elastic network to ectasia and periductal fibrosis.[38]

Most cases described are found in the perimenopausal age groups. There are also younger women who present with inflammation of the ducts in the region of the nipple, which may produce fissures and fistulas with connections from the nipple ducts to the skin at the edges of the areola. Whether these two conditions are linked is not absolutely clear. The presentation of fistulas in younger women seems to be straightforwardly connected with infection. The more classic appearance of duct ectasia in older women may be a more smoldering infection of the larger ducts, and infection as the basis of this condition has been strongly suggested but remains unproved for the majority of cases.[26] At least recent reports have added to our knowledge by indicating that there is no association with parity or lactation.[38]

As is the case with so many of these benign conditions of the breast, the greatest importance clinically is the mimicry of carcinoma. The pultaceous material that may be present in the dilated ducts can be seen by mammography and has been termed secretory disease. Also, the plaque-like calcifications that occur within the scarred wall are, of course, visible by mammography (Fig. 6–14). Usually these can be differentiated from the more irregular punctate calcifications of comedo carcinoma, but this is not always clear. Besides this frequent approximation to the mammographic appearance of comedo ductal carcinoma *in situ*, the localized scarring of duct ectasia can produce lumps that are fixed within

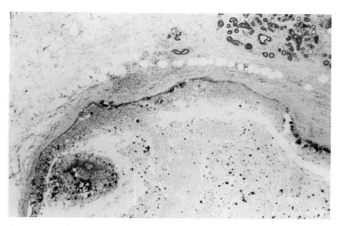

Figure 6–14. Large duct affected by duct ectasia. There is periductal fibrosis and inflammation. Note calcification in wall of duct. × 50.

inflamed scar in the breast. These mimic carcinoma quite completely upon occasion. One variant of this condition containing many plasma cells has been termed plasma cell mastitis in the past. This is probably not a separate condition but part of the spectrum of duct ectasia. This is known to be a close mimicker of breast carcinoma of lobular infiltrating type, both grossly and microscopically. Another synonym for duct ectasia, not utilized in several decades, is "comedo mastitis."[143] This term is useful in that it recalls the grumous material that may be present within the dilated ducts mimicking comedo carcinoma.

Fat Necrosis

This condition is relatively uncommon but may present in a most dramatic fashion mimicking a well-developed scirrhous carcinoma or even inflammatory carcinoma. In its late, scarred phase, fat necrosis may not have an identifiable preceding traumatic etiology; however, the mammographic appearance in the late stages is quite characteristic.[115] The great majority of cases seen in the more acute phases, with some inflammatory activity still apparent, will have an identifiable recent traumatic event.

The histology of fat necrosis in the breast is no different from its appearance in other organs. The characteristic active chronic inflammatory cells are usually evident, with lymphocytes and histiocytes predominating. In the unusual very acute cases presenting within approximately one week after an inciting event, polymorphonuclear leukocytes and free, oily, lipid material may be most apparent, particularly by needle aspiration. In this stage the clinical features of swelling, redness, and warmth will be present.

In the later stages collagenous scar is the predominant finding, with seemingly granular histiocytes surrounding "oil cysts" of varying size. These "oil cysts" contain the free lipid material released by lipocyte necrosis.

The greatest clinical importance of fat necrosis is in its mimicry of carcinoma as noted above. There is no known association with carcinoma or carcinoma risk.

MISCELLANEOUS CONDITIONS

Granulomatis Mastitis

Granulomatis mastitis should be understood as a descriptive diagnostic term only. Within the broad confines of such a descriptive designation there are variants of duct ectasia, granulomatous infectious diseases, and idiopathic granulomatous conditions. Idiopathic granulomatous mastitis may be difficult to distinguish from duct ectasia or from infectious granulomatous mastitis. Specific granulomatous infections such as tuberculosis may present in the breast, though uncommonly.[83, 145] Recognition of granulomatous inflammation at the time of frozen section should prompt a search for the etiological agent through culture. Granulomatous mastitis may be the presenting sign of a systemic disorder such as Wegener's granulomatosis.[36, 42] Sarcoidosis is another diagnostic consideration when granulomas are found in the breast.[14, 59] The associated features of duct ectasia should be absent in sarcoidosis. The variety of infectious and noninfectious granulomatous mammary conditions are listed by Symmers and McKeown.[141]

FIBROADENOMA AND PHYLLODES TUMOR

Fibroadenoma

Fibroadenomas (FA) often, if not invariably, have a characteristic clinical presentation with an easily movable mass, seemingly unfixed to surrounding breast tissue. The gross appearance of fibroadenomas is usually characteristic and often diagnostic. It is the sharp circumscription and smooth boundary with surrounding breast tissue, usually producing an elevation of the FA on cut section, that is characteristic. The cut surface is white, although one may identify the epithelial elements, if they are numerous, as light brown areas. The cut surface is shiny and occasionally may seem to present an almost papillary appearance if the clefts lined by epithelium are larger. There may be slight variation from one area to another, with more dense fibrosis in the stroma and, occasionally, calcification. The latter two features are more common in older women.

Traditionally, the risk for subsequent carcinoma in patients with typical fibroadenoma has not been considered to be higher than for the general population. By 1985, approximately 100 cases of carcinoma arising in fibroadenomas had been reported.[61, 124] In this setting, lobular carcinoma *in situ* is the predominant type.

Microscopically, fibrous tissue composes most of the fibroadenoma; either the stroma may surround rounded and easily definable ductlike epithelial structures or the epithelium may be stretched into curvilinear arrangements (Figs. 6–15 and 6–16). This latter pattern has been known as intracanalicular, with the former pattern known as pericanalicular. These two terms are still useful as descriptors but are of no practical or prognostic importance and therefore are not used to define sup-

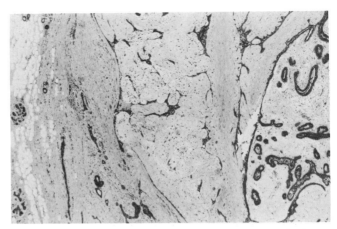

Figure 6–15. Fibroadenoma showing prominent intracanalicular pattern. × 30.

posed subtypes of fibroadenoma. Smooth muscle is an extremely rare component of fibroadenomas.[65] The epithelium within an FA may have the same appearance as elsewhere in the breast, including apocrine metaplasia.[8] Rarely, squamous metaplasia is present.[138]

Fibroadenomas that are allowed to grow after initial detection usually cease to grow when they reach 2 to 3 cm in diameter.[70] Blacks more commonly develop fibroadenomas compared with whites, and at a younger age as well. Fibroadenomas in blacks are also more likely to recur.[114] As fibroadenomas are more common in blacks, probably related lesions are also more common in blacks.[92] Infarcts of the breast may occur during pregnancy or lactation with a resultant discrete mass.[77] Approximately 1 of 200 fibroadenomas shows infarction.[98, 152] Pain and tenderness may occur during pregnancy, and an inflammatory reaction may be accompanied by lymphadenopathy, leading to the clinical impression of carcinoma.[37] Clinical features of typical fibroadenoma are presented in Table 6–2.

Fibroadenoma may also be regarded as a generic term, referring to any benign, confined tumor of the breast (mass-occupying lesion) that has a mixture of glandular and mesenchymal elements. When it is viewed as a more specific term, then special or specific variants of the general pattern are recognized as being separate entities. These latter are hamartoma, tubular adenoma, lactating adenoma, adenolipoma, juvenile fibroadenoma, and giant adenoma.

Hamartomas of the breast have received attention relatively recently. As with so many other breast lesions, the introduction of mammography led to enthusiasm about the creation of this entity.[55] The series of Hessler et al.[79] and Linell et al.[95] have been the most important in establishing the notation of hamartomas as first proposed by Arrigoni et al.[4] These are lesions made up of recognizable lobular units, often present at the sharply demarcated margins of these lesions. Fat is rare in fibroadenomas, which are also infrequently characterized by well-ordered lobular units throughout a majority of their substance. Another feature supporting the recognition of hamartomas as separate entities is that their

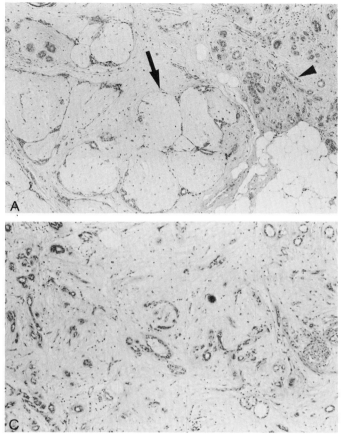

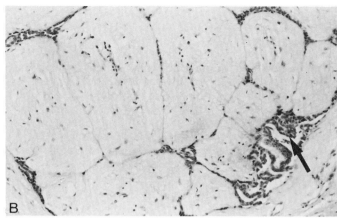

Figure 6–16. *A,* Fibroadenoma with irregular border. Both intracanalicular (*arrow*) and pericanalicular (*arrowhead*) patterns are well demonstrated. × 30. *B,* Higher power of *A.* Fixation artifact gives appearance of hyperplastic epithelium (*arrow*). × 125. *C,* Same case as *A.* Complex epithelial patterns are evident. × 50.

average age of presentation is almost two decades after that for fibroadenomas in general. It is the sharp, smooth borders of these lesions and their intermixture with fat that allows mammographic identification in pronounced examples. Duchatelle et al.[43] support the formation of these lesions as more likely to be developmental than neoplastic. A similar lesion is the adenolipoma.[47] These lesions are only one tenth as common as ordinary lipomas.[71]

Other types of fibroadenoma, perhaps better regarded as variants rather than as separate entities, are lesions tending to occur in women in the younger age range of fibroadenoma and characterized by increased cellularity of stroma and/or epithelium. Duray et al.[46] described cellular fibroadenomas most likely to occur in adolescents and more likely to recur locally as "adolescent cellular fibroadenoma." These lesions bear some resemblance to benign phyllodes tumors of some other classifications. Juvenile fibroadenoma is a diagnostic term that is predominantly predicated on clinical grounds.[5] Oberman[109] initially suggested the term "juvenile adenofibroma" in a review of breast lesions in juveniles. He felt that five to ten percent of the adenofibromas occurring in that age group were notable for rapid growth and large size. Pike and Oberman,[126] further elaborating "juvenile adenofibroma," characterized them by their tendency to occur around the time of menarche and to frequently have a ductal pattern of epithelial hyperplasia as well as the defining stromal

hypercellularity. Local recurrence was not felt to be a feature of these lesions. Mies and Rosen[103] have also described a series of patients with an average age of 26 years who had an unusual and atypical pattern of epithelial hyperplasia within fibroadenomas, which is likely to be misinterpreted as carcinoma *in situ.* No specific clinical feature was suggested. There is certainly no overlap between the latter series of patients and those described by Duray et al.,[46] whereas the cases of Pike and Oberman[126] appear to be somewhere in between. The practical utility of these interesting approaches to unusual fibroadenomas appears to be that rapidly growing lesions in juveniles are usually benign, often have a densely cellular stroma, and less often have prominent epithelial hyperplasia. The last characteristic may occur in older patients and is regularly benign, even if patterns closely mimic carcinoma *in situ.*

The histological definitions separating fibroadenoma from phyllodes tumors are even less well defined than are the definitions of benign vs. malignant within the phyllodes tumors (see following discussion). It seems clear that the term "phyllodes tumors" will be applied to most large fibroadenomas with any suggestion of hypercellularity. As long as the descriptor "benign" is added to the designation (particularly if the synonymous diagnostic phrase "benign cystosarcoma phyllodes" is used), no harm will come of this usage. Fechner[55] considers up to three mitoses per high power field as acceptable in fibroadenomas. Perhaps with the designation of cellular fibroadenomas,[46] indicating a slightly greater likelihood of local recurrence, the separation of phyllodes tumors from fibroadenomas may become more precise. In a carefully reported series of phyllodes tumors, Chua and Thomas[30] recognized 92 percent to be benign because of fewer than five mitoses per ten high power field, only mild stromal pleomorphism, and circumscribed tumor margins. An 18 percent local recurrence rate for these lesions is within the range of 15 percent cited for fibroadenomas alone, further evidence that clinical terminology for these lesions might be considered to be a matter of personal choice.

There remains the possibility that fibroadenomas may evolve into phyllodes tumors, but that is not well documented.[97] Certainly there has been a recent major change from the prior clinical dictum that any determinate mass had to be surgically removed from the breast. Recently many surgical groups have noted that characteristic 2- to 3-cm fibroadenomas could be watched clinically after careful notation; this being most appropriate in patients younger than 25 years and also appropriate in those aged 25 to 35 years, but probably not thereafter.[27] Also, needle aspiration with characteristic findings should document the fact that such lesions are fibroadenomas. The natural history of most fibroadenomas supports this approach.[153] A condition that may resemble fibroadenoma is fibromatosis.[2, 146] Fibromatosis is benign histologically, and recurrence is common.[134, 146]

Another variant of fibroadenoma is the tubular adenoma. These are quite uncommon and are recognized as having dominant tubular elements in a circumscribed mass with minimal supporting stroma.[78, 122] Grossly tubular adenomas have a fine nodularity.[104] Portions of otherwise characteristic fibroadenomas may have the appearance of a tubular adenoma.[111] Uniform tubular structures are seen, and lobular anatomy is usually not evident. The myoepithelial layer is subtle or inapparent. Tubular adenomas may have evidence of secretory activity, but when not occurring in association with pregnancy or lactation should not be termed "lactating adenomas." Lactating adenomas are certainly analogous in some ways to tubular adenomas, and may represent a physiologic response of the tubular adenoma to pregnancy.[111] In addition to showing lactational changes, the adenomas presenting in pregnancy have a more evident lobular anatomy than that seen in most tubular adenomas. James et al.[84] have recently supported the notion that the lesions arising in pregnancy, formerly termed "lactating adenomas," be termed "breast tumor of pregnancy" because they are distinct from tubular adenomas and should not be related to lactation (despite histological changes) because they arose during pregnancy and not during the time of breast feeding. The microscopic changes seen in the breast tumor of pregnancy are similar to those seen in the normal pregnant breast, but are variable in degree and are out of phase with the pregnancy changes of the normal breast.

Phyllodes Tumor

The series of mammary tumors known as phyllodes tumors continues to pose problems for the physician managing breast disease. Three problems remain incompletely resolved: (1) the confusing terminology of cystosarcoma phyllodes is still in frequent usage; (2) rarity of these lesions has made clear understanding of the borderline between benign and malignant difficult; and (3) there remain a fairly large number relative to the entire group of lesions that must continue to be regarded as of borderline malignancy, presenting obvious problems in patient management.

First, the replacement of the classic terminology that placed the suffix "sarcoma" on benign and malignant examples of these lesions is a necessary recognition of the evolution of the term sarcoma.[151] When first coined by Muller[106] in 1838, the term meant only a fleshy tumor. The general acceptance of the term to mean predicted malignant behavior did not come until decades later, and we may regard cystosarcoma as a vestigial example of the 19th century descriptive use of that term.[80]

Second, the rarity of these lesions has led them to be overdiagnosed in some settings, and, probably, underdiagnosed in others. Two differential diagnostic problems are represented by this situation; the separation of the benign phyllodes tumors from some similar, and probably closely related, unusual fibroadenomas, and the recognition of the malignant end of the spectrum of phyllodes tumors.

There is no reliable way to grossly differentiate a giant fibroadenoma or the so-called juvenile fibroadenoma from a benign phyllodes tumor. Indeed, the frequent tendency to recognize the large size as the dominant characteristic of phyllodes tumor has led to the frequent confusion of these entities. They may well be interrelated in any case. A classic gross pattern for a phyllodes tumor includes sharp demarcation from the surrounding normal breast tissue, with the latter obviously compressed. The connective tissue that makes up the greatest bulk of the mass is firm and varies from dense and white to glistening and edematous. Local areas of degeneration lead to cystic and discolored areas. The classic pattern that gave these tumors their name may be evident with smoothly contoured leaf-like areas separated from others by narrow, epithelial-lined spaces.[21]

The histological appearance of phyllodes tumors may be considered exactly that of large fibroadenomas unless some specific guidelines are accepted. Fechner feels that the stroma in phyllodes tumors should have greater cellularity and cell activity, but that up to three mitoses per high power field should be accepted within the definition of fibroadenoma.[55] Johnson et al.[87] have also accepted that approach and suggested that the close application of a particularly cellular connective tissue element of the basement membrane region of the epithelial element should be defining, and that size should have no part in the differential diagnosis of these mixed tumors of the breast (Fig. 6–17). The proliferating stroma is usually rich and cellular, regularly deforming the epithelium into extreme examples of the intracanalicular pattern seen in the more common fibroadenomas. The classic paper of Norris and Taylor[108] inaugurated the approach to documenting histological features as rigorously as possible. Later papers have supported

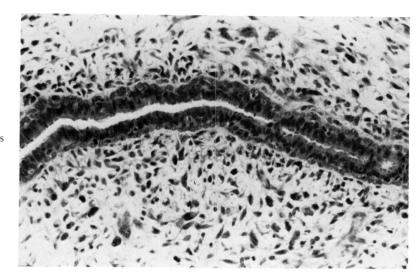

Figure 6–17. Phyllodes tumor. Hypercellular stroma shows nuclear pleomorphism and atypia. × 300.

counting mitoses and evaluating the margins with care to see if there is an infiltrating focus.[76, 107, 125] Evaluated in this way, Chua and Thomas[30] identified five borderline phyllodes tumors, two of which recurred after local excision. A predominantly circumscribed margin, five to ten mitoses per high power microscopic field, and moderate nuclear pleomorphism were felt defining in this group. Thus borderline lesions are unlikely to evidence truly malignant behavior and may be more likely to recur locally than the usual phyllodes tumor. Special note should be made of the fact that malignant behavior in phyllodes tumors of young women is extremely rare.[24] The majority of malignant phyllodes tumors reported in the literature which have metastasized have had overgrowth of an obvious sarcomatous element (Fig. 6–18). This malignant element has often been something other than fibrosarcoma (i.e., liposarcoma, rhabdomyosarcoma, etc.). Close examination of the stroma with multiple sections is mandatory. The truly malignant phyllodes tumor may be so only in a portion of the tumor where easily diagnostic foci of sarcoma may be evident. On the other hand, a richly cellular fibrosarcoma-like stroma present in many foci or diffusely throughout the tumor presents the greatest difficulty in differential diagnosis. This difficulty primarily leads to overdiagnosis of malignancy as evidenced by the 27 patients reported by Blumencranz and Gray[23] with 13 of the phyllodes tumors diagnosed as malignant because of any combination of increased mitotic activity, invasive borders, or marked pleomorphism. None of the women in this study developed recurrences or metastases.

Foci of calcification and necrosis may be seen in either

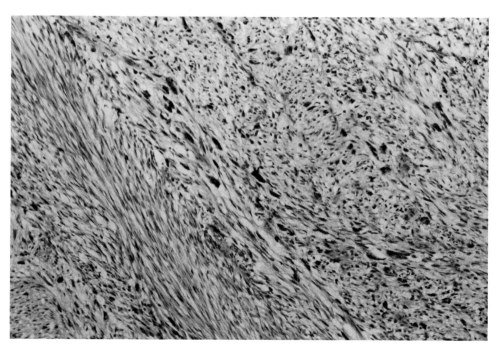

Figure 6–18. Phyllodes tumor. Low-grade fibrosarcomatous element is evident. × 110.

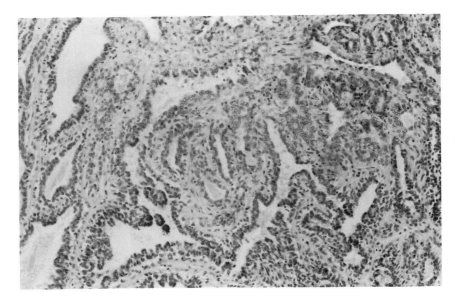

Figure 6–19. Delicate fibrovascular fronds of papilloma covered by single or double epithelial cell layers. × 280.

benign or malignant phyllodes tumors and are of no aid in differentiating the two major types of phyllodes tumor.

Although it is frequently stated that histological criteria are not reliable and that lesions appearing to be benign histopathologically may metastasize, these events are poorly characterized or poorly documented. With the use of a borderline category (tumors that usually do not act in a malignant fashion), this unpredictability is no longer completely true. Certainly even the tumors with diffuse features of low grade fibrosarcoma in the stroma rarely act in a malignant fashion. It is not even

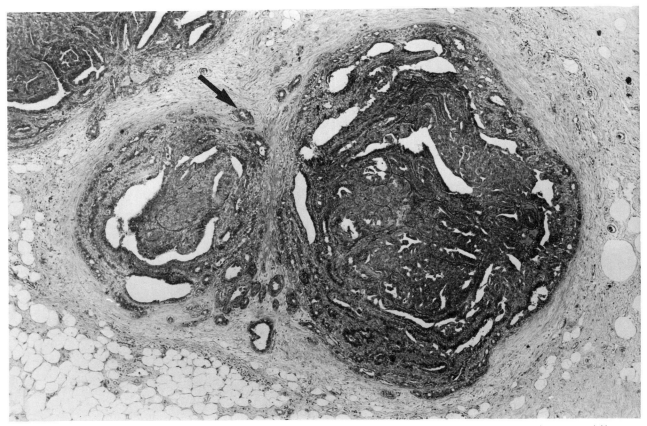

Figure 6–20. Proliferating glandular epithelium of a "ductal adenoma." Irregularities at the interface between adenotic elements and fibrous capsule simulate invasion (*arrow*). × 70.

clear that such "borderline" tumors reliably recur locally more often than other benign tumors. However, local recurrence has been reported in up to 59 percent of cases.[75, 94, 150] Other series have not found that the approximate 15 percent local recurrency figure accorded fibroadenomas was reliably different from that of phyllodes tumor. Very importantly, local recurrences have not been reported to evolve into malignant features if these were not present in the primary tumor.[99]

PAPILLOMA

The usual and classic solitary papilloma is a mass lesion of the large ducts and most often presents in the subareolar region. In the periphery, papillary lesions are often multiple and are continuous with hyperplastic alterations within lobular units, as shown by Ohuchi et al.[112] in three-dimensional reconstruction studies of papillomas. Particularly when extensive, these papillary lesions may be associated with atypical hyperplasia and ductal pattern carcinoma *in situ* within and adjacent to the papillomas.

There is an important clinical correlate of these lesions, and that is that they frequently present with a hemorrhagic discharge from the nipple which is usually unilateral.[12] This is true for the more central and larger lesions, but may be also seen in smaller, more peripheral lesions. A careful follow-up of women with a solitary papilloma showed an increased risk of subsequent development of carcinoma.[29] It was suggested that accompanying epithelial hyperplasia was responsible for further elevating the increased risk (see Table 6–3). Others have felt that women with multiple papillomas have an increased risk for subsequent carcinoma development.[72] The co-occurrence of highly atypical hyperplastic lesions (including carcinoma *in situ*) with these multiple papillomas has been illustrated.[73, 113, 137]

Histopathology

Papillomas are truly papillary lesions with a branching fibrovascular course surmounted by epithelium (Fig. 6–19). They are most often identified in careful gross examination as lying within dilated ductal spaces. The papillomas may attain several centimeters in size and when that large may appear encysted with the continuity of the duct within which they arose, less apparent than in smaller examples. Papillomas vary from a soft texture to being firm with dense sclerotic foci. Focal areas of necrosis and hemorrhage are a natural part of the basic elements of papillomas. Infarction may cause compression and distortion of epithelium to produce the appearance of carcinoma.[60] Squamous metaplasia may also be present.[127]

The epithelium lining in benign papillomas varies greatly, but is usually evidently and easily identified as benign (see Fig. 6–19). A double cell layer with more rounded cells adjacent to the basement membrane and surmounted by more columnar cells is frequently seen.

When the cell numbers are increased beyond that, the same rules for atypia and carcinoma *in situ* used for hyperplasia may be applied. Thus, there will be papillomas with focal atypia that may qualify for atypical hyperplasia. When the cell proliferation is quite uniform and attains the features seen in patterns in ductal carcinoma *in situ*, noninvasive papillary carcinoma is diagnosed (see Chapter 9).

Other lesions bearing resemblance to papilloma are discussed here for convenience, as they remain a portion of the differential diagnosis of those lesions. These are nipple adenoma (florid papillomatosis of the nipple) and nodular adenosis (ductal adenoma).

Nipple adenoma is a term used to describe quite a variety of appearances that may present in the nipple or immediately adjacent tissues. Patterns of hyperplasia with pseudoinvasion of dense stroma may be taken to be the basic features of these lesions. They may be misinterpreted as Paget's disease when presenting clinically because of irregularities of the surface of the nipple. However, they rarely ulcerate and therefore do not have the moist, red appearance of the eczematous features of Paget's disease. The greatest importance is to avoid calling these lesions of the nipple malignant. These lesions have localized areas of hyperplasia of slightly varying patterns intermixed with fibrous and cystic changes. Nipple adenomas or subareolar papillomatosis usually are diagnosed when approximately 1 cm or somewhat less in size. Patterns of papilloma are also mimicked. Careful histological sampling and complete excision are important, because foci of carcinoma have been described in such lesions but apparently are rare.[66, 133] These lesions frequently have nuclear hyperchromatism and a relatively high nuclear cytoplasmic ratio as well as fibrosis—features that may be worrisome.[123] Complex patterns of epithelial hyperplasia enveloped by fibrosis may lead to the mistaken diagnosis of malignancy. Careful attention to these features will avoid overdiagnosing malignancy.[110]

Nodular adenosis or *ductal adenoma* may be taken to be closely similar terms for an important group of lesions presenting a quite varied histology. These are most closely related to papillomas with unusual patterns of sclerosis and adenosis.[13] Because these lesions are characteristically surrounded by dense fibrous tissue within which epithelial cells are pseudoinvasive, they present problems for the overdiagnosis of malignancy by the unwary (Fig. 6–20).

References

1. Ackerman LV, Katzenstein AL: The concept of minimal breast cancer and the pathologist's role in the diagnosis of "early carcinoma." Cancer 39:2755–2763, 1977.
2. Ali M, Fayemi AO, Braun EV, Remy R: Fibromatosis of the breast. Am J Surg Pathol 3:501–505, 1979.
3. Anderson TJ, Battersy S: Radial scars of benign and malignant breasts: comparative features and significance. J Pathol 147:23–32, 1985.
4. Arrigoni MG, Dockerty MB, Judd ES: The identification and treatment of mammary hamartoma. Surg Gynecol Obstet 133:577–582, 1971.

5. Ashikari R, Farrow JH, O'Hara J: Fibroadenomas in the breast of juveniles. Surg Gynecol Obstet 132:259–262, 1971.
6. Ashikari R, Huvos AG, Snyde RE: A clinicopathologic study of atypical lesions of the breast. Cancer 33:310–317, 1974.
7. Azzopardi JG: Problems in Breast Pathology. Philadelphia, WB Saunders, 1979, pp 62–64.
8. Azzopardi JG: Problems in Breast Pathology. Philadelphia, WB Saunders, 1979, pp 25–56.
9. Azzopardi JG: Problems in Breast Pathology. Philadelphia, WB Saunders, 1979, pp 193–203.
10. Azzopardi JG: Problems in Breast Pathology. Philadelphia, WB Saunders, 1979, pp 72–91.
11. Azzopardi JG: Problems in Breast Pathology. Philadelphia, WB Saunders, 1979, pp 113–123, 213–233.
12. Azzopardi JG: Problems in Breast Pathology. Philadelphia, WB Saunders, 1979, pp 150–166.
13. Azzopardi JG, Salm R: Ductal adenoma of the breast: a lesion which can mimic carcinoma. J Pathol 144:11–23, 1984.
14. Banik S, Bishop PW, Ormerod LP, O'Brien TEB: Sarcoidosis of the breast. J Clin Pathol 39:446–448, 1986.
15. Bartow SA, Black WC, Waeckerlin RW, Mettler FA: Fibrocystic disease: a continuing enigma. Pathol Annu 17(2):93–111, 1982.
16. Bartow SA, Pathak DR, Black WC, Key CR, Teak SR: Prevalence of benign, atypical, and malignant breast lesions in populations at different risk for breast cancer. Cancer 60:2751–2760, 1987.
17. Battersby S, Anderson TJ: Myofibroblast activity of radial scars. J Pathol 147:33–40, 1985.
18. Black EM, Chabon AB: In-situ carcinoma of the breast. Pathol Annu 4:185–210, 1969.
19. Black MM, Barclay THC, Cutler SJ, Hankey BF, Asire AJ: Association of atypical characteristics of benign breast lesions with subsequent risk of breast cancer. Cancer 29:338–343, 1972.
20. Blichert-Toft M, Dyreborg U, Andersen J: Diagnostic strategy in the management of patients with breast symptoms. A recommended design and present experiences. Acta Oncol 27:597–600, 1988.
21. Blichert-Toft M, Hansen JPH, Hansen OH, Schidt T: Clinical course of cystosarcoma phyllodes related to histologic appearance. Surg Gynecol Obstet 140:929–932, 1975.
22. Bloodgood JC: The pathology of chronic cystic mastitis of the female breast; with special consideration of the blue-domed cyst. Arch Surg 3:445, 1921.
23. Blumencranz PK, Gray GF: Cystosarcoma phyllodes—clinical and pathological study. NY State J Med 78:623–627, 1978.
24. Briggs RM, Walters M, Rosenthal D: Cystosarcoma phyllodes in adolescent female patients. Am J Surg 146:712–714, 1983.
25. Bright RA, Morrison AS, Brisson J, Burstein N, Sadowsky NL, Kopans DB, Meyer JE: Histologic and mammographic specificity of risk factors for benign breast disease. Cancer 64:653–657, 1989.
26. Bundred NJ, Dixon JM, Lumsden AB: Are the lesions of duct ectasia sterile? Br J Surg 72:844–845, 1985.
27. Cant PJ, Madden MV, Close PM, Learmonth GM, Hacking EA, Dent DM: Case for conservative management of selected fibroadenomas of the breast. Br J Surg 74:857–859, 1987.
28. Carter CL, Corle DK, Micozzi MS: A prospective study of the development of breast cancer in 16,692 women with benign breast disease. Am J Epidemiol 128:467–477, 1988.
29. Carter D: Intraductal papillary tumors of the breast: a study of 78 cases. Cancer 39:1689–1692, 1977.
30. Chua CL, Thomas A: Cystosarcoma phyllodes tumors. Surg Gynecol Obstet 166:302–306, 1988.
31. Clement PB, Azzopardi JG: Microglandular adenosis of the breast—a lesion simulating tubular carcinoma. Histopathology 7:169–180, 1983.
32. D'Ardenne AJ: Use of basement membrane markers in tumour diagnosis. J Clin Pathol 42:449–457, 1989.
33. Davis HH, Simons M, Davis JB: Cystic disease of the breast: Relationship to carcinoma. Cancer 17:957, 1964.
34. Dawson EK: Carcinoma in the mammary lobule and its origin. Edinb Med J 40:57–82, 1933.
35. Dawson EK: A histological study of the normal mammal in relation to tumor growth. Early development to maturity. Edinb Med J 41:653–681, 1934.
36. Deininger HK: Wegener's granulomatosis of the breast. Radiology 154:59–60, 1985.
37. Delarue J, Redon H: Les infarctus des fibro-adenomes mammaires: probleme clinique et pathogenique. Sem Hop Paris 25:2991–2996, 1949.
38. Dixon JM, Anderson TJ, Lumsden AB, Elton RA, Roberts MM, Forrest APM: Mammary duct ectasia. Br J Surg 70:601–603, 1983.
39. Dixon JM, Lumsden AB, Miller WR: The relationship of cyst type to risk factors for breast cancer and the subsequent development of breast cancer in patients with breast cystic disease. Eur J Cancer Clin Oncol 21:1047–1050, 1985a.
40. Dixon JM, Miller WR, Scott WN, Forrest APM: The morphological basis of human breast cyst populations. Br J Surg 70:604–606, 1983.
41. Dixon JM, Scott WN, Miller WR: Natural history of cystic disease: importance of cyst type. Br J Surg 72:190–192, 1985.
42. Douglas AC, Anderson TJ, MacDonald M, Simpson JGG: Midline and Wegener's granulomatosis. Ann NY Acad Sci 278:618–635, 1976.
43. Duchatelle V, Auberger E, Amouroux J: Hamartomas du sein. Ann Pathol 6:335–339, 1986.
44. Dupont WD, Page DL: Risk factors for breast cancer in women with proliferative breast disease. N Engl J Med 312:146–151, 1985.
45. Dupont WD, Rogers LW, Vander Zwaag R, Page DL: The epidemiologic study of anatomic markers for increased risk of mammary cancer. Pathol Res Pract 166:471–480, 1980.
46. Duray PH, Holahan KP, Merino M, Risdall K: Adolescent cellular fibroadenomas: a clinical and pathologic study. Abstracts, annual meeting of IAP. Lab Invest 50:17A, 1984.
47. Dyreborg U, Starklint H: Adenolipoma mammae. Acta Radiol (Diagn) (Stockh) 16:362–366, 1975.
48. Ernster VL: The epidemiology of benign breast disease. Epidemiol Rev 3:184–205, 1981.
49. Ernster VL, Mason L, Goodson WH, Sickles EA, Sacks ST, Selvin S, Dupuy ME, Hawkinson J, Hunt TK: Effects of caffeine-free diet on benign breast disease. Surgery 91:263–267, 1982.
50. Eusebi V, Casadei GP, Bussolati G, Azzopardi JG: Adenomyoepithelioma of the breast with a distinctive type of apocrine adenosis. Histopathology 11:305–315, 1987.
51. Eusebi V, Foschini MA, Cook MG, Berrino F, Azzopardi JG: Long-term follow-up of in situ carcinoma of the breast with special emphasis on clinging carcinoma. Semin Diagn Pathol 6:165–173, 1989.
52. Eusebi V, Grassigli A, Grosso F: Lesioni focali scleroelastotiche mammarie simulant, il carcinoma infiltrante. Pathologica 68:507–518, 1976.
53. Ewing J: Neoplastic Disease. Philadelphia, WB Saunders, 1919, p 473.
54. Fechner RE: Epithelial alterations in the extralobular ducts of breast with lobular carcinoma. Arch Pathol 93:164–171, 1972.
55. Fechner RE: Fibroadenoma and related lesions. In Page DL, Anderson TJ: Diagnostic Histopathology of the Breast. Edinburgh, Churchill Livingstone, 1987, pp 72–88.
56. Fenoglio C, Lattes R: Sclerosing papillary proliferations in the female breast. Cancer 33:691–700, 1974.
57. Fisher ER: The pathology of breast cancer as it relates to its evolution, prognosis and treatment. Clin Oncol 1:703–734, 1982.
58. Fisher ER, Palekar S, Kotwal N, Lipana N: A nonencapsulated sclerosing lesion of the breast. Am J Clin Pathol 71:239–246, 1979.
59. Fitzgibbons PL, Simley DF, Kern WH: Sarcoidosis presenting initially as breast mass: report of two cases. Hum Pathol 16:851–852, 1985.
60. Flint A, Oberman HA: Infarction and squamous metaplasia of intraductal papilloma: a benign breast lesion that may simulate carcinoma. Hum Pathol 15:764–767, 1984.
61. Fondo EY, Rosen PP, Fracchia AA, Urban JA: The problem of carcinoma developing in a fibroadenoma. Recent experience at Memorial Hospital. Cancer 43:563–567, 1979.
62. Foote FW, Stewart FW: Comparative studies of cancerous versus noncancerous breasts. I. Basic morphologic characteristics. II.

Role of so-called chronic cystic mastitis in mammary carcinogenesis; influence of certain hormones on human breast structure. Ann Surg 121:6–53, 197–222, 1945.

63. Frantz VK, Pickren JW, Melcher GW, Auchincloss H Jr: Incidence of chronic cystic disease in so-called "normal breasts." A study based on 225 postmortem examinations. Cancer 4:762–783, 1951.

64. Geschicter CF: The early literature of chronic cystic mastitis. Bull Inst Histol Med 2:249–257, 1939.

65. Goodman ZD, Taxy JB: Fibroadenomas of the breast with prominent smooth muscle. Am J Surg Pathol 5:99–101, 1981.

66. Gudjonsdottir A, Hagerstrand I, Ostberg G: Adenoma of the nipple with carcinomatous development. Acta Pathol Microbiol Scand (A) 79:676–680, 1971.

67. Haagensen CD: The relationship of gross cystic disease of the breast and carcinoma. Ann Surg 185:375–376, 1977.

68. Haagensen CD: Diseases of the Breast, 3rd ed. Philadelphia, WB Saunders, 1986, pp 250–266.

69. Haagensen CD: Diseases of the Breast, 3rd ed. Philadelphia, WB Saunders, 1986, pp 106–124.

70. Haagensen CD: Diseases of the Breast, 3rd ed. Philadelphia, WB Saunders, 1986, p 268.

71. Haagensen CD: Diseases of the Breast, 3rd ed. Philadelphia, WB Saunders, 1986, pp 335–336.

72. Haagensen CD: Diseases of the Breast, 3rd ed. Philadelphia, WB Saunders, 1986, pp 136–191.

73. Haagensen CD, Bodian C, Haagensen DE Jr: Breast Carcinoma Risk and Detection. Philadelphia, WB Saunders, 1981, pp 83–105.

74. Haagensen CD, Lane N, Lattes R, Bodian C: Lobular neoplasia (so-called lobular carcinoma in situ) of the breast. Cancer 42:737–769, 1978.

75. Hajdu SI, Espinosa MH, Robbins GF: Recurrent cystosarcoma phyllodes: a clinicopathologic study of 32 cases. Cancer 38:1402–1406, 1976.

76. Hart WR, Bauer R, Oberman H: Cystosarcoma phyllodes: a clinicopathologic study of twenty-six hypercellular periductal stromal tumors of the breast. Am Clin Pathol 70:211–216, 1978.

77. Hasson J, Pope CH: Mammary infarcts associated with pregnancy presenting as breast tumors. Surgery 49:313–316, 1961.

78. Hertel BG, Zaloudek C, Kempson RL: Breast adenomas. Cancer 37:2891–2905, 1976.

79. Hessler C, Schnyder P, Ozzello L: Hamartoma of the breast: diagnostic observation of 16 cases. Radiology 126:95–98, 1979.

80. Hough AJ, Page DL: Prospectives on cartilaginous tumors: Nomenclature, nosology, and neologism. Hum Pathol. 20:927–929, 1989.

81. Hutter RVP: Editorial. N Engl J Med 312:179–181, 1985.

82. Hutter RVP, and others: Consensus meeting. Is "fibrocystic disease" of the breast precancerous? Arch Pathol Lab Med 110:171–173, 1986.

83. Ikard RW, Perkins D: Mammary tuberculosis: a rare modern disease. South Med J 70:208–212, 1977.

84. James K, Bridger J, Anthony PP: Breast tumour of pregnancy ("lactating adenoma"). J Pathol 156:37–44, 1988.

85. Jensen HM: Breast Pathology, emphasizing precancerous and cancer-associated lesions. In Bulbrook RD, Taylor DJ (eds): Commentaries on Research in Breast Disease, Vol 2. New York, Liss, 1981, pp 41–86.

86. Jensen RA, Page DL, Dupont WD, Rogers LW: Invasive breast cancer (IBC) risk in women with sclerosing adenosis (SA). Cancer. 64:1977–1983, 1989.

87. Johnson RL, Page DL, Anderson TJ: Sarcomas of the breast. In Page DL, Anderson TJ: Diagnostic Histopathology of the Breast. Edinburgh, Churchill Livingstone, 1987.

88. Kelsey JL, Berkowitz GS: Breast cancer epidemiology. Cancer Res 48:5615–5623, 1988.

89. Kersey P, Kriukov V, Shannon P, Boyd NF: Cyclical mastopathy: an evaluation of methods of assessment. J Clin Epidemiol 42:53–59, 1989.

90. Kiaer H, Neilsen B, Paulsen S, Sorensen IM, Dyreborg U, Blicher-Toft M: Adenomyoepithelial adenosis and low-grade malignant adenomyoepithelioma of the breast. Virchows Arch (A) 405:55–67, 1984.

91. Kodlin D, Winger EE, Morgenstern NL, Chen U: Chronic mastopathy and breast cancer. A follow-up study. Cancer 39:2603–2607, 1977.

92. Kovi J, Chu HB, Leffall LD Jr: Sclerosing lobular hyperplasia manifesting as a palpable mass of the breast in young black women. Hum Pathol 15:336–340, 1984.

93. Leinster SJ, Whitehouse GH, Walsh PV: Cyclical mastalgia: clinical and mammographic observations in a screened population. Br J Surg 74:220–222, 1987.

94. Lindquist KD, van Heerden JA, Weiland LH, Martin JK Jr: Recurrent and metastatic cystosarcoma phyllodes. Am J Surg 144:341–343, 1982.

95. Linell F, Ostberg G, Soderstrom J, Anderson I, Hidell J, Ljungqvist U: Breast hamartomas. An important entity in mammary pathology. Virchows Arch (A) 383:253–264, 1979.

96. Love SM, Gelman RS, Silen W: Fibrocystic "disease" of the breast—a nondisease? N Engl J Med 307:1010–1014, 1982.

97. Maier WP, Rosemond GP, Wittenburg P, Tassoni EM: Cystosarcoma phyllodes mammae. Oncology 22:145–158, 1968.

98. Majmudar B, Rosales-Quintana S: Infarction of breast fibroadenomas during pregnancy. JAMA 231:963–964, 1975.

99. Martin RG, Gallager HS: Sarcomas of the breast. In Gallager HS, Leis HP Jr, Snyderman RK, Urban JA (eds): The Breast. St. Louis, CV Mosby, 1978, p 539.

100. Mazoujian G, Pinkus GS, Davis S, Haagensen DE: Immunohistochemistry of a breast gross cystic disease fluid protein (GCDFP-15): a marker of apocrine epithelium and breast carcinomas with apocrine features. Am J Pathol 110:105–111, 1983.

101. McCarty KS Jr, Keterson GHD, Wilkinson WE, Georgiade N: Histologic study of subcutaneous mastectomy specimens from patients with carcinoma of the contralateral breast. Surg Gynecol Obstet 147:682–688, 1978.

102. McDivitt RW, Stewart FW, Berg JW: Tumors of the breast. Atlas of Tumor Pathology, second series, fascicle 2. Washington DC, Armed Forces Institute of Pathology, 1968, p 91.

103. Mies C, Rosen PP: Juvenile fibroadenoma with atypical epithelial hyperplasia. Am J Surg Pathol 11:184–190, 1987.

104. Moross T, Lang AP, Mahoney L: Tubular adenoma of breast. Arch Pathol Lab Med 107:84–86, 1983.

105. Moskowitz M, Gartside P, Wirman JA, McLaughlin C: Proliferative disorders of the breast as risk factors for breast cancer in a self-selected screened population: pathologic markers. Radiology 134:289–291, 1980.

106. Muller J: Über den feinern bau und die formen der krankhaften geschwulste. Berlin, G Reimer, 1838, pp 54–60.

107. Murad TM, Hines JR, Beal J, Bauer K: Histopathological and clinical correlations of cystosarcoma phyllodes. Arch Pathol Lab Med 112:752–756, 1988.

108. Norris HJ, Taylor HB: Relationship of histologic features to behavior of cystosarcoma phyllodes—analysis of 94 cases. Cancer 22:22–28, 1967.

109. Oberman HA: Breast lesions in the adolescent female. Ann Pathol 14:175–201, 1979.

110. Oberman HA: Benign breast lesions confused with carcinoma. In McDivitt RW, Oberman HA, Ozzello L, Kaufman N (eds): The breast. Baltimore, Williams and Wilkins, 1984, pp 1–33.

111. O'Hara MF, Page DL: Adenomas of the breast and ectopic breast under lactational influences. Hum Pathol 16:707–712, 1985.

112. Ohuchi N, Abe R, Takahashi T, Tezuka F: Origin and extension of intraductal papillomas of the breast: a three-dimensional reconstruction study. Breast Cancer Res Treat 4:117–128, 1984.

113. Ohuchi N, Rikiya A, Kasai M: Possible cancerous change of intraductal papillomas of the breast: a 3D reconstruction study of 25 cases. Cancer 54:605–611, 1984.

114. Organ CH Jr, Organ BC: Fibroadenoma of the female breast: a critical clinical assessment. J Natl Med Assoc 75:701–704, 1983.

115. Orson LW, Cigtay OS: Fat necrosis of the breast: characteristic xeromammographic appearance. Radiology 146:35–38, 1983.

116. Page DL: Cancer risk assessment in benign biopsies. Hum Pathol 17:871–874, 1986.

117. Page DL: Benign disorders of the breast. In Stein JH (ed):

Internal Medicine, ed 2. Boston, Little, Brown, 1987, pp 1994–1997.

118. Page DL, Dupont WD: Are breast cysts a premalignant marker? Eur J Cancer Clin Oncol 22:635–636, 1986.

119. Page DL, Dupont WD, Rogers LW: Ductal involvement by cells of atypical lobular hyperplasia in the breast. Hum Pathol 19:201–207, 1988.

120. Page DL, Dupont WD, Rogers LW, Rados MS: Atypical hyperplastic lesions of the female breast. A long-term follow-up study. Cancer 55:2698–2708, 1985.

121. Page DL, Vander Zwaag R, Rogers LW, Williams LT, Walker WE, Hartmann WH: Relation between component parts of fibrocystic disease complex and breast cancer. J Natl Cancer Inst 61:1055–1063, 1978.

122. Persaud V, Talerman A, Jordan RP: Pure adenoma of the breast. Arch Pathol 86:481–483, 1968.

123. Perzin KH, Lattes R: Papillary adenoma of the nipple (florid papillomatosis, adenoma, adenomatosis): a clinicopathology study. Cancer 54:605–611, 1984.

124. Pick PW, Iossifides IA: Occurrence of breast carcinoma within a fibroadenoma. A review. Arch Pathol Lab Med 108:590–594, 1984.

125. Pietruszka M, Barnes L: Cystosarcoma phyllodes: a clinicopathologic analysis of forty-two cases. Cancer 41:1974–1983, 1978.

126. Pike AM, Oberman HA: Juvenile (cellular) fibroadenoma. A clinicopathologic study. Am J Surg Pathol 9:730–736, 1985.

127. Reddick RL, Jennette JC, Askin FB: Squamous metaplasia of the breast. Am J Clin Pathol 84:530–533, 1985.

128. Rees BI, Gravelle IH, Hughes LE: Nipple retraction in duct ectasia. Br J Surg 64:577–580, 1977.

129. Riddell RH, Davies JD: Muscular hamartomas of the breast. J Pathol 111:209–211, 1973.

130. Rogers LW, Page DL: Epithelial proliferative disease of the breast. A marker of increased cancer risk in certain age groups. Breast Dis Breast 5:2–7, 1979.

131. Rogers LW, Page DL, Anderson TJ: Epithelial hyperplasia. *In* Page DL, Anderson TJ: Diagnostic Histopathology of the Breast. Edinburgh, Churchill Livingstone, 1987.

132. Rosen PP: Microglandular adenosis: a benign lesion simulating invasive mammary carcinoma. Am J Surg Pathol 7:137–144, 1983.

133. Rosen PP, Caicco JA: Florid papillomatosis of the nipple. A study of 51 patients, including nine with mammary carcinoma. Am J Surg Pathol 10:84–101, 1986.

134. Rosen PP, Ernsberger D: Mammary fibromatosis. A benign spindle-cell tumor with significant risk for local recurrence. Cancer 63:1363–1369, 1989.

135. Rosenblum MK, Parrazella R, Rosen PP: Is microglandular adenosis a precancerous disease? A study of carcinoma arising therein. Am J Surg Path 10:237–245, 1986.

136. Sakamoto G, Page DL, Anderson TJ: Infiltrating carcinoma: major histologic types. *In* Page DL, Anderson TJ: Diagnostic Histopathology of the Breast. Edinburgh, Churchill Livingstone, 1987, p 211.

137. Salhany KE, Dupont WD, Rogers LW, Page DL: Epithelial proliferative lesions in benign intraductal papillomas. Abstract. Lab Invest 58:80A, 1988.

138. Salm R: Epidermoid metaplasia in mammary fibroadenoma with formation of keratin cysts. J Pathol Bacteriol 74:221–222, 1957.

139. Sandison AT: An autopsy study of the adult human breast: with special reference to proliferative epithelial changes of importance in the pathology of the breast. Bethesda, National Cancer Institute monograph no. 8, June, 1962.

140. Siegel GP, Barsky SH, Terranova VP, Liotta LA: Stages of neoplastic transformation of human breast tissue as monitored by dissolution of basement membrane components. An immunoperoxidase study. Invas Metast 1:54–70, 1981.

141. Symmers W StC, McKeown KC: Tuberculosis of the breast. Br Med J 289:48–49, 1984.

142. Tavassoli FA, Norris HJ: Microglandular adenosis of the breast: a clinicopathologic study of 11 cases with ultrastructural observations. Am J Surg Pathol 7:731–737, 1983.

143. Tice GI, Dockerty MB, Harrington SW: Comedomastitis: a clinical and pathological study of data in 172 cases. Surg Gynecol Obstet 87:525–540, 1984.

144. Vilanova JR, Simon R, Alvarez J, Rivera-Pomar JM. Early apocrine change in hyperplastic cystic disease. Histopathology 7:693–698, 1983.

145. Wapnir IL, Pallan TM, Gaudino J, Stahl W: Latent mammary tuberculosis: a case report. Surgery 98:976–978, 1985.

146. Wargotz ES, Norris HJ, Austin RM, Enzinger FM: Fibromatosis of the breast. A clinical and pathological study of 28 cases. Am J Surg Pathol 11:38–45, 1987.

147. Warren JC: The surgeon and the pathologist. JAMA 100:1–17, 1905.

148. Wellings SR, Alpers CE: Apocrine cystic metaplasia: subgross pathology and prevalence in cancer-associated versus random autopsy breasts. Hum Pathol 18:381–386, 1987.

149. Wellings SR, Jensen HM, Marcum RG: An atlas of subgross pathology of the human breast with special reference to possible precancerous lesions. J Natl Cancer Inst 55:231–273, 1975.

150. West TL, Weiland JH, Clagett OT: Cystosarcoma phyllodes. Ann Surg 173:520–528, 1971.

151. WHO International Histologic Classification of Tumors, ed 2. Histologic Typing of Breast Tumours. Geneva, World Health Organization, 1981.

152. Wilkinson L, Green WO Jr: Infarction of the breast lesion during pregnancy and lactation. Cancer 17:1567–1572, 1964.

153. Wilkinson S, Anderson TJ, Rifkind E, Chetty U, Forrest APM: Fibroadenoma of the breast: a follow-up of conservative management. Br J Surg 76:390–391, 1989.

Chapter 7

GYNECOMASTIA

Kirby I. Bland, M.D. and David L. Page, M.D.

Gynecomastia (Greek: *gyne,* relationship to women; *mastos,* breast) denotes the presence of female type mammary glands in the male. Enlargement of the male breast is a common disorder, and most examples should not be considered a disease. The disorder may be categorized as physiological or endogenous, although in many patients it is idiopathic. In recent years, clinical, anatomical, and biochemical advances have largely clarified the etiology and natural history of gynecomastia.

INCIDENCE

Wilson and coworkers[428] considered gynecomastia so common as to be considered part of normal development. Gynecomastia develops in approximately 60 to 70 percent of pubertal boys and is estimated by Schydlower[353] to occur within 1.2 years following an increase in testicular size, the first sign of puberty. Typically, the clinical presentation occurs in normal boys during puberty at the age of 12 to 15 years.[63, 82] Usually, breast enlargement and tenderness, if present, regress spontaneously over a 12- to 24-month period. The diagnosis of *pubertal gynecomastia* is made by the clinical presence of breast enlargement in the otherwise healthy pubertal male. In contrast with the aforementioned physiological event, *prepubertal gynecomastia* is extraordinarily rare (only 41 cases being identified), with underlying causes that include the following: adrenal carcinoma (nine cases), testicular tumor (two cases), 11-β-hydroxylase deficiency (four cases), familial gynecomastia (two cases), tuberous sclerosis (two cases), and, in part, overlapping sexual precocity (four cases).[169] Nuttall[298] identified gynecomastia in 36 percent of 306 military reservists examined and noted a modest increase in prevalence with advancing age. Carlson[63] confirmed Nuttall's findings; in a study of 100 male veterans, he noted an overall prevalence of 32 percent for palpable gynecomastia (30 percent in 50 inpatients and 34 percent in 50 outpatients). These results correlate well with those of Ley et al.[245] and the autopsy study by Williams,[425] who noted gynecomastia in 40 percent of 447 aging men. In these three clinical series, all male subjects denied breast tenderness or pain, and all had been unaware of breast enlargement or the presence of any palpable breast tissue.

Rubens et al.[338] considered testicular failure with relative hypogonadism to occur in varying degrees in men beyond age 60 years as a consequence of (1) decreased concentrations of total and free serum testosterone, (2) escalations in serum luteinizing hormone (LH), and (3) maintenance of normal serum estradiol. Further, there is evidence that enhanced peripheral aromatization of androgens to estrogens with increasing adiposity contributes to *senescent gynecomastia* in aging males. Thus, the constellation of part or all of these endocrine and biological events leads to a predominant estrogen effect on the breast parenchyma and the clinical emergence of gynecomastia in the aging male. The etiology and clinical manifestations of gynecomastia in different age groups will be presented in a subsequent section.

PHYSIOLOGICAL GYNECOMASTIA

Male breast enlargement occurring in the absence of a known or precipitating cause is noted largely during three phases of life and is regarded as an alteration in steroid hormone physiology rather than a pathological event.

Neonatal Period

Palpable enlargement of the male breast in the neonate is considered normal and is to be distinguished from the rare clinical syndrome of prepubertal gynecomastia. This event almost assuredly occurs from the action of placental estrogens (estradiol, estriol) on neonatal breast parenchyma. Although this breast enlargement regresses within a few weeks, Bronstein and Cassorla[53] observed that it may persist for prolonged durations in exceptional circumstances.

Adolescence

Pubertal gynecomastia occurs in approximately two thirds of adolescent males.[428] Of 1855 boys of different ages examined at a Boy Scout camp, Nydick et al.[299] noted that 39 percent had gynecomastia and that 65 percent of boys aged 14 to 14.5 years were affected. The observation that virtually all males have gynecomastia at some time during puberty suggests that this is a transient physiological event. For many of these male patients, enlarged breasts are grossly asymmetrical, tender, and cosmetically and psychologically disturbing. By age 20, only a small number of men have palpable gynecomastia in one or both breasts.

This common pubertal variant of gynecomastia may best be explained by the physiological excess of plasma estradiol relative to the plasma testosterone.[40, 98, 226, 237, 245] As a consequence of this relative hyperestrogen state, physiological gynecomastia becomes manifest. Hemsell et al.[180] observed the production rate of androstenedione to be closely related to body surface area and plasma androstenedione to be the preferred substrate of the extraglandular aromatase system. Therefore, with maximal synthesis of this estrogen precursor during pubertal development and prior to maximal testosterone secretion by the testes, a relative excess of estrogen is produced.

Senescence

The review by Wilson and colleagues[428] states, "In the normal adult man, no breast tissue can be palpated." This implies that whenever palpable gynecomastia is present, a cause should be sought. The prevalence of gynecomastia increases with age and was observed in 57 percent of men over age 45 years by Nuttall.[298] In the report by Carlson,[63] the overall prevalence of gynecomastia was 32 percent in male veterans; however, no increase in incidence with age was observed. Williams[425] reported that 40 percent of elderly men have gynecomastia.

Niewoehner and Nuttall[292] examined 214 hospitalized adult men aged 27 to 92 years for the presence of palpable gynecomastia. The overall prevalence in this series was 65 percent. Gynecomastia was bilateral in all but 11 (5.1 percent) subjects. The prevalence was greatest in the 50 to 69 year group (72 percent); it was lowest in the 70 to 89 year group (47 percent, $p < 0.01$) and in the 30 to 49 year group (54 percent, $p < 0.05$). Importantly, the authors observed gynecomastia to increase with body mass index (BMI). More than 80 percent of those with a BMI of 25 kg/m² or greater had gynecomastia. Further, the diameter of breast tissue also increases with increasing BMI ($p < 0.001$). These authors consider the decreased prevalence of gynecomastia after the seventh decade to be best explained by the lower BMI in this group. It was concluded that palpable bilateral gynecomastia is present in most older men, is correlated with the amount of body fat, and does not require clinical evaluation unless symptomatic or of recent onset.

Wilson et al.[428] suggest that endocrine changes may result in breast enlargement and occur in virtually all aging men. As the plasma testosterone concentration begins to decline at approximately age 70, there is simultaneous elevation of the plasma testosterone-estrogen (sex hormone) binding globulin such that the level of unbound or free testosterone declines even further. Moreover, there is an associated rise in plasma luteinizing hormone (LH), as suggested by Snyder,[366] with an increase in the rate of conversion of androgens to estrogens in peripheral tissues (Fig. 7–1). The net effect

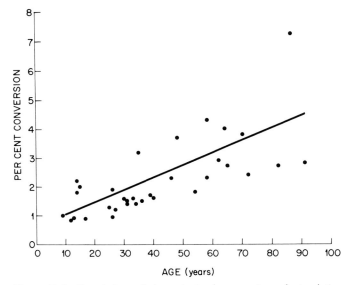

Figure 7–1. Correlation of the extent of conversion of circulating androstenedione to estrone in men as a function of age. (From Siiteri PK, MacDonald PC: Role of extraglandular estrogen in human endocrinology. *In* Greep RO, Astwood EB (eds): Handbook of Physiology. Washington, D.C., American Physiological Society, 1975. Reprinted by permission.)

is a static concentration or increase in plasma estradiol for elderly men. As the plasma testosterone falls, relative hyperestrinism is evident with the decreasing plasma androgen:estrogen ratio. Siiteri and MacDonald[362] further suggest that the development of obesity increases the rate for peripheral conversion of androgens to estrogens. These alterations in the normal elements of the aging process contribute to gynecomastia in the otherwise normal elderly male.

PHYSIOLOGY

Major mammary ductal systems are evident in the normal adult male breast with rare secondary ductal branching. However, with the clinical development of gynecomastia, enlargement of the subareolar portion of the breast is evident as a result of secondary ductal branching and proliferation of fibroblastic stroma. Poulsen[321] presented evidence of a trophic and stimulatory effect of estrogens on mammary epithelial tissues, while Turkington and Topper[401] demonstrated less importance for the inhibitory role of androgens. Thus, gynecomastia may emerge as a result of the alterations in balance between the influence of a relative (or absolute) excess of circulating estrogen in the presence of deficient circulating plasma androgen. Estrogens stimulate growth of ductal epithelium (see Chapter 3A); whereas androgens inhibit proliferation. Defective androgen receptors, as found in testicular insufficiency (feminization) and related syndromes, may likewise contribute via the loss of active androgenic influences on ductal breast epithelium. Testosterone, which is synthethesized by the testes, and dihydrotestosterone, which is converted from testosterone in the prostate,

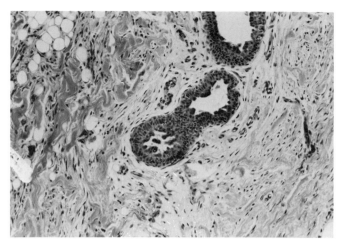

Figure 7–2. From the florid phase of gynecomastia, a tortuous duct passes through the center of the photograph. A richly vascular, loose connective tissue is present around the duct.

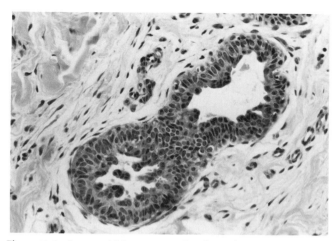

Figure 7–3. Seen at higher power, the duct (shown in Figure 7–2) demonstrates hyperplastic epithelium. Note increase in epithelial cell number over the usual two above the basement membrane.

skin, adipose tissue, and other peripheral sites, are the major active biological androgens. In contradistinction, estradiol is the major biologically active estrogen, the majority of which is synthesized from the peripheral conversion of testosterone or androstenedione, a weak androgen secreted by the adrenals. Testicular secretion of testosterone is primarily regulated by negative feedback inhibition of the pituitary gonadotropin luteinizing hormone (LH).

The loss of inhibitory androgenic influences on breast development as suggested by MacDonald et al.,[254, 255] greatly clarifies the effect of the hypoandrogenic state on the development of gynecomastia. The role of prolactin in promoting lactation is evident; however, its role in gynecomastia is uncertain. Turkington[400] noted normal serum prolactin values in most males with gynecomastia and observed that enlarged breasts do not develop in most subjects with *hyperprolactinemia*. However, the hyperprolactinemic state may contribute to impotence and gynecomastia by the indirect effects on gonadal and possibly adrenal function. Franks and associates[123] confirmed that prolactin may lead to alterations in the ratio of circulating estrogens to androgens, thus contributing to an imbalance of sex steroid hormones and, hence, to the emergence of gynecomastia.

HISTOPATHOLOGY

Without reference to the setting in which gynecomastia occurs, the gross and histological anatomy remains the same. Grossly, there is a relatively sharp margin between breast tissue and surrounding subcutaneous fat. The few ductal structures of the male breast enlarge, elongate, and branch along with an ensheathing connective tissue.[208, 291] This combined increase in glandular and stromal elements usually presents a regular distribution of each element throughout the enlarged breast. Often there is an increase in cell number relative to the basement membrane, which is discussed under hyperplasia. The changes in the connective tissue are quite

characteristic at different stages and are also discussed later.

This increased number of ducts is in such a pattern that cross sections are most common, but short longitudinal views, including branch points, are frequently present. The loose, edematous connective tissue that regularly outlines these ducts as a central feature of gynecomastia is prominent only in the earliest stage of the disease (Figs. 7–2 to 7–4). The fibroblasts within this loose tissue are relatively large but lack atypical features and are not clustered except so to appear slightly more frequent immediately adjacent to the basement membrane of the ducts. The epithelial lining cells are frequently increased to three or four in height. The cells are, for the most part, cuboidal without a prominence of basilar or apparent myoepithelial cells. With greater cell number there is a tendency toward a pattern mimicking "tufting"; these small areas, four to five cells in width, are the only foci of cell increase. This very slight hyperplasia, suggesting a papillary pattern, is often increased or enhanced to produce quite long, narrow

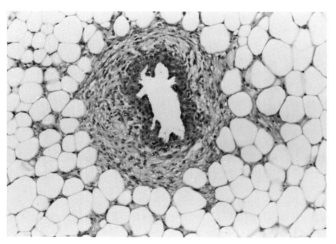

Figure 7–4. From the florid phase of gynecomastia, this duct has elongated into surrounding fat. Note the cellular, young fibrous tissue ensheathing the duct and insinuated between fat cells.

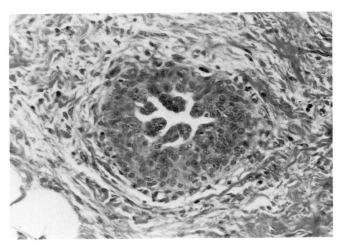

Figure 7–5. Hyperplasia of epithelial cells is evident in the many layers of cells. The micropapillary fronds that are present centrally are characteristic of the hyperplasia seen in gynecomastia.

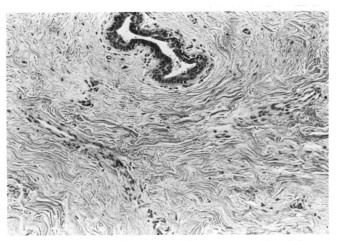

Figure 7–6. In the late or fibrous stage of gynecomastia, ductal elements are less prominent and a dense collagenous strome is predominant.

papillary proliferations of epithelial cells. These occasionally mimic atypical hyperplastic patterns except that the cells tend to have a regular placement, which differs from the pattern seen in the well-developed atypical hyperplasias (Figs. 7–3 and 7–5).

When frequent and evenly distributed throughout the sample, these micropapillae will not seem alarming. The micropapillary pattern is the most frequent hyperplastic pattern seen with gynecomastia. When present only focally, it may cause occasional concern because it resembles atypical hyperplasia or even carcinoma *in situ*. However, the presence of atypical ductal hyperplasia (ADH) in the male breast is not well studied nor are its clinical correlates known. Also, the cytological and histological forms are only reminiscent of ADH, not diagnostic of that condition. The rigid and bulbous character of micropapillary carcinoma *in situ* is lacking, despite the features that mimic it (see Chapter 8). Focal squamous metaplasia also may be found, with islands of quite obviously squamous metaplastic cells interspersed within the hyperplastic epithelial cells.[155] Foci of apocrine change are even less common but may be seen in the male breast.

The discovery of lobular units in the male breast is quite rare, being reported in 1 in 1000 cases.[19] This formation of lobular units has no known clinical correlate except that it seems to be somewhat more prevalent in the presumed later stage of gynecomastia, known as the florid type.

Fibrous gynecomastia is the term for the later stage of gynecomastia, which is clinically firmer and histologically has a very dense collagenous stroma that may contain relatively few fibroblasts (Figs. 7–6 to 7–8). This dense collagenous tissue is applied quite closely to delicate basement membrane regions surrounding sparse epithelial elements in which hyperplasia is usually absent. The loose "active" pattern of periductal stroma that characterizes the florid stage is lacking.

The histological differential diagnosis of gynecomastia is not necessary, particularly if the clinical setting is known to the histopathologist. It is relevant to note that

virtually any benign alteration found in the female breast may be found in the male, as noted above, although such changes are quite rare. This refers particularly to fibroadenoma and sclerosing adenosis.[38] These two changes may be present in somewhat altered form in the male breast but are best recognized as closely mimicking the female counterpart.

Certainly, differentiating carcinoma of the male breast from gynecomastia may occasionally be difficult clinically, but the problem is easily resolved by histological examination and usually by cytological examination from needle aspiration specimens. The carcinomas do not merge so smoothly with surrounding stroma and are indistinguishable from the female counterparts.

It is surprising that there is apparently no favored association between gynecomastia and the development of carcinoma in the male. At least, the association remains unproved. Whether the unusual but definite cases of atypical hyperplasia and carcinoma in the male breast, which present as a slightly enlarged breast, may

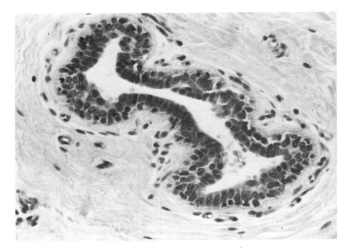

Figure 7–7. Higher magnification of Figure 7–5 demonstrates compact fibrous tissue applied almost directly on ductal basement membrane. There are fewer capillaries encircling the duct than in the more active earlier stages of gynecomastia.

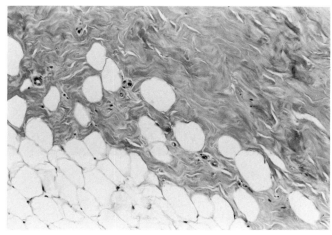

Figure 7–8. At the interface of mammary connective tissue with subcutaneous fat there is an intermingling of elements. Note density of connective tissue in this example of six years' duration.

have been preceded by gynecomastia is not known. The carcinoma *in situ* that are reported in the male breast are most often solid and comedo types of ductal carcinoma *in situ,* although complex cribriform patterns are also demonstrated.[203, 413]

PHYSICAL EXAMINATION AND DETECTION OF GYNECOMASTIA

The physician is often confronted with enlargement of the unilateral breast in the pubertal male who demonstrates allometric growth of breast tissue, typically between the ages of 12 and 15 years. The majority of these young men with gynecomastia are asymptomatic.[63, 82] In the aging male, prevalence appears to increase modestly, as demonstrated by Nuttall.[298] Niewoehner and Nuttall[292] suggest the following reliable technique for demonstration of gynecomastia: With the patient lying supine, the physician places the examining thumb at the inferior outer quadrant of the patient's breast and the index finger at the superior inner quadrant. He then elevates breast tissue up and off the chest wall in a pinching fashion for measurement. In the nonobese patient at least 2 cm of subareolar breast tissue must be present before gynecomastia can be said to exist. Should there be doubt about whether the tissue is glandular or adipose, its consistency should be compared with that of adipose tissue in the anterior or lateral axillary folds. Dershaw[95] and Jackson and Gilmore[196] cite the value of *xeromammography and ultrasonography* to differentiate ill-defined or indistinguishable surrounding fatty tissues from male breast lesions and soft tissue structure.

Dominant masses or local areas of firmness, irregularity, or asymmetry suggest the possibility of early *male breast carcinoma* in the aging patient. This site-specific cancer accounts for 0.2 percent of all cancer in male patients and approximately 1 percent of all breast cancer. Further, the presence of a bloody nipple discharge, fixation, ulceration, asymmetry, eccentric location, and

axillary adenopathy suggests a malignant process. Nuttall[298] considers it both impractical and unnecessary to perform biopsy on all patients with gynecomastia, as benign breast enlargement is quite common in the aging male. Gynecomastia does not appear to predispose the male breast to the development of cancer. In contrast, Scheike and coworkers[348] identify *Klinefelter syndrome* (47,XXY) as the only condition that is clearly associated with an enhanced risk for breast cancer in men.

PATHOPHYSIOLOGICAL MECHANISMS

I. Estrogen excess states
  A. Gonadal origin
   1. True hermaphroditism
   2. Gonadal stromal (nongerminal) neoplasms of the testis
     a. Leydig cell (interstitial)
     b. Sertoli cell
     c. Granulosa-theca
   3. Germ cell tumors
     a. Choriocarcinoma
     b. Seminoma, teratoma
     c. Embryonal carcinoma
  B. Nontesticular tumors
   1. Skin—nevus
   2. Adrenal cortical neoplasms
   3. Lung carcinoma
   4. Hepatocellular carcinoma
  C. Endocrine disorders
  D. Diseases of the liver—nonalcoholic and alcoholic cirrhosis
  E. Nutrition alteration states
II. Androgen deficiency states
  A. Senescent causes with aging
  B. Hypoandrogen states (hypogonadism)
   1. Primary testicular failure
     a. Klinefelter syndrome (XXY)
     b. Reifenstein syndrome (XY)
     c. Rosewater, Gwinup, Hamwi familial gynecomastia (XY)
     d. Kallmann syndrome
     e. Kennedy disease with associated gynecomastia
     f. Eunuchoidal males (congenital anorchia)
     g. Hereditary defects of androgen biosynthesis
     h. ACTH deficiency
   2. Secondary testicular failure
     a. Trauma
     b. Orchitis
     c. Cryptorchidism
     d. Irradiation
     e. Hydrocele
     f. Varicocele
     g. Spermatocele
  C. Renal failure
III. Drug-related conditions that initiate gynecomastia
IV. Systemic diseases with idiopathic mechanisms

A. Non-neoplastic diseases of the lung
B. Trauma (chest wall)
C. CNS-related causes from anxiety and stress
D. AIDS (autoimmune deficiency syndrome)

Estrogen Excess States

Increased secretion of estrogens into plasma can have origin from the testis. Wilson and colleagues[428] suggest that increased estrogen production (independent of pituitary gonadotropin) can be manifest by at least three pathophysiological mechanisms: (1) increased secretion by endocrine organs; (2) increased availability of substrate for peripheral conversion to estrogens, and (3) increased aromatase activity within peripheral tissues in the presence of normal substrate levels. Gynecomastia that results from the increase in estrogen formation and subsequent activity on breast parenchyma is depicted in Figure 7–9. Diagnostic approaches to the male patient with breast masses suspicious for gynecomastia are presented in the algorithm in Figure 7–10.

Gonadal Origin

True Hermaphroditism. This clinical syndrome occurs when both an ovary and a testis or gonad with mixed histological features of both organs (ovotestis) are present. As indicated by Van Niekerk,[406] four categories are recognized: (1) *bilateral*, with testicular and ovarian tissue (ovotestis) anatomically present on each side; (2) *unilateral*, in which an ovotestis is evident on one side and an ovary or testis on the contralateral side; (3) *lateral*, in which a testis is evident on one side and an ovary on the opposite side; and (4) *indeterminate*, in which the clinical syndrome is expressed but the location and type of gonadal tissue is uncertain. Approximately one half of cases are unilateral, one fourth are bilateral, one fourth are lateral, and the remainder are indeterminate.

Significant gynecomastia is evident at puberty in approximately 75 percent of individuals with true hermaphroditism. Approximately half these individuals menstruate. For the phenotypic male with true hermaphroditism, menstruation presents as cyclic hematuria. Hormonal activity has been noted by Gallegos et al.[139] and Aiman et al.,[4] who observed gonadal secretion of estradiol in phenotypic men with feminization (gynecomastia and menstruation). Aiman and associates[4] observed excess estradiol secretion relative to androgen production by the ovotestis.

Gonadal Stromal (Nongerminal) Neoplasms

Leydig Cell (Interstitial) Tumors of the Testis. Overall, Leydig cell neoplasms of the testis are relatively uncommon, constituting approximately 2 to 3 percent of all testicular neoplasms.[64] Such neoplasms are found in children as young as 2 years and in adults as old as 82 years.[180] Leydig cell tumors compose up to 39 percent of non–germ cell tumors of the testis and 12 percent of the testicular neoplasms of children.[54, 61, 283, 385] Approximately 25 percent of the Leydig cell tumors of adult

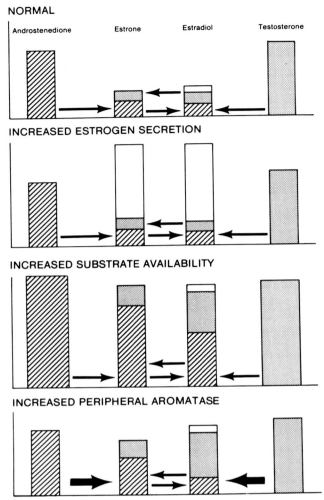

Figure 7–9. Gynecomastia as the result of increased estrogen formation can arise because of increased estrogen secretion into plasma by the adrenal or the testis, increased availability of substrate for peripheral conversion to estrogen, or an increased rate of aromatization tissues. (From Wilson JD, Aiman J, MacDonald PC: The pathogenesis of gynecomastia. *In* Stollerman GH, et al (eds): Advances in Internal Medicine, Vol. 25. © 1980 by Year Book Medical Publishers, Inc., Chicago.)

men secrete estrogens predominantly and in this setting usually produce gynecomastia.[281–283, 385] Veldhuis et al.[411] and Bercovici et al.[33] noted the effect of endogenous hyperestrogenism to be inhibitory for both gonadotropin secretion and testicular steroidogenesis. As Leydig cells are the principal source of estradiol biosynthesis, neoplasia and hyperplasia of these cells may initiate feminization as a consequence of estrogen hypersecretion.

Camin et al.[61] and Turner et al.[402] observed that Leydig cell tumors of the testis are most often unilateral. Although bilateral neoplasms have been reported, the differential diagnosis of hyperplasia with nodules in each testis from multiple neoplasms may be difficult. These neoplasms present in early to middle childhood; Brosman[54] observed the average age for diagnosis to be 4.7 years. Sexual precocity is usually observed in children with these tumors and is accompanied by an

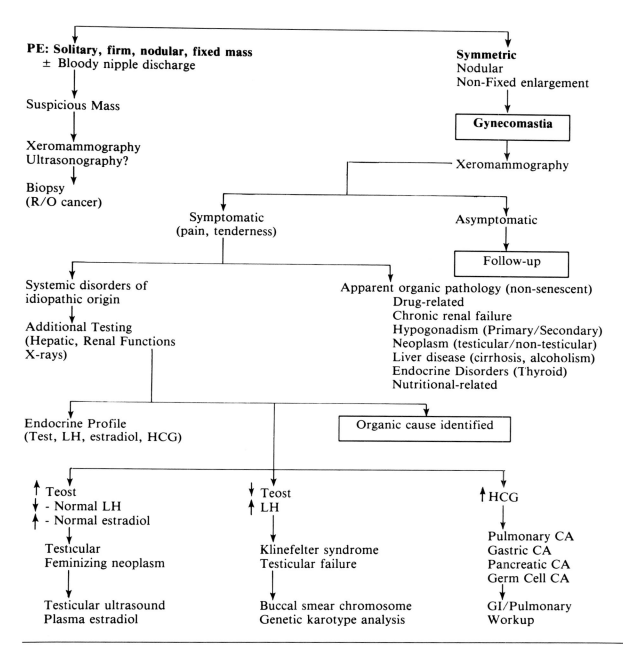

PE: Solitary, firm, nodular, fixed mass
± Bloody nipple discharge

Suspicious Mass

Xeromammography
Ultrasonography?

Biopsy
(R/O cancer)

Symmetric
Nodular
Non-Fixed enlargement

Gynecomastia

Xeromammography

Symptomatic
(pain, tenderness)

Asymptomatic

Follow-up

Systemic disorders of
idiopathic origin

Additional Testing
(Hepatic, Renal Functions
X-rays)

Apparent organic pathology (non-senescent)
Drug-related
Chronic renal failure
Hypogonadism (Primary/Secondary)
Neoplasm (testicular/non-testicular)
Liver disease (cirrhosis, alcoholism)
Endocrine Disorders (Thyroid)
Nutritional-related

Endocrine Profile
(Test, LH, estradiol, HCG)

Organic cause identified

↑ Teost
↓ - Normal LH
↑ - Normal estradiol

↓ Teost
↑ LH

↑ HCG

Testicular
Feminizing neoplasm

Klinefelter syndrome
Testicular failure

Pulmonary CA
Gastric CA
Pancreatic CA
Germ Cell CA

Testicular ultrasound
Plasma estradiol

Buccal smear chromosome
Genetic karotype analysis

GI/Pulmonary
Workup

HCG = human chorionic gonadotrophin
Teost = testosterone
LH = leuteinizing hormone
CA = cancer (carcinoma)
PE = physical exam

Figure 7–10. An algorithm for diagnostic approaches to the male patient with unilateral/bilateral breast mass suspicious for gynecomastia. (Modified from Lucas LM, Kumar KL, Smith DL: Postgrad Med 82:73, 1987.)

increase in muscle mass and stature with advanced bone age in the majority of patients. In children, Leydig cell tumors are almost uniformly benign. Many consider that therapy should be restricted to unilateral orchiectomy in children.[43, 54, 61, 86, 90, 189] Biopsy of the contralateral testis may be advisable if bilateral enlargement is evident, although bilateral neoplasms occur in only a minority of such patients.

In the adult, feminization is less frequent with these tumors, and painful gynecomastia and decreased libido are the most common endocrine manifestations. Caldamone et al.[58] observed endocrine signs in approximately 30 percent of adults. Symptoms may precede the onset of a palpable testicular mass, particularly with Leydig cell hyperplasia. Leydig cell hyperplasia is a rare and poorly understood condition, with interstitial cells between seminiferous tubules of each testis increasing in number and endocrine function. The diffuseness of the condition explains the delay between onset of symptoms and discovery of the testicular mass.[426]

Malignant behavior of Leydig cell tumors occurs in approximately 10 percent of such patients, the great majority being seen in adults.[131, 132]

The carcinomas of interstitial cells may require electron microscopy for certain diagnoses because of poor differentiation at the light microscopic level. Extensive smooth endoplasmic reticulum with tubular cristae in mitochondria are defining features in tumors of the testis.[112] Malignant clinical behavior is most common in tumors of older men. Abnormal estrogen or androgen levels are usually evident in malignant Leydig cell tumors.[91]

All signs of feminization associated with Leydig cell tumors are considered to develop secondary to estrogen secretion by these cells.[361] For patients with gynecomastia and increased circulating estrogen levels, pituitary suppression of LH release may initiate atrophy of the contralateral testis.[355] For some patients, gynecomastia may be observed despite normal serum estrogen and testosterone levels. In these patients, gynecomastia may occur secondary to *in situ* conversion of androstenedione to estrone in breast parenchyma, leading to increased local (tissue) estrogen values without elevating serum levels.[52, 118, 252, 316] Gynecomastia associated with Leydig cell tumors is more often seen when these tumors are benign, especially when 17-ketosteroid values are normal. Malignant Leydig cell tumors are associated more frequently with elevated estrogens and 17-ketosteroid levels without gynecomastia.[131, 132] Gabrilove and Furukawa[134] performed selective venous sampling of spermatic veins of the testis involved with the Leydig tumor and observed estrogen values to be 20- to 30-fold higher than in normal subjects. The feminizing effect of excess estradiol is reinforced by the associated hypogonadism. Veldhuis et al.[411] observed the inhibitory action of estradiol on testosterone production to occur at two principal sites: the pituitary and the testis. Gabrilove et al.[137] observed low-normal luteinizing hormone values for patients with Leydig cell tumors. Goh et al.[149, 150] demonstrated that estrogens inhibit gonadotropin secretion in castrated transsexuals, and

Veldhuis[411] noted a similar biological event in patients with feminizing adrenal tumors.

Mineur et al.[271] established that estrogen values decrease to normal values soon after tumor removal (orchiectomy). In a study of chronic hyperestrogenism on gonadal function in men who had estrogen-secreting Leydig cell tumors, these investigators observed men to have low plasma gonadotropin and testosterone levels before unilateral orchiectomy with concurrent increase in estradiol values. Before surgery, spermatogenesis was abnormal in some subjects. Testicular endocrine function and spermatogenesis did not return to normal after surgery. Estradiol values decreased to normal immediately after surgery but returned to upper normal limits in follow-up.[270] Mineur and associates[271] concluded that chronic hyperestrogenism produced hypothalamopituitary inhibition as well as direct steroidogenic blockade at the testicular level.

Other Nongerminal Testicular Neoplasms (Sertoli Cell and Granulosa-Theca Cell Tumors). The great majority of testicular neoplasms take origin from germ cells. Testicular neoplasms of nongerminal origin having endocrine function, besides the interstitial cell tumor (Leydig cell), are other tumors of specialized gonadal stroma.[185] This latter group of gonadal stromal lesions, including tumors of Sertoli, granulosa, theca cell origin,[280] all arise from the primitive gonadal mesenchyma.[281-283] Neoplasms of the testis are limited almost entirely to three age groups: infancy, late adolescence–young adulthood, and 50 years or greater.[118] The incidence of testicular tumors in the United States is 2.1 neoplasms per 100,000 males, of which only a small percentage occur in children.[279, 283]

The proportion of germinal to nongerminal tumors is greater in children.[189, 283] However, 30 percent of reported Sertoli cell tumors have been in infants and children under age 10 years.[132] A calcifying variant of Sertoli tumor has been described by Waxman et al.[418]

Hopkins and Parry[185] identified gynecomastia in 26 percent of patients with benign Sertoli cell tumors of the testis, the majority of which rapidly regressed following orchiectomy. Fligiel[118] identified five patients with malignant Sertoli cell tumors with evidence of gynecomastia, two of whom had elevated gonadotropin levels. In the majority of cases, there were no elevations of estrogen or testosterone values. Gabrilove and coworkers[132] noted that gynecomastia may reflect an alteration in the estrogen-androgen ratio with or without an increase in the actual estrogen plasma value.

Proppe and Scully[323] note that a variety of Sertoli cell tumors tend to be bilateral and familial and may be associated with precocious puberty, gynecomastia, and atrial myxomas. The report by Wilson et al.[427] confirmed multifocal Sertoli cell tumors associated with the autosomal dominant syndrome of Peutz-Jeghers in a six-year-old boy. The previous recognition of increased risk of gonadal tumors for females with Peutz-Jeghers syndrome was made by Scully.[354]

Mostofi and Price[282] and Teilum[390, 391] suggest that the classification, and consequently the frequency of each cell type, varies according to the degree of cellular differentiation and perceptions of individual observers. Neoplasms of Leydig and Sertoli cells make up the bulk of these nongerminal testicular lesions. Thus, neoplasms that are composed predominantly of ovarian cellular homologues—theca cell and granulosa cell—are infrequently observed in the testes. Some mixed gonadal stromal neoplasms (e.g., Sertoli-Leydig cell tumor) have been described as having undifferentiated gonadal stroma. Early reported cases of the testicular granulosa cell tumor claim a morphological similarity to the analogous ovarian neoplasm.[77, 232, 261, 265] These lesions are of great rarity, with fewer than ten examples recorded in men aged 20 to 53 years. Only recently has a distinct cystic variant of the granulosa cell tumor of the infant testis been recognized that is morphologically similar to the ovarian juvenile granulosa cell tumor.[84, 234, 324, 440]

Sertoli cell and other gonadal stromal tumors may exhibit malignant behavior after infancy. Rosvoll and Woodard[337] and Kaplan et al.[206] report males with distant metastatic disease. These older boys probably require aggressive therapy, including radical orchiectomy as well as retroperitoneal lymph node dissections. At present, neither chemotherapy nor irradiation has been utilized with sufficient frequency to predict salvageability for these tumors. No known tumor markers have been identified for the non–Leydig cell gonadal stromal tumors. Alpha-fetoprotein values (AFP) may be markedly elevated in normal infants.[272, 438] Masterson et al.[262] attribute these findings to the production and metabolism of alpha-fetoprotein by the infant, which appears to be unrelated to tumor activity. These authors observed elevated values of AFP in only two infants; findings were negative in five other boys, including one with metastatic disease.

Germinal Cell Tumors (Choriocarcinoma, Seminoma, Teratoma, and Embryonal Cell Carcinoma). Precise mechanisms for the pathogenesis of germinal cell testicular neoplasms have not been determined. It has been postulated by Pierce[314, 315] that any early germ cell has potential for malignant transformation if the factors integrating and controlling its development fail to function. Thus, neoplastic transformation of normal germ cells into *embryonal carcinoma* cells may occur. Neoplasms may be composed solely of the stem *embryonal carcinoma* cells or may differentiate along somatic and extraembryonic pathways,[314, 315] producing *teratoma* in the former case and trophoblastic tissue *(choriocarcinoma)* or yolk sac tissue *(yolk sac tumor)* in the latter.[309] *Seminoma* may take origin from the totipotent embryonal carcinoma cells.[101, 127] This theory of a common origin of germ cell tumors of the testis from embryonal carcinoma cells is supported by the ultrastructural studies of Pierce et al.[315] and the experimental production of teratoma from embryonal carcinoma explants by Stevens and Hummel.[377, 378] Reports suggest that patients with gynecomastia secondary to elevated estrogen plasma values have increased conversion of dehydroepiandrosterone to estradiol.[118, 284, 376, 414] While others[215, 254, 256] acknowledge that this event occurs with choriocarcinoma, this bioconversion plays a diminutive role in estrogen production for patients with testicular tumors

other than choriocarcinoma.[362] Estrogen effects in men with these neoplasms occur secondary to increased aromatization of testosterone and androstenedione into estrogens in peripheral sites because more of the estrogen percursors are synthesized or possibly because of an enhanced activity of aromatizing enzymes.[20] Androstenedione, which has low androgenicity and is readily aromatized to estrone peripherally, may also be produced in increased concentrations by some tumors with the result of enhanced estrogen production.[362]

Stephanas et al.[376] observed gynecomastia in patients with germ cell tumors to be correlated with a higher mortality than in patients without gynecomastia. Further, resolution of the gynecomastia in these subjects following orchiectomy indicates response of tumor and a good prognosis.

Ultrasonographic detection of malignant, nonpalpable germ cell tumors is well documented.[148, 240, 285, 313] Such tumors may be small focal lesions within the parenchyma of the testis. Testicular origin is often suggested by feminizing features, including gynecomastia, as well as peripheral lymphadenopathy. Use of testicular ultrasound for detection and localization of these early testicular masses manifested by gynecomastia is essential. Hendry et al[182] and Emory et al.[109] recommend that any young adult male with unexplained gynecomastia, loss of libido, or impotence have diagnostic testicular ultrasound for evaluation of occult tumors of this organ.

Nontesticular Tumors

Skin—Nevus. The onset of progressive gynecomastia following delivery of a normal fetus with a giant pigmented nevus (3 cm × 6.5 cm) has been documented by Leung et al.[242] The removal of this nevus resulted in regression of breast enlargement, suggesting that the association of these two seemingly unrelated problems may be more than coincidental. Nonendocrine tumors (including those of the skin) may result in hormonal imbalance and pathological signs that are well documented. Salassa et al.[342] confirmed hypophosphatemic osteomalacia associated with nonendocrine tumors; the removal of these nonendocrine neoplasms resulted in restoration of a normal metabolic state. It is possible that giant pigmented nevi may elaborate a mammotrophic substance that is capable of increasing target organ sensitivity to estrogen or may stimulate increased conversion of androstenedione and/or testosterone to estrogen.

In 1970 the review by Fienman and Yakovac[114] included a single case of male prepubertal gynecomastia among 46 patients with neurofibromatosis; since this report, only isolated cases have been documented.[14, 104, 119, 192, 204, 233, 258, 341] Etiological and pathogenetic associations are unproved.

Neoplasms of the Adrenal Cortex. Primary tumors of the adrenal cortex are rare.[199] Although nonfunctional tumors in the adrenal have been reported, the majority of pediatric patients have been initially evaluated for clinical signs of hormonal activity.[238] In a review by Hayles et al.,[178] it was determined that a majority of children had virilization or feminization as a preponderant sign, while one third had hyperadrenocorticism. Additionally, a variety of symptom complexes that include feminization and hyperaldosteronism have been documented by others.[15, 37, 83, 136, 138, 142, 190, 194, 212, 278, 365, 416, 424] Adrenocortical neoplasms have been associated with several congenital anomalies. These include astrocytoma, cutaneous lesions, hemihypertrophy, abnormalities of the contralateral adrenal gland, and the Beckwith-Wiedemann syndrome.[27, 423]

J.W. Ogle[300] reported the first childhood adrenal tumor in 1865. In the 48-year review of surgical experience at Roswell Park Memorial Institute by Didolkar et al.,[99] it was determined that adrenal tumors constitute only 0.04 percent of all cancer cases. Additionally, in a 20-year review of the pediatric population in Manchester, England, Stewart et al.[379] found neuroblastoma (a tumor of the adrenal medulla) to be 16 times more frequent than cortical tumors. In the review by Hayles et al. in 1966,[178] there were 222 cases of functional adrenocortical tumors of childhood. Thus, it appears that adrenocortical tumors are rare in the general population and are especially uncommon in the pediatric group. However, there is a bimodal age distribution favoring children and older adults.[304]

Adrenal neoplasms should be suspected in any child with premature or inappropriate signs of progressive virilization or feminization, especially if accompanied by evidence of hyperadrenocorticism or gynecomastia. Feminizing adrenal carcinomas are relatively uncommon.[434] Bittorf[41] reported, in 1919, the first estrogen-producing adrenal tumor in an adult male. Since that time, a relatively small number of patients have been documented by Gabrilove et al.[138] and Rose et al.[332] Of these additional patients documented by Gabrilove et al.,[136] an increase in estrogen production with an increased urinary excretion of estrogen was confirmed. Wohltmann and coworkers[434] concluded that the biological manifestations are a result of alterations in the ratio of estrogen-androgen levels rather than an absolute value of testosterone or estrogen. More recently, Nishiki et al.[293] confirmed preoperative elevations of urinary 17-ketosteroids and hydroxycorticosteroids; serum estrogens were dramatically reduced following treatment of the primary adrenal carcinoma.

Feminization with subsequent gynecomastia as a consequence of adrenal adenomas is rare in childhood, with only a few reports in young males.[235] The apparent benignity of physiological pubertal gynecomastia contrasts with the rare prepubertal gynecomastia that may point to an adrenal or testicular neoplasm. In patients documented by Sultan et al.,[383] the bilateral gynecomastia of an estrogen-producing adrenal adenoma had the unusual appearance of a ballooned areola with prominent venous vascularization. There appears to be overproduction of estrogen by the adrenal adenoma with consequent persistent adolescent gynecomastia and blockade of pubertal maturation. The gonadal insufficiency in these patients can be related to the negative feedback exerted by estrogens on the hypothalamopituitary axis.[227]

The observations of Itami et al.[194] as well as of Latorre and Kenny[233] confirmed that evidence of premature development of secondary sexual characteristics, such as enlarged penis, axillary hair, and pubic hair, may be seen in children with gynecomastia associated with tumors of the adrenal or testis.

Desai and Kapadia[96] documented the great infrequency of feminizing adrenocortical adenoma in comparison with the more common feminizing adrenocortical carcinomas of the male. In patients with adrenocortical carcinoma, a diverse pattern of symptoms may become evident during the course of disease such that feminization, Cushing's syndrome, and masculinization may predominate at different times in the clinical course.[44] Gabrilove et al.[136, 138] confirmed that estrogens may be the major functional product, with no evidence of Cushing's syndrome.

Most of the information about the occurrence of neoplasms of the adrenal cortex relates to a time prior to the introduction of computed tomography,[433] which has replaced other methods of studying the adrenals in situ. This sensitive test may present specific difficulties in the setting of gynecomastia, considering that somewhat enlarged adrenals are relatively common in the older age group. This will not present a problem in the pediatric age group, but older persons often have enlarged adrenals, which are perhaps analogous to nodular alteration of the thyroid and have no known physiological correlate.[304] These incidentally discovered masses have been called incidentalomas and certainly should occasion no concern in the absence of other indications if they are 3 cm or less in size. Some authors feel that one should operate only if the lesions are 6 cm in diameter or greater.[1, 31, 394]

The recent information of greatest interest with regard to malignancy in adrenocortical tumors is that those producing feminization in the pediatric age group are not as often malignant as previously thought.[289, 304] It is also quite clear that neoplasms producing mixed syndromes, such as feminization and Cushing's disease, in adult males are virtually always malignant.[304, 394] Careful histological analysis of adrenal tumors is extremely sensitive and specific with regard to indicating the likelihood or nonlikelihood of malignant behavior.[188] This contrasts sharply with what was thought to be the case prior to the mid-1970s.[136, 138] Most adrenocortical carcinomas are capable of rapidly producing death, with few modalities of effective therapy available. Occasional adrenocortical carcinomas have a more prolonged clinical course.[304]

Lung Carcinoma. Wilson and associates[428] acknowledge that carcinoma of the lung may initiate an increase in plasma chorionic gonadotropin values with a simultaneous escalation in estrogen secretion. Further, it appears that the volume of estrogen-induced breast tissue correlates with estrogen production. Fusco and Rosen[130] were the first to identify gonadotropin in the urine of male patients who died from bronchogenic carcinoma. In three of the four patients, gonadotropin was also present in tissue samples from the primary lung tumor.

The association of gynecomastia with bronchial carcinoma has previously been reviewed by Camiel et al.[60]; with the reports by Fusco and Rosen[130] and Becker and associates,[25] the most plausible explanation is stimulation of the testes, and possibly the adrenals, by chorionic gonadotropin (Fig. 7–11). This physiological event was previously observed by Fine et al.[115] and suggests that gonadotropin stimulation is responsible for the release of estrogens that initiate hyperplasia of the breast. The causative role of gonadotropin-producing bronchogenic carcinoma is apparent from the report by Faiman et al.,[110] who observed regression of the gynecomastia following excision of the primary lung neoplasm. Daily and Marcuse[85] propose that the detection of chorionic gonadotropin may be an aid in the diagnosis of bronchogenic carcinoma. These authors suggest that the appearance of gynecomastia in the adult male should nevertheless arouse the suspicion of carcinoma of the lung.

The ectopic production of hormones by bronchogenic carcinoma may also initiate *lactation,* as has been recorded in a single female patient with anaplastic carcinoma of the lung.[162] Behera et al.[28] reported the rare observation of *galactorrhea with gynecomastia* in a male patient with squamous carcinoma of the lung. This patient was also hypercalcemic with absence of documented skeletal metastasis. The authors postulate an osteoclast-activating factor or parathormone-like substance secreted by the primary tumor. Further, the abnormal lactation may be secondary to excess secretion of prolactin, as evident in the variance of lactation frequency (2 percent to one third of cases) seen in lung cancer.[28, 163] For cases in which prolactin values are normal, the intermittent secretion of prolactin or the excessive sensitivity of breast tissue to normal values may initiate clinical gynecomastia.

Hepatocellular Carcinoma. Hepatocellular carcinoma may initiate gynecomastia. As confirmed by Kew and associates,[213] feminization in primary liver carcinoma is the consequence of increased aromatase activity in the hepatic neoplasm.

Males develop hepatocellular carcinoma in the cirrhotic liver much more frequently than do females.[202] Furthermore, Andervont[9] determined that in animal models, male castration decreased the incidence of spontaneous hepatocellular carcinoma from 33 percent to 12 percent. The administration of testosterone to mice with chemically induced hepatic nodules significantly increased the rate of malignant transformation. Goodall and Butler[151] further determined that control rats fed a diet of aflatoxin B_1 (4 ppm) consistently developed hepatic neoplasms, whereas hypophysectomized animals were resistant to hepatic neoplastic transformation.

Although the mechanism of tumor development remains unknown, the presumptive sexual difference in steroid and drug metabolism is an obvious possibility.[290] A report by Stedman et al.[374] suggests that primary hepatic neoplasms contain estrogen receptors, as does normal hepatic parenchyma. More recently, Iqbal et al.[193] determined that these malignant neoplasms also contain androgen receptors, whereas normal liver parenchyma does not. The precise metabolic and biochemical interrelationship of receptors in hepatic tissue and alterations of the estrogen:testosterone ratio may have a definitive role in the initiation of gynecomastia, but this mechanism has not been clinically established.

Endocrine Disorders (Hyperthyroidism, Hypothyroidism)

In 1959, Hall[171] reviewed the English literature for gynecomastia that occurred in association with hyperthyroidism. This author found only 26 cases, and in most instances, gynecomastia appeared during hyperthyroidism and receded following establishment of the euthyroid state. This clinical observation suggests that coexistence of the two diseases is more than coincidental.[334, 373, 380] Further, the therapy of the hyperthyroid state has usually resulted in diminution or clinical disappearance of gynecomastia whether the therapy was by surgery (thyroidectomy),[231, 373, 397] by I-131 radioactiv-

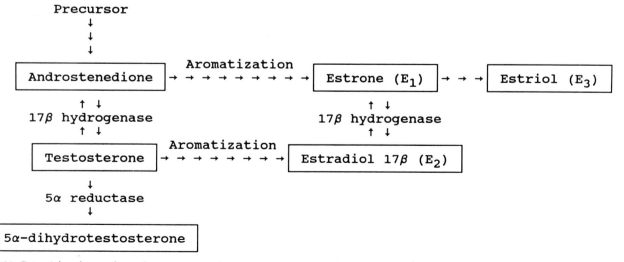

Figure 7–11. Potential pathways for androgen-estrogen interconversion in normal men. (Adapted from Gordon GG et al: J Clin Endocrinol Metab 40:1018, 1975.)

ity,[176, 231, 380] or by administration of antithyroid medication.[171, 334] In rare cases, gynecomastia may not regress after return to the euthyroid state; Larsson et al.[231] documented the need for bilateral mastectomy for gynecomastia that persisted for six months following control of the hyperthyroid condition. This author suggests that the diffuse toxic goiter of Graves' disease is the most frequent type of hyperthyroidism to occur in association with gynecomastia. Gynecomastia associated with thyroid disease usually presents clinically with grossly enlarged, tender breasts and, rarely, nipple discharge.[36] In most of the reported cases, gynecomastia is bilateral, although it may commence unilaterally.[231, 397] Rarely, gynecomastia remains unilateral[6, 26, 339]; the testes are usually normal in size and consistency, although isolated case reports by Larsson and associates[231] described small testes and others noted testicular atrophy.[6, 176, 373]

The pathogenesis of gynecomastia with associated thyroid disease remains enigmatic. Nydick and associates[299] observed that size and the occurrence of gynecomastia in clinically euthyroid adolescent boys correlates with the size of the thyroid gland. Further, the mammotrophic effects of thyroid hormone upon breast development has been demonstrated by the studies of Weichert and Boyd,[420] who fed thyroid hormones to pregnant rats and noted an earlier and more prominent hypertrophy of breasts than in pregnant controls. Fitzsimons[117] observed a reduction in gynecomastia following administration of exogenous estrogens, making it tempting to identify alterations in endogenous estrogen metabolism as instrumental in the genesis of gynecomastia in the hyperthyroid male. Chopra[70] confirmed that gynecomastia occurs frequently in men with hyperthyroidism who have high serum free estrogen values and normal free testosterone levels.[71] More recently, Nomura and associates[294] found elevated serum progesterone values in hyperthyroid men, which declined concomitant with serum thyroid hormone levels during antithyroid drug therapy.

The fact that progesterone enhances estrogen stimulation of mammary gland growth[125] strongly intimates that high serum progesterone levels in hyperthyroid men may contribute to the development of this clinical state in conjunction with the imbalance between estrogen and testosterone. Chopra[70] estimates that gynecomastia occurs in approximately 20 to 40 percent of men with hyperthyroidism. He noted that serum concentrations of total estradiol-17β, total testosterone, and luteinizing hormone are supranormal in these patients. Further, serum concentrations of sex hormone (testosterone and estrogen) binding globulin is high in hyperthyroidism. While serum unbound testosterone is normal, the serum unbound estradiol-17β is above normal in the hyperthyroid male. Further, this author suggests that the imbalance in relative concentrations of unbound gonadal steroids is apparently quite favorable to the development of gynecomastia in hyperthyroid states.[70] As a consequence, increased peripheral tissue metabolism of androgens to estrogens seems to be the major factor responsible for the high estradiol-17β value in this state;

increased glandular secretion of the hormone may also be important.

Galactorrhea rarely occurs in men, most cases being reported in patients with prolactin-secreting pituitary tumors.[116, 219] Kleinberg et al.[219] and Edwards and associates[106] have documented hyperprolactinemia and galactorrhea in the presence of *hypothyroidism* in women. More recently, Arnaout and associates[12] reported the occurrence of galactorrhea and gynecomastia in a patient with occult hypothyroidism, both of which resolved following thyroxin replacement therapy. This report is the first to document galactorrhea secondary to hypothyroidism in a male patient. Arnaout suggests that the differential diagnosis of galactorrhea in male patients should include hypothyroidism.[12]

Diseases of the Liver

While it has been accepted for several decades that the hyperestrogen state is commonly observed in *nonalcoholic cirrhosis of the liver,* it has only recently been determined that plasma concentrations and urinary excretion of estrogen are both increased. Previous reports confirmed that the peripheral conversion of plasma androgens to estrogens is increased in the cirrhotic state.[153, 154, 301]

Kley and associates[221] evaluted estrogen, testosterone, androstenedione, and cortisol values and percentage of binding of these steroids in plasma for normal, young, and old male subjects and in male patients with fatty liver, chronic hepatitis, and cirrhosis of the liver. Alterations of these steroids were most marked in the cirrhotic patients but were also evident to a lesser degree in patients with *fatty metamorphosis of the liver* and in normal *aging patients.* These authors determined a definite increase in estrone, a smaller escalation in estradiol, a decrease in testosterone, and a rise in luteinizing hormone for cirrhosis. Cortisol remained unchanged, whereas ratios of estradiol/testosterone and estrone/testosterone were augmented in cirrhotic patients and were higher than in healthy young subjects. These authors suggest that the combination of elevated estrone and estradiol and reduced testosterone, which was strongly bound by increased sex hormone–binding globulin, may be responsible for gynecomastia and hypogonadism in chronic liver diseases. As patients with hepatic disease and elderly men both are observed to have similar alterations of steroid plasma concentrations and the binding of these steroids to plasma proteins, these authors suggest that the etiological mechanism is similar, namely, altered hepatic parenchymal function. In 1985, Kley et al.[220] confirmed the absence of gynecomastia in patients with *idiopathic hemochromatosis,* including those with severe liver disease. The variance in clinical presentation of idiopathic hemochromatosis and *alcoholic cirrhosis* suggests that the mechanism of hepatic failure is accompanied by different abnormalities in sex hormone metabolism. Kley and associates[220] confirmed the clinical features of hypogonadism and normal estrogen activity in patients with idiopathic hemochromatosis. Conversely, in alcoholic cirrhosis, estradiol and estrone were significantly elevated and sex hormone–binding globulin was increased. In idiopathic hemochromatosis, sex hormone–binding globulin levels were in the same range as for normal men. For idiopathic hemochromatosis, the instantaneous conversion of plasma androstenedione to estrone and estradiol was normal, whereas that of plasma testosterone to plasma estrogen was decreased by about one half. The converse was observed in alcoholic cirrhosis, as the instantaneous conversion of plasma androstenedione to estrogen was greatly increased, and that of testosterone was within the normal range.

Farthing and associates[111] observed plasma progesterone values to be increased in 72 percent (36/50) of men with liver disease compared with 20 healthy male controls. The plasma progesterone values were significantly higher for men with nonalcoholic cirrhosis and gynecomastia than for those without gynecomastia; however, this hormonal relationship was not observed for men with alcoholic fatty change and alcoholic cirrhosis. Although hyperprolactinemia was observed in 14 percent of males with hepatic disease, it was felt that levels were unrelated to the presence of gynecomastia. The authors suggest that increased circulating values of progesterone and prolactin do not explain the development of gynecomastia in patients with liver disease, but these sex steroids may be a factor acting in concert with other hormones to initiate breast hypertrophy. Further, Johnson,[201] as well as other reviewers, has concluded that observed increases in estradiol are not great enough to contribute to the feminization seen in cirrhosis. These conclusions are drawn from results of free estradiol estimations that have been equally varied and from the fact that estrone is only a weak estrogen. Kley and coinvestigators[220, 221] confirmed the variations in free testosterone and estradiol values in controls and for patients with varying stages of hepatic cirrhosis (from well compensated to decompensated with ascites, variceal hemorrhage, gynecomastia, and testicular atrophy). The progressive rise in estradiol was marked, as was the reciprocal fall of free testosterone (Table 7–1). The progressive rise in steroid hormone–binding globulin

tends to escalate the profound feminizing aspects of alcoholic disease, as testosterone has a significantly higher affinity for sex hormone–binding globulin, thus enhancing the estrogen:testosterone ratio.

Gynecomastia in the Cirrhotic Male. Gynecomastia is observed in approximately 40 percent of cirrhotic men.[17, 18, 141, 251, 322, 384] Total plasma testosterone concentrations were lower than normal as identified by Van Thiel et al.[409] and by others.[72, 211, 220, 221, 317] Although this relative decrease in testosterone is significant, it is modest and is masked by the far greater fall in the non–protein bound (biologically active) fraction of plasma testosterone.[71, 72, 141, 286] This decrease appears to result from the increased concentration of sex hormone–binding globulin (SHBG) present in cirrhotic males.[333, 336, 412] Anderson[8] considers SHBG the most important plasma protein for determination of the protein binding of plasma testosterone. Biologically, the low plasma testosterone of cirrhotic men is initiated by a reduction in testosterone synthesis by the testes. Horton and Tait[187] and Gordon et al.[153, 154] have confirmed by kinetic studies that the atrophic testes of alcoholic cirrhotics contribute approximately one quarter of the normal concentrations of testosterone. Moreover, Gordon and associates[154] suggest that 15 percent of the testosterone produced in cirrhotic males is derived from peripheral conversion of circulating androstenedione, as indicated in Figure 7–11. Green[158] notes that unlike biochemical evidence of hypogonadism, the biochemical feminization of the cirrhotic male has not been adequately established. With the advent of sensitive assay methodology to evaluate plasma steroidal concentrations, the measurement of unconjugated plasma estrogens has centered around evaluation of plasma estradiol. In *alcoholic cirrhosis,* several investigators[141, 143, 158, 409] have noted that the total unconjugated plasma estradiol is normal, mildly elevated,[220, 221, 224, 312] or markedly increased.[66, 72, 301] Green[157, 158] recognized that there is equal disagreement about the role of unbound (biologically active) plasma estradiol in cirrhotic men, with reports of normal, marginally increased, or markedly increased free serum values of this sex steroid.

Temporal Effects of Alcohol Consumption in the Noncirrhotic Male

Short-Term Alcohol Consumption in Noncirrhotic Men. Gordon and associates[153] published a study of short-term (four-week) alcohol consumption with evidence of increased hepatic metabolism and enhanced metabolic clearance rates of testosterone from plasma. Further, the plasma testosterone values declined over the period of the study, as did the protein binding of the plasma testosterone. The authors observed no consistent change in serum luteinizing hormone and interpreted these findings as evidence of direct suppression of hypothalamic-pituitary and testicular function due to alcohol consumption.

Chronic Alcohol Consumption in the Noncirrhotic Male. The biochemical alterations evident in noncirrhotic chronic alcoholics are somewhat different from those of the short-term consumers. In the chronic alcohol user, plasma SHBG was observed to increase mark-

Table 7–1. CONCENTRATIONS OF FREE TESTOSTERONE AND FREE ESTRADIOL IN PLASMA IN HEALTHY MALES (n = 8) AND IN PATIENTS OF THE SAME AGE WITH ALCOHOL-INDUCED CIRRHOSIS OF THE LIVER

	Free Testosterone (pg/ml) >	Free Estradiol (pg/ml) >
Controls	124.7 ± 10.2	0.51 ± 0.06
Group 1	94.9 ± 9.9	0.55 ± 0.03
Group 2	57.8 ± 7.4	0.71 ± 0.05
Group 3	32.0 ± 4.0	1.14 ± 0.15

>Values are means ± SEM

Group 1: Well-preserved liver function. Group 2: Intermediate liver function. Group 3: Decompensated liver disease with ascites, episodes of variceal hemorrhage, gynecomastia, and testicular atrophy.

From Kley HK, Strohmeyer G, Krunkemper HL: Gastroenterology 76:235–241, 1979. Reprinted by permission.

edly, thus reducing the free fraction of plasma testosterone to below normal.[220, 221, 247, 384] Further, there is increasing evidence that many of these patients with fatty livers have augmented plasma gonadotropins[407-409] with marginally decreased concentration of free testosterone values.[157]

The hypothesis that explains the aforementioned changes of hypogonadism and overt feminization in men with chronic alcoholic liver disease cannot adequately explain the clinical and biochemical features found in these men. Green et al.[158] suggest that the pathogenesis of endocrine changes in the cirrhotic male is multifactoral and includes a combination of decreased hepatic clearance of several estrogenic compounds, an autoimmune-mediated primary testicular defect, and possibly a specific potentiation effect of alcohol consumption. While all these explanations are plausible, the precise mechanisms of endocrine, biochemical, and histological alterations are yet to be confirmed.

Johnson[201] presented data that cast doubt upon the hypothesis that chronic liver disease may lead to elevations of estrogen consequent upon failure of the liver to metabolize endogenously produced steroids, thereafter initiating low urinary androgen and high urinary estrogen excretion. Johnson[201] reasoned that these hypotheses are dubious, as metabolic clearance rates for estradiol and estrone are usually normal in male cirrhotics and the correlation between elevated estrogen values in gynecomastia is poor. This author notes the clinical parallels, such as Klinefelter syndrome (see p. 149), in which gynecomastia is also frequent despite normal to marginally increased estrogen values.[307]

Rose and associates[331] present data to suggest that *spironolactone* initiates gynecomastia via a blockade of the androgen receptor in the male breast that leads to the unopposed action of estrogen. As a consequence of this metabolic activity, perhaps, gynecomastia in cirrhosis most commonly occurs following the treatment of ascites with spironolactone. The biochemical and histopathological abnormalities induced by the drug are strikingly akin to those of cirrhosis. In this metabolic syndrome, testosterone is decreased, estrogen is increased, and the rate of conversion between the steroids is escalated.

Evidence of hypogonadism is common in men with advanced hepatic disease.[22, 32, 251, 276] Earlier, investigations explained this observation on the basis of an increased circulating level of estrogen and assumed that a prehepatic accumulation of female sex hormones results in hepatic inactivation or clearance of these hormones.[409] Using the technology of assay systems, investigators showed that plasma estradiol values, and presumably those of other steroidal estrogens, were not elevated in men with hepatic insufficiency.[72, 141, 211] Both total and free plasma levels of testosterone in males with cirrhosis has been uniformly reduced.[17, 18, 72, 80, 141, 211] Further, plasma values of luteinizing hormone and follicle-stimulating hormone were reported as normal or elevated for subjects in whom they were evaluated.[17, 18, 72, 141, 211] Van Thiel and associates[409] evaluated hypothalamic-pituitary-gonadal function in 40 men with a wide spectrum of alcoholic liver diseases in an effort to identify an anatomical location and biochemical mechanism responsible for the observed hypogonadism and feminization. Mean plasma testosterone values were lower (p <0.05) and associated with severe derangements of hepatic histology. Both follicle-stimulating hormone and luteinizing hormone concentrations were normal to moderately elevated when compared with those of normal men. These authors[409] confirmed that total plasma estradiol values were normal or reduced and that these mean values did not differ from normal. In contradistinction, plasma testosterone was reduced in over 50 percent of the men and differed significantly (p <0.01) from values for normal subjects.

Nutritional Alteration States

Gynecomastia produced by nutritional deprivation has been well documented. Case-control studies of World War II American prisoners of war determined that approximately 15 percent of males in Japanese prisoner camps developed gynecomastia.[197, 218, 441] Further, approximately one third of the cases of gynecomastia occurred during refeeding after release from prison, while other cases were associated with temporary increases in food supplied during imprisonment. In the majority of these subjects, gynecomastia was bilateral and disappeared within five to seven months following refeeding. A confounding variable to such studies is the potential for concurrent diseases (i.e., hepatic disease, infectious hepatitis), which may have played a significant role in the development of gynecomastia, as many of these prisoners had fatty infiltration of the liver and spider angiomas. Thus, the exact etiological mechanisms are not clarified, and similarities to primary liver disease are so close that pathogenesis is assumed to be secondary to the gynecomastia of hepatic disease.[197] Bardin[20] and Paulsen[307] suggest that *"refeeding gynecomastia"* may be related to a resumption of pituitary gonadotropin secretion following pituitary shutdown that initiates a secondary puberty as a consequence of protein deprivation.

Sattin and associates[346] documented an epidemic of gynecomastia among illegal Haitian entrants of the United States in 1981 and 1982. These authors postulated that the pattern of development of gynecomastia and its resolution among these detained Haitian entrants (in view of their probable nutritional deficiency) suggest that refeeding may have been the cause. Although refeeding gynecomastia has not been reported in other entrant or refugee populations, this is possibly related to the fact that the phenomenon is poorly understood and thus was not documented. The transient nature of refeeding gynecomastia with differences in geographical location, dietary practices, the indigenous population and available medical care may explain the discrepancies in previous reports.

The Influence of Aging in Initiating Gynecomastia

As noted under physiological gynecomastia, *senescent gynecomastia* (Fig. 7–12) appears to increase in inci-

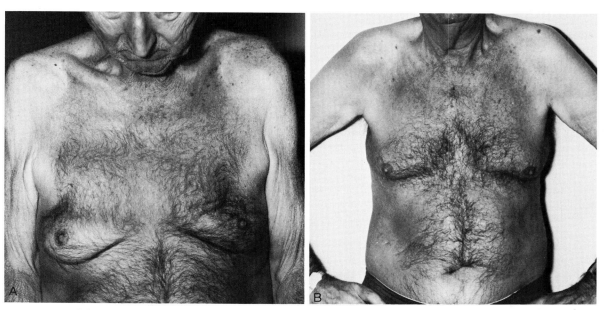

Figure 7–12. *A,* Senescent bilateral gynecomastia in an 85-year-old male. The patient had observed gradual increase in the size of both breasts over the past four years. There are no breast masses, and the patient takes no medication. *B,* Senescent bilateral gynecomastia in a 72-year-old male with progressive enlargement of breasts over a six-year period. The patient has no systemic diseases and takes no medications.

dence with advancing age; it was observed by Nuttall[298] in over half of the men greater than age 45 years. Further, Williams[425] noted that greater than 40 percent of elderly men have true gynecomastia. Plasma testosterone concentration values begin to diminish at approximately 70 years. In addition, there is concurrent elevation in the plasma testosterone-estrogen binding globulin such that the levels of free or unbound testosterone concentrations decline even further. Snyder[366] suggests that there is a simultaneous increase in plasma luteinizing hormone such that an increase in the rate of conversion of androgen to estrogen in peripheral tissues is a concurrent event. The net result is an effective increase in the relative plasma estradiol values for these elderly men with a synchronous fall in testosterone values secondary to the affinity of this molecule for testosterone-estrogen binding globulin. Overall, relative hyperestrinism is evident with a decrease in the plasma androgen:estrogen ratio. Because *senescent gynecomastia,* as the term implies, develops in the elderly male population, the lesion must be differentiated from carcinoma of the breast. Haagensen[168] suggests that *"senescent hypertrophy"* occurs most commonly in men between the ages of 50 and 70 years, and that, classically, the hypertrophy takes the form of a tender, 2 to 4 cm, discoid tumor beneath the areola. Its tenderness and bilateral occurrence, if present, are considered to be important physical findings that differentiate hypertrophy from carcinoma. In a great majority of such cases, the lesions are unilateral and the hypertrophy is located centrally beneath the areola with well-defined, smooth, tender margins. In contradistinction, *carcinoma of the male breast* (Fig. 7–13) is poorly defined clinically, with irregular edges and presenting as a hard, nontender mass that is fixed to the underlying fascia or skin, possibly with associated retraction of the nipple. The

identification of these ominous physical findings makes it incumbent upon the physician to biopsy suspicious lesions to exclude the presence of carcinoma.

Hypoandrogen States (Hypogonadism)

Primary Testicular Failure
Klinefelter Syndrome (XXY). The syndrome of 47,XXY karyotype was described more than four decades ago by Klinefelter.[223] The syndrome was first observed in adult phenotypic males with gynecomastia, hypergonadotropic hypogonadism and azoospermia. Only subsequently in the genetic evaluation of these

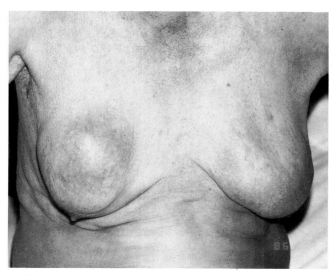

Figure 7–13. Advanced bilateral gynecomastia in a 70-year-old male. The patient also has a palpable, discrete mass of right breast confirmed mammographically and on biopsy to be a carcinoma.

patients was the syndrome found to be associated with the presence of the extra X chromosome. Further, as the condition was rarely diagnosed until late in life, little was known about the natural history of hypogonadism in young males with the karyotype. The chromosomal pattern XXY is common; Gerald[146] estimates that the syndrome occurs in approximately 1 in 600 live births. When the syndrome is associated with hypergonatropic hypogonadism and a negative buccal smear, a chromosomal analysis should be done to search for a mosaicism. If the buccal smear is positive, it should have a karyotype confirmation of the extra X chromosome. Tennes et al.[389] note that in addition to XXY, patients with Klinefelter syndrome may have multiple X (XXXY) or Y (XXYY) chromosomes or mosaic patterns (e.g., XXY/XY).

Klinefelter syndrome represents the most common variant of *male hypogonadism*. Children with the 47,XXY karyotype demonstrate relatively few clinical findings, although there may be an occasional patient who has reduced testicular size or penile length. The clinical picture of gynecomastia, eunuchoidism, and microorchidism does not usually emerge until well after midpuberty and may never be fully expressed. Testicular biopsy confirms a reduced number of spermatogonia; however, tubular fibrosis and hyalinization of seminiferous tubules are not observed until well after the onset of puberty.[113] Ahmad et al.[2] noted that the testes of adult patients revealed extensive fibrosis and hyalinization and that Leydig cell volume may be preserved. Biochemical findings confirm reduced levels of serum testosterone with high-normal or enhanced values of serum estradiol.[120] Gabrilove and associates[133] noted that this increased estradiol:testosterone ratio is maintained even in elderly patients despite the reduction in testicular function with aging.

Salbenblatt and coinvestigators[343] evaluated the serum concentrations of follicle-stimulating hormone (FSH), luteinizing hormone (LH), testosterone, and estradiol at intervals before and during puberty in 40 individuals with Klinefelter syndrome. Prior to the appearance of secondary sexual changes in these patients, basal serum hormone concentrations and acute responses to stimulation with gonadtropin-releasing hormone and human chorionic gonadotropin (HCG) was confirmed to be normal. Although onset of clinical puberty was normal in these patients, serum FSH and estradiol concentrations were significantly elevated. Early pubertal males showed initial testicular growth and normal serum testosterone values. By midpuberty, these authors confirm that Klinefelter subjects were uniformly hypergonadotropic and that testicular growth had ceased. Serum testosterone concentrations after age 15 remained in the low-normal range, while serum estradiol values were increased, irrespective of the presence or absence of gynecomastia. Drucker et al.[102] distinguished the primary nature of tubular atrophy in *myotonic dystrophy* and indicated that the testicular lesion differs morphologically and clinically from the seminiferous tubule dysgenesis of Klinefelter syndrome, with which it often has been confused.

Klinefelter[222] notes that mental deficiency, manic depressive psychoses, and schizophrenia do not occur more commonly in the syndrome than in control subjects and that most patients work regularly and lead normal lives except for their inability to procreate. There is no treatment for the sterility associated with the syndrome.

Therapy directed toward Klinefelter syndrome is both surgical and medical. Gynecomastia is best treated by excision of the hypertrophic breast tissue with preservation of the nipple-areola complex. This should not be done for cosmetic reasons but because *carcinoma of the breast*, as confirmed by Cole,[78] is 20 times more frequent in individuals with this condition than in normal men. Indeed, Jackson and associates[195] have suggested that breast carcinoma associated with the syndrome is 66.5 times more frequent than for normal controls. *Bilateral carcinoma of the breast* has also been reported in the syndrome by Robson et al.[329] In the presence of hypogonadism, treatment should include testosterone injections, which appears to be effective in the majority of patients. Further, Klinefelter[222] suggests that there is evidence that treatment of adolescent patients with testosterone may abrogate some of the personality traits and abnormalities that emerge in later life.

Reifenstein Syndrome (XY). In 1947, Reifenstein described hereditary familial hypogonadism with a characteristic phenotype that includes severe hypospadias, incomplete virilization at the time of expected puberty, and azoospermia associated with maturational arrest of spermatogenesis.[7, 326, 429] Patients with the syndrome present with profound gynecomastia. The family history suggests X-linkage of the phenotype. Endocrinological studies confirm elevated levels of plasma luteinizing hormone and estradiol with normal to high values of testosterone.[429] With this endocrine profile, feminization of affected subjects results from a combination of enhanced estradiol secretion and resistance to androgen action.[352] Schweikert et al.[352] suggest that the endocrine features of Reifenstein syndrome are the consequence of diminished feedback of testosterone on LH secretion with subsequent rise in the plasma LH and, consequently, an enhancement in mean secretion of estradiol and testosterone by the testes. These authors also confirm that plasma levels of free estradiol as well as free testosterone are elevated even in the presence of an elevated sex hormone–binding globulin. These findings further support the concept that the disorder is the result of a resistance to hormone action, rather than a defect in androgen physiology.

Rosewater, Gwinup, Hamwi Familial Gynecomastia (XY). In 1965, Rosewater and colleagues[335] described a family in which four males presented with gynecomastia as part of a syndrome previously unreported. In these patients, blood chemistries, including hepatic functions, were normal as were urinary 17-ketosteroids and 17-hydroxysteroids. Pituitary gonadotropins and luteinizing hormone were low or absent. Urinary estriol levels were within normal ranges for males. Patients demonstrated a defect in spermatogenesis. Testicular biopsies confirmed tubular maturation arrest and decreased numbers of Leydig cells. Breast tissue biopsy was compatible with estrogenic stimulation despite normal plasma 17-hydroxycorticosteroid and 17-ketosteroids and normal urinary 17-ketosteroids fraction. Estrone and estradiol values were within normal limits. Analysis of the family pedigree suggested that the syndrome resulted as a sex-linked recessive or sex-limited autosomal dominant defect. The authors concluded that *familial gynecomastia* is a genetic trait associated with a secondary suppression of gonadotropins and that the testes produced an adequate concentration of androgens but were a potential site of increased estrogen production. These patients have a normal XY buccal epithelium chromatin pattern. No enhanced risk of male breast carcinoma appears evident with this syndrome of familial gynecomastia.

More recently, Berkovitz et al.[35] reported a variant of the syndrome for a family in which gynecomastia occurred in five males over two generations. For each affected subject, gynecomastia and male sexual maturation began at an early age. The ratio of plasma concentration of estradiol to 17β-testosterone was elevated in each subject. For three siblings with gynecomastia, the transfer constant for conversion of androstenedione to estrone was ten times normal. Despite elevation in extraglandular aromatase activity, there was a normal response of the hypothalamic-pituitary axis to provocative stimuli. This documentation of familial gynecomastia, and the report in 1977 by Hemsell et al.,[180] note the association of gynecomastia with increased extraglandular aromatase activity. The report by Berkovitz et al.[35] was the first to document the defect as familial with a probable X-linked (autosomal dominant, sex-limited) mode of inheritance.

Kallmann Syndrome. Van Dop et al.[405] note that isolated *gonadotropin deficiency* comprises a heterogeneous group of disorders. The most common variant, Kallmann syndrome, is a familial deficiency of hypothalamic luteinizing hormone–releasing factor (LRF) that is transmitted as an autosomal dominant trait with variable penetrance. Described in 1944,[205] this syndrome occurs with a frequency of approximately 1 per 10,000 males and 1 per 50,000 females. A cardinal feature of the syndrome is an impairment or defect of the sense of smell *(hyposmia or anosmia)*[370] as a consequence of hypoplasia or aplasia of the rhinencephalon. Associated congenital anomalies are multiple and include the kidneys,[419] the skeleton,[47, 246] the reproductive system (testes),[21, 246] and the nasopharynx with associated cleft palate and congenital deafness.[345] Abnormalities commonly include gynecomastia and obesity.[47]

Patients with the syndrome (genito-olfactory dysplasia) have more associated anomalies than do patients with euosmia. Van Dop and coauthors[405] observed the occurrence of undescended testes in approximately half their patients, which is not surprising in view of the postulated role of gonadotropins to initiate testicular descent during embryogenesis.[164] The association of cryptorchidism with severe gonadotropin deficiency in the syndrome possibly has predictive value for evaluation of boys with cryptorchidism and hyposmia. In these males, treatment with testosterone is appropriate. However, the therapy for boys who are not clearly hypogo-

nadal may present various problems. Patients with delayed puberty and low serum gonadotropin in the absence of intracranial lesions should be examined closely for ocular and skeletal anomalies in addition to the assessment of olfactory function.[405] Replacement testosterone therapy should be initiated at an appropriate age to induce full virilization if the diagnosis of isolated gonadotropin deficiency is established in males with any of these anomalies.

Kennedy Disease with Associated Gynecomastia. In 1966, Kennedy et al.[209] described a condition that presents with muscle cramps, weakness, and atrophy of the limb girdles by age 30 to 40 years. All patients had diffuse fasciculations, especially of the chin and lips, dysarthria, and dysphagia. The clinical course of the disease was quite slow, such that life expectancy was unaffected. On electromyography and muscle biopsy, the condition was confirmed to be frankly neurogenic in origin. This clinical syndrome as described by Kennedy and coworkers[210] differs from other spinal muscle atrophies of adulthood and is considered to have an X-linked mode of inheritance. More recently, Guidetti et al.[166] described an X-linked adult-onset neurogenic muscular atrophy that was chiefly proximal, with late involvement of distal musculature and the medulla oblongata. Affected kindred all had gynecomastia, impotence, and essential tremor. Hormonal stimulation tests confirmed borderline low testicular response in the younger of two patients and a pathological response in older patients. Of the endocrine disturbances, gynecomastia has been cited as one of the signal features of the syndrome since Kennedy's first description. Hausmanowa-Petrusewicz[177] and Arbizu et al.[11] established the testicular origin of the deficit. These authors consider gynecomastia, which is not necessarily present, a symptom that occurs secondary to the peripheral transformation of testosterone into estrogen.[264]

Eunuchoidal Males (Congenital Anorchia). The eunuchoidal male has defective masculinity of appearance—usually as the cryptorchid individual. *Embryonic testicular regression* (congenital anorchia) is a disorder, often familial, in which the testes are absent in the phenotypically normal male with the 46, XY karyotype.[105, 170, 179, 216, 217] In this example of deficient testosterone production, gynecomastia results despite normal estrogen production rates in adult men. Levitt et al.[243] emphasize that the individuals are often considered to have bilateral cryptorchidism at birth; however, plasma testosterone values are undetectable following stimulation with pharmacologically active doses of chorionic gonadotropin. Further, no testes can be identified on abdominal or scrotal exploration. Kirschner and associates[216] confirmed that even when the testes cannot be located anatomically, Leydig cell remnants may be identified along the urogenital ridge and may secrete diminutive amounts of testosterone. It is estimated that approximately half the subjects who have anorchia develop gynecomastia.

Hereditary Defects of Androgen Biosynthesis. At least five enzymatic defects have been identified to occur in embryogenesis that result in defective androgen biosynthesis with incomplete virilization of the male embryo.[45, 161, 428, 430] The enzymes responsible for these failures in biosynthesis include 20,22-desmolase, 17,20-desmolase, 3β-hydroxysteroid dehydrogenase, 17α-hydroxylase, and 17β-hydroxysteroid dehydrogenase. Each enzyme represents a critical pathway for the conversion of cholesterol to testosterone. In addition, *congenital adrenal hyperplasia* (Fig. 7–14) may be associated with 20,22-desmolase, 3β-hydroxysteroid dehydrogenase, and 17α-hydroxylase deficiencies. As a consequence of the variability in the blockade of these enzymatic biochemical reactions, affected individuals manifest a profound escalation in gonadotropin secretion following negative feedback. For individuals with complete or partial deficiencies of 17β-hydroxysteroid dehydrogenase, feminization, which includes gynecomastia, develops at the time of expected puberty in the male. Presumably, the gynecomastia results from diminished testosterone biosynthesis in the presence of enhanced or normal estrogenic formation. Further, escalated estrogen biosynthesis may occur from increased availability of androstenedione for conversion to estrogen in peripheral tissues or may secondarily occur from increased estrogen secretion from the testes as a consequence of enhanced gonadotropin secretion.[428]

ACTH Deficiency. The association between gynecomastia and isolated ACTH deficiencies, an uncommon cause of adrenocortical insufficiency,[372] has only rarely been documented.[403, 439] Recently, Shimatsu and co-workers[360] described a patient with ACTH deficiency who had gynecomastia with elevated estrogens, luteinizing hormone, and prolactin serum values that normalized following replacement therapy with glucocorticoids. Similar cases of isolated deficiency of ACTH associated with gynecomastia have been reported by Uehra et al.[403]

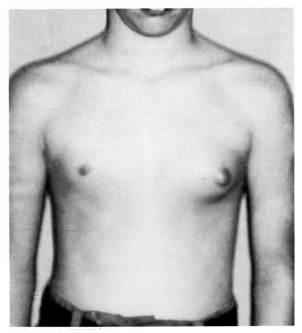

Figure 7–14. Congenital adrenal hyperplasia in an 11-year-old male patient with unilateral left gynecomastia evident at puberty.

and Yoshida and associates.[439] The etiology of gynecomastia in patients with ACTH deficiency remains enigmatic. In these subjects, normal values of thyroid hormone, testosterone, and human chorionic gonadotropins are evident. Low values of androstenedione and urinary 17-ketosteroid were seen in the subjects with high estrogen values. As a consequence of the high estrogen values with normal testosterone levels in the presence of elevated luteinizing hormone concentrations, a decreased testosterone:estrogen ratio is maintained and presumably is the cause of the breast enlargement. High luteinizing hormone values in the presence of normal testosterone suggest that patients have a compensated Leydig cell insufficiency. However, there is evidence that hyperreactive responses to luteinizing hormone may be, in part, related to glucocorticoid deficiency. The high estrogen levels may reflect increased peripheral conversion of estrogens. Further, these augmented values may occur with secretion of testicular estradiol following stimulation by elevated luteinizing hormone. The biochemical role of glucocorticoids in the regulation of estrogen metabolism in men remains to be elucidated.

Secondary Testicular Failure. Gynecomastia is common following the secondary testicular failure of *trauma, viral orchitis (mumps), or bacterial infections (e.g., tuberculosis, leprosy).* These causes of organic failure of the testes for active androgen biosynthesis are extraordinarily rare in the United States. *Bilateral testicular atrophy* may occur as a consequence of major direct trauma to the penis and testis and/or pelvic trauma. The progressive loss of androgen function relates to the deprivation of active testosterone secretion and biosynthesis by the devascularized testes secondary to massive hematoma and/or direct testicular injury. *Mumps* represents the most common cause of viral orchitis, although other viruses including *ECHO, lymphocytic choriomeningitis virus,* and *Group B arboviruses* have been implicated in secondary testicular failure.[328, 422] Bjorvatn[42] suggests that viral orchitis occurs secondary to the direct effects of the virus on testicular parenchyma, as the mumps virus has been isolated from the testes of affected subjects. This serious complication of mumps occurs in approximately one fourth of men infected with the virus; two thirds have unilateral orchitis. Atrophy appears secondary to the direct action of the virus on the seminiferous tubules or to the ischemia of pressure and edema within the tunica albuginea. There is no correlation of the clinical severity of the orchitis and the degree of atrophy of the testes. Atrophy occurs in approximately one third of subjects with viral orchitis and is bilateral in approximately one tenth of infected patients. In a survey of 2000 adult men, Werner[422] observed atrophy to occur in one or both testes in approximately 2 percent; in half these patients, the atrophy occurred secondary to mumps.

The utilization of *irradiation* and *chemotherapy* in children treated for malignancies may initiate gonadal failure secondary to the cancer therapy. Testicular biopsies have shown absence of spermatogenesis in azoospermic patients.[310, 311] Although prepubertal gonads were found to be less sensitive to toxicity,[92, 214, 305, 310] the testes of boys in early puberty are very sensitive to drug toxicity, as reflected by elevated basal levels of gonadotropins, normal testosterone concentration, and enhanced luteinizing hormone responses to gonadotropin-releasing hormone. Shalet et al.[356] suggest that for children with malignant disease, gonadal damage may occur secondary to the irradiation or chemotherapy that initiates these gonadotropin elevations. Further, irradiation to the hypothalamic-pituitary axis in children with brain tumors may ultimately result in gonadotropin deficiency or hyperprolactinemia, which, in turn, results in gonadal insufficiency. If the testicular damage in prepubertal males is transient, androgen function will return and the chemotherapy- or irradiation-induced gynecomastia will abate.

Testicular failure as a consequence of *hydrocele, varicocele,* or *spermatocele* is indeed rare and would be expected to have a higher frequency following *trauma* in the patient with unilateral *cryptorchidism.* In such patients, surgical treatment of the hydrocele, varicocele, or spermatocele may be indicated. The testicles should be salvaged if clinically possible, but for instances in which orchiectomy is necessary (e.g., major trauma), testosterone replacement with therapeutic doses is indicated.

Wilson and associates[428] point out that estrogen and androgen serum concentration dynamics have not been measured in these traumatic, therapeutic, and infectious states. Gynecomastia is also recognized with other causes of testicular failure, including *neurological diseases* in which testicular atrophy supervenes,[75, 79] *postcastration states,*[437] and *granulomatous diseases of the testes,* especially lepromatous leprosy.[89, 275]

Renal Failure

Gynecomastia is common in males who develop uremia. Further, data suggest that approximately half the patients undergoing chronic hemodialysis develop gynecomastia.[126, 167, 183, 287, 347, 350] Wilson et al.[428] noted that the endocrine changes of chronic renal failure are complex and that the relationships of these changes to the pituitary-testicular axis are only now being elucidated. Holdsworth and associates[183] observed that plasma luteinizing hormone and follicle-stimulating hormone values are increased approximately fourfold in men with creatinine clearance rates less than or equal to 4 ml per minute. Further plasma testosterone concentrations are 30 percent of normal for these subjects. These authors[183] cite evidence of histological damage to the testes, with hypospermia and a subnormal response for plasma testosterone secretion following chorionic gonadotropin administration.

Holdsworth et al.[183] further state that elevated plasma luteinizing hormone values occur secondary to a reduction in metabolic clearance from the renal failure; a secondary increase in the secretion of luteinizing hormone by the pituitary is evident. Wilson et al.[428] explain this sequence of renal failure and gynecomastia as a consequence of increased gonadotropin secretion following the subnormal response of Leydig cells to gonado-

tropin stimulation. The biochemical and histological transformation to gynecomastia remains enigmatic. To date, no studies have confirmed estrogen or androgen alterations that result from chronic renal failure. A plausible hypothesis for the development of gynecomastia is enhanced estradiol secretion by the testes following elevations of the plasma gonadotropins.

Drug-Related Conditions That Initiate Gynecomastia

The development of gynecomastia in the adult male is frequently recognized as a consequence of drug administration. In contrast to the development of gynecomastia in the pubertal or prepubertal male because of endogenous sex-steroid hormonal production from various organ sites, in the adult a specific inquiry into drug use and a review of the past history is essential. Table 7–2 identifies the categories in which exogenous drugs or their metabolic products initiate gynecomastia, including (1) drugs with estrogenic or estrogen-related activity, (2) drugs that inhibit the action and/or synthesis

Table 7–2. DRUGS ETIOLOGICAL FOR GYNECOMASTIA

Drugs with Estrogenic or Estrogen-Related Activity
Anabolic steroids (nandrolone, testosterone cypionate)
Clomiphene citrate
Diethylpropion hydrochloride
Diethylstilbestrol
Digitalis
Estrogens
Heroin
Oral contraceptives
Tetrahydrocannabinol (cannabis, marijuana)

Drugs that Inhibit the Action and/or Synthesis of Testosterone
Antineoplastic agents (vincristine, nitrosoureas, methotrexate)
Cimetidine
Cyproterone acetate
D-Penicillamine
Diazepam
Flutamide
Ketoconazole
Medroxyprogesterone acetate
Phenytoin
Spironolactone

Drugs that Enhance Estrogen Synthesis by the Testes
Human chorionic gonadotropin

Drugs with Idiopathic Mechanism for Induction of Gynecomastia
Amiodarone
Bumetanide
Busulfan
Domperidone
Ethionamide
Furosemide
Isoniazid
Methyldopa
Nifedipine
Reserpine
Sulindac
Theophylline
Tricyclic antidepressants
Verapamil

of testosterone, (3) drugs that enhance estrogen synthesis by the testes, and (4) drugs that have idiopathic mechanisms for induction of gynecomastia.

Drugs with Estrogenic or Estrogen-Related Activity. The administration of estrogens or compounds with estrogen-like activity can induce severe gynecomastia in males. The development of breast masses in men with prostate carcinoma is common following therapy with estrogen. Hendrickson and Robertson[181] reported gynecomastia following administration of *diethylstilbestrol (DES)* for prostate carcinoma, and Brandt et al.,[48] reporting on the use of oral contraceptives in hemophilia, identified rapid onset of gynecomastia with estrogen administration. Orentreich and Dur[303] described mammogenesis in transsexuals following administration of oral estrogen. Symmers[386] has identified transsexual males who develop metastasizing mammary adenocarcinoma following castration, augmentation mammoplasty, and administration of large doses of estrogen. In contrast, Holleb et al.[184] reported in 1968 on a survey of 17,000 patients with cancer of the prostate treated with estrogen by 150 urologists. Only two cases of carcinoma of the breast (incidence rate 0.012 percent) were observed. Holleb et al.[184] and Wilson and Hutchinson[431] conclude that it is highly improbable that a causal relationship exists between estrogen administration and breast carcinoma. Only six reported cases of primary breast carcinoma in males with prostate cancer have been reported in the English literature, which further supports this view.[431] Further, prepubertal gynecomastia has been described following topical inunction of estrogen-containing ointment,[173] and persistent gynecomastia has resulted from scalp inunction of estradiol.[104, 135] Beas et al.[24] and Landolt and Murset[228] note the extraordinary sensitivity of young men and boys to dermal ointments that contain estrogens.

Gynecomastia is a frequent consequence of *digitalis* administration[244]; Navab et al.[288] attribute gynecomastia induction from the estrogen-like activity of this cardiac glycoside. Wolfe[435] observed a 10 percent incidence of gynecomastia in patients who received digitalis preparations for 12 or more months. Stouffer and associates[382] reported that an increase in total serum estrogens and a decrease of plasma testosterone was evident in patients treated with digoxin. Novak et al.[295] suggest that the mechanism of initiating gynecomastia by digitalis is the estrogen or estrogen-precursor activity of the drug, similar to the estrogen effect evident in the vaginal mucosa of menopausal women.

Clomiphene citrate has been used to treat ovulatory disturbances in selected infertile women and, more recently, for the treatment of male infertility.[367] The administration of clomiphene has been shown to induce gynecomastia,[69] and gynecomastia has also been induced by withdrawal of the drug.[236]

With the current enthusiasm for use of the *anabolic steroids nandrolone* and *testosterone cypionate,* clinics have observed the induction of severe gynecomastia following administration of these injectible steroids. The report by Spano and Ryan[369] admonishes physicians to be cognizant of the potential deleterious application of

tamoxifen to prevent gynecomastia from a similar drug regimen.

Successful application of external radiation to the breast to prevent the estrogen-induced gynecomastia evident with the treatment of prostate cancer has been reported.[55, 121] For patients with prostate cancer receiving diethylstilbestrol, radiation to breast tissue was administered with superficial x-rays 4 mV ^{60}cobalt with doses from 1200 to 1500 cGy in three fractions. The majority of patients had satisfactory results in terms of prevention of gynecomastia and mammalgia.

Drug abuse in the form of intravenous *heroin* administration or *cannabis (marijuana) smoking* may induce gynecomastia as a consequence of depression of plasma androgen levels.[73, 174, 175, 266] Olusi[302] reported on the hyperprolactin state induced by cannabis smoking. While the etiological mechanism through which marijuana initiates gynecomastia is conjectural, there are structural resemblances between *tetrahydrocannabinol* (the metabolite of marijuana) and estradiol. Further, tetrahydrocannabinol has been observed to stimulate the development of breast tissue in rats.[174] However, epidemiological evidence to support an association between cannabis use and gynecomastia was not substantiated by Cates and Pope.[65]

Drugs that Inhibit the Action and/or Synthesis of Testosterone. The mechanisms of drug-induced gynecomastia are less ambiguous with regard to the effects of *spironolactone* on breast parenchyma in the male. This commonly used diuretic initiates a substantial incidence of gynecomastia when administered in high dosage.[260] Siiteri and MacDonald[362] confirm that the drug interferes with testosterone biosynthesis. A reduction in the relative concentration of free testosterone is evident, as the conversion of androstenedione and testosterone to estrone and estradiol is normal. Bellati and Ideo[30] and Dupont[103] have reported the disappearance of spironolactone-induced gynecomastia following treatment with *potassium canrenoate.* Although gynecomastia is rare following administration of potassium canrenoate or canrenone,[128, 259] 30 to 62 percent of patients on long-term spironolactone experienced this side effect.[128, 159, 191, 259] Rose et al.[331] note that spironolactone alters the peripheral metabolism of testosterone with resultant changes in the testosterone:estradiol ratio. These changes appear primarily from significant increases in the metabolic clearance of testosterone and in the rate of peripheral conversion of testosterone into estradiol following spironolactone therapy. Caminos-Torres et al.[62] postulate that spironolactone-induced gynecomastia does not occur from alterations in the serum concentrations of testosterone or estradiol. Rather, these investigators hypothesize that changes may be related to binding of canrenone to tissue androgen receptors. Therefore, it is plausible that the drug has at least two effects on androgen metabolism, i.e., inhibition of testosterone biosynthesis and binding of androgen to its receptor, thus effectively reducing the active androgenic effect of testosterone. At low-dose levels, it is possible that gynecomastia is induced by receptor blockade at testosterone binding sites. Conversely, following high-dose administration, inhibition of testosterone synthesis may initiate gynecomastia.

In 1979, Moerck and Magelund[273] reported a patient with gynecomastia related to abuse of *diazepam*. More recently, Bergman and associates[34] described five patients with gynecomastia related to diazepam use in therapeutic doses. Diazepam-induced gynecomastia that was associated with other endocrine and/or hepatic diseases was ruled out by laboratory tests. Of these five patients with elevated serum estradiol concentrations and normal hepatic and thyroid function, all had normal serum testosterone values. The discontinuance of diazepam was associated with fall of the estradiol levels to normal values and clinical improvement in the gynecomastia. These authors postulate that diazepam contributes to gynecomastia by three potential mechanisms: (1) enhanced conversion of testosterone to estradiol; (2) increased sex hormone–binding globulin; and (3) decreased peripheral metabolism or decreased excretion of estrogen.

While D-*penicillamine* therapy is associated with a wide variety of side effects, some occur more commonly in patients with rheumatoid arthritis.[253] *Breast gigantism* was reported in six women, five of whom suffered from rheumatoid arthritis, following therapy with penicillamine. Reid and associates[325] confirmed this clinical report with evidence of gynecomastia in a man with rheumatoid arthritis who was receiving penicillamine. The infrequent association of breast gigantism with penicillamine usage[97, 306, 388, 393] confirms the gynecomastia associated with this drug to be a rare adverse side effect. The gynecomastia usually disappears promptly following withdrawal of penicillamine and differs from the course observed in patients with breast gigantism. Desai[97] indicated the need for mastectomy and prosthetic surgery in one case and the successful administration of danazol to reverse D-penicillamine–induced breast gigantism in another.[388] It appears that breast gigantism and gynecomastia are initiated by stimulatory effects of D-penicillamine, which inhibits synthesis of testosterone in males and the augmentation of estrogenic activity in females.

Cimetidine is an effective drug for the healing of peptic ulcers and for preventing their recurrence. In vivo animal studies demonstrated that cimetidine can inhibit the binding of dihydrotestosterone to androgen receptors in the prostates of rats and the kidneys of mice.[51, 129, 308, 392, 432] Thereafter, gynecomastia[74, 93, 371] was observed especially in pathological hypersecretory states[172, 263] and was associated with impotence in patients treated with the drug.[268, 436] Jensen and associates[200] prospectively evaluated male patients with gastric hypersecretory states and examined the ability of cimetidine to initiate clinically important antiandrogen side effects. These investigators confirmed that impotence, breast tenderness, or gynecomastia developed in exactly half the patients and that these side effects disappeared when cimetidine was replaced by *ranitidine,* the newer antagonist of histamine H_2 receptors.[51, 392] Moreover, cimetidine has been shown to block testosterone synthesis.[229] These investigators confirmed low plasma testos-

terone values and elevated plasma gonadotropin concentrations that suggest a primary testicular disorder following administration of cimetidine hydrochloride. These alterations of sexual function improved and plasma testosterone values rose to normal following discontinuance of the drug. Further, readministration of cimetidine resulted in prompt recurrence of sexual problems and low testosterone values. Despite the reversal of gynecomastia following discontinuance of cimetidine and initiation of ranitidine, Tosi and Cagnoli[396] confirmed painful gynecomastia following ranitidine administration. Mignon and associates[268, 269] observed divergent effects of cimetidine and ranitidine on androgen receptors, pituitary hormones, and plasma testosterone levels. These data are in accord with the work by Brittain and Daly[50] and Edwards and associates[107] that suggest minimal effects of ranitidine on these sex hormone parameters. Other drugs such as *cyproterone acetate*[145] and *flutamide (glutamine)*[59] may cause gynecomastia by interference with the binding of androgens to their receptor proteins.

In attempts to find the technique of medical castration useful as therapy for prostate cancer without the side effects of estrogen or surgical castration, Geller and associates[144] conducted clinical trials with *megestrol acetate (Megace),* a progestational antiestrogen. Megace was well tolerated by patients and rarely initiated gynecomastia, thromboembolic events, or salt retention, in contrast to the side effects evident with high-dose *medroxyprogesterone acetate.* Medroxyprogesterone acetate will lower mean plasma testosterone values.[296, 297] Meyer et al.[267] have shown that the drug is effective in decreasing serum gonadotropin and plasma testosterone concentrations in males.

The oral antifungal *ketoconazole* has been shown to produce gynecomastia by transit blockade of testosterone synthesis and the adrenal response to corticotropin.[319, 320] Therapeutic doses of the drug will suppress serum testosterone concentrations markedly; serum estradiol values are suppressed to a much lesser extent. Neither bound nor free percentages of androgens and estrogens were significantly altered. It is postulated by Pont and associates[319, 320] that since gynecomastia appears to be the result of an elevated estradiol:testosterone ratio, selective hormonal effect is demonstrated following use of ketoconazole. Hormonal effects of the drug are generally unrelated to duration of therapy, and occasionally there may be partial reversal of gynecomastia with continual therapy. Side effects appear to be reversible with discontinuation of ketoconazole therapy. Patients receiving the drug should be considered potentially unable to mount an adrenal stress response and may require testosterone supplementation. Because the drug also has a propensity for hepatotoxicity, Moncada and Baranda[274] argue that indications for ketoconazole therapy are not completely established and suggest that it be reserved for cases of chronic deep mycoses in life-threatening situations, or perhaps in recalcitrant superficial mycoses. The treatment of trivial diseases susceptible to effect local therapy should not include this drug with its potential (and severe) side effects.

The commonly utilized anticonvulsant *phenytoin (Di-*

lantin), may initiate gynecomastia in men with epilepsy. Graybill and Drutz[156] noted resolution of gynecomastia when phenytoin was discontinued and suggested the causal of the drug to this clinical syndrome. It has been suggested by several investigators.[23, 87, 156, 330, 395] that a reduction in the circulating free testosterone concentrations occurs in patients receiving long-term therapy with various anticonvulsants. These data and the data of Graybill and Drutz[156] are consistent with the hypothesis that phenytoin therapy diminishes free testosterone concentrations, possibly as a result of increasing the concentration of sex hormone–binding globulin with induction of an increased conversion of testosterone to 17β-estradiol. Turkington and Topper[401] indicate that gynecomastia may result from either of these effects, or a combination, with a loss of libido and subfertility as a possible side effect of long-term therapy.

Antineoplastic (cytotoxic) drugs are recognized to initiate amenorrhea, disturbances of gonadal estrogen and androgen secretion, oligospermia, and increased plasma concentrations of gonadotropins.[13, 67, 68, 122, 417] Gynecomastia has been commonly observed in pubertal males following administration of cytotoxic chemotherapy[359] but is considered a rare event in adult men.[349, 357] Trump and associates[398, 399] described six men with painful gynecomastia following the administration of antineoplastic therapy, with sharp increases in levels of plasma follicle-stimulating hormone (FSH) and luteinizing hormone. Plasma testosterone concentrations were within or above normal ranges in the majority of subjects evaluated; plasma estradiol concentrations were modestly increased. These authors could not define the precise mechanisms responsible for gynecomastia following cytotoxic chemotherapy. Damage to germinal epithelium and Leydig cells as well as changes in peripheral metabolism of testosterone and estrogen may be important. It is clear that unilateral or bilateral tender gynecomastia may occur in adult men following therapy with cytotoxic drugs.[351] Moreover, gynecomastia seen in these patients does not necessarily indicate recurrent carcinoma following therapy with single or combination antineoplastic agents.

Gynecomastia induction may occur with administration of the chemotherapeutic agents *busulfan*,[140] *vincristine*,[363] *nitrosoureas*,[364] and *methotrexate*[94] as well as with *MOPP* (mechlorethamine, vincristine, procarbazine, and prednisone) *combination chemotherapy*.[357] Trump and Anderson[398] described painful gynecomastia in 8 percent of patients receiving cytotoxic chemotherapy for germ cell neoplasms of the testes.

A Danish study[39] reported a 4 percent incidence of gynecomastia in patients with Hodgkin's disease; several of the patients with breast enlargement had been treated with *alkylating agents*. The use of these chemotherapeutic agents in the treatment of lymphoma and various renal disorders is routinely associated with damage to the testicular germ cells and is manifested by elevation of serum FSH and oligospermia or azoospermia.[165, 198, 305, 357, 359, 410] These patients as a group often have reduced serum testosterone, although individual values are usually within normal ranges.[198, 230, 357, 359] It appears that the

testicular toxicity from chemotherapeutic agents could result in impaired androgen production; the resulting increase in serum estrogen:androgen ratio might then initiate gynecomastia.

Drugs that Enhance Estrogen Synthesis by the Testes. Smith[364] identified an adult patient with acquired gynecomastia who had elevated urinary estrogens, borderline to low FSH and LH, and borderline high serum estradiol. It was thought that the patient potentially had a semiautonomous lesion of the testis that led to an increase of estrogen production, with suppression of LH and FSH causing mild atrophic changes of the contralateral testis. Following administration of *human chorionic gonadotropin (HCG)*, there was a 300 percent increase in urinary estrogens. Morse et al.[277] gave a similar dose of HCG (5000 units IU daily for four days) to normal adult males and measured urinary estrogens on the third and fourth days. These authors confirm that the mean increase in estrogen excretion from baseline to the HCG-stimulated situation was 137 percent. Lipsett and associates[250] gave a similar dose of HCG per day to males and measured estradiol production rates initially and on the fourth day of HCG administration. Increase in estradiol production averaged 194 percent (range 119 to 265 percent). Therefore, it appears that urinary estrogen in these patients is more responsive to HCG than is usually the case among young adult males. These data are compatible with enhanced estrogen synthesis and secretion by the testes or an increased conversion of testosterone to estrogen. In the normal man, the majority of estradiol is thought to be produced by conversion from circulating testosterone.[16, 248]

Acquired feminization secondary to testicular neoplasms is seen most often with choriocarcinoma or other germ cell–derived neoplasms that are associated with high values of HCG (see Fig 7–3).[215, 307] The hyperestrogen state with associated gynecomastia may be due to any germ cell–derived neoplasm and can be ruled out by the low radioimmunoassay values for LH since HCG is measured by the same assay.[249] As noted earlier, Leydig cell, Sertoli cell, or gonadal mesenchymal tumors of the testes have been reported to be estrogen-producing. These neoplasms do not produce HCG, but patients frequently present with gynecomastia as the most prominent clinical finding. Maddock and Nelson[257] identified severe gynecomastia in adult men following administration of therapeutic doses of HCG. Similar effects can result in the pubertal male and are predictable, since HCG initiates an increase in secretion of estradiol and testosterone by the testes as was identified by Weinstein and associates.[421]

Clinical practice has recently witnessed the introduction of potent analogues of *gonadotropin hormone–releasing hormone (GnRH)* for use in patients with metastatic prostate cancer.[3] GnRH provides an effective alternative to the exogenous administration of pharmacological doses of estrogen or surgical castration. The advantage of GnRH over estrogen is primarily related to a decrease in the incidence of cardiovascular toxicity and gynecomastia. The therapeutic potential of GnRH was first suggested by the recognition that pituitary secretion of FSH and LH could be modulated by administration of exogenous GnRH. Clayton and Catt[76] determined that the effects of GnRH depend largely upon the dosage and schedule of administration of this hormone. Frequent low doses of GnRH and other agonists mimic physiological pulsatile secretion and thereafter activate gonadotropin secretion. Sandow noted the paradoxical effect seen with administration of high doses of GnRH either daily or by continuous infusion in causing inhibition of pituitary/gonadal function.[344] Prolonged treatment with GnRH to decrease levels of luteinizing hormone and testosterone to subnormal ranges that reach nadirs following four weeks of daily therapy have been noted.[2, 46, 415] Eisenberger et al.[108] suggest that these hormonal changes are consistent with a gradual physiological selective hypophysectomy and represent the basis for the oncological application of GnRH agonists.

Drugs with Mechanisms for Induction of Gynecomastia. As identified in Table 7–2, a variety of drugs may be etiological for gynecomastia by inexplicable pathophysiological mechanisms. Drugs with potential to initiate idiopathic gynecomastia include *amiodarone, bumetanide, busulfan, domperidone, ethionamide, furosemide, isoniazid, methyldopa, nifedipine, reserpine, sulindac, theophylline, tricyclic antidepressants, and verapamil.*[207] While the aforementioned mechanisms for drug-induced gynecomastia have not been elucidated for these medications, several authors have attempted to explain the basis of the clinical syndrome without exclusion of concurrent drugs that have the known side effect of gynecomastia. The medical literature does not conclusively exclude other established physiological causes of gynecomastia in patients using these medications.

Van der Steen et al.[404] identified gynecomastia in a male infant treated for nausea and vomiting with the investigational antiemetic *domperidone.* These authors postulate that the gynecomastia and galactorrhea seen in this infant produced a concomitant increase in serum levels of prolactin. Serum TSH and estradiol values were normal for this age group. This clinical syndrome was thought to be the consequence of activation of prolactin secretion by domperidone. A similar physiological effect was produced following calcium channel blocker therapy with *verapamil* and *nifedipine.* Tanner and Bosco[387] identified elevated prolactin values following verapamil treatment. This report is confounding, as most of these patients had concomitant therapy with other drugs, although the majority experienced amelioration of symptoms following discontinuation of the calcium channel blocker.

In the majority of patients with idiopathic gynecomastia related to drug therapy, discontinuance of the suspected drug(s) led to regression of the gynecomastia. Resolution of drug-induced gynecomastia following discontinuance of the medication has been confirmed for bumetanide,[100, 381] sulindac,[207] theophylline,[88] amiodarone,[10] and domperidone.[404]

Systemic Diseases with Idiopathic Mechanisms

As noted previously, the majority of male patients presenting with gynecomastia have documentable pathophysiological or drug-related causes to explain this clinical syndrome. For the prepubertal male, *idiopathic gynecomastia* may be differentiated by the normal values of estrogen, testosterone, 17-ketosteroids, and dehydroandrosterone (Table 7–3). Latorre and Kenny[233] differentiate adrenal and testicular etiology of prepubertal gynecomastia in boys who have normal circulating or urinary sex steroids. Male secondary sexual development is accelerated in patients with adrenal or testicular lesions but not in those with idiopathic gynecomastia. Urinary estrogen levels are consistently elevated with adrenal/testicular lesions and may be normal or high in the idiopathic variant. In contrast, urinary 17-ketosteroids and dehydroandrosterone are elevated for patients with adrenal abnormalities; patients with adrenal or testicular tumors will have elevated serum testosterone values (see Table 7–3).

While the English literature is replete with inconsistent and confounding reports that lack documentation for the etiology of gynecomastia, these explanations may be forthcoming in the future, following assessment of endocrine and pharmacological induction mechanisms.

Non-neoplastic Diseases of the Lung

Braude et al.[49] described transient gynecomastia in four of seven patients with *cystic fibrosis* having associated *hypertrophic osteoarthropathy.* Thereafter, Russi[340] reported a similar case in a 23-year-old male with cystic fibrosis of two years' duration. The gynecomastia seen with cystic fibrosis is usually transient and associated with severe mastalgia. In the majority of cases, patients were not taking drugs known to cause gynecomastia and had no evidence of liver or testicular disease. Lemen and associates[239] correlated digital clubbing with the severity of lung disease and elevation of the serum prostaglandin $F_2\alpha$ and E concentrations in these patients. Russi[340] suggests that the diseased lungs may incompletely metabolize these sex steroids and one may see an escalation in the estrogenic component of the circulating steroids.

Trauma (Chest Wall)

Although infrequent, unilateral, and rarely, bilateral gynecomastia may be observed following trauma to the chest wall. Such trauma is most commonly seen after blunt injury but also may be noted with penetrating damage of the chest wall. This idiopathic mechanism for gynecomastia may result as a consequence of (1) an increased secretion of gonadotropin-releasing hormone; (2) decreased testosterone synthesis and, thus an androgen-deficiency state; or (3) decreased metabolic clearance of estrogen-like compounds secreted endogenously or administered exogenously. The precise mechanism

Table 7–3. DIFFERENTIAL DIAGNOSIS OF PREPUBERTAL GYNECOMASTIA IN BOYS*

| Condition | Sexual Maturation | Circulating or Urinary Steroids | | | IVP and Retroperitoneal Pneumogram |
		Estrogens	*Testosterone*	*17-KS and DHA*	
Idiopathic	Preadolescent	Normal or High	Normal	Normal	Normal
Adrenal					
Feminizing tumor	Accelerated	Elevated	Normal	Elevated	May be normal or tumor may be seen
Isosexual tumor	Accelerated	Elevated	Normal or elevated	Elevated	
Testicular					
(Tumor usually palpable)					
Interstitial cell tumor	Accelerated	Elevated	Elevated	Normal	Normal
Choriocarcinoma†	Accelerated	Elevated	Normal	Normal	Normal

*Exposure to hormonal or nonhormonal drugs that may produce gynecomastia must be ruled out by careful history. Persistent elevation of estrogens or gonadotropins or both indicates need for exploratory laparotomy. (IVP = intravenous pyelogram.)
†Not yet reported in prepubertal age. Chorionic gonadotropin-levels are elevated.
From Latorre H, Kenny FM: Am J Dis Child 126: 772, 1973. Reprinted by permission.

by which trauma initiates gynecomastia has not been documented.

CNS-Related Causes from Anxiety and Stress

Endocrine responses to stress and psychological stimuli have been documented by Rose et al.[332] to increase secretion of growth hormone, prolactin, and cortisol with a concomitant decrease in testosterone production. An interaction of the latter two hormones has been proposed. The carefully documented report by Gooren and Daantje[152] correlated the occurrence of gynecomastia with psychological stress. These authors documented hormonal parameters during episodes of gynecomastia and regression in five men. These data provide evidence that stressful life events associated with increased adrenal secretion and a fall in testosterone production may initiate transitory gynecomastia. The gynecomastia resolved spontaneously (without therapy) when subjects were able to cope successfully with their environment. Thereafter, hormonal functions returned to normal values in all subjects.

Psychological stress may be an etiological factor to be considered in gynecomastia. Frantz and Wilson[124] found that in over 50 percent of the cases no underlying endocrine or pathological cause could be identified. Certainly, one has to consider the mechanism of "refeeding gynecomastia" (see under nutritional alteration states) in individuals who are stressed and have increased consumption of foodstuffs that contain compounds or metabolites with estrogenic or estrogen-like activity. Further, such confounding reports must also exclude concurrent administration of drugs that are known to cause gynecomastia.

AIDS (Autoimmune Deficiency Syndrome) Virus (HIV) Infection

Couderc and Clauvel[81] reported the association of *transient gynecomastia* in two patients with HIV (human immunodeficiency virus) infection. A 36-year-old homosexual intravenous drug abuser had serum antibodies to HIV detected by the enzyme-linked immunosorbent assay (ELISA) technique and Western blot. The patient developed unilateral, then bilateral, painless gynecomastia that resolved spontaneously six months following identification of AIDS. Another homosexual patient had generalized lymphadenopathy and bilateral gynecomastia that also resolved spontaneously. Both patients showed transient gynecomastia with normal plasma values of testosterone, estrone, estradiol, and prolactin. Unexplained gynecomastia in a young male homosexual with generalized lymphadenopathy suggests that the HIV infection should be suspected.

DRUGS UTILIZED IN THE TREATMENT OF GYNECOMASTIA

The medical therapy of gynecomastia is rarely of value except when a specific diagnosis has been established. For disorders of androgen deficiency, Hopwood[186] claims that testosterone administration will improve (decrease) the estradiol:testosterone ratio, with some regression of the gynecomastia. Conversely, on occasion, testosterone therapy will make the condition worse, especially when there is increased conversion of androgens to estrogens by the peripheral tissues. When breast diameter is less than 4 cm, very frequently the clinician can expect a spontaneous regression; only reassurance of the patient as well as a period of observation is indicated. In contrast, for large, progressive gynecomastia that is refractory to drug discontinuance or treatment of the appropriate endocrine defect (testicular, adrenal) the most effective therapy is *transareolar mastectomy* using the technique described for total glandular mastectomy. This relatively simply surgical procedure carries minimal morbidity and no mortality. Surgical therapy is reserved for idiopathic causes of gynecomastia in which exhaustive attempts to define endocrine, anatomical, metabolic, or drug-related causes have not availed.

LeRoith and associates[241] and Plourde et al.[318] report varying success in reducing the breast size of gyneco-

Table 7–4. RESPONSE OF GYNECOMASTIA TO TREATMENT WITH DANAZOL

Type of Patients	No. of Patients	Regression of Gynecomastia			
		Marked	*Moderate*	*Nil*	*Marked/Moderate Improvement (%)*
Adult idiopathic	17	8	5	4	77
Thyrotoxic	1	1			100
Spironolactone-induced	13	9	2	2	85
Pubertal	11	7	3	1	91
Total	42	25	10	7	83

From Buckle R: Drugs 19:356–361, 1980. Reprinted by permission.

mastia following therapy with the antiestrogen *clomiphene citrate*. However, clomiphene is known to act at the level of the hypothalamic-pituitary axis to increase gonadotropin secretion with its attendant side effects. Stephanas and associates[375] have reported on the use of clomiphene citrate to treat pubertal-adolescent gynecomastia, with a 95 percent success rate for the subjects treated. However, the side effects of clomiphene therapy were significant and included adverse gastrointestinal reactions, rashes, and visual impairment. At present, clomiphene citrate should be considered investigational in the therapy of gynecomastia and is not approved as a primary drug for the medical management of this disorder.

The report by Kuhn et al.[225] is encouraging for the use of percutaneous *dihydrotestosterone* therapy of idiopathic gynecomastia, but this agent requires prospective clinical trials to establish its efficacy and safety. The synthetic heterocyclic steroid *danazol (Danocrine)* is the 2,3,isoxazol derivative of 17α-ethyl testosterone. This compound is devoid of estrogenic or progestational activities but possesses well-defined antigonadotropic properties in man. Prolonged therapy with danazol for women with endometriosis has resulted in atrophy of breasts.[160, 350] Greenblatt et al.[160] were the first to report, in 1971, improvement in gynecomastia following danazol therapy; beneficial effects have been further described by Buckle.[57] More recently, Buckle[56] identified response rates for 77 to 100 percent of patients with gynecomastia induced by several causes (idiopathic, thyrotoxic, spironolactone, and pubertal); these results are depicted in Table 7–4. Overall, of 42 patients with gynecomastia treated with danazol, there was marked or moderate improvement in 83 percent. This author determined that danazol initiated a progressive diminution in plasma concentrations of follicle-stimulating hormone and luteinizing hormone over the 3- to 16-week duration of therapy with dose schedules of 300 to 600 mg per day in adults and 200 to 300 mg per day in adolescents. Side effects of danazol therapy relate primarily to the androgenic properties of the compound, which may result in acne and weight gain with fluid retention. Muscle weakness and muscle cramps and spasms occur in a small percentage of patients.

Ricciardi and Ianniruberto[327] used *tamoxifen citrate (Nolvadex)* as a treatment for benign breast disorders in 1979 under the assumption that benign breast lesions have estrogen receptors that may respond to hormonal influences. It has been suggested that tamoxifen may achieve its endocrine effect by competing for estrogen-receptor sites in target organs or possibly by decreasing the serum prolactin values of hormonally sensitive breast cancers. These authors determined that 71 percent of patients with symptomatic benign breast disease who were treated with tamoxifen experienced complete regression of symptoms and disappearance of the lesions as assessed by clinical examination and ultrasonography.

Recently, Alagaratnam[5] reported 80 percent complete regression of idiopathic gynecomastia in 61 Chinese men with an age range 25 to 74 years (median 35 years) treated with 40 mg of tamoxifen daily for one to four months (median two months). This author noted no long-term side effects of tamoxifen for patients observed through a median follow-up period of 36 months. Further, pain and tenderness disappeared by the end of the second week of therapy, although breast swelling required prolonged therapy to produce complete regression of the breast tissue. In 30 of 47 (64 percent) successfully treated patients, breast edema and mastalgia responded to tamoxifen within two months of initiating therapy. There was an inconsistent relationship between reduction in size of the gynecomastia and symptoms with the duration of therapy. Alagaratnam[5] questioned whether the response was a potential placebo effect. However, it is difficult to postulate that the observed rapid response to therapy with tamoxifen is the result of a placebo effect. Such therapy should be reserved exclusively for idiopathic gynecomastia following evaluation of exhaustive endocrine and metabolic profiles and comprehensive radiological evaluation of potential organ sites etiological for gynecomastia. Side effects, efficacy, and long-term toxicities associated with usage of tamoxifen in the medical therapy of gynecomastia have not been established.

References

1. Abecassis M, McLoughlin MJ, Langer B, Kudlow JE: Serendipitous adrenal masses: Prevalence, significance, and management. Am J Surg 139:783–788, 1985.
2. Ahmad KN, Dykes JRW, Ferguson-Smith MA, Lennox B, Mach WS: Leydig cell volume in chromatin-positive Klinefelter's syndrome. J Clin Endocrinol Metab 33:517, 1971.
3. Ahmad SR, Shalet SM, Brooman PJC, et al: Treatment of advanced prostatic cancer with LHRH analogue 118630: Clin-

ical response and hormonal mechanisms. Lancet 2:415–419, 1983.

4. Aiman J, Hemsell DL, MacDonald PC: Production and origin of estrogen in two true hermaphrodites. Am J Obstet Gynecol 132:401, 1978.

5. Alagaratnam TT: Idiopathic gynecomastia treated with tamoxifen: A preliminary report. Clin Ther 9:483–487, 1987.

6. Albright F, cited in Hall PH: Gynaecomastia. Monographs of the Federal Council of the British Medical Association in Australia No. 2, 1959.

7. Amrhein JA, Lingensmith GJ, Walsh PC, McKusick VA, Migeon CJ: Partial androgen insensitivity. The Reifenstein syndrome revisited. N Engl J Med 297:350–356, 1977.

8. Anderson DC: Sex-hormonal-binding globulin. Clin Endocrinol 3:69–96, 1974.

9. Andervont HB: Studies on the occurrence of spontaneous hepatomas in mice of strains C_3H and CBA. J Natl Cancer Inst 11:581–591, 1952.

10. Antonelli D, Luboshitzky R: Amiodarone-induced gynecomastia. N Engl J Med 315(24):1553, 1986.

11. Arbizu T, Santamaria J, Gomez JM, Quilez A, Serra JP: A family with adult spinal and bulbar muscular atrophy X-linked inheritance and associated testicular failure. J Neurol Sci 59:371–382, 1983.

12. Arnaout MA, Garthwaite TL, Krubsack AJ, Hagen TC: Galactorrhea, gynecomastia, and hypothyroidism in a man (Letter). Ann Intern Med 106:779–780, 1987.

13. Asbjornsen G, Molne K, Klepp O, et al: Testicular function after combination chemotherapy for Hodgkin's disease. Scand J Haematol 16:66–69, 1976.

14. August GP, Chandra R, Hung W: Prepubertal male gynecomastia. J Pediatr 80:259, 1972.

15. Bacon GE, Lowrey GH: Feminizing adrenal tumor in a 6-year-old boy. J Clin Endocrinol 25:1403, 1965.

16. Baird DT, Horton R, Longscope C, Tait JF: Steroid dynamics under steady-state conditions. Recent Progr Horm Res 25:628, 1969.

17. Baker HWG, Burger HG, de Kretser DM, Dulmanis A, Hudson B, O'Connor S, Paulsen CA, Purcell N, Rennie GC, Seah CS, Taft HP, Wang C: A study of the endocrine manifestations of hepatic cirrhosis. Q J Med 45:145–178, 1976.

18. Baker HWG, Dulmanis A, Hudson B, et al: Endocrine aspects of hepatic cirrhosis (abstr). Washington, DC, Fourth International Endocrine Congress, June 1972.

19. Bannayan GA, Hajdu SI: Gynecomastia: Clinicopathologic study of 351 cases. Am J Clin Pathol 57:431–437, 1972.

20. Bardin CW: Pituitary-testicular axis. In Yen SSC, Jaffe RB (eds): Reproductive Endocrinology. Philadelphia, WB Saunders, 1978, p 110.

21. Bardin CW, Ross GT, Rifkind AB, Cargille CM, Lipsett MB: Studies of the pituitary–Leydig cell axis in young men with hypogonadotropic hypogonadism and hyposmia: comparison with normal men, prepubertal boys, and hypopituitary patients. J Clin Invest 48:2046–2056, 1969.

22. Barr RW, Som SC: Endocrine abnormalities accompanying hepatic cirrhosis and hepatoma. J Clin Endocrinol Metab 17:1017–1029, 1957.

23. Barragry JM, Makin HLJ, Trafford DJH, Scott DF: Effects of anticonvulsants on plasma testosterone and sex hormone binding globulin levels. J Neurol Neurosurg Psychiatr 41:913–914, 1978.

24. Beas F, Varbas L, Spada RP, Merchak N: Pseudoprecocious puberty in infants caused by a dermal ointment containing estrogens. J Pediatr 75:127, 1969.

25. Becker KL, Cottrell J, Moore CF, Winnacker JL, Matthews MJ, Katz S: Endocrine studies in a patient with a gonadotropin-secreting bronchogenic carcinoma. J Clin Endocrinol Metab 28:809–818, 1968.

26. Becker KL, Winnacker JL, Matthews MJ, Higgins GA: Gynecomastia and hyperthyroidism. An endocrine and histological investigation. J Clin Endocrinol Metab 28:277–285, 1968.

27. Beckwith JB: Macroglossia, omphalocele, adrenal cytomegaly, gigantism and hyperplastic visceromegaly. Birth Defects 5:188, 1969.

28. Behera D, Kalra S, Nalini K, Malik SK, Jindal SK, Dash RJ: Galactorrhea with gynecomastia in a male with lung cancer. Indian J Chest Dis Allied Sci 29(2):112–114, 1987.

29. Behera D, Malik SK, Sharma BR, Dash RJ: Circulating hormones in lung cancer. Indian J Med Res 79:636–640, 1984.

30. Bellati G, Ideo G: Gynaecomastia after spironolactone and potassium canrenoate. Lancet 1:626, 1986.

31. Belldegrun A, Hussain S, Seltzer SE, et al: Incidentally discovered mass of the adrenal gland. Surg Gynecol Obstet 163:203–208, 1986.

32. Bennett HS, Baggenstoss AH, Butt HR: Testes, breast, and prostate of men who die of cirrhosis of liver. Am J Clin Pathol 20:814–828, 1950.

33. Bercovici JP, Nahoul K, Ducasse M, Tater D, Kerlan V, Scholler R: Leydig call tumor with gynecomastia: Further studies—the recovery after unilateral orchiectomy. J Clin Endocrinol Metab 61:957, 1985.

34. Bergman D, Futterweit W, Segal R, Sirota D: Increased oestradiol in diazepam related gynaecomastia. Lancet 2:1225–1226, 1981.

35. Berkovitz GD, Guerami A, Brown TR, MacDonald PC, Migeon CJ: Familial gynecomastia with increased extraglandular aromatization of plasma carbon 19 steroids. J Clin Invest 75:1763–1769, 1985.

36. Berson SA, Schreiber SS: Gynecomastia and hyperthyroidism (Letter). J Clin Endocrinol 13:1126–1128, 1953.

37. Bhettay E, Bonnici F: Pure oestrogen-secreting feminizing adrenocortical adenoma. Arch Dis Child 52:241, 1977.

38. Biagotti G, Kasznica J: Sclerosing adenoisis in the breast of a man with pulmonary oat cell carcinoma. Hum Pathol 17:861–863, 1986.

39. Bichel J: Gynecomastia in Hodgkin's disease. Dan Med Bull 4:157–158, 1957.

40. Bidlingmaier R, Knorr D: Plasma testosterone and estrogens in pubertal gynecomastia. Z Kinderheilkd 115:89, 1973.

41. Bittorf A: Nebennieren tumor and geschlechtsdrusenausfall beim mann. Berl Klin Wochenschr 56:776, 1919.

42. Bjorvatn B: Mumps virus recovered from testes by fine-needle aspiration biopsy in cases of mumps orchitis. Scand J Infect Dis 5:3, 1973.

43. Blundon KE, Russi S, Bunts RC: Interstitial cell hyperplasia or adenoma. J Urol 70:759–767, 1953.

44. Bondy PK: Disorders of the adrenal cortex. In: Wilson JD, Foster DW (eds): Williams' Textbook of Endocrinology. 7th ed. Philadelphia, WB Saunders, 1985, pp 816–890.

45. Bongiovanni AM: Congenital adrenal hyperplasia and related conditions. In Stanbury JB, Wyngaarden JB, Fredrickson DS (eds): The Metabolic Basis of Inherited Disease. New York, McGraw:Hill, 1978, p 868.

46. Borgmann V, Hardt W, Schmidt-Gollwitzer M, Adenauer H, Nagel R: Sustained suppression of testosterone production by the luteinizing hormone-releasing hormone agonist buserelin in patients with advanced prostatic cancer. Lancet 1:1097–1099, 1982.

47. Boyar RM, Finkelstein JW, Witkin M, Kapen S, Weitzman E, Hellman L: Studies of endocrine function in "isolated" gonadotropin deficiency. J Clin Endocrinol Metab 36:64–72, 1973.

48. Brandt NJ, Cohn J, Hilder M: Controlled trial of oral contraceptives in haemophilia. Scand J Haematol 11:225, 1973.

49. Braude S, Kennedy H, Hodson M, Batten J: Hypertrophic osteoarthropathy in cystic fibrosis. Br Med J 288(6420):822–823, 1984.

50. Brittain RT, Daly MJ: A review of the animal pharmacology of ranitidine: a new selective histamine H_2 antagonist. Scand J Gastroenterol 16:Suppl 69:1–8, 1981.

51. Brittain RT, Daly MJ, Jack D, Martin LE, Stables R, Sutherland M: The outline of the animal pharmacology of ranitidine. In Misiewicz JJ, Wormsley KJ (eds): The Clinical Use of Ranitidine. Medicine Publishing Foundation Symposium Series No. 5. Oxford, Medicine Publishing Foundation 1–10, 1982.

52. Brogard JM, Maurer C, Philippe E: Gynécomastie et tumeur á cellules de Leydig. Press Med 75:1253, 1967.

53. Bronstein IP, Cassorla E: Breast enlargement in pediatric practice. Med Clin North Am 30:121–133, 1946.

54. Brosman SA: Testicular tumors in prepubertal children. Urology 13:581–588, 1979.

55. Brown JS, Rubenfeld S: Irradiation in preventing gynecomastia induced by estrogens. Urology 3(1):51–53, 1974.
56. Buckle R: Danazol in the treatment of gynaecomastia. Drugs 19:356–361, 1980.
57. Buckle R: Studies on the treatment of gynaecomastia with danazol (danol). J Intern Med Res 5 (Suppl 3):114–123, 1977.
58. Caldamone AA, Altebarmakian V, Frank IN, Linke CA: Leydig cell tumor of the testis. Urology 14:39–43, 1979.
59. Caine M, Perlberg S, Gordon R: The treatment of benign prostatic hypertrophy with Flutamide (SCH 13521): a placebo-controlled study. J Urol 114:564–568, 1975.
60. Camiel MR, Benninghoff DL, Alexander LL: Gynecomastia associated with lung cancer. Dis Chest 52:445–451, 1967.
61. Camin AJ, Dorfman RI, McDonald JH, Rosenthal IM: Interstitial cell tumor of the testis in a seven-year-old child. Am J Dis Child 100:389–399, 1960.
62. Caminos-Torres R, Lisa MA, Snyder PJ: Gynecomastia and semen abnormalities induced by spironolactone in normal men. J Clin Endocrinol Metab 45:255–260, 1977.
63. Carlson HE: Gynecomastia. N Engl J Med 303:795–799, 1981.
64. Castle WN, Richardson JR Jr: Leydig cell tumor and metachronous Leydig cell hyperplasia: A case associated with gynecomastia and elevated urinary estrogens. J Urol 136:1307–1308, 1986.
65. Cates W Jr, Pope JN: Gynecomastia and cannabis smoking. Am J Surg 134:613–615, 1977.
66. Cedard L, Mosse A, Klotz HP: Les oestrogenes plasmatiques dans les gynecomasties et les hepatopathies. Ann Endocrinol 31:453–458, 1970.
67. Chapman RM, Sutcliffe SM, Malpas JS: Cytotoxic-induced ovarian failure in women with Hodgkin's disease. JAMA 242:1877–1881, 1979.
68. Chapman RM, Sutcliffe SB, Rees LH, et al: Cyclical combination chemotherapy and gonadal function. Lancet 1:285–286, 1979.
69. Check JH, Murdock MG, Caro JF, Hermel MB: Case report: cystic gynecomastia in a male treated with clomiphene citrate. Fertil Steril 30:713, 1978.
70. Chopra IJ: Gonadal steroids and gonadotropins in hyperthyroidism. Med Clin North Am 59:1109, 1975.
71. Chopra IJ, Tulchinsky D: Status of estrogen-androgen balance in hyperthyroid men with Graves' disease. J Clin Endocrinol Metab 38:269, 1974.
72. Chopra IJ, Tulchinsky D, Greenway FL: Estrogen-androgen imbalance in hepatic cirrhosis: Studies in 13 male patients. Ann Intern Med 79:198–203, 1973.
73. Cicero TJ, Bel RD, Wiest WG, et al.: Function of the male sex organs in heroin and methadone users. N Engl J Med 292:822, 1975.
74. Cimetidine Postmarket Surveillance Program. Philadelphia; Medical Affairs Department, Smith, Kline and French Laboratories, 1981.
75. Clarke BG, Shapiro S, Monroe RG: Myotonia atrophica with testicular atrophy. J Clin Endocrinol 16:1235, 1956.
76. Clayton RN, Catt KJ: Gonadotropin-releasing hormone receptors: Characterization, physiological regulation, and relationship to reproductive function. Endocr Rev 2:186–203, 1981.
77. Cohen J, Diamond I: Leiontiasis ossea, slipped epiphysis and granuloma cell tumor of the testis with renal disease. Arch Pathol Lab Med 56:488–500, 1953.
78. Cole EW: Klinefelter's syndrome and breast cancer. Johns Hopkins Med J 138:105–108, 1976.
79. Cooper IS, Ryanson EA, Bailey AA, MacCarty CS: The relation of spinal cord disease to gynecomastia and testicular atrophy. Proc Staff Meet Mayo Clin 25:320, 1950.
80. Coppage WS, Cooner AE: Testosterone in human plasma. N Engl J Med 273:902–907, 1965.
81. Couderc LJ, Clauvel JP: HIV-infection induced gynecomastia. Ann Intern Med 107(2):257, 1987.
82. Courtiss EH: Gynecomastia: Analysis of 159 patients and current recommendations for treatment. Plast Reconstr Surg 79(5):740–750, 1987.
83. Crane MG, Hollowary JE, Winsor WG: Aldosterone-secreting adenoma: Report of a case in a juvenile. Ann Intern Med 54:280, 1961.
84. Crump WD: Juvenile granulosa cell tumor in an infant. J Urol 129:1057–1058, 1983.
85. Dailey JE, Marcuse PM: Gonadotropin secreting giant cell carcinoma of the lung. Cancer 24:388–396, 1969.
86. Damjanov I, Katz SM, Jewett MAS: Leydig cell tumors of the testis. Ann Clin Lab Sci 9:157–163, 1979.
87. Dana-Haeri J, Oxley J, Richens A: Reduction of free testosterone by antiepileptic drugs. Br Med J 284:85–86, 1982.
88. Dardick KR: Gynecomastia associated with theophylline. J Fam Pract 18(1):141–142, 1984
89. Dass J, Murugesan K, Laumas KR, Deo MG, Kandhari KC, Bhutani LK: Androgenic status of lepromatous leprosy patients with gynecomastia. Int J Lepr 44:469, 1976.
90. Davis M, Floret D, Touraille P, Aguercif M, Freycon F, Jeune M: Adenome testiculaire à cellules de Leydig chez l'enfant. Pediatrie 31:457–472, 1976.
91. Davis S, DiMartino NA, Schneider G: Malignant interstitial cell carcinoma of the testis: Report of two cases with steroid profiles, response to therapy, and review of the literature. Cancer 47:425–431, 1981.
92. DeGroot GW, Faiman C, Winter JSD: Cyclophosphamide and the prepubertal gonad: A negative report. J Pediatr 84:123–125, 1974.
93. Delle Fave GF, Tamburrano G, deMagistris L, et al: Gynaecomastia with cimetidine. Lancet 1:1319, 1977.
94. Del Paine DW, Leek JC, Jakle C, Robbins DL: Gynecomastia associated with low dose methotrexate therapy. Arthritis Rheum, 26(5):691–692, 1983.
95. Dershaw DD: Male mammography. AJR 146(1):127–131, 1986.
96. Desai MB, Kapadia SN: Feminizing adrenocortical tumors in male patients: Adenoma versus carcinoma. J Urol 139:101–103, 1988.
97. Desai SN: Sudden gigantism of breasts: drug induced? Br J Plast Surg 26:371–372, 1973.
98. Dexter CJ: Benign enlargement of the male breast. N Engl J Med 254:996–997, 1956.
99. Didolkar MS, Bescher RA, Elias EG, et al: Natural history of adrenal cortical carcinoma: A clinicopathologic study of 42 patients. Cancer 47:2153, 1981.
100. Dixon DW, Barwolf-Gohlke C, Gunnar RM: Comparative efficacy and safety of bumetanide and furosemide in long-term treatment of edema due to congestive heart failure. J Clin Pharmacol 21:680–687, 1981.
101. Dixon FJ, Moore RA: Tumors of the male sex organs. In Dixon FJ, Moore RA (eds): Atlas of Tumor Pathology. Washington, DC, Armed Forces Institute of Pathology, Parts 31b and 32, 1952, p. 1.
102. Drucker WD, Blanc WA, Rowland LP, Grumbach MM, Christy NP: The testis in myotonic muscular dystrophy: A clinical and pathologic study with a comparison with the Klinefelter syndrome. J Clin Endocrinol Metab 23:59–75, 1963.
103. Dupont A: Disappearance of spironolactone-induced gynecomastia during treatment with potassium canrenoate. Lancet 2:731, 1985.
104. Edidin DV, Levitsky LL: Prepubertal gynecomastia associated with estrogen-containing hair cream. Am J Dis Child 136:587, 1982.
105. Edman CD, Winters AJ, Porter JC, Wilson JD, MacDonald PC: Embryonic testicular regression. A clinical spectrum of XY agonadal individuals. Obstet Gynecol 49:209, 1977.
106. Edwards CRW, Forsyth IA, Besser GM: Amenorrhea, galactorrhea, and primary hypothyroidism with high circulating levels of prolactin. Br Med J 3:462–464, 1971.
107. Edwards CRW, Yeo T, Delitala G, Al Dujaili EAS, Boscaro M, Besser GM: In vitro studies on the effects of ranitidine on isolated anterior pituitary and adrenal cells. Scand J Gastroenterol 16(Suppl 69):75–77, 1981.
108. Eisenberger MA, O'Dwyer PJ, Friedman MA: Gonadotropin hormone–releasing analogues: A new therapeutic approach for prostatic carcinoma. J Clin Oncol 4:3:414–424, 1986.
109. Emory TH, Charboneau JW, Raymond VR, Scheithauer BW, Grantham JG: Occult testicular interstitial-cell tumor in a patient with gynecomastia: Ultrasonic detection. Radiology 151(2):474, 1984.
110. Faiman C, et al: Gonadotropin secretion from bronchiogenic carcinoma: Demonstration by radioimmunoassay. N Engl J Med 277:1395–1399, 1967.

111. Farthing MJG, Green JRB, Edwards CRW, Dawson AM: Progesterone, prolactin, and gynaecomastia in men with liver disease. Gut 23:276–279, 1982.
112. Feldman PS, Kovacs K, Horvath E, Adelson GL: Malignant Leydig cell tumor: Clinical histologic and electron microscopic features. Cancer 49:714–721, 1982.
113. Ferguson-Smith MA: The prepubertal testicular lesion in chromatin-positive Klinefelter's syndrome (primary micro-orchidism) as seen in mentally handicapped children. Lancet 1:219, 1959.
114. Fienman NL, Yakovac WC: Neurofibromatosis in childhood. J Pediatr 76:339, 1970.
115. Fine G, Smith RW Jr, Pachter MR: Primary extragenital choriocarcinoma in a male subject: Case report and review of literature. Am J Med 32:776–794, 1962.
116. Finn JE, Mount LA: Galactorrhea in males with tumors in the region of the pituitary gland. J Neurosurg 35:723–727, 1971.
117. Fitzsimons MP: Gynecomastia in stilbestrol workers. Br J Ind Med 1:235–237, 1944.
118. Fligiel Z, Kaneko M, Leiter E: Bilateral Sertoli cell tumor of the testes with feminizing and masculinizing activity occurring in a child. Cancer 38:1853, 1976.
119. Fontaine G, Lacheretz M, Dupont A: Tumor de la corticosurrenale avec puberté précoce et gynecomastie chez un garcon de 3 ans 1/2. Ann Pediatr 17:463, 1970.
120. Forti G, Giusti G, Borghi A, Pazzagli M, Fiorelli G, Cabresi E, Manneli M, et al: Klinefelter's syndrome: A study of its hormonal plasma pattern. J Endocrinol Invest 2:149, 1978.
121. Foss D, Steinfield A, Brown J, Tessler A: Radiotherapeutic prophylaxis of estrogen-induced gynecomastia: A study of late sequelae. Int J Radiat Oncol Biol Phys 12:407–408, 1985.
122. Fossa SD, Klepp O, Aakvaag A: Serum, hormone levels in patients with malignant testicular germ cell tumours without clinical and/or radiological sign of tumour. Br J Urol 52:151–157, 1980.
123. Franks S, Jacobs HS, Martin N, Nabarro JDN: Hyperprolactinemia and impotence. Clin Endocrinol 8:277–287, 1978.
124. Frantz AG, Wilson JD: Endocrine disorders of the breast. In Wilson JB, Foster DW (eds): Williams' Textbook of Endocrinology. 7th ed. Philadelphia, WB Saunders, 1985, pp 403–421.
125. Freeman CS, Topper YG: Progesterone is not essential to the differentiative potential of mammary epithelium in the male mouse. Endocrinology 103:186–192, 1978.
126. Freeman RM, Lawton RL, Fearing MO: Gynecomastia: an endocrinologic complication of hemodialysis. Ann Intern Med 69:67, 1968.
127. Friedman NB, Moore RA: Tumors of the testis: A report on 922 cases. Milit Surg 99:573, 1946.
128. Fromantin M: Surveillance clinique et hormonale des traitements prolongés de l'hypertension arteriele par les anti aldosterones. Mises Jour Cardiol 11:95–98, 1980.
129. Funder JW, Mercer JE: Cimetidine, a histamine H_2 receptor antagonist, occupies androgen receptors. J Clin Endocrinol Metab 48:189–191, 1979.
130. Fusco FD, Rosen SW: Gonadotropin-producing anaplastic large-cell carcinomas of the lung. N Engl J Med 275:507–515, 1966.
131. Gabrilove JL: Some recent advances in virilizing and feminizing syndrome and hirsutism. Mt Sinai J Med 41:636, 1974.
132. Gabrilove JL, Freiberg EK, Leiter E, Nicolis GL: Feminizing and nonfeminizing Sertoli cell tumors. J Urol 124:757–767, 1980.
133. Gabrilove JL, Freiberg EK, Thornton JC, Nicolis GL: Effect of age on testicular function in patients with Klinefelter's syndrome. Clin Endocrinol 11:343, 1979.
134. Gabrilove JL, Furukawa H: Gynecomastia in association with a complex tumor of the testis secreting chorionic gonadotropin: Studies on the testicular venous effluent. J Urol 131:348–350, 1984.
135. Gabrilove JL, Luria M: Persistent gynecomastia resulting from scalp inunction of estradiol: A model for persistent gynecomastia. Arch Dermatol 114:1672–1673, 1978.
136. Gabrilove JL, Nicolis GL, Hausknecht RU, Wotiz HH: Feminizing adrenocortical carcinoma in a man. Cancer 25:153, 1970.
137. Gabrilove JL, Nicolis GL, Mitty HA, Sohval AR: Feminizing interstitial cell tumor of the testis: Personal observations and a review of the literature. Cancer 35:1184–1202, 1975.
138. Gabrilove JL, Sharma DC, Wotiz HH, Dorfman RI: Feminizing adrenocortical tumors in the male: A review of 52 cases including a case report. Medicine 44:37, 1965.
139. Gallegos AF, Guizar O, Armendares S, et al: Familial true hermaphroditism in three siblings: Plasma hormonal profile and in vitro steroid biosynthesis in gonadal structures. J Clin Endocrinol Metab 42:653, 1976.
140. Galton DAG, Till M, Wiltshaw W: Busulfan: Summary of clinical results. Ann NY Acad Sci 68:967–973, 1957.
141. Galvão-Teles A, Anderson DC, Burke CW, Marshall JC, Corker CS, Brown RL, Clark ML: Biologically active androgens and oestradiol in men with chronic liver disease. Lancet 1:173–177, 1973.
142. Ganguly A, Bergstein J, Grim CE, et al: Childhood primary aldosteronism due to an adrenal adenoma: Preoperative localization by adrenal vein catheterization. Pediatrics 65:605, 1980.
143. Geisthövel W, von zur Mühlen A: Studies on the pituitary-testicular axis in patients with chronic hepatic failure (Abstract). Acta Endocrinol (Suppl.) 199:256, 1975.
144. Geller J, Albert J, Yen SS, Geller S, Loza D: Medical castration with megestrol acetate and minidose of diethylstilbestrol. Urology 17:27–33, 1981.
145. Geller J, Vozakos G, Fruchtenay B, Newman H, Nakao K, Loh A: The effect of cyproterone acetate on advanced carcinoma of the prostate. Surg Gynecol Obstet 127:748, 1968.
146. Gerald PS: Sex chromosome disorders. N Engl J Med 294:707, 1976.
147. Glass AR, Berenberg J: Gynecomastia after chemotherapy for lymphoma. Arch Intern Med 139:1048–1049, 1979.
148. Glazer HS, Lee JKT, Melson GL, McClennan BL: Sonographic detection of occult testicular neoplasms. AJR 138:673–675, 1982.
149. Goh HH, Chew PCT, Karim SMM, Ratnam SS: Control of gonadotrophin secretion by steroid hormones in castrated male transsexuals. I. Effects of oesteradiol infusion on plasma follicle-stimulating hormone and luteinizing hormone. Clin Endocrinol 12:16, 1980.
150. Goh HH, Karim SMM, Ratnam SS: Control of gonadotrophin secretion by steroid hormones in castrated male transsexuals. II. Effects of androgens alone and in combination with oestradiol on the secretions of FSH and LH. Clin Endocrinol 15:301, 1981.
151. Goodall CM, Butler WH: Aflatoxin carcinogenesis: Inhibition of liver cancer induction in hypophysectomized rats. Int J Cancer 4:422–429, 1969.
152. Gooren LJG, Daantje CRE: Psychological stress as a cause of intermittent gynecomastia. Horm Metabol Res 18:424, 1986.
153. Gordon GG, Altman K, Southren AL, Rubin E, Lieber CS: Effect of alcohol (ethanol) administration on sex-hormone metabolism in normal men. N Engl J Med 295:793–797, 1976.
154. Gordon, GG, Olivo, J, Rafii, F, Southren AL: Conversion of androgens to estrogens in cirrhosis of the liver. J Clin Endocrinol Metab 40:1018–1026, 1975.
155. Gottfried MR: Extensive squamous metaplasia in gynecomastia. Arch Pathol Lab Med 110:971–973, 1986.
156. Graybill JR, Drutz DJ: Ketoconazole: A major innovation for treatment of fungal disease. Ann Intern Med 93:921–923, 1980.
157. Green JRB: Mechanism of hypogonadism in cirrhotic males. Gut 18:843–853, 1977.
158. Green JRB, Mowat NAG, Fisher RA, Anderson DC: Plasma oestrogens in men with chronic liver disease. Gut 17:426–430, 1976.
159. Greenblatt DJ, Koch-Weser J: Adverse reactions to spironolactone. JAMA 225:40–43, 1973.
160. Greenblatt RB, Dmowski WP, Mahesh VB, Scholer HFL: Clinical studies with an antigonadotrophin—danazol. Fertil Steril 22:102–112, 1971.
161. Griffin JE, Wilson JD: Hereditary male pseudohermaphrodism. Clin Obstet Gynecol 5:457, 1958.
162. Grillo IA: Endocrine manifestations of pulmonary carcinoma in a Nigerian. Br J Cancer 25:266–269, 1971.
163. Gropp C, Havemann K, Scheur A: Ectopic hormones in lung cancer patients at diagnosis and during therapy. Cancer 46:347–354, 1980.
164. Grumbach MM, Conte FA: Disorders of sex differentiation. In

Wilson JD, Foster DW (eds): Williams' Textbook of Endocrinology. Philadelphia, WB Saunders, 1985, pp 312–401.

165. Guersy P, Lenoir G, Broyer M: Gonadal effects of chlorambucil given to prepubertal and pubertal boys for nephrotic syndrome. J Pediatr 92:299–303, 1978.

166. Guidetti D, Motti L, Marcello N, Vescovini E, Marbini A, Dotti C, Lucci B, Solime F: Kennedy disease in an Italian kindred (Abstract). Eur Neurol 25:188–196, 1986.

167. Gupta D, Burdschu HD: Testosterone and its binding in the plasma of male subjects with chronic renal failure. Clin Chim Acta 36:479, 1972.

168. Haagensen CD: Abnormalities of breast growth, secretion and lactation. *In* Haagensen CD (ed): Diseases of the Breast. Philadelphia, WB Saunders, 1986, p 65.

169. Haibach H, Rosenholtz MJ: Prepubertal gynecomastia with lobules and acini: A case report and review of the literature. Am J Clin Pathol 80:252–255, 1983.

170. Hall JG, Morgan A, Blizzard RM: Familial congenital anorchia. Birth Defects 11:115, 1975.

171. Hall PH: Gynaecomastia. Monographs of the Federal Council of the British Medical Association in Australia, No. 2, 1959.

172. Hall WH: Breast changes in males on cimetidine. N Engl J Med 295:841, 1976.

173. Halperin DS, Sizonenko PC: Prepubertal gynecomastia following topical inunction of estrogen containing ointment. Helv Paediatr Acta 38:361–366, 1983.

174. Harmon J, Aliapoulios MA: Gynecomastia in marijuana users. N Engl J Med 287:936, 1972.

175. Harmon J, Aliapoulios MA: Marijuana induced gynecomastia: clinical and laboratory experience. Surg Forum 25:423–425, 1974.

176. Hartemann P, Dureux JB, Vaillant G, Ducas J.: Gynecomastie et hyperthyroidie. Rapport de deux observations. Ann Med Nancy 2:1104–1111, 1963.

177. Hausmanowa-Petrusewicz I, Barkowsky J, Janczewski Z: X-linked adult form of spinal muscular atrophy. J Neurol 229:175–188, 1983.

178. Hayles AB, Hahn HB, Sprague RC, et al: Hormone-secreting tumors of the adrenal cortex in children. Pediatrics 37:19, 1966.

179. Heller, CG, Nelson WO, Roth AC: Functional prepubertal castration in males. J Clin Endocrinol 3:573, 1943.

180. Hemsell DL, Edman CD, Marks JF, Siiteri PK, MacDonald PC: Massive extraglandular aromatization of plasma androstenedione resulting in the feminization of a prepubertal boy. J Clin Invest 60:455–464, 1977.

181. Hendrickson DA, Robertson WR: Diethylstilbestrol therapy. Gynecomastia. JAMA 213:468, 1970.

182. Hendry WS, Garview WHH, Ah-See AK, Bayliss AP: Ultrasonic detection of occult testicular neoplasms in patients with gynaecomastia. Br J Radiol 57:571–572, 1984.

183. Holdsworth MB, Atkins RC, de Kretzer DM: The pituitary testicular axis in men with chronic renal failure. N Engl J Med 296:1245, 1977.

184. Holleb AI, Freeman HP, Farrow JH: Cancer of the male breast. NY State J Med 68:544–553, 656–663, 1968.

185. Hopkins GB, Parry HD: Metastasizing Sertoli cell tumor. Cancer 23:463–467, 1969.

186. Hopwood NJ: Pathogenesis and management of abnormal puberty. Spec Top Endocrinol Metab 7:175–236, 1985.

187. Horton R, Tait JF: Androstenedione production and interconversion rates measured in peripheral blood and studies on the possible site of its conversion to testosterone. J Clin Invest 45:301–303, 1966.

188. Hough AJ Jr.: Flow cytometry and adrenal cortical tumors. J Urol 134:931–932, 1985.

189. House R, Izant RJ, Persky L: Testicular tumors in children. Am J Surg 110:876–892, 1965.

190. Howard CP, Takashashi H, Hayles AB: Feminizing adrenal adenoma in a boy. Proc Mayo Clin 52:354, 1977.

191. Huffman DH, Kampmann JP, Hignite CE, Azarnoff DL: Gynecomastia induced in normal males by spironolactone. Clin Pharmacol Ther 24:465–473, 1978.

192. Hung W, August GP, Glasgow AM: Pediatric Endocrinol. New York, Medical Examinations Publishing, 1978.

193. Iqbal MJ, Wilkinson ML, Johnson PJ, Williams R: Sex steroid receptor proteins in foetal, adult and malignant human liver tissue. Br J Cancer 48(16)791–796, 1983.

194. Itami RM, Amundson GM, Kaplan SA, Lippe BM: Prepubertal gynecomastia caused by an adrenal tumor. Am J Dis Child 136:584–586, 1982.

195. Jackson AW, Mudal S, Ockey CH, O'Connor PJ: Carcinoma of the male breast in association with the Klinefelter syndrome. Br Med J 1:223, 1965.

196. Jackson VP, Gilmore RL: Male breast carcinoma and gynecomastia: Comparison of mammography with sonography. Radiology 149(2):533–536, 1983.

197. Jacobs EC: Effects of starvation on sex hormones in the male. J Clin Endocrinol 8:228, 1948.

198. Jacobson RF, Sagel J, Distiller LA, et al: Leydig cell dysfunction in male patients with Hodgkin's disease receiving chemotherapy (abstract). Clin Res 26:437A, 1978.

199. Javadpour N, Woltering EA, Brennan MF: Adrenal neoplasms. Curr Probl Surg 17:1, 1980.

200. Jensen RT, Collen MJ, Pandol SJ, Allende HD, Raufman J, Bissonnette BM, Duncan WC, Durgin PL, Gillin JC, Gardner JD: Cimetidine-induced impotence and breast changes in patients with gastric hypersecretory states. N Engl J Med 308:883–887, 1983.

201. Johnson PJ: Sex hormones and the liver. Clin Sci 66:369–376, 1984.

202. Johnson PJ, Krasner N, Portmann B, Eddleston ALWF, Williams R: Hepatocellular carcinoma in Great Britain: Influence of age, sex, HBsAg status and aetiology of underlying cirrhosis. Gut 19:1022–1026, 1978.

203. Johnson RL: The male breast and gynaecomastia. *In* Page DL, Anderson TJ (eds): Diagnostic Histopathology of the Breast. New York, Churchill Livingstone, 1988, pp 30–42.

204. Johnstone G: Prepubertal gynecomastia in association with an interstitial tumor of the testes. Br J Urol 39:211, 1967.

205. Kallmann FJ, Schoenfeld WA, Barrera SE: The genetic aspects of primary eunuchoidism. Am J Ment Defic 48:203–236, 1944.

206. Kaplan GW, Cromie WJ, Panayotis PK, Silber I, Tank ES Jr: Gonadal stromal tumors: A report of the prepubertal testicular tumor registry. J Urol 136:300–302, 1986.

207. Kapoor A: Reversible gynecomastia associated with sulindac therapy. JAMA 250(17):2884–2885, 1983.

208. Karsner HT: Gynecomastia. Am J Pathol 22:235–313, 1946.

209. Kennedy WR, Alter M, Foreman RT: Hereditary proximal spinal muscular atrophy of late onset. Neurology 18:306–307, 1966.

210. Kennedy WR, Alter M, Sung JH: Progressive proximal spinal and bulbar atrophy of late onset. A sex linked recessive trait. Neurology 18:671–680, 1968.

211. Kent JR, Scaramuzzi RJ, Lammers W, Parlow AF, Hill M, Penardi R, Hilliard J: Plasma testosterone, estradiol and gonadotrophins in hepatic insufficiency. Gastroenterology, 64:111–115, 1973.

212. Kepler EJ, Walters W, Dixon RK: Menstruation in a child aged nineteen months as a result of tumor of the left adrenal cortex: Successful surgical treatment. Proc Mayo Clin 13:362, 1938.

213. Kew MC, Kirschner MA, Abrahams GE, Katz M: Mechanism of feminization in primary liver cancer. N Engl J Med 296:1084, 1977.

214. Kirkland RT, Bongiovanni AM, Cornfield D, McCormich JB, Parks JS, Tenore A: Gonadotropin responses to luteinizing releasing factor in boys treated with cyclophosphamide for nephrotic syndrome. J Pediatr 89:941–944, 1976.

215. Kirschner MA, Cohen FB, Jespersen D: Estrogen production and its origin in men with gonadotrophin-producing neoplasms. J Clin Endocrinol Metab 39:112, 1974.

216. Kirschner MA, Jacobs JB, Fraley EE: Bilateral anorchia with persistent testosterone production. N Engl J Med 289:240, 1970.

217. Kirschner MA, Wider JA, Rose GT: Leydig cell function in men with gonadotrophin producing testicular hormones. J Clin Endocrin Metab 30:504, 1970.

218. Klatskin G, Saltin WT, Humm FD: Gynecomastia due to malnutrition. Am J Med Sci 213:19, 1947.

219. Kleinberg DL, Noel GL, Frantz AG: Galactorrhea: A study of 235 cases, including 48 with pituitary tumors. N Engl J Med 296:589–600, 1977.

220. Kley HK, Niederau C, Stremmel W, Lax R, Strohmeyer G, Krüskemper HL: Conversion of androgens to estrogens in idiopathic hemochromatosis: comparison with alcoholic liver cirrhosis. J Clin Endocrinol Metab 61(1):1–6, 1985.

221. Kley HK, Nieschlag E, Wiegelmann W, Solbach HG, Krüskemper HL: Steroid hormones and their binding in plasma of male patients with fatty liver, chronic hepatitis and liver cirrhosis. Acta Endocrinol 79:275–285, 1975.

222. Klinefelter HF: Klinefelter's syndrome: Historical background and development. South Med J 79:(9)1089–1093, 1986.

223. Klinefelter HF, Reifenstein EC, Albright F: Syndrome characterized by gynecomastia, aspermatogenesis without aleydigism, and increased excretion of follicle-stimulating hormone. J Clin Endocrinol 2:615–627, 1942.

224. Korenman SG, Perrin LE, McCallum T: Estradiol in human plasma: demonstration of elevated levels in gynecomastia and in cirrhosis (Abstract). J Clin Invest 48:45a, 1969.

225. Kuhn JM, Roca R, Laudat MH, Rieu M, Lutton JP, Bricaire H: Studies on the treatment of idiopathic gynecomastia with percutaneous dihydrotestosterone. Clin Endocrinol 19:513–520, 1983.

226. LaFranchi SH, Parlow AF, Lippe BM, Coyotypa J, Kaplan SA: Pubertal gynecomastia and transient elevation of serum estradiol level. Am J Dis Child 129:927–931, 1975.

227. Landau RL, Stimmal BE, Humphrey E, Clark DE: Gynecomastia and retarded sexual development resulting from a long-standing estrogen secreting adrenal tumor. J Clin Endocrinol 14:1097, 1954.

228. Landolt R, Murset G: Premature signs of puberty as late sequelae of unintentional estrogen administration. Schweiz Med Wochenschr 98:638, 1968.

229. Lardinois CK, Mazzaferri EL: Cimetidine blocks testosterone synthesis. Arch Intern Med 145:920–922, 1985.

230. Large DM, Jones JM, Shalet SM, Scarffe JH, Gibbs ACC: Gynaecomastia complicating the treatment of myeloma. Br J Cancer 48:69–74, 1983.

231. Larsson O, Sundbom CM, Astedt B: Gynaecomastia and diseases of the thyroid. Acta Endocrinol 44:133, 1963.

232. Laskowski J: Feminizing tumors of the testis. General review with case report of granulosa cell tumor of the testis. Endokrynol Pol 3:337–343, 1952.

233. Latorre H, Kenny F: Idiopathic gynecomastia in seven preadolescent boys: Elevation of urinary estrogen secretion in two cases. Am J Dis Child 126:771–773, 1973.

234. Lawrence WD, Young RH, Scully RE: Juvenile granulosa cell tumor of the infantile testis. Am J Surg Pathol 9:87–94, 1985.

235. Leditschke JF, Arden F: Feminizing adrenal adenoma in a five-year-old boy. Aust Paediatr J 10:217, 1974.

236. Lee PA: The occurrence of gynecomastia upon withdrawal of clomiphene citrate treatment for idiopathic oligospermia. Fertil Steril 34:285, 1980.

237. Lee PA: The relationship of concentrations of serum hormones to pubertal gynecomastia. J Pediatr 86:212, 1975.

238. Lee PDK, Winter RJ, Green OC: Virilizing adrenocortical tumors in childhood: Eight cases and a review of the literature. Pediatrics 76(3):437–444, 1985.

239. Lemen RJ, Gates AJ, Waring WW, Hyman AL: Relationship among digital clubbing, disease severity, and serum prostaglandins F_{2A} and E concentrations in cystic fibrosis patients. Am Rev Respir Dis 117:639–646, 1978.

240. Leopold GR, Woo VL, Scheible FW, Nachtscheim D, Gosink BB: High-resolution ultrasonography of scrotal pathology. Radiology 131:719–722, 1979.

241. LeRoith D, Sobel R, Glick SM: The effect of clomiphene citrate on pubertal gynecomastia. Acta Endocrinol 95:177–180, 1980.

242. Leung A, McArthur RG, Birdsell DC, Amundson GM: Resolution of prepubertal male gynecomastia following removal of a giant pigmented nevus. Ann Plast Surg 15(2):167–169, 1985.

243. Levitt SB, Kogan SJ, Schneider KM, Becker JM, Sobel EH, Mortimer RH, Engel RME: Endocrine tests in phenotypic children with bilateral impalpable testes can reliably predict "congenital" anorchism. Urology 11:11, 1978.

244. LeWinn EB: Gynecomastia during digitalis therapy: Report of eight cases with liver function studies. N Engl J Med 248:316–320, 1953.

245. Ley SB, Mozzafarian GA, Leonard JM, Highley M, Paulsen CA: Palpable breast tissue versus gynecomastia as a normal physical finding (Abstract). Clin Res 28:24A, 1980.

246. Lieblich JM, Rogol AD, White BJ, Rosen SW: Syndrome of anosmia with hypogonadotropic hypogonadism (Kallmann syndrome). Clinical and laboratory studies in 23 cases. Am J Med 73:506–519, 1982.

247. Liegel J, Fabre LF, Howard PY, Farmer RW: Plasma testosterone and sex hormone binding globulin (SBG) in alcoholic subjects (Abstract). Physiologist 15:198, 1972.

248. Lipsett MB: In Bondy PK (ed): Diseases of Metabolism. 6th ed. Philadelphia, WB Saunders, 1969, p 1174.

249. Lipsett MB, Sarfaty GA, Wilson H, Bardin CW, Fishman LM: Metabolism of testosterone and related steroids in metastatic interstitial cell carcinoma of the testis. J Clin Invest 45:1700, 1966.

250. Lipsett MB, Wilson H, Kirschner MA, Korenman SG, Fishman LH, Sarfaty GA, Bardin CA: Studies in Leydig cell physiology and pathology: Secretion and metabolism of testosterone. Recent Prog Horm Res 22:245, 1966.

251. Lloyd CW, Williams RH: Endocrine changes associated with Laennec's cirrhosis of the liver. Am J Med 4:315–330, 1948.

252. Lucas LM, Kumar KL, Smith DL: Gynecomastia: A worrisome problem for the patient. Postgrad Med 82(2):73–81, 1987.

253. Lyle WH: Penicillamine. Clin Rheum Dis 5:569–601, 1979.

254. MacDonald PC, Edman O, Kerber IJ, Siiteri PK: Plasma precursors of estrogen. III. Conversion of plasma dehydroisoandrosterone to estrogen in young nonpregnant women. Gynecol Invest 7:165, 1976.

255. MacDonald PC, Madden JD, Brenner PF, Wilson JD, Siiteri PK: Origin of estrogen in normal men and women with testicular feminization. J Clin Endocrinol Metab 49:905–916, 1979.

256. MacDonald PC, Siiteri PK: The in vivo mechanisms of origin of estrogen in subjects with trophoblastic tumors. Steroids 8:589, 1966.

257. Maddock WO, Nelson WO: The effects of chorionic gonadotropin in adult men. J Clin Endocrinol 12:985, 1952.

258. Marchandise B, Lederer J: Gynecomastia par exces de dihydroepiandrosterone. Rev Fr Endocrinol Clin 7:383, 1966.

259. Marco J, Constans R, Alibeli MJ, Baradar G, Dardene P: Effets sexuels secondaire de la spironolactone: intérêt d'une thérapeutique substitutive par la canrenone. Nouv Presse Med 7:3668, 1978.

260. Marcus R, Korenman SG: Estrogens and the human male. Annu Rev Med 27:357–370 1976.

261. Marshall FF, Kerr WS, Kliman B, Scully RE: Sex cord–stromal (gonadal stroma) tumors of the testis: A report of 5 cases. J Urol 117:180–184, 1977.

262. Masterson JST, McCullough AR, Jeffs RD, Smith RL: Neonatal gonadal stromal tumor: Limitations of tumor markers. Presented at Annual Meeting of Section on Urology of the American Academy of Pediatrics, San Francisco, October 1983.

263. McCarthy DM: Report on the United States experience with cimetidine in Zollinger-Ellison syndrome and other hypersecretory states. Gastroenterology 74:453–458, 1978.

264. McFadyen IJ, Bolton AE, Cameron EHD, Hunter WM, Roab G, Forrest AMP: Gonadal-pituitary hormone levels in gynecomastia. Clin Endocrinol 13:77–86, 1980.

265. Melicow MM: Classification of tumors of the testis: A clinical and pathological study based on 105 primary and 13 secondary cases in adults and 8 primary and secondary cases in children. J Urol 73:547–574, 1955.

266. Mendelsohn JH, Kuehnle J, Ellingboe J, Babior RG: Plasma testosterone levels before, during and after chronic marijuana smoking. N Engl J Med 291:1051–1055, 1974.

267. Meyer WJ III, Walker PA, Wiedeking C, Money J, Howarski AA, Migeon CF, Borganonkaris D: Pituitary function in adult males receiving medroxyprogesterone acetate. Fertil Steril 28:1072–1076, 1977.

268. Mignon M, Vallot T, Mayeur S, Bonfils S: Rantidine and cimetidine in Zollinger-Ellison syndrome. Br J Clin Pharmacol 10:173–174, 1980.

269. Mignon M, Vallot T, Bonfils S: Gynaecomastia and histamine-2 antagonists. Lancet 2:499, 1982.

270. Mikuz G, Schwartz S, Hopfel-Kreiner I, Greber F: Leydig cell tumor of the testis. Morphological and endocrinological investigations in two cases. Eur Urol 6:293, 1980.

271. Mineur P, DeCooman S, Hustin J, Verhoeven G, DeHertogh R: Feminizing testicular Leydig cell tumor: Hormonal profile before and after unilateral orchiectomy. J Clin Endocrinol Metab 64:686–691, 1987.

272. Mizejewski GJ, Bellisario R, Carter TP: Birth weight and alpha-fetoprotein (AFP) levels in the newborn (Letter). Pediatrics 73:736, 1984.

273. Moerck HJ, Magelund G: Gynecomastia and diazepam abuse. Lancet 1:1344, 1979.

274. Moncada B, Baranda L: Ketoconazole and gynecomastia. J Am Acad Dermatol 7(4):557, 1982.

275. Morley JE, Distiller LA, Sagel J, Kok SH, Kay G, Carr P, Katz M: Hormonal changes associated with testicular atrophy and gynaecomastia in patients with leprosy. Clin Endocrinol 6:299, 1977.

276. Morrione TG: Effects of estrogens on testes in hepatic insufficiency. Arch Pathol 37:39–48, 1944.

277. Morse WI, Clark AF, MacLeod SC, Ernst WA, Gosse CL: J Clin Endocrinol 22:678, 1982.

278. Mosier HD, Goodwin WE: Feminizing adrenal adenoma in a seven-year-old boy. Pediatrics 27:1016, 1961.

279. Mostofi FK: Testicular tumors. Cancer 32:1186–1201, 1973.

280. Mostofi FK: Pathology of germ cell tumors of testis: A progress report. Cancer 45:1735–1754, 1980.

281. Mostofi FK, Price EB: Tumors of the testis. In Tumors of the Male Genital System, Atlas of Tumor Pathology, series 2, part 8. Washington DC, Armed Forces Institute of Pathology, 1973, pp 1–85.

282. Mostofi FK, Price EB: Tumors of specialized gonadal stroma. In Tumors of the Male Genital System, Atlas of Tumor Pathology, fasc. 8, Armed Forces Institute of Pathology, Washington DC, 1973, pp 86–94.

283. Mostofi FK, Price EB: Tumors of the testis in children. In Tumors of the Male Genital System, Atlas of Tumor Pathology, series 2, fasc 16. Armed Forces Institute of Pathology, Washington DC, 1973, pp 121–126.

284. Mostofi FK, Thiess EA, Ashley DJB: Tumors of specialized gonadal stroma in human male patients. Cancer 12:944–957, 1959.

285. Moudy P, Makhija JS: Ultrasonic demonstration of a non-palpable testicular tumor. J Clin Ultrasound 11:54–55, 1983.

286. Mowat NAG, Edwards CRW, Fisher R, McNeilly AG, Green JRB, Dawson AM: Hypothalamic-pituitary-gonadal function in men with cirrhosis of the liver. Gut 17:345–350, 1976.

287. Nagel TC, Freinkel N, Bell RH, Friesen H, Wilber JF, Metzger BE: Gynecomastia, prolactin, and other peptide hormones in patients undergoing chronic hemodialysis. J Clin Endocrinol Metab 36:428, 1973.

288. Navab A, Koss LG, LaDue JS: Estrogen-like activity of digitalis: Its effect on the squamous epithelium of the female genital tract. JAMA 194:30–32, 1965.

289. Neblett WW, Frexes-Steed M, Scott HW Jr.: Experience with adrenocortical neoplasms in childhood. Am Surg 53:117–125, 1987.

290. Neuberger J, Nunnerly HB, Portmann B, Laws JW, Williams R: Oral contraceptive–associated liver tumours: Occurrence of malignancy and difficulties in diagnosis. Lancet 1:273–276, 1980.

291. Nicolis GL, Modlinger RS, Gabrilove JL: A study of the histopathology of human gynecomastia. J Clin Endocrinol 32:173–178, 1971.

292. Niewoehner CB, Nuttall FQ: Gynecomastia in a hospitalized male patient. Am J Med 77(4):633–638, 1984.

293. Nishiki M, Amano K, Itoh H, Ezaki H, Miyachi Y: Feminizing adrenocortical carcinoma in man. Jpn J Surg 10(2):159–163, 1980.

294. Nomura K, Suzuki H, Saji M, Horiba N, Ujihara M, Tsushima T, Demura H, Shizume K: High serum progesterone in hyperthyroid men with Graves' disease. J Clin Endocrinol Metab 66(1):230–232, 1988.

295. Novak A, Kass LF, LaDue JS: Estrogen-like activity of digitalis. JAMA 194:142, 1965.

296. Novak E, Hendrix JW, Chen TT, Seckman CE, Royer GL, Rochi PE: Sebum production and plasma testosterone levels in man after high-dose medroxyprogesterone acetate treatment and androgen administration. Acta Endocrinol 95:265–270, 1980.

297. Novak E, Hendrix JW, Seckman CE: Effects of medroxyprogesterone acetate on some endocrine functions of healthy male volunteers. Curr Ther Res 21:320–326, 1977

298. Nuttall FQ: Gynecomastia as a physical finding in normal men. J Clin Endocrinol Metab 48(2):338–340, 1979.

299. Nydick M, Bustos J, Dale JH Jr., Rawson RW: Gynecomastia in adolescent boys. JAMA 178:449–454, 1961.

300. Ogle JW: Unusually large mass of carcinomatous deposit in one of the suprarenal capsules of a child. Trans Pathol Soc Lond 16:250, 1865.

301. Olivo J, Gordon GG, Rafii F, Southren AL: Estrogen metabolism in hyperthyroidism and in cirrhosis of the liver. Steroids 26:47, 1975.

302. Olusi SO: Hyperprolactinaemia in patients with suspected cannabis-induced gynaecomastia (Letter). Lancet 1:255, 1980.

303. Orentreich N and Dur NP: Mammogenesis in transsexuals. J Invest Dermatol 63:142, 1974.

304. Page DL, DeLellis RA, Hough AF Jr.: Tumors of the adrenal. In Atlas of Tumor Pathology. Second series, Fascicle 23. Washington, DC, Armed Forces Institute of Pathology, 1985.

305. Parra A, Santos D, Cervantes C, Sojo I, Carranco A, Cortes-Gallegos V: Plasma gonadotropins and gonadal steroids in children treated with cyclophosphamide. J Pediatr 92:117–124, 1978

306. Passas C, Weinstein A: Breast gigantism with penicillamine therapy. Arthritis Rheum 21:167–168, 1978.

307. Paulsen CA: The testes. In Williams RH (ed): Textbook of Endocrinology. 4th ed. Philadelphia, WB Saunders, 1968, p 449.

308. Pearce P, Funder JW: Histamine H_2 receptor antagonist: radioreceptor assay for antiandrogenic side effects. Clin Exp Pharmacol Physiol 7:442, 1980.

309. Pearson JC: Endocrinology of testicular neoplasms. Urology 17(2):119–125, 1981.

310. Pennisi AJ, Grushkin CM, Lieberman E: Gonadal function in children with nephrosis treated with cyclophosphamide. Am J Dis Child 129:315–318, 1975.

311. Penso J, Lippe B, Ehrlich R, Smith FG Jr: Testicular function in prepubertal and pubertal male patients treated with cyclophosphamide for nephrotic syndrome. J Pediatr 84:831–836, 1974.

312. Pentikäinen PJ, Pentikäinen LA, Azarnoff DL, Dujovne CA: Plasma levels and excretion of estrogens in urine in chronic liver disease. Gastroenterology 69:20–27, 1975.

313. Peterson LJ, Catalona WJ, Koehler RE: Ultrasonic localization of a nonpalpable testis tumor. J Urol 122:843–844, 1979.

314. Pierce GB Jr.: Ultrastructure of human testicular tumors. Cancer 19:1963, 1966.

315. Pierce GB Jr, Stevens LC, Nakane PK: Ultrastructural analysis of the early development of teratocarcinomas. J Natl Cancer Inst 39:755, 1967.

316. Pierrepoint CG: The metabolism in vitro of dehydroepiandrosterone and hydroepiandrosterone sulphate by Sertoli cell tumours of the testis of two dogs with clinical signs of hyperoestrogenism. J Endocrinol 42:99, 1968.

317. Pincus IJ, Rakoff AE, Cohn EM, et al: Hormonal studies in patients with chronic liver disease. Gastroenterology 19:735–754, 1951.

318. Plourde PV, Kulin HE, Santner SJ: Clomiphene in the treatment of adolescent gynecomastia. Am J Dis Child 137:1080–1082, 1983.

319. Pont A, Goldman ES, Sugar AM, Siiteri PK, Stevens DA: Ketoconazole-induced increase in estradiol-testosterone ratio. Arch Intern Med 145, 1429–1431, 1985.

320. Pont A, Graybill JR, Craven PC, Galgiani JN, Dismukes WE, Reitz RE, Stevens DA: High-dose ketoconazole therapy and adrenal and testicular function in humans. Arch Intern Med 144, 2150–2153, 1984.

321. Poulsen HS: Demonstration of hormonal sensitivity in gynaecomastic tissue by thymidine incorporation in vitro. Acta Pathol Microbiol Scand [A] 85:19–24, 1977.

322. Powell LW, Mortimer R, Harris OD: Cirrhosis of the liver—a comparative study of the four major aetiological groups. Med J Aust 1:941–950, 1971.

323. Proppe KH, Scully RE: Large-cell calcifying Sertoli cell tumor of the testis. Am J Clin Pathol 74:607, 1980.

324. Raju U, Fine G, Warrier R, Kini R, Weiss L: Congenital testicular juvenile granulosa cell tumor in a neonate with X/XY mosaicism. Am J Surg Pathol 10(8):577–583, 1986.

325. Reid DM, Martynoga AG, Nuki G: Reversible gynaecomastia associated with D-penicillamine in a man with rheumatoid arthritis. Br Med J 285:1083–1084, 1982.

326. Reifenstein EC Jr: Hereditary familial hypogonadism. Proc Am Fed Clin Res 3:86, 1947.

327. Ricciardi I, Ianniruberto A: Tamoxifen-induced regression of benign breast lesions. Obstet Gynecol 54(1):80–84, 1979.

328. Riggs S, Sanford JP: Viral orchitis. N Engl J Med 266:990, 1962.

329. Robson MC, Santiago Q, Huang TW: Bilateral carcinoma of the breast in a patient with Klinefelter's syndrome. J Clin Endocrinol 28:897–902, 1968.

330. Rodin E, Subramanian MG, Gilroy J: Investigation of sex hormones in male epileptic patients. Epilepsia 25:690–694, 1984.

331. Rose LI, Underwood RH, Newmark SR, Kisch ES, Williams GH: Pathophysiology of spironolactone-induced gynecomastia. Ann Intern Med 87:398–403, 1977.

332. Rose LI, Williams GH, Emerson K, Villee DB: Steroidal and gonadotropin evaluation of a patient with feminizing tumor of the adrenal gland. In vivo and in vitro studies. J Clin Endocrinol Metab 29:1526, 1969.

333. Rosenbaum W, Christy NP, Kelly WG: Electrophoretic evidence for the presence of an estrogen-binding β-globulin in human plasma. J Clin Endocrinol Metab 26:1399–1403, 1966.

334. Rosenthal FD, Lees F: Thyrotoxicosis with glucosuria and adrenocortical hyperactivity. Lancet 2:340–342, 1958.

335. Rosewater S, Gwinup G, Hamwi GJ: Familial gynecomastia. Ann Intern Med 63(3):377–385, 1965.

336. Rosner W: A simplified method for the quantitative determination of testosterone-estradiol-binding globulin activity in human plasma. J Clin Endocrinol Metab 34:983–988, 1972.

337. Rosvoll RV, Woodard Jr: Malignant Sertoli cell tumor of the testis. Cancer 22:8, 1968.

338. Rubens R, Dhont M, Vermeulen A: Further studies on Leydig cell function in old age. J Clin Endocrinol Metab 39:40–45, 1974.

339. Rupp J, Cantarow A, Rakoff AE, Paschkis KE: Hormone excretion in liver disease and in gynecomastia. J Clin Endocrinol 11:688, 1951.

340. Russi EW: Gynaecomastia in cystic fibrosis. Br Med J 288:1660, 1984.

341. Saenz CA, Bongiovanni AM: An outbreak of premature thelarche in Puerto Rico (Abstract). Pediatr Res 17:171A, 1983.

342. Salassa RM, Jowsey J, Arnaud CD: Hypophosphatomic osteomalachia associated with "non-endocrine" tumors. N Engl J Med 283:65, 1970.

343. Salbenblatt JA, Bender BG, Puck MH, Robinson A, Faiman C, Winter JSD: Pituitary-gonadal function in Klinefelter syndrome before and during puberty. Pediatr Res 19(1):82–86, 1985.

344. Sandow J: Clinical application of LHRH and its analogues. Clin Endocrinol 18:571–592, 1983.

345. Santen RJ, Paulsen CA: Hypogonadotropic eunuchoidism I. Clinical study of the mode of inheritance. J Clin Endocrinol Metab 36:47–54, 1973.

346. Sattin RW, Roisin A, Kafrissen ME, Dugan JB, Farer LS: Epidemic of gynecomastia among illegal Haitian entrants. Public Health Rep 99(5):504–510, 1984.

347. Sawin CT, Longcope C, Schmitt GW, Ryan RJ: Blood levels of gonadotropins and gonadal hormones in gynecomastia associated with chronic hemodialysis. J Clin Endocrinol Metab 36:988, 1973.

348. Scheike O, Visfeldt J, Peterson B: Male breast cancer. 3. Breast carcinoma in association with the Klinefelter syndrome. Acta Pathol Microbiol Scand [A] 81:352–358, 1949.

349. Schilsky RL, Lewis BJ, Sherins RF, et al: Gonadal dysfunction in patients receiving chemotherapy for cancer. Ann Intern Med 93:109–114, 1980.

350. Schmitt GW, Shehadeh I, Sawin CT: Transient gynecomastia in chronic renal failure during chronic intermittent hemodialysis. Ann Intern Med 69:73, 1968.

351. Schorer AE, Oken MM, Johnson GJ: Gynecomastia with nitrosourea therapy. Cancer Treat Rep 62:574–576, 1978.

352. Schweikert H, Weissbach L, Stangenberg C, Leyendecker G, Kley HK, Griffin JE, Wilson JD: Clinical and endocrinological characterization of two subjects with Reifenstein syndrome associated with qualitative abnormalities of the androgen receptor. Hormone Res 25:72–79, 1987.

353. Schydlower M: Breast masses in adolescents. Am Fam Physician 25(2):141–145, 1982.

354. Scully RE: Sex cord tumor with annular tubules: A distinctive ovarian tumor of the Peutz-Jeghers syndrome. Cancer 25:1107–1121, 1970.

355. Selvaggi FP, Young RT, Brown R, Kick AS: Interstitial cell tumor of the testis in an adult: Two case reports. J Urol 109:436, 1973.

356. Shalet SM, Beardwell CG, Morris-Jones PH, Pearson D, Orrell DH: Ovarian failure following abdominal irradiation in childhood. Br J Cancer 33:655, 1976.

357. Sherins RJ, DeVita VT: Effect of drug treatment for lymphoma on male reproductive capacity. Ann Intern Med 79:216–220, 1973.

358. Sherins RJ, Gandy HM, Thorslund TW, Paulsen CA: Pituitary and testicular function studies. 1. Experience with a new gonadal inhibitor, 17α-pregn-4-en-20-yno (2,3-d) isoxazol-17-01 (danazol). J Clin Endocrinol Metab 32:521–522, 1971.

359. Sherins RJ, Olweny CLM, Ziegler JL: Gynaecomastia and gonadal dysfunction in adolescent boys treated with combination chemotherapy for Hodgkin's disease. N Engl J Med 299:12–16, 1978.

360. Shimatsu A, Suzuki Y, Tanaka S: Gynecomastia associated with isolated ACTH deficiency. J Endocrinol Invest 10:127, 1987.

361. Shimp WS, Schultz AL, Hastings JR, Anderson WR: Leydig cell tumor of the testis with gynecomastia and elevated estrogen levels. Am J Clin Pathol 67:562, 1977.

362. Siiteri PK, MacDonald PC: Role of extraglandular estrogen in human endocrinology. In Greep RO, Aswood EB (eds): Handbook of Physiology, Section VII, Vol. II, Part 1. Baltimore, Waverly Press, 1973, pp 615–629.

363. Smith RH, Barrett O Jr: Gynecomastia associated with vincristine therapy. Calif Med 107:347–349, 1967.

364. Smith SR: Acquired gonadotropin-responsive hyperestrogenism in a male without evidence of neoplasia. J Clin Endocrinol Metab 32:77–82, 1971

365. Snaith AH: A case of feminizing adrenal tumor in a girl. J Clin Endocrinol 18:318, 1958.

366. Snyder PF: Effect of age on the serum LH and FSH responses to gonadotropin-releasing hormone. In Grayhack JT, Wilson JD, Scherbenske MJ (eds): Benign Prostatic Hyperplasia. Washington DC, DHEW Publication No. (NIH) 76-1113, 1976, p 161.

367. Sorbie PJ, Perez-Marrero R: The use of clomiphene citrate in male infertility. J Urol 131:425–429, 1984.

368. Southern AL, Gordon GG, Olivo J, et al: Androgen metabolism in cirrhosis of the liver. Metabolism 22:695–702, 1973.

369. Spano F, Ryan WG: Tamoxifen for gynecomastia induced by anabolic steroids? N Engl J Med 311:861–862, 1984.

370. Sparkes RS, Simpson RW, Paulsen CA: Familial hypogonadotropic hypogonadism with anosomia. Arch Intern Med 121:534–538, 1968.

371. Spence RW, Celestin LR: Gynaecomastia associated with cimetidine. Gut 20:154–157, 1979.

372. Stacpoole PW, Interlandi JW, Nicholson WE, Rabin D: Isolated ACTH deficiency: a heterogenous disorder. Medicine 61:13, 1982.

373. Starr P: Gynecomastia during hyperthyroidism. JAMA 104:1988, 1935.

374. Stedman KC, Moore GE, Morgan RT: Estrogen receptor proteins in diverse human tumours. Arch Surg 115:244–248, 1980.

375. Stephanas AV, Burnet RB, Harding PE, et al: Clomiphene in the treatment of pubertal-adolescent gynecomastia: A preliminary report. J Pediatr 90:651–653, 1977.

376. Stephanas AV, Samaan NA, Schultz PN, Holoye PY: Endocrine

studies in testicular tumor patients with and without gynecomastia. Cancer 41:369, 1978.
377. Stevens LC: Experimental production of testicular teratomas in
mice. Proc Natl Acad Sci USA 52:661, 1964.
378. Stevens LC, Hummel KP: A description of spontaneous congenital teratomas in strain 129 mice. J Natl Cancer Inst 18:719,
1957.
379. Stewart DR, Morris Jones PH, Jolleys A: Carcinoma of the
adrenal gland in children. J Pediatr Surg 9:59, 1974.
380. Stokes JF: Unexpected gynaecomastia. Lancet 2:911–913, 1962.
381. Stone WJ, Bennett WM, Cutler RE: Long-term bumetanide
treatment of patients with edema due to renal disease. Cooperative Studies. J Clin Pharmacol 21:587–590, 1981.
382. Stouffer SS, Hynes KM, Jiang NS, Ryan RJ: Digoxin and
abnormal serum hormone levels. JAMA 225:1643–1644, 1973.
383. Sultan C, Descomps B, Garandeau P. Bressot N, Jean R:
Pubertal gynecomastia due to an estrogen-producing adrenal
adenoma. J Pediatr 95(5):744–746, 1979.
384. Summerskill WHJ, Davidson CS, Dible JH, Mallory GK, Sher-
lock S, Turner MD, Wolfe SJ: Cirrhosis of the liver: a study
of alcoholic and nonalcoholic patients in Boston and London.
N Engl J Med, 262:1–9, 1960.
385. Symington T, Cameron KM: Endocrine and genetic lesions. In
Pugh RCB (ed): Pathology of Testes. Oxford, Blackwell, 1976,
p 259.
386. Symmers W St C: Carcinoma of breast in transsexual individuals
after surgery and hormonal interference with the primary and
secondary sex characteristics. Br Med J 2:83–85, 1968.
387. Tanner LA, Bosco LA: Gynecomastia associated with calcium
channel blocker therapy. Arch Intern Med 148, 379–380, 1988.
388. Taylor PJ, Cumming DC, Corenblum B: Successful treatment of
D-penicillamine-induced breast gigantism with danazol. Br
Med J 282:362–363, 1981.
389. Tennes K, Puck M, Orfanarkis D, Robinson A: The early
childhood development of 17 boys with sex chromosome
anomalies. A prospective study. Pediatrics 59:574, 1977.
390. Teilum G: Estrogen-producing Sertoli cell tumors of the human
testis and ovary. J Clin Endocrinol 9:301–319, 1958.
391. Teilum G: Classification of testicular and ovarian androblastoma
and Sertoli cell tumors. Cancer 11:769–782, 1958.
392. The H$_2$-receptor antagonist anthology: Worldwide Tagamet experience. Philadelphia, Smith, Kline and French International,
1982, pp 153–156.
393. Thew DCN, Stewart IM: D-Penicillamine and breast enlargement. Ann Rheum Dis 39:200, 1980.
394. Thompson NW, Cheung PSY: Diagnosis and treatment of functioning and nonfunctioning adrenocortical neoplasms including
incidentalomas. Surg Clin North Am 67:423–436, 1987.
395. Toone BK, Wheeler M, Nanjee M, Fenwick P, Grant RHE: Sex
hormones, sexual drive and plasma anticonvulsant levels in
male epileptics. In Parsonage M, Grant RHE, Craig AG,
Ward AA (eds): Advances in epileptology. IVth Epilepsy
International Symposium. New York, Raven Press, 1983, pp
313–317.
396. Tosi S, Cagnoli M: Painful gynaecomastia with ranitidine (Letter). Lancet 2:160, 1982.
397. Treves N: Gynecomastia. Cancer 11:1083–1102, 1958.
398. Trump DL, Anderson SA: Painful gynecomastia following cytotoxic therapy for testis cancer: A potentially favorable prognostic sign? J Clin Oncol I(7):416–420, 1983.
399. Trump DL, Pavy MD, Staal S: Gynecomastia in men following
antineoplastic therapy. Arch Intern Med 142:511–513, 1982.
400. Turkington RW: Serum prolactin levels in patients with gynecomastia. J Clin Endocrinol Metab 34:62–66, 1972.
401. Turkington RW, Topper YJ: Androgen inhibiting of mammary
gland differentiation in vitro. Endocrinology 80:329–336, 1967.
402. Turner WR, Derrick FC, Worltmann H: Leydig cell tumor in
identical twins. Urology 7:194–197, 1976.
403. Uehara Y, Hayashi T, Matsuoka H, Ishii A, Takeda T, Murao
O: A case of isolated ACTH deficiency associated with gynecomastia (Abstract). J Jpn Soc Intern Med 67:328, 1978.
404. Van der Steen M, Du Caju MVL, Van Acker KJ: Gynaecomastia
in a male infant given domperidone. Lancet 2:884–885, 1982.
405. Van Dop C, Burstein S, Conte FA, Grumbach MM: Isolated
gonadotropin deficiency in boys: Clinical characteristics and
growth. J Pediatr 111(5)684–692, 1987.
406. Van Niekerk WA: True hermaphroditism. An analytic view with
a report of three new cases. Am J Obstet Gynecol 126:890,
1976.
407. Van Thiel DH, Gavaler JS, Vaitukaitis J, Lester R: Evidence
for an isolated defect in pituitary secretion of LH in chronic
alcoholic men. Gastroenterology 71:40–93, 1976.
408. Van Thiel DH, Lester R: Alcoholism: its effect on hypothalamic-
pituitary-gonadal function. Gastroenterology 71:318–327,
1976.
409. Van Thiel DH, Lester R, Sherins RJ: Hypogonadism in alcoholic
liver disease; evidence for a double defect. Gastroenterology
67:1188–1199, 1974.
410. Van Thiel DH, Sherins RJ, Myers GH, et al: Evidence for a
specific seminiferous tubular factor affecting follicle-stimulating hormone secretion in man. J Clin Invest 51:1009–1019,
1972.
411. Veldhuis JD, Sowers JR, Rogol AD, Klein FA, Miller N, Dufau
ML: Pathophysiology of male hypogonadism associated with
endogenous hyperestrogenism. N Engl J Med 312:1371, 1985.
412. Vermeulen A, Verdonck L, Van der Straeten M, Orie N:
Capacity of the testosterone-binding globulin in human plasma
and influence of specific binding of testosterone on its metabolic clearance rate. J Clin Endocrinol Metab 29:1470–1480,
1969.
413. Visfeldt J, Scheike O: Male breast cancer. Histologic typing and
grading of 187 Danish cases. Cancer 32:985–990, 1973.
414. von Eyben FE: Biochemical markers in advanced testicular
tumors. Cancer 41:648, 1978.
415. Walker KJ, Turkes AO, Nicholson RI, et al: Therapeutic potential of the LHRH agonist, ICI 118630 in the treatment of
advanced prostatic carcinoma. Lancet 2:413–415, 1983.
416. Wallach S, Brown H, Englert E, et al: Adrenocortical carcinoma
with gynecomastia: A case report and review of the literature.
J Clin Endocrinol 17:945, 1957.
417. Wang C, Ng RP, Chan TK, et al: Effect of combination of
chemotherapy on pituitary-gonadal function in patients with
lymphoma and leukemia. Cancer 45:2030–2037, 1980.
418. Waxman M, Damjanov I, Khapra A, Landau SJ: Large cell
calcifying Sertoli tumor of the testis: Light microscopic and
ultrastructural features. Cancer 54:1574–1581, 1984.
419. Wegenke JD, Uehling DT, Wear JB Jr, et al: Familial Kallmann
syndrome with unilateral renal aplasia. Clin Genet 7:368–381,
1975.
420. Weichert CK, Boyd RW: Stimulation of mammary gland development in the pregnant rat under conditions of experimental
hyperthyroidism. Anat Rec 59:157, 1934.
421. Weinstein RL, Kelch RP, Jenner MR, et al: Secretion of unconjugated androgens and estrogens by the normal and abnormal
testis before and after human chorionic gonadotropin. J Clin
Invest 53:1–6, 1974.
422. Werner CA: Mumps orchitis and testicula atrophy. Ann Intern
Med 32:1066, 1950.
423. Wiedemann HR: Tumours and hemihypertrophy associated with
Wiedemann-Beckwith syndrome. Eur J Pediatr 141:129, 1983
424. Wilkins L: A feminizing adrenal tumor causing gynecomastia in
a boy of five years contrasted with a virilizing tumor in a five-
year-old girl. J Clin Endocrinol 8:111, 1948.
425. Williams MJ: Gynecomastia: Its incidence, recognition, and host
characterization in 447 autopsy cases. Am J Med 34:103, 1963.
426. Wilson BE, Netzloff ML: Primary testicular abnormalities causing precocious puberty Leydig cell tumor, Leydig cell hyperplasia, and adrenal rest tumor. Ann Clin Lab Sci 13(4):315–
320, 1983.
427. Wilson DM, Pitts WC, Hintz RL, Rosenfeld RG: Testicular
tumors with Peutz-Jeghers syndrome. Cancer 57:2238–2240,
1986.
428. Wilson JD, Aiman J, MacDonald PC: The pathogenesis of
gynecomastia. Prog Intern Med 25:1–32, 1980.
429. Wilson JD, Harrod MJ, Goldstein JL, Hemsell DL, MacDonald
PC: Familial incomplete male pseudohermaphroditism, type
1: evidence for androgen resistance and variable clinical manifestations in a family with the Reifenstein syndrome. N Engl
J Med 290:1097–1103, 1982.
430. Wilson JD, Goldstein JL: Classification of hereditary disorders
of sexual development. Birth Defects (Original Article Series).
11:1, 1975.

431. Wilson SE, Hutchinson WB: Breast masses in males with carcinoma of the prostate. J Surg Oncol 8:105–112, 1976.

432. Winters SJ, Banks JL, Loriaux DL: Cimetidine is an antiandrogen in the rat. Gastroenterology 76:504–508, 1979.

433. Wittenberg J: Computed tomography of the body (second of two parts). N Engl J Med 309:1224–1230, 1983.

434. Wohltmann H, Mathur RS, Williamson HO: Sexual precocity in a female infant due to feminizing adrenal carcinoma. J Clin Endocrinol Metab 50:186–189, 1980.

435. Wolfe CJ: Gynecomastia following digitalis administration. J Fla Med Assoc 62:54, 1975.

436. Wolfe MM: Impotence on cimetidine treatment. N Engl J Med 300:94, 1979.

437. Woodham CWB: Hyperplasia of the male breast. Lancet 2:307, 1938.

438. Wu JT, Book L, Sudar K: Serum alpha fetoprotein (AFP) levels in normal infants. Pediatr Res 15:50, 1981.

439. Yoshida T, Arai T, Sugano J, Yarita H, Yanagisawa H: Isolated ACTH deficiency accompanied by "primary hypothyroidism" and hyperprolactinemia. Acta Endocrinol 104:397, 1983.

440. Young RH, Lawrence DW, Scully RE: Juvenile granulosa cell tumor—Another neoplasm associated with abnormal chromosomes and ambiguous genitalia. A report of 3 cases. Am J Surg Pathol 9:737–743, 1985.

441. Zurbiran S, Gomez-Mont F: Endocrine disturbances in chronic human malnutrition. Vitam Horm 11:97, 1953.

Section IV

Pathology of Malignant Lesions

Chapter 8

NONINFILTRATING (IN SITU) CARCINOMA

David L. Page, M.D. and Hugo Japaze, M.D.

While the straightforward or fundamental definition of carcinoma *in situ* (CIS) is uncomplicated, its recognition in the breast is complex because of its heterogeneity of anatomical expression and natural history. The original definition of CIS was histologic only and recognized CIS as those samples that had cells appearing as cancer cells but without invasion into the stroma (i.e., highly abnormal cells within their normal sites of residence, the branching glandular and ductal elements of the breast).[13, 58] Thus by this definition the epithelial–connective tissue junction had not been broached by the "cancer cells." The practical prognostic, therapeutic, and biological implications of these lesions have been learned during many decades. Basic, reliable follow-up information was not available until the 1970s and early 1980s. Very important information is still being collected, but there is general agreement that CIS in the human breast is not an integrated entity but includes several different types.

The current changing approach toward and increased concern for CIS is the product of mammographic examination. The great majority of these lesions are found by mammography without the presence of a palpable mass.[88] Thus the incidence of recognition of CIS is greatly increased compared with the premammographic era.

Understanding of the nature of *in situ* disease has not been achieved in a uniform manner. Manifestation of the philosophic diversity may be seen by comparing recent comments concerning the characterization of CIS. Connolly et al.[21] indicate that *in situ* carcinoma of the breast is a "proliferation of potentially malignant cells within the lumen of the ductal system," a definition with which we would largely concur. However, Schwartz et al.,[81] when discussing ductal carcinoma *in situ* (DCIS) state that DCIS is a malignant neoplasm that is "not yet invasive." Whatever our individual or collective philosophical stance toward these lesions might be, they have become clinicopathologic entities each in their own right. They clearly occupy an intermediate position between hyperplasias and invasive carcinoma in clinical malevolence. They are lesions without concurrent metastatic potential, which mark an increased likelihood of that eventuality. Thus, they are not carcinoma in full definition, and they are not non-cancer; they are unique, they are carcinoma *in situ*.

Two major types of carcinoma *in situ* have been accepted for several decades. They are named for their supposed relationship to the two major histologic types of epithelial cells or anatomic structures present within the breast: the ducts and the secreting (or potentially so) cells of the lobular units.[58] Because the human breast is primarily found in its resting state rather than its secreting state, this differentiation has been confused. Considering also that markers of lactation such as the presence of milk products are found in "ductal" carcinoma, we recognize the term "ductal" to indicate patterns of lesions[63] and not necessarily site of origin or presentation. In most settings this approach recognizes as "ductal" lesions that have no other specific features to separate them from the most common patterns of neoplastic disease. "Ductal" includes the most common,[63] frequently observed lesions of "no special type." This approach allows the term "ductal," which has achieved acceptance widely throughout the world, to continue to be used in its accustomed clinical settings without confusion of altered terminology.

Various types or subtypes of carcinoma *in situ* of the breast constitute a complex and currently evolving body of anatomical and biological information. These subtypes are distinguished by unique features of histology, prognosis, and detectability. They aid in decision making with regard to the various therapeutic options available. The recognition of subtypes of CIS, beyond the major dichotomy of lobular and ductal CIS, is in a period of evolution. However, these subtypes are useful in providing guidelines for the several therapeutic options available. Therapeutic decisions in this specialized area of breast disease depend on careful documentation of histological tumor types and their extent as well as knowledge of the probabilistic nature of outcomes with different therapies. Accretion of knowledge concerning these conditions will be forthcoming from experience as well as through the use of various new modes of characterization, e.g., primarily genomic features including oncogene alterations, cell cycle kinetics, and other tumor markers applied to this special setting.

DUCTAL CARCINOMAS *IN SITU*

Terminology and Definitions

Ductal carcinoma *in situ* should be understood to represent all examples of *in situ* mammary epithelial cell proliferation recognized as carcinoma *in situ* other than those patterns designated as lobular carcinoma *in situ*. This follows the approach utilized for infiltrating lesions, in which the term "ductal" is used to apply to any pattern not otherwise having specific designation. Lobular carcinoma *in situ* usually occurs in pure form, but the various forms of ductal carcinoma *in situ* frequently occur in overlapping histological patterns. This is true with minor exceptions noted in the following discussion.

DCIS identifies a group of closely related diseases. Their recognition as a single entity with a single therapeutic alternative[36, 90] was accepted until the 1980s. The advent of mammography has produced two major changes in the mix of these lesions detected in patients and presented to surgical pathology laboratories: (1) a great increase in the number of DCIS cases and (2) a large change in their type or subtype. This latter change has been both in histologic pattern as well as in size of lesions. Average sizes of detected lesions has decreased from more than 3 to 4 cm in greatest dimension to approximately 1 cm. Gump et al.[43] have suggested that we recognize two types of DCIS: one palpable and one nonpalpable, detected by mammography or incidentally. The histologic patterns of non-comedo carcinoma now predominate over examples of comedo carcinoma.

With regard to types, they have been divided classically into three broad histologic patterns: comedo, cribriform, and micropapillary.[8, 58] The histologic patterns have recently been expanded to include comedo carcinoma, non-comedo carcinoma with necrosis (largely cribriform with necrosis), cribriform, micropapillary, and solid.[7, 22] The last category has also been considered to include "endocrine" or "microglandular" patterns (see following discussion). The acceptance of three broad groups—comedo, non-comedo, and an intermediate category that can be termed cribriform CIS with necrosis (recognized by lack of bizarre nuclear features in company with cellular necrosis)—is the most useful way to group these lesions.[50] This stratification might in the future be recognized by several parameters including special marker studies yet to be determined or measures of genetic alteration, genetic instability, or manifestation of specific oncogenes.

Any attempt to characterize DCIS as a single entity can only be misleading. Acceptance of their complexity and multiple types will foster understanding. When these lesions were rare and seen infrequently by any one management team or physician, the oversimplified approach of grouping DCIS together was appropriate, but now their heterogeneity must be dealt with and exploited for the patient's benefit. Some examples may be only millimeters in size, have no further determinate disease in the breast, and be cured by biopsy only. Whilst in other examples, the disease is widespread and, indeed, may fill most of the epithelial-lined spaces of the breast. The discussion that follows will highlight the heterogeneity of these conditions.

Anatomic Pathology of Non-Comedo DCIS

The varied patterns of DCIS, once recognized as a single entity, have gained wide acceptance as including different prognostic implications that determine widely different therapeutic options.

Comedo carcinoma *in situ* will be discussed in a separate section, because, at least in large (usual palpable) form, this subtype is associated with a particularly menacing prognosis and should not be considered along with the majority of ductal carcinoma *in situ* cases.

The three-dimensional extent of any ductal carcinoma *in situ* lesion is a major concern when considering therapy which conserves the breast. The categories of lesions presented by Andersen et al.[4] are (1) microfocal, (2) diffuse, and (3) tumor-forming, although it is evident that different combinations may occur. The microfocal category indicates one or several lobular units without notable changes of the surrounding stroma and less than 5 mm in greatest extent. The diffuse type was defined by the Copenhagen group as lesions larger than 5 mm. The tumor-forming group differs from the diffuse group in lacking normally distributed glands and ducts; instead, the glandular structures are approximated and separated only by a confluent fibrotic or otherwise altered and often inflammatory stroma. These lesions measure at least 5 mm. This is a useful approach to the categorization of these very diverse lesions, but there is no readily available, agreed-upon system of classification, and each individual lesion will need to be described in individual reports as carefully and completely as possible. Size is certainly a prime consideration, with the utility of separating gross from microscopic disease[43] now generally recognized. It will remain relatively easy to ascertain the prognostic and therapeutic significance of tiny, contained lesions without advanced nuclear atypia as opposed to lesions at the other end of the cytologic and gross size spectrum.

The non-comedo carcinomas *in situ* include predominantly the cribriform and micropapillary patterns (Figs. 8–1 through 8–10). These are frequently found to occur together but, less commonly, they are found in pure form, with the cribriform being more common. The solid pattern is less common and seldom occurs in pure form.

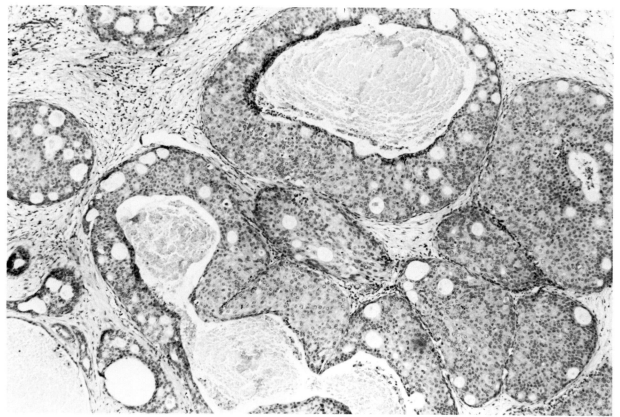

Figure 8–1. This low-power view of a common form of DCIS shows solid cellular masses distending basement membrane–bound spaces. Within these cellular masses are sharply defined, rounded secondary lumina. There are central areas of necrosis and evident distention and distortion of the involved spaces. × 75

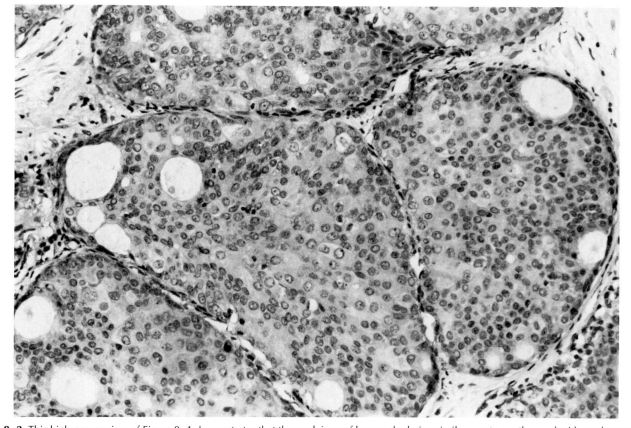

Figure 8–2. This high-power view of Figure 8–1 demonstrates that the nuclei are of low grade, being similar one to another and without demonstrated irregularity. The presence of necrosis and low-grade nuclei is indicative of a condition intermediate between well-developed comedo carcinoma and the usual ductal noncomedo carcinoma *in situ*. × 200

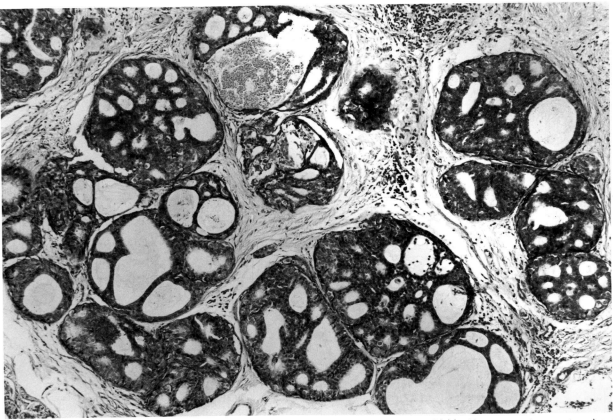

Figure 8–3. Here the extensiveness of change makes the diagnosis of ductal carcinoma *in situ* unavoidable. However, note some tapering of arches. This is cribriform ductal carcinoma *in situ.* × 75

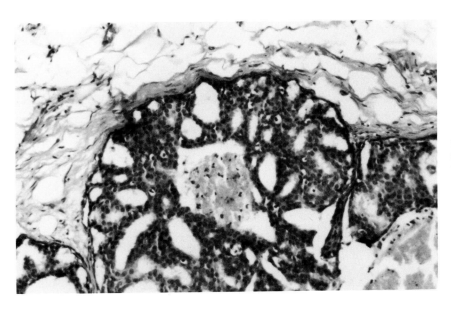

Figure 8–4. This example of DCIS is characterized by sinuous, interconnecting strands of hyperchromatic cells. Note few necrotic cells centrally. × 100

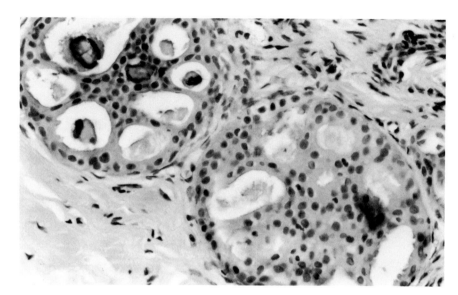

Figure 8–5. Rigid arches of a cribriform pattern variant of ductal carcinoma *in situ.* Note calcified material in central spaces is not indicative of cellular necrosis. × 225

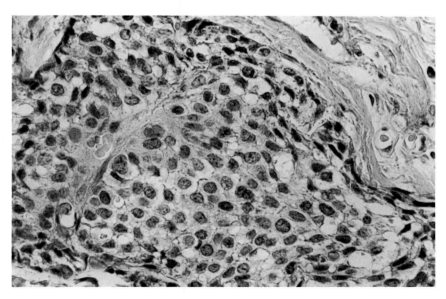

Figure 8–6. An example of a solid pattern variant of ductal carcinoma *in situ.* There are no evident intercellular spaces, and the slightly irregular placement of cells and sharply defined intercellular contours are not consistent with the lobular pattern of carcinoma *in situ.* × 450

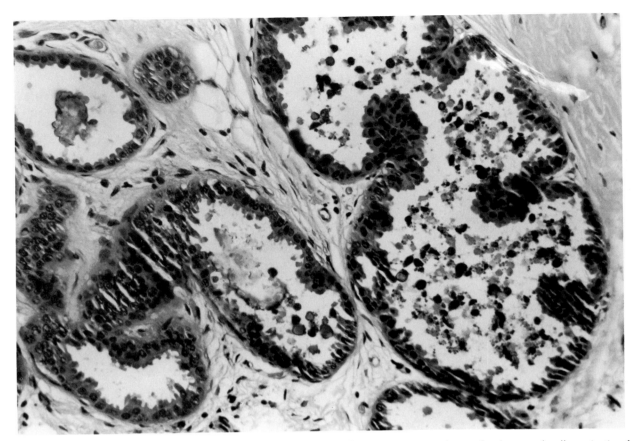

Figure 8–7. This example of micropapillary carcinoma *in situ* has small papillary projections made up of only several cells projecting from the intersurface of ductular spaces. Note that they are quite irregular and bulbous, with the area distant from the tether being broader than the base. Also notice extensive cellular necrosis with cellular debris and probably bits of calcified material present as well. × 175

The diagnostic criteria for recognition of non-comedo ductal carcinoma *in situ* of any of these patterns, and constructed to separate it from the atypical ductal hyperplasia (ADH) (Figs. 8–11 through 8–13) and related patterns noted in chapter 6 (Fig. 8–14), are as follows.

First, a uniform population of neoplastic-appearing cells should be present, completely populating at least two basement membrane–bound spaces.

Second, the classic geometric and sharply defined arches and punched-out secondary spaces defined by and present between the cells must be clearly and uniformly present. Note, micropapillary forms are also restricted as to form, involving a regularly repeating pattern of bulbous papillae. This also involves even or regular placement of the involved cells, necessitating the absence of the swirling or streaming patterns characteristic of usual florid hyperplasia.

Third, most examples have hyperchromatic nuclei. This is a helpful and not a mandatory feature of definition because it is occasionally absent in examples having the first two defining criteria. It is a feature helpful in identification of the small lesions on low-power scanning microscopy.

The solid type of DCIS is least common. The definitions listed previously also apply, except that there are no secondary spaces between the cells or the spaces are little larger than a single cell. The solid pattern is rarely present in pure form, but it frequently exists with cribriform foci or, more commonly, a very specific pattern of microglandular spaces. These are smaller than those of the cribriform pattern, and the bordering cells have a tendency to be oriented radially about the space in the manner of a rosette. In general, the presence of rosette-like cellular arrangements about intercellular spaces may be included within the diagnostic term "solid pattern," non-comedo DCIS. Also termed "endocrine" because of co-occurrence with apparent markers of endocrine or neuroendocrine differentiation,[7, 22] these cases are confined to a small area and are frequently incidental findings (i.e., not found by mammography).

One particularly valuable study has sought to accept the heterogeneity of histology and extent of disease in order to give guidelines for future clinical management as well as future studies.[68] Because the study is confined to correlates obtained with disease at mastectomy, it should be viewed in the context of the classic early studies of Lagios et al.[51] that reported serially sectioned mastectomy specimens. These study designs deal with concurrent disease and do not predict the evolution of clinical disease after biopsy alone. This statement may seem unnecessary and simplistic, but it is frequently unrecognized when such studies are cited. The heterogeneity of DCIS, at least in patterns present at time of

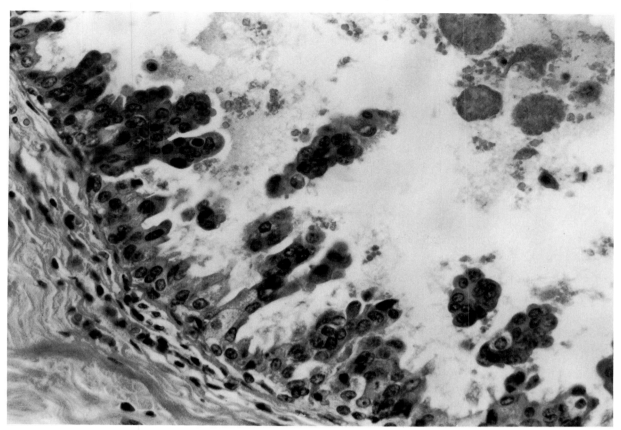

Figure 8–8. Micropapillary CIS with necrosis. Although some cells have lighter cytoplasm, the nuclear pattern is similar throughout. × 400

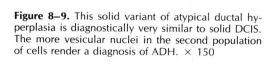

Figure 8–9. This solid variant of atypical ductal hyperplasia is diagnostically very similar to solid DCIS. The more vesicular nuclei in the second population of cells render a diagnosis of ADH. × 150

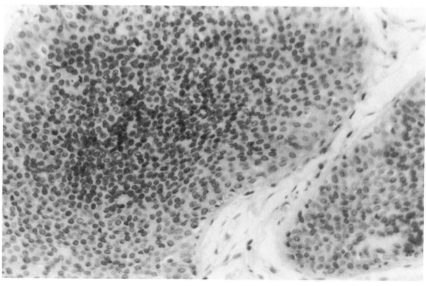

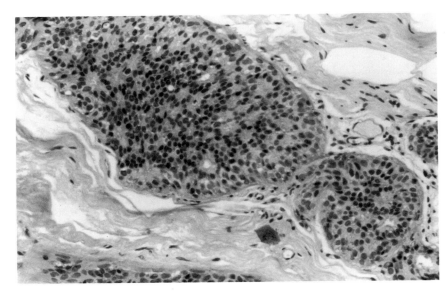

Figure 8–10. The microglandular or "endocrine" pattern of solid DCIS. × 150

initial diagnosis, is highlighted in the studies by Patchefsky et al.[68] This series is perhaps unusual in that 16 of 55 cases presented have foci of microinvasion, and the study identifies the patterns of *in situ* disease that are most frequently associated with microinvasion. Two of the 16 cases with foci of microinvasion also had lymph node metastasis involving only one or two lymph nodes. The method by which DCIS is detected is an important indicator of the extent of the lesion as determined by residual disease at subsequent mastectomy (Table 8–1) as well as the likelihood of microinvasion. Note from Table 8–2 that almost two thirds of the comedo carcinoma cases had minimal invasion, about one third of the micropapillary cases had associated minimal invasion, and none of the other types had associated minimal invasion. This favored association of the comedo carcinoma histologic pattern and large size with foci of microinvasion is also mirrored in the greater likelihood

of recurrence after treatment by partial mastectomy (see discussion of natural history). Note that specific and clearly presented criteria for microinvasion are not readily available, but disordered involvement of sclerotic lobules must be excluded, because microinvasion should indicate invasion into the interlobular stroma. In the absence of guidelines for measurement, we suggest that foci of invasion be recorded according to numbers of millimeters in extent.

Azzopardi has inaugurated a category of non-comedo carcinoma termed "clinging carcinoma."[8] As noted in the original description[9] other more completely developed patterns of DCIS may be present concurrently. We believe this pattern represents incompletely developed examples of DCIS in some form and that most of these cases can be included in the better developed cases of ADH as described in chapter 6. This contention is supported by natural history studies that have reported

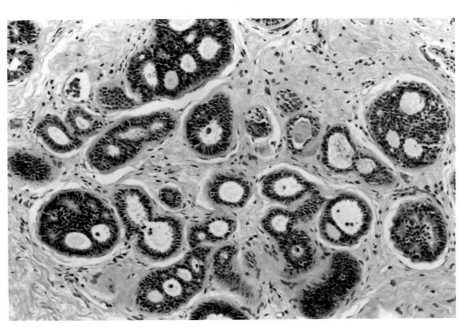

Figure 8–11. Low-power photograph demonstrating the full extent of the evidence supporting a diagnosis of atypical ductal hyperplasia. Note that there are only three or four spaces in which a central population of uniform cells may be seen. In the others, only narrow bars cross from one side to the other. Thus there are pattern and cell population features of ductal carcinoma *in situ*. However, in the three largest spaces involved, there are cells adjacent to the basement membrane that appear different, and thus a diagnosis of atypical ductal hyperplasia rather than ductal carcinoma *in situ* is made. × 75

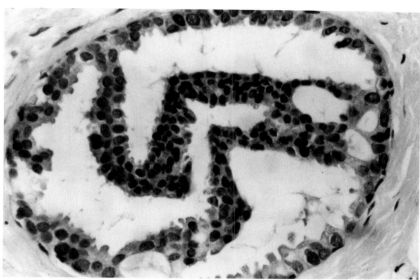

Figure 8–12. Atypical ductal hyperplasia with a dominant pattern of trabecular bars and without complete filling of the cells in this space by the hyperchromatic and neoplastic-appearing cellular population present in the bars. Note at the lower right a different population of cells with lighter nuclei and cytoplasmic staining. Although such central patterns may be found in cases otherwise fulfilling the diagnosis of ductal carcinoma *in situ* in other spaces, this incomplete filling of the basement membrane–bound space supports an atypical ductal hyperplasia diagnosis. × 400

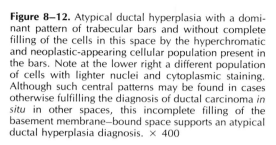

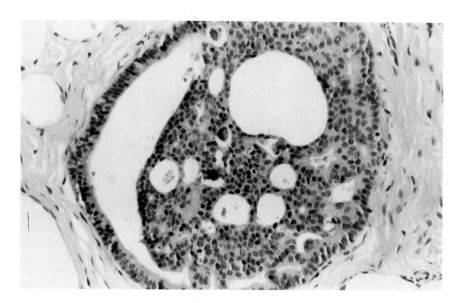

Figure 8–13. Photomicrograph exhibiting a detail of the polarization of luminal cells near the basement membrane that are quite different from the evenly placed and "suspicious" cells present in the central proliferation. This is atypical ductal hyperplasia. × 200

Figure 8–14. Collagenous spherulosis, a pattern sometimes confused with ADH or DCIS.[21] Note that the spaces are defined by a secreted material that may be seen faintly. The spaces are surrounded by a sparse population of cells that everywhere is tapered or thinned in its extent. Such a pattern is not recognized as atypical. × 150

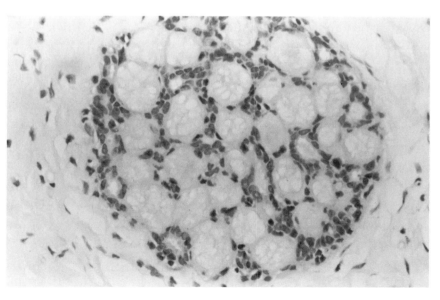

Table 8–1. DCIS PRESENTATION AND EXTENT

Method of Detection	Number of Cases	Avg. No. of Ducts	No. DCIS only	No. DCISM*	Residual†
Mammography	26	117	18	8	11
Incidental	10	7	10	0	0
Palpable Mass‡	19	110	11	8	13

*Ductal carcinoma *in situ* with minimal invasion.
†After mastectomy.
‡Also presenting with nipple signs.
From Patchefsky et al: Cancer 63:731–741, 1989.

a risk of subsequently developing carcinoma of four to five times that of the general population for patients with ADH[66] and those with clinging carcinoma.[29]

Mention has previously been made of intermediate categories of DCIS, particularly between non-comedo carcinoma and comedo carcinoma. Lagios et al. have approached this question by evaluating nuclei as well as cytoarchitecture and necrosis,[50] producing four categories of DCIS:

1. Comedo carcinoma
2. Cribriform with necrosis
3. Cribriform with anaplasia and rare or no necrosis
4. Uniform small cell type with delicate and cribriform and micropapillary architecture

Less than 20 percent of the DCIS cases reviewed by Lagios et al. were in the two intermediate categories, indicating that most DCIS cases may be placed clearly into comedo carcinoma or non-comedo carcinoma categories. Note that none of the 33 patients with the small-cell, non-comedo features had recurrence after local excision by tylectomy.[50]

An important associated condition of DCIS must be mentioned, but is covered in detail elsewhere. Paget's disease of the nipple is best regarded as an extension of subareolar DCIS to the nipple surface.[63] The associated disease within the breast is usually extensive and may even be invasive. However, between five percent and ten percent of patients with Paget's disease may have DCIS confined to the region of the nipple.[20, 52]

Mammographic Detection and Clinical Diagnosis

Mammographic detectability is a major concern in the management of DCIS. The fact that many examples of

Table 8–2. ASSOCIATIONS OF DCIS TYPE

Type of DCIS	Avg. No. ducts	% Microinvasion (No.)	% Multicentric (No.)
Comedo carcinoma	78	63 (12/19)	37 (7/19)
Micropapillary	198	30 (3/10)	80 (8/10)
Solid & Cribriform	20	0	27 (3/11)

From Patchefsky et al: Cancer 63:731–741, 1989.

DCIS are detectable by x-ray examination has produced a quantum leap in the frequency with which patients with this disease are detected. Prior to the widespread use of mammography, cases were only clinically detectable or incidentally discovered, but now mammographically detected cases are in the great majority. The mammographic patterns vary greatly[47] and are of importance in indicating extent of disease.[25, 61]

This ability of x-ray mammography to indicate the presence of DCIS is a direct result of the ability of these lesions to concentrate (or deposit) calcium salts in ductal and ductular locations between cells. These accretions are usually centered in the major lesion and associated with cellular debris. The latter association is itself closely allied to cellular necrosis and hence to the comedo carcinoma types of DCIS. Without calcification, there is no detectability; soft tissue deformity with noninvasive disease is rare, although it occasionally occurs.

Fortunately for the detectability of carcinoma *in situ*, calcification is not limited to the comedo carcinoma types in which it is best known and most frequent.[12, 60] The cribriform type of DCIS is also frequently associated with ductal calcifications, and these may be determinant because they are present wherever the disease is also present. This is a particularly important factor for the pathologist to document. The micropapillary type of DCIS may also have calcifications, but this is less common.

Few studies have been aimed directly at understanding the nature of calcification itself. The salts are usually hydroxyapatite or tricalcium phosphate and may contain other elements.[39]

In a recent screening series, 55 of 66 detected cases had microcalcification by mammography[6]; fibrosis with a disturbed architecture was present in seven cases. It should be noted that only 24 of these 66 cases were interpreted by the mammograph as probably or definitely malignant. Thus in many instances the mammographic pattern of calcification presented is not easily discriminated from patterns associated with benign disease. Some examples of DCIS will remain undetected by mammograms.[69]

Fine Needle Aspiration

In general, fine needle aspiration (FNA) should not be considered a reliable technique in the diagnosis of carcinoma *in situ*. In a great number of cases this technique is incapable of obtaining a diagnostic sample, thus producing many false-negative diagnoses. Also, the histologic patterns useful in the diagnosis of carcinoma *in situ* are not present in FNA samples, and misinterpretation of these cases as probably invasive may be frequent. Thus the most important consideration for FNA in carcinoma *in situ* is that both false-negative and false-positive (i.e., invasive) diagnoses are likely, necessitating careful correlation with clinical features.[78]

Natural History and Associated Disease

These subjects, including evolution to invasion and disease in the other breasts, are particularly difficult.

They may be pursued in a practical fashion as noted above if one accepts different postures or standpoints as follows:

1. Preceding disease, concurrent disease, and subsequent disease must be carefully separated and individually analyzed.

2. Clinically evident disease must be separated from focal or incidental disease.

Thus the cases designated as bilateral when there is a history of prior disease are misleading at least so far as clinical predictability is concerned. One study from the Medical College of Virginia[14] claims a certain percentage of bilaterality, but all but one case claimed as bilateral consisted of patients presenting with ductal carcinoma *in situ* who had a previous carcinoma in the other breast. These cases were documented predominantly before the use of mammography; only one patient out of 40 presented with a carcinoma in the contralateral breast after DCIS in the initial one. In another large investigation, the Connecticut tumor registry and the California tumor registry were utilized to determine the incidence of bilaterality.[89] That study demonstrated no greater incidence of later carcinoma in contralateral breast in patients with DCIS than in the general population.

Many of the avoidable pitfalls of accepting retrospective data without critical examination may be seen in the paper from the Medical College of Virginia.[14] The 52 cases originally diagnosed as DCIS became 40 cases on careful review. Eight of these cases were excluded as representing invasive disease. Without a targeted histologic re-review in such retrospective studies, we must assume that at least some cases recorded as ductal carcinoma *in situ* had focal invasion present originally. Also, the one patient after histologic re-review who had a solitary lymph node metastasis was also acknowledged to have had only two histologic sections taken from the ductal carcinoma *in situ*. This was acknowledged as a probably inadequate sample in order to rule out the possibility of invasive disease being present. Despite this, the abstract does not equivocate about one in 40 having nodal metastasis. The separate analysis of cases with microinvasion is strongly supported by the report of ten percent of such cases having axillary nodal metastases.[48]

What is the long-term outcome if a biopsy of breast tissue is performed, the specimen is found to contain a focus of DCIS, and the patient is not treated further? This is as close as we have been able to get to unraveling the natural history of DCIS. Thus the condition is identified at one point in time, and the evolution of disease may then be observed. This study design, an accident of the standard practice in the 1940s through the 1960s, allowed for the opportunity of small and incidental examples of DCIS to be undiagnosed at the time of biopsy and not further treated because they were not identified as carcinoma. Two remarkably similar studies have been carried out in this fashion;[10, 65] they are similar in case recruitment as well as outcome. Both studies involved small, non-comedo carcinoma examples, and the reproducibility of results is strong evidence of the reliability of this information. One study

was well under way when the second was published, and it is likely that the most important piece of information deriving from these studies was unexpected by either group. This fundamental fact is that later presentation of invasive carcinomas occurred locally in relation to the initial ductal carcinoma *in situ*. Thus this is a focal process and is likely amenable to extirpative surgery. It is likely that the end result of 25 percent to 30 percent incidence of developing invasive carcinomas would have been larger if biopsies had not been done. The biopsy procedure probably completely removed some lesions and may have interrupted the natural history of others.

In the largest series of patients treated by planned local excision without radiation, large size and comedo carcinoma type indicated a greater likelihood of local recurrence.[50] Determination of size was accomplished in this study by measuring the maximum extent of the lesions in a three-dimensional reconstruction of the sequentially embedded segments. However, even if this approach is used, postoperative mammographic examination is recommended. Lesions larger than 25 mm in maximum extent are most likely to recur. Very small lesions (less than 1 cm) can be determined with a less careful approach to measurement, but larger and definitive resections will demand very careful attention to the extent of the lesion and relationship to resection margins.

We can conclude that the natural history of this disease is not known, but by combining the information from concurrent mastectomy studies and follow-up after biopsy or regional excision,[10, 17, 50, 65, 76] we have the following guidelines:

1. After biopsy containing ductal carcinoma *in situ*, a mastectomy subsequently performed will be free of disease about 50 percent of the time, depending on size and method of detection.

2. If, after biopsy showing DCIS, no further surgery is done, slightly more than 25 percent of women develop invasive carcinoma in the same locality (Table 8–3).

3. We can conclude, as a good possibility and useful theoretical construct, that if 50 percent of women treated only by biopsy have foci of DCIS left behind, then one half of these foci do not evolve into clinically evident cancer.

4. Prior to the use of mammography, most later presenting cancers were invasive and occurred within 10 years of initial biopsy (Table 8–3). Most later presenting cancers after planned local excision and follow-up by mammography are noninvasive.[6, 15, 36, 50]

Comedo Carcinoma *In Situ*

Comedo carcinoma *in situ* has long been recognized and diagnosed as carcinoma and was treated by mastectomy at least as early as the 1890s. Prior to mammography, it constituted most examples of CIS, and by the 1930s[11] was recognized as a special type of breast cancer. The greater association of comedo carcinoma *in situ* with a palpable mass, usual greater extension in the breast, frequent association with microinvasive foci,[41] and occasional reports of lymph node involvement in

Table 8–3. PATIENTS WITH SUBSEQUENT INVASIVE CARCINOMA AFTER "INCIDENTAL" DCIS

Age	Location of Biopsy	Location of Infiltrative Carcinoma	Interval to Invasive Carcinoma (yr)	Size of Lesion	Lymph Nodes	Survival
33	LUOQ	Left massive	3	Massive	Positive	2 yr
38	RUOQ	RUOQ	7	2.5 cm	Negative	Living with disease 6 yr later
44	LUOQ	LUOQ	10	3 cm	Positive	3 yr
53	RUOQ	RUOQ	4	Unknown	Positive	1 yr
60	RUOQ	RLOQ	3	2 cm	Negative	Died of lymphoma 15 yr later
63	LUOQ	LUOQ	6	2 cm	Positive	Died of CVA 20 yr later
74	RUOQ	RUOQ	10	2.5 cm	(Simple mastectomy)	Died of heart disease 2 yr later

Abbreviations: CVA = cerebrovascular accident; LUOQ = left upper outer quadrant; RLOQ = right lower outer quadrant; RUOQ = right upper outer quadrant.
From Page et al: Cancer 49:751–758, 1982.

the axilla demonstrate its greater magnitude of clinical presence and menace compared with other types of CIS.

Incidence is usually presented as a percentage of cases diagnosed as carcinoma. Prior to the frequent use of mammography, about one percent to two percent of breast cancers were DCIS,[63, 73, 79] and most of these were of the comedo carcinoma type.[79] Their incidence in the general population is probably similar in the 1980s, but the lesion size is generally smaller, a reflection of earlier detection by both mammography and physical examination.

The firmness and resultant palpability with which such lesions often present clinically is the result of expanding preformed spaces with cells that are denser and more firm than the surrounding fat. Also there is frequently a fibrous reaction around the involved spaces. Thus a palpable mass as well as a mammographically dense lesion is produced.

In removed specimens, a gross cross section will reveal dots of 0.5 to 2 mm in diameter of pultaceous material rising from the cut surface. Their appearance is reminiscent of the common comedo, thus the name given to this lesion. They consist of necrotic debris present centrally in involved spaces. There is a great range in size from a few dots of focal disease in some mammogram-detected cases to diffuse disease present through much of the breast.

Of course, detection of smaller lesions must be aided by localization techniques using clinical and specimen radiography. These x-ray–produced images are frequently useful, because the necrotic material that gives these lesions their name is frequently calcified, or at least partially so.

The cells around the fields of intraluminal necrosis have no particular pattern but are usually large and irregularly placed and have very bizarre nuclear patterns. In many examples, few cell layers are present surrounding the basement membrane area, but in others, thick layers of cells may be present and may demonstrate, at least focally, the patterns of micropapillary or cribriform carcinoma *in situ*.

Most examples of comedo carcinoma *in situ* have frequent foci of necrosis (Figs. 8–15 to 8–19). However, there are also a great number of cases, usually detected by mammography, in which necrosis is present only focally in the lesion. Elsewhere the lesion is otherwise characteristic of solid or cribriform ductal carcinoma *in situ*. The work of Lagios et al.[50] has attempted to stratify these cases on the basis of nuclear atypia. Thus, despite the presence of necrosis, these cases would be separated from fully developed comedo carcinoma with its characteristic high-grade and bizarre nuclear patterns.

There are some cases recorded of local therapy of palpable comedo carcinoma disease.[40, 56] These are few, because the standard treatment for this condition for decades has been mastectomy, and when local extirpation was attempted, there was more than a 50 percent recurrence with invasive disease within 3 years. Note the striking difference in percentage, occurrence, and temporal evolution of disease from the non-comedo carcinoma cases described previously.

The extent of disease is not independent of histologic pattern, as comedo carcinoma cases tend to be the largest. However, there are cases in which the comedo carcinoma lesion may be very small, and the less bizarre examples of non-comedo carcinoma lesions may be fairly large. Size itself is positively associated with foci of microinvasion. Both Lagios et al.[51] and Carter and Smith[19] have recorded a greater incidence of microinvasion in cases involving lesions greater than 2.5 cm in maximum extent.

Encysted Papillary Carcinoma

Encysted papillary carcinoma is one of the most valuable recent additions to the diagnostic armamentarium in neoplastic breast disease. Here histologic staging

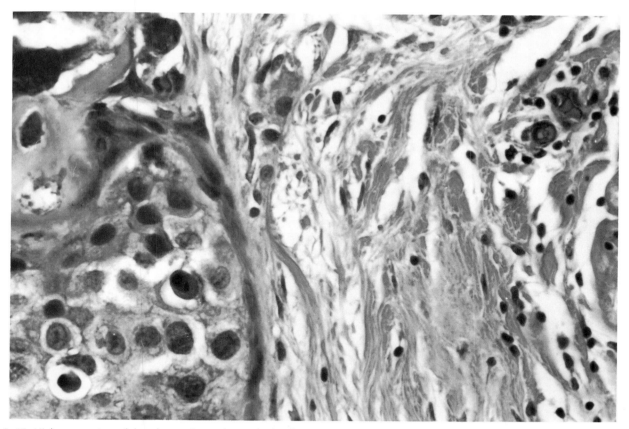

Figure 8–15. High-power view of ductal comedo carcinoma *in situ* demonstrating necrosis in the upper left hand corner. Note also that the stroma is altered about this area, which occurs frequently in this type of carcinoma *in situ.* × 700

and category of alteration are combined to give a clear indication of acceptable therapeutic options. Here lie the best current examples of the utility of histologic subcategorization in breast disease. The classic paper of Kraus and Neubecker[49] on papillary carcinoma is, in retrospect, an excellent example of the failure of the grouping together of various histologic elements rather than the reductionist approach in the understanding of neoplastic mammary disease. Focal areas of stromal invasion were included as one of the many histologic cues to malignancy, because the paper was produced at a time when cancer was perceived to be a yes or no proposition. In the attempt to clarify a very complex situation, there was no separate analysis of which features (including stromal invasion) were associated with the few cited[49] examples of lymph node metastases. This situation was clarified by the paper of Carter et al.[18] that introduced the concept of encysted papillary carcinoma and produced a clear conclusion: in the absence of adjacent DCIS in neighboring ducts, local excision of these lesions was curative. This is a very valuable study, because most of the women with these lesions are older (late post-menopausal), and avoidance of major surgical procedures in such patients will probably save more lives than will mastectomy.

Terminologic concerns are unavoidable in this area. Papillary carcinoma, not otherwise specified, may indicate an invasive process,[32, 35] and prior to the 1980s meant a very mixed group of lesions as indicated pre-

viously. The classic paper by Carter et al.[18] has produced critical follow-up information allowing prognostic stratification of these lesions. The notation of "papillary" indicates that these lesions are characterized by fibrovascular cores associated with the proliferating epithelium (Fig. 8–20). This must be differentiated from the "micropapillary" pattern discussed previously. The terms "noninvasive" and "intracystic" used to qualify papillary carcinoma should be understood to be largely synonymous with the latter (intracystic), indicating local confinement. If, however, DCIS extends beyond the local area, later recurrence after local excision is likely.[18]

Tumor Markers

Tumor markers and other nonhistologic indicators of these lesions are few but promising. Evaluation of genetic material by quantitating DNA per nucleus produces an indicator of gross genetic alteration. This information is reported as aneuploidy or diploidy depending on whether the normal (diploid) amount of genetic material is present. The aneuploid cases are more likely to be associated with foci of invasion.[16, 24] It is likely that the bizarre nuclei characteristic of comedo carcinoma are also very closely associated with aneuploidy, but this has not been carefully studied. Norris et al.[62] utilized Feulgen measurement of nuclear DNA and morphometry to separate DCIS lesions from atypi-

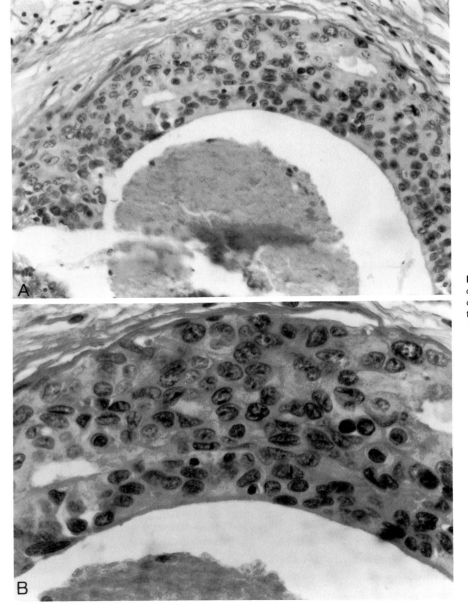

Figure 8–16. Two photographs from the same area of comedo carcinoma demonstrating central necrosis and a sufficiently varied nuclear population to support a diagnosis of comedo carcinoma. *A,* × 200; *B,* × 400.

cal hyperplasias without complete success. At best, 69 percent of well-differentiated DCIS lesions (probably non-comedo carcinoma) could be distinguished from atypical hyperplasia using a combination of DNA content and nuclear perimeter measurements.

The *erb-B-2 (Neu)* oncogene has been studied,[87] revealing that 42 percent of 45 cases of carcinoma *in situ* had overexpression of this oncogene. Of particular interest to the subtyping of CIS is the finding that all such cases with overexpression had comedo carcinoma microscopic features.

Both Norris et al.[62] and Carpenter et al.[16] have studied the cellular DNA content for the determination of aneuploidy or diploidy of the lesions in question. Carpenter et al.[16] utilized Feulgen staining of disaggregated tissue sections and classified the resulting histograms as diploid or aneuploid. Comparing proliferative atypia

(examples of atypical hyperplasia) with examples of ductal carcinoma *in situ* revealed no major differences between the two, although the number of cases were small. Roughly one third in each category were aneuploid. Almost 90 percent of cases of ductal carcinoma *in situ* associated with microinvasion were aneuploid, and the majority of cases in which the invasive component was analyzed were also aneuploid. However, four cases (25 percent) of microinvasive carcinomas had only diploid cells, whereas the adjacent *in situ* component of DCIS was aneuploid.

Thymidine labeling studies that indicate cell cycle kinetics, or at least the percentage of cells in the process of DNA synthesis, have also supported a stratification of different histologic types of carcinoma *in situ*.[59] The comedo carcinoma *in situ* cases had a labeling index of more than twice that of other lesions. The solid variant

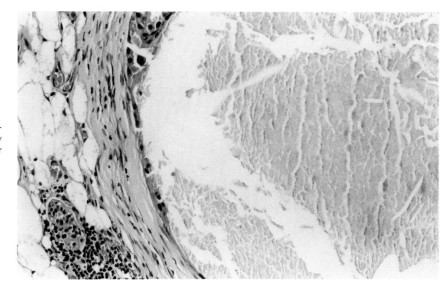

Figure 8–17. Occasionally cellular necrosis in comedo carcinoma *in situ* is so extensive that very few atypical cells remain. Indeed, the necrosis may appear to extend to the basement membrane. × 125

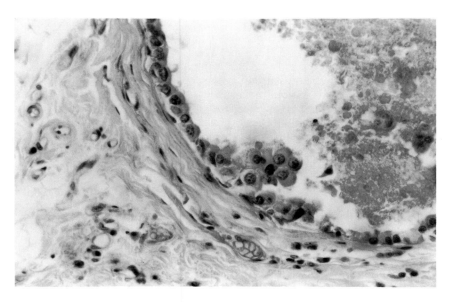

Figure 8–18. Photomicrograph from an area at the periphery of a comedo carcinoma *in situ*. There are probably some normal and reactive cells intermixed with the few cells of comedo carcinoma. The extensive flocculated, necrotic material should raise concern about the possibility of a diagnosis of comedo carcinoma *in situ*. × 250

Figure 8–19. Characteristic of more advanced and comedo carcinoma type examples of ductal carcinoma *in situ* is the spread of highly atypical cells into lobular units. Here this phenomenon of so-called "cancerization of lobules" is demonstrated. × 200

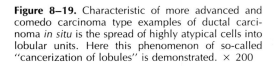

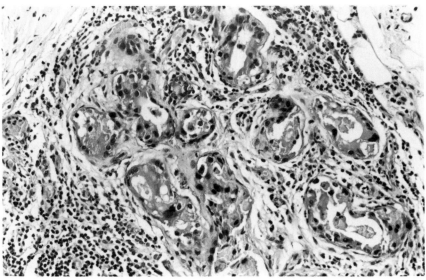

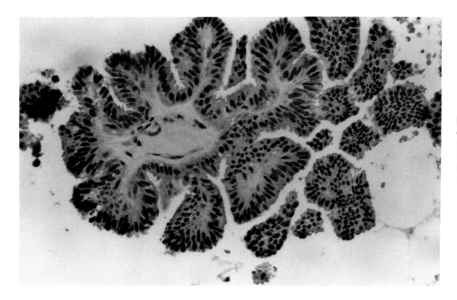

Figure 8–20. The presence of tall and hyperchromatic cells surmounting these papillary fronds supports the possibility of a diagnosis of encysted papillary carcinoma. Usually the epithelium is much more atypical and closely mimics that found in other ductal carcinoma *in situ* patterns. × 125

of non-comedo carcinoma *in situ* is rarely discussed in the literature but was one of the categories in the cell kinetics studies of Meyer.[59] With a low cellular growth fraction, the solid DCIS lesions were similar to other non-comedo carcinoma lesions.

DCIS: Summary

It must be emphasized that the diagnosis of ductal carcinoma *in situ*, not otherwise specified, relays very little information. The presenting lesion could be minuscule (i.e., less than a millimeter in diameter) and may in some systems of nomenclature be called atypical ductal hyperplasia. On the other hand, the lesion may be a palpable mass of comedo DCIS measuring more than 5 cm in diameter. The former has been demonstrated to confer a somewhat greater increased risk of subsequent carcinoma development and is discussed in chapters 6 and 14. The latter has long been recognized as a clear threat to life, although lymph node metastases at the time of detection are few. In the presence of a fairly large area of induration, the biopsy of only a portion showing extensive ductal comedo carcinoma *in situ* is associated with a fairly high incidence of foci of invasion elsewhere in the breast. The predictability and size of the initial biopsy specimen as well as the findings remaining within the breast will be the ultimate determinates of therapeutic decision making. With treatment failure being rare, several options are evident. Therapeutic trials are in progress, although many physicians have already embraced local excision with or without radiotherapy as an acceptable approach to the smaller lesions.[50]

Behind all of this diversity lies the fact that DCIS is, by definition, a noninvasive disease. Treatment failure is unusual even in the more marked examples of this group of conditions.[31, 43, 82] The comparison of treatment modalities by different means, combined with the heterogeneity of these conditions, produces a great difficulty in accruing a sufficient number of cases to ascertain the most acceptable form of treatment.

Much of the confusion enshrouding DCIS can be relieved by a redefinition which recognizes the different types and varying extent of disease. These patterns and their various natural histories will need to be further verified. However, the application of recent knowledge to prior studies allows us to arrive at a consistent interpretation of the probable natural history of the majority of these lesions and thus accrue consistent information. Although several recent reviews of this subject report a lack of knowledge, in fact the amount of knowledge we have on the different lesions of DCIS is much more certain than that which we have on others in which therapeutic certainty is thought to be available. The major complexity here is the diversity of therapeutic options, compounded by the fact that treatment failure is rare with any modality.

Small lesions (i.e., less than 3 to 4 mm) without the cytologic or necrotic character of comedo carcinoma are adequately treated by local therapy. It is also quite clear that when the comedo-type disease extends through most of two quadrants of the breast that a mastectomy is mandated because of frequent (over 50 percent) incidence of treatment failure after local excision (see below). Treating lesions in the intermediate area between these two extremes is the current challenge, and it must be understood that patient involvement in the decision making is essential. Continued analysis of different types of DCIS with the outcomes for different therapies is an immediate and continuing challenge.

LOBULAR CARCINOMA *IN SITU*

Terminology and Anatomical Pathology

The term "lobular carcinoma *in situ*" (LCIS) was coined and supported by Foote and Stewart[37] in 1941. This term is the preferred one, although "lobular neoplasia" has been appropriately and advantageously used to include both more intense or extensive examples of this phenomenon as well as lesser ones.[45]

Foote and Stewart's paper[37] did not discuss lesser examples of this phenomenon, an approach used subsequently in related papers from the same institution.[57, 77] Note that the category of atypical lobular hyperplasia (ALH) as discussed in chapter 6 was specifically instituted in order to place diagnostic boundaries on this spectrum of lobular neoplastic change. The difference in these approaches is highlighted in the following discussion.

The terminology of *lobular carcinoma in situ* (LCIS) and *atypical lobular hyperplasia* (ALH) is maintained here largely because of the dominance of the term "LCIS" in the literature and because ALH recognizes a lesser risk of invasive cancer. We would agree with the use of *lobular neoplasia* (LN) when discussing both atypical lobular hyperplasia and lobular carcinoma *in situ* in combination. We do hold with the notion that the full impact of the term "carcinoma" on many physicians who do not understand the special natural history of LCIS and ALH is avoided by the utilization of the diagnostic term "atypical lobular hyperplasia" for lesser examples of this phenomenon.

It is unfortunate that the word "carcinoma" remains in the diagnostic term "lobular carcinoma *in situ.*" Consistency is fostered by maintaining a well-understood entity, but we support the idea held by many others that LCIS is primarily a marker of increased risk.[1, 3, 46, 54] Whatever the theoretical bias, the unique biology of this entity (Table 8–4) must be accepted.[38]

A comment about the source of the term "lobular" should be made. The original describers[37] assumed that these lesions arose within the terminal and presumably functional portions of the breast, and thus the term "lobular" was used in contrast to the term "duct." Whether this dichotomy is actually true in all of its aspects is highly questionable. However, there is a close association between a specific pattern of infiltrating carcinoma (infiltrating lobular carcinoma) and these *in situ* patterns. Indeed, when single cell infiltration pattern of infiltrating lobular carcinoma (LC) is seen, the 60 percent to 70 percent incidence of coexisting lobular carcinoma *in situ* originally demonstrated by Foote and Stewart[37] has been consistent in later reports.[26] This association as a pattern and consistent co-occurrence should be seen as the backdrop and hallmark for these conditions.

The *anatomical pathology* of lobular carcinoma *in situ* is confined to a discussion of microscopy, because it is recognized microscopically only and is invisible to the naked eye as tissue is examined. There seems to be a positive association with local calcification,[71] but this is seldom within the foci of LCIS.

The histologic definition of lobular carcinoma *in situ* involves the presence of a lobular unit with its cluster of ductules or acini filled, distorted, and distended by cells of a characteristic pattern (Figs. 8–21 through 8–25). This has remained unchanged from the original description.[37] The nuclei are usually regularly rounded and are often but not always hyperchromatic. The nuclear chromatinic pattern is quite regular and never bizarre. The cytoplasm tends to be somewhat clear and frequently has clear vacuoles somewhat displacing the nucleus (Fig. 8–23). This last feature may be regarded as a helpful but not mandatory marker for both *in situ* and invasive lobular carcinoma. There is a remarkable similarity in cellular appearance and in the distance between individual cells without a discernable repeating pattern of cell placement. The evaluation of an area with the appearance of LCIS involves searching for the presence of intercellular spaces as well as the degree and extensiveness of distortion and distention of the involved acinar spaces. Lesser examples (ALH, chapter 6) of this phenomenon (Fig. 8–22) may be reproducibly separated from the fully developed examples by utilizing the following criterion: when more than 50 percent of the acini of a lobular unit have the complete criteria for the diagnosis, then lobular carcinoma *in situ* is diagnosed. This is true whether only one lobular unit is involved or many. The recognition of full distortion and distention is demonstrated in Figures 8–21 through 8–25. Note that we take the normal component of an acinus to be four cells in diameter from basement membrane to opposite basement membrane. This cell component of the acinar diameter should be at least five or six before distention is considered to be present.

The presence of clear vacuoles in the cytoplasm of cells of lobular neoplasia is a helpful marker.[5] Both these vacuoles and the uniformity of cytologic features are largely common to *in situ* and invasive disease (Fig. 8–25), a particularly important point when evaluating cytologic samples from fine needle aspiration specimens.[78] These cytoplasmic spaces are quite crisply defined with hematoxylin and eosin and are usually completely clear. Sometimes a small dot may be seen in the center of the larger, otherwise clear spaces. Electron microscopy demonstrates that these are lined by the same structures that normally line the lumen. Thus these vacuoles are often termed "intracytoplasmic lumina." The combined stain for neutral and acidic mucosubstances, Alcian blue and PAS, demonstrates these structures most clearly. Their frequent presence is virtually confined to examples of lobular neoplasia, although there are some examples of ductal pattern neoplasia that also have mucous globules in the cytoplasm.[33] Occasional demonstration of these vacuoles may be seen

Table 8–4. FEATURES OF LOBULAR CARCINOMA *IN SITU*

Multifocal, multicentric, bilateral

Decreasing incidence after menopause

Nonpalpable, incidental even to mammography
Indicates high risk of subsequent invasive carcinoma
    Relative risk: 8 to 11 times that of the general population
    Absolute risk: 20 to 25 percent in 15 years after diagnosis

Coexistence with infiltrating carcinoma of special types in increased frequency: lobular and tubular

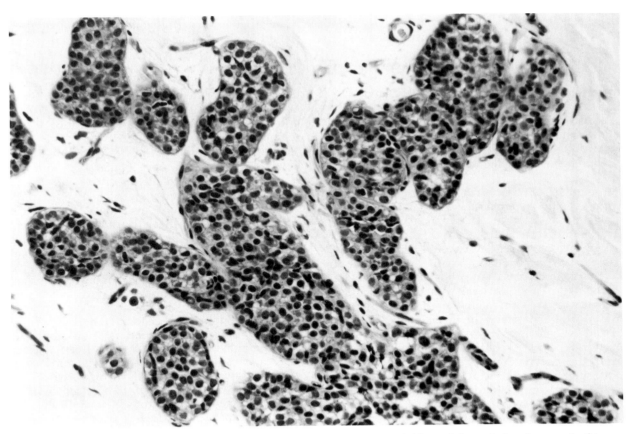

Figure 8–21. An example of lobular carcinoma *in situ* showing complete distention and filling of the majority of spaces in this area by the characteristic population of cells. × 200

in other situations; when rare, the presence of mucosubstances may actually indicate some form of degeneration. Thus, when present only rarely, vacuoles should not be regarded as diagnostic of any variant of lobular neoplasia.

Multicentricity is a prime feature of LCIS, with many cases having the disease demonstrable by biopsy in the contralateral breast at the time of initial diagnosis.[74] It is probable that the more extensive the disease in one part of the breast, the more likely it is to be extensive throughout other parts of either breast,[84] but that has yet to be proven in prospective studies.

In summary, a well-developed or "classic" case of LCIS would contain characteristic and similar cells throughout the majority of the acinar or ductular spaces of a lobular unit. The presence of apparent intercellular spaces and lack of apparent distention of involved spaces as well as intermixture of other cell types would support a diagnosis of atypical lobular hyperplasia rather than lobular carcinoma *in situ*. These diagnostic histologic criteria may be cited as follows:

1. The characteristic uniform cells must comprise the entire population of cells in the lobular unit.

2. All the acini (terminal ductules) must be filled (no interspersed, intercular spaces between cells).

3. There must be expansion and/or distortion of at least one half the acini in the lobular unit.

Involvement of solitary or apparent ductal spaces by a similar cell population may present specific difficulties in differential diagnosis. This spread within ducts was called "pagetoid" in the original description,[37] and this term has continued in clinical use. The characteristic cells with benign-appearing nuclei may be present, undermining a seemingly normal population of luminal cells, with the latter tending to be flattened. When well developed, these alterations may be recognized as either mural (when they are confined to the area adjacent to the wall of the ductal space) or solid (if they fill the entire space).[30] Although these patterns of ductal involvement are seen in the great majority of cases of lobular carcinoma *in situ*,[33] it is still a specific diagnostic problem when such patterns are present in less well developed form without characteristic changes in the lobular unit. It is the practice of most to follow a careful sampling of all the tissue available in order to establish more characteristic changes within the lobular units.[58] This approach has been advocated by Wheeler and Enterline in an excellent general discussion of lobular neoplasia including invasive disease.[91] Note here that the term "pagetoid" is particularly appropriate, as it designates a change similar to that seen in Paget's disease, although the cells in the pagetoid change tend to have continuity and are not distributed singly or in small groups interspersed within the "foreign" epithelium in which they reside (as is seen in Paget's disease of the nipple).

Involvement of lobular units by a more varied population of cells characteristic of ductal carcinoma *in situ*

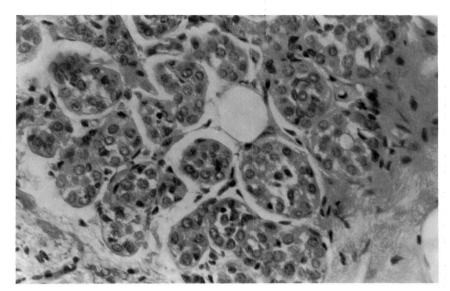

Figure 8–22. Portion of a lobular unit demonstrating some distention and little filling of the involved acini. This is atypical lobular hyperplasia. × 300

presents an important, although unusual, differential diagnostic problem. This pattern has been termed "cancerization of lobules" by Azzopardi.[8] Usually more characteristic ductal carcinoma *in situ* is present, and the differential diagnosis is relatively easy. However, any time that lobular units are distended, distorted, and filled by a group of more pleomorphic cells than is characteristic for lobular carcinoma *in situ,* a consideration should be given to the fact that the ductal pattern disease may be present.

Cells characteristic of lobular neoplasia may be seen in fibroadenomas. This condition is relatively uncommon but is of sufficient occurrence to demand citation. Indeed, the majority of cases described in the literature as "carcinoma" within fibroadenomas have been LCIS.[70] Characteristic lobular involvement is not usually present, because fibroadenomas usually lack lobules, but the extensiveness of the cellular population characteristic of LCIS usually makes the diagnosis relatively easy.

The discussion of microscopic pathology of lobular carcinoma *in situ* is not complete unless it mentions the necessity of searching with care for the possibility of invasive disease when the *in situ* disease is present. It has been known for as long as lobular disease has been diagnosed that the infiltrative type of lobular carcinoma may be very subtle. Presence of very few invasive cells in a single line is a pattern that the surgical pathologist should be aware of and sensitive to. It should be consciously searched for in situations of *in situ* disease because it is more often seen in this setting.

Incidence

Although we assume a female dominance in all breast malignancy, this is particularly true with LCIS. Even the 100:1 female-male ratio that exists for breast carcinoma in general is not present in LCIS. This disease is virtually nonexistent in males despite occasional case reports that are suggestive.

Because the diagnosis of LCIS is incidental to the obtaining of tissue for some other indication, the determination of precise incidence figures is difficult. The disease is clinically and largely mammographically silent.

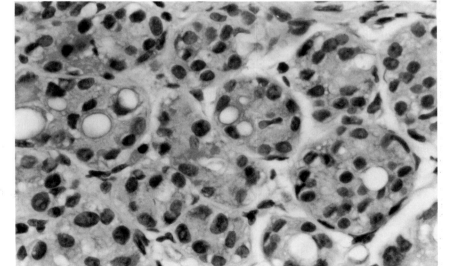

Figure 8–23. The vacuoles or globules in the cytoplasm are characteristic of lobular neoplasia. Note that some of the cells have the appearance of signet ring cells. × 400

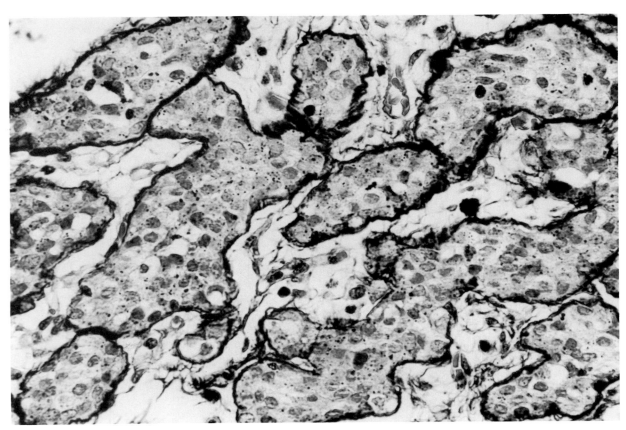

Figure 8–24. This example of lobular carcinoma *in situ* has been stained with a variant of the methenamine silver stain. Note that the basement membrane demonstrated by the black precipitate surrounds all the collections of cells. Silver also decorates the cytoplasm but is of unknown significance here. × 350

Most examples probably remain clinically silent because only about 25 percent of women diagnosed at biopsy go on to develop invasive carcinoma. Thus many who go undiagnosed at the stage of lobular carcinoma *in situ* die of some other disease, and LCIS remains undetected. Also, because the great majority of LCIS diagnoses are made in premenopausal women, there is a strong presumption that many LCIS lesions recede after menopause.[38]

It should also be realized that if there is no positive association of lobular carcinoma *in situ* with any other indicator for biopsy, then the incidence in any population undergoing biopsy would reflect the incidence in the general population. Thus if one percent to two percent of otherwise benign breast biopsy specimens have LCIS, then a similar incidence may be present in the general population.[9]

The apparent incidence of LCIS has changed during the past two or three decades primarily because of (1) the greater use of mammography and some slight association of LCIS with calcification; (2) a greater tendency for suspicious breast lesions to undergo biopsy, leading to a much greater number of biopsies performed; and (3) greater awareness of the importance of grossly invisible lesions and the much more complete and thorough sectioning of tissue sections by surgical pathologists in the past 10 to 12 years.

Another major consideration in determining the in-

cidence of LCIS is the variability of diagnostic criteria. Incidence figures approximating 2.5 percent have been found for all biopsies of the breast performed during a defined period of time.[42, 55] In retrospective series, particularly those done when multiple sections of benign breast biopsy specimens were not taken, the incidence should be lowered, because the amount of tissue sampled determines the incidence of this lesion in the biopsy population.[2, 23, 53] Both higher[92] and lower[80] incidences have been reported. Note that the incidence of lobular neoplasia in a classic series reported by Haagensen et al.[45] is quite a bit higher than that reported by Rosen et al.[75] A possible reason for the difference between these two series is that lesser examples of this phenomenon, otherwise diagnosed as atypical lobular hyperplasia, are included within the designation for lobular neoplasia used by Haagensen et al.[45] This contention at least provides some consistency to the observations, since other studies have demonstrated a lesser degree of risk of subsequent breast carcinoma with the atypical lobular hyperplasia lesions.[66]

As is true for other malignant-associated lesions of the breast as well as well-developed carcinomas, the incidence of LCIS is slightly higher in the left breast.[38] The incidence of LCIS is also more common in those areas in which there is the greatest amount of breast tissue (e.g., the central subareolar portion and the upper outer quadrant).[62]

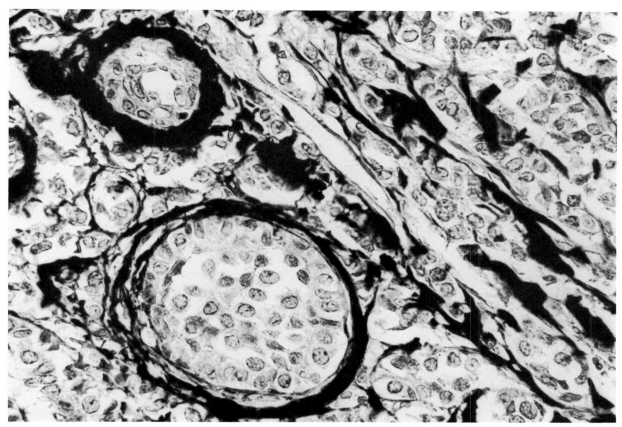

Figure 8–25. A methenamine silver stain demonstrates basement membrane around two *in situ* collections of lobular type cells. The infiltrating component of a mixed or pleomorphic lobular type is also demonstrated. Note the similarity of the nuclei in the *in situ* and infiltrating portions, which are all of low grade. × 350

The average age at detection of LCIS is 45 years. This is also the age for peak occurrence of benign breast lesions. However, based on the percentage of biopsies performed, LCIS decreases rapidly in incidence after menopause,[45, 46, 54, 75] which indicates that more than 90 percent of women with lobular carcinoma *in situ* as diagnosed at biopsy are premenopausal. The decreasing incidence as a percentage of biopsies performed after menopause indicates that at least some, if not many, of these lesions actually resolve or at least remain stable after menopause.[38] The reasons for this are unknown.

Multicentricity and Bilaterality

It is a well-accepted truism that of all breast lesions associated with malignancy (not including such changes as cysts), LCIS has the greatest indications of multicentricity and bilaterality. However, considerations of multicentricity and bilaterality should take into account the nature of the evidence. Specifically, concurrent demonstration of disease is less important as a predictor than is evidence obtained in follow-up studies. *In situ* or invasive disease, focal or multiple, at the time of initial diagnosis is very different and less relevant information for clinical management than is the information gained from following women after biopsy alone to see what the clinical evolution of disease might be. Most impor-

tantly, the end points of mortality and morbidity are more impelling evidence than the appearance of clinically occult disease that may remain so. However, if breast tissue is left in a woman with a diagnosis of lobular carcinoma *in situ,* then the risk of breast cancer occurring in that remaining tissue is increased over that of comparable breast tissue in women in the general population.

It is not the intent of management of lobular carcinoma *in situ* to necessarily be concerned with the multicentricity and bilaterality when the above comment is accepted. In any case, if lobular carcinoma *in situ* is found at the biopsy, the likelihood that there will be some foci remaining within the breast is somewhat over 50 percent, and the likelihood that there will be some remaining in the opposite breast if it is extensively biopsied approaches 50 percent.[74]

One of the most important studies of lobular carcinoma *in situ*[62] indicated that about 90 percent of all foci of lobular carcinoma *in situ* are found in the nipple and the upper outer quadrant. This determination may be somewhat altered by the changes that occur in breast tissue with postmenopausal involution.

Incidence of Coexisting Invasive Disease

If a mastectomy is performed soon after a diagnosis of LCIS, invasive disease may be concurrently present within the breast. This is less likely with the use of mammography and its greater sensitivity for detection of small lesions than it was in the premammography era. It is also important to note that many reports addressing these problems have excluded patients who had coincident invasive cancer. Indeed, this was part of the study design of one large follow-up study of carcinoma in situ[28, 65] in which any patient presenting with invasive disease within 6 months of the initial indicator biopsy was excluded from the analysis. This study design is occasioned by a desire to indicate predictability. Some of the cases in which later invasive disease became clinically evident would have had that invasive disease in occult form at the time of initial biopsy demonstrating LCIS. Thus at this time we can only record the experience of coincident invasive carcinoma from the premammography era. None of these series is very large, and the incidence range for a contralateral mastectomy specimen varies from zero to 13 percent. Carter and Smith found that three of 49 patients (six percent) with LCIS had invasive disease at mastectomy.[19] The combined series of Benfield et al.[9a] and Dall'Olmo et al.[23] found no evidence of invasive disease in a total of 36 patients. In a series of only 16 patients reported by Ringberg et al.[72] two patients (13 percent) had invasive carcinoma concurrently with LCIS at biopsy. This is counterbalanced by the larger series of Rosen et al.[76] in which two of 50 (4 percent) of patients had concurrent invasive disease.

We must conclude that there is a real but low risk that invasive disease is present in minimal form at the time of LCIS diagnosis and that the invasive disease might well be of the invasive lobular pattern with its attendant subtle presentation on mammography. There is also the possibility of coexisting invasive disease on the contralateral side, but this risk is apparently even lower. In the paper by Rosen et al.,[74] which recorded the results of sampling of the contralateral breast, there was an incidence of about ten percent (six of 63 biopsy specimens taken from the contralateral breast) of invasive carcinoma on the contralateral side. Note that patients who did not undergo biopsy did not have suspicious clinical findings. These results correspond to those reported by Urban[86] from the same medical center, in which ten of 26 patients with LCIS on one side had a positive biopsy result on the contralateral side, with invasive carcinoma found in only one of the ten.

Subsequent Risk of Invasive Cancer

It is as an indicator of subsequent invasive breast cancer presentation that lobular carcinoma in situ attains its greatest clinical impact. Beginning with two large follow-up series presented in 1978,[45, 75] there has been a general understanding that women who are not treated after detection of this disease at biopsy have a risk of developing invasive breast cancer about ten times that of the general population. The absolute risk of later cancer development approximates 20 percent to 25 percent at 15 to 20 years after biopsy. In the Rosen et al.

series,[74] more than a third of the patients presented with invasive carcinoma more than 20 years after the initial indicator biopsy. For the forseeable future there will remain a great deal of debate as to whether close clinical surveillance or some form of surgical treatment is appropriate in each individual patient.

As in DCIS, a review of various experiences with LCIS as recorded in the literature demands careful analysis of the recording biases. Occasionally this analytical approach may indicate interpretations that are enlightening and consistent with other data. For example, Tulusan et al.[85] reported a 16 percent incidence of invasive carcinoma within 24 months of LCIS diagnosis. However, this group selectively performed mastectomy when the LCIS was extensive, and these cases came from the performance of subcutaneous mastectomy in the absence of clinically evident disease. This experience indicates that (1) there was clinically occult invasive cancer coexistent with LCIS at biopsy, and (2) more extensive examples of LCIS[85] may be more likely to have such an association. However, this latter suggestion remains unproven as a predictor of subsequent invasion.[45, 75]

Type of Associated Invasive Disease

Whether present concurrently with LCIS or developing later, special types of invasive carcinoma, primarily tubular and lobular, have a positive association with LCIS.[44, 45, 57, 67, 92] There remains a greater frequency of no special type, or ductal, carcinoma in most series.[23, 34, 44, 75, 91] Patients with tubular carcinoma have a favorable prognosis, with death from breast cancer being very unusual.[27] Patients with invasive lobular carcinoma also have a somewhat better prognosis than average for breast cancer.[26] Thus, as has been stressed by others,[45, 91, 92] the prognosis of the particular malignancy that develops later and its metastatic capacity are more important than its absolute incidence. The remarkable survival rate of one series of patients with lobular neoplasia is attributed to a strict regimen of surveillance for early detection.[45, 54] This series as well as others[67] show an increased incidence of patients who later developed cancers with improved prognosis.

Ductal carcinoma in situ may occur with LCIS, concurrently or subsequently. In one review of 112 cases of CIS, six had "combined disease" (i.e., DCIS and LCIS),[83] and in a similar series, 16 percent of 150 patients with CIS had both LCIS and DCIS.[48] One follow-up study included later developing DCIS as a possible cancer event equal to that of invasive carcinoma.[45] Two large follow-up studies of patients with microscopic DCIS showed a five percent to ten percent incidence of co-occurrence of the two diseases at diagnostic biopsy.[10, 65] DCIS may be present with LCIS more frequently than by chance alone, but more precise numbers are unavailable. We conclude that LCIS is a marker of increased risk of any breast cancer type, with a greater percentage of invasive lobular and tubular carcinomas than are otherwise identified. The clinician is referred to chapter 35 for a comprehensive review of the historical and contemporary management perspectives for early (*in situ* and clinically occult) carcinoma of the breast.

References

1. Ackerman LV, Katzenstein AL: The concept of minimal breast cancer and the pathologist's role in the diagnosis of "early carcinoma." Cancer 39:2755–2763, 1977.
2. Andersen JA: Lobular carcinoma in situ. A long-term follow-up in 52 cases. Acta Pathol Microbiol Scand (A) 82:519–533, 1974.
3. Andersen JA, Lattes R, Rosen PP: Lobular carcinoma in situ: (Lobular neoplasia) of the breast (a symposium). Pathol Annu 14(2):193–223, 1980.
4. Andersen JA, Neilsen M, Bilchert-Toft: The growth pattern of in situ carcinoma in the female breast. Acta Oncol 27:739–743, 1988.
5. Andersen JA, Vendelboe ML: Cytoplasmic mucous globules in lobular carcinoma in situ. Am J Surg Pathol 5:251–255, 1981.
6. Arnesson LG, Fagerberg G, Grontoft O: Follow-up of two treatment modalities for ductal cancer in situ of the breast. Br J Surg 76:672–675, 1989.
7. Ashworth MT, Haqqani MT: Endocrine variant of ductal carcinoma in situ of breast: ultrastructural and light microscopical study. J Clin Pathol 39:1355–1359, 1986.
8. Azzopardi J: Problems in breast pathology. Philadelphia, W.B. Saunders, 1979, pp 113, 266.
9. Bartow SA, Pathak DR, Black WC, Key CR, Teaf SR: Prevalence of benign, atypical, and malignant breast lesions in populations at different risk for breast cancer. Cancer 60:2751–2760, 1987.
9a. Benfield JR, Fingerhut AG, Warner NE: A multidiscipline view of lobular breast carcinoma. Am J Surg 38:115–116, 1972.
10. Betsill WL Jr, Rosen PP, Lieberman PH, Robbins GF: Intraductal carcinoma. Long-term follow-up after treatment by biopsy alone. JAMA 239:1863–1867, 1978.
11. Bloodgood JC: Comedo carcinoma (or comedo-adenoma) of the female breast. Am J Cancer 22:842–849, 1934.
12. Bouropoulou V, Anastassiades OT, Kontogeorgos G, Rachmanides M, Gogas I: Microcalcifications in breast carcinomas—a histological and histochemical study. Pathol Res Pract 179:51–58, 1984.
13. Broders AC: Carcinoma in situ contrasted with benign penetrating epithelium. JAMA 99:1670–1674, 1932.
14. Brown PW, Silverman J, Owens E, Tabor DC, Terz JJ, Lawrence WJ: Intraductal 'non-infiltrating' carcinoma of the breast. Arch Surg 111:1063–1067, 1976.
15. Carpenter R, Boulter PS, Cooke T, Gibbs N: Management of screen detected ductal carcinoma in situ of the female breast. Br J Surg 76:564–567, 1989.
16. Carpenter R, Gibbs N, Matthews J, Cooke T: Importance of cellular DNA content in pre-malignant breast disease and pre-invasive carcinoma of the female breast. Br J Surg 74:905–906, 1987.
17. Carter D: Intraductal papillary tumors of the breast: a study of 78 cases. Cancer 39:1689–1692, 1977.
18. Carter D, Orr SL, Merino MJ: Intracystic papillary carcinoma of the breast. After mastectomy, radiotherapy or excisional biopsy alone. Cancer 52:14–19, 1983.
19. Carter D, Smith RRL: Carcinoma in situ of the breast. Cancer 40:1189–1193, 1977.
20. Chaudary MA, Millis RR, Lane EB, Miller NA: Paget's disease of the nipple: a ten year review including clinical, pathological, and immuno-histochemical findings. Breast Cancer Res Treat 8:139–146, 1986.
21. Connolly JL, Boyages J, Schnitt SJ, Recht A, Silen W, Sadowsky N, Harris JR: In situ carcinoma of the breast. Annu Rev Med 40:173–180, 1989.
22. Cross AS, Azzopardi JG, Krausz T, van Noorden S, Polak JM: A morphological and immunocytochemical study of a distinctive variant of ductal carcinoma in situ of the breast. Histopathology 9:21–37, 1985.
23. Dall'Olmo CA, Ponka JL, Horn CR, Riu R: Lobular carcinoma of the breast in situ. Arch Surg 110:537–542, 1975.
24. DePotter CR, Praet MM, Slavin RE, Verbeeck P, Roels HJ: Feulgen DNA content and mitotic activity in proliferative breast disease. A comparison with ductal carcinoma in situ. Histopathology 11:1307–1319, 1987.
25. Dershaw DD, Abramson A, Kinne DW: Ductal carcinoma in situ: mammographic findings and clinical implications. Radiology 170:411–415, 1989.
26. Dixon JM, Anderson TJ, Page DL, Lee D, Duffy SW: Infiltrating lobular carcinoma of the breast. Histopathology 6:149–161, 1982.
27. Dixon JM, Page DL, Anderson TJ, Lee D, Elton RA, Stewart HJ, Forrest AP: Long-term survivors after breast cancer. Br J Surg 72:445–448, 1985.
28. Dupont WD, Page DL: Risk factors for breast cancer in women with proliferative breast disease. N Engl J Med 312:146–151, 1985.
29. Eusebi V, Foschini MA, Cook MG, Berrino F, Azzopardi JG: Long-term follow-up of in situ carcinoma of the breast with special emphasis on clinging carcinoma. Semin Diagn Pathol 6:165–173, 1989.
30. Fechner RE: Epithelial alterations in the extralobular ducts of breasts with lobular carcinoma. Arch Pathol 93:164–171, 1972.
31. Fentiman IS, Fagg N, Millis RR, Hayward JL: In situ ductal carcinoma of the breast: implications of disease pattern and treatment. Eur J Surg Oncol 12:261–266, 1986.
32. Fisher ER: The pathology of breast cancer as it relates to its evolution, prognosis and treatment. Clin Oncol 1:703–734, 1982.
33. Fisher ER, Brown R: Intraductal signet ring carcinoma: a hitherto undescribed form of intraductal carcinoma of the breast. Cancer 55:2533–2537, 1985.
34. Fisher ER, Fisher B: Lobular carcinoma of the breast: an overview. Ann Surg 195:377–385, 1977.
35. Fisher ER, Palekar AS, Redmond C, Barton B, Fisher B: Pathologic findings from the national surgical adjuvant breast project (protocol no. 4). VI. Invasive papillary cancer. Am J Clin Pathol 73:313–322, 1980.
36. Fisher ER, Sass R, Fisher B, Wickerman L, Paik SM: Pathologic findings from the National Surgical Adjuvant Breast Project (Protocol 6). I. Cancer 57:197–208, 1986.
37. Foote FW, Stewart FW: Lobular carcinoma in situ. Am J Pathol 17:491–495, 1941.
38. Frykberg ER, Santiago F, Betsill WL, O'Brien PH: Lobular carcinoma in situ of the breast. Surg Gynecol Obstet 164:285–301, 1987.
39. Galkin BM, Feig SA, Patchefsky AS, Rue JW, Gamblin WJ, Gomèz DG, Marchant LM: Ultrastructure and microanalysis of "benign" and "malignant" breast calcifications. Radiology 124:245–249, 1977.
40. Geschickter CF: Diseases of the Breast. Philadelphia, JB Lippincott, 1943, p 502.
41. Gillis DA, Dockerty MB, Clagett OT: Pre-invasive intraductal carcinoma of the breast. Surg Gynecol Obstet 110:555–562, 1960.
42. Giordano JM, Klopp CT: Lobular carcinoma in situ: incidence and treatment. Cancer 31:105–109, 1973.
43. Gump FE, Jicha DL, Ozello L: Ductal carcinoma in situ (DCIS): A revised concept. Surgery 102:790–795, 1987.
44. Haagensen CD, Lane N, Bodian C: Coexisting lobular neoplasia and carcinoma of the breast. Cancer 51:1468–1482, 1983.
45. Haagensen CD, Lane N, Lattes R, Bodian C: Lobular neoplasia (so-called lobular carcinoma in situ) of the breast. Cancer 42:737–769, 1978.
46. Hutter RVP: The management of patients with lobular carcinoma in situ of the breast. Cancer 53:798–802, 1984.
47. Ikeda DM, Andersson I: Ductal carcinoma in situ: atypical mammographic appearances. Radiology 172:661–666, 1989.
48. Kinne DW, Petrek JA, Osborne MP, Fracchia AA, DePalo AA, Rosen PP: Breast carcinoma in situ. Arch Surg 124:33–36, 1989.
49. Kraus FT, Neubecker RD: The differential diagnosis of papillary tumours of the breast. Cancer 15:444–455, 1962.
50. Lagios MD, Margolin FR, Westdahl PR, Rose MR: Mammographically detected duct carcinoma in situ. Cancer 63:618–624, 1989.

51. Lagios MD, Westdahl PR, Margolin FR, Roses MR: Duct carcinoma in situ. Relationship of extent of noninvasive disease to the frequency of occult invasion, multicentricity, lymph node metastases, and short-term treatment failures. Cancer 50:1309–1314, 1982.

52. Lagios MD, Westdahl PR, Rose MR, Concannon S: Paget's disease of the nipple: alternative management in cases without or with minimal extent of underlying breast carcinoma. Cancer 54:545–551, 1984.

53. Lambird PA, Shelley WM: The spatial distribution of lobular in situ mammary carcinoma. JAMA 210:689–693, 1969.

54. Lattes R: Lobular neoplasia (lobular carcinoma in situ) of the breast—a histological entity of controversial clinical significance. Pathol Res Pract 166:415–429, 1980.

55. Letton AJ, Mason ME: Routine breast screening: survival after 10.5 years follow-up. Ann Surg 203:470–473, 1986.

56. Lewis D, Geschickter CF: Comedo carcinomas of the breast. Arch Surg 36:225–244, 1938.

57. McDivitt RW, Hutter RVP, Foote FW, Stewart FW: In situ lobular carcinoma: a prospective follow-up study indicating cumulative patient risks. JAMA 201:96–100, 1967.

58. McDivitt RW, Stewart FW, Berg JW: Tumors of the breast. Atlas of Tumor Pathology, second series, fascicle 2. Washington, DC, Armed Forces Institute of Pathology, 1968.

59. Meyer JS: Cell kinetics of histological variants of in situ breast carcinoma. Breast Cancer Res Treat 7:171–180, 1986.

60. Millis RR, Davis R, Stacey A: The detection and significance of calcifications in breast: a radiological and pathological study. Br J Radiol 49:12–26, 1976.

61. Mitnick JS, Roses DF, Harris MN, Feiner HD: Circumscribed intraductal carcinoma of the breast. Response. Radiology 172:579–580, 1989.

62. Norris HJ, Bahr GF, Mikel UV: A comparative morphometric and cytophotometric study of intraductal hyperplasia and intraductal carcinoma of the breast. Anal Quant Cytol Histol 10:1–9, 1987.

63. Page DL, Anderson TJ, Rogers LW: Carcinoma in situ (CIS). *In* Page DL, Anderson TJ: Diagnostic Histopathology of the Breast. Edinburgh, Churchill Livingstone, 1988, p 157.

64. Page DL, Dupont WD: Anatomic markers of human premalignancy and risk of breast cancer. Cancer 1991, in press.

65. Page DL, Dupont WD, Rogers LW, Landenberger M: Intraductal carcinoma of the breast: follow-up after biopsy only. Cancer 49:751–758, 1982.

66. Page DL, Dupont WD, Rogers LW, Rados MS: Atypical hyperplastic lesions of the female breast. A long-term follow-up study. Cancer 55:2698–2708, 1985.

67. Page DL, Kidd TE, Dupont WD, Rogers LW: Lobular neoplasia of the breast (LN) has varying magnitudes of risk for subsequent invasive carcinoma (IBC). (Abstract) Lab Invest 58:69A, 1988.

68. Patchefsky AS, Schwartz GF, Finkelstein SD, Prestipino A, Sohn SE, Singer JS, Feig SA: Heterogeneity of intraductal carcinoma of the breast. Cancer 63:731–741, 1989.

69. Peeters PHM, Verbeek ALM, Hendriks JHCL, Holland R, Mravunac M, Vooijs GP: The occurance of interval cancers in the Nijmegen screening programme. Br J Cancer 59:929–932, 1989.

70. Pick PW, Iossifides IA: Occurrence of breast carcinoma within a fibroadenoma. A review. Arch Pathol Lab Med 108:590–594, 1984.

71. Pope TL, Fechner RE, Wilheim MC, Wanebo HJ, deParedes ES: Lobular carcinoma in situ of the breast: mammographic features. Radiology 168:63–66, 1988.

72. Ringberg A, Palmer B, Linell F: The contralateral breast at reconstructive surgery after breast cancer operation—a histological study. Breast Cancer Res Treat 2:151–161, 1982.

73. Rosen PP: The pathological classification of human mammary carcinoma: past, present and future. Ann Clin Lab Sci 9:144–156, 1979.

74. Rosen PP, Braun DW Jr, Lyngholm B, Urban JA, Kinne DW: Lobular carcinoma in situ of the breast: preliminary results of treatment by ipsilateral mastectomy and contralateral breast biopsy. Cancer 47:813–819, 1981.

75. Rosen PP, Lieberman PH, Braun DW Jr, Kosloff C, Adair F: Lobular carcinoma in situ of the breast: detailed analysis of 99 patients with average follow-up of 24 years. Am J Surg Pathol 2:225–251, 1978.

76. Rosen PP, Senie R, Schottenfeld D, Ashikari R: Non-invasive breast carcinoma. Frequency of unsuspected invasion and implications for treatment. Ann Surg 189:377–382, 1979.

77. Ross PM: Apparent absence of a benign precursor lesion: implications for the pathogenesis of malignant melanoma. J Am Acad Dermatol 21:529–538, 1989.

78. Salhany KE, Page DL: Fine-needle aspiration of mammary lobular carcinoma in situ and atypical lobular hyperplasia. Am J Clin Pathol 92:22–26, 1989.

79. Schnitt SJ, Silen W, Sadowsky NL, et al: Ductal carcinoma in situ (intraductal carcinoma) of the breast. N Engl J Med 318:898–903, 1988.

80. Schwartz GF, Feig SA, Rosenberg AL: Staging and treatment of clinically occult breast cancer. Cancer 53:1379–1384, 1984.

81. Schwartz GF, Patchefsky AS, Finklestein SD, Sohn SH, Prestipino A, Feig SA, Singer JS: Nonpalpable in situ ductal carcinoma of the breast. Arch Surg 124:29–32, 1989.

82. Silverstein MJ, Rosser RJ, Gierson ED, et al: Axillary lymph node dissection for intraductal breast carcinoma—is it indicated? Cancer 59:1819–1824, 1987.

83. Sunshine JA, Moseley HS, Fletcher WS, Krippaehne WW: Breast carcinoma in situ: a retrospective review of 112 cases with a minimum 10 years follow-up. Am J Surg 150:44–51, 1985.

84. Tulusan AH, Egger H, Ober KG: Lobular carcinoma in situ and its relation to invasive breast cancer. *In* Zander J, Baltzer J (eds). Early Breast Cancer. Berlin, Springer-Verlag, 1985, 48–51.

85. Tulusan AH, Egger H, Schneider ML, Willgeroth F: A contribution to the natural history of breast cancer: lobular carcinoma in situ and its relation to breast cancer. Arch Gynecol 231:219–226, 1982.

86. Urban JA: Bilaterality of cancer of the breast. Cancer 20:1867–1870, 1967.

87. VanDeVijver MJ, Peterse JL, Mooi WJ, Wisman P, Lomans J, Dalesio O, Nusse R: Neu-protein overexpression in breast cancer: association with comedo-type ductal carcinoma in situ and limited prognostic value in stage II breast cancer. N Engl J Med 319:1239–1245, 1988.

88. von Rueden DG, Wilson RE: Intraductal carcinoma of the breast. Surg Gynecol Obstet 158:105–111, 1984.

89. Webber BL, Heise H, Neifeld JP, Costa J: Risk of subsequent contralateral breast carcinoma in a population of patients with in situ breast carcinoma. Cancer 47:2928–2932, 1981.

90. Westbrook KC, Gallager HS: Intraductal carcinoma of the breast: a comparative study. Am J Surg 130:667–670, 1975.

91. Wheeler JE, Enterline HT: Lobular carcinoma of the breast in situ and infiltrating. Pathol Annu 11:161–188, 1976.

92. Wheeler JE, Enterline JT, Roseman JM: Lobular carcinoma in situ of the breast: long term follow-up. Cancer 34:554–563, 1974.

Chapter 9

MALIGNANT NEOPLASIA OF THE BREAST: INFILTRATING CARCINOMAS

K Kendall Pierson, M.D. and Edward J. Wilkinson, M.D.

Invasive epithelial mammary neoplasms are a major cause of cancer morbidity and mortality in Western countries. This chapter will review the pathology of principal types of invasive breast cancer, emphasizing the relationship of morphology and prognosis. Sarcomas of the breast are extensively reviewed in chapter 10. Lesions with significant proliferative atypia, both cytological and architectural, have been the subject of study and conjectural debate for many years.[96] Recently, a large study has clearly established a significant breast cancer risk for those patients afflicted with atypical hyperplastic diseases, a situation compounded if close relatives have had breast cancer.[36]

The prognosis and management of the high-risk patient for the development of breast cancer are discussed in chapters 14 and 52. Fully evolved noninvasive breast carcinoma takes one of two histopathological forms—intraductal or intralobular carcinoma *in situ*. Intraductal carcinoma presents any of four microscopic patterns of growth, which are often intermixed; micropapillary, cribriform or sievelike, solid, or solid centrally necrotic (comedocarcinoma).[45, 99]

Less than 5 percent of breast carcinomas can be placed in one of these pure noninvasive categories. The majority are of mixed histology or are associated with invasive adenocarcinoma. Mammographic screening has significantly increased the detection of preinvasive lesions.[5] Mammography often detects preinvasive and invasive mammary carcinomas before they can be palpated (see chapter 24.)

Approximately three quarters of infiltrating carcinomas of the breast have been included in the imprecise "infiltrating ductal" or adenocarcinoma, not otherwise specified, category. Several authors have suggested that the term "adenocarcinoma, not otherwise specified" (NOS) be preferred to "ductal carcinoma" because the exact anatomical site of origin of the most common form of breast adenocarcinoma remains indeterminate. With the exception of better differentiated lesions that clearly resemble or contain ductal structures, this designation is largely arbitrary and subjective. Approximately half these tumors are associated, or mixed, with specific types of morphological carcinoma (Tables 9–1 and 9–2). Wellings and coworkers, in 1973,[97] reported

that 40 to 60 percent of cancerous breasts contain multiple foci of in situ carcinoma within the terminal epithelial structure and designated their anatomical subunit the terminal ductal lobular unit. The terminal ductal lobular unit remains the most likely site of origin of breast adenocarcinoma. Based upon pure morphology, there has been no clinically significant difference observed between the less differentiated "unspecified" breast carcinomas and the mixed variants, unless qualified by objective assessment of nuclear and architectural degrees of differentiation, i.e., grading.

Tumors exhibiting extreme histopathological deviation from their normal tissues of origin are often associated with aggressive clinical behavior. Attempts to objectively quantify these observations have focused on (1) cytological features emphasizing nuclear morphology and (2) architectural growth patterns of cell groupings. *Nuclear grading* as advocated by Black et al.[19, 20] and Cutler et al.[31] has received wide, though not universal, acceptance. Confusion arises with application of their terminology, i.e., Grade 3 for well-differentiated, Grade 2 for moderate differentiation, and Grade 1 for poor differentiation. Other authors[42, 98] have modified this grading so that higher grades of tumor are reflected on higher grading scores. We prefer to avoid numerical

Table 9–1. HISTOLOGICAL TYPES OF INVASIVE BREAST CANCER

Infiltrating Duct Carcinoma	Approximate Incidence (%)
Usual type—not otherwise specified	50
Combined with other distinctive types	25
Medullary carcinoma	6
Colloid carcinoma	2
Paget's disease	2
Less common specific types (tubular, papillary, adenoid cystic, invasive cribriform)	2
Rare combined types	<2
Infiltrating lobular carcinoma	5
Combined lobular/ductal	6
Malignant stromal tumors	<1

Modified from Fisher E, et al.: Cancer 36:1, 1975.

Table 9–2. COMPARATIVE RECENT SERIES OF INVASIVE BREAST CARCINOMA BY TYPE

Rosen (1979)[75] NYC	Fu et al. (1981)[49] Ohio	Wallgren et al. (1976)[94] Stockholm	Sakamoto et al. (1981)[85, 86] Tokyo	Anderson (1987)[66a] Edinburgh
75% Ductal	53% NOS*	64% NST†	47% Common (scirrhous)	70% NST†
3% Minimally invasive	13% Predominantly intraductal	—	—	3% Minimally invasive
10% Lobular	11% Lobular	14% Lobular	2% Lobular	10% Lobular (7% variants)
10% Medullary	15% Medullary (10% variants)	6% Medullary	2% Medullary	5% Medullary (3% variants)
1% Tubular	7% Tubular	7% Tubular	—	3% Tubular
2% Colloid	2% Mucinous		4% Mucinous	2% Mucinous
			—	1% Papillary
0.55% Papillary	2% Papillary	9% Cribriform or papillary	22% Papillotubular	4% Cribriform
	5% Combined		20% Solid tubular	2% Combined

*Not otherwise specified
†No special type
Modified from Page DL, Anderson TJ: Diagnostic Histopathology of the Breast. New York, Churchill Livingstone, 1987.

designators and use three less ambiguous descriptive terms: well, moderately, and poorly differentiated. These correspond to Black's low, intermediate, and high grades. *Well-differentiated* nuclear morphology is characterized by small, relatively uniform, rounded nuclei with few nucleoli and rare mitoses (Fig. 9–1). *Moderately differentiated* tumors present increased nuclear size, pleomorphism, and chromatin/DNA variability. Mitoses are numerous and nuclei contain prominent nucleoli, often with irregular shapes (Fig. 9–2). *Poorly differentiated* nuclei are usually large with vesicular and variable chromatin patterns, prominent nucleoli, and conspicuous, often atypical, mitotic figures (Fig. 9–3).

Architectural grading has also contributed useful prognostic information. Architectural grading is generally described in terms that refer to the extent of tubuloacinar formation that resembles the terminal ductal lobular unit.[42, 96] Typically, well-differentiated breast carcinoma presents as a dominant tubular architectural pattern. Intermediate grades usually display easily identifiable tubular or acinar structures, though the dominant pattern may be small groups, different-sized nests, or cords

of variably differentiated cells. Poorly differentiated patterns rarely present recognizable tubular or acinar structures and most often grow as sheets of syncytial cells, as frequently seen in medullary carcinoma or infiltrating carcinomas composed of smaller cells arranged in single files, which is typical of invasive lobular carcinoma.

Nuclear and architectural grades are often congruent within a given tumor; however, divergent grades of differentiation between the nuclear and architectural grades are not unusual. Nuclear and architectural grading are generally combined to establish the tumor histological grading, because neither can be consistently utilized alone as an independent variable.[93] For greatest usefulness, histological grading must be combined with other features in determining prognosis.[21, 22, 37, 48]

Gross observations of tumor size and appearance, particularly the degree of circumscription, add valuable prognostic information. Small tumors with sharply delineated, well-defined borders have generally been recognized as biologically less aggressive in a variety of organ systems. Larger lesions (over 2 cm in diameter) pre-

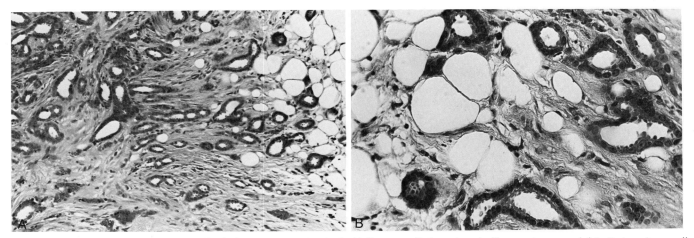

Figure 9–1. *A*, Invasive, well-differentiated tubular carcinoma (× 100). Uniform small ducts invade fibrous stroma and fat. *B*, Invasive, well-differentiated, tubular carcinoma (× 250). Single small cuboidal cells line the ducts.

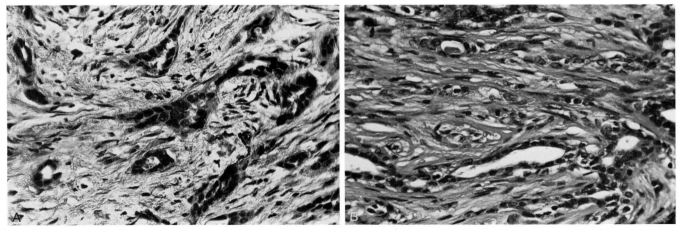

Figure 9–2 *A,* Invasive adenocarcinoma, not otherwise specified (NOS) (× 250). Poorly formed ductlike elements are seen, which, for the most part, have a single cell lining. *B,* Invasive moderately differentiated adenocarcinoma, NOS (× 250). This tumor also contains poorly formed ducts; however, cells can be seen arranged singly in the so-called Indian file pattern of growth. Marked stromal desmoplasia is present.

senting ill-defined infiltrative margins, as a group, are associated with poorer prognoses.[98] Notable exceptions do occur. Color and consistency are less reliable but represent important features that often suggest particular specific types of tumors. Tumor necrosis is frequently seen in the common forms of breast adenocarcinoma. Necrosis is often apparent on cross section of the breast tumor. Within breast parenchyma, tumor necrosis presents as chalky white or yellowish streaks, forming a conspicuous radiating pattern in classic scirrhous carcinomas of the breast. As an independent observation, microscopic or small areas of necrosis do not have a significant impact on prognosis. Focal necrosis in tumors with poorly defined borders, however, is associated with a higher morbidity and mortality. Carter et al., in 1978,[26] reported a ten-year survival rate of only 35 percent for patients whose tumors had poorly defined borders and were necrotic, as compared with 50 percent for those with non-necrotic tumors. Furthermore, 63 percent of

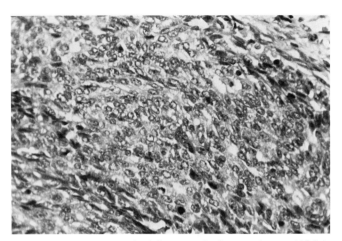

Figure 9–3. Invasive, poorly differentiated adenocarcinoma, NOS (× 250). This tumor is composed almost entirely of tumor cells with little intervening stroma. Some small secondary neoplastic glands are seen within the more solid tumor.

the patients with necrosis had axillary lymph node metastases, in contrast to a 42 percent frequency of node metastases for those without tumor necrosis. The influence on survival in those patients with axillary nodal metastases was most significant. In comparing actuarial survival rates related to the presence or absence of tumor necrosis and axillary node metastasis, less than 20 percent of those patients with tumor necrosis and axillary metastases survived ten years. Conversely, the ten-year survival was 43 percent for women with axillary metastases but without tumor necrosis.

Combined clinical and pathological staging, complemented by histological grading, provides the most informative prognostic information.[6] Clinical staging is discussed in detail in chapter 17 and can be summarized as follows: Stage I includes patients with small tumors, 2 cm or less in maximal dimension and negative axillary lymph nodes. Stage II includes tumors 2 to 5 cm in diameter in patients whose axillary lymph nodes are positive for metastatic disease but with freely movable local and regional lesions. Smaller tumors (2 cm or less in diameter) with clinically or pathologically positive lymph nodes are also included in this group. Stage III patients present with more extensive local disease and/or regional nodal spread. Stage IV includes any patient with distant metastasis regardless of local or regional extent of tumor spread.

Although the biological outcome of an individual patient's disease is difficult to predict with precision, general principles do apply. The principal, and most reliable, indicators of outcome are the presence or absence of axillary metastases and the number, size, and location of lymph nodes involved by tumor.[40] Secondary features that significantly contribute to prognosis include tumor size, circumscription, the presence or absence of necrosis, and the histological grade, as previously described.[41, 82]

The presence of vascular, lymphatic, or blood vessel invasion portends a lower survival rate and shorter disease-free interval.[83] For example, inflammatory carcinoma of the breast characteristically has clinical and microscopic involvement of the dermal lymphatics by adenocarcinoma, heralding a poor prognosis with presentation as an adenocarcinoma of the breast (Figs. 9–4 and 9–5). As many as 15 percent of patients free of axillary metastasis are found to have microscopic tumor emboli in tissues surrounding the primary tumor. This is especially significant in patients with small tumors, since one third ultimately die of their disease.[81] Furthermore, 17 percent of Stage I cases initially interpreted as

having no evidence of metastatic tumors within the lymph nodes have occult axillary metastases to those nodes when the nodes are re-examined by detailed sectioning methods.[98] The finding of the occult metastases in lymph nodes, however, does not appear to influence overall survival.[80, 98]

Lymphoplasmacytic infiltrates in and about the tumor are required for the diagnosis of medullary carcinoma and may contribute to a more favorable prognosis in other tumors. The presence of breast stromal fibrous

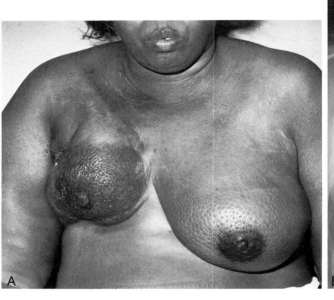

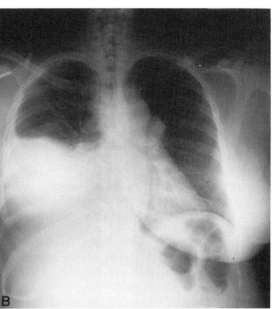

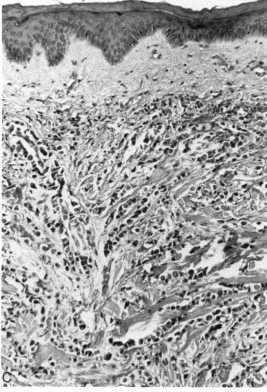

Figure 9–4. *A,* Clinical presentation of advanced inflammatory carcinoma of the right breast in a 38-year-old female. There is en cuirasse fixation to the chest wall with development of ipsilateral extremity lymphedema. The left breast has secondary infiltration from the opposite breast with development of peau d'orange. *B,* Posteroanterior chest radiograph of same patient at initial clinical presentation with large right pleural effusion. There is associated hilar adenopathy. *C,* Inflammatory carcinoma of the breast (× 100). Within the dermis infiltrating adenocarcinoma, NOS, can be seen. Note that the tumor does not involve the epithelium, as seen in Paget's disease.

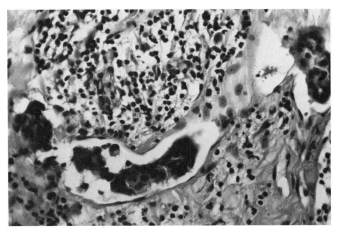

Figure 9–5. Inflammatory carcinoma of the breast (× 250). Nests of adenocarcinoma cells can be seen in endothelium-lined vascular spaces within the dermis—a characteristic of inflammatory carcinoma. A moderate chronic inflammatory infiltrate within the stroma is seen adjacent to the tumor.

response within and around malignant breast neoplasms has been of interest for many years.[2] Poorly circumscribed breast adenocarcinomas have not shown prognostically significant differences related to their specific fiber content. Increased elastic fibers, particularly the poorly defined entity "elastosis," have been seen in tumors containing estrogen receptors. Immunohistochemical procedures have been applied to a variety of breast neoplasms.[56, 68, 69] Perineural invasion, as an independent prognostic variable, has not proved to be of clinical significance.

The past decade has witnessed increasing interest in nuclear DNA content and morphometry. Atkin and Kay[13] performed microspectrophotometric DNA measurements on Feulgen-stained tumor imprints and demonstrated that tumors exhibiting *diploid* DNA content were associated with longer survivals than those exhibiting quantitative differences consistent with *aneuploidy*.[14, 15] The application of flow cytometry has further refined and clarified these observations and has been applied to a wide variety of hematological and solid neoplasms. Demonstration of DNA content in neoplasms has proved to be a reliable indicator of biological behavior and aggressiveness in assessing many of these neoplasms.[12, 56] The majority of breast carcinomas studied by flow cytometric techniques have revealed DNA aneuploidy, specifically bimodal hyperdiploid peaks.[17] Recent observations have also demonstrated a relationship between histological grading and the nuclear DNA abnormalities demonstrated by flow cytometry. The proportion of cells in active DNA synthesis has been studied by thymidine-indexing technique. This technique provides an objective indication of DNA synthesis and the proportion of cells in S-phase. Tumors with high S-phase activity tend to be hormone-receptor negative.[18] This laborious technique has recently been simplified by the application of monoclonal antibodies, such as KI-67, that demonstrate cells in active synthesis by utilizing immunoperoxidase or flow cytometric methodologies.

COMMON ADENOCARCINOMA OF THE BREAST

Table 9–3 summarizes common types of breast tumors and their associated prognosis.[60] Three quarters of invasive breast adenocarcinomas fall within a heterogeneous group variously termed ductal carcinoma, scirrhous carcinoma, adenocarcinoma, not otherwise specified, or simply adenocarcinoma of the breast, to list only a few (see Figs. 9–1 to 9–3). Approximately one third of these neoplasms have recognizable elements of a specific histological type of breast carcinoma; however, the presence of a specific tumor type in small amounts does not appear to favorably or unfavorably affect the prognosis. The prototypical common adenocarcinoma of the breast presents in a perimenopausal woman in her sixth decade as a firm, ill-defined, solitary mass.[77, 78, 88] On pathological examination, the cut surface of the mass reveals the central radiating stellate tumor with chalky white or yellow streaks extending into the surrounding breast tissues. The tumor characteristically has a poorly defined visible border that is frequently better defined by palpation than by inspection. The histology of this group of tumors is extremely variable. Tumor nests, sheets, cords, trabeculae, and often, imperfectly formed glandlike spaces are present in variable amounts. Specific types of growth, such as papillary, mucinous, and medullary, are seen associated with the tumor in about one third of the cases. If a specific tumor type does not dominate or constitutes one quarter or less of the tumor, its effect upon prognosis is negligible. It appears prudent, therefore, when pathologically classifying such tumors, to use the designation "adenocarcinoma of breast, not otherwise specified" and to describe the histological features present in the nondominant areas. The relative volume of invasive and in situ carcinoma should also be recorded by the pathologist, since size of the neoplasm has impact on the prognosis when one or the other is clearly dominant (Figs. 9–6 and 9–7). This largest group of breast carcinomas is generally composed of moderately to poorly differentiated tumors.[42] As noted above, inflammatory carcinoma of the breast is a clinicopathological term applied to a distinctive inflamed appearance of the skin of the breast occurring secondary to involvement of the dermal lymphatics by intramammary spread of adenocarcinoma of the breast (see Figs. 9–4C and 9–5).

PAGET'S DISEASE

Paget's disease of the nipple and areola is found in approximately 2 percent of patients with breast carcinoma. The characteristic clinical presentation of this disease as described by Sir James Paget is a chronic, moist, erythematous or scaly eczematous areolar and periareolar eruption, which in the great majority of cases is associated with an underlying intraductal or invasive carcinoma of the breast (Fig. 9–8A and B). Ashikari et al.[9] reported a large series in which half the women presenting with typical clinical mammary Paget's

Table 9–3. COMPARISON OF HISTOLOGICAL TYPES AND OUTCOME

Histological Type	Infiltrating Duct Carcinoma	Infiltrating Lobular Carcinoma	Medullary Carcinoma	Mucinous (Colloid) Carcinoma	Papillary Carcinoma
Node involvement	60%	60%	44%	32%	17%
Crude survival					
5 years	54%	50%	63%	73%	83%
10 years	38%	32%	50%	59%	56%
Actuarial survival					
5 years	59%	57%	69%	76%	89%
10 years	47%	42%	68%	72%	65%
20 years	38%	34%	62%	62%	65%

Modified from McDivitt RW, Stewart FW, Berg JW: Tumors of the breast. Atlas of Tumor Pathology. Series 2, Fascicle No 2. Washington DC, Armed Forces Institute of Pathology, 1968.

disease did not have an associated palpable mass in the breast. Approximately two thirds of these patients were subsequently proved to have an associated intraductal carcinoma, and one third had infiltrating adenocarcinoma. In this study, 95 percent of those patients who had negative axillary lymph nodes survived ten years. The survival of a given patient with Paget's disease associated with a palpable breast mass closely conforms to the prognosis for the underlying breast neoplasm. Both infiltrating and in situ lobular carcinoma have been reported in association with Paget's disease, although these are infrequent associations.

Microscopically, Paget's disease presents as an intraepithelial neoplasm composed of single or small groups of clear cells with large vesicular nuclei and prominent nuclei (Fig. 9–8C). Intracellular mucin can be demonstrated on occasion but is an inconsistent finding. Recently, the application of immunohistochemistry, specifically demonstrating carcinoembryonic antigen (CEA) within the Paget cells, has greatly aided in the diagnosis of mammary Paget's disease. The troublesome differential diagnosis between pagetoid intraepithelial malignant melanoma and Paget's disease is simplified by demonstrating S-100 protein, or melanoma-specific antigen immunoreactivity within most cells of malignant melanoma. These antigens are absent in the cells of Paget's disease. Melanoma cells, on the other hand, do not contain CEA, which can be identified within Paget cells.

Although the origin of the Paget cell remains controversial, there are two hypotheses: first, *epidermotropism* of underlying tumor cells, and second, *intraepithelial carcinomatous metaplasia*. It is important to emphasize that mammary Paget's disease not associated with underlying palpable invasive adenocarcinoma is highly curable if appropriately treated, the cure rate with palpable lesions being essentially the same as that of the associated underlying *in situ* or invasive adenocarcinoma.[11]

MEDULLARY CARCINOMA

Medullary carcinoma accounts for less than 10 percent of malignant breast tumors. The term has been used for

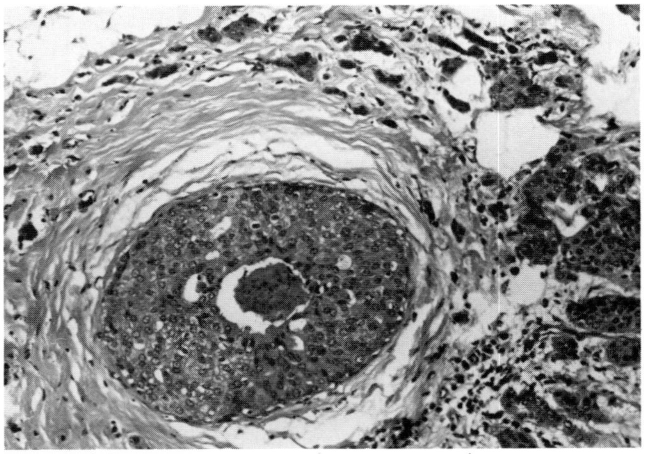

Figure 9–6. Intraductal carcinoma with adjacent invasive adenocarcinoma, NOS (× 100). The intraductal carcinoma nearly fills the duct. Cribriform growth is seen within the duct. Debris is noted within the ductal lumen. Invasive adenocarcinoma with adjacent desmoplastic fibrous stroma.

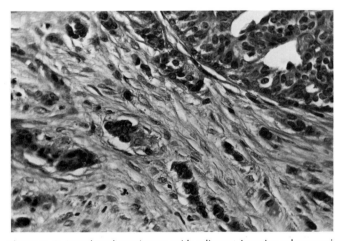

Figure 9–7. Intraductal carcinoma with adjacent invasive adenocarcinoma, NOS (× 250). At this magnification the cribriform nature of the intraductal component can be seen. The adjacent adenocarcinoma is surrounded by fibrous stroma.

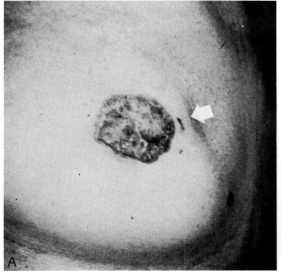
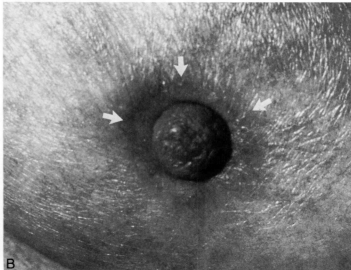
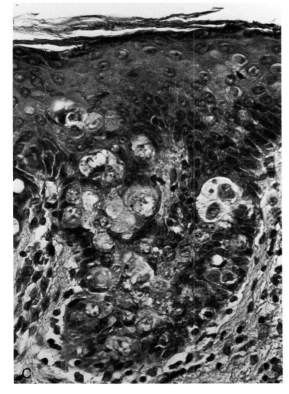

Figure 9–8. Two clinical presentations of Paget's disease. *A*, Paget's disease of the left breast. Note the clinical presentation of a moist, erythematous, scaly eczematoid nipple-areola complex with periareolar eruption. An invasive carcinoma of the subareolar parenchyma was evident *(arrow)*. *B*, Paget's disease of the right breast, presenting with profound erythematous halo of areola *(arrows)* that surrounds an encrusted, eczematoid, retracted nipple. An occult invasive ductal cancer was evident on biopsy. *C*, Paget's disease (× 250). Within the epithelium large cells are seen with relatively clear cytoplasm, as compared with the adjacent keratinocytes. These are the Paget cells. Note that they have large nuclei with prominent nucleoli.

many years and was originally applied to large, bulky breast neoplasms without regard to histology.[71] The histological definition was provided by Geschickter in 1945,[51] and by Moore and Foote in 1949.[63] The latter authors noted that the majority of patients with medullary carcinoma were less than 50 years of age, a finding subsequently confirmed by others.[58, 60] Large size, circumscription, and occasionally cystic change (cystification) are often noted. Bilaterality has been reported in as much as 18 percent, and less than 10 percent of these neoplasms contain detectable estrogen or progesterone receptors. The growth rate of medullary carcinomas is among the fastest recorded for breast carcinomas.[62]

The diagnosis of medullary carcinoma is made by application of precise histological criteria.[63, 77] Tumors that display some, but not all, of the morphological features of medullary carcinoma are best described as atypical medullary carcinomas, denoting a more guarded prognosis for these patients. The typical medullary carcinoma has a circumscribed nodular architecture and a softer, bulkier consistency than do commoner variants of breast carcinoma. Cyst formation and hemorrhagic necrosis are occasionally seen. Microscopically, these tumors display (1) a dense lymphoreticular infiltrate composed predominantly of lymphocytes and variable numbers of plasma cells; (2) large pleomorphic nuclei

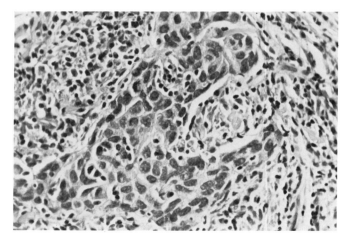

Figure 9–9. Medullary carcinoma of the breast (× 250). The tumor cells are present within a stroma densely infiltrated by small inflammatory cells consisting predominantly of lymphocytes. The nuclei of the tumor cells are large and pleomorphic.

(poorly differentiated) accompanied by numerous cells in active mitosis; and (3) a syncytial sheetlike growth pattern with little or no tendency toward tubuloacinar differentiation (Fig. 9–9). Nearly half these neoplasms are associated with intraductal carcinoma, the intraductal component characteristically being present at the periphery of the tumor mass. The host lymphoreticular response may engulf these intraductal areas as well as the main tumor mass. Squamous metaplasia is identified in approximately one sixth of these tumors. Rarely, mesenchymal metaplasia and/or anaplastic transformation may be found.

Patients with medullary carcinoma have a more favorable prognosis than do individuals with common adenocarcinoma of the breast. This is a somewhat surprising fact in view of the characteristically large size of the tumor mass at presentation and the histologically poor differentiation that is frequently evident. The presence of axillary nodal metastases, as in commoner forms of breast cancer, remains the primary prognostic determinant for patients with medullary carcinoma. The intense lymphohistiocytic response in and about the tumor is often associated with benign enlargement of the lymph nodes in the axilla and often contributes to erroneous clinical staging of the disease.

TUBULAR CARCINOMA

This well-differentiated type of breast carcinoma has been recognized for many years and has a reported incidence in the range of 2 percent.[32, 92] This tumor is being detected mammographically with apparent increasing frequency. Tubular carcinoma has been reported in one fifth of the women whose breast carcinomas were detected by mammography.[4] Controversy exists concerning the precise pathological definition of tubular carcinoma. As discussed, tubular differentiation may be seen in the common adenocarcinoma of the breast, and unless of the dominant tumor type, this

growth pattern does not imply a favorable prognosis. Clinically, tubular carcinoma is found in younger-than-average patients with breast carcinoma. The latter half of the fifth decade is the most commonly observed age group in which the neoplasm is diagnosed. Further, tubular carcinomas are often discovered when small, typically 1 cm or less in maximum dimension.[24, 25]

Microscopically, well-differentiated tubular carcinoma is distinctive. Low magnification reveals a haphazard array of small, randomly arranged tubular structures (Figs. 9–1 and 9–10). The small glandular (tubular) pattern, angulation, and single-cell lining of the neoplastic tubules are important histological features. The absence of myoepithelial cells and well-defined basement membranes serve to distinguish this neoplasm from common proliferative microglandular and sclerosing adenosis.[46, 74] The association with, and putative derivation from, intraductal carcinoma also aids in diagnosis. The associated intraductal carcinoma often contains microcalcification, which facilitates mammographic recognition. Pathological criteria for well-differentiated tubular carcinomas require that three quarters or more of the tumor be composed of typical tubular adenocarcinoma, as described above. Approximately 10 percent of patients with the typical tubular adenocarcinoma will develop axillary metastases. The metastases are generally confined to small numbers of lower axillary lymph nodes. On review of the literature, Rosen found recurrences in approximately 3.5 percent of patients treated surgically for tubular carcinoma.[76]

MUCINOUS CARCINOMA (COLLOID CARCINOMA)

Breast tumors associated with abundant mucin production account for approximately 2 percent of breast carcinomas. This variant of breast cancer was first de-

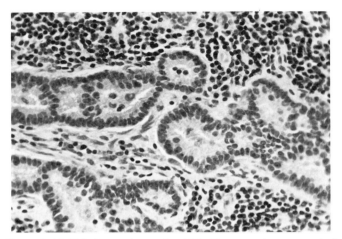

Figure 9–10. Tubular carcinoma (× 100). The tumor is composed of small, relatively uniform glands that are separated by a fibrovascular stroma. There is minimal glandular branching, and the gland lumens are well formed, open, and lined by a single layer of epithelium. Some intraductal bridging is present. There is no myoepithelial layer, and mild nuclear pleomorphism is evident. The inflammatory cells within the stroma in this case are not a distinctive feature.

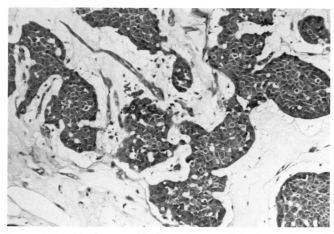

Figure 9–11. Mucinous (colloid) carcinoma of the breast (× 100). Nests of tumor cells are seen surrounded by mucus and an edematous fibrovascular stroma.

scribed in 1852 by Robinson.[72] Mucinous carcinoma generally presents as a palpable mass in the breast of a woman in her sixth or seventh decade. However, smaller, clinically nonpalpable mucinous carcinomas are being recognized with increasing frequency in younger women, challenging the belief that bulky, mucinous tumors are largely confined to older patients. The pathological features of mucinous carcinomas are quite distinctive. The tumors present a glairy, glistening, gelatinous cut surface. Fibrosis is variable and, when abundant, may impart a firm consistency to the neoplasm. The characteristic microscopic appearance of mucinous carcinoma must be seen in virtually all the tissues examined to establish this diagnosis. Large pools of mucin are found to surround variable groups of tumor cells (Figs. 9–11 and 9–12). The tumor cells may not be detectable in all sections of the neoplasm. *Signet-ring cells* are generally not seen in this form of mucin-producing adenocarcinoma, in contrast to the presence

of these cells in malignancies of the upper digestive tract. Approximately two thirds of pure mucin-producing adenocarcinomas contain detectable estrogen receptors. Argyrophilia and ultrastructural features suggesting neuroendocrine differentiation have been described in up to one half of mucinous carcinomas. The presence of argyrophilic granules may indicate a poorer prognosis.[30] Pure mucinous carcinoma is associated with a more favorable prognosis, although late recurrences and death can be seen in a significant proportion of women.[84]

PAPILLARY CARCINOMA

Pure papillary carcinoma accounts for less than 2 percent of breast carcinoma in most series and generally presents in the seventh decade of life. This carcinoma has been observed in a disproportionate number of non-Caucasian patients in one study.[44] Papillary carcinomas are generally small, rarely larger than 2 to 3 cm in maximal diameter, and are well circumscribed. Microscopically, papillary differentiation in the form of papillae with well-defined fibrovascular stalks, which have multilayered epithelium with moderately pleomorphic cells, is required for the diagnosis (Fig. 9–13).[66–69] Although many of these patients have palpable axillary lymph nodes, and up to one third have axillary metastatic disease, the disease-free survival is very similar to that for mucinous and tubular carcinoma. The data suggest that even with axillary metastases, papillary carcinoma may be a more indolent, slowly progressive disease than common breast adenocarcinoma.[33]

ADENOID CYSTIC CARCINOMA

Pure adenoid cystic carcinoma is exceedingly rare, accounting for less than 0.1 percent of the types of breast carcinomas.[100] The histology is generally indistin-

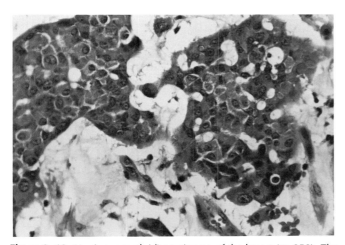

Figure 9–12. Mucinous (colloid) carcinoma of the breast (× 250). The tumor groupings are composed of cells containing relatively large amounts of cytoplasm and having relatively small nuclei. Mucin is present adjacent to the cell groupings as well as within some of the small glandlike structures within the groupings.

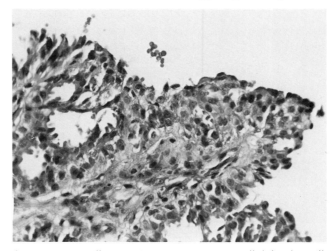

Figure 9–13. Papillary carcinoma (× 100). A well-defined papillary structure, with a fibrovascular core and covered with a stratified neoplastic epithelium, is seen. Some cribriform growth is seen adjacent to the base of this papillary growth and is commonly observed in papillary carcinoma. Moderate nuclear pleomorphism is evident.

guishable from that of the more common tumor found in the salivary glands (Fig. 9–14). The age distribution of patients with this neoplasm does not differ from that of common adenocarcinoma of the breast. Most adenoid cystic carcinomas of the breast are relatively small, measuring between 1 and 3 cm in diameter. These cancers characteristically have circumscribed, well-defined margins. The disproportionate interest in this rare tumor is probably explained by the striking microscopic similarity to common cribriform intraductal carcinoma.[7] Close inspection of adenoid cystic carcinoma discloses characteristic dense mucoid type material within glandular spaces that ultrastructurally resembles the lamina densa of the basement membrane. These small, well-differentiated, uniform, basiloid tumor cells show ultrastructural myoepithelial features. Distinguishing this rare tumor from more common forms of breast carcinoma is extremely important, because only a single case of axillary metastasis has been reported in association with breast adenoid cystic carcinoma.[57] Seven deaths from pulmonary metastases with origin from this tumor have been reported.[65]

APOCRINE CARCINOMA

Apocrine metaplasia is commonly present in benign breast diseases.[8] However, the presentation of breast neoplasms with malignant pure apocrine carcinoma histology is exceedingly uncommon. Apocrine carcinoma is so named because of its resemblance to normal apocrine glands that are concentrated in the anogenital area, axilla, and groin.[73] Similar glandular appendages are also found in the eyelid, external auditory canal, and beneath the areola of the breast. Normal apocrine glands are generally associated with the pilosebaceous apparatus. Histopathologically, their apocrine structures characteristically are composed of granular eosinophilic

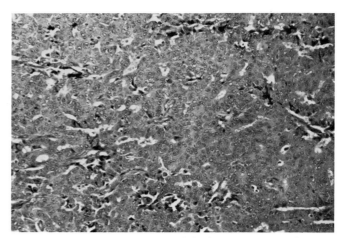

Figure 9–15. Apocrine carcinoma of the breast (× 100). The tumor contains secondary neoplastic glandlike spaces. The adjacent fibrovascular stroma is scant.

cells that produce merocrine secretions histologically termed apocrine "snouts." Cytoplasmic eosinophilia is attributable to the numerous mitochondria in the cytoplasm of apocrine cells.[27]

Apocrine carcinoma commonly presents a ductal or acinar growth pattern and has an unusual tendency to involve the lobular epithelium. These tumors are generally quite well differentiated histologically, with rounded vesicular nuclei and prominent nucleoli; they have a very low mitotic rate and little cytomorphological variability is evident (Figs. 9–15 and 9–16). Although numbers are small, four of six patients with apocrine carcinoma in one study had axillary metastases, indicating a potentially aggressive biological behavior.[64] Of interest, all six patients' neoplasms had low to absent levels of estrogen and progesterone receptors.

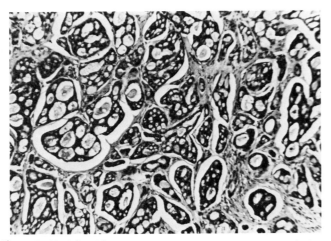

Figure 9–14. Adenoid cystic carcinoma (× 40). Prominent cribriform formation is seen with intraluminal bridging. The neoplastic cells reveal minimal stratification and are hyperchromatic with mild nuclear pleomorphism. Many of the glandlike lumens contain eosinophilic acellular material that is PAS positive. The stroma is fibrotic and relatively hypocellular. Trabecular and solid areas of tumor growth may also occur.

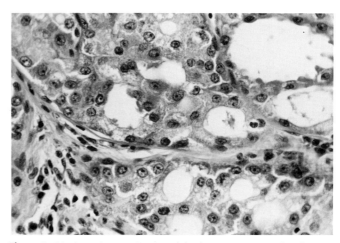

Figure 9–16. Apocrine carcinoma of the breast (× 250). The glandlike spaces within the tumor, some of which contain secretion, are apparent. The tumor cells have prominent cytoplasm, which is somewhat granular, similar to that of apocrine glands. The tumor nuclei are relatively uniform, and many contain prominent small nucleoli. The adjacent stroma contains some lymphocytes.

METAPLASTIC CARCINOMA

The transformation of one adult tissue into another variant is termed metaplasia. In rare instances, otherwise common adenocarcinomas of the breast undergo histological regression to a more primitive (undifferentiated) type. Metaplastic change in mammary carcinoma generally takes two forms. The first transformation involves an alteration of variably differentiated glandular epithelium into recognizable squamous elements. The second demonstrates mesenchymal differentiation, often in the form of bone or cartilage.[55, 91] Squamous metaplasia may be seen in up to 2 percent of otherwise unremarkable breast carcinomas. This histopathological feature is unusually frequent in medullary carcinoma, in which up to one sixth of the tumors show areas of squamous differentiation. Confusion exists in using the term "carcinosarcoma," since squamous carcinomas may present as a malignant spindle cell, pseudosarcomatous pattern. Clinically, the prognosis for patients with metaplastic carcinoma appears not to differ significantly from that of others with high-grade neoplasms. Immunohistochemical techniques that demonstrate epithelial and mesenchymal differentiation are useful in separating and rendering a definitive diagnosis in difficult cases. The prognosis for this group of rare metaplastic carcinomas is indeterminate at this writing. Poorly differentiated, predominantly spindle cell lesions tend to be most aggressive. The rare, pure squamous cell carcinoma of breast may represent a totally metaplastic carcinoma. In such cases an occult primary tumor, such as squamous cell carcinoma of the lung, metastatic to breast, must be excluded.

SECRETORY CARCINOMA

McDivitt and Stewart, in 1966,[59] described secretory carcinoma of the breast, a rare form of carcinoma that is, however, the most common variant of breast carcinoma occurring in children. Subsequent studies have clearly established that secretory carcinoma is not found exclusively in children, although younger age groups do predominate. Patients generally present with a painless breast mass that is circumscribed and is often of long duration. Circumscription is especially common in younger patients. The histology is that of a low-grade microcystic neoplasm. The neoplastic glandular lumen contains abundant mucin-positive secretions that can also be identified within the granular cytoplasm of lining cells. Akhtar et al., in 1983,[3] reviewed the literature and added three adult cases, one of which demonstrated axillary metastases. Because of the rarity of metastases in children, local excision has been recommended as adequate therapy.

MAMMARY CARCINOMA WITH OSTEOCLAST-LIKE GIANT CELLS

Agnantis and Rosen, in 1979,[1] described eight cases of mammary carcinoma associated with osteoclast-like giant cells. These tumors characteristically present a well-defined margin and an unusual dark brown or red-brown cut surface. Pigmentation may be so intense as to suggest metastatic melanoma. Aside from the presence of the osteoclast-like giant cells, the histological appearance is not unusual. The association of tumor admixed with giant cells in metastatic deposits may lead to erroneous diagnoses unless giant cells are recognized in the primary tumor. High levels of progesterone receptors have been reported in these tumors.[53]

INFILTRATING LOBULAR CARCINOMA

In 1865, Cornil[29] illustrated a variant of invasive breast carcinoma with a distinctive linear and target-like growth pattern, which is now commonly accepted as invasive lobular carcinoma. Foote and Stewart, in 1941,[47] provided their classic description of lobular carcinoma *in situ*. Invasive lobular carcinoma characteristically permeates a desmoplastic stroma in a linear fashion that has been termed Indian filing (Figs. 9–17 and 9–18). There is also a tendency for single-file linear groups of cells to surround the terminal ductal lobular unit in concentric circles. The term "targetoid" is in common usage for this growth pattern. Clinically, patients with infiltrating lobular carcinoma are in the same general age range as those with common adenocarcinoma ("infiltrating ductal") and constitute a reported frequency of 5 to 10 percent of breast carcinoma. This invasive neoplasm has a reported frequency of bilaterality approaching 30 percent in some series, bilateral occurrence being approximately twice that seen in common adenocarcinomas.

The gross appearance of infiltrating lobular carcinoma deserves special consideration. These tumors vary from clinically inapparent, microscopic lesions to those totally replacing the entire breast with a poorly defined, somewhat firm lesion. The tumor may grossly mimic inflammatory and benign disease in many instances. Because

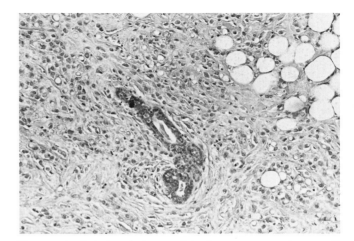

Figure 9–17. Lobular carcinoma of the breast (× 100). Tumor cells, which are relatively small and uniform, can be seen about fat and a preformed breast duct. A prominent desmoplastic stromal response is seen about the tumor cells.

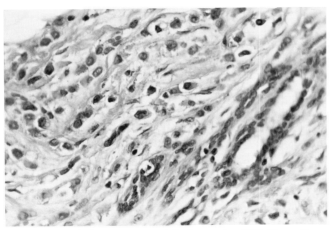

Figure 9–18. Lobular carcinoma of the breast. (× 250). The uniform, relatively small tumor cells of lobular carcinoma are seen arranged in a single file orientation ("Indian filing"). Adjacent benign duct elements are seen, lined by uniform ductal epithelium, with small dark myoepithelial cells present immediately beneath the epithelial cells.

infiltrating lobular carcinoma has a high propensity for multicentricity and multifocality, these neoplasms can present perplexing problems to surgeons attempting to perform subtotal mammary resections (see chapters 15, 35, and 36).

Efforts to subclassify infiltrating lobular carcinoma within the confines of its current restrictive definition have proved to be difficult, if not impossible.[90] Dixon et al., in 1982,[34] described approximately 100 cases of infiltrating lobular carcinoma, of which they found that 30 percent conformed to the classic histological pattern. Twenty-nine percent of the lesions presented as a mixture of growth patterns, 22 percent were classified as solid, and 19 percent were designated an alveolar variant. The pure or classic type may have a somewhat better prognosis than its variants. The lack of recognition and separation of these forms may account for the poorer prognosis reported in the past (see Table 9–3). Our approach has been to avoid an unequivocal or unqualified diagnosis of infiltrating lobular carcinoma in the absence of either associated lobular carcinoma *in situ* or the classic histological features accepted and described above.[35, 38, 43]

The histopathological features of lobular carcinoma include characteristic small cells with rounded nuclei, inconspicuous nucleoli, and scanty, indistinct cytoplasm (see Figs. 9–17 and 9–18). Special stains for mucin give variable results but, not infrequently, reveal intracytoplasmic mucin. When intracytoplasmic mucin is abundant and displaces the nucleus laterally, the resemblance to signet-ring carcinoma of the gastrointestinal tract becomes apparent and the designation "infiltrating lobular carcinoma, signet-ring type" is appropriate.[23, 50, 61] Dense-core neurosecretory granules have occasionally been described in otherwise typical infiltrating lobular carcinomas.

Patterns of metastatic spread for lobular carcinoma are often distinctive. *Meningeal carcinomatosis* is typically seen, in contradistinction to the nodular metastatic

deposits evident within the brain from metastatic (common) adenocarcinoma. This tendency toward diffuse membrane involvement is also seen with *peritoneal* and *pulmonary serosal metastases*. Diffuse *retroperitoneal spread*, with thickening and desmoplasia of the retroperitoneal tissues, has also been described. The diagnostic dilemma that this type of metastatic spread presents for clinicians and pathologists may be insoluble. The presence of estrogen and progesterone receptors in the tumor cells favors the diagnosis of metastatic lobular breast carcinoma rather than gastrointestinal signet-ring carcinoma. Metastatic deposits have been confused with a variety of histiocytic lesions and even confused with chalazion of the eyelid.[95] There is considerable controversy concerning the prognosis of infiltrating lobular carcinoma. The overall prognosis as a group probably does not differ greatly from that for common adenocarcinomas of the breast of equivalent stage.[10, 28, 79]

MAMMARY CARCINOMA WITH ENDOCRINE FEATURES

Rosen has focused attention on a heterogeneous group of mammary tumors that contain detectable amounts of human chorionic gonadotropin, calcitonin, and adrenocortical hormone as well as epinephrine.[76] These hormonally active substances are rarely produced by breast tumors in quantities sufficient to produce clinical symptoms. Detection relies upon biochemical analysis or immunohistochemistry of the tumor. An interesting morphological correlate is the demonstration of dense-core, membrane–bound neurosecretory type granules in a variety of breast carcinomas.[39, 87] Argyrophilia has been demonstrated in a small percentage of infiltrating common breast adenocarcinomas as well as lobular, mucinous, intraductal, and small cell neuroendocrine carcinomas (Figs. 9–19 and 9–20). The clinical implications of these interesting observations remain to be established.[16, 54]

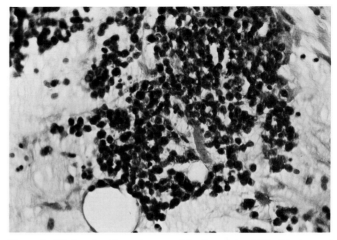

Figure 9–19. Small cell carcinoma of the breast (× 100). The tumor is composed of relatively uniform small cells within a fibrous stroma.

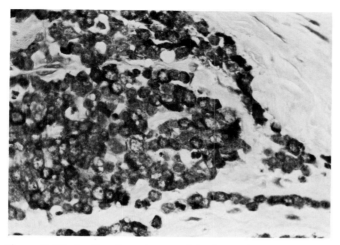

Figure 9–20. Small cell carcinoma of the breast (× 250). Neuron-specific enolase immunoperoxidase stain of the tumor demonstrates cytoplasmic staining, seen as darkened cytoplasm here. The tumor growth is in both nests and cords of single cells. The adjacent fibrous stroma reveals little inflammatory response.

CARCINOMA OF THE BREAST PRESENTING IN THE AXILLA

The axillary tail of Spence normally extends well into the axilla. However, heterotopic breast tissue, including fully functional breasts with the nipple, is infrequently identified in the axilla (see chapter 4). Primary carcinomas may therefore arise in this axillary breast tissue. Confident separation of a primary axillary breast tumor from nodal metastases of occult breast cancer occasionally presents a dilemma to the diagnostician and the surgeon.[52] The recognition of small portions of unequivocal residual lymph node, especially cortical sinuses and germinal centers, is of great value in making this distinction, as is the recognition of in situ ductal carcinoma associated with axillary adenocarcinoma within adjacent axillary breast tissue. Poorly differentiated tumors must be distinguished from malignant lymphomas and metastases from other primary sites, particularly cutaneous malignant melanoma. As previously noted, immunohistochemical techniques now provide an objective state-of-the-art means of determining histogenesis in many poorly differentiated neoplasms. The presence of putative carcinoma of the breast in an axillary lymph node in the absence of palpable or mammographically detectable primary breast cancer is an uncommon but difficult problem.

Patel et al., 1981,[70] described 29 cases of adenocarcinoma presenting in the axillae of women in the absence of clinically evident primary breast neoplasms. No extramammary primary tumors were detected. Mammographic lesions were found in 17 of the 29 patients. Mastectomy confirmed the presence of breast carcinoma in 16 of the 17 patients (94 percent). Of particular interest is that only 5 percent of these patients were free of disease at ten years. In the 13 patients in whom no primary breast carcinoma was found, 30 percent were free of disease after ten years. The authors observed that survival correlates best with the number of axillary lymph nodes involved by tumor rather than with the demonstration (anatomically and pathologically) of the presence of a primary breast carcinoma. Since no additional primary tumors developed in these women, these authors concluded that patients with axillary lymph nodes containing adenocarcinoma compatible with breast origin can probably be cured by mastectomy with axillary dissection.

PATHOLOGICAL EXAMINATION OF BREAST SPECIMENS

Procurement and processing of tissues for histological examination remains the standard method for establishing diagnoses in breast diseases. Adequate tissue must be surgically excised atraumatically to avoid crush or cautery artifact. Newer diagnostic techniques require increasing quantities of very fresh tumor tissue to provide reliable prognostic information derived from immunochemical and histochemical analyses. Principal among these are the quantitative measurements of steroid hormone receptors (estrogen and progesterone) and the quantitation and characterization of nuclear DNA. Ideally, all tissue should be delivered to the pathology laboratory in the fresh state immediately following gentle surgical excision. The receipt of breast tissue in the fresh, nonfixed state will provide the greatest number of diagnostic procedural options.

Conventional diagnostic techniques, such as mammography, identify very small carcinomas. These small lesions mandate preoperative consultation between the clinician, the radiologist, and the pathologist in order to plan and obtain the greatest amount of pathological and prognostic information for the individual patient. For detailed technical and historical reviews the reader is referred to recent works by Schmidt[89] and Rosen.[76]

The Biopsy

Nonpalpable lesions that are detected mammographically are virtually all removed by *excisional biopsy* techniques that utilize needle localization and specimen radiology to confirm complete removal. Small (1 to 10 mm) to intermediate (1 to 2 cm) sized lesions are commonly removed by total excision, and the surgical pathologist is requested to determine the adequacy of the surgical margins. Surgical margins can be readily evaluated microscopically if the intact surfaces of the margins of excision are coated with India ink or other easily identified soluble particulate substances, such as tattoo pigments. Larger tumors, generally those larger than 2 cm in diameter, are often initially approached by *incisional biopsy*. The indications and techniques for breast biopsy are extensively reviewed in chapter 28. Orientation of the tumor surface margin is the responsibility of the operating surgeon; it is best accomplished by providing a clear diagram of the lesion and marking with sutures of different lengths to indicate superior, inferior, medial, and lateral margins. Should difficulty with orientation of the tumor and soft tissues become evident at the time of request of pathology review, the surgeon should personally discuss the specimen with the pathologist to ensure accuracy of orientation and surgical margins. Following orientation of the exterior surface and recording of the three-dimensional metric measurements of the specimen, the lesion should be bisected to expose the cut surface of the neoplasm. Appropriate samples are then submitted for hormone-receptor analysis, DNA analysis/flow cytometry, and histology. In all cases of minimal breast cancer (< 1 cm) or small lesions (< 2 cm), the *priority for diagnostic tissue procured from breast biopsies must be given to histology.* An accurate gross description of cut surfaces and the borders of the neoplasm, with three-dimensional measurements of the neoplasm, is essential to any complete pathological examination.

Each patient should be considered individually and should participate in the development of her treatment goals and objectives. Documented patient discussions and concurrence with treatment plans are essential for good medical care and avoidance of medicolegal entanglements.

The role of frozen-section analysis of tissues in the management of breast diseases has changed somewhat in the past decade. The primary role of the frozen section is to establish the diagnosis at operation such that therapeutic decisions can be initiated intraoperatively; however, the current focus is on determining the adequacy of the tissue for the newer studies previously described. In most institutions, definitive operations are delayed until all prognostic tests are completed. The conservation and allocation of tissues for diagnostic procedures (immunohistochemical, hormone receptor analysis) other than traditional frozen-section diagnoses is a major new responsibility of the pathologist.

SEGMENTAL, SUBTOTAL, AND SIMPLE MASTECTOMY

The efficacy of chemotherapy and/or radiotherapy to control subclinical or microscopic residual breast cancer, as well as a better understanding of the general biology of breast neoplasia, has resulted in major technical alterations of the formerly accepted radical mastectomy. Subtotal or segmental resection is performed in a number of centers throughout the world. Although controversy still exists concerning the long-term adequacy of lesser procedures, the results are comparing favorably with the radical mastectomy. Patients selected for more conservative procedures generally have smaller tumors (≤ 3 to 4 cm) and clinically negative axillary lymph nodes. The subcutaneous (total glandular) mastectomy or simple mastectomy is usually reserved for patients with severe atypia or multifocal proliferative intraductal and lobular disease, especially if there is an associated family history of breast carcinoma.

Simple (total) mastectomy has previously been reserved for those patients with large, fungating breast carcinomas for which palliation, rather than cure, is the

therapeutic intent. The complete simple mastectomy removes all the glandular breast tissue with the exception of breast mesenchyma adherent to the skin flaps. Currently, low axillary nodal sampling (Levels I and II) is usually added. Often the term "simple mastectomy" is confusing, and we rely upon detailed descriptions of the tissues received, as examined and recorded by the pathologist.

Pathology Assessment of Radical and Modified Radical Mastectomy Specimens

The Radical Mastectomy

The standard radical mastectomy has largely been replaced by lesser surgical procedures described in chapter 29. The modified radical mastectomy spares a portion of the pectoral musculature and breast skin, thus enabling more acceptable cosmesis and the potential for better breast reconstruction. All standard and modified radical mastectomies include contents of the axillae, the lymph nodes of which must be clearly marked by the operating surgeon as to their precise anatomical origin (levels, groups).

The presence of attached pectoral muscles often enables approximate orientation of large radical mastectomy specimens. Accurate pathology assessment often becomes difficult or impossible with subtotal, modified procedures unless specimens are appropriately tagged by the surgeon. Following orientation and removal of the pectoral muscle, palpable lesions are best identified by placing the specimen skin side down and completing a series of 1 cm parallel incisions down to the skin surface. The cut surface of tumors displayed by this technique should be measured, described, and recorded. If mastectomy specimens are delivered to the laboratory immediately following their removal, hormone receptor analyses and other special procedures can be performed.

Pathology Assessment of Axillary Lymph Nodes

The presence or absence of axillary lymph node metastases as well as their number, size, and location is the most significant independent prognostic determinant in malignant breast diseases. Establishing the anatomical location of resected lymph nodes in the absence of orientation by the operating surgeon is imprecise, if not impossible. Careful dissection of unfixed axillary fat with digital examination on a hard surface will detect the vast majority of clinically significant lymph nodes. Previously, great attention has been paid to obtaining the largest possible number of lymph nodes from axillary dissections. Wide variation in the number of lymph nodes recovered has been reported. The wide range of numerical variability probably results from biological variability of the disease process, although the diligence of the pathologist examining the specimen has always been open to question. Wilkinson et al., in 1982,[98] studied 525 cases of invasive breast carcinomas whose axillary lymphatics had initially been reported to be free of metastatic tumor. These patients were followed for a minimum of five years. Re-examination of the axillary lymph nodes, employing serial and step section techniques, revealed 89 occult tumor metastases (17 percent) within the lymph nodes originally determined to be free of tumor. Of particular importance is the fact that this observation did not significantly influence the overall survival of these patients. Because of these observations, we recommend that the axillary lymph nodes be sliced into 2 mm sections, parallel to their long axes, and that all lymph node tissue be submitted for sectioning. To maximize the probability of detecting metastasis, at least two sections (slides) should be cut from each nodal slice, preferably one superficial section from the face of the block and one deeper section approximately half way into the block. These superficial and deep sections of the lymph node material will allow optimal examination of the nodes at approximately 1 mm intervals and enable detection of micrometastases greater than 1 mm in diameter.

References

1. Agnantis NT, Rosen PP: Mammary carcinoma with osteoclast-like giant cells. Am J Clin Pathol 72:383–389, 1979.
2. Ahmed A: Ultrastructural aspects of human breast lesions. Pathol Annu 15 (Pt:2):411–443, 1980.
3. Akhtar M, Robinson C, Ali MA, Godwin JT: Secretory carcinoma of the breast in adults. Light and electron microscopic study of three cases with review of the literature. Cancer 51:2245–2254, 1983.
4. Andersson I: Breast cancer screening in Malmö. Recent Results Cancer Res 90:114–116, 1984.
5. Andersson I, Andrén L, Hildell J, Linell F, Ljungqvist U, Pettersson H: Breast cancer screening with mammography. A population-based randomized trial with mammography as the only screening mode. Radiology 132:273–276, 1979.
6. Andersen JA, Fischermann K, Hou-Jensen K, Henriksen E, Andersen KW, Johansen H, Brincker H, Mouridsen HT, Castberg T, Rossing N, North M: Selection of high risk groups among prognostically favorable patients with breast cancer. Analysis of the value of prospective grading of tumor anaplasia in 1048 patients. Ann Surg 194:1–3, 1981.
7. Anthony PP, James PD: Adenoid cystic carcinoma of the breast: Prevalence, diagnostic criteria and histogenesis. J Clin Pathol 28:647–655, 1975.
8. Archer F, Omar M: Pink cell (oncocytic) metaplasia in a fibro-adenoma of the human breast: Electron microscope observations. J Pathol 99:119–124, 1969.
9. Ashikari R, Hajdu SI, Robbins, GF: Intraductal carcinoma of the breast (1960–1969). Cancer 28:1182–1187, 1971.
10. Ashikari R, Huvos AG, Urban JA, et al: Infiltrating lobular carcinoma of the breast. Cancer 31:110, 1973.
11. Ashikari R, Park K, Huvos AG, Urban JA: Paget's disease of the breast. Cancer 26:680–685, 1970.
12. Atkin NB: Modal deoxyribonucleic acid value and survival in carcinomas of the breast. Br Med J 1:271–272, 1972.
13. Atkin NB, Kay R: Prognostic significance of modal DNA value and other factors in malignant tumors, based on 1465 cases. Br J Cancer 40:210–221, 1979.
14. Auer GU, Caspersson TO, Gustafsson SA, Humla SA, Ljung BM, Nordenskjöid BA, Silfvergwärd C, Wallgren AS: Relationship between nuclear DNA distribution and estrogen receptors in human mammary carcinomas. Anal Quant Cytol Histol 2:280–284, 1980.
15. Auer GU, Fallenius AG, Erhardt KY, Sundelin BS: Progression of mammary adenocarcinomas as reflected by nuclear DNA content. Cytometry 5:420–425, 1984.
16. Azzopardi JG, Muretto P, Goddeeris P, Eusebiv J, Eusebiv J, Lauweryns JM: Carcinoid tumors of the breast: The morphological spectrum of argyrophil carcinomas. Histopathology 6:549–569, 1982.
17. Bedrossian CWM, Raber M, Barlogie B: Flow cytometry and cytomorphology in primary resectable breast carcinomas. Anal Quant Cytol Histol 3:112–116, 1981.
18. Bichel P, Paulsen HS, Andersen J: Estrogen receptor content and ploidy of human mammary carcinomas. Cancer 50:1771–1774, 1982.
19. Black MM, Barclay THC, Hankey BF: Prognosis in breast cancer utilizing histologic characteristics of the primary tumor. Cancer 36:2048–2055, 1975.
20. Black MM, Speer FD: Nuclear structure in cancer tissues. Surg Gynecol Obstet 105:97–102, 1957.
21. Bloom HJG: Prognosis in carcinoma of the breast. Br J Cancer 4:259–288, 1950.
22. Bloom HJG, Richardson WW: Histological grading and prognosis in breast cancer. A study of 1049 cases, of which 359 have been followed 15 years. Br J Cancer 11:359–377, 1957.
23. Breslow A, Brancaccio ME: Intracellular mucin production by lobular breast carcinoma cells. Arch Pathol Lab Med 100:620–621, 1976.
24. Carstens PHB: Tubular carcinoma of the breast. A study of frequency. Am J Clin Pathol 70:204–210, 1978.
25. Carstens PHB, Greenberg RA, Francis D, Lyon H: Tubular carcinoma of the breast. A long term follow-up. Histopathology 9:271–280, 1985.
26. Carter D, Pipkin RD, Shepard RH, Elkins RC, Abbey H: Relationship of necrosis and tumor border to lymph node metastases and 10 year survival in carcinoma of the breast. Am J Surg Pathol 2:39–46, 1978.
27. Charles A: An electron microscopic study of the human axillary apocrine gland. J Anat 93:226–232, 1959.
28. Cormier WJ, Gaffey TA, Welch JM, Welch JS, Edmonson JH: Linitis plastica caused by metastatic lobular carcinoma of the breast. Mayo Clin Proc 55:747, 1980.
29. Cornil AV: Contributions à l'histoire du developpement histologique des tumeurs épithéliales (squirrhe, encephaloide, et.) J Anat Physiol 2:266–276, 1865.
30. Cubilla AL, Woodruff JM, Erlandson RA: Comparative clinicopathologic study of endocrine-like and ordinary mucinous carcinomas of the breast. Lab Invest 50:14A, 1984.
31. Cutler SJ, Black MM, Mork T, Harvei S, Freeman C: Further observations on prognostic factors in cancer of the female breast. Cancer 24:653–667, 1969.
32. Deos PH, Norris HJ: Well-differentiated (tubular) carcinoma of the breast. Am J Clin Pathol 78:1–7, 1982.
33. Devitt JE, Barr JR: The clinical recognition of cystic carcinoma of the breast. Surg Gynecol Obstet 159:130–132, 1984.
34. Dixon JM, Anderson TJ, Page DL, Lee D, Duffy SW: Infiltrating lobular carcinoma of the breast. Histopathology 6:149, 1982.
35. Dixon JM, Anderson TJ, Page DL, Lee D, Duffy SW, Stewart HJ: Infiltrating lobular carcinoma of the breast: An evolution of the incidence and consequence of bilateral disease. Br J Surg 70:513–516, 1983.
36. Dupont WD, Page DL: Risk factors for breast cancer in women with proliferative breast disease. N Engl J Med 312:146–151, 1985.
37. Elston CW: Grading of invasive carcinoma of the breast. In Page DL, Anderson TJ (eds): Diagnostic Histopathology of the Breast. New York, Churchill-Livingstone, 1987, pp 300–311.
38. Fechner RE: Histologic variants of infiltrating lobular carcinoma of the breast. Hum Pathol 6:373–378, 1975.
39. Fetissof F, Dubois MP, Arbeille-Brassart B, Lansac J, Jobard P: Argyrophilic cells in mammary carcinoma. Hum Pathol 14:127–134, 1983.
40. Fisher B, Bauer M, Wickerham L, Redmond CK, Fisher ER: Relation of number of positive axillary nodes to the prognosis of patients with primary breast cancer. NSABP update. Cancer 52:1551–1557, 1983.
41. Fisher B, Slack NH, Bross IDJ, et al: Cancer of the breast: Size of neoplasm and prognosis. Cancer 24:1071–1080, 1969.
42. Fisher ER, Gregorio RM, Fisher B, Redmond C, Vellios F, Sommers SC: The pathology of invasive breast cancer. A

syllabus derived from findings of the National Surgical Adjuvant Breast Project (No. 4). Cancer 36:1–85, 1975.

43. Fisher ER, Gregorio RM, Redmond C, Fisher B: Tubulolobular invasive breast carcinoma: A variant of lobular invasive cancer. Hum Pathol 8:679–683, 1977.

44. Fisher ER, Palekar AS, Redmond C, Barton B, Fisher B: Pathologic findings from the National Surgical Adjuvant Breast Project (Protocol No. 4) VI. Invasive papillary cancer. Am J Clin Pathol 73:313–322, 1980.

45. Fisher E, Sass R, Fisher B, Wickerham L, Paik SM, et al: Pathologic findings from the National Surgical Adjuvant Breast Project (Protocol 6). I. Intraductal carcinoma (DCIS). Cancer 57:197–208, 1986.

46. Flotte TJ, Bell DA, Greco MA: Tubular carcinoma and sclerosing adenosis. The use of basal lamina as a differential feature. Am J Surg Pathol 4:75–77, 1980.

47. Foote FW Jr, Stewart FW: Lobular carcinoma in situ: A rare form of mammary cancer. Am J Pathol 17:491–496, 1941.

48. Freedman LS, Edwards DN, McConnell EM, Downham DY: Histological grade and other prognostic factors in relation to survival of patients with breast cancer. Br J Cancer 40:44–45, 1979.

49. Fu YS, Marksem JA, Hubay CA, et al: The relationship of breast cancer morphology and estrogen receptor protein status. *In* Fenoglio CM, Wolff M (eds): Progress in Surgical Pathology, Vol III. New York, Masson, 1981, pp 65–76.

50. Gad A, Azzopardi JG: Lobular carcinoma of the breast: A special variant of mucin secreting carcinoma. J Clin Pathol 28:711–716, 1975.

51. Geschickter CF: Disease of the Breast: Diagnosis, Pathology, Treatment. 2nd ed. Philadelphia, JB Lippincott, 1945, pp 565–575.

52. Haupt HM, Rosen PP, Kinne DW: Breast carcinoma presenting with axillary lymph node metastasis: An analysis of specific histopathologic features. Am J Surg Pathol 9:165–175, 1985.

53. Holland R, van Haelst UJ: Mammary carcinoma with osteoclast-like giant cells. Additional observations on six cases. Cancer 53:1963–1973, 1984.

54. Jundt G, Schulz A, Heitz PU, Osborn M: Small cell neuroendocrine (oat cell) carcinoma of the male breast. Virchows Arch [Pathol Anat] 404:213–221, 1984.

55. Kahn LB, Uys CJ, Dale J, Rutherfoord S: Carcinoma of the breast with metaplasia to chondrosarcoma: A light and electron microscopic study. Histopathology 2:93–106 1978.

56. Lee AK, Rosen PP, DeLellis RA, Saigo PE, Gangi MD, Groshen S, Bagin R, Wolfe HJ: Tumor markers expression in breast carcinomas and relationship to prognosis. An immunohistochemical study. Am J Clin Pathol 84:687–696, 1985.

57. Lim SK, Kovi J, Warner OG: Adenoid cystic carcinoma of breast with metastasis: A case report and review of the literature. J Natl Med Assoc 71:329–330, 1979.

58. Maier WP, Rosemond GP, Goldman LI, et al: A-ten year study of medullary carcinoma of the breast. Surg Gynecol Obstet 144:695–698, 1977.

59. McDivitt RW, Stewart FW: Breast carcinoma in children. JAMA 195:388–390, 1966.

60. McDivitt RW, Stewart FW, Berg JW: Tumors of the breast. Atlas of Tumor Pathology, Series 2, Fascicle No 2. Washington DC, Armed Forces Institute of Pathology, 1968, pp 89–90.

61. Merino MJ, LiVolsi VA: Signet ring carcinoma of the female breast: A clinicopathologic analysis of 24 cases. Cancer 48:1830–1837, 1981.

62. Meyer JS, McDivitt RW, Stone KR, Prey MU, Bauer WC: Practical breast carcinoma cell kinetics: Review and update. Breast Cancer Res Treat 4:79–88, 1984.

63. Moore OS Jr, Foote FW Jr: The relatively favorable prognosis of medullary carcinoma of the breast. Cancer 2:635–642, 1949.

64. Mossler J, Barton TK, Brinkhouse AD, McCarty KS, Moylan JA, McCarty KS Jr: Apocrine differentiation in human mammary carcinoma. Cancer 46:2463–2471, 1980.

65. Nayer HR: Cylindroma of the breast with pulmonary metastases. Dis Chest 31:324–327, 1957.

66. Ohuchi N, Abe R, Kasai M: Possible cancerous change in intraductal papillomas of the breast. A 3-D reconstruction study of 25 cases. Cancer 54:605–611, 1984.

66a. Page DL, Anderson TJ: Diagnostic Histopathology of the Breast. New York, Churchill Livingstone, 1987, p 194.

67. Page DL, Vander Zwagg R, Rogers LW, Williams LT, Walker WE, Hartmann WH: Relation between component parts of fibrocystic disease complex and breast cancer. J Natl Cancer Inst 61:1055–1063, 1978.

68. Papotti M, Eusebi V, Gugliotta P, Bussolati G: Immunohistochemical analysis of benign and malignant papillary lesions of the breast. Am J Surg Pathol 7:451–561, 1983.

69. Papotti M, Gugliotta P, Ghiringhello B, Bussolati G: Association of breast carcinoma and multiple intraductal papillomas: An histological and immunohistochemical investigation. Histopathology 8:963–975, 1984.

70. Patel J, Nemoto T, Rosner D, Dao TL, Pickren JW: Axillary lymph node metastasis from an occult breast cancer. Cancer 47:2923–2927, 1981.

71. Richardson WW: Medullary carcinoma of the breast. A distinctive tumor type with a relatively good prognosis following radical mastectomy. Br J Cancer 10:415–423, 1956.

72. Robinson RR: Gelatinous cancer of the breast. Trans Pathol Soc Lond 4:275, 1852.

73. Roddy HJ, Silverberg SG: Ultrastructural analysis of apocrine carcinoma of the human breast. Ultrastruct Pathol 1:385–393, 1980.

74. Rosen PP: Microglandular adenosis, a benign lesion simulating invasive mammary carcinoma. Am J Surg Pathol 7:137–144, 1983.

75. Rosen PP: The pathological classification of human mammary carcinoma: Past, present and future. Ann Cli Lab Sci 9:144–156, 1979.

76. Rosen PP: The pathology of breast carcinoma. *In* Harris J, Hellman S (eds): Breast Diseases. Philadelphia, JB Lippincott, 1987, pp 147–209.

77. Rosen PP, Lesser ML, Kinne DW: Breast carcinoma at the extremes of age: A comparison of patients younger than 35 years and older than 75 years. J Surg Oncol 28:90–96, 1985.

78. Rosen PP, Lesser ML, Kinne DW, Beattie EJ: Breast carcinoma in women 35 years of age or younger. Ann Surg 199:133–142, 1984.

79. Rosen PP, Kosloff C, Lieberman PH, Adair F, Braun DW Jr: Lobular carcinoma in situ of the breast. Detailed analysis of 99 patients with average follow-up of 24 years. Am J Surg Pathol 2:225–251, 1978.

80. Rosen PP, Saigo PE, Braun DW Jr, Beattie EJ Jr, Kinne DW: Occult axillary lymph node metastases from breast cancers with intramammary lymphatic tumor emboli. Am J Surg Pathol 6:639–641, 1982.

81. Rosen PP, Saigo PE, Braun DW Jr, Weathers E, DePalo A: Predictors of recurrence in Stage I (T1N0M0) breast carcinoma. Ann Surg 193:15–25, 1981.

82. Rosen PP, Saigo PE, Braun DW Jr, Weathers E, Kinne DW: Prognosis in Stage II (T1N1M0) breast cancer. Ann Surg 194:576–584, 1981.

83. Rosen PP: Tumor emboli in intramammary lymphatics in breast carcinoma: Pathologic criteria for diagnosis and clinical significance. Pathol Annu 18 (Pt2):215–232, 1983.

84. Rosen PP, Wang TY: Colloid carcinoma of the breast. Analysis of 64 patients with long-term follow-up. Am J Clin Pathol 73:304, 1980.

85. Sakamoto G: Histological classification of breast cancer. Jpn J Cancer Clin 32 (Suppl 1):197–204, 1986.

86. Sakamoto G, Sugano H, Hartmann WH: Comparative pathological study of breast carcinoma among American and Japanese women. *In* McGuire WL (ed): Breast Cancer. Advances in Research and Treatment, Vol 4. New York, Plenum, 1981, pp 211–231.

87. Sariola H, Lehtonen E, Saxen E: Breast tumors with a solid and uniform carcinoid pattern. Ultrastructural and immunohistochemical study of two cases. Pathol Res Pract 178:405–411, 1985.

88. Schaefer G, Rosen PP, Lesser ML, Kinne DW, Beattie EJ Jr: Breast carcinoma in elderly women: Pathology prognosis and survival. Pathol Annu 19 (Pt1):195–219, 1984.

89. Schmidt WA: Principles and Techniques of Surgical Pathology. New York, Addison-Wesley, 1983.

90. Shousha S, Backhous CM, Alaghband-Zadeh J, Burn I: Alveolar variant of invasive lobular carcinoma of the breast. Am J Clin Pathol 85:1–5, 1986.
91. Smith BH, Taylor HB: The occurrence of bone and cartilage in mammary tumors. Am J Clin Pathol 51:610–618, 1969.
92. Taylor HB, Norris HJ: Well differentiated carcinoma of the breast. Cancer 25:687–692, 1970.
93. Thoresen S: Histological grading and clinical stage at presentation in breast carcinoma. Br J Cancer 46:457–458, 1982.
94. Wallgren A, Silversward C, Eklund G: Prognostic factors in mammary carcinoma. Acta Radiol 15:1–16, 1976.
95. Weinstein GW, Goldman JN: Metastatic adenocarcinoma of the breast masquerading as chalazion. Am J Ophthalmol 56:960, 1963.
96. Wellings SR, Alpers CE: Subgross pathologic features and incidence of radial scars in the breast. Hum Pathol 15:475–479, 1984.
97. Wellings SR, Jensen HM: On the origin and progression of ductal carcinoma in the human breast. J Natl Cancer Inst 50:1111–1116, 1973.
98. Wilkinson EJ, Hause LL, Hoffman RG, Kuzma JF, Rothwell DJ, Doengan WL, Clowry LJ, Almagro UA, Choi H, Rimm AA: Occult axillary lymph node metastases in invasive breast carcinoma: Characteristics of the primary tumor and significance of the metastases. Pathol Annu (Pt2)17:67–91, 1982.
99. World Health Organization: Histological Typing of Breast Tumours. 2nd ed. International Histological Classification of Tumours No 2, p 19. Geneva, World Health Organization, 1981.
100. Zaloudek C, Oertel YC, Orenstein JM: Adenoid cystic carcinoma of the breast. Am J Clin Pathol 81:297–307, 1984.

Chapter 10

MESENCHYMAL INFILTRATING TUMORS

John Reynolds, M.D., Carolyn Mies, M.D., and John M. Daly, M.D.

Soft tissue sarcomas are rare, constituting 0.7 percent of all cancers.[15] Breast sarcomas represent less than 5 percent of all sarcomas, and it is estimated that they make up less than 1 percent of all breast malignancies.[75] The rarity of sarcomas limits our knowledge regarding their natural history and precludes the performance of prospective clinical trials to determine optimal treatment.

Mammary sarcomas are histologically identical to comparable soft tissue tumors in other anatomical sites. These neoplasms have origin from the stroma and fat of the breast and lack a neoplastic epithelial component. Angiosarcoma and lymphoma, the latter once referred to as lymphosarcoma, are two distinct clinicopathological entities that are usually excluded from the general group of mammary sarcomas even though they are nonepithelial neoplasms. Stewart-Treves syndrome represents the development of angiosarcoma of the skin and soft tissue in the presence of postmastectomy lymphedema and will be discussed separately. Cystosarcoma phyllodes, a tumor arising from the unique, hormonally responsive intralobular stroma of the breast, is also considered as a separate entity with its own distinctive histomorphology and clinical behavior.

SARCOMA: AN OVERVIEW

The term *sarcoma* (from the Greek "sarkoma," meaning fleshy growth) denotes tumors that have arisen from the primitive mesenchyme. The term sarcoma classically refers to nonepithelial growths and includes tumors derived from vascular and lymphatic endothelium, as both arise from the mesoderm and behave biologically like other soft tissue sarcomas. Soft tissue sarcomas tend to arise unifocally and to spread along a path of least resistance, in general respecting anatomical boundaries. Surrounding normal tissue is compressed into a layered edematous and neovascularized rim of pseudocapsule that often contains invasive projections of malignant tissue. Sarcomas have a propensity to metastasize by the hematogenous route, usually to the lungs or bone. Ten percent of patients presenting with high-grade soft tissue sarcomas have metastases evident at the time of presentation. Regional lymph node involvement is rare and may be prognostically equivalent to metastatic disease.[74]

Pathological classification of soft tissue sarcoma is currently based on the putative cell of origin of each tumor rather than on the predominant cell type.[25] Currently, malignant fibrous histiocytoma (MFH), heretofore rarely recognized as a distinct entity, constitutes 20 to 30 percent of sarcomas in most series. There remains, however, a large percentage of "unclassifiable" sarcomas (10 to 20 percent) and a great variation of reported subtypes from different institutions, undoubtedly reflecting differences in pathological opinion rather than true differences in frequency. Pathologists often disagree on the histological grade of sarcomas, because the criteria used to grade these tumors are not readily quantifiable (nuclear morphology, mitoses, anaplasia, pleomorphism, presence of necrosis). Grade is incorporated into the system of staging developed by the American Joint Committee for Cancer Staging.[74] G1 represents low malignancy, G2 moderate malignancy, and G3 high malignancy. Table 10–1 indicates the criteria for assignment of a tumor to Stages I to IV. This staging has been criticized for four reasons: First, the criteria for grading set down by the Task Force is imprecise and does not lead to consensus among expert pathologists; second, site (whether intracompartmental or extracompartmental) is arguably more important than size; third, nodal metastases carry a poor prognosis and may best be included along with M1; and fourth, the inclusion of local disease (T3N0M0) in the same stage as M1 is strongly disputed.[24, 46]

Clinically, sarcomas are usually asymptomatic at presentation, and because they generally arise in compressible tissues, they may attain a large size. An incisional biopsy should be performed for diagnosis, with the line of incision in such a location as not to compromise subsequent definitive excision. Pulmonary metastatic evaluation is recommended using CT scan, which is preferred to conventional tomography.[59] The extent of local involvement is best determined by CT or magnetic resonance imaging, with arteriography indicated in selected situations.[38]

The mainstay of treatment is wide excision in a tissue plane external to the sarcoma. Lymph node dissection is unnecessary unless nodal tissues are grossly involved. Perioperative radiation therapy results in a lessening[85] of local recurrence, which occurs in 20 to 50 percent of patients who undergo wide local excision alone.[14] Distant

T	Primary tumor T_1 Tumor less than 5 cm T_2 Tumor 5 cm or greater T_3 Tumor that grossly invades bone, vessel, or major nerve
N	Regional lymph nodes N_0 No histologically verified metastases in regional lymph nodes N_1 Histologically verified regional lymph node metastasis
M	Distant metastasis M_0 No distant metastasis M_1 Distant metastasis
G	Histologic grade of malignancy G_1 Low G_2 Moderate G_3 High

Stage I	
Stage Ia $G_1T_1N_0M_0$	Grade 1 tumor less than 5 cm in diameter with no regional lymph nodes or distant metastases
Stage Ib $G_1T_2N_0M_0$	Grade 1 tumor 5 cm or greater in diameter with no regional lymph nodes or distant metastases
Stage II	
Stage IIa $G_2T_2N_0M_0$	Grade 2 tumor less than 5 cm in diameter with no regional lymph nodes or distant metastases
Stage IIb $G_2T_2N_0M_0$	Grade 2 tumor 5 cm or greater in diameter with no regional lymph nodes or distant metastases
Stage III	
Stage IIIa $G_3T_1N_0M_0$	Grade 3 tumor less than 5 cm in diameter with no regional lymph nodes or distant metastases
Stage IIIb $G_3T_2N_0M_0$	Grade 3 tumor 5 cm or greater in diameter with no regional lymph nodes or distant metastases
Stage IIIc $G_{1-3}T_{1-2}N_2M_0$	Tumor of any grade or size (no invasion) with regional lymph nodes, but no distant metastases
Stage IV	
Stage IVa $G_{1-3}T_3N_{0-1}M_0$	Tumor of any grade that grossly invades bone, major vessel, or major nerve with or without regional lymph node metastases but without distant metastases
Stage IVb $G_{1-3}T_{1-3}N_0M_1$	Clinically diagnosed distant metastases

From Russell WO, Cohen J, Enzinger F, et al: Cancer 40:1562–1570, 1977. Reprinted by permission.

recurrence, usually pulmonary, occurs in 50 percent of cases.[70] Effective adjuvant therapy is therefore desirable for high-grade sarcomas. Rosenberg et al.[73] demonstrated prolongation of disease-free survival using doxorubicin and cyclophosphamide following operative resection of primary extremity soft tissue sarcomas, but other trials[23] have not confirmed these results. For established pulmonary metastases, aggressive pulmonary resection is recommended, as up to 20 percent of patients with resectable metastases can be cured.[51] For unresectable metastases, response rates of up to 20 percent have been reported for regimes containing doxorubicin.[8] Rosenberg et al. recently reported responses of metastatic sarcoma to treatment with a combination of lymphokine-activated killer cells and high–dose interleukin 2.[72] It is likely that future improvement in the management of high-grade soft tissue sarcomas will be through effective adjuvant chemotherapy or immunotherapy.

BREAST SARCOMA

Mammary Sarcoma

Sarcomas of the breast are a heterogeneous[3] group of tumors, not a single entity. Some common clinical and pathological features are shared by this diverse group of neoplasms, which include fibrosarcoma, fibromatosis (low-grade fibrosarcoma or desmoid tumor), malignant fibrous histiocytoma, liposarcoma, leiomyosarcoma, osteogenic sarcoma, and chondrosarcoma. Stromal sarcoma is a term introduced in 1962 by Berg and his colleagues[6] to describe mammary tumors other than lymphoma, angiosarcoma, and cystosarcoma phyllodes. This nonspecific term obscures the diversity of this group of neoplasms, which are histologically identical to comparable soft tissue tumors arising in other anatomical sites; its use is not advocated except for sarcomas arising in the unique hormone-responsive stroma of the mammary lobules.[13]

For a variety of reasons, a clear picture of the morphological and clinical spectrum of each specific type of sarcoma has been slow to emerge. First, these mammary tumors are rare. Second, the histological classification of sarcoma has undergone considerable change over the last few decades. Certain tumor types, such as malignant fibrous histiocytoma, were not recognized as specific entities until relatively recently. Thus, discriminating true sarcomas from metaplastic carcinoma, an important pathological differential diagnosis, can be difficult. Accurate classification of spindle cell neoplasms has been greatly facilitated by immunohistochemistry and electron microscopy.

Survival data from previous studies of mammary sarcoma are difficult to interpret because of the aforementioned confounding variables. Because most reported patients have been treated with mastectomy of some type, it is difficult to gain a clear picture of the relationship between pathological features and the risk of local recurrence complicating less extensive disease.

Clinical Features. Clinical presentation is typically with a large painless breast mass. Barnes and Pietruska,[3] reviewing 100 patients, report that the mean age at the time of presentation was 52 and that the median tumor size was 5.3 cm. In most series, over 50 percent of patients were aware of their tumors for more than six months, and sought medical attention because of a sudden rapid growth phase. Routine mammography does not appear to be a useful diagnostic aid.

Pathological Features. Grossly, most mammary sarcomas are solid tumors, although small cysts and degenerated areas are occasionally noted. They lack the "cut cabbage" or leafy, laminated appearance of cystosarcoma phyllodes. Some tumors are well circumscribed, whereas others have an ill-defined, infiltrative margin.

In general, sarcomas of the breast are histologically similar to their more common counterparts in the skin and soft tissues of other parts of the body.[6, 13, 62] Essentially, they are spindle cell neoplasms growing as expansile, solid masses with a microscopic margin that may be sharp and pushing or infiltrative. In the latter instance, tumor cells invade fat and tend to grow between the glandular structures of the breast, separating individual lobules and expanding the intralobular space, a common morphological feature shared with angiosarcoma and lymphoma. These tumors are graded in the same way as extramammary sarcomas; cellularity, the degree of cellular pleomorphism and nuclear atypia, mitotic activity, and evidence of differentiation are the features generally considered. Neoplastic glands or epithelium are never seen in mammary sarcoma.

Fibrosarcoma

Primary mammary fibrosarcoma is a neoplastic proliferation of fibroblasts. Fibrosarcomas are composed of spindle-shaped cells of fibroblastic origin. These tumor cells have little cytoplasm and grow in long, sweeping fascicles. In the classic example, fibrosarcoma usually forms a herringbone pattern. The collagen formed by the tumor cells is variable in amount and is found in the intercellular space in the form of wavy or solid hyaline material. Mitoses are often seen; they may be numerous and appear abnormal in poorly differentiated tumors. Multinucleated giant cells are not a feature of fibrosarcoma. Occasionally, small foci of osseous or cartilaginous metaplasia are seen in tumors rich in collagen.[25]

Ultrastructurally, the cells composing fibrosarcoma have features of fibroblasts, i.e., irregularly shaped nuclei and abundant rough endoplasmic reticulum. Cells with intracytoplasmic microfilaments and basal lamina, characteristic of myofibroblasts, are also a frequent component of fibrosarcoma.[25]

Fibromatosis (Low-Grade Fibrosarcoma)

Mammary fibromatosis or desmoid tumor is an unusual lesion of the breast that has become recognized as a distinct clinicopathological entity in recent years. Previously, it may have been grouped with mammary fibrosarcoma, which it resembles histologically. It is a low-grade neoplasm that can be locally aggressive but does not metastasize; it should be distinguished from frank fibrosarcoma.[1, 89]

The gross appearance of mammary fibromatosis is somewhat different from that of other types of sarcoma. It varies depending on the composition of the tumor

itself and the breast in which it arises. These tumors are characteristically firm and poorly circumscribed. They average 2 to 3 cm in diameter, although larger lesions have been described. In some instances, the tumor blends with the fibrofatty tissue of the breast and can be difficult to grossly distinguish from normal tissue (Fig. 10–1A).

In histomorphology, mammary fibromatosis resembles the usual fibrosarcoma in that it is composed of an infiltrative proliferation of spindle-shaped cells forming sweeping fascicles (Fig. 10–1B). It differs in having low cellularity, inconspicuous mitotic activity, and usually abundant intercelluar collagen. Necrosis, hemorrhage, cytological atypia, and aberrant mitoses are features of frank fibrosarcoma and not of the nonmetastasizing fibromatosis.[89]

Mammary fibromatosis, on rare occasions, spontaneously regresses, unlike frank fibrosarcoma. More characteristically, it tends to recur locally, although this tendency is not as pronounced as it is for fibromatosis in other anatomical sites. Pathological features other than a positive resection margin have not been found to correlate with clinical behavior.[32, 89] In general, the prognosis of this mammary soft tissue tumor is excellent.

Malignant Fibrous Histiocytoma

Malignant fibrous histiocytoma (MFH) arising in the mammary parenchyma is uncommon.[13, 25] It is a neoplasm composed of cells expressing features of differentiated fibroblasts and histiocytes, the former producing collagen and the latter exhibiting phagocytosis. In its classic form (Fig. 10–2), MFH comprises bundles of spindle-shaped cells disposed in small fascicles forming a pinwheel or storiform pattern about small vessels. The spindle cells have the features of fibroblasts and produce collagen to a variable degree. Larger, more rounded fibroblasts, irregularly shaped histiocytic cells, and multinucleated tumor giant cells are the other cellular constituents of this tumor. These are densely cellular neoplasms, and mitoses are commonly observed. There is an accompanying inflammatory infiltrate of lymphocytes, plasma cells, and so-called xanthoma cells, which are benign, fat-laden histiocytes.[25, 45]

Ultrastructurally, there are no findings specific for MFH. The constituent cells have features of fibroblasts, myofibroblasts (a related cell type), and histiocytes, as would be expected from the light microscopic appearance of these tumors.

Liposarcoma

Primary mammary liposarcomas arise either as de novo neoplasms or as malignant components within cystosarcoma phyllodes. Rare occurrences in men have been described.[2] Grossly, liposarcomas unassociated with cystosarcoma phyllodes resemble other primary mammary sarcomas except that they tend to be larger. Austin and Dupree[2] reported an average size of 8 cm among their 13 cases. Four major histological subtypes are recognized in other soft tissue sites: well-differen-

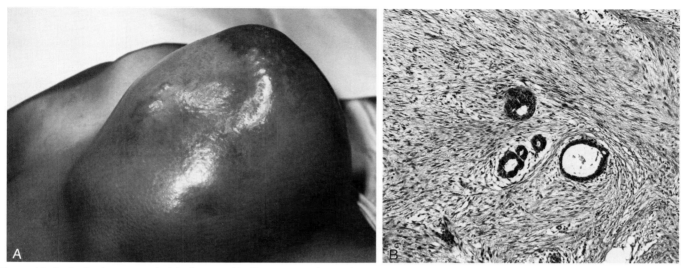

Figure 10–1. *A,* Replacement of right breast with fibromatosis (desmoid tumor) in an 18-year-old gravid black female. Because this poorly circumscribed neoplasm infiltrated the pectoralis major muscle, a Halsted radical mastectomy was necessary. A second focus of fibromatosis was identified in the right retroperitoneum and pelvis. *B,* Mammary fibromatosis (desmoid tumor). Sweeping fascicles of fibroblasts envelop an atrophic mammary lobule. (H & E, × 100.)

tiated, myxoid, pleomorphic, and round cell.[25] In the best documented series[2] the first three subtypes have been described as occurring in breast.

Well-differentiated liposarcoma has histological features suggestive of lipoma or mature adipose tissue. Its malignant character, however, is betrayed by variations in cell size and shape uncharacteristic of normal adipocytes, fibrous septa dividing the fat into irregular lobules, the presence of hyperchromatic lipocyte nuclei, and most importantly, the presence of lipoblasts, which are immature adipose cells.[2, 25]

Myxoid liposarcoma is more readily recognized and consists of a proliferation of lipoblasts, a characteristic plexiform proliferation of capillary-sized blood vessels,

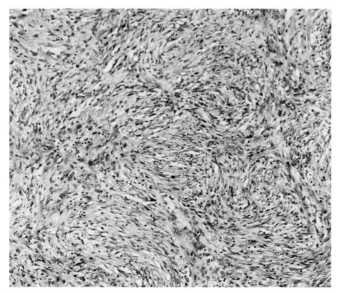

Figure 10–2. Malignant fibrous histiocytoma. Short fascicles of tumor cells arranged in the characteristic storiform pattern. (H & E, × 100.)

and a rich mucopolysaccharide matrix in a pattern reminiscent of fetal fat. The lipoblasts most often appear as lipid-containing, vacuolated cells with a signet ring configuration. More primitive-appearing mesenchymal cells and fibroblast-like spindle cells are other constituents. Mitotic figures are scarce in both myxoid and well-differentiated liposarcoma.[2, 25]

Pleomorphic liposarcoma, as the name suggests, consists of a highly cellular proliferation of atypical cells of many shapes and sizes. Bizarre giant cells, many containing lipid droplets, are a prominent feature of this histological subtype. Mitotic activity is often pronounced, and hemorrhage and necrosis frequently complicate these tumors.[2, 25]

The ultrastructure of liposarcoma reflects the morphological variability observed with the light microscope. In appearance, liposarcoma cells run the gamut from the undifferentiated spindle cell containing few organelles to the highly differentiated lipoblast bearing cytoplasmic lipid droplets. Intermediate cells with features of fibroblasts are also seen. Desmosomes and other types of intercellular junctions are not observed.[40]

A relationship of the pathological features of liposarcoma to outcome is suggested by the work of Austin and Dupree.[2] Metastatic disease developed in 3 of their 13 patients with pure mammary liposarcoma but in none of the seven patients with liposarcoma arising in a cystosarcoma phyllodes; three of these patients had been initially treated with mastectomy. Local recurrence occurred in only two patients, one initially treated with local excision and the other by mastectomy. All recurrences were noted within one year of initial treatment. These data are inconclusive but suggest that the risk of recurrence, either local or distant, is higher in those patients with the pleomorphic subtype of liposarcoma and when the microscopic tumor margins are infiltrating rather than circumscribed or pushing. Overall, the prognosis for patients with mammary liposarcoma is good, with an overall recurrence rate of 20 percent.

Leiomyosarcoma

Primary mammary leiomyosarcoma is rare, and only a few cases have been reported to date. The smooth muscle structures of the nipple-areola complex are the site of many of these malignant tumors, which have been described in both men[36] and women.[25, 60] The prognosis of patients with these tumors appears to be good; however, a tendency to late distant recurrence after intervals of more than ten years has been noted.[17, 60] This clinical behavior differs from that of the more common mammary sarcoma, usually recurring within one to two years of treatment if progressive disease develops.

The histomorphology of mammary leiomyosarcoma is identical to that of leiomyosarcomas occurring at other sites. The tumor is formed of interlacing fascicles of spindle-shaped cells with abundant cytoplasm and blunt-ended nuclei. Small perinuclear vacuoles may be seen. Long fascicles of cells with a tendency to intersect at right angles characterize the best differentiated examples of this tumor. Multinucleated and bizarre giant cell forms have been observed. Mitotic activity varies from sparse to abundant.[36, 60]

Ultrastructurally, the cells of mammary leiomyosarcoma have the features expected of smooth muscle differentiation. Important features include clefted nuclei, cytoplasmic myofilaments with condensations called dense bodies, and a basal lamina at the cell periphery in the best differentiated cells. Pinocytic vesicles and interconnections are other features.[25, 36]

Immunohistochemistry can be helpful in confirming evidence of smooth muscle differentiation in these neoplasms. Muscle-specific actin antibody stains most smooth muscle tumors, although it is not specific for these lesions. Sarcomas containing differentiated myofibroblasts also show focal faintly positive staining.[87]

Osteogenic Sarcoma and Chondrosarcoma

Bone and cartilage-forming tumors of the breast are quite unusual. In most instances, the bone or cartilage formation is merely one component in a metaplastic carcinoma rather than a feature of a true sarcoma. Hence, the diagnostic criteria for mammary osteogenic sarcoma and chondrosarcoma are the identification of bone and cartilage formation, respectively, with malignant-appearing stromal cells and absence of a neoplastic epithelial element.[56] Numerous sections must be taken of any bone- or cartilage-forming mammary tumor to avoid sampling error. Immunohistochemical evaluation of epithelial markers is valuable to exclude the diagnosis of metaplastic carcinoma.

Examples of genuine primary osteogenic sarcoma and chondrosarcoma of the breast are rare. Osteogenic sarcoma is composed of malignant mesenchymal cells that produce calcified or nonmineralized osteoid either in organized trabeculae or as an amorphous intercellular material (Fig. 10–3). Cellular pleomorphism and nuclear atypia are typical and mitoses are usually abundant, as in their extramammary counterparts. Multinucleated giant cells are commonly found at the edge of the neoplastic bone.[48]

Mammary chondrosarcoma differs in gross appearance from other types of sarcoma. Cartilage formation imparts a gelatinous consistency to these tumors, which tend to be multinodular and bosselated. Foci of calcification are also common as they are in cartilaginous tumors at other sites. In better differentiated examples, the tumor cells lie in lacunae in a hyaline matrix that resembles normal hyaline cartilage. Cellular pleomorphism, nuclear hyperchromasia, and atypia are often observed.[5] More poorly differentiated tumors have less cartilage formation, greater mitotic activity, and more degenerative changes in the form of necrosis and cysts. Very immature appearing cartilage is formed by some tumors. Immunohistochemical staining for S-100 protein is positive in the cartilage-forming cells of mammary chondrosarcoma. Although not unique to chondrosarcoma, the finding of this antigen is confirmatory evidence in tumors with appropriate histological features.[44]

Management of Mammary Sarcoma. The diagnosis should be established by open incisional biopsy for large tumors (> 2 cm) and excisional biopsy for small tumors. Primary treatment for mammary stromal sarcoma is wide excision, which often requires a total mastectomy. It is clear from the literature that the principles of sarcoma surgery should not be compromised in order to avoid mastectomy. Berg et al.,[6] for instance, reported a 53 percent local recurrence rate in 32 patients treated by local excision compared with an 8 percent local recurrence rate in 71 patients treated by total mastectomy. Nodal dissection is not indicated unless nodes are clinically involved.[39] An exception may be made for mammary liposarcoma, in which a 10 percent incidence of metastases to the axillary nodes has been observed.

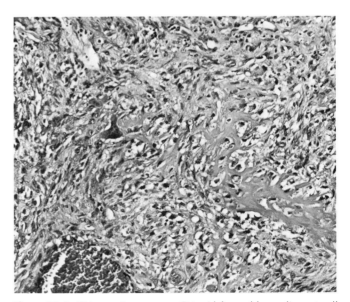

Figure 10–3. Osteogenic sarcoma. Osteoid formed by malignant cells is seen on the right. (H & E, × 160.)

As with sarcoma in other sites, the value of adjuvant radiotherapy and chemotherapy is under investigation.

Prognosis is not clearly related to structure or size of the primary tumor. A poorer prognosis has been noted when the tumor margin is infiltrating adjacent tissues, when more than eight mitoses per high power field are found, and when moderate to severe stromal nuclear atypia is present.[3] In Berg's study, the five-year survival averaged 60 percent.[6]

Mammary Angiosarcoma

Primary angiosarcoma of the breast is extremely rare.[17] The relative incidence of angiosarcoma among breast sarcomas is 2.7 to 7.9 percent.[58] Up to 15 percent of all angiosarcomas occur in the breast. Breast angiosarcoma is notable for two reasons. First, it is frequently initially misdiagnosed as being benign; and second, it carries the poorest prognosis of all the malignant tumors of the breast, with frequent fulminant metastatic extension of the tumor over the course of two to three months.

Clinical Features. Age at presentation ranges from 14 to 82 years, with a mean age of 35 years.[17] The clinical presentation is most frequently with a painless mass in the breast, although diffuse enlargement and violaceous or black discoloration of the overlying skin may be present (Fig. 10–4A). As with other breast sarcomas, the mean size at presentation is greater than 5 cm. A number of authors have identified a correlation between the size of the primary tumor and prognosis; patients with small tumors, i.e., less than 3 cm in diameter, fare better than do those with larger masses.[21, 83] Chen et al.[17] noted that 11 of 87 patients were pregnant at the time of diagnosis and suggested that these tumors are hormonally influenced. In support of this, receptors for estrogen, progesterone, and glucocorticoids were iden-

tified in tissue sections of angiosarcoma, but the diagnostic and therapeutic relevance of these findings is currently unknown.[10, 21]

Pathological Features. Mammary angiosarcoma may appear histologically benign and yet have extreme malignant potential. Chen et al.,[17] in a review of 87 cases, noted that 37 percent were misdiagnosed as lymphangiomas, hemangiomas, and hematomas. The gross pathological features of primary mammary angiosarcoma are variable. Most are soft hemorrhagic masses with an ill-defined margin. However, these tumors occasionally appear only as a thickened or indurated area in the breast.[21] A honeycomb appearance, dilated vascular channels, or pools of blood characterize some tumors.

Angiosarcoma of the breast is a morphologically heterogeneous process as viewed under the microscope. There is histological variability both within a given tumor and between cases. It is imperative that all vascular tumors of the breast be thoroughly sampled and examined by the surgical pathologist, both to exclude benign vascular proliferations and to accurately classify malignant ones. Frozen section has a role only in discriminating these lesions from carcinoma.

Primary mammary angiosarcoma, by definition, arises within the breast parenchyma itself, although there may be secondary involvement of overlying skin or the pectoralis muscles in advanced cases. Histologically, all these tumors are composed of proliferating endothelial cells forming interanastomosing vascular channels that infiltrate the glandular structures and fat of the breast. Microscopic extension of the process some distance from the grossly observed margin is typical and can thwart the efforts of the surgeon attempting to encompass the lesion in a wide excision.[17, 21, 83]

An early attempt by Steingaszner et al.[83] to correlate the histomorphology of mammary angiosarcoma with

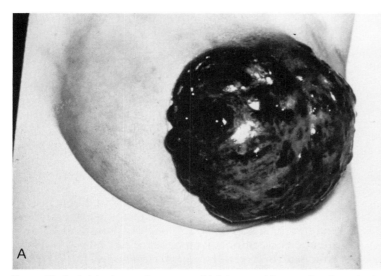
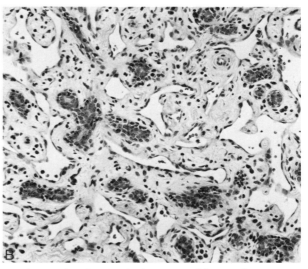

Figure 10–4. *A,* Massive angiosarcoma of left breast with extension through nipple-areola complex. Despite the large size of the neoplasm (15 cm), this low-grade, well-differentiated lesion was not fixed to the pectoralis major muscle. Further, the axilla had no evidence of disease. The patient was managed with total mastectomy and split-thickness skin graft of the large defect. (Courtesy of Dr. Condict Moore, Department of Surgery, University of Louisville.) *B,* Group I, well-differentiated angiosarcoma. Irregularly shaped, dilated vascular structures infiltrating a mammary lobule. (H & E, × 200.)

clinical outcome identified mitotic activity as the only feature to have any relationship to prognosis. The growth patterns of angiosarcoma comprise a histological spectrum ranging from a well-differentiated vessel-forming pattern to a poorly differentiated solid spindle cell proliferation.[21, 53]

A three-tiered system for classifying these lesions in a meaningful way has been developed. Tumors growing in the Group I or well-differentiated pattern are characterized by infiltrating, well-formed, interanastomosing vascular channels involving the glandular structures of the breast (Fig. 10–4B). The mammary gland architecture is preserved as the proliferating vascular structures grow and expand the intralobular stroma. Neoplastic endothelial cells tend to be flat and show little, if any, tufting and capillary formation. Nuclear hyperchromasia without conspicuous pleomorphism is typical. Identifiable mitotic activity is minimal or absent.[21, 53] It is this innocuous-appearing growth pattern that is most commonly misinterpreted as benign.

The intermediate Group II or moderately differentiated tumors show many of features of the Group I lesions but differ in that endothelial tufting with focal capillary proliferation is always seen. Furthermore, mitotic activity is often noted in these regions. A rare solid or spindle cell focus, characteristic of the higher grade lesions, is identified in some Group II tumors.[21]

Group III or poorly differentiated angiosarcomas are notable for areas, often very extensive, of solid spindle cell growth with prominent mitotic activity. Nuclear abnormalities are conspicuous, and necrosis and hemorrhage are salient features of many of these tumors. Coexistent foci of Groups I and II growth are nearly always identified and provide the clue to the diagnosis of angiosarcoma in the least differentiated examples of the neoplasm.[21, 53]

Significantly, the Group I pattern is seen at the peripheral infiltrating margin of virtually all mammary angiosarcomas; the less differentiated components are more often found centrally.[21] This underscores the need for thorough pathological sampling to ensure accurate classification.

Immunohistochemistry rarely has a practical role in the pathological assessment of mammary angiosarcoma. Factor VIII–related antigen and *Ulex europaeus* agglutinin-1 (UEA-1) are markers of normal as well as neoplastic endothelial cells except for the least differentiated examples in the latter category.[12, 53] Thus, their identification within cells of a vascular neoplasm cannot be used to discriminate benign from malignant processes. Furthermore, as indicated above, even the most poorly differentiated mammary angiosarcoma has better differentiated areas readily identified as vascular in nature.

Management. The principle of management is wide excision of the tumor, which generally involves a total mastectomy. Axillary node involvement by angiosarcoma is rare. In view of its aggressiveness and poor prognosis, adjuvant chemotherapy and radiotherapy should be strongly considered. Donnell et al.[21] reported that 8 of 11 patients treated with adjuvant actinomycin D were free of disease at two years.

In recent series the prognosis of patients with angiosarcoma of the breast is better than that shown in earlier reports but is poor compared with that of patients with carcinoma. Donnell et al.[21] reported the most complete series of patients and noted disease-free survival rates of 41 percent and 33 percent at three and five years, respectively, for their group of 40 women. The average survival of those who died was two years.

Further analysis correlating survival with pathology demonstrates differences among the three histological subgroups. The majority (12/13) of women with Group I or well-differentiated lesions were alive, ten without recurrent disease, after an average of five years. In contrast, most (14/18) patients with Group III or poorly differentiated tumors died of metastatic sarcoma. Two long-term survivors after mastectomy and chemotherapy (actinomycin D) were, however, seen in this group. The survival rate of the intermediate Group II patients was lower but not statistically different from that of Group I patients.[21, 71]

Merino and colleagues[53] found a similar correlation between histomorphology and survival in their smaller series of 15 patients, with the exception that the survival of their intermediate group was more like that of the patients with poorly differentiated, or Group III, angiosarcomas. The discrepancy may have resulted from differences in histological criteria between the two studies.

Postmastectomy Angiosarcoma (Stewart-Treves Syndrome)

In 1948, Stewart and Treves reported the first six cases of lymphangiosarcoma in patients with lymphedematous arms after radical mastectomy.[84] Since then, over 200 cases have been reported in the literature, with an overall incidence of 0.45 percent in patients living five years after radical mastectomy.[78] Although initially described as lymphangiosarcoma, a distinction from hemangiosarcoma is usually not apparent, and therefore the term "angiosarcoma" is best adopted.

The existence of this entity has on occasion been challenged. Salm[76] suggested that all the cases reported can be explained as retrograde metastases from a breast carcinoma. While there is no doubt that such a sequence of events can occur and the lesion can be mistakenly interpreted as a malignant endothelial tumor, the condition described by Stewart and Treves is a definite pathological entity: (1) Miettinen et al.,[54] using a specific immunocytochemical marker (anti–Factor VIII antibody) for endothelial cells, demonstrated conclusively the endothelial origin of postmastectomy angiosarcoma; and (2) angiosarcoma has been reported to arise in situations of chronic lymphedema secondary to benign lymphatic obstruction (e.g., from filariasis).[22, 28, 35, 92]

It has been suggested that the etiology of tumor arising in a lymphedematous extremity may be secondary to impaired immune mechanisms in the affected limb.[80] Stark et al.,[82] in support of this, noted that rejection of homograft skin is markedly delayed in lymphedematous extremities. The probable mechanism is an interruption of the afferent limb of the immune response such that putative spontaneously arising tumor cells may not be properly processed by the immune system with resultant failure of the host to reject the tumor.

The average interval between mastectomy and onset of angiosarcoma has been reported to be 10.5 years.[92] In over 60 percent of cases, postoperative radiotherapy had been administered. Radiotherapy is considered to be a factor in the development of angiosarcoma only in the respect that it contributes to the development of lymphedema. The overall incidence of postoperative lymphedema after radical mastectomy has been cited at 15 to 25 percent compared with a 5.5 percent incidence after modified radical mastectomy.[30, 31] The trend toward less ablative surgery will undoubtedly reduce the incidence of lymphedema in the future. It must be noted, however, that angiosarcoma has been reported to arise even 30 years after radical mastectomy.[50]

Clinical Features. Clinically, postmastectomy angiosarcoma usually appears initially as an innocuous-looking painless bruise or bruises. Over 75 percent appear in the upper arm, with other sites including the forearm, elbow, chest wall, and shoulder. Some tumors are soft, spongy, and hemorrhagic, whereas others grow as firm solid masses. Hemorrhagic tumors have been mistaken clinically for the lesions of Kaposi's sarcoma. The lesions may ulcerate or penetrate through the chest wall to the lungs and pleura.[49]

Pathological Features. The histomorphology of postmastectomy angiosarcoma is similar to that of angiosarcoma arising de novo in the skin and soft tissues, except for an associated diffuse proliferation of lymphatic channels, so-called lymphangiomatosis, that characterizes chronic lymphatic obstruction of all types and may constitute a premalignant change.[25, 81]

Tumor involves the dermis and subcutis in all cases of postmastectomy angiosarcoma. Ulcerated lesions characteristically show tumor at the base. Dermal masses of tumor cells elevate the overlying epidermis, which is sometimes hyperkeratotic, in grossly nodular and papular lesions. Diffuse tumor infiltration with ill-defined borders within the dermis corresponds to grossly observed indurated lesions. Skin appendages may be preserved even in the presence of extensive tumor, which often grows around or pushes aside these structures without destroying them.[49]

Postmastectomy angiosarcoma displays a great deal of histological heterogeneity, especially within individual patients. A spectrum of differentiation is apparent in most examples of this tumor. Small capillary-sized vessels formed by atypical endothelial cells characterize the best differentiated component. Less well differentiated tumor grows as a complex papillary proliferation of malignant-appearing cells forming interanastomosing vascular channels. The most poorly differentiated examples grow as solid nests and masses of either spindle-shaped or epithelioid cells, the former mimicking Kaposi's sarcoma and the latter carcinoma.[49, 81] Exuberant mitotic activity, necrosis, and hemorrhage are common features of the higher grade tumors.

Superficial skin biopsies performed on the postmastectomy patient with cutaneous lesions may be misleading or difficult to interpret. As in mammary angiosarcoma, the well-differentiated component of these tumors can be mistaken for benign processes. Furthermore, the poorly differentiated components can be mistaken for other neoplasms, such as recurrent mammary carcinoma, melanoma, or other types of sarcoma.[54, 81] A search for the better differentiated, recognizable vessel-forming components of the tumor will often solve the diagnostic problem in a biopsy of adequate size.

Immunocytochemistry can be useful in the diagnostic interpretation of malignant tumors occurring in the postmastectomy state. Factor VIII–related antigen, a protein produced by endothelial cells, has been identified in postmastectomy angiosarcoma and constitutes a reliable marker for these tumors.[16, 54] Although not useful in distinguishing between benign and malignant vascular proliferations, the demonstration of Factor VIII in an anaplastic cutaneous neoplasm excludes the diagnoses of carcinoma and melanoma.[34]

The ultrastructural features of postmastectomy angiosarcoma are identical to those of other types of angiosarcoma. Specifically, intercellular junctions, pinocytic vesicles, and a partial basal lamina at the antiluminal borders of the cells surrounding vascular lumens are characteristic features. Weibel-Palade bodies, pathognomonic for vascular endothelium, have been demonstrated in some instances. All these features are found less frequently in poorly differentiated tumors, limiting the usefulness of electron microscopy in cases of very anaplastic tumors in this setting.[16, 54]

Management. The prognosis for patients with angiosarcoma has been dismal, with a median survival of 19 months.[92] No correlation has been observed between histology and survival. Interpapulothoracic amputation appears to offer the best hope of long-term survival. Sordillo et al.[81] reported that patients receiving primary amputation had a median survival of 48 months, and a review of the literature indicates that the majority of long-term survivors had undergone amputation. Reports on the use of chemotherapy are variable. Yap et al.[93] reported a 42 percent partial or complete response rate in patients receiving systemic chemotherapy and found a median survival of 26.5 months in responders compared with 4 months in nonresponders.

Cystosarcoma Phyllodes

Cystosarcoma phyllodes (CSP) of the breast is a stromal tumor with a generally good but unpredictable prognosis. It resembles the much more common fibroadenoma both histologically and pathogenetically, apparently arising from the unique hormone-responsive intralobular and periductal mammary stroma.[13, 90] The diagnosis of CSP is entirely pathological, and both an epithelial and a stromal component must be identified.

Clinical Features. Cystosarcoma phyllodes is rare. It accounts for about 0.5 percent of all breast tumors. The tumors are often very large, averaging 6 to 8 cm, and are usually nodular, nontender, and mobile.[29, 79] Between 3 and 12 percent of all patients have metastasis,[7, 26, 86] with the risk of metastasis from malignant CSP between 40 and 50 percent. The distinction between benign and malignant is based on histological criteria.[86] However, histologically "benign" cystosarcomas can metastasize and histologically "malignant" cystosarcomas can have an excellent prognosis.[61] The average age of patients presenting with cystadenoma is 43 years. Most present with a painless mass in one breast. Rapid tumor growth and pain have not consistently predicted the biological behavior of the tumor. Interestingly, skin fixation and ulceration are rarely observed but, when present, are more often associated with benign than with malignant lesions.[86]

Pathology. Muller[57] coined the term "cystosarcoma phyllodes" in 1838 for what appeared to him to be, literally, a cystic, fleshy, leafy tumor of the breast. While some of the large, bulky examples of the neoplasm have these gross characteristics, many grow as solid, expansile, rubbery or firm solid masses without a conspicuous cystic component. CSP often has a rounded, bosselated contour and typically appears well delineated from the surrounding breast.[52, 86] The cut surface may appear solid but more commonly contains numerous slits separating solid lamina of tumor, somewhat resembling a cut cabbage. Foci of necrosis or hemorrhage may be grossly observed, more often a manifestation of infarction than of malignancy.[52, 61]

The histological appearance of the benign variant of CSP (Fig. 10–5) most closely resembles that of fibroadenoma but differs in having greater cell density. It is a neoplasm of the mammary stroma; the accompanying epithelial component is an intrinsic part of the overall biological picture but is benign. The proliferating spindle cells have the light microscopic and ultrastructural features of fibroblasts and grow as nodular masses that may protrude into a cystic space or compress other, adjacent

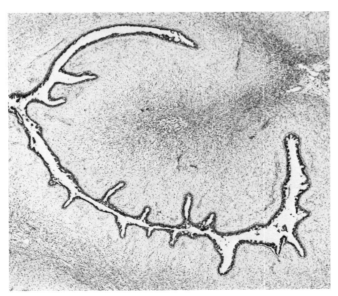

Figure 10–5. Histologically benign cystosarcoma phyllodes. (H & E, × 40.)

expanding tumor nodules to form the grossly observed lamina.[52, 69] The character and the density of the stroma varies considerably between patients and in individual instances. The stroma may have a myxoid, edematous quality, and focal lipomatous metaplasia is seen in some cases.[63]

The epithelium associated with CSP is generally the low cuboidal type that is characteristic of breast. Apocrine or squamous metaplasia of the epithelium is a secondary change seen in some cases. Epithelial hyperplasia and, rarely, coexistent carcinoma may complicate CSP.

Attempts to correlate the histological features of CSP with clinical outcome date back to some of the earliest studies of this neoplasm.[46, 76] Efforts have centered on classifying individual tumors as histologically benign, malignant, or "borderline" but have had only limited success in solving the vexing problem of prognostication. The occasional lesion with a completely benign histological appearance metastasizes, whereas many patients with what appear to be frank sarcomas never develop metastatic disease.[9, 88] While the overall good prognosis of CSP must be emphasized, there are some pathological correlates of increased risk of disease recurrence.

The pathological features of interest in CSP are the degree of stromal cellularity, cytological atypia, mitotic atypia, and the character of the tumor border. No single feature is predictive of outcome, but a composite assessment of these attributes can be useful in estimating prognosis.[33, 61, 65, 88] Specifically, tumors that are densely cellular, composed of highly atypical cells containing hyperchromatic aberrant nuclei, and exhibiting abundant mitotic activity have the highest likelihood of recurrence (Fig. 10–6). Tumors with an infiltrative rather than a pushing border at the interface with the surrounding breast have a greater propensity to recur.[61, 65] Evidence of stromal overgrowth, i.e., marked expansion of the spindle cell component to the point of partial obliteration of the characteristic fibroepithelial configuration that we recognize as CSP, is another poor prognostic feature.[33, 88]

Tumors at the highly malignant end of the histological spectrum most commonly display features of fibrosarcoma. Instances of liposarcoma and rhabdomyosarcoma arising within the context of CSP have also been described.[4, 63, 66] Metastatic lesions typically resemble the spindle cell component of the primary tumor; the benign epithelial component of CSP does not undergo malignant change, nor does it metastasize.

Hormone receptor evaluation of a small number of cases of CSP has verified the presence of estrogen[43, 64] and progesterone[67] receptors, the latter being a more typical finding. These findings support the view that these neoplasms arise from the hormone-responsive lobular stroma of the breast. The therapeutic potential of this finding has not yet been explored.[67]

Management. As with all sarcomas, the diagnosis should be made by incisional biopsy with careful placement of the incision so as not to compromise subsequent therapy. Definitive local treatment is with operative resection. Owing to the fact that the tumor, with rare

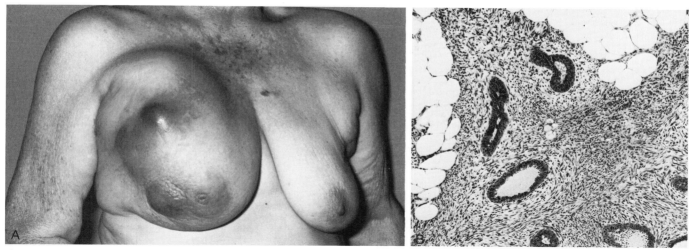

Figure 10–6. *A,* Malignant cystosarcoma phyllodes of right breast in a 68-year-old white female. The breast is totally replaced with the bulky, multicentric, fleshy tumor that gives the "teardrop" contour. Treatment included a total mastectomy with 3 cm margins and skin graft of the chest wall defect. *B,* Histologically malignant cystosarcoma phyllodes. Densely cellular tumor infiltrates the mammary fat. (H & E, × 100.)

exceptions,[77] is unifocal and does not involve lymphatics,[55] local management should follow the previously mentioned principle of a wide excision with at least a 3 cm margin on each side of the tumor. Since these tumors are often large at presentation, this often requires a total mastectomy.[19] Unless axillary lymph nodes are clinically involved, there is no indication for axillary dissection.

Local recurrences[7, 79] (15 to 60 percent) usually indicate inadequate initial excision and can be cured by re-excision. Adjuvant chemotherapy is not routine for malignant cystosarcomas, which tend to be low grade. The treatment of metastases to date has been unsuccessful. In view of the fact that hormone receptors are usually present within these tumors, hormonal manipulation will undoubtedly merit evaluation in adjunctive therapy.

MALIGNANT LYMPHOMA OF THE BREAST

Primary breast lymphoma is extremely rare.[27, 91] Brustein et al.,[11] in recently reported Memorial Sloan Kettering Cancer Center experience of 53 patients from 1949 to 1984, noted that only 207 cases had been reported in the literature from 1930 to 1985.

Clinical Features. Mammary lymphomas tend to be larger at diagnosis than do adenocarcinomas, with a mean size of 4 cm. The mean age at diagnosis is 60 years, and there appears to be a peculiar predominance of right-sided lesions, in contrast to the left-sided predominance in all other breast carcinomas. DeCosse et al.[20] reported a high incidence of tumor-positive axillary lymph nodes; in these cases it is not always easy to ascertain whether the tumor is primary within the breast.

Pathological Features. Structurally, mammary lymphomas do not differ from other malignant lymphomas, with tumor cells densely infiltrating the breast tissue in the gross lesion and irregularly infiltrating the paren-

chyma at the periphery of the mass for a variable distance. Using the Rappaport system of classification,[68] Brustein et al.[11] noted a relative predominance of diffuse histiocytic lymphoma (26/53 patients), consistent with the usual breakdown of subtypes of extranodal lymphomas. They noted a relatively higher number (5/53) of cases classified as diffuse mixed lymphoma than had previously been observed.

Management. Total mastectomy and axillary node sampling is advocated for large primary lymphomas of the breast. Recurrent local disease and accessible regionalized nodal disease should be managed with radiotherapy, and systemic or multiregional disease with chemotherapy using current regimens for non-Hodgkin's lymphoma. Prognosis is favorable, with five-year survival rates of 74 percent and a ten-year survival rate of 51 percent in Brustein's series.[11]

References

1. Ali M, Fayemi AO, Braun EV, et al: Fibromatosis of the breast. Am J Surg Pathol 12:501–505, 1979.
2. Austin RM, Dupree WB: Liposarcoma of the breast: A clinicopathological study of 20 cases. Hum Pathol 17 (9):906–913, 1986.
3. Barnes L, Pietruzka M: Sarcomas of the breast: A clinicopathological analysis of ten cases. Cancer 40:1577–1585, 1977.
4. Barnes L, Pietruzka M: Rhabdomyosarcoma arising within a cystosarcoma phyllodes: Case report and review of the literature. Am J Surg Pathol 2:423–429, 1978.
5. Beltaos E, Banerjee TK: Chondrosarcoma of the breast: Report of two cases. Am J Clin Pathol 71(3):345–349, 1979.
6. Berg JW, DeCosse JJ, Fracchia AA, et al: Stromal sarcomas of the breast: A unified approach to connective tissue sarcomas other than cystosarcoma phyllodes. Cancer 13:418–424, 1962.
7. Blichert-Toft M, Hansen JPH, Hansen OH, et al: Clinical course of cystosarcoma phyllodes related to histologic appearance. Surg Gynecol Obstet 140:929–938, 1975.
8. Blum RH: An overview of studies with Adriamycin (NSC 123127) in the United States. Cancer Chemother Rep 6:247–251, 1975.
9. Blumencranz PW, Gray GF: Cystosarcoma phyllodes: A clinical and pathological study. NY State J Med 78:623–627, 1978.

10. Brenatani MM, Pacheco MM, Oshima CTF: Steroid receptors in breast angiosarcoma. Cancer 51:2105–2111, 1983.

11. Brustein S, Kimmel M, Lieberman PH, et al: Malignant lymphoma of the breast. A study of 53 patients. Ann Surg 205:144–149, 1987.

12. Burgdorf WHC, Mukai K, Rosai J: Immunohistochemical identification of Factor VIII related antigen in endothelial cells of cutaneous lesions of alleged vascular structure. Am J Clin Pathol 75:167–171, 1981.

13. Callery CD, Rosen PP, Kinne DW: Sarcoma of the breast: A study of 32 patients with reappraisal of classification and therapy. Ann Surg 201 (4):527–532, 1985.

14. Cantin J, McNeer P, Chu FC, et al: The problem of local recurrence after treatment of soft tissue sarcoma. Ann Surg 168:47–53, 1968.

15. Cancer Patient Survival: Report No 5. Washington DC, US Department of Health, Education and Welfare, Publication No. (NIH) 77–992, 1976.

16. Capo V, Ozzello L, Fenoglio CM, et al: Angiosarcomas arising in lymphedematous extremities: Immunostaining of Factor VIII-related antigen and ultrastructural features. Hum Pathol 16:144–150, 1985.

17. Chen KTK, Kirkegaard DD, Bocian JJ: Angiosarcoma of the breast. Cancer 46:368–371, 1980.

18. Chen KTK, Kuo TT, Hoffman KD: Leiomyosarcoma of the breast: A case of long survival and late hepatic metastasis. Cancer 47:1883–1886, 1981.

19. Contarini O, Urdaneta LF, Hagan W, et al: Cystosarcoma phyllodes of the breast: A new therapeutic proposal. Am Surg 48:157–166, 1982.

20. DeCosse J, Berg J, Fracchia A, et al: Primary lymphosarcoma of the breast. A review of 14 cases. Cancer 15:1264–1268, 1962.

21. Donnell RM, Rosen PP, Lieberman PH, et al: Angiosarcoma and other vascular tumors of the breast. Am J Surg Pathol 7(1):53–60, 1981.

22. Eby CS, Brennan MJ, Fine G: Lymphangiosarcoma: A lethal complication of chronic lymphedema. Report of two cases and review of the literature. Arch Surg 94:223–230, 1967.

23. Edmonson JH, Fleming TR, Ivins JC, et al: Randomized study of systemic chemotherapy following complete excision of non-osseous sarcomas. Proc Am Soc Clin Oncol 45:182, 1982.

24. Enneking WF, Spannier SS, Goodman MA: The surgical staging of musculoskeletal sarcoma. J Bone Joint Surg 62A:1027–1039, 1980.

25. Enzinger FM, Weiss SW: Soft Tissue Tumors. St Louis, CV Mosby, 1983.

26. Fernandez BB, Hernandez KJ, Spindler W: Metastatic cystosarcoma phyllodes. A light and electron microscopic study. Cancer 37:1737–1741, 1976.

27. Fischer M, Chideckel N: Primary lymphoma of the breast. Breast 10:7–10, 1984.

28. Francis KG, Lindquist HD: Lymphangiosarcoma of the lower extremity involved with chronic lymphedema. Am J Surg 100:617–622, 1960.

29. Gogas JG: Cystosarcoma phyllodes: A clinicopathological analysis of 14 cases. Int Surg 64:77–82, 1979.

30. Goldsmith HS: Disorders of the lymphatic system. In Sabiston DS Jr (ed.): Textbook of Surgery. 12th ed. Philadelphia, WB Saunders, 1981, p 1805.

31. Golematis BC, Delikaris PG, Balarutsos C, et al: Lymphedema of the upper limb after surgery for breast cancer. Am J Surg 129:286–288, 1975.

32. Gump FE, Steinchein MJ, Wolff M: Fibromatosis of the breast. Surg Gynecol Obstet 153:57–60, 1981.

33. Hart WR, Bauer RC, Oberman HA: Cystosarcoma phyllodes: A clinicopathologic study of twenty-six hypercellular periductal stromal tumors of the breast. Am J Clin Pathol 70:211–216, 1978.

34. Hashimoto K, Matsumoto M, Eto H, et al: Differentiation of metastatic breast carcinoma from Stewart-Treves angiosarcoma. Arch Dermatol 121:742–746, 1985.

35. Hermann JB: Lymphangiosarcoma of the chronically edematous extremity. Surg Gynecol Obstet 121:1107–1115, 1965.

36. Hernandez FJ: Leiomyosarcoma of male breast originating in the nipple. Am J Surg Pathol 3:299–304, 1978.

37. Hoover CH, Trestioreau A, Ketcham AS: Metastatic cystosarcoma phyllodes in an adolescent girl, an unusually malignant tumor. Ann Surg 181:279–282, 1975.

38. Hudson TM, Haas G, Enneking WF, et al: Angiography in the management of musculoskeletal tumors. Surg Gynecol Obstet 141:11–21, 1975.

39. Ii K, Hizawa K, Okazaki K, et al: Liposarcoma of the breast—fine structural and histochemical study of a case and review of 42 cases in the literature. Tokushima J Exp Med 27:45, 1980.

40. Kanemoto K, Nakamura T, Matsuyama A: Liposarcoma of the breast: Review of the literature and report of a case. Jpn J Surg 11(5):381–384, 1981.

41. Kerns LL, Simons MA: Surgical theory, staging, definitions and treatment of musculoskeletal sarcomas. Surg Clin North Am 63:671–696, 1983.

42. Kessinger A, Foley JF, Lemon HM, et al: Metastatic cystosarcoma phyllodes: a case report and review of the literature. J Surg Oncol 4:131–137, 1972.

43. Kesterson GHN, Georgiade N, Seigler HF, et al: Cystosarcoma phyllodes: A steroid receptor and ultrastructure analysis. Ann Surg 190:640–645, 1979.

44. Ladefoged C, Nielsen BB: Primary chondrosarcoma of the breast: A case report and review of the literature. Breast 10:26–28, 1984.

45. Langham MR, Mills AS, DeMay RM, et al: Malignant fibrous histiocytoma of the breast: A case report and review of the literature. Cancer 54:558–563, 1984.

46. Lester J, Stout AP: Cystosarcoma phyllodes. Cancer 7:335–353, 1954.

47. Lindquist KD, van Heerden JA, Weiland LH, et al: Recurrent and metastatic cystosarcoma phyllodes. Am J Surg 144:341–345, 1982.

48. Lumsden AB, Harrison D, Chetty U: Osteogenic sarcoma—a rare primary tumor of the breast. Eur J Surg Oncol 11:183–186, 1985.

49. Maddox JC, Evans HL: Angiosarcoma of the skin and soft tissues. A study of forty-four cases. Cancer 48:1907–1921, 1981.

50. Martin MB, Kon ND, Kawamoto WH, et al: Postmastectomy angiosarcoma. Am Surg 50:541–545, 1984.

51. Martini N, McCormick PM, Bains MS, et al: Surgery for solitary and multiple pulmonary metastasis. NY State J Med 78:1711–1713, 1978.

52. McDivitt RW, Urban JA, Farrow JH: Cystosarcoma phyllodes. Johns Hopkins Med J 120:33–45, 1967.

53. Merino MJ, Carter D, Berman M: Angiosarcoma of the breast. Am J Surg Pathol 7(1):53–60, 1983.

54. Miettinen M, Lehto V–P, Virtanen I: Post-mastectomy angiosarcoma (Stewart-Treves syndrome). Light microscopic, immuno-histological and ultrastructural characteristics of two cases. Am J Surg Pathol 7:329–339, 1983.

55. Mincowitz S, Zeichner M, DiMaio V, et al: Cystosarcoma phyllodes: A unique case with multiple unilateral lesions and ipsilateral axillary metastases. J Pathol 96:514–518, 1968.

56. Muffarij AA, Feiner HD: Breast sarcoma with giant cells and osteoid. A case report and review of the literature. Am J Surg Pathol 11(3):225–230, 1987.

57. Muller J: Uber den feinern Ban und die Formen der Krankafter Geschwulste. Lfg. I. Berlin, Reimer, 54, 1838.

58. Myerowitz RL, Pietruszka M, Barnes EL: Primary angiosarcoma of the breast. JAMA 239:403–408, 1978.

59. Neifeld JP, Walsh JW, Lawrence W Jr: Computerized tomography in the management of soft tissue sarcoma. Surg Gynecol Obstet 155:535–540, 1982.

60. Nielsen BB: Leiomyosarcoma of the breast with late dissemination. Virchows Arch [Pathol Anat] 403:241–245, 1984.

61. Norris HJ, Taylor HB: Relationship of histologic features to behaviour of cystosarcoma phyllodes: Analysis of ninety-four cases. Cancer 20(12):2090–2099, 1967.

62. Norris HJ, Taylor HB: Sarcomas and related mesenchymal tumors of the breast. Cancer 22:22–28, 1968.

63. Oberman HA, Nosanchuk JS, Finger JE: Periductal stromal tumors of the breast with adipose metaplasia. Arch Surg 98:384–387, 1969.

64. Palshof T, Blichert-Toft M, Daehnfeldt L, et al: Estradiol binding protein in cystosarcoma phyllodes of the breast. Eur J Cancer 16:591–593, 1980.

65. Pietruzka M, Barnes L: Cystosarcoma phyllodes: A clinicopathologic analysis of 42 cases. Cancer 41:1974–1983, 1978.
66. Quisilbash AH: Cystosarcoma phyllodes with liposarcomatous stroma. Am J Clin Pathol 65:321–327, 1976.
67. Rao BR, Meyer JS, Fry CG: Most cystosarcomas phyllodes and fibrosarcomas have progesterone receptor but lack estrogen receptor: Stromal localization of progesterone receptor. Cancer 47:2016–2021, 1981.
68. Rappaport H: Tumors of the hematopoietic system. In Atlas of Tumor Pathology, Section 111, Fascicle 8. Washington, DC, Armed Forces Institute of Pathology, 1966.
69. Reddick RL, Shin TK, Sawney D, et al: Stromal proliferations of the breast: An ultrastructural and immunohistochemical evaluation of cystosarcoma phyllodes, juvenile fibroadenoma, and fibroadenoma. Hum Pathol 18:45–49, 1987.
70. Ronsdahl MM, Lindberg RD, Martin RG: Patterns of failure after treatment of soft tissue sarcoma. Cancer Treat Symp 2:251–258, 1983.
71. Rosen PP, Kimmel M, Ernsberger D: Mammary angiosarcoma: The prognostic significance of histologic grading. Cancer. In press.
72. Rosenberg SA, Lotze MJ, Buul LM, et al: A progress report on the treatment of 157 patients with advanced cancer using lymphokine-activated killer cells and interleukin-2 or high-dose interleukin-2 alone. N Engl J Med 316(15):889–897, 1987.
73. Rosenberg SA, Tepper J, Glatstein E, et al: Prospective randomized evaluation of adjuvant chemotherapy in adults with soft tissue sarcomas of the extremities. Cancer 52:424–434, 1983.
74. Russell WO, Cohen J, Enzinger FM, et al: A clinical and pathological staging system for soft tissue sarcomas. Cancer 40:1562–1570, 1977.
75. Sailer S: Sarcoma of the breast. Am J Cancer 31:183–206, 1937.
76. Salm R: The nature of the so-called post-mastectomy lymphangiosarcoma. J Pathol Bacteriol 85:445–456, 1963.
77. Salm R: Multifocal histogenesis of a cystosarcoma phyllodes. J Clin Pathol 31:897–903, 1978.
78. Schirger A: Postoperative lymphedema: Etiologic and diagnostic factors. Med Clin North Am 46:1045–1050, 1962.
79. Schmidt B, Lantsberg L, Goldstein J, et al: Cystosarcoma phyllodes. Isr J Med Sci 17:895–900, 1981.
80. Schreiber H, Barry FM, Russell WC: Stewart-Treves syndrome: a lethal complication of post-mastectomy lymphedema and regional immune deficiency. Arch Surg 114:82–85, 1979.
81. Sordillo PP, Chapman R, Hajdu S, et al: Lymphangiosarcoma. Cancer 48:1674–1679, 1981.
82. Stark RB, Dwyer EM, DeForest M: Effect of surgical ablation of regional lymph nodes on survival of skin homografts. Ann NY Acad Sci 87:140–148, 1960.
83. Steingaszner LC, Enzinger FM, Taylor HB: Hemangiosarcoma of the breast. Cancer 18(3):352–361, 1965.
84. Stewart FW, Treves N: Lymphangiosarcoma in postmastectomy lymphedema: a report of six cases in elephantiasis chirurgica. Cancer 1:64–81, 1948.
85. Suit HD: Patterns of failure after treatment of sarcoma by radical surgery or by conservative surgery and radiation. Cancer Treat Symp 2:241–246, 1983.
86. Treves N, Sunderland DA: Cystosarcoma of the breast: A malignant and a benign tumor. Clinicopathological study of seventy-five cases. Cancer 4:1286–1332, 1951.
87. Tsukada T, McNutt MA, Ross R, et al: HHF35, a muscle actin-specific monoclonal antibody. Am J Pathol 127(2):389–402, 1987.
88. Ward RM, Evans HL: Cystosarcoma phyllodes: A clinicopathologic study of 26 cases. Cancer 58:2282–2289, 1986.
89. Wargotz ES, Norris HJ, Austin RM, et al: Fibromatosis of the breast: A clinical and pathological study of 28 cases. Am J Surg Pathol 11:38–45, 1987.
90. West TL, Weiland LH, Clagett OT: Cystosarcoma phyllodes. Ann Surg 173:520–528, 1971.
91. Wiseman C, Liao K: Primary lymphoma of the breast. Cancer 29:1705–1712, 1972.
92. Woodward AH, Ivins JC, Soule EA: Lymphangiosarcoma arising in chronically lymphedematous extremities. Cancer 30:562–572, 1972.
93. Yap B-S, Yap H-J, McBride CM, et al: Chemotherapy for postmastectomy lymphangiosarcoma. Cancer 47:853–856, 1981.

Chapter 11

BENIGN AND MALIGNANT EPITHELIAL NEOPLASMS AND DERMATOLOGICAL DISORDERS

Lori J. Shehi, M.D. and K Kendall Pierson, M.D.

In most industrialized countries, the female breast is covered and protected by supportive garments, and less effectively, by the force of (diminishing) social taboos. Clothing has reduced exposure to environmental agents such as sunlight but provided innumerable opportunities for contact dermatitis from dyes, sizing agents, and rubber products. Perfumes, applied directly or in myriad toiletries, also are often implicated in a variety of contact/irritant reactions and photosensitivities involving the skin covering and surrounding the breast.

With the exception of Paget's disease of the nipple and areola, benign tumors and primary epithelial malignancies are uncommon. Malignant melanoma is not frequently encountered in the skin of the female breast. When this tumor occurs, the pathologist should search for remnants of dysplastic nevi; if found, the clinician should be alerted to the possibility of the *dysplastic nevus syndrome* with the attendant high probability that the patient will develop a second primary melanoma.

INFLAMMATORY AND INFECTIOUS CONDITIONS

Contact dermatitis can occur on the breast and skin of the trunk owing to textiles used in brassieres and sportswear. Areas covered by the elastic parts of the garments develop an eczematous dermatitis, usually beginning about three days after exposure.[47] This sensitization can be due to mercaptobenzthiazole contained in rubber or to unknown substances in polyurethane elastomers known as Spandex. Some patients have cross-reacting sensitivity to both agents. Patch tests elicit classic hypersensitivity patterns.

Dermatitis related to substances in contact with skin of the breast is generally divided into (1) primary irritant reactions, those caused directly by local toxic effects of the offending agent; and (2) Type IV delayed hypersensitivity. Cell-mediated delayed reactions (Type IV) result from intraepidermal uptake, processing, and presentation of complexed antigens by Langerhans cells to lymphocytes. The resulting differentiated lymphocytes evolve in at least two directions: (1) long-lived memory cells, and (2) effector cells that initiate acute contact dermatitis. The latter require interleukin-1 (IL-1), secreted by macrophage-like Langerhans cells. This facilitates interleukin-2 (IL-2 or T-cell growth factor) production by helper T cells, resulting in amplification of the immune inflammatory response. For an in-depth description the reader is referred to the extensive review by Cohen.[9]

Factitial or artifactual breast disorders are created by the patient through complicated, often clandestine, repetitive actions that have origin from basic psychosocial or mental disorders. Possible presentations include excoriation and ulceration, puncture wounds, foreign bodies that must be surgically removed, intermittent bleeding from the nipple, or nipple discharge leading to recurrent eczema.[40] These problems may extend over long periods of time, be recurrent, lead to multiple surgical procedures, and result in long-term disability or cosmetic problems due to tissue destruction. Occasionally, the sequelae may be life-threatening. Malignancy must be ruled out by mammography followed by biopsy to exclude the coexistence of a malignant process.

Factitial disorders of the breast should be considered in the differential diagnosis of unusual breast lesions when the clinical situation does not conform to common pathological entities. Artifactual breast disease must be considered when the patient exhibits inappropriate affect or requests a mastectomy. Once the diagnosis is confirmed and a serious underlying organic pathological process is ruled out, further surgery should be avoided. The patient should be reassured that her condition is not life-threatening, cannot be helped by further surgery, and eventually will heal if further intervention is avoided.

A form of *cutaneous herpes simplex* can present as painful, burning, vesicular lesions of the nipple or areola. Axillary lymphadenopathy is commonly associated with this herpetic lesion. In a few reported cases, the source of infection was herpetic gingivostomatitis in a nursing baby. As reported by Dekio and associates,[12] the diagnosis can be confirmed by a Tzanck smear from the vesicle, revealing multinucleate giant cells with viral intranuclear inclusions. Viral cultures are more sensitive and specific but incur additional expense.

Another viral infection of the nipple, *condyloma acuminatum*, caused by human papillomavirus, is often seen in sexually permissive societies. The papillary lesions tend to occur on genital or anal squamous mucosa and on the adjacent skin. In immunosuppressed patients, Wood[49] observed other areas of skin to be affected. Clinically, the lesions are soft verrucous papules that coalesce into cauliflower-like masses. Histologically, the lesions reveal marked acanthosis and papillomatosis with mild hyperkeratosis (Fig. 11–1). The keratinocytes of the upper epidermis have distinct perinuclear vacuoles and are called koilocytes. The dermis is usually chronically inflamed, often with dilated capillaries.

Disciform erythrasma of the breast presents as a well-demarcated, reddish brown patch with fine scaling and sometimes a shiny atrophic-looking surface.[45] Typically, erythrasma occurs in intertriginous areas, especially the web spaces of the toes. A generalized form is most commonly observed in diabetics and black women who live in humid climates. Involvement of the nonintertriginous skin is termed disciform erythrasma. The lesion is caused by *Corynebacterium minutissimum*. Porphyrins produced by the organism initiate a coral red fluorescence under the ultraviolet Wood's light. Diagnosis is confirmed by demonstrating rodlike coccoid or filamentous bacteria on Giemsa, PAS, or Gram stain of scrapings or tissue. The potassium hydroxide (KOH) preparation is negative for fungi. Treatment consists of the administration of topical antibiotics.[45]

Other common infectious diseases of the breast include *tinea corporis* (dermatophytosis or "ringworm"), bacterial folliculitis, and abscess formation. In developing countries, tuberculosis remains a problem (see chapter 5).

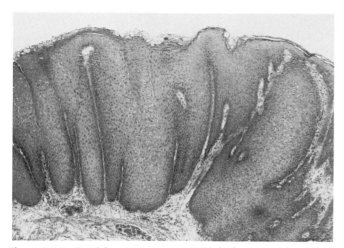

Figure 11–1. Condyloma acuminatum with koilocytes in the midepidermis (× 40).

BENIGN CONDITIONS

Hyperkeratosis of the nipple and areola is a rare benign condition that occurs most often in two subsets of the population. One group of this bimodal patient population is women in the childbearing years; the other is men receiving estrogen therapy, especially diethylstilbestrol, for prostatic cancer.[30] In both groups, estrogens or their metabolites are thought to induce the characteristic changes.

Clinically the nipple and areola are hyperpigmented, thickened, and verrucous with occasional itching and malodorousness. Some lesions are white rather than hyperpigmented and are termed leukokeratosis.[29] Histological findings include minimal hyperkeratosis, marked papillomatosis, regular acanthosis, keratin plugging, and frequent intraepidermal microabscesses. The dermis shows mild perivascular chronic inflammation.

Hyperkeratosis of the nipple and areola can be (1) associated with ichthyosis, where it is bilateral and in both sexes; (2) associated with epidermal nevis, unilateral in both sexes; (3) nevoid hyperkeratosis of the nipple, the most common form, which occurs in women during the childbearing years and is bilaterally symmetrical; and (4) acquired as a result of hormone therapy.

Treatment of hyperkeratosis with keratolytic agents, topical steroids, retinoids, and cryotherapy has been attempted with variable effectiveness.[23, 30, 44, 48]

Necrosis of skin of the breast has been reported secondary to anticoagulant therapy (see chapter 5). Skin necrosis is an unpredictable consequence of Coumadin therapy, occurring in 0.1 percent of patients,[20] and is a less common side effect than cutaneous hemorrhage. It is important to differentiate these two conditions because the prognosis and treatment are different. When skin necrosis does occur, the presentation and course are extremely consistent. The usual patient is an obese woman who develops pain in an area of abundant subcutaneous fat, especially buttocks, thighs, and breast, after three to six days of treatment. Examination of the skin confirms a well-defined maplike ecchymosis with a halo of erythema. There is progression to bullous formation and frank skin necrosis with extensive subcutaneous induration.

The areas of breast necrosis may heal spontaneously with time; otherwise, debridement and skin grafting may be indicated. Occasionally, with extensive involvement of skin of the breast, mastectomy has been necessary. The prothrombin time is usually within a therapeutic range. Other coagulation studies are normal, and the continuation of anticoagulant therapy does not cause progression of existing lesions or the development of new areas of necrosis.[7]

The etiology of Coumadin-related skin necrosis of the breast is thought to be a direct toxic effect of Coumadin on vascular endothelium. Capillaries and venules of the involved tissues are thrombosed and show histological evidence of vasculitis while the arterioles are spared. Thereafter, the skin undergoes ischemic necrosis.

Another variant of skin necrosis that may involve the breast is *pyoderma gangrenosum*. The condition may arise de novo; however, surgical procedures and minor (innocuous) trauma may elicit the lesions in predisposed individuals. The painful cutaneous ulcer characteristically has a mucopurulent base, an advancing rim of purple discoloration, and a surrounding zone of erythema. The histological appearance of pyoderma gangrenosum is not diagnostic. In early lesions, circumscribed abscesses with abundant neutrophils or multilocular intraepidermal bullae are identified. The fully developed ulcer has an absent epidermis, acute inflammation and necrosis in the upper dermis, and chronic inflammation of the lower dermis. The border of the ulcer reveals epidermal hyperplasia with underlying lymphocytic vasculitis. Fibrinoid necrosis of vessel walls with thrombosis may be seen.

The cause of breast pyoderma gangrenosum is not infectious. Rand et al.[39] consider the condition to result from altered host immunity, including hypersensitivity, altered cell-mediated immunity, and inappropriate neutrophil response to antigens. In over 80 percent of patients, pyoderma gangrenosum is associated with systemic illness; between 40 percent and 60 percent have ulcerative colitis.[39] Other underlying diseases include Crohn's disease, peptic ulcer, perforated appendix, chronic active hepatitis, diverticulitis, rheumatoid arthritis, leukemia, bronchitis, empyema, and hypogammaglobulinemia.

When other causes of acute and chronic skin ulceration are excluded and antibiotic therapy fails to improve the lesions, treatment consists of appropriate therapy aimed at the underlying illness, high-dose corticosteroids (optional), and local wound care. Recently, split-thickness skin grafting and administration of hyperbaric oxygen therapy have been successful.[39]

Mondor's disease, or mammary subcutaneous phlebitis, presents as a painful superficial cord beneath the skin of the breast. The lesion occurs secondary to superficial thoracic vein thrombophlebitis and is reviewed in chapter 5B. Microscopically, subcutaneous veins are thrombosed, leading to secondary fibrosis of the vein wall.

Primary osteoma cutis is a rare condition characterized by de novo formation of osseous nodules without the skin. The nodules may be single or multiple, are hard, are usually asymptomatic, and are located in the deep dermis or subcutaneous fat. The overlying skin is usually normal but may be erythematous, atrophic, pigmented, excoriated, or ulcerated.[22] Microscopically, well-formed mature bone spicules are seen. Secondary, or metaplastic, bone formation can be associated with fibroadenomas, trauma, epidermoid cysts, pigmented nevi, acne, syphilis, scleroderma, or systemic lupus erythematosus.[22]

Silicone granuloma should be considered in nodular or subcutaneous plaque-like lesions of the breast, upper chest, and upper arm. A history of breast implants or silicone injection is commonly, but not always, elicited. The diagnosis is made by persistent inquiry and a confirmatory biopsy. Pure silicone is inert and should initiate minimal tissue reaction. Oils and fatty acids may be added to induce scarring and will thereafter decrease migration of the silicone from the site of rupture of the breast implant (see chapter 5). The route of spread of the polymer to the chest and arm is through the vascular sheath around axillary vessels.[26]

Microscopically oval cavities of various sizes are surrounded by foamy macrophages and foreign body giant cells. The cavities may contain a film or droplets of oily material that shows no birefringence with polarized illumination. The adjacent tissue reaction is that of a mixed granuloma with histiocytes, lymphocytes, eosinophils, and multinucleate giant cells.

Since 1964, more than 30 cases of connective tissue diseases have been reported that developed in patients after cosmetic silicone injection of Silastic implants.[6] Some of these diseases are *autoimmune-like syndromes* and some are classic collagen vascular diseases such as systemic lupus erythematosus, rheumatoid arthritis, scleroderma, and mixed connective tissue disease.[32] These disorders occur in response to foreign substances such as paraffin and silicone and are known as human adjuvant disease.

Scleroderma or morphea may involve the breast, unrelated to foreign material. Clinical findings include depigmentation, thickening, and contraction of the skin. Tissue examination reveals atrophy of the epidermis and its appendages, thickened dermis with large sclerotic and hyalinized collagen bundles, and reduced dermal vascularity. The glandular breast tissue may be atrophic and surrounded by dense fibrosis and sclerotic collagen.

Recently, a case of scleroderma localized to the breast was reported.[17] The patient had no obvious signs of systemic disease. However, the involvement of the breast skin was progressive and systemic manifestations were expected to develop.

Amyloidosis of the nipple may present as long-standing intermittent pruritus.[14] The nipple may enlarge slightly during attacks of pruritus but otherwise appears normal. Microscopically the amyloid is deposited in the papillary dermis as globules, similar to the colloid bodies of lichen planus, or as homogeneous material that fills the entire papillary dermis. Extensive pigment deposition is commonly associated with this entity. Crystal violet and congo red stains demonstrate the amyloid.

CONGENITAL LESIONS

Unilateral hypoplasia of the female breast has been associated with congenital melanotic spots.[50] In this association, the small hypoplastic breast and small areola are covered by a hyperpigmented irregular spot that may extend to cover part of the back. The melanotic spot is present from birth with no change in size or color with time. Involved skin contains the normal number of melanocytes, but increased melanin pigment is evident. Assuming that the two findings are related, the abnormality may be genetically determined early in embryogenesis. Ectoblast, of ectodermal origin, gives rise to the neural crest and the epiblast. While melanocytes originate from the neural crest, the epiblast is the source of skin, including the mammary ridges and ultimately the breast. This abnormality of development may occur as a consequence of embryological maldevelopment of both components.

Becker's melanosis can be associated with hypoplasia of the breast and pectoralis major muscle.[31] Becker's melanosis is an acquired hypermelanosis and hypertrichosis appearing on the shoulder or arm and sometimes on the breast.[15] Identification of these lesions may be a marker for underlying structural abnormalities, especially in females. The hyperpigmented area shows moderate elongation of rete ridges, variable acanthosis and hyperkeratosis, increased melanin in the basal layer, and enlarged pilar apparati. The common associated anomalies include lumbar spina bifida and hypoplasia of the ipsilateral breast, areola, and nipple. Less commonly observed associations are absence of the pectoralis major muscle and a decrease in size of the ipsilateral arm.

Hereditary acrolabial telangiectasia, as described by Millns and Dicken[28] in 1979, is a rare familial syndrome demonstrating diffuse blue discoloration of the lips, nipples, areolae, and nail beds; telangiectases of the elbows, chest, and dorsa of the hands; varicosities of the lower legs; and migraine headaches. The presence of blue lips and nail beds at birth is commonly interpreted by the physician as cyanosis. In actuality, the blue coloration of these areas occurs secondary to an extensive network of thin-walled vessels high in the papillary dermis. Variable numbers of smaller vessels are present in the reticular dermis. Despite widespread vascular telangiectasia, no serious sequela such as hemorrhage, stroke, or hypertension has developed in individuals with the syndrome.[28]

BENIGN EPITHELIAL NEOPLASMS

Papillary adenoma of the nipple, also known as *erosive adenomatosis* of the nipple or *florid papillomatosis*, is a most important benign lesion of the breast. Typically the disorder occurs on the female breast as an erosion, ulceration, or mass of the nipple accompanied by serous or bloody discharge. In the early phase of presentation, differentiation from Paget's disease may be clinically impossible. Eczematous dermatitis is another common clinical disorder that may be confused with papillary adenoma.

Histologically, two patterns are observed. One pattern includes an *adenomatous* growth with proliferation of round, oval, or irregularly shaped ducts within normal, fibrotic, or hyalinized stroma. The ducts are lined by an inner columnar epithelium and an outer flattened to cuboidal myoepithelial layer. In most cases, the columnar cells show focal apocrine "snouts" and dense eosinophilic material in some duct lumens.

The second pattern is *papillomatous.* Although there is proliferation of ductlike structures, the ducts are larger, oval or round, and almost solidly filled with cells. The outer myoepithelial layer persists. The inner columnar cell layer shows prominent intraluminal growth that essentially occludes the lumen, except for slitlike spaces at the periphery. Though individual cases show a predominance of one pattern, there is considerable overlap.

Other microscopic features include a direct connection between the surface squamous epithelium and the columnar epithelium of the tumor; superficial keratin and debris-filled cysts, occasionally with foreign body giant cell reactions; and an inflammatory infiltrate that is rich in plasma cells.[5] True epithelium-lined papillae with connective tissue cores are not present. Benign papillary adenoma must be differentiated from primary breast cancer or breast cancer that is metastatic to the skin. All malignant cases show hypercellular atypical neoplastic glands irregularly dispersed within a cellular fibrotic stroma. Patterns typical of breast cancer are cribriforming, Indian-filing, and growth in cords. Surrounding myoepithelial cells are absent. Cytological malignancy is characterized by enlarged hyperchromatic nuclei, prominent nucleoli, and mitotic figures.

The typical papillary adenoma occurs in perimenopausal women who present with a history of nipple erosion, discharge, or a mass over the interval of a few months to several years. The lesion is biologically benign and simple resection is indicated.

A major pitfall in diagnosis is confusion of the papillary adenoma with sweat gland tumors. Features supporting the diagnosis of adenoma include superficial keratocyst, intraluminal giant cells, and intraductal papillomatosis.[5]

Clear cell hidradenoma (eccrine acrospiradenoma) is a skin appendage tumor that may occur beneath the areola. It usually presents as a solitary intradermal nodule, 0.5 to 2 cm in diameter, with an intact covering of skin, although some tumors show superficial ulceration and serous discharge. Microscopically, the tumor is well circumscribed and may appear encapsulated. Lobulated masses within the dermis, and possibly into the subcutaneous fat, have tubular lumens and cystic spaces. The tubular lumens are lined by cuboidal duct cells or columnar secretory cells, which occasionally show decapitation secretion. The wide cystic spaces are usually bordered by tumor cells with no particular orientation, which suggests that the cysts form as a result of degeneration. In the solid parts of the tumor there are also two types of cells. One is polygonal or spindled with a round nucleus and basophilic cytoplasm. The other is round with a distinct cell membrane and clear cytoplasm containing glycogen. Usually the tumor lobules have no connection to the surface epidermis. The lesion is benign. Simple excision is adequate therapy.

Eccrine poroma is a benign skin appendage tumor that is firm, raised, often pedunculated, asymptomatic, and less than 2 cm in diameter. The usual location is feet or hands, but the lesion may arise in breast skin. The typical eccrine poroma begins within the lower epidermis and extends downward as broad, anastomosing bands. The tumor cells are distinctive. They are smaller than squamous cells, are uniform and cuboidal, have a round dark nucleus, are connected by intercellular bridges, do not keratinize, and contain a large amount of glycogen. In most patients, the poroma has narrow duct lumens; sometimes cystic spaces are found in the tumor bands. These spaces and ducts are lined by an eosinophilic cuticle similar to that in the eccrine sweat ducts and by a single row of cells.

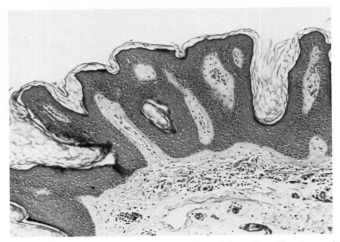

Figure 11–2. Seborrheic keratosis. Note the epidermal proliferation and keratin-filled horn cysts (× 100).

Poromas located entirely within the epidermis as discrete aggregates are known as *hidroacanthoma simplex*. They present in adult life and resemble seborrheic keratoses.[36]

Pilomatrixoma has occurred in the male breast and may be clinically indistinguishable from breast carcinoma.[16] These tumors present as a painless hard mass adjacent to the nipple that produces ulceration of the overlying skin. Grossly, the tumor is circumscribed and has a gritty, calcified, friable center. Histologically, the lesion presents in deep dermis and sometimes extends into the subcutaneous fat. Islands of small basaloid cells at the periphery gradually blend in with islands of densely eosinophilic ghost cells with absent nuclei. Calcification and cholesterol clefts are prominent. This lesion is benign and requires simple excision.

Seborrheic keratoses are very common lesions that occur primarily on the trunk or face, appearing in middle age. These benign epithelial lesions are sharply demarcated, brown, and elevated so that they appear stuck on the skin surface. Some are verrucous with a friable surface; others are smooth with keratin plugs. They become crusted after trauma and may be pedunculated, especially on the neck and upper chest.

There are many variants of seborrheic keratosis. All have in common the features of hyperkeratosis, acanthosis, and papillomatosis (Fig. 11–2). The acanthosis is due entirely to the upward (vertical) growth phase so that the base of the lesion is level with the skin surface. Both squamous cells and small basaloid cells proliferate. Horny invaginations of the surface appear as pseudo-horn cysts. The lesions may contain increased melanin pigment.

The hyperkeratotic seborrheic keratosis shows marked, often digitate, hyperkeratosis and papillomatosis with minimal acanthosis. Numerous epidermis-lined papillae resemble church spires. An irritated seborrheic keratosis contains numerous whorls or eddies of flattened squamous cells in poorly delineated horn pearls. This lesion may also show modest downward proliferation from the base of the epithelial growth, into

the dermis. Other variants are the reticulated type and the clonal type.

Epidermal cysts occur mostly on the face, scalp, neck, and trunk but may be seen on skin of the breast. They are slow-growing, elevated, round, firm to fluctuant intradermal or subcutaneous masses. The cyst wall is composed of true epidermis with a granular cell layer. The cyst is filled with laminated orthokeratin. If the cyst ruptures, an intense foreign body reaction results.

Trichilemmal cysts (sebaceous cysts) are clinically indistinguishable from epidermal cysts. They are less common than epidermal cysts. Ninety percent occur on the scalp. These cysts are frequently multiple. The wall of the cyst is composed of epithelial cells with no intercellular bridges. There is often peripheral palisading. The luminal epithelial cells are swollen and pale, with no granular layer, and demonstrate abrupt keratinization. Nuclear remnants and ghostlike cells are present in the homogeneous eosinophilic contents. Focal calcification is common, and rupture produces a prominent foreign body reaction. Then, incision and drainage is appropriate initial management. Following resolution of the inflammatory phase with discharge of the eosinophilic contents, simple excision is recommended.

Basal cell epitheliomas occur almost exclusively on hair-bearing, sun-exposed skin, such as on the head and neck. The most common form is noduloulcerative, which begins as a small, waxy nodule with small telangiectatic vessels on the surface. The epithelioma slowly increases in size and often ulcerates centrally. The typical lesion has a progressively enlarging crater with a pearly rolled border, termed a *rodent ulcer*. Other clinical types include *pigmented basal cell epithelioma, morphea-like or fibrosing basal cell epithelioma, superficial basal cell epithelioma*, and *fibroepithelioma*.

Microscopically, masses of basaloid cells proliferate from the basal layer of the epidermis as nests and cords with peripheral palisading (Fig. 11–3). The nuclei are slightly larger and darker than normal basal cells. The cell borders are indistinct, and intercellular bridges are inconspicuous. Mitoses are variable. The connective tissue stroma proliferates with the tumor, is arranged in

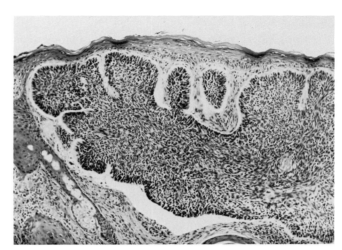

Figure 11–3. Basal cell carcinoma (× 100).

bundles around the tumor masses, and tends to detach from the tumor after fixation. Basal cell epitheliomas may show differentiation resembling hair structures, sebaceous glands, and apocrine or eccrine glands.

Basosquamous cell epitheliomas, or *metatypical epitheliomas*, have malignant features with squamous differentiation. These epithelial tumors are thought to have a greater propensity to invade and metastasize than do pure basal cell epitheliomas. The more common basal cell epithelioma does not typically spread widely, and those reported to metastasize are usually large, ulcerated, locally invasive, destructive recurrent lesions. One case of basal cell epithelioma of the nipple seen in a 54-year-old male metastasized to 3 of 20 axillary lymph nodes four years after simple excision of the primary lesion.[42]

Cutaneous leiomyomas, arising from the mammillary muscles, may occur on the nipple and areola. Approximately 20 cases of cutaneous leiomyoma of the nipple, 17 of which were in women, have been reported.[46] The leiomyoma presents as an enlargement of the nipple that is often a painful, elastic, firm mass adherent to the skin. The lesion is unattached to the underlying soft tissue. The dermal tumor is unencapsulated and connected to the normal smooth muscle bundles of the breast. It is composed of irregular interlacing elongated bundles of spindle cells with long, blunt-ended nuclei. Occasionally remnants of dilated breast ducts are entrapped. A Masson trichrome stain identifies pink smooth muscle cells with varying amounts of green collagen. Mitoses are absent.

Granular cell tumors, originally called *granular cell myoblastomas*, are benign lesions most commonly of the tongue, skin, and subcutaneous tissues. The granular cell tumor of the skin of the breast presents as a well-circumscribed, often raised, firm nodule 0.5 to 3 cm in diameter. It may be tender or pruritic and sometimes has a verrucous surface.

Histologically, the dermal tumor cells are large and often elongated, with a distinct cell membrane. The cytoplasm is pale and eosinophilic with fine granules. The nuclei are small, round, and central. Mitoses are rare. The overlying epidermis frequently demonstrates pseudoepitheliomatous hyperplasia, which may be mistaken for squamous cell carcinoma. The granules are PAS-positive and diastase-resistant. The immunoperoxidase stain for S-100 is positive. On electron microscopy the granules are seen to be complex phagolysosomes. Simple excision is curative. Granular cell tumors in glandular tissues of the breast are easily mistaken for adenocarcinoma on mammography and clinical examination, owing to the stellate, radiographic configuration of the lesion and the solid, elastic, firm features of the mass.

MALIGNANT TUMORS

One of the most important malignancies of the skin of the breast is *Paget's disease*. Almost all cases of mammary Paget's disease have an underlying *ductal adenocarcinoma*. This malignant epithelial lesion must be differentiated from extramammary Paget's disease, in which underlying sweat gland carcinoma is present in less than one third of patients. The cells of mammary Paget's disease are believed to originate in adenocarcinomas of the lactiferous ducts that ascend to involve the epidermis. Only very rarely does *adenocarcinoma in situ* of the nipple, areola, or skin of the breast arise without underlying ductal carcinoma. Some argue that the carcinoma will invariably be discovered if searched for exhaustively.

Dabski and Stoll[10] determined that in 20.9 percent of the cases, Paget's disease presented as a nipple lesion *without* a palpable breast mass; in 48.9 percent of cases as a nipple lesion *with* a palpable mass at the first examination; and in 10.2 percent as a palpable breast tumor with Paget's disease identified only on microscopic examination. The gross lesion of the nipple, areola, or adjacent skin is a persistent eczematous dermatitis with erythema, scaling, oozing, and crusting. Occasionally a bloody or purulent discharge is noted. One reported case of mammary Paget's disease presented with thick hard keratinized material forming a cutaneous horn.[10] It has been pointed out that one half of cutaneous horns of the breast are benign, but a histological examination is warranted in every case.[10]

Paget described large pale-staining cells within the epidermis, generally above the basement membrane (Fig. 11–4). They have a large nucleus and abundant cytoplasm. Frequently the basal epidermal cells are flattened between the Paget's cells and the dermis. Paget's cells are PAS-positive and diastase-resistant and are positive for carcinoembryonic antigen (CEA) by immunoperoxidase techniques. Only 40 percent of samples stain positively for mucin and then only weakly.[43] In extramammary Paget's disease, 90 percent of the lesions are strongly mucin-positive.

Paget's disease can be identified within the large ducts beneath the nipple. This lesion may arise against a background of other chronic skin disease. Any non-healing nipple lesion should be biopsied, even in the

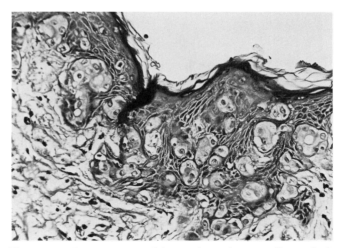

Figure 11–4. Paget's disease of the nipple. Malignant cells invade the epidermis ($\times$ 400).

presence of another well-documented skin disorder (e.g., pemphigus vulgaris).[37]

Additionally, Paget's disease may arise in ectopic breast tissue adjacent to a supernumerary nipple.[21] Underlying ductal carcinoma should be searched for, as in the normal breast (see chapter 9).

Other skin abnormalities may be associated with carcinoma of the breast. Four variants of cutaneous metastases are observed to disseminate via the lymphatics: *inflammatory carcinoma, telangiectatic carcinoma, nodular carcinoma, and carcinoma-en-cuirasse*. More than one type may be present in the same patient.

Inflammatory carcinoma results when dissemination of tumor cells occurs through the lymphatics of the entire dermis and possibly into the subcutaneous tissue. The skin is red, warm, and slightly indurated in an area with well-demarcated borders. Histology reveals invasion of dermal and often subcutaneous lymphatics by groups of tumor cells that are similar in appearance to the primary tumor (Figs. 11–5 and 11–6). Associated capillary congestion, edema, and perivascular chronic inflammation are seen.

If dissemination of tumor occurs only through the superficial lymphatics and blood vessels of the dermis, it produces *telangiectatic carcinoma*. The skin is covered by numerous purple papules and hemorrhagic vesicle-like lesions that resemble hemangiomas. Dilated small blood vessels and lymphatics in the upper dermis are permeated by tumor. The blood vessels contain red blood cells as well as tumor cells.

With the clinical presentation of nodular carcinoma and carcinoma-en-cuirasse, the tumor cells infiltrate along tissue planes and to a lesser extent directly via lymphatics. In *nodular carcinoma*, asymptomatic firm nodules are evident on palpation in the skin and subcutis. Superficial lesions may ulcerate. Microscopically, groups of tumor cells in the dermis are surrounded by dense fibrosis. With *carcinoma-en-cuirasse*, the breast skin is diffusely thickened and indurated. Histologically, these indurated areas reveal fibrosis with sparse tumor cells. The tumor cells may be single, in small groups, or in single cell rows (Indian-filing) between thickened collagen fibers.

Hematogenous dissemination of breast carcinoma to skin usually produces single, but sometimes multiple, elevated nodules. A common site of metastasis is the scalp, where the loss of hair follicles produces a condition known as *alopecia neoplastica*.

The development of *angiosarcoma* in an area of *postmastectomy lymphedema* was first described in 1948 by Stewart and Treves (*Stewart-Treves syndrome*). Cutaneous and subcutaneous nodules may develop several years after radical mastectomy in the edematous tissues of the ipsilateral arm. The nodules are bluish, often demonstrate rapid growth rates, and may ulcerate. Death often occurs within one to two years of the diagnosis of metastases. The most common cause of death is pulmonary failure secondary to diffuse lung metastases. The angiosarcomas are often very undifferentiated, invasive, and more aggressive clinically than the typical angiosarcomas that occur on the face or scalp of the elderly. Complex, anastomosing vascular structures are lined by proliferative, atypical endothelial cells. Solid areas of spindle cell proliferation are identifiable

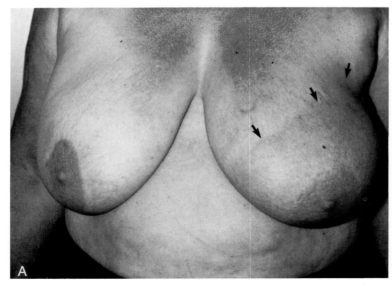

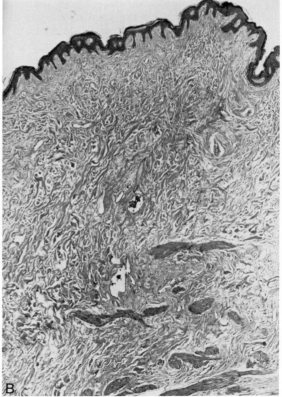

Figure 11–5. *A*, Sixty-six-year-old white female with inflammatory carcinoma of the left breast. A 3 cm lesion was palpable in the subareola and was visualized on mammography. The skin is red (arrows), warm, and indurated. *B*, Photomicrograph of inflammatory carcinoma in the same patient. Tumor cells are present in dermal lymphatics (× 40).

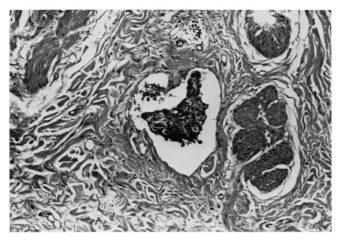

Figure 11–6. Inflammatory carcinoma. The malignant cells in the lymphatics are the same as those in the primary tumor (× 400).

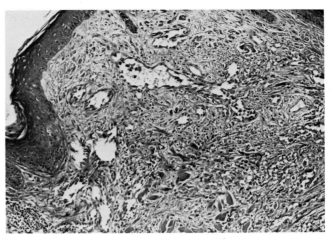

Figure 11–8. Angiosarcoma. Irregular vascular spaces are lined by neoplastic endothelium (× 100).

at the center of the lesion, and can be seen infiltrating collagen (Figs. 11–7 and 11–8). The vascular origin of the tumor cells can be verified by immunostaining for Factor VIII or *Ulex europaeus* antigen (UEA).

Primary *melanoma* of the skin of the breast accounts for 1.8 to 5.0 percent of all melanomas.[24, 41] Ariel and Caron[1] noted that the average age of occurrence in their series was 36 years.[1] Melanoma can arise in the skin or glandular tissues of the breast, although the latter is quite rare. The origin of approximately 25 percent of all melanomas is the trunk, with only 5 percent identified

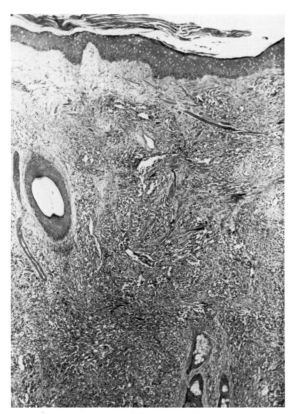

Figure 11–7. Angiosarcoma. Solid portions of the tumor are composed of spindled cells (× 40).

on the anterior chest wall or breast.[24] Women have a preponderance of lesions on the lower extremity, less often have melanomas of the trunk, and even less frequently lesions of the breast.

Conditions that cause patients to seek medical advice and treatment of the primary lesion include increase in size, change in pigmentation, ulceration, bleeding, enlargement during pregnancy, lateral spread of the lesion, and pruritus.[1] Signs that should alert the physician to the possibility of malignancy include irregular borders; variation in color including not only tan, brown, and black but pink, blue, and gray; depigmentation in surrounding areas indicating spontaneous regression; nodularity; induration; and ulceration.

The initial evaluation of a suspicious pigmented lesion should include a biopsy. Since an accurate diagnosis is much more likely when the entire lesion is studied, excisional biopsy is recommended. When the lesion is large (>2cm) or in a location where total excision poses cosmetic problems with closure (e.g., contiguous with nipple-areola), an incisional biopsy inclusive of a representative section of tumor and normal skin is appropriate. However, controversy exists concerning incisional biopsies and the possibility[19, 38] that they may cause metastatic spread. European studies[19, 38] suggest decreased five-year survival after incisional biopsy, whereas American studies[2, 13] have demonstrated no adverse effect on survival when punch biopsy was utilized. A shave biopsy or curettement is absolutely contraindicated. Accurate diagnosis and determination of depth of invasion of the tumor are essential for prognosis and treatment strategy and are significantly compromised by the absence of adequate intact tissue from the primary neoplasm.

Four histopathological variants of malignant melanoma are widely recognized: (1) *lentigo maligna*, occurring on sun-exposed skin; (2) *superficial spreading*; (3) *acral lentiginous*, occurring on palm, soles, and periungual areas; and (4) *nodular melanoma*.[8] The two most common types are superficial spreading (Fig. 11–9) and nodular melanoma (Fig. 11–10), accounting for 70 percent and 15 percent of all melanomas, respectively.

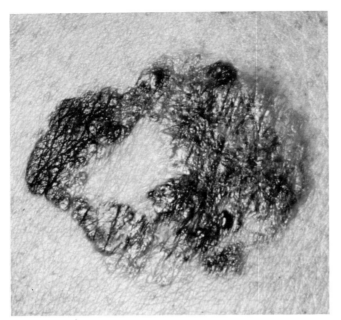

Figure 11–9. Superficial spreading malignant melanoma on skin of the sun-exposed breast.

These are the two types that most often occur on the breast. The most common sites for the development of melanoma are the upper back in men and the lower leg in women.

Microscopically, early melanoma appears as pleomorphic, irregular junctional nevomelanocytic proliferation composed of single units, nests, or theques of cells with hyperchromatic nuclei and variable nucleoli (Fig. 11–11). These atypical cells extend upward into the epidermis in a pagetoid fashion and later invade downward into the dermis. The epidermis may show irregular downward acanthotic proliferation of the rete ridges. The tumor cells may be large and epithelioid, small and

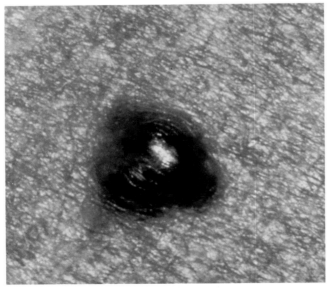

Figure 11–10. Nodular variant of malignant melanoma of the breast skin. Note surrounding actinic injury of skin.

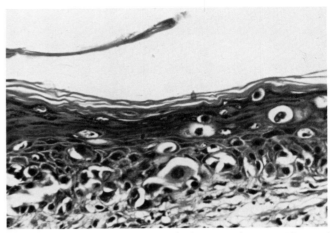

Figure 11–11. Superficial spreading malignant melanoma with prominent pagetoid epidermal invasion (× 100).

nevoid, or spindle-shaped. Mitotic figures are usually present in small numbers. The amount of melanin pigmentation is variable, and a significant number of lesions are amelanotic. The chronic inflammatory infiltrate that occurs in response to the tumor is also variable. Early lesions typically have a bandlike lymphoid infiltrate at the base of the tumor. In deeply invasive tumors, this is often less pronounced and mixed with the malignant melanocytes.

Some consider important the distinction between superficial spreading and nodular melanoma and claim that the prognosis is much different. In nodular melanoma the pagetoid upward spread of melanoma cells is limited to epidermis immediately overlying the dermal tumor infiltrate (Fig. 11–12). In the superficial spreading variant of melanoma, pagetoid spread occurs lateral to the invading main tumor mass and is termed the radial growth phase.

In superficial spreading melanoma, invasiveness is heralded by the development of papules, nodules, or induration. Ulceration is a late occurrence. Prognosis depends on staging and, most importantly, depth of invasion. The overall five-year survival of Stage I pa-

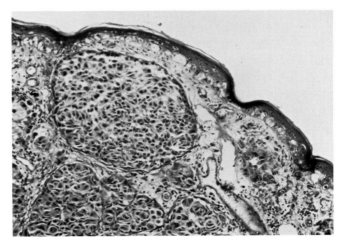

Figure 11–12. Nodular melanoma with large mass of malignant cells in the dermis (× 100).

tients is approximately 70 percent and is improving with early recognition and appropriate treatment. Nodular melanoma begins as an elevated nodule that invades rapidly with vertical growth and often ulcerates. Because of more rapid and deeper invasion it often has a poorer prognosis; Stage I has a 50 to 60 percent five-year survival.[27]

Prognosis of malignant melanoma largely depends upon stage of disease, which directly correlates with depth of invasion. For patients in Stage I (those *without* palpable lymph node involvement), prognosis is directly proportional to tumor thickness. Originally, depth of invasion was assessed only by Clark's levels.[8]

Level I: Melanoma cells confined to the epidermis and skin appendages.
Level II: Extension into but not filling the papillary dermis.
Level III: Extension throughout the papillary dermis, filling and often expanding it, and impinging upon the reticular dermis.
Level IV: Invasion of the reticular dermis.
Level V: Invasion of subcutaneous fat.

Clark originally reported the five-year mortality to be 8 percent in Level II, 35 percent in Level III, 46 percent in Level IV, and 52 percent in Level V.

In 1970 Breslow objectively measured tumor thickness with an ocular micrometer.[4] The depth of invasion is measured from the top of the granular layer to the deepest extent of vertical extension of the tumor, or from the ulcer base to the deepest point in ulcerated lesions. He observed that melanomas less than 0.76 mm thick rarely metastasize and do not require prophylactic lymph node dissection, an observation confirmed by many investigators.[3] For melanomas greater than 1.5 mm thick, prophylactic regional lymph node dissection doubled the survival. Melanomas from 0.76 to 1.5 mm thick were inconclusive as to the value of lymph node dissection.[3]

Clinical factors that favorably affect prognosis include female gender and location of the tumor on hair-bearing portions of the extremities rather than on the trunk. Adverse effects are related to rapid growth rate of the tumor and include advancing age of the patient, diameter of the lesion, and ulceration.

Histological factors also affect the prognosis. Nodular melanoma has a poorer survival rate than does superficial spreading melanoma, as the former tends to grow more rapidly and patients more commonly present with advanced disease. These two variants have similar mortalities for equivalent depth of invasion. A high mitotic rate, vascular or lymphatic invasion, and absence of melanin suggest a less differentiated neoplasm and a guarded prognosis. Further, these factors usually best correlate with tumor thickness. A lymphocytic infiltrate at the base of the tumor is considered to be favorable, although some authors disagree. Satellite nodules around the primary tumor are a form of metastasis and indicate a guarded prognosis. Regional lymph node involvement increases with increasing tumor thickness.

It is generally accepted that tumors less than 0.76 mm thick do not require regional lymph node dissection. Lymph node dissection significantly improved five-year survival in one series[3] (from 37 percent to 83 percent) when tumor depth was 1.5 mm to 4 mm. In those patients with tumors greater than 4 mm thick, lymph node dissection serves as a *staging* rather than a *therapeutic* procedure. Patients with tumors 0.76 mm to 1.5 mm thick have not received disease-free or survival benefit from regional lymph node dissection.[4] Thus, tumors of intermediate thickness, 1.5 mm to 4 mm, remain therapeutically controversial, and treatment should be individualized. The prognosis of patients with clinical Stage I disease is affected by the number of nodes found to be pathologically positive following regional lymph node dissection. Day et al.[11] noted that involvement of less than 20 percent of the resected nodes with tumor thickness less than 3.5 mm is prognostically more favorable.

Metastases generally occur via the regional lymph nodes and through hematogenous routes. Major sites of metastasis include lungs, brain, dura, spinal cord, gastrointestinal tract, heart, liver, peritoneum, and adrenals. Late metastases to the skin and subcutaneous tissue are common.

Treatment of malignant melanoma of the breast has aroused some controversy. In the past, guidelines for the surgical management of melanoma of the breast were similar to the treatment of carcinoma of the breast. Therapy formerly consisted of mastectomy, although the underlying glandular tissue was rarely invaded, with axillary node dissection. Additionally, primary melanomas of the medial quadrants were managed with extended radical mastectomy, which incorporated internal mammary nodes in the dissection.[34] Most older studies recommend wide and deep re-excision of the biopsy site, including 5 cm skin margins and subcutaneous tissue down to the fascia of the pectoralis major or serratus muscles.[24, 34, 35, 41] Those who recommend prophylactic axillary lymph node dissection suggest a 10 to 20 percent increase in survival when lymphadenectomy is routinely performed for stage I melanoma.[24] An elective axillary node dissection, in continuity with the breast excision when possible, has been recommended for all melanomas of Clark's Level III or greater and/or a thickness of 1.5 mm or more. When the regional lymph nodes are clinically positive, a therapeutic axillary (Patey, Levels I to III) dissection is mandatory. Internal mammary node dissection has not enhanced local or regional disease control in several studies.[1, 23, 33] Supraclavicular lymph node dissection should be considered for lesions within 3 cm of the clavicle.[34] It appears that breast melanomas do not differ from other primary cutaneous melanomas with regard to prognosis and regional node status as related to levels of tumor microinvasion (mm). Therapeutic rules similar to those that obtain for primary melanoma in other anatomical sites should be applied to the breast.[34]

Primary melanomas of the nipple and areola are extremely rare. These lesions have a better prognosis and lower incidence of nodal metastasis than do other breast melanomas (28 percent axillary node metastasis as opposed to 60 percent overall).[33] Axillary lymph node dissection is recommended for Clark's Level III or deeper.

Premalignant melanocytic lesions of the breast may include benign and *dysplastic nevi*. Histologically, remnants of nevus are found in about 35 percent of all malignant melanomas.[25] Despite the rarity of malignant melanoma of the skin of the breast, one author suggests that any nevus at a site of irritation by clothing or around the areola should be excised.[1]

Dysplastic nevi occur as part of the *dysplastic nevus syndrome* and as sporadic events. Those patients with multiple dysplastic nevi and the syndrome have a 100 percent lifetime risk for the development of malignant melanoma. The incidence of melanoma in patients who develop sporadic dysplastic nevi is not known but may be higher than that of the general population. Dysplastic nevi tend to occur more frequently on the thorax and buttocks (Fig. 11–13), thus, dispelling the notion of actinic exposure's being etiological in the syndromal or sporadic variant.

Clinically, dysplastic nevi present as minimally elevated lesions of relatively larger size (usually 5 mm or more) with irregular indefinite borders in various shades of brown and tan (Fig. 11–14). Histologically, dysplastic nevi are *junctional* or *compound nevi* with single melanocytes and nests that demonstrate cytological atypia.

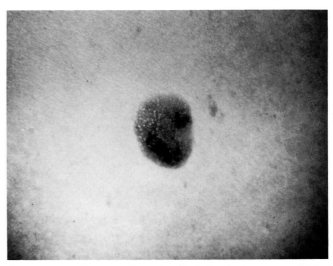

Figure 11–14. Close-up view of typical dysplastic nevus, which is minimally elevated with indefinite borders and various tones of tan-brown.

Individual melanocytes and groups are largely confined to the basal layers of the epidermis. The nests extend downward from the basal layer into the upper dermis, often with the long axis of the cellular nests paralleling the dermal-epidermal junction. The atypical melanocytes are frequently spindled but may be epithelioid and variably pigmented. Most nests of nevus cells in the dermis are not atypical and diminish in size with their descent, i.e., demonstrate "maturation." Eosinophilic and lamellar fibrosis of the upper dermis hugs the base of the junctional nests. Sparse perivascular lymphoid infiltrates are commonly present. The lesion that progresses to *melanoma in situ* often displays intraepidermal pagetoid spread of the atypical melanocytes.

An unusual malignancy of the breast is *leiomyosarcoma of the nipple*. As with leiomyomas, smooth muscle tumors of the skin usually arise from erector pili muscles or the smooth muscle of blood vessels. However, the breast nipple and areola contain mammillary muscles that may give rise to neoplasms. Leiomyosarcoma of the breast is extremely rare.

The tumor presents as a slightly tender nodule of the nipple and underlying breast tissue. Thereafter, the skin becomes fixed to the tumor without associated dimpling. The lesion is composed of a mass of nodules of varying sizes that present with interlacing fascicles of malignant smooth muscle cells with cigar-shaped nuclei and frequent mitoses. Multinucleate bizarre tumor giant cells can be present. At the edge of the lesion a transition to the benign smooth muscle of the mammillary muscle can sometimes be observed. It is suggested that the criteria generally applied for malignancy in extrauterine leiomyosarcomas be used, i.e., five or more mitoses per ten high power fields.[18] Men and women are equally affected by this sarcoma, and the prognosis is quite good. The treatment of choice is complete wide excision or mastectomy, if necessary to allow clear margins of resection. Axillary lymph node dissection is *not* done for this sarcoma, which spreads hematogenously.

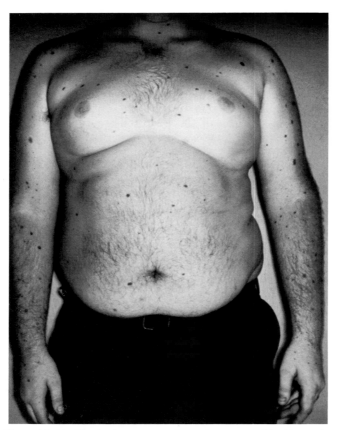

Figure 11–13. Dysplastic nevus syndrome in 23-year-old white male. Multiple dysplastic nevi cover the arms and trunk.

References

1. Ariel IM, Caron AS: Diagnosis and treatment of malignant melanoma arising from the skin of the female breast. Am J Surg 124:384–390, 1972.
2. Bagley FH, Cady B, Lee A, et al: Changes in clinical presentation and management of malignant melanoma. Cancer 47:2126–2134, 1981.
3. Balch CM, Murad TM, Soong SJ, et al: Tumor thickness as a guide to surgical management of clinical Stage I melanoma patients. Cancer 43:883–888, 1979.
4. Breslow A: Tumor thickness level of invasion and node dissection in Stage I cutaneous melanoma. Ann Surg 182:572–575, 1975.
5. Brownstein MH, Phelps RG, Magnin PH: Papillary adenoma of the nipple: Analysis of fifteen new cases. J Am Acad Dermatol 12:707–715, 1985.
6. Byron MA, Venning VA, Mowat AG: Post-mammoplasty human adjuvant disease. Br J Rheumatol 23:227–229, 1984.
7. Caldwell EH, Stewart S: Skin necrosis as a consequence of Coumadin therapy. Plast Reconstr Surg 72:231–233, 1983.
8. Clark WH, From L, Bernardino EH, et al: Histogenesis and biologic behavior of primary human malignant melanoma of the skin. Cancer Res 29:705–727, 1969.
9. Cohen S: Symposium on cell-mediated immunity. Hum Pathol 17(2):111–168, 1986.
10. Dabski K, Stoll HL: Paget's disease of the breast presenting as a cutaneous horn. J Surg Oncol 29:237–239, 1985.
11. Day CL, Sober AJ, Lew RA, et al: Malignant melanoma patients with positive nodes and relatively good prognosis. Cancer 47:955–962, 1981.
12. Dekio S, Kawasaki Y, Jidoi J: Herpes simplex on nipples inoculated from herpetic gingivostomatitis of a baby. Clin Exp Dermatol 11:664–666, 1986.
13. Epstein E, Bragg K, Linden G: Biopsy and prognosis of malignant melanoma. JAMA 208:1369–1371, 1969.
14. Ganor S, Dollberg L: Amyloidosis of the nipple presenting as pruritus. Cutis 31:318, 1983.
15. Glinick SE, Alper JC, Bogaars H, Brown JA: Becker's melanosis: Associated abnormalities. J Am Acad Dermatol 9:509–514, 1983.
16. Hamilton A, Young GI, Davis RI: Pilomatrixoma mimicking breast carcinoma. Br J Dermatol 116:585–586, 1987.
17. Harrison GO, Elliott RL: Scleroderma of the breast: Light and electron microscopy study. Am Surg 53:528–531, 1987.
18. Hernandez FJ: Leiomyosarcoma of male breast originating in the nipple. Am J Surg Pathol 2:299–304, 1978.
19. Ironside P, Pitt TTE, Rank BK: Malignant melanoma; some aspects of pathology and prognosis. Aust NZ J Surg 47:70–75, 1977.
20. Kahn S, Stern HD, Rhodes GA: Cutaneous and subcutaneous necrosis as a complication of coumadin-congener therapy. Plast Reconstr Surg 48:160, 1971.
21. Kao GF, Graham JH, Helwig EB: Paget's disease of the ectopic breast with an underlying intraductal carcinoma: report of a case. J Cutan Pathol 13:59–66, 1986.
22. Katz M, Weinrauch L: Primary osteoma cutis. Cutis 36:477, 1985.
23. Kuhlman DS, Hodge SJ, Owen LG: Hyperkeratosis of the nipple and areola. J Am Acad Dermatol 13:596–598, 1985.
24. Lee YN, Sparks FC, Morton DL: Primary melanoma of skin of the breast region. Ann Surg 185:17–22, 1977.
25. Lopansri S, Mihm MC Jr: Clinical and pathological correlation of malignant melanoma. J Cutan Pathol 6:180–194, 1979.
26. Mason J, Apisarnthanarax P: Migratory silicone granuloma. Arch Dermatol 117:366–367, 1981.
27. McGovern VJ: The classification of melanoma and its relationship with prognosis. Pathology 2:85–98, 1970.
28. Millns JL, Dicken CH: Hereditary acrolabial telangiectasia. Arch Dermatol 115:474–478, 1979.
29. Millns, JL, Randle HW, Dicken CH: Benign leukokeratosis of the areolae and abdomen. Arch Dermatol 116:353–354, 1980.
30. Mold DE, Jegasothy BV: Estrogen-induced hyperkeratosis of the nipple. Cutis 26:95–96, 1980.
31. Moore JA, Schosser RH: Becker's melanosis and hypoplasia of the breast and pectoralis major muscle. Pediatr Dermatol 3:34–37, 1985.
32. Okano Y, Nishakai M, Sato A: Scleroderma, primary biliary cirrhosis, and Sjögren's syndrome after cosmetic breast augmentation with silicone injection: a case report of possible human adjuvant disease. Ann Rheum Dis 43:520–522, 1984.
33. Papachristou DN, Kinne DW, Ashikari R, Fortner JG: Melanoma of the nipple and areola. Br J Surg 66:287–288, 1979.
34. Papachristou DN, Kinne DW, Rosen PP, Ashikari R, Fortner JG: Cutaneous melanoma of the breast. Surgery 85(3):322–328, 1979.
35. Pressman PI: Malignant melanoma and the breast. Cancer 31:784–788, 1973.
36. Price ML, Forman L: Hidroacanthoma simplex. J R Soc Med 77(Suppl):35–36, 1984.
37. Rae V, Gould E, Ibe MJ, Penneys NS: Coexistent pemphigus vulgaris and Paget's disease of the nipple. J Am Acad Dermatol 16:235–237, 1987.
38. Rampen FHJ, Van Houten WA, Hop WCJ: Incisional procedures and prognosis in malignant melanoma. Clin Exp Dermatol 5:313–320, 1980.
39. Rand RP, Brown GL, Bostwick J: Pyoderma gangrenosum and progressive cutaneous ulceration. Ann Plast Surg 20:280–284, 1988.
40. Rosenberg MW, Hughes LE: Artefactual breast disease: a report of three cases. Br J Surg 72:539–541, 1985.
41. Roses DF, Harris MN, Stern JS, Gumport SL: Cutaneous melanoma of the breast. Ann Surg 189:112–115, 1979.
42. Shertz WT, Balogh K: Metastasizing basal cell carcinoma of the nipple. Arch Pathol Lab Med 110:761–762, 1986.
43. Sitakalin C, Ackerman AB: Mammary and extramammary Paget's disease. Am J Dermatopathol 7:335–340, 1985.
44. Soden CE: Hyperkeratosis of the nipple and areola. Cutis 32:69–71, 74, 1983.
45. Tschen JA, Ramsdell WM: Disciform erythrasma. Cutis 31:541–542, 547, 1983.
46. Tsujioka K, Kashihara M, Imamura S: Cutaneous leiomyoma of the male nipple. Dermatologica 170:98–100, 1985.
47. Van Dijk D: Contact dermatitis due to Spandex. Acta Derm Venereol 48:589–591, 1968.
48. Vestey JP, Bunney MH: Unilateral hyperkeratosis of the nipple: The response to cryotherapy. Arch Dermatol 122:1360–1361, 1986.
49. Wood C: Condyloma acuminatum of the nipple. J Cutan Pathol 5:88–89, 1978.
50. Zubowicz V, Bostwick J: Congenital unilateral hypoplasia of the female breast associated with a large melanotic spot: Report of two cases. Ann Plast Surg 12:204–206, 1984.

Section V

Epidemiology and Natural History of Breast Cancer

Chapter 12

EPIDEMIOLOGY AND PRIMARY PREVENTION OF BREAST CANCER

Epidemiology of Breast Cancer

David Mant, M.B. and Martin P. Vessey, M.D.

Breast cancer is becoming an increasingly important disease in all parts of the world. It is estimated that more than 500,000 new cases were diagnosed in 1975, and by the year 2000 the world total may well exceed 1,000,000 new cases each year. The highest rates are seen in the industrialized nations of Europe and North America, but the rate of increase in the incidence of breast cancer is much slower in industrial nations than in the economically developing nations of Asia and South America. The challenge to the epidemiologist is to identify the causes of this global epidemic, which appear to be closely linked to industrial development.

Epidemiologists have responded to this challenge by producing a vast and daunting scientific literature. However, a recent authoritative review, particularly of the role of endogenous hormones, has been written by Henderson et al.[23] In addition, the consensus of a recent International Union Against Cancer (U.I.C.C.) meeting on the "epidemiology, aetiology and prevention" of breast cancer was reported in 1986 by Miller and Bulbrook[40] and provides a useful summary of current issues. Finally, a rapid introduction to the literature can be gained from the annotated bibliography published by the National Cancer Institute.[41] The purpose of this chapter is to present the results of epidemiological research in an accessible format, to indicate areas of current debate, and to demonstrate the contribution of epidemiology to the prevention of breast cancer.

DEMOGRAPHY OF BREAST CANCER

Age and Sex

In every country of the world, breast cancer is rare in men and in young people. The female:male ratio is approximately 100 to 1 in almost all areas except those with a very low incidence of breast cancer, such as East Africa, where Clifford and Bulbrook have demonstrated high levels of urinary estrogen secretion in men.[8] It has been suggested that this may be related to the prevalence of bilharzia, a disease associated with hepatic cirrhosis and male gynecomastia.[31]

Again, in all countries, the age-specific incidence rates for breast cancer increase sharply up to the age of the menopause. Thereafter, the rates depend on the underlying incidence of breast cancer in the country concerned. In high risk countries such as the UK and the USA, incidence rates continue to increase but at a slower rate; in countries with intermediate breast cancer rates, such as those in central Europe, the incidence tends to level off; and in low risk countries, such as Japan, the incidence declines. Annual age-specific breast cancer incidence rates for the United States and the United Kingdom are shown in Figure 12–1. The overall reported incidence of breast cancer is higher in the United States. The rates shown for the United States are for all races; racial differences in age-specific incidence are discussed in the next section.

International Differences

There is at least a fivefold variation in the incidence of breast cancer reported among different countries, although this difference appears to be narrowing. Table 12–1 gives the approximate lifetime risk of breast cancer for women living in different parts of the world. As previously mentioned, women living in less industrialized nations tend to have lower rates than those living in industrialized countries, although Japan is an obvious exception to this rule. Table 12–1 also demonstrates that there can be considerable differences in rates within countries (although variations in the efficiency of registration may contribute to these differences). For example, the incidence of breast cancer in British Columbia is approximately twice that in Newfoundland, and the incidence in Los Angeles is nearly 50 percent more than the incidence in New York State. Age-standardized female breast cancer mortality ratios are presented in Figure 12–2. These ratios show that although breast cancer mortality in the United States and Canada is four times greater than in Japan, an even higher ratio is seen in the United Kingdom. This is paradoxical in view of the lower registration rate in the UK than in the United States or Canada (Fig. 12–1), and it is unclear whether this reflects the effect of better treatment or more accurate cancer registration (or perhaps other less obvious factors) in North America.

Buell reported in 1977 that established Polish and

	Age-Standardized Rate (per 100,000)	Cumulative Rate* (%)
Table 12–1. INTERNATIONAL VARIATION IN THE ANNUAL INCIDENCE OF CANCER OF THE FEMALE BREAST		
JAPAN (Osaka)	12.1	1.3
NIGERIA (Ibidan)	15.3	1.7
INDIA (Bombay)	20.1	2.2
CUBA	28.0	3.1
FINLAND	32.9	3.7
NORWAY	44.4	4.9
SWEDEN	52.4	5.8
NEW ZEALAND	52.5	5.8
UK (Oxford)	54.5	5.9
USA (NY)	57.2	6.2
USA (LA whites)	79.9	8.9
CANADA (Alberta)	57.4	6.2
CANADA (British Columbia)	80.3	8.8
SWITZERLAND (Geneva)	70.6	7.5

*Approximates cumulative lifetime risk.

From Waterhouse J, et al: Cancer Incidence in Five Continents. Scientific Publication No 15, Lyon, IARC, 1976. Reprinted by permission.

Japanese migrants to the United States were exhibiting the breast cancer incidence rates associated with their adopted country rather than their country of origin.[5] Figure 12–3 gives the age-specific incidence rates for Japanese women in Okayama, Hawaii, and San Francisco, and for white women in San Francisco. In those younger than 50 years, the incidence of breast cancer in Japanese women in Okayama is about one fifth that of white women in San Francisco, whereas Japanese-American women have rates approaching those in whites. In those older than 50 years, the rates in Okayama are about one tenth the rates in Los Angeles whites, while the rates in Japanese Americans are intermediate. Buell also noted that Japanese immigrants to the United States took longer to exhibit a high breast cancer risk than Polish immigrants who had arrived at the same time, and he suggested that this reflected the rate of cultural assimilation of the two nationalities.

Race

The preceding discussion of breast cancer in immigrants leads to the question of variation in rates between different racial groups within each country. For example, in 1968–72 the age-standardized incidence rates for female breast cancer (per 100,000) in the different racial groups in Hawaii were as follows: White, 80.3; Hawai-

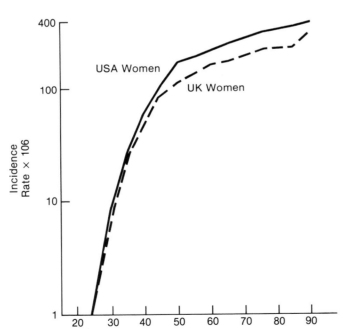

Figure 12–1. Annual age-specific incidence of cancer of the female breast in the UK (1983) and USA (1973–1977). (Data taken from SEER Incidence & Mortality Data. NCI Monograph No 57, 1981, and Cancer Statistics: incidence survival and mortality in England and Wales. Series SMPS No 43. OPCS/CRC. HMSO, 1981.)

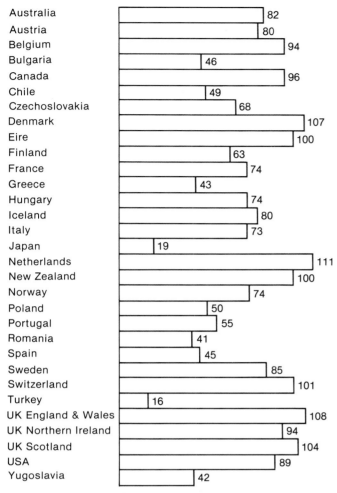

Australia	82
Austria	80
Belgium	94
Bulgaria	46
Canada	96
Chile	49
Czechoslovakia	68
Denmark	107
Eire	100
Finland	63
France	74
Greece	43
Hungary	74
Iceland	80
Italy	73
Japan	19
Netherlands	111
New Zealand	100
Norway	74
Poland	50
Portugal	55
Romania	41
Spain	45
Sweden	85
Switzerland	101
Turkey	16
UK England & Wales	108
UK Northern Ireland	94
UK Scotland	104
USA	89
Yugoslavia	42

Figure 12–2. Mortality from breast cancer in women: Age-standardized mortality ratios (base = 100) for various countries (1971–1975). (From Alderson M: International Mortality Statistics. London, MacMillan, 1981. Reprinted by permission.)

ian, 66.2; Chinese, 54.2; Japanese, 44.2; and Filipino, 21.5.[53]

In the United States as a whole, the major racial comparison is between black and white women. Table 12–2, taken from a paper by Gray et al.,[19] reports the ratio of female breast cancer incidence rates in blacks and whites and demonstrates that although white women have a higher overall rate of breast cancer than black women, this is not apparent until the age of 40, and the difference is marked only after the age of menopause. The authors argue that much of this difference can be attributed to known risk factors (early menarche, late menopause, and late age at first full-term pregnancy) that are discussed later.

Social Status

There have been at least 12 studies relating breast cancer to social status; these are summarized in a recent publication by the International Agency for Research on Cancer (I.A.R.C.).[36] Table 12–3 abstracted from this

source, shows that mortality from breast cancer is greatest in the higher socioeconomic groups (whether based on income, education, or occupation) and smallest in the lower socioeconomic groups. Four studies are also reported that looked at incidence rather than mortality rates, and once again, the same positive relationship between high incidence and high social status was documented.

Secular Trends

In the United States and the United Kingdom there has been little change in the incidence of or mortality from breast cancer during the past three decades. The annual age-adjusted incidence rates per 100,000 women in the United States, as determined by the national cancer surveys of 1947–48 and 1969–71, were 73.6 and 73.3 (white), and 50.4 and 53.7 (non-white), respectively. The change in breast cancer mortality in the UK between 1951 and 1981 is shown in Figure 12–4. It can be seen that there has been a small upward trend in all age groups.

As previously mentioned, the small increase in breast cancer mortality seen in all high incidence countries contrasts markedly with the rapidly increasing rate in many Asian, central European, and some South American countries. Moreover, in some countries of low

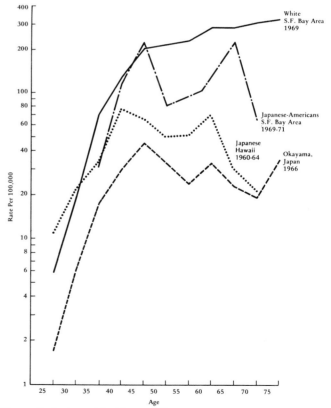

Figure 12–3. Annual incidence of breast cancer per 100,000 women, by area of residence and ethnic origin. (From Buell P: Changing incidence of breast cancer in Japanese-American women. J Natl Cancer Inst 51:1480, 1973. Reprinted by permission.)

Table 12-2. RATIO OF BREAST CANCER INCIDENCE RATES OF BLACK FEMALES TO THOSE OF WHITE FEMALES IN THE UNITED STATES

Rates from	Ratio at the Following Ages (yr)										
	20-24	*25-29*	*30-34*	*35-39*	*40-44*	*45-49*	*50-54*	*55-59*	*60-64*	*65-69*	*70-74*
Third National Cancer Survey (1969-1971)	2.27	1.23	1.30	1.06	0.90	0.76	0.78	0.76	0.72	0.66	0.64
Los Angeles County Cancer Surveillance Program (1972-1976)	3.75	0.95	1.12	1.19	0.79	0.71	0.68	0.69	0.66	0.65	0.67

From Gray GE, Henderson BE, Pike MC: J Natl Cancer Inst 64(3):462, 1980. Reprinted by permission.

incidence, such as Japan and Singapore, the rise in incidence has been predominantly in women younger than 50 years. As increases in risk appear to persist throughout life, the U.I.C.C. study group on breast cancer has predicted a major increase in breast cancer incidence in these countries in 20 to 30 years' time.[40] Although a proportion of the increase in reported breast cancer must be a result of improvements in the efficiency of cancer registration and the introduction of screening programs, the U.I.C.C. group felt that these factors could not explain the major increases seen in countries with previously low rates.

RISK FACTORS

Family and Medical History

There is no doubt that if a woman has a family history of breast cancer she is herself at increased risk. Ottman et al. have published a practical guide for estimating this risk, in the form of a set of probability tables.[42] Relatives of patients with bilateral premenopausal breast cancer are shown to be at highest risk; for example, a 30-year-old sister of such a patient has a 51 percent chance of developing breast cancer before age 70. However, the risk among relatives of women with unilateral breast cancer is less: most case-control studies indicate a relative risk of two- to threefold in first degree relatives, corresponding to a lifetime risk of about 20 percent. There is conflicting evidence on whether the risk to relatives is higher if a woman develops unilateral breast cancer before menopause; although reported in some studies, this was not shown in Ottman's data. Finally, Anderson has suggested that susceptibility to breast cancer occurs through both the paternal and the maternal lines and that risk is proportional to the number of relatives affected.[1]

The risk of developing a second primary breast cancer after suffering a first is reported to be up to five times the general risk and is inversely related to age at presentation of the first primary cancer.[7] About 0.5

Table 12-3. BREAST CANCER MORTALITY ACCORDING TO INDICES OF SOCIAL STATUS

Country	Year(s)	Units	Population at Risk	Social Status Indices		
				Average Income		
				$400 and Over	*$200-$399*	*Less Than $200*
Hong Kong	1971	Death rate per 100,000	Women, 35-64	46.6	28.8	15.4

				Education Level			
				College	*High School*	*Elementary School*	*Less Than 8 Years' Education*
USA	1960	SMR	White women 25-64	111	103	98	87

				Social Class				
				I	*II*	*III*	*IV*	*V*
Scotland	1959-1963	SMR	Married women, 20-64;	115	111	101	89	102
			single women, 20-64	135	81	123	114	98

From Logan WPD: IARC Scientific Publication No 36, OPCS Studies on Medical and Population Subjects No 44, 1982. Reprinted by permission.

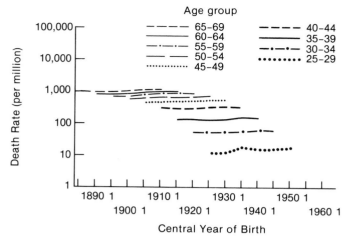

Figure 12–4. Breast cancer mortality in England and Wales: trend in age-specific rates between 1951 and 1981. (From Osmond C, Gardner MJ, Acheson ED, Adelstein AM: Trends in cancer mortality 1951–1980. OPCS/MRC Environmental Epidemiology Unit 1983 [Series DHI No 11]. Reprinted by permission.)

percent of women with a previous history of unilateral breast cancer will be expected to develop a second primary breast cancer each year for at least the next 15 years.[26] Primary ovarian or endometrial cancer is also associated with an increased risk of breast cancer, but this risk is probably less than two times that of the general population.

Benign breast disease consists of a number of quite different pathological and epidemiological entities. The most common type of benign breast disease is fibrocystic disease, commonly diagnosed in middle-aged women. In general terms, this condition seems to be associated with about a twofold increase in the risk of breast cancer, although Dupont and Page have provided data indicating that the excess risk is particularly related to lesions with epithelial hyperplasia and histological evidence of calcification.[11] Fibroadenoma is the second most common type of benign breast lesion and is diagnosed most frequently in young women. Here any associated increase in breast cancer risk is less well established. In addition there is a general problem with "detection bias" in determining the relative risk of breast cancer associated with benign breast disease; this is demonstrated and discussed in a recent paper by Silber and Horwitz.[47]

The mammographic patterns described by Wolfe may also be interpreted as describing a type of benign breast disease associated with an increased risk of cancer.[59] Although the very high relative risks described by Wolfe himself have not been widely replicated, there is some support for an increased risk of two- to threefold in women whose mammograms show dysplasia (DY pattern) or a greater than normal amount of prominent ducts (P2 pattern).[6]

A summary of the risks associated with the family and past medical history are shown in Table 12–4.

Menstrual and Reproductive Factors

Most studies have found that an early onset of menarche is associated with a modest increase in breast cancer risk (twofold or less). This effect decreases with age and is small after menopause. In a recent study by Henderson et al., it was found that breast cancer cases established regular menstrual cycles more rapidly than controls, and that the combination of early menarche (age 12 years) and early establishment of regular cycles (within 1 year of menarche) was associated with a more than threefold increase in risk.[22]

The rate of increase in the incidence of breast cancer slows sharply at the time of menopause, and for the individual woman, menopause before the age of 45 leads to a twofold reduction in risk compared with menopause occurring after age 55.[49] Artificial menopause induced by medical treatment has a protective effect similar to that of natural menopause.

Our understanding of the role of reproductive factors in determining the risk of breast cancer relies heavily on the collaborative case-control study in seven countries with markedly different breast cancer rates carried out in 1970 by MacMahon et al.,[37] which drew attention to the important protective effect of early first term birth. This study also demonstrated that the protective effect of bearing a large number of children was explained by the high negative correlation between age at first term birth and total parity, and that the protection conferred by early first term birth persisted in women at all subsequent ages, even in those older than 75 years. More recently, it has been shown that there is some additional protective effect of high parity,[35] which may be important in developing countries where high parity is common, but in general MacMahon et al.'s findings have stood the test of time.

There is still some discussion about the effect of incomplete pregnancies before the first full-term pregnancy. Two recent studies have suggested that first trimester abortion before first full-term pregnancy is associated with a substantial increased risk of breast cancer.[21, 43] However, this finding has not been replicated in other studies.[3, 52] Abortions after the first full-term pregnancy do not carry any increased risk.

There is also continuing debate about the independent effect of lactation on risk. Early studies, such as that by MacMahon et al., had suggested that there was no protective effect of lactation. However, a relative risk of premenopausal breast cancer of 0.49 for women who had breast-fed a child was recently reported from the Cancer and Steroid Hormone (CASH) study.[39] Byers et al.,[4] who have also reported a protective effect of lactation, have hypothesized that this effect may be the result of an association between high breast cancer risk and failure of lactation.

Table 12–5 summarizes the risk factors associated with menstrual and reproductive history.

Ionizing Radiation

There is direct evidence of the carcinogenic effect of radiation on the breast from follow-up data on survivors of the atomic bomb explosions in Japan and from women exposed medically to high doses of ionizing radiation for the treatment of mastitis and tuberculosis.[28] The

Table 12–4. RISK FACTORS FOR BREAST CANCER ASSOCIATED WITH FAMILY OR MEDICAL HISTORY

Factor	High Risk	Low Risk	Magnitude of Relative Risk <2	2–4	>4
Family history of breast cancer in first degree relative	Positive	Negative		X	
Family history of premenopausal bilateral breast cancer	Positive	Negative			X
Previous breast cancer	Positive	Negative			X
Fibrocystic disease of breast	Positive	Negative		X	
Previous ovarian cancer	Positive	Negative	X		
Previous endometrial cancer	Positive	Negative	X		

Adapted from Kalache A, Vessey M: Clin Oncol, 1(3):661–678, WB Saunders, 1982.

extent of the risk is directly proportional to the dosage of radiation and inversely proportional to the age of the woman at time of exposure. This relationship between radiation and breast cancer risk has raised anxieties about the widespread use of mammography for breast cancer screening. However, extrapolating the dose-response relationship observed in the high dose studies mentioned, the probability of a middle-aged woman developing breast cancer as a result of a single mammographic screening examination is estimated as 1 in 2,000,000. This level of risk is too small to detect by standard epidemiological methods and is far outweighed by the potential benefits of screening.[16]

Weight and Diet

Most case-control studies, and at least one prospective study, indicate that breast cancer risk is directly proportional to relative weight, with obese women experiencing an increased risk of 1.5- to twofold. However, this increased risk is restricted to postmenopausal women. In fact, some studies have shown a protective effect of high relative weight in premenopausal women, but Willett et al. have argued that this may be, at least in part, the result of easier diagnosis of tumors in lean women.[55] The size of the increase in risk in postmenopausal women is not sufficient to allow clear delineation between the effects of weight and body mass; however, it is interesting to note that the rapid increase in breast

cancer mortality in Japan has been paralleled by an increase in both height and weight in Japanese women.

Population correlation studies, both cross-sectional and of time trends, suggest that animal fat or meat consumption may be of primary importance in determining breast cancer risk.[45] However, individual case-control studies have produced, at best, weak confirmatory evidence, and a prospective study of 89,000 nurses has failed to show a relationship between fat intake and subsequent breast cancer during the first 4 years of follow-up.[56] This could be caused by the small size of the studies, by a lack of precision of dietary methodology, or by the fact that only recent or current diet has been measured. Studies on migrants and on special religious groups including nuns and Seventh Day Adventists have also produced equivocal results. A useful review of the experimental as well as the epidemiological evidence linking dietary fat and breast cancer has been written by Wynder et al.[60]

A summary of the relative risk associated with ionizing radiation and body build appears in Table 12–6.

Hormone Use for Contraception and Medical Treatment

Combined oral contraceptives have no effect at all on breast cancer risk when used by women in the middle of reproductive life (i.e., between the ages of 25 and 39 years), even if they are taken for many years.[30] However,

Table 12–5. RISK FACTORS FOR BREAST CANCER ASSOCIATED WITH MENSTRUAL OR REPRODUCTIVE HISTORY

Factor	High Risk	Low Risk	Magnitude of Relative Risk <2	2–4	>4
Age at menarche	Early	Late	X		
Age at natural menopause	Late	Early	X		
Oophorectomy	Not done or done late	Done early		X	
Parity	Nulliparous	Parous	X		
Parous women: age at first full-term pregnancy	Old	Young		X	
Parous women: number of children	Small	Large	X		

Adapted from Kalache A, Vessey M: Clin Oncol 1(3):661–678, WB Saunders, 1982.

Table 12–6. OTHER RISK FACTORS FOR BREAST CANCER

Factor	High Risk	Low Risk	Magnitude of Relative Risk		
			>2	2–4	<4
Ionizing radiation	Irradiated	Not irradiated		X	
Body build	Fat	Thin	X		

Adapted from Kalache A, Vessey M: Clin Oncol 1(3):661–678, WB Saunders, 1982.

it is still possible that there is an adverse effect of combined oral contraceptives on breast cancer risk when they are taken for long periods at a very early age[35] or before the first full-term pregnancy.[38] Among the problems hindering the resolution of this controversy are (1) the relatively recent adoption of oral contraceptives on a widespread basis by very young women, (2) the possibility of a long latent interval between oral contraceptive use and the onset of cancer, and (3) the changing estrogen and progestogen content of oral contraceptive preparations over the past 20 years.

Limited data are available on the effects of injectable contraceptives. The World Health Organization (WHO) study suggests that the risk of breast cancer from the use of depot medroxy-progesterone acetate (DMPA) is neither increased nor decreased.[10]

The epidemiological literature on the prolonged use of estrogens by peri- and postmenopausal women (on hormone replacement therapy) suggests that such use may very slightly increase the risk of breast cancer.[50] This risk may be accentuated in women with preexisting benign breast disease. Having said this, the possibility remains that at least some of the excess risk is attributable to more complete diagnosis of breast cancer in women using estrogens than in other women. This point of view is supported by the favorable stage distribution of breast cancers in estrogen users reported by Brinton et al.[2] and Hunt et al.[29] Unfortunately, almost nothing is known about the effects of products containing both an estrogen and a progestogen, and in view of the probable latent period of 10 to 20 years, it may be some time before conclusive data become available about the forms of hormone replacement therapy now most commonly administered in the UK and United States.

Alcohol

The relationship between alcohol consumption and breast cancer is still a matter for debate. Strongest

Table 12–7. POSSIBLE RISK FACTORS FOR BREAST CANCER

High alcohol consumption
High fat diet
High meat consumption
Oral contraceptive use before first pregnancy
Injectable contraceptive use (DMPA)
Hormone replacement therapy
Mammographic pattern
Lactation

support for an adverse effect comes from case-control studies based on hospital populations, and it has been suggested that this reflects relative abstinence by the controls rather than excess drinking by breast cancer cases.[12] Community-based case-control studies have not, in general, reported an excess risk. However, three recent cohort studies, in which alcohol consumption was recorded at the outset and the women were subsequently followed up to see who would develop breast cancer, have reported an increased overall risk of approximately 60 percent, with the exact risk being proportional to the amount of alcohol consumed. The earliest cohort study, by Hiatt and Bawol,[24] has been criticized for the lack of adequate information about other factors that influence breast cancer risk and, along with the later study by Willett et al.,[57] for following an unrepresentative group of women of relatively high social status. The third study, by Schatzkin et al.,[46] followed a representative sample, but the number of cases was small. In view of the conflict between the results of these studies and the essentially negative results of large and well-conducted case-control studies such as the CASH study,[54] it is difficult to reach a firm conclusion. Indeed, some authorities have questioned whether the suggestion of increased risk with the low levels of alcohol consumption reported from the cohort studies is biologically plausible. However, at least one commentator has argued that women at high risk of breast cancer by virtue of other factors should be advised to curtail alcohol consumption, pending further scientific inquiry.[18]

A summary of possible risk factors, including alcohol and exogenous hormones, is given in Table 12–7.

NON-RISK FACTORS

A large number of factors have been considered as possible indicators of increased breast cancer risk but should perhaps now be considered as "non-risk factors" (Table 12–8). These include exposure to diazepam, reserpine, and hair dyes, and the occurrence of chole-

Table 12–8. NON-RISK FACTORS FOR BREAST CANCER

Diazepam
Reserpine
Cholecystectomy
Thyroid disease
Hair dyes
Psychological stress

cystectomy and thyroid disease. The inclusion of psychological stress in this category is more contentious, not least because of the methodological difficulties involved in studying it, but six reasonably well-conducted case-control studies since 1966 have failed to show a clear detrimental effect.[13]

Finally, it is necessary to mention cigarette smoking. This is a non-risk factor, but it should not be considered as a protective factor. Although smoking is related to earlier menopause, the balance of evidence does not suggest that smoking prevents breast cancer.[25]

CAUSAL EXPLANATIONS

Initiators and Promoters

It is almost certainly wrong to think of breast cancer as having a single cause. The development of the disease is a multi-stage process that is probably influenced by different factors at each stage of development. In the simplest analysis, a clear distinction should be made between the *initiation* and *promotion* of cancer. However, this does not exclude the possibility that the same substance could act as an initiator at one stage and a promoter at a later stage; this is probably true of ionizing radiation.

It is also known that the risk associated with exposure to certain factors is dependent on the age of the woman and the stage of development of the breast at the time of exposure. The effect of radiation in increasing the risk of breast cancer is maximal in adolescence and in early adult life and appears to fall with increasing age. Recent work shows that women irradiated in childhood have as great a susceptibility to the effects of radiation as those irradiated in adolescence or early adult life, but little or no risk has been found in women after the age of 40.[48]

The "estrogen window" hypothesis is also based on a model that assumes differential susceptibility at different ages. This hypothesis was suggested by Korenman in 1980, who proposed that estrogenic stimulation in the absence of progesterone is the most favorable state for breast cancer induction.[33] Hence, he suggested that the periods around menarche and menopause, when irregular anovulatory cycles are common, are the prime determinants of risk. However, Henderson et al. have demonstrated that breast cancer cases establish regular cycles more rapidly than controls,[22] and Coulam et al. reported no excess breast cancer risk in 1270 patients with "chronic anovulation syndrome."[9] A recent update on this debate can be found in a paper by La Vecchia et al.; these authors also report that frequent ovular cycles impart greater risk than anovular cycles.[34]

A number of other authors have also attempted to draw together the known etiological facts and produce an overall model for the development of breast cancer. An example of this is the hormonal model devised by Henderson et al., which is summarized in Figure 12–5. The implication of this particular model is that the prevention of breast cancer depends primarily on the modification of secretion and metabolism of estrogens and prolactin. A further discussion of the hormonal mechanisms implicated in the development of breast cancer can be found in the review paper by Henderson et al.[23]

Nature and Nurture

The risk of breast cancer in first degree relatives of breast cancer patients and the difference in breast cancer rates between different racial groups living within the same country do suggest some genetic influence in the development of breast cancer. However, it can also be argued that a proportion of the familial risk is related to shared environmental influences, and the tendency of immigrants to exhibit the incidence rates of their adoptive countries supports this view.

Hoel et al.[27] set out to examine the extent to which known behavioral and environmental risk factors could account for the difference in breast cancer rates between Japanese and American women. They demonstrated profound differences in reproductive factors, particularly age at menarche, which could account for between one third and one half of the difference in premenopausal breast cancer rates. However, Pike et al.[44] have argued that the difference in postmenopausal breast cancer rates could be completely accounted for by the much greater postmenopausal weight of American women. They have developed a theoretical model relating hormonal risk factors, breast tissue age, and weight, that appears to explain about 85 percent of the difference in rates between Japanese and American women. They also suggest that the missing factors could be low intake of dietary fat during childhood and delay in the onset of regular cycles in Japanese women, but little evidence is available to assess these suggestions, and studies of hormone secretion in relation to young people who have diets with very different fat intake have not been very revealing.[20]

In a small number of families, it has been shown that the observed distribution of breast cancer is compatible with the transmission of an autosomal dominant gene with incomplete penetrance.[58] Recent developments in DNA technology may well allow further advances to be made in our understanding of the genetics of breast cancer within the next ten years. At the present time there is no doubt that the balance of evidence strongly suggests that environmental factors are more important than genetic susceptibility in determining breast cancer risk.

Endocrine Status

In view of the importance of menstrual and reproductive history in the determination of the risk of breast cancer, an understanding of the role of estrogens and progesterone is essential. The most important endogenous estrogen is estradiol (E2), but in postmenopausal women estrone (E1) may also have a significant effect.

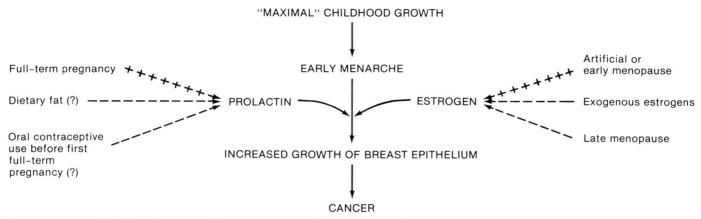

Figure 12–5. A model of the pathogenesis of breast cancer (+ indicates protective effect). (From Henderson BE, Pike MC, Ross RK, Bonadonna G (eds): Epidemiology and Risk Factors in Breast Cancer: Diagnosis and Management. New York, John Wiley, 1984. Reprinted by permission.)

A large number of studies have examined the relationship between breast cancer and both plasma and urinary estrogens. Recent studies have concentrated on the plasma concentration of non–protein-bound (or "free") E2. This work follows the suggestion that the risk of breast cancer may be positively related to the amount of plasma estrogen that is unbound (free E2), or only loosely bound (albumin-bound E2), to plasma proteins. Most estrogen in the plasma is bound to sex hormone–binding globulin (SHBG). Apart from the difficulty of measuring free E2, an additional problem in characterizing the biological effect of both estrogen and progesterone is the marked variation in levels according to time of day and the stage of the menstrual cycle.

Key and Pike[32] have provided a very useful review of case-control studies carried out between 1964 and 1987 that measured hormone status in breast cancer cases and controls. In postmenopausal breast cancer, there seems little doubt that women with breast cancer have higher endogenous estrogen levels than do controls. All eight studies reviewed, which measured either total free E2 or percentage free E2, found a higher level in cases than in controls. Of two additional studies that examined blood taken before breast cancer was diagnosed (and therefore in which elevated estrogen levels could not be said to have been caused by breast cancer), one study did not report E2 concentrations and the other (Wysowski et al.[61]) found no difference in total E2 between cases and controls.

In premenopausal women results have been far less consistent, although four out of five studies measuring percentage free E2 have reported a higher plasma concentration in cases. However, only one of these studies was prospective. This study has shown a decrease in the magnitude of the case-control difference over time, perhaps indicating improvements in study design and, in particular, in matching of cases and controls on storage time.

Key and Pike have also reviewed a number of studies of plasma progesterone (or urinary pregnanediol) in premenopausal women.[32] They report that all studies reviewed are consistent with a decreased progesterone exposure in breast cancer cases, although there have been only three prospective studies, and these were all extremely small (accumulating only 30 cases among them). Nevertheless, the finding of a possible protective effect of progesterone is perhaps surprising in view of reports that cell multiplication in the breast is most frequent in the luteal phase of the cycle, and that progesterone enhances the effect of prolactin, which is known to promote the growth of breast cancer in rodents. Conversely, the findings are consistent with the estrogen window hypothesis.

Finally, very little is known of the relationship between testosterone and breast cancer, but case-control studies that have measured testosterone have invariably reported higher levels in cases. The biological significance of this observation is unclear, and this area may merit further study.

IMPLICATIONS FOR PREVENTION

To what extent do the epidemiological findings we have discussed help us prevent breast cancer? It is very unlikely that many women will decide to have a large number of children or to bear their first child shortly after menarche in order to avoid the risk of breast cancer. Similarly, early bilateral oophorectomy or mastectomy in women with a strong family history are equally unacceptable from a social perspective. However, epidemiological research has identified three areas where there is some scope for prevention.

Primary Prevention

The scope for primary prevention, in the absence of major social change, is limited: unnecessary radiation of the thorax or breast can be prevented, breast-feeding can be encouraged, and a reduction in the fat content of the diet can be recommended. Of these three actions, only the last holds much hope of a significant reduction in the incidence of breast cancer, and this is by no means certain. This recommendation is a lot easier to make because of the increasingly clear evidence that the

Table 12–9. KEY ISSUES IN ASSESSING VALUE OF SELECTIVE SCREENING

Table 12–9. KEY ISSUES IN ASSESSING VALUE OF SELECTIVE SCREENING

Is the risk factor strongly predictive?
Is the risk factor easily and reliably identifiable?
Is the risk factor commonly found?
How is the risk factor related to other risk factors?

very high intake of fat, particularly saturated fat, in Western nations is largely responsible for the epidemic of coronary heart disease.

It is by no means clear whether the use of oral contraceptives before first term pregnancy is associated with an increased risk, and therefore it is not possible to state at the present time whether the avoidance of oral contraception at this stage of life would have any influence at all on breast cancer mortality. Clearly there are considerable social implications from such a recommendation. There is better evidence that the use of estrogen alone as a hormone replacement therapy at the time of menopause can slightly increase risk, but current practice is to use preparations containing both estrogen and progestogen, and as with oral contraceptive use at an early age, we do not know whether this is harmful. As hormone replacement therapy has major benefits both in terms of symptomatic relief and prevention of bone disease, it would also be wrong to recommend its avoidance as a means of preventing breast cancer. Finally, it is interesting to note that Key and Pike have suggested that it should be possible to synthesize a contraceptive pill that actually reduces breast cancer risk.[32] This leads to the discussion of prophylactic therapy.

Prophylactic Therapy

It has been suggested that the anti-estrogen tamoxifen could be used as a prophylactic agent in women at high risk of breast cancer, such as those with a history of bilateral premenopausal cancer. Although tamoxifen is relatively free from side effects when used for the treatment of breast cancer, it clearly has side-effects that are inseparable from its anti-estrogenic activity and that might be unacceptable in healthy premenopausal women. Nevertheless, it has been suggested that a reduction in risk approximating 30 percent might be achieved, and a trial has been suggested for women at

high risk. However, even if such a trial was successful, there would clearly be difficulties in implementing such preventive activity at a population level, in part because of problems in identifying the high risk patients who should be treated. Moreover, if the definition of high risk was limited to women with a first degree relative with premenopausal breast cancer, the overall reduction in breast cancer incidence and mortality that could be achieved in the population as a whole would be considerably less than one percent, because so few women with breast cancer exhibit this risk factor. A useful discussion of the issues involved can be found in Gazet.[17]

Screening

An important epidemiological contribution to the introduction of population screening in order to detect breast cancer at an early and curable stage lies in the definition of high risk groups. Age and sex are obviously the primary risk factors that must be used, and the major trials of breast cancer screening have indeed concentrated on older women. However, the efficiency of screening could potentially be improved further by the employment of other risk factors as indicators of potential yield. Kalache and Vessey proposed four key issues that should be considered when assessing the possible value of risk factors in selective screening; these are displayed in Table 12–9.[31] If these four issues are applied to the risk factors discussed earlier, only two (apart from age, sex, and country of residence) are associated with a relative risk greater than four. These are (1) a very high risk family history and (2) a previous history of breast cancer in the woman herself. Most clinicians already follow up the latter group with great care, and again, they are a group that may well be considered for long-term prophylactic therapy in the future.

Factors that are weakly predictive of breast cancer (i.e., associated with a relative risk of less than two) are of little use for selective screening because they discriminate poorly between cases and healthy women. This leaves those factors associated with a relative risk of two to four. If irradiation of the breast is excluded as too rare to be of much interest, then this leaves three factors (family history, fibrocystic disease, and age at a first-term birth) to be considered. The potential value of these factors can be assessed by reference to the results of a case-control study conducted by Vessey et al.,[51] the

Table 12–10. RISK OF BREAST CANCER IN RELATION TO RISK FACTORS OTHER THAN AGE THAT MIGHT BE USED FOR SELECTIVE SCREENING

Risk Factor	Cases		Controls		Relative Risk*
	No.	%	No.	%	
Breast cancer in mother and sister	63	10.1	31	5.0	2.1
History of breast biopsy	50	8.1	25	4.0	2.1
Age at first term birth 26 years +	239	44.9	139	26.1	2.3

*Relative to women without risk factor.

Table 12–11. MULTIVARIATE ANALYSIS OF RISK FACTORS IN THE GUERNSEY COHORT STUDY

No. of Positive Risk Factors	Normal Women		Women Developing Cancer	
	No.	*%*	*No.*	*%*
≥0	1400	100	45	100
≥1	1260	90	45	100
≥2	770	55	37	82
≥3	238	17	21	47
≥4	28	2	3	7

Risk factors: Low aetiocholanolone excretion; age at menarche before 14th birthday; age at first term birth after 25th birthday, or no children; positive family history. From Farewell VT: Cancer 40:931–936, 1977. Reprinted by permission.

relevant data from which are presented in Table 12–10. This shows that by screening five percent of women with a history of breast cancer in a first degree relative, ten percent of cancers might be identified; by screening the four percent of women with a history of a breast biopsy, it will be possible to detect 8 percent of breast cancer cases; and by screening the 26 percent of women who had their first child at age 26 or more, it will be possible to detect 45 percent of the breast cancer cases. None of these factors is therefore of great individual value, and for this reason some investigators have considered using risk factors in combination. The results of a cohort study set up in Guernsey[14] are shown in Table 12–11. It is clear that they do not meet the selective screening criterion of Forrest and Roberts,[15] which states that a method of identification of those at risk should isolate 80 percent of the cancers in less than 30 percent of the population. It can be seen that the best discrimination achieved in Guernsey was 82 percent of the cancers in 55 percent of the population, and this was achieved only by including data on urinary excretion of steroids. It appears that we must conclude that selective screening on the basis of factors other than age or sex is unlikely to be productive.

Nevertheless, it is possible to end on an optimistic note. Breast cancer screening by mammography is effective in reducing mortality in women older than 50 years by about 30 percent, and it seems that screening on the basis of age alone is feasible and will lead to an overall ten percent reduction in mortality from breast cancer in North America and Europe within the next decade.

References

1. Anderson DE: Genetic study of breast cancer: identification of a high risk group. Cancer 34:1090–1097, 1974.
2. Brinton LA, Hoover R, Fraumeni JF: Epidemiology of minimal breast cancer. JAMA 249(4):483–487, 1983.
3. Brinton LA, Hoover R, Fraumeni JF: Reproductive factors in the aetiology of breast cancer. Br J Cancer 47(6):757–762, 1983.
4. Byers T, Graham S, Rzepka T, et al: Lactation and breast cancer. Am J Epidemiol 121(5):664–674, 1985.
5. Buell P: Changing incidence of breast cancer in Japanese-American women. J Natl Cancer Inst 51(5):1479–1483, 1973.
6. Carlile T, Kopecky KJ, Thompson DJ, et al: Breast cancer prediction and the Wolfe classification of mammograms. JAMA 254(8):1050–1018, 1985.
7. Chaudary MA, Millis RR, Hoskins EO, et al: Bilateral primary breast cancer: a prospective study of disease incidence. Br J Surg 71:711–714, 1984.
8. Clifford P, Bulbrook RD: Endocrine studies in African males with nasopharyngeal cancer. Lancet i:1228–1231, 1966.
9. Coulam CB, Annegers JF, Kranz JS: Chronic anovulation syndrome and associated neoplasia. Obstet Gynecol 61(4):403–407, 1983.
10. DMPA and cancer: report from a WHO meeting, September 1985. Bull WHO 64(4):375–382, 1986.
11. Dupont WD, Page DL: Risk factors for breast cancer in women with proliferative breast disease. New Engl J Med 312:146–151, 1985.
12. Editorial: does alcohol cause breast cancer? Lancet i:1311–1312, 1985.
13. Ewertz M: Bereavement and breast cancer. Br J Cancer 53:701–703, 1986.
14. Farewell VT: The combined effect of breast cancer risk factors. Cancer 40:931–936, 1977.
15. Forrest AP, Roberts MM: Screening for breast cancer. Br J Hosp Med 2:18–22, 1980.
16. Forrest P, et al: Breast cancer screening: report to the health ministers of England, Scotland and Northern Ireland, Appendix D. Department of Health and Social Security/Her Majesty's Stationery Office (DHSS/HMSO), 1987.
17. Gazet JC: Tamoxifen prophylaxis. Lancet i:263, 1986.
18. Graham S: Alcohol and breast cancer. N Engl J Med 316(19):1211–1212, 1987.
19. Gray GE, Henderson BE, Pike MC: Changing ratio of breast cancer incidence rates with age of black females compared with white females in the United States. J Natl Cancer Inst 64(3):461–463, 1980.
20. Gray GE, Pike MC, Henderson BE: Diet and hormone profiles in teenage girls in four countries at different risk for breast cancer. Prev Med 11:108–113, 1982.
21. Hadjimichael OC, Boyle CA, Meigs JW: Abortion before first livebirth and risk of breast cancer. Br J Cancer 53:281–284, 1986.
22. Henderson BE, Pike MC, Casagrande JT: Breast cancer and the oestrogen window hypothesis. Lancet ii:363–364, 1981.
23. Henderson BE, Pike MC, Ross RK: Epidemiology and risk factors. In Bonadonna G (ed): Breast Cancer: Diagnosis and Management. New York, John Wiley, 1984.
24. Hiatt RA, Bawol RD: Alcoholic beverage consumption and breast cancer incidence. Am J Epidemiol 120:676–683, 1984.
25. Hiatt RA, Fireman BH: Smoking, menopause and breast cancer. J Natl Cancer Inst 76(5):833–838, 1986.
26. Hislop TG, Elwood JM, Coldman AJ, et al: Second primary cancers of the breast: incidence and risk factors. Br J Cancer 49:79–85, 1984.
27. Hoel DG, Wakabayashi T, Pike MC: Secular trends in the distribution of the breast cancer risk factors—menarche, firstbirth, menopause and weight in Hiroshima and Nagasaki, Japan. Am J Epidemiol 118(1):78, 1983.
28. Howe GR: Epidemiology of radiogenic breast cancer. Prog Cancer Res Ther 26:119–129, 1984.
29. Hunt K, Vessey M, McPherson K, Coleman M: Long-term surveillance of mortality and cancer incidence in women receiving hormone replacement therapy. B J Obstet Gynaecol 94:620–635, 1987.
30. Kalache A, McPherson K, Barltrop K, et al: Oral contraceptives and breast cancer. Br J Hosp Med 30:278–283, 1983.
31. Kalache A, Vessey M: Risk factors for breast cancer. Clin Oncol 1(3):661–678, 1982.
32. Key TJ, Pike MC: The role of oestrogens and progestagens in the epidemiology and prevention of breast cancer. Eur J Cancer Clin Oncol 24(1):29–43, 1988.
33. Korenman SG: The oestrogen window hypothesis of the aetiology of breast cancer. Lancet i:700–701, 1980.
34. La Vecchio C, Decarli A, De Pietro S, et al: Menstrual cycle patterns and the risk of breast cancer. Eur J Cancer Clin Oncol 21:417–422, 1985.
35. Lipnick, Speizer FE, Bain C, et al: Case control study of risk indicators among women with premenopausal and early post menopausal breast cancer. Cancer 53:1020–1024, 1984.

36. Logan WPD: Cancer mortality by occupation and social class 1851–1971. IARC Scientific Publication No 36/OPCS Series SMPS No 44, London, HMSO, 1982.
37. MacMahon B, Cole P, Lin TM, et al: Age at first birth and breast cancer risk. Bull WHO 43:209–212, 1970.
38. McPherson K, Neil A, Vessey MP, Doll R: Oral contraceptives and breast cancer. Lancet ii:1414–1415, 1983.
39. McTiernan A, Thomas DB: Evidence for a protective effect of lactation on the risk of breast cancer in young women. Am J Epidemiol 124(3):353–358, 1986.
40. Miller AB, Bulbrook RD: UICC multidisciplinary project on breast cancer: the epidemiology, aetiology and prevention of breast cancer. Int J Cancer 37:173–177, 1986.
41. Moore DH, Kuncio GS (eds): Oncology Overview: Breast Cancer Demography. National Cancer Institute/International Cancer Research Data Bank, 1986.
42. Ottman R, Pike MC, King M-C, Henderson BE: Practical guide for estimating risk for familial breast cancer. Lancet ii:556–558, 1983.
43. Pike MC, Henderson BE, Casagrande JT, et al: Oral contraceptive use and early abortion as risk factors for breast cancer in young women. Br J Cancer 43:72–76, 1981.
44. Pike MC, Krailo MD, Henderson BE, et al: Hormonal risk factors, breast tissue age and the age-incidence of breast cancer. Nature 303:767–770, 1983.
45. Rose DP, Boyar AP, Wynder EL: International comparisons of mortality rates for cancer of the breast, ovary, prostate, colon and per capita food comsumption. Cancer 58:2363–2371, 1986.
46. Schatzkin A, Jones DY, Hoover RN: Alcohol consumption and breast cancer in the epidemiological follow-up of the 1st national health and nutrition survey. N Engl J Med 316(19):1169–1173, 1987.
47. Silber ALM, Horwitz RI: Detection bias and relation of benign breast disease to breast cancer. Lancet i:638–641, 1986.
48. Tokunaga M, Land CE, Yamamoto T, et al.: Breast cancer among atomic bomb survivors. Prog Cancer Res Ther 26:45–56, 1984.
49. Trichopolous D, MacMahon B, Cole P, et al: The menopause and breast cancer risk. J Natl Cancer Inst 48:605–613, 1972.
50. Vessey MP: Exogenous hormones in the aetiology of cancer in women. J Roy Soc Med 77:542–549, 1984.
51. Vessey MP, Doll R, Jones K, et al: An epidemiological study of oral contraceptives and breast cancer. Br Med J i:1757–1760, 1979.
52. Vessey MP, McPherson K, Yeates D, et al: Oral contraceptive use and abortion before first term pregnancy in relation to breast cancer risk. Br J Cancer 45:327–331, 1982.
53. Waterhouse J, et al: Cancer Incidence in Five Continents. Scientific Publication No 15, Lyon, IARC, 1976.
54. Webster LA, Layde PM, Wingo PA, Ory HW: Cancer and Steroid Hormone Study Group. Alcohol consumption and risk of breast cancer. Lancet 2:724–726, 1983.
55. Willett WC, Browne ML, Bain C: Relative weight and risk of breast cancer among premenopausal women. Am J Epidemiol 122(5):731–740, 1985.
56. Willett WC, Stampfer MJ, Colditz GA: Dietary fat and the risk of breast cancer. N Engl J Med 316:22–28, 1987.
57. Willett WC, Stampfer MJ, Colditz GA, et al: Moderate alcohol consumption and the risk of breast cancer. N Engl J Med 316(19):1174–1175, 1987.
58. Williams WR, Anderson DE: Genetic epidemiology of breast cancer: segregation analysis of 200 Danish pedigrees. Genet Epidemiol 1:7–20, 1984.
59. Wolfe JN: Risk for breast cancer development determined by mammographic parenchymal patterns. Cancer 37:2486–2492, 1976.
60. Wynder EC, Rose DP, Cohen LA: Diet and breast cancer in causation and therapy. Cancer 58:1804–1813, 1986.
61. Wysowski DK, Comstock GW, Helsing KJ: Sex hormone levels in serum in relation to the development of breast cancer. Am J Epidemiol 125(5):791, 1987.

Primary Prevention of Breast Cancer

Michael P. Osborne, M.D., M.S., and Nitin T. Telang, Ph.D.

The primary prevention of breast cancer remains an ideal. Prevention strategies can be approached by applying methodology derived from epidemiological or laboratory research. These leads, if considered to be both safe and potentially effective, can be applied to humans to observe the biological effect of cancer rate reduction in those with a defined risk of developing the disease. Success in such defined risk groups may lead to application in the general population. However, many complex problems arise in the implementation of such approaches; the major issues include toxicity, safety, feasibility, design and statistical considerations, compliance, duration of study, and ethical concerns. The difficulties faced are derived from the fact that the cause of breast cancer is very poorly understood; the disease has a relatively low risk in the general population and in addition, the definition and measurement of risk is inadequate. It is estimated that approximately one in ten women (10%) have a lifetime risk of developing

breast cancer. It has also been noted that only 25% of women developing the disease have an identifiable risk factor. Given the incidence of the disease, statistical considerations of sample size will make implementation of a preventive trial a difficult problem. Initial efforts should be directed at defined risk populations such as those at risk because of a genetic influence or with tissue markers identified on a breast biopsy.[100, 159] A paradigm exists in the preventive studies conducted by the Heart, Blood and Lung Institute (HBLI) of the National Institutes of Health (NIH), which demonstrated a reduction in myocardial infarction by a specific intervention, using the intermediate marker of risk, blood cholesterol levels.[75] The development of intermediate markers for breast cancer is an important research priority.

Currently, the only known method of preventing breast cancer is bilateral mastectomy. This drastic and mutilating approach has very limited indications in individuals with defined high risk, such as those with a family history of hereditary breast cancer and/or premalignant lesions determined to be present on a breast biopsy. Clearly, safe interventions that will reduce the risk of developing breast cancer are a much more attractive alternative, to both the high risk and the general population. This chapter considers the laboratory and epidemiological basis for breast cancer prevention in the future and examines the possibility of applying interventions in the context of clinical trials.

POTENTIAL PREVENTIVE INTERVENTIONS

Dietary Fat Reduction

The Committee on Diet, Nutrition and Cancer of the National Academy of Sciences published a report concluding that of all dietary components studied, the combined epidemiological and experimental evidence is suggestive of a causal relationship between dietary fat intake and the incidence of breast cancer.[93] The committee recommended that research should try to establish more convincing links between diet and the development of cancer. Epidemiological research in this field continues to accumulate circumstantial evidence of a significant effect of dietary fat intake on the development of breast cancer. This relationship does not exclude the possibility of other agents influencing the evolution of the disease. Establishing an association between diet and breast cancer requires evaluation of the evidence by the following criteria:[45]
1. Consistency
2. Strength
3. Specificity
4. Temporal relationship
5. Coherence

Consistency. The consistency of the data indicating a link between dietary fat and breast cancer has been shown in a number of studies. For example, a study compared dietary fat intake in Seventh Day Adventists developing breast cancer to Seventh Day Adventist controls who did not develop breast cancer.[105] The results showed that those patients who ate fried foods frequently, when compared to those who did so less frequently, had approximately twice the risk of developing breast cancer. A study of five different ethnic groups in Hawaii demonstrated a strong correlation between breast cancer incidence and average daily intake of total fats, animal fats, saturated fats, or unsaturated fats.[72] Calculation of fat intake in premenopausal and postmenopausal patients with breast cancer showed that there was an elevated risk ratio compared to controls for total fat and selected types of fat intake; this association was for fat and not for total calories.[87] A study conducted by the National Cancer Institute compared the dietary fat intake for breast cancer patients to that of controls[78] and showed that individuals in the highest quartile for beef or pork consumption had a risk of developing breast cancer 2.7 times that of those in the lowest quartile. Elevated risk was also found in the upper quartile of women who ate cream and desserts or animal fats.

Strength. The strength of the association between dietary fat and breast cancer can be determined by examination of the relative risk ratios for developing the disease. Epidemiological research comparing the variation in dietary fat ingestion and age-adjusted breast cancer mortality in various countries correlates closely with fat consumption.[161] The national level of dietary fat intake is directly proportional to the age-adjusted breast cancer mortality. The strength of the association was such that those countries with half the levels of dietary fat intake had a mortality rate half that of those countries in which dietary fat intake is high. It has been suggested that halving the dietary calories derived from fat, which is estimated to be 40 percent in the United States,[108] might more than halve the breast cancer mortality rate.

The association between fat intake and breast cancer must be carefully evaluated; both the quality and quantity of dietary fat may influence the incidence of this disease. Epidemiological evidence indicates that both Japanese women and Greenland Eskimo women have a low incidence of breast cancer,[34, 73, 97] yet Greenland Eskimos have a high fat diet. Eskimo and Japanese diets traditionally included a large amount of omega-3 fatty acids which are unique to the marine-derived lipids—eicosapentaenoic acid (EPA) (C20:5 omega-3) and docosahexaenoic acid (DHA) (C22:6 omega-3).[124] However, in both populations the situation has been changing in recent years. In Japan, the number of annual deaths from breast cancer doubled in the 20-year period from 1955 to 1975; over this same period the Japanese diet became more akin to that of Western countries, primarily among the younger, more affluent, urban segments of the population.[55] This change in dietary practices has particularly affected fat consumption. The typical Japanese diet includes large quantities of fish, so that approximately 10 percent of the total fat is comprised of long chain fatty acids. In contrast, the dietary intake of long chain fatty acids in the U.S. is only about 1 percent of the total. Epidemiological evidence suggests that the change in breast cancer incidence among Eskimos may be caused by an increased exposure to western influence. One of the consequences of modernization has been a change in dietary habits; imported foods have become more accessible, resulting in an increased consumption of saturated and unsaturated omega-6 fatty acids. At the beginning of this century, approximately half the caloric intake of Eskimos consisted of fats of marine origin. The meat of seal, whale, and fish is rich in unsaturated omega-3 fatty acids.[124, 131] Because of an increase in dietary fat in a 20-year period from 1933 to 1953,[131] the ratio of omega-3 unsaturated fatty acids to total fat intake is still higher in Eskimo women than in women in highly industrialized countries such as Denmark.

In addition, an extremely low incidence of atherosclerotic heart disease in Eskimos has stimulated researchers to study the relationship between intakes of marine oil and incidence of atherosclerosis.[51, 113, 114] This should be translated to studies of human breast carcinogenesis.

Specificity. The specificity of dietary fat in causing breast cancer raises difficult problems. There is a lack of good alternative hypotheses other than the small cohort of patients who clearly have an autosomal dominant pattern of inheritance of the disease. A considerable amount of further research is required to examine interacting influences, such as genetics, dietary macro- and micronutrients, and the impact of these factors on steroid hormone synthesis and metabolism.

Temporal Relationship. The temporal relationship between dietary fat and breast cancer is manifested by the fact that dietary patterns are well established for a long period of time before development of the disease in the late premenopausal or postmenopausal period.

Coherence. The coherence of evidence for dietary fat being related to the evolution of breast cancer is further supported by a number of experimental studies. The classic study by Tannenbaum[134] showed that mice with high incidence of mammary tumor virus–induced breast cancer had a higher breast cancer rate when on a high-fat diet compared to mice on low-fat diets. Since that time, detailed studies by Carroll,[17, 18] Carroll and Hopkins,[19] and Carroll and Khor[20, 21] have confirmed these findings in rats with carcinogen-induced breast cancer and are supported by other investigators.[23–26, 54, 58, 152] These investigators showed that the effects were most marked at low levels of carcinogen and that the primary mechanism of dietary fat was promotional. This finding is of particular interest in application to humans, as the effect worked after the exposure to an initiating agent.

The term "polyunsaturated fatty acids" covers a wide range of agents having 18, 20, and 22 carbon chains length, with two to six methylene-interrupted double bonds with the *Cis* configuration. Linoleic acid (18:2 omega-6) and alpha-linoleic acid (18:3 omega-3) are required for normal cellular growth and function. These parent essential fatty acids (EFA) undergo chain elongation and desaturation to produce long chain derivatives of 20 and 22 carbon chain lengths with 3, 4, 5, and 6 double bonds. The result is two families (omega-6 and omega-3) of EFA that are required for prostaglandin synthesis. It has been reported that promotional effect of polyunsaturated fat on carcinogen-induced mammary tumorigenesis may in part be mediated via increased synthesis of prostaglandins,[22, 54] and this effect of fat can be blocked by indomethacin, an inhibitor of prostaglandin synthesis.[22] In vitro experiments on cell and organ cultures of mouse mammary glands have shown that the omega-6 fatty acid, arachidonic acid (ARA, C20:4, omega-6) enhances the incidence of putative preneoplastic lesions.[141, 143] Indomethacin can also block the enhancement of preneoplasia.[141] More recent in vitro experiments have shown that omega-6 fatty acids also enhance the expression of the mammary tumor virus and of the cellular *ras* proto-oncogene, the two critical molecular events for tumorigenic transformation of mammary gland.[139] In contrast, the omega-3 fatty acid, EPA, and the saturated fatty acid, stearic acid, were found to downregulate the two molecular events. As expected, modulation of the molecular events was seen to be reflected in a parallel alteration in the frequency of mammary lesions, the cellular end point of preneoplastic transformation. The two in vitro studies taken together suggest that selected fatty acids, by virtue of their influence on molecular and cellular events of preneoplastic transformation, may be effective chemopreventive agents against mammary tumorigenesis. Arachidonic acid (ARA C20:4 omega-6) has also been demonstrated to enhance cell proliferation and mutant expression in mammary epithelial cells exposed to the carcinogen 7,12-dimethylbenz[a]anthracene (DMBA).[136, 143] These observations are particularly important, since the dietary intake of unsaturated fat (omega-6) has significantly increased in recent years.[108] Omega-3 fatty acids have also been shown to inhibit established tumor prostaglandin synthesis,[68, 70] and therefore these agents may exert antipromotional effects through this mechanism.

Evidence supporting the contention that omega-3 fatty acids may exert a protective effect on mammary tumorigenesis comes from recent studies. Cohen et al.[30] found that the brown seaweed *Laminaria augusta* effectively blocked the tumor-promoting effect of a high-fat (20 percent corn oil) diet on mammary tumors induced with *N*-nitroso-*N*-methylurea. When a control diet was supplemented with five percent seaweed, there was a delay in the appearance of tumors induced with DMBA and a reduction in the number of tumors.[135] This brown kelp seaweed, although low in fat content, has half of its fat as EPA.[69] Whether the chemopreventive effect of this seaweed is related to its content of EPA has not been determined.

Dietary Prevention Studies

The Women's Health Trial, a prevention trial based on the hypothesis that a greater-than-50 percent reduction in dietary fat may halve breast cancer incidence, was proposed[10] but was subsequently cancelled.

Measurement of compliance to low-fat diets poses a number of problems, but detailed methodology is being developed.[10]

Modification of Dietary Fat

It can be argued that it is not just a question of the amount of dietary fat that is a risk factor for breast cancer; qualitative considerations may also be of importance (see earlier sections of this chapter). A Cancer Control Science Program Project, funded by the National Cancer Institute, was piloted at Memorial Sloan-Kettering Cancer Center. These exploratory studies are evaluating the modifying effects of omega-3 fatty acids in the normal American diet on estrogen metabolism. It is suggested that abnormalities of estrogen metabolism may correlate with the risk of developing breast cancer[9, 37, 115] in defined populations, such as those with particular types of family history of breast cancer or those who have undergone a biopsy with pathological changes indicating an elevated level of risk.[99] The intervention pilot trial is an attempt to favorably perturb estrogen metabolism toward normal.[101] In addition, detailed genetic, endocrine, pathological, and psychosocial studies are being carried out in the defined population at risk.

Despite the compelling evidence, derived from studies undertaken on animal models, that dietary fat influences the development of breast cancer, direct effects of fat on tumorigenic transformation of human mammary tissue have not been established. Clearly, this lack of information seriously limits the clinical relevance of dietary fat–induced modulation of human breast cancer. In our attempts to eliminate this limitation, we have developed an in vitro model using explant cultures of human mammary terminal duct lobular units (TDLU), the presumptive precursor tissue for human breast carcinoma. In our initial studies performed on TDLU explants obtained from mammoplasty and mastectomy specimens, we have identified a specific molecular marker (cellular *ras* proto-oncogene expression) and a metabolic marker (estradiol-16α-hydroxylation) with which relative risk for developing breast cancer could be evaluated.[11, 102] These experiments revealed substantially higher constitutive levels of both the molecular and metabolic markers in TDLU-HR (obtained from "high-risk" mastectomy samples, i.e., from patients undergoing surgery for breast cancer) in comparison to TDLU-LR (obtained from "low-risk" mammoplasty specimens that lacked clinicopathological evidence for breast cancer). In a separate study, we examined the ability of selected fatty acids to modulate the molecular and metabolic marker. Treatment of explant cultures with the polyunsaturated omega-6 fatty acid linoleic acid induced a parallel enhancement of both the markers, while treatment with the polyunsaturated omega-3 fatty acid eicosapentaenoic acid resulted in a suppression of the two markers. These experiments indicate that *ras* expression and estradiol-16α-hydroxylation may constitute useful markers for risk identification, and that selected fatty acids can directly modulate the two markers in human mammary tissue.[103]

Having obtained the evidence about intrinsic differences in the constitutive levels for *ras* expression and estradiol metabolism in TDLU from mammoplasty and mastectomy specimens, it was important to examine whether chemical carcinogens can alter the two markers, and if so, whether these alterations are susceptible to modulation by fatty acids. Treatment of TDLU explant cultures with *N*-nitroso-*N*-methylurea (NMU) and benzo[a]pyrene (BP) was found to enhance *ras* expression.[138] Furthermore, BP exposure was found to induce a parallel enhancement in *ras* expression and estradiol-16α-hydroxylation. The relative extents of these two markers were positively modulated by omega-6 fatty acid and negatively modulated by omega-3 fatty acid.[140] This study provides evidence that *ras* expression and estradiol-16α-hydroxylation may constitute sensitive measures of target tissue susceptibility to carcinogenic insult and of tissue sensitivity to dietary modulators of carcinogenesis.

Vitamin A and its Derivatives (Retinoids)

Vitamin A (Retinol) and its analogues, the retinoids, have profound effects on the general growth and differentiation of epithelial tissues. Since, in many respects, breast cancer is fundamentally a disease of abnormal differentiation of breast epithelial cells, retinoids may be considered as agents with potential for arresting or preventing cancer.

The relationship between vitamin A and cancer was discovered in the 1920s when Fujimaki[40] detected the development of carcinoma in the stomach of rats fed a vitamin A–deficient diet. In their classic paper describing the cellular effects of vitamin A deficiency in the rat, Wolbach and Howe[160] noted increased mitotic activity in metaplastic de-differentiated epithelia of vitamin A–deficient animals, and pointed out this common feature shared by truly malignant lesions. The landmark study by Lasnitzki[74] showed that malignant transformation of mouse prostate cells induced by a chemical carcinogen could be inhibited by vitamin A. Subsequently the chemopreventive effects of retinoids were demonstrated by Saffioti et al.[111] in the squamous metaplasia model of the trachea.

Abels et al.[1] conducted the first epidemiological study of vitamin A and cancer. They measured plasma vitamin levels in patients with gastrointestinal cancer in New York City and found significantly lower values in patients with malignancy when compared to controls. A recent study of breast cancer and its relationship to vitamins[47] showed that an increased risk for breast cancer in women 55 years of age or older correlated with a decreased intake of foods containing vitamin A. Unfortunately many epidemiological and dietary studies are flawed by confounding variables and the difficulties of retrospective dietary analysis.

Retinoids have been shown to be potentially effective mammary cancer chemopreventive agents based on experimental evidence in vivo and in vitro. Less success has been encountered in investigations of retinoid-induced inhibition of growth in established tumors.[95, 102] Most human cancers, including breast cancer, arise in the epithelial tissues that depend on retinoids for normal cellular differentiation.[91, 151] As significant biological regulators of orderly epithelial cell development, retinoids would appear to be the ideal agents potentially capable of modifying aberrant epithelial proliferation such as occurs in carcinogenesis. Many retinoids, both natural and synthetic, have been tested in the chemoprevention of breast cancer in the laboratory.[88, 89, 126, 127] Retinoids with a preventive action are all found at various concentrations in the breast tissue. Among them, the synthetic retinoid retinyl methyl ether accumulates at higher concentrations in the mammary gland than does retinyl acetate[126] and is also more effective than retinyl acetate in prevention of mammary carcinogenesis.[48] The synthetic retinoid *N*-(4-hydroxyphenyl)retinamide (HPR) similarly concentrates at a higher level in the mammary gland of the rat when compared to retinyl acetate, although it is less effective than retinyl acetate for prevention of breast cancer in chemically induced mammary carcinogenesis.[90] It is not clear whether the concentration in the mammary gland is in fat or epithelium.

One of the main obstacles to long-term use of retinoids is their toxicity. Most retinoids, such as retinyl acetate, are stored in the liver and have the potential to cause hepatotoxicity.[90] Synthetic retinoids used in the prevention of cancer in animals have been shown to be less toxic than natural ones.[126] Hydroxyphenyl retinamide (HPR) may be one such efficacious and relatively nontoxic cancer chemopreventive agent. In both in vitro and in vivo experiments, it has been shown to prevent carcinogenesis.[27, 90]

Chemopreventive Effect of HPR

It has been demonstrated that mammary glands from 4-week-old BALB/c female mice, primed by daily injections of estradiol-17β and progesterone, develop preneoplastic nodule-like alveolar lesions (NLAL) when they are incubated in a lactogenic hormone–supplemented medium initially, then in a medium containing a carcinogen such as diethylnitrosamine (DENA) or 7,12-dimethylbenz[a]anthracene (DMBA), and lastly in the lactogenic hormone–free medium. Carcinogen-induced NLAL, because of their ability to survive in the absence of lactogenic hormones, are easily detectable in the predominantly ductal parenchyma of the organ cultured mammary gland.[137] The NLAL induced by DMBA in organ culture produce mammary carcinomas after transplantation into gland-free mammary fat pads of syngeneic virgin hosts.[137] The induction of NLAL in carcinogen-exposed mammary glands may therefore represent an in vitro marker for mammary preneoplasia.[7] The ability of HPR to reduce the incidence of NLAL, which are considered preneoplastic, was assessed. Cultures of DENA-treated mammary glands during 4 to 10 days of incubation in the presence of HPR resulted in 61 percent inhibition of NLAL incidence.[27] The ability of HPR to inhibit the expression of NLAL appears to be reduced in the presence of estrogen and progesterone. In a medium containing insulin, prolactin, hydrocortisone, and aldosterone, HPR caused 68 percent inhibition of NLAL incidence in DMBA-treated mammary gland cultures.

The addition of estrogen and progesterone to the medium reduced the inhibitory action of HPR to 15 percent. Although both ovarian hormones reduced the inhibitory action of HPR on the frequency of NLAL, the antagonistic action of estrogen was more pronounced.[27] HPR has also been shown to favorably affect transformed cells in the murine mammary tumor cell culture model.[15, 16]

The chemopreventive effect of HPR against preneoplastic transformation has also been examined using an adult mouse mammary explant culture system. In a mouse strain (R III), highly susceptible to murine mammary tumor virus–induced mammary cancer, emergence of overt adenocarcinoma is preceded by foci of alveolar hyperplasia, the mammary alveolar lesions (MAL). These MAL-containing mammary explant cultures were incubated with HPR for 14 days. Following HPR exposure, there was a 60 percent to 70 percent reduction in the number of lesions per gland.[142]

HPR has also been shown to be effective in the prevention of both NMU-[90] and DMBA-induced rat mammary carcinoma.[82, 125] Moon et al.[90] originally described a rat mammary carcinoma rate reduction of 50 percent using high-dose HPR with a low-dose NMU induction schedule, and a 35 percent rate reduction using high-dose HPR with a high-dose NMU schedule (Table 12–12). A low dose of HPR was not as effective in reducing the cancer rate. These experiments demonstrated that HPR was much less toxic than retinyl acetate (RA), but it is unknown whether doses equitoxic to RA would be equally effective. There was no accumulation of HPR in the liver, but accumulation was observed in the mammary gland. In another study of carcinogen-induced mammary cancer, the administration of a 782 mg/kg diet of HPR was begun 29 days before, 2 days before, or 2 days after treatment with NMU. The retinoid was given for 12 to 17 weeks post-induction, and the animals sacrificed at 28 weeks post-induction. The only significant inhibition of tumor incidence was found in the group of rats fed 2 days prior to NMU.[125] Similar trends, which were not significant, were observed in other HPR-treated groups.

These data suggest that retinoids can reduce the frequency of subsequent cancer, with improved survival. Whether this represents the benefit derived from delay in metachronous cancer or a direct antitumor action is unclear.

Welsch et al.[153] used a diet containing 391 mg/kg of HPR in C3H mice. This synthetic retinoid had an inhibitory action in the genesis of spontaneous mammary gland tumors in nulliparous mice, but no inhibition occurred in the genesis of mammary tumors in multiparous mice. In the latter, unlike young nulliparous C3H mice, many hyperplastic alveolar nodules (HAN) are already present. HAN are precursors to mammary tumors in this species,[33] and this suggests that HPR acts at an earlier stage of neoplastic development.[153]

Mechanisms of Action of Retinoids. The mechanism of action of retinoids in controlling cellular differentiation is poorly understood. Target epithelia contain receptors for retinoids [the cytosolic retinoic acid–binding protein (cRABP)],[28] and it has been suggested that there are strong similarities between the action of retinoids and hormones.[129] Retinoids have been described as having antiproliferative properties[90] or, alternatively, a role in the control of differentiation.[5] In vivo studies

Table 12–12. PERCENT OF RATS DEVELOPING MAMMARY CARCINOMA

Agent	Dose/kg (mmol)	Carcinogen (NMU)	
		15 mg/kg (%)	50 mg/kg (%)
None	—	30	100
HPR	1	30	80
HPR	2	15	65
RA	1	13	67
RA	2	0	13

Abbreviations: HPR = N-(4-hydroxyphenyl) retinamide; RA = Retinyl acetate.
From Moon RC, et al: Cancer Res 39:1339–1346, 1979. Reprinted by permission.

cannot easily distinguish these mechanisms. As stated by Sporn and Roberts[129] in their recent review, the key issue is which specific genes retinoids control. The molecular mechanism by which retinoids modify gene expression is of importance. It is known that retinoids control the expression of constituents of the cytoskeleton such as keratins.[39] These and other markers are being used to measure cell differentiation. One example of the gene-regulatory property of retinoic acid has been demonstrated in the HL60 system where physiological levels of all-*trans* retinoic acid suppress the expression of the *myc* oncogene.[156]

Apart from influences on gene control, other factors may also be considered. The ability of retinoids to block polypeptide growth factors that control cell proliferation and differentiation[128, 146] may also be influential in prevention.

The role of prostaglandin synthesis in tumorigenesis has been discussed earlier in this chapter. HPR has been shown to have an inhibitory action on PGE2. Brickerhoff et al.[12] have reported that 10^{-6} mol/L HPR prevented the increase in PGE2 induced by phorbol myristate acetate (PMA) in rabbit synovial fibroblast cultures. Trenthan and Brickerhoff[147] have shown that the in vitro addition of 10^{-6} mol/L HPR to cells cultured from arthritic rats was as effective as 10^{-7} mol/L indomethacin in suppressing PGE2 production. Similarly, in organ cultures of mouse mammary glands, arachidonic acid induces increased prostaglandin production, which is inhibited by 10^{-6} mol/L indomethacin.[141] PGE2 production was also significantly reduced in in vivo studies. HPR was given to rats with collagen arthritis at concentrations of 243 mg/kg or 486 mg/kg for 21 days. PGE2 production by synovial cells was significantly decreased when compared to rats that had received a control diet.[42]

Tamoxifen

The simple hydrocarbon triphenylethylene was noted to have a weak estrogenic action. Derivatives from these nonsteroidal compounds were initially explored for their effects on fertility, but the observation of an antiestrogenic activity of tamoxifen suggested its use in the therapy of advanced breast cancer. Its lack of toxicity and its efficacy in treatment have led to widespread use in more than 80 countries; tamoxifen has also been registered as a treatment for infertile women to induce ovulation.[79] Experimental and epidemiological evidence points to a major role of estrogens in the pathogenesis of human breast cancer.[80] The only known intervention likely to reduce the risk of breast cancer, other than prophylactic mastectomy, is ovariectomy before the age of 45.[64]

The experimental evidence that tamoxifen can retard or prevent DMBA-induced mammary cancer[76] suggests that this agent may be a feasible approach to prevention.

In Vitro Studies

Research on the subcellular aspects of tamoxifen's action has been carried out on human breast cancer cell lines. Tamoxifen can induce an inhibitory effect on ^{3}H-thymidine incorporation,[36] on DNA polymerase activity,[57] and can reduce DNA content in the *MCF7* cell line.[29] These findings have been observed in two other cell lines *(CG5 and ZR751)* and are dependent on the presence of estrogen receptors.[65]

Little work has been recorded on the in vitro effects of tamoxifen on precursor lesions in culture in contrast to tumor explants.

In Vivo Studies

Tamoxifen has been demonstrated to cause regression of established tumors.[76] Large doses of tamoxifen, when given synchronously with the carcinogen, almost completely inhibit the appearance of tumors. More relevant to the clinical situation, it has been shown that tamoxifen is inhibitory to tumorigenesis after exposure to the initiator but before overt tumors appear.[66] A long continuous course of tamoxifen is superior to a short (fewer than 30 days) course.[67] It is possible that continuous tamoxifen therapy is superior to ovariectomy. Ovariectomy 30 days after DMBA administration delayed the appearance of tumors, but eventually 50 percent of animals developed tumors. In contrast, continuous treatment with tamoxifen prevented tumor appearance in approximately 90 percent of animals after 200 days.[66, 155] The greater efficacy of tamoxifen may be its ability to antagonize all estrogens, whether from the ovaries or from peripheral aromatization of adrenal androgens.[79, 80] Welsch et al.[155] administered tamoxifen for 66 days, starting 33 days before administration of DMBA, and reduced the incidence of mammary carcinoma by 49 percent. Treatment with tamoxifen for 66 days, starting 33 days after DMBA initiation, reduced the incidence of carcinoma by 65 percent.

The efficacy of tamoxifen in rat mammary carcinoma chemoprevention has been reproduced in the NMU-induced mammary carcinoma model described by Gullino et al.[49] Treatment was initiated on the first day of carcinogen administration and continued for 145 days; it exerted a similar effect to ovariectomy.[44]

Mechanisms of Preventive Action

The mechanisms of action postulated in the carcinogen-initiated models include (1) prevention of local tissue activation of DMBA; (2) induction of cellular biochemistry so as to render the target organ refractory; and (3) inhibition of prolactin essential to rat mammary carcinogenesis.[79]

Some experiments have suggested that tamoxifen may act independently of estrogen receptors and can be inhibitory in estrogen receptor negative *(BT20)* cell lines[32] or tumor explants.[107] The proposed mechanism is alteration of prostaglandin concentrations.[41, 98]

Role in Human Breast Cancer Prevention

No study of breast cancer prevention using an antiestrogen has yet been undertaken. In a randomized study evaluating the adjuvant properties of tamoxifen against micrometastatic disease after mastectomy, a modest statistically significant beneficial effect in relapse-free survival was observed.[120] In this adjuvant trial, three of 876 patients receiving tamoxifen developed contralateral breast cancer, compared to 12 of 892 controls ($p = 0.03$).[71]

The epidemiological finding that ovariectomy before the age of 45 years reduces the risk of breast cancer suggests that tamoxifen might be required during the premenopausal years. This carries the theoretical problems relating to the acceleration of osteoporosis. Weak estrogen agonist effects on the endometrium may also carry risks for endometrial cancer[84] and for a known low but significant incidence of side effects such as hot flashes, nausea, menstrual irregularity, dry vagina, and skin rashes.[79]

Chemopreventive Effect of Tamoxifen and HPR in Combination

Preliminary studies have examined the effect of ovariectomy in combination with HPR.[83] Female rats had mammary cancer induced with either 50 mg/kg NMU or 20 mg/kg of DMBA. One week later, the animals were divided into four groups: control, ovariectomy, diet containing 782 mg/kg of HPR, and diet with 782 mg/kg of HPR along with ovariectomy. Following both carcinogens, ovariectomy was more effective than HPR in the reduction of incidence of mammary cancer, and the combination of ovariectomy and HPR was significantly more active than either therapy alone (Table 12–13). This indicated a synergistic action on mammary cancer inhibition and demonstrated that HPR inhibition of mammary carcinogenesis did not involve an influence mediated through ovarian hormones.

To further investigate the interaction between retinoids and estrogens, an experiment was carried out using HPR and tamoxifen. Fifty female rats were given NMU (50 mg/kg body weight). Seven days later, the animals were divided into four groups; one group was placed on a placebo diet, and the other three groups were given HPR alone or combined with subcutaneous injections of either 10 or 100 µg tamoxifen three times

Table 12–13. INFLUENCE OF N-(4-HYDROXYPHENYL) RETINAMIDE (HPR) AND OVARIECTOMY (OVEX) ON RAT MAMMARY CARCINOGENESIS

	Therapy			
	None (%)	*HPR* (%)	*Ovex* (%)	*HPR + Ovex*
NMU % with Carcinoma	100	92	18	2
T25 (d)	48	68	274	—*
DMBA % with Carcinoma	91	85	50	50
T25 (d)	64	75	225	—*

*Group never reached 25 percent cancer incidence.
From McCormick DL, et al: Cancer Res 42:508–512, 1982. Reprinted by permission.

a week. Tamoxifen was found to inhibit the appearance of mammary tumors in a dose-related manner; this inhibition was enhanced by HPR.[83] This effect was found to be additive, not synergistic.

Selenium

The trace element selenium is a factor that has been identified by researchers as a potential modulator of the process of carcinogenesis. Selenium was first identified by John Jacob Berzelius (1779–1848) in 1817. Selenium belongs to the same group of elements as sulfur and is found widely distributed in soil, grasses, and grain. The agent is used industrially to decolorize glass and in the manufacture of photoelectric cells and dandruff shampoo. The main source of industrial selenium is copper refining, in which selenium occurs as a by-product. Selenium is found in biological products in organic and inorganic forms. These forms include selenite, selenate, selenocystine, and selenonethionine. Selenium is a toxic chemical but is also an essential nutrient for both human and animal systems. It plays a role in the activity of selenoenzyme glutathione peroxidase. A deficiency in animals will result in impaired growth, and in murine species, sparse hair coats and cataracts. Chicks deficient in selenium develop a bleeding tendency and muscular dystrophy. Primates have been shown to exhibit liver, muscular, cardiac, and renal damage. Selenium deficiency has been reported in association with total parenteral nutrition. The adequate and safe intake of selenium for an adult is considered to be 50 µg to 200 µg per day. The role of selenium in cancer prevention has been well reviewed by Helzlsouer.[52]

Carcinogenesis

Selenium has been described to induce cancer in early experiments, but some of these experiments did not have adequate control groups, and the vehicle in which selenium was administered may be incriminated in its carcinogenic effect.[50, 96, 132, 148] Subsequent major clinical toxicity studies in rats by Harr[50] did not reveal any incidence in cancer of the breast in 1437 experimental animals. In addition, a study of selenium toxicity in 5000 workers exposed to selenium industrially did not show any evidence of excessive mortality resulting from cancer.[43]

Epidemiological Evidence

Epidemiological studies, both within the United States and internationally, have suggested a correlation between the selenium content of soil and forages. Shamberger and Willis[123] have examined the age-adjusted cancer mortality rates in various states by the selenium content in forage crops. Cancer mortality for breast cancer was decreased in high and medium selenium–containing areas when compared with low selenium–containing areas. The authors noted a similar pattern within states that contained both high and low selenium counties.

Selenium Levels and Carcinogenesis

Schrauzer et al.[119] calculated the dietary selenium intake in 27 countries and found it to be inversely correlated with overall cancer mortality. This observation was applied to breast, ovarian, and large bowel cancer. Additional supporting evidence was obtained by determining blood selenium levels in blood bank collections in 19 centers in the United States.[4] In a study of the serum selenium levels in 35 breast cancer patients, a significantly lower mean serum concentration was found in the cancer patients when compared to control patients with nonmalignant disease.[81, 122] This did not confirm a previous negative study with small numbers.[13] A number of other studies have suggested an inverse relationship between blood selenium levels and cancer risk.[61, 110, 158] Caution should always be observed in interpreting the results of serum selenium levels in patients who either have or have been treated for cancer; low levels are more significant if they precede the diagnosis of cancer.[158] It has been suggested that low selenium levels are a consequence of illness and are not related to the cause of cancer.

Chemopreventive Effects

Several experimental studies have shown that spontaneous (virally induced) mammary carcinoma as well as carcinogen-induced mammary carcinoma in murine systems can be reduced by exposure to selenium. Selenium-mediated inhibition of virally-induced murine mammary carcinoma has been demonstrated with both SeO_2 and organic selenium in the diet. Using SeO_2, an 88 percent reduction in tumor incidence was observed,[117] and with organic selenium, a 65 percent reduction in tumor incidence was observed.[118] Similar observations have been made[86] in which the extent of the reduction of tumor incidence was directly proportional to the concentration of sodium selenite in drinking water. A 2-ppm concentration resulted in a 41 percent reduction of tumor incidence, and a 6-ppm concentration resulted in an 85 percent reduction in tumor incidence. Medina and Shepherd[86] observed similar effects in DMBA-induced mouse mammary tumorigenesis. Studies of the rat mammary carcinoma model using either DMBA[60, 154] or NMU[145] demonstrated a similar cancer-preventive effect of selenium.

Recently, the combined effect of selenium and the polyamine synthesis inhibitor difluoromethylornithine (DFMO) has been studied on DMBA-induced mammary carcinoma in the rat.[144] This study demonstrated that selenium and DFMO exhibited an additive effect on DMBA-induced mammary carcinoma that was potentiated by a low methionine diet.

The evidence for selenium as an anticarcinogenic agent has been well reviewed by several authors.[46, 62, 121]

Potential Hazards. Selenium is a group VI metalloid. The group VI metalloid subgroup VIA includes oxygen, sulfur, selenium, tellurium, and polonium. Selenium is the most toxic member of this group.[150] This trace element is essential for mammalian life, but an excess of 3–10 ppm in the diet will cause toxicity to animals. The therapeutic-to-toxic–dose ratio is 1:100, and toxicity may be exacerbated by vitamin E deficiency. The toxic effects of selenium have been recently reviewed in detail by Wilber[157] and Buell.[14] In summary, selenosis has been well documented in horses and livestock who have grazed on seleniferous plants; this was even observed by Marco Polo in 1295. This phenomenon may have had an historical effect in the wars against the Indians in the United States, but it was not until the 1930s that it was established that selenium in grains and grasses and certain weeds was the agent that resulted in livestock toxicity.

The Food and Nutrition Board of the National Research Council has had difficulty in defining quantitatively the human requirements for selenium.[94] It has been established that for most mammalian species a selenium concentration of 0.1 μg (ppm) is adequate for satisfactory performance, growth, and reproduction. Human diet can be assumed to be satisfactory with a daily intake of 50 μg selenium, and a general range between 50 μg and 200 μg per day has been established. The Food and Nutrition Board has stated that "a maximal dietary intake of 200 μg per day should not be exceeded habitually if the risks of long-term chronic exposure are to be avoided." This is a conservative estimate, and observations in Japanese fishermen have suggested that no adverse effect has been noted from chronic ingestion of approximately 500 μg/d.[112]

Toxicity in Humans. Selenite is detoxified in the liver and excreted in the urine. When toxic levels are approached, detoxification in the form of dimethylselenide increases. This volatile substance is excreted by the lungs and is characterized by garlic breath or other symptoms in humans, including indigestion and the ill-defined sociopsychological effects of lassitude and irritability. The major occurrence of selenium toxicity in the human population has been reported from China.[162] Because of a period of drought, the population ate alternative cereals and vegetables high in selenium. The selenium toxicity was characterized by loss of hair and nails, skin lesions on the backs of the hands and feet and outsides of the legs, and the symptoms and signs of a chronic toxic polyneuritis. Selenium in both organic and inorganic forms is transmitted through the placenta to the fetus, and high levels have been associated with teratogenic effects in animal embryos. Miscarriage and a congenital deformity have been described in female laboratory workers exposed to high levels of selenite powder.[109] Clearly, a considerable amount of further experimental and epidemiological evidence needs to be accumulated before selenium can be seriously considered as a possible chemopreventive agent for human breast cancer.

Mechanisms of Action

A number of mechanisms have been proposed by which selenium acts as a chemopreventive agent. It is possible that one or several of these modes of action may be involved in preventing carcinogenesis. In the models utilizing injected chemical carcinogens, it is possible that selenium may alter the mode of metabolism of the carcinogenic agent. This clearly is not the sole method of action, as selenium has been shown to reduce the incidence of tumor when given several weeks after carcinogen exposure.[59, 117] It is possible that selenium, through its involvement in the selenoenzyme glutathione peroxidase, inhibits carcinogenesis by preventing the free oxygen radical oxidative damage to DNA. Apart from its anti-oxidant properties, selenium also enhances immune response and, in the Ames test, decreases mutagenicity of a carcinogen.[63] However, selenite has by itself been shown to induce DNA fragmentation, chromosome aberration, and DNA repair synthesis.[56] Selenate has been observed to give rise to base pair substitution.[77]

STRATEGIES FOR BREAST CANCER PREVENTION

In 1982, the National Cancer Institute (NCI) undertook comprehensive reorganization and reformulation of its programs under the Division of Cancer Prevention and Control (DCPC). A strategic model for coordinating promising research leads was evolved. It was determined that cancer prevention efforts should be directed chiefly toward those cancers of the greatest mortality and morbidity and should include cancers for which the potential risk factors associated with known common exposures have been determined. While documented environmental exposure, such as that that applies to lung cancer, has yet to be demonstrated for breast cancer, promising approaches have evolved from epidemiological and laboratory evidence that genetic, endocrine, and dietary factors may be involved. These principles have been discussed in depth by Greenwald,[45] who has reviewed the research phases for cancer prevention strategy and discussed the potential for these strategies in human prevention trials. In summary, the methodology to implement cancer prevention is as follows:

PHASE NUMBER	PHASE TITLE
I	Hypothesis development
II	Methods development
III	Controlled intervention trials
IV	Defined population studies
V	Demonstration and implementation

The phases of prevention strategy are sequential, one leading to the next.

Phase I: Hypothesis Development

Compilation of epidemiological and/or laboratory research evidence may suggest a potential intervention that could be applied to reduce a particular type of cancer. An hypothesis is then formulated to test the effectiveness of the specific intervention(s). The hypothesis will allow testing, by clinical trial, of the efficacy of the method in reducing cancer incidence morbidity and mortality rates in a defined population.

Phase II: Methods Development

A prerequisite of initiating any large-scale clinical trial is the development of suitable methodology to ensure that accurate and valid procedures are used in the trial. Pilot studies in phase II include (1) the development of an approach to recruitment and obtaining consent to the prevention trial; (2) identification of the psychosocial factors influencing this process and adherence to the trial; and (3) the development of strategies to enhance adherence during the conduct of the trial. To ensure the appropriateness and accuracy of data collected, a considerable amount of methodological research is required in the setting up of psychosocial instruments and development of questionnaires. Because prevention studies may be conducted in relatively healthy populations, side effects and toxicity are of critical importance. The handling of toxicity reporting requires the development of comprehensive computerized data bases, and the structuring of appropriate personnel to ensure quality control and the transmission of important information to the investigators. The pilot testing of specific interventions emphasizes safety in particular, because it is expected that such interventions will be used in large numbers of healthy women over long periods of time. The phase II studies allow the investigators a chance to evolve the specific methods intended for use and demonstrate their ability to manage large population studies.

Phase III: Controlled Intervention Trials

The controlled trials in a phase III study test hypotheses developed in phase I using the methodology validated in phase II. The trials test the efficacy of the specific preventive intervention in a group of individuals who have been selected to allow the interpretation of efficacy. The general principle is that the defined population in phase III studies may be more homogeneous and chosen for the ability of the investigators to study them in detail. This group may not be entirely representative of the general population. Phase III trials are instituted, preferably in a randomized fashion, to allow comparison of the intervention group to the controls. In a dietary intervention trial, for example, the controls may have no dietary advice given to them. In this case, the number of "drop-ins" (controls who adopt the dietary intervention) becomes considerably important. This may necessitate the geographical separation of the treatment group from the control group so that contamination is reduced. Alternatively, if an additive is given to the diet, a placebo arm is required.

Phase IV: Defined Population Studies

Phase IV studies measure quantitatively the impact of an efficacious intervention applied as a carefully controlled trial in a defined population. Large, distinct, well-characterized populations are chosen in such a way that the study subjects and results are representative of the ultimate target population. It is important to define the population of the study carefully so that valid inferences can be made from results and subsequently generalized to the entire target population.

In the case of breast cancer, appropriate defined populations could, for example, be chosen by risk factors, such as type of family history or breast biopsies indicating elevation of risk. Alternatively, epidemiological risk factors such as age at first pregnancy, age at menarche, or age at menopause could be used. The larger scale of phase IV studies requires broad eligibility criteria and considerable input by the community to enhance participation.

Phase V: Demonstration and Implementation

Once an intervention has proved to be efficacious in a phase IV study, it is possible to implement the intervention throughout the community and measure the public health impact of it. This phase can be reached only after prolonged and careful research studies in the preceding phases have provided results that justify such an approach. At the conclusion of phase V studies, it should be possible to demonstrate that there has been reduction, in a population with known characteristics, of both cancer morbidity and mortality.

A number of preventive approaches have sufficient epidemiological and experimental bases to allow phase II and III testing and are discussed in the remainder of this chapter.

CLINICAL TRIALS OF CANCER PREVENTION

The elements of design[35, 92] and issues relating to sample size,[31, 92] recruitment,[53] and compliance[92, 130] have been reviewed at a Chemoprevention Clinical Trials Workshop sponsored by the Chemoprevention Branch of the Division of Cancer Prevention and Control, National Cancer Institute.[106]

Design

In its most simplistic design, the trial setting out to demonstrate a reduction in cancer incidence and mortality should be controlled, randomized, and double-blind. The principles of trial design have been discussed in detail by Peto.[104] The sample size should be sufficiently large to yield a high capability for detecting worthwhile treatment effects. In addition, adequate sample size relates to achieving control of confounding factors, be they known or unknown. Sufficient numbers will ensure distribution of confounding variables between the randomized groups. The power of a trial is proportional not only to the number of participants but also to two other critical factors: the number of "events" occurring between the treatment arms and the difference in compliance between the two groups. In order to enhance the number of sufficient "events" in the trial, two approaches could be taken: observing a very long period of follow-up or, alternatively, selecting a high risk population to study where "events" are likely to occur more frequently. Difficulties arise in the planning of such trials, because it has been noted that individuals enrolling in trials (for example, the Multiple Risk Factor Intervention Trial (MRFIT)[92]) have somewhat less morbidity and mortality than those who do not enroll in trials. In addition, there may be changes in the overall disease rate occurring in any given population or geographical area. As end points accumulate exponentially rather than arithmetically, prolonged follow-up can lead to the observation of a statistically significant fact that might not have been apparent in the earlier phases of the trial. Recruitment of high risk individuals to a trial can be proposed as an attractive means of increasing the number of events likely to be observed in the time frame of the trial. Not only do the risk factors themselves need to be taken into account, but also the age of the population being studied must be considered. It is also advantageous to have measurable biochemical parameters that will correlate with the risk. There is an urgent need to develop such biochemical parameters in relation to the risk of breast cancer. An analogy could be drawn with the Coronary Primary Prevention Trial, wherein the high risk population was defined on the basis of a biochemical parameter.[31] An alternative strategy is that utilized by the Physicians Health Study,[130] in which prerandomization blood specimens were drawn from a proportion of the participating physicians. Baseline biochemical levels of the appropriate micronutrients may enhance the ability, in this trial, to define which groups are or are not benefiting from treatment.

The design of a randomized trial is crucial in maximizing the amount of information available from the sample size. The use of a fixed sample size in relation to a factorial design may be beneficial.[130] A 2×2 factorial design randomizes participants between treatment A or treatment B to specifically address one question and then within each treatment group a further randomization occurs to treatment alpha or beta to address a second scientific question. Design of this type is used in the Physicians' Health Study (PHS). The major advantage of a factorial design is the ability to answer two unrelated questions in a single trial without a large increase in costs. It is also possible to study more than two treatments simultaneously. An additional advantage exists for the use of a factorial design that may have an impact on compliance by trial participants. It is a difficult ethical question to balance the investigator's desire to test a hypothesis and the potential results of the trial, which may fill a gap in our knowledge of accepted medical practice. It is therefore essential that there is sufficient doubt about the agent being tested to allow the use of a placebo arm or an arm from which treatment is withheld in half the subjects. Such an argument might have applied to beta-carotene, which many individuals regard to be beneficial, and therefore it might become unfeasible to study it as a single agent. The introduction of an additional agent into the trial (such as aspirin in the case of the PHS study) may help to overcome some of these problems.[53]

Sample Size

In determining the sample size required for any given trial, it is necessary for the statistician, in conjunction with the clinician, to guess the likely outcome or at least to specify the smallest outcome that would be of clinical and medical importance (i.e., that the trialist would like to have a reasonable power of detecting as statistically significant). The sample size and stopping rules for clinical trials have been discussed by Beauman et al.[8] The discussions between statisticians and physicians planning to run a study must be comprehensive and detailed. It has been shown that of 71 trials reporting negative treatment results published between 1960 and 1977, 80 percent had power of less than 50 percent to detect a 25 percent reduction in the rate of end points under study.[116] It is illogical to design a trial with a power of less than 50 percent, because it is as likely to miss detecting important differences as it is to find one. Most clinical trials should strive to achieve a power of 80 percent to 90 percent to detect a clinically worthwhile and significant difference.

A sample size is dependent, in the first place, on the type of prevention study being undertaken. There are three types of prevention studies: (1) treatment trials of precancerous lesions or *in situ* lesions, seeking to observe regression; (2) intervention trials in high risk populations; and (3) trials carried out in the general population, although that population may be defined by age and/or sex. Each of these three studies requires a larger number of trial participants than the previous study in order to demonstrate the desired effect. It is clear that even modest improvements in cancer rate reduction are worthwhile. The level to which a cancer rate can be reduced can, to some extent, be calculated from the levels that can be expected based on epidemiological studies or from levels observed in laboratory studies. It would appear in the field of breast cancer prevention that a rate reduction of 20 percent to 25 percent would be very worthwhile and feasible. A particular problem arising in prevention trials is the prevalent cases; that is, cancers already present at the initiation of the study but not detectable at that time. It would be unreasonable to expect to prevent such preexistent cancers, and they will tend to dilute true differences between the treatment groups, if there are any. This can be overcome in three ways: by a concerted effort to eliminate such cases in the beginning (this is

Table 12–14. ACTUARIAL 30-YEAR RISKS OF A CONTRALATERAL BREAST CANCER (155)

Years After First Breast Cancer	Percentage
0–4	3.8
5–9	3.1
10–14	2.9
15–19	3.8
20–24	2.4
25–29	1.6
Mean risk/year	0.6

From Adair F, et al: Cancer 33:1145–1150, 1974. Reprinted by permission.

feasible in the area of breast cancer by admitting patients who have only normal clinical examination and mammography); by increasing the sample size to such a level that the dilutional effects of prevalent cases to incident cases do not occur; and by omitting from the analysis those cases in which cancer appears in the early part of the study.

The numbers of subjects required to show a statistically significant reduction in a specific high risk group (e.g., those who have already had unilateral breast cancer but are at risk for contralateral breast cancer) can be calculated from the known incidence of this event. The actuarial 5-year risk of a second breast cancer after treatment of an initial unilateral breast cancer has been well documented in a 30-year follow-up study by Adair et al.[2] (Table 12–14).

These defined actuarial risks can be used to calculate the number of subjects required in the randomized study design to show the ultimate effect of a cancer rate reduction. The sample sizes required to demonstrate a statistically significant rate reduction with "drop-outs" and "drop-ins" leading to sample dilution are indicated in Table 12–15, assuming a cancer rate for the normal population of 3/1000/year and a 20 percent dropout rate.[38]

Recruitment

In order to attain the sample sizes predicted for large cancer prevention trials, it is inevitable that multicenters will be required. Difficulty exists in recruitment for

Table 12–15. NUMBER OF SUBJECTS PROJECTED TO BE REQUIRED IN A TWO-ARM RANDOMIZED STUDY OF BREAST CANCER PREVENTION

| Rate Reduction from 3.0 | Power | |
	0.8	0.9
2.5	72,000	102,000
2.0	16,000	22,000
1.5	7,000	9,500

From Zelen M: Cancer Res 44:3151–3154, 1984. Reprinted by permission.

clinical trials of individuals known to be suffering from a specific disease; the history of such difficulty goes back to 1948, in one of the earliest randomized multicenter trials conducted in England by the Medical Research Council. The trial was designed to investigate the use of streptomycin in the treatment of pulmonary tuberculosis.[85] Since that time there have been few advances in recruitment for clinical trials. The pool of potential participants in any clinical trial is defined as the subset of the population that meets the preliminary study requirements.[8] Individuals identified within this pool are termed "contacts." The source of these contacts is from the medical institution conducting the trial, other associated institutions, outside medical agencies, patient groups, and screening programs. The contacts are subsequently subjected to a preliminary visit to ensure that they meet the study criteria. The major difficulties exist in the steps between identifying eligible patients and selecting the actual study subjects. The yield of study subjects from the contacts approached is small; it is not surprising that many trials do not achieve the requisite size and can frequently overrun the projected time period for recruitment. As a result, in order to be realistic, the number of cases promised in any clinical study must be divided by a factor of at least ten;[3, 116] in addition, the time stated to accomplish this trial should be doubled.

Investigators usually overestimate the number of patients who will qualify for a trial because they fail to consider the impact of the exclusionary criteria in the trial and the lack of willingness of the patients to participate. In the case of multicenter trials, there may be marked differences among the centers, such as variations in the types of patients seen, the numbers of patients, and their socioeconomic level, and diversity in organizational approaches in subject participation.

The methods that should be used in recruitment have been well described by Tangrea.[133] The following four major elements are required to develop a coordinated and successful recruitment with participating medical centers:

1. Formulation of a comprehensive recruitment scheme
2. Development of an organizational structure to support recruitment effort
3. Establishment of viable recruitment goals
4. Monitoring and feedback on recruitment progress

Attention to these areas allows detailed estimates of the magnitude of the recruitment effort, the identification of investigators in the coordinating center and its affiliated centers, the setting of long-term and interim recruitment goals, and rapid feedback of recruitment data to each center concerning its progress in the context of the trial. The latter course allows each center to examine its recruitment policy and alter it as appropriate. Attention to these areas of recruitment will allow investigators to overcome the major hindrance to the conduction of clinical trials in breast cancer prevention.

Compliance: Drop-in and Drop-out Rates

Noncompliance within the clinical trials can occur in two ways: the nonintervention group can put themselves on the specific intervention ("drop-ins") or, those randomized to either the intervention or, if appropriate, a placebo, can stop the intervention ("drop-outs"). These factors must be estimated with care so that the sample size is appropriately chosen.[116] Compliance in a clinical trial can be improved by randomizing only subjects who are likely to be compliant or by encouraging compliance during the trial by specific interventions designed by the investigators. The use of a run-in, that is a 1-month trial period of placebo before randomization, is a possible means to identify those who are noncompliant. They can then subsequently be excluded. In addition, it is important that the trial participants identify with the trial rather than with the agent under study. Although this concept is abstract, it will reduce focus on the proposed intervention, which would encourage individuals to "drop in." Probably the most important factor is the communication between the investigators and the study participants. Compliance may be measured by self-report questionnaires, pill counts, and, best of all, biochemical monitoring.

Organization

An ideal source to recruit subjects interested in participating in prevention trials is to be found in either screening or early detection centers [for example, the Breast Cancer Detection Demonstration Project (BCDDP), as set up by the American Cancer Society and the National Cancer Institute].[6, 133] For individual institutions, special surveillance breast programs can be set up[100] where selected risk factors can be studied in a computerized breast cancer risk registry.

The development of pilot breast cancer prevention studies and subsequent major trials will lead to a better understanding of the consent process and adherence. A great deal is known about adherence in therapeutic trials, but our knowledge of adherence to preventive medical regimens in unaffected populations remains small. Ultimately these preventive approaches may have a more profound effect on breast cancer control than the past century of therapy for the established disease.

CONCLUSIONS

At the present time no finite advice can be given regarding primary prevention. While it may seem prudent to reduce fat in the diet and increase fiber intake, there is no available evidence that this will reduce breast cancer rate. It is unwise to prescribe any of the agents discussed in this chapter until further evidence of safety and efficacy is forthcoming. Prime importance must continue to be attached to secondary prevention using breast self-examination and mammography.

References

1. Abels JC, Gorham AT, Pack GT, Rhoads CD: Metabolic studies in patients with cancer of the gastrointestinal tract. 1. Plasma vitamin A levels in patients with malignant neoplastic disease,

particularly of the gastrointestinal tract. J Clin Invest 20:749–764, 1941.

2. Adair F, Berg G, Joubert L, Robbins GF: Long-term follow up of breast cancer patients: the 30-year report. Cancer 33:1145–1150, 1974.

3. Agras WS, Bradford RM. Recruitment: an introduction. Circulation 66(suppl 1V):1V-2–1V-5, 1982.

4. Allaway WH, Kubota J, Losee F, Roth M: Selenium, molybdenum and vanadium in human blood. Arch Environ Health 16:342–348, 1968.

5. Astrup EG, Paulsen JE: Effect of retinoic acid pretreatment on 12-0-tetradecanoylphorbol-13-acetate-induced cell population kinetics and polyamine biosynthesis in hairless mouse epidermis. Carcinogenesis (London) 3:312–320, 1982.

6. Baker LH: Breast cancer detection demonstration project. Five year summary report. Cancer J Clin 32:194–225, 1982.

7. Banerjee MR: An in vitro model for neoplastic transformation of epithelial cells in an isolated whole mammary organ of the mouse. In Weber MM (ed): In Vitro Models for Cancer Research, vol. III. Boca Raton, FL, CRC Press, 1986, pp 69–114.

8. Beauman JE, Lowenson RB, Gullen WH: Corrolaries. Biometrics Note No. 4. Bethesda, MD, Office of Biometry and Epidemiology, National Eye Institute, NIH, 1974.

9. Bloch G: Nutrition assessment in-clinical trials. In Sestili M (ed): Chemoprevention Clinical Trials. Publication #85-2715. Bethesda, MD, NIH, 1984, pp 50–57.

10. Boyd NF, Cousins ML, Bayuss SE, et al: Diet modification in clinical trials: behavioral issues in the prevention of cancer. In Burish TG, Levy SM, Meyerowitz BE (eds): Nutrition, Taste Aversion and Cancer: A Biobehavioral Perspective. Hillsdale, NJ, Lawrence Erlbaum Associates (in press).

11. Bradlow HL, Michnovicz JJ: A new approach to the prevention of breast cancer. Proc Roy Soc Edin 95B:77–86, 1989.

12. Brickerhoff CE, Nagase H, Nogel JE, Harris ED: Effects of all trans-retinoic acid and 4-hydroxyphenylretinamide on synovial cells and articular cartilage. J Am Acad Dermatol 6:591–602, 1982.

13. Broghamer WL, McKonnell KP, Blotcky KP: Relationship between serum selenium levels and patients with carcinoma. Cancer 37:1384–1388, 1976.

14. Buell DN: Potential hazards of selenium as a chemopreventive agent. Semin Oncol 10:311–321, 1983.

15. Bunk MJ, Kinahan JJ, Sarkar NH: Biotransformation and protein binding of N-(4-hydroxyphenyl) retinamide in murine mammary epithelial cells. Cancer Lett 26:319–326, 1985.

16. Bunk MJ, Telang NT, Higgins PJ, Traganos F, Sarkar NH: Effect of N-(4-hydroxyphenyl)retinamide on murine mammary tumor cells in culture. Nutr Cancer 7:105–115, 1985.

17. Carroll KK: Experimental evidence of dietary factors and hormone-dependent cancers. Cancer Res 35:3374, 1975.

18. Carroll KK: Lipids and carcinogenesis. J Environ Pathol Toxicol 3:253–271, 1980.

19. Carroll KK, Hopkins GJ: Dietary polyunsaturated fat versus saturated fat in relation to mammary carcinogenesis. Lipids 14:155–158, 1979.

20. Carroll KK, Khor HT: Effects of dietary fats and dose level of 7,12-dimethylbenz(a)anthracene on mammary tumor incidence in rats. Cancer Res 30:2260–2264, 1970.

21. Carroll KK, Khor HT: Effects of level and type of dietary fat on incidence of mammary tumor induced in female Sprague-Dawley rats by 7,12-dimethylbenz(a)anthracene. Lipids 6:415–420, 1971.

22. Carter CA, Milholland RJ, Shea W, Margot M: Effect of prostaglandin synthetase inhibitor indomethacin on 7,12-dimethylbenz(a)anthracene-induced mammary tumorigenesis in rats fed different levels of fat. Cancer Res 43:3559–3562, 1983.

23. Chan PC, Cohen L: Dietary fat and growth promotion of mammary tumors. Cancer Res 35:3384–3386, 1975.

24. Chan PC, Dao TL: Enhancement of mammary carcinogenesis by a high-fat diet in Fischer, Long-Evans and Sprague-Dawley rats. Cancer Res 41:164–167, 1981.

25. Chan PC, Didato F, Cohen L: High dietary fat, elevation of serum prolactin and mammary cancer. Proc Soc Exp Biol Med 149:133–139, 1975.

26. Chan PC, Head JF, Cohen LA, Wynder EL: Influence of dietary fat on the induction of rat mammary tumors by N-nitrosomethylurea: strain differences and associated hormonal changes. J Natl Cancer Inst 59:1279–1283, 1977.

27. Chatterjee M, Banjerjee MR: N-nitrosodiethylamine-induced nodule-like alveolar lesion and its prevention by a retinoid in BALB/c mouse mammary glands in the whole organ in culture. Carcinogenesis 3:801–807, 1982.

28. Chytil F, Ong DE: Cellular retinol and retinoic acid-binding proteins in vitamin A action. Fed Proc 38:2510–2514, 1979.

29. Coezy E, Borgna JL, Rochefort H: Tamoxifen and metabolites in MCF7 cells: correlation between binding to estrogen receptor and inhibition of cell growth. Cancer Res 42:317–323, 1982.

30. Cohen LA, Thompson DO, Teas J: Seaweed blocks the mammary tumor promoting effects of high fat diets. Denver, Breast Cancer Research Conference, March, 1983, Poster #52.

31. Coronary Drug Project Research Group: Influence of adherence to treatment and response of cholesterol on mortality in the Coronary Drug Project. New Engl J Med 303:1038–1041, 1980.

32. Dao TL, Sinha DK, Nemoto T, Patel J: Effect of estrogen and progesterone on cellular replication of human breast tumors. Cancer Res 42:359–362, 1982.

33. DeOme KB, Faulkin LJ, Bern HA, Blair PB: Development of mammary tumors from hyperplastic alveolar nodules transplanted into gland-free mammary fat pads of female c3H mice. Cancer Res 19:515–520, 1959.

34. Drasar BS, Irving D: Environmental factors and cancer of the colon and breast. Br J Cancer 27:167–172, 1973.

35. Edwards BK: Overview: design issues in chemoprevention trials. In Sestili MA: Chemoprevention Trials: Problems and Solutions. NIH Publication No. 85–2715, pp 59–61, 1984.

36. Edwards DP, Murthy SR, McGuire WL: Effects of estrogen and anti-estrogen on DNA polymerase in human breast cancer. Cancer Res 40:1722–1726, 1980.

37. Fishman J, Bradlow HL, Fukushima DH, O'Connor I, Rosenfeld R, Gracpel GJ, Elston R, Lynch H: Abnormal estrogen conjugation in women at risk for familial breast cancer at the preovulatory stage of the menstrual cycle. Cancer Res 43:1884–1890, 1983.

38. Freiman JA, Chalmers TC, Smith H Jr, Kuebler RR: The importance of beta, type II error and sample size in the design and interpretation of the randomized control trial: survey of 71 "negative" trials. N Engl J Med 299:690–694, 1978.

39. Fuchs E, Green H: Regulation of terminal differentiation of cultured human keratinocytes by vitamin A. Cell 25:617–625, 1981.

40. Fujimaki Y: Formation of carcinoma in albino rats fed on deficient diets. J Cancer Res 10:469–477, 1926.

41. Furr BJA: Future prospects in the treatment of hormone responsive cancer. Clin Oncol 1:289–307, 1982.

42. Furr BJA, Jordan VC: The pharmacology and clinical uses of tamoxifen. Pharm Ther 25:127–205, 1984.

43. Glover JR: Selenium and its industrial toxicology. Industr Med 39:50–54, 1970.

44. Green MD, Whybourne AM, Taylor LW, et al: Effects of antiestrogens on the growth and cell cycle kinetics of cultured human mammary carcinoma cells. In Sutherland RL, Jordan VC (eds): Nonsteroidal Antiestrogens. Sydney, Academic Press, 1981, pp 397–412.

45. Greenwald P: Prevention of cancer. In DeVita V, Hellman S, Rosenberg S (eds): Principles and Practice of Oncology, ed 2. Philadelphia, Lippincott, 1983.

46. Griffin AC: Role of selenium in the chemoprevention of cancer. Adv Cancer Res 29:419–442, 1979.

47. Groham S, Marshall J, Mettlin C, Rzepka T, Nemoto T, Byers T: Diet in the epidemiology of breast cancer. Am J Epidemiol 116:68–75, 1982.

48. Grubbs CJ, Moon RC, Sporn MB, Newton DL: Inhibition of mammary cancer by retinyl methyl ether. Cancer Res 37:599–602, 1977.

49. Gullino PM, Pettigrew HM, Grantham FH: N-nitrosomethylurea as mammary gland carcinogen in rats. J Natl Cancer Inst 54:401, 1975.

50. Harr JR: Selenium toxicity in rats. In Muth OH (ed): Selenium in Biomedicine. Westport, CT, AV1, 1967, pp 153–178.

51. Hay CRM, Durber AP, Saynor R: Effect of fish oil on platelet kinetics in patients with ischaemic heart disease. Lancet i:1269–1272, 1982.
52. Helzlsouer KJ: Selenium and cancer prevention. Semin Oncol 10:305–310, 1983.
53. Hennekens CH, Eberlein K: Physicians Health Study Research Group: A randomized trial of aspirin and beta-carotene among US Physicians. Prevent Med 14:165–168, 1985.
54. Hillyard LA, Abraham S: Effect of dietary fatty acids in growth of mammary adenocarcinomas in mice and rats. Cancer Res 39:4430–4437, 1979.
55. Hirayama T. Epidemiology of breast cancer with special reference to the role of diet. Prevent Med 7:173–195, 1978.
56. Ho LW, Koropotneck J, Stich HF: The mutagenicity and cytotoxicity of selenite, "activated" selenite and selenate for normal and DNA repair-deficient human fibroblasts. Mutat Res 49:305–312, 1978.
57. Horwitz, KB, McGuire WL: Nuclear mechanisms of estrogen action. J Biol Chem 253:8185–8191, 1978.
58. Ip C: Ability of dietary fat to overcome the resistance of mature female rats to 7,12-dimethylbenz(a)anthracene-induced mammary tumorigenesis. Cancer Res 40:2785–2789; 1980.
59. Ip C: Factors influencing the anticarcinogenic efficacy of selenium in dimethylbenz(a)anthracene-induced mammary tumorigenesis in rats. Cancer Res 41:2683–2686, 1981.
60. Ip C: Prophylaxis of mammary neoplasia by selenium supplementation in the initiation and promotion phases of chemical carcinogenesis. Cancer Res 41:4386–4390, 1981.
61. Ip C: Selenium inhibition of chemical carcinogenesis. Fed Proc 44:2573–2578, 1985.
62. Jacobs MM: Effects of selenium on chemical carcinogenesis. Rev Med 9:362–367, 1980.
63. Jacobs MM, Matney TS, Griffin AC: Inhibitory effects of selenium on the mutagenicity of 2-acetylaminofluorene (AAF) and AAF derivatives. Cancer Lett 2:319–322, 1977.
64. Jordan VC: Effect of tamoxifen (ICI 46,474) on initiation and growth of DMBA-induced rat mammary carcinomata. Eur J Cancer Clin Oncol 12:419–424, 1976.
65. Jordan VC: Use of DMBA-induced rat mammary carcinoma system for the evaluation of tamoxifen treatment as a potential adjuvant therapy. Revs Endocr Cancer Oct suppl:49–55, 1978.
66. Jordan VC, Allen KE, Dix CJ: Pharmacology of tamoxifen in laboratory animals. Cancer Treat Rep 64:745–759, 1980.
67. Jordan VC, Dix CJ, Allen KE: Effects of antiestrogens in carcinogen-induced rat mammary cancer. In Sutherland RL, Jordan VC (eds): Non-steroidal Antiestrogens. Sydney, Academic Press, 1981, pp 260–280.
68. Karmali RA: Lipid nutrition, prostaglandins and cancer. In Lands WEM (ed) Biochemistry of Arachidonic Acid Metabolism. Boston, Martinus Nijihoff, 1985, pp 203–212.
69. Karmali RA, Cohen LA: Personal communication (unpublished).
70. Karmali RA, Marsh J, Fuchs C: Effect of omega-3 fatty acids on growth of rat mammary tumor. J Natl Cancer Inst 73:457–461, 1984.
71. Killackey NW, Hakes TB, Pierce VK: Endometrial adenocarcinoma in breast cancer patients receiving antiestrogens. Cancer Treat Rep 69:237–238, 1985.
72. Kolonel LN, Hankin JH, Lee J, Chusy, Nomura A, Hinds MW: Nutrient intakes in relation to cancer incidence in Hawaii. Br J Cancer 44:332–339, 1981.
73. Krogh A, Krogh M: A study of the diet and metabolism of Eskimos undertaken in 1908 on an expedition to Greenland. Medd Groenl 51:1–52, 1913.
74. Lasnitzki I: The influence of a hyper-vitaminosis on the effects of 20-methylcholanthrene on mouse prostate glands grown in vitro. Br J cancer 9:438–439, 1955.
75. Lipid Research Clinics Program: The Lipid Research Clinics Coronary Primary Prevention Trial results, 1. Reduction of incidence of coronary heart disease. JAMA 251:351–364, 1984.
76. Lippman ME, Bolan G, Huff K: The effects of estrogens and antiestrogens on hormone responsive human breast cancer in long-term tissue culture. Cancer Res 36:4595–4601, 1976.
77. Lofroth G, Ames BN: Mutagenicity of inorganic compounds in salmonella typhirium: arsenic, chromium and selenium. Mutat Res 53:65–66, 1978.
78. Lubin JH, Burns PE, Blot WJ, Ziegler RG, Lees AW, Fraumeni JF Jr: Dietary factors and breast cancer risk. Int J Cancer 28:685–689, 1981.
79. MacMahon B, Cole P: The ovarian etiology of human breast cancer. Rec Results Cancer Res 39:185–192, 1972.
80. MacMahon B, Cole P, Brown J: Etiology of human breast cancer: a review. J Natl Cancer Inst 50:21–42, 1973.
81. McConnell KP, Jager RM, Bland KI, Blotcky AJ: The relationship of dietary selenium and breast cancer. J Surg Oncol 15:67–70, 1980.
82. McCormick DL, Menta RG, Thompson CA, Dinger N, Caldwell JA, Moon RC: Enhanced inhibition of mammary carcinogenesis by combined treatment with N-(4-hydroxyphenyl)-retinamide and ovariectomy. Cancer Res 42:508–512, 1982.
83. McCormick DL, Moon RC: Retinoid-tamoxifen interaction in mammary cancer chemoprevention. Carcinogenesis 7:193–196, 1986.
84. McCormick DL, Sowell ZL, Thompson CA, Moon RC: Inhibition by retinoid and ovariectomy of additional primary malignancies in the rat following surgical removal of the first mammary cancer. Cancer 51:594–599, 1983.
85. Medical Research Council: Streptomycin treatment of pulmonary tuberculosis. Br Med J 11:769–782, 1948.
86. Medina D, Shepherd F: Selenium-mediated inhibition of 7,12-dimethylbenz(a)anthracene-induced mouse mammary tumorigenesis. Carcinogenesis 2:451–455, 1981.
87. Miller A, Kelley A, Choi N, Matthews V, Morgan RW, Munan L, Burch JD, Feather J, Howe GR, Jain M: A study of diet and breast cancer. Am J Epidemiol 107:499–509, 1978.
88. Moon RC, Grubbs CJ, Sporn MB: Inhibition of 7,12-dimethylbenz(a)anthracene-induced mammary carcinogenesis by retinyl acetate. Cancer Res 36:2626–2630, 1976.
89. Moon RC, Grubbs CJ, Sporn MB, Goodman DG: Retinyl acetate inhibits mammary carcinogenesis induced by N-methyl-N-nitrosourea. Nature 267:620–621, 1977.
90. Moon RC, Thompson HJ, Becci PJ, Grubbs CJ, Gander RJ, Newton DL, Smith JM, Phillips SL, Henderson WR, Mullen LT, Brown CC: N-(4-hydroxyphenyl)retinamide, a new retinoid for prevention of breast cancer in the rat. Cancer Res 39:1339–1346, 1979.
91. Moore T: Vitamin A. New York, Elsevier, 1957.
92. Multiple Risk Factor Intervention Trial: Risk factor changes and mortality results. JAMA 248:1465–1477, 1982.
93. National Academy of Sciences, Committee on Diet, Nutrition and Cancer: Dietary factors in cancer. Washington, DC, National Academy Press, 1982, p 496.
94. National Research Council Food and Nutrition Board: Recommended daily allowances, 9: 1980, pp 162–163.
95. Nettesheim P: Inhibition of carcinogenesis by retinoids. Can Med Assoc J 122:757–766, 1980.
96. Nelson AA, Fitzhugh OG, Calvery HO: Liver tumors following cirrhosis caused by selenium in rats. Cancer Res 3:230–236, 1943.
97. Nielsen NH, Hansen JPH: Breast cancer in Greenland—selected epidemiological, clinical and histological features. Eur J Cancer Res Clin Oncol 98:287–299, 1980.
98. Novaldex Adjuvant Trial Organization: Controlled trial of tamoxifen as adjuvant agent in management of early breast cancer. Lancet 1:257–261, 1983.
99. Osborne MP, Bradlow HL, Hershcopf R, Fishman J: A potential marker for the risk of breast cancer: abnormal 16-alpha-hydroxylation of estradiol. Society of Surgical Oncology, 37th Annual Meeting, New York, 1984, Abstract 36.
100. Osborne MP, Crowe JP: The identification of enhanced risk patients and their management in a special surveillance breast clinic. In Ariel IM, Cleary JB (eds): Breast Cancer: Diagnosis and Treatment. New York, McGraw Hill, 1987.
101. Osborne MP, Karmali RA, Hershkopf RJ, Bradlow HL, Kourides JA, Williams WR, Rosen PP, Fishman J: Omega-3 fatty acids: Modulation of estrogen metabolism and potential for breast cancer prevention. Cancer Invest 8:629–631, 1988.
102. Osborne MP, Telang NT, Kurihara H, Bradlow HL: Risk-enhanced metabolism of estradiol in explant cultures of benign human mammary tissue. Proc Am Assoc Cancer Res 29:4071, 1988.

103. Osborne MP, Telang NT, Wong GY, Modak MJ, Bradlow HL: Breast cancer-dependent elevation in constitutive ras proto-oncogene expression and estradiol 16 alpha-hydroxylation in benign human mammary tissue: Modulation by fatty acids. Proc Am Assoc Cancer Res 30:900, 1989.

104. Peto R: Statistical aspects of cancer trials. *In* Halnan KE (ed): Treatment of Cancer. London, Chapman and Hall, 1982, pp 867–870.

105. Phillips RL: Role of life-style and dietary habits in risk of cancer among Seventh Day Adventists. Cancer Res 35:3513–3522, 1975.

106. Pocock SJ: Size of cancer clinical trials and stopping rules. Br J Cancer 38:757–766, 1978.

107. Ritchie G: The direct inhibition of prostaglandin synthetase of human breast cancer tumour tissue by Novaldex. Revs Endocr Cancer Oct suppl:35–39, 1978.

108. Rizek RL: Food supply studies and consumption survey statistics on fat in United States diets. Cancer Res 41:3729–3730, 1981.

109. Robertson DSE: Selenium—possible teratogen. Lancet 1:518–519, 1970.

110. Robinson MF, Godfrey PJ, Thomson CD, Rea HM, van Rij AM: Blood selenium and glutathione peroxidase activity in normal subjects and in surgical patients with and without cancer in New Zealand. Am J Clin Nutr 32:1477–1485, 1979.

111. Saffiotti U, Montesano R, Sellakumr AR: Experiments in cancer of the lung. Inhibition by vitamin A of the induction of tracheobronchial squamous metaplasia and squamous cell tissues. Cancer 20:857–864, 1967.

112. Sakurai H, Tsuchiya K: A tentative recommendation for the maximum daily intake of selenium. Environ Physiol Biochem 5:107–118, 1975.

113. Sayner R, Verel D: Eicosapentaenoic acid, bleeding time and serum lipids. Lancet ii:272, 1982.

114. Sayner R, Verel D: Eskimos and their diets. Lancet i:1335, 1983.

115. Schneider J, Kinne D, Fracchia A, Pierce V, Anderson KE, Bradlow HL, Fishman J: Abnormal oxidative metabolism of estradiol in women with breast cancer. Proc Natl Acad Sci 79:3047–3051, 1982.

116. Schork MA, Remington RD: The determination of sample size in treatment-control comparisons for chronic disease studies in which drop-out or non-adherence is a problem. J Chron Dis 20:233–239, 1967.

117. Schrauzer GN, Ishmael D: Effects of selenium and of arsenic on the genesis of spontaneous mammary tumors in inbred C3H mice. Ann Clin Lab Sci 4:441–447, 1974.

118. Schrauzer GN, McGinness JE, Kuehn K: effects of temporary selenium supplementation on the genesis of spontaneous mammary tumors in inbred female C3H/St mice. Carcinogenesis 1:199–201, 1980.

119. Schrauzer GN, White DA, Schneider CJ: Cancer mortality correlation studies. III. Statistics associated with selenium intakes. Bioinorg Chem 7:23–34, 1977.

120. Scott M: Workshop on the Role of Novaldex in the Treatment of Non-Malignant Conditions and in the Prevention of Breast Cancer. Washington DC, September 12–13, 1985.

121. Shamberger RJ: Relationship of selenium to cancer: Inhibitory effect of selenium on carcinogenesis. J Natl Cancer Inst 44:931–936, 1970.

122. Shamberger RJ, Rukovena E, Longfield AK, Tytko SA, Deodhar S, Willis CE: Antioxidants and cancer. 1. Selenium in the blood of normals and cancer patients. J Natl Cancer Inst 50:867–870, 1973.

123. Shamberger RJ, Willis CE: Selenium distribution and human cancer mortality. CRC Crit Rev Lab Sci 2:211–221, 1971.

124. Shukla VKS, Clausen J, Egsgaard H, et al: The content of fat and polyenoic and dienoic fatty acids in sources of the arctic diet. Fette Seifen Anstrichmittel 82:193, 1980.

125. Silverman J, Katayama S, Radok R, Levenstein MJ, Weisburger JH: Effect of short-term administration of N-(4-hydroxy-phenyl)-all-trans-retinamide on chemically induced mammary tumors. Nutr Cancer 4:186–191, 1983.

126. Sporn MB, Dunlop NM, Newton DL, Smith JM: Prevention of chemical carcinogenesis by vitamin A and its synthetic analogs (retinoids). Fed Proc 35:1332–1338, 1976.

127. Sporn MB, Newton DL: Chemoprevention of cancer with retinoids. Fed Proc 38:2528–2534, 1979.

128. Sporn MB, Newton DL, Roberts AB: Retinoids and suppression of the effects of polypeptide transforming factors—a new molecular approach to chemoprevention in cancer. *In* Sartorelli AC, Laso S, Bertino JR (eds): Molecular Actions and Targets for Cancer Chemotherapeutic Agents. New York, Academic Press, 1981, pp 541–544.

129. Sporn M, Roberts AB: Role of retinoids in differentiation and carcinogenesis. Cancer Res 43:3034–3040, 1983.

130. Stampfer M, Buring J, Willett W, Rosner B, Eberlein K, Hennekens CH: The 2x2 factorial design: its application to a randomized trial of aspirin and carotene in US Physicians. Stat Med 4:111–116, 1985.

131. Stefansson V: Cancer: Disease of Civilization? New York, Hillard Wang, 1960.

132. Sufler JW, Ehrich WE, Hudyma G, Muellen G: Thyroid adenomas in rats receiving selenium. Science 103:762, 1946.

133. Tangrea JA: Recruitment: A perspective for multicenter clinical trials. *In* Sestili A (ed): Chemoprevention Clinical Trials. Publication # 85–2715. Bethesda, MD, NIH 1984, pp 44–48.

134. Tannenbaum A: The genesis and growth of tumors. III. Effects of a high fat diet. Cancer Res 2:468–475, 1942.

135. Teas T, Harbison ML, Gelman RS: Dietary seaweed as a protective factor in DMBA induced mammary carcinogenesis. Breast Cancer Research Conference, Denver, March, 1983, poster 53.

136. Telang NT: Fatty acid-induced modifications of mouse mammary epithelium as studied in an organ culture and cell culture system. *In* Ip C, Birt DF, Rogers AE, Mettlin C (eds): Dietary Fat and Cancer. New York: Alan R Liss, 1986, pp 707–728.

137. Telang NT, Banerjee MR, Iyer AP, Kundu, AB: Neoplastic transformation of epithelial cells in whole mammary gland in vitro. Proc Natl Acad Sci 76:5886–5890, 1979.

138. Telang NT, Basu A, Kurihara H, Axelrod D, Modak M, Osborne MP: Molecular effects of chemical carcinogens on explant cultures of human mammary terminal duct lobular units (TDLU). Breast Cancer Res Treat 9:28, 1987.

139. Telang NT, Basu A, Kurihara H, Osborne MP, Modak MJ: Modulation in the expression of murine mammary tumor virus, ras proto-oncogene and of alveoler hyperplasia by fatty acids in mouse mammary explant-cultures. Anticancer Res 8:971–976, 1988.

140. Telang NT, Basu A, Modak MJ, Bradlow HL, Osborne MP: Fatty acid-induced modulation of molecular and metabolic markers of chemical carcinogenesis in human mammary explant cultures. Proc Am Assoc Cancer Res 30:694, 1989.

141. Telang NT, Bockman RS, Sarkar NH: Fatty acid-induced modification of mouse mammary alveolar lesions in organ culture. Carcinogenesis 5:1123–1127, 1984.

142. Telang NT, Sarkar NH: Long-term survival of adult mouse mammary glands in culture and their response to a retinoid. Cancer Res 43:4891–4900, 1983.

143. Telang NT, Sarkar NH: Effects of modulators of mammary tumorigenesis on a drug resistant mouse mammary epithelial cell line. Proc Am Assoc Cancer Res 27:93, 1986.

144. Thompson HJ, IP C: New strategies for cancer chemoprevention by diffluoro methylornithene (DFMO) and selenite. Proc Am Assoc Cancer Res 30:173, 1989.

145. Thompson HJ, Becci PJ: Selenium inhibition of N-methyl-N-nitrosourea-induced mammary carcinogenesis. J Natl Cancer Inst 65:1299–1301, 1980.

146. Todaro GJ, Delarco JE, Sporn MB: Retinoids block phenotypic cell formation produced by sarcoma growth factor. Nature (Lond) 276:272–274, 1978.

147. Trentham DE, Brinckerhoff CE: Augmentation of collagen arthritis by synthetic analogues of retinoic acid. J Immunol 129:2668–2672, 1982.

148. Tscherkes LA, Volgarev MN, Aptehar SG: Selenium caused tumors. Acta Chir Intern Contra Cancrum 19:632–633, 1963.

149. Turcot-Lemay L, Kelly P: Characterization of estradiol, progesterone, and prolactin receptors in nitrosomethylurea-induced mammary tumors and effect of antiestrogen treatment on the development and growth of these tumors. Cancer Res 40:3232–3240, 1980.

150. Venugopal B, Luckey TD: Toxicity of Group VI metals and metalloids: metal toxicity in mammals. Semin Oncol 10:311–321, 1983.

151. Verma AK, Shapas BG, Rice HM, Boutwell RK: Correlation of the inhibition by retinoids of tumor promoter-induced mouse epidermal ornithine decarboxylase activity and of skin tumor promotion. Cancer Res 39:419–425, 1979.
152. Welsch CW, Aylsworth CF: Enhancement of murine mammary tumorigenesis by feeding high levels of dietary fat: a hormonal mechanism? J Natl Cancer Inst 70:215–221, 1983.
153. Welsch CW, DeHoog JV, Moon RC: Inhibition of mammary tumorigenesis in nulliparous C3H mice by chronic feeding of the synthetic retinoid N-(4-hydroxyphenyl)retinamide. Carcinogenesis 4:1185–1187, 1983.
154. Welsch CW, Goodrich-Smith M, Brown CK, Green HD, Hamel EJ: Selenium and the genesis of murine mammary tumors. Carcinogenesis 2:519–522, 1981.
155. Welsch CW, Goodrich-Smith M, Brown CK, Mackie D, Johnson D: 2-bromo-alpha-ergocryptine (CB-154) and tamoxifen (ICI 46,474) induced suppression of the genesis of mammary carcinomas in female rats treated with 7,12-dimethylbenzanthracene DMBA: a comparison. Oncology 39:88–92, 1982.
156. Westin EH, Song-Staal F, Gelman ET, Favera RD, Papas TS, Lautenberger JA, Eva A, Reddy EP, Tronick SR, Aaronson SA, Gallo RC: Expression of cellular homologues of retroviral oncogenes in human hematopoietic cells. Proc Natl Acad Sci 79:2490–2494, 1982.
157. Wilber CG: Toxicology of selenium. Rev Clin Toxicol 17:171–230, 1980.
158. Willett WC, Polk BF, Morris SJ, Stampfer MJ, Pressel S, Rosner B, Taylor JO, Schneider K, Hames CG: Prediagnostic serum selenium and risk of cancer. Lancet ii:130–133, 1983.
159. Williams WR, Osborne MP: Familial aspects of breast cancer. In Harris JR, Hellman S, Henderson IC, Kinne DW (eds): Breast Diseases. Philadelphia, JB Lippincott, 1987, pp 109–120.
160. Wolbach SB, Howe PR: Tissue changes following deprivation of fat soluble A vitamin. J Exp Med 42:753–777, 1925.
161. Wynder EL, MacCormick F, Hill P, Cohen LA, Chan PC, Weisburger JH: Nutrition and the etiology and prevention of cancer. Cancer Detect Prev 1:293–310, 1976.
162. Yang G, Wang S, Zhou R, Sun S: Endemic selenium intoxication of humans in China. Am J Clin Nutr 37:872–881, 1983.
163. Zelen M: Workshop on chemoprevention of breast cancer. Cancer Res 44:3151–3154, 1984.

Chapter 13

FAMILIAL BREAST CANCER, FAMILY CANCER SYNDROMES, AND PREDISPOSITION TO BREAST NEOPLASIA

Henry T. Lynch, M.D., Joseph N. Marcus, M.D., Patrice Watson, Ph.D., and Jane Lynch, B.S.N., R.N.

Study of the causes of breast cancer has received greater attention than that given to the causes of any other form of cancer in humans. Its familial aggregation was first reported in the Roman medical literature of 100 A.D.[53] In the 1860s, Paul Broca described an excess of breast cancer in combination with gastrointestinal tract cancer in multiple generations of his wife's family (Fig. 13–1).[9]

Breast cancer's etiology is exceedingly complex. Factors that are generally agreed to increase breast cancer (BC) risk include early age of menarche, late menopause, late age at first pregnancy (with protection afforded by full-term pregnancy prior to age 20), nulliparity, obesity, personal history of unilateral BC with corresponding risk to the contralateral breast, a personal history of a benign breast biopsy with histological features showing atypical epithelial hyperplasia, the presence of lobular carcinoma *in situ* and intraductal carcinoma, mammographic evidence of severe dysplasia, high animal fat and protein diet, and finally, a positive family history of BC.

We will attempt to provide a frame of reference for comprehending breast cancer etiology in the context of genetic factors, although our knowledge of the role of primary genetic factors in breast cancer etiology is extremely limited.

SPORADIC, FAMILIAL, AND HEREDITARY BREAST CANCER

Definition

Our series of more than 350 breast cancer patients undergoing treatment in our oncology clinic, all of them with thorough family histories, has provided a valuable resource of cases with a well documented negative family history [*sporadic* cases of breast cancer (SBC)] and cases with a positive family history evidencing *familial* or *hereditary* breast cancer (FBC or HBC). We define SBC, FBC, and HBC as follows:

Sporadic breast cancer: A breast cancer case with no family history of breast carcinoma through two generations involving siblings, offspring, parents, aunts and uncles, and both sets of grandparents.

Familial breast cancer: A breast cancer case with a family history including one or more first or second degree relatives with breast cancer that does not fit the hereditary breast cancer definition.

Hereditary breast cancer: A breast cancer case with a positive family history of breast cancer and, sometimes, related cancers (e.g., ovary) with high incidence and a distribution in the pedigree that is consistent with an autosomal dominant, highly penetrant, cancer susceptibility factor. Other factors that support the HBC classification include frequent early age at onset (premenopausal onset), an excess of bilateral breast cancer, and other multiple primary cancer expression.

Frequency of Sporadic, Familial, and Hereditary Breast Cancer

Using the consecutive series of patients with histologically verified breast cancer in our oncology clinic, we attempted to comprehend the frequency of sporadic, familial, and hereditary breast cancer.[52] Figure 13–2 depicts the change in frequency of the respective sporadic, familial, and hereditary breast cancer categories following an intensive follow-up of the original cohort of 225 consecutive breast cancer patients. This updated cohort plus 103 new patients revealed that 68 percent of 328 probands studied were sporadic, 23 percent were familial, and 9 percent were hereditary.[51]

These estimates are tentative and may considerably underestimate the frequency of hereditary breast cancer. The sporadic set includes cases with very few female relatives and cases with little or no information on the

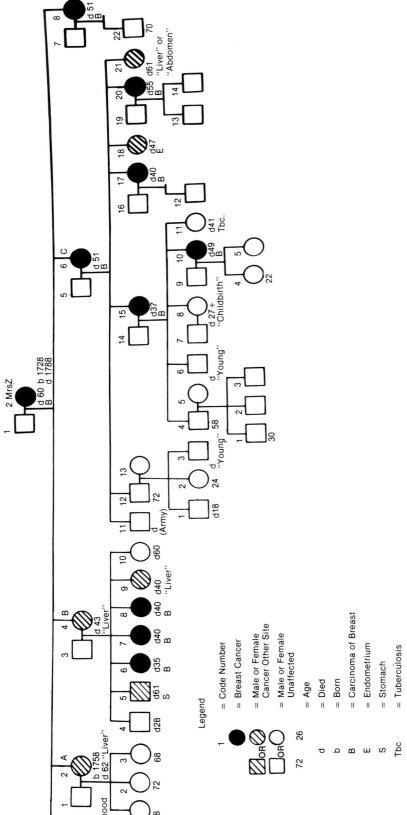

Figure 13–1. Pedigree chart of Broca's family constructed from a review of his original paper published in 1866. (From Lynch HT, et al: JAMA 222:1631, 1972. Reprinted by permission.)

Legend

1	= Code Number
●	= Breast Cancer
◐or◙	= Male or Female Cancer Other Site
□or○	= Male or Female Unaffected
72 26	= Age
d	= Died
b	= Born
B	= Carcinoma of Breast
E	= Endometrium
S	= Stomach
Tbc	= Tuberculosis

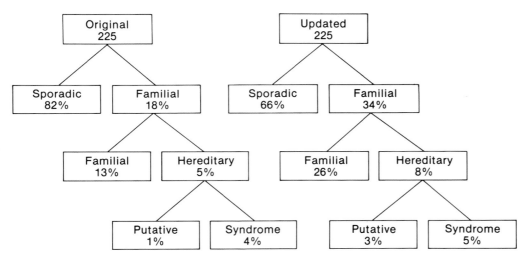

Figure 13–2. Schematic depicting frequency of sporadic, familial, and hereditary breast cancer as originally documented in a consecutively ascertained series of patients and with findings (updated) after intensive follow-up of these same patients. (From Lynch HT, Lynch JF: Cancer Genet Cytogenet 22:369, 1986. Reprinted by permission.)

medical history of family members (for example, cases in which the proband was adopted, cases in which family members were uncooperative with the family study, and cases in which family members were uninformed about predecessors' medical histories). The familial group includes several cases in which the cancer incidence in the family was suggestive of HBC but insufficient to actually classify the family as HBC. On the other hand, the HBC group may include some families that represent fortuitous aggregations of breast cancer in a pattern consistent with segregation of a dominant susceptibility gene. We hope to recontact and restudy all the families in the future to determine the extent to which the classification system is effective in indicating breast cancer risk. This will allow revision of the estimate of the frequency of HBC. We predict that the estimate will be increased during this revision process, since new information will be more likely to move a family into the HBC group than out of it.

RISK FACTORS IN FAMILIAL AND HEREDITARY BREAST CANCER

Increased Risk with Positive Family History

Studies by investigators from all parts of the world have shown so-called familial aggregations of breast cancer.[46, 57] Consensus suggests that the presence of breast cancer in a first degree relative increases a woman's risk of developing breast cancer by two- to three-fold.[80] Sattin et al.[90] found that the relative risk (RR) to a woman with an affected first degree relative was 2.3; to women with an affected second degree relative, it was 1.5; and to women with both an affected mother and sister, the RR was 14. Ottman et al.[77] studied breast cancer risk to sisters of breast cancer patients in a population-based series of patients diagnosed in Los Angeles County between 1971 and 1975. They observed that sisters of patients with bilateral breast cancer diagnosed at age 50 years or younger had an RR = 5; the risk increased for sisters of bilateral patients diagnosed at age 40 years or younger (RR = 10.5). Sisters of

unilateral patients diagnosed at 50 years or younger did not show a significantly increased breast cancer risk. However, sisters of unilateral patients diagnosed at age 40 years or younger had an RR = 2.4. These studies clearly indicate the existence of families in the general population who show a statistical predisposition to breast cancer.

These epidemiological studies of risk associated with a positive family history have not assumed any specific type of genetic mechanism to account for these results.

Heterogeneity in Risk Factors

We believe that breast cancer risk is heterogeneous in both the positive family history group and the negative family history group. In the latter group, most individuals will have a low risk for breast cancer, but a few will be at very high risk. For example, a woman might have no breast cancer–affected first degree relatives, but her father might be a member of an hereditary breast cancer (HBC) family. If his mother and/or sisters were affected, in the context of an HBC family, he would have a 50 percent chance of carrying the HBC trait, although it might not affect his cancer risk. If he were carrying the gene, he would have a 50 percent chance of transmitting it to his daughters, resulting in high breast cancer risk to his daughters despite their "negative" family history. The positive family history group contains members of HBC families at very high risk for breast cancer, as well as women who are very unlikely to carry any genetic traits associated with high risk. We would infer a great difference in risk between two women with breast cancer–affected daughters, one with breast cancer–affected sisters and mother, and the other with breast cancer–affected sisters-in-law and mother-in-law. These sorts of distinctions in risk status can only be made at present through genetically informed studies of extended families; we believe that they are crucial to the process of understanding the etiology of breast cancer.

There is considerable confusion in the BC literature with respect to the manner in which host factors may interact with other risk factors in BC etiology. We are confident that in some families, there is a genetically transmitted breast cancer susceptibility segregating as an autosomal dominant trait. Is there increased BC risk associated with a positive family history of BC in families lacking evidence for such a major gene effect? In HBC cases and/or other positive family history cases, is the age-specific BC risk dependent on the age of BC onset in affected family members? Do environmental risk factors such as diet and reproductive history have the same impact on HBC gene carriers as they do in noncarriers? Knowledge on these issues is crucial to developing targeted surveillance, prevention, and management programs. However, we are not aware of any well-designed, genetic/epidemiological investigations that have adequately appraised these BC risk factors in the context of HBC to enable calculation of a valid and reliable BC risk factor profile.

For genetic/epidemiological purposes, simplifying family history to the point of a dichotomy (positive vs. negative) obscures essential pedigree information. An empirical risk estimate, based on the presence of one or more BC-affected close relatives, does not take into consideration such important features as the age of onset of BC, the presence or absence of bilaterality, the paternal family history of BC, or the presence of other forms of cancer in the family. The fact of the matter is that the familial or genetic risk for BC shows extraordinary heterogeneity.

First Term Pregnancy and HBC Risk

In an attempt to determine whether age at first pregnancy might influence age of onset of BC and its risk in patients with HBC, we studied the age at first pregnancy and age of onset of BC among 162 females at 50 percent genetic risk for HBC, 72 of whom had already developed the disease.[54] We then compared these patients to the then 154 consecutively ascertained BC patients from the Creighton Cancer Center.

Findings showed that within the hereditary subset, early age at first term pregnancy did not demonstrate a "protective" effect; that is, age at first pregnancy did not show a significant positive correlation with the proportion of females affected by the disease (Fig. 13–3). Among the females from the HBC population who had been diagnosed with the disease, early age at first full-term pregnancy was not significantly correlated with an early onset of BC, whereas those from the consecutive series did show a significantly earlier age at diagnosis with an earlier age at first pregnancy (Figs. 13–4 and 13–5). Age at diagnosis of BC in the hereditary subset was not significantly different in parous vs. nulliparous females.

While based on a limited sample, our results illustrate significant differences between HBC and breast cancer in the population at large with regard to the effects of pregnancy. First, the generally accepted dictum of an early first term pregnancy providing a protective effect against the development of breast cancer may not be applicable to the hereditary population. Second, although Woods et al.[108] reported an earlier age at breast cancer diagnosis with an earlier age of first term pregnancy, and an earlier age of diagnosis in nulliparous than in parous females, these relationships were not found in the hereditary population. These observations together give more credence to our hypothesis of distinct biological differences between hereditary and sporadic forms of breast cancer.

Age of Onset and HBC Risk

Breast cancer diagnosis in young women from the general population is rare.[28] One hundred and thirty thousand women in the United States manifested breast cancer (BC) in 1987.[94] Interpolation of age of onset distribution from the SEER tumor registry indicates that approximately 6 percent (7800) of these patients were younger than age 40 at time of diagnosis, and 2 percent of patients were younger than age 30 at time of diagnosis.[109]

It has long been recognized that members of HBC pedigrees show a significantly earlier age of BC onset (approximately age 44 years) when compared to BC patients from the general population (approximately age 62).[28] We have recent experience in the study of families who were noteworthy for clustering of remarkably early onset breast cancer, with multiple cases occurring in patients in their 20s and 30s. In some of these pedigrees, these extraordinarily early onset BC occurrences ranged through three and four generations. These rather unusual observations prompted us to investigate the age of onset of breast cancer in 329 breast cancer probands who were consecutively ascertained from our oncology clinic. In order to avoid bias of ascertainment, patients with known proneness to BC in their families prior to their initial clinic visit were excluded from this analysis. BC incidence and age of onset in their female relatives were the primary foci of this study.

We observed that a family history of early onset BC was associated with a higher risk of early onset BC among high risk relatives. A family history of early onset BC occurred significantly more frequently among young (<40 years of age) BC probands than among older (≥40 years of age) BC probands. This relationship was particularly evident when the analysis was restricted to the HBC probands. We also observed a positive family history of BC (at any age) significantly more frequently in young BC probands than in older BC probands.

These findings assume major clinical importance for surveillance/management programs of affected and/or at risk relatives from HBC kindreds showing significantly early age of onset of BC. They are evidence of heterogeneity in HBC's age of onset (namely, extremely early age of onset clustering in certain HBC kindreds). Thus, while HBC differs remarkably in tumor combinations (e.g., the hereditary breast/ovarian carcinoma and the SBLA syndrome) and by cutaneous stigmata (e.g., Cowden's disease) some families, and others to be discussed subsequently, may now be characterized by remarkably

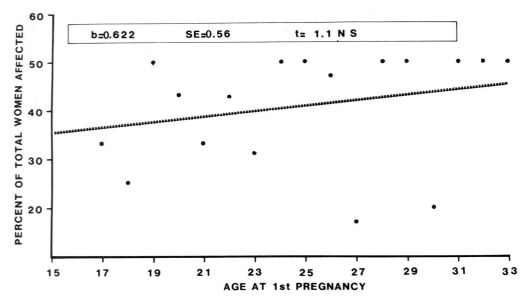

Figure 13–3. Percentage of females affected with breast cancer as a function of age at first pregnancy in the Creighton Hereditary Breast Cancer Family Resource. (From Lynch HT, et al: J Med Genet 21:96, 1984. Reprinted by permission.)

early age of onset criteria (Fig. 13–6). On the other hand, some HBC kindreds may have a much *later* age of onset of BC than the average age of HBC onset.

The implications from this research are of major clinical importance, particularly in the time for initiation of surveillance. Research results also imply heterogeneity in the etiology of HBC. For example, it would seem unlikely that the same environmental factors would be effectively perturbing the deleterious genotype in the earlier onset HBC cohorts as in later age HBC cohorts. Specifically, there would be less time available for such endogenous and exogenous risk factors as early age at menarche, early age of first pregnancy, habitus, cigarette smoking, and alcohol consumption to materially perturb the HBC-prone genotype in the early age of onset cohort. Late natural menopause would be of no etiolog-

ical consequence in these patients since they show premenopausal onset of BC.

HBC Risk in Males and Transsexuals

Familial breast cancer in males has been recently reviewed by Kozak et al.[36] They describe breast cancer in two related males, an uncle and a nephew. In their review of breast cancer occurring in families, including its association with cancers in other family members, they noted ten such families, including their own, from whom they believed that sufficient information was obtained. Six of these families (60 percent) had females affected with breast cancer; they concluded that there are some families in whom males as well as females show an increased risk of developing breast cancer.

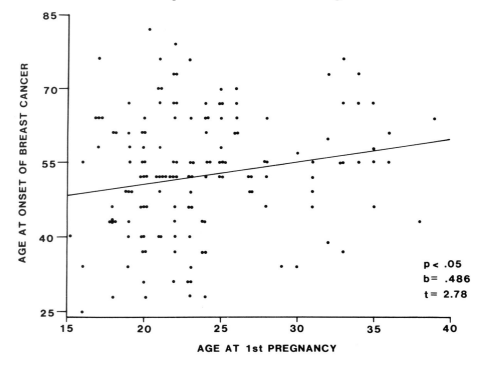

Figure 13–4. Age of diagnosis of breast cancer as a function of age at first pregnancy in our consecutively ascertained series. (From Lynch HT, et al: J Med Genet 21:96–98, 1984. Reprinted by permission.)

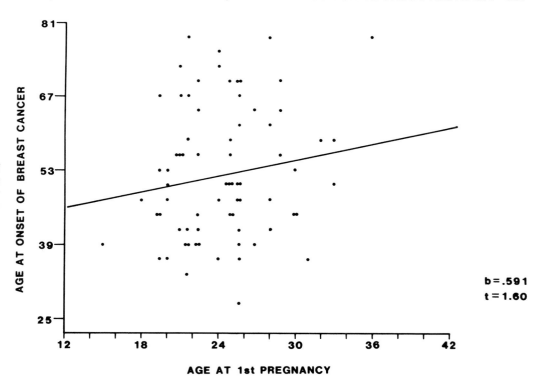

Figure 13–5. Age of diagnosis of breast cancer as a function of age at first term pregnancy in the hereditary subset. (From Lynch HT, et al: J Med Genet 21:96, 1984. Reprinted by permission.)

Klinefelter's syndrome patients have shown an excess risk of breast cancer. A positive family history of BC may accentuate the risk in a Klinefelter's patient.[61] In our own extensive experience in the study of breast cancer–prone families, we have only rarely encountered males with breast cancer.

Pritchard et al.[81] reported the occurrence of breast cancer in a male-to-female transsexual patient ten years following the sexual reassignment. He had received oral estrogens for a prolonged period for maintenance of secondary female characteristics. It was of interest that this patient's mother had breast cancer. No other detail of the family history was given. It was postulated that the development of carcinoma in this patient may have been etiologically related to the positive family history of breast cancer in concert with the long-term estrogen administration. This report shows the importance of recording family history in all patients with breast cancer. The authors note that there have been two other reports of breast cancer occurring in transsexual men who also had prolonged exposure to oral estrogens. The family histories in those cases were not provided.

HBC in Non-whites

Epidemiological studies of HBC have been almost exclusively of white populations, but the disease is present in other races as well. Siraganian et al.,[96] describing two black families showing an excess of breast cancer, were unaware of any case reports of black families with apparent excess of breast cancer, a fact that they suggested could be explained by the true low incidence of familial breast cancer in blacks; another reason may have been difficulty in ascertaining and verifying medical histories in black kindreds. In one of the black families they reported, there was an excess of other types of tumors. Significantly, in this family, there were at least five gynecologic malignancies, including two ovarian cancers. In the second family, breast cancer appeared to be more aggressive. Thus there is a suggestion of heterogeneity with respect to tumor combinations as well as to breast cancer's prognosis. We have ongoing an investigation of a black family with extraordinarily early onset breast cancer that shows clinical features

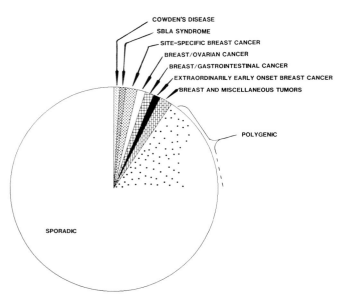

Figure 13–6. Schematic depicting heterogeneity in breast cancer.

similar to those in the families reported by Siraganian et al.[96]

A recent study of 534 histologically verified incident cases of breast cancer in Shanghai, which used age- and sex-matched comparison white controls, showed that the Chinese population had similar risk factors, including increased risk of BC if there was a personal history of benign breast disease and history of BC in a first degree relative.[32]

Enhanced Risk with Atypical Hyperplasia and Family History

Dupont and Page[14, 15] and Page et al.[79] have described an excess BC risk in women with proliferative breast disease (see Chapter 14). When atypia is present, the risk becomes four times that for a woman who had a breast biopsy for benign disease but who lacked histological features of proliferative disease with atypia. Furthermore, a woman with proliferative breast disease with atypia and a positive family history (defined as a mother, sisters, or daughter with breast cancer) was found to have a risk that was about 11 times that for a woman who lacked these features. In contrast, McDivitt et al.[70] found a slight, but not significant, increased risk (4.4 times) in women with hyperplasia with atypia and a positive BC history as compared to those with atypical hyperplasia without a positive family history (3.2 times) (D. Gersell, personal communication). In this latter study, positive family history was defined more expansively as breast cancer in either a first or second degree relative, a factor that may have diluted differences between the positive and negative family history groups.

Rosen et al.[84, 87] have recently described juvenile papillomatosis as a special type of hyperplasia occurring at earlier ages. Nine of the 180 patients in their registry presented concurrently or subsequently with *in situ* or invasive carcinoma. Of these, five (56 percent) had a positive family history of BC compared to 44 of 171 juvenile papillomatosis patients (26 percent) without BC. While these numbers are suggestive, they appear too small as yet to statistically associate juvenile papillomatosis and family history, and as the authors point out,[87] additional cases are needed.

HETEROGENEITY IN HBC: SYNDROMES

Detailed medical/genetic studies of breast cancer–prone families with meticulous pathology verification initiated by Lynch[44] and Lynch and Krush[48] in the mid 1960s have been continuous and now involve several hundred kindreds. They have aided in the comprehension of breast cancer genetics and have disclosed the earlier age of onset,[63] heterogeneous tumor associations (see Fig. 13–6), and improved survival of breast cancer in HBC patients when compared to sporadic breast cancer.[46, 53, 54] These studies have demonstrated certain differences between HBC and sporadic breast cancer; they have also indicated phenotypic heterogeneity within

HBC subsets. This heterogeneity involves age of onset[60] and the occurrence of associated tumors.[6–8, 29, 46, 64] It is unknown whether all or most phenotypic variants of HBC involve an abnormality at one locus (possibly with a variety of defective alleles) or whether several loci are involved, one in each etiological subset of families.

Site-Specific Breast Cancer

As we have previously discussed, the bulk of earlier investigations of HBC pertained only to queries about site-specific BC in BC-prone families. Because of this bias, discussions about proneness to BC were necessarily restricted to BC risk among the relatives of BC probands. We have noted pedigrees in which the proneness to cancer did appear to be restricted to BC (Fig. 13–7). We suspect that the majority of HBC is of the site-specific variety, but the data are too limited to provide a reliable estimate as to the relative frequency of site-specific BC vs. other heterogeneous forms of this disease.

Breast/Ovarian Cancer Syndrome

The hereditary breast/ovarian cancer syndrome is characterized by an excess of carcinoma of the breast in association with ovarian carcinoma.[46, 60] As in all hereditary cancer syndrome identification, the workup required to arrive at a secure diagnosis often necessitates extension of the pedigree.

Figure 13–8 provides an example of the manner in which breast/ovarian cancer syndrome might be recognized, beginning with the combination of these lesions in the nuclear portion of the kindred. Further substantiation of this pattern emerges with extension of the kindred. It is important to attempt to verify medical and tumor history through second degree and even more distant relatives. Helpful features include early age of onset of cancer, bilaterality in the case of paired organs, and multiple primary cancer associations as evident in patients with the breast/ovarian cancer syndrome.

An example of the necessity for such extension beyond the modified nuclear pedigree (MNP) is seen in Figure 13–8. Note that the patient with bilateral BC later developed ovarian carcinoma. Two of her sisters manifested BC. Her father was cancer free, and her mother had colon cancer at age 72. Her mother's family history was negative. Had we restricted our investigation to the father, we would not have been able to establish the hereditary breast/ovarian cancer syndrome. However, note that when extending our search to the father's mother, we find that she manifested ovarian cancer by history. Extending the history further, we find that the father's mother had sisters with ovarian cancer, and they in turn had daughters with ovarian cancer as well as BC. Those findings in this pedigree show a significant excess of breast and ovarian cancer with direct transmission in accord with an autosomal dominant inherited

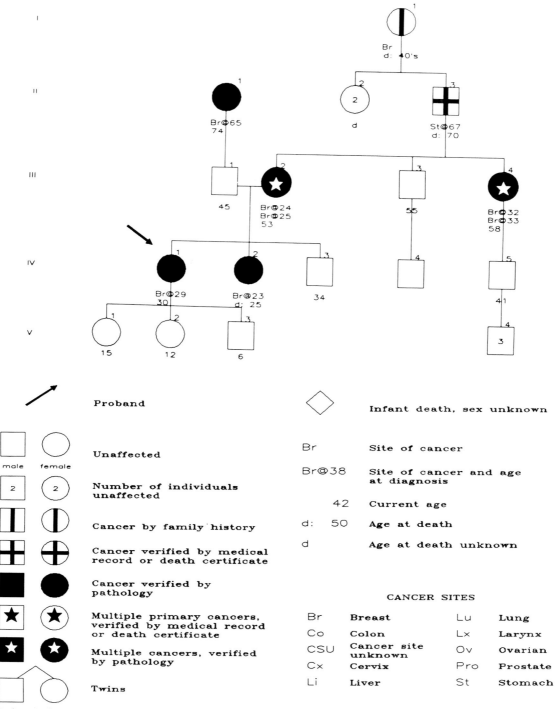

Figure 13–7. Pedigree of a site-specific hereditary breast cancer family. This is a black family wherein breast cancer showed early age of onset in the proband, her sister, her mother, and her maternal aunt. Note that a paternal grandmother had breast cancer at age 65, and that the maternal great-grandmother had breast cancer and died from this disease in her 40s.

mechanism. In this case, the cancer-free father is a putative obligate carrier of the deleterious gene.

Lynch and Krush[49] and Lynch et al.[58] and, subsequently, Fraumeni et al.[24] reported clustering of breast and ovarian cancer in extended pedigrees. In order to define the breast/ovarian cancer syndrome further, Lynch et al.[60] studied 12 families who showed clustering

of breast/ovarian cancer among female relatives (Figs. 13–9, 13–10, and 13–11). These pedigrees were analyzed from a medical/genetic standpoint, and the findings revealed significant linear decline in estimates of cumulative breast/ovarian cancer risk for females with diminishing genetic relationship to probands and index cases. There was a lack of excessive site-specific cancer risk to

Text continued on page 274

B119

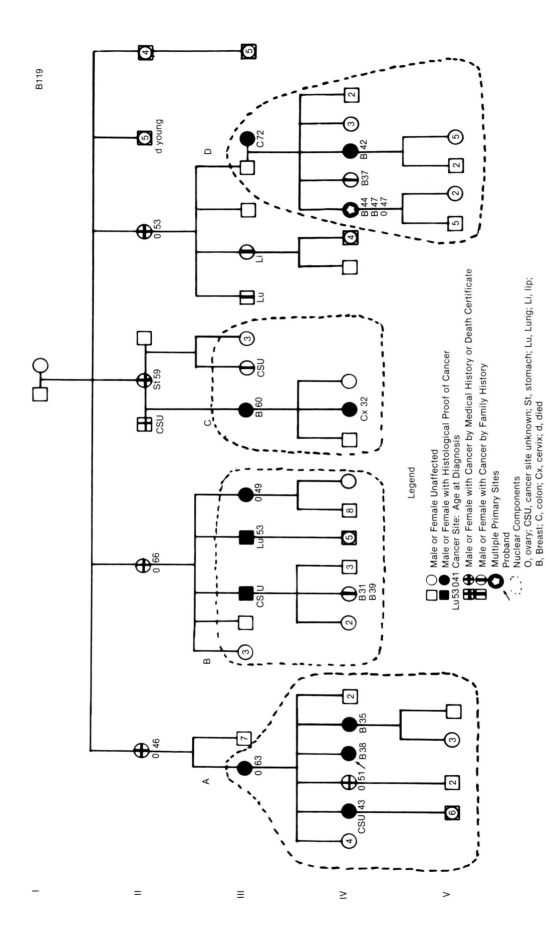

Figure 13–8. Pedigree of a breast/ovarian cancer family, which emphasizes the need to extend the pedigree for accurate syndrome identification. (From Lynch HT, et al: Arch Surg 113:1061, 1978. Reprinted by permission.)

Legend

○ □ Male or Female Unaffected
● ■ Male or Female with Histological Proof of Cancer
Lu53041 Cancer Site: Age at Diagnosis
⊕ ⊞ Male or Female with Cancer by Medical History or Death Certificate
▣ ▢ Male or Female with Cancer by Family History
⬡ Multiple Primary Sites
Proband
⊞ ⊞ Nuclear Components
⸺ O, ovary; CSU, cancer site unknown; St, stomach; Lu, Lung; Li, lip;
B, Breast; C, colon; Cx, cervix; d, died

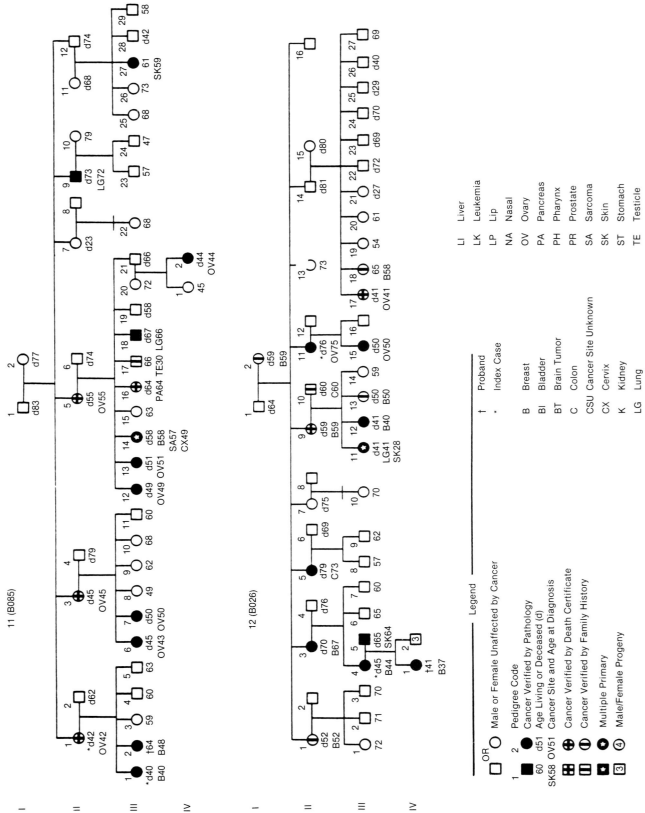

Figure 13–9. Pedigree of breast/ovarian cancer family. This reflects the need to conduct surveillance programs for women at high genetic risk for both breast and ovarian cancer. (From Lynch HT, et al: Cancer 41:1543, 1978. Reprinted by permission.)

Legend

□ OR ○	Male or Female Unaffected by Cancer
1 2	Pedigree Code
60 d51 SK58 OV51	Age Living or Deceased (d) / Cancer Site and Age at Diagnosis
● ■	Cancer Verified by Pathology
⊕ ⊖	Cancer Verified by Death Certificate
⊞ ⊟	Cancer Verified by Family History
✸	Multiple Primary
③	Male/Female Progeny

†	Proband
*	Index Case

B	Breast	LI	Liver
BI	Bladder	LK	Leukemia
BT	Brain Tumor	LP	Lip
C	Colon	NA	Nasal
CSU	Cancer Site Unknown	OV	Ovary
CX	Cervix	PA	Pancreas
K	Kidney	PH	Pharynx
LG	Lung	PR	Prostate
		SA	Sarcoma
		SK	Skin
		ST	Stomach
		TE	Testicle

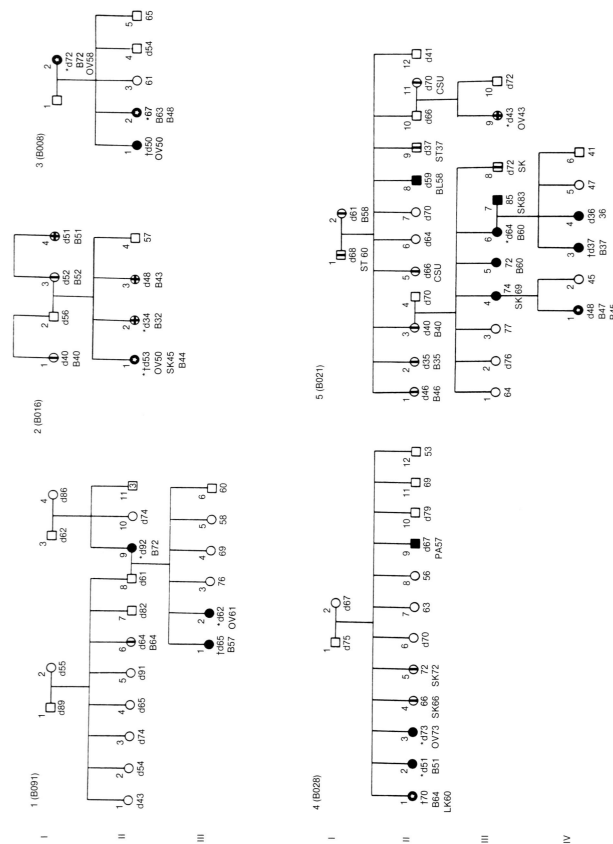

Figure 13–10. Pedigree of breast/ovarian cancer family. This reflects the need to conduct surveillance programs for women at high genetic risk for both breast and ovarian cancer. (From Lynch HT, et al: Cancer 41:1543, 1978. Reprinted by permission.)

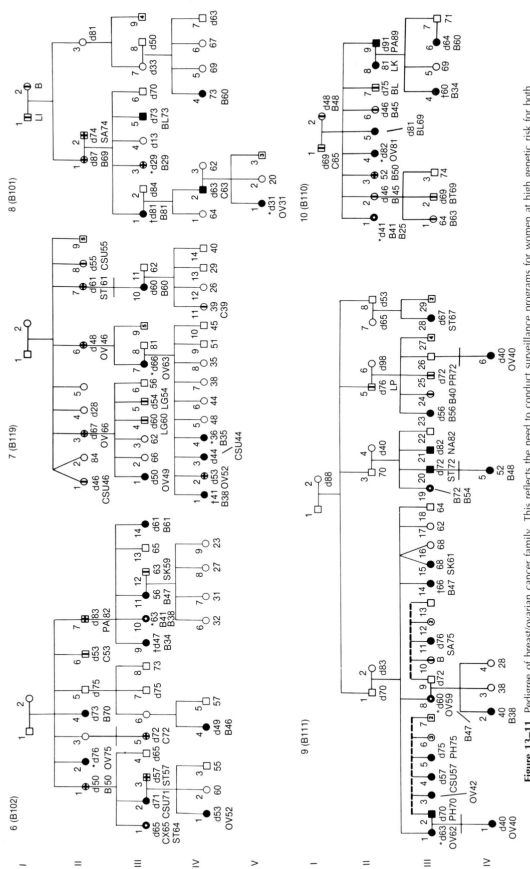

Figure 13–11. Pedigree of breast/ovarian cancer family. This reflects the need to conduct surveillance programs for women at high genetic risk for both breast and ovarian cancer. (From Lynch HT, et al: Cancer 41:1543, 1978. Reprinted by permission.)

male relatives, a phenomenon that supported a sex-limited genetic etiology. Breast/ovarian cancer onset typically occurred at an early age (mean = 50.6 years) in these kindreds compared to the general population (mean = 62 years), which is characteristic of hereditary cancer. Examples of apparent mother-to-daughter and father-to-daughter genetic transmission of proclivity for breast/ovarian carcinoma were prevalent in the 12 pedigrees.

Excluding probands and index cases, the estimated cumulative risk of breast/ovarian cancer to female progeny of affected mothers was 46 percent for those aged 20 to 80 years, suggesting that affected mothers in the pedigrees were transmitting the deleterious cancer-predisposing gene to one half of their daughters. Eight sibships involving putative carrier males contained a total of 15 female progeny older than age 20. Of these, six have manifested breast cancer, and five have had ovarian cancer. These results underscore the need for physicians to be cognizant of both males and females as potential transmitters of cancer in this familial tumor association. In addition, surveillance and management implications must involve both breast and ovarian cancer in women at increased genetic risk in these families.

SBLA Syndrome

Lynch et al.[64] described an extended kindred that showed a broad spectrum of cancer: namely, *S*arcoma, *B*reast cancer and brain tumors, *L*ung and laryngeal cancer and leukemia, and *A*drenal cortical carcinoma, (SBLA syndrome). A limited description of the elements of this syndrome had previously been recognized in four nuclear kindreds by Li and Fraumeni,[39] who subsequently published a prospective observation of these families that covered a 12-year time frame (1969 through 1981).[40, 41] Of interest was the fact that in 31 surviving family members, 16 additional cancers developed (the expected number was 0.5). Five of these were carcinomas of the breast, four were soft tissue sarcomas, and seven were cancers of other anatomic sites. Eight of the patients had multiple primary cancers. Four cancers occurred at sites of prior radiotherapy (three soft tissue sarcomas and one mesothelioma). The SBLA syndrome has also been appropriately referred to as the Li-Fraumeni syndrome.

We have continued to follow the original SBLA syndrome kindred that we described in 1978.[64] We republished the pedigree (Fig. 13–12) after a 5-year-old boy in the fifth generation (V-5) developed a rhabdomyosarcoma and his sister (V-1) died at age 11 years with a glioblastoma.[62] Subsequently, a third sibling was born; this child developed a medulloblastoma at age 2 years and died from this disease at age 2.5 years.

This is obviously an exceedingly complex syndrome and requires intensive investigation of cancer of *all* anatomic sites with a vigorous effort toward histopathological verification of cancer. Problems in pedigree analysis in the SBLA syndrome are compounded by the fact that in addition to reduced penetrance of the deleterious

gene, two age-specific modes of cancer expression are encountered, one in childhood and the second in adult life. For example, in the previously described family, the affected siblings' 39-year-old father (Fig. 13–12, IV-15) was in the direct genetic lineage but has not yet manifested cancer. Nevertheless, two of his five children (V-1 and V-5 and, as mentioned, the subsequently born child) manifested cancers consonant with the SBLA syndrome. Thus each of the remaining children are at 50 percent risk for the development of cancer. The father of these syndrome cancer–affected children is considered to be an obligate gene carrier. Their mother (IV-16) and her relatives have been cancer free.

Cowden's Disease

Brownstein[10] and Brownstein et al.[11] described in detail a cancer-associated genodermatosis known as Cowden's disease. This disorder involves multiple trichilemmomas, the presence of which appear to be pathognomonic for Cowden's disease. These cutaneous lesions are often located on the face and are multiple (Fig. 13–13). Skin lesions are also common on the dorsal and ventral aspects of the hands, feet, and forearms of patients with Cowden's disease. These are hyperkeratotic, slightly brownish lesions, but show the histological pattern of benign keratoses. The stratum corneum is thick, compact, and largely orthokeratotic. The granular layer is prominent; the malpighian layer is papillomatous, acanthotic, and well-differentiated, but shows no distinguishing features. The importance of these cutaneous findings is the fact that breast cancer, often bilateral, occurs with increased frequency in Cowden's disease. In addition to the susceptibility to breast cancer, at-risk women may show virginal hypertrophy of the breasts. Affected males and females may also manifest thyroid goiter, thyroid adenoma, or hypothyroidism, as well as carcinoma of the thyroid. Gastrointestinal polyps are relatively common and have been observed throughout the gastrointestinal tract, including the esophagus. The risk for carcinoma of the colon in Cowden's disease–affected patients is yet to be clearly defined. Cowden's disease is inherited as an autosomal dominant. A comprehensive coverage of the subject of Cowden's syndrome is contained in the monograph by Starink.[98]

Extraordinarily Early Onset Breast Cancer

We have identified a subset of HBC in which remarkably early onset of breast cancer occurs. This study involved the relationship between age of onset of breast cancer in 328 breast cancer probands (consecutively ascertained patients from our oncology clinic) and breast cancer incidence and age of onset in their female relatives (Table 13–1). We found that a family history of early onset breast cancer was associated with higher risk of early onset breast cancer. A family history of early onset breast cancer occurred more frequently among young (<40 years old) breast cancer probands than

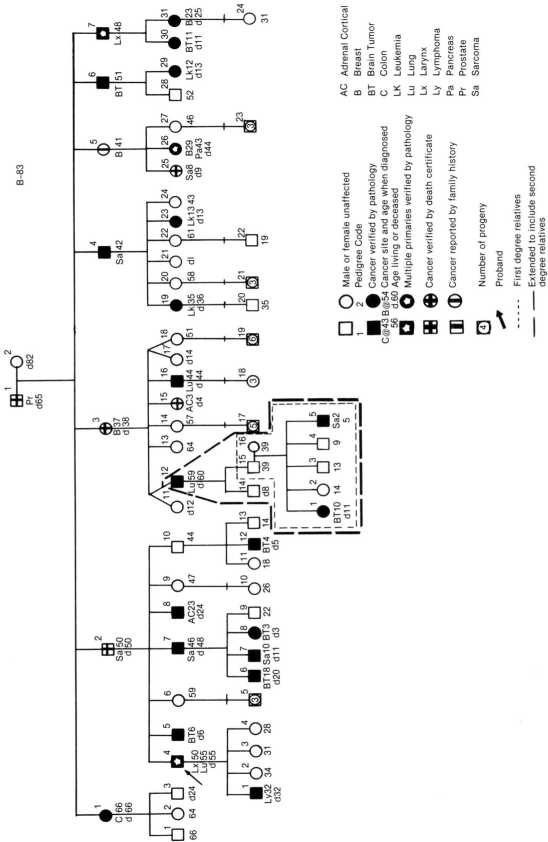

Figure 13–12. An updated SBLA kindred showing cancer occurrences through five generations. (From Lynch HT, et al: AJDC 139:134, 1985. Reprinted by permission.)

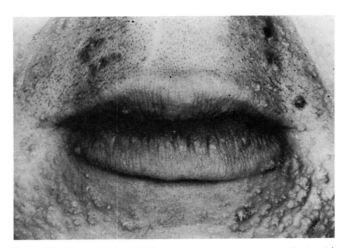

Figure 13–13. Multiple trichilemmomas as seen in a patient with Cowden's disease, which is frequently associated with breast cancer. (From Brownstein MH. *In* Lynch HT [ed]: Genetics and Breast Cancer. New York, Van Nostrand Reinhold, 1981, pp 187–195. Reprinted by permission.)

among older (>40 years old) breast cancer probands ($p<0.001$; odds ratio [OR] = 23). This relationship was particularly evident when the analysis was restricted to the hereditary breast cancer probands ($p<0.001$; OR = 33). We also observed a positive family history of breast cancer (at any age) more frequently in young breast cancer probands than in older breast cancer probands ($p<0.001$; OR = 2.9). These observations

Table 13–1. BREAST CANCER INCIDENCE IN FEMALE RELATIVES* OF 328 CONSECUTIVE BREAST CANCER PROBANDS

	Probands	
	Young	*Old*
Family history of breast cancer†		
Negative		
Sporadic	20 (0/164)	196 (0/1356)
Familial	15 (13/124)	67 (70/553)
Positive		
Hereditary	11 (30/100)	20 (46/223)
Family history of early breast cancer‡		
Negative	37 (0)	280 (0)
Familial	2 (2)	2 (2)
Positive		
Hereditary	7 (11)	1 (1)

*Includes sisters, mothers, grandmothers, and aunts.

†Values given are number of probands (number of relatives with BC/number of female relatives). Note that more probands were young in the family history positive group than in the sporadic group ($p<0.01$; OR = 2.9); the same relationship was seen when the familial group was compared to the sporadic ($p<0.03$; OR = 2.2).

‡Values given are number of probands with a family history of early onset BC (number of relatives with BC < age 40). Note that more probands were young in the family history positive group than in the negative group ($p<0.001$; OR = 23); the same relationship was observed when hereditary cases only were included ($p<0.001$; OR = 33).

From Lynch HT, et al: Breast Cancer Research and Treatment, 1988. Reprinted by permission of Kluwer Academic Publishers, The Netherlands.

have important pragmatic implications for surveillance. We recommend intense surveillance for breast cancer, initiated earlier, for women with close relatives diagnosed with early onset breast cancer.[56]

We have described seven families from our Hereditary Cancer Consultation Center (HCCC) and the Creighton Oncology Clinic who are noteworthy for extraordinarily early age of onset (Figs. 13–7, 13–14 to 13–19). This appears to be an additional example of heterogeneity in HBC and may represent the first account of this remarkable subset. The manner in which age of onset can be incorporated with other aspects of natural history for expecting diagnosis has been discussed in greater detail in Lynch et al.[55]

COMPILING AN INFORMATIVE FAMILY HISTORY: PEDIGREE DEVELOPMENT

Pattern recognition of the several natural history facets of hereditary breast cancer facilitates genetic diagnoses and provides one of the most powerful methods for identification of cancer risk.[46] Nevertheless, there remains the vexing problem of not being able to determine the precise cancer risk (cancer-prone genotype affected vs. unaffected) for specific, asymptomatic, unaffected women in the direct lineage of a well defined hereditary breast cancer kindred. A biomarker is desperately needed that can identify the presence or absence of the deleterious genotype in at-risk individuals. The etiological and cancer control implications of such an advance in knowledge would be legion. Meanwhile, until such a biomarker is discovered, we must continue to rely on a complete family history for prediction of genetic risk status. Paradoxically, the cancer family history is one of the most neglected portions of the medical workup of cancer-affected individuals. This is surprising since this knowledge can be used effectively for highly targeted surveillance and management through the identification of patients whose predictability to cancer of specific organ sites exceeds that of any other known risk factors.[46]

Thus a definitive compilation of a patient's family history is one of the most powerful methods for identification of cancer risks. In a research setting such as ours, we extensively develop the family history for accurate syndrome identification.

Methods of Family Study

Initially, information is gathered on first degree relatives and selected maternal/paternal second degree relatives (grandparents, aunts, and uncles), which is referred to as a "modified nuclear pedigree" (Fig. 13–20). These older relatives are more informative than younger individuals, because most cancers are adult onset, making phenotype expression more likely in older relatives than in more youthful relatives (progeny, cousins, nephews, and nieces of probands).

Relatives of the proband are sent a letter explaining

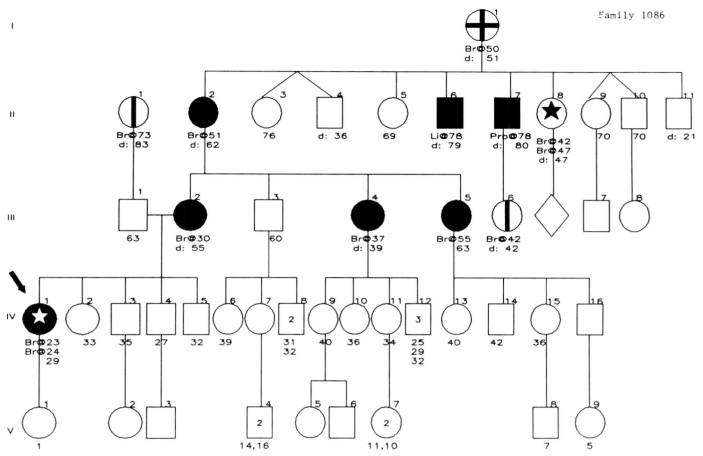

Figure 13–14. Proband with bilateral breast cancer of extremely early onset (age 23) with breast cancer manifested through four generations. Please refer to the symbol legend in Figure 13–7.

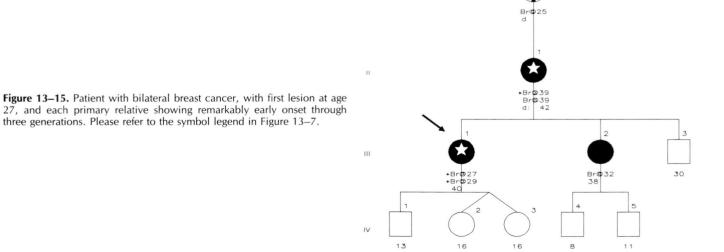

Figure 13–15. Patient with bilateral breast cancer, with first lesion at age 27, and each primary relative showing remarkably early onset through three generations. Please refer to the symbol legend in Figure 13–7.

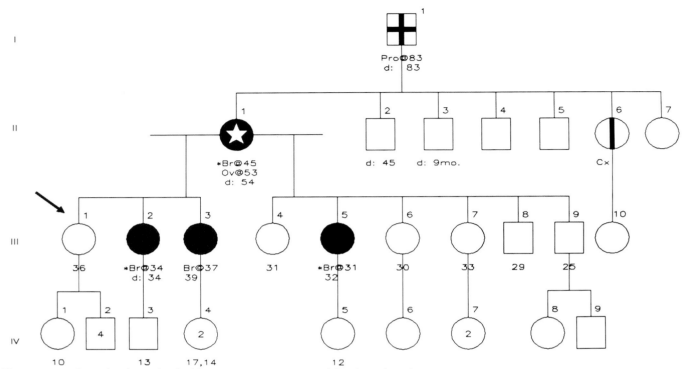

Figure 13–16. The proband's mother had breast cancer at age 45, and daughters through two separate marriages manifest early-onset breast cancer. Please refer to the symbol legend in Figure 13–7.

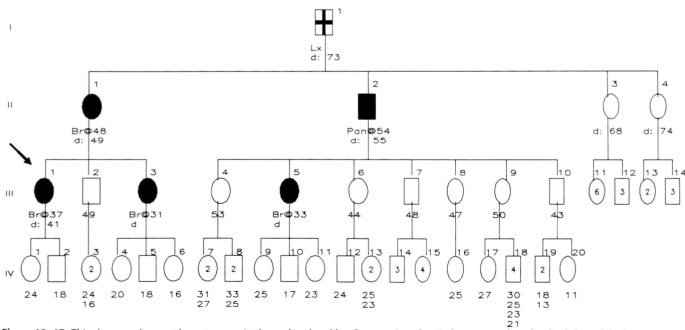

Figure 13–17. This shows early-onset breast cancer in the proband and her first cousin, wherein her maternal uncle, the father of the breast cancer–affected cousin, manifested pancreatic carcinoma. Please refer to the symbol legend in Figure 13–7.

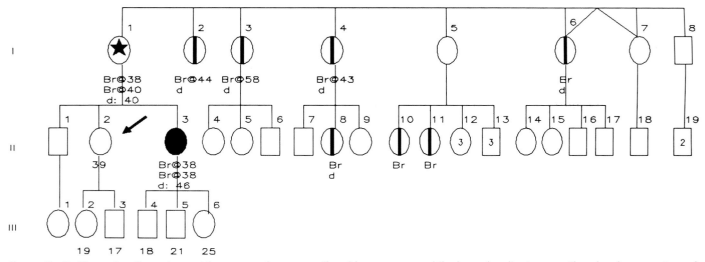

Figure 13–18. The proband's mother and four maternal aunts manifested breast cancer, while the proband's sister manifested early onset. Ages of her cousins are not known. The pedigree is noteworthy in that one of the maternal aunts (I-5) appears to be an obligate gene carrier in that two of her daughters (II-10, II-11) are affected with breast cancer, but ages of onset not available. Please refer to the symbol legend in Figure 13–7.

the purpose of the family study. Accompanying the letter is a questionnaire and a medical record permission release form. All family members are given assurances of confidentiality. Family wishes are followed expressly, and requests to resign from further study are accommodated. However, cooperation of family members is usually excellent, and large informative pedigrees can often be constructed from the questionnaires.

Cancer verification procedures are initiated immediately on return of the questionnaire and the signed permission form. A cover letter and the signed release of information form is sent to the appropriate hospital, requesting pathology reports and other medical documents on the cancer-affected family members. Surviving spouses, children, or closely related individuals are contacted to give permission to access the records of deceased family members. When records are not available because of destruction or other problems, death certificates are utilized as a last resort.

These family studies are coordinated by registered nurses or research associates who have the experience and training to solve the various problems that arise. These problems include "lost" and alienated family members, grief, anger, concerns about confidentiality, and questions about cancer risk and surveillance. Many of our clinical colleagues have assigned this responsibility to their office nurse, thereby enabling their own time to be more effectively and economically employed in the analysis of the family pedigree.

An Example of Pedigree Development

The initial ascertainment of a pedigree may, in certain circumstances, provide invaluable clues relevant to the potential for an HBC diagnosis. Such an example is shown in Figure 13–19 (insert A), in which the proband (III-2) had histologically verified breast cancer at age 35. Note that her father died at age 59 and was cancer free. However, two of her father's sisters (II-5 and II-10) had breast cancer at ages 42 and 59, respectively. The paternal grandmother had unverified ovarian cancer at age 84. Thus, with this initial ascertainment, we might preliminarily consider the father to be a putative obligate gene carrier by virtue of his having two sisters affected with breast cancer, one at early age (age 42), and the markedly early onset (age 35) in his daughter. The occurrence of ovarian carcinoma at an advanced age in his mother is not too informative at this stage of the evaluation.

However, we note in the updated part of this pedigree (Fig. 13–19, insert B), following some 4 years of follow-up, that it now portrays findings that are wholly consistent with HBC. Note particularly that there are two potential cancer-prone lineages emanating from the proband's paternal grandmother and paternal aunt, in which multiple descendents of these progenitors show early onset breast cancer, including bilaterality (Fig. 13–19(B), II-5, III-5). Examples depict direct line of descent of breast cancer with markedly early onset, as in the two previously mentioned bilateral occurrences, and in the case of the woman in Figure 13–19(B), II-10, with breast cancer occurring at 43, who had a daughter (III-11) with breast cancer at the extraordinarily early age of 28. Examples of putative obligate gene carrier patients are II-13, who had a daughter (III-13) with breast cancer at age 30, and II-15, who had a daughter (III-17) with breast cancer at age 34.

There were also three cases of early onset uterine cervical carcinoma (IV-1, IV-5, and IV-10). There were also occurrences of early onset Hodgkin's disease and childhood tumor (Wilms' tumor) in patients from generation IV (IV-12 and IV-14). The significance of these lesions within this kindred remain enigmatic. Recent investigations of childhood cancers occurring in children of mothers with breast cancer or who ultimately develop breast cancer may have a bearing on this phenomenon. For example, in a previous population-based study, Birch et al.[4] evaluated families of young children with

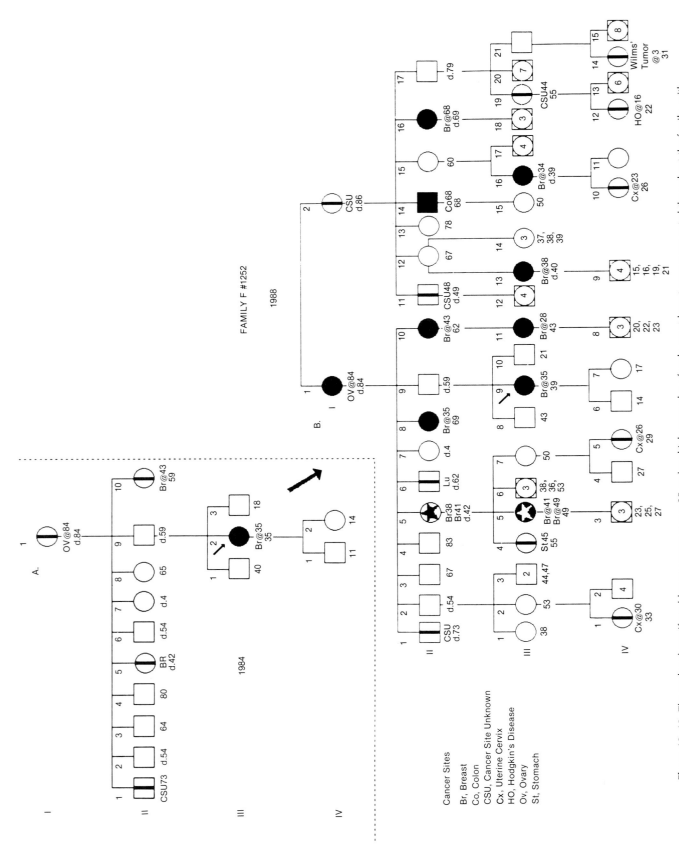

Cancer Sites

Br, Breast
Co, Colon
CSU, Cancer Site Unknown
Cx, Uterine Cervix
HO, Hodgkin's Disease
Ov, Ovary
St, Stomach

Figure 13–19. The proband manifested breast cancer at age 35 and multiple examples of early onset breast cancer are noted throughout the family, with putative transmission through a carrier male (II-9). Pedigree in insert A shows the initial family information that was obtained from the proband. This amount of information enabled us to recommend an intensive surveillance program. Insert B reflects the pedigree after it was updated and extended. The findings are consistent with a hereditary breast cancer diagnosis. Please refer to the symbol legend in Figure 13–7.

280

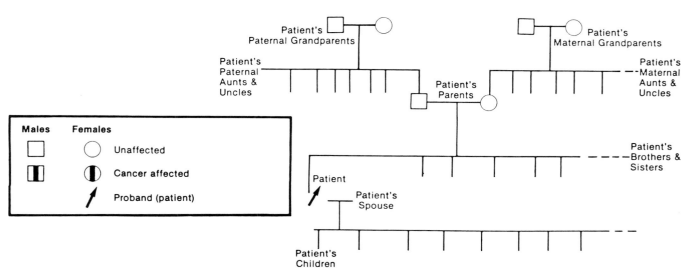

PATIENT'S MODIFIED NUCLEAR PEDIGREE

Figure 13–20. Diagram portraying a modified nuclear pedigree, the minimum information needed to evaluate cancer family history. (From Lynch HT, et al: Surv Dig Dis 2:244–260, 1984. Reprinted by permission.)

soft tissue sarcoma, predominantly rhabdomyosarcomas. They observed that breast cancer incidence in the mothers of these cancer-affected children was significantly increased. Findings in some of the patients were suggestive of the SBLA syndrome. More recently, Thompson et al.[99] evaluated parental cancer in 326 children who were referred to a single pediatric oncology unit. They observed a significant increase in breast cancer incidence in the mothers of children with solid tumors. Specifically, the cancer occurrences were 8.9 times the expected number. They could not identify any known risk factors for breast cancer that could explain this cancer excess. We have noted many anecdotal examples of childhood cancers reflecting a large variety of hereditary cancer syndromes in individuals in the direct genetic lineage of many of our pedigrees. It would be prudent to study extended pedigrees with documentation of cancer of all anatomic sites in a sufficiently large population of consecutively ascertained patients with childhood cancer.

In summary, this example traces some of our typical experience in breast cancer genetic investigations. We are frequently able to utilize information at initial ascertainment, as seen in Figure 13–19(A), for clinical purposes, such as recommending intensive surveillance/management programs. For example, in the initial ascertainment [Figure 19(A)], we see a patient in the fourth generation (IV-2); namely, the daughter of a patient with early onset breast cancer, who would tentatively be considered to be at 50 percent risk for breast cancer. We would begin an educational program for this young woman, using tact, discretion, and considerable empathy in the hope of persuading her to objectively view her genetic risk status for breast cancer and to comply with our surveillance recommendations. In the updated portion of the pedigree [Fig. 19(B)], we see more clearly that our supposition about her increased

risk has been fortified by events that were discovered and more thoroughly documented over a period of 4 years follow-up of the family. The follow-up of families prone to breast cancer (as well as all other forms of hereditary cancer) is a dynamic process that encompasses constant updating once new medical information accrues. This does not have to be restricted to a formal research setting. For example, in one of the authors' (HTL) medical oncology practice, during the course of the follow-up of patients, new information is constantly brought forth relevant to the pedigree and entered on the chart.

Pragmatic Implications: An HBC Clinical Vignette

The primary objectives of the Hereditary Cancer Consultation Center at Creighton University School of Medicine and the AMI/St. Joseph Hospital pertain to the diagnosis, surveillance, and management of patients who are at high risk for all forms of hereditary cancer. In order to demonstrate some of the practical implications of HBC diagnosis and management, we provide an example: a family who was recently seen in the HCCC.

The proband [Fig. 13–21(B), III-7] is a 29-year-old white female who was self-referred because of her concern about her risk for breast cancer, prompted by the striking excess of this disease in her family. She was interviewed by a nurse specially trained in genetics, following which a family study was carried out. The proband's two sisters manifested breast cancer at ages 26 [Fig. 13–21(A), III-1] and 34 (III-4), and a maternal aunt (II-5) had breast cancer at age 28. Note that the proband's mother (II-2, age 59) was unaffected. The proband's maternal grandmother (I-1) had cancer, site

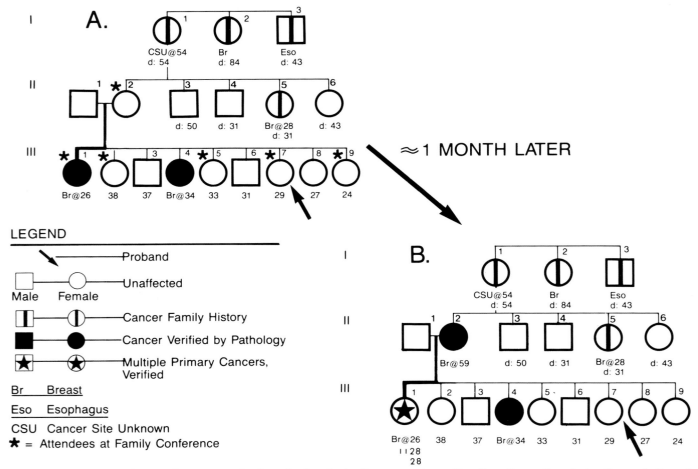

Figure 13–21. Pedigree A depicts a breast cancer family at the time the family was seen in our Hereditary Cancer Consultation Center. Pedigree B reflects the family one month later. Note that the obligate gene carrier II-2, and her daughter III-1, following our counseling and surveillance recommendations, were diagnosed with breast cancer.

unknown, at age 54. The remarkably early onset of breast cancer in the proband's two sisters and their maternal aunt indicated that the proband's mother, by virtue of her position in the pedigree, was a putative obligate gene carrier of a breast cancer susceptible genotype.

Those members of the family indicated by asterisks on the pedigree met together in the HCCC following the workup of their pedigree. A detailed educational session was provided, highlighting the breast cancer occurrences in their family and the important facets of its natural history, particularly the early age of onset, bilateral expression, and the surveillance/management strategies deemed important by us. These recommendations were responsive to HBC's natural history and included initiation of mammography by age 25 (or 5 years younger than the earliest age of expression of breast cancer in a patient's primary relative), monthly competent breast self-examination (BSE), and physician examination of their breasts semiannually. These aspects of our surveillance strategy were further emphasized during an unstructured group therapy session in which each of the individuals was able to ask questions freely. This type of session allowed family members to express

concerns that they freely admitted had previously been difficult to discuss with their own physicians. All family members were instructed in BSE.

Each of these women was examined by one of us (HTL), and mammograms were performed. Two patients were of particular concern; namely, the proband's mother [Fig. 13–21(A), II-2] and one of her sisters (III-1).

The proband's mother's breasts were normal on inspection and physical examination. She had not had a prior mammogram. Screening mammography showed a primarily fat-replaced breast with a clump of calcifications in the 3 o'clock position of the left breast. Initial mammographic interpretation was that the clump calcifications represented benign disease. Because the patient was considered an obligate gene carrier for HBC, the mammogram was reviewed. Several fine dot-dash type calcifications were seen extending from the cluster toward the nipple. These were felt to be worrisome and further focal compression mammography was recommended, followed by a needle-directed biopsy. Histology showed both invasive adenocarcinoma and intraductal carcinoma. A left modified radical mastectomy and prophylactic right total mastectomy with axillary sampling was performed. Lymph nodes were negative. Estrogen receptors were positive (33 fmol/mg protein) and progesterone receptors were negative (<5 fmol/mg protein).

The proband's sister [Fig. 13–21(A), III-1] had a prior diagnosis of comedocarcinoma of the left breast at age 26. Estrogen receptors were negative (<3 fmol/mg protein) and progesterone receptors were negative (<5 fmol/mg protein). A modified radical mastectomy had been performed, and all of the lymph nodes were free of tumor. On our examination, we noted a 2-cm, well-defined nodule in the upper outer quadrant of the right breast. The patient stated that she had been aware of this lesion but thought that it was changing in size with her menstrual cycle and that it most probably was "fibrocystic disease of the breast." She underwent an excisional biopsy; histological diagnosis was infiltrating ductal carcinoma [Fig. 13–21(B), III-1]. A right modified radical mastectomy was performed. All of her axillary nodes were negative for metastases. Estrogen receptors were negative (<3 fmol/mg protein) and progesterone receptors were negative (<5 fmol/mg protein).

This family clearly illustrates the need for intensive surveillance and follow-up of relatives who are at inordinately high risk for HBC. The risk is of sufficient magnitude to require greater attention than would be given to patients who are not members of HBC families.

The radiologist must be made fully aware of the genetic risk status of HBC patients so that extra attention can be given to their mammograms. This attention contributed to early diagnosis of an otherwise subtle lesion, resulting in a Stage I diagnosis of breast cancer in the proband's mother. In turn, a more obvious lesion was detected in the proband's sister's contralateral breast. Contralateral breast cancer occurs with a frequency of 46 percent during a 20-year time frame following initial cancer in HBC.[29]

The cornerstone for optimal patient and family compliance with surveillance/management recommendations is the patient's understanding of the genetic risk, natural history, and the potentially hopeful aspects of early detection in HBC.[25, 46, 51] This information must be imparted to each family member, preferably in a setting where there is sufficient time for patients to ask questions and to freely discuss their concerns. Thus their fears, anxieties, apprehensions, and inadequacies in their knowledge base can be more effectively discussed and interpreted. Discussing the pedigree as a family unit is particularly valuable in that each of the relatives is able to see firsthand the manner in which he or she fits into the overall risk status in the pedigree. As a group, this family was able to discuss concerns freely with each other, and all members were provided an empathetic listening ear by the interested nurse and physician.

In summary, we have described virtually concurrent breast cancer diagnoses in a mother and her daughter that were heavily prompted by knowledge of HBC's natural history and its occurrence in this kindred. This family approach to cancer control can be achieved in the clinical practice setting with efficiency of time, effort, and economy.

BIOMARKERS AND HBC

Biomarkers may be used to characterize neoplastic or non-neoplastic tissue with the goal of distributing cancer patients into clinically significant groups or non-cancer patients into genetic risk categories. The range of markers is quite diverse, from tumor protein expression to qualitative and quantitative changes in its DNA and chromosomes. The recent capability to study allelic differences in nontumor (germline) DNA provides an especially powerful tool to study linkage, discussed in the subsequent section. In the case of breast cancer, surprisingly little is known about biomarkers in the hereditary form of this disease. However, there is ample reason to believe that given the distinctiveness of HBC, biomarkers may one day be identified that will discriminate between it and sporadic breast cancers. Such findings would supplement pedigree information in diagnosing HBC. We are also hopeful that genetic linkage markers will be identified. These would have great clinical importance in assessing BC risk in unaffected members of HBC families.

Histopathology and Proliferative Characteristics

The histopathology of breast cancer is a biomarker that is easily obtained, but no sensitive or specific pathological characteristic is recognized for FBC and HBC at the present time. Some studies in the past decade have implicated an excess of some of the rarer histological subtypes in familial breast tumors. Lagios et al.[37] found some predilection for tubular carcinoma histology in patients with a positive family history (six of 15 vs. 31 of 186 in those without a family history; $p<0.05$). Anderson[3] earlier had shown an excess of the medullary carcinoma subtype in patients with sisters, but not mothers, with breast cancer, while Rosen et al.[86] observed that women with medullary carcinoma are more likely to have mothers with breast cancer. Each of these studies concerned FBC.

Mulcahy and Platt[76] studied HBC and found an excess of medullary carcinoma with or without lymphoid stroma when compared to SBC controls (12 of 75 vs. two of 53; $p<.05$). The patients in this study, however, were not age matched, which becomes a significant problem, because both medullary breast carcinoma and HBC are known to occur at younger ages. Marcus et al.[67] have been performing a double-blind, case-control study of breast cancer histopathology among affected individuals from additional, clearly defined, HBC-prone kindreds using age-matched and race-matched SBC controls. Medullary carcinoma [Fig. 13–22(A)] was classified as "typical" or "atypical" after the criteria of Ridolfi et al.[82] With the age-matched criterion relaxed, we could confirm a persistent excess of medullary or atypical medullary carcinoma histology (12 of 52 HBC mastectomies vs. three of 40 SBC mastectomies; $p<0.05$). However, with the age-matched criterion in force, five of 31 in the HBC group had a medullary subtype,

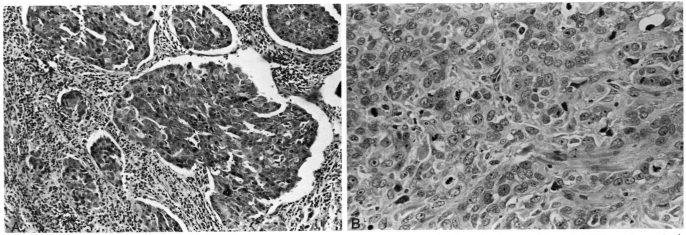

Figure 13–22. Medullary breast carcinoma *(A)* in a 24-year-old woman who, one year later, developed a "no special type" (NST) carcinoma in the contralateral breast. Note the expansive islands of large tumor cells with intervening stroma filled with lymphocytes (× 125). *B,* NST carcinoma with a high mitotic rate in the mother (× 375). These two patients are part of a site-specific HBC pedigree (III-2 and IV-1, respectively) shown in Figure 13–7 that illustrate many of the features of HBC, including young ages of onset, excess bilaterality, and possible age-independent excesses of medullary carcinoma histology and NST high mitotic grade.

compared to three of 31 in the SBC group. The result has no statistical significance, but since the number of cases in this ongoing study is currently small, the question of an age-independent excess of medullary carcinoma in HBC appears unresolved. In neither the age-matched nor non–age-matched datasets did we find any trends toward tubular carcinoma or other histopathological subtypes, but again, the case numbers are small and the possibility of such excesses cannot be ruled out.

Marcus et al. also examined histological grade, defined as a composite of scores for tubule formation, nuclear pleomorphism, and mitotic rate.[17] While there was no difference in total histological grade between HBC and SBC, a significantly increased mitotic grade [Fig. 13–22(B)] was observed in HBC (22 of 35 were mitotic grades 2 and 3 vs. 11 of 33 in SBC; not age-matched; $p<0.02$). Since only "no special type" (NST, or infiltrating ductal type) carcinomas were scored, the result is independent of the effect of the presence of any excess medullary carcinoma, which has a very high mitotic grade. However, as with medullary histology, proliferative rates appear to be higher in breast cancers in younger age groups, as evidenced by higher thymidine labeling indices,[74] which should be expected to correlate to mitotic grade. When we looked at age-matched HBC/SBC pairs, a trend toward higher mitotic grade in HBC persisted in our data (16 of 27 vs. 10 of 27 for SBC), although the result is not formally statistically significant in this small sample ($p<0.18$).

Clearly, more work needs to be done. Higher proliferative rates in breast cancer correlate to shorter disease-free intervals and survival times.[23, 72] HBC, on the other hand, does not appear to behave more aggressively than SBC; if there is any clinical difference, its behavior may actually be less aggressive.[1] A higher mitotic grade in HBC, if borne out, would thus be somewhat paradoxical. Future approaches to the study of proliferative rates in HBC could include flow cytometric analysis of DNA-stained tumor cells to assess the *fraction in S phase,* which correlates highly to the mitotic rate.[70] These studies could be prospective, using fresh tumor tissue, or retrospective, using formalin-fixed, paraffin-embedded archival tumor.[107] Such data, however, are currently lacking.

Tumor Cell DNA Content and Other Markers

The DNA content of tumor cells, most frequently measured by flow cytometry, is loosely termed "diploid" if normal or "aneuploid" if abnormal. Many recent DNA flow cytometry studies have shown that aneuploidy correlates to more aggressive behavior in breast cancer.[13, 18, 23, 30, 68] At the present time, there has been no study that stratifies HBC, FBC, or SBC with respect to ploidy. The only major hereditary cancer to be so stratified, hereditary nonpolyposis colorectal cancer (Lynch syndromes I and II), appears to have a lesser incidence of aneuploidy than sporadic colon cancer.[35]

Hormone Receptors

There are no current studies that stratify HBC, FBC, and SBC with respect to tumor cell content of estrogen or progesterone receptors.

Endocrine Studies

Endocrine studies were also informative on our HBC resource. We performed a case-control study of endocrine profiles involving 30 premenopausal white women at 50 percent risk from HBC-prone kindreds and compared them with 30 meticulously matched controls who had negative family histories of breast cancer through at least two generations.[20–22] Urine samples were collected every 12 hours through an entire monthly menstrual cycle. Blood was collected every other day. Findings from this study showed that (1) plasma androsterone sulfate was significantly lower in our high-risk patients; (2) urinary estrone and estradiol glucuronide, but not estriol glucuronide, were significantly lower in the high-risk patients; and (3) estrogen conjugation occurred at a specific time of the ovulatory cycle: during the periovulatory period. These results merit testing on a larger number of patients at risk for hereditary breast cancer.

Reverse Transcriptase

In a solitary report, reverse transcriptase activity has recently been detected in cultured peripheral blood monocytes from patients with breast cancer, but not in control patients without cancer.[2] Reverse transcriptase is strong evidence for the presence of a retrovirus, as the activity was associated with particles of a density similar to that of known retroviruses. This finding, if verified, would be of particular interest, since a retroviral etiology for breast cancer is known in mice and has been suggested in humans. If there is a retroviral etiology for human breast cancer, it would seem more likely to be associated with FPC or HBC than with SBC; the former two would be associated with vertical transmission, and the latter with horizontal transmission of virus. This report is preliminary and needs further investigation.

Oncogene Expression

Various oncogenes or oncogene products, such as Harvey *ras* p21[100] and *erb*-2b[12] are expressed in breast carcinomas. Oncogenes themselves may be amplified (i.e., present in increased copies) in the genome of tumors. In the case of *HER2/neu*, such amplification is associated with poorer prognosis,[97] and amplifications or deletions of other oncogenes also are associated with poorer prognosis in breast cancer.[12] In no case has expression or amplification of oncogenes yet been correlated to HBC or FBC status, however.

Polymorphic Oncogene Alleles

Since Lidereau[42] had reported an excess of rare alleles of the highly polymorphic c-Ha-*ras*-1 oncogene in breast cancer patient germline DNA compared to normal controls, we have examined this and other polymorphic oncogenic loci in collaboration with the Laboratory of Tumor Immunology and Biology at the National Cancer Institute.[51] We have looked for differences in germline allele frequencies between normals and members of HBC families, and between affected and unaffected members within HBC families. Since the possibility exists that the defect underlying HBC involves a specific germline deletion of genetic materials that would in-

crease the chance of a specific deleterious somatic mutation in an oncogene on the homologous chromosome, we are also examining nearby polymorphic loci, searching for loci with a diminution of heterozygosity. Since somatic alterations of certain oncogenes have been shown to occur in various types of cancer, including breast cancer, and to be related to certain clinical aspects of the disease, we hoped to compare genotypes for oncogene loci between germline (lymphocyte) DNA and somatic (tumor) DNA.

In the loci so far studied,[51] we have found no differences between the affected and unaffected members of the HBC families. Comparing the pooled set of HBC cases to published gene frequencies based on a series of normal and/or non-HBC breast cancer cases (see Table 13–2), we found that the relative frequency of "rare" c-Ha-*ras*-1 alleles was intermediate between previously ascertained frequencies in a normal (unaffected) series of cases and those in non-HBC breast cancer cases, and that there was a slightly decreased frequency of the *a* allele and a slightly elevated frequency of the *b* (shorter) allele of *erb-a*-2 compared to a series of normal cases. Since the numbers of cases are so small, and since no differences were found between affected and unaffected cases, we consider these results to be inconclusive. Similarly, for the three loci studied so far, no reductions in germline heterozygosity have been observed.

We investigated whether the breast cancer–affected members of the HBC families show any alterations of DNA structure at these oncogene loci in formalin-fixed, paraffin-embedded, archival tumor tissue, relative to fresh lymphocyte DNA (we did not have a sufficient number of fresh tumor specimens to study). Unfortunately, we were not successful in extracting high molecular weight DNA from the great majority of these fixed tumors. We recommend archiving fresh breast cancer specimens from patients with HBC.

Cytogenetics

The cytogenetic evaluation of human solid tumors has received significantly less attention than that of the human leukemias.[101] Mitelman,[75] in an extensive review of this subject, has shown that less than 10 percent of the total cytogenetic studies of human cancer pertained to carcinomas. However, among solid tumors, breast cancer has received relatively frequent attention by cytogeneticists. Sandberg[88] reported that in the majority of primary and metastatic breast cancer cases, the chromosomal picture, regardless of modal chromosome number, was extremely abnormal; diploid cells were rare, and most of the breast cancers were aneuploid with markers. In a study of HBC kindreds, we have observed an excess of hyperdiploidy in cultured skin fibroblasts,[53] a result that needs further investigation.

In breast cancer cases investigated by chromosome banding analysis, Trent[102] states that those chromosomes most commonly altered were numbers 1, 6, 7, and 11. Of special interest is the fact that these chromosomes serve as the site for various c-*onc* sequences. For ex-

Table 13–2. FREQUENCIES OF RFLP ALLELES OF THREE PROTO-ONCOGENES IN HEREDITARY BREAST CANCER CASES AND THEIR FIRST DEGREE RELATIVES

Locus Name	Allele(s)	Non-HBC Frequencies*		HBC Gene Frequencies†	
		Unaffected (%)	*BC Affected (%)*	*Unaffected (%)*	*BC Affected (%)*
c-Ha-*ras*-1	Common	91	58	70	73
	Rare	9	42	30	27
	a	61	59	59	52
int-2	a	67	66	76	67
	b	33	34	24	33
erb-A-2	a	44	26	23	
	b	56	74	77	

*Non-HBC comparison gene frequencies are taken from:
  (*ras*) Lidereau R, et al: J Natl Cancer Inst 77:697, 1986;
  (*int*) Unpublished results of series of cases studied at NCI;
  (*erb*) Middleton PG, et al: Nucl Acids Res 14:1925, 1986.
†HBC gene frequencies are based on 63 cases (26 affected and 37 unaffected relatives).

ample, three oncogenes have now been mapped to chromosome 1: c-B-*lym*-1, c-N-*ras*, and c-*sk*; the c-*myb* is on chromosome 6; the c-*erb*-b is localized on 7p; and on chromosome 11, two c-*onc* genes are present, the c-H-*ras* (on 11p) and c-*ets* (on 11q).

Ferti-Passantonopoulou and Panani[19] studied the cytogenetics, using G-banding on direct tumor preparations, from five patients with breast cancer. Aberrations in chromosomes, according to frequency, were 1, 11, 3, 6, 5, and 17. In all of the cases abnormalities of chromosomes 1 and 11 were observed. In each patient chromosome 1 was involved in at least two different situations. In four of the patients abnormalities of chromosome 11 showed nonrandom involvement of q22-23. These investigators concluded that ". . . band 11q22-23, which has been reported to be an inheritable fragile site and is a specific breakpoint in acute leukemia, also may be specific in a group of breast cancer. Thus, correlation of an inheritable fragile site and a malignant disease with familial incidence seems possible."

The study of a variety of cytogenetic markers of specific tumors has shown that while most are acquired somatically by the tumor, a certain fraction are known to be constitutional, such as the 11p13 deletion of Wilms' tumor and the 13q14 deletion in hereditary retinoblastoma. The subsequent deletion of the normal allele may then unmask an otherwise recessive cancer allele. Lundberg et al.[43] described tumor loss of heterozygosity occurring specifically and nonrandomly on chromosome 13 in a small number of cases of ductal carcinoma. These data indicated the possibility that in these cases pathogenesis involved a somatic deletion of genetic material that unmasked a recessive breast cancer–predisposing allele.

NEW OBSERVATIONS IN MOLECULAR GENETICS OF BREAST CANCER

Restriction fragment length polymorphism (RFLP) analysis has identified allelic loss involving loci on several chromosomes in breast cancer. Ali et al.[1a] reported allelic loss at loci on the short arm of chromosome 3 in breast cancer. The region involved on 3p contains two oncogenes, c-*erb*AB and c-*erb*A2, that are members of the steroid/thyroid hormone receptor family. Deletions on 3p have also been described in small cell lung cancer and renal cell carcinoma. This finding is consistent with a model of a suppressor gene as described to occur in retinoblastoma.

In 1986, Theillet et al.[98a] reported allele loss of chromosome 11 in 27 percent of informative breast carcinomas. Ali et al.[1b] reported that chromosome 11 allelic loss has significant association with tumors that lack estrogen and progesterone receptors, grade III tumors, and distal metastases.

Loss of heterozygosity on chromosome 13 in ductal breast cancer occurring in premenopausal women suggested that these occurrences of breast cancer may involve the same genetic locus that has been implicated in retinoblastoma.[43] Lee et al.[38a] suggest that the Rb gene is inactivated in some breast cancer cell lines.

Mackay et al.[66a] studied fresh tumor tissue and blood leucocyte DNA from 100 consecutive patients undergoing surgical resections for primary breast cancer. The highest frequency of allele loss, namely 61 percent, was identified with the probe YNZ22, which detects a sequence on the short arm of chromosome 17 (p13.3). These investigators postulate that the putative breast tumor suppressor gene on 17p may be the same as that noted for sporadic colon and lung cancers.

Using classical genetics, Anderson et al.[2a] found evidence of linkage between the Rh locus on the 1p32-36 region and tumor development in breast/ovarian cancer families. By employing molecular probes for this region to examine DNAs from normal and tumor tissue, they detected loss of heterozygosity in five of ten patients with informative alleles and, in another, detected alterations in 20 of the 38 DNAs. It is now clear that chromosomes 1, 3, 11, 13, and 17 must be considered as candidates for linkage studies in HBC kindreds.

LINKAGE

The ultimate objective of research in genetic linkage in breast cancer is to localize the site of the deleterious gene(s) on one of the chromosomes. Once gene localization has been accomplished we will then be in a better position to identify at-risk individuals and to study the pathogenetic mechanisms that may be responsible for variance in HBC subsets. At the present time, however, no linkage markers are known for HBC.

Previous Studies of HBC Genetics

A major gene hypothesis for hereditary cancer was tested by Go et al.[25] using segregation analysis on 18 families from our breast cancer family resource. In two of these families, the cancer appeared to be of nongenetic origin, while in two others, there was an excess of childhood cancers (fitting the diagnosis of the SBLA syndrome). The remaining 14 families were divided into two groups based on family mean age of diagnosis: Group I (ten families, 1548 individuals) with a mean age at diagnosis of less than 52 years; and Group II (four families, 463 individuals) with a mean age at diagnosis of more than 54. It was tentatively concluded that in the Group I families, there was a dominant segregating gene that increased susceptibility to either breast or ovarian cancer. Female carriers of the gene in these families had an estimated lifetime risk of 0.9 to either of the two cancers, whereas noncarriers of the gene had a trivially small risk of these two cancers. In the Group II families, on the other hand, it was estimated that female carriers of the dominant gene were completely susceptible; i.e., they had a lifetime risk of unity, if they lived long enough, to either breast cancer or endometrial cancer.

Linkage studies were also performed on HBC families from our resource[33] using 21 polymorphic genetic markers and analyzing for linkage to postulated dominant and recessive cancer susceptibility alleles. The strongest lod score for linkage was between a dominant susceptibility allele and GPT (glutamic pyruvic transaminase) in a subset of families with premenopausal HBC; this lod score was small and considered preliminary by the authors.

Prospective Linkage Studies and Implications

Major advances in biomolecular genetic technology during the past decade have made successful human linkage studies more likely. For example, the growing number of DNA polymorphisms that have become available for genetic linkage studies has enabled the construction of detailed maps of the human genome.[106] These resultant linkage maps are constantly being refined for a variety of chromosome regions.[38] Cancer-prone families will make linkage studies possible; selection of the most informative families will make these research ef-

forts more cost effective. Finding genetic linkage will have immediate relevance to genetic counseling and for the detection of disease heterogeneity.

Major applications for the use of DNA probes for detection of linkage between a restriction fragment length polymorphism (RFLP) and a mutated locus has resulted in the successful mapping of several inherited diseases, including Duchenne type muscular dystrophy; Huntington's chorea; polycystic kidney disease; cystic fibrosis; and multiple endocrine neoplasia, type IIa (MEN IIa). Linkage data, for example, have shown that in some kindreds, the predisposing mutation in MEN IIa maps relatively close to the centromere of chromosome 10, which is where the interstitial retinol-binding protein gene is located (10p11.2-q11.2),[69] a finding also confirmed by Simpson et al.[95] In another precancer hereditary disorder, Bodmer et al.[5] employed the C11p11 probe in a study of 124 members from 13 FPC families. Six of the families, which included 79 individuals, yielded a combined maximum lod score of 3.26 at a recombination fraction of $\theta = 0$. In situ hybridization localized the probe on chromosome 5 to 5q21-q22.

The ideal family for linkage investigation would be one in whom the phenotype has been clearly defined in the light of the natural history facets of hereditary cancer. Such a family should contain a large number of affected and at-risk subjects who are available for typing, with multiple generations and an extended kindred in which several sibships include affected members.

While advances in the recognition of breast cancer–prone families through clinical and pedigree analyses have been prodigious during the past two decades, there remain many problem areas. Linkage studies of HBC families may be confounded by (1) a sporadic occurrence; (2) incomplete penetrance and variable expressivity of the gene; (3) limited number of at-risk women; (4) paternal transmission; (5) deaths of key relatives before the onset of breast cancer; and (6) the occurrence of cancer at nonbreast sites that has an uncertain etiological association with the breast cancer susceptibility in a given family. It is unclear whether breast cancer–prone families differing in typical age of onset,[57] typical histological type of cancer, or the frequent occurrence of cancer at a particular nonbreast site represent etiologically distinct syndromes, or whether a single major genetic susceptibility defect underlies them.

The search for biomarkers that can predict genotypic status in cancer-prone families may assist in resolving many of the perplexities in the multistep process of carcinogenesis. Knowing who will and who will not manifest cancer in one of the more than 100 hereditary cancer and precancer-prone disorders afflicting man will have profound implications for cancer surveillance programs. Would at-risk patients want to be tested, and if so, when? Would third party carriers use this information to deny insurance or to find an opportunity to cancel a given patient's policy? Would society come to the rescue of at-risk patients by providing financial support for biomarker assessment and, in turn, for highly targeted surveillance and management programs? These are just a few of the many vexing issues and questions that will have to be addressed by physicians and policy makers once linkage for HBC is established.

SURVEILLANCE AND THERAPEUTIC CONSIDERATIONS

There has been much controversy surrounding the time for instituting mammographic screening. Opinions have ranged from performing baseline mammography at age 35 for women in the general population to recommendations by the American Cancer Society and the National Cancer Institute for initiation of mammography at age 40 years, with repeat mammograms every 2 years through age 50 and then annually thereafter. More recently, serious questions were raised about performance of mammography among individuals younger than 50 years from the general population. Specifically, Eddy et al.[16] has provided evidence that healthy asymptomatic women between ages 40 and 49 do not show sufficient health or economic benefit from mammography to offset the costs and risks. They contend that the costs for screening this cohort are high and relatively few lives would be saved. Their data indicate that mammography screening in the fourth decade would carry a risk of radiation-induced cancer of the breast of about one in 25,000. They conclude that a more prudent approach is to initiate mammography at age 50.

The matter of hereditary breast cancer was totally ignored in these reports. This is surprising, since HBC accounts for approximately nine percent of the total number of breast cancer cases[51] and its average age of onset is approximately 44 years.[46, 59] Indeed, as mentioned, we have recently described a subset of HBC that is characterized by extraordinarily early age of breast cancer onset, typically in the 20s and 30s.[56] We therefore recommend that HBC family members initiate mammography by age 25 years. HBC family members are one component of a group of women who are at much higher risk for breast cancer prior to age 50 than are average "healthy asymptomatic" women. In this group of women, we believe that the health and economic benefits of mammography far outweigh the costs and risks.

Mammograms can be interpreted, albeit with greater difficulty as a result of dense parenchyma, in younger women. While the majority of women younger than 35 will have dense breast parenchyma, it has been demonstrated that 20 percent will exhibit considerable fatty replacement.[73] Discriminants of breast parenchymal patterns are likely multifactorial. Several studies have shown that detection of early breast cancer in women with dense breast parenchymal patterns is clearly possible.[91, 92] Sickles reviewed mammograms on 300 nonpalpable breast cancers. Slightly less than half of the patients had breast parenchymal patterns identified as dense (Wolf's classification P2 and DY).[92] Mammographic features present to suggest malignancy were composed of calcifications in 42 percent of all patients, masses in 39 percent of all patients, and indirect signs such as architectural distortion or asymmetry in 19 percent of all patients. While not specifically addressed, it can be assumed that each of these features that suggested malignancy were seen in the dense as well as the fatty breast parenchymal pattern.[92]

We are concerned about the manner in which the genral public, as well as physicians, may interpret the findings of Eddy et al.,[16] particularly because they have been reported by the lay press. These reports may discourage many HBC and other high-risk patients from coming forward for mammography screening at appropriate early ages.

A second controversial question in HBC management concerns the use of prophylactic mastectomy to prevent breast cancer development.[65] This is sometimes recommended in two types of cases. Women with unilateral breast cancer, diagnosed at a treatable stage, are frequently encouraged to have prophylactic contralateral mastectomy because of the high risk of developing cancer in the opposite breast.[29]

Cancer-free HBC family members may be considered for prophylactic bilateral total mastectomy based on the following highly selective criteria:

1. The clear establishment of the patient's family as an HBC family and the 50 percent risk status of the patient based on her pedigree position.

2. Clear and careful presentation of the risk situation to the patient, with stress on the fact that while she has a 50 percent chance of carrying the high-risk gene, she also has a 50 percent chance of not carrying the gene and thus of being at normal risk for breast cancer. We find that the majority of our patients in this situation opt for intensive follow-up rather than prophylactic surgery.

3. The presence of additional factors that indicate a higher than 50 percent risk to the patient (such as the case of an HBC family member with both affected sisters and daughters, who would be presumed to be an obligate gene carrier, with a breast cancer risk approaching 100 percent and other factors (such as severe cancer phobia or breasts that are difficult to examine clinically or radiographically and on biopsy show proliferative disease with atypical hyperplasia).

For the purposes of both surveillance and therapy, it is extremely important to gather as much scientific evidence as possible about the impact differing risk factors might have on BC-prone genotype(s). One obvious point of clinical importance is that if certain risk factors significantly perturbed BC risk in women who are considered to be at 50 percent risk within an HBC pedigree, then appropriate control measures (e.g., avoiding such risk factors) should then be exercised in the interest of cancer control. Regarding therapy, hypotheses to be tested pertain to whether or not patients with HBC might be more or less responsive to such well-known chemotherapeutic protocols as cytoxan, methotrexate, and 5-fluorouracil (CMF), to adriamycin, or to the antiestrogen tamoxifen. We should also search for differences in response to radiation therapy, either as a single agent or in concert with chemotherapy and surgery. We should even assess the effectiveness of differing surgical approaches to BC (i.e., lumpectomy, simple mastectomy, modified radical mastectomy, and axillary node dissection in concert with HBC). While axillary node dissection is a standard course of action for these surgeries, including lumpectomy, it would be of value to determine whether there might be a differential response with respect to axillary lymph nodes; i.e., retaining or resecting them for a "protective" vs. "nonprotective" impact in BC occurrence in hereditary vs. nonhereditary cohorts. As far as we can determine, these types of data are nonexistent since chemotherapy, radiation therapy, and surgical protocols have failed to stratify patients relevant to positive family history (HBC) vs. negative family history (SBC), thereby assessing the host factor influence on outcome in context with these specific therapeutic modalities.

SUMMARY AND CONCLUSIONS

Familial breast cancer has been known for nearly two millenia; recent studies indicate that it comprises one third of the total number of breast cancer cases. About one fourth of FBC falls into the special subset of hereditary breast cancer, characterized by an additional combination of factors that may include a family history of breast and other cancers in an autosomal dominant susceptibility pattern, early age of onset, and an excess of bilateral breast cancer and other multiple primary cancers. The risk of developing a hereditary breast cancer is determined by the pedigree, appears to be independent of age at first pregnancy, and is enhanced when a biopsy shows atypical hyperplasia. Particularly early ages of onset are seen when other HBC pedigree members have early onset breast cancer. HBC is a heterogeneous entity, with site-specific, breast/ovarian, SBLA syndrome, and Cowden's disease variants currently recognized. The most important tool in the diagnosis and management of HBC and FBC at the present time is epidemiological: the importance of obtaining a thorough family history cannot be overemphasized. Unfortunately, biomarkers at present do not sensitively or specifically identify HBC individuals before the cancer is expressed. Ultimately, genetic linkage analysis of alleles polymorphic in DNA restriction fragment lengths should identify site(s) on chromosomes associated with HBC. This knowledge should identify individuals who will develop HBC. Until then, a careful and complete family pedigree and close surveillance with frequent physical examinations and mammograms must suffice to identify and follow individuals at risk and to gauge therapy.

References

1. Albano WA, Recabaren JA, Lynch HT, et al: Natural history of hereditary cancer of the breast and colon. Cancer 50:360–363, 1982.
1a. Ali IU, Lidereau R, Callahan R: Presence of two members of c-*erb*A receptor gene family (c-*erb*AB and c-*erb*A2) in smallest region of somatic homozygosity on chromosome 3p21-p25 in human breast carcinoma. JNCI 81:1815–1820, 1989.
1b. Ali IU, Lidereau R, Theillet C, Callahan R: Reduction to homozygosity of genes on chromosome 11 in human breast neoplasia. Science 238:185–188, 1987.
2. Al-Sumidaie AM, Leinster SJ, Hart CA, Green CD, McCarthy K: Particles with properties of retrovirus in monocytes from patients with breast cancer. Lancet i:5–8, 1988.
2a. Anderson DE: Clinical characteristics of the genetic variety of cutaneous melanoma in man. Cancer 28:721–725, 1971.
3. Anderson DE: Genetic study of breast cancer: identification of a high risk group. Cancer 34:1090–1097, 1974.
4. Birch JM, Hartley AL, Marsden HB, Harris M, Swindell R: Excess of breast cancer in mothers of children with soft tissue sarcomas. Br J Cancer 49:325–331, 1984.
5. Bodmer WF, Bailey CJ, Bodmer J, Bussey HJR, et al: Localization of the gene for familial adenomatous polyps on chromosome 5. Nature 328:614–616, 1987.
6. Bottomley RH, Condit PT: Cancer families. Cancer Bull 20:22–24, 1968.
7. Bottomley RH, Condit PT, Chanes RE: Cytogenetic studies in familial malignancy. Clin Res 15:334, 1967.
8. Bottomley RH, Trainer AL, Condit PT: Chromosome studies in a "cancer family." Cancer 28:519–528, 1971.
9. Broca P: Traite' des Tumeurs, vols. 1 and 2. Paris, Asselin, 1866.
10. Brownstein MH: Breast cancer in Cowden's syndrome. *In* Lynch HT (ed): Genetics and Breast Cancer. New York, Van Nostrand Reinhold, 1981, pp 187–195.
11. Brownstein MH, Wolf M, Bikowski JB: Cowden's disease: a cutaneous marker of breast cancer. Cancer 41:2393–2398, 1978.
12. Cline MH, Battifora H, Yokata J: Proto-oncogene abnormalities in human breast cancer: correlations with anatomic features and clinical course of disease. J Clin Onc 5:999–1006, 1987.
13. Coulson PB, Thornthwaite JT, Wooley TW, et al: Prognostic indicators including DNA histogram type, receptor content, and staging related to human breast cancer patient survival. Cancer Res 44:4187–4196, 1984.
14. DuPont WD, Page DL: Risk factors for breast cancer in women with proliferative breast disease. N Engl J Med 312:145–151, 1985.
15. DuPont WD, Page DL: Breast cancer risk associated with proliferative disease, age at first birth, and a family history of breast cancer. Am J Epidemiol 125:769–779, 1987.
16. Eddy D, Hasselblad V, McGivney W, Hendee W: The value of mammography screening in women under age 50 years. JAMA 259:1512–1519, 1988.
17. Elston CW: Grading of invasive carcinoma of the breast. *In* Page DL, Anderson TJ (eds): Diagnostic Histopathology of the Breast. Edinburgh, Churchill Livingstone, 1987.
18. Ferenc MJ, Naus GJ: Predictive value of flow cytometric DNA content analysis of paraffin-embedded tissue in carcinoma of the breast. Lab Invest 54:19A, 1986.
19. Ferti-Passantonopoulou AD, Panani AD: Common cytogenetic findings in primary breast cancer. Cancer Genet Cytogenet 27:289–298, 1987.
20. Fishman J, Bradlow HL, Fukushima D, et al: Abnormal estrogen conjugation in women at risk for familial breast cancer is concentrated at the periovulatory stage of the menstrual cycle. Cancer Res 43:1884–1890, 1983.
21. Fishman J, Fukushima D, O'Connor J, et al: Plasma hormone profiles of young women at risk for familial breast cancer. Cancer Res 38:4006–4011, 1978.
22. Fishman J, Fukushima D, O'Connor J, Lynch HT: Low urinary estrogen glucuronides in women at risk for familial breast cancer. Science 204:1089–1091, 1979.
23. Fraschini G, Johnson T, Raber M, et al: Prediction of breast cancer relapse by ploidy, proliferative activity, and estrogen receptor content (ER). (Abstract) Proc Am Soc Cancer Res 27:158, 1986.
24. Fraumeni JF, Grundy GW, Creagan ET, Everson RB: Six families prone to ovarian cancer. Cancer 36:364–369, 1975.
25. Go RCP, King M-C, Bailey-Wilson JE, et al: Genetic epidemiology of breast cancer and associated cancers in high risk families, part I. J Natl Cancer Inst 71:455–461, 1983.
26. Greene GL, Gilna P, Waterfield M, et al: Sequence and expres-

sion of human estrogen receptor complementary DNA. Science 231:1150–1154, 1986.

27. Green S, Walter P, Kumar V, et al: Human oestrogen receptor cDNA: sequence expression and homology to v-*erb*-A. Nature 320:134–139, 1986.

28. Haagensen CD, Haagensen DE Jr, Bodian C: Risk and Detection of Breast Cancer. Philadelphia, WB Saunders, 1981, pp 10–13.

29. Harris RE, Lynch HT, Guirgis HA: Familial breast cancer: risk to the contralateral breast. J Natl Cancer Inst 60:947–955, 1978.

30. Hedley DW, Rugg CA, Ng ABP, Taylor IW. Influence of cellular DNA content on disease free survival of stage II breast cancer patients. Cancer Res 44:5395–5398, 1984.

31. Henderson BE, Pike MC, Ross RK: Epidemiology and risk factors. In Bonadonna G (ed): Breast Cancer: Diagnosis and Management. Chichester, MA, John Wiley and Sons, 1984, pp 15–33.

32. Jian-Min Y, Yu MC, Ross RK, Yu-Tang G, Henderson BE: Risk factors for breast cancer in Chinese women in Shanghai. Cancer Res 48:1949–1953, 1988.

33. King M-C, Go RCP, Lynch HT, et al: Genetic epidemiology of breast cancer associated cancers in high risk families, part II. J Natl Cancer Inst 71:463–467, 1983.

34. Kokal W, Shebani K, Terz J, Harada R: Tumor DNA content in the prognosis of colorectal carcinoma. JAMA 255:3123–3127, 1986.

35. Kouri M, Laasonen A, Mecklin JP, Pyrhonen S. DNA ploidy of hereditary nonpolyposis colorectal cancer. (Abstract) Cytometry 8:54, 1987.

36. Kozak FK, Hall JG, Baird PA: Familial breast cancer in males: a case report and review of the literature. Cancer 58:2736–2739, 1986.

37. Lagios MD, Rose MR, Margolin FR: Tubular carcinoma of the breast: association with multicentricity, bilaterality, and family history of mammary carcinoma. Am J Clin Path 23:25–30, 1980.

38. Lathrop GM, Lalouel JM, White RL: Construction of human linkage maps: likelihood calculations for multilocus linkage analysis. Genet Epidemiol 3:39–47, 1986.

38a. Lee EYH, To H, Shew JY, Bookstein R, Scully P, Lee WH: Inactivation of the retinoblastoma susceptibility gene in human breast cancers. Science 241:218–221, 1988.

39. Li FP, Fraumeni JF: Soft tissue sarcomas, breast cancer, and other neoplasms: a familial syndrome? Ann Int Med 71:747–752, 1969.

40. Li FP, Fraumeni JF: Familial breast cancer, soft-tissue sarcomas, and other neoplasms. Ann Int Med 83:833–834, 1975.

41. Li FP, Fraumeni JF: Prospective study of a family cancer syndrome. JAMA 247:2692–2694, 1982.

42. Lidereau R, Escot C, Theillet C, et al: High frequency of rare alleles of the human c-Ha-*ras*-1 proto-oncogene in breast cancer patients. J Natl Cancer Inst 77:697–701, 1986.

43. Lundberg C, Skoog L, Cavenee WK, Nordenskjold M: Loss of heterozygosity in human ductal breast tumors indicates a recessive mutation on chromosome 13. Proc Natl Acad Sci 84:2372–2376, 1987.

44. Lynch HT: Hereditary Factors in Carcinoma: Recent Results in Cancer Research, vol 12. New York, Springer-Verlag, 1967, p 186.

45. Lynch HT: Cancer Genetics. Springfield, IL, Charles C Thomas, 1976.

46. Lynch HT: Genetics and Breast Cancer. New York, Van Nostrand Reinhold, 1981.

47. Lynch HT, Fusaro RM: Cancer-Associated Genodermatoses. New York, Van Nostrand Reinhold, 1982.

48. Lynch HT, Krush AJ: Heredity and breast cancer: implications for cancer detection. Med Times 94:599–605, 1966.

49. Lynch HT, Krush AJ: Carcinoma of the breast and ovary in three families. Surg Gynecol Obstet 133:644–648, 1971.

50. Lynch PM, Lynch HT: Colon Cancer Genetics. New York, Van Nostrand Reinhold, 1985.

51. Lynch HT, Lynch JF: Breast cancer genetics in an oncology clinic: 328 consecutive patients. Cancer Genet Cytogenet 22:369–371, 1986.

52. Lynch HT, Albano WA, Danes BS, et al: Genetic predisposition to breast cancer. Cancer 53:612–622, 1984.

53. Lynch HT, Albano WA, Heieck JJ, et al: Genetics, biomarkers, and breast cancer: a review. Cancer Genet Cytogenet 13:43–92, 1984.

54. Lynch HT, Albano WA, Layton MA, et al: Breast cancer, genetics, and age at first pregnancy. J Med Genet 21:96–98, 1984.

55. Lynch HT, Conway T, Fitzgibbons RJ Jr, et al: Age of onset heterogeneity in hereditary breast cancer: minimal clues for diagnosis. Br Cancer Res Treat 12:275–285, 1988.

56. Lynch HT, Conway T, Watson P, Schreiman J, Fitzgibbons RJ Jr: Extremely early onset hereditary breast cancer (HBC): surveillance/management implications. Nebr Med J 73:97–100, 1988.

57. Lynch HT, Fain PR, Goldgar D, et al: Familial breast cancer and its recognition in an oncology clinic. Cancer 47:2730–2739, 1981.

58. Lynch HT, Guirgis HA, Albert S, Brennan M, Lynch J, Kraft C, Pocekay D, Vaughn C, Kaplan A: Familial association of carcinoma of the breast and ovary. Surg Gynecol Obstet 138:717–724, 1974.

59. Lynch HT, Guirgis HA, Brodkey F, et al: Early age of onset in familial breast cancer: genetic and cancer control implications. Arch Surg 111:126–131, 1976a.

60. Lynch HT, Harris RE, Organ CH, et al: Familial association of breast/ovarian cancer. Cancer 41:1543–1548, 1978.

61. Lynch HT, Kaplan AR, Lynch JF: Klinefelter's syndrome, genetically transmitted cancer diathesis, and breast cancer: a family study. JAMA 229:809–811, 1974.

62. Lynch HT, Katz D, Bogard PJ, Lynch JF: The sarcoma, breast cancer, lung cancer, and adrenocortical carcinoma syndrome revisited. AJDC 139:134–136, 1985.

63. Lynch HT, Krush AJ, Lemon HM, et al: Tumor variation in families with breast cancer. JAMA 222:1631–1635, 1972.

64. Lynch HT, Mulcahy GM, Harris RE, et al: Genetic and pathologic findings in a kindred with hereditary sarcoma, breast cancer, brain tumors, leukemia, lung, laryngeal, and adrenal cortical carcinoma. Cancer 41:2055–2064, 1978.

65. Lynch HT, Watson P, Conway T, Fitzsimmons ML, Lynch J: Breast cancer family history as a risk factor for early onset breast cancer. Br Cancer Res Treat 11:263–267, 1988.

66. Lynch HT, Watson P, Marcus JN, et al: Hereditary breast cancer: search for biomarkers. J Tumor Mark Oncol 2:153–159, 1987.

66a. Mackay J, Steel CM, Elder PA, Forrest AP, Evans HJ: Allele loss on short arm of chromosome 17 in breast cancers. Lancet ii:1384–1385, 1988.

67. Marcus J, Page D, Watson P, Conway T, Lynch HT: High mitotic grade in hereditary breast cancer. Lab Invest 58:61A, 1988.

68. Masters JRW, Camplejohn RS, Millis RR, Rubens RD. Histologic grade, elastosis, DNA ploidy and the response to chemotherapy of breast cancer. Br J Cancer 55:455–457, 1987.

69. Mathew CGP, Chin KS, Easton DF, et al: A linked genetic marker for multiple endocrine neoplasia type 2A on chromosome 10. Nature 328:527–528, 1987.

70. McDivitt RW, Rubin GL, Wingo PA, et al: Benign breast disease histology and the risk of breast cancer. Lab Invest 58:62A, 1988.

71. McDivitt RW, Stone KR, Craig B, Palmer JO, Meyer JS, Bauer WC. A proposed classification of breast cancer based on kinetic information. Cancer 57:269–276, 1986.

72. Meyer JE, Friedman E, McCrate MM, Baver WC: Prediction of early course of breast carcinoma by thymidine labeling. Cancer 51:1879–1886, 1983.

73. Meyer JE, Kopans DB, Oot R: Breast cancer visualized by mammography in patients under 35. Radiology 147:93–94, 1983.

74. Meyer JS, Prey MV, Babcock DS, McDivitt RW: Breast carcinoma cell kinetics, morphology, stage, and host characteristics: a thymidine labeling study. Lab Invest 54:41–51, 1986.

74a. Middleton PG, Angelis CD, Weir-Thompson EM, Steel CM: RFLP for the human erbA₂ gene. Nucl Acids Res 14:1925, 1986.

75. Mitelman F: Catalogue of chromosome aberrations in cancer. Cytogenet Cell Genet 36:1–516, 1983.

76. Mulcahy GM, Platt R: Pathology aspects of familial carcinoma of the breast. *In* Lynch HT (ed): Genetics and Breast Cancer. New York, Van Nostrand Reinhold, 1981, p 65.
77. Ottman R, Pike MC, King M-C, Casagrande JT, Henderson BE: Familial breast cancer in a population-based series. Am J Epidemiol 123:15–21, 1986.
78. Page DL, Anderson TJ: Diagnostic Histopathology of the Breast. Edinburgh, Churchill Livingstone, 1987.
79. Page DL, Dupont WD, Rogers LW, Rados MS: Atypical hyperplastic lesions of female breast: long-term followup study. Cancer 55:2698–2708, 1985.
80. Petrakis NL, Ernster V, King M-C: Breast cancer. *In* Schottenfeld DS, Fraumeni JF Jr (eds): Cancer Epidemiology and Prevention. Philadelphia, WB Saunders, 1981, pp 855–870.
81. Pritchard TJ, Pankowsky DA, Crowe JP, Abdul-Karim FW: Breast cancer in a male-to-female transsexual: a case report. JAMA 259:2278–2280, 1988.
82. Ridolfi RL, Rosen PP, Port A, et al: Medullary carcinoma of the breast. Cancer 40:1365–1385, 1977.
83. Rosen N, Israel MA: Genetic abnormalities as biological tumor markers. Semin Oncol 14:213–231, 1987.
84. Rosen PP, Ashikari R, Thaler H, et al: A comparative study of some pathologic features of mammary carcinoma in Tokyo, Japan and New York, USA. Cancer 39:429–434, 1977.
85. Rosen PP, Cantrell B, Mullen DL, DePalo A: Juvenile papillomatosis (Swiss cheese disease) of the breast. Am J Surg Pathol 4:3–12, 1980.
86. Rosen PP, Lesser ML, Senie RT, Kinne DW: Epidemiology of breast carcinoma, III: a clinicopathologic study with a 10 year followup. Cancer 50:171–179, 1982.
87. Rosen PP, Holmes G, Lesser ML, Kinne DW, Beattie EJ: Juvenile papillomatosis and breast carcinoma. Cancer 55:1345–1352, 1985.
88. Sandberg AA: The Chromosomes in Human Cancer and Leukemia. New York, Elsevier, 1980, p 485.
89. Sap J, Munoz A, Damm K, et al: The c-*erb*-A protein is a high affinity receptor for thyroid hormone. Nature 324:635–640, 1986.
90. Sattin RW, Rubin GL, Webster LA, et al: Family history and the risk of breast cancer. JAMA 253:1908–1913, 1985.
91. Seidman H, Gelb SK, Silverberg E, LaVerda N, Lubera JA: Survival experience in the breast cancer detection demonstration project. Cancer 37:258–290, 1987.
92. Sickles EA: Mammographic features of 300 consecutive nonpalpable breast cancers. AJR 146:661–663, 1986.
93. Silverberg E: Cancer statistics, 1984. Cancer 34:7–23, 1984.
94. Silverberg E, Lubera JA: Cancer statistics, 1987. Cancer 37:2–19, 1987.
95. Simpson NE, Kidd KK, Goodfellow PJ, et al: Assignment of multiple endocrine neoplasia type 2A to chromosome 10 by linkage. Nature 328:528–530, 1987.
96. Siraganian PA, Levine PH, Madigan P, Mulvihill JJ: Familial breast cancer in black Americans. Cancer 60:1657–1660, 1987.
97. Slamon DJ, Clark GM, Wong SG, et al: Human breast cancer: correlation of relapse and survival with amplification of the HER-2/*neu* oncogene. Science 235:177–182, 1987.
98. Starink TM: The Cowden syndrome and other familial multiple hair follicle tumor syndromes. Amsterdam, Free University Press, 1986.
98a. Theillet C, Lidereau R, Escot C, et al.: Loss of a c-H-*ras*-1 allele and aggressive human primary breast carcinomas. Cancer Res 46:4776–4781, 1986.
99. Thompson EN, Dellamore NS, Brook DL: Parent cancer in an unselected cohort of children with cancer referred to a single center. Br J Cancer 57:127–129, 1988.
100. Thor A, Ohuchi N, Horan-Hand P, et al: *Ras* gene alterations and enhanced levels of *ras* p21 expression in a spectrum of benign and malignant human mammary tissues. Lab Invest 55:603–615, 1986.
101. Trent J: Chromosomal alterations in human solid tumors: implications of the stem cell model to cancer cytogenetics. *In* Rowley JD (ed): Chromosomes and Oncogenes in Human Cancers, vol. 3. (Bristol Myers Cancer Symposium Series). New York, Academic Press, 1984, p 395.
102. Trent JM: Cytogenetic and molecular biologic alterations in human breast cancer: a review. Br Cancer Res Treat 5:221–229, 1985.
103. Van de Vijver M, van de Bersselaar R, Devilee P, et al: Amplification of the *neu* (c-*erb*-B2) oncogene in human mammary tumors is relatively frequent and is often accompanied by amplification of the linked c-*erb*-A oncogene. Molec Cell Biol 7:2019–2023, 1987.
104. Venter DJ, Tuzi NL, Kumar S, Gullick WJ: Overexpression of the c-*erb*B-2 oncoprotein in human breast carcinomas: immunohistological assessment correlates with gene amplification. Lancet ii:69–72, 1987.
105. Weinberger C, Thompson CC, Ong ES, et al: The c-*erb*-A gene encodes a thyroid hormone receptor. Nature 324:641–646, 1986.
106. White R, Leppert M, Bishop DT, et al: Construction of linkage maps with DNA markers for human chromosomes. Nature 313:101–105, 1985.
107. Witzig TE, Barlow JF (principal investigators): A retrospective study of the value of the tumor cell kinetic parameters DNA ploidy and %S in patients with breast cancer. North Central Cancer Treatment Group Protocol Study 86-30-52, 1986.
108. Woods KL, Smith SR, Morson JM: Parity and breast cancer: evidence of a dual effect. Br Med J 281:1349–1350, 1980.
109. Young JL, Percy CL, Asire AJ: Surveillance, epidemiology, and end results program: incidence and mortality data 1973–1977. NCI Monogr 57:1–1082, 1981.

Chapter 14

RISK FACTORS FOR BREAST CARCINOMA IN WOMEN WITH PROLIFERATIVE BREAST DISEASE

William D. Dupont, Ph.D. and David L. Page, M.D.

Warren[35] was among the first investigators to observe that women who have undergone biopsy revealing benign breast tissue are at increased risk of breast cancer. This finding has been confirmed many times since 1940.[1, 3, 4, 6–8, 11, 15, 16, 21, 23, 25, 26, 28–30, 33, 34] The histology of benign breast biopsies is highly variable, and biopsied tissue may vary from the physiologically normal at one extreme through *in situ* carcinoma at the other. It was thus natural to subdivide these lesions into biologically meaningful categories and to attempt to determine the cancer risk associated with these different categories. This task has proved to be difficult, as the studies must be large and there have been almost as many classification schemes as there have been studies addressing this question. Many of these authors[12, 13, 18, 22, 31, 32] have performed concurrent studies in which the malignant potential of benign lesions was judged by the frequency of their association with breast carcinoma in the same biopsy. The problem with such studies is that it is impossible to infer whether the implicated benign lesions are true precursor lesions for cancer, are markers of risk elevation, or are themselves a consequence of the malignancy. Thus to prove that a benign lesion increases a woman's breast cancer risk it is necessary to establish a temporal relationship between the occurrence of the benign lesion and the development of breast cancer. Several investigators have performed such studies, most notably Kodlin et al.,[21] Black et al.,[1] Hutchinson et al.,[16] and ourselves.[8, 28, 29] These studies will be discussed later.

Another problem with studies of premalignant breast disease is that of establishing reproducible and biologically meaningful diagnoses. Our approach to this problem has been, first, through extensive pretesting, to devise a preliminary classification scheme that can distinguish between fine differences in breast morphology and cytology and yet be reproducible. This classification scheme was applied to over 10,000 benign breast biopsies, and follow-up from a suitable sample of the biopsied women was obtained. Relative risk estimates associated with the different benign lesions were derived and compared. Our published benign disease categories represent groupings of preliminary classifications that are associated with consistent levels of cancer risk and that are readily explained to surgical pathologists. These categories and the cancer risks associated with them have been endorsed by the College of American Pathologists (CAP).[17] The results of our studies are discussed in the next section. The relationship between our results and those of other investigators will be described subsequently.

THE NASHVILLE STUDIES

We re-evaluated 10,366 consecutive benign breast biopsies that were performed between 1950 and 1968 at three hospitals in Nashville, Tennessee.[8] Follow-up was obtained on 3303 of these women, representing 84 percent of eligible subjects. This sample was weighted in favor of patients with proliferative disease. The median length of follow-up was 17 years. Relative risks of breast cancer were calculated with respect to women from the Third National Cancer Survey from Atlanta.[5] These risks are adjusted for the patients' age at biopsy and length of follow-up. These analyses indicated that 70 percent of women who undergo biopsy revealing benign breast tissue are not at increased risk of breast cancer. The remaining 30 percent of the 10,000 evaluated biopsies contained proliferative disease. These lesions are characterized by at least moderate hyperplasia[27] and are associated with an approximate twofold increase in breast cancer risk. The lesions within this disease category include, most prominently, hyperplasia of usual type (ductal) of moderate and florid degree as well as sclerosing adenosis and papillomas. Also constituting a minor component of this category are mild or poorly developed examples of atypical hyperplasia (AH). This latter category was created primarily to provide a clear lower boundary for the criteria needed to diagnose AH. Mild hyperplasia of usual type is excluded from the proliferative disease category because it is not associated

Table 14–1. RELATIVE RISK OF BREAST CANCER IN WOMEN WHO HAVE UNDERGONE BENIGN BREAST BIOPSY

	No. of Women	No. of Cancers	Relative Risk*	95% Confidence Interval	P Value
All women	3303	134	1.5	1.3–1.8	<0.0001
Proliferative disease	1925	103	1.9	1.6–2.3	<0.0001
No proliferative disease	1378	31	0.89	0.62–1.3	0.51
Family history†	369	26	2.5	1.7–3.7	<0.0001
No family history	2934	108	1.4	1.2–1.7	0.0007
Proliferative disease and					
Family history	234	22	3.2	2.1–4.9	<0.0001
No family history	1691	81	1.7	1.4–2.2	<0.0001
Calcification	359	23	2.4	1.6–3.6	<0.0001
No calcification	1566	80	1.8	1.5–2.3	<0.0001
Age‡ 20–45	1205	57	1.9	1.5–2.5	<0.0001
Age 46–55	563	35	1.9	1.3–2.6	0.0002
Age >55	157	11	2.2	1.2–4.0	0.007
No proliferative disease and					
Family history	135	4	1.2	0.43–3.1	0.78
No family history	1243	27	0.86	0.59–1.3	0.43
Calcification	174	4	0.80	0.30–2.1	0.66
No calcification	1204	27	0.90	0.62–1.3	0.59
Age 20–45	1025	23	0.99	0.66–1.5	0.96
Age 46–55	247	7	0.83	0.40–1.8	0.63
Age >55	106	1	0.30	0.04–2.2	0.21
Family history and					
Cysts	246	21	3.0	1.9–4.5	<0.0001
No cysts	123	5	1.6	0.65–3.7	0.32
No family history and					
Cysts	1808	73	1.5	1.2–1.9	0.0008
No cysts	1126	35	1.2	0.88–1.7	0.23

Adapted from Dupont WD, Page DL: N Engl J Med 312:146, 1985.
*Risk relative to women from Atlanta survey[5] adjusted for age at biopsy and length of follow-up.
†Mother, sister, or daughter with breast cancer.
‡Age at benign breast biopsy.

with increased cancer risk and thus is not considered a disease.

The proliferative lesions can be further dichotomized into those with and without atypia. The former, denoted atypical hyperplasia, are characterized by meeting some but not all the criteria needed for a diagnosis of carcinoma *in situ*. These lesions are rare, having a prevalence of 4 percent in our consecutive series of benign biopsies, and are associated with a four- to fivefold increase in breast cancer risk. There are two morphologically distinct subtypes of atypical hyperplasia, denoted lobular (ALH) and ductal (ADH) (see Chapter 6). However, women with these lesions have roughly comparable breast cancer risks.[28] Minor differences include a shorter average period between biopsy and invasive carcinoma diagnosis for ADH (8 years) than for ALH (12 years). There are also differences in the age distribution,[28] with both types predominating in the perimenopausal period but with ALH even less common in younger and older women. Proliferative disease without atypia (PDWA) was associated with a 60 percent increase in breast cancer risk (1.6 times) when compared with women from the Third National Cancer Survey and was associated with a 90 percent increase (1.9 times) when compared with women without such changes from our study. The CAP Consensus Conference[17] stated that this slight elevation in risk ranged from 1.5 to 2 times that of the general population.

Tables 14–1 and 14–2 are adapted from Dupont and Page.[8] In reading these tables it is important to bear in mind that the estimated relative risks may differ from their true values owing to chance by the amount indicated in the 95 percent confidence intervals. The *P* values given in these tables are with respect to the null hypothesis that the true relative risk equals 1. Table 14–1 shows the effect of family history, calcification, and age on breast cancer risk in women with and without proliferative disease. Study subjects with a mother, sister, or daughter who developed breast cancer were at 2.5 times the risk of women in the general population, while study subjects without such a history had only a 40 percent increase in cancer risk. This 40 percent increase reflects the average of our entire study group. A family history of breast cancer had little effect on breast cancer risk in women without proliferative disease. However, among women with proliferative disease a family history almost doubled breast cancer risk. This interaction is much stronger for atypical hyperplasias (Table 14–2). Similarly, the presence of calcification was of some importance in women with proliferative disease but had no effect on cancer risk among women lacking proliferative lesions.

Table 14–2. RELATIVE RISK OF BREAST CANCER IN WOMEN WITH PROLIFERATIVE BREAST DISEASE

	No. of Women	No. of Cancers	Relative Risk*	95% Confidence Interval	P Value
Proliferative disease without atypia	1693	73	1.6	1.3–2.0	0.0001
Atypical hyperplasia	232	30	4.4	3.1–6.3	<0.0001
Calcification	533	27	1.8	1.3–2.7	0.001
Proliferative disease without atypia and					
Family history†	195	12	2.1	1.2–3.7	0.009
No family history	1498	61	1.5	1.2–1.9	0.002
Calcification	321	16	1.9	1.2–3.1	0.012
No calcification	1372	57	1.5	1.2–1.9	0.002
Atypical hyperplasia and					
Family history	39	10	8.9	4.8–17	<0.0001
No family history	193	20	3.5	2.3–5.5	<0.0001
Calcification	38	7	6.5	3.1–14	<0.0001
No calcification	194	23	4.0	2.7–6.1	<0.0001

Adapted from Dupont WD, Page DL: N Engl J Med 312:146, 1985.
*Risk relative to women from Atlanta survey,[5] adjusted for age at biopsy and length of follow-up.
†Mother, sister, or daughter with breast cancer.

The interaction between proliferative disease and age at biopsy is particularly interesting. Women with proliferative disease are at approximately twice the breast cancer risk of women of similar age from the general population regardless of whether they are in the premenopausal, perimenopausal, or postmenopausal age group. In contrast, the relative breast cancer risk falls with increasing age among patients lacking proliferative disease, with postmenopausal patients having about one third the risk of postmenopausal women in general. This result suggests that women undergoing senile involution whose breasts lack any hyperplastic activity may be at reduced risk of developing breast cancer.

Table 14–2 shows how breast cancer risk varies among women with proliferative breast disease. Note the profound interaction between family history and atypical hyperplasia.

Figure 14–1 shows the absolute risk of breast cancer

associated with the disease categories discussed above as a function of time since benign biopsy. These curves emphasize the considerable variation in cancer risk associated with these lesions. Note that patients with both atypical hyperplasia and a family history have a breast cancer risk comparable to that of women with *in situ* carcinoma (see Chapter 52). Traditionally, all patients in our study cohort would have been diagnosed as having fibrocystic disease. It is clear from Figure 14–1 that this term has little prognostic value and should be replaced by more precise terminology. When an imprecise indication is useful, the term fibrocystic change may be preferred.

THE RELATIONSHIP BETWEEN THE HISTOLOGICAL CLASSIFICATION SCHEMES OF DIFFERENT AUTHORS

The results of our study must be compared with those of Black et al.,[1] Kodlin et al.,[21] and Hutchinson et al.[16] Black et al.[1] and Kodlin et al.[21] use a scheme devised by Black and Chabon[2] that classifies the lesions by their location in the breast and by their degree of proliferation. Lesions in the Black and Chabon system are located in primary ducts, in terminal interlobular ducts, in intralobular ducts, or in individual acini. Their method of grouping lesions by location has not proved to be useful in distinguishing between different levels of breast cancer risk, and those authors who have used their system have emphasized their scoring system for degree of proliferation. This system consists of an atypia score in which 1 denotes normal epithelium, 2 denotes hyperplasia, 3 and 4 denote different degrees of atypia, and 5 denotes *in situ* carcinoma. Black et al.,[1] in a case-control study of Saskatchewan women, found a remarkable fivefold difference in cancer risk between women with atypia scores of 3 or 4 as compared with those having scores of 1 or 2. Kodlin et al.,[21] in a retrospective

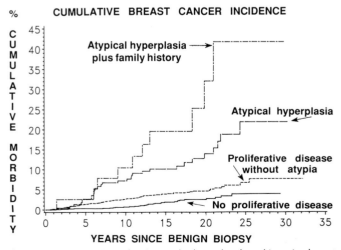

Figure 14–1. Proportion of patients who have developed invasive breast cancer as a function of time since their benign breast biopsy. (Adapted from Dupont WD, Page DL: Hum Pathol. 20:723–725, 1989.)

Table 14–3. SUMMARY OF RESULTS FROM TWO LARGE COHORT STUDIES OF HISTOLOGICALLY DEFINED BENIGN BREAST DISEASE

Histological Diagnoses	No. of Patients	Relative Risk*
Kodlin et al.[21]		
Entire group	2931	2.7
Black-Chabon atypia score 4	49	6.0
Black-Chabon atypia score 3	262	2.4
Black-Chabon atypia score 1–2	2092	2.3
Fibroadenoma	849	7.0
Adenosis or fibrosing adenosis	177	5.0
Intraductal papilloma	80	5.0
Hutchinson et al.[16]		
Entire group	1356	2.2
Epithelial hyperplasia or papillomatosis	466	2.8
With atypia	33	2.9
Without atypia	433	2.8
With calcification†	102	5.3
Without calcification†	190	2.8
Fibroadenoma with fibrocystic disease	122	3.8

*Calculated with respect to the general population. Different external reference populations were used in each study.

†Women with main lesion type other than epithelial hyperplasia or papillomatosis excluded.

cohort study of women in a health maintenance organization, found far less variation in cancer risk associated with the Black-Chabon atypia scores. The major results in their study are summarized in Table 14–3. It is important to note that 11 percent of their patients had atypia scores of 3 or 4 as compared with 4 percent of our patients with atypical hyperplasia. Thus, it is clear that the criteria for atypia in the Black-Chabon system are broader than those in our own. It would appear, however, that their Grade 4 atypia is roughly comparable to our atypical hyperplasia. As a group, the patients in Kodlin's cohort were at considerably higher breast cancer risk than the women in our study. This discrep-

ancy may be due to several factors, including different selection biases between the studies.

Table 14–3 also shows the results of the retrospective cohort study by Hutchinson et al.[16] In this study, as in Kodlin's and our own, the study patients' benign breast biopsies were reanalyzed using a predefined classification scheme. The discussion of the classification scheme is brief, making it difficult to compare their results with those of other investigators. They found a threefold elevation in cancer risk associated with epithelial hyperplasia or papillomatosis. This risk was not appreciably affected by the presence or absence of atypia. They did find that calcification substantially increased the risk of breast cancer associated with epithelial hyperplasia or papillomatosis. This result is consistent with our finding of increased risk associated with calcification and proliferative disease.

Haagensen et al.[14] have reported an increased risk of breast cancer associated with cysts. This result is in partial agreement with our finding, in that the presence of cysts increased cancer risk among women with a first-degree family history of breast cancer. This association was not present among women without such a history (see Table 14–1).

INTERACTION BETWEEN PROLIFERATIVE BREAST DISEASE AND OTHER VARIABLES ON BREAST CANCER RISK

Interesting interactions have also been observed between the effects of proliferative breast disease, age at first childbirth, and family history on breast risk.[9] The results were obtained from the same cohort of women discussed previously. However, the relative risks presented here are derived with respect to women from the cancer in Connecticut database and are adjusted for calendar age of biopsy as well as age at biopsy and

Table 14–4. EFFECT OF REPRODUCTIVE HISTORY AND PROLIFERATIVE DISEASE ON BREAST CANCER RISK

	No. of Women	No. of Cancers	Relative Risk*	95% Confidence Interval	P Value
No proliferative disease and					
AFB† ≤ 20	317	4	0.50	0.19–1.3	0.15
AFB 21–29	569	11	0.71	0.39–1.3	0.25
AFB ≥ 30	114	3	0.85	0.27–2.6	0.78
Nulliparous	294	9	0.96	0.50–1.8	0.89
PDWA‡ and					
AFB ≤ 20	330	9	0.95	0.50–1.8	0.89
AFB 21–29	720	28	1.3	0.90–1.9	0.17
AFB ≥ 30	156	8	1.5	0.77–3.1	0.22
Nulliparous	379	18	1.4	0.90–2.3	0.13
Atypical hyperplasia and					
AFB ≤ 20	42	2	1.6	0.39–6.30	0.52
AFB > 20	110	16	4.5	2.7–7.3	<0.0001
Nulliparous	68	11	4.9	2.7–8.9	<0.0001

Adapted from Dupont WD, Page DL: Am J Epidemiol 125:769, 1987.

*Risk relative to women from Atlanta survey[5] adjusted for age at biopsy and length of follow-up.

†AFB: Age at first birth.

‡PDWA: Proliferative disease without atypia.

Table 14–5. EFFECT OF A FAMILY HISTORY* OF BREAST CANCER AND REPRODUCTIVE HISTORY ON BREAST CANCER RISK

	No. of Women	No. of Cancers	Relative Risk†	95% Confidence Interval	P Value
No family history and					
AFB‡ ≤ 20	620	14	0.83	0.49–1.4	0.48
AFB 21–29	1219	43	1.2	0.90–1.6	0.19
AFB ≥ 30	251	8	0.98	0.49–2.0	0.95
Nulliparous	645	29	1.4	0.97–2.0	0.076
Family history and					
AFB ≤ 20	69	1	0.53	0.08–3.8	0.52
AFB 21–29	61	10	2.1	1.1–3.9	0.015
AFB ≥ 30	38	5	4.0	1.7–9.6	0.0008
Nulliparous	96	9	2.7	1.4–5.2	0.002

Adapted from Dupont WD, Page DL: Am J Epidemiol 125:769, 1987.
*Mother, sister, or daughter with breast cancer.
†Risk relative to women from Atlanta survey[5] adjusted for age at biopsy and length of follow-up.
‡AFB: Age at first birth.

length of follow-up. These relative risks are very close to the analogous risks derived with respect to women from the Third National Cancer Survey. Table 14–4 shows the effect of age at first birth or nulliparity and proliferative disease on breast cancer risk. MacMahon et al.[24] as well as other investigators[20] have found that breast cancer risk increases with increasing age at first birth; nulliparous women and women who first give birth after age 30 have comparable breast cancer risks. Our results show a similar trend. Women without proliferative disease were not at elevated cancer risk regardless of their reproductive history, whereas women with proliferative disease who were nulliparous or who gave birth after age 30 had an appreciable increase in

cancer risk. Women with atypical hyperplasia who were nulliparous or who gave birth after age 20 were at almost three times the breast cancer risk of women with atypia who gave birth by age 20; they were at over ten times the risk of women without proliferative disease who gave birth by age 20.[9]

Table 14–5 shows the effect of a first-degree family history of breast cancer and reproductive history on breast cancer risk. The effect of reproductive history on breast cancer risk is fairly modest among women without a first-degree family history. Nulliparous women have only a 40 percent increase in breast cancer risk, and there is no effect of age at first birth. In contrast, among patients with a family history, the relative risk of breast

Table 14–6. EFFECT OF BREAST SIZE, PROLIFERATIVE DISEASE, AND FAMILY HISTORY* ON BREAST CANCER RISK

	No. of Women	No. of Cancers	Relative Risk†	95% Confidence Interval	P Value
Small breasts	773	23	1.0	0.69–1.6	0.84
Medium breasts	1741	60	1.1	0.87–1.4	0.38
Large breasts	402	18	1.5	0.96–2.4	0.070
No proliferative disease and					
Small breasts	298	6	0.75	0.34–1.7	0.47
Medium breasts	743	14	0.65	0.38–1.1	0.098
Large breasts	183	4	0.80	0.30–2.1	0.66
Proliferative disease and					
Small breasts	475	17	1.2	0.75–2.0	0.43
Medium breasts	998	46	1.4	1.1–1.9	0.012
Large breasts	219	14	2.1	1.2–3.5	0.006
No family history and					
Small breasts	681	19	0.97	0.62–1.5	0.91
Medium breasts	1548	47	1.0	0.75–1.3	0.97
Large breasts	342	13	1.3	0.76–2.3	0.33
Family history and					
Small breasts	92	4	1.6	0.58–4.1	0.37
Medium breasts	193	13	2.0	1.2–3.5	0.008
Large breasts	60	5	2.7	1.1–6.5	0.022

*Mother, sister, or daughter with breast cancer.
†Risk relative to women from Atlanta survey[5] adjusted for age at biopsy and length of follow-up.

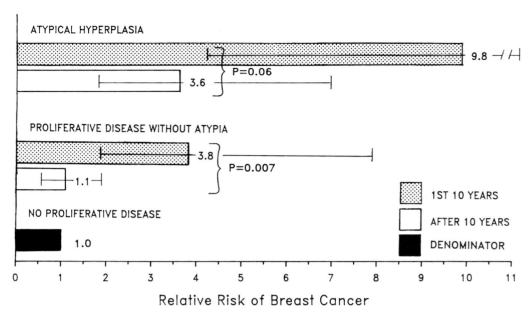

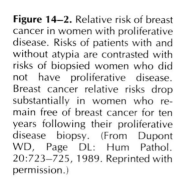

Figure 14–2. Relative risk of breast cancer in women with proliferative disease. Risks of patients with and without atypia are contrasted with risks of biopsied women who did not have proliferative disease. Breast cancer relative risks drop substantially in women who remain free of breast cancer for ten years following their proliferative disease biopsy. (From Dupont WD, Page DL: Hum Pathol. 20:723–725, 1989. Reprinted with permission.)

cancer varies from 0.53 for women who give birth by age 20 up to 4.0 for women who give birth after age 20.

We also looked at the interaction between breast size, proliferative disease, and a family history of breast cancer (Table 14–6). Breast size had little effect on breast cancer risk among women without proliferative disease or without a family history of breast cancer. However, breast cancer risk did increase with greater breast size among patients with either of these risk factors.

EFFECT OF TIME SINCE BIOPSY ON BREAST CANCER RISK

Most relative risk estimates from longitudinal studies are derived under the assumption that each patient's relative risk remains constant over time. It is possible, however, for the relative risk of an individual patient to vary as a function of either age or time since initial diagnosis. An example of such a change can be found in our studies of benign breast disease. We have previously reported that women who have undergone breast biopsy revealing atypical hyperplasia have 5.3 times the breast cancer risk of biopsied women who lacked proliferative disease, and that the corresponding relative risk for women with proliferative disease without atypia (PDWA) is 1.9.[8] These results were obtained using a proportional hazards regression model that assumes that relative risk remains constant over time. Figure 14–2, however, shows an alternative analysis of these same data. The risk estimates were derived from a hazard regression model that uses time-dependent covariates.[10, 19] Figure 14–2 shows that the breast cancer risk for women with both atypical hyperplasia and proliferative disease without atypia (PDWA) is greatest in the first ten years after benign breast biopsy. Women with PDWA who remain free of breast cancer for ten years are at no greater risk than are women of similar age

who do not have such a history. The relative risk of breast cancer in women with atypical hyperplasia is halved if they remain free of breast cancer for ten years following their initial biopsy. This supports the hypothesis that the atypical hyperplasias are not obligate precursor lesions for breast cancer and that these lesions may progress to cancer, remain unchanged, or possibly regress over a substantial period. Their presence at time of biopsy may be best regarded as a marker of increased risk.

The absolute risk for all the women in this study group[8] seems to be approximately evenly distributed over the 17-year period of follow-up (see Fig. 14–1). The knowledge that invasive carcinomas were fairly evenly distributed over this time, combined with the fact that approximately half the invasive carcinomas had occurred by year 10, would have led us to predict the finding just described. Thus, an approximately constant cancer incidence over a 17-year age span, together with a rising age-specific incidence in women without proliferative disease (the denominator of the relative risk statistic), implies that a woman's relative risk of breast cancer must fall with increasing time since biopsy. Whether relative risk will continue to drop with further follow-up is, of course, yet to be determined. This time-dependent analysis does suggest that one should not presume the constancy of relative risk figures through an entire lifetime when making clinical decisions.

References

1. Black MM, Barclay THC, Cutler SJ, Hankey BF, Asire AJ: Association of atypical characteristics of benign breast lesions with subsequent risk of breast cancer. Cancer 29:338–343, 1972.
2. Black MM, Chabon AB: In situ carcinoma of the breast. Pathol Annu 4:185–210, 1969.
3. Brinton LA, Williams RR, Hoover RN, Stevens NL, Feinleib M, Fraumeni JF Jr.: Breast cancer risk factors among screening program participants. J Natl Cancer Inst 62:37–44, 1979.
4. Coombs LJ, Lilienfeld AM: A prospective study of the relation-

ship between benign breast diseases and breast carcinoma. Prev Med 8:40–52, 1979.

5. Cutler SJ, Young JL Jr (eds): Third National Cancer Survey: Incidence data. Bethesda, National Cancer Institute, 1975, p 230. (DHEW publication no. (NIH) 74–787.)

6. Davis HH, Simons M, Davis JB: Cystic disease of the breast: relationship to carcinoma. Cancer, 17:957–978, 1964.

7. Donnelly PK, Baker KW, Carney JA, O'Fallon WM: Benign breast lesions and subsequent breast carcinoma in Rochester, Minnesota. Mayo Clin Proc 50:650–656, 1975.

8. Dupont WD, Page DL: Risk factors for breast cancer in women with proliferative breast disease. N Engl J Med 312:146–151, 1985.

9. Dupont WD, Page DL: Breast cancer risk associated with proliferative disease, age at first birth, and a family history of breast cancer. Am J Epidemiol 125:769–779, 1987.

10. Dupont WD, Page DL: Relative risk of breast cancer varies with time since diagnosis of atypical hyperplasia. Hum Pathol 20:723–725, 1989.

11. Ernster VL: The epidemiology of benign breast disease. Epidemiol Rev 3:184–202, 1981.

12. Foote FW, Steward FW: Comparative studies of cancerous versus noncancerous breasts. Ann Surg 121:197–222, 1945.

13. Frantz VK, Pickren JW, Melcher GW, Auchingloss H, Jr: Incidence of chronic cystic disease in so-called "normal breasts." Cancer 4:762–783, 1951.

14. Haagensen CD, Bodian C, Haagensen DE Jr: Breast Cancer Risk and Detection. Philadelphia, WB Saunders, 1981, pp 70–75.

15. Helmrich SP, Shapiro S, Rosenberg L, Kaufman DW, Slone D, Bain C, Miettinen OS, Stolley PD, Rosenshein NB, Knapp RC, Leavitt T Jr, Schohenfeld D, Engle RL Jr, Levy M: Risk factors for breast cancer. Am J Epidemiol 117:35–45, 1983.

16. Hutchinson WB, Thomas DB, Hamlin WB, Roth GJ, Peterson AV, Williams B: Risk of breast cancer in women with benign breast disease. J Natl Cancer Inst 65:13–20, 1980.

17. Hutter RVP, et al: Consensus meeting. Is "fibrocystic disease" of the breast precancerous? Arch Pathol Lab Med 110:171–173, 1986.

18. Jensen HM, Rice JR, Wellings SR: Preneoplastic lesions in the human breast. Science 191:295–297, 1976.

19. Kalbfleisch JD, Prentice RL: The Statistical Analysis of Failure Time Data. New York, Wiley, 1980.

20. Kelsey JL, Hildreth NG, Thompson WD: Epidemiologic aspects of breast cancer. Radiol Clin North Am 21:3–12, 1983.

21. Kodlin D, Winger EE, Morgenstern NL, Chen U: Chronic mastopathy and breast cancer: A follow-up study. Cancer 39:2603–2607, 1977.

22. Kramer WM, Rush BF Jr: Mammary duct proliferation in the elderly. A histopathologic study. Cancer 31:130–137, 1973.

23. Love SM, Gelman RS, Silen W: Fibrocystic "disease" of the breast: A non-disease. N Engl J Med 307:1010–1014, 1982.

24. MacMahon B, Cole P, Lin TM, Lowe CR, Mirra AP, Ravnihar B, Salber EJ, Valaoras VG, Yuasa S: Age at first birth and breast cancer risk. Bull WHO 43:209–221, 1970.

25. Monson RR, Yen S, Warren S: Chronic cystic mastitis and carcinoma of the breast. Lancet 2:224–226, 1976.

26. Moskowitz M, Gartside P, Wirman JA, McLaughlin C: Proliferative disorders of the breast as risk factors for breast cancer in a self-selected screened population: Pathologic markers. Radiology 134:289–291, 1980.

27. Page DL, Anderson TJ, Rogers LW: Epithelial hyperplasia. In Diagnostic Histopathology of the Breast. Edinburgh, Churchill Livingstone, 1987, pp 120–156.

28. Page DL, Dupont WD, Rogers LW, Rados MS: Atypical hyperplastic lesions of the female breast: A long term follow-up study. Cancer 55:2698–2708, 1985.

29. Page DL, Vander Zwaag R, Rogers LW, Williams LT, Walker WE, Hartman WH: Relation between component parts of fibrocystic disease complex and breast cancer. J Natl Cancer Inst 61:1055–1063, 1978.

30. Potter JF, Slimbaugh WP, Woodward SC: Can breast carcinoma be anticipated?: A follow-up of benign breast biopsies. Ann Surg 167:829–838, 1968.

31. Sandison AT: An autopsy study of the adult human breast. National Cancer Institute Monograph 8, DHEW PHS, US GPO, Washington, DC, 1962.

32. Sasano N, Tateno H, Stemmerman GN: Volume and hyperplastic lesions of breasts of Japanese women in Hawaii and Japan. Prev Med 7:196–204, 1978.

33. Shapiro S, Strax P, Venet L, Fink R: The search for risk factors in breast cancer. Am J Public Health 58:820–835, 1968.

34. Veronesi U, Pizzocaro G: Breast cancer in women subsequent to cystic disease of the breast. Surg Gynecol Obstet 126:529–532, 1968.

35. Warren S: The relation of "chronic mastitis" to carcinoma of the breast. Surg Gynecol Obstet 71:257–273, 1940.

Chapter 15

MULTICENTRICITY OF *IN SITU* AND INVASIVE CARCINOMA

Philip L. Dutt, M.D., J.D. and David L. Page, M.D.

Multicentricity refers to the occurrence of two or more physically separate foci of breast carcinoma. The term does not necessarily indicate tumors of independent origin and is usually confined to tumors within the same breast. Bilaterality, the occurrence of carcinoma in the contralateral breast, is usually excluded by definition and is discussed separately in Chapter 48. Also excluded is concurrence of breast carcinoma and sarcoma, which is reviewed in Chapters 9 and 10, respectively.

The terms *multicentricity* and *multifocality* have been used for decades to indicate seeming or real multiplicity of cancer throughout an individual breast. The terms have no intrinsically different meaning, but have in recent years been interpreted as follows: "multicentricity" indicates multicentric origin, usually in sites remote or relatively so from the initially identified neoplasm; "multifocality" indicates foci of the same tumor, relatively close to each other, usually in the same quadrant. Earlier studies reviewed by Fisher et al.[6] were concerned with establishing the concept of multicentric origin and were not specifically concerned with whether foci of tumor apart or separable from the primary neoplasm were either adjacent to or remote from the dominant mass. One of the first studies distinguishing between cancerous foci in the vicinity of the primary mass and those that may be regarded as distant was that of Qualheim and Gall.[23] They found that 54 percent of mastectomy specimens contained multiple foci of carcinoma, but their study was limited to one or two large sections of the breast without three-dimensional examination to exclude the possibility that apparently separate foci were connected. This approach obviously maximizes the apparent incidence of multicentricity. One study that analyzed grossly inapparent disease within radical mastectomy specimens found seven percent of cases to have "precancerous or early intraductal carcinomatous lesions."[12] Thus many of these studies are hampered by failing to indicate the precise location as well as by leaving unclear the distinction between cancers and atypical hyperplasia. Some studies, for example, indicate only that the distant carcinomas were "microscopic."

The observations of multicentricity of the National Surgical Adjuvant Breast Project (NSABP) by Fisher et al., which are separated by about 10 years,[6, 7] are particularly illuminating. A standard definition of multicentricity was established in these studies and indicated the determination of cancer in a quadrant other than the one in which the dominant mass is located. These studies produced an admitted conservative estimate of separated cancer sites, because cases in which the dominant mass was present in the tail of the breast or beneath the nipple were excluded from analysis. Thus multicentricity was operationally defined as having some distance between it and the dominant mass (i.e., not being immediately adjacent in the same quadrant even if separable). Others have inaugurated and utilized the term "multifocal" for lesions appearing to be separate from the dominant mass but not in a different quadrant. The studies of Holland et al.,[11] reviewed in later sections, have used a more rigorous definition of distance from the primary mass by actually measuring this distance. This is of course only possible in studies performed under careful prospective guidance.

More recent studies have been concerned with practical questions that are precisely defined in space, such as the occurrence of cancer in remote quadrants, whereas the concept of multicentric origin was the focus of earlier studies.[6] Other recent studies have added both the elements of time and biology (natural history) by observing the evolution (or nonevolution) of clinical disease in the living breast after partial mastectomy. These have given a clear focus and better understanding to our clinical decisions as these empirical observations relative to various therapeutic strategies are recorded.

DEFINITION AND ANATOMY

A perfect definition of multicentricity referable to all settings is either unobtainable or of practical impossibility because of the inherent difficulties in understanding and studying the three-dimensional microanatomy of the breast. Distinguishing between separate breast carcinomas and intramammary spread of breast carcinoma, particularly along ducts, is difficult and would require microscopic three-dimensional reconstruction. Therefore any definition of multicentricity is necessarily arbitrary and will be situationally confined (i.e., bound by the method utilized for detection).

The breast is a branching (racemose) gland with 15 to 20 collecting (lactiferous) ducts exiting at the nipple. Each of these ductal systems or lobes subserves hundreds of lobular units, which are collections of acinar elements. Although the lobes are not defined anatomical units separated by septa, at least only adjacent radiating lobar units may overlap (Fig. 15–1). Apparent multicentricity caused by spread along ducts of the originating lobe will be preferentially arranged in a radial fashion from nipple to periphery in whatever quadrant it appears. Thus the irregular branching system of breast ducts in three dimensions easily explains why those numerous breast cancers that spread along the ducts appear as separate foci in the two-dimensional slides routinely utilized.

HISTORICAL REVIEW

Cheatle and Cutler[3] first defined multicentricity as two lesions separated by normal breast tissue. Since then, most authors have adhered to the "quadrant rule," which defines multicentric lesions as second tumors lying in a *different* quadrant from that in which the primary or dominant lesion is located. In this chapter, the lesion

that attracted attention clinically or mammographically and led to diagnostic procedures will be called the primary or dominant lesion, and other malignant lesions will be called secondary lesions. Some authors treat lesions lying in the subareolar region as a fifth mammary area, separate from the four quadrants. Others place subareolar lesions in the most closely associated quadrant. Note also that the quadrant rule accepts the radial anatomy of the breast and implies that if two foci are in the same quadrant, the same radially arranged ductal unit(s) are likely involved.

In addition to the quadrant rule, some authors have used a "distance rule," with varying distances ranging from 5 cm down to 2 cm having been applied. It should be noted that the basis for the 5-cm distance rule used by Lagios[13] was that using such a distance would generally place a second lesion in a different quadrant.

Each of these definitions has shortcomings. Cheatle and Cutler's rule is surely overly inclusive, whereas the quadrant rule will underestimate the prevalence of multicentric lesions. A distance rule is less arbitrary but may still underestimate, particularly if tumors of different histological type are involved. For example, it is difficult to understand why two distinct, discrete lesions of different histological type lying within the same quadrant within 2 cm of each other should not be counted as a multicentric lesion, but under either the quadrant rule or the distance rule this will not be

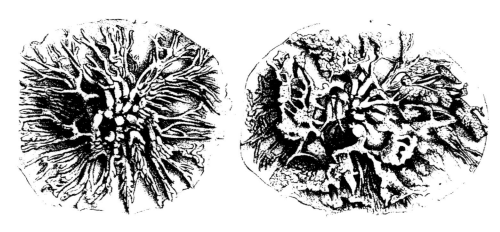

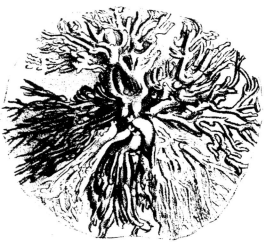

Figure 15–1. Lobar, radiating anatomy of the ductal system of the breast. (From Cooper A: The Anatomy and Diseases of the Breast. Philadelphia, Lea and Blanchard, 1845, plate VI.)

counted as a case of multicentricity. Thus clinical and current therapeutic relevance is emphasized, because the currently relevant question is how much of the breast may be conserved? The example just cited is of more theoretical than practical interest, because adjacent lesions of greatly different histological patterns are rare.

Egan and McSweeney[4] offered a possible solution to this problem by employing multiple criteria: (1) wide separation of foci grossly, radiographically, and microscopically; (2) a pattern of multiple areas scattered throughout much of the breast; or, (3) sharp delineation of different histological types. Although the first criterion is subjective and fails to define "wide," this definition attempts to introduce flexibility by combining the various definitions and seeking a multifactorial definition of multicentricity, particularly when different histological types are present or lesions are distinctly circumscribed.

Holland et al.[11] cleverly avoided the problems of both the rule of quadrants and the arbitrary distance definitions of multicentricity by measuring the distance from the secondary foci to the dominant lesion and graphing the frequencies at which invasive and noninvasive foci were located at various distances from the edge of the dominant lesion. Their approach minimizes the problem of defining multicentricity and has important therapeutic implications regarding how generous the margins around tumors should be in lumpectomy specimens. However, it does not specifically allow for the plane in which the distances occur, which may be of practical relevance (e.g., occurring within the same quadrant).

On balance, it should be remembered that the quadrants rule is the most frequently used definition and is also attractive because it conforms most closely to protocols used in surgical pathology for the examination of mastectomy specimens and is therefore suitable to large retrospective studies.

A study of the phenomenon of multicentricity has at least the potential for yielding implications about the etiology of breast carcinoma. However, it is more important when viewed as a practical measure of prognosis and efficacy of different therapeutic regimens. Thus multicentricity, however defined, may worsen the patient's prognosis by indicating an increased risk of recurrence or subsequent development of invasive carcinoma.

CASE 1. A 46-year-old woman underwent a modified radical right mastectomy for a 2 × 1.7 × 1.3 cm mass in the lower inner quadrant. Histologically this was an infiltrating mammary carcinoma of predominantly lobular type with an extensive intraductal component (Fig. 15–2). Sampling of the upper inner quadrant revealed a separate 0.7 × 0.5 × 0.5 cm focus of infiltrative lobular carcinoma with extensive lobular carcinoma *in situ* (Fig. 15–3).

CASE 2. An 87-year-old woman had two clinically apparent masses in her left breast. The decision to perform mastectomy was based on a diagnosis of carcinoma made on material obtained with fine needle aspiration of a mass in the upper inner quadrant. The left mastectomy specimen contained an 8 × 5 × 4 cm mass in the upper inner quadrant that histologi-

cally was invasive mammary carcinoma of no specific type (Fig. 15–4). The upper outer quadrant contained a separate, smaller 3.5 × 3 × 2.5 cm mass with a similar histological appearance (Fig. 15–5). Biopsy of a lesion in the right breast at the time of mastectomy revealed ductal carcinoma *in situ* (Fig. 15–6).

CASE 3. A 47-year-old woman underwent mastectomy. The mastectomy specimen contained invasive mammary carcinoma of no specific type (Fig. 15–7). Elsewhere in the most remote sites were extensive areas with mucinous histological appearance (Fig. 15–8).

CASE 4. A mammogram revealed three lesions in a single quadrant in a 43-year-old woman (Fig. 15–9). All three were invasive carcinomas with extensive intraductal components. Tissue sampled between each of the lesions demonstrated *in situ* carcinoma only. This case demonstrates the importance of ductal carcinoma *in situ* in the occurrence of multiple carcinomas within one breast.

Recording of such a case in which these lesions are separately identifiable and separately measurable should emphasize the largest lesion (*Manual for Staging of Cancer*, edition 3, American Joint Committee on Cancer, 1988). As is frequently the case, each invasive focus appeared histologically similar.

PREVALENCE

Partly because of difficulties with definitions of multicentricity, the exact prevalence of multicentricity is uncertain but is more frequent with some forms of carcinoma. The reported prevalences of multicentricity have ranged from 9 percent to 75 percent.[15] In a complete review of these diverse studies, McDivitt[19] concluded that the prevalence of multicentricity probably is between 25 percent and 50 percent, with approximately five percent to ten percent of secondary lesions being invasive. This tremendous disparity in prevalence rates is attributable to many variables, including (1) definition of multicentricity used, (2) method of examining mastectomy specimens employed, (3) number of quadrants sampled and number of sections from each quadrant examined, (4) subsets of patients included in or excluded from the study, (5) whether the lesions were detected clinically or mammographically, and (6) the age of patients in the group, among others.

One should be aware of the method used to study breasts in a series looking for multicentricity. The most thorough method involves combined examination of breast tissue using radiographs, a dissecting microscope, and microscopic examination of whole tissue sections from breasts that have been frozen and serially sectioned at 2.5-mm intervals.[13, 15] This method is thorough and best captures the three-dimensional anatomy of the breast; however, it uses technology that may not be available at all centers and may force investigators to elect between examining large numbers of slides on a small number of specimens and examining a smaller number of less extensive sections of a much larger sample.[8]

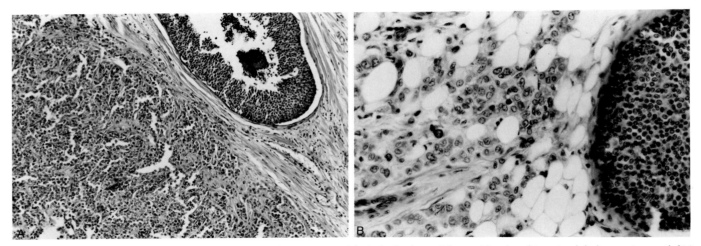

Figure 15–2. A and B, Extension of prominent intraductal component (right in both pictures) beyond border of invasive lobular carcinoma (left) in lower inner quadrant mass of Case 1. (A, × 60, B, × 200)

Associated Factors

Numerous authors have considered various factors associated with increased risk of multicentricity. The presence of a lesion in the nipple or subareolar area is perhaps the most clearly and consistently demonstrated risk factor for multicentricity.[6] Rosen et al.[24] found an 80 percent rate of multicentricity with subareolar lesions, compared with a 25 percent to 35 percent risk of multicentricity if the primary lesion lay in one of the quadrants of the breast away from the nipple. Andersen and Pallesen[1] found carcinoma lying within 1 cm of the areolar epidermis in 50 percent of mastectomy specimens, with cases of carcinoma *in situ* alone slightly outnumbering cases of invasive carcinoma with or without carcinoma *in situ*. Nearly all had carcinoma lying within 6 mm of the areolar epidermis. Luttges et al.[18] found that 38 percent of patients with multicentricity had nipple involvement. The strong relationship be-

tween presence of an extensive intraductal component and multicentricity[6, 10] is discussed in a later section.

The relationship of tumor size to multicentricity is an interesting and controversial question, with somewhat conflicting and even paradoxical results. Fisher et al.[6] initially reported that tumors larger than 5 cm were associated with an increased risk of multicentricity. Rosen et al.[24] showed that there was a 38 percent rate of multicentricity for tumors larger than 2 cm, vs. a 26 percent rate of multicentricity for tumors smaller than 2 cm in greatest extent. Other studies have also shown a relationship between tumor size and multicentricity.[16, 30] Lagios et al.[15] found that lesions larger than 25 mm were more likely to be multicentric and to be associated with occult invasion. On the other hand, some studies have shown no relationship between tumor size and multicentricity.[25, 32] In seeming paradox, some studies have even shown that smaller invasive carcinomas are more likely to be multicentric than large lesions.[11, 13, 21] Perhaps the

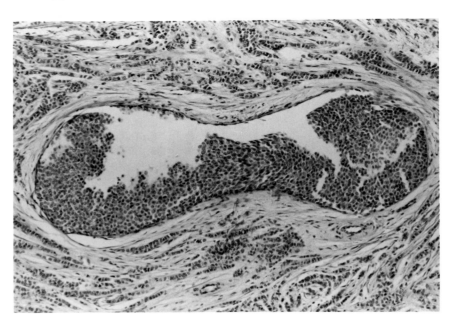

Figure 15–3. Separate upper inner quadrant lesion from Case 1 contains infiltrating lobular carcinoma with extensive *in situ* lobular component involving the duct in the center of picture. (× 180)

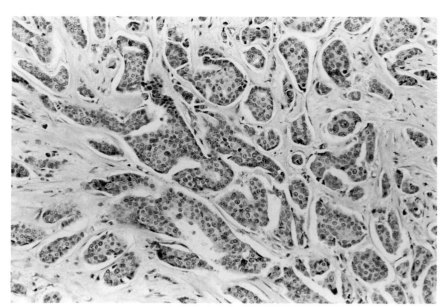

Figure 15–4. (Case 2) Infiltrating mammary carcinoma of no specific type (invasive ductal carcinoma) found in larger mass in the upper inner quadrant. (× 250)

explanation for these disparate conclusions is that tumor size may be a risk factor for some but not all subsets of breast carcinoma. For example, Gump et al.[8] showed that increased tumor size was associated with greater rates of multicentricity for invasive ductal carcinomas but not for invasive lobular lesions.

Most authors have concluded that there is no relationship between age and multicentricity.[6, 16, 32] One study found that only those patients aged 71 to 80 years had an increased incidence of multicentricity.[25]

Positive family history for breast carcinoma indicates an increased risk of multicentricity in some studies but not in others. It is at least fairly clear that the risk of homolateral multicentricity is little affected by familial history of breast cancer, whereas the risk of bilateral disease is greater when there is a positive family history (see chapter 48). Rosen et al.[24] found that there was

generally no correlation between positive family history and multicentricity, but they did find an increased risk with a positive family history in patients with multicentric tumors if the primary was smaller than 2 cm. Sarnelli and Squartini[25] found a relationship between positive family history and multicentricity and noted that other authors had shown associations between multicentricity and positive family history for breast carcinoma in their study of the rate of multicentricity.[15]

Lesser et al.[16] found that patients with axillary nodal metastases were more likely to have multicentric disease; Sarnelli and Squartini[25] found no relationship between axillary metastases and multicentricity of invasive carcinoma. Other studies have shown no relationship between nodal status and multicentricity.[6, 32]

Among other factors investigated that have been shown to have no relationship with an increased risk of

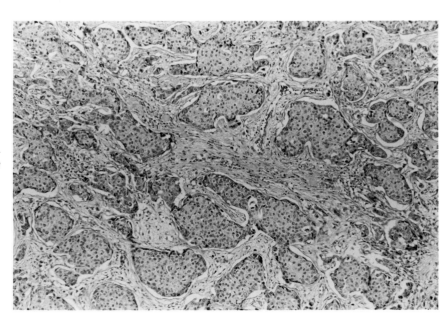

Figure 15–5. Similar histological features were present in the smaller upper outer quadrant lesion in Case 2. (× 180)

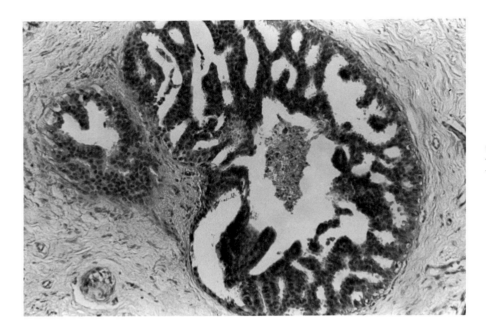

Figure 15–6. This ductal carcinoma *in situ* was found simultaneously in the breast contralateral to the one containing the lesions in Figures 15–4 and 15–5. (× 200)

multicentricity are estrogen receptor status, height, weight, parity,[16] which breast or quadrant is involved, amount of necrosis,[6] nuclear grade, preexisting or concurrent benign breast disease,[6, 32] and bilaterality[32] (Table 15–1).

In Situ *Lesions*

The prevalence of multicentricity can vary depending on whether the primary lesion is an *in situ* or invasive lesion and on the histological type of the primary lesion. The risk of multicentricity associated with lobular carcinoma *in situ* is discussed in Chapter 8 and will not be repeated here.

Ductal carcinoma *in situ* (DCIS) is often multicentric, but perhaps less frequently than is lobular carcinoma *in situ* (LCIS).[23] Ductal carcinoma *in situ* also produces proportionally more ipsilateral concurrent breast neoplasia than does lobular carcinoma *in situ* (LCIS).[23] This is true for clinically evident disease, as the multiple foci of LCIS are inapparent to mammography. Lagios et al.[15] noted that ductal carcinoma *in situ* had been reported to have rates of multicentricity ranging from 30 percent to 33 percent, and found in his own concurrent series that 29 percent of *in situ* ductal lesions were multicentric. Of his cases of ductal carcinoma *in situ*, 19.5 percent were associated with occult foci of invasion. All lesions with multicentric foci were larger than 25 mm, and two thirds of those were larger than 50 mm in greatest extent. Conversely, 47 percent of specimens with lesions larger than 25 mm contained multicentric foci. Gump et al.[8] found an extremely high rate (81

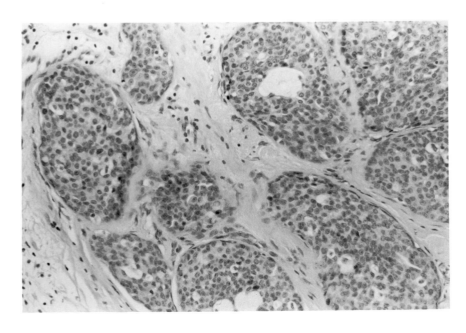

Figure 15–7. Invasive mammary carcinoma of no specific type described in Case 3. (× 200)

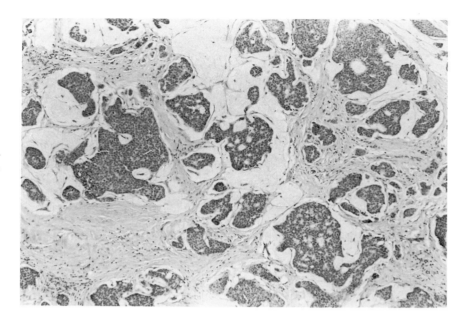

Figure 15–8. Mucinous carcinoma present elsewhere in breast of patient described in Case 3. (× 75)

percent) of multicentricity associated with ductal carcinoma *in situ*. In a study of lesions detected only by mammography, 45.5 percent of *in situ* ductal lesions were multicentric.[29]

Patchefsky et al.[22] examined the incidence of multicentricity associated with various subsets of ductal carcinoma *in situ*, finding that multicentricity was greatly increased with the micropapillary type of ductal carcinoma *in situ* and was much less common with the cribriform and solid types of ductal carcinoma *in situ* (see chapter 8).

Invasive Lesions

Although invasive mammary carcinoma of no specific type (invasive ductal carcinoma) is the most common type of invasive mammary carcinoma, fortunately invasive ductal carcinoma is also associated with one of the lowest rates of multicentricity. Gump et al.[8] found that it was least likely to have multicentric disease, accounting for a 19 percent rate of multicentricity, compared with a rate of 27 percent for all types. The rate of multicentricity increases when other factors are present. For example, the rate of multicentricity associated with minimally invasive ductal carcinoma is apparently greater than that associated with usual invasive ductal carcinoma.[29] This may not be related to the small size of the invasive component per se but rather to the regular presence in such cases of extensive DCIS. The rate of multicentricity is also increased approximately twofold when infiltrating ductal carcinoma is associated with *in situ* lobular carcinoma.[16]

Infiltrating lobular carcinoma is associated with ele-

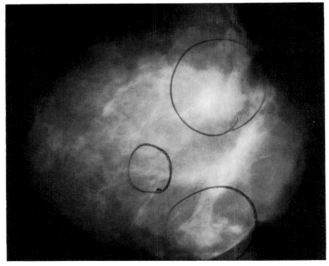

Figure 15–9. Mammogram described in Case 4 showing three radiographic lesions within the circles. Each contained invasive carcinomas of similar histological pattern with extensive intraductal components. Note that all three are linked by connective tissue strands that histologically contained ductal carcinoma *in situ*. (Courtesy of L. Ming Hang, M.D., Escondido, California.)

Table 15–1. RELATIONSHIP OF VARIOUS PARAMETERS TO MULTICENTRICITY

Strong correlation with multicentricity
  Involvement of nipple/areolar area by carcinoma[1, 6]
  Presence of extensive intraductal component[6, 10]
  Certain histological types, especially lobular[6]

Controversial association
  Tumor size[6, 11, 16, 32]
  Family history of breast carcinoma[15, 16, 24, 25]
  Axillary node status[6, 16, 25, 32]

Little or no correlation with multicentricity
  Age[6, 16, 32]
  Nuclear grade[6, 32]
  Bilaterality[32]
  Estrogen receptor status[16]
  Parity[16]
  Whether right or left breast involved[6]
  Quadrant of breast involved[6]
  Benign breast disease[6, 32]
  Amount of necrosis[6]
  Intralymphatic carcinoma[6]

vated rates of multicentricity.[16] Fisher et al.[6] showed that invasive lobular carcinoma was more frequently associated with invasive secondary lesions but not with noninvasive secondary lesions. Some authors have pointed out that most of the secondary lesions lie near the primary and probably represent recurrence or spread of the original invasive lobular carcinoma rather than true multicentricity.[28]

Ascertaining accurate rates of multicentricity for special types of invasive mammary carcinoma is difficult because of small sample sizes. Lagios et al.[14] reported that 56 percent of tubular carcinomas were multicentric. In a study of minimal invasive carcinoma (lesions 10 mm or less in diameter), 59 percent of small tubular carcinomas were multicentric.[15] Other studies have shown much lower rates of multicentricity.[20] Despite this variation in rates, tubular carcinoma probably has an increased rate of multicentricity compared with the average for all cancers.

In studies with both large[16] and small[24] numbers of examples, medullary carcinoma has been shown to have one of the lowest rates of multicentricity. In Rosen et al.'s study,[24] multicentric lesions occurred only if the primary lesion was larger than 2 cm.

It is difficult to draw conclusions about the rate of multicentricity associated with colloid or mucinous carcinoma because of the small numbers involved.[15, 24]

Combined Invasive and In Situ Carcinoma

Several authors have noted that multicentricity is more likely if invasive carcinoma coexists with a significant amount of intraductal carcinoma. The early studies of the NSABP found that the rate of multicentricity was higher in patients with a moderate or marked intraductal component or noninvasive carcinoma in the vicinity of the primary lesions.[6]

RECENT STUDIES

The collaborative study between medical schools at Nijmegen and Harvard represents the best clinically relevant information presently available.[10] A large group of unselected patients were studied with a three-dimensional reconstructive technique. A correlated radiological-pathological mapping technique was utilized, and the precise distribution, type, and extent of additional tumor foci in the mastectomy specimen were identified. These findings were correlated with the characteristics of the excisional biopsy specimen preformed previously. Thus the study design is predicated on a practical clinical question: given an excisional biopsy, what is its ability to predict tumor within the remaining breast? Dominant initial carcinomas were separated into two groups on the basis of the extensiveness of ductal carcinoma *in situ*.

These concurrent data are consistent with several studies that had analyzed the same information relevant to the initial carcinoma and had reported on clinical lesions presenting within the remaining breast that were radiated and not surgically removed. These correlates between follow-up studies after irradiation and concurrent studies of the entire breast demonstrate an important complementarity. Studies restricted to concurrent demonstration of multicentricity can never answer questions as to predictability of success with conserving surgery.

This concurrent study of Holland et al.[10] indicates that primary tumors with an extensive intraductal component (EIC +) often have cancer found beyond the edge of the primary tumor. This tumor present beyond the major borders of the primary tumor is largely of intraductal carcinoma type. Forty-four percent of the EIC + cases as judged from the biopsy specimens had a prominent intraductal carcinoma component in the mastectomy specimen. (For the purposes of this study, a prominent component of DCIS was defined as representing six or more low-power microscopic fields of tumor; each low field measured 6 mm in diameter.) In remarkable contrast, only three percent of the EIC − cases had a prominent DCIS component in the subsequent mastectomy specimen. Fourteen percent of patients with EIC + tumors had a prominent DCIS component 4 or more centimeters away from the edge of the primary tumor, compared with only one percent of patients with EIC − primary tumors (Fig. 15–10). These figures for a 2-cm distance from the primary tumor border were 33 percent and 2 percent, respectively.

The EIC + patients were also more likely to have additional foci of invasive carcinoma remaining within the breast at time of mastectomy. However, this difference was small and only reached statistical significance within the immediate vicinity of the primary tumor (within 2 cm of the margin of the primary tumor). The major difference, then, between the EIC positive and negative tumors was in the extensiveness of the *in situ* disease of ductal type within the remainder of the breast. Intralymphatic channel tumor involvement was not different between the two tumor types characterized by presence or absence of EIC.

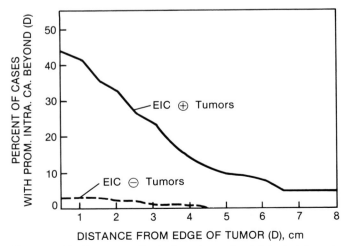

Figure 15–10. Frequency distribution of prominent intraductal carcinoma at various distances from the edge of the primary tumor. (From Holland R, et al.: J Clin Oncol 8:113–118, 1990. Reprinted with permission.)

The definition of an extensive intraductal component (EIC) for this specific study was similar to that in a previous study by Schnitt et al.[26] and consisted of two criteria: (1) DCIS was present prominently within the infiltrating tumor, and (2) DCIS was present clearly extending beyond the infiltrating margin of the tumor. Note that tumors that were predominantly intraductal with little invasion were included. Also, the selection process for this study involved exclusion of tumors greater than 5 cm in diameter and exclusion of about 23 percent of tumors in the original series because they had special type histology (i.e., the invasive component was not "ductal"). The other features of this carefully studied group of 282 mastectomy specimens have been previously reported.[11]

The Holland et al. study on the predictive capability of EIC produced results compatible with those of the initial studies on this phenomenon from the Joint Center for Radiation Therapy in Boston.[9, 26] One of these supportive studies described the histological elements in reexcision specimens from 71 patients with infiltrating ductal carcinoma who initially underwent a limited excision of tumor.[27] Residual carcinoma on reexcision was present in 88 percent of patients with EIC, with one half of these having a considerable quantity of residual DCIS. Only two percent of patients without EIC on initial biopsy had subsequent biopsies with extensive DCIS. These histological findings mirror very closely the predictability of EIC with regard to local recurrence after local excision and radiotherapy as definitive therapy for breast cancer. In these latter studies, most of the local recurrences within 5 years of follow-up were predicted by EIC. These clinical follow-up studies of the predictive utility of EIC have been confirmed in studies from Amsterdam[2] and London.[17]

Two studies have not agreed with the predictive utility of EIC with regard to local treatment failure. This disparity may be explained by the fact that one of these studies employed a large resection[31] and the other required tumor-free margins.[5] These wider initial resections are accompanied by a lower rate of local failure and may well largely negate the importance of EIC and its predictive value, because little or no DCIS is left behind in the breast. All of these observations are compatible with the contention that residual foci of DCIS left within the breast at the time of radiation after local resection of primary breast cancer are largely responsible for local recurrence.

SUMMARY

We have seen the concept of multicentricity evolve from a time when it was merely a phenomenon to be observed to the present, when the importance of multicentricity lies solely in its ability to predict treatment success or failure.

Although we may believe that multicentricity and bilaterality are related in some respects, and although both breasts may be viewed simplistically as a single organ system, these beliefs break down in the face of actual rates of occurrence of breast carcinoma. Multicentricity is strongly related to involvement of the nipple, presence of an extensive intraductal component, and presence of certain histological types, particularly lobular histology; of these three factors, only lobular histology is also predictive of bilateral disease. Discovery of a focus of invasive carcinoma more than 4 cm from the edge of a definable invasive carcinoma is uncommon, and many of these may actually be separate primaries. Their rate of occurrence is approximately that of separate primaries in the opposite breast. Even so, the rate of truly separate ipsilateral primaries does not account for all, or even the majority, of multicentric lesions.

The observation that multiple foci may frequently be found in one breast seems now to be largely the product of spread of carcinoma along the duct system. The evidence for this has been given previously and depends largely on observations that approximately 90 percent of recurrences following local removal of a carcinoma from a breast are found in the vicinity of the original carcinoma (see chapter 29). Moreover, some breast carcinomas are more confined than others, and the degree of confinement is somewhat predictive of the extensiveness of the carcinoma beyond the bounds of the original biopsy.

It should be emphasized that multicentricity must now be defined in quantitative terms. Difficulties in defining multicentricity absolutely should not obscure recognition that multicentricity is a relative term, having importance only insofar as it has predictive value for treatment success or failure.

References

1. Andersen JA, Pallesen RM: Spread to the nipple and areola in carcinoma of the breast. Ann Surg 189:367–372, 1979.
2. Bartelink JH, Borger JH, vanDongen JA, Peterse JL: The impact of tumor size and histology on local control after breast-conserving therapy. Radiother Oncol 11:279–303, 1988.
3. Cheatle GL, Cutler M: Tumors of the breast: their pathology, symptoms, diagnosis and treatment. Philadelphia, JB Lippincott, 1931, p 1.
4. Egan RL, McSweeney MB: Multicentric breast carcinoma. Recent Results Cancer Res 90:28–35, 1984.
5. Fisher B, Redmond C, Poisson R, Margolese R, Wolmark N, Wickerham L, Fisher E, Deutsch M, Caplan R, Pilch Y, Glass A, Shibata H, Lerner H, Terz J, Sidorovich L: Eight-year results of a randomized clinical trial comparing total mastectomy and lumpectomy with or without irradiation in the treatment of breast cancer. N Engl J Med 320:822–828, 1989.
6. Fisher ER, Gregorio R, Redmond C, Velljos F, Sommers SC, Fisher B: Pathologic Findings from the National Surgical Adjuvant Breast Project (protocol no. 4), I. Observations concerning the multicentricity of mammary cancer. Cancer 35:247–254, 1975.
7. Fisher ER, Sass R, Fisher B, Wickerman L, Paik SM: Pathologic findings from the National Surgical Adjuvant Breast Project (protocol 6), I. Cancer 57:197–208, 1986.
8. Gump FE, Habif DV, Logergo P, Shikora S, Kister S, Estabrook A: The extent and distribution of cancer in breasts with palpable primary tumors. Ann Surg 204:384–388, 1986.
9. Harris JR, Connolly JL, Schnitt SJ, Cohen RB, Hellman S: Clinical-pathologic study of early breast cancer treated by primary radiation therapy. J Clin Oncol 1:184–189, 1983.
10. Holland R, Connolly JL, Gelman R, Mravunac M, Hendriks JHCL, Verbeek ALM, Schnitt SJ, Silver B, Boyages J, Harris JR: The presence of an extensive intraductal component (EIC) following a limited excision correlates with prominent residual

disease in the remainder of the breast. J Clin Oncol 8:113–118, 1990.

11. Holland R, Veling SH, Mravunac M, Hendriks JHCL: Histologic multifocality of Tis, T1–2 breast carcinomas: implications for clinical trials of breast-conserving surgery. Cancer 56:979–990, 1985.

12. Kern WH, Brooks RN: Atypical epithelial hyperplasia associated with breast cancer and fibrocystic disease. Cancer 24:668–675, 1969.

13. Lagios MD: Multicentricity of breast carcinoma demonstrated by routine correlated serial subgross and radiographic examination. Cancer 40:1726–1734, 1977.

14. Lagios MD, Rose MR, Margolin FR: Tubular carcinoma of the breast association with multicentricity, bilaterally, and family history of mammary carcinoma. Am J Clin Pathol 73:25–30, 1980.

15. Lagios MD, Westdahl PR, Rose MR: The concept and implications of multicentricity in breast carcinoma. Pathol Ann 16 (pt 2):83–102, 1981.

16. Lesser ML, Rosen PP, Kinne DW: Multicentricity and bilaterality in invasive breast carcinoma. Surgery 91:234–240, 1982.

17. Lindley R, Bulman A, Parsons P: Histologic features predictive of an increased risk of early local recurrence after treatment of breast cancer by local tumor excision and radical radiotherapy. Surgery 105:13–20, 1989.

18. Luttges J, Kalbfleisch H, Prinz P: Nipple involvement and multicentricity in breast cancer. A study on whole organ sections. Cancer Res Clin Oncol 113:481–487, 1987.

19. McDivitt RW: Breast cancer multicentricity. In McDivitt RW, Oberman HA, Ozzello L, Kaufman N (eds): The Breast. Baltimore, Williams and Wilkins, 1984, p 139.

20. McDivitt RW, Boyce W, Gersell D: Tubular carcinoma of the breast clinical and pathological observations concerning 135 cases. Am J Surg Pathol 6:401–411, 1982.

21. Morgenstern L, Kaufman PA, Friedman NB: The case against tylectomy for carcinoma of the breast. Am J Surg 130:251–258, 1975.

22. Patchefsky AS, Schwartz GF, Finkelstein SD, Prestipino A, Sohn SE, Singer JS, Feig SA: Heterogeneity of intraductal carcinoma of the breast. Cancer 63:731–741, 1989.

23. Qualheim RE, Gall EA: Breast carcinoma with multiple sites of origin. Cancer 10:460–468, 1957.

24. Rosen PP, Fracchia AA, Urban JA, Schottenfeld D, Robbins G: "Residual" mammary carcinoma following simulated partial mastectomy. Cancer 35:739–747, 1975.

25. Sarnelli R, Squartini F: Multicentricity in breast cancer: a submacroscopic study. Pathol Ann 21(pt 1):143–158, 1986.

26. Schnitt SJ, Connolly JL, Harris JR, Hellman S, Cohen RB: Pathologic predictors of early local recurrence in stage I and II breast cancer treated by primary radiation therapy. Cancer 53:1049–1057, 1984.

27. Schnitt SJ, Connolly JL, Khettry U: Pathologic findings on re-excision of the primary site in breast cancer patients considered for treatment by primary radiation therapy. Cancer 59:675:681, 1987.

28. Schnitt SJ, Connolly JL, Recht A, Silver B, Harris JR: Influence of infiltrating lobular histology on local tumor control in breast cancer patients treated with conservative surgery and radiotherapy. Cancer 64:448–454, 1989.

29. Schwartz GF, Patchefsky AS, Feig SA, Shaber GS, Schwartz AB: Multicentricity of non-palpable breast cancer. Cancer 45:2913–2916, 1980.

30. Squartini F, Sarnelli R: Structure, functional changes, and proliferative pathology of the human mammary lobule in cancerous breasts. J Natl Cancer Inst 67:33–46, 1975.

31. VanLimbergen E, Van den Bogaert W, Van der Schueren E, Rijnders A: Tumor excision and radiotherapy as primary treatment of breast cancer. Analysis of patient and treatment parameters and local control. Radiother Oncol 8:1–9, 1987.

32. Westman-Naeser S, Bengtsson E, Eriksson O, Jarkrans T, Nordin B, Stenkvist B: Multifocal breast carcinoma. Am J Surg 142:255–257, 1981.

Chapter 16

PATTERNS OF RECURRENCE IN BREAST CANCER

John T. Hamm, M.D. and Warren E. Ross, M.D.

The recurrence patterns of breast cancer reveal much about its natural history and the success or failure of therapeutic interventions. Recurrence patterns are the distribution of failures by site. Recurrence rates are the percentage of patients failing therapy regardless of site. The failure rate depends upon intrinsic factors such as tumor size, presence of axillary nodes, tumor grade, and oncogene expression as well as on extrinsic factors such as the type of surgery and the administration of radiotherapy or adjuvant chemotherapy. Knowledge of these patterns influences the choice and rationalization of current therapy. This chapter will examine recurrence patterns and how they vary according to these prognostic indicators.

The concept of breast cancer as a local disease developed in the 1700s. Breast cancer was considered to arise in the breast, spreading by direct invasion and regional lymphatics. The regional lymphatics were viewed as a filter through which tumor cells must pass to disseminate systemically. Any residual tumor cells in the local region were considered responsible for later dissemination. Removal of all regional lymphatics was considered essential for cure. Failure occurred because the regional lymphatics were not adequately resected, thus the development of aggressive surgery, such as radical mastectomy. This was followed by attempts to improve survival even more with operations such as the supraradical mastectomy. With this operation, the intramammary nodes were noted to be positive in 17 to 20 percent of the patients, thus providing a rationale for continued intramammary node dissection. In retrospective comparisons, these radical operations appeared to improve survival results. Not until the 1960s and 1970s were large prospective randomized trials undertaken, which showed equivalent survival for patients treated with radical mastectomy and for those treated with extended radical mastectomy. There was no difference in local control; patients were dying because of distant metastasis.

NATURAL HISTORY

Valagussa et al.[15] reported the relapse in survival patterns following radical mastectomy and extended radical mastectomy in 716 consecutive patients. The ten-

year relapse rate for Stage I patients was 27.9 percent; Stage II with one to three positive nodes, 66.5 percent; and with greater than three nodes positive, 83.6 percent. The corresponding ten-year survival rates were 81.9 percent, 53.7 percent, and 25.6 percent. The sites of first relapse were similar for Stage I and Stage II patients. The ten-year cumulative first relapse rate for Stage II patients was as follows: local/regional disease only, 17.8 percent; bone, 14.4 percent; viscera, 10.9 percent; soft tissue, 2.9 percent; local/regional disease plus distant metastasis, 9.1 percent; multiple distant metastases, 14.2 percent; and contralateral breast, 6.2 percent of all patients. Thus, the majority of patients experienced recurrence with distant failures. Interestingly, the median time to first relapse varied by the site of the first relapse. For Stage II patients, the median time to first relapse was 1.6 years for local/regional recurrences, 2.4 years for bone lesions, and 2.6 years for distant organs.

By the time of death, patients frequently have widespread dissemination of metastasis. Hagemeister et al.[7] reported the results of autopsy on 166 patients who died with metastatic breast cancer. Metastases were found in the following distribution: soft tissue, 36 percent; respiratory, 75 percent; osseous, 67 percent; hepatic, 71 percent; CNS, 30 percent; gastrointestinal, 35 percent; endocrine, 35 percent; renal and bladder, 22 percent; and orbital, less than 1 percent. These patients represented advanced states of disease and do not necessarily indicate the pattern at initial occurrence. However, if one accepts that most of these metastatic sites were seeded prior to diagnosis and definitive therapy, this would emphasize that breast cancer metastasizes widely to sites not commonly considered.

RECURRENCE FOLLOWING SURGERY

With the recognition that radical surgery did not cure more patients than the modified radical mastectomy, the emphasis began to shift to less aggressive surgery. Several studies comparing radical mastectomy with modified radical mastectomy have found little difference in the outcome or recurrence patterns. Local/regional recurrences represented only a small percentage of failures. Distant metastases were present in the majority of patients with recurrences. The most common distant site of recurrence was bone, followed by lung, soft tissues, liver, CNS, and other sites.

Donegan and Skibba[3] retrospectively reviewed the results of 951 patients treated with different mastectomies, comparing radical mastectomies, modified radical mastectomies, and simple mastectomies. There was no difference in five-year survival or disease-free survival among the groups. There was a trend toward increased initial recurrence in the local site with less extensive surgery; however, this was not statistically significant. This was accompanied by a percentage increase recurrence at distant sites with more extensive surgery—also not statistically significant. It is important to note that this was not a randomized trial and thus was susceptible to selection bias. Of the 246 patients with documented recurrences, the following patterns were noted: local only, 14.6 percent; local plus regional only, 7.3 percent; and distant only, 68.7 percent. The cumulative percentages of patients with each of the following initial sites of recurrence were as follows: local, 20.7 percent; regional, 14.4 percent; and distant, 74.2 percent. The sites of distant metastasis are broken down as follows: bone, 54 percent; lung and pleura, 36 percent; soft tissues, 14 percent; liver, 10 percent; brain, 4 percent; other, 7 percent; and multiple sites, 24 percent. Comparing Stages I, II, and III patients, there was no observed increase in local recurrence with increased size of tumors or with axillary involvement. Radiation decreased the occurrence of local/regional failures, with the resulting relative increase in distant failures, but the disease-free survival and prognosis were not affected.

Fisher et al.[6] reported the ten-year results of the NSABP Trial (B-04) comparing radical mastectomy and total mastectomy, with or without radiation. There were 1665 eligible patients randomly assigned to one of three treatments: radical mastectomy, total mastectomy with radiotherapy, and total mastectomy followed by axillary dissection only if nodes were later clinically positive. Patients presenting with clinically positive axillary nodes were randomized only between radical mastectomy and mastectomy with radiotherapy. There was no observed survival or disease-free survival advantage with the different therapies. There was a difference noted in the first recurrences being local/regional failure among the clinically node-negative groups: radical mastectomy, 7.7 percent; total mastectomy plus radiotherapy, 4.5 percent; and total mastectomy alone, 12.6 percent. These differences in local control did not translate into statistically significant differences in either disease-free survival or survival at ten years. When the axillary nodes were clinically negative, supraclavicular nodal recurrence was relatively uncommon. Of patients with clinically positive nodes, there was a difference in supraclavicular nodal recurrence between the therapy groups: 5.8 percent with radical mastectomy, compared with no supraclavicular recurrences in the total mastectomy and radiotherapy group. On the other hand, patients with clinically positive nodes treated with radical mastectomy had a lower incidence of ipsilateral recurrences (1.0 percent) than did patients treated with total mastectomy

and radiotherapy (11.9 percent). The failure rate for patients with clinically negative nodes was 55 percent; for clinically positive nodes it was 72 percent. The pattern of distant metastasis did not vary significantly with the therapies. As a percentage of all patients on study, distant recurrences were as follows: skeletal, 8 to 11.6 percent; pulmonary, 6 to 9.2 percent; hemic and lymphatic, 1.7 to 2.3 percent; nervous system, 0 to 1 percent; and multiple sites, 3.9 to 6.5 percent.

The next generation of trials examined recurrence rates and patterns following lumpectomy with or without radiotherapy and modified radical mastectomy. Patients treated with lumpectomy and radiotherapy or with modified radical mastectomy had a low local recurrence rate, which ranged from 8 to 11 percent. Patients treated with lumpectomy and no radiotherapy had a much higher (28 percent) local recurrence rate than did the other groups. Thus, by minimizing surgery to lumpectomy without radiotherapy, the recurrence pattern was shifted to include more local recurrences, though the rate and pattern of distant metastasis and overall survival were unaffected.

NSABP Trial B-06[4] asked if even smaller breast operations would affect survival or recurrence patterns. The study randomized 1843 women with operable breast cancer to one of three treatments: total mastectomy, segmental mastectomy, or segmental mastectomy followed by breast irradiation. By life-table analysis, the five-year local recurrence rate was projected at 28 percent in the group that had segmental mastectomy alone, but 8 percent in those receiving irradiation. Patients treated with total mastectomy or segmental mastectomy alone had similar local recurrence rates. Despite this finding, distant metastasis and five-year survival were similar in all treatment groups.

Calle et al.[1] reviewed the results of 514 patients with operable breast cancer. There were 120 patients with tumors less than 3 cm in size and clinically negative nodes who were treated with lumpectomy and radiotherapy. There were 394 patients with tumors greater than 3 cm in size or clinically positive axillary nodes who were treated with radiotherapy alone. Of the patients treated with lumpectomy and radiotherapy, five- and ten-year disease-free survivals were 85 percent and 75 percent, respectively. Of the patients with recurrences at five years, 11 percent were local only and 72 percent were distant only. Of the patients with advanced lesions treated with radiotherapy alone, 59 percent required secondary surgery for either disease persistence following radiation or recurrence at the site of the primary lesion. The causes of ultimate failure at five years for this group with advanced disease were local recurrence alone, 14 percent; local plus distant, 9 percent; distant disease, 60 percent; contralateral tumor, 6 percent; secondary primary, 5 percent; and other causes, 8 percent. These results agree with the results of other studies, indicating that, regardless of primary therapy, the ultimate cause of failure is usually distant metastasis.

Veronesi et al.[16] reviewed the results of a randomized trial comparing radical mastectomy and quadrantectomy with axillary dissection and radiotherapy in 701 patients with primary breast tumors less than 2 cm in size and clinically negative axillary nodes. There was no difference noted in survival or disease-free survival at five years between the two therapy groups. Of patients treated with radical mastectomy who failed therapy, local recurrences were 8 percent, contralateral breast tumors 13 percent, and distant metastasis 79 percent. In the quadrantectomy group, local recurrences were 3 percent, ipsilateral primary breast tumors 11 percent, contralateral breast tumors 25 percent, and distant metastasis 61 percent. The distribution of distant metastasis for all patients was respiratory, 38 percent; bone, 50 percent; liver, 15 percent; lymph nodes or skin, 27 percent; CNS, 4 percent; and other sites, 8 percent.

A SWOG chemotherapy trial[8] reported sites of first recurrence. Of the 213 women with first recurrence, the involved sites were reported according to whether the patient was premenopausal, postmenopausal, or castrated. The range of percent involvement was bone, 56 to 63 percent; skin and lymph nodes, 50 to 55 percent; lung, 13 to 26 percent; pleura, 9 to 23 percent; liver, 4 to 18 percent; and other, 5 to 14 percent, with a mean number of sites of 1.57 to 1.78.

ADJUVANT TRIALS

Trials of adjuvant therapy offer an opportunity to observe both the natural history of recurrences and the effects of therapy on the sites of recurrence. Although many trials demonstrate decreased recurrence rates with adjuvant therapy compared with controls, the pattern of recurrence does not change.

Tormey et al.[14] reported the results of an ECOG trial of adjuvant therapy in 776 patients with node-positive breast cancer treated with cyclophosphamide, methotrexate, and 5-fluorouracil (CMF); with CMF plus prednisone (CMFP); with CMFP plus tamoxifen; with observation. Of the premenopausal patients with 54 months' median follow-up, sites of first recurrence were as follows: local only, 6 percent; regional ± local, 7 percent; distant and local and/or regional, 5 percent; distant only, 25 percent; no relapse, 60 percent. Postmenopausal patients with 59 months' median follow-up had a similar distribution but a higher percentage of recurrences: local only, 11 percent; regional ± local, 7 percent; distant and local and/or regional, 6 percent; distant only, 31 percent; and no relapse, 45 percent. Although there were minor differences in recurrence patterns between the observation and treatment groups, these were not significant.

The Ludwig Breast Cancer Study Group[9] reported results of a randomized trial of adjuvant chemoendocrine therapy in node-positive patients. In the control group of 156 patients with a median follow-up of 36 months, there was a failure rate of 36 percent. The distribution was mastectomy scar alone, 4 percent; contralateral breast alone, <1 percent; other regional or local disease without distant recurrence, 3 percent; distant recurrence or distant disease plus other sites, 27

percent; second primary, 1 percent; and death without recurrence, 1 percent. The Ludwig Group[10] also reported results of adjuvant therapy in a premenopausal group of patients; the recurrence rate was 46 percent, but the distribution of recurrence was similar to that in the postmenopausal group.

The NSABP has reported results of adjuvant trials in women with operable breast cancer. Trial B-05[5] postoperatively randomized 380 patients with axillary nodal involvement to receive either L-Pam or no further therapy. In the placebo group, 29 percent were alive and disease-free at ten years. The cumulative incidences of first events in the placebo group were: local, 14 percent; regional, 10 percent; distant, 34 percent; second cancer, 1 percent; and other, 5 percent. The event-free survival in the treatment group was 36 percent. The failures were as follows: local, 10 percent; regional, 4 percent; distant, 35 percent; second cancer, 4 percent; death from other cause, 6 percent. Thus, in the chemotherapy group there were fewer local and regional treatment failures but nearly identical distant failure rates.

The Nolvadex Adjuvant Trial Organization (NATO) reported the results of a randomized trial[11] of 1285 patients with operable breast cancer randomized to receive tamoxifen for two years or no further therapy. With a median follow-up of 45 months, the tamoxifen group had a 27 percent failure rate distributed as follows: local/regional or new primary, 7.5 percent; distant metastasis, 15 percent; and death without previously confirmed recurrence, 4.4 percent. In the group receiving no adjuvant therapy, the failure rate was 39 percent: local/regional or new primary, 13.8 percent; distant metastasis, 18.2 percent; and death without previously confirmed recurrence, 6.9 percent. Tamoxifen appeared to decrease both local/regional and distant metastasis, although the largest percentage change was in local/regional recurrences.

OTHER STUDIES

Clinical studies of recurrence often fail to emphasize the extent to which breast cancer can metastasize because they frequently report the first site of recurrence, which is limited by the technical ability to detect metastasis. Pandya and others[12] reviewed data from ECOG adjuvant breast trials and found that 73.7 percent of recurrences were detected by history and physical examination, only 5 percent by routine chest x-rays, 8 percent by bone scans, and 12 percent by blood chemistries. Other approaches emphasize the frequent multiorgan involvement in breast cancer. Several studies have reported monoclonal antibody techniques to examine bone marrow aspirates for metastatic breast cancer cells. In patients with Stages I and II breast cancer, bone marrow involvement has been found. Porro et al.[13] examined bone marrow aspirates taken at the time of surgery in women with operable breast cancer and clinically negative axillary nodes. The marrow was tested by immunofluorescence to MBr1 antibody. Of patients with histologically negative nodes, 17 percent had evidence of bone marrow involvement by this technique.

Cote et al.[2] utilized monoclonal antibodies to membrane and cytoskeletal antigens to examine bone marrow aspirates in 51 patients with operable breast cancer. Thirty-five percent of patients had evidence of bone marrow involvement. Of patients with negative axillary nodes, 27 percent had positive marrows, while 41 percent of those with positive axillary nodes had marrow metastasis. Long-term follow-up will be necessary to determine the significance of this observation.

SUMMARY

Most of the studies reviewed emphasize the sites where a tumor is most likely to occur first, but patients frequently have multiple metastatic lesions or subsequently develop metastasis at other sites. The autopsy study by Hagemeister et al.[7] and the bone marrow studies cited earlier indicate that most patients have subclinical lesions in other sites that are simply not detected. From these studies it is possible to draw the conclusion that breast cancer, even in early stages, is frequently a systemic disease. It metastasizes hematogenously, early, and widely. Analyzing patterns of recurrence has modified the surgical approach: Lumpectomy followed by radiotherapy is now widely practiced, allowing conservation of the breast. Aggressive surgery offers no advantage over modified radical mastectomy or lumpectomy with radiotherapy. Radiotherapy, with the exception of its use following lumpectomy, alters the course of this disease little. Adjuvant therapy, which decreases the overall recurrence rate, does not appear to alter the distribution of recurrences. By following patterns of recurrence, it is hoped that we will be able to further refine our therapy in the future.

References

1. Calle R, Pilleron J, Schlienger P, Vilcoq J: Conservative management of operable breast cancer. Cancer 42:2045–2053, 1978.
2. Cote RJ, Rosen PP, Hakes TB, Sedira M, Bazinet M, Kinne D, Old L, Osborne M: Monoclonal antibodies detect occult breast carcinoma metastases in the bone marrow of patients with early stage disease. Am J Surg Pathol 12:333–340, 1988.
3. Donegan W, Skibba J: Patterns of survival and disease recurrence after mastectomy for carcinoma of the breast. Cancer Treat Symp 2:107–116, 1983.
4. Fisher B, Bauer M, Margolese R, Poisson R, Pilch Y, Redmond C, Fisher E, Wolmark N, Deutsch M, Montague E, Saffer E, Wickerham L, Lerner H, Glass A, Shibata H, Deckers P, Ketcham A, Oishi R, Russell I: Five-year results of a randomized clinical trial comparing total mastectomy and segmental mastectomy with or without radiation in the treatment of breast cancer. N Engl J Med 312:665–673, 1985.
5. Fisher B, Fisher E, Redmond C: Ten-year results from the National Surgical Adjuvant Breast and Bowel Project Clinical Trial evaluating the use of L-phenylalanine mustard (L-PAM) in the management of primary breast cancer. J Clin Oncol 4:929–941, 1986.
6. Fisher B, Redmond C, Fisher E, Bauer M, Wolmark N, Wickerham L, Deutsch M, Montague E, Margolese R, Foster R: Ten-year results of a randomized trial comparing radical mastectomy and total mastectomy with or without radiation. N Engl J Med 312:674–681, 1985.
7. Hagemeister FB, Buzdar A, Luna M, Blumenshein G: Causes of death in breast cancer. Cancer 46:162–167, 1980.
8. Hoogstraten B, Gad-el-Mawla N, Maloney T, Fletcher W, Vaughn C, Tranum B, Athens J, Costanzi J, Foulkes M: Combined modality therapy for first recurrence of breast cancer, a Southwest Oncology Group Study. Cancer 54:2248–2256, 1984.
9. Ludwig Breast Cancer Study Group: Randomized trial of chemo-endocrine therapy, endocrine therapy, and mastectomy alone in postmenopausal patients with operable breast cancer and axillary node metastasis. Lancet 1:1256–1260, 1984.
10. Ludwig Breast Cancer Study Group: Chemotherapy with or without oophorectomy in high-risk premenopausal patients with operable breast cancer. J Clin Oncol 3:1059–1067, 1985.
11. Nolvadex Adjuvant Trial Organization: Controlled trial of tamoxifen as single adjuvant agent in management of early breast cancer. Lancet 1:836–839, 1985.
12. Pandya K, McFadden E, Kalish L, Carbone P: Frequency and patterns of early disease recurrence and method of detection in operable breast cancer with pathologically positive axillary lymph nodes in ECOG adjuvant studies—a preliminary report. Cancer Treat Symp 2:117–122, 1983.
13. Porro G, Menard S, Tagliabue E, Drefice S, Sawadori B, Squicciarini P, Andreola S, Rilke F, Colnaghi M: Monoclonal antibody detection of carcinoma cells in bone marrow biopsy specimens from breast cancer patients. Cancer 61:2407–2411, 1988.
14. Tormey D, Gray R, Taylor S, Knuiman M, Olson JE, Cummings FJ: Postoperative Chemotherapy and Chemohormonal Therapy in Women with Node-Positive Breast Cancer. NCI Monographs 1, Adjuvant Chemotherapy and Endocrine Therapy for Breast Cancer. 1986, pp 75–80.
15. Valagussa P, Bonadonna G, Veronesi U: Patterns of relapse and survival following radical mastectomy. Cancer 41:1170–1178, 1978.
16. Veronesi U, Saccozzi R, Del Vecchio M, Banfi A, Clemente C, DeLena M, Gallus G, Greco M, Luini A, Marubini E, Muscolino G, Rilke F, Salvadori B, Zecchini A, Zucali R: Comparing radical mastectomy with quadrantectomy, axillary dissection, and radiotherapy in patients with small cancers of the breast. N Engl J Med 305:6–11, 1981.

Clinical and Pathological Staging of Breast Cancer and Prognostic Factors

Chapter 17

STAGING OF BREAST CANCER

Timothy J. Yeatman, M.D. and Kirby I. Bland, M.D.

PURPOSE OF STAGING

The purpose of cancer staging is to determine the anatomical extent of current disease and the tendency for tumor progression such that appropriate therapy may be instituted. This process requires objective analysis of pertinent, well-organized clinical and pathological data. "They are called wise who put things in their right order" is a quotation from Saint Thomas Aquinas that has been appropriately applied to this meticulous process of staging cancer.

In the past, cancer staging was quite simplistic. Neoplasms were staged on the basis of clinical evaluation alone as either operable or inoperable, and classified as local, regional, or metastatic. Because of the limitations of clinical staging, the importance of deriving more sophisticated and prognostic staging systems based on objective, pathological data has been realized.

Despite the inclusion of pathological factors, however, current staging systems are still limited by their ability to assess the future biological behavior of a cancer. Neoplasms in different patients progress at different rates despite being initially classified as the same histological type. This rate of progression is probably dependent on a myriad of factors, many of which are still poorly understood. In a sense, staging in its current form is quite primitive, because its predictive power is largely derived from simple physical measurements such as size or extent of anatomical spread of disease. These measurements are static and permit only limited evaluation of an ever changing, heterogeneous neoplasm that often has been in existence for years prior to the initiation of the staging process.

There are several universal requisites for any effective staging system. First and foremost, the staging methodology must provide an accurate estimate of the extent of disease. This estimation must in turn yield accurate prognostic information that can be used to guide therapy. A staging system should be simplistic and "user-friendly" so that data can be easily compiled, analyzed, and transmitted from one physician or institution to another for use in prospectively randomized, multi-institutional trials that derive their statistical power from numbers. These sorts of studies are possible only through the adjunctive use of universally accepted staging systems that permit comparisons between groups of patients. Lastly, a staging system should be flexible and revisable. As new information is derived, better ways to estimate prognosis are identified and should be incorporated. In this sense, a staging system should be dynamic, providing the means for its own evolution.

THE CHANGING BIOLOGY OF BREAST CANCER

Long before the true biological nature of breast cancer was established, Galen (circa 100 A.D.) proposed that cancer was a systemic illness from the onset. Although he did not understand the meaning of the term "carcinoma," he suggested that cancers were incurable by any operation.[36] Consequently, surgery was not a treatment option until the eighteenth century.

Halstedian surgical principles of breast cancer management were derived from concepts supported long ago by surgeons such as Valsalva (1704), LeDran (1757), and Morgagni (1769), who suggested that breast cancer was a local process that spread in an orderly fashion to regional lymph nodes and only then to distant sites.[36] These anatomical principles led to the development of surgical therapy for breast cancer, with the Halsted radical mastectomy being the most aggressive form.

Only recently have we begun to realize that Galenian principles, rather than those of Halsted, might better

RELATIVE SURVIVAL OF BREAST CANCER PATIENTS (ALL STAGES)

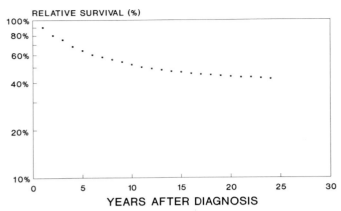

Figure 17–1. Despite attempts at curative therapy, breast cancer patients continue to die from their disease up to 20 or more years after initial diagnosis. (Adapted from Fox MS: JAMA 241:489–494, 1979.)

approximate the truth regarding breast cancer progression. In fact, we now know that breast cancer may often be systemic from the time of initial diagnosis. This concept is well illustrated by the findings that greater than 30 percent of patients with small, non-palpable breast cancers (mammogram positive) may have lymph node metastases at the time of diagnosis[74] and that breast cancers may recur distantly up to 20 or more years after curative therapy (Fig. 17–1).[38] Furthermore, despite many changes in management, the absolute death rate for breast cancer in the United States for the past 25 years has not been affected.[52]

Fisher et al.[22] developed a more progressive theory of breast cancer management that in many ways departs from classical Halstedian principles and has been partly responsible for the return to conservativism in the surgical treatment of this disease. The findings of the National Surgical Adjuvant Bowel and Breast Project (NSABP) supported a biologically-based hypothesis suggesting that variations in local/regional treatment would not affect distant, undetected disease or survival. These projections have, in part, been borne out by clinical trials demonstrating equivalent survivorship for patients treated by radical mastectomy versus more surgically conservative treatment modalities. Other unique biological principles (diametrically opposed to those of Halsted) have been derived from clinical observations, such as the importance of regional lymph nodes as prognostic indicators of disease progression instead of simply as harbingers of local/regional disease that require surgical excision (Table 17–1).

Contemporary management principles are still limited by a superficial understanding of the biology of breast cancer. Although breast cancer may be systemic and rapidly progressing from its inception or presentation, it may also have a prolonged natural history. This biological heterogeneity is well documented by longitudinal studies by Bloom et al.[9] of patients who went untreated but survived for many years. Ultimately, improvements in survivorship will depend on therapy adjunctive to surgery that might control systemic disease. We have recently seen the promising, beneficial effects of hormonal and/or chemotherapy in patients with node-negative breast cancer.[3] These effects support the need for the development of new therapies directed at a disease that may already be beyond the reach of the surgeon's knife at the time of diagnosis.

Table 17–1. DIVERGENT HYPOTHESES OF TUMOR BIOLOGY

Halstedian	Fisher
Tumors spread in an orderly defined manner based on mechanical considerations.	There is no orderly pattern of tumor cell dissemination.
Tumor cells traverse lymphatics to lymph nodes by direct extension supporting en bloc dissection.	Tumor cells traverse lymphatics by embolization challenging the merit of en bloc dissection.
The positive lymph node is an indicator of tumor spread and is the instigator of distant disease.	The positive lymph node is an indicator of a host-tumor relationship which permits development of metastases rather the instigator of distant disease.
Regional lymph nodes (RLNs) are barriers to the passage of tumor cells.	Regional lymph nodes are ineffective as barriers to tumor cell spread.
RLNs are of anatomic importance.	RLNs are of biologic importance.
The blood stream is of little significance as a route of tumor dissemination.	The blood stream is of considerable importance in tumor dissemination.
A tumor is autonomous of its host.	Complex host-tumor interrelationships affect every facet of the disease.
Operable breast cancer is a local disease.	Operable breast cancer is a regional systemic disease.
The extent and nuances of operation are the dominant factors influencing patient outcome.	Variations in local/regional therapy are unlikely to substantially affect survival.

From Fisher B, et al: Cancer 46:1009–1025, 1980. Reprinted by permission.

CLINICAL AND PATHOLOGICAL CORRELATES WITH PROGNOSIS

Central to any staging system are identifiable objective tumor and host characteristics that are prognostic of tumor progression. A large number of clinical and histopathological factors have been identified that may predict long-term outcome after surgical therapy. Although clinical parameters have historically been used to predict survival potential, pathological evaluation of the primary tumor and its local/regional lymph nodes has recently become the "gold standard." Both clinical and pathological factors predicting tumor progression and survival are essential components in determining prognosis and therapy and are best incorporated in the current TNM staging system.

Clinical Factors

Tumor Characteristics

Clinical evaluation of tumor size[24, 48, 73] and fixation[15] by physical examination have been included in many staging systems because both features are easily assessable and may be indicators of advanced disease. It has been elegantly demonstrated by Koscielny et al.[48] that metastasis correlates directly with tumor size (Fig. 17–2) and does not occur in 50 percent of the cases until the primary tumor attains the size of 3.6 cm in diameter. Similarly, Nemoto et al.[62] determined a distinct relationship between increasing tumor size and probability of axillary node metastasis in addition to a reduction in 5-year survivorship. These investigators demonstrated that tumor size must reach 3.1–4.0 cm in diameter to generate axillary metastases in 50 percent of patients (Table 17–2). Fisher et al.[28] have likewise shown that tumor size correlates with disease-free survival at 10 years, even when controlled for nodal metastases (Fig. 17–3). It is also true, however, that more than one third of patients with tumors greater than 6 cm in palpable diameter have negative lymph nodes, thus demonstrating the limited predictiveness of tumor size alone.[24]

The location of the primary tumor within the breast may have some prognostic importance for patients with negative nodes. While the risk of axillary lymph node metastasis is greater for lateral versus medial breast cancers, two studies have shown that patients with medial tumors fare more poorly than those with lateral tumors secondary to greater risks of local recurrence.[23, 61] These data have led us to recommend adjunctive radiotherapy for primary tumors of the medial half of the breast.

Lymph Node Metastasis

Once the diagnosis of breast cancer has been established, the single most predictive factor of 10- and 20-year survival is the absolute number of lymph nodes involved with tumor (see section on pathological factors).[20] Physical examination, however, is notoriously inaccurate to preoperatively determine the presence of lymph node metastasis. In fact, microscopic evidence of tumor can be demonstrated in one third of patients in the absence of palpable axillary lymph nodes.[84] False-

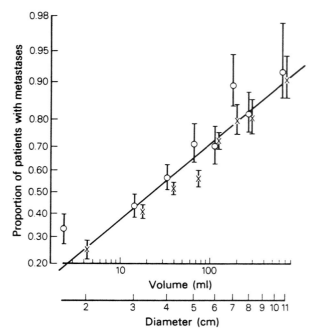

Figure 17–2. A linear relationship exists between tumor size (volume or diameter) and potential for metastasis. (From Koscielny S, et al: Br J Cancer 49:709–715, 1984. Reprinted by permission.)

Tumor Diameter (cm)	No. of Patients	Axillary Node-Negative (%)	Axillary Node-Positive (%)
0.1–0.5	147	71.4	28.6
0.6–1.0	960	75.3	24.7
1.1–2.0	4044	65.9	34.1
2.1–3.0	3546	57.3	42.1
3.1–4.0	1917	49.9	50.1
4.1–5.0	1135	43.5	56.5
> 5.0	1232	35.5	64.5

Table 17–2. RELATIONSHIP BETWEEN TUMOR SIZE AND AXILLARY METASTASES

Adapted from Nemoto T, et al: Cancer 45:2917–2924, 1980.

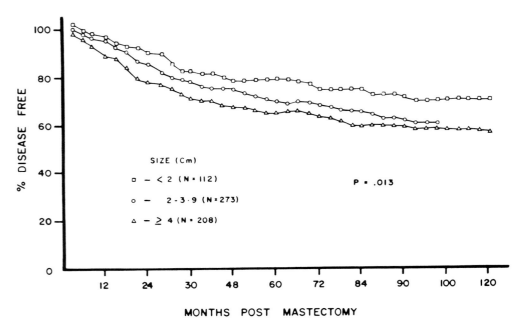

Figure 17–3. Primary tumor size correlates with disease-free survival in patients undergoing curative surgery. (From Fisher ER: NCI Monogr 1:29–34, 1986. Reprinted by permission.)

positive rates for detection of axillary metastases range from 25 percent to 31 percent, and false-negative rates range from 27 percent to 33 percent.

Delay in Diagnosis

Studies of the relationship between survival and the length of time between first symptoms and diagnosis have shown that tumors diagnosed early (within 3 months) have a better prognosis than those diagnosed after a longer delay (3 to 6 months).[7] With even longer delays, however, survival improves. These observations suggest that improved survival may be associated with tumors that are detected earlier and, perhaps more importantly, with tumors that are slow growing. Tumors that are diagnosed after a long interval of delay may possess slower growth kinetics, which in turn may enhance prognosis.

Endocrine Factors

Data concerning the effects of pregnancy and menopausal status are contradictory. Pregnancy in and of itself does not adversely affect breast cancer prognosis; however, studies suggest that patients treated earlier in pregnancy fair better than those treated during the second and third trimesters.[39, 67] While one extensive study of premenopausal patients versus postmenopausal patients has reported better survivorship[54], others have failed to confirm this.[46]

Physical Factors

Age, race, and body weight have been implicated to affect survival in breast cancer. Studies of age as it relates to breast cancer survival have been controversial. Although older studies are contradictory, this disease generally carries a more favorable prognosis in younger women, especially when follow-up is continued past 20 years. Hibberd et al.,[42] in a study of more than 2000 patients with breast cancer, found that women aged 20–34 years had survival rates of 37 percent, 35 percent, and 35 percent at 10, 20, and 30 years, respectively, whereas those aged 55–64 years had reduced levels of survivorship of 35 percent, 22 percent, and 19 percent at these same intervals. Others have found that there is a correlation between age and stage, with older patients presenting with more advanced disease.[72] When patients <55 years of age were compared with those ≥55 years, younger patients more frequently presented with Stage I disease (64 percent) than older patients (45 percent). This was also true for Stages II (32 percent vs. 20 percent) and III (28 percent vs. 14 percent) disease. Studies of very young patients (<30 years) have, however, suggested that disease-free survival in this group (43 percent) is worse than in older patients (59 percent).[63] The effect of age on breast cancer prognosis is most likely multifactorial. For example, young patients are generally premenopausal and have fewer estrogen receptor–positive tumors than older, postmenopausal women. Additionally, tumor cell kinetics (growth rates) may be directly related to the age of the patient and affect overall survival.

Race may adversely affect prognosis in breast cancer. Findings by Natarajan et al.[59] for the American College of Surgeons have shown that black women present with more advanced stages than white women. Whites were generally diagnosed more frequently than blacks with smaller tumors (T1 lesions) (45 percent vs. 35 percent) and with negative lymph nodes (58 percent vs. 48 percent).

Both body weight and cholesterol levels have been correlated with survival. Obese patients tend to have reduced 5-year survival rates in comparison to patients

Table 17–3. SURVIVAL OF PATIENTS WITH BREAST CANCER RELATIVE TO HISTOLOGICAL STAGE

Histological Staging	Crude Survival (%)		5-Yr Disease-Free Survival (%)
	5 Yr	*10 Yr*	
All patients	64	46	60
Negative	78	65	82
Positive axillary lymph nodes	46	25	35
1–3 positive axillary lymph nodes	62	38	50
>4 positive axillary lymph nodes	32	13	21

Adapted from Henderson IC, Canellos GP: N Engl J Med 302(1):17–30, 1980.

weighing less than 150 pounds (49 percent vs. 67 percent) and have even worse survivorship (32 percent) when cholesterol levels are elevated.[80] Similarly, these overweight patients have an increased incidence of positive lymph nodes (44 percent vs. 35 percent) and tumor recurrence (41 percent vs. 8 percent) in comparison to age-matched, normal-weight patients.[17]

Pathological Factors

Lymph Node Metastasis

Once the diagnosis of invasive breast cancer has been made, the single most predictive factor of 10- and 20-year survival is the number of lymph nodes found to contain metastatic tumor on histological examination.[20] These data are important not only for prognostic reasons (probability and interval of recurrence), but also for determining when systemic adjuvant therapy is warranted. Clinical evaluation of the axilla is fraught with error in one third of all patients examined; the importance of axillary dissection for staging purposes is clear. In a 10-year clinical trial, Fisher et al.,[25] reporting for the NSABP, found that crude and disease-free survival correlated directly with the number of positive lymph nodes. Patients with negative axillary lymph nodes had 5- and 10-year survival rates of 78 percent and 65 percent, whereas those with four or more positive lymph nodes had survival rates of 32 percent and 13 percent, respectively (Table 17–3). Similarly, the number of positive nodes correlated with the percent of 5- and 10-year treatment failures. Zero positive nodes were associated with a 20 percent treatment failure rate at 10 years while more than four positive lymph nodes were associated with a 71 percent treatment failure rate. More than 13 positive nodes increased the failure rate even further to 87 percent (Table 17–4).

While routine pathological examination of lymph nodes is more accurate than physical examination, exhaustive studies of lymph nodes with thin section techniques have demonstrated occult micrometastases in patients with lymph nodes initially reported as histologically negative.[31] Similarly, it has been estimated by Wilkinson and Lawrence[86] that commonly employed methods of sectioning lymph nodes can result in a greater than 30 percent false-negative rate. The prognostic implication of micrometastases, however, is not yet clear because the survival of patients with these lesions is not different from that of patients with negative nodes using the same pathological techniques. Recent studies concerning the treatment of node-negative patients with chemotherapy or hormonal therapy has further complicated this issue. These data suggest that there may be patients with occult micrometastases who would benefit from adjuvant therapy despite the absence of axillary metastases on routine pathology (Table 17–5).[21, 53, 56, 60]

Other indices that portend an unfavorable prognosis for breast cancer relate to the presence of gross rather than microscopic disease in the lymph nodes[2] and/or the presence of extranodal tumor.[55] Similarly, the location of the positive lymph nodes is important. Involvement of apical axillary (level III) lymph nodes[1, 35] carries a grim prognosis.

Another issue is the number and level of axillary lymph nodes that must be removed in order to obtain accurate prognostic information. Certainly, complete dissection of all three levels of lymph nodes (Patey dissection) not only provides the maximum amount of prognostic information but also clears the axilla of gross disease and obviates the need for axillary radiotherapy. In fact, total axillary clearance has been supported by some authors as the only acceptable method of assessing axillary nodal status.[15a] Several studies, however, have addressed this topic and have concluded that, in certain

Table 17–4. NODAL STATUS AND 5- AND 10-YEAR TREATMENT FAILURE

No. of Positive Nodes	No. of Patients (N = 614)	% Treatment Failure	
		5 Yr	*10 Yr*
0	279	13	20
1–3	160	39	47
4 +	175	69	71
4–6	65		59
7–12	55		69
13 +	55		87

Adapted from Fisher ER: NCI Monogr 1:29–34, 1986.

Table 17–5. EFFECT OF TAMOXIFEN AND/OR CHEMOTHERAPY ON NODE-NEGATIVE BREAST CANCER

Study	No. Patients	ER	Therapy	Control* (%)	Study* (%)	P
B-13*†	679	−	Chemotherapy	71	80	0.003
B-14*†	2644	+	Tamoxifen	77	83	0.00001
INT-0011‡	536	±	Chemotherapy	69	84	0.00001
Ludwig-V§	1275	±	Chemotherapy	73	77	0.04

*Disease-free survival after 3–4 years of follow-up.
†NSABP study. Fisher B, et al: N Engl J Med 320(8):479–484, 1989.
‡Intergroup study [Eastern Cooperative Oncology Group, Southwest Oncology Group (SWOG), and Cancer and Leukemia Group B (CALGB)]. Mansour EG, et al: N Engl J Med 320(8):485–490, 1989.
§Ludwig Breast Cancer Group: N Engl J Med 320(8):491–496, 1989.
Abbreviation: ER = estrogen-receptor status.

cases, a Level I dissection can be predictive of the actual involvement of the residual axillary contents. Boova et al.[10] examined the contents of 200 consecutive mastectomy and total axillary dissection specimens. The average number of lymph nodes recovered from each level was 14 at Level I, 11 at Level II, and 8 at Level III. Forty percent of patients had axillary metastases, with one half of these involving only Level I (Table 17–6). Interestingly, seven patients (3.5 percent of all patients or 8.7 percent of patients with lymph node metastases) had positive nodes at Level II and/or III without positive nodes at Level I. These authors concluded that Level I dissections can be accurate predictors of the status of the entire axillary chain, assuming an adequate number of lymph nodes has been sampled. Fisher et al.[26] have also suggested that dissection of Levels I and II is more than adequate in most cases to accurately predict systemic spread of disease. Their report found that qualitative disease (positive vs. negative) in the axilla could be determined equally well by studying three to five or ≥27 lymph nodes; however, to quantitatively determine true axillary involvement, sampling of more than ten lymph nodes was required.

Inclusion of internal mammary lymph nodes in routine dissections has not been warranted, although sampling this nodal basin may be important for cases where the primary tumor is medial in location or when axillary nodes are negative. Positive internal mammary lymph nodes may be found in up to 8.9 percent of cases when axillary nodes are negative and in as many as 26 percent of cases when the primary tumor location is medial.[58]

Supraclavicular lymph node involvement always indicates the presence of advanced disease (Stage IV) and implies distant dissemination of tumor. Routine scalene lymph node biopsy is generally not indicated. In the pre-chemotherapy era, scalene lymph node biopsy was done to determine operability of breast cancer patients with advanced local disease but without demonstrable distant metastases. It was noted by Papaioannou and Urban, however, that when scalene lymph nodes were pathologically positive, despite the use of radical mastectomy with adjuvant radiotherapy, no patients were disease free after 1 year, and >50 percent were dead with disease in 3 years.[65] These data once again suggest that metastases to lymph node beds other than regional (axillary and internal mammary) suggest the presence of distant, systemic disease.

Histological Classification and Grade

The most frequently utilized classification of tumor types is seen in Table 17–7. Tumors have been classified by the World Health Organization into six major groups, with epithelial tumors being the most common. Of the malignant epithelial tumors, there are three subtypes: noninvasive, invasive, and Paget's disease of the nipple. Next to inflammatory carcinoma, which has a 5-year survival rate of 11 percent, the invasive ductal carcinoma (most common subtype) carries the worst prognosis, with 5-year survival rates of approximately 59 percent.[82] Medullary, papillary, and colloid subtypes portend a better prognosis than do ductal invasive cancers (Table 17–8).

Attempts have been made to stage tumors based on histological characteristics alone. Hoge et al.[44] described four classes of tumors after analyzing tumor specimens from 3902 patients. Class A tumors (5 percent of total) included all in situ lesions and carried a 5-year survival rate of 91 percent. Class B tumors (medullary, mucinous, tubular, and adenoid cystic carcinomas) occurred

Table 17–6. PATTERNS OF AXILLARY NODAL INVOLVEMENT: LEVELS I, II, AND III

Node Status	Number of Patients	Percentage
All levels negative	120	60.0
Level I positive	39	19.5
Level I and II positive	19	9.5
Level I, II, and III positive	11	5.5
Level I and III positive	4	2.0
Level II positive*	5	2.5
Level III positive*	1	0.5
Level II and III positive*	1	0.5

*skip metastasis group.
From Boova RS, et al: Ann Surg 196(6):642–644, 1982. Reprinted by permission.

Table 17–7. HISTOLOGICAL CLASSIFICATION OF BREAST TUMORS

I. Epithelial tumors
  A. Benign
    1. Intraductal papilloma
    2. Adenoma of the nipple
    3. Adenoma
      a. Tubular
      b. Lactating
  B. Malignant
    1. Noninvasive
      a. Intraductal carcinoma
      b. Lobular carcinoma in situ
    2. Invasive
      a. Invasive ductal carcinoma
      b. Invasive ductal carcinoma with a predominant intraductal component
      c. Invasive lobular carcinoma
      d. Mucinous carcinoma
      e. Medullary carcinoma
      f. Papillary carcinoma
      g. Tubular carcinoma
      h. Adenoid cystic carcinoma
      i. Secretory (juvenile) carcinoma
      j. Apocrine
      k. Carcinoma with metaplasia
        i. Squamous type
        ii. Spindle-cell type
        iii. Cartilaginous and osseous type
        iv. Mixed type
      l. Others
    3. Paget's disease of the nipple
II. Mixed connective tissue and epithelial tumors
  A. Fibroadenoma
  B. Phyllodes tumor (cystosarcoma phyllodes)
  C. Carcinosarcoma
III. Miscellaneous tumors
  A. Soft tissue tumors
  B. Skin tumors
  C. Tumors of hematopoietic and lymphoid tissues
IV. Unclassified tumors
V. Mammary dysplasia/fibrocystic disease
VI. Tumor-like lesions
  A. Duct ectasia
  B. Inflammatory pseudotumors
  C. Hamartoma
  D. Gynecomastia
  E. Others

From WHO International Histological Classification of Tumors, No. 2 Histological Typing of Breast Tumors, ed 2. Geneva, World Health Organization, 1981. Reprinted by permission.

developed.[6] Hutter[45] has reviewed this topic and reports that overall survivorship is related to differentiation of tumor cells. Survival at 20 years was estimated to be 41 percent for Grade I (well differentiated), 29 percent for Grade II (moderately differentiated), and 21 percent for Grade III (poorly differentiated). Fisher et al.[30] have examined histological grade in relationship to 5-year treatment failures and found that there is a significant correlation between these two factors in patients with absent nodal metastases or with four or more positive lymph nodes.

Histological Characteristics

In 1975, Fisher et al.[29] examined the relationship of 32 pathological and seven clinical characteristics to 5-year survival in 1000 patients treated by radical mastectomy. Although they found that pathological nodal status was the most dominant influence on treatment failure rates and corresponding survivorship, they also identified a number of other important predictors of short-term (<24 months) treatment failure (Table 17–9). Characteristics such as noncircumscription, perineural invasion, tumor necrosis, the absence of sinus histiocytosis, and other parameters correlated with poor long-term survival.

Other histological characteristics have also been found to bear prognostic importance. These include blood vessel invasion, lymphatic extension, elastosis, glycogen staining, and the presence or absence of numerous host inflammatory responses. These and other histological characteristics can frequently be identified in many patients. Unfortunately, histological criteria can rarely be used to modify the management of a patient by stratification into different substages; when these characteristics are present, the prognosis is usually guarded.

Steroid Receptors and Response to Endocrine Therapy

Both estrogen (ER) and progesterone (PR) receptors have been shown to be significant prognostic indicators in the treatment of breast cancer and should be obtained

in 41 percent of patients and were associated with a 75 percent survival rate. Class C tumors (85 percent of total) included the most common tumor types (e.g., infiltrating ductal, infiltrating lobular, etc.) and had a reduced 5-year survival rate of 66 percent. Class D tumors (4.3 percent of total) consisted of high-risk lesions such as inflammatory and undifferentiated carcinoma and had the worst survival rate (33 percent).

Histological grading based on criteria established by Bloom and Richardson[8] incorporates cytoplasmic and nuclear characteristics such as size, shape, and hyperchromatism along with the percent and number of mitotic figures and tubules. Other systems of grading based on nuclear characteristics alone have also been

Table 17–8. AMERICAN COLLEGE OF SURGEONS 1979 SURVEY OF INFILTRATING BREAST CANCER

	No. of Cases	% of Total	% 5-Yr Survival
Histological type			
Lobular	700	3	70
Ductal	2,845	56	59
Paget's	122	0.5	61
Scirrhous	2,438	11	60
Medullary	735	3	66
Colloid	442	2	69
Comedo	236	1	65
Inflammatory	117	0.5	11
All cases	22,989	100	58

Adapted from Hutter RVP: Cancer 46:961–976, 1980.

Table 17–9. FACTORS ASSOCIATED WITH SHORT-TERM TREATMENT FAILURE

Feature	Time to Failure (months)
Clinically positive axillae	6, 12, 18, 24
>4 pathologically positive nodes	6, 12, 18, 24
Size >4.1 cm	6, 12, 18, 24
Noncircumscribed (gross and micro)	12, 18, 24
Lymphatic extension in quadrants	12, 18
Proliferative fibrocystic disease in quadrants	12, 18
Age 20–54 years	18, 24
Nipple involvement	6
Absent or slight/moderate cell reaction to tumor	6
Absent sinus histiocytosis	12
Skin involvement	12
Perineural extension	18
Black race	18
Nuclear Grade 1	24
Marked tumor necrosis	24
Glycogen present	24

Adapted from Fisher ER, et al: Cancer 46:908–918, 1980.

on all tumor specimens when feasible. ER and PR receptor positivity generally correlates with a better prognosis and a better response to chemotherapy with or without the concomitant use of tamoxifen. Knight et al.,[47] Stewart and Rubens,[79] and Osborne and McGuire[64] have shown that ER status affects survival and is independent of axillary nodal status.

Similarly, other studies have demonstrated longer survivorship for PR positive than PR negative patients.[69] Recently, reports of the beneficial use of chemotherapy and/or tamoxifen have suggested that receptor status may be important in patients with known systemic disease as well as in patients without axillary metastases.[60]

Tumor Growth Rate and Kinetics

Anatomical methods for staging breast cancer have withstood the test of time and remain the "gold standard"; however, these methods often provide only a static or instantaneous view of what is actually occurring at the cellular level. Attempts at measuring dynamic characteristics (clinical and pathological) have also been predictive of tumor progression. Clinical measurements of flux of tumor volume over time and pathological determinations of cell kinetics have both been useful as well.

Charlson and Feinstein[12] developed a clinical index of growth rate based on the first clinical manifestation of disease and then on subsequent unfavorable transition events. Their methods were used in conjunction with the anatomic TNM system to better predict which subgroups of patients would have predictably good 10-year survival rates despite poor anatomical status. Conversely, patients with rapidly progressing lesions could be identified despite favorable anatomical staging.

Measurement of tumor doubling time, although not clinically practical, has been shown to correlate with prognosis (see Section VIII, Chapter 25). Multiple studies have demonstrated a wide range of doubling times, not only between patients but also within the same patient over time.[32, 50, 68] This heterogeneity is typical of breast cancer. Serial mammography has also been used for this purpose and has shown that shorter doubling times correlate with diminished survivorship.[41]

Studies of tumor cell kinetics through the use of tritium-labeled thymidine (^{3}H-TdR) incorporation into DNA have demonstrated some promise in their ability to identify aggressive, rapidly growing tumors. This method is more sensitive than standard histological tests that enumerate the relative number of mitoses. Tumor cells are sampled from the specimen and then incubated with ^{3}H-TdR, which is taken up by cells in the DNA synthetic or S phase. Measuring ^{3}H-TdR uptake then permits the estimation of the percentage of cells in the S phase (labeling index). Tubiana et al.[81] demonstrated a correlation between the thymidine labeling index and the long-term prognosis in 128 patients. Labeling indices signifying a low level of cell replication (<0.25) were predictive of low rates of relapse (25 percent) and death (30 percent) at 10 years, whereas high indices (≥3.84) correlated with high rates of relapse (62 percent) and death (37 percent). Using multivariate analysis, the labeling index has been found to be independent of clinical and pathological staging factors such as the presence of axillary node involvement and primary tumor size. This index does, however, correlate with histological characteristics such as tumor grade and may be important in the staging of node-negative patients.[76]

Because ^{3}H-TdR uptake assays can be tedious and time consuming, flow cytometry has been recently used to estimate cellular kinetics and to detect the presence of aneuploidy. Flow cytometry permits rapid, single-cell analysis of DNA content per cell, enabling the determination of the fraction of cells within the S phase and the ploidy levels within a tumor cell population. This sort of analysis has been used in multiple studies to predict future survival.[18, 37, 57]

Knowing that 50 percent to 60 percent of patients with breast cancer have disease confined to the breast at the time of diagnosis, Clark et al.[13] studied 395 specimens of node-negative breast cancer using aliquots of frozen breast tissue. Sixty-eight percent of these tumors were aneuploid, with an associated 5-year survival of 74 percent, while 32 percent were diploid, with an 88 percent survival rate (Fig. 17–4). The S-phase fraction of cells was also an important predictor of disease-free survival in patients with diploid tumors. Five-year survival rates of 90 percent and 70 percent were measured for tumors with low and high S-phase fractions, respectively.

Biological Markers

With the development of monoclonal antibody technology, antibodies specific for breast cancer have been developed.[11] These antibodies can be used to detect microscopic disease not easily seen on routine histopa-

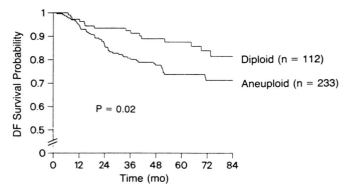

Figure 17–4. Aneuploid tumors have poorer disease-free survival probabilities than diploid tumors. (From Clark GM, et al: N Engl J Med 320:627–633, 1989. Reprinted by permission.)

thology through immunoperoxidase technology and radioimmunoassay. They may be useful in accurately staging the anatomical extent of axillary disease and distant disease such as tumor infiltration of bone marrow.[71] Newer technology may also permit preoperative staging of the axilla and the internal mammary chain through the use of hand-held probes that detect radiolabeled tumor cells.

Tumor markers, such as carcinoembryonic antigen (CEA), pregnancy-associated glycoprotein, human tissue polypeptide antigen, and C-reactive protein, are not very specific for breast cancer and are unpredictably secreted by heterogeneous breast carcinomas.[43]

Oncogenes may be related to the complex phenomenon of human breast cancer initiation and progression through the processes of gene amplification, mutation, chromosomal breakage, or insertion of retroviral promoters near oncogenes.[14] With current technology, both their number and their expressed gene products may be measured. Amplification of the *HER-2/neu* oncogene has recently been found to portend a poor prognosis, correlating with axillary lymph node and steroid receptor status along with the nuclear grade.[5, 77] This oncogene, however, has prognostic significance only in patients with node-positive breast cancer.[77] Other oncogenes, such as *c-myc*, are also under current study and have been associated with poor prognosis.[83] The reader is referred to chapters 19 and 20 for a more comprehensive discussion of oncogenes and growth regulation of normal breast and breast cancer.

EVOLUTION OF STAGING

Early staging systems for breast cancer were based on the feasibility of operative intervention. Simplistically, most tumors were classed as either operable or inoperable; however, this grouping did not offer any significant prognostic information. In 1905, Steinthal[78] recommended three different classifications for patients with breast cancer: (1) tumors not larger than "a plum" and clinically not associated with skin or axillary lymph node involvement; (2) large tumors adherent to the skin with palpably enlarged axillary lymph nodes; and (3) large tumors diffusely involving the breast with skin, deep muscle, and supraclavicular lymph node involvement. This classification was based on clinical factors that were perceived as important in predicting prognosis. Early on, it was clear that surgeons had identified some of the most ominous prognostic indicators for breast cancer. It is also interesting to note the inclusion of primary tumor size in this primitive staging scheme.

An unpopular but insightful system was proposed by Lee and Stubenbord[49] in 1928 that included an index of the rate of tumor growth. This method was the first to attempt assessment of the biology of individual tumors and their potential for progression.

In 1940, the four-stage Manchester classification was introduced (Table 17–10).[66] It permitted staging based solely on clinical criteria, including the extent of local involvement by the primary tumor, the presence and mobility of palpably enlarged axillary lymph nodes, and the presence of distant metastases. Neither pathological information nor tumor size were included in this system.

In 1943, Portmann[70] described a staging system that incorporated clinical, pathological, and roentgenographic characteristics of breast cancers and evaluated each lesion based on three categories: skin involvement, location and mobility of the primary tumor, and the extent of local and distant metastases (Table 17–11).

Haagensen and Stout[35] evaluated 568 patients with breast cancer who were treated by radical mastectomy. In 1943, they published the following criteria of inoperability, which were based on the clinical characteristics of patients who were clearly incurable by aggressive surgery alone:

1. Extensive edema of the skin overlying the breast or edema of the arm.
2. Satellite nodules of the breast or parasternal tumor nodules.
3. Inflammatory carcinoma.
4. Supraclavicular or distant metastases.

Table 17–10. THE MANCHESTER SYSTEM

Stage I:	The tumor is confined to the breast. Involvement of the skin may be present, provided the area is small in relation to the size of the breast.
Stage II:	The tumor is confined to the breast and associated lymph nodes are present in the axilla.
Stage III:	The tumor extends beyond the breast as demonstrated by: a. Skin invasion or fixation of a large area in relation to the size of the breast or skin ulceration b. Tumor fixation to the underlying muscle or fascia; mobile axillary nodes
Stage IV:	The tumor extends beyond the breast as shown by: a. Fixation or matting of the axillary nodes b. Fixation of tumor to chest wall c. Deposits in supraclavicular nodes or in the opposite breast d. Satellite nodules or distant metastases

From Patterson R: The Treatment of Malignant Disease by Radium and X-rays. London, Edward Arnold, 1948.

5. Two or more of the "grave signs" of locally advanced cancer:
   a. Breast skin edema.
   b. Breast skin ulceration.
   c. Tumor fixation to chest wall.
   d. Axillary lymph node fixation to skin or deep tissues.
   e. Enlarged axillary lymph nodes >2.5 cm in diameter.

Haagensen and Stout also advocated the use of biopsy material in the determination of inoperability. Their proposed "triple biopsy" included sampling the primary tumor, apical axillary nodes, and internal mammary nodes as part of the pretreatment evaluation. This represented the first attempt at including pathological data in the staging process.

Although largely derived from Haagensen and Stout's criteria of inoperability, the Columbia Clinical Classification (CCC) ignored the use of tumor size and any biopsy material or other pathological data. It has, however, been successfully used to separate different groups of patients with distinctly different survival rates.[34] Patients were staged on the basis of physical examination and other roentgenographic information in an attempt to simplify and streamline the staging process. Four stages were defined (Table 17–12). Stages A and B were both used to describe operable cancers, but stage B patients had palpably enlarged, unfixed axillary lymph nodes (presumed to represent regional metastases). Based on the five "grave signs" listed previously, Stage C defined a group of patients with cancers that were locally advanced. Stage D patients were considered inoperable as defined by the "criteria of inoperability."

Table 17–11. PORTMANN CLASSIFICATION

Stage I:
(−)	Skin—not involved.
(+)	Tumor—localized to breast, mobile.
(−)	Metastases—none.

Stage II:
(−)	Skin—not involved.
(+)	Tumor—localized to breast, mobile.
(+)	Metastases—few axillary lymph nodes involved on microscopic evaluation; no other metastases.

Stage III:
(−)	Skin—edematous; brawny red induration and inflammation not obviously caused by infection; extensive ulceration; multiple secondary nodules.
(+ +)	Tumor—diffusely infiltrating breast; fixation of tumor or breast to chest wall; edema of breast; secondary tumors.
(+ +)	Metastases—many axillary lymph nodes involved or fixed; no clinical or roentgenologic evidence of distant metastases.

Stage IV:
(+/−)	Skin—involved or not involved.
(+/+ +)	Tumor—localized or diffuse.
(+ + +)	Metastases—axillary and supraclavicular lymph nodes extensively involved, and clinical or roentgenological evidence or more distant metastases.

Adapted from Portmann UV: Cleveland Clin Q 10:41–47, 1943.

Table 17–12. COLUMBIA CLINICAL CLASSIFICATION

Stage A	No skin involvement or fixation of the tumor to the chest wall. Axillary nodes are not palpable.
Stage B	No skin involvement or fixation of the tumor to the chest wall. Clinically palpable nodes, but less than 2.5 cm in transverse diameter and not fixed to overlying skin or deeper structures of the axilla.
Stage C	Any one of the five grave signs of advanced breast carcinoma: (1) Limited edema of the skin involving less than one third of the skin over the breast (2) Skin ulceration (3) Fixation of the tumor to the chest wall (4) Massive involvement of axillary lymph nodes measuring 2.5 cm or more in transverse diameter (5) Fixation of the axillary nodes to overlying skin or deeper structures of the axilla.
Stage D	Any patients with signs of advanced breast carcinoma: (1) A combination of any two or more of the five grave signs listed under Stage C (2) Extensive edema of the skin (involving more than one third of the skin over the breast) (3) Satellite skin nodules (4) The inflammatory type of carcinoma (5) Clinically involved supraclavicular lymph nodes (6) Internal mammary metastases as evidenced by a parasternal tumor (7) Edema of the arm (8) Distant metastases.

From Haagensen CD: *In* Diseases of the Breast. Philadelphia, WB Saunders, 1986.

Stage A and B patients were treated with radical mastectomy, while stage C and D patients underwent radiation therapy.

Despite initial acceptance, the CCC has since been replaced by the current TNM system, which incorporates the use of both clinical and pathological features. This system was adopted for many reasons, including its initial simplicity, clinical applicability, and universal utility. Moreover, it is clear that in the last decade, because of the widespread use of screening mammography and public education, breast cancers are being detected earlier, with smaller delays in diagnosis. This has necessarily shifted the contemporary population of patients being studied to earlier stages at diagnosis. In turn, the need for elaborate classification schemes based on generally advanced clinical criteria has become obsolete. At present, patients need to be stratified into groups based on more subtle, less advanced characteristics of disease progression. This is necessary not only because many women now present with small or even non-palpable tumors, but also because not all small tumors have the same biological behavior (e.g., growth, metastases, etc.).

The TNM system for classification of malignant tumors was first conceived by Denoix in 1943.[16] In 1958, the International Union Against Cancer (UICC) described the first recommendations for the staging of breast cancer and for the presentation of results. Since that time, four separate editions of the TNM manual for classification of malignant tumors have been published. Simultaneously, the American Joint Committee for Cancer Staging and End Results Reporting (AJCC) has produced three editions of their *Manual for Staging of Breast Cancer*. The proposals of the AJCC have undergone somewhat parallel and confluent evolutionary changes to those of the UICC such that in 1987, for the first time, a truly universal staging system was developed. The current UICC[40] and AJCC[4] staging systems for breast cancer are now identical. This alliance will now hopefully permit collaboration in multi-institutional trials on an international level.

RATIONALE BEHIND THE TNM SYSTEM

The TNM system was originally conceived to be a simplistic system that would class patients into various groups, each with a different survival rate and prognosis. There were binary choices for each evaluable patient/tumor characteristic: T0 represented the absence of tumor; T1 represented the presence of tumor. Similarly, N0/M0 and N1/M1 represented the absence or presence of regional or distant metastatic disease. Thus, using three different determinants (T, N, and M) with two possible choices (0 or 1), 2^3 ($=8$) permutations were possible. Any patient could be rapidly classified into one of eight possible groups that could then be stratified into any number of stages based on observed survival frequencies. Such a classification system would have been simple, logical, and easy to commit to memory for future use.

Although the TNM system was originally simplistic in design, modifications were necessary to improve prognostic power and stage definition. A large number of clinical and pathological prognostic indicators have been identified since the inception of the TNM system (see section on Clinical and Pathological Correlates of Prognosis). The TNM staging system, to date, is the only system that has successfully incorporated many of these factors. For this reason, despite the observation that this method of staging for breast cancer is the most complicated, it is also highly practical and adaptable. It provides more prognostic information and better stratifies patients for the purpose of guiding therapy than do other systems based largely on clinical criteria alone.

The more precisely the clinician is able to define specific groups of patients who should undergo equivalent therapeutic regimens, the greater the probability that medical scientists should be able to reduce the number of patients with aggressive disease who are undertreated and those with limited disease who are overtreated. As more and more prognostic indices are identified and successful therapeutic modalities discovered, more subcategories will be required, and for this reason, binary choices have become quaternary (N0, N1, N2, N3) or greater (T0, Tis, T1, T2, T3, T4). Further delineation within each subcategory has also been added. For example, T1 is now divided into a, b, and c and T4 has been separated into a, b, c, and d. Similarly, the pN1 category has two subdivisions into

N1a and N1b, with N1b being further subdivided into i–iv.

CURRENT STAGING

Present System

The TNM system for the staging of breast cancer is not simplistic and is considered quite cumbersome and difficult to use without a written manual. Nevertheless, it is currently the most popular staging system in use, because losses in simplicity have been surpassed by gains in prognostic power and accuracy in grouping for appropriate therapeutic intervention.

The updated system represents the culmination of many years of evolution through the combined efforts of the AJCC and the UICC. Despite these unified efforts, however, the current system will certainly undergo future changes. Clearly, the best staging system will be flexible and continue to evolve with new prognostic data. Unfortunately, each addition or change tends to result in further complexity.

The current TNM staging system requires that microscopic confirmation and histological typing of disease be obtained (either by biopsy or any definitive surgical procedure) prior to attempting any stage classification. Any patient with documented breast cancer may then be staged by clinical criteria (preoperatively) and/or by pathological criteria (postoperatively) designated by a "p" prefix.

The clinical-diagnostic staging process requires a complete physical examination with determination of the extent of ipsilateral and contralateral neoplastic involvement of the skin, breast tissue, regional and distant lymph nodes, and underlying muscles. The microscopic diagnosis of breast cancer must be confirmed by examination of breast tissue. Routine laboratory examinations, chest roentgenograms, and bilateral mammograms are also recommended.

The pathological classification utilizes all of the data employed in clinical staging; however, this more definitive staging system can only be implemented after resection of the primary tumor and regional lymph nodes. It requires that no gross tumor be present at the margins of resection and that at least the Level I axillary lymph nodes (usually six or more in number) be resected and histologically examined. Should tumor be present at the margins on gross examination of the resected specimen, the code TX is applied, indicating that the pathological stage cannot yet be determined.

The clinical and pathological TNM systems are essentially identical with the exception of the N (lymph node) category (Tables 17–13 and 17–14). The T and pT categories are both divided into TX (primary tumor not assessed), T1 (primary tumor ≤ 2 cm in greatest dimension), T2 (tumor > 2 cm but ≤ 5 cm), T3 (tumor > 5 cm), and T4 (any tumor size with skin or chest wall, excluding pectoral muscle, extension). T1 is subdivided into T1a (primary tumor ≤ 0.5 cm in greatest dimension) T1b (tumor > 0.5 cm but ≤ 1.0 cm), and T1c (tumor

Table 17–13. TNM CLINICAL CLASSIFICATION

TX	Primary tumor cannot be assessed
T0	No evidence of primary tumor
Tis	Carcinoma in situ: intraductal carcinoma, or lobular carcinoma in situ, or Paget's disease of the nipple with no tumor
T1	Tumor ≤ 2 cm in greatest dimension
	T1a: ≤0.5 cm
	T1b: >0.5–1.0 cm
	T1c: 1–2.0 cm
T2	Tumor >2–5.0 cm in greatest dimension
T3	Tumor >5.0 cm in greatest dimension
T4	Tumor of any size with direct extension to chest wall* or skin
T4a	Extension to chest wall
T4b	Extension to chest wall
T4b	Edema (including peau d'orange), or ulceration of the skin of the breast, or satellite skin nodules confined to the same breast
T4c	Both 4a and 4b, above
T4d	Inflammatory carcinoma†

N—Regional Lymph Nodes

NX	Regional lymph nodes cannot be assessed (e.g., previously removed)
N0	No regional lymph node metastasis
N1	Metastasis to moveable ipsilateral axillary node(s)
N2	Metastasis to ipsilateral axillary node(s) fixed to one another or other structures
N3	Metastasis to ipsilateral internal mammary lymph node(s)

M—Distant Metastasis

MX	Presence of distant metastasis cannot be assessed
M0	No distant metastasis
M1	Distant metastasis (includes metastasis to supraclavicular lymph nodes)

The category M1 may be further specified according to the following notation:

Pulmonary	PUL	Bone marrow	MAR
Osseous	OSS	Pleura	PLE
Hepatic	PEP	Peritoneum	PER
Brain	BRA	Skin	SKI
Lymph nodes	LYM	Other	OTH

*Chest wall includes ribs, intercostal muscles, and serratus anterior muscle, but not pectoral muscle.

†Inflammatory carcinoma of the breast is characterized by diffuse, brawny induration of the skin with an erysipeloid edge, usually with no underlying palpable mass. If the skin biopsy is negative and there is no localized, measurable primary cancer, the T category is pTX when pathologically staging a clinical inflammatory carcinoma (T4d). When classifying pT the tumor size is a measurement of the invasive component. If there is a large in situ component (e.g., 4 cm) and a small invasive component (e.g., 0.5 cm) the tumor is coded pT1a. Dimpling of the skin, nipple retraction or other skin changes, except those in T4, may occur in T1, T2, or T3 without affecting the classification.

Compiled from Hermanek P, Sobin LH (eds): TNM Classification of Malignant Tumors, ed 4. Berlin, Springer-Verlag, 1987; and Beahrs OH, et al (eds): Manual for Staging of Cancer, ed 3. Philadelphia, JB Lippincott, 1988.

> 1.0 cm but ≤ 2.0 cm). T4 has also been subdivided into T4a (chest wall extension), T4b (edema/ulceration of breast skin, or satellitosis), T4c (presence of both T4a and T4b characteristics), and T4d (inflammatory breast cancer as documented by dermal lymphatic invasion by malignant cells).

The T and pT categories differ only slightly in that measurements are either made clinically or histologi-

cally. The clinical T measurement may be based on physical exam or on mammographic estimations of size; the measurement that is deemed most accurate is used. The pT measurement of tumor size is based on the size of the invasive tumor component. Tumors with large in situ components but with coexisting invasive components are coded pT1–pT4, instead of pTis, based on the size of the invasive tumor.

For the clinical TNM system, the N category is divided into four groups. NX refers to regional lymph nodes that cannot be assessed (previously resected). N0 represents no palpable lymph node metastases, while N1 (moveable ipsilateral axillary), N2 (fixed ipsilateral axillary), and N3 (ipsilateral internal mammary) refer to palpably enlarged, regional lymph node basins. Intramammary and infraclavicular lymph nodes are considered regional, whereas supraclavicular, cervical, and contralateral internal mammary lymph nodes are classified as distant.

Table 17–14. pTNM PATHOLOGICAL CLASSIFICATION

pT—Primary Tumor

The pathological classification requires the examination of the primary carcinoma with no gross tumor at the margins of resection. A case can be classified pT if there is only microscopic tumor in a margin.

The pT categories correspond to the T categories.

pN—Regional Lymph Nodes

The pathological classification requires the resection or examination of at least the low axillary lymph nodes (Level I). Such a resection will ordinarily include six or more lymph nodes.

pNX		Regional lymph nodes cannot be assessed (not removed for study or previously removed)
pN0		No regional lymph node metastasis
pN1		Metastases to moveable ipsilateral axillary node(s)
	pN1a	Only micrometastasis (none larger than 0.2 cm)
	pN1b	Metastasis to lymph node(s), any larger than 0.2 cm
	pN1bi	Metastasis in 1–3 lymph nodes, any more than 0.2 cm and all less than 2.0 cm in greatest dimension
	pN1bii	Metastasis to four or more lymph nodes, any more than 0.2 cm and all less than 2.0 cm in greatest dimension
	pN1biii	Extension of tumor beyond the capsule of a lymph node metastasis less than 2.0 cm in greatest dimension
	pN1biv	Metastasis to a lymph node 2.0 cm or more in greatest dimension
pN2		Metastasis to ipsilateral axillary lymph nodes that are fixed to one another or to other structures
pN3		Metastasis to ipsilateral internal mammary lymph node(s)

pM—Distant Metastasis

The pM categories correspond to the M categories.

Compiled from Hermanek P, Sobin LH (eds): TNM Classification of Malignant Tumors, ed 4. Berlin, Springer-Verlag, 1987; and Beahrs OH, et al (eds): Manual for Staging of Cancer, ed 3. Philadelphia, JB Lippincott, 1988.

The pathological TNM system differs from the clinical system only in group N1, where pN1 is divided into pN1a (micrometastases: tumor diameter ≤ 0.2 cm) and pN1b (gross metastases: tumor diameter > 0.2 cm). The pN1b is further subdivided into four groups based on the number and/or size of lymph node metastases: pN1bi (one to three lymph nodes involved with metastatic tumor <2.0 cm in greatest dimension), pN1bii (four or more lymph nodes involved with tumor <2.0 cm), pN1biii (invasion of lymph node capsule by tumor <2.0 cm), and pN1biv (lymph node with large deposit of metastatic tumor ≥ 2.0 cm).

The clinical and pathological systems for staging distant metastases are identical. MX refers to the presence of distant metastases that cannot be assessed. M0 signifies no distant metastases at the time of staging, whereas M1 represents the presence of distant metastases that now include metastases to supraclavicular lymph nodes. M1 may be further amended by site specifications for distant metastases (i.e., pulmonary, osseous, hepatic, brain).

While certain recorded data are not directly utilized in the staging process, these characteristics may become important in the future and will be readily accessible. The axillary level (I, II, or III) and anatomical location of lymph node metastases and distant metastases, if present, should be recorded. Primary tumors may also be assigned to one of five "G" categories (histopathological grade) (Table 17–15) as well as to one of three basic histopathological types (ductal, lobular, or nipple) (Table 17–16). The "R" classification, signifying the presence or absence of residual tumor after treatment, may further be assigned.

There are five stage groupings (0, I, II, III, IV) in the new TNM system, with Stages II and III being subdivided into A and B (Table 17–17). Stage 0 tumors carry the best prognosis and are essentially 100 percent curable, whereas stage IV cancers are generally beyond cure secondary to distant metastases. Stage I cancers are localized to the breast and are small in size. Stage II is reserved for cases with regional lymph node metastases and carries a worse prognosis than I and 0 but better than III or IV.

Stage 0 (Tis, N0, M0) refers to pre-invasive cancers (tumor in situ) that have yet to penetrate the basement membrane of the ductule or lobule. There are no regional or distant metastases.

Table 17–15. HISTOPATHOLOGICAL GRADING

GX	Grade of differentiation cannot be assessed
G1	Well differentiated
G2	Moderately differentiated
G3	Poorly differentiated
G4	Undifferentiated

Compiled from Hermanek P, Sobin LH (eds): TNM Classification of Malignant Tumors, ed 4. Berlin, Springer-Verlag, 1987; and Beahrs OH, et al (eds): Manual for Staging of Cancer, ed 3. Philadelphia, JB Lippincott, 1988.

Table 17–16. HISTOPATHOLOGICAL TYPES

Cancer, NOS*
Ductal
    Intraductal (in situ)
    Invasive with predominant intraductal component
    Comedo
    Inflammatory
    Medullary with lymphocytic infiltrate
    Mucinous (colloid)
    Papillary
    Scirrhous
    Tubular
    Other
Lobular
    In situ
    Invasive with predominant in situ component
    Invasive
Nipple
    Paget's disease, NOS*
    Paget's disease with intraductal carcinoma
    Paget's disease with invasive ductal carcinoma

*Not otherwise specified.
Compiled from Hermanek P, Sobin LH (eds): TNM Classification of Malignant Tumors, ed 4. Berlin, Springer-Verlag, 1987; and Beahrs OH, et al (eds): Manual for Staging of Cancer, ed 3. Philadelphia, JB Lippincott, 1988.

Stage I (T1, N0, M0) refers to invasive tumors without metastases.

Stage IIA describes undetectable (T0, N1, M0) or small tumors (T1, N1, M0) with regional metastases and larger primary tumors without metastases (T2, N0, M0). Stage IIB includes large tumors without metastases (T3, N0, M0). The inclusion of the T3, N0, M0 tumors in Stage II represents a recent change based on 76 percent 5-year survival statistics derived from the Surveillance Epidemiology and End Results (SEER) study.[4]

Stage IIIA includes the most permutations or subgroups. Tumors in this category may be any size and

Table 17–17. STAGE GROUPING

Stage 0	Tis	N0	M0
Stage I	T1	N0	M0
Stage IIA	T0	N1	M0
	T1	N1*	M0
	T2	N0	M0
Stage IIB	T2	N1	M0
	T3	N0	M0
Stage IIIA	T0	N2	M0
	T1	N2	M0
	T2	N2	M0
	T3	N1, N2	M0
Stage IIIB	T4	Any N	M0
	Any T	N3	M0
Stage IV	Any T	Any N	M1

*Note: The prognosis of patients with pN1a is similar to that of patients with pN0.
Compiled from Hermanek P, Sobin LH (eds): TNM Classification of Malignant Tumors, ed 4. Berlin, Springer-Verlag, 1987; and Beahrs OH, et al (eds): Manual for Staging of Cancer, ed 3. Philadelphia, JB Lippincott, 1988.

are generally associated with fixed regional lymph nodes. Stage IIIB includes locally advanced tumors (T4) and cases with internal mammary lymph node metastases (N3).

Finally, stage IV is reserved for cases of documented distant metastases or supraclavicular lymph node involvement.

Because of the complex nature of the current TNM system, the reader is referred to Table 17–18 and Figure 17–5 for rapid reference for the clinical or pathological staging of patients with breast cancer.

Classification in Unique Clinical Situations

Previously, nonpalpable breast cancers did not fall into any clear stage grouping and were often classified as T0. Recent changes in the staging systems have recommended that these tumors be measured in their largest dimension on mammography and then staged after needle localization biopsy to confirm malignancy. An appropriate T category may then be assigned. This change has been supported by data suggesting that a significant percentage of nonpalpable tumors are malignant and are associated with lymph node metastasis. Schwartz et al.[74] recently reported a study of 1059 patients who underwent 1132 biopsies for nonpalpable lesions of the breast (mammograph positive). Almost 30 percent of these biopsies proved to be malignant, and 32.9 percent of the invasive cancers detected were associated with at least one positive lymph node.

When multiple simultaneous ipsilateral tumors occur, the T classification should be assigned on the basis of the size (volume) of the largest cancer. Synchronous bilateral breast cancers should be staged independently.

Inflammatory carcinoma is diagnosed by physical (dif-

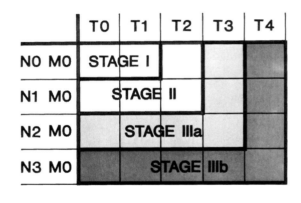

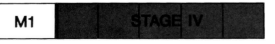

Figure 17–5. Breast cancer TNM staging: Correlation of tumor size and nodal status to stage of disease. (From Donegan WL, Spratt JS: Cancer of the Breast, ed 3. Philadelphia, WB Saunders, 1988. Reprinted by permission.)

fuse brawny induration of skin), radiological (skin thickening and/or a breast mass), and pathological characteristics (the presence of tumor embolization in dermal lymphatics for microscopic confirmation). T4d is the appropriate class for this tumor.

Paget's disease of the nipple is classified according to the presence or absence of an associated tumor. Without any associated mass or microscopic invasive cancer, Paget's disease is classed Tis. When Paget's disease is diagnosed in the presence of a palpable breast mass or an invasive carcinoma, the tumor is staged according to its size.

Table 17–18. CLASSIFICATION SUMMARY

Tis	In situ		
T1	≤ 2 cm		
T1a	≤ 0.5 cm		
T1b	> 0.5 to 1 cm		
T1c	> 1 to 2 cm		
T2	> 2 to 5 cm		
T3	> 5 cm		
T4	Chest wall/skin		
T4a	Chest wall		
T4b	Skin edema/ulceration, satellite skin nodules		
T4c	Both 4a and 4b		
T4d	Inflammatory carcinoma		
N1	Moveable axillary	pN1	
		pN1a	Micrometastasis only ≤0.2 cm
		pN1b	Gross metastasis
		i	1–3 nodes/> 0.2 to <2 cm
		ii	≥4 nodes/>0.2 cm to <2 cm
		iii	through capsule/<2 cm
		iv	≥2 cm
N2	Fixed axillary	pN2	
N3	Internal mammary	pN3	

Compiled from Hermanek P, Sobin LH (eds): TNM Classification of Malignant Tumors, ed 4. Berlin, Springer-Verlag, 1987; and Beahrs OH, et al (eds): Manual for Staging of Cancer, ed 3. Philadelphia, JB Lippincott, 1988.

Limitations

Both clinical and pathological staging systems are useful. The clinical system may serve to guide initial therapy based on all available preoperative data that include history, physical and laboratory examinations, and biopsy material. The pathological system, because of its ability to precisely define the extent of disease, is certainly more important for predicting prognosis and planning subsequent secondary therapeutic interventions after primary surgical therapy.

NSABP STAGING

Because a large amount of valuable data have been and are still currently being derived and assessed by the National Surgical Adjuvant Bowel and Breast Project (NSABP), knowledge of their staging system for breast cancer is important. The NSABP system resembles the CCC system in that skin changes are important but tumor size is irrelevant, largely because lymph node metastasis is the most important prognostic indicator that has been identified to predict tumor progression. This system also depends heavily on pathological data for analysis.

There are four stages in the NSABP system. Stage I represents all patients with primary tumors in the absence of axillary metastasis. Stage II includes tumors confined to the breast with no evidence of skin adherence but with ipsilateral axillary lymph node metastases. Stage III tumors are locally advanced with skin adherence, and are associated with positive supraclavicular nodes or positive matted axillary nodes. Stage IV includes all cases with distant metastases.

ADJUNCTS TO STAGING

Mammography

Mammographic evaluation prior to breast biopsy may provide invaluable information that may ultimately affect treatment plans.[19] For this reason, bilateral mammograms are recommended *prior to surgery* when the suspicion of a breast lesion has been raised. Obtaining mammograms prior to the operative procedure avoids the complication of detecting a confounding image related to edema and hemorrhage in the wound. The utility of screening mammography has already been established and has permitted the detection of nonpalpable breast cancers through needle localization techniques.

Bone Scans

The use of bone scans in the staging of primary breast cancer is controversial.[51] These radionuclide tests are quite sensitive but often not very specific for the presence of metastatic disease. Inflammation associated with degenerative joint disease or overlying soft tissue often results in false-positive scans. Similarly, previous fractures and bone islands can yield misleading results.

Positive bone scans are generally associated with advanced states of regional disease or systemic disease. This fact has led to the recommended use of these scans in a cost-effective manner for patients with cancers other than T1, T2, and T1N1. Scans should also be obtained on any patient with bone pain, positive skeletal roentgenograms, and palpable regional or metastatic disease.

CT Scan/MRI

Computed tomographic (CT) scanning and magnetic resonance imaging (MRI) are diagnostic modalities that are equivalent, if not superior, to extracavitary ultrasound or radionuclide scans in detecting hepatic metastases.[19] Although their preoperative use in the initial staging process is controversial, patients who have suspected distant metastatic disease as evidenced by specific symptomatology, supraclavicular adenopathy, abnormal roentgenograms, elevated liver enzymes, or bony metastases, deserve CT and/or MRI scanning. These modalities may be used for the detection of brain, chest, liver, abdomen, and pelvic metastases. They may also be useful to confirm bony metastases. Suspected sites of distant metastatic disease, in order of decreasing frequency include: bone, liver, lung, skin, extra-regional lymphatics and brain.

Hormone Receptors

Because a strong correlation exists between the presence of estrogen receptor (ER) and progesterone receptor (PR) activity in freshly resected tumor specimens and the potential clinical response to endocrine therapy, all tissues should be analyzed when adequate volumes are available. Greater than 60 percent of ER positive tumors will respond to adjunctive hormonal therapy. Similarly, high response rates are obtained for tumors that are PR positive, even when ER negative (see Section XVII, Chapter 43).

Internal Mammary Lymph Node Dissection

Because patients with lymph node metastases are at a significantly increased risk for recurrent systemic disease, identifying the patients with these metastases will ultimately affect prognosis and permit appropriate therapeutic intervention. Controversy exists as to when internal mammary lymph nodes should be scanned, sampled, or resected.

Lymphoscintigraphy has been reported as a method for detecting internal mammary lymph node metastases. This method, however, has been shown clearly to be non-specific for the presence of tumor and can predict metastasis at a rate (66 percent) only marginally improved over that afforded by physical examination (55 percent).[75]

A recent review of 7070 patients with breast cancer in whom the axillary and internal mammary lymph nodes were resected and examined histologically found that five percent to ten percent of patients studied had internal mammary lymph node metastases in the *absence* of axillary metastases.[58] Tumors beneath the nipple and in the inner (medial) quadrants of the breast were most likely to metastasize to the internal mammary lymph nodes. These patients were possible candidates for both chemotherapy and localized radiotherapy (for incomplete dissections). Some authors, therefore, support the excision of visible lymph nodes in the ipsilateral second, third, and fourth intercostal spaces for medial primary tumors (see chapter 29B-3). Although TNM staging does not require internal mammary lymph node sampling or dissection, provisions have been made for inclusion of this sort of data in stage classification. Trends toward the use of chemotherapy in "node-negative" patients and radiotherapy to the internal mammary lymph nodes for medial quadrant tumors may, however, ultimately obviate the need for these dissections and biopsies.

FUTURE TRENDS

The continued evolution of a universal staging system is a desirable, albeit ambitious, goal essential to the proper classification of breast cancer, providing clinicians a practical, biologically reproducible methodology on which future therapies are based. While constant revisions are often quite confusing and cumbersome, these modifications are needed to keep pace with new diagnostic technology and therapeutic strategies. For example, it would make little biological sense to base staging solely on the size of the primary tumor when lymph node metastases were present and evaluable.

The influx of new technology has permitted us to detect hormone receptors in the cytosol of breast tumor cells and thus to predict certain functional characteristics. Flow cytometry has been extensively utilized to study both cell surface and nuclear characteristics of tumor cells with resultant prognostic implications. We can now also detect certain specific or associated tumor surface antigens with monoclonal antibodies. Using these antibodies, it is plausible that their role in defining the precise anatomic extent of tumor (through radiolabeled antibody scanning modalities) may be expanded.

Other modifications of staging that have been proposed include the application of clinical measurements of the primary tumor growth rate and the percentage of malignant involvement of the breast as prognostic indices. Certainly, any reproducible and predictive prognostic index should be considered for inclusion in future staging systems.

References

1. Adair F, Berg J, Joubert L, Robbins GF: Long term follow-up of breast cancer patients: the 30 year report. Cancer 33:1145–1150, 1974.
2. Attiyeh FF, Jenson M, Huvos AG, Fracchia A: Axillary micrometastasis and macrometastasis in carcinoma of the breast. Surg Gynecol Obstet 144:839–842, 1977.
3. Balch CE, Singletary SE: Adjuvant therapy for node-negative breast cancer patients. Who benefits? Arch Surg 123:1189–1190, 1988.
4. Beahrs OH, Henson DE, Hutter RVP, et al (eds): American Joint Committee on Cancer. Manual for Staging of Breast Cancer, ed 3. Philadelphia, JB Lippincott, 1988, pp 145–150.
5. Berger MS, Locher GW, Saurer S, Gullick WJ, Waterfield MD, Groner B, Hynes NE: Correlation of c-erbB-2 gene amplification and protein expression in human breast carcinoma with nodal status and nuclear grading. Cancer Res 48:1238–1243, 1988.
6. Black MM, Speer FD: Nuclear structure in cancer tissues. Surg Gynecol Obstet 105:97–102, 1957.
7. Bloom HJ: The influence of delay on the natural history and prognosis of breast cancer. A study of cases followed for five to twenty years. Br J Cancer 19:228–262, 1965.
8. Bloom HJG, Richardson WW: Histological grading and prognosis in breast cancer. A study of 1409 cases of which 359 have been followed 15 years. Br J Cancer 11:359–377, 1957.
9. Bloom HJG, Richardson WW, Harrier EJ: Natural history of untreated breast cancer (1805–1933). Br Med J 2:213–221, 1962.
10. Boova RS, Roseann B, Rosato F: Patterns of axillary nodal involvement in breast cancer. Predictability of level one dissection. Ann Surg 196:642–644, 1982.
11. Buckman R, Coombes RC, Dearnaley DP, et al: Some clinical uses of biological markers. *In* Bonadonna G (ed.): Breast Cancer: Diagnosis and Management. Chichester, John Wiley, 1984, pp 109–126.
12. Charlson ME, Feinstein AR: A new clinical index of growth rate in the staging of breast cancer. Am J Med 69:527–536, 1980.
13. Clark GM, Dressler LG, Owens MA, Pounds G, Oldaker T, McGuire WL: Prediction of relapse or survival in patients with node negative breast cancer by DNA flow cytometry. N Engl J Med 320:627–633, 1989.
14. Cline MJ, Battifora H, Yokota J: Proto-oncogene abnormalities in human breast cancer: correlations with anatomic features and clinical course of disease. J Clin Oncol 5:999–1006, 1987.
15. Cutler SJ: The prognosis of treated breast cancer. *In* Forrest AP, Kunkler PB (eds.): Prognostic Factors in Breast Cancer. Edinburgh, Churchill Livingstone, 1968, pp 20–31.
15a. Davies GC, Rosemary RM, Hayward JL: Assessment of axillary lymph node status. Ann Surg 192:148–151, 1980.
16. Denoix PF: Bull Inst Nat Hyg (Paris) 1:1–69, 1944.
17. Donegan WL, Hartz AJ, Rimm AA: The association of body weight with recurrent cancer of the breast. Cancer 41:1590–1594, 1978.
18. Ewers SB, Langstrom E, Baldetorp B, Killander D: Flow-cytometric DNA analysis in primary breast carcinomas and clinicopathological correlations. Cytometry 5:408–419, 1984.
19. Feig SA: The role of new imaging modalities in staging and follow-up of breast cancer. Semin Oncol 13:402–414, 1986.
20. Fisher B, Slack NH: Number of lymph nodes examined and prognosis of breast carcinoma. Surg Gynecol Obstet 131:79–88, 1970.
21. Fisher B, Constantino J, Redmond C, et al: A randomized clinical trial evaluating tamoxifen in the treatment of patients with node-negative breast cancer who have estrogen-receptor-positive tumors. N Engl J Med 320(8):479–484, 1989.
22. Fisher B, Redmond C, Fisher ER, et al: The contribution of recent NSABP clinical trials of primary breast cancer therapy to an understanding of tumor biology—an overview of findings. Cancer 46:1009–1025, 1980.
23. Fisher B, Slack NH, Ausman RK, Bross IDJ: Location of breast carcinoma and prognosis. Surg Gynecol Obstet 129:705–716, 1969.
24. Fisher B, Slack NH, Bross IDJ, et al: Cancer of the breast: size of neoplasm and prognosis. Cancer 24:1071–1080, 1969.
25. Fisher B, Slack N, Katrych D, Wolmark N: Ten-year follow-up results of patients with carcinoma of the breast in a cooperative clinical trial evaluating surgical adjuvant chemotherapy. Surg Gynecol Obstet 140:528–534, 1975.

26. Fisher B, Wolmark N, Bauer M, Redmond C, Gebhardt M: The accuracy of clinical nodal staging and of limited axillary dissection as a determinant of histologic nodal status in carcinoma of the breast. Surg Gynecol Obstet 152:765–772, 1981.
27. Fisher ER: Prognostic and therapeutic significance of pathological features of breast cancer. NCI Monogr 1:29–34, 1986.
28. Fisher ER, Gregorio RM, Fisher B: Pathologic findings from the National Surgical Adjuvant Breast Project (protocol no. 4). Discriminants for five-year treatment failure. Cancer 46:908–919, 1980.
29. Fisher ER, Gregorio RM, Fisher B: The pathology of invasive breast cancer. A syllabus derived from the findings of the National Surgical Adjuvant Breast Project (protocol no. 4). Cancer 36:1–85, 1975.
30. Fisher ER, Redmond C, Fisher B: Pathologic findings from the National Surgical Adjuvant Breast Project (protocol no. 4). VI. Discriminants for five-year treatment failure. Cancer 46:908–918, 1980.
31. Fisher ER, Swamidoss S, Lee CG, Rockette H, Redmond C, Fisher B: Detection and significance of occult axillary node metastases in patients with invasive breast cancer. Cancer 42:2025–2031, 1978.
31a. Fox MS: On the diagnosis and treatment of breast cancer. JAMA 241:489–494, 1979.
32. Gershon-Cohen J, Berger SM, Klickstein HS: Roentgenography of breast cancer moderating the concept of biologic predeterminism. Cancer 16:961–964, 1963.
33. Haagensen CD: Clinical classification of the stage of advancement of breast carcinoma. *In* Diseases of the Breast. Philadelphia, WB Saunders, 1986.
34. Haagensen CD, Cooley E, Miller E, Handley RS, Thackray AC, Butcher HR Jr, Dahl-Inversen E, Tobiassen T, Williams EG, Stone J, Kaae S, Johansen H: Treatment of early mammary carcinoma. A cooperative international study. Ann Surg 170(6):875–878, 1969.
35. Haagensen CD, Stout AP: Carcinoma of the breast. Criteria for operability. Ann Surg 118:859–870, 1943.
36. Hayward OS: The history of oncology. I. Early oncology and the literature of discovery. Surgery 58:460–468, 1965.
37. Hedley DW, Friedlander ML, Taylor IW: Application of DNA flow cytometry to paraffin-embedded archival material for the study of aneuploidy and its clinical significance. Cytometry 6:327–333, 1985.
38. Henderson IC, Canellos GP: Cancer of the breast. The past decade. N Engl J Med 302(1):17–30, 1980.
39. Herbsman H, Feldman J, Seldera J, Gardner B, Alfonso AE: Survival following breast cancer surgery in the elderly. Cancer 47:2358–2363, 1981.
40. Hermanek P, Sobin LH (eds): UICC TNM Classification of Malignant Tumors, ed 4. Berlin, Springer-Verlag, 1987, pp 94–99.
41. Heuser LS, Spratt JS, Kuhns JG, Chang AF-C, Polk HC Jr, Buchanan JB: The association of pathologic and mammographic characteristics of primary human breast cancers with "slow" and "fast" growth rates and with axillary lymph node metastases. Cancer 53:96–98, 1984.
42. Hibberd AD, Harwood LJ, Wells JE: Long term prognosis of women with breast cancer in New Zealand: study of survival to 30 years. Br Med J 286:1777–1779, 1983.
43. Hillyard JW, Keyser JW, Newcombe RG, Webster DJT, Teasdale C, Fifield R, Watkins GL, Fish R, Worwood M, Groom G: Biochemical aids to the staging of breast cancer. Clin Biochem 15:9–12, 1982.
44. Hoge A, Asal N, Owen W, Anderson P: Histologic and staging classification of breast cancer: implications for therapy. South Med J 75:1329–1334, 1982.
45. Hutter RVP: The influence of pathologic factors on breast cancer management. Cancer 46:961–976, 1980.
46. Hyman B, Myers MM, Schottenfeld D: The relationship of menstrual status and other risk factors of recurrence to carcinoma of the breast. Am J Epidemiol 36:173–182, 1972.
47. Knight WA III, Livingston RB, Gregory EJ, McGuire WL: Estrogen receptor as an independent prognostic factor for early recurrence in breast cancer. Cancer Res 37:4669–4671, 1977.
48. Koscielny S, Tubiana M, Le MG, Valleron AJ, Mouriesse H, Contesso G, Sarrazin D: Breast cancer: relationship between the size of the primary tumor and the probability of metastatic dissemination. Br J Cancer 49:709–715, 1984.
49. Lee BJ, Stubenbord JG: Clinical index of malignancy for carcinoma of the breast. Surg Gynecol Obstet 47:812–814, 1928.
50. Lee YT: The lognormal distribution of growth rates of soft tissue metastases of breast cancer. J Surg Oncol 4:81–88, 1972.
51. Lee YT: Bone scanning in patients with early breast carcinoma: should it be a routine staging procedure? Cancer 47:486–495, 1981.
52. Lippman ME, Chabner BA: Editorial overview. NCI Monogr 1:5–10, 1986.
53. The Ludwig Breast Cancer Study Group: Prolonged disease-free node-negative breast cancer. N Engl J Med 320(8):491–496, 1989.
54. MacMahon B, List ND, Eisenberg P: Relationship of survival of breast cancer patients to parity and menopausal status. *In* Forrest AP, Kunkler P (eds.): Prognostic Factors in Breast Cancer. Edinburgh, Churchill Livingstone, 1968, pp 56–64.
55. Mambo NC, Gallagher HS: Carcinoma of the breast. The prognostic significance of extranodal extension of axillary disease. Cancer 39:2280–2285, 1977.
56. Mansour EG, Gray R, Shatila AH, Osborne CK, Tormey DC, Gilchrist KW, Cooper MR, Falkson G: Efficacy of adjuvant chemotherapy in high-risk node-negative breast cancer. N Engl J Med 320(8):485–490, 1989.
57. Moran RE, Black MM, Alpert L, Straus MJ: Correlation of cell-cycle kinetics, hormone receptors, histopathology, and nodal status in human breast cancer. Cancer 54:1586–1590, 1984.
58. Morrow M, Foster RS: Staging of breast cancer. A new rationale for internal mammary node biopsy. Arch Surg 116:748–751, 1981.
59. Natarajan N, Nemoto T, Mettlin C, Murphy GP: Race-related differences in breast cancer patients. Cancer 56:1704–1709, 1985.
60. National Cancer Institute Clinic Alert, May 18, 1988. *In* McGuire WL (ed.): Breast Cancer Res Treat 12:3–5, 1988.
61. Nemoto T, Natarajan N, Bedwani R, Vana J, Murphy GP: Breast cancer in the medial half: results of the 1978 National Survey of the American College of Surgeons. Cancer 51:1333–1338, 1983.
62. Nemoto T, Vana J, Bedwani RN, Baker HW, McGregor FH, Murphy GP: Management and survival of female breast cancer: results of a national survey by the American College of Surgeons. Cancer 45:2917–2924, 1980.
63. Noyes RD, Spanos WJ, Montague ED: Breast cancer in women aged 30 and under. Cancer 49:1302–1307, 1982.
64. Osborne CK, McGuire WL: Current use of steroid hormone receptor assays in the treatment of breast cancer. Surg Clin North Am 58:777–788, 1978.
65. Papaioannou AN, Urban JA: Scalene node biopsy in locally advanced primary breast cancer of questionable operability. Cancer 17:1006–1011, 1964.
66. Patterson R: The Treatment of Malignant Disease by Radium and X-rays. London, Edward Arnold, 1948.
67. Peters MV: The effect of pregnancy in breast cancer. *In* Forrest AP, Kunkler P (eds.): Prognostic Factors in Breast Cancer. Edinburgh, Churchill Livingstone, 1968, pp 65–80.
68. Phillippe E, Le Gal Y: Growth of 78 recurrent mammary carcinomas. Cancer 21:461–467, 1968.
69. Pichon MF, Pallud C, Brunet M, Milgrom E: Relationship of the presence of progesterone receptors to progress in early breast cancer. Cancer Res 40:3357–3360, 1980.
70. Portmann UV: Clinical and pathologic criteria as a basis for classifying cases of primary cancer of the breast. Cleveland Clin Q 10:41–47, 1943.
71. Redding WH, Coombes RC, Monaghan P, Clink McDH, Imrie SF, Dearnaley DP, Ormerod MG, Sloane JP, Gazet J-C, Powies TJ, Neville AM: Detection of micrometastases in patients with primary breast cancer. Lancet ii:1271–1273, 1983.
72. Rutqvist LE, Wallgren A, Nilsson B: Is breast cancer a curable disease? Cancer 56:898–902, 1985.
73. Schottenfeld D, Nash AG, Robbins GF, Beattie EJ Jr: Ten-year

results of the treatment of primary operable breast carcinoma: a summary of 304 patients evaluated by the TNM system. Cancer 38:1001–1007, 1976.

74. Schwartz GF, Feig SA, Patchefsky AS: Significance and staging of nonpalpable carcinomas of the breast. Surg Gynecol Obstet 166:6–10, 1988.

75. Shibata HR: Lymphoscintigraphy in the staging of breast cancer. Can J Surg 26:487–488, 1983.

76. Silvestrini R, Daidone MG, Gasparini G: Cell kinetics as a prognostic marker in node-negative breast cancer. Cancer 56:1982–1987, 1985.

77. Slamon DJ, Clark GM, Wong SG, Levin WJ, Ullrich A, McGuire WL: Human breast cancer: correlation of relapse and survival with amplification of the HER2/*neu* oncogene. Science (Washington, DC) 235:177–182, 1987.

78. Steinthal CF: Zue Dauerheilung des Brustkrebses. Beitr z klin Chir 47:226–239, 1905.

79. Stewart JF, Rubens RD: General prognostic factors. *In* Bonadonna G (ed.): Breast Cancer: Diagnosis and Management. Chichester, John Wiley, 1984, pp 141–167.

80. Tartter P, Papatestas AE, Ionnovich S: Cholesterol and obesity as prognosticators in breast cancer. Cancer 47:2222–2227, 1981.

81. Tubiana M, Pejovic MH, Chavaudra N, Contesso G, Malaise EP: The long-term prognostic significance of the thymidine labeling index in breast cancer. Int J Cancer 33:441–445, 1984.

82. Vana J, Bedwani R, Nemoto T, Murphy GT (eds.): American College of Surgeons Commission on Cancer. Final report on long-term patient care evaluation study for carcinoma of the female breast. American College of Surgeons, Chicago, 1979.

83. Varley JM, Swallow JE, Brammar WJ, Whittaker JL, Walker RA: Alterations to either c-*erbB*-2 *(neu)* or c-myc protooncogenes in breast carcinomas correlate with poor short-term prognosis. Oncogene 1:423–430, 1987.

84. Wallace IWJ, Champion HR: Axillary nodes in breast cancer. Lancet 1:217–218, 1972.

85. WHO International Histological Classification of Tumors, No. 2. Histological Typing of Breast Tumors, ed 2. Geneva, World Health Organization, 1981.

86. Wilkinson EJ, Lawrence H: Probability in lymph node sectioning. Cancer 33:1269–1274, 1974.

Chapter 18

PROGNOSTIC PARAMETERS FOR BREAST CARCINOMA

Henry Patrick Leis, Jr., M.D.

MAGNITUDE OF THE BREAST CANCER PROBLEM

The magnitude of the breast cancer problem emphasizes the need to determine the best possible predictors of prognosis so that appropriate therapy can be selected on an individual basis for women suffering from this common and dreaded disease.

In the United States, breast cancer is the most common malignant neoplasm occurring in women, accounting for 28 percent of the total. There is an increasing number of breast cancers. In 1965 it was projected that 1 out of every 17 women, or about 6 percent, would develop breast cancer, and there were about 68,000 new cases. In 1989 the projection for breast cancer development is one in ten, or about 10 percent. The estimated number is 142,900, 142,000 of which will occur in women. This is chiefly due to the fact that there are more women and that they are living longer into the cancer-prone years. In addition, there is an increasing incidence rate per 100,000 women. In 1965 the incidence rate was 69 per 100,000 women, whereas now it is about 107 per 100,000. This increasing incidence is predominately in women under 55 years of age and in black women. Among the possible reasons are earlier diagnosis, better statistical reporting, changes in dietary and socioeconomic habits and hormonal milieu, increasing exposure to carcinogens, and decreasing immunocompetence.[68, 162, 180, 188]

In the United States, breast cancer was the leading cause of cancer death in women for many years. Currently, it is responsible for 18 percent of these deaths. In 1985 it was surpassed by lung cancer, which now accounts for 21 percent of cancer deaths in women. Breast cancer remains the leading cause of death due to all causes in women aged 40 to 44 years. Every 15 minutes there is one death from breast carcinoma. In 1989 in the United States alone, 43,300 deaths were projected, 43,000 of which were in women, as compared with 49,000 projected lung cancer deaths in women.[188]

While the mortality rates in some cancers have decreased, e.g., cancers of the uterus, stomach, and colon, and increased in others, e.g., cancers of the ovaries and lungs, the incidence has remained relatively unchanged for breast cancer for over half a century and averages approximately 26 cancers per 100,000. The increasing

incidence rate per 100,000 women and this fixed mortality rate per 100,000 can only reflect better cure rates for earlier staged lesions and does not support the pessimistic view so often expressed about breast cancer.[68, 162, 180, 188]

The incidence figures for breast cancer, as well as for all other cancers, are only estimates, since there is no national office in the United States that records every new cancer case. Prior to 1974, estimates were based on data from two state registries. From 1974 through 1978, incidence rates were derived from the National Cancer Institute's Third National Cancer Survey (1969–1971) of nine major areas in the United States. Beginning in 1979, incidence information has been based on data from 11 population-based registries through a program, started by the National Cancer Institute in 1973, called SEER (Surveillance, Epidemiology and End Results).[4]

The National Center for Health Statistics, Department of Health and Human Services, has been the constant source for mortality statistics over the years. The 1989 figures are estimates based on the latest available information, which includes mortality data through 1983. Beginning in 1981, mortality rates per 100,000 population were age-adjusted to the 1970 census population, rather than the 1940 census population. Attempts to compare current figures with those of previous years may indicate false trends.[4]

Divergent Hypotheses of Breast Tumor Biology

For almost 100 years, the nineteenth century "halstedian" hypothesis on breast tumor biology was the basis for breast cancer therapy. It was a mechanistic concept postulating that cancer spread in an orderly fashion, progressing in a centrifugal manner from the breast to the regional lymph nodes and ultimately to distant sites. It postulated that breast cancers were local at the time of onset, that regional nodes served as a barrier to local spread, that removal of involved regional nodes influenced the survival of the patient, and that the type of local-regional therapy employed affected the survival of the patient. Implicit in this hypothesis was the concept that cancer could be held up for a time in the lymph nodes and that adequate removal of the breast with en bloc dissection of the regional lymph nodes could effect a "cure." This theory supported the use of the radical and extended radical mastectomies, sometimes with adjuvant radiotherapy, as the best means of obtaining local-regional control. The role of direct hematogenous spread was not considered important, and so systemic therapy was not included in the concept.[107]

This hypothesis was challenged by MacDonald[147, 148] in 1951, who suggested that human breast cancer was biologically predetermined from its onset. He stated that he had failed to find any evidence that early diagnosis, size of the tumor, or type of surgery had any influence on the outcome in mammary carcinoma. This was followed by a period of marked pessimism regarding this form of cancer.

In the 1970s an alternative hypothesis to the "halstedian" one, based on animal experiments and the failure of some clinical trials to demonstrate the superiority of en bloc dissection, was advanced by Fisher.[79] This hypothesis stressed the importance of hematogenous dissemination of the cancer and postulated that breast cancers were systemic at the time of onset, that regional nodes were not effective as barriers to systemic spread but rather were only indicators of biological behavior and metastatic potential as determined by a complex tumor-host interaction, that the removal of involved nodes had little influence on survival, and that the type of local-regional therapy did not substantially affect survival. It suggested that the only impact that could be made on breast cancer was by effective systemic therapy. It supported the use of lesser surgical procedures, with or without radiation, the use of adjuvant systemic chemoendocrine therapy, and the performance of axillary node dissections for staging purposes only.

Neither of these hypotheses can be accepted in its entirety. Both have elements of truth and are involved in explaining observed events. They should not be considered as mutually exclusive. Some cancers are very aggressive, producing early disseminated metastases, and require adjuvant systemic therapy in addition to the local-regional removal of the tumor burden. Others are much less aggressive, rarely making a transition to metastatic disease, and can be treated adequately by local-regional therapy without systemic adjuvant therapy. Osborne[170] stated: "It is far from clear that there is a unified hypothesis to explain the biology of breast cancer, which is a complex and heterogeneous disease. It is naive, in this heterogeneous and poorly understood neoplasm, to propose one."

Neither the theory of biological predetermination nor the concept that breast cancer is systemic from its inception is supported by several data sets. Reports by Adair et al.,[3] Duncan and Kerr,[71] and Koscielny et al.[127] have shown a definite relationship between tumor size and survival, noting a decrement in survival with increasing tumor diameter. The trial by the Health Insurance Plan of Greater New York[187] found that the early detection of breast cancer by combined physical examination and mammography screening reduced mortality by approximately one third. These findings were essentially confirmed in a trial supported by the Swedish National Board of Health[198] utilizing screening by mammography alone. Schwartz[186] noted a statistically significant reduction in breast cancer mortality in a screened population, without significant contribution from lead time and length basis. This supports the concept that there probably is a time phase in the early detection of breast cancer by mammography when the disease is not systemic.

The balance of currently available data does not support the concept that breast cancer is necessarily a systemic disease from its inception. Rather it supports the concept that adequate local treatment can reduce local-regional recurrences and thus systemic disease rates, since the possibility exists that these local-regional recurrences can act as a source of tertiary spread. Further support for the need of adequate local-regional therapy comes from a 20-year analysis of survival data by Leak et al.,[132] who noted not only a difference with various types of operations but also a definite difference in comparisons of good and poor surgical techniques with the same procedure, with a noteworthy increase in survival in the former. The principle of adequate local-regional treatment must not be abandoned for systemic approaches. Leaving tumor behind in the breast or regional nodes increases the tumor volume. Results from tumor-cell kinetic experimental models suggest that the best outcomes with adjuvant systemic therapy are obtained in patients with low tumor burdens.[170]

Dynamic Interplay of Prognostic Parameters

There are a number of valuable parameters for determining the prognosis for patients with breast cancer, including the size of the tumor, the status of the axillary nodes as related to metastatic involvement, the invasive status of the neoplasm, multicentricity, histological type, nuclear grade, estrogen-progesterone receptor levels, and immunological competence of the host.[26, 35, 84, 137, 138]

Even better predictors of prognosis are constantly being sought. In 1980, the National Institutes of Health re-emphasized the importance of prognostic factors by establishing grants to stimulate studies that search for parameters based on histological, histochemical, immunochemical, or other methods that would permit a more precise prediction of prognosis for patients with breast cancers. The ultimate goal is to be able to select the individual patients who can be treated adequately by breast conservation procedures, without any systemic adjuvant therapy, and to define the best type of treatment, both local-regional and systemic, for all other patients so as to offer them the best possible results.

In general, the prognosis for patients with breast cancer seems to be based on a dynamic interplay between the anatomical extent of the cancer, time of diagnosis, and the growth potential or virulence of the cancer, on one side, versus the degree of host immunocompetence and appropriate therapy, on the other.[26, 35, 137, 138]

ANATOMICAL EXTENT OF THE CANCER

The anatomical extent of the cancer refers to the stage and location of the tumor. It relates to the size of the cancer, to the extent of local advancement, to the regional node status, to the location of the tumor, and to distant metastases (systemic spread).

Staging

Cancer staging is representative of the anatomical extent or degree of advancement of the cancer when diagnosed. Celsus,[49] a Roman scholar of the early first century A.D., was probably the first to classify breast carcinoma, dividing it into three stages: cocethis, scirrhous, and ulcerative. He also suggested the first criterion of inoperability by advising that no surgical extirpation should be attempted when the cancer had reached the ,stage of ulceration. Since then, many different systems for staging breast cancers have been advocated.[135]

The American Joint Committee on Cancer (AJCC) and the Union Internationale Contre le Cancer (UICC) have recently agreed on a new TNM system for the classification and staging of cancer.[117] This system offers details regarding the tumor (T), the nodes (N), and any distant metastases (M). It can be used for clinical diagnostic (cTNM), surgical evaluation (sTNM), or postsurgical pathological (pTNM) staging.

The TNM system classifies tumors by their anatomical extent using designations and then combines these groups into prognostically similar categories called stages. The stages are numbered from the best (Stage 0) to the poorest (Stage IV) regarding prognosis based on survival rates: i.e., Stage 0, carcinoma *in situ*; Stage I, localized cancer; Stage II, limited local or regional spread; Stage III, extensive local or regional spread; and Stage IV, distant metastasis.

It is imperative that such a uniform system for classification and staging of cancer be used, not only in the United States but throughout the world, so that data can be properly compared. The system allows for the collection of uniform data that will be helpful in selecting appropriate treatments, in evaluating new treatment results, in acquiring uniform data for statistical analysis, and in estimating prognosis.

There are noteworthy differences in the TNM system for classification and staging of breast cancers between those recommended in the second edition of the Manual for Staging of Cancer of the American Joint Committee on Cancer (AJCC) (1983)[6] and those in the third edition (1988).[7] The current recommended TNM system for classification is presented in Tables 18–1 to 18–3, and for staging in Table 18–4. In the author's staging system there are some modifications, but the meanings of each stage are defined by the TNM classification (Table 18–5).

The following changes are reflected in the third edition of the AJCC Manual: (1) inclusion of a Stage 0 for *in situ* cancers (Tis, N0, M0); (2) Ta, N0, M0 cancers were

Table 18–1. STAGING OF TUMOR (T) ACCORDING TO TNM SYSTEM

Tx	Primary tumor cannot be assessed.
T0	No evidence of primary tumor.
Tis	Carcinoma *in situ*: clinical Paget's disease of the nipple with no tumor mass. Pathological intraductal carcinoma, lobular carcinoma *in situ,* or Paget's disease with no invasive component.
T1	Tumor 2.0 cm or less in greatest dimension.
T1a	0.5 cm or less in greatest dimension.
T1b	More than 0.5 cm but not more than 1.0 cm in greatest dimension.
T1c	More than 1.0 cm but not more than 2.0 cm in greatest dimension.
T2	Tumor more than 2.0 cm but not more than 5.0 cm in greatest dimension.
T3	Tumor more than 5.0 cm in greatest dimension.
T4	Tumor of any size with direct extension to chest wall or skin. Chest wall includes ribs, intercostal muscles, and serratus anterior muscle but not pectoral muscle.
T4a	Extension to chest wall.
T4b	Edema (peau d'orange) or ulceration of skin of the breast, or satellite skin nodules confined to the same breast.
T4c	Both *a* and *b* above.
T4d	Inflammatory carcinoma.

Adapted from American Joint Committee on Cancer: Manual for Staging of Cancer. 3rd ed. Philadelphia, JB Lippincott, 1988.

previously Stage II and are now Stage IIA; (3) T3, N0, M0 cancers were previously Stage IIIA and are now Stage IIB; (4) ipsilateral supraclavicular lymph node metastases, which were juxtaregional, formerly were classified as N3 and are now M1; (5) fixation to the pectoral fascia is no longer recorded, since its presence or absence does not influence staging; (6) inflammatory carcinoma, previously considered separately, is now classified as T4d; and (7) clinical, surgical, and pathological stage classifications have been redefined.

The vast majority of patients with breast cancer show a direct relationship between the stage of the cancer when diagnosed and the length of survival. Currently, with appropriate local-regional and adjuvant systemic therapy, ten-year, crude, absolute, NED (no evidence of disease) survival rates should approach 100 percent for patients with Stage 0, *in situ* cancers. It should be about 90 to 95 percent for those with occult, invasive Stage I cancers, 70 to 75 percent for those with overt invasive Stage I cancers, 40 to 45 percent for those with Stage II cancers, 10 to 15 percent for those with Stage III cancers, and practically zero for those with Stage IV cancers, based on the author's TNM system (Table 18–5).

In a series of 2437 patients with potentially curable breast cancer treated at New York Medical College Affiliated Hospitals from 1950 to 1983 predominately by modified mastectomies,[138, 139, 142] 1692 have been followed for ten or more years. A crude, absolute, NED

Table 18–2. STAGING OF NODES (N) ACCORDING TO TNM SYSTEM

	Clinical			Pathological
Nx	Regional nodes cannot be assessed.	Nx		Regional nodes cannot be assessed.
N0	No regional lymph node metastasis.	N0		No regional lymph node metastasis.
N1	Metastasis to movable ipsilateral axillary lymph node(s).	N1		Metastasis to movable ipsilateral axillary lymph node(s).
		N1a		Only micrometastasis (less than 0.2 cm).
		N1b		Metastasis to lymph node(s), any larger than 0.2 cm.
		N1bi		Metastasis to one to three lymph nodes.
		N1bii		Metastasis to four or more lymph nodes.
		N1biii		Extension of tumor beyond the capsule of the lymph node.
		N1biv		Metastasis to lymph node 2.0 cm or more in greatest dimension.
N2	Metastasis to ipsilateral axillary lymph nodes that are fixed to one another or to other structures.	N2		Metastasis to ipsilateral axillary lymph nodes that are fixed to one another or to other structures.
N3	Metastasis to ipsilateral internal mammary lymph node(s).	N3		Metastasis to ipsilateral internal mammary lymph node(s).

Adapted from American Joint Committee on Cancer: Manual for Staging of Cancer. 3rd ed. Philadelphia, JB Lippincott, 1988.

Table 18–3. STAGING OF METASTASIS (M) ACCORDING TO TNM SYSTEM

Mx	Presence of distant metastasis cannot be assessed.
M0	No distant metastasis.
M1	Distant metastasis (includes metastasis to ipsilateral supraclavicular node(s).

Adapted from American Joint Committee on Cancer: Manual for Staging of Cancer. 3rd ed. Philadelphia, JB Lippincott, 1988.

Table 18–4. TNM SYSTEM OF CLASSIFICATION AND STAGING

Stage	Tumor (T)	Classification Node (N)	Metastasis (M)
0	Tis	N0	M0
1	T1	N0	M0
11A	T0	N1	M0
	T1	N1*	M0
	T2	N0	M0
11B	T2	N1	M0
	T3	N0	M0
111A	T0	N2	M0
	T1	N2	M0
	T2	Na	M0
	T3	N1, N2	M0
111B	T4	Any N	M0
	Any T	N3	M0
1V	Any T	Any N	M1

*The prognosis for patients with classification N1a is similar to that for patients with classification N0.
Adapted from American Joint Committee on Cancer: Manual for Staging of Cancer. 3rd ed. Philadelphia, JB Lippincott, 1988.

ical staging was 32 percent. Smart et al.[191] in their review of 8587 cases of breast cancer, reported that 35 percent of clinically negative lymph nodes had metastases detected by pathological examination, whereas 87 percent of those considered clinically positive contained metastases.

The prognostic difference of clinical and pathological staging was emphasized by Cutler et al.[61] They reported five- and ten-year survival rates of 84 percent and 70 percent, respectively, for patients with pathologically negative nodes; for those with clinically negative nodes, the rates were, respectively, 74 percent and 58 percent. In the pathologically positive group, the five- and ten-year survival rates were 52 percent and 33 percent, and in the clinically positive group, 58 percent and 38 percent. These investigators also noted that patients with

survival rate of 99.1 percent was noted for those with Stage 0 *in situ* cancers, 94.9 percent for those with occult invasive Stage I cancers, 73.9 percent for those with overt invasive Stage I cancers, and 43.7 percent for those with Stage II cancers. (The author's TNM staging system was used.)

For proper staging, a pathological rather than clinical evaluation of the nodes is mandatory. Clinical appraisal is notoriously inaccurate, with a difference of about 33 percent in clinical and pathological evaluation of nodes. Cutler and Connelly[60] found that in patients having clinically negative nodes, 38 percent were positive on pathological examination, and in those with clinically positive nodes, 37 percent were pathologically negative. Fisher et al.[84, 86] reported that the false positive and false negative evaluation of the axilla was 24 percent and 39 percent, respectively, and that the overall error in clin-

Table 18–5. LEIS TNM SYSTEM CLASSIFICATION AND STAGING

Stage	Classification		
0	Noninvasive *(in situ)*		
	Tis	N0	M0
I	Invasive—negative ipsilateral axillary nodes		
	Occult (tumors < 1 cm)		
	T1a < 0.5 cm	N0	M0
	T1b 0.5–0.9 cm	N0	M0
	Overt (tumors > 1 cm)		
	T1c 1.0–1.9 cm	N0	M0
	T2 2.0–5.0 cm	N0	M0
	T3 Over 5.0 cm	N0	M0
II	Invasive—positive ipsilateral axillary nodes		
	Any T	N1	M0
III	Invasive—locally advanced		
	T4	Any N	M0
	Any T	N2 or N3	M0
IV	Invasive—distant metastasis		
	Any T	Any N	M1

bilateral palpable axillary nodes had better survival rates than did those with unilateral. Black and Asire[23] correlated this with a host defense mechanism.

Tumor Size

Several data sets and studies indicate a strong relationship between the size of the cancer and prognosis, with a definite decrement in survival associated with an increasing tumor diameter.[3, 71, 127, 186, 187, 198] The American College of Surgeons Survey in 1979[5] showed that as the size of the cancer increased, the frequency of axillary metastasis increased and the survival rate decreased. There is no question that tumor size is an important determinant for prognosis, but size estimated on clinical judgment is subject to considerable error and so pathological size, i.e., the maximum diameter as measured in centimeters in the pathology laboratory, should be used.

Fisher et al.[80] showed in their studies an inverse relationship between tumor size and survival rate. Goldenberg et al.[98] reported a higher tumor size and survival rate for breast cancer patients with small tumors regardless of the microscopic status of the axillary nodes. Eggers et al.[73] reported a 75 percent five-year survival rate for patients with tumors less than 2 cm in size, 24 percent for those with tumors from 3 to 6 cm, and 16 percent for those with tumors larger than 7 cm.

Gallager and Martin[92] defined minimal breast cancers as lobular carcinoma *in situ*, noninvasive intraductal carcinoma, and invasive cancers up to 0.5 cm in maximum diameter. They estimated a ten-year (or more) survival rate of over 90 percent. Using this definition, Frazier et al.[88] calculated a 20-year estimated survival rate of 93 percent. Others, among them Wanebo et al.,[211] Hutter and Rickert,[119] and Leis et al.,[141] have been more liberal with the definition of minimal breast cancer and have included cancers that measure up to 1 cm in size; the first two authors have also included some favorable histological types. Wanebo et al.[24] reported a ten-year survival rate of 95 percent, and Leis et al.[141] a ten-year, absolute, NED survival rate of 96.2 percent. The current figures on 220 patients are 97.2 percent (99.1 percent for *in situ* cancers and 94.9 percent for invasive cancers less than 1 cm in size).

The poor prognosis for patients with breast cancers over 5 cm in diameter is emphasized by the fact that the American Joint Committee on Cancer Staging, using 1983 TNM criteria,[6] classified these tumors as Stage IIIA. In the 1988 Staging Manual, they are classed as Stage IIB. Fisher et al.[80] calculated that, "If all tumors 2.0 cm or larger (70% of the total) had been removed when they were 1.0 to 1.9 cm. in size, at the end of five years the recurrence rate for all patients entered might have decreased by 10% to 18%, and the overall survival might have increased 11% to 20%." Nodal involvement is also related to tumor size. Johnstone[123] noted that almost three quarters of patients with tumors larger than 5 cm harbor nodal metastases when first seen. Berg[15] reported that the larger the primary tumor, the higher the level of axillary node metastasis. Tumors larger than 6 cm had ten times the incidence of Level III node metastases as compared with tumors less than 2 cm.

Tumor Margins

Clinically and mammographically, the appearance of the tumor margin (contour or configuration) has also been reported to be of prognostic significance. Lane et al.[131] noted that patients whose cancers had an irregular contour (who constitute up to 75 percent of their cases) had a 38 percent ten-year survival rate, while the remaining 25 percent of patients whose cancers had a rounded spherical contour had an 80 percent survival rate. Silverberg et al.[189] found that breast cancers with "pushing margins" were less likely to be associated with extensive lymph node metastases. In a study of tumor margins by mammography, Gold et al.[97] noted that the axillary metastatic rate was 56 percent for tumors with highly infiltrative margins compared with 21 percent for those with slightly infiltrative margins.

Axillary Node Status

Hutter[118] has emphasized that one of the most significant discriminants in predicting prognosis is the presence or absence of axillary node metastasis. Not only is the involvement important, but also the determination of whether the metastases are microscopic or macroscopic, the number of nodes involved, the levels at which they are involved, and whether there is extension through the lymph node capsule.

Berg[15] has shown that the number of axillary nodes involved is inversely proportional to the patient's survival. The greater the number of nodes involved, the worse the prognosis. Carbone[45] stated that when one to three nodes were involved the ten-year survival rates were in the range of 38 percent to 54 percent, but that this diminished to 13 percent when four or more nodes were involved. A five-year survival rate of 49 percent for patients with positive nodes was reported by Fisher et al.[80] They found that when one to three nodes were involved survival was 62 percent, but for four or more nodes with metastases this rate was 35 percent. The American College of Surgeons Survey[5] reported on survival rates related to pathologically positive axillary nodes in 8248 patients. There was a progressive decline in five-year cure rates from 48 percent to 38 percent as the involvement increased from one to four lymph nodes, respectively; the rate dropped sharply to 29 percent when five lymph nodes were involved.

Not only is the number of nodes involved important, but also the level of nodal metastases. Adair[2] reported a five-year survival rate of 65.2 percent for patients with Level I involvement, 44.9 percent for those with Level II involvement, and 28.4 percent for those with Level III involvement. The distribution of axillary nodes from the lowest to the highest levels was reported by Berg[15] to be 45 percent, 35 percent, and 20 percent, respectively. The respective distribution of metastases, however, was 61 percent, 31 percent, and 9 percent. In general terms, the mortality for patients with Level III involvement was twice that for Level II, which in turn was twice that for Level I. Smith et al.,[192] in an analysis of total lymph node involvement versus level of metastases, reported that survival seemed to be more closely related to the total number of metastatic nodes than to the levels involved.

Lane et al.[131] noted that the prognosis was much better if metastatic node involvement was microscopic rather than macroscopic. Huvos et al.[120] defined micrometastases as smaller than 2 mm and macrometastases being larger than this and generally visible grossly. In a study of 227 patients from Memorial Sloan Kettering Cancer Center, these investigators concluded that the prognosis for Level I nodal disease was as good with micrometastases as that for tumors lacking pathological evidence of nodal involvement. For Level III, the eight-year survival rate for patients with axillary node micrometastases was 59 percent as compared with 29 percent for those with macrometastases. These findings were reconfirmed by Attiyeh et al.[9] in some of these same patients with 10- and 14-year follow-ups. The 14-year survival for patients with metastases at Level I was 64 percent. It was 67 percent for those with micrometastases at any level and 36 percent for those with macrometastases at any level. No patient with micrometastases only had more than three lymph nodes involved.

Fisher et al.[86] reported that the extension of tumor through the capsule of the lymph node was associated with a 47 percent recurrence rate at 22 months compared with 30 percent for those with metastases confined within the capsule. They also found that involvement of extracapsular blood vessels was a poor prognostic parameter. A difference in ten-year survival rates depending on lymph node morphology was noted by Tsakraklides et al.,[205] the rates being 75 percent for patients whose nodes had lymphocyte predominance, 54 percent for those whose nodes had germinal center predominance, 33 percent for whose nodes had lymphocyte depletion, and 39 percent for those whose nodes were unstimulated.

Tumor Location

Reports on the relationship between the location of the cancer in the breast and prognosis have not been uniform. Location certainly does not carry the same prominent prognostic significance as tumor size and nodal involvement. Urban[206] noted that central and medial cancers have a worse prognosis than do those in the outer aspect of the breast. Most reports support the concept that cancers in the lateral aspect of the breast carry a better prognosis than those located medially. Berkson et al.,[17] in an analysis of 9649 patients, found a five-year survival rate of 70.7 percent for those with medial lesions and 84.2 percent for those with lateral lesions. Goldenberg et al.[98] found a higher survival rate for lateral lesions regardless of whether there was axillary node metastasis. A five-year survival rate of 52.1 percent for medial-half lesions and 64.6 percent for outer-half ones was reported by Hawkins.[109] Donegan[70] noted that in a collected series of 2742 cases from eight surgeons performing various types of internal mammary node resections, cancers in the central and medial quad-

rants metastasized to the internal mammary nodes in 28 percent of patients but in only 18 percent of those with lateral lesions. If there was axillary node metastasis, there was internal mammary node metastasis in 25 percent of the patients with lateral lesions and in 50 percent of those with medial or central lesions. When the axillary nodes were negative, positive internal mammary nodes were found in 4 percent of the patients with lateral lesions and in 13 percent of those with medial or central lesions. Fisher et al.,[81] however, in a study of 1665 breast cancers did not find that the site of the primary cancer itself influenced survival, and Cutler and Axtell[59] reported that among cancers classified according to nuclear grade and sinus histiocytosis, survival was not significantly influenced by location.

TUMOR GROWTH POTENTIAL (AGGRESSIVENESS OR VIRULENCE)

Breast cancer is a complex and heterogeneous disease. Despite all the research related to neoplasms of this organ it is still poorly understood, as is evidenced by the divergent hypotheses about breast tumor biology. There seem to be two different types of breast cancer, with some lesions having little virulence and a slow growth pattern. These lesions are not aggressive and rarely make a transition to metastatic disease. Others are markedly aggressive with a rapid growth pattern resulting in early disseminated disease and death.

Analysis of survival data by Bergson and Gage,[16] Cutler and Axtell,[59] and Fox[91] indicates that there are two prominent breast cancer population groups, with a striking difference in their mortality rates. Based on their studies, about 40 percent of accurately diagnosed patients with breast cancer would die at an exponential rate of 25 percent per year, whereas the remaining 60 percent would die at a rate of only 2.5 percent per year. As previously discussed, patients with axillary node metastasis have a worse prognosis than do those with negative nodes. However, one third of the patients with regional disease were found to have a low mortality in this analysis, again emphasizing the concept of a difference in tumor growth potential.

Invasive Quality

Smart et al.,[191] in a study of SEER data on 8587 breast cancers registered in 1975, reported an incidence rate for noninvasive (in situ) cancers of only 5 percent. In the author's series of 2437 breast cancers, there were 172 in situ cancers (7 percent). Beahrs et al.,[12] reporting on the National Cancer Institute and American Cancer Society–sponsored Breast Cancer Demonstration Detection Project (BCDDP), which screened asymptomatic women with mammography and physical examination, found an incidence of noninvasive cancers of 25 percent, which was a frequency exceeding the expectation based on incidence figures by the National Institutes of Health.[167]

Noninvasive cancer, defined as cancer of the breast confined within the basement membrane by light microscopy, may be lobular carcinoma *in situ* arising from the epithelium of the lobules or intraductal carcinoma arising from ductal epithelium.[141] The latter may be cribriform, intracystic, noninvasive Paget's, papillary, or solid (comedo).[213] The characteristics and treatment of these lesions are discussed by Leis et al.[141] They have an excellent prognosis; with appropriate treatment, ten-year, crude, absolute, NED survival rates should approach 100 percent. Farrow[76] collected a series of 403 patients with noninvasive cancers over a 16-year period from the Memorial Sloan Kettering Cancer Center. He reported that no clinical evidence of recurrence was observed in any of the patients treated by simple mastectomy and partial axillary gland dissection. Appropriate therapy for patients with these lesions is certainly moot, but lesser procedures, including those of breast conservation, are being employed today.[141]

Multicentricity

The current trend toward procedures aimed at preserving part or all of the breast makes the subject of multicentricity one of clinical significance as related to recurrence and prognosis.[99, 141, 170] There is no question but that breast cancer is multicentric. The incidence and biological significance of multicentricity, however, have been questioned by Fisher et al.[85] Gallager and Martin,[92] in their classic study, observed the extent of multicentricity by subserial whole-organ sectioning. They found a 74 percent incidence of multicentricity, 37 percent with concurrent multicentric invasive cancer and 37 percent with multicentric *in situ* cancer. The high incidence of multicentricity in breast cancer has been confirmed by Rosen et al.,[178] who showed a relationship to tumor size, and by Lesser et al.,[144] who found a relationship to histological type.

Fisher et al.[85] reported a low level of multicentricity (13.4 percent) in the National Surgical Adjuvant Breast Project, B-04; this is probably due to the limited extent of examination of any residual breast tissue following surgery.

There is well-documented evidence that operations designed to preserve the breast without other therapy, e.g., wide local excision, segmental or partial mastectomy, and quadrantectomy, may result in high local recurrence rates, ranging from 18 percent to 37 percent,[58, 70, 100, 101, 199] which obviously would influence survival. There was a 28 percent local recurrence rate, at a mean follow-up time of only 39 months, in the NSABP trial (B-06)[77] in patients treated by segmental resection only. In the arm in which treatment was with segmental resection and radiation the local recurrence rate fell to 8 percent, indicating the influence of radiation in retarding growth of multicentric disease. Long periods of time must elapse before these results can be properly assessed, since radiation may only delay rather than permanently reduce local recurrences.[99, 170]

Histological Types

Most reports indicate that certain histological types of breast cancer, even though they are invasive, are *prognostically* more *favorable*, e.g., adenoid cystic, colloid (gelatinous or mucinous), medullary with lymphoid infiltrate, papillary, and tubular.[83] Black and Kwon[26] emphasize that such lesions constitute only one fifth of the breast cancers seen in the United States and most Western countries. They also point out that distinct histological structural characteristics or growth patterns can vary in different areas of the same primary tumor and that they are often lacking in metastatic foci.

A number of classifications aimed at grouping breast cancers according to their histological growth pattern structural characteristics have been developed,[83, 134, 175] with some including histological grading as well as growth patterns. A histological type of classification has been recommended by the American Commission on Cancer Staging (Table 18–6). The one used by the author divides breast cancers into two main types, i.e., the uncommon *lobular,* arising from the epithelium of the lobules, and the common *ductal,* arising from the ductal epithelium. Each is divided into the less common in situ or noninvasive type, in which the cancer is confined within the basement membrane on light microscopy, and the more common invasive type (Table 18–7).

Adenoid cystic carcinoma is a rare form of mammary carcinoma, exhibiting patterns similar to those of cancers of the nasopharyngeal area and salivary glands, which clinically has a favorable prognosis.[1, 44, 50, 89, 93, 103, 110, 118, 185, 194] The histological picture is one of island-like and

Table 18–6. AJCC HISTOLOGICAL TYPE OF CANCER

Check predominant type:
( ) Cancer, NOS (Not otherwise specified)
Ductal
    ( ) Intraductal *(in situ)*
    ( ) Invasive with predominant intraductal component
    ( ) Invasive, NOS
    ( ) Comedo
    ( ) Inflammatory
    ( ) Medullary with lymphoid infiltrate
    ( ) Mucinous (colloid)
    ( ) Papillary
    ( ) Scirrhous
    ( ) Tubular
    ( ) Other
        Specify _____
Lobular
    ( ) *In situ*
    ( ) Invasive with predominant in situ component
    ( ) Invasive
Nipple
    ( ) Paget's disease, NOS
    ( ) Paget's disease with intraductal carcinoma
    ( ) Paget's disease with invasive ductal carcinoma
Other
        Specify _____

Adapted from American Joint Committee on Cancer: Manual for Staging of Cancer. 3rd ed. Philadelphia, JB Lippincott, 1988.

Table 18–7. HISTOLOGICAL GROWTH PATTERN CLASSIFICATION

( ) Cancer, NOS (not otherwise specified)
Lobular
   ( ) *In situ*
   ( ) Invasive
Ductal
   ( ) *In situ*—intraductal
   ( ) Cribriform ( ) ( ) Intracystic ( ) Paget's
   ( ) Papillary ( ) Solid or comedo
   ( ) Invasive
   ( ) Adenoid cystic
   ( ) Apocrine
   ( ) Colloid (mucinous)
   ( ) Comedo
   ( ) Inflammatory
   ( ) Medullary with lymphoid infiltrate
   ( ) No special type (NST)
   ( ) NOS
   ( ) Scirrhous
   ( ) Paget's
   ( ) Papillary
   ( ) Tubular
   ( ) With predominant intraductal component
( ) Other
     Specify _____

trabecular cell complexes that contain slitlike or round cavities filled with an amorphous PAS-positive secretion, with a loose edematous stroma separating the cell complexes.[194]

Colloid carcinoma, also referred to as mucinous or gelatinous carcinoma, is a glandular papillary or glandular cystic tumor of a high degree of maturity, with the cell aggregates lying in pools of mucin. It can occur in a pure form or in association with other types of cancer.[83, 194] The pure form, which accounts for only one to two percent of all breast cancers, has a good prognosis, whereas the mixed forms are more common and prognostically less favorable.[83, 96, 105, 118, 161, 166, 168, 190, 194]

Medullary carcinoma is a parenchyma-rich tumor of marrow-like consistency with little stroma that shows a striking lymphoid infiltrate, prompting the term "medullary carcinoma with lymphoid infiltrate." These tumors show a high degree of cellular pleomorphism and a large number of mitoses, which is in direct contrast to their good prognosis.[40, 118, 164, 166, 173, 174] They are large, well-circumscribed tumors, accounting for some 5 to 7 percent of all breast cancers. Because of their size, two thirds of these lesions were classified as Stage IIIA cancers according to the 1983 Staging System.[6] Ridolfi et al.[174] reported an 84 percent ten-year survival rate for patients with these tumors as compared with 63 percent for nonmedullary carcinomas. Bloom et al.,[40] in a 20-year follow-up, reported a 74 percent survival rate for patients with these cancers as compared with 14 percent for those with other types. Rosen et al.,[177] in a study comparing pathological features of breast cancers in Tokyo and New York City, found a higher frequency of colloid and medullary carcinomas in the Japanese women. This greater number of cancers with good prognoses may explain the better survival rates for Japanese women.

True infiltrating *papillary carcinoma* is a rare neoplasm, accounting for only 0.3 to 1.5 percent of all breast cancers. However, intraductal papillary growth is a not uncommon component of various histological types of invasive mammary carcinomas.[83, 194] Histologically there are branched papillary extensions within ectatic ducts and microcystic cavities, the papillae usually lacking vascular stroma. These lesions must be distinguished from benign intraductal papillomas, to which their origin is credited by some authors.[69, 108, 128] Most reports indicate a good prognosis,[69, 108, 153, 203] but Kraus and Neubecker[128] found no difference in their prognosis as compared with other ordinary breast cancers. Carter et al.[47] reported a good prognosis for patients with intracystic papillary carcinomas but noted that this prognosis deteriorated when there was an accompanying papillary intraductal carcinoma.

Tubular carcinoma, also referred to as orderly carcinoma by McDivitt et al.,[153] is regarded as having an excellent prognosis.[46, 153, 200] Although it is a relatively infrequent type of breast cancer, Cooper et al.[56] reported an incidence of 2 percent in 636 patients with breast cancer, and Patchefsky et al.[171] noted that 10 percent of breast cancers detected in a screening clinic were tubular. The histological picture is of tubular structures typically lined by a single layer of well-differentiated epithelial cells.

Histological Grading

Grading is a measurement of the degree to which the tumor tissue lacks normal histological differentiation; this may be recorded as a general grade (GG) or a nuclear grade (NG). Grading is recorded by numbers from 1 to 3, but unfortunately, GG and NG are numbered in opposite directions. In general, the better the differentiation or grade, the better the prognosis. GGIII, NGI indicates a poorly differentiated cancer with a poor prognosis; GGII, NGII a moderately well-differentiated cancer with an intermediate prognosis; and GGI, NGIII a well-differentiated cancer with a good prognosis.

Von Hansemann in 1893 is generally credited as being the first to call attention to a possible relationship between the behavior of malignant neoplasms and their degree of anaplasia,[104] but Tough et al.[204] noted that a similar correlation was suggested even earlier by Dennis in 1891.

In 1925 Greenough[102] developed a technique for the general grading of mammary carcinomas that is the basis for general grading systems used by most investigators today. He divided tumors into three grades of anaplasia, i.e., low, medium, and high malignancy. In this first attempt at grading breast cancer he found a striking relationship between the grade of anaplasia and curability. Current general histological grading is usually based on the criteria established by Bloom.[37–39] These include the degree of tubule formation, the size and shape of the cells and their nuclei, and the frequency of hyperchromasia and mitosis. Survivorship was related to histological differentiation: Grade I, well-differentiated; Grade II, moderately differentiated; and Grade III, poorly differentiated. Survival rates at 5 and 20 years, respectively, were: Grade I, 81 percent and 41 percent; Grade II, 54 percent and 29 percent; and Grade III, 34 percent and 21 percent. The value of general grading as related to prognosis has been emphasized by a number of other investigators.[3, 11, 51, 69, 86, 115, 196] In the study by Fisher et al.,[86] Grade I, well-differentiated tumors were found to be correlated with older age, absence of nodal involvement, and good-prognosis histological type. Davis et al.[63] evaluated the prognostic significance of general histological tumor grade in 1537 women. They concluded that histological grade can be determined by any pathologist and enables selection of a subpopulation of breast cancer patients at high risk for early mortality.

Broders,[43] in his classic paper published in 1920 on squamous epithelioma of the lip, was the first to stress the importance of the characteristics of nuclei in estimating the degree of malignancy. Black et al.[26, 30–32] have emphasized the relatively simple technique of nuclear, rather than general, grading, which eliminates differences due to the fragility of the cytoplasm. Unlike the characteristics used in general grading, the nuclear characteristics of individual cancers are the same throughout the primary tumor and throughout the course of the disease. These investigators showed that nuclear grading is an independent variable correlating with prognosis. The essentials in the grading system relate to the nuclei alone—variations in size and shape, prominent nucleoli, chromatin clumping, and frequency of mitotic figures. Nuclear grades are divided into four groups. NG0, indicating anaplasia, and NGI, indicating poor differentiation, are commonly put into one group, NGI.[83] NGII indicates intermediate or moderate differentiation and NGIII, well-differentiated nuclei, (these numbers being in reverse order of general grading). Cutler and Axtell,[59] in a study of 1067 women with proven breast cancers, reported a definite correlation between patient survival and nuclear grade. Fisher et al.[78] noted that the prognostic value as to outcome for patients with breast cancer was similar for nuclear grade, estrogen receptor, and progesterone receptor. The Cox regression analyses,[57] however, indicate that a more accurate assessment of outcome can be obtained when more than one marker is used. Fisher[82] endorses the prognostic significance of both general and nuclear histological grading.

Growth Rate—Cell Kinetics

Gershon-Cohen et al.,[95] in their classic paper on biologic predeterminism, first reported on the doubling times or rate of growth of breast cancers. These doubling times ranged from 23 to 209 days, with the average tumor doubling in 100 days. Based on this, a tumor with a doubling time of 23 days would take only two years to reach the size of 1 cm, whereas one with a doubling time of 209 days would take 17 years to reach this size. Despite the valid observation that postoperative sur-

vival tends to have an inverse relationship to the size of the primary tumor when diagnosed, it has long been known that some patients having large tumors experience prolonged survival after therapy, whereas others with smaller tumors die from rapidly disseminating disease.

Clinical studies suggest that the rapidity of growth may be biologically more significant than the absolute size. Denoix[65] emphasized that "the important fact is how long a tumor takes to reach a certain size, not time or size alone." When breast cancers were divided into stationary, slow-growing, and fast-growing, it was predictably established that the slow-growing neoplasms had favorable survival characteristics, whereas the fast-growing lesions connoted unfavorable survival.

Breast cancers with a history of rapid growth and peritumor edema have been designated as "evolving" cancers (PEV).[165] The five-year survival without recurrence for PEV I lesions was 35 percent, for PEV II lesions 11 percent, and for PEV III lesions 0 percent. Mourali et al.[165] went on to report that PEV lesions made up a significant proportion of breast cancers seen in Tunisia, accounting for 55 percent. Black and Kwon[26] concluded that small, slow-growing tumors have a low percentage of nodal involvement and favorable survival rates.

The next generation of prognostic markers may well be in the field of cell kinetics, measuring tumor growth rate and aggressiveness. In this regard, the technique of flow cytometry provides two important pieces of information. First, it tells how rapidly the tumor is dividing by measuring the percentage of cells in the S phase of the DNA replication cycle. Second, it indicates the malignant aggressiveness of the tumor by assessing the aneuploidy or total amount of extra DNA in the tumor cell.[8, 10, 157, 159]

Stat et al.[193] found in a comparative study of static cytofluorometry and flow cytometry that both techniques were useful for the estimation of DNA ploidy and replication in human breast cancer. Meyer et al.[163] reported that the S-phase fraction (SPF) measured by flow cytometry of DNA is like the thymidine-labeling index (TLI), which is measured autoradiographically, insofar as both indicate the proportion of cancer cells currently synthesizing DNA and thus reflect the rate of proliferation or growth. It would seem that high SPF and aneuploidy should have a prognostic significance like that of the thymidine-labeling index regarding tumor aggressiveness. Meyer and Province[163a] reported that thymidine labeling seemed to have a prognostic power independent of stage or of estrogen and progesterone receptor status. Flow cytometry has a substantial front end cost, but it can be performed on paraffin-embedded tissue, and by using multicolor probes it can also measure receptor levels on a cellular basis.[157]

McGurrin et al.[160] assessed cell proliferation in invasive breast cancers by an immunoperoxidase procedure using the monoclonal antibody Ki-67, which reacts with a nuclear antigen in proliferating cells. Tumors with a high mitotic rate, high nuclear grade, high histological grade, and negative estrogen receptors as well as those in premenopausal women had high numbers of Ki-67–positive cells. These findings are similar to those reported for other measurements of cell cycle kinetics, such as the thymidine-labeling index, and suggest that this technique may provide prognostically significant cell cycle information.

Tumor growth factors (TGFs) are substances secreted by cells that mediate transformation of normal cells to cancer cells via a self-stimulating mechanism. Growth factors are similar in many properties to TGFs, but they are mitogenic and not transforming. Both act via a cell surface receptor mechanism. Some oncogene products have been found to be growth factors, but their role in either mammary cell differentiation or neoplastic transformation is unknown. Active research is needed into the relationship of oncogenes, growth factors, and the action of hormones and hormone antagonists on breast cancer cells in the hope of discovering a new approach in the control of growth of breast cancer cells.[184]

Steroid Hormone Receptors

The knowledge that some breast cancers are hormone-dependent dates to more than 90 years ago, when Sir George Beatson,[13] a Scottish surgeon, reported that inoperable mammary carcinoma in women could be induced to regress by excision of the ovaries. Jensen et al.[122] in 1967 reported on the presence in breast cancers of a specific estrogen receptor (ER) that correlated well with the response to endocrine therapy. Since then, a progesterone receptor (PR) has been identified. Currently, the value of estrogen and progesterone assays of breast cancers in predicting response to hormone manipulations has been generally accepted.[155] About 60 percent of patients with estrogen receptors respond to such therapy, with the rate increasing to about 80 percent if the tumor has both estrogen and progesterone receptors.[118] The biochemical assay method for determining the presence of steroid hormone receptors, although very valuable, is expensive and time-consuming. Results are expressed in femtomoles (1×10^{-15}) per mg of protein with levels above 10 fm per mg being considered receptor-positive.[87] Immunofluorescent histochemical techniques requiring little tissue have been developed using cryostat-prepared frozen sections.[133, 171] Compared with the assay method, the immunofluorescent procedure is relatively inexpensive, and sections can be prepared at the time of surgery for later use.

Brigati et al.[42] suggest that steroid hormone receptor analyses be performed routinely on all patients. The value of these assays in patients with axillary metastases from occult cancers has been reported by Bhatia et al.[18] This analysis provides information regarding the identity of the primary tumor and may well represent the sole opportunity to determine receptor status. In a similar vein, knowing that only tumors of the breast, ovary, and endometrium contain significant amounts of estrogen receptors, Kiang and Kennedy[125] have stressed the importance of doing receptor assays on any areas of metastasis when the primary lesion is occult.

More recently, the prognostic implications for patients with positive or negative hormone receptors have initiated great interest. Based on the evidence that a receptor-negative status is seen with poorly differentiated cancers,[78, 152] indicating a poor prognosis, a number of reports have shown that patients whose cancers have positive receptors have less aggressive tumors with a better prognosis and with statistically longer survival rates.[19, 53, 67, 78, 182]

When used alone, estrogen receptor, progesterone receptor, and nuclear grade each offers significant information in breast cancer prognosis.[78] Each seems to have an independent influence on outcome, however, and their combined use offers a more accurate assessment of prognosis.[57, 78] ER and PR levels are excellent prognostic factors. Both should be assayed, since patients with discordant values have a midway survival prognosis between both positive and both negative values and PR status enhances the predictive power of ER.[157]

Monoclonal antibodies are also being employed in immunohistopathology to establish the phenotype of carcinoma lesions. The use of various monoclonal antibodies for estrogen receptor studies is being evaluated in comparison with immunoassays of tumor extracts. Immunochemical assays have the advantage of defining reactivity to specific cell types and overcome the criticism that values obtained from standard assays of tumor extracts may be more reflective of the percentage of tumor cells present in the sample than the actual amount of estrogen receptor per tumor cell.[184]

Biological Markers

There has been an intense search in recent years for biological markers for breast cancer. Many different types of materials have been found, sometimes elevated, in the body fluid of breast cancer patients, some of which hold prognostic significance. Of the solitary markers, specific patterns of serial carcinoembryonic antigen (CEA) measurements are helpful in predicting recurrence, but combinations of markers seem to enhance the probability of predicting prognosis.[210, 214]

Patterns of multiple biomarkers have the capability of defining specific response characteristics better than does any single biomarker alone when assessed by multivariate regression analysis.[214] Coombes et al.,[55] after studying 19 different markers in combination, found that the ones that were most frequently elevated in patients with metastatic disease were CEA, ferritin, C-reactive protein, acid glycoprotein, alkaline phosphatase, sialyl transferase, and urinary hydroxyproline/creatinine ratio. More recently, Coombes et al.[54] reported in a study of ten biomarkers that three of these seemed to be most useful in detecting recurrence, namely CEA, alkaline phosphatase, and 2-glutamyltranspeptidase. These three tests identified approximately 50 percent of patients who developed metastases, with a lead time of about three months. Haagensen et al.[106] reported that the combination of plasma carcinoembryonic antigen (CEA) and gross cystic disease fluid protein (GCDFP) were abnormally elevated in 48 percent of patients who developed metastases, but only rarely were both markers elevated.

Monoclonal Antibodies

The methodologies of gene cloning procedures and hybridoma monoclonal antibody technology, introduced in the 1970s, have been breakthroughs in both molecular biology and immunological research. Their use in breast cancer research is throwing new light on considerations regarding the etiology, detection, treatment, and prognosis of this disease. The identification and characteristics of proto-oncogenes, oncogenes, antioncogenes, and other cellular genetic elements have brought a new perspective to the etiology and pathogenesis of human mammary carcinoma. Monoclonal antibodies are being used to define and detect breast cancer–associated antigens. Growth factors, tumor growth factors, and other biological response modifiers are being investigated as to the role they play in the maintenance of the transformed phenotype.[184]

The identification of tumor-associated antigens and the development of specific immunological reagents against these tumors have long been sought. With the methodology of gene cloning it has been possible to clone fused cell products. These cloned cell populations, called hybridomas, can be assayed to select for homogeneous populations of immunoglobulins with the desired reactivity. As a result of this, numerous monoclonal antibodies have been generated that are reported to bind to normal and malignant cell surfaces or intracellular organelles. At least a dozen of these monoclonal antibodies are against human mammary carcinoma. Studies are continuing to seek out tumor-specific antigens in breast cancer cells. The monoclonal antibodies thus far identified and future generations of them show great promise for use in the diagnosis, treatment, and prognosis of patients with breast cancer.[129, 146, 156, 184, 210]

There is preliminary evidence that monoclonal antibodies are useful in determining the state of differentiation of a given breast cancer. It is well recognized that the degree of differentiation or grade of a breast cancer is a significant prognostic factor. With antibody reactivity also reflecting the state of differentiation of breast tumors, it should serve as an aid in prognosticating the outcome of patients with this disease. The problem is in obtaining large amounts of material for either retrospective or prospective studies because of the many variables that are associated with breast cancer.[129, 146, 156, 210]

Thompson et al.[202] have reported on the development of two murine monoclonal antibodies against the human breast carcinoma cell line MCF-7. One antibody detects a 100-kD antigen that is distinct from the well-characterized protein antigens of normal breast tissue. In a screening of over 4000 primary hybridoma cultures by Colcher et al.,[52] 11 monoclonal antibodies were identified that reacted with human mammary cells and not

with normal human tissue. One antibody (B6.2) has been shown to detect a cell surface tumor–associated antigen of 90 kD in 75 percent of the primary and metastatic breast lesions examined.[130]

There have been reports in which specific monoclonal antibodies have been shown statistically to be indicators of breast cancer prognosis. Kufe et al.[129] reported on a murine monoclonal antibody MAb, designated DF-3, that they developed, which reacts with a 300-kD human mammary epithelial antigen expressed on apical borders of secreting mammary epithelial cells and in the cytosol of less differentiated malignant cells. Preliminary reports indicate that this antibody does reflect the state of differentiation of the tumor. Lundy et al.[146] evaluated human mammary tumors for levels of DF-3 and correlated this value with other clinicopathological parameters, i.e., the degree of tumor differentiation, nuclear grade, and estrogen receptor status. They concluded that DF-3 reacts to a differentiation antigen present in some human breast cancers and that this correlates well with the other parameters. It suggests that DF-3 histochemistry may serve as a prognostic indicator and as a useful alternative in assessing estrogen receptor status of small breast cancers, when there is an insufficient amount of tumor present for biochemical assay of hormone receptor levels.

A study of two monoclonal antibodies, GB-3 and GB-5, on breast tissues by indirect immunofluorescence was also done. GB-3 detects the epithelial membrane, and GB-5 reacts with the junctional substances between the epithelial cells.[218] These investigators[218] found that normal epithelial antigens recognized by these two monoclonal antibodies were diminished in intraductal carcinomas and lost in them in infiltrating carcinomas. The data suggested to them that these antigens may contribute to the interaction of the epithelium with the extracellular matrix and the intercellular binding between the epithelial cells. The loss of these antigens may facilitate the wide dissemination of tumor cells and therefore be of prognostic importance.

Looking into the future one can see the possibility of using a series of monoclonal antibodies to assay sections of the mammary cancer of a specific patient to help define the likelihood of metastases and hence prognosis.

The predictive value of tumor metastases in regional nodes is well recognized, but at present this entails removing at least the axillary nodes to detect the presence of metastases; also, about 25 percent of axillary node–negative patients still develop metastatic breast cancer.

In the future it may be possible to assay all regional nodes, i.e., axillary and internal mammary, for metastases by a noninvasive technique such as lymphoscintigraphy. Radiolabeled monoclonal antibodies could theoretically be administered regionally, and the patient could then be monitored by scanning with a gamma camera for concentrations of radionuclide-coupled monoclonal antibody in tumor-bearing lymph nodes. One can also foresee the use of radionuclide-conjugated monoclonal antibody to a breast tumor-associated antigen, administered intravenously at regular intervals, as a means of defining the appearance and location of metastatic lesions.[184]

Tumor Necrosis

Carter et al.[48] noted that tumor necrosis was associated with a greater rate of axillary metastases and mortality, and that tumors with necrosis and an infiltrative border were clinically more aggressive. Patients who had cancer with an infiltrating border and necrosis had a 75 percent rate of axillary metastases and a 29 percent ten-year survival, whereas those whose cancer had smoothly circumscribed borders and no necrosis had a 30 percent rate of axillary metastases and a 61 percent ten-year survival.

Pathological findings from the National Surgical Adjuvant Breast Project (Protocol B-04) were reported by Fisher et al.[79] regarding discriminants for prognosis. Thirty-six pathological and six clinical characteristics were evaluated. Tumor necrosis was one of the discriminants that heralded a poor outcome. The investigators noted that there were two kinds of necrosis. The most common, which involves the intraductal component of the cancer, was designated the comedo type. Its appearance seemed to be less ominous than the less frequent type of infarct-like necrosis observed in areas of invasive cancers. The degree of necrosis (slight, moderate, or marked) was also significant, with the last having the most unfavorable prognosis.

Blood Vessel Invasion

Blood vessel invasion is noted most frequently in veins and venules adjacent to uninvolved arteries. Its incidence has been reported as ranging from a low of 4.7 percent by Fisher et al.[84, 86] to a high of 46 percent by Friedell et al.,[90] with both groups indicating that it carries a poor prognosis. A number of other authors have also reported that blood vessel invasion has a negative effect on survival.[14, 64, 126, 150, 181, 183, 201]

Friedell et al.[90] stated that they found blood vessel invasion to be of prognostic significance only in the presence of nodal metastases. The reports by Fisher et al.[84, 86] noted that blood vessel invasion was more likely to be associated with a severe cell reaction in the tumor, lymphatic invasion, mestastases to four or more axillary nodes, necrosis, and a poor nuclear grade. Martin et al.,[150] in a study of histological sections from patients with infiltrating duct cell carcinomas by immunohistochemical staining with antibody against human Factor VIII–related antigen, found that a positive correlation exists between vascular invasion and lymph node metastases. Sampat et al.,[183] in a series of 242 patients, reported that the five-year survival was 98 percent with no blood vessel invasion or axillary node metastasis; survival was reduced to 59 percent with blood vessel invasion, and only 12 percent survived five years when there was both vascular invasion and axillary metastasis.

Lymphatic Invasion

Lymphatic invasion, as well as invasion of veins and venules by cancer cells, is evidence of probable dissemination.[118] It may be limited to the area of the primary cancer, diffused throughout the breast substance, or in the dermal lymphatics as seen in inflammatory carcinoma, with a corresponding ominous outcome. Fisher et al.[84, 86] reported that their studies strongly implied that lymphatic invasion is an unfavorable pathological finding in relationship to patient survival. They found it to be more often associated with noncircumscribed large tumors of poor histological grade and no special histological type, with blood vessel and perineural space invasion and nipple involvement. When present, there was an association with early tumor recurrence at 6 to 18 months.

Perineural Space Invasion

Perineural space involvement with tumor cells was present in 104 of 378 cases studied by Fisher et al.[84, 86] in which such structures were recognized, representing an incidence of 27.8 percent. They found that tumors with perineural space invasion were more likely to be associated with lymphatic invasion, nipple involvement, and metastases in the axillary lymph nodes. Early tumor recurrence (within 18 months) was also noted more frequently when there was perineural space involvement. Clinical and pathological features were evaluated as to their relationship to long-term disease-free survival in a selected group of 207 breast cancer patients with tumor-free axillary nodes by van de Velde et al.[208] Of the four pathological features that appeared to have significance, one was the presence of neoplastic cells in intramammary lymphatic vessels.

Elastosis

The exact biological significance and histogenesis of elastosis in patients with mammary carcinomas have not been determined and are open to question. Some studies[151, 207] have reported that elastosis in the tumor bed may indicate a more favorable five-year survival, possibly being a sign of slow growth of the cancer and therefore favorable prognosis.

Abnormal Thermogram

There is a definite relationship between growth rate and metabolic heat production. Thermography offers a safe, noninvasive method of evaluating the amount of heat produced by a cancer. Gautherie and Gros[94] developed a thermogram staging system of Th I to Th V based on an increasing heat pattern. The heat production is high, as represented in thermogram readings of Th IV and Th V, in cancers that have a rapid growth rate. Even small lesions with an abnormal, high thermal reading are indicative of a rapid growth rate. As previously discussed, patients whose cancers have a rapid growth rate have a poor prognosis, and the measurement of heat produced by the cancer with thermography offers another method of determining prognosis.[94]

Psychological Factors

At least four psychological factors have been reported as influencing the survival rates of patients with breast cancers.[121] The first is that longevity is related to how well the patient adjusts to her illness.[62, 176] Second, Derogatis et al.[66] found that patients who expressed their emotions about the disease lived longer. They proposed that "fighters" have a better chance of surviving than do "compliers." The "will to live" has been reported as being an important third factor in patient survival.[124, 149, 195] Finally, Weisman and Worden[212] reported that increased emotional stress contributes to short-term survival. Jamison et al.,[12] however, felt that their data suggest that for breast cancer patients with metastatic disease, disease-related variables probably outweigh the influence of select psychosocial factors in determining length of survival.

The role of psychological factors in human disease is emphasized in the quotation by Francis W. Peabody[197]: "Disease in man is never exactly the same as the same disease in an experimental animal, for in man the disease at once affects and is affected by what we call the emotional life."

HOST RESISTANCE—IMMUNOCOMPETENCE

The ultimate outcome of a patient with breast cancer is reflected in the interaction between the growth potential (virulence or aggressiveness) of the primary cancer and the immunologically mediated tumor-retarding response of the host.[21, 26, 34, 35, 137, 138] The prognosis of the patient deteriorates as measurements to determine immunocompetence decrease from marked to moderate to slight and finally to immunological incompetence.

Tumor cells have antigens associated with them that are not apparent on normal cells.[169] Immunological responses (immunogenicity) involve stimulation of the appropriate lymphoid cells by an immunogenic antigen determinant.[35]

The primary importance of lymphoid cells in tumor immunity has been well demonstrated in experimental animal systems.[111] The responsive cells undergo a complex sequence of proliferation and differentiation in the *lymphoreticuloendothelial (LRE) system.* One line of differentiation, of course, involves the thymus gland and leads to the development of T cells that mediate cellular immune reactions. A subpopulation of T lymphocytes has been described that forms "active" E-rosettes.[216] These have been reported to be depressed in patients with cancer.[215]

The lymphoid cells that have undergone differentia-

tion in the LRE system are recognizable as focal accumulations of lymphoid cells at the site of the reference antigen, in the tumor, and as distinct morphological patterns in antigen-draining lymph nodes.

An accumulation of lymphoid cells can occur around the tumor as a *lymphoid infiltrate (LI)* or as a *perivenous infiltrate (PVI)* in sections cut through the tumor. LI is most vividly demonstrated in medullary carcinomas with lymphoid infiltrates, which have a good prognosis. PVI can occur with or without simultaneous diffuse infiltrations, predominately of the plasmacytoid type, around the cancerous ducts. Approximately 80 percent of patients with *in situ* carcinomas have lymphoid cellular responses in the region of their cancers,[35] and about 33 percent of patients with atypical proliferative lesions designated as precancerous mastopathies have demonstrable lymphatic infiltration.[22, 25] The relative frequency of LRE responses to invasive breast cancers is lower than it is to *in situ* cancer. Reactivity to invasive cancer foci appears to be dependent upon reactivity to coexisting foci of *in situ* carcinoma. Black and Zachrau[35] noted that in an appreciable minority of invasive breast cancer patients (33 percent) such antigenicity was not expressed. They found that while the prognostically favorable influence of LRE responses to breast cancer was demonstrated even among patients who were unselected as to nuclear grade (NG), the prognostically favorable effect was most apparent among patients with NGI and NGII cancers, the prognosis of NGIII cancers being so good that any improvement related to LRE response would be minimal.

Another LRE measurement of the host's immunocompetence is a distinctive type of regional node reactivity characterized by paracortical lymphoid cellular hyperplasia and intrasinusoidal accumulations of large histiocytes whose ultrastructure is similar to that of epithelial cells.[20, 25, 35, 113] This accumulation of histiocytes in the sinusoids of the regional lymph nodes is called *sinus histiocytosis (SH).* Black and Zachrau[35] reported that more than 80 percent of in situ carcinomas were associated with SH, supporting their similar findings of lymphoid cellular responses as determined by LI and PVI to these cancers. As with lymphoid cellular responses, the relative frequency of LRE responses to invasive cancers determined by SH is lower than it is with *in situ* cancer. The prognostically favorable influence of SH is similar to that of LI and PVI. The conclusions reached by Black et al.[24, 35] on the prognostic significance of the interactions between nuclear differentiation and LRE reactivity were based on observations of approximately 3000 breast cancer patients who were followed more than five years or until death.

Lymphoreticuloendothelial responses as measured by LI, PVI, and SH allow for the determination of the host's immunocompetence at the time of surgery. Other tests are available that offer an ongoing method of measuring the reactive immunocompetence of the host.

Cell-mediated immunity (CMI) to specific antigens can be measured by in vitro test procedures. One such procedure is the *leukocyte migration inhibition (LMI) assay,* adapted to measure reactivity of healthy individuals and cancer patients to microscopically characterized areas of breast tissue.[29] Another in vitro procedure is the determination of reactivity to RIII-Gp55, which is the major envelope glycoprotein of the RIII strain murine mammary tumor tissue.[36, 219]

In vivo CMI is commonly evaluated by means of skin testing, which involves the development of erythema and induration 24 to 48 hours after the intradermal injection of an antigen. Black and Leis[27, 28] have modified Redbuck's[172] skin window (SW) procedure by using specific tumor-related antigens on the SW. To date, approximately 2000 SW tests have been performed on several hundred patients over a wide range of postoperative intervals, using cryostat sections of autologous breast cancer tissue and purified Gp55 as targets.[22] Response patterns to autologous breast cancer tissue by SW are characterized by prominent, compact accumulations of histiocytic cells and/or aggregates of lymphoblastoid cells.

The majority of Stage 0 cancer patients are reactive to autologous and homologous in situ carcinomas within the first three postoperative years as determined by LMI assays, but normotypic breast tissue does not show such reactivity.[22, 35, 212] Positive SW responses were found in 78 percent of patients with Stage 0 breast cancers tested against autologous cancer tissue within the first three postoperative years. Response patterns were inversely correlated with the subsequent development of metastatic disease among breast cancer patients.[34] The SW procedure also demonstrated that Stage 0 breast cancer patients typically responded in simultaneous tests to autologous breast cancer and to Gp55 in a similar fashion, both qualitatively and quantitatively.[35] Negative response to Gp55 in patients with invasive breast cancer was usually accompanied by a lack of reactivity to autologous breast cancer tissue. Positive SW reactivity to Gp55 in association with simultaneous reactivity to autologous invasive breast cancer tissue occurred in 58 percent of the patients tested. When patients react against their autologous cancers, these cancers are obviously antigenic. Failure of response may be due to lack of tumor antigenicity and/or specific host cell-mediated immunity. SW testing should be done against both Gp55 and autologous breast cancer tissue. Patients who have positive SW tests to autologous breast cancer tissue have a reduced risk of developing recurrent disease. There are some patients who have negative SW responses to autologous breast cancer tissue but positive responses to Gp55 who should also be at reduced risk.

Positive SW reactivity to NG-classified autologous breast cancers, 1 to 12 months postoperatively, was associated with a reduced risk of systemic metastases within the next four years independent of the tumor size or stage at the time of diagnosis.[35] Black and Zachrau[35] felt that their studies indicated that prognostically different subpopulations of breast cancer patients could be identified according to tumor-host interactions in individual patients. They concluded that the evaluation of host CMI against autologous breast cancer and Gp55 was pertinent to the assessment of the patient's risk for developing recurrent disease.

TREATMENT

Despite the pessimistic attitude promoted by such suggestions as McDonald's, that human breast cancer is biologically predetermined from its onset, there is no question that treatment is far better than no treatment. A baseline for assessing the value of therapy in patients with primary breast cancer is provided by the clinical course of this disease when it is untreated. A number of authors have published on this subject. Vermund[209] assembled data from six of these studies. The survival rates in this collected series of 1308 patients, dated from the beginning of the disease, was 19 percent for five years and 5 percent for ten years. Bloom et al.,[41] in a review of 250 untreated cases from the cancer charity ward at the Middlesex Hospital in England, found an absolute survival rate of 18 percent at five years and 4 percent at ten years. Bloom[38] reviewed reports of other authors and together with the aforementioned cases collected a total of 1728 untreated breast cancers with a mean survival rate of 39.9 months. Absolute survival rates varied from 12 percent to 22 percent at five years and from 3.6 percent to 6.6 percent at ten years. He estimated that slightly more than 5 percent of patients with breast cancers in England between 1950 and 1962 were untreated.

Everson and Cole,[74] in a unique book entitled *Spontaneous Regression of Cancer,* reviewed the world literature from 1900 to 1965 and studied cases described in personal communications. They were able to find only 176 cases that they considered to adequately document criteria for spontaneous cancer regressions. Six of these were breast cancers. In the tumor-host relationship, it seems that biological control of cancer without therapy is a possibility, although this would be an extreme rarity.

Despite the possibility that the data pertaining to untreated cases may be biased as to case selection, there is a dramatic difference in survival rates of treated versus untreated cancer patients. Currently, crude, absolute, NED survival rates for patients with potentially curable breast cancers (Stages 0, I and II) should be in the range of 60 to 65 percent, at ten years. In evaluating the reported survival rates obtained with different therapeutic regimens, the statistical method used for determining the figures must be clearly understood. To properly compare the results of various types of treatment, the same methods of statistical evaluation must be used. There are considerable differences in survival rates depending on the method of reporting, i.e., observed or crude, relative or NED. There are also differences in observed and crude survival rates depending on whether they are reported as absolute, actuarial (life-table), or Kaplan-Meier (product limit) results.[143]

As to appropriate therapy, surgery is the primary modality offering diagnostic accuracy, the removal of the tumor volume, and tissues for prognostic evaluation tests. Humphrey et al.[116] emphasized that a large tumor burden has a deleterious effect on immune responsiveness, resulting in a stage of immunosuppression or tumor enhancement; this emphasizes the importance of complete removal of the primary cancer and any metastatic regional nodes. It should also be noted that the best results of adjuvant systemic therapy are obtained in individuals with minimal tumor burden.[170]

Today radical and extended radical mastectomies are rarely utilized, and the main options for patients with potentially curable breast cancer are either some type of modified mastectomy with selected breast reconstruction[138, 142] or a breast conservation procedure utilizing local excision, axillary dissection, and primary radiotherapy.[138, 140, 170] At present the latter seems to offer a viable alternative to mastectomy in selected patients with early cancers, with equivalent ten-year survival results.[138] However, long periods of observation with extended analyses must elapse before the results with local excision and radiotherapy for breast conservation can be properly assessed, since local recurrences and other adverse effects can occur many years after this type of therapy.[170] It must also be emphasized that some 25 to 30 percent of women are not good candidates for breast conservation procedures and radiotherapy.[27] Data from some of the prospective clinical trials support the concept that adequate local treatment will reduce recurrences, and hence systemic spread, suggesting that this principle should not be abandoned at the present time.[170]

As previously stated, there is well-documented evidence to show that operations designed to preserve the breast *without* adjuvant therapy (radiotherapy and/or chemotherapy) result in high local recurrence rates that range from 18 percent to 37 percent,[58, 77, 100, 101, 199] and that deleteriously influence survival rates.

Regardless of their value, surgery and radiotherapy can only enhance local-regional control. Adjuvant chemotherapy,[112, 145, 158] endocrine therapy,[112, 145, 158] immunotherapy,[33, 35, 72] and even dietary therapy[154, 217] offer important systemic approaches to the management of this disease.[138] The reported gains derived from modern adjuvant therapy programs strongly suggest that this approach be utilized in patients who are identified, by prognostic parameters, as having an increased risk for systemic disease.

The patient's age and constitutional physiological status are factors that may influence the type of treatment and prognosis. The outcome for patients with breast cancers is worse in younger women (under 35 years of age), in older patients (over 75 years of age), and in patients in poor physiological condition (i.e., concurrent cardiovascular pulmonary diseases). The poor prognosis in older patients and those with a compromised status from concurrent systemic disease is, in large part, secondary to less aggressive treatment, but the poor prognosis in younger patients is evident even when other good prognostic factors are present and when the treatment plan is excellent.[75, 114]

CONCLUSIONS

To date, despite changing concepts, there is no unified hypothesis to explain the biology of breast cancer, which is a complex and heterogeneous disease. Parameters for tumor aggressiveness measurements are mandatory for determining the prognosis of patients with breast cancer, both for disease-free survival and for overall survival. These parameters also serve as predictors regarding results obtainable by various types of local-regional therapies and systemic therapies, enabling the selection of appropriate therapeutic modalities for individual patients.

It is of the utmost importance to continue the search for more sensitive, readily reproducible, and reliable prognostic parameters as to the aggressiveness of specific breast cancers so as to determine appropriate therapy. Since noninvasive, *in situ* cancers are virtually 100 percent curable by total mastectomy, many centers advocate this treatment. Lesser procedures are rejected on the basis of this cure rate, as well as on the frequent multicentricity of these lesions and their high rate of developing into invasive cancers when treated by excision only. In the same way, most centers do not use segmental or partial mastectomy alone, without radiation, since the local recurrence rate is unacceptably high. Better prognostic parameters could identify which patients could be treated safely by lesser procedures.[137a]

In an effort to determine whether simple excision of a noninvasive or invasive cancer was adequate therapy, Nieroda et al.[166a] developed a surgical detection method that uses a hand-held gamma detecting probe, following the injection of the radiolabeled monoclonal antibody B72.3, to study the remaining breast. Their preliminary data indicate that this technique can identify residual, subclinical, and multicentric deposits of carcinoma in the remaining breast tissue, which offers hope for identifying patients who might be adequately treated by simple excision.

It is well recognized that one of the most important discriminants in predicting prognosis is the presence or absence of axillary node metastases. Both of the current main treatment options for women with invasive breast cancer require axillary gland dissection for staging, i.e., modified mastectomy or breast conservation with radiotherapy, with a resulting increase in cost and morbidity to the patient, especially as related to arm edema. Furthermore, nothing is learned about the status of the internal mammary nodes. One of the most exciting future prospects avoids this axillary dissection. Both the axillary and the internal mammary nodes are assayed by regionally administering radiolabeled monoclonal antibodies and scanning the nodal areas with a gamma camera for signs of metastasis.[91a, 137a, 184, 194a]

Beyond the need for better prognostic parameters to identify those women with *in situ* and early invasive breast cancers that could be safely managed with lesser procedures, there is a similar need to determine which patients need adjuvant systemic chemoendocrine therapy. Although the percentage of improvement in overall survival is currently being questioned,[137a] there is general agreement that adjuvant systemic therapy in women with Stage II breast cancer improves disease-free survival (DFS) and overall survival (OS). There also seems to be agreement that a six-month course of adjuvant chemotherapy with CMF should be standard treatment for node-positive premenopausal women and that tamoxifen should be the standard therapy for postmenopausal node- and hormone receptor–positive women, administered over a five-year period.[137a]

The use of adjuvant systemic therapy in node-negative women is a much more debatable issue. The "clinical alert" issued by the NCI in 1988[51a] reported that data from three clinical trials showed that adjuvant hormonal or cytotoxic chemotherapy resulted in a statistically significant improvement in disease-free survival in both pre- and postmenopausal node-negative patients. This report caused clinicians to prematurely give adjuvant therapy to all node-negative patients, a group that increases by about 70,000 new cases yearly in the United States. Since some 70 to 75 percent of patients in this group have a good prognosis, it is of paramount importance to identify the subgroup of patients who could be benefited, based on good prognostic parameters, rather than to give adjuvant therapy to all node-negative women. The majority would not be benefited, and at best, one could only estimate a very small percentage improvement in overall survival.[137a, 138]

McGuire[155a] feels that even at the present time it is possible to identify over 50 percent of node-negative patients who fall into a very favorable prognostic group and who should not receive any adjuvant therapy (i.e., 42 percent who have tumors less than 2 cm in size with a relative survival rate at five years of 96.3 percent, and 28 percent who have tumors with normal DNA and a slow growth rate who have a 90 percent disease-free survival at five years). It is also possible to identify 30 to 40 percent of these patients who have high-risk profiles for recurrence and who could be benefited by adjuvant therapy.

The standard prognostic parameters, including the invasive status of the tumor as well as its size, growth rate, nuclear grade, multicentricity, and histologic type, and the axillary nodal status, have been supplemented by cell-mediated immunity studies, i.e., skin window tests of autologous breast cancer tissue and purified Gp-55, and by measurements of estrogen and progesterone levels. Now flow-cell cytometry can indicate how aggressive or virulent a tumor is and how rapidly it is growing by determining its ploidy (amount of DNA in the cells) and the level of the S-phase fraction (percentage of new DNA being made by the cells). Thymidine labeling offers a proliferative index with a prognostic power independent of stage and estrogen and progesterone receptor status. The importance of the degree of differentiation of a tumor, as determined by its nuclear grade, is well recognized, and now monoclonal antibody studies, such as the monoclonal antibody DF-3, offer independent determinations of the degree of differentiation of a cancer. Genetic cloning and research hold great promise for the future. Currently, the human homologue of the transforming gene *neu* has been cloned and is referred to as HER-2/*neu* oncogene protein. It is a significant independent predictor of both disease-free survival and overall survival in node-positive breast cancer patients.[199a] All available prognostic indicators should be used, whenever possible, in order to determine the most appropriate form of therapy.

References

1. Ackerman LV: Surgical Pathology. 4th ed. St. Louis, CV Mosby, 1968.
2. Adair FE: Surgical problems involved in breast cancer. Ann R Coll Surg Engl 4:360–380, 1949.
3. Adair F, Berg J, Joubert L, Robbins GF: Long term follow up of breast cancer patients: The 30-year report. Cancer 33:1145–1150, 1974.
4. American Cancer Society: Cancer Facts & Figures—1989. New York, American Cancer Society, 1989.
5. American College of Surgeons Commission on Cancer: Final Report on Long-Term Patient Care Evaluation Study for Carcinoma of the Female Breast. ACS Bulletin, 1979, pp 1–42.
6. American Joint Committee on Cancer: Manual for Staging of Cancer. 2nd ed. Philadelphia, JB Lippincott, 1983.
7. American Joint Committee on Cancer: Manual for Staging of Cancer. 3rd ed. Philadelphia, JB Lippincott, 1988.
8. Atkin NB, Kay R: Prognostic significance of modal DNA value and other factors in malignant tumors based on 1,465 cases. Br J Cancer 40:210–221, 1979.
9. Attiyeh FF, Jensen M, Huvos AG, Frachia A: Axillary micrometastases and macrometastases in carcinoma of the breast. Surg Gynecol Obstet 144:839–842, 1977.
10. Barlogie B, Raber MN, Schumann J, Johnson TS, Drewinko B, Swartzendruber DE, Göbde W, Andreeff M, Freireich EJ: Flow cytometry in clinical cancer research. Cancer Res 43:3982–3997, 1983.
11. Barnett RN, Eisenberg H: Histologic grading in breast cancer. Conn Med 28:123, 1964.
12. Beahrs OH, Shapiro S, Smart S: Report of the working group to review NCI/ACS Breast Cancer Demonstration Detection Projects. September 1977.
13. Beatson GT: On the treatment of inoperable carcinoma of the mammary: Suggestion of a new method of treatment with illustrative case. Lancet 2:104–107, 1896.
14. Bell JR, Friedell GH, Goldenberg IS: Prognostic significance of pathologic findings in human breast carcinoma. Surg Gynecol Obstet 129:258–262, 1969.
15. Berg JW: The significance of axillary node levels in the study of breast cancer. Cancer 8:776–778, 1955.
16. Bergson J, Gage RP: Survival curve for breast cancer patients following treatment. J Am Stat Assoc 47:501, 1952.
17. Berkson JS, Harrington SW, Clagett OT, et al: Mortality and survival in surgically treated cancer of the breast. Proc Mayo Clin 32:645–670, 1957.
18. Bhatia SK, Saclarides J, Witt TR, Bonomi PD, Anderson KM, Economou SG: Hormone receptor studies in axillary metastases from occult breast cancers. Cancer 59:1170–1172, 1987.
19. Bishop HM, Blamey RW, Elston CW, Haybittle JL: Relationship of estrogen receptor status to survival in breast cancer. Lancet 2:283–287, 1979.
20. Black MM: Cellular and biologic manifestations of immunogenicity in precancerous mastopathy. Natl Cancer Inst Monogr 35:73–82, 1972.
21. Black MM: Human breast cancer: A model for cancer immunology. Isr J Med Sci 9:284–299, 1973.
22. Black MM: Structural, antigenic and biological characteristics of precancerous mastopathy. Cancer Res 36:2596–2604, 1976.
23. Black MM, Asire AJ: Palpable axillary lymph nodes in cancer of the breast. Cancer 23:251–259, 1969.
24. Black MM, Barclay THC, Hankey BF: Prognosis in breast cancer utilizing histologic characteristics of the primary tumor. Cancer 36:2048–2055, 1975.
25. Black MM, Chabon AB: In situ carcinoma of the breast. Pathol Annu 4:185, 1969.
26. Black MM, Kwon S: Prognostic factors in breast cancer. *In* Gallager HG, Leis HP Jr, Snyderman RK, Urban JA (eds): The Breast. St. Louis, CV Mosby, 1978, p 297.
27. Black MM, Leis HP Jr: Human breast carcinoma. Cellular responses to autologous breast cancer: Skin window procedure. NY State J Med 70:2583–2589, 1970.
28. Black MM, Leis HP Jr: Cellular responses to autologous breast

cancer tissue: Sequential observations. Cancer 32:384–389, 1973.

29. Black MM, Leis HP Jr, Shore B, Zachrau RE: Cellular hypersensitivity to breast cancer: Assessment by a leukocyte migration procedure. Cancer 33:952–958, 1974.

30. Black MM, Opler SR, Speer FD: Survival in breast cancer cases in relation to the structure of the primary tumor and regional lymph nodes. Surg Gynecol Obstet 100:543–551, 1955.

31. Black MM, Speer FD: Nuclear structure in cancer tissues. Surg Gynecol Obstet 105:97, 1957.

32. Black MM, Speer FD, Opler SR: Structural representations of tumor-host relationship in mammary carcinoma. Biologic and prognostic significance. Am J Clin Pathol 26:250–265, 1956.

33. Black MM, Zachrau RE: Immunotherapy of breast cancer? *In* Gallager HS, Leis HP Jr, Snyderman RK, Urban JA (eds): The Breast. St. Louis, CV Mosby, 1978, p 393.

34. Black MM, Zachrau RE: Antitumor immunity in breast cancer patients. J Reprod Med 23:21, 1979.

35. Black MM, Zachrau RE: Immune mechanisms: Prognostic, therapeutic and preventive significance. *In* Ariel IM, Cleary JB (eds): Breast Cancer: Diagnosis and Treatment. New York, McGraw-Hill, 1987, p 128.

36. Black MM, Zachrau RE, Shore B, Dion AS, Leis HP Jr: Cellular immunity to autologous breast cancer and RIII-murine mammary tumor virus preparations. Cancer Res 38:2068–2076, 1978.

37. Bloom HJG: Prognosis in carcinoma of the breast. Br J Cancer 4:259–288, 1950.

38. Bloom HJG: Survival of women with untreated breast cancer—past and present. *In* Forrest APM, Kumkler PB, (eds): Prognostic Factors in Breast Cancer. Baltimore, Williams & Wilkins, 1968, p 3.

39. Bloom HJG, Richardson WW: Histologic grading and prognosis in breast cancer. A study of 1,409 cases of which 359 have been followed fifteen years. Br J Cancer 11:359, 1957.

40. Bloom HJG, Richardson WW, Field JR: Host resistance and survival in carcinoma of the breast—study of 104 cases of medullary carcinoma in a series of 1,411 cases of breast cancer followed for twenty years. Br Med J 3:181, 1970.

41. Bloom HJG, Richardson WW, Harris EJ: Natural history of untreated breast cancer (1805–1933). Comparison of untreated and treated cases according to histological grade of malignancy. Br Med J 2:213, 1962.

42. Brigati J, Bloom N, Tobin B, et al: Morphologic methods of steroid hormone receptor analysis in human breast cancer: A review. Breast 5:27, 1979.

43. Broders AC: Squamous-cell epithelioma of the lip. Study of 537 cases. JAMA 74:656, 1920.

44. Cammoun H, Contesso G, Rouesse J: Les adenocarcinomes cylindromateaux du sein. Ann Anat Pathol 17:143, 1972.

45. Carbone PP: Options in breast cancer therapy. Hosp Pract 1:53, 1981.

46. Carstens PHB, Huvos AG, Foote FW Jr, et al: Tubular carcinoma of the breast—a clinicopathologic study of thirty-five cases. Am J Clin Pathol 58:231, 1972.

47. Carter D, Orr SL, Merino MJ: Intracystic papillary carcinoma of the breast. Cancer 52:14, 1983.

48. Carter D, Pipkin RD, Shepard RH, et al: Relationship of necrosis and tumor border to lymph node metastases and ten-year survival in carcinoma of the breast. Am J Surg Pathol 2:39, 1978.

49. Castiglioni A: A History of Medicine: A.C. Celsus. New York, Alfred A. Knopf, 1941, p 204.

50. Cavanzo RJ, Taylor HB: Adenoid cystic carcinoma of the breast. Cancer 24:740, 1969.

51. Champion HR, Wallace IW, Prescott RJ: Histology in breast cancer prognosis. Br J Cancer 26:129, 1972.

52. Colcher D, Haand PH, Nuti M, et al: A spectrum of monoclonal antibodies reactive with human mammary tumor cells. Proc Acad Sci USA 78:3199, 1981.

53. Cooke T, George D, Shields R, Maynard P, Griffiths K: Estrogen receptors and prognosis in early breast cancer. Lancet 1:995–997, 1979.

54. Coombes RC, Deanally DP, Ellioson ML, et al: Markers in breast and lung cancers. Ann Clin Biochem 19:263, 1982.

55. Coombes RC, Gazet JC, Sloane JP, et al: Biochemical markers in breast cancer. Lancet 2:132, 1977.

56. Cooper HS, Patchefsky AS, Krall RA: Tubular carcinoma of the breast. Cancer 42:2334, 1978.

57. Cox DR: Regression models and life-tables. J R Stat Soc (B) 34:187, 1972.

58. Crile GC Jr: The incidence of local recurrences of carcinoma of the breast. Surg Gynecol Obstet 156:497–498, 1983.

59. Cutler SJ, Axtell LM: Portioning of a patient population with respect to different mortality risks. J Am Stat Assoc 58:701, 1963.

60. Cutler SJ, Connelly RE: Mammary cancer trends. Cancer 23:767, 1969.

61. Cutler SJ, Zipin C, Asire AJ: The prognostic significance of palpable lymph nodes in breast cancer. Cancer 23:243, 1969.

62. Davies RK, Quinlan DM, McKegney P, Kimball CP, Chase P: Organic factors and psychologic adjustment in advanced cancer patients. Psychosom Med 35:464–471, 1973.

63. Davis BW, Gelber RD, Goldhirsch A, Hartmann WH, Locher GW, Reed R, Golouh R, Säve-Söderbergh J, Holloway L, Russell I, Rudenstam CM: Prognostic significance of tumor grade in clinical trials of adjuvant therapy for breast cancer with axillary lymph node metastasis. Cancer 58:2662–2670, 1986.

64. Delbert P, Mendaro A: Les Cancers du Sein. Paris, Masson, 1927.

65. Denoix P: Treatment of Malignant Breast Tumors. New York, Springer-Verlag, 1970.

66. Derogatis LR, Abeloff MD, Melisaratos N: Psychological coping mechanisms and survival time in metastatic breast cancer. JAMA 242:1504–1508, 1979.

67. De Sombre ER, Jensen EV: Estrophilin assays in breast cancer. Cancer 46:2783, 1980.

68. Devesa SS, Silverman DT: Cancer incidence and mortality trends in the United States: 1935–1974. Natl Cancer Inst 60:545–571, 1978.

69. Dockerty MB: The grading and typing of carcinoma of the breast. J Iowa Med Soc 54:289–294, 1964.

70. Donegan WL: Primary treatment options and end results. *In* Spratt JS, Donegan WL (eds): Cancer of the Breast. Philadelphia, WB Saunders, 1979, p 267.

71. Duncan W, Kerr GR: The curability of breast cancer. Br Med J 2:781, 1976.

72. Durant JR: Immunotherapy of cancer: The end of the beginning? N Engl J Med 316:939–941, 1987.

73. Eggers C, deCholnoky T, Jesup DS: Cancer of the breast. Ann Surg 113:321–340, 1941.

74. Everson TC, Cole WH: Spontaneous Regression of Cancer. Philadelphia, WB Saunders, 1966.

75. Falkson G, Gelman RS, Pretorius FJ: Age as a prognostic factor in recurrent breast cancer. J Clin Oncol 4:663–671, 1986.

76. Farrow JH: Late recurrence of breast cancer. JAMA 195:157, 1966.

77. Fisher B, Bauer M, Margolese R, Poisson R, Pilch Y, Redmond C, Fisher E, Wolmark N, Deutsch M, Montague E, Saffer E, Wickerham L, Lerner H, Glass A, Shibata H, Deckers P, Ketcham A, Oishi R, Russell I: Five-year results of a randomized clinical trial comparing total mastectomy and segmental mastectomy with or without radiation in the treatment of breast cancer. N Engl J Med 312:665–673, 1985.

78. Fisher B, Fisher ER, Redmond C, et al: Tumor nuclear grade, estrogen receptor, and progesterone receptor: Their value alone or in combination as indicators of outcome following adjuvant therapy for breast cancer. Breast Cancer Res Treat 7:147, 1986.

79. Fisher B, Redmond C, Fisher ER, and participating NSABP investigators: The contribution of recent NSABP clinical trials of primary breast cancer therapy to an understanding of tumor biology. An overview of findings. Cancer 46:1009–1025, 1980.

80. Fisher B, Slack NH, Bross IDJ: Cancer of the breast. Size of neoplasm and prognosis. Cancer 24:1071, 1969.

81. Fisher B, Wolmark N, Redmond C, Deutsch MD, Fisher E, and participating NSABP investigators: Findings from NSABP Protocol No. B-04. Cancer 48:1863, 1981.

82. Fisher ER: The pathologist's role in the diagnosis and treatment of invasive breast cancer. Surg Clin North Am 58:705, 1978.

83. Fisher ER, Gregorio RM, Fisher B: The pathology of invasive breast cancer: A syllabus derived from the findings of the National Surgical Adjuvant Breast Project (Protocol No. 4). Cancer 36:1, 1975.

84. Fisher ER, Gregorio R, Fisher B: Prognostic significance of histopathology. *In* Stoll BA (ed): Risk Factors in Breast Cancer. London, Heinemann Medical Books, 1976, p 83.

85. Fisher ER, Gregorio R, Redmond C, Vellios F, Sommers SC, Fisher B, Sheldon C: Pathologic findings from the NSABP trial (B-04). Observations concerning the multicentricity of mammary cancer. Cancer 35:247–254, 1975.

86. Fisher ER, Gregorio RM, Redmond C, Sunkim WHA, Fisher B: Pathologic findings from the National Surgical Adjuvant Breast Project (Protocol No. 4). Am J Clin Pathol 65:439–444, 1976.

87. Fisher ER, Sass R, Fisher B: Pathologic findings from the National Surgical Adjuvant Project. Cancer 59:1554–1559, 1987.

88. Frazier TG, Copeland EM, Gallager HS, Paulus DD Jr, White EC: Prognosis and treatment in minimal breast cancer. Am J Surg 133:697–699, 1977.

89. Friedman BA, Oberman HA: Adenoid cystic carcinoma of the breast. Am J Clin Pathol 54:1–14, 1970.

90. Friedell GH, Betts A, Sommers SC: The prognostic value of blood vessel invasion and lymphocyte infiltrates in breast carcinoma. Cancer 18:164, 1965.

91. Fox MS: On the diagnosis and treatment of breast cancer. JAMA 241:489, 1979.

92. Gallager HS, Martin JF: The study of mammary carcinoma by mammography and whole organ sectioning: Early observations. Cancer 23:855, 1969.

93. Galloway JR, Woolner LB, Clagett OT: Adenoid cystic carcinoma of the breast. Surg Gynecol Obstet 122:1289, 1966.

94. Gautherie M, Gros SM: Breast thermography and cancer risk prediction. Cancer 45:51, 1980.

95. Gershon-Cohen J, Berger SM, Klockstein HS: Roentgenography of breast cancer moderating concept of biologic predeterminism. Cancer 16:961, 1963.

96. Geschickter CF: Gelatinous mammary cancer. Ann Surg 108:321, 1938.

97. Gold RH, Main G, Zippin C, Annes GP: Infiltration of mammary carcinomas as an indicator of axillary metastases. Cancer 29:35–40, 1972.

98. Goldenberg IS, Bailar JC III, Hayes MA, Lowry R: Female breast cancer re-evaluation. Ann Surg 154:397–407, 1961.

99. Goodson WH III: The incidence and significance of local recurrence. *In* Ariel IM, Cleary JB (eds): Breast Cancer: Diagnosis and Treatment. New York, McGraw-Hill, 1987, p 300.

100. Greening WP, Montgomery AC, Growing NF: Report on a pilot study of treatment of breast cancer by quadrantic excision with axillary dissection and no other therapy. J R Soc Med 71:261, 1978.

101. Greening WP, Montgomery AC, Growing NF: Treatment of breast cancer by quadrantic excision with axillary dissection. J R Soc Med 72:710, 1979.

102. Greenough RB: Varying degrees of malignancy in cancer of the breast. J Cancer Res 9:453, 1925.

103. Groshong LE: Adenocystic carcinoma of the breast. Arch Surg 92:424, 1966.

104. Haagensen CD: The bases for the histologic grading of carcinoma of the breast. Am J Cancer 19:285, 1933.

105. Haagensen CD: Diseases of the Breast. Philadelphia, WB Saunders, 1971.

106. Haagensen DE, Kister SJ, Panick J, Giannola T, Hansen HJ, Wells SA: Comparative evaluation of carcinoembryonic antigen and gross cystic disease fluid protein as plasma markers for human breast carcinoma. Cancer 42:1642–1646, 1978.

107. Halsted WS: Operations for carcinoma of the breast. Johns Hopkins Hosp Rep 2:227, 1890–1.

108. Hart D: Intracystic papillomatous tumors of the breast, benign and malignant. Arch Surg 14:783, 1927.

109. Hawkins JW: Evaluation of breast cancer therapy as a guide to control programs. J Natl Cancer Inst 4:445, 1944.

110. Hayes JA, Brooks V: Adenoid cystic carcinoma of the breast. Arch Surg 94:134–135, 1967.

111. Hellstrom KE, Hellstrom I: Lymphocyte-mediated cytotoxicity and blocking serum activity to tumor antigens. Adv Immunol 18:209–227, 1974.

112. Henderson IC: Adjuvant chemotherapy and endocrine therapy in patients with operable breast cancer. *In* Cancer: Principles and Practice of Oncology Updates. Philadelphia, JB Lippincott, 1(3), 1987.

113. Hirschl S, Black MM, Kwon CS: Ultrastructural characteristics of sinus histiocytic reaction in lymph nodes draining various stages of breast cancer. Cancer 38:807, 1976.

114. Host H, Lund E: Age as a prognostic factor in breast cancer. Cancer 57:2217–2221, 1986.

115. Hultborn KA, Tornberg B: Mammary carcinoma: The biologic character of mammary cancer studied in 517 cases by a new form of malignant grading. Acta Radiol (Suppl) 196:1, 1960.

116. Humphrey LJ, Singla O, Volenec FJ: Immunologic responsiveness of the breast cancer patient. Cancer 46:893–898, 1980.

117. Hutter RVP: At last—worldwide agreement on the staging of cancer. Arch Surg 122:1235, 1987.

118. Hutter RVP: The influence of pathologic factors on breast cancer management. Cancer 46:961–976, 1980.

119. Hutter RVP, Rickert RR: The pathologic basis for therapeutic considerations in minimal lesions of the breast. J Breast 2:26, 1976.

120. Huvos AG, Hutter RVP, Berg JW: Significance of axillary macrometastases and micrometastases in mammary cancer. Am Surg 173:44–46, 1971.

121. Jamison RN, Burish TG, Wallston KA: Psychogenic factors in predicting survival of breast cancer patients. J Clin Oncol 5:768–772, 1987.

122. Jensen EV, DeSombre R, Jungblut PW: Estrogen receptors in hormone responsive tissues and tumors. *In* Wissler RN, Dao TL, Wood S Jr (eds): Endogenous Factors Influencing Host-Tumor Balance. Chicago, University of Chicago Press, 1967.

123. Johnstone FR: Carcinoma of the breast: Influence of size of primary lesion and lymph node involvement based on selective biopsy. Am J Surg 124:158–164, 1972.

124. Kennedy BJ, Tellegen A, Kennedy H, Havernick N: Psychological response of patients cured of advanced cancer. Cancer 38:2184–2191, 1976.

125. Kiang DT, Kennedy BJ: Estrogen receptor assay in the differential diagnosis of adenocarcinoma. JAMA 233:32–34, 1977.

126. Kister SJ, Sommers SC, Haagensen CD, Cooley E: Re-evaluation of blood vessel invasion as a prognostic factor in carcinoma of the breast. Cancer 19:1213–1218, 1966.

127. Koscielny S, Tubiana M, Lekle MG, Valleron AJ, Mouriesse H, Contesso G, Sarrazin D: Breast cancer: Relationship between the size of the primary tumor and the probability of metastatic dissemination. Br J Cancer 49:709–715, 1984.

128. Kraus FT, Neubecker RD: The differential diagnosis of papillary tumors of the breast. Cancer 15:444–455, 1962.

129. Kufe D, Inghirami G, Abe M, et al: Differential reactivity of monoclonal antibody (DF-3) with human malignant versus benign breast tumors. Hybridoma 3:223, 1984.

130. Kufe D, Nadler L, Sargent L, Shapiro H, Hand P, Austin F, Colcher D, Schlom J: Biological behavior of human breast carcinoma–associated antigens expressed during cellular proliferation. Cancer Res 43:851–857, 1983.

131. Lane N, Goskel H, Salerno A, Haagenson CD: Clinicopathologic analysis of the surgical curability of breast cancers. A minimal ten-year study of personal cases. Ann Surg 153:483–498, 1961.

132. Leak GH, Berg J, Wesp EH, Robbins GF: Primary treatment of patients with resectable breast cancer. Surg Gynecol Obstet 129:953–959, 1969.

133. Lee SH: Cytochemical study of estrogen receptor in human mammary cancer. Am J Clin Pathol 70:197, 1978.

134. Leis HP Jr: Prognosis and recurrence of breast cancer. *In* Leis HP Jr: Diagnosis and Treatment of Breast Lesions. Flushing NY, Medical Examination Publishing Co, 1970, p 121.

135. Leis HP Jr: Staging of breast cancer. *In* Leis HP Jr: Diagnosis and Treatment of Breast Lesions. Flushing NY, Medical Examination Publishing Co. 1970, p 168.

136. Leis HP Jr: Criteria and standards for evaluation of treatment results in breast cancer. *In* Gallager HS, Leis HP Jr, Snyderman RK, Urban JA (eds): The Breast. St. Louis, CV Mosby, 1978, p 195.

137. Leis HP Jr: Prognosis in breast cancer. *In* Stromeck JO, Rosato FO (eds): Surgery of the Breast: Diagnosis and Treatment of Breast Diseases. New York, Georg Thieme Verlag, 1986, p 119.

137a. Leis HP Jr: Current methods for biopsy and treatment of potentially curable breast cancer. Int Surg 75:1–7, 1990.

138. Leis HP Jr: The role of prevention, early detection, and appropriate therapy in the war against breast cancer. Contemp Surg 34:11, 1989.

139. Leis HP Jr, Cammarata A: Modified radical mastectomy: The moderate selective surgical approach. *In* Feig SA, McLelland R (eds): Breast Carcinoma: Current Diagnosis and Treatment. New York, Masson Publishing USA, 1983, p 445.

140. Leis HP Jr, Cammarata A, LaRaja RD: Update in primary potentially curable breast cancer therapy. Contemp Surg 26:13, 1985.

141. Leis HP Jr, Cammarata A, La Raja RD: The management of clinically nonpalpable breast cancer. *In* Ariel IM, Cleary JB (eds): Breast Cancer: Diagnosis and Treatment. New York, McGraw-Hill, 1987, p 205.

142. Leis HP Jr, Greene FL, Cammarata A, et al: The modified radical mastectomy: What does it mean? Contemp Surg 30:35, 1987.

143. Leis HP Jr, Robbins GF, Greene FL, et al: Breast cancer statistics: Use and misuse. J Intens Surg 71:237, 1986.

144. Lesser ML, Rosen PP, Kinne DW: Multicentricity and bilaterality in invasive breast carcinomas. Surgery 91:234, 1982.

145. Lippman ME: The NIH Consensus Development Conference on adjuvant chemotherapy for breast cancer. Breast Cancer Res Treat 6:195, 1985.

146. Lundy J, Thor A, Maenza R, et al: Monoclonal antibody DF-3 correlates with tumor differentiation and hormone receptor status in breast cancer patients. Breast Cancer Res Treat 5:269, 1985.

147. MacDonald I: Biological predeterminism in human cancer. Surg Gynecol Obstet 92:443, 1951.

148. MacDonald I: The natural history of mammary carcinoma. Am J Surg 111:435, 1966.

149. Maguire PL: The will to live. *In* Stoll BA (ed): Mind and Cancer Prognosis. New York, Wiley, 1979, p 169.

150. Martin SA, Perez-Reyes N, Mendelsohn G: Angioinvasion in breast carcinoma. Cancer 59:1918–1922, 1987.

151. Martinez-Hernandez A, Francis DJ, Silverberg SG: Elastosis and other stromal reactions in benign and malignant breast tissue. Cancer 40:700, 1977.

152. Maynard PV, Daview CJ, Blamey RW, Griffiths K, Elston W, Johnson J: Relationship between estrogen receptor content and histologic grade in human primary breast tumors. Br J Cancer 38:745–748, 1978.

153. McDivitt RW, Stewart FW, Berg JW: Tumors of the breast. Atlas of Tumor Pathology. Washington DC, Armed Forces Institute of Pathology, 1968.

154. McDougall JA: Preliminary study of diet as an adjuvant for breast cancer therapy. J Breast (Dis Breast) 10:18, 1984.

155. McGuire WL: Current status of estrogen receptors in human breast carcinoma. Cancer 36:638, 1975.

155A. McGuire WL: Adjuvant therapy of node-negative breast cancer. N Engl J Med 320:525, 1989.

156. McGuire WL, Ceriani RL, Schlom J, et al: Monoclonal antibodies, benign breast disease and cancer. Breast Cancer Res Treat 6:37, 1985.

157. McGuire WL, Clark GM, Fisher ER, et al: Predicting recurrence and survival in breast cancer. Breast Cancer Res Treat 9:27, 1987.

158. McGuire WL, Lippman ME, Buzdar A, Tormet DC: Combining endocrine and chemotherapy—any true benefits? A panel discussion. Breast Cancer Res Treat 4:251, 1984.

159. McGuire WL, Meyer JS, Kute TE: Impact of flow cytometry on predicting recurrences and survival in breast cancer patients. Breast Cancer Res Treat 5:117, 1985.

160. McGurrin JF, Doria MI Jr, Dawson PJ, Franklin WA, Karrison T, Stein HO: Assessment of tumor cell kinetics by immunohistochemistry in carcinoma of breast cancer. Cancer 59:1744–1750, 1987.

161. Melamed MR, Robbins GF, Foote FW Jr: Prognostic significance of gelatinous mammary carcinoma. Cancer 14:699, 1961.

162. Mersheimer WL, Heise HW: End results in breast cancer. *In* Cutler SJ (ed): End Results in Cancer. National Cancer Institute. Washington DC, US Government Printing Office, Report No. 3, 1968.

163. Meyer JS, McDivitt RW, Stone KR, et al: Practical breast cancer kinetics: Review and update. Breast Cancer Res Treat 4:79, 1984.

163a. Meyer JS, Province M: Proliferative index of breast carcinoma by thymidine labeling. Breast Cancer Res Treat 12:191, 1988.

164. Moore OS, Foote FW Jr: The relatively favorable prognosis of medullary carcinoma of the breast. Cancer 2:635, 1949.

165. Mourali N, Tabbane F, Hoerner GV, et al: Choice of treatment according to rate of growth. Int Cong 353:5, 1974.

166. Nemoto T, Vana J, Bedwani RN, Baker HW, McGregor FH, Murphy GP: Management and survival of female breast cancer: Results of a national survey by the American College of Surgeons. Cancer 45:2917–2924, 1980.

166a. Nieroda CA, Mojzsik C, Sardi A, Farrar WB, Hinkle G, Siddiqi MA, Ferrara PJ, James A, Schlom J, Thurston MO, Martin ED Jr: Staging carcinoma of the breast using a hand-held detecting probe and monoclonal antibody B72.3. Surg Gynecol Obstet 169:35–40, 1989.

167. NIH: Correlation Between Microscopic Characteristics of Primary Breast Tumors and Subsequent Patient Survival. NIH Guide For Grants and Contracts. Vol 9(8). Bethesda MD, June 6, 1980.

168. Norris HJ, Taylor HB: Prognosis of mucinous (gelatinous) carcinoma of the breast. Cancer 18:879, 1965.

169. Old LJ: Cancer immunology: The search for specificity—GHA Clowes Memorial Lecture. Cancer Res 41:361, 1981.

170. Osborne MP: The biologic basis for breast cancer treatment options. Bull Am Coll Surgeons 71:1, 1986.

171. Patchefsky AS, Shaber GS, Schwartz GF, Feig SA, Nerlinger RE: The pathology of breast cancer detected by mass population screening. Cancer 40:1659–1670, 1977.

172. Redbuck JW: Cytology of acute inflammation in man by two original technical procedures with particular reference to the role of lymphocytes. Doctoral thesis, University of Minnesota, 1947.

173. Richardson WW: Medullary carcinoma of the breast—a distinctive tumor type with a relatively good prognosis following radical mastectomy. Br J Cancer 10:415, 1956.

174. Ridolfi RL, Rosen PP, Port A, Kinne D, Mike V: Medullary carcinoma of the breast. A clinicopathologic study with a ten-year follow-up. Cancer 40:1365–1385, 1977.

175. Robbins GF, Leis HP Jr, Hutter RVP: A rational approach to end-result reporting of women with breast carcinoma. J Breast 3:9, 1977.

176. Rogentine G, Van Kammen D, Fox B, Docherty JP, Rosenblatt JE, Boyd SC, Bunney WE Jr: Psychological factors in the prognosis of malignant melanoma: A prospective study. Psychosom Med 41:647, 1979.

177. Rosen PP, Ashikari R, Thaler H, Isikawa S, Hirota T, Abe O, Yamamoto H, Beattie EJ, Urban JA, Mike V: A comparative study of some pathologic features of mammary carcinoma in Tokyo, Japan and New York, USA. Cancer 39:429–434, 1977.

178. Rosen PP, Fracchia AA, Urban JA, Schottenfeid P, Robbins GF: "Residual" mammary carcinoma following simulated partial mastectomy. Cancer 35:739–747, 1975.

179. Rosenberg SA, Lotzer MT, Muul LM, et al: Observation on the systemic administration of autologous lymphokine-activated killer cells and recombinant interleukin-2 to patients with metastatic cancer. N Engl J Med 313:1485, 1985.

180. Ross WL: The magnitude of the breast cancer problem. Cancer 24:1106, 1969.

181. Ruiz U, Babeu S, Schwartz MS, Soto E, McAuley RA, Friedell GH: Blood vessel invasion and lymph node metastases: Two factors affecting survival in breast cancer. Surgery 73:185, 1973.

182. Samaan NA, Buzdar AU, Aldinger KA, Schultz PN, Yang KP, Romsdahl MM, Martin R: Estrogen receptor: A prognostic factor in breast cancer. Cancer 47:554–560, 1981.

183. Sampat MB, Sirsat MV, Gangadharan P: Prognostic significance of blood vessel invasion in carcinoma of the breast in women. J Surg Oncol 8:623, 1977.

184. Schlom J: Future prospects in breast cancer research and management. *In* Lippman ME, Lichter AS, Danfort DN Jr (eds): Diagnosis and Management of Breast Cancer. Philadelphia, WB Saunders, 1988, p 549.
185. Schulenburg CA, Pepler WJ: Adenoid cystic carcinoma of the breast. Br J Surg 56:395, 1969.
186. Schwartz M: Estimates of lead time and length bias in a breast cancer screening program. Cancer 46:844, 1980.
187. Shapiro S, Venet W, Strax P, et al: Ten to fourteen-year effect of screening on breast cancer mortality. J Natl Cancer Inst 69:349, 1982.
188. Silverberg E, Lubera J: Cancer statistics 1988. Cancer 38:3, 1989.
189. Silverberg SG, Chitale AR, Levitt SH: Prognostic significance of tumor margins in mammary carcinoma. Arch Surg 102:450, 1971.
190. Silverberg SG, Kay S, Chitale AR, et al: Colloid carcinoma of the breast. Am J Clin Pathol 55:355, 1971.
191. Smart CR, Myers MH, Gloeckler LA: Implications from SEER data on breast cancer management. Cancer 41:787, 1978.
192. Smith JA, Gamez-Araujo JJ, Gallager HS, White EC, McBride CM: Carcinoma of the breast: Analyses of total lymph node involvement versus level of metastases. Cancer 39:527–532, 1977.
193. Stat O, Klinyenberg C, Franzen G, et al: A comparison of static cytofluorometry and flow cytometry for the estimation of ploidy and DNA replication in human breast cancer. Breast Cancer Res Treat 7:15, 1986.
194. Stegner HE: Pathology of malignant diseases of the breast. *In* Strombeck JO, Rosato FE (eds): Surgery of the Breast: Diagnosis and Treatment of Breast Diseases. New York, George Thieme Verlag, 1986, p 66.
194a. Sterns EE, Cochran JJ: Monoclonal antibodies in the diagnosis and treatment of carcinoma of the breast. Surg Gynecol Obstet 169:81, 1989.
195. Stoll BA: Is hope a factor in survival? *In* Stoll BA (ed): Mind and Cancer Prognosis. New York, Wiley, 1979, p 183.
196. Stout AP: Tumor grading. *In* Haagensen CD (ed): Diseases of the Breast. Philadelphia, WB Saunders, 1956, p 527.
197. Straus MB: Familiar Medical Quotations. Boston, Little Brown, 1968.
198. Tabar L, Fagerberg CJC, Gad A, et al: Reduction in mortality from breast cancer after mass screening with mammography. Randomized trial from the Breast Cancer Screening Working Group of the Swedish National Board of Health and Welfare. Lancet 1:829, 1985.
199. Tagert REB: Partial mastectomy for breast cancer. Br Med J 2:1268, 1978.
199a. Tandon AK, Clark GM, Chamness GC, et al: HER-2/neu oncogene protein and prognosis in breast cancer. J Clin Oncol 7:1120, 1989.
200. Taylor HB, Norris HJ: Well-differentiated carcinoma of the breast. Cancer 25:687, 1970.
201. Teel P, Sommers SC: Vascular invasion as a prognostic factor in breast cancer. Surg Gynecol Obstet 118:1006, 1964.
202. Thompson CH, Jones SL, Witehead RH, et al: A human breast tissue–associated antigen detected by monoclonal antibody. J Natl Cancer Inst 70:409, 1983.
203. Tomic S, Vukecevic S, Vidovic Z: Hostoloski drugi faktori u prognozi raka dojke i histoloski tip raka dojke i prognoza. Med Arch 26:3, 1972.
204. Tough IC, Carter DC, Fraser J, et al: Histologic grading in breast cancer. Br J Cancer 23:294, 1969.
205. Tsakraklides V, Olsen P, Kersey JH, et al: Prognostic significance of the regional lymph node histology in cancer of the breast. Cancer 20:1259, 1974.
206. Urban JA: Clinical experience and results of excision of the internal mammary lymph node chain in primary operable breast cancer. Cancer 12:14, 1959.
207. Van Bogaert LJ, Maldague P: Histologic variants of lipid secreting carcinoma of the breast. Virchows Arch Pathol Anat 375:345, 1977.
208. van de Velde CJH, Gallager HS, Giacco GG: Prognosis in node negative breast cancer. Breast Cancer Res Treat 8:189, 1986.
209. Vermund L: Trends in radiotherapy of breast cancer. *In* Proceedings of the Fifth National Cancer Conference. Philadelphia, JB Lippincott, 1964.
210. Waalkes TP, Enterline JP, Shaper JH, et al: Biological markers for breast cancer. Cancer 53:644, 1984.
211. Wanebo HJ, Huvos AG, Urban JA: Treatment of minimal breast cancer. Cancer 33:349, 1974.
212. Weisman AD, Worden JW: Psychosocial analysis of cancer deaths. Omega 6:61, 1979.
213. Westbrook KC, Gallager HS: Intraductal carcinoma of the breast, a comparative study. Am J Surg 130:667, 1975.
214. Woo KB, Waalkes TP, Ahmann DL, Tormey DC, Gehree CW, Oliverio VT: A quantitative approach to determining disease response during therapy using multiple biologic markers: Application to carcinoma of the breast. Cancer 41:1685–1703, 1978.
215. Wybran J, Belohradsky BH, Fudenberg HH: Unmasking by antimetabolites of receptors for sheep red blood cells on human lymphocytes. Cell Immunol 14:359, 1974.
216. Wybran J, Fudenberg HH: Thymus derived rosette forming cells. N Engl J Med 288:1072, 1973.
217. Wynder EL: Dietary factors related to breast cancer. Cancer 46:899, 1980.
218. Yeh CG, Hsi B, Ettore F: Normal epithelial antigens recognized by GB3 and GB5 are diminished in intraductal and lost in infiltrating human breast carcinomas. Breast Cancer Res Treat 8:117, 1986.
219. Zachrau RE, Black MM, Dion AS, Shore B, Williams CJ, Leis HP Jr: Specificity of the simultaneous cell-mediated immune reactivity to RIII-murine mammary tumor virus glycoprotein 55 and human breast cancer tissues. Cancer Res 38:3413, 1978.

Section VII

Mechanisms of Breast Oncogenesis and Metastases

Chapter 19

ROLE OF ONCOGENES IN HUMAN BREAST CANCER

Edward P. Gelmann, M.D. and Marc E. Lippman, M.D.

Proto-oncogenes, the cellular homologues of genes transduced or activated by transforming retroviruses, may be important in the etiology of a number of human cancers. Cellular transformation can be caused by point mutation,[20, 30, 82] gene truncation,[66] transcriptional activation,[73] gene rearrangement,[6, 94] or gene amplification[3, 25, 89] of proto-oncogenes. More than 20 proto-oncogenes, falling into five general categories, have been identified: (1) growth factors (e.g., *sis*[108] and perhaps *int-2*[31]; (2) growth factor and hormone receptors (e.g., *erbB*,[35] *fms*,[93] and *erbA*[88]); (3) intracellular tyrosine (e.g., *src*[90]) and serine (e.g., *mos*[14]) kinases; (4) nuclear associated oncogenes (e.g., *fos*,[87] *myc*,[79] *myb*,[59] and *jun*[16]); and (5) G protein–like molecules (e.g., *ras*[48]).

This chapter will review studies of the known c-*onc* genes and their expression or activation in human breast cancer. We will summarize information on proto-oncogenes identified in the murine mammary tumor virus model system. We will also discuss results of transfection experiments designed to identify dominant transforming genes in cancerous tissues. Lastly, we will discuss the effect of expression of known *onc* genes on the phenotype of mammary epithelial cells in vitro and the ability of *onc* genes to affect the development of mammary cancer in transgenic mice.

The discovery that acutely transforming retroviruses had transduced *onc* genes from their host cell genomes led to the identification and characterization of corresponding cellular proto-oncogenes.[12] Great effort was dedicated to defining roles for these proto-oncogenes both as normal elements in cellular physiology and as mediators in the development of neoplasia. In a few cases, proto-oncogenes have been implicated in the etiology of specific human malignancies. Two examples are Burkitt's lymphoma, in which c-*myc* gene activation is associated with chromosomal translocations affecting chromosome 8,[66] and chronic myelogenous leukemia, in

which the Philadelphia chromosome translocation, t(9;22)[3, 48] alters the structure of the c-*abl* gene transcript and protein product.[60, 94] In both these cases, the proximity of the implicated proto-oncogenes to the breakpoint of the characteristic chromosomal translocations provided important clues for molecular analysis of these diseases. Similar investigations of most carcinomas and sarcomas have not uncovered unambiguous correlations between proto-oncogenes and specific tumor types.

Despite insights into enzymatic activities and subcellular localization of proto-oncogene products, we do not know the specific physiological role for most of these proteins. Exceptions include proto-oncogenes that correspond to known growth factors, such as the c-*sis* gene, which codes for the polypeptide B-chain of the platelet-derived growth factor (PDGF),[108] and growth factor receptor genes, such as c-*erbB* and c-*fms*, which code for the epidermal growth factor receptor (EGFR)[35] and for the receptor for colony stimulating factor-1, respectively.[93] Like growth factors and their receptors, these proto-oncogenes may affect cell growth and differentiation and may contribute to the establishment or maintenance of a malignant phenotype. The entire field of growth factors, growth factor receptors, and their roles in breast cancer will be reviewed in Chapter 20.

Serendipitous insertion of a proviral genome near a proto-oncogene can also contribute to neoplasia. Mammary tumorigenesis by the mouse mammary tumor virus (MMTV) is mediated by insertional activation of at least one of several genes by enhancer sequences in the MMTV proviral long terminal repeat (LTR). These target proto-oncogenes appear to be unrelated but may share the common characteristic of coding secreted proteins. Characterization of these MMTV-induced genes will be discussed in detail.

Experiments utilizing DNA-mediated gene transfer provided an important means of detecting transforming

351

oncogenes in tumor tissues and cell lines. Theoretically, it seemed that uptake of human tumor cell DNA by NIH/3T3 mouse fibroblasts and subsequent expression of a transmitted dominant tumor gene would provide insight into a broad spectrum of novel oncogenes. As researchers began to identify the genes that were able to transform NIH/3T3 cells, it became clear that this assay was particularly sensitive for the *ras* family of oncogenes. Even though activated *ras* genes were found in a wide variety of human tumor cell lines as well as in primary cancers, the results with human breast cancer samples were largely negative.[80] A number of transfection experiments with human breast cancer cell DNA have been described in the literature and will be reviewed here.

Studies of tumor tissues and cell lines have not definitively linked known oncogenes to the pathogenesis of human breast cancer. To further the approach to this problem, different transforming genes were introduced into mammary cells that were either not adapted for in vitro growth or had limited malignant potential. Such experiments have, in one case, identified genes capable of immortalizing or transforming mammary epithelial cells and, in another case, identified genes capable of conferring a fully malignant potential to a mammary carcinoma cell line that was hormone-dependent. Animal models for mammary tumorigenesis have employed oncogenes linked to organ-specific promoter sequences for use as transgenes in recipient mice. These experiments have permitted the study of tissue-specific expression of potent oncogenes subsequent to their stable integration into early mouse embryos. The last section of the chapter will discuss these experiments and their relevance to the search for breast cancer oncogenes.

PROTO-ONCOGENES IN HUMAN BREAST CANCER

Onc Gene Expression in Tumor Tissues

Comprehensive surveys have been conducted with v-*onc* gene probes to analyze fresh human tumor specimens for expression of the corresponding c-*onc* genes. One such study of 54 various tumor specimens included four samples of breast cancer.[97] These were found to express *fes, fos, fms, myb* (two of the four samples), and *myc, ras*[H], and *ras*[K] (three of four samples). This pattern of expression was very similar to that of nearly all other classes of tumor examined.

A larger survey of 101 tumor samples, many of which were paired with adjacent normal tissue specimens, included ten cases of breast cancer.[111] Of 11 *onc* genes analyzed by Southern blotting, three (*myc, myb,* and *ras*[H]) had structural alterations in tumor specimens compared with their normal controls. The breast cancer samples displayed, in one case, the loss of a c-*ras*[H] allele and, in a second case, an alteration in the ratio of the two c-*myb* alleles in a metastasis that was not present in the primary tumor or normal tissue. Two of the breast cancer specimens contained amplifications of c-*myc*

gene. Further studies on allelic retention of a c-*ras*[H] gene will be discussed below.

Expression of the *Ras* Gene Family in Human Breast Cancer

There are at least four distinct *Ras* genes in the human genome. These code for proteins whose amino-termini and specific internal regions are highly conserved among the group and whose carboxy-terminal ends are more variable. The four well-characterized human genes are *ras*[H] on chromosome 11,[75, 86] *ras*[K] on chromosome 12,[75, 86] *ras*[N] on chromosome 1,[42] and *ras*[R] on chromosome 19.[69] The *Ras* genes have similar exon structures, suggesting that they arose from an ancestral precursor.

Ras genes have been identified in yeast[28, 55, 103] and *Dictyostelium discoidium*[83] as well as in higher organisms. The primary structure of the yeast *Ras* genes shows remarkable preservation of amino-terminal protein sequence when compared with the *Ras* genes of higher organisms.[81] Yeast has two genes, *ras1* and *ras2,* both of which appear to play a role in the activation of yeast adenylate cyclase.[17, 106] Genetic experiments have suggested that deletion of both yeast *ras* genes is lethal. However, the human *ras*[H] proto-oncogene can rescue a yeast with both *ras* alleles deleted.[29, 54] Despite the structural conservation of *ras* during evolution, its function has changed somewhat, since in higher organisms *ras* p21 does not interact directly with adenylate cyclase.[11]

Structure and Expression of ras in Human Breast Cancer

Activated *ras* oncogenes have been detected in a number of human tumors as assayed by tumor DNA transformation of NIH/3T3 cells. The transformed cells lose contact inhibition and can form tumors in nude mice. The activation of *ras* may be achieved by point mutation or by enhanced gene expression.[22] Point mutations in *ras* genes have been detected in a wide variety of human cancers, but breast cancers have been underrepresented on this list. No breast carcinoma has been found to have a point mutation in the *ras*[H] proto-oncogene. A cell line from a breast carcinosarcoma, HS578T, contains an *asp*[12] mutation.[63]

Although *ras*[K] mutations in breast cancer have not been reported to date, the use of oligonucleotide-specific probes may reveal *ras*[K] mutations in breast cancer specimens, as has been indicated by some preliminary observations in breast cancer cell lines. The *ras*[K] proto-oncogene extends over 40kb and as a result is inefficiently integrated in an intact state during gene transfer experiments.[70] Sequence-specific oligonucleotide probes can distinguish between normal and mutated regions of the *ras*[K] gene by Southern analysis, obviating the need for a successful *ras*[K] gene transfer. Mutated *ras*[N] genes have not been identified in breast cancer.

High levels of *ras* proto-oncogene expression also can transform NIH/3T3 cells and cause them to become tumorigenic but to a lesser degree than with the mutated *ras* genes.[22] In the face of largely negative data for *ras* mutations in breast cancer, attention has been focused on the levels of expression of *ras* p21 in tumor specimens and cultured cells.

Expression of ras p21 in Breast Cancer Tissues and Cell Lines

Since inappropriate expression of the *ras* gene could be important for malignancy, Spandidos and Agnantis examined breast tumor tissue and adjacent normal tissue for the expression of the c-*ras*[H] gene.[98] In each of 12 tumors there was an apparent 4- to 15-fold increase in c-*ras*[H] mRNA compared with adjacent normal tissue as determined by dot blot analysis. For comparison, the expression of c-*sis* was also examined and found not to differ between the tumor and normal tissues. Unlike the dot blot data, Northern blot analysis of a number of RNA samples in this series did not clearly demonstrate the differences in expression. A follow-up study by the same group sought to correlate the amount of c-*ras*[H] gene expression with clinical parameters, but the study lacked the rigorous statistical analysis to support the contention that elevated c-*ras* expression correlated with more advanced histological grades.[1]

Another group examined the expression of the *ras* p21 protein in breast cancer tissues, benign breast tumors, and normal mammary glands.[27] Levels of p21 were determined by Western blotting analysis to be elevated in each of seven hormone-responsive breast cancer specimens and in five of six hormone-independent tumors. Normal breast tissue and three fibroadenomas had very low or undetectable levels of p21. Using a photoaffinity label, the authors also showed that the elevated levels of p21 were accompanied by high GTPase activity, the enzymatic function associated with the *Ras*[H] protein. Expression of *ras* p21 was also examined in paraffin-embedded sections of benign and malignant breast tissue by immunohistochemical staining with monoclonal antibodies prepared against p21 peptides.[44] The antibodies clearly reacted with malignant mammary cells in 19 of 30 samples but did not show binding to most of the benign tissues tested, of which only 3 of 21 were positive.

In a more recent study, high levels of expression of *ras* p21 were detected using protein blotting and immunostaining in a variety of fresh human tumor specimens, including gastrointestinal, ovarian, lung, liver, kidney, and lymph node as well as breast tissues.[102] Two of the antibodies used in these experiments were designed to react with both *ras*[K] and *ras*[N], and one was specific for *ras*[H]. Eight of ten breast cancer samples reacted with one or the other cross-reactive anti-p21 sera, but none reacted with the specific anti-p21 *ras*[H] serum. The conclusion that breast tissues express p21 species different from *ras*[H] is a novel finding. Specific data to the contrary were obtained in a Northern blot analysis of mRNA from 22 invasive ductal carcinomas, of which c-*ras*[H] was expressed by 16 but c-*ras*[K] and *ras*[N] were expressed at low levels or not at all.[104]

A more comprehensive study of *ras* p21 expression in mammary tissues reinforced many presumptions about the role of normal *ras* genes in breast neoplasia.[76] In agreement with other reports, *ras* p21 expression was found by immunohistochemistry to be elevated in invasive mammary carcinoma as compared with hyperplastic lesions. An example of the results is shown in Figure 19–1. Expression of p21 in mammary cancers was heterogeneous among primary and metastatic lesions. Although there was a trend toward higher expression in postmenopausal patients, there was no correlation of p21 expression with estrogen receptor status. Among 18 patients with hyperplastic lesions who had been followed for up to 15 years, p21 expression tended to decrease slightly over time. Of the 18 mammary hyperplasia patients, the five who developed carcinoma had significantly higher levels of p21 expression at the time of first biopsy than did the 13 patients who did not develop carcinoma. The authors concluded that p21 expression may contribute to the establishment of cancer but probably is not essential for its maintenance.

Structure of the Ras Gene in Human Breast Cancer

Lidereau and coworkers identified structural heterogeneity in the 3' flanking region of the human c-*ras*[H] gene. They classified a number of common and rare alleles by means of restriction fragment length polymorphism (RFLP) analysis of Southern blots with human tumor DNA.[67] Four common and 16 rare alleles were identified in the study population, which included breast cancer patients and normal control subjects. The distribution of common and rare alleles differed significantly between the groups of normal controls and breast cancer patients. Common RFLPs represented 91 percent of the *ras*[H] alleles in normal subjects and 59 percent of the *ras*[H] alleles in breast cancer patients. The 104 breast cancer patients in this survey had a much lower frequency of possessing two common alleles.

The state of the c-*ras*[H] gene in breast cancers has also been examined with respect to genomic structure and allelic exclusion. Southern analysis of DNA from 104 breast cancer samples failed to disclose any instances of rearrangement or amplification of c-*ras*[H].[104] The c-*ras*[H] gene has been shown, however, to have frequent BamHI restriction fragment length polymorphisms (RFLP). Of the 51 patients who were heterozygous for these polymorphic sites, 14 exhibited allelic exclusion of one of the two *ras* alleles in the tumor tissue. Loss of an allele did not alter p21 expression, although allelic exclusion did correlate significantly with advanced histological grade, lack of hormone receptors, and subsequent occurrence of distant metastases. Such a correlation in the presence of negative protein expression data may reflect general chromosomal instability, which may coincide with a more undifferentiated tumor. This notion is supported by the observation that other regions of chromosome 11p are frequently deleted in breast cancer cells. The deleted regions most often include the c-*ras*[H] and beta globin loci.[2] Moreover, located nearby at 11p13

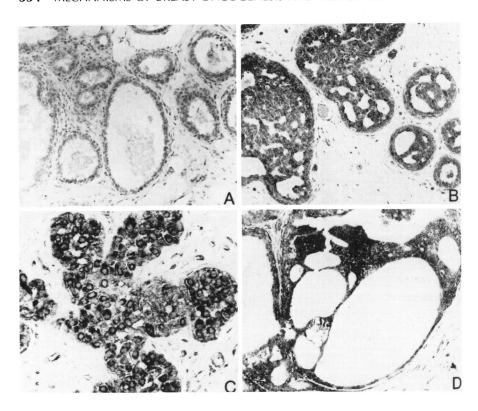

Figure 19–1. Immunohistochemical staining of formalin-fixed, paraffin-embedded human mammary tissue sections with MAb RAP-5. *A*, Non-hyperplastic tissue, showing cystic change. No staining of epithelial cells. × 130. *B*, Atypical ductal hyperplasia. Atypical hyperplastic epithelium reacted with MAb RAP-5 expressing cytoplasmic *ras* p21. × 150. *C*, Atypical lobular hyperplasia. Over one half of the terminal portions of lobular unit were expanded by severe atypical epithelial cells positive for reactivity with MAb RAP-5. × 330. *D*, Ductal carcinoma in situ, showing cribriform structure. Note that the early carcinoma lesion reacted strongly with MAb RAP-5. × 150. Sections were counterstained with hematoxylin. (From Ohuchi N, et al: Cancer Res 46:2511, 1986. Reprinted by permission.)

is a heritable fragile site[46], and also adjacent, but not deleted, is the locus for Wilms' tumor.[61]

There are considerably fewer data on the roles of other members of the *ras* family of oncogenes in human breast cancer. One cell line, MCF-7, has an amplified ras^N gene.[39] The extent of ras^N amplification in different substrains of these cells correlates with the level of ras^N mRNA. However, a survey of other human mammary carcinoma cell lines and of several fresh tissues showed no evidence that ras^N amplification is a general phenomenon in breast cancer.

Protein Kinase Activity of c-*src* in Human Mammary Carcinoma

Many of the known proto-oncogenes code for proteins with tyrosine kinase activity. The best characterized tyrosine kinase gene is c-*src*, which codes for a 60kd phosphoprotein, pp60[c-src]. This protein phosphorylates some of its own tyrosine residues and those of a number of cellular proteins. Studies with the viral transforming gene v-*src* have shown that this kinase activity is crucial for the transforming potential of the protein.[90] Although many natural substrates for pp60[c-src] phosphorylation have been identified, none has been linked directly to the enzyme's transforming potential.

Jacobs and Rubsamen assayed pp60[c-src] activity in 21 human mammary carcinoma specimens.[50] To assay protein kinase activity they exploited the ability of the pp60[c-src] molecule to phosphorylate the immunoglobulin used to perform the immunoprecipitation. Nearly half the breast carcinomas tested (10 of 21) had elevated levels of pp60[c-src] activity. Comparison was made with

only three samples of normal mammary tissue, and in only one case was a normal tissue specimen adjacent to a tumor sample available for study. In that one case the breast tumor showed markedly elevated kinase activity. This study contained no data regarding the amount of pp60[c-src] protein present in tissue samples and therefore left unclear whether the enhanced kinase activity in the assays resulted from an altered *src* protein or from increased levels of normal protein.

Some of the deficiencies of this study were addressed in a study by Rosen et al.[85] Utilizing assays of both pp60[c-src] autophosphorylation and phosphorylation of casein, they found that three hormone-dependent breast cancer cell lines, but not two hormone-independent lines, had elevated kinase activity. They performed Western blot analysis of the cellular proteins to show that pp60[c-src] protein concentrations did not differ between the cells with high and low kinase activity. Moreover, analysis of a breast cancer tissue specimen and adjacent normal tissue showed that the samples had the same levels of pp60[c-src] protein but that the tumor had markedly elevated kinase activity. This finding was not unique to mammary carcinoma, being found in neuroectodermal tumors and colon carcinoma although many other cancers were negative. The apparent increase in the specific activity of an oncogenic protein in breast carcinoma suggests a role for pp60[c-src] in at least some breast cancers.

Amplification of c-*erbB2 (neu)* in Breast Cancer Cells

A gene closely related in structure to the epidermal growth factor receptor (EGFR) gene, but probably distinct in function, is c-*erbB2*. It appears that c-*erbB2* is a transmembrane protein with an extracellular ligand binding site and an intracellular tyrosine kinase domain.[24] The corresponding ligand for this putative receptor protein has not been identified. The gene *erbB2* was originally cloned from an EMS-induced murine neural tumor, in which the gene was activated by point mutation in the hydrophobic transmembrane domain of the molecule.[8]

The c-*erbB2* gene is amplified in several human mammary carcinoma cell lines, including MAC117,[58] SK-Br-3, MDA-MB-330, MDA-MB-361, and BT-474[62] (Fig. 19–2). In other mammary carcinoma cell lines, increased expression in the absence of gene amplification has been observed. In a preliminary survey of fresh tumor tissues that included eight primary breast cancer specimens and two metastases, one of the primary tumors and one metastasis had an amplified c-*erbB2* copy number.[110] Subsequently, substantial numbers of breast cancer tumor specimens have been screened for c-*erbB2* amplification. Whereas it was initially thought that nearly 30 percent of breast cancer specimens contained amplified copies of c-*erbB2*,[96] more carefully controlled experiments suggested that this fraction is between 15 and 20 percent.[107] Simultaneous assessment of the copy number of c-*erbB2* and the closely linked *erbA* gene has shown that both genes are often amplified coincidentally in breast cancer tissues. Although there is often increased expression of c-*erbB2* in tissues in which the gene is amplified, no *erbA* expression was seen. Some investi-

gators have suggested that c-*erbB2* amplification is an independent variable predictive of shorter disease-free survival and time to relapse in breast cancer.[113]

Alterations of c-*myc* in Breast Cancer Cell Lines

The codes of c-*myc* for one of several related nuclear proteins have been implicated in neoplasia. The c-*myc* gene itself is consistently altered in Burkitt's lymphoma.[66] The gene c-*myc* is also expressed normally during the transition in the cell cycle from G_0 to G_1.[5, 15, 45, 105] Questions about the state of c-*myc* in breast cancer arose when the gene for glutamate-pyruvate transaminase (GPT), which is linked to a genetic locus for familial predisposition to human breast cancer, was found to be located on chromosome 8,[57] the same chromosome as c-*myc*. Kozbor and Croce examined the state of the c-*myc* gene in five human breast cancer cell lines.[114] Of the five lines, SKBR-5, SKBR-3, Cama-1, MCF-7, and BT-20, they found that SKBR-3 had a c-*myc* gene amplification of four to eight fold. Three of the cell lines had a somewhat elevated level of c-*myc* expression, but the significance of this was not clear.

Another human breast cancer cell line, SW 613-S, has amplified copies of the c-*myc* gene located both in double minute chromosomes and in normal chromosomes.[71] Passage of the cells as tumors in nude mice resulted in an increase in c-*myc* copy number in this cell line. Since further c-*myc* amplification appeared to be coincident with the capacity for tumor growth in vivo, these results imply a role for c-*myc* in the growth of these breast carcinoma cells.

A comprehensive study of the c-*myc* gene was conducted in 121 primary breast cancers.[36] This survey of c-*myc* genomic structure and expression revealed that the gene was amplified 2 to 15 fold in 32 percent of the samples tested and that in five cases there was a non–germ line restriction enzyme fragment. Alterations of the c-*myc* gene correlated with invasive ductal histology and more advanced patient age. Ninety-five of the 121 specimens were from invasive ductal carcinomas, and 40 of those had alterations of c-*myc*.

ONCOGENES ACTIVATED BY RETROVIRAL INTEGRATION IN MURINE MAMMARY CARCINOMAS

Mammary tumors in mice have long been associated with infection by several strains of MMTV. The MMTV genome does not contain a transduced oncogene. Rather, MMTV occasionally integrates next to genes, resulting in their transcriptional activation in mammary tumor cells. Transcription is stimulated by enhancer sequences in the viral long terminal repeat sequence (LTR). Viral integration may take place in any orientation with respect to the activated oncogene, since an enhancer sequence can influence transcription regardless of its position relative to the affected gene.

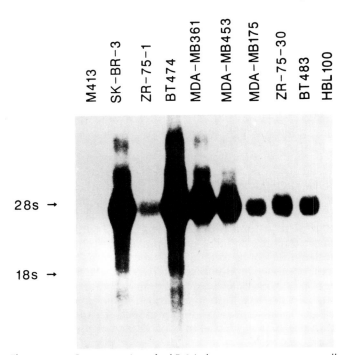

Figure 19–2. Overexpression of *erbB*-2 in human mammary tumor cell lines. Northern blot analysis. Total cellular RNA (10 μg) of mammary tumor cell lines, normal human fibroblasts M413 and HBL100 was hybridized with a cDNA probe derived from the 5′ end of the *erbB*-2 coding region. M413 and HBL100 cells contain *erbB*-2 specific mRNA detectable after longer autoradiographic exposures. (From Krays MH, et al: EmBo J 6:605, 1987. Reprinted by permission.)

The *int-1* Gene

The *int-1* gene was first identified by Nusse and Varmus[74] to be adjacent to a common MMTV proviral integration site in C3H mice. The *int-1* gene was always next to the integration site but was never itself the site for integration. The pattern of proviral insertion in relation to the *int-1* gene is shown in Figure 19–3. The *int-1* expression is restricted to mammary tumors and is not found in normal breast tissue.[74] The only other adult cells expressing *int-1* are developing spermatids of the male. In the mouse embryo, *int-1* is transcribed in the brain and spinal cord during days 9 to 14 of development.[92] The *int-1* codes for a 36kd protein that is glycosylated to higher molecular weight forms, the largest being 44kd. Subcellular fractionation experiments have shown that the *int-1* protein is associated primarily with the membrane and perhaps is sequestered in cytoplasmic vesicles.[19, 78] Although this would suggest that the *int-1* protein is secreted from the cell, no evidence for this has been found.

The *int-1* oncogene causes morphological transformation of cultured mammary epithelial cells but is unable to transform fibroblasts in vitro. In search of functional counterparts to *int-1* in lower animals, the *Drosophila int-1* gene was cloned and found to be the *wingless* gene, first identified by a mutation that resulted in the absence of wing development and the duplication of part of the thorax.[84] The *Drosophila* and murine proteins are 54 percent similar in their primary structure. In *Drosophila* the *int-1* counterpart belongs to the segment polarity class of developmental genes. The functional correlation between murine *int-1* and *wingless* is somewhat obscure. The *int-1* in the mouse is not expressed in a segmental fashion in the embryo. There is no evidence thus far that *wingless* is expressed during spermatid development. However, it may be important that a protein believed to be a secreted peptide may be involved both in normal embryonic developmental signals and in pathological epithelial cell transformation.

The *int-2* Gene

The analysis of MMTV proviral integration in mammary tumors of BALB/c mice identified a common integration site in this mouse strain that differed from the *int-1* locus and was called *int-2*.[32] Approximately 50 percent of virus-induced tumors have proviral integration at this locus. The *int-2* gene is transcriptionally activated in tumors but is not expressed in normal mammary tissue.

Primary structure analysis of cloned *int-2* DNA suggested a similarity with peptides of the fibroblast growth factor (FGF) family.[31] This family includes acidic FGF, basic FGF, and *hst*. Each member resembles the other in a central domain. In the central *int-2* exon, 19 of 32 amino acids are identical to those in a similar region in basic FGF. Overall, these peptides share 37 to 42 percent similarity in their primary structure.

The *int-2* oncogene is believed to code for a growth factor whose expression is restricted in adult tissues and present early in the developing mouse embryo. To date, no example of *int-2* expression has been found in human tissues.

THE POSSIBLE ROLE FOR A RETROVIRUS IN HUMAN MAMMARY CANCER

Research into the possible viral etiology of human breast cancer has been inspired by the murine model of retrovirus-induced mammary tumorigenesis. To date, there is no conclusive evidence identifying a human mammary tumor virus. Experiments aimed at finding such an agent have focused on three areas. First, endogenous human genomic sequences that have sequence similarity with the MMTV have been identified. None of these putative endogenous retroviral genomes contained a full-length proviral sequence. Moreover, there is no conclusive proof that they are expressed in normal or malignant tissues.

A second avenue of investigation has focused on geographical or ethnic groups who have a higher incidence of breast cancer or who have breast cancer with unusual characteristics. Rapidly progressive breast cancer (PEV) in Tunisian women represents a unique concentration of aggressive, rapidly fatal cases of inflammatory carcinoma of the breast.[101] Its unusual clinical characteristics and its geographical concentration suggest a role for a unique etiological factor. Women of the Parsi sect in Bombay, India, have the highest incidence of breast cancer of the many ethnic groups residing in that city.[51] In the early 1970s, several studies collected evidence for the presence of retrovirus-like particles in the breast milk of Parsi women.[26, 72] However, no virus particles have ever been isolated or transmitted from any human breast tissues. Currently, there is no conclusive evidence from studies of these groups that an infectious agent contributes to the pathogenesis of human breast cancer.

Attempts at isolating retroviruses from human breast cancer cell lines have been largely unsuccessful, except

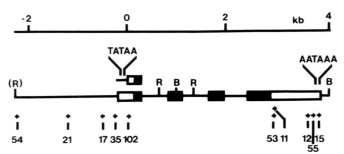

Figure 19–3. Structure of the *int*-1 gene. The intron-exon structure as determined by nuclease S1 mapping and DNA sequencing is shown. Exons are indicated by blocks; coding sequences are black. The putative polyadenylation signal (AATAAA) at the 3' end of the gene and a putative RNA polymerase initiation signal (TATAA) are indicated. Sites and orientations of proviral integrations in tumors having an integration in the depicted area are represented by arrows. Tumor numbers are below arrows. B: Bam HI; R: Eco RI. The Eco RI site in brackets is not present in the chromosomal DNA but derived from DNA cloning. (From van Ooyen A, Nusse R: Cell 39:233, 1984. Reprinted by permission.)

in one case. Keydar and coworkers, using clonal derivatives of the T47D cell line, have identified a particulate fraction from culture supernatant that contains 70s RNA, reverse transcriptase activity, and antigens that are cross-reactive with MMTV gp52.[56] Proteins cross-reactive with this putative viral protein are also found in human breast cancer specimens but not in normal samples.[91] The rigorous identification of this particulate fraction as a virus still requires both ultrastructural examination and molecular cloning of the 70s RNA genome. It is also remarkable that samples of the T47D cell line in other laboratories have not been found to contain the same particulate material.

ONCOGENES IDENTIFIED BY TRANSFECTION WITH BREAST CANCER DNA

Showing that transfer of tumor cell DNA to normal cells could confer a tumorigenic phenotype was the experimental tour de force that gave rise to a new area of oncogene research. It soon became clear that the indicator cells, NIH/3T3 fibroblasts, formed detectable foci in response to a limited number of transforming genes. New assays were developed that increased the sensitivity of the detection system and provided a second end-point, tumor formation, with which to score oncogenes.[13] Moreover, transfection studies with diploid fibroblasts demonstrated not only their more complex requirements for focus formation but also that NIH/3T3 cells are not entirely "normal" and may have already bypassed the need for certain oncogenic functions by their establishment as an immortal cell line.[64] The results with this new in vitro model of diploid fibroblast transformation supported the hypothesis that more than one step was needed to achieve the mature tumor phenotype.

Extensive transfection studies to identify a dominant transforming gene from human breast cancer cells have been, at best, inconclusive. In fact, one group found no codon 12 mutations of the c-ras^H and c-ras^K genes, respectively, in 32 and 64 breast tumors.[104] The first data to suggest that breast cancers would score positive in the transfection assay came from the work of Cooper and coworkers, using MCF-7 mammary carcinoma DNA.[65] These experiments were done in parallel with transfection of MTV-induced murine mammary tumor DNA into the NIH/3T3 cells. Both the human and the murine tumor DNAs contained putative oncogenes with the same restriction enzyme inactivation profile. A subsequent report described a tumor-specific 86kd glycoprotein present on the NIH/3T3 cells that had received the human mammary tumor DNA.[26] There have been no further reports of this protein, and its identity is unclear. No evidence has been presented to identify the transforming gene as the coding region for this 86kd protein.

Other groups have had difficulty reproducing the transfection results with the MCF-7 cells. Wigler and coworkers, having been frustrated in these attempts,

adapted the nude mouse tumor assay to try to identify MCF-7 transforming genes.[37] After exhaustive passage of tumors in nude mice, they identified three human genes that caused murine tumors: *N-ras*, which is amplified and not mutated in MCF-7 cells; a *c-ros* rearranged artifactually during the transfection;[112] and a third gene whose identity and genomic organization in the parental MCF-7 DNA is unknown. Thus far there has been no unequivocal identification of a pathogenic oncogene in human mammary carcinoma using DNA-mediated gene transfer. There may be some other molecular basis for an inherited predisposition to breast cancer. Recessive oncogenes, similar to those identified in pediatric malignancies, possibly may play a role in families in whom one of the two alleles is defective. These genes would not be detected by an assay designed to detect a dominant transforming mutation.

ALTERING MAMMARY CELLS BY INTRODUCTION OF ONCOGENES

The role of oncogenes in mammary carcinogenesis has been addressed via a third experimental approach, the transfer of cloned oncogenes. The transfection of viral or cellular transforming genes, individually or in combination, has allowed the in vitro propagation of mammary epithelial cells and has been used to alter the phenotype of hormone-dependent breast carcinoma cells. This approach has helped to define roles for different classes of genes in the abnormal growth of mammary cells. Moreover, the development of transgenic strains of mice with tissue-specific promoters directing transcription of oncogenes primarily in breast tissue has provided great insight into mammary carcinogenesis. The choice of agents for transfection or for use as transgenes has been directed in large part by the work of Weinberg and coworkers, who illustrated complementary functions of oncogenes playing an early or a late role in in vitro transformation.[64]

The *ras* Gene Transfection of MCF-7 Cells

MCF-7 human breast cancer cells are estrogen-dependent in that they require estrogen supplementation for efficient in vitro growth and for tumor formation in nude mice. The estrogen-treated cells secrete peptide growth factors, including a factor related to tumor-derived growth factor-α (TGF-α),[9] insulin-like growth factor I (IGF-I),[47] platelet-derived growth factor (PDGF),[18] an epithelial cell colony stimulating factor,[100] mammary-derived growth factor,[7] and autocrine motility factor.[68] Production of many of these factors is responsive to estrogen supplementation. When supported with concentrated serum-free conditioned medium supplementation (via minipumps) instead of estrogen, MCF-7 cell implants in nude mice grow to tumors of limited size and then regress. Peptide growth factor secretion appears to be an important element in mediating estradiol-induced growth effects, in that the growth-promoting activity of the concentrated conditioned medium is abrogated by heating or trypsin treatment. Furthermore, infusions of EGF and/or IGF-I also support limited tumor growth.[34]

Whereas hormone-dependent breast cancer cells respond to estrogen with growth factor production that accompanies alterations in growth properties, hormone-independent breast cancer cells produce constitutively a number of the same growth factors. To try to clarify whether the hormone-independent state was phenotypically similar to the hormone-induced state, Kasid et al. constructed an estrogen-independent MCF-7 cell line by transfecting MCF-7 with a v-ras^H DNA clone.[53] The ras gene was chosen because it is activated by point mutation in many human carcinomas and because it provides the second-stage transformation function in models of two-step oncogenesis.[64] The resultant MCF-7$_{ras}$ cells expressed the mutant p21^{ras} protein, had a shorter doubling time in vitro than the parental MCF-7 cells, were resistant to growth inhibitory effects of antiestrogens, and formed tumors in nude mice independent of exogenous estrogen supplementation.

This new hormone-independent cell line exhibited constitutive secretion of the identical peptide growth factors whose production was stimulated by estrogen in the parental MCF-7 cells.[33] Moreover, tumor implants of the MCF-7$_{ras}$ cells were able to support limited growth of MCF-7 cell implants at sites distant from the site of the MCF-7$_{ras}$ cells.[52] This implied that secreted growth factors supported limited tumor growth similar to the growth effects of conditioned medium from estrogen-treated MCF-7 cells. The MCF-7$_{ras}$ cells retained the expression of estrogen receptors, and their function remained intact as evidenced by the estrogen induction of progesterone receptor. In this derivative cell line, the introduction of a single mutated oncogene was accompanied by growth alterations that bypassed the hormone-dependent tumorigenic phenotype without inactivating the hormone-response mechanism.

Oncogenes Used to Immortalize Mammary Epithelial Cells

The introduction of specific oncogenes into cultured primary mammary epithelial cells can result in their immortalization and/or their transformation. Primary cultures of murine,[77] lapin,[41] and human[43] mammary epithelial cells have been described. Results of gene transfer experiments in three different animal systems indicate that at least a two-step transformation process is required for the expression of experimental tumorigenesis. A mouse mammary epithelial cell line that was not tumorigenic was changed into a tumorigenic line by transfection with EJ-c-ras^H.[49] Primary rabbit mammary epithelial cells were immortalized after microinjection with simian virus 40 DNA.[38] The rabbit cells were not tumorigenic in nude mice unless an activated human c-ras^H gene was injected in addition to the SV40 DNA. Lastly, human mammary epithelial cells, which can be passed in serum-free media,[109] were immortalized by the

combination of SV40 T-antigen and v-ras^H transferred into the cells in retroviral vectors. Neither gene alone was sufficient to immortalize the cells for long-term passage in vitro. Tumorigenicity studies of these cells are still under way.[23]

ONCOGENE-INDUCED MAMMARY CARCINOGENESIS IN TRANSGENIC MICE

The production of transgenic mice that faithfully express foreign genes has generated enthusiasm for the study of oncogene regulation in vivo. Coupling an oncogene to a promoter whose activity is subject to tissue-specific regulation allows the targeting of potential oncogenic effects to the tissue in question.

To this end, constructs of the MMTV LTR, which contains a steroid hormone–inducible promoter,[21] were fused to the c-myc gene and used as a transgene.[99] Of 13 strains of transgenic mice that carried different fusions of promoter and c-myc, depending on the extent of normal c-myc promoter that was deleted, two strains with substantial c-myc promoter deletions developed spontaneous mammary adenocarcinomas. There was no obvious effect of the transgene during early or pubertal development in the mice. Tumors appeared only after females had experienced two or three pregnancies. Examples of these mammary tumors are shown in Figure 19–4.

Subsequently, transgenic mice were constructed using an MMTV-v-ras^H fusion construct.[95] These mice developed hyperplasia of the harderian gland, an apocrine lacrimal organ located in the murine orbit, and later demonstrated malignancies of mammary, salivary, and lymphoid tissue. The appearance of malignant tumors was stochastic, apparently requiring other somatic events for expression of the malignant phenotype. The results with the MMTV-v-ras^H construct have been independently reproduced by P. Jolicoeur, who has found a similar predisposition of the MMTV-v-ras^H transgenic mice to form tumors of apocrine organs, including breasts and salivary glands (personal communication, 1989).

Female mice arising from F$_1$ crosses of the MMTV-v-ras^H mice with the MMTV-c-myc mice developed mammary tumors earlier after puberty and with a higher frequency than either of the parental transgenic strains.[95] Thus, the expression of two oncogenes accelerated and improved the efficiency of tumor formation.

The whey acidic protein (WAP) promoter region has also been fused to a mutated c-ras^H gene and used as a transgene.[4] WAP is expressed selectively in mammary epithelial cells in response to lactogenic hormones. Therefore, the promoter conferred mammary specificity to the expression of the oncogene. After a long latency period (9 to 12 months), mammary and salivary gland tumors developed in the transgenic mice. These were also the two tissues to express the transgene.

Transgenic experiments suggest that a mutated ras^H oncogene can contribute to the development of mammary carcinoma, but expression of the oncogenic trans-

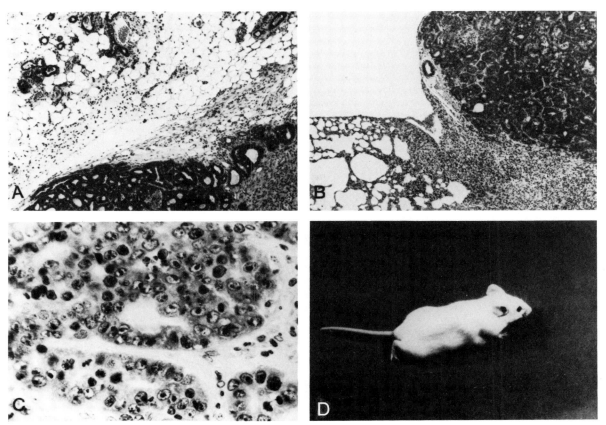

Figure 19–4. Histologic appearance of spontaneous mammary tumor occurring in founder mouse 141-3 and gross morphologic appearance of tumor in female progeny 141-3-38. Virtually identical microscopic histologies were observed in founder mouse 164-4 and progeny 141-3-38. *A*, Low-power view of primary tumor, demonstrating a moderately well differentiated, locally invasive adenocarcinoma arising in and involving subcutaneous mammary tissue. Note the residual, uninvolved, nonneoplastic breast tissue. *B*, Lower power view of lung, demonstrating a large subpleural nodule of metastatic adenocarcinoma. *C*, High-power view of primary mammary tumor, demonstrating malignant epithelial glands. Note the piled and heaped-up appearance of the dysplastic epithelial cells, which also exhibit nuclear atypia, prominent large nucleoli, and a high mitotic rate. Mouse 141-3, hematoxylin and eosin: subcutaneous mammary tissue, 70× (*A*); lung, 70× (*B*); subcutaneous mammary tissue, 640× (*C*). (*D*) Female offspring of 141-3 founder animal (141-3-38) at 131 days. Note tumor mass in right axillary nipple line. Animal had delivered one litter and was pregnant for the second time. (From Stewart TA, et al: Cell 38:627, 1984. Reprinted by permission.)

gene must be accompanied by other somatic events to generate tumors. Even the addition of a second activated oncogene did not guarantee the formation of carcinomas in 100 percent of progeny animals.

CONCLUSIONS AND SPECULATIONS

Much has been learned about oncogene expression in breast cancer and the role that oncogenes may play in mammary carcinogenesis. Thus far, most of the information accumulated has served to remove candidate oncogenes from consideration as essential participants in breast cancer development. We are therefore limited to making only the most general statements about genes whose function may account for the tumorigenic phenotype in some subsets of breast cancer.

Most of the data implicating various oncogenes in the progression of mammary cancer are based on surveys of tumor tissues or cell lines for gene alteration or expression. On the one hand, it is not surprising that genes such as *c-myc* and *c-ras*[H], which appear to have roles in

the growth of normal cells, are expressed at higher levels in cancer cells and at the highest levels in aggressive cancer cells. We must be cautious about overinterpreting these data. Except in examples of retrovirus-induced neoplasia, there has never been proof that oncogene amplification, rearrangement, or increased expression causes cancer rather than maintains the phenotype or is a concomitant phenomenon resulting from the metabolic state of the neoplastic cells.

There are other known oncogenes that may play a still unclarified role in human breast cancer. Although there was much enthusiasm about possible expression of *int-1* and *int-2* in human mammary carcinoma, data supporting a role for these genes have been elusive. Lastly, the recent molecular cloning of the glucocorticoid[109] and estrogen receptors[40] and recognition of their homology with another oncogene, *erbA*, raises the intriguing possibility that they have the potential to be oncogenes. Perhaps they become altered and acquire oncogenic activity similar to the way in which other receptor genes become altered and acquire oncogenic activity as a result. For the present, we must conclude that the mammary carcinoma oncogene, if it exists, has not yet been found.

References

1. Agnantis NJ, Parissi P, Anagnostakis D, Spandidos DA: Comparative study of Harvey ras oncogene expression with conventional clinicopathologic parameters of breast cancer. Oncology 43:36–39, 1986.
2. Ali IU, Lidereau R, Theillet C, Callahan R: Reduction to homozygosity of genes on chromosome 11 in human breast neoplasia. Science 238:185–188, 1987.
3. Alitalo K, Schwab M, Lin C, Varmus H, Bishop J: Homogeneously staining chromosomal regions contain amplified copies of an abundantly expressed cellular oncogene (c-myc) in malignant neuroendocrine cells from a human colon carcinoma. Proc Natl Acad Sci USA 80:1707–1711, 1982.
4. Andres A-C, Schonenberger C-A, Groner B, Hennighausen L, LeMeur M, Gerlinger P: Ha-ras oncogene expression directed by a milk protein gene promoter: tissue specificity, hormonal regulation, and tumor induction in transgenic mice. Proc Natl Acad Sci USA 84: 1299–1303, 1987.
5. Armelin HA, Armelin MCS, Kelly K, Stewart T, Leder P, Cochran BH, Stiles CD: Functional role for c-myc in mitogenic response to platelet-derived growth factor. Nature 310:655–660, 1984.
6. Bakhshi A, Jensen JP, Goldman P, Wright JJ, McBride OW, Epstein EL, Korsmeyer SJ: Cloning the chromosomal breakpoint of t(14;18) human lymphomas: Clustering around JH on chromosome 14 and near a transcriptional unit on 18. Cell 41:899–906, 1985.
7. Bano M, Salomon DS, Kidwell WR: Purification of a mammary-derived growth factor from human milk and mammary tumors. J Biol Chem 260:5745–5752, 1986.
8. Bargmann CI, Hung M-C, Weinberg RA: Multiple independent activations of the neu oncogene by a point mutation altering the transmembrane domain of p185. Cell 45:649–657, 1986.
9. Bates S, Dickson R, McManaway M, Lippman ME: Characterization of estrogen-responsive transforming activity in human breast cancer cell lines. Cancer Res 46:1703–1717, 1986.
10. Becker D, Lane M-A, Cooper GM: Identification of an antigen associated with transforming genes of human and mouse mammary carcinomas. Proc Natl Acad Sci USA 79:3315–3319, 1982.
11. Becker SK, Hattori S, Shih TY: The ras oncogene product p21 is not a regulatory component of adenylate cyclase. Nature 317:71–72, 1985.
12. Bishop JM: Exploring carcinogenesis with retroviral and cellular oncogenes. Prog Med Virol 32:5–14, 1985.
13. Blair DG, Cooper CS, Oskarsson MK, Eader LA, Vande Woude GF: New method for detecting cellular transforming genes. Science 281:1122–1125, 1982.
14. Blair DG, Oskarsson MK, Seth A, Dunn KJ, Dean M, Zweig M, Tainsky MA, Vande Woude GF: Analysis of the transforming potential of the human homolog of mos. Cell 46:785–794, 1986.
15. Blanchard J-M, Piechaczyk M, Dani C, Chambard J-C, Franchi A, Pouyssegur J, Jeanteur P: c-myc gene is transcribed at high rate in GO-arrested fibroblasts and is post-transcriptionally regulated in response to growth factors. Nature 317:443–445, 1985.
16. Bohmann D, Bos TJ, Admon A, Nishimura T, Vogt PK, Tjian R: Human proto-oncogene c-jun encodes a DNA binding protein with structural and functional properties of transcription factor AP-1. Science 238:1386–1392, 1987.
17. Broek D, Samily N, Fasano O, Fujiyama A, Tamanoi F, Northrup J, Wigler M: Differential activation of yeast adenylate cyclase by wild-type and mutant ras proteins. Cell 41:763–769, 1985.
18. Bronzert D, Pantazis P, Antoniades H, Kasid A, Davidson N, Dickson RB, Lippman ME: Synthesis and secretion of platelet-derived growth factor by human breast cancer cell lines. Proc Natl Acad Sci USA 84:5763–5767, 1987.
19. Brown AMC, Papkoff J, Fung YKT, Shackleford GM, Varmus HE: Identification of protein products encoded by proto-oncogene int-1. Mol Cell Biol 7:3971–3977, 1987.
20. Capon DJ, Chen EY, Levinson AD, Seeburg PH, Goeddel DV: Complete nucleotide sequence of the T24 human bladder carcinoma oncogene and its normal homologue. Nature 302:33–37, 1983.
21. Chandler VL, Maler BA, Yamamoto KR: DNA sequences bound specifically by glucocorticoid receptor in vitro render a heterologous promoter hormone responsive in vivo. Cell 33:489–499, 1983.
22. Chang EH, Furth ME, Scolnick EM, Lowy DR: Tumorigenic tranformation of mammalian cells induced by a normal human gene homologous to the oncogene of Harvey murine sarcoma virus. Nature 297:479–483, 1982.
23. Clark R, Stampfer MR, Milley R, O'Rourke E, Walen KH, Kriegler M, Kopplin J, McCormick F: Transformation of human mammary epithelial cells by oncogenic retroviruses. Cancer Res 48:4689–4694, 1988.
24. Coussens L, Yang-Feng TL, Liao Y-C, Chen E, Schlessinger J, Francke U, Levinson A, Ullrich A: Tyrosine kinase receptor with extensive homology to EGF receptor shares chromosomal location with neu oncogene. Science 230:1132–1139, 1985.
25. Dalla Favera R, Wong-Staal F, Gallo RC: Onc gene amplification in promyelocytic leukaemia cell line HL-60 and primary leukaemic cells of the same patient. Nature 299:61–63, 1982.
26. Das MR, Vaidya AB, Sirsat SM, Moore DH: Polymerase and RNA studies on milk virions from women of the Parsi community. J Natl Cancer Inst 48:1191–1196, 1972.
27. DeBortoli ME, Abou-Issa H, Haley BE, Cho-Chung YS: Amplified expression of p21 ras protein in hormone-dependent mammary carcinomas of humans and rodents. Biochem Biophys Res Commun 127: 699–706, 1985.
28. Defeo-Jones D, Scolnick E, Koller R, Dhar R: ras-Related gene sequences identified and isolated from Saccharomyces cerevisiae. Nature 306:707–709, 1983.
29. Defeo-Jones D, Tatchell K, Robinson LC, Sigal IS, Vass WC, Lowy DR, Scolnick EM: Mammalian and yeast ras gene products: Biological function in their heterologous systems. Science 228: 179–184, 1985.
30. Dhar R, Ellis R, Shih TY, Oroszlan S, Shapiro B, Maizel J, Lowy D, Scolnick E: Nucleotide sequence of the p21 transforming protein of Harvey murine sarcoma virus. Science 217:934–936, 1982.
31. Dickson C, Peters G: Potential oncogene product related to growth factors. Nature 326:833, 1987.
32. Dickson C, Smith R, Brookes S, Peters G: Tumorigenesis by mouse mammary tumor virus, proviral activation of a cellular gene in the common integration region int-2. Cell 37:529–536, 1984.
33. Dickson RB, Kasid A, Huff KK, Bates SE, Knabbe C, Bronzert D, Gelmann EP, Lippman M: Activation of growth factor secretion in tumorigenic states of breast cancer induced by 17B-estradiol or v-Ha-ras oncogene. Proc Natl Acad Sci USA 84:837–841, 1987.
34. Dickson RB, McManaway ME, Lippman ME: Estrogen-induced factors of breast cancer cells partially replace estrogen to promote tumor growth. Science 232:1540–1543, 1986.
35. Downward J, Yarden Y, Mayes E, Scrace G, Stockwell P, Ullrich A, Schlessinger J, Waterfield MD: Close similarity of epidermal growth factor receptor and v-erb-B oncogene protein sequences. Nature 307:521–527, 1984.
36. Escot C, Theillet C, Lidereau R, Spyratos F, Champene M-H, Gest J, Callahan R: Genetic alterations of the c-myc protooncogene (MYC) in human primary breast carcinomas. Proc Natl Acad Sci USA 83:4834–4838, 1986.
37. Fasano O, Birnbaum N, Edlund L, Fogh J, Wigler M: New human transforming genes detected by a tumorigenicity assay. Mol Cell Biol 4:1695–1705, 1984.
38. Garcia I, Sordat B, Rauccio-Farinon E, Dunand M, Kraehenbuhl J-P, Diggelmann H: Establishment of two rabbit mammary epithelial cell lines with distinct oncogenic potential and differentiated phenotype after microinjection of transforming genes. Mol Cell Biol 6:1974–1982, 1986.
39. Graham KA, Richardson CL, Minden MD, Trent JM, Buick

RM: Varying degrees of amplification of the N-ras oncogene in the human breast cancer cell line MCF-7. Cancer Res 45:2201–2205, 1985.

40. Green S, Walter P, Kumar V, Krust A, Bornert J-M, Argos P, Chambon P: Human estrogen receptor cDNA; sequence, expression, and homology to v-erb-A. Nature 320:134–139, 1986.

41. Haeuptle M-T, Suard YLM, Bogenmann E, Reggio H, Racine L, Kraehenbuhl JP: Effect of cell shape change on the function and differentiation of rabbit mammary cells in culture. J Cell Biol 96:1425–1434, 1983.

42. Hall A, Marshall CJ, Spurr NK, Weiss RA: Identification of transforming gene in two human sarcoma cell lines as a new member of the ras family located on chromosome 1. Nature 303:396–400, 1983.

43. Hammond SL, Ham RG, Stampfer MR: Serum-free growth of human mammary epithelial cells: Rapid clonal growth in defined medium and extended serial passage with pituitary extract. Proc Natl Acad Sci USA 81:5435–5439, 1984.

44. Hand PH, Thor A, Wunderlich D, Muraro R, Caruso A, Schlom J: Monoclonal antibodies of predefined specificity detect activated ras gene expression in human mammary and colon carcinomas. Proc Natl Acad Sci USA 81:5227–5231, 1984.

45. Hann SR, Thompson CB, Eisenman RN: c-myc Oncogene protein synthesis is independent of the cell cycle in human and avian cells. Nature 314:366–369, 1985.

46. Hecht F, Glover TW: Cancer chromosome breakpoints and common fragile sites induced by aphidicolin. Cancer Genet Cytogenet 13: 185–188, 1984.

47. Huff KK, Lippman ME, Spencer EM, Kaufman D, Dickson RB: Human breast cancer cells secrete an insulin-like growth factor I–related polypeptide. Cancer Res 46:4613–4619, 1986.

48. Hurley JB, Simon MI, Teplow DB, Robishaw JD, Gilman AG: Homologies between signal transducing G proteins and ras gene products. Science 226:860–862, 1984.

49. Hynes NE, Jaggi R, Kozma SC, Ball R, Muellener D, Wetherall NT, Davis BW, Groner B: New acceptor cell for transfected genomic DNA: Mol Cell Biol 5:268–272, 1985.

50. Jacobs C, Rubsamen H: Expression of pp60c-src protein kinase in adult and fetal human tissue: high activities in some sarcomas and mammary carcinomas. Cancer Res 43:1696–1702, 1983.

51. Jussawalla DJ, Deshpande VA, Haenszel W, Natekar MV: Differences observed in the site incidence of cancer, between the Parsi community and the total population of greater Bombay: a critical appraisal. Br J Cancer 24:56–66, 1970.

52. Kasid A, Knabbe C, Lippman ME: Effect of v-rasH oncogene transfection on estrogen-independent tumorigenicity of estrogen-dependent human breast cancer cells. Cancer Res 47:5733–5738, 1987.

53. Kasid A, Lippman ME, Papageorge AG, Lowy DR, Gelmann EP: Transfection of v-rasH DNA into MCF-7 human breast cancer cells bypasses dependence on estrogen for tumorigenicity. Science 228: 725–728, 1985.

54. Kataoka T, Powers S, Cameron S, Fasano O, Goldfarb M, Broach J, Wigler M: Functional homology of mammalian and yeast RAS genes. Cell 40:19–26, 1985.

55. Kataoka T, Powers S, McGill C, Fasano O, Strathern J, Broach J, Wigler M: Genetic analysis of yeast RAS1 and RAS2 genes. Cell 37: 437–445, 1984.

56. Keydar I, Ohno T, Nayak R, Sweet R, Simoni F, Weiss F, Mesa-Tejada R, Spiegelman S: Properties of retrovirus-like particles produced by a human breast carcinoma cell line: immunological relationship with mouse mammary tumor virus proteins. Proc Natl Acad Sci USA 81:4188–4192, 1984.

57. King MC, Go RC, Elston RC, Lynch HT, Petrakis NL: Allele increasing susceptibility to human breast cancer may be linked to glutamate-pyruvate transaminase locus. Science 208:406–408, 1980.

58. King CR, Kraus MH, Aaronson SA: Amplification of a novel v-erbB-related gene in a human mammary carcinoma. Science 229:974–976, 1985.

59. Klempnauer K-H, Symonds G, Evan GI, Bishop JM: Subcellular localization of proteins encoded by oncogenes of avian myeloblastosis virus and avian leukemia virus E26 and by the chicken c-myb gene. Cell 37:537–547, 1984.

60. Konopka JB, Watanabe SM, Singer JW, Collins SJ, Witte ON: Cell lines and clinical isolates from Ph-positive chronic myelogenous leukemia patients express c-abl proteins with a common structural alteration. Proc Natl Acad Sci USA 82:1810–1814, 1985.

61. Koufos A, Hansen MF, Lampkin BC, Workman ML, Copeland NG, Jenkins NA, Cavenee WK: Loss of alleles at loci on human chromosome 11 during genesis of Wilms' tumour. Nature 309:170–172, 1984.

62. Kraus MH, Popescu NC, Amsbaugh SC, King CR: Overexpression of the EGF receptor-related proto-oncogene erbB-2 in human mammary tumor cell lines by different molecular mechanisms. EMBO J 6:605–610, 1987.

63. Kraus MH, Yuasa Y, Aaronson SA: A position 12-activated H-ras oncogene in all HS578T mammary carcinosarcoma cells but not normal mammary cells of the same patient. Proc Natl Acad Sci USA 81:5384–5388, 1984.

64. Land H, Parada L, Weinberg R: Tumorigenic conversion of primary embryo fibroblasts requires at least two cooperating oncogenes. Nature 304:596–602, 1983.

65. Lane M-A, Sainten A, Cooper GM: Activation of related transforming genes in mouse and human mammary carcinomas. Proc Natl Acad Sci USA 78:5185–5189, 1981.

66. Leder P, Battey J, Lenoir G, Moulding C, Murphy W, Potter H, Stewart T, Taub R: Translocations among antibody genes in human cancer. Science 222:765–771, 1983.

67. Lidereau R, Escot C, Theillet C, Champeme M-H, Brunet M, Gest J, Callahan R: High frequency of rare alleles of the human c-Ha-ras-1 proto-oncogene in breast cancer patients. J Natl Cancer Inst 77: 697–701, 1986.

68. Liotta L, Mandler R, Murano G, Katz D, Gordon R, Chiang P, Schiffman E: Tumor cell autocrine motility factor. Proc Natl Acad Sci USA 83:3302–3306, 1986.

69. Lowe DG, Capon DJ, Delwart E, Sakaguchi A, Naylor SL, Goeddel DV: Structure of the human and murine R-ras genes, novel genes closely related to ras proto-oncogenes. Cell 48:137–146, 1987.

70. McGrath JP, Capon DJ, Smith DH, Chen EY, Seeburg PH, Goeddel DV, Levinson AD: Structure and organization of the human Ki-ras proto-oncogene and a related processed pseudogene. Nature 304:501–505, 1983.

71. Modjtahedi N, Lavialle C, Poupon MF, Landin RM, Cassingena R, Monier R, Brison O: Increased level of amplification of the c-myc oncogene in tumors induced in nude mice by a human breast carcinoma cell line. Cancer Res 45:4372–4379, 1985.

72. Moore DH, Charney J, Kramarsky B, Lasfargues EY, Brennan MJ, Sirsat SM, Paymaster JC, Vaidya AB: Search for a human breast cancer virus. Nature 229:611–615, 1971.

73. Nishikura K: Sequences involved in accurate and efficient transcription of human c-myc genes microinjected into frog oocytes. Mol Cell Biol 6:4093–4098, 1986.

74. Nusse R, van Ooyen A, Cox D, Fung YKT, Varmus H: Mode of proviral activation of a putative mammary oncogene (int-1) on mouse chromosome 15. Nature 307:131–136, 1984.

75. O'Brien SJ, Nash WG, Goodwin JL, Lowy DR, Chang EH: Dispersion of the ras family of tranforming genes to four different chromosomes in man. Nature 302:839–842, 1983.

76. Ohuchi N, Thor A, Page DL, Hand PH, Halter S, Schlom J: Expression of the 21,000 molecular weight ras protein in a spectrum of benign and malignant human mammary tissues. Cancer Res 46:2511–2519, 1986.

77. Owens RB, Smith HS, Hackett AJ: Epithelial cell cultures from normal glandular tissues of mice. J Natl Cancer Inst 53:261–266, 1974.

78. Papkoff J, Brown AMC, Varmus HE: The int-1 proto-oncogene products are glycoproteins that appear to enter the secretory pathway. Mol Cell Biol 7:3978–3984, 1987.

79. Persson H, Leder P: Nuclear localization and DNA binding properties of a protein expressed by human c-myc oncogene. Science 225:718–721, 1984.

80. Perucho M, Goldfarb M, Shimizu K, Lama C, Fogh J, Wigler M: Human tumor-derived cell lines contain common and different transforming genes. Cell 27:467–476, 1981.

81. Powers S, Kataoka T, Fasano O, Goldfarb M, Strathern J,

Broach J, Wigler M: Genes in S. cerevisiae encoding proteins with domains homologous to the mammalian ras proteins. Cell 36:607–612, 1984.

82. Reddy EP, Reynolds RK, Santos E, Barbacid M: A point mutation is responsible for the acquisition of transforming properties by the T24 human bladder carcinoma oncogene. Nature 300:149–152, 1982.

83. Reymond CD, Gomer RH, Mehdy MC, Firtel RA: Developmental regulation of a Dictyostelium gene encoding a protein homologous to mammalian ras protein. Cell 39:141–148, 1984.

84. Rijsewijk F, Schuermann M, Wagenaar E, Parren P, Weigel D, Nusse R: The Drosophila homolog of the mouse mammary oncogene int-1 is identical to the segment polarity gene wingless. Cell 50:649–657, 1987.

85. Rosen N, Bolen JB, Schwartz AM, Cohen P, DeSeau V, Israel MA: Analysis of pp60c-src protein kinase activity in human tumor cell lines and tissues. J Biol Chem 261:13754–13759, 1986.

86. Ryan J, Barker PE, Shimizu K, Wigler M, Ruddle F: Chromosomal assignment of a family of human oncogenes. Proc Natl Acad Sci USA 80:4460–4463, 1983.

87. Sambucetti LC, Curran T: The fos protein complex is associated with DNA in isolated nuclei and binds to DNA cellulose. Science 234:1417–1419, 1986.

88. Sap J, Munoz A, Damm K, Goldberg Y, Ghysdael J, Leutz A, Beug H, Vennstrom B: The c-erb-A protein is a high-affinity receptor for thyroid hormone. Nature 324:635–640, 1986.

89. Schwab M, Ellison J, Busch M, Rosenau W, Varmus H, Bishop JM: Enhanced expression of the human gene N-myc consequent to amplification of DNA may contribute to malignant progression of neuroblastoma. Proc Natl Acad Sci USA 81:4940–4944, 1984.

90. Sefton BM, Hunter T, Beemon K, Eckhart W: Evidence that the phosphorylation of tyrosine is essential for transformation by Rous sarcoma virus. Cell 20:807–816, 1980.

91. Segev N, Hizi A, Kirenberg F, Keydar I: Characterization of a protein, released by the T47D cell line, immunologically related to the major envelope protein of mouse mammary tumor virus. Proc Natl Acad Sci USA 82:1531–1535, 1985.

92. Shackleford GM, Varmus HE: Expression of the proto-oncogene int-1 is restricted to postmeiotic germ cells and the neural tube of mid-gestational embryos. Cell 50:89–95, 1987.

93. Sherr CJ, Rettenmeier CW, Sacca R, Roussel MF, Look AT, Stanley ER: The c-fms proto-oncogene product is related to the receptor for the mononuclear phagocytic growth factor, CSF-1. Cell 41:665–676, 1985.

94. Shtivelman E, Lifshitz B, Gale RP, Canaani E: Fused transcript of abl and bcr genes in chronic myelogenous leukemia. Nature 315: 550–554, 1985.

95. Sinn E, Muller W, Pattengale P, Tepler I, Wallace R, Leder P: Coexpression of MMTV/v-Ha-ras and MMTV/c-myc genes in transgenic mice: Synergistic action of oncogenes in vivo. Cell 49:465–475, 1987.

96. Slamon D, Clark GM, Wong SG, Levin WJ, Ullrich A, McGuire WL: Human breast cancer: Correlation of relapse and survival with amplification of the HER-2/neu oncogene. Science 235:177–182, 1986.

97. Slamon DJ, deKernion JB, Verma IM, Cline MJ: Expression of cellular oncogenes in human malignancies. Science 224:256–262, 1984.

98. Spandidos DA, Agnantis NJ: Human malignant tumors of the breast, as compared to their respective normal tissue, have elevated expression of the Harvey ras oncogene. Anticancer Res 4:269–272, 1984.

99. Stewart TA, Pattengale PK, Leder P: Spontaneous mammary adenocarcinomas in transgenic mice that carry and express MTV/myc fusion genes. Cell 38:627–637, 1984.

100. Swain S, Dickson R, Lippman ME: Anchorage-independent epithelial colony-stimulating activity in human breast cancer cell lines. Proc Am Assoc Cancer Res 27:844, 1986.

101. Tabbane F, Muenz L, Jaziri M, Cammoun M, Belhassen S, Mourali N: Clinical and prognostic features of a rapidly progressing breast cancer in Tunisia. Cancer 40:376–382, 1977.

102. Tanaka T, Slamon D, Battifora H, Cline MJ: Expression of p21 ras oncoproteins in human cancers. Cancer Res 46:1465–1470, 1986.

103. Tatchell K, Chaleff D, Defeo-Jones D, Scolnick E: Requirement of either of a pair of ras-related genes of Saccharomyses cerevisiae for spore viability. Nature 309:523–527, 1984.

104. Theillet C, Lidereau R, Escot C, Hutzell P, Brunet M, Gest J, Schlom J, Callahan R: Loss of a c-H-ras-1 allele and aggressive human primary breast carcinomas. Cancer Res 46:4776–4781, 1986.

105. Thompson CB, Challoner PB, Neiman PE, Groudine M: Levels of c-myc oncogene mRNA are invariant throughout the cell cycle. Nature 314:363–366, 1985.

106. Toda T, Uno I, Ishikawa T, Powers S, Kataoka T, Broek D, Cameron S, Wigler M: In yeast, RAS proteins are controlling elements of adenylate cyclase. Cell 40:27–36, 1985.

107. van de Vijver M, van de Bersselaar R, Devilee P, Cornelisse C, Peterse J, Nusse R: Amplification of the neu (c-erbB-2) oncogene in human mammary tumors is relatively frequent and is often accompanied by amplification of the linked c-erbA oncogene. Mol Cell Biol 7:2019–2023, 1987.

108. Waterfield MD, Scrace G, Whittle N, Stroobant P, Westermark B, Heldin C-H, Huang JS, Deuel TF: Platelet-derived growth factor is structurally related to the putative transforming protein of simian sarcoma virus. Nature 304:35–39, 1983.

109. Weinberger C, Hollenberg SM, Rosenfeld MG, Evans RM: Domain structure of the human glucocorticoid receptor and its relationship to the v-erb-A oncogene product. Nature 318:670–672, 1985.

110. Yokota J, Toyoshima K, Sugimura T, Yamamoto T, Terada M, Battifora H, Cline MJ: Amplification of c-erbB-2 oncogene in human adenocarcinomas in vivo. Lancet 1:765–766, 1986.

111. Yokota J, Tsunetsugu-Yokota Y, Battifora H, Le Fevre C, Cline MJ: Alterations of myc, myb, and rasH proto-oncogenes in cancers are frequent and show clinical correlation. Science 231:261–265, 1986.

112. Young D, Waitches G, Birchmeier C, Fasano O, Wigler M: Isolation and characterization of a new cellular oncogene encoding a protein with multiple potential transmembrane domains. Cell 45:711–719, 1986.

113. Zhou D, Battifora H, Yokota J, Yamamoto T, Cline MJ: Association of multiple copies of the c-erbB-2 oncogene with spread of breast cancer. Cancer Res 47:6123–6125, 1987.

114. Kozbor D, Croce CM: Amplification of the c-myc oncogene in one of five human breast carcinoma cell lines. Cancer Res 44:438–441, 1984.

Chapter 20

GROWTH REGULATION OF NORMAL AND MALIGNANT BREAST EPITHELIUM

Robert B. Dickson, Ph.D. and Marc E. Lippman, M.D.

GROWTH REGULATION: ENDOCRINE, AUTOCRINE, AND PARACRINE MECHANISMS

Since the 1940s it has been established that the progression of normal to cancerous tissue depends on interactions of inherited genetic factors, exposure to chemical carcinogens, damaging radiation, oncogenic viruses, and mitogenic hormones and other promotional agents.[31] While studies in experimental animal model systems[468] have allowed considerable insight into the mechanisms at work in the action of each component, few human cancers have a completely known etiology. The seminal work by Huggins[201] linking testicular secretions (androgen) to prostatic carcinoma and by Beatson[25] linking ovarian secretions (estrogens) to breast carcinoma represented critical insights into hormonal control of cancer. One focus of this chapter is to consider the mechanisms of systemic (or endocrine) actions of estrogen in the breast cancer process.[217] A second area of emphasis will be mechanisms of loss of endocrine control of breast cancer, commonly observed during chemo-hormonal therapy.[258]

That a fundamental mechanism such as estrogenic control of breast cancer growth can be lost during malignant progression implies the existence of other growth control processes that take over in its place. Indeed, work on locally acting, diffusible growth regulatory substances known as growth factors has provided a model for how additional growth controls might be exerted on mammary epithelial cells ranging from normal, to hormone-dependent intraductal, to metastatic, and finally to states of resistance to hormonal and chemotherapeutic agents.[118] In some case, these hormones are autostimulatory or "autocrine." In addition, a number of cancer-associated genes known as oncogenes[327, 392] have been described. Some of these oncogenes code for growth factors or their receptors. Others appear to code for defective, cell membrane–bound growth factor receptors that are enzymatically active even though they lack extracellularly exposed ligand-binding sites. One oncogene codes for a protein with homology to nuclear receptors for steroid and thyroid hormones. Still other oncogenes appear to act more distally on growth regulatory pathways, some directly modulating transcriptional complexes in the cell nucleus.[33, 420] Genetic events probably involve activation of dominant oncogenes and inactivation of dominant cancer-suppressive genes. The mutation of cellular proto-oncogenes (at least some of which appear to be functional in physiological growth control of normal tissue) to highly active oncogenes is now known to be extremely important in chemical- and radiation-induced carcinogenesis.[327, 392]

Though incompletely defined at present, malignant progression of breast cancer through its various stages probably involves multiple elements, including underlying genetic predisposition, mutation, and mitogenesis in response to estrogen, growth factors, and overexpressed growth factor receptors.[78, 121] On a cellular level, the actual mechanisms involved in malignant progression remain conjectural. Although the entire tumor could undergo progressive, malignant changes, this is not the most likely scenario. Rather, most observations suggest that subpopulations of ever-changing cancer cells continuously arise within the tumor. These subpopulations may be genetically altered; a small proportion tend to survive and overtake other less progressed tumor and normal cells. Surviving subpopulations are mitigated by selective pressures: host defenses, competition for nutrients, survival of chemo-hormonal therapeutic agents, and altered environment after metastatic spread.[306, 314]

Growth control processes in breast cancer are not limited to the cancerous tissue itself. Cancer depends on an intimate interrelationship with non-tumor tissues of the host. The cancer must thwart host immune surveillance and nourish itself as its mass increases.[336] The processes of angiogenesis (blood vessel invasion) and desmoplasia (stromal proliferation), commonly observed in breast cancer, are probably involved to some extent in these processes.[161] Potential soluble mediators of such processes are known as "paracrine"-acting hormones. Some of these hormones may also be coded for by oncogenes.[400, 403] The cancer can eventually invade the host, first via passage across the basement membrane, and then by local invasion, infiltration of blood vessels and lymphatics, and reseeding in distant metastatic sites. Development of metastatic potential probably also involves both oncogene- and mitogenic-mediated processes.

Estrogen is clearly one of the most important endocrine influences for the development and mitogenic control of breast cancer, but it appears to trigger multiple local influences on the cancer. What kinds of hormones might act in local autocrine or paracrine fashions? A well-established system for the identification of mediators of growth control has been provided by rodent fibroblasts in vitro. Studies were initially carried out in cell monolayers on plastic surfaces. Smith et al., among others, identified "restriction points" in the cell cycle of normal (but immortalized) fibroblasts.[393] Various polypeptide growth factors abrogate these restriction points, allowing the cell cycle to progress.[393] Platelet-derived growth factor (PDGF), a "competence" growth factor, allows cells to pass a restriction point in early G1. As PDGF acts to initiate the cell cycle, several genes known as proto-oncogenes are sequentially induced. Among these are c-*fos* and c-*myc*, in the nucleus, and c-*ras* in the plasma membrane (reviewed in Heldin and Westermark[189]). Epidermal growth factor (EGF), or the related transforming growth factor α (TGFα), acts later, while insulin-like growth factor I (IGF-I), also known as somatomedin C, and other hormones act still later in G1. A 68-kDa protein of unknown function (and c-*ras*) is induced during this time. EGF and IGF-I are termed "progression growth factors." Sometimes one growth factor induces another one, which acts further along in the cell cycle. For example, human diploid fibroblasts treated with PDGF, EGF, or growth hormone secrete their own IGF-I. Secreted IGF-I is capable of self-stimulation to promote mitogenesis; anti–IGF-I antibodies block growth hormone stimulation of DNA synthesis.

A number of investigators have noted that when fibroblasts and other cells are transformed with various tumor viruses, oncogenes, chemicals, or radiation, they lose some requirements for exogenous growth factors and produce more of their own.[36, 69, 189, 486] Thus malignant transformation was proposed to result from ectopic production of growth factors, abolishing both competence and progression points in a cell's own cycle. This may reflect the decreased serum requirement of some cancer cells.[98, 405]

In an attempt to generate a more cancer-specific growth assay for growth factor effects, an "anchorage-independent" growth assay has been developed. It had been observed that the ability of some cells to grow in colonies under anchorage-independent conditions (growth suspended in agar or agarose) was correlated with their tumorigenicity or state of malignant "transformation."[163] At least four growth factor activities have been identified that together can reversibly induce this transformed phenotype of murine fibroblasts: PDGF, EGF (or TGFα), IGF-I (or IGF-II, a different somatomedin activity), and an additional growth factor, transforming growth factor β (TGFβ).[12, 276, 405] An important aspect of TGFβ's action as a transforming agent appears to be its induction of basement membrane components,

such as collagen and fibronectin,[205] and the c-*sis* proto-oncogene.[247] Results from studies using anchorage-independent growth assays suggest that these growth factors are likely to be involved in cancer growth control, but little direct evidence for an in vivo role in tumor growth has yet emerged. Conclusions drawn from the murine fibroblast model system may not necessarily apply to cancers of other tissue or species or origin.

The principal restriction points, if any, for epithelial cell cycles are unknown. However, it is now clear that normal human mammary epithelial cells require hydrocortisone (a glucocorticoid), insulin, EGF, PGE$_1$ (a prostaglandin), transferrin, (the iron-carrying serum protein), and an incompletely defined pituitary component to proliferate in serum-free medium.[181] In contrast to the fibroblast model, TGFβ is a growth inhibitor for many types of normal and malignant epithelial cells, including breast.[349, 439] While some of the same growth factors may facilitate traverse of the cell cycle in both fibroblasts and epithelial cells, control of anchorage-independent growth may involve other growth factors. A candidate for such an epithelial transforming growth factor is provided by the work of Halper and Moses.[179] They have identified an adrenal carcinoma cell line (SW13) that is extremely sensitive for anchorage-independent cloning to a mitogen found in epithelial cancers or cell lines. Basic pituitary fibroblast growth factor (FGF) can also subserve such a function in cloning of SW13, and the epithelial cancer-derived growth factor may be a new member of the FGF family. Using an independent model system (SV40T oncogene–transfected, immortalized human mammary epithelial cells) TGFα, EGF, and FGF can also be shown to have transforming activity.[72, 442] In MCF-7 human breast cancer cells, estrogen is capable of inducing anchorage-independent growth.[261, 423] Biochemical mechanisms have not yet emerged to explain the transformed phenotype in malignant human epithelial cells. Perhaps estrogenic control of growth factors and basement membrane components will be found to contribute to steroid control of the malignant phenotype.

ROLE OF ESTROGEN AND ITS RECEPTOR IN CARCINOGENESIS AND GROWTH CONTROL OF MAMMARY EPITHELIUM

Estrogen Receptor

In the late 1950s, work by Jensen focused attention on high-affinity, estrogen-binding components in estrogen target tissues.[215] Initial cell localization studies utilizing radiolabeled estrogen demonstrated long-term retention of estrogen by the rodent uterus. The principal binding component, the estrogen receptor, has been characterized. Many studies have also localized the estrogen receptor to neural and many other nonreproductive organs of both male and female mammals (reviewed in Dickson and Clark[115]). The estrogen receptor appears to be a necessary mediator of estrogen action, initiating diverse developmental and physiological roles in many tissues.[418]

Based on subcellular fractionation results, early studies proposed that the unoccupied estrogen receptor was located in the cellular cytoplasm. Following ligand binding, the receptor affinity for chromatin increased (a process called activation or transformation) and a "translocation" to the nucleus was proposed to occur.[216] However, Zava and McGuire observed "unoccupied" nuclear receptors in MCF-7 breast cancer cells, a finding inconsistent with the translocation hypothesis.[485] Although work by Edwards et al.[132] called into question the existence of unoccupied nuclear receptors in the intact cells, this receptor form is now generally accepted based on two other lines of evidence. Following characterization of monoclonal antiestrogen receptor antibodies, King and Greene reported nuclear immunolocalization of the unoccupied estrogen receptor, further suggesting that the nuclear translocation model was incorrect.[233] Similar results were obtained by Gorski's group using a cell enucleation procedure.[469]

Though still controversial, both unoccupied and occupied estrogen receptors are now believed to reside largely in the nucleus, though probably in different biochemical complexes. Whether the estrogen receptor translocates to the nucleus in response to ligand occupancy, it must traverse the nuclear membrane at some point in its existence, since it is most likely synthesized on cytoplasmic ribosomes. Indeed, its primary sequence encodes two short series of amino acid residues with significant homology to nuclear transfer domains found on SV40T antigen (also a nuclear protein). The role of these sequences, however, has not been tested in the estrogen receptor.[476] However, in the glucocorticoid receptor, the hypothesis has been supported.[334]

The precise nature of the estrogen receptor–nuclear interaction is unknown. Presumably the receptor interacts both with DNA and chromosomal proteins. Nuclear "acceptor" binding proteins have been isolated for the uterine estrogen receptor[337] and other steroid receptors.[398] In addition, the estrogen receptor forms a complex with the nuclear matrix,[17] a chromatin scaffolding structure that may be involved in regulation of transcription and replication of DNA.[328, 352] Schuh et al.[379] have also shown that receptors for estrogen and other steroids associate (at least in vitro) with a 90-kDa heat shock protein. This heat shock protein also associates with the Rous sarcoma virus–transforming protein pp60$^{v\text{-}src}$, a plasma membrane protein.

The role of the 90-kDa protein in receptor function and hormone action is not yet known. However, Groyer et al. have suggested that it suppresses DNA binding of at least the glucocorticoid receptor.[177] Another protein, a 29-kDa phosphoprotein, may also associate with the estrogen receptor. Its function is unknown, but its presence in breast cancer appears to correlate with hormone responsivity.[52]

Walter et al. have obtained cDNA clones of the estrogen receptor from MCF-7 cells.[462] The mRNA codes for a 66-kDa protein that contains a long 3′ untranslated region (like the glucocorticoid receptor).[167]

The DNA binding domain of the receptors for estrogen, glucocorticoid, mineralocorticoids, vitamin D, progesterone, retinoic acid, and some unknown ligands share a strong homology with one of the transforming proteins of avian erythroblastosis virus (v-erb-A).* Studies have shown that the cellular homologue of v-erb-A, known as c-erb-A, is a receptor for thyroid hormones.[374, 467] The functional significance of this homology is not yet known, though the DNA binding region of each is the most highly conserved portion.[265] Following expression in transfected cells or after in vitro translation, the protein product of the estrogen receptor gene is able to bind estrogen with high affinity.[126, 462] The in vitro translation experiments, coupled with detailed sequence analysis, strongly suggest that the estrogen receptor is not a protein kinase and does not require post-transcriptional modifications such as phosphorylation for binding activity.

A possible role of phosphorylation in the action of the estrogen receptor remains to be fully evaluated. Auricchio et al.[13] and Migliaccio et al.[289] have purified tyrosine kinase and phosphatase activities from calf and rodent uteri and demonstrated that the purified estrogen receptor is a substrate. The state of tyrosine phosphorylation is associated with the ability of the receptor to bind E_2 in in vitro assays.[290] These investigators have proposed that a phosphorylation-dephosphorylation cycle might exist in intact cells to regulate receptor binding and nuclear localization. Another study has reported that cAMP decreased and cGMP increased estrogen binding in cytosol fractions of endometrial cancer cells.[158] However, this study did not directly evaluate receptor phosphorylation. Later work by other investigators using intact MCF-7 cells and estrogen receptor immunoprecipitation following metabolic labeling with radioactive phosphate, has failed to detect either phosphotyrosine or changes in receptor binding following treatment of cells with activators of adenylate cyclase. However, phorbol ester treatment of MCF-7 cells resulted in a reduction of estrogen receptor binding activity and cell proliferation and was associated with a loss of estrogen inducibility of proliferation and progesterone receptor.[90, 235] Phosphorylation of the estrogen receptor appeared to occur much more rapidly than did receptor loss.[379] Reported differences among investigations concerning identity, inducibility, and function of amino acid phosphorylation in the estrogen receptor remain to be resolved.

Studies of the estrogen receptor have been greatly facilitated in breast cancer biopsies by the availability of monoclonal antibodies directed against the receptor.[174] These antibodies, some available in commercial detection kits, allow radioimmunoassay in cytosolic or nuclear extracts of tissue and also allow detection of receptor-positive cells in tissue sections. One important caveat of these assay systems would appear to be their selectivity for estrogen-occupied receptor over ligand-unoccupied receptor.[338] Nevertheless, numerous studies have demonstrated the comparability of ligand binding assays and

---

*References 9, 107, 144, 168, 169, 172, 173, 281, and 430.

antibody detection assays for the estrogen receptor.[123, 280] Use of the immunohistochemical assay has supported the conclusion that normal breast epithelium is quite low (but with intermittent positive cells) in estrogen receptor content.[232] Another important advance in receptor analysis has been the development of two radioactive affinity labels for the estrogen receptor: tamoxifen aziridine (an antiestrogen) and ketononestrol aziridine (an estrogen).[140, 293] Both of these compounds attach to and label the same 66-kDa estrogen receptor in receptor-containing tissue extracts. Furthermore, tamoxifen aziridine and one monoclonal antibody (H222/Spγ) recognized the same 6-kDa tryptic fragment and 28-kDa V8 protease fragment of the receptor.[224]

The Control of Normal Glandular Growth by Estrogen

Some of the most complete studies of the developing mammary gland have been made in the mouse. The embryonic mammary epithelium develops as a "bud" within the mammary fat pad. Fetal development is thought to proceed through epithelial-stromal (mesenchymal) interactions, with little hormonal involvement.[15, 339] A primitive gland duct is formed by day 19 of the embryo but does not further develop until the postnatal period.[15] In the male, in contrast, the developing fetal testes secretes testosterone, which inhibits epithelial development between days 13 and 15 through a stromal-epithelial interactive process.[124, 340] Receptors for both androgen and estrogen are present in the stromal but not in the epithelial components at this time.[124, 300]

In contrast to nonsexual organs, most of the development of the mammary gland occurs in subadult and adult life in response to a combination of interactions among systemic hormones and local mesenchymal cells. After birth, the mouse mammary gland consists of the primary duct and a few branching ducts. Development occurs with the onset of puberty and with cyclical growth, and regression occurs during successive reproductive cycles. Mammary ducts further develop (lobulo-alveolar development) during pregnancy and lactation. Glands partially regress at the termination of this phase.

From studies in both mice and women, estradiol is known to be essential for the ductal phases of mammary gland development.[238, 299] The end buds of the developing ducts appear to be the most rapidly proliferating regions. When estradiol is administered systemically to castrated female mice, quiescent ductal end buds have been shown to synthesize DNA and effect ductal elongation.[37] In contrast, if the same experiment is carried out in animals whose ovaries as well as pituitary glands have been removed, this result is not obtained.[251, 270] Such experiments have inspired hypotheses that estrogen does not act directly on mammary tissue but indirectly, through a systematically acting substance such as growth hormone.[251, 270, 299, 390] Estrogen and growth hormone partially reverse end bud regression in animals whose ovaries, pituitaries, and adrenals have been removed.[299]

Studies in vitro with normal mammary epithelial cell cultures have supported such a hypothesis of indirect action of estrogen with cells of either mouse or human origin.[409, 479] Estrogen-induced epithelial proliferation has been observed only when epithelial cells are cocultured with mammary stromal cells.[187, 282] Such experiments support an indirect but local mechanism of estrogen action involving a close communication between stromal and epithelial components.

In vivo studies have also supported this theory. Application of estrone to one nipple area of a mammary gland of monkeys, rabbits, and guinea pigs promotes lobulo-alveolar growth at the site of application but not in untreated glands.[62, 271, 304] Other studies in mice with plastic, estrogen-containing pellets implanted into the developing gland have also supported a local-acting and not a systemic-acting mechanism for estrogen-induced lobulo-alveolar development. Local, but not distant, end bud growth was observed.[88] In the same study, autoradiographical localization of estrogen receptors was observed in ductal epithelium, stroma, and luminal cells of the end bud but not in the proliferative cap cells of the end bud. For obvious ethical reasons, similar studies have not yet been carried out to localize the estrogen receptor in developing glands of pubescent girls. However, normal nonlactating biopsy samples from women have been subjected to immunocytochemistry to localize the estrogen receptor.[333] In this study, stromal cells were negative for estrogen receptor, and only seven percent of epithelial cells were positive. The positive cells were scattered, with highest frequency in lobules.

If estrogen might have local but indirect mediators, what is the nature of such mediating substances? In vivo organ culture studies have begun to cast light on this problem. If prepubescent female mice are "primed" with estrogen and progesterone, their glands are capable of lobulo-alveolar development in vitro in response to a combination of hormones and growth factors. Insulin, prolactin, aldosterone, and hydrocortisone can act along with an extract of estrogen-progesterone–primed gland to induce in vitro development in organ culture. The gland extract contains an EGF receptor–binding component, and either EGF or the closely related TGFα can substitute for the activity supplied by the gland extract. TGFα and EGF are both able to promote local lobulo-alveolar development in vitro when implanted in slow-release pellets into the mammary gland.[457, 458] Isolated ductal end buds from mice also have a requirement of EGF for in vitro growth.[345] The site of action of EGF is still problematic; one report has demonstrated that in intact, prepubescent mice, EGF receptors are predominant in the stromal cells surrounding the growing end buds.[87] Thus, although one local mediator of proliferation in normal ductal development appears to be a TGFα- or EGF-related growth factor, it is not yet clear whether this mediator acts directly on the epithelium. A similar system also appears to be operative in estrogen-induced uterine growth. In that organ, estradiol-stimulated growth may depend on both induction of EGF receptor and an EGF-related growth factor.[110, 253]

In vitro studies with cell lines derived from normal

breast sources have supported the notion that the epithelium is not directly responsive to mitogenic stimulation by estrogen. Normal lines of epithelial[406] and myoepithelial origin[178] and epithelial lines immortalized spontaneously,[38] by carcinogens[407] or by SV40T oncogene,[55, 64, 65] have not been reported to contain the estrogen receptor or to respond to estrogens. However, proliferative normal cultures express high levels of the GF receptor and TGFα.[249, 364] As mentioned, in low-density culture, these cells require multiple hormones: EGF (or TGFα), insulin, transferrin, isoproterenol (or cholera toxin, PGE_1, or phosphodiesterase inhibitors, which stimulate cAMP production or accumulation), hydrocortisone, and bovine pituitary extract (whose active ingredient is not yet known).[181, 409]

In summary, estrogen appears to interact with multiple hormones, some of which are pituitary in origin, to stimulate the growth of normal gland. While some evidence for estrogen receptors in the epithelium exists, it is not yet clear that growth responses of the normal epithelium are direct responses to estrogen. Rather, stromal-epithelial interaction and growth factor mediators (such as TGFα) appear to be involved.

Hormonal Carcinogenesis

Epidemiology and Pathology

Breast cancer is a frighteningly common disease, striking approximately one in 12 women in North America. Epidemiological data have suggested that familial, environmental, and hormonal factors all play a role. Pathologically, breast cancer arises "multifocally." Numerous premalignant and malignant lesions occur in an afflicted woman. Eventually, a single cellular lineage usually takes over as the disease progresses.[153, 291] The multifocal nature of breast cancer in susceptible individuals suggests that a single, local insult is not important in early-stage cancer. Rather, there is a high frequency of premalignant lesions that become malignant with increasing exposure to estrogen (during and after puberty). Breast cancer occurs in men, or in women who have never had functional ovaries, with only one percent of the frequency of that in women with intact ovaries.

The correlation with ovarian function has been further demonstrated in studies of the victims of the Hiroshima and Nagasaki bombings in World War II.[283] The highest incidence of breast cancer occurred in women who were 10 to 19 years of age at the time of this radiation exposure. As mentioned in the previous section, normal mammary tissue responds to elevations in estrogens at puberty. Thus estrogens appear to have a stimulatory role in both normal and neoplastic breast epithelium. Estrogenic hormones may play multiple roles in neoplastic progression of breast cancer as carcinogens and as permissive, promotional, and tumor growth–inducing agents.

Breast tissue may be directly damaged by estrogens. Hormonal damage, along with damage caused by diet and other environmental factors, may combine with hereditary defects to yield premalignant cells. Hormonal stimulation of premalignant cells may then yield multifocal lesions. The proportion of early breast cancer lesions that are hormone dependent is unknown but almost certainly very high, given the nearly complete dependence of disease on ovarian function at puberty. At the time of clinical detection, two thirds of breast cancers contain the estrogen receptor; one half of this number contain the progesterone receptor and respond to initial therapy directed toward blockade of estrogenic stimulation.[246]

As breast cancer proceeds from multifocal premalignant lesions, cells are selected for rapid growth. When treatment is begun, tumor cells are further selected for resistance to chemotherapeutic and antihormonal agents. These phases may be associated with greater efficiency of estrogen to stimulate growth or with the appearance of alternate growth stimulatory pathways. This progression of malignancy may involve progressive overexpression or mutation of proto-oncogenes, as well as progressive loss of estrogen-controlled pathways. Ultimately, unless the cancer is excised and aggressively treated with pharmacological agents, radiation at an early (intraductal) stage, or both, the patient stands a very good chance of developing advanced metastatic disease. In the worst scenario, breast cancer widely metastasizes to the brain, bone, and viscera and can no longer be controlled by surgical, radiation, antihormonal, or chemotherapeutic strategies. We systematically address the roles of hormone stimulation and proto-oncogene expression in this and the next sections of this chapter.

The observation that estrogenic exposure is associated with experimental mammary cancer was first made in mice by Bittner (reviewed in Henderson et al.[190]). He proposed that hormones can directly increase the incidence of neoplasia (i.e., act as carcinogens). Considerable epidemiological evidence in women now suggests that the length of estrogenic exposure of the mammary glands, among other dietary, genetic, and environmental factors, is proportional to breast cancer risk. Long-term exposure to endogenous estrogens (early menarche; late menopause; late age at first full-term pregnancy; and being overweight, leading to increased aromatization of circulating androgens to estrogens) appears to increase cancer risk. Risk is decreased with early menopause (natural or artificial) and childbearing. However, first-trimester abortion increases risk.[190] Surprisingly, oral contraceptive use does not appear to be a major risk factor, although this is currently controversial.[51]

A few studies have suggested that while not a primary mitogen in breast tissue, prolactin enhances the mitogenic effects of estrogen.[295] Also, since breast epithelial mitoses peak in the luteal phase of the menstrual cycle (when progesterone is highest and estrogen lowest), some investigators have suggested that a role for progesterone should not be overlooked.[146] Estrogenic exposure has been associated with vaginal adenocarcinoma,[191] endometrial cancer,[218] and liver tumors.[444] From the cumulative observations, the strongest hypothesis of hormonal carcinogenesis in breast cancer invokes the "total cumulative exposure of breast tissue to bioavailable estrogens and the associated cumulative mitotic activity" as an etiological factor.[190]

Direct Damage of Cells by Estrogen

An alternative hypothesis on hormonal carcinogenesis has proposed that estrogens also act directly to damage cells. This hypothesis has received strong impetus from the well-known carcinogenic effects of diethylstilbesterol (DES) in daughters of women who took DES in hope of preventing spontaneous abortions. DES is metabolized by a peroxidase-mediated oxidation. It appears that epoxide and semiquinone intermediates are short lived but carcinogenic. Though DES is genotoxic, no clear evidence of purine or pyrimidine adduct formation has yet been published. Perhaps DES-DNA adducts are unstable, or perhaps the mechanism of damage involves some other lesion.[285] One intriguing possible alternate mechanism for such damage involves interaction of DES with the spindle apparatus, partially disrupting cellular mitosis. DES is thought to induce cellular aneuploidy by this action.[438]

Steroidal estrogens are thought to act as carcinogens by alternate metabolic transformations. Estradiol and the oral contraceptive ethinylestradiol are susceptible to reactive hydroxylated intermediates (2 OH and 16 OH). These compounds are also thought to be genotoxic through reactive semiquinone formation. Both DNA and proteins may be substrates of such damage.[96, 155, 287] Interestingly, both types of reactive intermediates bind the estrogen receptor[114, 424a] and the 16α OH form of estradiol appears to form a covalent adduct with the estrogen receptor.[156] Several investigators have shown that estradiol-16α hydroxylation is increased in women with a high inherited risk of developing breast cancer or who have developed breast cancer.[35, 378] It may be that carcinogenicity of estrogens involves both a mitogenic component of action and a component of action requiring metabolism to a reactive species. For example, in a model rodent system (Syrian hamster) 2-fluoro-estradiol does not induce renal cancer, but estrodiol itself does. Both compounds have identical estrogenicity in vivo and in vitro for several cell types, including kidney and uterus. However, only estradiol is metabolized to a reactive 2 OH intermediate. Mitogenicity and carcinogenicity of estrogens are clearly separable characteristics.[252]

Hormonal Interactions with Carcinogens and Oncogenes

The carcinogen-induced rat mammary tumor model has been especially useful for pinpointing a cell of origin for mammary cancer.[368] Based on retrospective human surgical studies, the intralobular terminal duct has been proposed as the principal site of origin of breast cancer. Detailed carcinogen/oncogene induction studies in rodent model systems have come to the same general conclusion but have focused more critically on especially early events.

In the rat, progressive stimulation by each estrus cycle facilitates progressive growth and differentiation of club-shaped, terminal end buds of mammary ducts into "alveolar buds." Hormonal stimulation of the gland occurs from the onset of estrus (days 35 to 42) until approximately 6 months later. During this time, inoculation of rats with the carcinogen 7,12-dimethylbenz[a]anthracene (DMBA) is maximally effective at inducing cancer. DMBA induces many terminal end buds to develop into "intraductal proliferations" instead of alveolar buds; these lesions can develop into intraductal carcinoma.

Since mammary gland development is rather asynchronous in the rat, some terminal end buds (later called terminal ducts) are still available as targets for DMBA–induced transformation in older animals. If terminal end buds are allowed to undergo differentiation to alveolar buds, they are refractory to DMBA–induced carcinogenesis. They are more likely to develop into nonmalignant hyperplastic alveolar nodules, tubular adenomas, or cystic dilatations. Thus, in this model, carcinomas arise from more undifferentiated structures, whereas more benign lesions arise from structures that were more differentiated during the interval of carcinogen exposure. The rat mammary gland is composed of myoepithelial cells and so-called light, dark, and intermediate epithelial cells. Morphologically, DMBA–induced tumors appear to arise from the intermediate cells, the most rapidly proliferating cell type in the gland. In general, DMBA–sensitive terminal and bud cells are more proliferative than the more differentiated, less DMBA–sensitive, alveolar buds.

In the rat model, pregnancy induces a rapid growth and differentiation of terminal end buds to alveolar buds and further (through lobulo-alveolar development) to secretory ducts. This transition is associated with an inhibition of susceptibility to DMBA carcinogenesis. Experimentally, similar inhibition of DMBA carcinogenesis is obtained in rats with mammary growth and development stimulated by hypothalamic lesions or pituitary grafts (both of which elevate secretion of many pituitary hormones, including prolactin and growth hormones). The placental hormone human chorionic gonadotropin (hCG) or progestational hormones (in early reproductive life) have a similar protective effect. Human placental lactogen (hPL), another pregnancy hormone, has no protective effect. While incidence of ductal carcinoma decreases with pregnancy, the incidence of benign fibroadenomas doubles, as would be expected based on increased differentiation of the gland. These studies suggest that mammary differentiation strategies could be attempted in high-risk women. We discuss cancer prevention strategies later in the section on antiestrogens, which are also preventative of DMBA tumorigenesis in rats.

The carcinogen-induced rat mammary cancer model has also been useful for pinpointing a critical genotoxic lesion, activation of the c-H-*ras* oncogene. The carcinogens DMBA and *N*-methylnitrosurea (NMU) reproducibly activate this oncogene. The possible etiological importance of this oncogene has been highlighted by transgenic mouse studies. In these studies, the activated *ras* oncogene was placed under the control of a mammary lactation-specific promoter known as the whey acidic protein promoter. Use of this promoter targets expression of *ras* oncogene for lactating mammary glands. The transgenic model allowed gene insertion in developing blastocyst and eventual expression and mammary tumor development after pregnancy.[7] Similar studies have also implicated the c-*myc* oncogene as possibly important in tumorigenesis,[413] and a combination of *myc* and *ras* expression under lactation-specific promoters led to a synergistic enhancement of pregnancy-dependent tumors.[389]

These studies together have allowed a proof that oncogenes can act, in combination with appropriate hormonal stimulation of the gland, to induce breast cancer. A firm proof of this hypothesis in human breast cancer, however, is lacking at present. A difficulty with these transgenic models is that they have not allowed study of proto-oncogene–estrogen interaction, the presumed interaction giving rise to human cancer. Instead, these transgenic models require pregnancy and lactation to induce the oncogenes. As previously mentioned, pregnancy-lactation is usually considered protective for breast cancer. Future use of tissue-specific promoters of proto-oncogenes or oncogene expression that do not depend on a lactational stimulus would appear to be warranted.

Human Cell Culture Models

Testing etiological hypotheses of human breast carcinogenesis requires development of in vitro models. Ideally, with such models it would be possible to explore the varied roles of such putative etiological factors as hormones, radiation, and carcinogens. Several normal lines have been developed: diploid Hs578Bst (a myoepithelial morphology),[178] and a series of diploid epithelial lines from reduction mammoplasty patients. These lines eventually undergo terminal squamous differentiation.[181, 367, 409] Another approach, utilizing a medium with a low concentration of calcium, has allowed maintenance of the diploid phenotype without expressing terminal differentiation.[389] A spontaneously immortalized, near-diploid epithelial line, HMT-3522, has also been established from fibrocystic breast tissue.[38]

An interesting aspect of normal epithelial cells in culture[367] is that their growth requirements have been defined: insulin, glucocorticoid, EGF, isoproterenol (or other stimulator of cAMP), bovine pituitary extract, and transferrin. Two of these components, the glucocorticoid and EGF, are less critical when the cells are in mass culture than when they are at low density, suggesting autoproduction and crossfeeding of either a growth factor (in the case of EGF or TGFα) or other unknown factors. The pituitary extract components are not yet identified, but two agents of likely importance are bFGF and TGFα. Transferrin, glucocorticoid, and insulin appear to be the necessary serum components, whereas TGFα appears to be a necessary autocrine factor that must be externally supplied if cells are not of sufficient density.[410] A TGFα–like component also appears to be made by myoepithelial cells.[366] The requirement for cAMP is interesting in light of the production of PGE$_2$ (a stimulator of cAMP) by stromal cells.[366] PGE$_2$–stimulated cAMP may contribute to stromal epithelial growth controls. Thus the culture of normal cells appears to require replacement of the natural hormones initially present in serum and made by the surrounding stromal and myoepithelial elements of the gland. Malignant progression appears to involve gradual abrogation of these requirements.

The normal mammary epithelial cell in culture has been an imperfect model in the study of carcinogenic factors in cancer. Its most important deficit is that no estrogen or progesterone receptors are present, and no experiments have successfully utilized estrogens in vitro as carcinogens or co-carcinogens. The lack of these receptors is not yet understood. Possibilities include a lack of proper stromal epithelial interactions, a subpopulation of cells without the estrogen receptor reproducibly adapts to tissue culture, and a critical component of the medium is missing. In addition, carcinogen treatment alone has failed to induce full malignant transformation. However, immortalized human mammary epithelial cell cultures have been obtained by treatment of cells with benzo[a]pyrene,[18] SV40 virus,[397] or low Ca^{++} medium.[63] The molecular basis of the carcinogen and low Ca^{++} effects is not yet understood.

A partially malignant state has been obtained by benzo[a]pyrene immortalization coupled with SV40 treatment. These cells form anchorage-independent colonies in the presence of TGFα/EGF or bFGF.[408] Full malignancy was obtained by superinfecting these same cells with v-H-*ras* oncogene. It thus appears possible to obtain full hormone-independent malignancy with a three-step treatment of human mammary epithelial cells.[65, 408] There is a need to develop in vitro model systems that also allow for study of estrogen interactions in mammary carcinogenesis.

Chromosomal and Oncogene Abnormalities in Human Breast Cancer

Chromosomal Alterations. It has become clear that breast cancer etiology has familial and environmental components in addition to hormonal ones. From the genetic point of view, recurring chromosomal alterations in breast tumors have involved chromosomes 1, 3, 6, 7, 9, and 11.[436] In particular, loss of variable lengths of one allele of chromosome 11 are significantly associated with breast tumors lacking estrogen and progesterone receptors, grade III histology, and distal metastasis. This pattern has been associated with the loss of an inhibitory gene in other conditions, such as retinoblastoma.[6] In addition, cellular aneuploidy is related to increased rates of tumor proliferation and estrogen receptor negativity.[154] In some other diseases, such as lymphoma, characteristic chromosomal translocations have been associated with activation of dominant acting, cancer-causing genes known as oncogenes.[85]

Oncogenes were originally identified as the genes

conferring transforming potential to RNA tumor viruses (retroviruses).[448] It was subsequently determined that these elements were mutated forms of genes (proto-oncogenes) that had been stolen or "transformed" from the host cell DNA. Proto-oncogenes are thought to be involved in control of normal growth and development and to contribute to carcinogenesis when their function, structure, or both are altered.[448]

Oncogenes have been suggested to be more important in some naturally occurring (nonbreast) human tumors through several lines of evidence. This evidence includes their ability (after isolation) to transform cultured mouse 3T3 fibroblast cells, their rearrangement, overexpression, or both, consistent with well-known chromosomal translocations of cancer, and amplification of the proto-oncogene copy number in the chromosome. Most of the tumor genes characterized by these criteria are human homologues of transduced retroviral oncogenes.

In breast cancer, no consistent pattern of oncogene activation by these criteria has yet emerged. Instead, increased expression of a variety of proto-oncogenic proteins has been associated with breast carcinogenesis and tumor progression. The functional consequences are currently under investigation, but as mentioned earlier other factors such as loss of inhibitory gene products[8] and direct effects of estrogen are probably also important in breast cancer. It is also likely that our current assays for oncogenes are inadequate to define all of the genes important for epithelial carcinogenesis, invasion, metastasis, phenotypic progression, and other aspects of tumor development.

Known oncogene and proto-oncogene products fall into several functional classes, including nuclear proteins that may act as transcriptional activators, growth factors, transmembrane tyrosine kinases that function as growth factor receptors, intracellular serine and tyrosine kinases, and membrane-bound G-protein analogues. Members of each class of proto-oncogenes are overexpressed in subsets of human breast cancer. For the most part, the functional significance of such overexpression is unknown. Proto-oncogenes, like their activated oncogene homologues, are thought to regulate replication, transcription, and hormonal signal transduction processes. Their coordinated overexpression in cancer could contribute to a more rapidly growing tumor as well as to invasiveness and metastases.[448]

Proto-oncogene c-*myc*. One of the most widely studied proto-oncogenes, classified with a family of nuclear-localized oncogenes, is known as c-*myc*. Its expression appears to be necessary in the cell cycle; it is induced by growth factor treatment of quiescent fibroblasts just prior to S-phase entry, and it is reported to be a component of the DNA replication complex.[134] In mutated form, *myc* exists as an avian retroviral oncogene (v-*myc*) and is commonly affected by characteristic chromosomal translocations, as in Burkitt's lymphoma.[448] A study has shown that in human breast cancer, c-*myc* is quite commonly rearranged, amplified, or both, and its RNA may be overexpressed in primary tumors, when compared with hyperplastic and normal breast controls.[274] In this study c-*myc* protein levels were not

addressed, and no relationship was observed between c-*myc* changes and tumor content of estrogen receptors. It is not yet known whether c-*myc* expression bears a causal relationship to malignant progression of breast cancer, although as previously mentioned, animal models suggest this possibility.

Tyrosine Kinases. One of the more interesting proto-oncogenes expressed in breast cancer is c-*erb-B*, the epidermal growth factor (EGF) receptor (a ligand-activated tyrosine kinase). It is commonly overexpressed in estrogen receptor–negative tumors with especially poor prognosis and a high degree of invasiveness.[369] The mechanism of overexpression appears to be at the transcriptional level.[94] However, one breast cancer cell line has a c-*erb-B* gene amplification. This line has allowed an interesting subclone analysis of sublines that have lost varying levels of c-*erb-B*; loss of c-*erb-B* amplification and expression led to decreased tumor growth rate but no change in tumor frequency in the nude mouse model system.[150] Similar conclusions were reached in an independent study with a vulvar carcinoma cell line.[373] Thus c-*erb-B* expression may be a relatively late lesion in tumorigenesis, allowing increased tumor growth rate and invasion in the estrogen receptor–negative, especially poor prognosis subgroup. The c-*erb-B* can act as an oncogene, provided a source of TGFα or EGF is available,[122, 450] and c-*erb-B* expression in human breast tumor biopsy specimens is reported to correlate with ^{3}H-thymidine labeling index.[399]

Whether c-*erb-B* activity is independent of ligand occupancy or requires TGFα (or EGF) to increase tumor growth is not yet clear. EGF and TGFα are known to act as oncogenes in EGF receptor–containing cell lines.[358, 412] Moreover, TGFα is commonly synthesized and secreted by human breast cancer, and EGF induces transient tumor formation by MCF-7 cells in vivo.

A recently discovered oncogene known as c-*erb-B₂* (*neu* or *HER2*) may also help to complete the process of malignant progression, conferring metastatic capacity to carcinogen-induced rat neuroblastomas. It is structurally similar to the receptor for EGF (c-*erb-B*), including an intracellular tyrosine kinase domain. The physiological ligand, if any, for this putative transmembrane receptor is unknown.

In a study on human breast cancer biopsy specimens, c-*erb-B₂* gene amplification and protein expression were significantly correlated with the number of lymph nodes invaded (an indicator of metastatic spread). No relationship has been observed between estrogen receptor content and c-*erb-B₂* oncogene amplification or expression.

Activity of the oncogene known as c-*src* may be associated with expression of the estrogen receptor. It is the proto-oncogene of the earliest described transforming protein, known as v-*src*; it is also a tyrosine kinase but not a receptor. Like its amino terminal truncated retroviral oncogene homologue v-*src*, c-*src* is associated with the inner plasma membrane and transforms fibroblasts by phosphorylation of tyrosine residues on as yet unknown substrates.[211]

One study with human breast tumors noted that nearly half had increased c-*src* kinase activity compared to normal control tissue. A later study in breast cancer cell lines reported the same conclusion, additionally noting that estrogen receptor–containing lines had signficantly higher activity than did receptor-negative ones.[356] Future studies with tumor biopsy specimens will be required to determine if this correlation in cell lines is of general significance and if c-src functionally replaces c-erb-B or c-erb-B$_2$ in more differentiated cancers.

The ras Family. V-ras-H was initially detected in a retrovirus (Harvey murine sarcoma virus).[448] Transformation of NIH 3T3 cells can result from expression of the mutated v-H-ras or overexpression of the unmutated c-H-ras.[68] Traversal of the cell cycle in fibroblasts in culture appears to require ras expression (as well as myc), and myc and ras can cooperate or synergize to allow complete transformation of rat embryo fibroblasts. Ras is associated with the inner plasma membrane and is at least superficially similar to the receptor-response coupling, GTP-binding G proteins. It appears to activate phospholipase C,[448] possibly by direct interaction or receptor coupling.

While not commonly activated in human breast cancer, the c-H-ras proto-oncogene is commonly overexpressed in tumors when compared with normal or benign lesion controls.[316] At the genetic level, breast cancer is often characterized by decreased frequency of normal c-H-ras alleles and increased rare alleles, suggesting rearrangements. No relationship has been detected between ras gene rearrangements and estrogen receptor content.[250] Nevertheless in vitro studies suggest that ras expression may contribute to increased tumor invasion metastasis,[176] polypeptide growth factor output,[448] and genetic mutability,[411] all potentially leading to increased malignant progression. When the v-H-ras gene was inserted and overexpressed in MCF-7 estrogen-dependent breast cancer cells, the cells gained the capacity to form tumors in the nude mouse in the absence of estrogen,[223] increased their capacity for invasion of an artificial basement membrane in vitro,[5] and elevated their secretion of polypeptide growth factors.[117, 222] Ras expression may act at many stages of the tumorigenic process and cooperate with other oncogenes and hormones. A study has identified an unusual, difficult-to-detect c-K-ras oncogene mutation in a human cell line, MDA-MB-231. Perhaps future studies will also find more widespread ras activation of diverse types in primary human tumors.[237]

The genes c-myc and c-H-ras may mediate or substitute for receptor-induced mitogenic events; c-erb-B, c-erb-B$_2$, and the estrogen receptor itself (distant c-erb-A homology)[34] may be more proximal, receptor-classed regulators, whereas growth factors themselves (such as TGFα and PDGF or c-sis)[41, 330, 358] may also have oncogenic potential. Clearly, more study is required to sort out the relative importance of these diverse receptor-related proto-oncogenic expressions, as well as other factors such as stimulation by estrogen that may underlie the development of breast cancer.

Growth Control of Cancer

An estrogenic component of neoplastic growth control would appear to be a modified remnant of a normal mechanism of mammary epithelial proliferation and differentiation during puberty (and possibly during fetal development). While estrogens are mitogens for both normal and malignant breast epithelium, the hypothalamus-pituitary axis is indirectly in control of ovarian estrogen secretion by virtue of GnRH and gonadotropin stimulation.[359] In addition, the pituitary gland (or other organs) may also secrete other direct- or indirect-acting mitogens[133, 473] such as IGF-II, FGF, or LH-RH. Studies of murine model systems have shown that estrogen can control breast tumor growth by inducing pituitary synthesis and secretion of prolactin. Ikeda et al. have employed the term "estromedin" for other analogous, but still hypothetical, estrogen-induced, endocrine-acting mitogens.[207]

Other investigators have proposed that estrogen acts by allowing breast cancers to overcome growth inhibitory agents in their environment or by synergy with another stimulatory agent.[108, 268, 395] These interacting components could be serum-derived, produced by the cancer itself, or produced by nearby tissues. Studies of hormonal control of breast cancer have been facilitated by the availability of cancer cell lines, usually derived from pleural or ascites fluids of patients. Several estrogen-responsive lines exist, including MCF-7, T47D, MDA-MB-134, ZR-75-1, PMC42, and CAMA-1, with the best characterized of these being MCF-7.* MCF-7 has an absolute requirement for estrogenic stimulation to form tumors in the athymic (nude) mouse model in vivo.[396] Experimental findings obtained using these cell lines must be regarded with some circumspection. After years in laboratory culture, subclonings, and assorted selective pressures, the hope is that data derived from these cell lines may prove relevant to understanding of tumorigenesis in vivo. This hope can be fulfilled only by eventual in vivo clinical verification.

Initial studies on in vitro hormone responsivity of MCF-7 cells produced disparate reports concerning the growth responses to estrogen. We and others succeeded in demonstrating receptors for[45, 261] and direct proliferative responses to physiological doses of estradiol-17β (E$_2$) in vitro† and in vivo in the nude mouse.[141, 225] However, a number of groups failed to observe such responses.[48, 108, 130, 268, 395] One problem appears to have been that countless groups were working with an incorrectly identified or contaminated MCF-7 cell line.[324] Other discrepancies in experiments with properly identified MCF-7 cells have now been largely resolved with a more complete understanding of relevant variables in culture conditions. Serum is a rich source of estrogenic compounds, including sulfate conjugates, that must be removed to observe maximal effects of exogenous estrogen in vitro.[48, 91, 326] Furthermore, it is now known that a component in phenol red, commonly present in culture medium as a pH indicator, can produce estrogenic effects.[29, 303] Growth factors (particularly of the insulin family) in the cellular environment can critically govern estrogen responses.[48]

---

*References 29, 45, 48, 60, 91, 131, 141, 225, 248, 261, 302, 326, 344, 388, 396, and 466.

†References 29, 60, 91, 225, 261, 302, 326, 388, and 466.

PMC42, a well-differentiated estrogen-responsive breast cancer cell line, has been described. Monoclonal antibodies prepared against surface antigens of this line cross-reacted with intraductal (early stage) breast cancer biopsy specimens.[102, 472] At the other end of the spectrum, numerous estrogen-independent breast cancer lines exist[48] such as the adenocarcinoma MDA-MB-231 and the carcinosarcoma Hs578T. Although existing cell lines can be ordered according to their estrogen receptor states, nearly all were derived from metastatic sites in patients and are fully malignant in that sense. Thus controls on metastatic behavior have been difficult to address. We will return to considerations of metastases further on in this chapter.

Throughout this chapter we summarize the literature addressing the hypothesis that estrogens can directly interact with receptor-containing breast cancer cells to modulate gene expression and phenotypic properties. In addition we propose that polypeptide growth factors may be common mediators of growth control for normal breast, estrogen-regulated breast cancer, and autonomous breast cancer. By stressing direct effects of estrogens on cancer cells in vitro, we in no way imply that growth control of tumors in vivo might not be a much more complex phenomenon resulting from many more interactions among other cell types, hormones, proteases, and basement membrane components.

Estrogen induces a large number of enzymes and other proteins involved in nucleic acid synthesis, including DNA polymerase, c-*myc* proto-oncogene,[127] thymidine and uridine kinases, thymidylate synthetase, carbamyl phosphate synthetase, aspartate transcarbamylase, dihydroorotase, glucose-6-phosphate dehydrogenase, and dihydrofolate reductase.[2, 3, 113, 130] Physiological concentration of estrogen stimulates DNA synthesis by both scavenger and de novo biosynthetic pathways. For example, estrogen regulates thymidine kinase and dihydrofolate reductase at the mRNA level.[83, 221] Regulation of thymidine kinase mRNA also occurs at the transcriptional level.[221]

Though increases in global transcription appear to be tightly coupled to estrogen action,[4] no study has yet identified the most critically regulated gene or genes. The existence of "second message" regulatory systems in the growth induction process is also possible but has not yet been proven. In MCF-7 cells, E_2-induced stimulation of phosphotidyl inositol turnover to generate diacylglycerol and inositol trisphospate occurs with an exceptionally long lag time.[164] In contrast, in a variety of other polypeptide growth factor- or protease-induced model systems, this metabolic effect is quite rapid (within minutes as opposed to hours for estrogenic effects) and tightly coupled to growth control.[54, 309] Thus, phosphatidyl inositol turnover, with its associated stimulation of Ca^{++} fluxes by inositol trisphosphate and of protein kinase C by Ca^{++} and diacylglycerol,[309] could serve as a metabolic mediator of mitogenic effects of estrogen-induced growth factors, protease, or both.

One potential target for protein kinase C is the Na^+/H^+ antiport. The Na^+/H^+ antiport is activated in a number of mitogen-triggered proliferation systems. Evidence has been presented that its inhibition with the antidiuretic amiloride prevents proliferative responses in some systems.[95] Protein kinase C is not an oncogene; however, its expression can lead to disordered morphology of fibroblasts.[194, 332]

Additionally, it has been demonstrated that the enzyme ornithine decarboxylase (ODC) is covalently linked to cellular membranes through inositol. This bond is cleared by a phosphatidylinositol-specific phospholipase C, activating the ODC enzyme.[297] ODC activity has been associated with induction of proliferation in numerous cellular systems, including breast cancer.[273] The actual contribution to growth control by any of these potential mediators (protein kinase C, ODC, Ca^{++}, Na^+/H^+ antiport) remains to be determined.

The progesterone receptor is also induced by estrogen.[193] However, progestins are partially growth inhibitory for human breast cancer while inducing specific protein of 48 kDa.[59] The presence of the progesterone receptor is generally coupled to functional growth regulation by estrogens in vivo and in vitro. Thus progesterone receptor content of breast tumors is used in addition to the estrogen receptor as a marker for estrogen and anti-estrogen responsiveness of tumors in clinical therapy.[260] Widespread exceptions to the coexpression of these two receptors do, however, exist in vitro [193, 344] (for example, T47D and MD-MB-134) and in vivo in some patient tumors.[260] Estrogen appears to induce the progesterone receptor at the mRNA level.[301, 341]

Both estrogens and antiestrogens alter the cellular synthesis, secretion of several other proteins, or both, but their role in growth control is unclear. These proteins include various plasminogen activators and collagenolytic enzymes. These proteases are thought to contribute to tumor progression and growth, allowing the tumor to digest and traverse encapsulating basement membrane.[49, 199, 257, 428] While this is likely, it is conceivable that proteases may serve additional roles such as facilitating release of mitogenic growth factors like IGF-I (somatomedin C) from carrier proteins, processing inactive precursor growth factors and proteases to active species,[226] or interacting directly with their own cellular receptors.[305, 416]

In addition, several relatively abundant breast cancer cells secrete proteins of 24 kDa,[71] 52 and 160 kDa,[470, 471] 37–39 kDa, 32 kDa,[42, 383] and 7 kDa (initially identified by detection of an estrogen-induced mRNA species termed pS2).[213, 314] Four other mRNA species (termed pNR 1 to pNR 4[279]) and the cytoplasmic enzyme LDH[47] are also under estrogen regulation. The 52-kDa glycoprotein, one of the major secreted proteins, has cathepsin D–like activity in purified form; it is also mitogenic for MCF-7 cells in vitro.[53, 454]

The nature of the 160-, 37- to 39-, 32-, 24-, and 7-kDa proteins are unknown at present, but the 160-, 52-, and 7-kDa secreted proteins may be dissociated from estrogen and antiestrogen modulation of MCF-7 cell growth using two MCF-7 clonal variants.[40, 43, 93] These three protein species are decreased by antiestrogen to the same extent in both MCF-7 and LY2, the latter being a stable antiestrogen-resistant variant of MCF-7.

In I-13, an MCF-7 clonal variant that is growth arrested by physiological concentrations of estrogen, the same three proteins are induced to the same extent as in MCF-7. These observations suggest that a significant reduction in secretion of these major proteins has no impact on growth in the case of LY2, and their induction does not affect I-13.

It has been demonstrated that estrogen induces the cell surface "receptor" or binding protein for laminin in MCF-7 cells.[5, 431] The laminin receptor is thought to mediate attachment of cells to basement membrane laminin,[257, 428] to contribute to invasiveness by tumor cells, and to promote colonization of new host tissues. Estrogen treatment of MCF-7 cells increases I^{125}-laminin binding; cell attachment to artificial, laminin-coated membranes; and migration of the same cells across an artificial membrane toward a diffusible source of laminin.[431] Estradiol treatment of MCF-7 cells also induces marked rearrangements of cytoskeletal and adhesion structures[375] and alterations in the plasma membrane microvilli as observed by scanning electron microscopy.[455]

In summary, estrogens exert a considerable number of influences in vivo that may indirectly alter breast cancer progression.[313] Direct effects of estrogens on isolated breast cancer cells are also well established. These effects include growth regulation as well as modulation of enzymes and other agents thought to mediate mitogenic, metastatic, and differentiated status. Some of these agents are secreted and can be detected as products of the normal gland (i.e., in milk).[56, 489]

BIOLOGY AND MOLECULAR BIOLOGY OF GROWTH FACTORS IN NORMAL AND MALIGNANT MAMMARY CELLS

Transforming Growth Factor (TGFα)/ Epidermal Growth Factor (EGF) Families

TGFα Regulation and Function in Breast Cancer

Though initially described as a product of oncogene-transformed rodent fibroblasts,[98, 350] TGFα has now been identified in many proliferating normal and malignant human tissues. Similarly, EGF was initially characterized from rodent salivary glands[81] but now appears to be more widely expressed in human tissues. The human form was originally known as urogastrone, a placental product. TGFα is known to exist in 25-kDa, 21-kDa, and 17- to 19-kDa precursor forms[39] and is usually processed to a 7-kDa form. EGF appears to be processed from a very large precursor (130 kDa) formed with multiple polypeptide products.[380] EGF, TGFα, and a related protein from vaccinia virus all appear to form a functional family of growth factors that utilize the "EGF receptor" to carry out their many functions.[57]

A number of studies now suggest that breast cancer cells produce TGF. Conditioned medium from MCF-7 cells, other breast cancer cell lines, and extracts of breast tumors have been studied to identify the growth stimulatory activities present. The cell lines secrete stimulatory factors for MCF-7 and murine 3T3 fibroblast monolayer cultures as well as "transforming growth activity" (TGF) determined by stimulation of anchorage-independent colonies of rodent NRK and AKR/2B fibroblasts in soft agar culture.[20, 21, 116, 308, 372] Breast cancer cells produce a 30-kDa apparent molecular weight species of transforming activity for NRK fibroblasts.

This species comigrates chromatographically with a peak of MCF-7 autostimulatory activity and is the principal species of EGF receptor competing activity.[21, 116] Antisera specific to TGFα react with this species.[331] Thus this activity may be related to TGFα, but it appears to be significantly larger than the cloned and sequenced 6-kDa species from transformed rodent fibroblasts.[106] It is not yet certain if this protein is related to the 17- to 19-kDa TGFα precursor protein observed in transformed fibroblasts,[39, 166, 204] whether it is modified by glycosylation or palmitoylation,[39] or whether it is the product of alternative mRNA splicing. The precursor species is thought to be membrane bound in cell lines that express it.[39, 166, 204] It cannot be ruled out at present that the breast cancer–derived TGFα might be the product of a novel TGFα–related gene. The 30-kDa TGFα–like species is induced by estrogen treatment of estrogen receptor–positive MCF-7, T47D, and ZR-75-1 cells from two- to fourteenfold, depending on cell type and culture conditions.[21, 116, 117, 119, 331, 371]

An expected 4.8-Kb TGF mRNA species has been detected in MCF-7 and other human breast cancer cell lines and breast tumors,[20, 104] ranging from low to high estrogen receptor content. No correlation of TGFα mRNA expression was observed with estrogen receptor status; at least 70 percent of the adenocarcinomas contained TGFα mRNA.[20] One breast cancer cell line, the estrogen receptor–negative carcinosarcoma Hs578T, does not contain detectable levels of TGFα protein or its mRNA.[20, 21]

The mechanism and possible functional relevance of TGFα induction has been further examined. When MCF-7 cells were treated with estradiol in vitro, TGFα mRNA was induced in 6 hours.[20] Similar observations have been made in mouse mammary tumors.[263] Studies using antibodies directed against either TGFα or its receptor (the EGF receptor) have noted growth suppression of MCF-7 cells grown as anchorage-independent colonies or as estrogen-stimulated, high-density monolayer cultures.[20] TGFα is currently one of the most likely growth factors to exert a positive autocrine effect in breast cancer. It has also been detected as a tumor burden marker in the urine of patients and nude mice having breast and other tumors.[230, 419] Thus it may be a marker for tumor burden, disease progression, or risk of malignancy. Detection of urinary TGFα has been complicated by the presence of very high levels of EGF–related growth factors present even in normal control urine.[230]

TGFα in Normal Mammary Epithelium

The possible biological roles for TGFα expression have been analyzed by genetic manipulations of normal fibroblasts, resulting in TGFα overexpression. Several studies have reported that normal fibroblasts do not make significant levels of TGFα.[20, 104, 405] Rosenthal et al.[358] have found that the TGFα gene expressed under an SV40 promoter in murine fibroblasts can act as an oncogene to induce anchorage-independent growth in vitro and tumor formation in nude mice. The in vitro transformation results were confirmed in NRK fibroblasts by Watanabe et al.[464] Furthermore, EGF regulated by a MoMULV promoter can also act as an oncogene in fibroblasts to induce their tumor formation in nude mice.[412] In contrast, Finzi et al. reported the failure of the TGFα gene to induce a malignant phenotype in mouse 3T3 cells, though the transfected cells proliferated more rapidly at high density.[152] The disparities among these reports remain to be resolved, but TGFα expression is clearly contributory to proliferation.

A large body of literature also exists demonstrating that EGF has tumor promotional activity (reviewed in Stoschek and King[417]). In studies investigating mouse mammary carcinogenesis, Kurachi et al. have demonstrated a likely role of EGF in both mammary tumor onset and subsequent growth support.[240] Using a mouse strain highly susceptible to spontaneous mammary tumors, removal of the submandibular glands (sialoadenectomy) reduced the incidence of tumor formation, the rate of growth of the breast tumors allowed to form, or both.[319] The submandibular gland is known to be a source of EGF in mammals. Reinfusion of EGF into sialoadenectomized mice returned tumor incidence and growth rate of tumors to their normally high level. Thus TGFα– and EGF–like activities (like estrogen) may have endocrine functions in tumor onset and support. As the data with MCF-7 cells show, one mechanism of tumor progression might involve local production of TGFα under estrogenic stimulation. Clearly, TGFα– or EGF–like growth factors are likely to be important regulators of mammary tumor progression by a variety of possible mechanisms.

Is TGFα a breast tumor– or early development– specific growth factor? A number of studies have failed to detect TGFα in normal epithelial tissue biopsy specimens,[104] although it has been reported in rat embryonic tissue. A report using in situ hybridization has localized the embryo-associated TGFα mRNA to the closely associated maternal decidua tissue rather than the rat embryo itself.[183] The hypothesis that TGFα is an oncofetal marker is further shaken with the discovery that normal bovine anterior pituitary cells proliferating in culture produce TGFα.[236] Furthermore, a TGFα–like growth factor has been detected in mouse mammary glands undergoing reproductive hormone–induced lobulo-alveolar development. In addition, EGF or TGFα implants in the mammary fat pads were able to induce lobulo-alveolar development.[433, 456]

It is also now known that normal human mammary epithelial cells rapidly proliferating in culture secrete high quantities of TGFα and produce its expected mRNA species.[408] Thus TGFα may contribute to growth control processes of normal as well as malignant breast tissue. It is possible that the response of breast tissue to TGFα or EGF rather than the absolute levels of its production might distinguish the cancer from normal in vitro. In addition, MCF-7 cells grown as tumors in nude mice responded to 2 to 4 weeks of infusion of estrogen-, EGF-, or breast cancer cell–conditioned medium with tumor formation; normal rodent breast tissue in situ did not form a tumor under these treatment conditions.[120]

Might TGFα have roles other than for proliferation or transformation of breast epithelium? Following secretion by the normal gland into milk, TGFα and EGF may act on neonatal development; the best known example is in eyelid opening. TGFα appears to also have roles in epithelial wound healing and angiogenesis (possibly tumor angiogenesis). Processes such as these are probably quite complex, involving a variety of hormones and other components (in addition to TGFα) that stimulate chemotaxis and mitogenesis of several cell types. In breast cancer, TGFα/EGF may also mediate or contribute to desmoplasia, a fibrotic, stromal proliferative response sometimes seen surrounding the tumor, and to hypercalcemia secondary to bone resorption. It is known that growth factors such as EGF and TGFα can be immunosuppressive in model systems, acting to counter host immune rejection of cancer cells.[371, 417]

EGF Receptor Function

The exact chemical nature of the interaction of TGFα with its receptor is not known but appears to require an intact, complete TGFα molecule.[426] Studies with point mutated TGFα species seem, however, to implicate the extreme carboxy terminus of the protein as the most critical receptor-binding domain.[243] The point of interaction of EGF with the EGF receptor has also been determined.[14, 242]

Both EGF and TGFα can act via the EGF receptor, a ligand-inducible tyrosine kinase, on both normal and cancerous cell lines. The EGF receptor has been detected in human and rodent mammary tumor biopsy specimens and malignant cell lines.[94, 157, 239, 370] In one breast cancer cell line (MDA-MB-468), Kudlow et al. have observed that EGF induces the biosynthesis of its own receptor;[239] in another (T47D), progestins induced the receptor.[296] The receptor observed in breast cancer cells appears to be very similar to the cloned and sequenced human EGF receptor. The apparent molecular size is 170 kDa, and the kinase domain is unaltered as determined by S1 ribonuclease analysis.[370] However, the state of phosphorylation or the tyrosine kinase activity of the receptor and the physiological substrates of the receptor kinase in breast cancer are unknown.

A study has shown that EGF induces phosphorylation of lipocortin (a phospholipase inhibitor) in A431 carcinoma cells.[377] The relevance of this effect to other EGF/TGFα actions remains to be determined. EGF also is known to induce trans-acting nuclear factors that appear to regulate transcription of responsive genes[135] (the genes known as transin[278] and fos[474]) and phosphorylation of the ribosomal protein known as S6.[312] The exact role of these functions is unknown; for instance, phosphorylation of all identifiable substrates has been dissociated from transformation in studies with the *src* oncogene.[212, 220] EGF also induces phosphoinositide turnover[335] and cell attachment proteins.[432]

How might the EGF receptor be associated with control of malignant growth? As mentioned, overexpression of the receptor is closely associated with poor prognosis breast cancer and with tumor growth rate in experimental systems. These may occur because receptor overexpression in the presence of TGFα/EGF may increase receptor self-association (dimerization or oligomerization) leading to activation of the tyrosine kinase.[381] Overexpression of the EGF receptor may be important in generating a tumor immunological response since several tumor specific antigens have been detected in the EGF-receptor carbohydrate structures.[19]

Mechanisms other than receptor overexpression may determine whether the EGF receptor mediates normal or malignant mitogenic effects. For instance, the c-*src* oncogene increases coupling of the EGF receptor to an anchorage-dependent mitogenic response.[19] The SV40T oncogene couples the receptor to an anchorage-independent or transformed growth response.[408]

Insulin and Insulin-Like Growth Factors and Their Receptors

The insulin family of growth factors presents a complex array of cross-reacting ligands, receptors, and serum-borne binding proteins. Insulin is a two-chain disulfide-linked growth factor processed from a single gene product whose primary site of synthesis is the pancreas. In contrast, the single-chain (uncleaved, 7.5-kDa size) IGF-I and IGF-II growth factors (somatomedins) are synthesized by many body tissues (including the liver) and are under quite different hormonal regulation, particularly growth hormone.[92, 276] Several other growth factors, such as relaxin (important in parturition) and lentropin (which controls lens fiber formation), appear to be members of an even larger insulin-related family.[26] Alternative splicing of mRNA of the insulin-like growth factors (particularly IGF-I[361]) also contributes to the complexity of members of this diverse family.

As noted previously, somatomedins are required for both anchorage-dependent and -independent proliferation of fibroblast model systems. They may also play a role in breast cancer. IGF-I is mitogenic for some breast cancer cells in culture.[165, 197] Using radioimmunoassay, we and others have also noted that an IGF-I (somatomedin C)–related species is secreted by all human breast cancer cells examined to date.[24, 197] After partial purification from MCF-7 cell–conditioned medium, this growth factor comigrates on gel exclusion chromatography with authentic human serum–derived IGF-I. Acid ethanol extraction is required to partially disrupt a high-molecular-weight form of the growth factor.

A complex series of IGF-I–cross-reacting mRNA species are also detected with northern blot analysis using a cDNA probe to authentic IGF-I.[197] However, none of these mRNA species are identifiable as IGF-I nuclease protection analysis of mRNA.[482] Complex species of

IGF-I cross-hybridizing mRNAs have been previously described for the human fetus.[182] No estrogenic induction of secreted IGF-I–like molecules is observed under standard culture conditions of MLF-7 cells using phenol red–containing medium. Subsequent studies, utilizing the more substantially estrogen-depleted phenol red–free medium have revealed a three- to six-fold induction of IGF-I–like growth factor with estrogen, TGFα, EGF, or insulin treatment.[198] Secretion of IGF-I–related factors is inhibited by growth inhibitory antiestrogens (in phenol red–containing medium), TGFβ, and glucocorticoids.

While growth hormone is a strong stimulus for IGF-I production by liver, fibroblasts, and other normal tissues, it is without effect on production of IGF-I–like growth factors by MCF-7 breast cancer cells.[75, 77, 103, 198, 214] Breast cancer cell in culture may have a unique hormonal specificity for its regulation of secretion of IGF-I–related factors. The production and regulation of IGF-I normal human breast epithelium has not yet been examined. As mentioned, IGF-I–related polypeptides are secreted by fibroblasts and smooth muscle and contribute to autocrine growth control in these cell types.[75-77] It remains to be seen whether IGF-I produced by breast cancer acts primarily on breast cancer itself in an autostimulatory mode or on surrounding stroma to promote chemotaxis and growth. However, studies have shown that an antibody that blocks the IGF-I receptor[159] is capable of inhibiting MDA-MB-231 breast cancer cloning in vitro[355] and tumor growth in vivo.[10]

IGF-I mitogenesis is thought to be mediated by its receptor, a close homologue of the insulin receptor, though it also weakly binds to the insulin receptor. The IGF-I receptor in a variety of cell types consists of a 450-kDa complex (two chains of 130 kDa and two β chains of 85 kDa).[357] The receptor has been purified, cloned, and sequenced; it is strongly homologous to the insulin receptor and possesses tyrosine kinase activity.[342, 357, 441] Its mechanism of action is unclear, but IGF-I binding has been hypothesized to stimulate growth by a posttranscriptional mechanism.[50] Alternatively, it has been shown to induce transcription of several specific mRNA species, including ribosomal RNA.[421, 488]

The results of site-directed mutagenesis studies with the highly homologous insulin receptor[138] suggest that IGF-I receptor function might also be mediated by activation of the tyrosine kinase activity. In addition, the insulin receptor appears to have the capacity to function as an oncogene when truncated and fused with the extracellular domain of the partially homologous v-*ros* oncogene.[139, 477] Although the IGF-I receptor is not yet known to bear a strong relationship to an oncogene, future studies will certainly address this possibility.

Receptors for IGF-I of the expected size have been detected by cross-linking studies on human breast cancer cell lines.[99, 165] Research on IGF-I receptors has been somewhat hampered by the presence of secreted, non-receptor-binding proteins that interfere in ligand binding assays.[74, 99, 109, 125] The binding proteins, however, may also influence the biological properties of IGF-I.[137] The binding proteins have been suggested to be both non-covalently and covalently linked with various IGF species.[245]

At the present time insufficient information is available to fully evaluate the structure, regulation, and function of breast cancer–derived IGF-I–related proteins and compare them to those produced by embryonic and adult tissues.[310, 447] The mechanisms of IGF-I induction and its possible biological role in breast cancer are not yet known. Since insulin synergizes with estrogen in promoting growth breast cancer cell lines in vitro and in vivo in the nude mouse, it is possible that somatomedins principally act by interacting with estrogen to promote breast tumor growth.[200, 446]

It has also been reported that IGF-II–related gene products are produced by normal and malignant tissue.[86] IGF-II appears to bind to multiple receptors (insulin, IGF-II, and IGF-I). All of these receptors, including the IGF-II receptor, have been detected in human breast cancer[99, 165] as well as lactational states of normal breast.[97] While IGF-II interaction with IGF-I insulin receptors may stimulate cellular response, IGF-II receptors may be primarily involved in IGF-II degradation. The IGF-II receptor is a multifunctional protein, previously described as the mannose-6-phosphate receptor for lysosomal enzymes.[264, 294] IGF-I mRNA has been reported in other human tumors (tumors in the lung and colon, and liposarcoma),[292, 298, 437] and IGF-II has been observed to be overproduced in Wilms' tumor.[343] Somatomedins appear to be among the most ubiquitous growth factors, produced by nearly all normal tissues[310, 342, 447] and found in the blood[415] and urine.[192]

Transforming Growth Factor β (TGFβ) and Its Receptor

Transforming growth factor beta (TGFβ) is a 25-kDa polypeptide initially purified from platelets and various normal tissues. It is required (along with other growth factors) for full induction of the transformed phenotype in fibroblasts. TGFβ is also produced autonomously in fibroblasts transformed by oncogenes.[404] TGFβ is a member of a multigene family that includes müllerian inhibiting substance, inhibins, and activins,[58, 404] a T cell–suppressor factor,[478] and a *Drosophila* morphogenesis-controlling gene known as decapentaplegic.[325] In contrast to TGFα and many other growth factors, TGFβ is growth inhibitory, differentiating-promoting, or both, for most epithelial cells.[61, 349, 439] Possibly as one aspect of its growth modulatory actions, TGFβ influences the differentiated state of many cell types. For example, it inhibits myogenic differentiation,[275, 320] inhibits normal hepatocyte growth more extensively than malignant liver cell growth, and prevents dedifferentiation of other epithelial cell types.[284, 347] In addition, it stimulates differentiated behavior of other cell types such as vascular smooth muscle[272] and normal breast epithelial cultures.[461]

Normal mammary epithelial cells are induced by TGFβ to synthesize milk fat globule antigen. In addition, growth of these cells in culture is arrested, and the morphology is markedly altered; TGFβ changes the cobblestone-like epithelial appearance to an elongated spindle shape.[461] TGFβ also appears to be extremely potent in vivo in the neonatal mouse. Implants of TGFβ in slow-release capsules near developing mammary ducts result in complete cessation of mammary ductal development. No effects of TGFβ are seen on surrounding stromal tissue or on more distant mammary glands.[387] TGFβ may play a role, along with other hormones (such as estrogen) and growth factors (such as EGF and TGFα),[458] in the delicately balanced process of mammary development. TGFβ (along with a plethora of other growth factors) is also a component of human milk.[311]

Several investigators have concluded that breast cancer, like normal breast epithelium, is inhibited by TGFβ. TGFβ might be an autocrine inhibitory type substance (chalone)[463] in breast cancer. Breast cancer cells have been shown to contain and secrete a TGFβ–related activity.[21, 105, 234, 349] Conditioned medium from an estrogen-responsive human breast cancer cell line (MCF-7) has been fractionated by gel exclusion chromatography and analyzed. The major peak of activity binds to TGFβ receptors, transforms AKR-2B and NRK fibroblasts, and comigrates with platelet-derived TGFβ.[234] SDS gel electrophoresis of metabolically labeled, immunoprecipitated material confirms its close similarity to TGFβ in size and antigenicity.

All breast cancer cell lines reported to date express the expected 2.5-Kb mRNA species, based on studies with other cell types that express TGFβ.[104, 234, 463] TGFβ secretion is inhibited by treatment of MCF-7 cells with mitogens (for example, estrogen and insulin[234]), but growth inhibitory antiestrogens and glucocorticoids strongly stimulate its secretion. Intracellular TGF does not appear to change in concentration following treatment with mitogens or growth inhibitors.[234] TGFβ from antiestrogen–induced MCF-7 cells strongly inhibits the growth of an estrogen receptor negative cell line MDA-MB-231. This growth inhibition was reversed in the presence of a polyclonal antibody directed against native TGFβ.[234] In addition to a possible role as an antiestrogen–induced chalone, antiestrogen–induced TGFβ in hormone responsive breast cancer might act to expand the growth inhibitory potential of antiestrogens in vivo. Breast cancers exist as mixtures of estrogen receptor–positive and –negative tumor cells.[175, 232]

Since breast cancers do not appear to become TGFβ unresponsive as they become antiestrogen unresponsive, TGFβ may act in tumors with such mixed cell populations to make antiestrogen more effective than might otherwise be expected based only on blockade of estrogen action.[234] We have observed that in LY2, an MCF-7 variant stepwise selected in vitro for antiestrogen resistance, TGFβ is no longer induced by antiestrogen, but the cells still retain the TGFβ receptor and response.[234] Neither the mechanism of TGFβ induction in MCF-7 cells nor its loss in LY2 cells is fully defined, but it is not at the regulation of steady-state TGFβ mRNA level. Among other possibilities, it may involve both synthesis of protein and conversion of a latent form to an active form of TGFβ.[234] Apparently in contrast to other cell types,[192, 241] there is significant active TGFβ present in breast cancer conditioned medium. The biochemical details of the conversion of a secreted inactive to active TGFβ remain to be elucidated. Inactive TGFβ may be activated in impure form by acidification or by addition of proteases. A 62-kDa precursor can be cleaved by plasmin to yield the 25-kDa mature species.[229, 269] The precursor appears to undergo phosphorylation and glycosylation prior to its final cleavage.[46] Further regulation of TGFβ activity appears to occur in the presence of the serum component α_2-macroglobulin. This protein covalently binds and inactivates TGFβ.[196, 317]

TGFβ is proposed to act through a high-molecular-weight (615-kDa) receptor complex, the receptor subunits being two 280-kDa species. In addition, 65-kDa and 85-kDa binding components have been reported.[66] The TGFβ receptor does not appear to "down regulate" from the cell surface following ligand occupancy. It appears to rapidly recycle and not to follow a lysosomal degradation pathway taken by tyrosine kinase–containing receptors such as insulin, IGF-I, EGF, and platelet derived growth factor (PDGF). Presumably, it follows an endocytosis-recycling pathway (like transferrin) or is rapidly replenished, following endocytosis from a large intracellular store.[112, 277] This receptor has not yet been purified, cloned, or sequenced but is reported not to have tyrosine kinase activity.[171]

An alternate gene for TGFβ (known as TGFβ$_2$) exists.[208] The gene product forms either a homodimeric complex or heterodimeric complex with TGFβ and appears to bind to the same 280-kDa receptor species as TGFβ but has lower affinity for the 65-kDa and 85-kDa receptor species.[67, 382] Although equipotent in inhibiting epithelial cell proliferation and adipogenic differentiation, TGFβ, but not TGFβ$_2$, has been reported to inhibit hematopoietic progenitor cell proliferation.[318]

In breast cancer cell lines the expected high-affinity receptor has been observed. High-affinity receptors appear to be present in greater numbers and more commonly in estrogen receptor–negative breast cancer. However, both estrogen receptor–positive and estrogen receptor–negative cells have been reported to contain receptors and to be inhibited by both TGFβ and TGFβ$_2$.[234, 349, 487] Though the presence of TGFβ receptors is generally associated with an inhibitory response to breast cancer, this is not necessarily the case. Transformation of immortalized normal breast epithelium with the oncogenes v-H-*ras* and SV40T can completely eliminate the cellular response to TGFβ, in association with malignant transformation, without abolishing high-affinity receptors.[443]

The mechanisms of action of TGFβ are unknown. Initial studies on mechanisms of TGFβ action focused on understanding its ability to synergize with EGF (or TGFα) in promotion of anchorage-independent growth of fibroblasts. In these studies it was observed that TGFβ induced the receptor for EGF/TGF.[11] In cells where TGFβ is inhibitory, however, this effect does not seem to explain the actions of TGFβ. For example, in rat hepatocytes,[385] TGFβ inhibits growth and still stimulates EGF/TGFα receptor expression.

In one human breast cancer cell line, MDA-MB-468, EGF is paradoxically growth inhibitory. In this line, TGFβ also induces EGF-receptor mRNA.[148] In breast epithelial organoid cultures, the TGFα–receptor system is further dissociated from the inhibitory actions of TGFβ. TGFβ inhibits organoid proliferation but does not induce EGF receptor mRNA or TGFα mRNA.[442] Thus it is likely that inhibitory actions of TGFβ in breast epithelium do not simply involve interruption of a positive autocrine pathway of growth control. Rather, other aspects of cellular metabolism might be involved.

In fibroblasts, TGFβ induces the mRNA for c-*sis* proto-oncogene, the B chain of PDGF.[247] Since PDGF, in addition to TGFβ, is a requirement for anchorage-independent growth of fibroblasts, it has been proposed that c-*sis* induction may mediate some of TGFβ's effects to induce the transformed phenotype in fibroblasts. Studies in mammary epithelial cells, however, suggest other roles for c-*sis*. In normal and immortalized mammary epithelial cells, TGFβ inhibits proliferation and still stimulates c-*sis* mRNA production (in contrast, PDGF A chain is constitutively expressed).[22] In these cells, as in other epithelial cells, PDGF has no known receptor and no known function. Perhaps intracellular c-*sis* serves some as yet unknown, receptor-independent function in TGFβ action.

Finally, TGFβ has been reported to induce production of the basement membrane components fibronectin and collagen in fibroblasts and epithelial cells.[205, 404] Since anchorage-independent growth of fibroblasts is also induced by fibronectin (in the absence of TGFβ), and anti-fibronectin antibodies interrupted TGFβ-induced anchorage-independent colony formation of fibroblasts, it has been proposed that fibronectin mediates at least some of the actions of TGFβ.[205] Thus a model has been proposed by Ignotz and Massague whereby a critical growth factor for anchorage-independent growth may act by stimulating production of basement membrane. TGFβ also decreases secretion of a variety of proteases and stimulates the production of protease inhibitors.[44, 58, 131] Such effects could further enhance accumulation of basement membrane. TGFβ stimulates the expression of receptors for fibronectin.[266] Multiple mechanisms appear to converge to mediate TGFβ effects on cell–basement membrane interaction. It is conceivable that in anchorage-independent states, basement membrane synthesis, accumulation, or assembly might be rate-limiting for cell growth.

Many current studies are beginning to address the functions of TGFβ in embryonic development. TGFβ and fibroblast growth factor (FGF) appear to be present at an extremely early stage of development in frog embryos. These two growth factors have been suggested to be the natural inducers of mesoderm development through their effects on actin expression.[206] Other studies in developing mouse embryo have localized TGFβ in differentiating mesenchymal tissues (bone muscle, blood vessels, and blood cells) and epithelial tissues. TGFβ also mediates inflammation and repair as it is released by degranulation of platelets, macrophages, and T lymphocytes in the adult. TGFβ can also accelerate wound healing but appears to inhibit certain aspects of the immune response.[404, 478]

The functions of TGFβ as it is produced by breast cancer in situ are not yet known. As mentioned, it might act to help mediate inhibitory effects of antiestrogens. Like PDGF, TGFα, and IGF-I, TGFβ produced by tumor cells might have paracrine effects on surrounding tissue. TGFβ may contribute to the marked stromal proliferation and basement membrane deposition commonly observed in breast tumors.[231] It also has been reported that TGFβ can induce bone resorption.[401] In the context of endothelial regeneration, TGFβ inhibits replication of angiogenesis and endothelial cells in vitro.[188, 427] However, Takehara et al. have proposed that TGFβ acts in vivo to promote fibrosis and angiogenesis.[425] TGFβ might indirectly induce angiogenesis by stimulating macrophage chemotaxis to the site of the tumor and degranulation.[162, 351, 404, 442]

Perhaps the inhibitory and differentiating effects of TGFβ on mammary epithelium can be utilized in the treatment of breast cancer. Though the in vivo, mammary inhibitory effects of TGFβ are only established at present on normal developing mammary ducts,[387] sufficient amounts of TGFβ applied locally may have some impact on cancer. Difficulties to be encountered in such studies undoubtedly will include the extremely rapid hepatic clearance of TGFβ[459] and its stromal proliferative,[231] bone-resorptive,[401] angiogenic effects.[425]

Platelet-Derived Growth Factor (PDGF) and Its Receptor

PDGF is a heterodimeric growth factor of approximately 30 kDa that, as the name implies, is found in high concentrations in platelets. PDGF-like–related growth factors are also produced by a variety of transformed murine fibroblast lines and by some human tumors of diverse origins. Some human tumors (sarcomas and glioblastomas) were derived from PDGF-responsive cell types, while others (hepatoma, T-cell leukemia, bladder carcinoma, and erythroleukemia) were derived from PDGF-unresponsive epithelial or white blood cell hematopoietic cell types. The v-sis oncogene is related to PDGF-B (or 2) chain homodimer and can transform PDGF-receptor–containing cell types. Consequently, PDGF could subserve an autocrine role in such tumors. However, this role has not yet been directly proven, and the PDGF receptor is no longer present (presumably "downregulated") in such tumors. In tumors derived from cell types initially lacking the PDGF receptor, v-sis is not transforming, and PDGF presumably functions in stromal proliferation (desmoplasia) and chemotaxis and degranulation of monocytes and neutrophils.[79]

Transformation of fibroblastic cells with simian sarcoma virus (SSV) provides a model system for investigation of the function of PDGF in initially responsive cell types. In such a system, the PDGF-B chain–related protein encoded by the virus forms a homodimer and is sometimes secreted by the cell. In such cases, antibodies directed against PDGF have been reported to exert antiproliferative and antitransforming activity.[79] However, in many instances the PDGF is largely cell associated and presumably already bound to its receptor. Thus anti-PDGF antisera have been only partially effective as antiproliferative reagents.[360] The subcellular origin or fate of PDGF in such instances remains to be fully characterized; however, immunoreactive PDGF has been observed in the cell nucleus in SSV–transformed cells.[195] PDGF is known to encode a short peptide sequence within its linear primary structure that is capable of directing the molecule across the nuclear pore complex.[484] It has been proposed that PDGF may exert autocrine growth control through both intracellular and extracellular mechanisms of action.[244]

Many breast cancer cell lines that have been examined to date secrete a PDGF–related activity detected by anchorage-dependent growth stimulation of mouse 3T3 fibroblasts in the presence of platelet-poor plasma. This is known as a "competency" assay for early mitogenic signals.[227] The 28-kDa and 16-kDa species were observed by immunoprecipitation of metabolically labeled MCF-7, MDA-MB-231, and other breast cancer cell extracts and medium. The 28-kDa species (the unreduced form) was biologically active after elution from nonreducing SDS–polyacrylamide gels, and its activity was blocked with anti-PDGF antiserum. On examination of poly A–selected mRNA from either cell line, transcripts of both PDGF A(1) and B(2) chains are observed.[30, 41, 362, 363] A and B chains have been reported to be widely expressed in breast cancer and other cell lines.[162, 188, 351, 424] While the B chain is homologous to the v-sis oncogene, the A chain is not known to have a retroviral oncogene homologue. The A and B chain share substantial sequence homology to each other,[434] and the A chain shows evidence of alternative mRNA splicing.[481] It is not yet known how A and B chains assemble in breast cancer cells.

PDGF acts through a 195-kDa glycoprotein receptor on a variety of mesenchymal cell types that encode a ligand-inducible tyrosine kinase similar to that of EGF, IGF-I, and insulin. The receptor has been purified, sequenced, and cloned, but does not appear to be expressed in any human mammary carcinoma cell lines.[30, 41, 228, 362, 363]

PDGF is known to mediate proliferation of stromal cells such as fibroblasts in vitro and possibly in such physiological and pathological conditions as wound healing, vasoconstriction, atherosclerosis, embryonic development, myeloproliferative diseases, and desmoplasia. PDGF circulates bound to at least one carrier protein, α_2-macroglobulin.[79] In model fibroblast systems, PDGF is known to act (similar to fibroblast growth factor) as a "competency" growth factor.[227] That is, it acts to allow density-arrested fibroblasts in platelet-poor plasma to respond to "progression" factors such as EGF or IGF-I. The presence of both competency and progression factors allows fibroblasts to fully traverse G_1 and enter the S phase of the cell cycle.

PDGF is known to rapidly induce both the turnover of phosphatidylinositol and the release of prostaglandins

PGI_2 and PGE_2.[227] Prostaglandins mediate vasodilatory and bone resorption functions.[79] In fibroblasts, PDGF induces proliferation, collagenase, and collagen secretion[79, 227] and induces production of an IGF-I–related growth factor.[75] IGF-I is autocrine-acting in such a system. PDGF induces mitogenic stimulation in cultured human fibroblasts and porcine aortic smooth muscle cells, being largely abolished in the presence of anti–IGF-I antibodies.[75]

Such observations make it likely that in breast cancer, estrogen-induced PDGF (along with other growth factors such as $TGF\alpha$) acts in a paracrine manner on fibroblasts and possibly other surrounding tissue. This action could result in the proliferation of fibroblasts and further enhanced tumor growth by released fibroblast mediators such as IGF-I. It is possible that fibroblast-derived IGF-I might be one of the stromal factors that are required in vivo to initiate all the estrogenic effects observed on epithelial proliferation. One report has suggested a correlation between PDGF mRNA expression and degree of stromal desmoplasia in primary breast cancer.[348]

Fibroblast Growth Factors (FGF) and Their Receptors

The fibroblast growth factors, like PDGF, were initially classified as "competency" factors acting early in the G1 phase of the cell cycle to stimulate the growth of mesenchymal cells. More recently, though, they have been appreciated as more widely functional in normal and malignant growth controls in mammary epithelium. The members of the family include acidic and basic FGF[142] (aFGF and bFGF), Kaposi FGF (kFGF—otherwise known as *hst,* for human stomach tumor oncogene),[100] and *int*-2[111] (a mouse mammary cancer oncogene already mentioned). A more distant homology also exists with interleukin-1 (IL-1).[429] It is not yet known how many receptors exist for this diverse class of ligands. However, both aFGF and bFGF bind a 140- to 210-kDa receptor and stimulate tyrosine phosphorylation of a 90-kDa protein.[82] bFGF is capable of acting on an oncogene when expressed in fibroblasts.[354, 376]

FGF has been shown to be a requirement for normal mouse mammary cells in culture. It is present in pituitary extract used for culture of mouse and human mammary myoepithelial and epithelial cells.[181, 394] FGF is also a potent angiogenic substance.[429] The FGF family is characterized by a binding site for heparin.[142] This finding has facilitated purification attempts and may allow for strategies to interrupt or otherwise modulate FGF action through binding of various polyanionic substances such as suramin to this site.[80] bFGF does not possess a signal peptide in its primary sequence,[1] giving rise to the hypothesis that it is secreted, but in an unusual fashion; after binding to heparin proteoglycan as it is synthesized by the cell, it is secreted as a part of the basement membrane.[142]

Some uncertainty exists as to the principal target of FGF in the normal mammary glands. Rudland has proposed that effects are restricted to myoepithelium and stroma,[365] but Riss and Sirbasku have found that MCF-7 and T47D human breast carcinoma cells respond. bFGF appears to bind α_2-macroglobulin in serum; serum-free conditions favor mitogenic responses of cells to this growth factor.[346] A 60-kDa, heparin-binding, FGF-related molecule is produced by human breast cancer cells in culture; its function could encompass autocrine and paracrine effects.[180, 424]

Pituitary Hormones, Steroids, and Other Growth Modulatory Hormones

This chapter has so far presented evidence for the production of autocrine and paracrine growth factors by breast cancer. The situation is undoubtedly more complex in vivo; for example, it is possible that in vivo growth factors, estrogen, or both act in concert with other systemic mitogens to promote tumor growth. Dembinski et al. have isolated a pituitary-derived activity that potentiates the mitogenic effects of E_2 on MCF-7 cells.[101] One pituitary factor has already been identified as IGF-II.[386] In addition, pituitary-derived GnRH may also directly interact with breast cancer to inhibit its proliferation,[133] while prolactin is stimulatory for some cell lines.[32]

Many groups have shown growth regulation of MCF-7 cells in monolayer culture by a variety of lipid-soluble trophic hormones in addition to estrogen. These include glucocorticoids, iodothyronine, androgens, and retinoids (reviewed in Lippman[259]). MCF-7 cells have receptors but are not growth-stimulated by progesterone or vitamin D.[59, 136, 259, 418] Progesterone induces a specific protein[59] and can be growth inhibitory in vitro (reviewed in Rochefort[353]). Other inhibitory hormones include somatostatin,[414] interleukin-1 and interleukin-6, tumor necrosis factor (TNF), and interferon (reviewed in Sporn and Roberts[402]). Receptors and metabolic effects, but little cellular growth response, have been demonstrated for other hormones, such as growth hormone, glucagon, and calcitonin.[259]

Transferrin, the serum iron delivery molecule, is required for proliferation of normal and malignant mammary cells;[185] its receptor is increased in estrogen-independent breast cancer compared with estrogen-dependent breast cancer.[435] The multiplicity of growth modulatory hormones for in vitro breast cancer systems suggests the possibility that many serum-borne or locally produced modulators of growth may play important regulatory roles in vivo. Alternatively, or additionally, growth factors with a similar spectrum of activities could be elaborated by the breast cancer cells themselves.

TUMOR HOST INTERACTIONS, INCLUDING METASTASES

In the nude (athymic) mouse model system, estrogen is an absolute tumor growth requirement for two human cell lines, MCF-7 and T47D, and a growth stimulator for a third cell line, ZR-75-1. Huseby et al. have further defined this system by showing that estrogen need not enter the systemic circulation in nude mice to promote MCF-7 tumorigenesis; elevation of local estrogen concentration was sufficient to promote local but not distant tumor growth.[202] This finding suggests that although estrogens might be required to induce a host of regulatory factors required by the tumor, the production and action of such regulated factors are probably restricted to the local area of the tumor.

What are these local, estrogen-induced events that contribute to tumor growth? The mammary stroma is likely to provide as yet unidentified contributory factors in vivo for full mitogenicity of estrogen.[209] In culture, normal mouse mammary epithelial cells require exposure to mammary fibroblasts for estrogen effects.[282] Estrogen induction of progesterone receptor requires the presence of glutaraldehyde-killed fibroblasts, type I (stromal) collagen, or conditioned medium from fibroblasts. This effect may be mediated by a basement membrane or by the substratum effect of fibroblasts. In contrast, estrogen-dependent DNA synthesis in normal mammary epithelium occurs only when live fibroblasts were in coculture.[186] These observations imply that a labile, secreted, fibroblast-derived material was permissive for estrogen-induced growth. Furthermore, fibroblasts proliferate in response to combinations of E_2 and mammary epithelial cells but not to estrogen alone. Taken together, these data provide evidence for intimate or paracrine communication between stromal and epithelial cells, each requiring the presence of the other for growth in response to estrogen.

In embryonic development of the male, androgen treatment of the receptor-containing mesenchyme results in necrosis of the epithelium.[129] Thus the stromal cells may contribute both negative and positive growth modulation of epithelium. A wide range of possible mechanisms exists for such communication including secretion of soluble mediators or basement membrane or even exchange of cell surface components. A cancer-specific basement membrane component, known as tenascin, has also been identified.[70]

At least one growth factor, known as MDGF-1, acts by promoting deposition of basement membrane collagen.[16] It is possible that cancer may represent a partial escape from dependence on a stromal requirement or an abnormally strong response to a stromal component.

A late step in tumor progression is metastasis. This is the process whereby the tumor trasverses the basement membrane and colonizes the host. It is thought that important events in this process include attachment of tumor cells to basement membrane laminin through a "laminin receptor," proteolytic digestion of the membrane with a variety of enzymes, and motility of the cells.[255, 431] Cells invade locally and enter lymph ducts and blood vessels to eventually seed other organs. Hormonal control of this process is poorly understood. However, Liotta et al. have isolated a 55-kDa "tumor cell autocrine motility factor" from a variety of cancer types; this activity may play an additional role in tumor invasion of basement membrane and metastases.[256]

Other major tumor-host interactions include desmoplasia (presumably mediated by a large number of growth factors) and angiogenesis. Angiogenic agents, as mentioned in the previous section, include TGFα and FGF.[351]

ANTIESTROGENS AND THEIR INTERACTIONS WITH CHEMOTHERAPEUTIC AGENTS

Among the first antiestrogen compounds utilized were ethamoxytriphetol (MER-25) and clomiphene. The triphenylethylene antiestrogen tamoxifen has subsequently become a mainstay of therapy both in advanced disease and stage II disease in postmenopausal women. In contrast to cytotoxic chemotherapy agents, antiestrogens appear to be cytostatic rather than cytocidal and have a low incidence of significant side effects. Many investigators have noted the close correlation between the initial clinical response to antiestrogens and the presence of the estrogen receptor (and its induced product, the progesterone receptor).[262]

Since antiestrogens and their active metabolites have a high affinity for the estrogen receptor, the most likely mechanism of antiestrogen action appears to be simple antagonism of the growth-promoting effects of estrogen.[219] However, alternate views involving other microsomal binding sites for antiestrogen can have direct antimitogenic effects mediated through the estrogen receptor but independent of estrogen occupancy.[353, 465] It is possible that an alternative receptor confirmation, chromosomal localization, or both may mediate such effects. In addition, high doses of antiestrogen inhibit both calmodulin and protein kinase C,[219, 315] but the physiological relevance of these observations is not yet certain.

Antiestrogen treatment of estrogen-dependent breast cancer leads to cell cycle blockade (early G_1) of most of the cells in vitro and to reduction in tumor growth in vivo.[219, 321, 323, 422] It had been initially observed that MCF-7 cells responded in vitro to both estrogens and antiestrogens under normal cell culture conditions.[261] These experiments were initially interpreted to suggest that antiestrogens could act to arrest growth independently of an occupied estrogen receptor complex. However, as previously mentioned, work by Berthois et al. has clearly shown that high concentrations of phenol red present in the culture medium of the cells in these studies produced estrogenic effects.[29] Removal of phenol red, whose structure resembles that of certain nonsteroidal estrogens, abrogated antiestrogen action on MCF-7 cells and dramatically enhanced the responsiveness of the cells to estrogen induction of cell growth and progesterone receptor. At the present time it appears that antiestrogens act at physiological doses primarily by direct antagonism of the initiation of signals generated by an agonist-occupied receptor.

The principal clinical limitation to the utility of antiestrogens is the gradual resistance that develops in tumors treated with these agents. While in some cases, antiestrogen-resistant tumors lack the estrogen receptor, it is unlikely that loss of the estrogen receptors fully explains the loss of antiestrogen sensitivity during clinical treatment.[384] At least 40 percent of all breast cancers contain the estrogen receptor.[329] Furthermore, a stable clone of MCF-7 cells (LY2, as well as other less stable resistant clones, R3 and R27), selected stepwise in vitro for antiestrogen resistance, still contains high levels of the estrogen receptor.[40]

Another limitation to the antineoplastic efficacy of antiestrogens has been the partial estrogenic (or agonist) activity characteristic of the compounds in clinical use. For instance, studies in the nude mouse model system with MCF-7 cells have only achieved modest inhibition of tumor growth with tamoxifen.[89] Tamoxifen and some other antiestrogens are weakly stimulatory for uterine growth in rodent model systems. However, novel 7-alkyl amide derivatives of estradiol have been reported as pure antiestrogens and are devoid of uterine growth-promoting potential. Such compounds might have greater clinical utility than tamoxifen in the suppression of breast tumor growth.[307, 460]

For patients with breast cancer, durable remissions may be achieved by treatment with cytotoxic drugs or hormonal agents, either singly or in combination. The anthracycline adriamycin is the single most frequently used drug for the treatment of this disease. Unfortunately, although initial response rates to these agents are usually high, most patients will eventually relapse. In the setting of relapse, most breast tumors are resistant to antineoplastic agents. Moreover, in common with tumors derived from other tissues, tumors of relapsed breast cancer patients are frequently cross-resistant to agents to which they have never been exposed.

In order to develop an in vitro model to study mechanisms of resistance to antineoplastic drugs, a number of laboratories have developed drug-resistant cell lines. Analogous to the clinical development of drug resistance, such lines are selected for resistance to single agents but display cross-resistance to a number of drugs that are dissimilar both in structure and in proposed mechanism of action. Drugs associated with multidrug resistance (MDR) phenotype include the anthracyclines, epipodophyllotoxins, *Vinca* alkaloids, and actinomycin D.[170, 453] Cells exhibiting MDR usually have decreased drug accumulation in association with the resistance phenotype. This alteration is frequently associated with the overexpression of a surface glycoprotein known alternatively as P-170, gp140–180, P-glycoprotein, or the *mdr* gene product. The expression of P-170 in multidrug resistance and the putative role of this protein as a drug efflux pump have been reviewed.[170, 453] Identifying biochemical and genetic changes associated with MDR in addition to P-170 overexpression has been an active area of research, and alterations in the levels of a number of proteins, including protein kinase C,[147, 151] sorcin,[445] and glucose-6-phosphate dehydrogenase.[483]

Probing of normal tissues and tumor samples have shown that while tumors derived from tissues that normally express relatively high levels of P-170 (e.g., kidney, adrenal gland, and colon) may increase their levels of this protein,[329] no clear association can be made between the general development of clinical drug resistance and the overexpression of P-170.[89, 307, 329] In the case of breast cancer, there are no examples of this disease being associated with increased levels of P-170, although this is an area of active, current investigation.

In order to determine the mechanisms associated with the development of MDR in breast cancer, an adriamycin-resistant MCF-7 human breast cancer cell line has been selected (MCF-7/Adr^R).* This cell line is 200-fold resistant to adriamycin and displays the phenotype of MDR. Resistance in MCF-7/Adr^R is associated with a two- to threefold decrease in drug accumulation and a 45-fold increase in the expression of P-170. Overexpression of P-170 in this cell line is associated with amplification of the P-170 gene, a gene that has been mapped to chromosome 7q21.1.[145] Detailed analysis of the biochemical characteristics of MCF-7/Adr^R has revealed that, in addition to overexpression of P-170, this cell line has alterations in the levels of a number of proteins, including drug-metabolizing enzymes.[23, 84, 147, 210, 445] These enzymes, which include glutathione-*S*-transferase (GST), UDP-glucoronyl transferase, and sulfotransferase, conjugate the products of the phase I reactions with hydrophilic moieties such as glutathione or glucuronide. The resulting conjugates are very soluble and readily excreted from the cell. In MCF-7/Adr^R cells, the activities of the phase II drug-conjugating enzymes glucuronyl transferase and GST are increased two- and 45-fold, respectively.[23, 84]

GST represents a class of at least 13 isozymes that vary in structure, isoelectric point, and substrate specificity. The increased GST activity in MCF-7/Adr^R is a result of the overexpression of only one of these isozymes, the anionic form (GST-π). In addition to increased activity of phase II enzymes, MDR in MCF-7/Adr^R is associated with down regulation of the phase I enzyme arylhydrocarbon hydroxylase (AHH), the product of the P450IA1 gene.[210] While the possible roles of GST and AHH in resistance to melphalan,[128] mitoxantrone,[415] BCNU,[143] and a number of carcinogens[84] have been defined, the role of these enzymes in resistance to drugs associated with MDR is under investigation. However, the alterations in drug-metabolizing enzymes and other proteins in MCF-7/Adr^R emphasize that the development of MDR in breast cancer is associated with multiple biochemical changes.

Because breast cancer may be successfully treated by both cytotoxic drugs and hormonal agents, it was of interest to determine whether the development of multidrug resistance in MCF-7/Adr^R results in any alteration in hormonal sensitivity. As mentioned, MCF-7 cells are an excellent model system for the study of hormone-responsive breast cancer, as they contain receptors for both estrogen and progesterone and respond to estrogen by increases in both the rate of cell proliferation and the synthesis of specific proteins. The development of MDR in the MCF-7/Adr^R cell line is associated with a loss of response of these cells to estrogen with respect

---

*References 147, 151, 170, 445, 453, 460, and 483.

to both growth stimulation and the induction of several estrogen-regulated proteins, including the progesterone receptor and secreted proteins of molecular weights 7 kDa and 52 kDa. In addition to the loss of responsiveness to estrogen, MCF-7/Adr[R] cells are cross-resistant to the antiestrogen 4-hydroxytamoxifen. Furthermore, while wild-type MCF-7 cells require estrogen to form tumors in athymic mice, the alterations in hormonal sensitivity in MCF-7/Adr[R] have resulted in the cells being able to form tumors equally well in the absence or presence of estrogen.[452]

Resistance to hormonal agents can apparently occur through a number of mechanisms.[89, 452] The development of hormonal insensitivity in MCF-7/Adr[R] is associated with loss of the estrogen receptor.[452] In contrast, this cell line displays a 100-fold increase in levels of the EGF receptor, which is associated with a loss of mitogenic response to EGF.[452] A similar inverse relationship between EGF receptor content and mitogenic effect of EGF has been reported in other cell lines. Other multidrug-resistant cell lines have also been shown to have increased levels of EGF receptor.[288]

What regulates the expression of both estrogen and EGF receptors in MCF-7/Adr[R], and why alterations in the levels of these receptors occurred during the selection for resistance to adriamycin, is unknown. Previous studies have shown that acute treatment of cells with cytotoxic drugs can decrease levels of the estrogen receptor and increase levels of the EGF receptor.[73, 480] Although associated with cytotoxicity, these effects were rapidly reversible on removal of drug from the medium. It remains unclear whether the mechanism responsible for these transient alterations in receptor levels bears any relationship to the stable receptor alterations induced in MCF-7/Adr[R] following chronic drug treatment. It is clear, however, that the development of multidrug resistance in the MCF-7/Adr[R] breast cancer cell line is associated with the development of hormonal insensitivity and increased tumorigenicity.

In addition to providing an in vitro model of multidrug resistance in breast cancer, the development of hormonal insensitivity in MCF-7/Adr[R] bears analogies to the clinical progression of breast cancer. It is well established that patients with estrogen receptor– and progesterone receptor–negative tumors have a poorer prognosis.[258, 262, 329, 369] Selection of MCF-7/Adr[R] has therefore resulted in the progression from estrogen receptor– and progesterone receptor–negative, hormone-responsive breast cancer cells to cells displaying features of the poorest prognosis breast tumors (estrogen receptor– and progesterone receptor–negative, increased levels of the EGF receptor, resistance to drugs and hormonal agents, and increased tumorigenicity).

CONCLUSIONS

We have reviewed the recent literature highlighting the multiple roles of both steroidal (primarily estrogen and progesterone) and polypeptide regulators of mammary epithelial cell growth. Effects of both classes are complex, probably involving multiple interactions with non-tumor, host tissue. Estrogen may induce growth-regulatory polypeptide growth factors and interact with them in hormone-dependent breast cancer. Progression of hormone-dependent breast cancer to hormone independence may involve multiple genetic mechanisms of oncogene activation, loss of the estrogen receptor, loss of tumor repressor genes, or loss of hormone responsivity of other gene products. Initial carcinogenesis and progression of mammary epithelium to cancer probably also requires both proliferative stimuli (estrogen, polypeptide growth factors) and genetic damage, leading to qualitatively different hormonal responses (hormone-responsive cancer). Future therapies could be designed to better block hormonal stimulation and to better monitor indicators of malignant progression such as oncogenes or polypeptide growth factor receptor systems. Perhaps interference with local growth factor regulators of proliferation and differentiation could also be used in cancer prevention, therapy, or both.

References

1. Abraham JA, Whang JL, Tumolo A, Mergia A, Friedman J, Gospodorowicz D, Fiddles JC: Human basic fibroblast growth factor: nucleotide sequence and genomic organization. Eur Mol Biol Organ J 5:2523–2528, 1986.
2. Aitken SC, Lippman ME: Hormonal regulation of de novo pyrimidine synthesis and utilization in human breast cancer cells in tissue culture. Cancer Res 43:4681–4690, 1983.
3. Aitken SC, Lippman ME: Effect of estrogens and antiestrogens on growth-regulatory enzymes in human breast cancer cells in tissue culture. Cancer Res 45:1611–1620, 1985.
4. Aitken SC, Lippman ME, Kasid A, Schoenberg DR: Relationship between the expression of estrogen regulated genes and estrogen-stimulated proliferation of MCF-7 mammary tumor cells. Cancer Res 45:2608–2615, 1985.
5. Albini A, Graf JO, Kitten T, Kleinman HK, Martin GR, Veillette A, Lippman ME: Estrogen and v-ras[H] transfection regulate the interactions of MCF-7 breast carcinoma cells to basement membrane. Proc Natl Acad Sci (USA) 83:8182–8186, 1986.
6. Ali IU, Liderau R, Theillet C, Callahan R: Reduction to homozygosity of genes on chromosome 11 in human breast neoplasia. Science 238:185–188, 1987.
7. Andrea AC, Schoenberger CA, Grover B, Hennighausen L, Le Maur M, Gerlinger P: Ha-ras oncogene expression directed by a milk protein gene promoter: tissue specificity, hormonal regulation and tumor induction in transgenic mice. Proc Natl Acad Sci (USA) 84:1299–1303, 1987.
8. Armelin HA, Armelin MCS, Kelly K, Stewart T, Leder P, Cochran BN, Stiles CO: Functional role for c-myc in mitogenic response to platelet-derived growth factor. Nature 310:655–660, 1984.
9. Arriza JL, Weinberger C, Cerelli G, Glaser TM, Handelin BL, Housman DE, Evans RM: Cloning of human mineralocorticoid receptor complementary DNA: structural and functional kinship with the glucocorticoid receptor. Science 237:268–275, 1987.
10. Arteaga CL, Kitten L, Coronado E, Jacobs I, Kull F, Osborne CK: Blockade of the type I somatomedin receptor inhibits growth of estrogen receptor negative human breast cancer cells in athymic nude mice. (Abstract 683) Proceedings of the Annual Meeting of the Endocrine Society, New Orleans, LA, 1988.
11. Assoian RK, Frolik CA, Roberts AB, Sporn MB: Transforming growth factor beta controls receptor levels for epidermal growth factor in NRK fibroblasts. Cell 36:35–41, 1984.
12. Assoian RK, Grotendorst GR, Miller DM, Sporn MB: Cellular

transformation by coordinated action of three peptide growth factors from human platelets. Nature (London) 309:804–806, 1984.

13. Auricchio F, Migliaccio A, Castoria G, Rotondi A: Regulation of hormone binding of 17β-estradiol receptor by phosphorylation-dephosphorylation of receptor on tyrosine. *In* Auricchio F (ed): Sex Steroid Receptors. Rome, Field Educational Italia Acta Medica, pp 98–107, 1985.

14. Bajaj M, Waterfield MD, Schlessinger J, Taylor WR, Blondell T: On the tertiary structure of the extracellular domains of the epidermal growth factor and insulin receptors. Biochim Biophys Acta 916:220–226, 1987.

15. Balinsky BI: On the pre-natal growth of the mammary gland rudiment in the mouse. J Anatomy 84:227–235, 1950.

16. Bano M, Salomon DS, Kidwell WR: Purification of a mammary derived growth factor from human milk and human mammary tumors. J Biol Chem 260:5745–5752, 1985.

17. Barrack ER, Coffey DS: The specific binding of estrogen and androgens to the nuclear matrix of sex hormone responsive tissues. J Biol Chem 255:7265–7275, 1980.

18. Bartley JC, Bartholomew JC, Smith HS, Bartley J: Metabolism of benzo(a)pyrene by human mammary epithelial cells: toxicity and DNA adduct formation. Proc Natl Acad Sci (USA) 78:6251–6255, 1982.

19. Basu A, Murthy A, Rodeck U, Herlyn M, Mattes J, Das M: Presence of tumor-associated antigens in epidermal growth factor receptors from different human carcinomas. Cancer Res. 47:2531–2536, 1987.

20. Bates SE, Davidson NE, Valverius E, Freter C, Dickson RB, Tam JD, Kudlow JE, Lippman ME, Salomon DS: Expression of transforming growth factor alpha and its messenger ribonucleic acid in human breast cancer: its regulation by estrogen and its possible functional significance. Molec Endocrinol 2:543–555, 1988.

21. Bates SE, McManaway ME, Lippman ME, Dickson RB: Characterization of estrogen responsive transforming activity in human breast cancer cell lines. Cancer Res 46:1707–1713, 1986.

22. Bates SE, Valverius EM, Ennis BW, Bronzert DA, Sheridan JP, Stampfer MR, Mendelsohn J, Lippman ME, Dickson RB: Expression of the transforming growth factor α/epidermal growth factor receptor pathway in normal human breast epithelial cells. Endocrinology 126:596–607, 1990.

23. Batist G, Tulpule A, Sinha BK, Katki AG, Myers CE, Cowan KH: Overexpression of a novel asionic glutathione transferase in multidrug-resistant human breast cancer cells. J Biol Chem 261:15,544–15,549, 1986.

24. Baxter RC, Maitland, JE, Raisur RL, Reddel R, Sutherland RL: High molecular weight somatomedin-C (IGF-I) from T47D human mammary carcinoma cells: immunoreactivity and bioactivity. *In* Spencer EM (ed): Insulin-like Growth Factors/Somatomedins. Berlin, Walter deGruyter, pp 615–618, 1983.

25. Beatson GT: On the treatment of inoperable cases of carcinoma of the mamma; suggestions for a new method of treatment with illustrative cases. Lancet 2:104–107, 162–165, 1896.

26. Beebe DC, Silver MH, Belcher KS, Van Wyk JJ, Svoboda ME, Zelenka PS: Lentropin, a protein that controls less fiber formation, is related functionally and immunologically to the insulin-like growth factors. Proc Natl Acad Sci (USA) 84:2327–2330, 1987.

27. Bell DR, Gerlach JH, Kartner N, Buick RN, Ling V: Detection of P-glycoprotein in ovarian cancer: a molecular marker associated with multidrug resistance. J Clin Oncol 3:311–315, 1985.

28. Berger MS, Locher GW, Saurer S, Gullick WJ, Waterfield MD, Grover B, Hynes NE: Correlation of c-erb B2 gene amplification and protein expression in human breast carcinoma with nodal status and nuclear grading. Cancer Res 48:1238–1243, 1988.

29. Berthois Y, Katzenellenbogen JA, Katzenellenbogen BS: Phenol red in tissue culture media is a weak estrogen: implications concerning the study of estrogen-responsive cells in culture. Proc Natl Acad Sci (USA) 83:2496–2500, 1986.

30. Betsholtz C, Hohnsson A, Heldin CH, Westermark B, Lind P, Urdea MS, Eddy R, Shows TB, Philpott K, Mellor AL, Knott TJ, Scott J: cDNA sequence and chromosomal localization of human platelet derived growth factor A chain and its expression in tumor cell lines. Nature 320:695–700, 1986.

31. Bishop JM: The molecular genetics of cancer. Science 235:305–311, 1987.

32. Biswas R, Vonderhaar BK: Role of serum in the prolactin responsiveness of MCF-7 human breast cancer cells in long-term tissue culture. Cancer Res 47:3509–3514, 1987.

33. Bohmann D, Bos TJ, Admon A, Nishimura T, Vogt PK, Tjian R: Human protooncogene c-jun encodes a DNA binding protein with structural and functional properties of transcription factor AP-1. Science 238:1386–1392, 1987.

34. Bourne HR, Sullivan KA: Signal transducers GTPases, and cyclic AMP mammalian G proteins: models for ras proteins in transmembrane signalling. Cancer Surv 5:257–274, 1986.

35. Bradlow HL, Hershcopf RE, Fishman J: Oestradiol 16α-hydroxylase: a risk marker for breast cancer. Cancer Surv 5:573–583, 1986.

36. Bradshaw GL, Dubes GR: Polyoma virus transformation of rat kidney fibroblasts results in loss of requirement for insulin and retinoic acid. J Gen Virol 64:2311–2315, 1984.

37. Bresciani F: Topography of DNA synthesis in mammary gland of the C3H mouse and its control by ovarian hormones: an autoradiographic study. Cell Tissue Kinet 1:51–63, 1968.

38. Brian P, Petersen DW, Van Deurs B: A new diploid non-tumorigenic human breast epithelial cell line isolated and propagated in chemically defined medium. In Vitro Cell Dev Biol 23:181–188, 1987.

39. Bringman TS, Lindquist PB, Derynck R: Different transforming growth factor species are derived from a glycosylated and palmitolated transmembrane precursor. Cell 48:429–440, 1987.

40. Bronzert DA, Greene GL, Lippman ME: Selection and characterization of breast cancer cell line resistant to the antiestrogen LY 117018. Endocrinology 117:1409–1417, 1985.

41. Bronzert DA, Pantazis P, Antoniades HN, Kasid A, Davidson N, Dickson RB, Lippman ME: Synthesis and secretion of PDGF-like growth factor by human breast cancer cell lines. Proc Natl Acad Sci (USA), 84:5763–5767, 1987.

42. Bronzert DA, Silverman S, Lippman ME: Estrogen inhibition of a Mr 39,000 glycoprotein secreted by human breast cancer cells. Cancer Res 47:1234–1238, 1987.

43. Bronzert DA, Triche TJ, Gleason P, Lippman ME: Isolation and characterization of an estrogen-inhibited variant derived from the MCF-7 breast cancer cell line. Cancer Res 44:3942–3951, 1984.

44. Bronzert DA, Valverius E, Bates SE, Stampfer M, Dickson RB: Production of alpha and beta chains of platelet derived growth factor by human mammary epithelial cells. New Orleans, Annual Meeting of the Endocrine Society, 1988.

45. Brooks SC, Locke ER, Soule HD: Estrogen receptor in a human breast cell line (MCF-7) from breast carcinoma. J Biol Chem 248:6251–6261, 1973.

46. Brunner AM, Gentry LE, Cooper JA, Purchio AF: Recombinant Type I transforming growth factor β precursor produced in Chinese hamster ovary cells is glycosylated and phosphorylated. Molec Cell Biol 8:2229–2232, 1988.

47. Burke RE, Harris SC, McGuire WL: Lactate dehydrogenase in estrogen responsive human breast cancer cells. Cancer Res 38:2773–2780, 1978.

48. Butler WB, Kelsey WH, Goran N: Effects of serum and insulin on the sensitivity of the human breast cancer cell line MCF-7 to estrogens and antiestrogens. Cancer Res 41:82–88, 1981.

49. Butler WB, Kirkland WL, Jorgensen TL: Induction of plasminogen activator by estrogen in a human breast cancer cell line (MCF-7). Biochem Biophys Res Comm 90:1328–1334, 1979.

50. Campisi J, Pardee AB: Post-transcriptional control of the onset of DNA synthesis by an insulin-like growth factor. Molec Cell Biol 4:1807–1814, 1984.

51. Cancer and steroid hormone study of the Centers for Disease Control and the National Institute of Child Health and Human Development. Oral contraceptive use and the risk of breast cancer. New Engl J Med 315:405–411, 1986.

52. Cano A, Coffey AI, Adatia R, Willis RR, Rubens RD, King RJB: Histochemical studies with an estrogen receptor-related protein in human breast tumors. Cancer Res 46:6475–6480, 1986.

53. Capony F, Morisset M, Barrett AJ, Capony JP, Broquet P, Vignon F, Chambon M, Louisot P, Rochefort H: Phosphorylation, glycosylation, and proteolytic activity of the 52-kD estrogen-induced protein secreted by MCF-7 cells. J Cell Biol 104:253–262, 1987.

54. Carney DH, Scott DL, Gordon EA, LaBelle EF: Phosphoinositides in mitogenesis: neomycin inhibits thrombin-stimulated phosphoinositide turnover and initiation of cell proliferation. Cell 42:479–488, 1985.

55. Caron de Fromentel C, Nardeaux PC, Soussi T, et al: Epithelial HBL-100 cell line derived from milk of an apparently healthy woman harbours SV40 genetic information. Exp Cell Res 160:83–94, 1985.

56. Carpenter G: Epidermal growth factor is a major growth promoting agent in human milk. Science 210:198–199, 1980.

57. Carpenter G, Stoscheck CM, Preston YA, Delarco JE: Antibodies to the epidermal growth factor receptor block the biological activities of sarcoma growth factor. Proc Natl Acad Sci (USA) 80:5627–5630, 1983.

58. Carter RL, Mattallano RJ, Hession C, Trizard R, Farber NM, Cheung A, Ninfa EG, Frey AZ, Gash DJ, Chow EP, Fisher RA, Bertonis JM, Tower G, Wallner BP, Ramachandran KL, Ragin RC, Manganaro TF, MacLaughlin DE, Donahoe PK: Isolation of the bovine and human genes for Mullerian inhibiting substance and expression of the human gene in animal cells. Cell 45:685–698, 1986.

59. Chablos D, Rochefort H: Dual effects of progestin R5020 on proteins released by the T47D human breast cancer cells. J Biol Chem 259:1231–1238, 1984.

60. Chablos D, Vignon F, Keydar I, Rochefort H: Estrogens stimulate cell proliferation and induce secretory proteins in a human breast cancer cell line (T47D). J Clin Endocrinol Metab 55:276–283, 1982.

61. Chakrapbarty S, Toborn A, Varani J, Brattain MG: Induction of carcinoembryonic antigen secretion and modulation of protein secretion/expression and fibrometron laminin expression in human colon carcinoma cells by TGFβ. Breast Cancer Res 48:4059–4064, 1988.

62. Chamberlin TL, Gardener WU, Allen E: Local responses of the sexual skin and mammary glands of monkeys to cutaneous application of estrogen. Endocrinology 28:753–757, 1941.

63. Chang SE: *In vitro* transformation of human breast epithelial cells. *In* Rich MA, Hager JC, Taylor-Papadimitrious J (eds): Breast Cancer: Origins, Detection, and Treatment. Boston, Martinus Nijhoff, 1985, pp 205–206.

64. Chang SE: In vitro transformation of human epithelial cells. Biochem Biophys Acta 823:161–180, 1986.

65. Chang SE, Keen J, Lane EB, Taylor-Papadimitriou J: Establishment and characterization of SV40 transformed human breast epithelial cell lines. Cancer Res 42:2040–2053, 1982.

66. Cheifetz S, Like B, Massague J: Cellular distribution of Type I and Type II receptors for transforming growth factor β. J Biol Chem 261:9972, 1986.

67. Cheifetz S, Wentherbee JA, Tsang MSS, Anderson JK, Mole JE, Lucas R, Massague J: The transforming growth factor β system, a complex pattern of cross-reactive ligands and receptor. Cell 48:409–415, 1987.

68. Cheng EH, Furth ME, Scolnick EM, Lowy DR: Nature 297:479–483, 1982.

69. Cherington PV, Smith BL, Pardee AB: Loss of epidermal growth factor requirement and malignant transformation. Proc Natl Acad Sci (USA) 76:3937–3942, 1979.

70. Chiquet-Ehrismann R, Mackie EJ, Pearson CA, Sakakura T: Tenascin: an extracellular matrix protein involved in tissue interactions during fetal development and oncogenesis. Cell 47:131–139, 1986.

71. Ciocca DR, Adams DJ, Edwards DP, Bjerke RJ, McGuire WL: Distribution of an estrogen induced protein with a molecular weight of 24,000 in normal and malignant human tissues and cells. Cancer Res 43:1204–1210, 1983.

72. Clark R, Stampfer MR, Milley R, O'Rourke E, Walen KH, Kriegler M, Kopplin J, McCormick F: Transformation of human mammary epithelial cells by oncogenic retroviruses. Cancer Res, 1988, in press.

73. Clarke R, Morwood J, van den Berg HW, Nelson J, Murphy RF: Effect of cytotoxic drugs on estrogen receptor expression and response to tamoxifen in MCF-7 cells. Cancer Res 46:6116–6119, 1986.

74. Clemmons DR, Elgin RG, Han VKM, Casella SJ, D'Ercole AJ, Van Wyk JJ: Cultured fibroblast monolayers secretage a protein that alters the cellular binding of somatomedin-C/insulin-like growth factor I. J Clin Invest 77:1548–1556, 1986.

75. Clemmons DR, Shaw DS: Variables controlling somatomedin production by cultured human fibroblasts. J Cell Physiol 115:137–143, 1983.

76. Clemmons DR, Shaw DS: Purification and biological properties of fibroblast somatomedin. J Biol Chem 261:10293–10298, 1986.

77. Clemmons DR, Van Wyk JJ: Evidence for a functional role of endogenously produced somatomedin-like peptides in the regulation of DNA synthesis in cultured human fibroblasts and porcine smooth muscle cells. J Clin Invest 75:1914–1918, 1986.

78. Cline MJ, Buttitora H, Yokota J: Protooncogene abnormalities in human breast cancer: correlations with anatomic features and clinical course of disease. J Clin Oncol 5:999–1006, 1987.

79. Coffey RJ, Kost LJ, Lyons RM, Moses HL, LaRusso NF: Hepatic processing of transforming growth factor β in the rat. J Clin Invest 80:705–757, 1987.

80. Coffey RJ, Leof EB, Shipley GD, Moses HL: Suramin inhibition of growth factor receptor binding and mitogenicity in AKR-2 cells. J Cell Physiol 132:143–148, 1987.

81. Cohen S: Isolation of a mouse submaxillary gland protein accelerating incisor eruption and eyelid opening in the newborn animal. J Biol Chem 237:1555–1562, 1962.

82. Coughlin SR, Barr PJ, Cousens LS, Fretto LJ, Williams LT: Acidic and basic fibroblast growth factors stimulate tyrosine kinase activity *in vivo*. J Biol Chem 263:988–993, 1988.

83. Cowan K, Levine R, Aitken S, Goldsmith M, Douglass E, Clendeninn N, Nienhuis A, Lippman ME: Dihydrofolate reductase gene amplification and possible rearrangement in estrogen-responsive methotrexate resistant human breast cancer cells. J Biol Chem 257:15,079–15,086, 1982.

84. Cowan KH, Batist G, Tulpule A, Sinha BK, Myers CE: Similar biochemical changes associated with multidrug resistance in human breast cancer cells and carcinogen-induced resistance to xenobiotics in rats. Proc Natl Acad Sci (USA) 83:9328–9332, 1986.

85. Croce CM: Role of chromosome translocations in human neoplasia. Cell 49:155–156, 1987.

86. Cullen KJ, Yee D, Paik S, Hampton B, Perdue JF, Lippman ME, Rosen N: Insulin-like growth factor II expression and activity in human breast cancer. (Abstract 947). Proceedings of the 79th Annual Meeting of the American Association for Cancer Research, New Orleans, LA, 1988.

87. Daniel CW, Silberstein GP: Postnatal development of the rodent mammary gland. *In* Daniel CW, Neville MC (eds): The Mammary Gland: Development, Regulation, and Function. New York, Plenum, 1988, in press.

88. Daniel CW, Silberstein GB, Strickland P: Direct action of 17β estradiol in mouse mammary ducts analyzed by sustained release implants and steroid autoradiography. Cancer Res 47:6052–6057, 1987.

89. Darbre P, King RJB: Progression to steroid insensitivity can occur irrespective of the presence of functional steroid receptors. Cell 41:521–528, 1987.

90. Darbon J-M, Valette A, Bayard F: Phorbol esters inhibit the proliferation of MCF-7 cells. Biochem Pharmacol 35:2683–2686, 1986.

91. Darbre P, Yates J, Curtis S, King RJB: Effect of estradiol on human breast cancer cells in culture. Cancer Res 43:349–354, 1983.

92. Daughaday WH, Hall K, Salmon WD, Van den Brande JL, Van Wyk JJ: On the nomenclature of the somatomedins and insulin-like growth factors. Endocrinology 121:1911–1912, 1987.

93. Davidson NE, Bronzert DA, Chambon P, Gelmann EP, Lippman ME: Use of two MCF-7 cell variants to evaluate the growth regulatory potential of estrogen-induced products. Cancer Res 46:1904–1908, 1986.

94. Davidson NE, Gelmann EP, Lippman ME, Dickson RB: EGF

receptor gene expression and its relation to the estrogen receptor in human breast cancer cell lines. Mol Endocrinol 1:216–223, 1987.

95. Davis S, Pouyssegur J: Pertussis toxin inhibits thrombin-induced activation of phosphoinositide hydrolysis and Na$^+$/H$^+$ exchange in hamster fibroblasts. EMBO J 5:55–60, 1986.

96. Degen GH, Metzler M: Sex hormone and neoplasia: genotoxic effects in short term assays. Arch Toxicol Vol 10(supplement):264–278, 1987.

97. Dehoff MH, Elgin RG, Collier RJ, Clemmons DR: Both type I and II insulin-like growth factor receptor binding increase during lactogenesis in bovine mammary tissue. Endocrinology 122:2412–2417, 1988.

98. Delarco JE, Todaro GJ: Growth factors from murine sarcoma virus-transformed cells. Proc Natl Acad Sci (USA) 75:4001–4005, 1978.

99. De Leon DD, Bakker B, Wilson DM, Hintz RL, Rosenfeld RG: Demonstration of insulin-like growth factor (IGF-I and -II) receptors and binding protein in human breast cancer cell lines. Biochem Biophys Res Comm 152:398–405, 1988.

100. Delli Bovi P, Gurutola AM, Kern FG, Greco A, Ittmann M, Basilico C: An oncogene isolated by transfection of Kaposi sarcoma DNA encodes a growth factor that is a member of the FGF family. Cell 50:729–737, 1987.

101. Dembinski TC, Leung CHK, Shiu RPC: Evidence for a novel pituitary factor that potentiates the mitogenic effect of estrogen in human breast cancer cells. Cancer Res 45:3038–3089, 1985.

102. Dempsey PJ, Feleppa FP, Brown RW, deKretser TA, Whitehead RH, Jose DG: Development of monoclonal antibodies to the human breast carcinoma cell line PMC42. J Natl Cancer Inst 77:1–15, 1986.

103. D'Ercole AJ, Applewhite GT, Underwood LE: Evidence that somatomedin is synthesized by multiple tissues in the fetus. Dev Biol 75:315–328, 1980.

104. Derynck R, Goeddel DV, Ullrich A, Gutterman JU, Williams RD, Bringman TS, Berger WH: Synthesis of messenger RNAs for transforming growth factor α and β and the epidermal growth factor receptor by human tumors. Cancer Res 47:707–712, 1987.

105. Derynck R, Jarrett JA, Chen EY, Eaton DH, Bell JR, Assoian RK, Roberts AB, Sporn MB, Goeddel DV: Human transforming growth factor β: complementary DNA sequence and expression in normal and transformed cells. Nature 316:701–705, 1985.

106. Derynck R, Roberts AB, Winkler ME, Chen EY, Goeddel DV: Human transforming growth factor α—precursor structure and expression in E. coli. Cell 38:287–297, 1984.

107. de The H, Marchio A, Tiollais P, Dejean A: A novel steroid thyroid hormone related gene inappropriately expressed in human hepatocellular carcinoma. Nature 330:667–669, 1987.

108. Devleeschouwer N, Legros N, Oleu-Serrano N, Pariduens R, Leclercq G: Estrogen conjugates and serum factors mediating the estrogenic trophic effect on MCF-7 cell growth. Cancer Res 47:5883–5887, 1987.

109. Devroede MA, Tseng LMH, Katsyannis PG, Nissley SP, Rechler MM: Modulation of insulin-like growth factor I binding to human fibroblast monolayers by insulin-like growth factor carrier proteins released to the incubation media. J Clin Invest 77:602–610, 1986.

110. DiAugustine RP, Petrusz P, Bell GI, Brown CF, Kovach KS, McLachlan JA, Teng CT: Influence of estrogens on mouse uterine epidermal growth factor precursor protein and messenger ribonucleic acid. Endocrinology 122:2355–2363, 1988.

111. Dickson C, Peters G: Potential oncogene product related to growth factors. Nature 326:833, 1987.

112. Dickson RB: Endocytosis of polypeptides and their receptors. Trends Pharmacol Sci 6:164–167, 1985.

113. Dickson RB, Aitken S, Lippman ME: Assay of mitogen-induced effects on cellular thymidine incorporation. In Barnes D, Sirbasku DA (eds): Methods in Enzymology, 46. Hormone Action Part II: Peptide Growth Factors. New York, Academic Press, 1987, pp 327–340.

114. Dickson RB, Aten RF, Eisenfeld AJ: Receptor bound estrogens and their metabolites in the nucleus of isolated parenchymal cell. Mol Pharmacol 18:215–223, 1980.

115. Dickson RB, Clark CR: Estrogen receptors in the male. Arch Androl 7:205–217, 1981.

116. Dickson RB, Huff KK, Spencer EM, Lippman ME: Induction of epidermal growth factor related polypeptides by 17-beta estradiol in MCF-7 human breast cancer cell lines. Endocrinology 118:138–142, 1986.

117. Dickson RB, Kasid A, Huff KK, Bates S, Knabbe C, Bronzert D, Gelmann EP, Lippman ME: Activation of growth factor secretion in tumorigenic states of breast cancer induced by 17-beta estradiol or v-ras^H oncogene. Proc Natl Acad Sci (USA) 84:837–841, 1987.

118. Dickson RB, Lippman ME: Estrogen regulation of growth and polypeptide growth factor secretion in human breast carcinoma. Endocr Rev 8:29–43, 1986.

119. Dickson RB, Lippman ME: Role of estrogen in malignant progression of breast cancer; perspectives. Trends Pharmacol Sci 7:294–296, 1986.

120. Dickson RB, McManaway M, Lippman ME: Estrogen induced factors of breast cancer cells partially replace estrogen to promote tumor growth. Science 232:1540–1543, 1986.

121. Dickson RB, Rosen N, Gelmann EP, Lippman ME: Receptor and signal transduction-related protooncogenes in breast cancer. Trends Pharmacol Sci 8:372–375, 1987.

122. Di Fiore PP, Pierce JH, Fleming TP, Hazan R, Ullrid A, King CR, Schlessinger J, Aaronson SA: Overexpression of the human EGF receptor confers on EGF-dependent transformed phenotype to NIH 3T3 cells. Cell 51:1063–1070, 1987.

123. DiFronzo G, Clemente C, Cappelletti V, Miodini P, Coradini D, Ronchi E, Andreola S, Rilke F: Relationship between ER-ICA and conventional steroid receptor assays in human breast cancer. Breast Cancer Res Treat 8:35–43, 1986.

124. Drews U, Drews U: Regression of mouse mammary gland antigen in recombinants of Tfm and wild-type tissue: testosterone acts via the mesenchyme. Cell 10:401–404, 1977.

125. Drop SLS, Kortlene DJ, Guyda HJ: Isolation of a somatomedin-binding protein from preterm amniotic fluid; development of a radioimmunoassay. J Clin Endocrinol Metab 59:899–910, 1984.

126. Druege PM, Klein-Hitpass L, Green S, Stock G, Chambon P, Ryffell GU: Introduction of estrogen-responsiveness into mammalian cell lines. Nucl Acids Res 14:9329–9337, 1986.

127. Dubik D, Dembinski TC, Shiu RP: Stimulation of c-myc oncogene expression associated with estrogen-induced proliferation of human breast cancer cells. Cancer Res 47:6517–6521, 1987.

128. Dulik DM, Hilton J, Fenselau C: Characterization of melphal-anglutathione adducts whose formation is catalyzed by glutathione-S-transferases. Biochem Pharmacol 35:3405–3408, 1986.

129. Durnberger H, Heuberger B, Schwartz P, Wasner G, Kratochwil K: Mesenchyme-mediated effect of testosterone on embryonic mammary epithelium. Cancer Res 38:4066–4070, 1978.

130. Edwards DP, Murphy SR, McGuire WL: Effect of estrogen and antiestrogen on DNA polymerase in human breast cancer. Cancer Res 40:1722–1726, 1980.

131. Edwards DR, Murphy G, Reynolds JJ, Whitham SE, Doherty JP, Angel P, Heath JK: Transforming growth factor beta modulates the expression of collagenase and metalloproteinase inhibitor. EMBO J 6:1899–1904, 1987.

132. Edwards PP, Martin PJ, Horwitz KB, Chamness GC, McGuire WL: Subcellular compartmentalization of estrogen receptors in human breast cancer cells. Exp Cell Res 127:197–213, 1980.

133. Eidne KA, Flanagan CA, Miller RP: Gonadotropin-releasing hormone binding sites in human breast carcinoma. Science 229:989–991, 1985.

134. Eisenman RN, Thompson CB: Oncogenes with potential nuclear function: myc, myb, and fos. Cancer Surv 5:309–328, 1986.

135. Eisholtz HP, Mangalam HJ, Potter E, Albert VR, Supowit S, Evans RM, Rosenfeld MG: Two different cis-active elements transfer the transcriptional effects of both EGF and phorbol esters. Science 235:1552–1557, 1986.

136. Eisman JA, Martin TJ, MacIntyre I, Framtin RJ, Moseley JM, Whitehead R: 25-dihydroxy vitamin D$_3$ receptor in a cultured human breast cancer cell line (MCF-7 cells). Biochem Biophys Res Comm 93:9–18, 1980.

137. Elgin RG, Busby WH, Clemmons DR: An insulin-like growth factor (IGF) binding protein enhances the biological response to IGF-I. Proc Natl Acad Sci (USA) 84:3254–3258, 1987.

138. Ellis L, Clauser E, Morgan DO, Ederg M, Roth RA, Rutter WJ: Replacement of insulin receptor tyrosine residues 1162 and 1163 compromises insulin-stimulated kinase activity and uptake of 2-deoxyglucose. Cell 46:721–732, 1986.

139. Ellis L, Morgan DO, Jong S-M, Wong L-H, Roth RA, Rutter WJ: Heterologous transmembrane signalling by a human insulin receptor-v-ras hybrid in Chinese hamster ovary cells. Proc Natl Acad Sci (USA) 84:5101–5105, 1987.

140. Elliston JF, Zablocki JA, Katzenellenbogen BS, Katzenellenbogen JA: Ketonestrol aziridine, an agonistic estrogen receptor affinity label: study of its bioactivity and estrogen receptor covalent labeling. Endocrinology 121:667–676, 1987.

141. Engle LW, Young NW: Human breast carcinoma cells in continuous culture: a review. Cancer Res 38:4327–4339, 1978.

142. Esch F, Baird A, Ling N, Ueno N, Hill F, Denoroy L, Kleppner K, Gospodarowicz D, Bohlen P, Guillemin R: Primary structure of bovine pituitary growth factor (FGF) and comparison with the amino terminal sequence of bovine brain acidic FGF. Proc Natl Acad Sci (USA) 82:6507–6511, 1985.

143. Evans CG, Bodell WJ, Tokuda K, Doane-Setzer P, Smith M: Glutathione and related enzymes in rat brain tumor cell resistance to 1, 3-bis (2-chloroethyl)-1-nitrosurea and nitrogen mustard. Cancer Res 47:2525–2530, 1987.

144. Evans RM: The steroid and thyroid hormone receptor superfamily. Science 240:887–895, 1988.

145. Fairchild CR, Ivy SP, Kao-Shan C-S, Whang-Peng J, Rosen N, Israel MA, Melera PW, Cowan KH, Goldsmith ME: Isolation of amplified DNA sequences associated with pleiotropic drug resistance from human breast cancer cells. Cancer Res 47:5141–5148, 1987.

146. Ferguson DJP, Anderson TJ: Morphological evaluation of cell turnover in relation to the menstrual cycle in the nesting human breast. Br J Cancer 44:177–181, 1981.

147. Ferguson PJ, Cheng Y-C: Transient protection of cultured human cells against antitumor agents by 12-0-tetradecanoylphorbol-13 acetate. Cancer Res 47:433–441, 1987.

148. Fernandez-Pol JA, Klos DJ, Hamilton PD, Talkad VD: Modulation of epidermal growth factor receptor gene expression by transforming growth factor β in a human breast carcinoma cell line. Cancer Res 47:4260–4265, 1987.

149. Fidler IJ, Gersten DM, Hart IR: The biology of cancer invasion and metastasis. Adv Cancer Res 28:149–160, 1978.

150. Filmus J, Trent JM, Polak MN, Buick RN: Epidermal growth factor gene-amplifier MDA-468 cell line and its non-amplified variants. Molec Cell Biol 7:251–257, 1987.

151. Fine RL, Patel J, Chabner BA: Phorbol esters induce multidrug resistance in human breast cancer cell. Proc Natl Acad Sci (USA) 85:582–586, 1988.

152. Finzi E, Fleming T, Segatto O, Pennington CY, Bringman TS, Derynck R, Aaronson SA: The human transforming growth factor type α coding sequence is not a direct-acting oncogene when overexpressed in NIH 3T3 cells. Proc Natl Acad Sci (USA) 84:3733–3737, 1987.

153. Fisher ER: The pathology of breast cancer as it relates to its evolution, prognosis and treatment. Clin Oncol 1:703–750, 1982.

154. Fisher ER, Gregorio RM, Fisher B: The pathology of invasive breast cancer. Cancer 36:1–75, 1975.

155. Fishman J: Aromatic hydroxylation of estrogens. Ann Rev Physiol 45:61–72, 1983.

156. No reference.

157. Fitzpatrick SL, LaChance MP, Schultz GS: Characterization of epidermal growth factor receptor and action on human breast cancer cells in culture. Cancer Res 44:3442–3447, 1984.

158. Fleming H, Blumenthal R, Gurpide E: Rapid changes in specific estrogen binding elicited by cGMP or cAMP in cytosol from human endometrial cells. Proc Natl Acad Sci (USA) 80:2486–2490, 1983.

159. Flier JS, Usher P, Moses AE: Monoclonal antibody to the type I insulin-like growth factor (IGF-I) receptor blocks IGF-I receptor-mediated DNA synthesis: clarification of the mitogenic mechanisms of IGF-I and insulin in human skin fibroblasts. Proc Natl Acad Sci (USA) 83:664–668, 1986.

160. Fojo AT, Ueda K, Slamon DJ, Poplack DG, Gottesman MM, Pastan I: Expression of a multidrug-resistance gene in human tumors and tissues. Proc Natl Acad Sci (USA) 84:265–269, 1987.

161. Folkman J: How is blood vessel growth regulated in normal and neoplastic tissue. Cancer Res 216:467–473, 1986.

162. Folkman J, Klagsbrun M: Angiogenic factors. Science 235:442–447, 1987.

163. Freedman VH, Shin S: Cellular tumorigenicity in nude mice: correlation with cell growth in semi-solid medium. Cell 3:355–359, 1974.

164. Freter CE, Lippman ME, Cheville A, Zinn S: Alterations in phosphoinoritide metabolism association with 17B-estradiol and growth factor treatment of MCF-7 breast cancer cells. Mol Endocrinol 2:159–166, 1988.

165. Furlanetto RW, DiCarlo JN: Somatomedin C receptors and growth effects in human breast cells maintained in long-term culture. Cancer Res 44:2122–2128, 1984.

166. Gentry LE, Twardzik DR, Lim GJ, Ranchalis JE, Lee DC: Expression and characterization of transforming growth factor precursor protein in transfected mammalian cells. Molec Cell Biol 7:1585–1591, 1987.

167. Giguere SM, Hollenberg SM, Rosenfeld MG, Evans RM: Functional domains of the human glucocorticoid receptor. Cell 46:645–652, 1986.

168. Giguere V, Ong ES, Segui P, Evans RM: Identification of a receptor for the morphogen retinoic acid. Nature 330:624–629, 1987.

169. Giguere V, Yang N, Segui P, Evans RM: Identification of a new class of steroid hormone receptors. Nature 331:91–97, 1988.

170. Gottesman MM, Pastan I: Resistance to multiple chemotherapeutic agents in human cancer cells. Trends Pharmacol Sci 9:54–58, 1988.

171. Goustin AS, Leof EB, Shipley GD, Moses HL: Growth factors and Cancer. Cancer Res 46:1015–1029, 1986.

172. Green S, Walter P, Kumar V, Krust A, Bornertt J-M, Argos P, Chambon P: Human oestrogen receptor cDNA: sequence, expression and homology to v-erb A. Nature 320:134–139, 1986.

173. Greene GL, Gilna P, Waterfield M, Baker H, Hort Y, Shine J: Sequence and expression of human estrogen receptor complementary DNA. Science 231:1150–1154, 1986.

174. Greene GL, Jensen EV: Monoclonal antibodies as probes for estrogen receptor detection and characterization. J Steroid Biochem 16:353–359, 1982.

175. Greene GL, Sobel NB, King WJ, Jensen EV: Immunological studies of estrogen receptors. J Steroid Biochem 20:51–56, 1984.

176. Greig RG, Koestler TP, Trainer DL, Corwin SP, Miles L, Kline T, Sweet R, Yokoyama S, Poste G: Proc Natl Acad Sci (USA) 82:3698–3701, 1985.

177. Groyer A, Schwiezer-Groyer G, Cadepond F, Mariller M, Baulieu EE: Antiglucocorticosteroid effects suggest why steroid hormone is required for receptors to bind DNA in vivo but not in vitro. Nature 328:624–627, 1987.

178. Hackett AJ, Smith HS, Springer EL, Owens RB, Nelson-Rees WA, Riggs JL, Gardner MB: Two syngeneic cell lines from human breast tissue: the aneuploid mammary epithelial (Hs578T) and the diploid myoepithelial (Hs578Bst) cell line. J Natl Cancer Inst 58:1795–1806, 1977.

179. Halper J, Moses HL: Epithelial tissue-derived growth factor-like polypeptides. Cancer Res 43:1972–1979, 1983.

180. Halper J, Moses HL: Purification and characterization of a novel transforming growth factor. Cancer Res 47:4552–4559, 1987.

181. Hammond SL, Ham RG, Stampfer MR: Serum-free growth of human mammary epithelial cells: rapid clonal growth in defined medium and extended serial passage with pituitary extract. Proc Natl Acad Sci (USA) 81:5435–5439, 1984.

182. Han VK, D'Ercole AJ, Lund PK: Cellular localization of somatomedin (insulin-like growth factor) messenger RNA in the human fetus. Science 236:193–197, 1987.

183. Han VKM, Hunter ES, Prott RM, Zendegni JG, Lee DC: Expression of rat transforming growth factor alpha mRNA during development occurs predominantly in the maternal decidua. Molec Cell Biol 7:2335–2343, 1987.

184. Hanover JA, Dickson RB: The possible link between receptor phosphorylation and internalization. Trends Pharmacol Sci 6:164–167, 1985.

185. Hanover JA, Dickson RB: Transferin: receptor-mediated endocytosis and iron delivery. *In* Pastan IH, Willingham ME (eds): Endocytosis. New York, Plenum, 1985, pp. 131–161.

186. Haslam SZ: Mammary fibroblast influence on normal mouse mammary epithelial cell responses to estrogen *in vitro*. Cancer Res 46:310–316, 1986.

187. Haslam SZ, Lively ML: Estradiol responsiveness of normal mouse epithelial cells in primary culture: association of mammary fibroblasts with estradiol regulation of progesterone receptors. Endocrinology 116:1835–1844, 1985.

188. Heimark RL, Twardzik DR, Schwartz SM: Inhibition of endothelial regeneration by type-beta transforming growth factor from platelets. Science 233:1078–1080, 1986.

189. Heldin CH, Westermark B: Growth factors: mechanism of action and relations to oncogenes. Cell 37:9–20, 1984.

190. Henderson BE, Ross R, Bernstein L: Estrogens as a cause of human cancer. The Richard and Hinda Rosenthal Foundation Award lecture. Cancer Res 48:246–253, 1988.

191. Herbst AL, Ulfelder H, Poskanzer DC: Adenocarcinoma of the vagina: association of maternal stilbesterol therapy with tumor appearance in young women. New Engl J Med 284:878–881, 1971.

192. Hizuka N, Takano K, Tanaka I, Asakawa K, Miyakawa M, Horikawa R, Shizumi K: Demonstration of insulin-like growth factor I in human urine. J Clin Endocrinol Metab 64:1309–1316, 1987.

193. Horwitz KB, McGuire WL: Estrogen control of progesterone receptor in human breast cancer. J Biol Chem 253:2223–2228, 1978.

194. Housley GM, Johnson MD, Wendy-Hsiao WL, O'Brian CA, Murphy JP, Kirschmeier P, Weinstein IB: Overproduction of protein kinase C causes disordered growth control in rat fibroblasts. Cell 52:343–354, 1988.

195. Huang JS, Huang SS, Deuel TF: Transforming protein of simian sarcoma virus stimulates autocrine growth of SSV-transformed cells through PDGF cell surface receptors. Cell 39:79–87, 1984.

196. Huang SS, O'Grady P, Huang JS: Human transforming growth factor α-2-macroglobulin complex is a latent form of transforming growth factor β. J Biol Chem 263:1535–1541, 1988.

197. Huff KK, Kaufman D, Gabbay KH, Spencer EM, Lippman ME, Dickson RB: Human breast cancer cells secrete an insulin-like growth factor-1-related polypeptide. Cancer Res 46:4613–4619, 1986.

198. Huff KK, Knabbe C, Lindsay R, Lippman ME, Dickson RB: Multihormonal regulation of insulin-like growth factor-I-related protein in MCF-7 human breast cancer cells. Mol Endocrinol 2:200–208, 1988.

199. Huff KK, Lippman ME: Hormonal control of plasminogen activator secretion in ZR-75-1 human breast cancer cells in culture. Endocrinology 114:1665–1671, 1984.

200. Huff KK, McManaway M, Paik S, Brunner N: In vivo effects of insulin-like growth factor-I (IGF-I) on tumor formation by MCF-7 human breast cancer cells in athymic mice. (Abstract 878) Proceedings of the 70th Annual Meeting of the Endocrine Society, New Orleans, LA, 1988.

201. Huggins C, Clark PJ: Quantitative studies of prostatic secretion. J Exp Med 72:747–762, 1940.

202. Huseby RA, Maloney TM, McGrath CM: Evidence for a direct growth-stimulating effect of estradiol on human MCF-7 cells in vivo. Cancer Res 44:2654–2659, 1984.

203. Hynes MA, Van Wyk JJ, Brooks PJ, D'Ercole AJ, Jansen M, Lund PK: Growth hormone dependence of somatomedin C/insulin-like growth factor-I and insulin-like growth factor-II messenger ribonucleic acids. Mol Endocrinol 1:233–242, 1987.

204. Ignotz RA, Kelly B, Davis RJ, Massague J: Biologically active precursor for transforming growth factor type α released by retrovirally transformed cells. Proc Natl Acad Sci (USA) 83:6307–6311, 1986.

205. Ignotz RA, Massague J: Transforming growth factor β stimulates the expression of fibronectin and collagen and their incorporation into the extracellular matrix. J Biol Chem 261:4337–4345, 1986.

206. Ignotz RA, Massague J: Cell adhesion protein receptors as targets for transforming growth factor β action. Cell 51:189–197, 1987.

207. Ikeda T, Danielpour D, Sirbasku BA: Isolation and properties of endocrine and autocrine type mammary tumor cell growth factors (estromedins). *In* Bresciani F, King RJB, Lippman ME, Namer M, Raynaud JP (eds): Progress in Cancer Research and Therapy, vol 31. New York, Raven Press, 1983, pp 171–186.

208. Ikeda T, Lioubin MN, Marquardt H: Human transforming growth factor β₂: production by a prostatic adenocarcinoma cell line, purification and initial characterization. Biochemistry 26:2406–2410, 1987.

209. Ikeda T, Sirbasku DA: Purification and properties of a mammary-uterine-pituitary tumor cell growth factor from pregnant sheep uterus. J Biol Chem 259:4049–4964, 1984.

210. Ivy SP, Tulpule A, Fairchild CR, Averbuch SD, Myers CE, Nebert DW, Baird WM, Cowan KH: Altered regulation of P450 1A1 expression in a multidrug resistant MCF-7 human breast cancer cell line. J Biol Chem, in press.

211. Jacobs C, Rubsumen H: Expression of pp60c-src protein kinase in adult and fetal human tissue: high activities in some sarcomas and mammary carcinomas. Cancer Res 43:1696–1672, 1983.

212. Jakobovits EB, Majors JE, Varmus HE: Hormonal regulation of the rous sarcoma src gene via a heterologous promoter defines a threshold dose for cellular transformation. Cell 38:757–765, 1984.

213. Jakolew SB, Breathneck R, Jeltsch J, Chambon P: Sequence of the pS2 mRNA induced estrogen in the human breast cancer cell line MCF-7. Nucl Acids Res 12:2861–2874, 1984.

214. Jansen M, Van Schaik FMA, Ricker AT, Bullock B, Woods PE, Gabbay KH, Nussbaum AL, Sussenback JS, Vander Branch JR: Sequence of cDNA encoding human insulin-like growth factor I precursor. Nature (London) 306:609–611, 1983.

215. Jensen EV: Studies of growth phenomenon using tritium-labeled steroids. Proceedings of the 4th International Congress of Biochem, vol 15. Vienna, Pergamon Press, 1958, p 119.

216. Jensen EV, DeSombre ER: Mechanism of action of the female sex hormones. Ann Rev Biochem 41:203–230, 1972.

217. Jensen EV, Polley TZ, Smith S, Block GE, Ferguson DT, DeSombre ER: Prediction of hormone dependence in human breast cancer. *In* McGuire WL, Carbone PP, Vollmer EP (eds): Estrogen Receptors in Human Breast Cancer. New York, Raven Press, 1975, pp 37–56.

218. Jick H, Walker AM, Rothman KJ: The epidemic of endometrial cancer: a commentary. Am J Pub Health 70:264–267, 1980.

219. Jordan VC: Biochemical pharmacology of antiestrogen action. Pharmacol Rev 36:245–276, 1984.

220. Kamps MP, Buss BM, Sefton JF: Rous sarcoma virus transforming protein lacking myristic acid phosphorylates known polypeptide substrates without inducing transformation. Cell 45:105–112, 1986.

221. Kasid A, Davidson N, Gelmann E, Lippman ME: Transcriptional control of thymidine kinase gene expression by estrogens and antiestrogens in MCF-7 human breast cancer cells. J Biol Chem 261:5562–5567, 1986.

222. Kasid A, Knabbe C, Lippman ME: Effect of v-rasᴴ oncogene transfection on estrogen-dependent human breast cancer cells. Cancer Res 47:5733–5738, 1987.

223. Kasid A, Lippman ME, Papageorge AG, Lowy DR, Gelmann EP: Transfection of v-rasᴴ DNA into MCF-7 cells bypasses their dependence on estrogen for tumorigenicity. Science 228:725–728, 1985.

224. Katzenellenbogen BS, Elliston JF, Monsama FJ, Springer PA, Ziegler YS: Structural analysis of covalently labeled estrogen receptors by limited proteolysis and monoclonal antibody reactivity. Biochemistry 26:2364–2373, 1987.

225. Katzenellenbogen BS, Norman MJ, Eckert RL, Peltz SW, Mangel WF: Bioactivities, estrogen receptor interactions, and plasminogen activator-inducing activities of tamoxifen and hydroxy-tamoxifen isomersin MCF-7 human breast cancer cells. Cancer Res 44:112–119, 1983.

226. Kaufman U, Zapf J, Torretti B, Froesch ER: Demonstration of a specific serum carrier protein of nonsuppressible insulin-like activity in vivo. J Clin Endocrinol Metab 44:160–166, 1977.

227. Keating MT, Lewis LT: Autocrine stimulation of intracellular PDGF receptors in v-sis-transformed cells. Science 239:914–916, 1988.

228. Keating MT, Williams LT: Processing of the platelet-derived growth factor receptor. J Biol Chem 16:7932–7937, 1987.

229. Keski-Oja J, Lyons RM, Moses HL: Immunodetection and modulation of cellular growth with antibodies against native transforming growth factor. Cancer Res 47:6451–6458, 1987.

230. Kimball ES, Bohn WH, Cockley KD, Warren TC, Sherwin SA: Distinct high performance liquid chromatography pattern of transforming growth factor activity in urine of cancer patients as compared with that of normal individuals. Cancer Res 44:3613–3619, 1984.

231. Kimelman D, Kirschner M: Synergistic induction of mesoderm by FGF and TGFβ and the identification of an mRNA coding for actin in the early xenopus embryo. Cell 51:869–877, 1987.

232. King WJ, DeSombre ER, Jensen EV, Greene GL: Comparison of immunocytochemical and steroid binding assays for estrogen receptor in human breast tumors. Cancer Res 45:294–304, 1985.

233. King WJ, Greene GL: Monoclonal antibodies localize estrogen receptor in the nuclei of target cells. Nature 307:745–749, 1984.

234. Knabbe C, Lippman ME, Wakefield L, Flanders K, Kasid A, Derynck R, Dickson RB: Evidence that TGFβ is a hormonally regulated negative growth factor in human breast cancer. Cell 48:417–428, 1987.

235. Knabbe CK, Lippman ME, Greene GL, Dickson RB: Phorbol ester induced phosphorylation of the estrogen receptor in intact MCF-7 human breast cancer cells. (Abstract 2437) Fed Proc 45:1899, 1986.

236. Kobrin MS, Samosondar J, Kudlow JE: α-transforming growth factor secreted by untransformed bovine anterior pituitary cells in culture. J Biol Chem 261:14,414–14,419, 1986.

237. Kozma SC, Bogaard ME, Buber K, Saurer SM, Bos JL, Grover B, Hynes NE: The human c-kirsten ras gene is activated by a novel mutation in codon 13 in the breast carcinoma line MDA-MB231. Nucl Acids Res 15:5963–5971, 1987.

238. Kratochwil K: Epithelium-mesenchyme interactions in the fetal mammary gland. In Medina D, Kidwell W, Heppner G, Anderson E (eds): Cellular and Molecular Biology of Mammary Cancer. New York, Plenum, pp 1–8.

239. Kudlow JE, Cheung CYM, Bjorge JD: Epidermal growth factor stimulates the synthesis of its own receptor in a human breast cancer cell line. J Biol Chem 261:4134–4138, 1986.

240. Kurachi H, Okamoto S, Oka T: Evidence for the involvement of the submandibular gland epidermal growth factor in mouse mammary tumorigenesis. Proc Natl Acad Sci (USA) 81:5940–5943, 1985.

241. Lawrence DA, Pircher R, Krycene-Martineirie A, Lullien P: Normal embryo fibroblasts release transforming growth factors in a latent form. J Cell Physiol 121:184–188, 1984.

242. Lax I, Burgess WH, Bellot F, Ullrich A, Schlessinger J, Gival D: Localization of a major receptor-binding domain for epidermal growth factor by affinity labeling. Molec Cell Biol 8:1831–1834, 1988.

243. Lazar E, Watanabe S, Dalton S, Sporn MB: Transforming growth factor α: mutation of aspartic acid 47 and leucine 48 result in different biological activities. Molec Cell Biol 8:1247–1252, 1988.

244. Lee BA, Maher DW, Hannink M, Donoghue DJ: Identification of a signal for nuclear targeting in platelet-derived growth-factor-related molecules. Molec Cell Biol 7:3527–3537, 1987.

245. Lee PDK, Powell DR, Li CH, Bohn H, Liu F, Hintz R: High molecular weight forms of insulin-like growth factor II and its binding protein identified by immunoblotting. Biochem Biophys Res Comm 152:1131–1137, 1988.

246. LeMaistere CF, McGuire WC: Progesterone receptor determinations: a refinement of predictive tests for hormone dependency of breast cancer. In Jordan VC (ed): Estrogen/antiestrogen Action and Breast Cancer Therapy. Madison, University of Wisconsin Press, 1986, pp 341–356.

247. Leof EB, Proper JA, Goustin AJ, Shipley GD, Dicorleto PE, Moses HL: Induction of c-sis mRNA and activity similar to platelet-derived growth factor: A proposed model for indirect mitogenesis involving autocrine activity. Proc Natl Acad Sci (USA) 83:2453–2457, 1986.

248. Leung BS, Qureshi S, Leung JS: Response to estrogen by the human mammary carcinoma cell line CAMA-1. Cancer Res 42:5060–5066, 1982.

249. LeVay-Young BK, Imagawa W, Yang J, Richards JE, Guzman RC, Nandi S: Primary culture systems for mammary biology studies. In Medina D, Kidwell W, Heppner G, Anderson E (eds): Cellular and Molecular Biology of Mammary Cancer. New York, Plenum Press, 1987, pp 181–204.

250. Liderau R, Escot C, Thillet C, Champone MH, Brunet M, Best J, Callahan R: High frequency of rare alleles of the human c-Ha-ras-1 protooncogene in breast cancer patients. J Natl Cancer Inst 77:699–701, 1986.

251. Lieberman ME, Maurer RA, Gorski J: Estrogen control of prolactin synthesis in vitro. Proc Natl Acad Sci (USA) 75:5946–5949, 1978.

252. Liehr JG, Stancel GM, Chorich LP, Bousfield GR, Ulubelen AA: Hormonal carcinogenesis: separation of estrogenicity from carcinogenicity. Chem-Biol Interact 59:173–184, 1986.

253. Lingham RB, Stancel GM, Loose-Mitchell DS: Estrogen regulation of epidermal growth factor messenger ribonucleic acid. Mol Endocrinol 2:230–235, 1988.

254. Liotta LA: Mechanisms of cancer invasion and metastases. In DeVita VT, Hellman A, Rosenberg S (eds): Progress in Oncology, 1. New York, J.B. Lippincott, 1985, pp 28–41.

255. Liotta LA: Tumor invasion and metastases—role of the extracellular matrix. Rhoads Memorial Award Lecture. Cancer Res 46:1–7, 1986.

256. Liotta LA, Mandler R, Murano G, Katz DA, Gordon RK, Chiang PK, Schiffman E: Tumor cell autocrine motility factor. Proc Natl Acad Sci (USA) 83:3302–3306, 1986.

257. Liotta LA, Rao CN, Weiner UM: Biochemical interactions of tumor cells with the basement membrane. Ann Rev Biochem 55:1037–1057, 1986.

258. Lippman ME: Efforts to combine endocrine and chemotherapy in the management of breast cancer: do two and two equal three? Breast Cancer Res Treat 3:117–127, 1983.

259. Lippman ME: Definition of hormones and growth factors required for optimal proliferation and expression of phenotype response in human breast cancer cells. In Barnes DW, Sirbasku DA, Sato GH (eds): Cell Culture Methods for Molecular and Cell Biology, vol 2. New York, Alan R Liss, 1984, pp 183–200.

260. Lippman ME: Endocrine responsive cancers of man. In Williams RH (ed): Textbook of Endocrinology. Philadelphia, WB Saunders 1985, pp 1309–1326.

261. Lippman ME, Bolan G, Huff K: The effects of estrogens and antiestrogens on hormone-response human breast cancer in long term tissue culture. Cancer Res 36:4595–4601, 1976.

262. Lippman ME, Buzdar A, Tormey DC, McGuire WL: Combining endocrine and chemotherapy any true benefits? Breast Cancer Res Treat 4:251–259, 1985.

263. Liu SC, Sanfilippo B, Perroteau I, Derynck R, Salomon DS, Kidwell WR: Expression of transforming growth factor α (TGFα) in differentiated rat mammary tumors: estrogen induction of TGF production. Mol Endocrinol 1:683–692, 1987.

264. Lobel P, Dahms NM, Breitmeyer J, Chirgwin JM, Kornfeld S: Cloning of the bovine 215-kDa cation-independent mannose six phosphate receptor. Proc Natl Acad Sci (USA) 84:2233–2238, 1987.

265. Lumar V, Green S, Stark A, Chambon P: Localization of the oestrodiol-binding and putative DNA-binding domains of the human oestrogen receptor. EMBO J 5:2231–2236, 1986.

266. Lund LP, Ricico A, Andreasan PA, Nielsen LS, Kristensen P, Laiko M, Saksela O, Blasi F, Dano K: Transforming growth factor β is a strong and fast acting positive regulator of the level of type-1 plasminogen activator inhibitor mRNA in WI-38 human lung fibroblasts. EMBO J 6:1281–1286, 1987.

267. Luttrell DK, Luttrell LM, Parson JJ: Augmented mitogenic responsiveness to epidermal growth factor in murine fibroblasts that overexpress pp60c-src. Mol Cell Biol 8:497–501, 1988.

268. Lykkesfeldt AE, Briand P: Indirect mechanism of estradiol stimulation of cell proliferation of human breast cancer cell lines. Br J Cancer 53:29–35, 1986.

269. Lyons RM, Keski-Oja J, Moses HL: Cleavage of a transforming growth factor β (TGFβ)—immunoreactive 62 kDa polypeptide by plasmin yields a TGFβ-like 25 kDa polypeptide. (Abstract 1652) Proceedings of the Annual Meeting of the American Society for Cell Biology, Washington, D.C., The Rockefeller University Press, 1986, p 443a.

270. Lyons WR: Hormonal synergism in mammary growth. Proc Roy Soc 149:303–325, 1958.

271. Lyons WR, Suko Y: Direct action of estrone on the mammary gland. Rec Progr Hormone Res 14:398–401, 1940.

272. Majack RA: Beta-type transforming growth factor specifies organizational behavior in vascular smooth muscle cell cultures. J Cell Biol 105:465–471, 1987.

273. Manni A, Wright C, Feil P, Baranao L, Demers L, Garcia M, Rochefort H: Autocrine stimulation by estradiol-regulated growth factor of rat hormone-responsive mammary cancer: interaction with the polyamine pathway. Cancer Res 46:1594–1600, 1986.

274. Mariami-Costantini R, Escot C, Theillet C, Gentile A, Merlo G, Liderau R, Callahan R: In situ c-myc expression and genomic status of the c-myc locus in infiltrating ductal carcinoma. Cancer Res 48:199–205, 1988.

275. Massague J, Cheifetz S, Endo T, Nadal-Ginard B: Type transforming growth factor β is an inhibitor of myogenic differentiation. Proc Natl Acad Sci (USA) 83:8206–8210, 1986.

276. Massague J, Kelly B, Mottola C: Stimulation by insulin-like growth factors is required for cellular transformation by type transforming growth factor. J Biol Chem 260:4551–4554, 1985.

277. Massague J, Kelly BJ: Internalization of transforming growth factor β and its receptor in BALB/c 3T3 fibroblasts. J Cell Physiol 128:216–222, 1986.

278. Matrison CM, Leroy P, Ruhlmann C, Gesnel MC, Breathnach R: Isolation of the oncogene and epidermal growth factor-induced transin gene: complex control in rat fibroblasts. Mol Cell Biol 6:1679–1686, 1986.

279. May FEB, Westley BR: Cloning of estrogen-regulated messenger RNA sequences from human breast cancer cells. Cancer Res 46:6034–6040, 1986.

280. McCarty KS Jr, Miller LS, Cox EB, Konrath J, McCarty KS Sr. Estrogen receptor analyses. Arch Pathol Lab Med 109:716–721, 1985.

281. McDonnell DP, Mangelsdorf J, Pike W, Haussler MR, O'Malley BW: Molecular cloning of complementary DNA encoding the avian receptor for vitamin D. Science 235:1214–1217, 1987.

282. McGrath CM: Augmentation of the response of normal mammary epithelial cells to estradiol by mammary stroma. Cancer Res 43:1355–1360, 1983.

283. McGregor DH, Land CE, Choi K, Tokuoka S, Liu PI, Wakabayashi I, Beebe GW: Breast cancer incidence among atomic bomb survivors. Hiroshima and Nagasaki, 1950–1969. J Natl Cancer Inst 59:799–807, 1977.

284. McMahon JB, Richards WL, del Campo AA, Song M-K, Thorgeirsson SS: Differential effects of transforming growth factor beta on proliferation of normal and malignant rat liver epithelial cells in culture. Cancer Res 46:4665–4671, 1986.

285. Metzler M: Biochemical toxicology of diethylstilbestrol. In Hodgson E, Bend JR, Philpst RM (eds): Reviews in Biochemical Toxicology. New York, Elsevier, 1984, pp 191–220.

286. Metzler M: Metabolism of stilbene estrogens and steroidal estrogens in relation to carcinogenicity. Arch Toxicol 55:104–109, 1984.

287. Metzler M: Metabolic activation of xenobiotic stilbene estrogens. Fed Proc 46:1855–1857, 1987.

288. Meyers MB, Merluzzi VJ, Spengler BA, Biedler JL: Epidermal growth factor receptor is increased in multidrug resistant Chinese hamster and mouse tumor cells. Proc Natl Acad Sci (USA) 83:5521–5525, 1986.

289. Migliaccio A, Rotondi A, Auricchio F: Calmodulin-stimulated phosphorylation of 17β-estradiol receptor on tyrosine. Proc Natl Acad Sci (USA) 81:5921–5925, 1985.

290. Migliaccio A, Rotondi A, Auricchio F: Estradiol receptor: phosphorylation on tyrosine in uterus and interaction with anti-phosphotyrosine antibody. EMBO J 5:2867–2872, 1986.

291. Miller AB: Breast cancer epidemiology, etiology, and prevention. In Harris JR, Henderson IC, Hellman S, Kinne DW

(eds): Breast Diseases. Philadelphia, JB Lippincott, 1987, pp 87–150.

292. Minuto F, Del Monte PD, Baweca A, Fortini P, Cariola G, Catarambone G, Giordano G: Evidence for an increased somatomedin C/insulin-like growth factor I content in primary human lung tumors. Cancer Res 46:985–988, 1986.

293. Monsama JJ Jr, Katzenellenbogen BS, Miller MA, Ziegler YS, Katzenellenbogen JA: Characterization of the estrogen receptor and is dynamics in MCF-7 human breast cancer cells using a covalently-attaching antiestrogen. Endocrinology 115:143–153, 1984.

294. Morgan DO, Edman JC, Standring DN, Fried VA, Smith MC, Roth RA, Rutter WJ: Insulin-like growth factor II receptor as a multifunctional binding protein. Nature 329:301–308, 1987.

295. Muldoon TG: Interplay between estradiol and prolactin in the regulation of steroid hormone receptor levels, nature and functionality in normal mammary tissue. Endocrinology 109:1339–1346, 1981.

296. Murphy LJ, Sutherland RI, Stead B, Murphy LC, Lazarus L: Progestin regulation of epidermal growth factor receptor in human mammary carcinoma cells. Cancer Res 46:728–734, 1986.

297. Mustelin T, Poso H, Lapinjoki SP, Gynther J, Andersson LC: Growth signal transduction: rapid activation of covalently bound ornithine decarboxylase during phosphatidylinositol breakdown. Cell 49:171–176, 1987.

298. Nakanishi Y, Mulshine JL, Kasprzyk PG, Natale RB, Maneckjee R, Avis I, Treston AM, Gasdar AF, Minna JD, Cuttitta F: Insulin-like growth factor-I can mediate autocrine proliferation of human small cell lung cancer cell lines in vitro. J Clin Invest 82:354–359, 1988.

299. Nandi S: Endocrine control of mammary gland development in the C3H/He Crgl mouse. J Natl Cancer Inst 21:1039–1063, 1958.

300. Narbaitz R, Stumpf WE, Sur M: Estrogen receptors in mammary gland primordia of fetal mouse. Anat Embryol 158:161–166, 1980.

301. Nardulli AM, Greene GL, O'Malley BW, Katzenellenbogen BS: Regulation of progesterone receptor messenger ribonucleic acid and protein levels in MCF-7 cells by estradiol: analysis of estrogen's effect on progesterone receptor synthesis and degradation. Endocrinology 122:935–944, 1988.

302. Natoli C, Sica G, Natoli V, Serra A, Iacobelli S: Two new estrogen-supersensitive variants of the MCF-7 human breast cancer cell line. Breast Cancer Res Treat 3:23–32, 1983.

303. Nelson JN, Clarke R, McFerran NV, Murphy RF: Morphofunctional effects of phenol red on oestrogen-sensitive breast cancer cells. Biochem Soc Trans 15:244, 1987.

304. Nelson W: Growth of the mammary gland following local application of estrogenic hormone. Am J Physiol 133:398–401, 1941.

305. Neufeld EF, Ashwell G: In Lennarz WJ (ed): The Biochemistry of Glycoproteins and Proteoglycans. New York, Plenum Press, 1980, pp 241–266.

306. Nicholson GL: Tumor cell instability, diversification, and progression to the metastatic phenotype: from oncogene to oncofetal expression. Cancer Res 47:1473–1479, 1987.

307. Nicholson RI: Oestrogen deprivation in breast cancer using LH-RH antagonists and antioestrogen. In Furr BJA, Wakeling AE (eds): Pharmacology and Clinical Uses of Inhibitors of Hormone Secretion and Action. London, Bulliere-Tindull, 1987, pp 60–86.

308. Nickell KA, Halper J, Moses HL: Transforming growth factors in solid human malignant neoplasms. Cancer Res 43:1966–1971, 1983.

309. Nishizuka Y: Protein kinases in signal transduction. Trends Biochem Sci 9:163–171, 1984.

310. Nissley SP, Rechler MM: Insulin-like growth factors: biosynthesis receptors and carrier proteins. In Li CH (ed): Hormonal Proteins and Peptides, vol XII. New York, Academic Press, 1984, pp 128–203.

311. Noda K, Umeda M, Ono T: Transforming growth factor activity in human colostrum. Gann 75:109–112, 1984.

312. Novak-Hofer I, Kung W, Fabbro D, Eppenberger U: Estrogen stimulates growth of mammary tumor cells ZR-75 without

activation of S6 kinase and S6 phosphorylation. Eur J Biochem 164:445–451, 1987.

313. Nowell PC: Mechanisms of tumor progression. Cancer Res 46:2203–2207, 1986.

314. Nunez AM, Jakolew S, Briand JP, Gaire M, Krust A, Rio MC, Chambon P: Characterization of the estrogen-induced pS2 protein secreted by the human breast cancer cell line MCF-7. Endocrinology 121:1758–1765, 1987.

315. O'Brian CA, Liskamp RM, Solomon DH, Weinstein IB: Inhibition of protein kinase C by tamoxifen. Cancer Res 45:2462–2465, 1985.

316. Ochuchi N, Thor A, Page DL, Hand PH, Halter S, Schlom J: Expression of the 21,000 molecular weight ras protein in a spectrum of benign and malignant human mammary tissues. Cancer Res 46:2511–2519, 1986.

317. O'Connor-McCourt MD, Wakefield LM: Latent transforming growth factor β in serum. J Biol Chem 262:14,090–14,099, 1987.

318. Ohta M, Greenberger JS, Anklesaria P, Bassols A, Massague J: Two forms of transforming growth factor β distinguished by multipotential hematopoietic progenitor cells. Nature 239:539–541, 1987.

319. Oka T, Tsutsumi O, Kurachi H, Okamoto S: The role of epidermal growth factor in normal and neoplastic growth of mouse mammary cells. In Lippman ME, Dickson RB (eds): Breast Cancer: Cellular and Molecular Biology. Kluwer Academic Press, Norwell, MA. 1988, pp 343–362.

320. Olson EN, Sternberg E, Hu JS, Spizz G, Wilcox C: Regulation of myogenic differentiation by type β transforming growth factor. J Cell Biol 103:1799–1805, 1986.

321. Osborne CK, Boldt DH, Clark CM, Trent JM: Effects of tamoxifen on human breast cancer cell cycle kinetics: accumulation of cells in early G_1 phase. Cancer Res 43:3583–3585, 1983.

322. Osborne CK, Hamilton B, Titus G, Livingston RB: Epidermal growth factor stimulation of human breast cancer cells in culture. Cancer Res 40:2361–2366, 1980.

323. Osborne CK, Hobbs K, Clark GM: Effects of estrogens and antiestrogens on growth of human breast cancer cells in athymic nude mice. Cancer Res 45:584–590, 1985.

324. Osborne CK, Hobbs K, Trent JM: Biological differences among MCF-7 human breast cancer cell lines from different laboratories. Breast Cancer Res Treat 9:111–121, 1987.

325. Padgett RW, St Johnson RD, Gelbart WM: A transcript from a Drosophila pattern gene predicts a protein homologous to the transforming growth factor beta family. Nature (London) 325:81–84, 1987.

326. Page MJ, Field JK, Everett NP, Green CD: Serum-regulation of the estrogen responsiveness of the human breast cancer cell line MCF-7. Cancer Res 43:1244–1249, 1983.

327. Pardee AD: Molecules involved in proliferation of normal and cancer cells. Cancer Res 47:1488–1491, 1987.

328. Pardoll DM, Vogelstein B, Coffey DS: A fixed site of DNA replication in eucaryotic cells. Cell 19:527–536, 1980.

329. Paridaens RJ, Piccart MJ: Chemo-hormonal treatment of breast cancer: the state of the art. In Sluyser M (ed): Growth Factors and Oncogenes in Breast Cancer. Chichester, England, Ellis Harwood, 1987, pp 193–206.

330. Peres R, Betsholtz C, Westermark B, Heldin CH: Frequent expression of growth factors for mesenchymal tissue for human mammary carcinoma cell lines. Cancer Res 47:3425–3429, 1987.

331. Perroteau E, Salomon D, Debortali M, Kidwell W, Hazarika P, Pardue R, Dedman J, Tam J: Immunologic detection and quantitation of alpha transforming growth factors in human breast carcinoma cells. Breast Cancer Res Treat 7:201–210, 1986.

332. Persons DA, Wilkerson WO, Bell RM, Finn OJ: Altered growth regulation and enhanced tumorigenicity of NIH 3T3 fibroblasts transfected with protein kinase C-1 cDNA. Cell 52:447–458, 1988.

333. Petersen DW, Hoyer PE, Van Deurs P: Frequency and distribution of estrogen receptor-positive cells in normal non-lactating human breast tissue. Cancer Res 47:5748–5751, 1987.

334. Picard D, Yamamoto KR: Two signals mediate hormone dependent nuclear localization of the glucocorticoid receptor. EMBO J 6:3333–3340, 1987.

335. Pike LJ, Eakes AT: Epidermal growth factor stimulates the production of phosphatidyl inositol monophosphates and the breakdown of polyphosphoinositides in A431 cells. J Biol Chem 262:1644–1651, 1987.

336. Prehn RT, Prehn LM: The autoimmune nature of cancer. Cancer Res 47:927–932, 1987.

337. Puca GA, Sica V, Nola E: Identification of a high affinity nuclear acceptor site for estrogen receptor of calf uterus. Proc Natl Acad Sci (USA) 171:979–983, 1974.

338. Raam S, Vrabel DM: Evaluation of an enzyme immunoassay kit for estrogen receptor measurements. Clin Chem 32:1496–1503, 1986.

339. Raynaud A: Recherches experimentales sur le development de l'appareil genital et functionnement des glandes endocrines des foetus de souris et de mulot. Arch Anat Microse Morphol Exp 39:518–576, 1950.

340. Raynaud A: Morphogenesis of the mammary gland. In Kon SA, Cowie AT (eds): Milk, the Mammary Gland and its Secretion, vol 1. New York, Academic Press, 1961, pp 3–46.

341. Read LD, Snider CE, Miller JS, Greene GL, Katzenellenbogen BS: Ligand modulated regulation of progesterone receptor messenger ribonucleic acid and protein in human breast cancer cell lines. Mol Endocrinol 2:263–271, 1988.

342. Rechler MM, Nissley SP: Insulin-like growth factor (IGF)/somatomedin receptor subtypes: structure, function and relationships to insulin and IGF carrier proteins. Hormone Res 24:152–159, 1986.

343. Reeve AE, Eccles MR, Wilkins RJ, Bell GI, Millon LJ: Expression of insulin-like growth factor II transcripts in Wilms tumor. Nature 317:258–260, 1985.

344. Reiner GCA, Katzenellenbogen BS: Characterization of estrogen and in MDA-MB-134 human breast cancer cells. Cancer Res 46:1124–1131, 1986.

345. Richards J, Guzman R, Konrad M, Yang J, Nandi S: Growth of mouse mammary gland end buds cultured in a collagen gel matrix. Exp Cell Res 141:4333–4343, 1982.

346. Riss TL, Sirbasku DA: Growth and continuous passage of COMMA-D mouse mammary epithelial cells in hormonally defined serum-free medium. Cancer Res 47:3776–3782, 1987.

347. Rizzino A: Appearance of high affinity receptors for type β transforming growth factor during differentiation of murine embryonal carcinoma cells. Cancer Res 47:4386–4390, 1987.

348. Ro JY, Holoye PY, Gutterman JU, Blick MB. c-sis expression in primary human breast carcinoma. (Abstract 74) Atlanta, Proceedings of the 78th Annual Meeting of the American Association for Cancer Research, 1987.

349. Roberts AB, Anzano MA, Wakefield LM, Roche NS, Stern DF, Sporn MB: Type β transforming growth factor: a bifunctional regulator of cellular growth. Proc Natl Acad Sci (USA) 82:119–123, 1985.

350. Roberts AB, Sporn MB: Growth factors and transformation. Cancer Surv 5:405–412, 1986.

351. Roberts AB, Sporn MB, Assoian RK, Smith JM, Roche NS, Wakefield LM, Heine UI, Liotta LA, Falanga V, Kehrl JH, Fauci A: Transforming growth factor type β: rapid induction of fibrosis and angiogenesis in vivo and stimulation of collagen formation in vitro. Proc Natl Acad Sci (USA) 83:4167–4171, 1986.

352. Robinson SI, Nelkin BD, Vogelstein B: The ovalbumin gene is associated with the nuclear matrix of chicken oviduct cells. Cell 28:99–106, 1985.

353. Rochefort H: Do antiestrogens and antiprogestins act as hormone antagonists or receptor-targeted drugs in breast cancer? Trends Pharmacol Sci 8:126–128, 1987.

354. Rogel S, Weinberg RA, Fanning P, Klagsbrun M: Basic fibroblast peptide transforms cells. Nature 331:173–175, 1988.

355. Rohlik QT, Adams D, Kull FC, Jacobs S: An antibody to the receptor for insulin-like growth factor I inhibits the growth of MCF-7 cells in tissue culture. Biochem Biophys Res Comm 149:276–281, 1981.

356. Rosen N, Bolen JB, Schwartz AM, Cohen P, Deseau V, Israel MA: Analysis of pp60c-src protein kinase activity in human tumor cell lines and tissues. J Biol Chem 261:13,754–13,759, 1986.

357. Rosen OM: After insulin binds. Science 237:1452–1458, 1987.
358. Rosenthal A, Lindquist PB, Bringman TS, Goeddel DV, Derynck R: Expression in rat fibroblasts of a human transforming growth factor α and cDNA results in transformation. Cell 46:301–309, 1986.
359. Ross GT, Vande Wiele RL, Frantz AG: The ovaries and the breasts. In Williams RH (ed): Textbook of Endocrinology. Philadelphia, WB Saunders, 1981, pp 355–411.
360. Ross R, Raines EW, Bowen-Pope DF: The biology of platelet-derived growth factor. Cell 46:155–169, 1986.
361. Rotwein P: Two insulin-like growth factor I messenger RNAs and expressed in human liver. Proc Natl Acad Sci (USA) 83:77–81, 1986.
362. Rozengurt E: Early signals in the mitogenic response. Science 234:161–166, 1986.
363. Rozengurt E, Sinnett-Smith J, Taylor-Papadimitriou J: Production of PDGF-like growth factor by breast cancer lines. Int J Cancer 36:247–252, 1985.
364. Rudland PS: Stem cells in mammary development and cancer. In Medina D, Kidwell W, Heppner G, Anderson E (eds): Cellular and Molecular Biology of Mammary Cancer. New York, Plenum Press, 1987, pp 9–28.
365. Rudland PS: Stem cells and the development of mammary cancers in experimental rats and humans. Cancer Metastatis Rev 6:55–83, 1987.
366. Rudland PS, Smith JA: Growth factors and the control of cell proliferation in cultured fibroblasts and mammary epithelial cells. (Abstract 7) J Endocrinol 117(supplement), 1988.
367. Russo J, Russo I: Role of differentiator on transformation of human breast epithelial cells. In Medina D, Kidwell W, Heppner G, Anderson E (eds): Cellular and Molecular Biology of Breast Cancer. New York, Plenum Press, 1987, pp 399–418.
368. Russo J, Russo IH: Biological and molecular bases of mammary carcinogenesis. Lab Invest 57:112–137, 1987.
369. Sainsbury, JRC, Farndon JR, Needham GK, Malcolm AJ, Harris AL: Epidermal growth factor receptor status of human breast cancer is related to early recurrence and death. Lancet i:1398–1402, 1987.
370. Sainsbury JRC, Malcolm AJ, Appleton DR, Farndon JR, Harris AL: Presence of epidermal growth factor receptors as an indicator of poor prognosis in patients with breast cancer. J Clin Pathol 38:1225–1228, 1985.
371. Salomon DS, Kidwell WR, Kim N, Ciardiello F, Bates SE, Valverius E, Lippman ME, Dickson RB, Stampfer M: Modulation by estrogen and growth factor of transforming growth factor alpha (TGFα) expression in normal and malignant human mammary epithelial cells. Rec Results Cancer Res 113:57–69, 1988.
372. Salomon DS, Zweibel JA, Bano M, Losonczy I, Felnel P, Kidwell WR: Presence of transforming growth factors in human breast cancer cells. Cancer Res 44:4069–4077, 1984.
373. Santon JB, Cronin MT, Macleod CL, Mendelsohn J, Masui H, Gill GN: Effects of epidermal growth factor concentration on tumorigenicity of A431 cells in nude mice. Cancer Res 46:4701–4705, 1986.
374. Sap J, Munoz A, Damm K, Goldberg U, Ghysdael J, Leutz A, Beug H, Vennstrom B: The c-erb A protein is a high-affinity receptor for thyroid hormone. Nature 234:635–640, 1986.
375. Sapino A, Peitribiasi F, Bussolati G, Marchiso PC: Estrogen- and tamoxifen-induced rearrangement of cytoskeletal and adhesion structures in breast cancer MCF-7 cells. Cancer Res 46:2526–2531, 1986.
376. Sasada R, Kurokawa T, Iwnane M, Igarashi K: Transformation of mouse BALB/c 3T3 cells with human basic fibroblast growth factor cDNA. Molec Cell Biol 8:588–594, 1988.
377. Sawyer ST, Cohen S: Epidermal growth factor stimulates the phosphorylation of the calcium-dependent 35,000-dalton substrate in intact A-431 cells. J Biol Chem 260:8233–8236, 1985.
378. Schneider J, Kinne D, Fracchia A, Pierce V, Anderson KE, Bradlow HL, Fishman J: Abnormal oxidative metabolism of estradiol in women with breast cancer. Proc Natl Acad Sci (USA) 79:3047–3051, 1982.
379. Schuh S, Yamemoto W, Brugge J, Bauer VJ, Riehl RM, Sullivan WP, Toft DO: A 90,000 dalton binding protein common to both steroid receptors and the rous sarcoma virus transforming protein pp60^{v-src}. J Biol Chem 260:14,292–14,296, 1985.
380. Scott J, Urdea M, Quirogu M: Structure of a mouse submaxillary messenger RNA encoding epidermal growth factor and seven related proteins. Science 221:236–240, 1983.
381. Schlessinger J: Allosteric regulation of the epidermal growth factor receptor kinase. J Cell Biol 103:2067–2072, 1986.
382. Segarini PR, Roberts AB, Rosen DM, Seyedin SM: Membrane binding characteristics of two forms of transforming growth factor β. J Biol Chem 262:14,655–14,662, 1987.
383. Sheen YY, Katzenellenbogen BS: Antiestrogen stimulation of the production of a 37,000 molecular weight secreted protein and estrogen stimulation of the production of a 32,000 molecular weight secreted protein in MCF-7 human breast cancer cells. Endocrinology 120:1140–1151, 1987.
384. Sheth SP, Allegra JC: What role for concurrent chemohormonal therapy in breast cancer? Oncology 1:19–27, 1987.
385. Shiota K, Nakamura T, Ichihara A: Distinct effects of transforming growth factor on EGF receptors and EGF-induced DNA synthesis in primary cultured rat hepatocytes. Biochem Int 13:893–901, 1986.
386. Shiu RPC, Murphy LC, Aigal Y, Dembinski TC, Tsuyuki D, Iwasiow BM: Actions of pituitary prolactin and insulin-like growth factor II in human breast cancer. In Lippman ME, Dickson RB (eds): Breast Cancer: Cellular and Molecular Biology. Boston, Klewer, 1988, pp 167–184.
387. Silberstein GB, Daniel CW: Reversible inhibition of mammary gland growth by transforming growth factor β. Science 237:291–295, 1987.
388. Simon WE, Albrecht M, Trams G, Dietel M, Holzer F: In vitro growth promotion of human mammary carcinoma cells by steroid hormones, tamoxifen, and prolactin. J Natl Cancer Inst 73:313–321, 1984.
389. Sinn E, Muller W, Pattengale P, Tepler I, Wallace R, Leder P: Coexpression of MMTV/v- Ha-ras and MMTV/c-myc genes in transgenic mice: synergistic action of oncogenes in vivo. Cell 49:465–475, 1987.
390. Sirbasku DA: New concepts in control of estrogen-responsive tumor cell growth. Banbury Rep 8:425–443, 1981.
391. Slamon J, Clark GM, Wong SG, Levin WJ, Ullrich A, McGuire WL: Human breast cancer: correlation of relapse and survival with amplification of the HER-2/new oncogene. Science 235:177–182, 1987.
392. Slamon DJ, DeKernion JB, Verma IM, Cline MJ: Expression of cellular oncogenes in human malignancies. Science 224:256–262, 1984.
393. Smith HS, Scher CD, Todaro GJ: Induction of cell division in medium lacking serum growth factor by SV40. Virology 44:359–370, 1971.
394. Smith JA, Winslow DP, Rudland PS: Different growth factors stimulate cell division of rat mammary epithelial myoepithelial and stromal cell lines in culture. J Cell Physiol 119:320–326, 1984.
395. Soto A, Sonnenschein C: Cell proliferation of estrogen-sensitive cells: the case for negative control. Endocr Rev 8:44–52, 1987.
396. Soule HD, McGrath CM: Estrogen responsive proliferation of clonal human breast carcinoma cells in athymic mice. Cancer Lett 10:177–189, 1980.
397. Soule HD, McGrath A: Simplified method for passage and long term growth of human mammary epithelial cells. In Vitro Cell Devel Biol 22:6–12, 1986.
398. Spelsberg TC, Webster RA, Pikler GM: Chromosomal proteins regulate steroid binding to chromatin. Nature 262:65–67, 1976.
399. Spitzer E, Grosse R, Kunde D, Schmidt EH: Growth of mammary epithelial cells in breast cancer biopsies correlates with EGF binding. Int J Cancer 39:279–282, 1987.
400. Sporn MB, Roberts AB: Autocrine, paracrine and endocrine mechanisms of growth control. Cancer Surv 4:627–632, 1985.
401. Sporn MB, Roberts AB: Peptide growth factors and inflammation, tissue repair and cancer. J Clin Invest 78:329–332, 1986.
402. Sporn MB, Roberts AB: Peptide growth factors are multifunctional. Nature 332:217–219, 1988.
403. Sporn MB, Roberts AB, Driscoll JS: Principles of cancer biology growth factors and differentiation. In DeVita VT, Hellman S, Rosenberg SA (eds): Cancer: Principles and Practice of Oncology, ed 2. Philadelphia, JB Lippincott, 1985, pp 49–65.

404. Sporn MB, Roberts AB, Wakefield LM, de Crombrugghe B: Some recent advances in the chemistry and biology of transforming growth factor beta. J Cell Biol 105:1039–1045, 1987.

405. Sporn MB, Todaro GJ: Autocrine secretion and malignant transformation of cells. New Engl J Med 303:878–880, 1980.

406. Stampfer MR: Isolation and growth of human mammary epithelial cells. J Tissue Cult Methods 9:107–115, 1985.

407. Stampfer MR, Bartley JC: Induction of transformation and continuous cell lines from normal human mammary epithelial cells after exposure to benzo(a)pyrene. Proc Natl Acad Sci (USA) 82:2394–2398, 1985.

408. Stampfer M, Bartley JC: Development of human mammary epithelial cell culture systems for studies of carcinogenesis and differentiation. In Sekley L, Webber M (eds): In Vitro Models for Cancer Research, vol 3. Cleveland, OH, CRC Press, 1986, pp 11–29.

409. Stampfer MR, Bartley J: Growth and transformation of human mammary epithelial cells in culture. In Medina D, Kidwell W, Heppner G, Anderson E (eds): Cellular and Molecular Biology of Mammary Cancer. New York, Plenum Press, 1987, pp 419–436.

410. Stampfer MR, Bartley JC: Human mammary epithelial cells in culture: differentiation and transformation. In Lippman ME, Dickson RB (eds): Breast Cancer: Cellular and Molecular Biology. Boston, Klewer, 1988, pp 1–24.

411. Steinman G, Delorme EO, Law CC, Sager R: Transfection with plasmid PSV2gpt EJ induces chromosome rearrangements in CHEF cells. Proc Natl Acad Sci (USA) 84:184–188, 1987.

412. Stern DF, Hare DL, Cecchini MA, Weinberg RA: Construction of a novel oncogene based on synthetic sequences encoding epidermal growth factor. Science 235:321–324, 1987.

413. Stewart TA, Pattengale PK, Leder P: Spontaneous mammary adenocarcinoma in transgenic mice that carry and express MTV/myc fusion genes. Cell 38:627–637, 1984.

414. Steyono HB, Henkelman MS, Foekens JA, Klijn JGM: Direct inhibitory effects of somatostatin (analogues) on the growth of human breast cancer cells. Cancer Res 47:1566–1570, 1987.

415. Stiles CD, Capone GT, Scher CD, Antoniades HN, Van Wyk J, Pledger WJ: Dual control of cell growth by somatomedins and platelet derived growth factor. Proc Natl Acad Sci (USA) 76:1279–1283, 1979.

416. Stoppelli MP, Tacchetti C, Cubellis MV, Corti A, Hearing VJ, Cassani G, Appella E, Blasi F: Autocrine saturation of prourokinase receptors on human A431 cells. Cell 45:675–684, 1986.

417. Stoscheck CM, King LE: Role of epidermal growth factor in carcinogenesis. Cancer Res 46:1030–1037, 1986.

418. Strobl JS, Thompson EB: Mechanism of steroid action. In Auricchio F (ed): Sex Steroid Receptors. Rome, Field Educational Halia Acta Medica, 1985, pp 9–36.

419. Stromberg K, Hudgins WR, Dorman LS, Henderson LE, Sowder RE, Shewell BJ, Mount CD, Orth DN: Human brain tumor-associated urinary high molecular weight transforming growth factor: a high molecular weight form of epidermal growth factor. Cancer Res 47:1190–1196, 1987.

420. Studzinski GP, Brelvi ZS, Feldman SC, Watt RA: Participation of c-myc protein in DNA synthesis of human cells. Science 234:467–470, 1986.

421. Surmacz E, Kaczmarek L, Ronning O, Baserga R: Activation of the ribosomal DNA promoter in cells exposed to insulin-like growth factor I. Molec Cell Biol 7:657–673, 1987.

422. Sutherland RL, Hall RE, Taylor IW: Cell proliferation kinetics of MCF-7 human mammary carcinoma cells in culture and effects of tamoxifen on exponentially growing and plateau phase cells. Cancer Res 43:3998–4006, 1983.

423. Sutherland RL, Reddel RR, Murphy LC, Taylor IW: Effects of antiestrogens on cell cycle progression. In Jordan JC (ed): Estrogen/Antiestrogen Action and Breast Cancer Therapy. Madison, University of Wisconsin Press, 1986, pp 93–114.

424. Swain S, Dickson RB, Lippman ME: Anchorage independent epithelial colony stimulating activity in human breast cancer cell lines. (Abstract 844) Los Angeles, Proceedings of the Annual Meeting of the American Association for Cancer Research, Annual Meeting, 1986.

424a. Swaneck GE, Fishman J: Covalent binding of endogenous estrogen 16α-hydroxyesterone to estradiol receptor in human breast cancer cells: characterization and intranuclear localization. Proc Natl Acad Sci (USA) 85:7831–7835, 1988.

425. Takehara K, LeRoy EC, Grotendorst GR: TGFβ inhibition of endothelial cell proliferation alteration of EGF binding, and EGF-induced growth regulatory (competence) gene expression. Cell 49:415–422, 1987.

426. Tam JP: Structure-activity studies of transforming growth factor. In Peptides: Chemistry and Biology. Proceedings of the 10th Annual Peptide Symposium, New York, 1988, pp 561–565.

427. Tasjian AH, Voelkel EF, Lazzaro M, Singer FR, Roberts AB, Derynck R, Winkler ME, Levine L: α and β human transforming growth factors stimulate prostaglandin production and bone resorption in cultured mouse calvaria. Proc Natl Acad Sci (USA) 82:4535–4538, 1985.

428. Terranova VP, Hujanen ES, Martin GR: Basement membrane and the invasive activity of metastatic tumor cells. J Natl Cancer Inst 177:311–316, 1986.

429. Thomas KA, Rios-Comdelloves M, Gremenez-Gallego G, DiSalvo J, Bennett C, Rodkey J, Fitzpatrick S: Pure brain-derived acidic fibroblast growth factor is a potent angiogenic vascular endothelial cell mitogen with sequence homology to interleukin 1. Proc Natl Acad Sci (USA) 82:6409–6423, 1985.

430. Thompson CC, Weinberger C, Lebo R, Evans RM: Identification of a novel thyroid hormone receptor expressed in the mammalian central nervous system. Science 237:1610–1614, 1987.

431. Thompson EW, Reich R, Martin GR, Albini A: Factors regulating basement membrane invasion by tumor cells. In Lippman ME, Dickson RB (eds): Breast Cancer: Cellular and Molecular Biology. Boston, Klawer, 1988, pp 239–250.

432. Thorne HJ, Jose DG, Zhang HY, Dempsey PJ, Whitehead RH: Epidermal growth factor stimulates the synthesis of cell attachment proteins in the human breast cancer cell line PMC42. Int J Cancer 40:207–212, 1987.

433. Tonelli QJ, Sorof S: Epidermal growth factor requirement for development of cultured mammary gland. Nature 285:250–252, 1980.

434. Tong BD, Auer DE, Jaye M, Kaplan JM, Ricca G, McConathy E, Drohan W, Deuel TF: cDNA clones reveal differences between human glial and endothelial platelet-derived growth factor A-chains. Nature 328:619–621, 1987.

435. Tonik SE, Shindelman JE, Sussman HH: Transferin receptor is inversely correlated with estrogen receptor in breast cancer. Breast Cancer Res Treat 7:71–76, 1986.

436. Trent JM, Yang JM, Thompson FH, Leibovitz A, Villar H, Dalton WS: Chromosomal alterations in human breast cancer. In Sluyser M (ed): Growth Factors and Oncogenes in Breast Cancer. Chichester, England, Ellis Hovwood, 1987, pp 142–151.

437. Tricoli JV, Rall LB, Karakousis CP, Herrera L, Petrelli N, Bell GI, Shows TB: Enhanced levels of insulin-like growth factor messenger RNA in human colon carcinomas and liposarcomas. Cancer Res 46:6169–6173, 1986.

438. Tsutsui T, Maizumi H, McLachlan JA, Barrett JC: Aneuploidy induction and cell transformation by diethylstilbestrol: a possible chromosomal mechanism in carcinogenesis. Cancer Res 43:3814–3821, 1983.

439. Tucker RF, Shipley GD, Moses HL, Holley RW: Growth inhibitor from BSC-1 cells closely related to platelet type β transforming growth factor. Science 226:705–707, 1984.

440. Uenter DJ, Tuzi NC, Kumar S, Gullick WJ: Overexpression of the c-erb B2 oncoprotein in human breast carcinomas: immunohistological assessment correlates with gene amplification. Lancet, July 11, pp 69–72, 1987.

441. Ullrich A, Gray A, Tam AW, Yang Feng T, Tsubokawa M, Collins C, Henzel W, Le Bon T, Kathuria S, Chen E, Jacobs S, Francke U, Ramachandran J, Fujita-Yamaguchi Y. Insulin-like growth factor I receptor primary structure: comparison with insulin receptor suggests structural determinants that define functional specificity. EMBO J 5:2503–2512, 1986.

442. Valverius E, Bates S, Stampfer M, Clarke R, McCormick F, Salamon D, Lippman ME, Dickson RB: Transforming growth factor alpha production and EGF receptor expression in human mammary epithelial cells: oncogenic influence on function EGR of receptor. Mol Endocrinol, 3:203–214, 1988.

443. Valverius EM, Walker-Jones D, Bates SE, Stampfer MR, Clark R, McCormick F, Dickson RB, Lippman ME: Production and responsiveness to transforming growth factor beta in normal and oncogene-transformed human mammary epithelial cells. Cancer Res 49:6269–6274, 1989.

444. Vana J, Murphy GP, Arnoff BL, Baker HW: Survey of primary liver tumors and oral contraceptive use. J Toxicol Environ Health 5:255–273, 1979.

445. Van der Blieck AM, Meyers MB, Biedler JL, Hes E, Borst P: A 22 Kd protein (sorcin/V19) encoded by an amplified gene in multidrug resistant cells is homologous to the calcium-binding light chain of calpain. EMBO J 5:3201–3208, 1986.

446. Van der Burg B, Rutteman GR, Blankenstein MA, de Laat SW, Van Zoelen EJJ: Mitogenic stimulation of human breast cancer cells in a growth factor-defined medium: synergistic action of insulin and estrogen. J Cell Physiol 134:101–108, 1988.

447. Van Wyk JJ: Somatomedins: biological actions and physiological control mechanisms. *In* Li CH (ed): Hormonal Proteins and Peptides, vol XII. New York, Academic Press, 1984, pp 82–125.

448. Varmus H, Bishop JM: Introduction. Cancer Surv 5:153–158, 1986.

449. Varley JM, Swallow JE, Brammar WJ, Whittaker JL, Walker RA: Alterations to either c-erb B2 (neu) or c-myc protooncogenes in breast carcinomas correlate with poor short term prognosis. Oncogene 1:423–430, 1987.

450. Velu TJ, Beguinot L, Vass WC, Willingham MC, Merlino GT, Pastan I, Lowy DR: Epidermal growth factor-dependent transformation by a human EGF receptor proto-oncogene. Science 238:1048–1050, 1987.

451. Vickers PJ, Dickson RB, Cowan KH: Multidrug resistance in breast cancer. Trends Pharmacol Sci 9:443–445, 1988.

452. Vickers PJ, Dickson RB, Shoemaker R, Cowan KH: Multidrug resistant breast cancer cells exhibit cross-resistance to antiestrogens and hormone independent growth in vivo. Mol Endocrinol 2:886–892, 1988.

453. Vickers PJ, Townsend AJ, Cowan KH: Mechanisms of resistance to antineoplastic drugs. *In* Glazer RI (ed): CRC Crit. Rev. Developments in Cancer Chemotherapy, vol. 2. In press.

454. Vignon F, Capony F, Chambon M, Freiss L, Garcia M, Rochefort H: Autocrine growth stimulation of the MCF-7 breast cancer cell by the estrogen regulated 52K protein. Endocrinology 118:1537–1545, 1986.

455. Vignon F, Derocq DF, Chambon M, Rochefort H: Estrogen induced proteins secreted by the MCF-7 human breast cancer cells stimulated their proliferation. CR Acad Sci Paris Endocrinol 296:151–157, 1983.

456. Vonderhaar BK: Hormones and growth factors in mammary development. *In* Veneziale CM (ed): Control of Cell Growth and Proliferation. Princeton, NJ, Van Nostrand-Reinhold, 1984, pp 11–13.

457. Vonderhaar BK: Local effects of EGF, -TGF, and EGF-like growth factors on lobuloalveolar development of the mouse mammary gland in vivo. J Cell Physiol 132:581–584, 1987.

458. Vonderhaar BK: Regulation of development of the normal mammary gland by hormones and growth factors. *In* Lippman ME, Dickson RB: (eds): Breast Cancer: Cellular and Molecular Biology. Boston, Klewer, 1988, pp 251–266.

459. Wahl SM, Hunt DA, Wakefield LM, McCartney-Francis N, Wahl LM, Roberts AB, Sporn MB: Transforming growth factor type β induces monocyte chemotaxis and growth factor production. Proc Natl Acad Sci (USA) 84:5788–5792, 1987.

460. Wakeling AE, Bowler J: Steroidal pure antiestrogens. J Endocrinol (March) 112:R7–R10, 1987.

461. Walker-Jones D, Valverius EM, Stampfer MR, Lippman ME, Dickson RB: Transforming growth factor beta (TGFβ) stimulates expression of epithelial membrane antigen in normal and oncogene-transformed human mammary epithelial cells. Cancer Res 49:6407–6411, 1990.

462. Walter P, Green S, Greene G, Krust A, Bornert JM, Jeltsch J-M, Straub A, Jensen E, Scrace G, Waterfield M, Chambon P: Cloning of the human estrogen receptor cDNA. Proc Natl Acad Sci (USA) 82:889–893, 1985.

463. Wang JL, Hsu YM: Negative regulators of cell growth. Trends Biochem Sci 11:24–26, 1986.

464. Watanabe S, Lazar E, Sporn MB: Transformation of normal rat kidney (NRK) cells by an infectious retrovirus carrying a synthetic rat type α transforming growth factor gene. Proc Natl Acad Sci (USA) 84:1258–1262, 1987.

465. Watts CKW, Murphy LC, Sutherland RL: Microsomal binding sties for nonsteroidal antiestrogens in MCF-7 human mammary carcinoma cells. J Biol Chem 259:4223–4229, 1984.

466. Weichselbaum RW, Hellman S, Piro A, Nove JJ, Little JB: Proliferation kinetics of a human breast cancer cell line in vitro following treatment with 17β-estradiol and 1-B-o-arabinofuranasylcytosine. Cancer Res 38:2339–2342, 1978.

467. Weinberger C, Thompson CC, Ong ES, Lebo R, Gruol DJ, Evans RM: The c-erb A gene encodes a thyroid hormone receptor. Nature 234:641–646, 1986.

468. Welsch CW: Rodent models to examine in vivo hormonal regulation of mammary gland tumorigenesis. *In* Medina D, Kidwell W, Heppner G, Anderson E (eds): Cellular and Molecular Biology of Mammary Cancer. New York, Plenum Press, 1987, pp 153–179.

469. Welshons WV, Lieberman ME, Gorski J: Nuclear localization of unoccupied estrogen receptors. Nature 307:747–749, 1984.

470. Westley B, Rochefort H: A secreted glycoprotein induced by estrogen in human breast cancer cell lines. Cell 20:353–362, 1980.

471. Westley BR, May FEB: Oestrogen regulates cathepsin D mRNA levels in oestrogen responsive human breast cancer cells. Nucl Acids Res 15:3773–3780, 1987.

472. Whitehead RH, Quirk SJ, Vitali AA, et al: A new human breast carcinoma cell line (PMC42) with stem cell characteristics. III. Hormone receptor status and responsiveness. J Natl Cancer Inst 73:643–648, 1984.

473. Wilding G, Chen M, Gelmann EP, Miller WR: LHRH agonists and human breast cancer cells. Nature 329:770, 1987.

474. Wilding G, Lippman ME, Gelmann EP: Effects of steroid hormones and peptide growth factors on protooncogene c-fos expression in human breast cancer cells. Cancer Res 48:802–805, 1988.

475. Wolf CR, Macpherson JS, Smyth JF: Evidence for the metabolism of mitozantrone by microsomal glutathione transferase and 3-methylcholanthrene-inducible glucaronosyltransferases. Biochem Pharmacol 35:1577–1581, 1986.

476. Wolff B, Dickson RB, Hanover JA: A nuclear localization signal in steroid hormone receptors? Trends Pharmacol Sci 8:119–121, 1987.

477. Wong LH, Lin B, Jong S-M, Dixon D, Ellis L, Roth RA, Rutter WJ: Activation of transforming potential of the human insulin receptor gene. Proc Natl Acad Sci (USA) 84:5725–5729, 1987.

478. Wrann M, Bodmer S, de Martin R, Siepl C, Hofer-Warbinek R, Frei K, Hofer E, Fontana A: T cell suppressor factor from human glioblastoma cells is a 12.5 Kd protein closely related to transforming growth factor β. EMBO J 6:1633–1636, 1987.

479. Yang J, Guzman R, Richards J, Nandi S: Primary culture of mouse mammary tumor epithelial cells inbedded in collagen gels. In Vitro (Rockville) 16:502–506, 1980.

480. Yang K-P, Samaan NA: Reduction of estrogen receptor concentration in MCF-7 cells following exposure to chemotherapeutic drugs. Cancer Res 43:3534–3538, 1983.

481. Yarden Y, Escobedo JA, Kwang WJ, Yang-Feng TL, Daniel R, Tremble PM, Chen EY, Ando ME, Harkins RN, Franks U, Fried VA, Ullrich A, Williams LT: Structure of the receptor for platelet-derived growth factor helps define a family of closely related growth factors. Nature 323:226–232, 1986.

482. Yee D, Favori RE, Huff KK, Paik S, Dickson RB, Lebovic GS, Schwartz A, Lippman ME, Rosen N: Insulin like growth factor I (IGF-I) expression and a novel IGF-I-related activity in human malignancy. New Orleans, Annual Meetings of the American Association for Cancer Research, 1988.

483. Yeh GC, Occhipinti SJ, Cowan KH, Chabner BA, Myers CE: Adriamycin resistance in human tumor cells associated with marked alterations in the regulation of the hexose monophosphate shunt and its response to oxidant stress. Cancer Res 47:5994–5999, 1987.

484. Yeh HJ, Pierce GF, Deuel TF: Ultrastructure localization of a platelet-derived growth factor/v-sis-related protein(s) in cytoplasm and nucleus of simian sarcoma virus-transformed cells. Proc Natl Acad Sci (USA) 84:2317–2321, 1987.

485. Zava DT, McGuire WL: Estrogen receptor: unoccupied sites in nuclei of a breast tumor cell line. J Biol Chem 252:2703–2708, 1977.

486. Zhan X, Goldfarb M: Growth factor requirements of oncogene-transformed NIH 3T3 and Balb/c 3T3 cells cultured in defined media. Mol Cell Biol 6:3541–3544, 1986.

487. Zugmaier G, Knabbe C, Deschauer B, Lippman ME, Dickson RB: Inhibition of anchorage-independent growth of estrogen receptor–positive and estrogen receptor–negative breast cancer cell lines by TGFβ_1 and TGFβ_2. J Cell Physiol 141:353–361, 1989.

488. Zumstein P, Stiles CD: Molecular cloning of gene sequences that are regulated by insulin-like growth factor I. J Biol Chem 262:11,252–11,260, 1987.

489. Zwiebel JA, Bano M, Nexo E, Salomon P, Kidwell WR: Partial purification of transforming growth factors from human milk. Cancer Res 46:933–939, 1986.

Chapter 21

CONCEPTS AND MECHANISMS OF BREAST CANCER METASTASIS

Isaiah J. Fidler, D.V.M., Ph.D. and Garth L. Nicolson, Ph.D.

Once breast cancer has been diagnosed, the most crucial question is whether the cancer is confined to the breast or whether it has already spread to distant sites. The reason for this concern is simple: metastasis, the spread of cells from the primary neoplasms to and growth at distant sites, is the most likely cause of death in breast cancer patients. Although our understanding of the pathogenesis of metastasis has increased considerably during the past decade, comparable improvements in the treatment of metastatic disease have, for the most part, not occurred. Despite major advances in general patient care, surgical techniques, and adjuvant therapies, the majority of deaths from cancer are still caused by the growth of metastases that are resistant to therapy.[47, 51, 109, 124] The major obstacle to the successful treatment of metastases is that the cancer cells in primary and secondary neoplasms are biologically heterogeneous.[29, 47, 51, 71, 109] For example, primary tumors and their metastases contain multiple cell populations exhibiting a wide range of genetic, biochemical, immunological, and biological characteristics, such as cell surface components and receptors, stored and released enzymes, karyotypes, cell morphologies, growth properties, sensitivities to various therapeutic agents, and abilities to invade and metastasize.[29, 39, 42, 47, 51, 71, 101, 109]

The ability to detect tumors and their metastases before significant cellular diversification into heterogeneous cell subpopulations has occurred is a major problem. By the time they are diagnosed, metastases can be of considerable size and heterogeneity. At the lower limit of detection, a tumor mass measures approximately one cm^3 and thus can contain about one billion cells. Even if 99.9 percent of these cells can be destroyed, a remarkable therapeutic achievement, one million cancer cells will remain to proliferate, invade, and produce further metastases.[29, 39, 42, 47, 101, 109]

Because metastasis is a major cause of death from cancer, a primary goal is to better understand the mechanisms of cancer metastasis in patients and to develop more effective therapy. In this chapter, we discuss some findings on mechanisms of tumor progression and metastasis and development of biological heterogeneity. We emphasize those data that have important relevance to metastatic breast carcinomas.

PATHOGENESIS OF METASTASIS

The process of invasion and metastasis consists of a dynamic sequence of interrelated steps (Fig. 21–1). If a disseminating tumor cell fails to complete one of these steps, it fails to form a detectable metastasis. Thus the malignant cells that eventually develop into growing metastases have survived a sequential series of limiting or potentially lethal interactions. The outcome of this process depends on both the intrinsic properties of the tumor cells and host responses or factors.[39, 42, 101, 156]

Metastasis begins with the local invasion of the surrounding host stroma by either single cells or clumps of cells from the primary tumor and penetration of vascular or lymphatic channels adjacent to the primary tumor. These malignant cells can grow at or near the sites of penetration, or they can detach as single cells or cell aggregates and be transported in the lymphatics or circulatory systems. Malignant cells in the lymphatics arrive at draining lymph nodes, where they can proliferate, pass through to adjacent lymph nodes, or enter the blood. In the lymphatics, as well as in the blood, circulating tumor emboli must survive host nonimmune and immune defenses, such as mechanical stress, and nonspecific and specific interactions with lymphocytes, monocytes, natural killer cells, and other effector cells. In the blood, surviving tumor cells and emboli implant in the capillary beds of distant organs and tissues. Malignant cells can remain at these sites, or they can detach and recirculate to the other organ sites. When they have undergone successful implantation, usually in the small blood vessels by adhesion to the vessel walls, the tumor cells penetrate the endothelium and underlying basement membrane and invade the organ tissue, where they must survive and proliferate. To continue growing, the micrometastases must develop a vascular network and evade the host immune system. Once the secondary tumor cells begin to proliferate, they can again invade, penetrate blood vessels, and enter the circulation, thus producing additional metastases.

Local Growth and Angiogenesis

The growth of tumors beyond the size of a few millimeters in diameter is dependent on the develop-

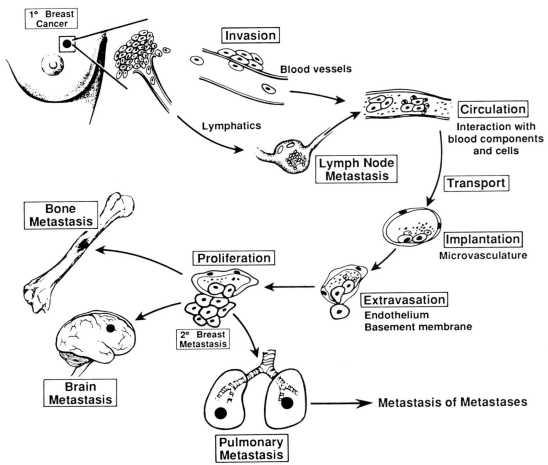

Figure 21–1. The pathogenesis of breast cancer metastasis. The process of cancer metastasis is sequential and requires that metastatic cells complete all the steps of highly selective events.

ment of an adequate blood supply.[57] In a variety of experimental tumor systems, tumor growth appears to be linked to capillary ingrowth into the tumor. Histological examination of cancers reveals that tumor cells often surround capillary blood vessels in a cylindrical configuration with a radius not exceeding about 200 μm—the critical diffusion distance for oxygen.[58] These data prompted Folkman to hypothesize that "once a tumor take has occurred, every increase in the tumor cell population must be preceded by an increase in new capillaries that converge upon the tumor."[58]

The process of capillary formation, or angiogenesis, was first recognized in studies of wound healing and then in experimental tumors. Although the process has been studied for more than 50 years, only relatively recently have several angiogenic factors been fully identified and purified.[59] Essentially, the process of angiogenesis is a normal host response to injury, and as such it is an integral part of host homeostatic mechanisms. It is therefore not surprising that tumor angiogenesis is influenced and controlled by products of both tumor cells and those of normal host cells. Regardless of their source, angiogenic factors may be amenable to therapeutic manipulation. The effectiveness of this approach may well depend on whether metastatic cells have in-

vaded and disseminated to distant sites. Although their growth at secondary sites might be inhibited by antiangiogenesis agents, once these agents are removed, tumor cell growth should occur.

Tumor Invasion

Tumor cell invasion can result in the direct spread of cancer to adjacent tissues or migration into body coelomic cavities.[156, 160] Several mechanisms may be responsible for the invasion of tissues surrounding a neoplasm. For example, mechanical pressure produced by the rapid proliferation of neoplasms may force cords of tumor cells along tissue planes of least resistance, leading to pressure atrophy.[65] Even for the many invasive tumors with slow growth rates, their tumor cells are fully capable of infiltrating tissues, despite the absence of pressure factors.[65, 88]

Cell motility may also play a role in tumor cell invasion. Tumor cells possess the necessary cytoplasmic machinery for active locomotion.[137, 149] Yet the inhibition of cell motility by certain drugs can prevent invasion in only some tumors. Increased cell motility is neither a requirement of malignancy nor is it unique to malignant cells. During fetal development, for example, normal cells migrate extensively, and in adult organisms cell locomotion of many normal cells is well recognized.[137] Metastatic mammary tumor cells can produce their own motility factors that appear to stimulate tumor cell movement and invasion.[3]

Less uncertainty surrounds the involvement of specific tissue-destructive enzymes in tumor invasion. Destruction of host tissue by degradative enzymes, aided by pressure from an expanding tumor mass, probably facilitates neoplastic cell infiltration. Many malignant neoplasms express higher levels of lytic enzymes than do benign tumors or corresponding normal tissues. For example, many malignant tumors produce elevated levels of lysosomal enzymes, such as cathepsin B[134] and plasminogen activator.[82]

During local tumor invasion and distant metastasis, blood-borne malignant cells penetrate blood vessels and extravasate into surrounding tissues. Tumor cells that invade blood vessels or exit capillaries at distant sites must penetrate a surrounding basement membrane. Dissolution of the basement membrane, suggestive of enzymatic action, has been observed in areas adjacent to arrested tumor cells. Basement membranes and connective tissues contain primarily four major groups of molecules: collagens, elastin, glycoproteins, and proteoglycans. The quantity of each of these differs among different tissues and basement membranes.[85, 145, 162] These extracellular matrix constituents are stabilized and organized by a variety of protein-protein and polysaccharide-protein interactions that can become destabilized by degradative enzymes.

Favored sites of tumor cell attachment and destruction of basement membranes are the collagen, glycoprotein, and proteoglycan components. Metastatic tumor cells can preferentially attach to the major collagen class, type IV collagen, of basement membranes,[85, 145, 162] and they often secrete high amounts of a collagenase specific for type IV collagen.[86, 162] Various metastatic tumor cells can also produce high amounts of enzymes capable of cleaving the major proteoglycan (heparan sulfate proteoglycan) of basement membranes.[95] These enzymes appear to be excellent markers for highly metastatic cells.[96]

Lymphatic Metastasis

Early clinical observations led to the impression that carcinomas spread mainly by the lymphatic route and mesenchymal tumors spread mainly by means of the blood stream. It is now known, however, that the lymphatic and vascular systems have numerous connections,[27] and that disseminating tumor cells may pass from one system to the other.[20] Therefore, the division of metastasis into lymphatic spread and hematogenous spread is arbitrary.

During tumor cell invasion, the process of infiltration and expansion into host tissues results in the penetration of small lymphatic vessels. Once inside the lymphatics, tumor cells and tumor cell emboli can become detached and passively transported in the lymph. Tumor emboli may be trapped in the first lymph node encountered on their route or they may traverse lymph nodes or bypass them to form distant nodal metastases ("skip metastasis"). Although this phenomenon was first recognized in the late 1800s,[118] its implications were frequently ignored in the development of surgical approaches to treat cancers.[42, 124, 156]

Although the view that the lymphatics are the primary route for spread of carcinomas is an oversimplification, the role that the draining lymph nodes may play in the control of metastatic spread is of prime importance. Regional lymph nodes (RLN) in the area of a primary neoplasm may become enlarged because of hyperplasia or growth of tumor cells in the node. Although the worth of lymph node appearance as a criterion for assessing prognosis is debatable, lymphocyte-depleted RLN may be indicative of a less favorable prognosis than those demonstrating reactive morphologies.[13] Hyperplastic responses of RLN could indicate reactivity to autochthonous tumors, which could be of benefit to the host.

Role of Regional Lymph Nodes in Metastasis

The role of RLN in metastasis is as controversial as it is important. Because the RLN may be involved immunologically in host responses to neoplasms, Crile,[24] in 1965, challenged the classic concept of complete resection of primary breast tumors and their RLN. He advocated simple mastectomy and preservation of the RLN in order to maintain a high level of systemic antitumor immunity, which theoretically could aid in preventing the growth of disseminated micrometastases.[25] Subsequent clinical trials by Fisher et al.[53] and by Fisher and Wolmark[55] comparing simple and radical mastectomy showed no improvement in survival rate of patients and an increased incidence of axillary lymph node metastasis in those who underwent simple mastectomy.[54]

Whether the RLN can serve as a temporary "barrier" for metastatic tumor cells is unclear. In experimental animal tumor systems used to investigate this question, we found that metastasis of mammary tumors implanted in the mammary fat pads of rats could be delayed considerably by prior ablation of RLN.[111] However, the lymph nodes were subjected to a sudden challenge with a large number of tumor cells, a situation that may not be analogous to RLN at the early stages of cancer spread in humans, in which small numbers of cancer cells are released continuously into the lymphatics.

The issue of a metastasis barrier is important because of practical considerations for surgical management of metastasis. Is there a justification for elective-prophylactic lymph node dissection for the treatment of micrometastases? The biological justification for elective lymph node dissection presumes that metastases of some cancers spread from the primary tumor site via lymphatics to RLN and grow there. Only at a later time do tumor cells gain access to the circulation to reach distant organs. If such is the case, and RLN can act as a temporary barrier to the spread of cancer, removing the RLN with micrometastases could clearly increase the cure rate in subgroups of patients with certain tumors, such as melanoma, breast, colon, and head and neck cancers. Indeed, in colorectal cancers, more radical operations that include removal of RLN have been associated with improved survival rates.[35] In contrast, in breast cancer, removal of the axillary lymph nodes in a randomized prospective study was not associated with improved survival rates.[54] In a third tumor system, melanoma, not all patients benefit from elective lymph node dissection, but there is some evidence that patients with intermediate thickness melanomas (1 to 4 mm) do.[4] Similarly, some data suggest that in head and neck cancers an improved survival rate can be achieved in selected patients by elective lymph node dissection or local treatment with x-irradiation.[17, 56]

As stated, many clinicians are convinced that carcinomas metastasize via lymphatics, whereas sarcomas metastasize via blood vessels. Although this oversimplified idea is not correct, it has had a significant impact on surgical oncology. The presence of lymph node metastases may merely indicate that systemic metastasis has occurred, and if that is the case elective lymph node dissection may be of little therapeutic consequence. In contrast, metastases of some tumors first develop in RLN, and only then can tumor cells gain entrance to the general circulation. In this case, elective lymph node dissection will remove micrometastases prior to further dissemination. This issue cannot be settled definitively, because most patients with clinically detectable cancers, even those cancers in which the first site of metastasis is the RLN, may already have disease beyond the RLN. For example, in a breast cancer trial, no improvement in survival rate of patients undergoing lymph node dissection was reported.[54]

The exact role of the RLN draining a primary tumor in the control of metastatic spread remains uncertain. Determining this role is important, since the decision to surgically excise the RLN must be based on the estimated risk of lymph node metastasis and the potential role that the RLN plays in the metastatic process.

Hematogenous Metastasis

During hematogenous metastasis, tumor cells must survive transport in the circulation, adhere to small blood vessels or capillaries, and invade the vessel wall. The mere presence of tumor cells in the circulation does not in itself constitute metastasis, since most cells released into the blood stream are eliminated rapidly.[38, 157] Using radiolabeled tumor cells, we have observed that by 24 hours after entry into the circulation, less than one percent of the cells are still viable, and less than 0.1 percent of tumor cells placed into the circulation eventually survive to produce metastases.[38] Observations such as this prompted us to question whether the 0.1 percent of the circulating cells responsible for the development of metastases survived at random, or whether

these cells represented the selective survival and growth of preexisting subpopulations of cells, ones endowed with special properties that enabled them to survive the process.

The first experimental evidence for nonrandom hematogenous metastasis demonstrated that tumor cells were heterogeneous for blood-borne implantation, invasion, survival, and growth.[48] Employing a modified fluctuation assay,[87] we showed that different tumor cell clones, each derived from individual cells isolated from the same parent tumor, varied dramatically in their abilities to form pulmonary nodules following intravenous injection into syngeneic mice. Control subcloning procedures demonstrated that the diversity in metastatic properties was not a consequence of the cloning procedure.[48] These findings have since been confirmed in numerous laboratories using a wide range of experimental animal tumors of different histories and histological origins,[39, 42, 47, 101, 109] including mammary tumors.[71, 109] Moreover, using young nude mice as models in the study of metastasis in human neoplasms, we have also demonstrated that human tumors, such as colon carcinoma, renal cell carcinoma, and melanoma, are biologically heterogeneous and contain subpopulations of cells with widely differing metastatic properties.[41]

Although most tumor cells are quickly destroyed within the blood stream, it appears that the greater the number of cells released by a primary tumor, the greater the probability that some cells will survive to form metastases.[38, 48] Thus the number of tumor emboli in the circulation appears to correlate well with the size and clinical duration of the primary tumor.[42, 51] The development of necrotic and hemorrhagic areas within large tumors may facilitate this process by providing tumor cells easier access to the circulation.[156, 157]

The rapid death of most circulating tumor cells is probably, to a large degree, a result of simple mechanical factors, notably blood turbulence. However, nonmechanical mechanisms that increase the chance of tumor cell survival also exist. For example, tumor cells can aggregate with each other (homotypic aggregation)[148] or with host cells (heterotypic aggregation) such as platelets[66] and lymphocytes.[43] Formation of such multicellular emboli enhances the survival of tumor cells in the circulation. The ability of circulating malignant cells to undergo deformation in the microcirculation and survive is another important factor in their ability to recirculate after initial lodgement. Indeed, drugs that disrupt cytoskeletal organization and modify cell deformability can alter tumor cell lodgement, detachment, and recirculation.[105]

Once metastatic cells reach the microcirculation, they can interact with cells of the vascular endothelium. These interactions include nonspecific mechanical lodgement of tumor cell emboli as well as formation of stable adhesions between tumor cells and small vessel endothelial cells. The organ distribution of metastatic foci is thought to be caused, in part, by the ability of blood-borne malignant cells to adhere to specific endothelia.[99] Once bound to endothelial cells, tumor cells elicit endothelial cell retraction, exposing the underlying basement membrane. This exposure can lead to platelet adherence, degranulation, and further retraction of the endothelium.[66] Since metastatic cells preferentially bind to exposed basement membrane, this process enhances tumor cell arrest.[84]

The formation of fibrin clots at sites of tumor cell arrest in the microcirculation can result in blood vessel damage.[33] However, fibrin deposits are not always found around tumor cell emboli,[152] and in some tumor systems, fibrin formation is not essential for tumor cell implantation or metastasis formation.[152] Increased coagulability is commonly observed in patients with advanced cancers and could be related to the high levels of thromboplastin found in certain tumors or to production of high levels of procoagulant-A activity, which can directly activate factor X in the clotting process.[23] The resulting reduced blood flow could lead to increased trapping of circulating tumor cells and perhaps to their increased survival. The use of anticoagulants to treat or control metastasis is based on the consideration of such factors.[76]

Extravasation of arrested tumor cells is thought to occur by mechanisms similar to those responsible for local invasion.[85, 109] Tumor cells can grow and destroy the surrounding vessel, invade by penetrating endothelial basement membrane, or follow extravasating white blood cells.[36] The ability of malignant cells to extravasate into surrounding tissues of particular organs appears to be caused, in part, by their selective adherence to and invasion of certain tissues.[104] Malignant cells frequently penetrate thin-walled capillaries but rarely invade arteries or arteriole walls, which are rich in elastin fibers.[20, 152] This resistance to invasion is not necessarily mediated by vessel mechanical strength or presence of undegradable surrounding materials. Connective tissues have been shown to produce protease inhibitors, and these may block enzyme-dependent processes of invasion.[80] In the case of metastasizing mammary tumors, evidence indicates that the tumor cells produce and secrete fully active basement membrane–degrading enzymes in relation to their spontaneous metastatic potential.[97]

The invasion, survival, and growth of malignant cells at particular secondary sites also involve their responses to tissue or organ factors. Tumor cells can recognize tissue-specific motility factors that direct their movement and invasion.[119] Once they are inside tissue at a secondary site, malignant cells must also respond to organ-specific factors that determine their survival and growth properties.[103] Since malignant tumors at secondary sites cannot produce a blood vessel system, their growth will ultimately be limited unless they can induce the ingrowth of new capillaries from host tissue by the release of angiogenesis factors.[57–59]

Throughout the process of tumor dissemination, malignant cells are susceptible to destruction by host-specific (lymphocytes, antibodies) and nonspecific (natural killer cell, macrophages) defense mechanisms.[49] In mammary tumors, susceptibility to host effector mechanisms can correlate with metastasis. The most metastatic mammary tumor cells can be the least sensitive to host cellular defense mechanisms.[112]

PATTERNS OF METASTASIS

Clinical observations of cancer patients have revealed that certain tumors have a marked predilection for metastasis to specific organs independent of vascular anatomy, rate of blood flow, and number of tumor cells delivered to each organ. Interest in factors that determine the pattern of breast cancer metastasis is not new. In 1889, Paget analyzed 735 autopsy records of patients with breast cancer. The nonrandom pattern of breast cancer visceral metastases suggested to Paget that the process was not a result of chance but, rather, that certain tumor cells (the "seeds") had a specific affinity for the milieu provided by certain organs (the "soils"). Metastases resulted only when the seed and soil were matched.[118] This "seed-and-soil" hypothesis has received considerable support.

Studies using experimental animal tumor systems have demonstrated that the formation and anatomical locations of metastases are determined by host factors and tumor cell properties.* The distribution and fate of hematogenously disseminated radiolabeled tumor cells in experimental rodent systems clearly reveal that tumor cells reach the microvasculature of many organs. The specific arrest, invasion, and proliferation of tumor cells occur in only some organs, but the mere presence of viable tumor cells in a particular organ does not always predict that metastasis will develop.†

Experimental data supporting the "seed-and-soil" hypothesis of Paget were derived from studies on the preferential invasion and growth of B16 melanoma metastases in specific organs. Following the intravenous (I.V.) injection of B16 melanoma cells into syngeneic C57BL/6 mice, tumor growths developed in the lungs and in fragments of pulmonary or ovarian tissue implanted intramuscularly into the quadriceps femoris. In contrast, metastatic lesions did not develop in control-implanted renal tissue or at the site of surgical trauma.[70] The formation of tumors in the transplanted organ could have been caused by the arrest and growth of tumor cells immediately following intravenous injection (i.e., "initial metastases"). Alternatively, tumor cells injected intravenously could have been arrested in the lungs, where metastasis developed. Once metastases were established, tumor cells could enter the circulation to be arrested at other organs and produce "secondary metastases." To distinguish between these possibilities, we performed several experiments with parabiotically joined mice.[50] Two weeks after normal, tumor-free mice were joined parabiotically to tumor-bearing animals, no evidence was found of any tumor growth in the "guest" animals. However, when the parabiotic animals were allowed to survive for 4 weeks after separation from the tumor-bearing animals, many developed lung metastases.

In vitro experiments demonstrating organ-selective adhesion, invasion, and growth also support the "seed-and-soil" hypothesis. Using the B16 melanoma system,

---

*References 29, 39, 42, 47, 51, 101, 109, and 124.
†References 29, 39, 42, 69, 100, 101, and 124.

organ-selective adhesion to and invasion of target organ tissues has been documented,[104] and experiments with organ tissue–derived soluble growth factors indicate that soil factors can have profound effects on certain tumor cell subpopulations.[103] Such organ or soil effects have also been seen in metastatic mammary tumors.[77]

In an alternative proposal, Ewing suggested that metastasis occurs merely as a consequence of mechanical factors, such as anatomical and hemodynamic factors of the vasculature.[36] Although circulatory anatomy may indeed influence the dissemination of many malignant cells,[155] it cannot fully explain the patterns of distribution of numerous tumors.

Ethical considerations rule out the experimental analysis of cancer metastasis in patients. The introduction of peritoneovenous (PV) shunts for palliation of malignant ascites has, however, provided an opportunity to study some of the factors affecting metastatic spread in humans. Tarin and colleagues[136, 143, 144] have described the outcome of ascitic fluids of patients with malignant ascites draining into the circulation, with the resulting entry of viable tumor cells into the jugular veins. Good palliation with minimal complications was reported for 29 patients with different neoplasms.[136] The autopsy findings in 15 patients substantiated the clinical observations that PV shunts do not increase the risk of significant metastasis. In eight patients, micrometastases were found in extraabdominal organs (most commonly, the lung). In seven patients, no evidence was found of tumor colonies outside the abdomen, even in cases where the PV shunt was operational for many months.[136] The negative findings in half of these patients are important because the studies provide clinical verification of the nearly century-old "seed-and-soil" hypothesis.

INFLUENCE OF ORGAN ENVIRONMENT ON THE BEHAVIOR OF METASTATIC CELLS

Tumor cell properties contribute significantly to organ arrest, invasion, and growth patterns. Organ-specific variant lines have been selected from parental tumor cell populations,[100, 109] and the modification of tumor cell properties can lead to alterations in their metastatic patterns.[69, 100, 126] The effect of host tissues on tumor development is not as well documented. Preferential growth in certain organs has been explained by the effects of local immune defenses,[81, 129–131] and it has also been suggested that diffusible inhibitors of tumor growth may be released by certain tissues.[9, 78, 103]

Individual cells within a neoplasm are exposed to different microenvironments, differences that can be attributed to variability in the concentrations of nutrients, oxygen, growth factors, hormones, enzymes, ions, inducers, and other regulatory factors (Fig. 21–2).[101] Clinical observations have suggested that the response of metastases in women with breast cancer is influenced by the anatomical location of the lesions.

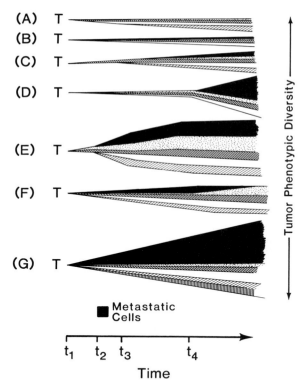

Figure 21–2. Schematic examples of tumor cell diversification. Tumor cells proliferate and diversify to yield a benign tumor (A) or low-grade malignant tumor (B). Malignant cell populations result from the process of diversification (C,D). Occasionally, a malignant neoplasm may revert to a benign tumor with the loss of metastatic subpopulations (F). In highly malignant neoplasms, diversification occurs at rapid rates (E, G), but in some malignancies, "interactions" between malignant cells limit diversification and the rate at which new metastatic variants are generated (E). From Nicolson GL: Cancer Res 47:1473–1487, 1987. (Reprinted by permission.)

With few exceptions, the patients with metastases in lymph nodes and skin have a better prognosis and treatment response than those with skeletal or pulmonary metastases.[16, 19, 133] Differential response of metastatic lesions in different organs to different cytotoxic drugs have also been reported.[30, 32, 138] Although the differences in the response of metastases to chemotherapy can be a result of heterogeneity in the tumor cell population, the influence of the organ environment cannot be ignored. Subcutaneous transplanted mouse neoplasms were sensitive to three cytotoxic agents, whereas the same tumor cells implanted intracerebrally were not.[32]

The viability and growth of tumor cells depends on an adequate source of nutrients. The degree of tumor vascularity can control the delivery of nutrients, the clearance of metabolites, and the delivery of cytotoxic drugs to a lesion. Measurements of blood flow in subcutaneous tumors of rats reveal a lack of autoregulation in response to infusions of angiotensin II. The selective increase in tumor blood flow, with no increase in normal tissues, could enhance chemotherapeutic drug delivery.[138] In addition, growing tumors are often extensively infiltrated by lymphocytes, granulocytes, mast cells, and macrophages. When such cells are in close contact with tumor cells, they may have profound effects on cell growth and phenotype. For example, tumor-infiltrating macrophages can either destroy tumor cells[40] or release substances that may cause chromosomal changes, leading to the generation of drug-resistant variants.[163]

BIOLOGICAL DIVERSIFICATION AND HETEROGENEITY OF MALIGNANT NEOPLASMS

Controversy is no longer associated with the concept that neoplasms are composed of diverse cell populations that are heterogeneous for a wide variety of characteristics, including many of those once thought to be expressed homogeneously among tumor cells.* The heterogeneous expression of such properties is thought to be transmittable to progeny cells, at least for several generations, although apparently a number of factors, such as organ microenvironmental efforts, can alter the expression of particular components in individual tumor cells.[39, 101]

An intriguing aspect of tumor heterogeneity is the ability of one tumor cell subpopulation to influence the properties of other subpopulations.[73] These interactions can modify neoplastic cell growth,[90] immunological[91] and metastatic properties,[93, 123] sensitivity to chemotherapeutic agents,[92] and expression of cell surface components.[93] Not all tumors cells, however, appear to be capable of influencing the properties of other tumor cells, and this characteristic also appears to be expressed heterogeneously among neoplastic cells.

Cellular heterogeneity is not unique to transformed cells. Normal cells and tissues are also heterogeneous for a wide variety of properties. What makes cancers different from normal tissues, however, is that the degree of tumor cellular heterogeneity is usually more pronounced. For example, a cell surface epithelial antigen of $M_r \sim 400,000$ was found to be expressed with a greater degree of cell-to-cell variation on breast carcinoma cells than on normal breast epithelial cells.[120] Differences in cell cycle fraction and differentiation status do not explain such widespread cellular heterogeneity in malignant neoplasms.[102]

Evolution of Heterogeneous Neoplasms

Most naturally occurring and induced neoplasms develop as a proliferation of single cells.[37, 113] Even in tumors with diversified heterogeneous cellular phenotypes, evidence of such clonal origin still exists. It is not difficult to understand the source of cellular diversity in neoplasms of multicellular origin; they are probably populated by the progenies of several transformed cells. It is more difficult to perceive the source of heterogeneity in neoplasms of unicellular origin. Clinical and

histological observations of neoplasms suggested to Foulds[60, 61] that tumors undergo a series of changes during the course of the disease. For example, a mammary tumor that was initially diagnosed as benign can, over a period of many months or even years, evolve into a malignant tumor.[128] To explain the process of tumor evolution and progression, Nowell[113] suggested that acquired genetic variability within developing clones of tumors, coupled with host selection pressures, can bring about the emergence of new clonal sublines of increased growth autonomy or malignancy.

Tumor heterogeneity is achieved because phenotypic diversification of individual neoplasms yields heterogeneous combinations of cellular phenotypes.[102] A hypothetical scheme for the progression of benign and malignant neoplasms to phenotypically diverse cells is shown in Figure 21–2. A benign tumor would be expected to exhibit minimal or some phenotypic diversification (Fig. 21–2A), whereas malignant tumors would be expected to diversify phenotypically at various rates (Fig. 21–2B to G), including some that may diversify at later times in their natural history (Fig. 21–2D). In addition, a few tumors may actually diversify while reverting to a less malignant phenotype (phenotypically diverse, but with relatively fewer metastatic cells, Fig. 21–2F). Certain neoplasms may show alterations in their rates of phenotypic diversification (Fig. 21–2E), which could be caused by tumor cell-tumor cell interactions that stabilize cellular diversification within the tumor.[102] In addition to the relatively slow rates of change shown in Figure 21–2, changes in the individual properties of malignant cells can occur quite suddenly; this has been termed "phenotypic drift"[98] or "dynamic heterogeneity."[74] Such rapid changes can also be modulated by cell-cell interactions.[73, 90–93, 123]

The phenotypic changes found in malignant cells are not always related to states of progression and malignancy. Properties that are not relevant to tumor cell survival, growth, and malignancy may be lost or diminish in importance in the later stages of tumor progression. Simple relationships, however, probably do not exist among the loss, reduction, or modulation of certain cellular components or their activities and their "loss of differentiation" observed in some malignant neoplasms.[102, 110]

Important questions for the clinical management of cancers are as follows: When do metastatic variants arise in a primary neoplasm? Do metastatic cells arise early or late in the development of a malignant neoplasm [c.f. Fig. 21–2(D,G)]? Do metastatic cells have a growth advantage over nonmetastatic cells so that, with the passage of time, metastatic cells constitute the majority of cells in a neoplasm [Fig. 21–2(G)]? Answers to some of these questions are now becoming available and may help oncologists make decisions critical to the timing and sequence of multimodality treatments for primary tumors and metastases. Tumors of unicellular origin may exhibit metastatic heterogeneity at early stages in their development. We base this conclusion on data generated by our studies of the in vivo behavior of murine fibroblasts transformed by an oncogenic virus[46]

---

*References 29, 39, 42, 46, 51, 71, 101, 109, 124, and 153.

where, by 6 weeks after initial transformation and despite its single-cell origin, the tumor contained subpopulations of cells with different metastatic properties. These data demonstrate that the generation of metastatic heterogeneity in neoplasms does not require a prolonged latent period.

Genetic and Epigenetic Instability

During tumor progression, increasing genetic alterations generated by random, somatic mutational events can be responsible for the emergence of tumor cell subpopulations with different properties.[102, 113, 114] Evidence for such genetic instability in malignant neoplasms has been obtained by examining gross chromosomal alterations,[161] mitotic errors, and rates of spontaneous mutations in highly metastatic cells as compared with low metastatic or nonmetastatic cells.[22] As tumors progress, chromosomal abnormalities or alterations in chromosome morphologies, banding patterns, or ploidy may progressively increase in frequency.[161]

Genetic instability has been estimated by determining the spontaneous rates of gene mutation in animal cells of various metastatic potentials. When several cell clones of differing metastatic potentials were examined for rates of spontaneous mutation to drug resistance, the more metastatic cells possessed rates approximately six to seven times higher than that of spontaneous mutation.[22] This finding is also heterogeneous, since it is not a universal finding in metastatic systems.[83]

Even taking into account the possible enhanced spontaneous mutation rates of highly malignant cells, their chromosome instability, and their selection by host responses, the rates of cellular phenotypic diversification found in many malignant neoplasms cannot be explained merely by genetic instability–host selection mechanisms. The highest rates of expected spontaneous gene mutation are orders of magnitude less than the rates of phenotypic variation found in many tumor systems. One explanation could be that gene mutation occurs at regulatory sites,[101] or that the critical modifications are in the transcriptional machinery.[102] These possibilities are reasonable because most changes in gene products associated with the malignant phenotype appear to be quantitative rather than qualitative.[106] In addition, analysis of certain metastatic models indicates that the effective rate of reversion of the metastatic phenotype can be as high as 10^{-2} to 10^{-1} per cell per generation, a rate that appears to be modulated by cell-cell interactions in the diversified tumor cell population.[164]

Epigenetic modifications of cells can also explain the high rates of cellular diversification found in many malignant neoplasms.[63, 102] Epigenetic changes in tumor cells could be mediated by such diverse mechanisms as DNA methylation, posttranscriptional modifications, nonmutational chromosomal rearrangements, and other mechanisms that may be sensitive to tumor cell microenvironments. Microenvironmental changes resulting in discrete modifications in gene expression could be important in generating diversification and heterogeneity in malignant neoplasms. One example of the type of microenvironmental signal that could stimulate tumor cells as well as normal cells is mediated by interactions with stromal and tissue matrix components.[12] Tumor cells may be capable of responding to a particular stromal environment (see following section). These responses could mimic some of the normal cell responses that occur during cellular differentiation and embryonic development.[101, 102]

Origin of Biological Diversity in Metastases

Tumor diversity is not restricted to primary neoplasms. Multiple metastases proliferating in the same organ or different organs can also exhibit heterogeneity with regard to many characteristics such as metastatic capacity, hormone receptors, marker enzymes, growth rate, antigenicity, and response to various chemotherapeutic agents.[39, 42, 101] This diversity could result from the process of tumor evolution and the nature of the secondary environment.

Metastases, like primary tumors, may have a unicellular or a multicellular origin. To determine whether individual metastases are clonal and whether different metastases can be produced by different progenitor cells, a series of experiments was carried out utilizing irradiation of tumor cells to induce random chromosome breaks and rearrangements.[140] The karyotype composition of 21 individual metastases was analyzed after cultivation of cells from individual lesions. Unique karyotypic patterns of abnormal, marker chromosomes were found in most of the lines established from metastases, suggesting that each metastasis originated from a single progenitor cell.[52] Similar results have been obtained in other rodent tumor systems.[79, 117, 141] These studies revealed that the majority of metastases are of clonal origin and that variant clones with diverse phenotypes are formed rapidly, resulting in the generation of significant cellular diversity within individual metastases.[127, 139] Collectively, these observations indicate that different metastases arise from different progenitor cells and account for the well-documented differences in the behavior of individual metastases in the same patient, including differences in response to therapy (i.e., interlesional heterogeneity). However, even within individual metastases of proven clonal origin, heterogeneity can rapidly develop by genetic and epigenetic mechanisms to create significant intralesional heterogeneity.[42, 139]

CLINICAL CHALLENGE OF METASTASES HETEROGENEITY

The major obstacle to the treatment of established metastases may well be their diversification and resulting heterogeneity resulting from their continuing evolution.

The three areas in which the heterogeneity of neoplasms is proving to be of practical importance are in the detection of tumor deposits using monoclonal antibodies or tumor cell markers, in the design of screening procedures for new therapeutic modalities, and in the application of therapeutic regimens other than surgical resection.

Cancer Detection

Several clinical observations demonstrate the impact of tumor cell heterogeneity on attempts to detect primary and metastatic tumor foci. For example, small cell carcinomas of the lung, medullary carcinomas of the thyroid, and carcinoid tumors can often be detected by elevation of serum levels of certain markers such as calcitonin, histaminase, and L-dopa decarboxylase. When Baylin et al.[7, 8] simultaneously sampled primary tumors and metastases for these markers, they found variable patterns of expression. Although primary tumors produced detectable levels of each marker, many of the metastases produced either low or undetectable levels of the enzymes. Heterogeneity in expression and release of tumor cell markers is well documented for other neoplasms as well.[26, 34, 68, 75] Findings such as these cast doubt on the feasibility of using any tumor cell product for the quantitation of disseminated disease.

Heterogeneous Response to Therapy

Many reports have presented the differences in drug sensitivity among tumor cell populations in various human neoplasms, such as melanoma, colon adenocarcinoma, breast carcinoma, lymphoma, and lung cancer.[5, 6, 11] Even more important, differences in drug response between tumor cells that populate metastases and those isolated from the primary neoplasm have also been reported.* Similar to the heterogeneous drug responses of cells populating primary tumors and their metastases, radiation sensitivities of cell populations in animal and human tumors are also heterogeneous.[94, 154, 158]

Although the growth inhibition of tumor cells in vitro by a drug does not always correlate with drug sensitivity in vivo, the development of in vitro assays of tumor cell response to cytotoxic agents to predict the outcome of cancer therapy in individual patients has been vigorously pursued. If such assays are to be meaningful, however, they must employ a sample representative of the cells populating the tumor. The introduction of the tumor stem cell assay was based on the rationale that the drug sensitivity or resistance of freshly isolated human tumor cells might more accurately predict clinical response to antineoplastic agents than cells from rodent tumors subjected to unknown selection pressures during prolonged serial passage. However, the isolation of cells

*References 1, 31, 64, 135, 142, 146 and 147.

from only one region of a solid tumor, which could be zonally heterogeneous,[45] coupled with the low cloning efficiency of most human tumor cells, may render such assays unusable for most clinical samples.[10, 15] In addition, clonal interactions between various subpopulations of tumor cells can influence their drug sensitivities,[73, 90–93, 123, 125] and the cells that proliferate in such assays may not represent the highly malignant tumor cell subpopulations that pose a risk for metastasis.[107]

Stimulation of the rate of formation of tumor cell variants by restriction of subpopulation diversity may provide an explanation for the rapid evolution of cellular diversity within individual metastases.[125, 127, 139] First, in the primary tumor, interactions between the heterogeneous constituent cell subpopulations impose relative phenotypic stability and restrict the rate of formation of tumor cell variants. However, for a single cell in a newly established metastasis, these interactions would be absent. The tumor diversification would thus be stimulated, quickly converting the initially clonally homogeneous metastasis to a clonally heterogeneous lesion.[127] Second, if a particular therapy could kill most of the cells in a heterogeneous tumor cell population, this could stimulate the formation of new tumor cell variants from the surviving subpopulations (iatrogenic stimulation of heterogeneity).[123]

The heterogeneous nature of the response of malignant tumor cell subpopulations to cytotoxic drugs and other therapeutic modalities coupled with the iatrogenic stimulation of surviving tumor cell diversification makes it unlikely that single or multiple treatment regimens will be able to kill all of the cells in a tumor, even if several agents are used simultaneously or sequentially. Clinically, repeated cycles of cytotoxic therapies with different agents followed by intervening recovery periods often result in the eventual emergence of highly resistant and increasingly malignant tumor cell populations. Suggested improvements on such schemes include truncation of recovery periods to limit surviving tumor cell diversification[122] and inhibition of tumor cell diversification during the recovery periods by cytostatic agents, such as differentiation modulators, hormones, growth factors, vitamin analogues, and other substances.[108]

Antigenic Heterogeneity

Over the years, numerous investigators have studied the possibility that enhancement of host immune mechanisms could control cancer metastases. In practice, there seem to be at least three major factors determining the success of immunological techniques in controlling cancer metastasis: (1) the heterogeneous nature of malignant neoplasms; (2) the intrinsic antigenicity of metastatic tumor cells; and (3) the ability of the primary host to recognize and destroy susceptible tumor cells. The heterogeneous nature of animal and human primary neoplasms and metastases with regard to antigenicity, immunogenicity, and susceptibility to lymphocyte-mediated lysis is now well recognized.[2, 18, 72, 89, 91, 116] In addition, studies have shown that the antigenicity of primary tumors and their metastases and antigenicity among different metastatic lesions can also differ.[62, 67, 89, 121, 159] Such variations may greatly influence the likelihood of success of specific immunotherapeutic modalities.

Another important issue is whether the relative antigenicity of malignant cells influences their metastatic potential. Experimental studies on the role of the immune response in cancer metastasis have yielded contradictory results. In some tumor systems, depression of immunological reactivity was shown to increase the incidence of both spontaneous and experimental metastasis, whereas in other systems, depression of host immunity was shown to decrease or prevent formation of metastases. In yet another series of tumors, alterations of immunological reactivity did not seem to influence the growth of local or disseminated tumors.[44, 49] We have made a systematic study of the role of tumor cell immunogenicity and host immune status in the formation of experimental and spontaneous metastases and have concluded that the role of the immune system in experimental metastasis varies for different tumors and that no generalizations regarding the role of host immunity that will predict the outcome of metastasis can be made from a single tumor system.[44] The data, however, suggest that the immunogenic properties of the tumor will determine, to some extent, the nature and degree of the influence of the immune system on the metastatic process.[49]

Active-specific immunotherapy, although more promising than classic nonspecific immunotherapy, also has its problems. Adoptive immunization of tumor-bearing animals using T lymphocytes sensitized to tumor cells has been only partially successful in antitumor therapy.[14, 21, 28, 62, 115] One reason is the cotransfer of suppressor T lymphocytes into the tumor-bearing host or the direct generation of these suppressor T lymphocytes by the tumor. Protocols to eradicate suppressor T lymphocytes generated in the host (irradiation or low-dose cyclophosphamide) may help, but still another potential problem needs to be resolved: the high probability of selecting for antigen-loss tumor cell variants, which could escape immune destruction.[14, 62] Given the overwhelming data on the instability of tumor cells and their rapid diversification during therapy, the generation of such antigen-loss variants may be a major obstacle to specific immunotherapy. An additional possibility for the further improvement of specific active immunotherapy is the use of cultured long-term lymphocyte lines expanded with interleukin-2.[132]

Other areas of active research for the immunotherapy of metastases are the use of monoclonal antibodies or immunoconjugates. Monoclonal antibodies alone may be useful to block specific steps in the pathogenesis of metastasis.[150, 151] In addition, immunoconjugates are being used in hope that monoclonal antibodies can be targeted to the sites of metastatic foci, allowing the linked toxic agent to kill tumor cells while preventing their systemic toxicity. Although promising, this therapeutic strategy relies on the cells in every metastatic deposit to display the specific antigen to which the monoclonal antibody is directed. As discussed previously, biochemical markers, including tumor cell surface antigens, are heterogeneously expressed by both experimental and human tumor cells. To circumvent the problem of heterogeneity with monoclonal antibody therapy, different combinations of monoclonal antibodies targeted to different target antigens may have to be used.

CONCLUSIONS

Metastasis of breast cancer is a highly selective process that depends on both unique tumor cell properties and specific host factors. It can be best understood in the context of the "seed-and-soil" hypothesis of Paget.[118] In breast and other cancers, the role of regional lymph nodes and distant organ sites in the pathogenesis of metastasis is beginning to be appreciated, and recent clinical and experimental data indicate that specific cellular mechanisms exist for implantation, invasion, survival, and growth of malignant cells at secondary sites. An important aspect of malignancy is the instability of individual tumor cells and their ability to undergo diversification to form heterogeneous cellular populations. Tumor diversification and heterogeneity appear to be driven by genetic and epigenetic events that can also be modulated by cell-cell interactions and host microenvironments.

The recognition that breast cancers do not consist of uniform entities but contain subpopulations of cells with diverse biological properties requires a critical reappraisal of the mechanisms of metastasis and the testing of new approaches for the treatment of metastasis.

References

1. Abe I, Suzuki M, Hori K, Saito S, Sato H: Some aspects of size-dependent differential drug response in primary and metastatic tumors. Cancer Metastasis Rev 4:27–40, 1985.
2. Albino AP, Lloyd KO, Houghton AN, Oettgen HF, Old LJ: Heterogeneity in surface antigen and glycoprotein expression of cell lines derived from different melanoma metastases of the same patient. J Exp Med 154:1764–1778, 1981.
3. Atnip KD, Haney L, Nicolson GL, Dubbons MK: Chemotactic response of rat mammary adenocarcinoma cell clones to tumor-derived cytokines. Biochem Biophys Res Commun 146: 996–1002, 1987.
4. Balch CM, Cascinelli N, Milton GW, Sim FH: Surgical decisions regarding lymph node dissection for stage I melanoma patients: pros and cons of immediate vs. delayed lymphadenectomy. In Balch CM, Milton GW (eds): Cutaneous Melanoma: Clinical Management and Treatment Results Worldwide. Philadelphia, JB Lippincott, 1985.
5. Barranco SC, Drewinko B, Humphrey RM: Differential response by human melanoma cells to 1,3-bis(2-chloroethyl)-1-nitrosourea and bleomycin. Mutat Res 19:277–280, 1973.
6. Barranco SC, Hanenelt BR, Gee EL: Differential sensitivities of five rat hepatoma cell lines to anticancer drugs. Cancer Res 38:656–660, 1978.
7. Baylin SB. Clonal selection and heterogeneity of human solid

neoplasms. *In* Fidler IJ, White RJ (eds): Design of Models for Testing Cancer Therapeutic Agents. New York, Van Nostrand Reinhold, 1982, pp 50–63.

8. Baylin SB, Weisburger WR, Eggleston JC, Mendelshon G, Beaven MA, Abeloff MD, Ettinger DS: Variable content of histaminase, L-dopa decarboxylase and calcitonin in small-cell carcinoma of the lung. Biologic and clinical implications. N Engl J Med 299:105–110, 1978.

9. Bellamy D, Hinsull SM: Influence of lodgement site on the proliferation of metastases of Walker 256 carcinoma in the rat. Br J Cancer 37:81–85, 1978.

10. Bertelsen CA, Sondak VK, Mann BD: Chemosensitivity testing of human solid tumors. A review of 1582 assays with 258 clinical correlations. Cancer 53:1240–1245, 1984.

11. Biorklund A, Hakansson L, Stenstarn B, Trope C, Akerman M: Heterogeneity of non-Hodgkin's lymphomas as regards sensitivity to cytostatic drugs: an in vitro study. Eur J Cancer 16:647–654, 1980.

12. Bissell MJ, Hall HG, Parry G: How does the extracellular matrix direct gene expression? J Theor Biol 99:31–68, 1983.

13. Black MM, Freeman C, Mork T, Harvei S, Cutler SJ: Prognostic significance of microscopic structure of gastric carcinomas and their regional lymph nodes. Cancer 27:703–710, 1971.

14. Boon T, Van Snick J, Pel AV, Uyttenhove C, Marchand M: Immunogenic variants obtained by mutagenesis of mouse mastocytoma P815. II. T lymphocyte mediated cytolysis. J Exp Med 152:1184–1193, 1980.

15. Bradley EC, Issell BF, Hellman R: The human tumor colony-forming chemosensitivity assay: a biological and clinical review. Invest New Drugs 2:59–70, 1984.

16. Brambilla C, Delena M, Rossi A, Valagussa P, Bonadonna G: Response and survival in advanced breast cancer after two non-cross resistant drug combinations. Br Med J 1:801–804, 1976.

17. Byers RM: Modified neck dissection: a study of 967 cases from 1970 to 1980. Am J Surg 150:414–421, 1985.

18. Bystryn JC, Bernstein P, Lui P, Valentine F: Immunophenotype of human melanoma cells in different metastases. Cancer Res 45:5603–5607, 1985.

19. Canellos GP, Devita VT, Gold GL, Chabner BA, Schein PS, Young RC: Cyclical combination chemotherapy for advanced breast carcinoma. Br Med J 1:218–220, 1974.

20. Carr I: Lymphatic metastasis. Cancer Metastasis Rev 22:307–319, 1983.

21. Cheever MA, Greenberg PD, Fefer A: Potential for specific cancer therapy with immune T lymphocytes. J Biol Response Mod 3:113–127, 1984.

22. Cifone MA, Fidler IJ: Increasing metastatic potential is associated with increasing genetic instability of clones isolated from murine neoplasms. Proc Natl Acad Sci USA 78:6949–6952, 1981.

23. Cliffton EE, Grossi CE: The rationale of anticoagulants in the treatment of cancer. J Med 5:107–116, 1974.

24. Crile G: Rationale of simple mastectomy without radiation for clinical stage 1 cancer of the breast. Surg Gynecol Obstet 120:975–982, 1965.

25. Crile G: Possible role of uninvolved regional nodes in preventing metastasis from breast cancer. Cancer 24:1283–1289, 1969.

26. Czerniak B, Darzynkiewicz Z, Staiano-Coico L, Herz F, Koss LG: Expression of Ca antigen in relation to the cell cycle in cultured human tumor cells. Cancer Res 44:4342–4346, 1984.

27. del Regato JA: Pathways of metastatic spread of malignant tumors. Semin Oncol 4:33–38, 1977.

28. Dennis JW, Laferte S, Man MS, Elliot BE, Kerbel RS: Adoptive immune therapy in mice bearing poorly immunogenic metastases, using T lymphocytes stimulated *in vitro* against highly immunogenic mutant sublines. Int J Cancer 34:709–716, 1984.

29. Dexter DL, Leith JT: Tumor heterogeneity and drug resistance. J Clin Oncol 4:244–257, 1986.

30. Donelli MG, Colombo T, Broggini M, Garattini S: Differential distribution of antitumor agents in primary and secondary tumors. Cancer Treat Rep 61:1319–1324, 1977.

31. Donelli MG, Colombo T, Dagnino G, Madonna D, Garattini S: Is better drug availability in secondary neoplasms responsible for better response to chemotherapy. Eur J Cancer 17:201–209, 1981.

32. Donelli MG, Rosso R, Garattini S: Selective chemotherapy in relation to the site of tumor transplantation. Int J Cancer 2:421–424, 1967.

33. Dvorak HF, Seneger DR, Dvorak AM: Fibrin as a component of the tumor stroma: origins and biological significance. Cancer Metastasis Rev 2:41–75, 1983.

34. Edwards PAW: Heterogeneous expression of cell surface antigens in normal epithelia and their tumors, revealed by monoclonal antibodies. Br J Cancer 51:149–160, 1985.

35. Enker E, Laffer UT, Block GE: Enhanced survival of patients with colon and rectal cancer is based upon wide anatomic resection. Ann Surg 190:350–360, 1979.

36. Ewing J: Neoplastic Diseases, ed 6. Philadelphia, WB Saunders, 1928.

37. Fialkow PJ: Clonal origin of human tumors. Ann Rev Med 30:135–176, 1979.

38. Fidler IJ: Metastasis: quantitative analysis of distribution and fate of tumor emboli labeled with ^{125}I-5-iodo-2′-deoxyuridine. J Natl Cancer Inst 45:773–782, 1970.

39. Fidler IJ: The evolution of biological heterogeneity in metastatic neoplasms. *In* Nicolson GL, Milas L (eds): Cancer Invasion and Metastasis: Biologic and Therapeutic Aspects. New York, Raven Press, 1984, pp 5–30.

40. Fidler IJ: Macrophages and metastasis—a biological approach to cancer therapy. Presidential address. Cancer Res 45:4714–4726, 1985.

41. Fidler IJ: Rationale and methods for the use of nude mice to study the biology and therapy of human cancer metastasis. Cancer Metastasis Rev 5:29–49, 1986.

42. Fidler IJ, Balch CM: The biology of cancer metastasis and implications for therapy. Curr Prob Surg 24:137–209, 1987.

43. Fidler IJ, Bucana C: Mechanism of tumor cell resistance to lysis by syngeneic lymphocytes. Cancer Res 37:3945–3956, 1977.

44. Fidler IJ, Gersten DM, Kripke ML: Influence of immune status on the metastasis of three murine fibrosarcomas of different immunogenicities. Cancer Res 39:3816–3821, 1979.

45. Fidler IJ, Hart IR: Biological and experimental consequence of the zonal composition of solid tumors. Cancer Res 41:3266–3267, 1981.

46. Fidler IJ, Hart IR: The origin of metastatic heterogeneity in tumors. Eur J Cancer 17:487–494, 1981.

47. Fidler IJ, Hart IR: Biological diversity in metastatic neoplasms: Origins and implications. Science 217:998–1003, 1982.

48. Fidler IJ, Kripke ML: Metastasis results from pre-existing variant cells within a malignant tumor. Science 197:893–895, 1977.

49. Fidler IJ, Kripke ML: Tumor cell antigenicity, host immunity and cancer metastasis. Cancer Immunol Immunother 7:201–205, 1980.

50. Fidler IJ, Nicolson GL: Organ selectivity for implantation survival and growth of B16 melanoma variant tumor lines. J Natl Cancer Inst 57:1199–1202, 1976.

51. Fidler IJ, Poste G: The cellular heterogeneity of malignant neoplasms: Implications for adjuvant chemotherapy. Semin Oncol 12:207–221, 1985.

52. Fidler IJ, Talmadge JE: Evidence that intravenously derived murine pulmonary metastases can originate from the expansion of a single tumor cell. Cancer Res 46:5167–5171, 1986.

53. Fisher B, Bauer M, Margolese R: Five-year results of a randomized clinical trial comparing total mastectomy and segmental mastectomy with or without radiation in the treatment of breast cancer. N Engl J Med 312:665–673, 1985.

54. Fisher B, Redmond C, Fisher E, Bauer M, Wolmark N, Wickermen L, Deutsch M, Montague E, Margolese R, Foster R: Ten-year results of a randomized clinical trial comparing radical mastectomy and total mastectomy with or without radiation. N Engl J Med 312:674–681, 1985.

55. Fisher B, Wolmark N: New concepts in the management of primary breast cancer. Cancer 36:627–632, 1975.

56. Fletcher GH, Jesse RH: The place of irradiation in the management of the primary lesion in head and neck cancers. Cancer 39:862–867, 1977.

57. Folkman J: Angiogenesis: initiation and modulation. *In* Nicolson GL, Milas L (eds): Cancer Invasion and Metastasis: Biologic and Therapeutic Aspects. New York, Raven Press, 1984, pp 201–209.

58. Folkman J: How is blood vessel growth regulated in normal and neoplastic tissue? GHA Clowes Memorial Award Lecture. Cancer Res 46:467–473, 1986.

59. Folkman J, Klagsburn M: Angiogenic factors. Science 235:444–447, 1987.

60. Foulds L: Neoplastic Development, vol 1. London, Academic Press, 1969.

61. Foulds L: Neoplastic Development, vol 2. London, Academic Press, 1975.

62. Frost P, Kerbel RS: Immunology of metastasis: can the immune response cope with disseminated tumor? Cancer Metastasis Rev 2:239–256, 1983.

63. Frost P, Kerbel RS: On the possible epigenetic mechanism(s) of tumor cell heterogeneity. Cancer Metastasis Rev 2:375–378, 1983.

64. Fugmann RA, Anderson JC, Stoli R, Martin DS: Comparison of adjuvant chemotherapeutic activity against primary and metastatic spontaneous murine tumors. Cancer Res 37:496–500, 1977.

65. Gabbert H: Mechanisms of tumor invasion: evidence from *in vivo* observations. Cancer Metastasis Rev 4:283–310, 1985.

66. Gasic GJ: Role of plasma, platelets and endothelial cells in tumor metastasis. Cancer Metastasis Rev 3:99–114, 1984.

67. Giorgio P, Cavaliere R, Bigotti A, Nicotra MR, Russo C, Ng AK, Giacomini P, Ferrone S: Antigenic heterogeneity of surgically removed primary and autologous metastatic human melanoma lesions. J Immunol 130:1462–1466, 1983.

68. Gold DV, Shochat D, Primus FJ, Dexter DL, Calabresi P, Goldenberg DM: Differential expression of tumor-associated antigens in human colon carcinomas xenografted into nude mice. J Natl Cancer Inst 71:117–124, 1983.

69. Hart IR: "Seed and soil" revisited: mechanisms of site-specific metastasis. Cancer Metastasis Rev 1:5–17, 1982.

70. Hart IR, Fidler IJ: Role of organ selectivity in the determination of metastatic patterns of B16 melanoma. Cancer Res 41:1281–1287, 1981.

71. Heppner G: Tumor heterogeneity. Cancer 214:2259, 1984.

72. Heppner GH, Miller BE: Tumor heterogeneity: biological implications and therapeutic consequences. Cancer Metastasis Rev 2:5–25, 1983.

73. Heppner GH, Miller BE, Miller FR: Tumor subpopulation interactions in neoplasms. Biochim Biophys Acta 695:215–226, 1984.

74. Hill RP, Chambers AF, Ling V: Dynamic heterogeneity: rapid generation of metastatic variants in mouse B16 melanoma cells. Science 224:998–1001, 1984.

75. Hockey MS, Stokes HJ, Thompson H, Woodhouse CS, Macdonald F, Fielding JWL, Ford CHJ: Carcinoembryonic antigen (CEA) expression and heterogeneity in primary and autologous metastatic gastric tumours demonstrated by a monoclonal antibody. Br J Cancer 49:129–133, 1984.

76. Hoover HC, Ketcham AS, Millar RC, Gralnick HR: Osteosarcoma: improved survival with anticoagulation and amputation. Cancer 41:2475–2480, 1978.

77. Horak E, Darling DL, Tarin D: Analysis of organ-specific effects on metastatic tumor formation by studies *in vitro*. J Natl Cancer Inst 76:913–922, 1986.

78. Houck JC, Hennings H: Chalones. Specific endogenous mitotic inhibitors. FEBS Lett 32:1–8, 1973.

79. Hu F, Wang RY, Hsu TC: Clonal origin of metastasis in B-16 murine melanoma: a cytogenetic study. J Natl Cancer Inst 78:155–163, 1987.

80. Hujanen ES, Terranova VP: Migration of tumor cells to organ-derived chemoalteractants. Cancer Res 45:3517–3521, 1985.

81. Ioachim HL, Pearse A, Keller SE: Role of immune mechanisms in metastatic patterns of hemopoietic tumors in rats. Cancer Res 36:2854–2862, 1976.

82. Jones PA, DeClerck YA: Extracellular matrix destruction by invasive tumor cells. Cancer Metastasis Rev 4:289–319, 1982.

83. Kendall WS, Frost P: Metastatic potential and spontaneous mutation rates: Studies with two murine cell lines and their recently induced metastatic variants. Cancer Res 46:6131–6135, 1986.

84. Kramer RH, Gonzalez R, Nicolson GL: Metastatic cells adhere preferentially to extracellular matrix of vascular endothelial cells. Int J Cancer 26:639–645, 1980.

85. Liotta LA: Tumor invasion and metastases—role of the extracellular matrix. Rhoads memorial award lecture. Cancer Res 46:1–7, 1986.

86. Liotta LA, Rao CN, Barsky SH: Tumor invasion and the extracellular matrix. Lab Invest 49:636–649, 1983.

87. Luria SE, Delbruck M: Mutations of bacteria from virus sensitivity to virus resistance. Genetics 28:491–511, 1943.

88. Mareel MM: Invasion in vitro: methods of analysis. Cancer Metastasis Rev 2:201–219, 1983.

89. McCune GS, Schapira DV, Henshaw EC: Specific immunotherapy of advanced renal carcinoma. Evidence for the polyclonality of metastases. Cancer 47:1984–1987, 1981.

90. Miller BE, Miller FR, Leith J, Heppner GH: Growth interaction in vivo between tumor subpopulations derived from a single mouse mammary tumor. Cancer Res 40:3977–3981, 1980.

91. Miller FR: Intratumor immunologic heterogeneity. Cancer Metastasis Rev 1:319–335, 1982.

92. Miller FR: Tumor subpopulation interactions in metastasis. Invasion Metastasis 3:234–242, 1983.

93. Miner KM, Kawaguchi T, Uba GW, et al: Clonal drift of cell surface, melanogenic and experimental metastatic properties in in vivo-selected, brain meninges-colonizing murine B16 melanoma. Cancer Res 42:4631–4638, 1982.

94. Morstyn G, Russo A, Carney DN, Karawya E, Wilson SH, Mitchell JB: Heterogeneity in the radiation survival curves and biochemical properties of human lung cancer cell lines. J Natl Cancer Inst 73:801–807, 1984.

95. Nakajima M, Irimura T, Di Ferrante DT, Di Ferrante N, Nicolson GL: Heparan sulfate degradation correlates with tumor invasive and metastatic properties of B16 melanoma sublines. Science 220:611–613, 1983.

96. Nakajima M, Irimura T, Nicolson GL: Heparanases and tumor metastasis. J Cell Biochem 36:157–167, 1988.

97. Nakajima M, Welch DR, Belloni PN, Nicolson GL: Degradation of basement membrane type IV collagen and lung subendothelial matrix by rat mammary adenocarcinoma cell clones of differing metastatic potentials. Cancer Res 47:4869–4876, 1987.

98. Neri A, Nicolson GL: Phenotypic drift of metastatic and cell surface properties of mammary adenocarcinoma cell clones during growth in vitro. Int J Cancer 28:731–738, 1981.

99. Nicolson GL: Metastatic tumor cell attachment and invasion assay utilizing vascular endothelial cell monolayer. J Histochem Cytochem 30:214–220, 1982.

100. Nicolson GL: Organ colonization and the cell surface properties of malignant cells. Biochim Biophys Acta 695:113–176, 1982.

101. Nicolson GL: Generation of phenotypic diversity and progression in metastatic tumors. Cancer Metastasis Rev 3:25–42, 1984.

102. Nicolson GL: Tumor cell instability, diversification, and progression to the metastatic phenotype: from oncogene to oncofetal expression. Cancer Res 47:1473–1487, 1987.

103. Nicolson GL, Dulski KM: Organ specificity of metastatic tumor colonization is related to organ-selective growth properties of malignant cells. Int J Cancer 38:289–294, 1986.

104. Nicolson GL, Dulski K, Basson C, Welch DR: Preferential organ attachment and invasion *in vitro* by B16 melanoma cells selected for differing metastatic colonization and invasive properties. Invasion Metastasis 5:144–158, 1985.

105. Nicolson GL, Fidler IJ, Poste G: The effects of tertiary amine local anesthetics on the blood-borne implantation and cell surface properties of metastatic melanoma cells. J Natl Cancer Inst 76:511–519, 1986.

106. Nicolson GL, La Biche RA, Frazier ML, Blick M, Tressler RJ, Irimura T, Rotter V: Differential expression of metastasis-associated cell surface glycoproteins and mRNA in a murine large cell lymphoma. J Cell Biochem 31:305–312, 1986.

107. Nicolson GL, Lembo TM, Welch DR: Growth of rat mammary adenocarcinoma cells in semisolid clonogenic medium not correlated with spontaneous metastatic behavior: heterogeneity in the metastatic, antigenic, enzymatic and drug sensitivity properties of cells from different sized colonies. Cancer Res 48:399–404, 1988.

108. Nicolson GL, Lotan R: Preventing diversification of malignant tumor cells during therapy. Clin Exp Metastasis 4:231–235, 1986.

109. Nicolson GL, Poste G: Tumor cell diversity and host responses

in cancer metastasis. I. Properties of metastatic cell. Curr Probl Cancer 6:4–83, 1982.

110. Nicolson GL, Van Pelt C, Irimura T, Kawaguchi T: Stabilities and characteristics of brain meninges-colonizing murine melanoma cells. Prog Exp Tumor Res 29:17–35, 1985.

111. North SM, Nicolson GL: Effect of host immune status on the spontaneous metastasis of clonal cell lines of the 13762NF rat mammary adenocarcinoma. Br J Cancer 52:747–755, 1985.

112. North SM, Nicolson GL: Heterogeneity in the sensitivities of 13762NF rat mammary adenocarcinoma cells to cytolysis mediated by extra- and intratumoral macrophages. Cancer Res 45:1453–1458, 1985.

113. Nowell PC: The clonal evolution of tumor cell populations. Science 194:23–28, 1976.

114. Nowell PC: Tumor progression and clonal evolution. The role of genetic instability. *In* German J (ed): Chromosome Mutation and Neoplasia. New York, Alan R Liss, 1983, pp 413–432.

115. Oldham RK: Biologicals and biological response modifiers: design of clinical trials. J Biol Response Mod 4:117–128, 1985.

116. Olsson L: Phenotypic diversity in leukemic cell populations. Cancer Metastasis Rev 2:153–163, 1983.

117. Ootsuyama A, Tanaka K, Tanooka H: Evidence by cellular mosaicism for monoclonal metastasis of spontaneous mouse mammary tumors. J Natl Cancer Inst 78:1223–1227, 1987.

118. Paget S: The distribution of secondary growths in cancer of the breast. Lancet 1:571–573, 1889.

119. Pauli BU, Schwartz DE, Thonar EJM, Kuttner KE: Tumor invasion and host extracellular matrix. Cancer Metastasis Rev 2:129–153, 1983.

120. Peterson JA, Ceriani RL, Blank EW, Osvaldo L: Comparison of rates of phenotypic variability in surface antigen expression in normal and cancerous breast epithelial cells. Cancer Res 43:4291–4296, 1983.

121. Pimm MV, Embleton MJ, Baldwin RW: Multiple antigenic specificities within primary 3-methylcholanthrene-induced rat sarcomas and metastases. Int J Cancer 25:621–629, 1980.

122. Poste G: Pathogenesis of metastatic disease: implications for current therapy and for the development of new therapeutic strategies. Cancer Treat Rep 70:183–199, 1986.

123. Poste G, Doll J, Fidler IJ: Interactions among clonal subpopulations affect stability of the metastatic phenotype in polyclonal populations of B16 melanoma cells. Proc Natl Acad Sci USA 78:6226–6230, 1981.

124. Poste G, Fidler IJ: The pathogenesis of cancer metastasis. Nature 283:139–146, 1979.

125. Poste G, Greig R, Tzeng J, Koestler T, Corwin S: Interactions between tumor cell subpopulations in malignant tumors. *In* Nicolson GL, Milas L (eds): Cancer Invasion and Metastasis: Biologic and Therapeutic Aspects. New York, Raven Press, 1984, pp 223–249.

126. Poste G, Nicolson GL: Modification of the arrest of metastatic tumor cells in the microcirculation after treatment with plasma membrane vesicles from highly metastatic cells. Proc Natl Acad Sci USA 77:399–403, 1980.

127. Poste G, Tzeng J, Doll J, Greig R: Evolution of tumor cell heterogeneity during progressive growth of individual lung metastases. Proc Natl Acad Sci USA 79:6574–6578, 1982.

128. Prehn RT: Tumor progression and homeostasis. Adv Cancer Res 23:203–236, 1976.

129. Proctor JW: Rat sarcoma model supports both "soil and seed" and "mechanical" theories of metastatic spread. Br J Cancer 34:651–654, 1976.

130. Proctor JW, Auclair BG, Stokowski L: Endocrine factors and the growth and spread of B16 melanoma. J Natl Cancer Inst 57:1197–1198, 1976.

131. Reif A: Evidence for organ specificity of defense against tumors. *In* Water H (ed): The Handbook of Cancer Immunology, vol 1. New York, Garland STPM Press, 1978, pp 174–240.

132. Rosenberg S: Lymphokine-activated killer cells: a new approach to immunotherapy of cancer. J Natl Cancer Inst 75:595–603, 1985.

133. Slack NH, Bross JBJ: The influence of site of metastasis on tumor growth and response to chemotherapy. Br J Cancer 32:78–86, 1975.

134. Sloane BF, Honn KV: Cysteine proteinase and metastasis. Cancer Metastasis Rev 3:249–265, 1984.

135. Smith KA, Begg AC, Denekamp J: Differences in chemosensitivity between subcutaneous and pulmonary tumours. Eur J Cancer Clin Oncol 21:249–256, 1985.

136. Souter RG, Tarin D, Kettlewell MGW: Peritoneovenous shunts in the management of malignant ascites. Br J Surg 70:478–481, 1983.

137. Strauli P, Haemmerli O: The role of cancer cell motility in invasion. Cancer Metastasis Rev 3:127–143, 1984.

138. Suzuki M, Hori K, Abe I, Saito S, Sato H: A new approach to cancer chemotherapy: selective enhancement of tumor blood flow with angiotensin II. J Natl Cancer Inst 67:663–669, 1981.

139. Talmadge JE, Benedict K, Madsen J, Fidler IJ: The development of biological diversity and susceptibility to chemotherapy in cancer metastases. Cancer Res 44:3801–3805, 1984.

140. Talmadge JE, Wolman SR, Fidler IJ: Evidence for the clonal origin of spontaneous metastasis. Science 217:361–363, 1982.

141. Talmadge JE, Zbar B: Clonality of pulmonary metastases from the bladder 6 subline of the B16 melanoma studied by southern hybridization. J Natl Cancer Inst 78:315–320, 1987.

142. Tanigawa N, Mizuno Y, Hashimura T, Hondo K, Satomura K, Hikasa Y, Niwa O, Sugahara T, Yoshida O, Kern DH, Morton DL: Comparison of drug sensitivity among tumor cells within a tumor, between primary tumor and metastases, and between different metastases in the human tumor colony-forming assay. Cancer Res 44:2309–2312, 1984.

143. Tarin D, Price JE, Kettlewell MGW, Souter RG, Vass ACR, Crossley B: Clinicopathological observations on metastasis in man studied in patients treated with peritoneovenous shunts. Br Med J 288:749–751, 1984.

144. Tarin D, Price JE, Kettlewell MGW, Souter RG, Vass ACR, Crossley B: Mechanisms of human tumor metastasis studied in patients with peritoneovenous shunts. Cancer Res 44:3584–3592, 1984.

145. Terranova VP, Hujanen ES, Martin GR: Basement membrane and the invasive activity of metastatic tumor cells. J Natl Cancer Inst 77:311–316, 1986.

146. Trope C, Aspergen K, Kullander S, Astredt B: Heterogeneous response of disseminated human ovarian cancers to cytostasis *in vitro*. Acta Obstet Gynecol Scand 58:543–546, 1979.

147. Tsuruo T, Fidler IJ: Differences in drug sensitivity among tumor cells from parental tumors, selected variants, and spontaneous metastases. Cancer Res 41:3058–3064, 1981.

148. Updyke TV, Nicolson GL: Malignant melanoma lines selective *in vitro* for increased homotypic adhesion properties have increased experimental metastatic potential. Clin Exp Metastasis 4:231–235, 1986.

149. Volk T, Geiger B, Raz A: Motility and adhesive properties of high and low-metastatic murine neoplastic cells. Cancer Res 44:811–824, 1984.

150. Vollmers HP, Birchmeier W: Monoclonal antibodies inhibit the adhesion of mouse B16 melanoma cells *in vitro* and block lung metastasis *in vivo*. Proc Natl Acad Sci USA 80:3729–3733, 1983.

151. Vollmers HP, Birchmeier W: Monoclonal antibodies that prevent adhesion of B16 melanoma cells and reduce metastases in mice: cross reaction with human tumor cells. Proc Natl Acad Sci USA 80:6863–6867, 1983.

152. Warren BA: Origin and fate of blood-borne tumor emboli. Cancer Biol Rev 2:95–169, 1981.

153. Weber G: Key enzymes and tumor cell heterogeneity. Antibiot Chemother 28:53–61, 1980.

154. Weichselbaum RR, Dahlberg W, Little JB: Inherently radioresistant cells exist in some human tumors. Proc Natl Acad Sci USA 82:4732–4735, 1985.

155. Weiss L: Cancer cell traffic from the lungs to the liver: an example of metastatic inefficiency. Int J Cancer 25:385–392, 1980.

156. Weiss L: Principles of Metastasis. Orlando, Academic Press, 1985.

157. Weiss L: Metastatic inefficiency: causes and consequences. Cancer Rev 3:1–24, 1986.

158. Welch DR, Milas L, Tomasovic SP, Nicolson GL: Heterogeneous response and clonal drift of sensitivities of metastatic

13762NF mammary adenocarcinoma clones to γ-radiation *in vitro*. Cancer Res 43:6–10, 1983.

159. Wikstrand CJ, Grahmann FC, McComb RD, Bigner DD: Antigenic heterogeneity of human anaplastic gliomas and glioma-derived cell lines by monoclonal antibodies. J Neuropathol Exp Neurol 44:229–241, 1985.

160. Willis RA: The Spread of Tumors in the Human Body. London, Butterworth, 1972.

161. Wolman SR: Karyotypic progression in human tumors. Cancer Metastasis Rev 2:257–293, 1983.

162. Woolley DE: Collagenolytic mechanisms in tumor cell invasion. Cancer Metastasis Rev 3:361–372, 1984.

163. Yamashina K, Miller BE, Heppner GH: Macrophage-mediated induction of drug-resistant variants in a mouse mammary tumor cell line. Cancer Res 46:2396–2401, 1986.

164. Young SD, Hill RP: Dynamic heterogeneity. Isolation of murine tumor cell populations enriched for metastatic variants and quantification of unstable expression of the phenotype. Clin Exp Metastasis 4:153–176, 1986.

165. Yung WKA, Shapiro JR, Shapiro WR: Heterogeneous chemosensitivities of subpopulations of human glioma cells in culture. Cancer Res 42:992–998, 1982.

Chapter 22

EXAMINATION TECHNIQUES: ROLE OF THE PHYSICIAN AND PATIENT IN EVALUATING BREAST DISEASES

Francis E. Rosato, M.D. and Anne L. Rosenberg, M.D.

Breast cancer is now a curable disease, thanks to earlier diagnosis and the advances in surgical technique, chemotherapy, and radiation. Although the prognosis for earlier stages of breast cancer is excellent, all of the new developments have done little to change the survival rate in later stages of the disease. Several combined modality protocols show promise for those patients with locally advanced disease, but the main thrust in the treatment of breast cancer has been toward earlier diagnosis. The patient has a role in diagnosis by performing monthly breast self-examination, obtaining routine screening mammography, and seeing a physician for regular examinations.

DIAGNOSIS

The symptoms of breast disease are generally localized, often with obvious physical findings, because the breast is so easily accessible for both inspection and palpation. Although up to 50 percent of patients presenting with breast complaints have no evidence of breast pathology, 65 percent or more of all breast lumps are discovered by the patient.[15]

A lump in the breast is the most common presentation for a carcinoma of the breast, and is often an accidental discovery. Another presenting symptom is breast pain. Preece et al.[30] and River et al.[31] studied the significance of breast pain. Although the frequency they observed may be higher than that seen by others, most likely because of their interviewing techniques, they reported a 15 percent to 24 percent incidence of breast pain in patients with cancer versus five percent seen by Haagensen and the Yorkshire Group (Table 22–1). The pain associated with cancer is usually described as "sticking" or "stabbing" and is localized and nonradiating.

Other presenting symptoms of breast cancer that occur much less frequently include breast enlargement, nipple discharge or epithelial changes in the nipple, retraction or changes in breast contour, ulceration, erythema, an axillary mass, and rarely, back or bone pain.

Unfortunately, although women may recognize these symptoms, too many delay seeking medical attention. This delay may adversely affect their prognosis, and any means of shortening this delay may therefore mean treating more patients at an earlier stage. In his experience, Haagensen found that although this delay was somewhat shorter in the 1970s than in the 1950s, even in the 1970s only 50 percent of patients sought attention within 1 month, and after 1 year, 20 percent still had not sought the advice of a physician.[15] Although there are fewer of these patients available for evaluation, patients with Paget's disease delayed up to 120 weeks, probably because of the subtle physical findings.

The reasons for delay must be identified if we are to minimize this interval. There seem to be three groups of factors responsible for the delay: economic factors, lack of education, and psychological factors. The costs of medical attention are significant for the poor, those with inadequate insurance coverage, and those with other financial obligations. Many older women were not

Table 22–1. FREQUENCY OF INITIAL SYMPTOMS OF BREAST CARCINOMA REPORTED BY PATIENTS

Author and Year of Report	Harnett (1948)	Donegan (1967)	Yorkshire Group* (1983)	Haagensen† (1983)
Period Included in Report	1938–1939	1940–1958	1976–1981	1943–1980
Lump	77.4%	66.5%	76%	65.3%
Pain	10.0%	11.0%	5%	5.4%
Enlargement of the breast		1.0%		1.0%
Skin of breast retraction			1%	3.1%
Nipple flattening or retraction	2.0%	3.0%	4.0%	2.1%
Skin of breast ulceration				0.2%
Edema of skin of breast		1.0%		0%
Redness of skin of breast		1.0%		0.8%
Nipple discharge	2.2%	9.0%	2.0%	1.8%
Nipple itching				0.4%
Redness and thickening of the epithelium of the nipple				0.1%
Nipple crusting and erosion	2.7%	2.0%		1.1%
Axillary tumor	0.8%		1.0%	2.0%
No symptoms—carcinoma found by previous examiner	1.6%			14.1%
Number of patients	2,529	774	1,205	2,198

*The Yorkshire report did not include patients with Paget's carcinoma.

†During the last 13 years carcinoma was found by mammograms in 10 patients who had not had any symptoms of breast disease. (From Haagensen CD: Diseases of the Breast. Philadelphia, WB Saunders, 1986, p. 502.)

taught to recognize the significance of a breast mass or the other presenting symptoms, since few books for the average person describe the physical characteristics of benign and malignant breast disease. Many women think that as long as pain is not present, there is nothing wrong. The most in-depth study about the psychological reasons for delaying diagnosis was done by Gold.[13] He identified six psychological causes for the delay in seeking medical attention:

1. Fear of cancer, mutilation, or a change in the relationship with the husband.
2. Shyness or false modesty regarding examination of the breast.
3. Negativism; some women raised in a hostile environment may become introverted and delay attention until the process is advanced.
4. Depression, causing the woman to ignore her health.
5. Compulsion toward another goal so that all other aspects of one's life are ignored.
6. Lack of breast tactilism; in Gold's study, 47 percent of women never experienced emotional sensations associated with their breasts and tended to ignore them, and therefore were not likely to discover an abnormality.

Even when patients present with a specific complaint or abnormal physical finding, there may be a delay in diagnosis because of the physician; this incidence can be as high as 18 percent in some series.[16] A study in the 1950s by the American Institute of Public Opinion revealed that of women who saw a doctor and requested a complete physical examination, only 70 percent had their breasts examined. In addition, the physician often did not examine the breasts at the time of an examination for another problem. Also, the physician may be unable to palpate the abnormality discovered by the patient and therefore may dismiss her without the ap-

propriate follow-up. Only ten percent to 20 percent of all breast masses are initially diagnosed by the physician (Table 22–2) without the patient being aware of the abnormality. Therefore, an area that the patient feels is abnormal must be evaluated thoroughly. If the physician is unable to appreciate any lesion, the patient should return for reexamination in a few months. Physicians must be educated about the cyclic changes in the breasts caused by the menstrual cycle and exogenous hormones. Engorgement, fullness, and increased sensitivity, seen especially in the upper outer quadrants, may be persistent and asymmetrical. Exogenous estrogens taken after menopause often cause the reappearance of cysts, breast tenderness, and fullness. Patients should be reexamined 5 to 8 days after the onset of the menstrual cycle or about 1 week after exogenous hormones have been discontinued.

HISTORY

Each physician examining a patient should take advantage of the accessibility of the breast for examination

Table 22–2. SUMMARY OF THOMAS JEFFERSON UNIVERSITY HOSPITAL EXPERIENCE IN 100 CASES AND EXPERIENCE IN A MUCH LARGER SAMPLE COMPILED BY THE AMERICAN COLLEGE OF SURGEONS

Tumor Discovered By	TJUH		All Hospitals	
	Number	%	Number	%
Patient	64	64.0	13,945	70.3
Physician	14	14.0	4128	20.8
Mammography	12	12.0	875	4.4
Not reported	10	10.0	893	4.5

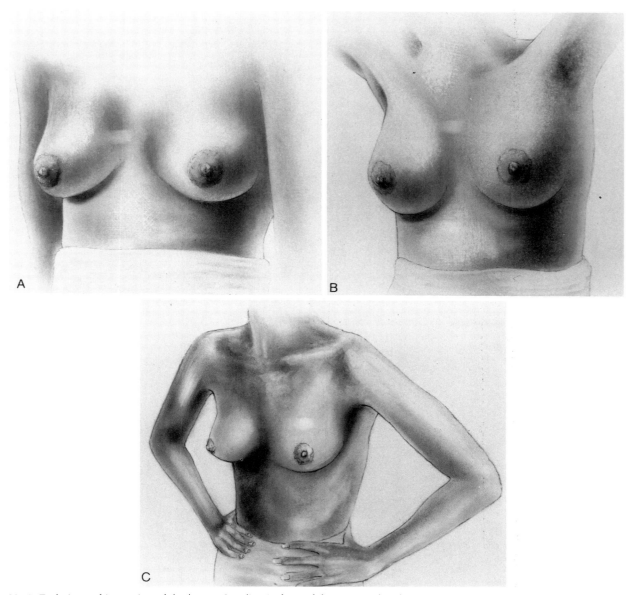

Figure 22–1. Technique of inspection of the breast. Standing in front of the patient, the physician should inspect the patient with her arms at the sides *(A)*; arms straight up in the air *(B)*; and hands on hips *(C)*.

and should learn to recognize signs of breast disease. A thorough history should be part of every evaluation. In addition to symptomatology, it is important to note the menstrual history (onset, regularity, menopause, gynecological surgery), reproductive history (number, times, problems with delivery or conception), the use of hormones, a family history of breast cancer, and a personal history of breast cancer or breast disease. The history and physical examination are critical to differentiating between benign and malignant breast pathology. Of all patients presenting with breast symptomatology, only about 20 percent have carcinoma. The majority (50 percent) have no evidence of intrinsic breast disease, 20 percent have evidence of cystic disease, and most of the rest have fibroadenomas.

PHYSICAL EXAMINATION

The American Cancer Society has outlined recommendations for the frequency of physical examinations by a physician: for women younger than 40 years, one examination every 3 years, and after 40, every year.

The technique of examination of the breast should include inspection and palpation of the entire breast and lymph node–bearing areas. The physician, standing in front of the patient, should first inspect the breasts with the patient's arms by her sides [Fig. 22–1*(A)*], with her arms straight up in the air [Fig. 22–1*(B)*], and with her hands on her hips with and without pectoral contraction (pressing in on the hips). [Fig. 22–1*(C)*]. The general shape, size, and symmetry of the breasts should be

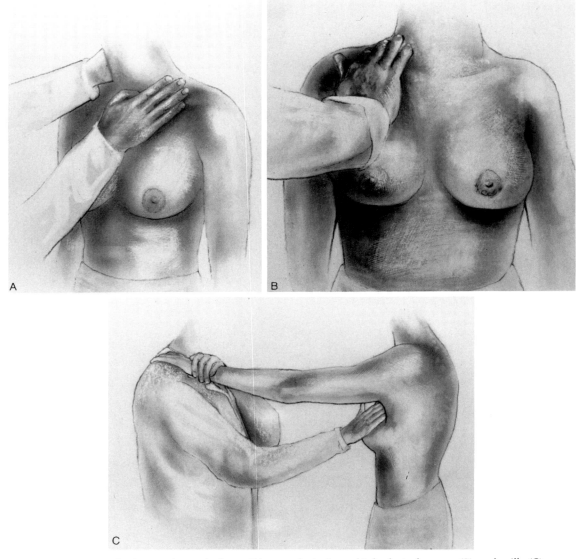

Figure 22–2. Technique of palpating the cervical area *(A)*; supraclavicular and infraclavicular areas *(B)*; and axilla *(C)*.

noted as well as any edema (peau d'orange), erythema, nipple inversion or change, and skin retraction. With the arms extended forward, the patient should then be asked to lean forward, once again to check for retraction. The node-bearing areas include the cervical area [Fig. 22–2(A)], the supra- and infraclavicular areas [Fig. 22–2(B)], and the axilla [Fig. 22–2(C)]. Each of these regions should be carefully palpated and any adenopathy noted. Any node that is firm and more than 5 mm in diameter should be suspect. The examination of the patient in the supine position is best performed with the benefit of a pillow under the shoulder on the side being examined (Fig. 22–3). This allows the breast to be flattened along the chest wall and facilitates palpation. The examiner should gently palpate the breast from the ipsilateral side, making certain to examine the entire breast from the sternum to the clavicle, posteriorly to the latissimus, and inferiorly to the rectus sheath. Baby powder may help to allow the examining

fingers to glide over the breast without friction from the patient's skin. The exam is performed with the palmar fingers flat, never grasping or pinching. The breast can also be molded or cupped in the examiner's hand, once again to check for retraction. The nipple-areola complex should be carefully inspected for subtle changes in the epithelium, retroareolar masses, and nipple discharge.

An accurate record of any significant physical findings should be carefully documented. Many physicians use a written description incorporated in the progress notes. A diagram or photograph may be more objective and accurate in relating the findings. Photographs may be useful in following the progression or regression of advanced lesions that have skin changes that are difficult to describe. Diagrams [Fig. 22–4(A, B)] are quite useful to record the location of a mass or nodularity. The size, shape, consistency, mobility, and delineation of any palpable mass should be noted.

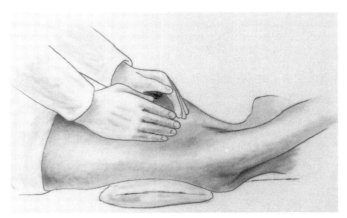

Figure 22–3. Palpation of the breast with the patient in the supine position.

DIAGNOSTIC TESTS

Having completed the history and physical examination, there are several noninvasive and invasive tests available for further evaluation of any suspected pathology.

Noninvasive Tests

Mammography

Mammography was used as early as 1913 by Salomon, a German surgeon, who radiographed 3000 operative specimens and described the radiographic abnormalities. Mammography has been used in the United States since the 1960s and has generated a wealth of literature. Several classic atlases have been published.[25, 42, 44] The techniques have been modified and improved using grids and compression to produce better image quality (see Chapter 24).

In addition to providing films that are more easily read, the change from xeromammography to film screen mammography was accompanied by reduction to a minimal radiation dose. Mammography utilizing a low-dose film/screen technique delivers as low as 0.1 rad per study.[4, 27] By comparison, a chest roentgenogram delivers 0.025 rads per study. Based on the observation that women exposed to high doses of radiation could develop breast cancers, investigators speculated as to the risk associated with mammography. There have been no cases reported of breast cancer developing as a consequence of screening mammography, and the benefit of detecting a small cancer, which is often curable with current therapeutic modalities, far outweighs any theoretical risk.[6, 7] According to Feig:

This risk estimate of 3.5 cancers per million women per year per rad means that if one million women aged 30 or older each received a mean breast dose of one rad there would, after a minimal latent period of 10 years, be an excess incidence of 3.5 cancers each year in the population. Examination with current low-dose technique (mean breast dose of 0.3 rad for a two view study) would carry a hypothetical risk of about one excess cancer case per year per million women examined. If

there were a 50 percent breast cancer mortality, the hypothetical risk would be one excess death per two million women examined. This level of risk (hypothetical), one death per two million women per year, is extremely small and can be equated with the following: 200 miles travelled by air, 30 miles travelled by car, smoking one half of one cigarette, 3/4 of a minute of mountain climbing, and ten minutes of being a man aged 60.[6]

Despite the fact that the majority of physicians agree that mammography is an effective screening tool, only eight percent to 15 percent of asymptomatic women have this study as part of a routine annual evaluation. In fact, only 15 percent to 20 percent of women older than 50 years have ever had a mammogram.[20] Data from the Health Insurance Plan and Breast Cancer Detection Demonstration Project studies suggest that mammography (with physical examination) was effective in diagnosing nonpalpable lesions, with a survival advantage resulting from the earlier stage at detection.[1, 20, 39]

There are indications for mammography in both a screening and diagnostic setting. Patients with tumors

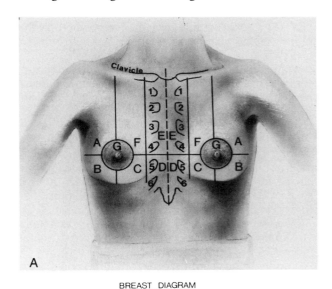

BREAST DIAGRAM

PATIENT:_____ DATE:_____

AGE:_____ MED REC NO:_____

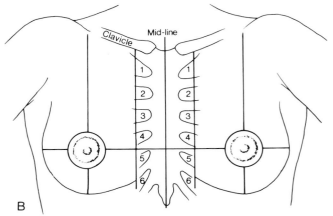

Figure 22–4. A and B, Diagrams of the breast to record location of a mass or nodulation.

or areas of asymmetry, nipple discharge, skin retraction or axillary adenopathy should be evaluated by mammography. It is not very useful in the teenage group because of the density of the breast but is indicated if a malignant process is suspected. The false-negative rate is about ten percent to 15 percent, and therefore the physician must be vigilant with the physical examination and not make a therapeutic decision based entirely on a negative mammogram.

All patients with a history of lobular neoplasia or carcinoma of the breast, a family history of carcinoma of the breast, intraductal papillomatosis, or gross cystic disease should have mammography at routine intervals. In addition, the American Cancer Society and American College of Radiology have outlined recommendations regarding screening mammography for asymptomatic women: for those between the ages of 35 and 39, a baseline study should be obtained; for women 40 to 49, studies should be obtained every 12 to 24 months; and for those older than 50, annual mammography is recommended. The National Institutes of Health recommends that these guidelines be applied to women younger than 50 years who are in high-risk groups (i.e., with personal or family histories of breast carcinoma). For women older than 50, they recommend annual screening. The American College of Obstetricians and Gynecologists recommends a baseline study in women between the ages of 35 and 50, followed by studies at intervals determined by the physician (Table 22–3).

Even with the general agreement that screening mammography can be beneficial in diagnosing smaller lesions, there are potential problems with the rapid institution of large-scale programs. As outlined by Hall,[18] these problems include the cost and availability of radiologists and facilities capable of producing high-quality, low-cost studies as well as the ability to interpret subtle findings and make recommendations for biopsy or follow-up.

Mammographic abnormalities that warrant further evaluation include masses, microcalcifications,[36] stellate densities or architectural distortion, and a "changing mammogram."[43] Biopsy specimens of these suspicious findings reveal carcinoma in 20 percent to 30 percent of cases, depending on the institution.[23, 24, 33]

Ultrasound

Ultrasound has been used since the early 1950s. It is most helpful and accurate[2] in the evaluation of the dense breast and in differentiating between cystic and solid masses.[29] The technique involves two parts: an automated whole breast section scanner and a hand-held real-time sector scanner. Unfortunately, masses that are smaller than 5 to 10 mm may not be visualized, and masses in fatty breasts are also difficult to visualize. Its advantages are that there is no radiation, and it is essentially painless.

Thermography

Thermography is mentioned for historical perspective, as it is no longer used in detecting breast lesions. Lawson[23a] first described the technique in a report in 1956. The technique takes advantage of temperature patterns in the breast set up by the natural infrared rays from tissues. It was hoped that this would be an ideal screening test, since it is painless and simple and a large number of patients can be studied in a short period of time. Unfortunately, it was not as sensitive as originally hoped, especially for deeper lesions.

Transillumination

Transillumination is not currently used but was described in the 1920s. It was an attempt to differentiate cystic and solid lesions using light transmitted through the breast.

CAT and MRI Scans

The use of computerized axial tomography (CAT) and magnetic resonance imaging (MRI) for the evaluation of breast disease is now being investigated. These techniques may play a role in evaluating the axilla, mediastinum, and supraclavicular areas for adenopathy and may aid in clinical staging of malignant processes.

Invasive Tests

Aspiration Cytology

Aspiration cytology involves using a fine needle (20-gauge or smaller) with a syringe to aspirate cells from a suspicious area, smear them on a glass slide, fix immediately to prevent air drying, and then stain for cytologic evaluation. If specimens are obtained correctly, this is extremely accurate (see section VIII, chapter 26 for a comprehensive review of fine-needle aspiration cytopathology techniques and results). However, specific

Table 22–3. MAMMOGRAPHY RECOMMENDATIONS FOR ASYMPTOMATIC WOMEN

	Recommended Interval by Age in Years		
Recommending Institution	*35–39*	*40–49*	*50 +*
American College of Radiology	Baseline	12–24 months	Annual
American Cancer Society	Baseline	12–24 months	Annual
NIH (high-risk patients only)	Baseline	12–24 months	Annual
American College of Obstetricians and Gynecologists	←————Baseline————→		Annual or as per M.D.

histological diagnosis may be impossible because of the inability to maintain architectural patterns with aspiration. Stereotactic techniques for sampling nonpalpable lesions have been described, although they are not commonly used in this country.[12, 28, 41] Another limitation with this technique is the inability to accurately determine estrogen and progesterone receptors on a specimen of such small size. Methods of determining receptor status on these specimens are being developed but are not uniformly available in surgical pathology laboratories.[37, 38]

Core Needle Biopsy

Needle biopsies using larger bore needles are rarely used. They are more invasive than needle aspiration with similar accuracy and inability to perform receptor determinations.

Open Biopsy

Excisional. Excisional biopsy refers to removal of all gross evidence of disease, usually with a small rim of normal breast tissue. It is important to plan all incisions carefully, in anticipation of the need for a subsequent surgical procedure should the lesion be malignant. Generally, it is preferable to use a circumareolar (incision G) or curvilinear incision (incisions A through I) along Langer's lines (Fig. 22–5). Most biopsies can be performed under local anesthesia on an outpatient basis with good patient acceptance and comfort. Frozen section may be performed, and a portion of the specimen can then be preserved for estrogen and progesterone receptor tests.

Incisional. For larger lesions not amenable to excisional biopsy, an incisional biopsy should be performed.

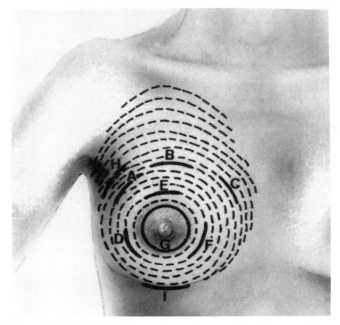

Figure 22–5. Excisional biopsy using a circumareolar (G) or curvilinear (A–I) incision parallel to Langer's lines.

This can also be performed under local anesthesia and on an outpatient basis without discomfort for the patient. Similar considerations for subsequent surgical procedures should be made when planning the incision. Usually 1 cc of tumor is required for receptor determination.

Needle-guided. Screening mammography is responsible for demonstrating many suspicious lesions before they are clinically apparent. The technique of needle localization was developed to permit biopsies to be performed by precisely removing the lesion without sacrificing normal surrounding breast tissue. The patient is taken to the mammography unit where, based on the original films, a needle is introduced into the breast and directed toward the lesion. Repeat mammography is then performed with the needle secured to confirm the proximity of the needle to the suspicious area. The needle can be left in place or replaced with a variety of hook wires[19, 21, 22, 24, 33,] and the patient is sent up to the operating room.

The surgeon then performs a biopsy of the area localized by the needle. The specimen should then be radiographed to confirm the presence of the abnormality. If the specimen does not contain the lesion, another piece of tissue should be submitted until the lesion has been removed (see section X, chapter 28).

Ultrasound-guided. For lesions that are nonpalpable but are visualized on ultrasound evaluation, ultrasound-guided biopsy may be used intraoperatively for localization. With the patient in the supine position, the breast is scanned using a hand-held transducer. The skin overlying the lesion is marked with a marking pencil, and then the biopsy is performed in the standard fashion. Covered by a sterile sheath, the transducer can also be introduced into the operating room to aid the surgeon in locating the lesion and also to confirm that the area has been excised by rescanning the area after the specimen has been removed. Cyst aspiration can also be performed under ultrasound guidance.[29]

Nipple Discharge Smear

After eliciting nipple discharge, the secretions can be smeared on a glass slide, fixed, and submitted for cytologic evaluation. These are often inaccurate, and the decision to perform a biopsy should therefore be based more on clinical evaluation than on cytologic evaluation of the smear.

Nipple Biopsy

Changes in the epithelium of the nipple, often associated with itching or nipple discharge, often warrant nipple biopsy. A wedge of the nipple-areolar complex can be excised under local anesthesia, reapproximating the edges with minimal deformity.

Galactography

Injection of contrast into one of the ducts through the orifice at the areola may demonstrate ductal ectasia,

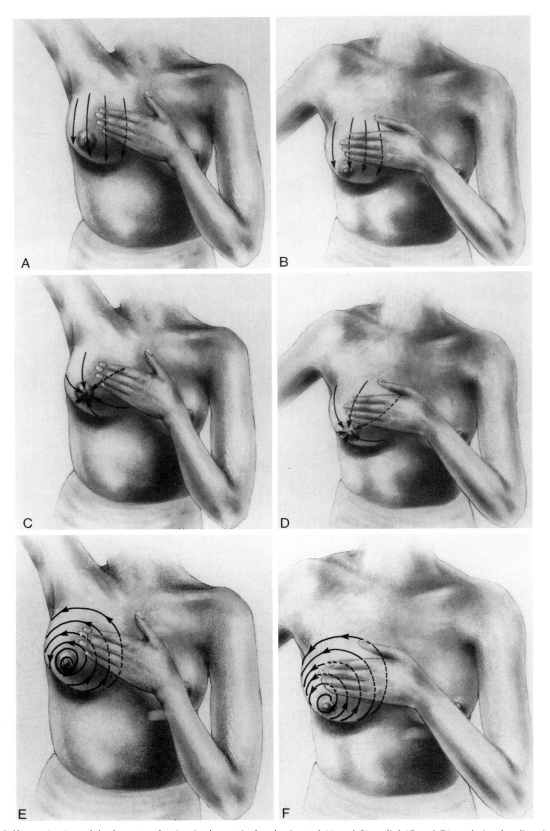

Figure 22–6. Self-examination of the breast; palpation in the vertical or horizontal *(A and B)*, radial *(C and D)*, and circular directions *(E and F)*.

obstruction, or a filling defect. This test is rarely used because it is time consuming and often painful and requires a repeat mammogram after the injection.

Pneumocystography

Pneumocystography, or injection of air into a cyst cavity after aspiration of the cyst, is another test that is rarely, if ever, used at the present time.

BREAST SELF-EXAMINATION

Since 70 percent to 80 percent of all breast masses are discovered by patients, even with regular examinations by a physician, breast self-examination may be a way to detect more cancers at an earlier and more treatable stage.[9, 34] Although Foster et al.[11] found an association between frequent breast self-examination and more favorable clinical stage of disease, the influence of this on survival was unclear. A report by Greenwald et al.[14] supports the fact that lesions discovered by breast self-examination tend to be smaller (by approximately 0.6 cm) than those found accidentally. Unfortunately, according to Foster and a Gallup Poll from 1973[45,] only 23 percent of women routinely examine their own breasts. Approximately 50 percent of women have never performed breast self-examination.

Breast self-examination has been advocated since 1949, when Haagensen[17] made a movie describing the technique for the American Cancer Society.

Technique

Breast self-examination is a three-step method: (1) inspection in front of a mirror with the arms by the sides, straight up in the air overhead, and on the hips, looking for changes in contour, skin color or texture, and nipple changes; (2) palpation in the shower; and (3) palpation in the supine position on a couch or bed, with a pillow under the shoulder on the side being examined.

Palpation can be done in several directions: horizontal or vertical [Fig. 22–6(A, B)], radial [Fig. 22–6(C, D)], or circular [Fig. 22–6(E, F)]. A study designed to evaluate the relative effectiveness of these three patterns determined that the vertical pattern was most thorough in examining the most breast tissue. Patients also need to be taught to discern a lump from "lumpiness."

Patients should start breast self-examination in their late 20s to early 30s and continue for the rest of their lives. The self-examination is best done 5 to 10 days after the onset of menses. Postmenopausal women should be instructed to do the examination on the same day of every month.

Despite all of the publicity about breast cancer and education about breast self-examination, only one fourth of women routinely perform breast self-examination. There is a need to disseminate information to increase participation of patients. There does seem to be a

positive effect on survival for tumors discovered by breast self-examination.[11] Most probably, this is related to the earlier stage of disease in patients performing routine examinations.[10, 11]

References

1. Baker LH: Breast Cancer Detection Demonstration Project: a five year summary report. CA 32:194–225, 1982.
2. Cole-Beuglet C, et al: Ultrasound mammography—a comparison with radiographic mammography. Radiology 139:693–698, 1981.
3. Dodd GP: Present status of thermography, ultrasound and mammography in breast cancer detection. Cancer 39:2796–2805, 1977.
4. Dodd GD: Mammography, state of the art. Cancer 53:652–657, 1984.
5. Feig SA: Low dose mammography, application to medical practice. JAMA 242:2107–2109, 1979.
6. Feig, SA: Assessment of the hypothetical risk from mammography and evaluation of the potential benefit. Radiol Clin North Am 21:173, 1983.
7. Feig SA: Radiation risk from mammography: is it clinically significant? Am J Radiol 143:469–475, 1984.
8. Feig SA, et al: Thermography, mammography and clinical examination in breast cancer screening. Review of 16,000 studies. Radiology 122:123–127, 1977.
9. Feldman JG: Breast self-examination, relationship to stage of breast cancer at diagnosis. Cancer 47:2740, 1981.
10. Foster RS, et al: Breast self-examination practices and breast cancer stage. New Engl J Med 299:265–270, 1978.
11. Foster RS, et al: Breast self-examination practices and breast cancer survival. Cancer 53:999–1005, 1984.
12. Gent HJ: Stereotaxic needle localization and cytological diagnosis of occult breast lesions. Ann Surg 204:580–584, 1986.
13. Gold MA: Causes of patients' delay in diseases of the breast. Cancer 17:564, 1964.
14. Greenwald P, et al: Estimated effect of breast self-examination and routine physician examinations on breast cancer mortality. New Engl J Med 299:271–273, 1978.
15. Haagensen CD: Diseases of the Breast. Philadelphia, WB Saunders, 1986, pp 502, 505, 574.
16. Haagensen CD: Breast Cancer: Risk and Detection. Philadelphia, WB Saunders, 1981, p 461.
17. Haagensen CD: Self-examination of the breasts. JAMA 149:356, 1952.
18. Hall FM: Screening mammography—potential problems on the horizon. N Engl J Med 314:53, 1986.
19. Herman G, et al: Percutaneous localization of nonpalpable breast lesions. Breast Dis Breast 9:4–6, 1983.
20. Howard J: Using mammography for cancer control: an unrealized potential. CA 37:33–48, 1987.
21. Kalisher L: An improved needle for localization of nonpalpable breast lesions. Radiology 128:815–817, 1978.
22. Kopans DB, et al: A modified needle-hookwire to simple preoperative localization of occult breast lesions. Radiology 134:781, 1980.
23. Landercasper J, et al: Needle localization and biopsy of nonpalpable lesions of the breast. Surg Gynocol Obstet 162:399–403, 1987.
23a. Lawson R: Implications of surface temperatures in the diagnosis of breast cancer. Can Med Assoc J 75:309–310, 1956.
24. Marrujo G, et al: Nonpalpable breast cancer: needle-localized biopsy for diagnosis and considerations for treatment. Am J Surg 151:599, 1986.
25. Martin JE: Atlas of Mammography: Histologic and Mammographic Correlations. Baltimore, Williams & Wilkins, 1982.
26. Moskowitz M, et al: Lack of efficacy of thermography as a screening tool for minimal and stage one breast cancer. N Engl J Med 295:249–252, 1976.
27. National Council on Radiation Precaution and Measurements: Mammography: a user's guide. Bethesda, 1986, pp 14–32.
28. Nordenstrom B, Azjicek J: Stereotaxic needle biopsy and preop-

erative indications of nonpalpable mammary lesions. Acta Cytol 21:350–351, 1977.

29. Pearce RB: Ultrasound, a useful adjunct to breast mammography. Diagn Imag, pp 114–119, September 1986.

30. Preece PE, et al: Importance of mastalgia in operable breast cancer. Br Med J 284:1299, 1982.

31. River L, et al: Carcinoma of the breast: the diagnostic significance of pain. Am J Surg 82:733, 1951.

32. Rosato FE, Thomas J, Rosato EF: Operative management of nonpalpable lesions detected by mammography. Surg Gynecol Obstet 137:491–493, 1973.

33. Rosenberg AL, et al: Clinically occult breast lesions: localization and significance. Radiology 162:167–170, 1987.

34. Saltzstein SL: Potential limitations of physical examination and breast self-examination in detecting small cancers of the breast. Cancer 54:1443, 1984.

35. Saunders KJ: Increased proficiency of search in breast self-examination. Cancer 58:2531–2537, 1986.

36. Sickles EA: Breast calcifications: mammographic evaluation. Radiology 160:289–293, 1986.

37. Silversward C, Humla SA: Estrogen receptor analysis on needle aspirates from human mammary cancer. Acta Cytol 24:54–57, 1980.

38. Silversward C, et al: Estrogen receptors—analysis on fine needle aspirates and on histologic biopsies from human breast cancer. Eur J Cancer 16:1351–1357, 1980.

39. Strax P, et al: Value of mammography in reduction of mortality from breast cancer in mass screening. Am J Roentgenol 117:686–689, 1973.

40. Strombeck JO, Rosato FE (eds): Surgery of the Breast. New York, Georg Thieme Publishers, 1986, p 39.

41. Svane G: Stereotaxic needle biopsy of nonpalpable breast lesions: a clinical and radiological follow-up. Acta Radiol Diag 24:385–390, 1983.

42. Tabar L, Dean P: Teaching Atlas of Mammography, ed 2. New York, Georg Thieme Publishers, 1985.

43. Wilhelm MC: The changing mammogram: a primary indication for needle localization biopsy. Arch Surg 121:1311–1314, 1986.

44. Wolfe JN: Xeroradiography of the Breast, ed 2. Springfield, IL, Charles C Thomas, 1983.

45. Women's Attitudes Regarding Breast Cancer: The Gallup Poll. Princeton, NJ, Gallup Organization, November 1973.

Chapter 23

SCREENING AND DETECTION

Anthony B. Miller, M.B.

In the absence of major advances in treatment, screening seems to have the most immediate potential for control of breast cancer, as there is a long delay before primary prevention of breast cancer could have a major impact.[30] Because of screening's potential importance in the control of breast cancer, many studies, including several large controlled trials, have been undertaken to evaluate the impact of screening. Although some of these have not yet reported results, the information available on the effectiveness of breast cancer screening is considerable, enabling some assessment of its impact on control of breast cancer. However, before presenting the results available from completed and ongoing studies, the problems and pitfalls in the evaluation of effectiveness of early detection will first be discussed.

In screening for breast cancer, the clinician is seeking the cancer as distinct from an identified precursor. However, as discussed later in this chapter, the available screening tests for breast cancer detect the cancer at a fairly late stage in its natural history. Because of this, it cannot be assumed that the "early" detection of a case of breast cancer by a screening test will be beneficial, even though such cases have a much better distribution of stage of disease than those diagnosed in the absence of screening.[36] Furthermore, it is not possible to base conclusions on effectiveness on better survival from the time of diagnosis than in a clinical series. This is because of four biases inseparable from screening for any cancer: lead time, length bias, (self) selection, and overdiagnosis bias.

Lead time is the amount of time the point of diagnosis has been advanced by the application of a screening test. Survival will inevitably be improved by at least this interval. Therefore, if survival of a group of screen-detected cases is compared with the survival of a group of cases diagnosed clinically, the comparison will be biased. Lead time will vary from case to case, depending on the rate of growth of that particular case and the time in relation to that case's natural history that the test was applied. When screening tests are applied in a population, therefore, there will be a range or distribution of lead times, ranging from a day to several years. Early estimates of lead time for breast cancer screening were a mean of about 1 year;[28] more recent estimates using more modern screening tests suggest longer periods, with distributions of up to 4 or more years, the mean lead time being shorter for younger than for older women.[48]

Length bias relates to the fact that fast-growing tumors will progress rapidly through the preclinical detectable phase of their natural history and will thus be less likely to be detected by screening tests applied relatively infrequently (e.g., annually or less frequently) than slow-growing tumors. Hence the tumors detected by screening tests will have a better prognosis than those not detected, possibly particularly those that present in the period just before screening is introduced and those that occur soon after a screening test has been applied.

Selection bias relates to the inevitable self-selection for attendance at breast screening programs. Various factors cause women to volunteer for screening. These include a perceived perception of increased risk for the disease (such as a positive family history) and some awareness of approaches they can take to improve their health care. These individuals may be more likely to present themselves promptly for treatment if they develop symptoms. In the absence of screening, therefore, their outcome is likely to be better than that of the general population. Part of this effect is offset by the self-selection of individuals with increased risk. It has been well documented that women who accept invitations to attend breast screening are at higher risk of developing breast cancer but at lower risk of dying of other causes than those who decline the invitations.[10]

Overdiagnosis bias results from the detection by screening of lesions of questionable malignancy that might never have been diagnosed in its absence. This has been a particular concern for some of the small or in situ cancers detected on mammography. Although it is clear that these lesions have a very good prognosis, it is not clear how many cancers that would otherwise result in death go through such a detectable phase. Furthermore, many, in the absence of screening, might never have progressed. Therefore the extent to which they should be actively sought by screening will probably only be determined by a controlled trial such as the one now ongoing in Canada.[32]

Because of these four biases, there is great difficulty in assessing the effectiveness of breast screening unless a control group is an integral part of the design of the study, with mortality (the number of deaths occurring in the population screened), rather than survival or case fatality, as the end point.[2]

It should be noted that surrogate measures that are known in the clinical situation to relate to outcome (e.g., distribution of cases by stage of disease, lymph node involvement, and size of tumor) are all influenced by the same biases. The measure closest to mortality is the rate or absolute number of cases of advanced disease occurring in the total population to whom screening is offered.[33] Evaluation of any approach to breast screening therefore has to be performed by a methodology that avoids these biases, such as in a controlled trial.

It is important to bear in mind the distinction between evaluation of screening tests for breast cancer and evaluation of screening programs. Screening tests are evaluated by their ability to detect cancer, using measures such as sensitivity (the proportion of people detected who have the disease), specificity (the proportion of people who do not have the disease regarded as negative), acceptability, and cost. Performance in a population is measured by a test's predictive value, both positive (the proportion of people with positive tests found to have disease) and negative (the proportion of people with negative tests found not to have disease). A screening program is not likely to be effective unless a good screening test as defined by these measures is used. Yet although good screening tests are necessary for a successful screening program, effectiveness in reducing mortality from breast cancer cannot be assumed from them; it has to be determined directly.

CLINICAL TRIALS OF BREAST CANCER SCREENING

Approaches for Evaluation of Screening

Because of the biases associated with the usually accepted clinical assessment measures, improvement in case survival or stage distribution cannot be accepted as sufficient evidence of effectiveness of screening, although they can both be anticipated in an effective program. Reduction in mortality from breast cancer (the preferred outcome) can best be demonstrated by randomized controlled trials.[36] These may be conducted to demonstrate either the efficacy of screening in individuals or the effectiveness of the program in a defined population.[21] The Canadian trial[32] is an *efficacy* trial designed to assess efficacy of screening in individuals who volunteer to participate in screening. The remaining trials discussed subsequently are *effectiveness* trials, based on defined populations, in which the randomization was to be invited to attend screening. This latter design more closely mirrors the situation if screening were to become part of routine cancer control, but there may be difficulty in assessing biological (explanatory) issues. The distinction will become clearer as the various trials are discussed.

Health Insurance Plan Study

The Health Insurance Plan (HIP) Study, based on contributors to the Health Insurance Plan (HIP) of Greater New York, was the first randomized controlled trial to evaluate screening for any site of cancer.[38, 39] The screening modalities evaluated were the combination of mammography, using the Eagan technique,[19] and phys-

ical examination of the breasts by skilled examiners. Sixty-two thousand women were included in the study and randomized to study or control groups by a pairwise allocation procedure. Of the 31,000 women allocated to the study group, 65 percent attended one or more of the four annual screening examinations scheduled. The investigators compared the outcome in the total study group to that in the control group, as they could not have identified within the control group those who would have refused screening if it had been offered to them. Hence a policy of inviting women to attend for screening was evaluated, and this can be regarded as an effectiveness trial within the defined population of HIP. All women received the routine care available in HIP. Follow-up was through HIP and other agencies. The wisdom of the controlled trial approach, and as a corollary the difficulty of evaluating screening without an appropriate control group, was emphasized when it became apparent that mortality from causes other than breast cancer was substantially lower in those who accepted the invitation to attend for screening than in the control group.[10] Indeed, the percentage reduction in mortality from breast cancer in those screened compared to the controls was less than the reduction in mortality from all causes other than breast cancer. This apparent paradox was resolved when it was appreciated that the women who accepted the invitation to attend for screening had a higher incidence of breast cancer than those who refused.[10] In assessing the results of this trial, many observers have tended to assume that the benefit obtained was largely a result of the use of mammography. This impression was heightened by the early reports of the trial, which showed much better survival in the cases detected on mammography alone than in those detected on physical examination alone or detected by both modalities. However, there was a differential lead time between those cases identified by mammography, those identified by physical examination, and those identified by both modalities. Such a differential confounds attempts to use survival as a measure of outcome in determining the relative contribution of the modalities used in screening programs.

Confining our attention therefore to comparisons of mortality between the study and control groups, two striking features emerged as a result of the analyses. The first was that although there were no differences between study and control groups in deaths from breast cancer in the first 2 years after initiating screening, a differential was seen beginning at 3 years and becoming maximal at 7 years.[40] Walter and Day[48] modeled the lead time distribution and found a best fit with an exponential distribution. This gave an estimate of a mean lead time of 1.7 years (20 months), with approximately 44 percent of cases having a duration less than 1 year and five percent with a duration of more than 5 years. It seems unlikely that cases with a much longer-than-average lead time, many of which were probably identified by mammography, could have contributed to an early mortality reduction. The implication is that screening for breast cancer improves the prognosis of cases detected somewhat late in their natural history.

One other observation supports the inference that the reduction in mortality was a result of the earlier detection of advanced disease. This is that the survival in the stage II (involved node) cases in the study group was better than the survival of those with the same stage in the control group. Thus the physical examination component of the screen probably made a contribution to the overall reduction in mortality. It has been calculated that this contribution might amount to as much as 70 percent of the mortality reduction.[6, 11]

The other striking aspect of the study was an initial apparent differential in effectiveness of screening at different ages. The initial analyses of the study related to breast cancer deaths in the first 5 years following entry. All the mortality reduction occurred in women older than 50 years, with no difference between the study and control groups in breast cancer deaths for women aged 40 to 49 years. However, after 14 years this had changed, and the lack of difference by age at entry has now been confirmed by the 18-year follow-up of the study.[41]

Habbema et al.,[27] in their analysis of the 14-year results of the study, have pointed to the lack of statistical heterogeneity of the results by 5-year age-at-entry groups. Furthermore, the number of person-years of life saved by screening is similar for women who entered the program in their forties or later. Nevertheless, the detailed 18-year results show clearly that the time of onset of beneficial effect varied by age.[41] Thus for women aged 50 to 59, a reduction in deaths from cancer occurred beginning at 3 years from entry and was significant by 5 years, though subsequently the absolute difference became less. For women aged 45 to 49, an effect was not seen until after 5 years, and for women aged 40 to 44, no effect was seen until after 8 years. This delay in seeing an effect of screening in women younger than 50 was unexpected but appears to be replicated in the results of other studies, as discussed in the following sections.

Kaiser Permanente Study

The use of mammography was evaluated as part of a controlled trial of multiphasic screening in the Kaiser Permanente Program in California in women aged 45 or more, with follow-up from 1964 to 1980.[14, 24] The results of this trial showed no mortality differential for breast cancer. Fourteen deaths from breast cancer were reported in each of the two groups when compared at 11 years, with 21 deaths in the study group and 24 in the control group at 16 years. Nevertheless, three fourths of the subjects were younger than 50 when the study began. Thus, although this study did not have sufficient power to refute the HIP findings, it reinforced the desirability of not extrapolating from the HIP findings without further study.

Swedish Trials

In Sweden three large trials of mammography alone have been in progress for some years; a fourth (in Stockholm) was started more recently. In two, single-view mammography is being used with control groups selected by randomization on a cluster sampling basis.[43] When single-view mammography is used alone, the oblique projection is the only view, an approach for which an adequate sensitivity is claimed.[29] The third project (in Malmö) uses two-view mammography and is based on randomization of individuals.[5] In this study it is known that the controls have access to mammography outside the screening center, and there is some concern over dilution. In the fourth study in Stockholm, randomization is also based on individuals, and single-view mammography is used.

Results have been reported on mortality from the first two trials using single-view mammography conducted in the counties of Kopparberg and Ostergotland. Two examinations of the population were planned at 35- to 36-month intervals during a 5-year period that commenced in 1977, but it proved possible to offer three screening rounds to younger women at an interval of about 21 months. A total of 162,981 women aged 40 or more who resided in the two counties were entered into the study. Participation by women aged 75 or older was less than 50 percent, and this group was excluded from the analysis. Among women aged 40 to 74 at the date of randomization, participation of those invited to screening was approximately 90 percent at the first screening round and only slightly lower at the second round. In this group, the estimate of relative risk of death from the two counties combined was 0.69 (95 percent confidence interval 0.51–0.92)[42] and, with an additional 2 years follow-up, 0.68.[16] However, no reduction in mortality in women aged 40 to 49 has been reported. In women aged 50 to 74 on entry, breast cancer mortality was 40 percent less in the screened group than in the control.

Mortality results from the Malmö trial show no significant benefit overall, but confirm a reduction in breast cancer mortality compatible with the other Swedish trials in women over age 55.[5a]

The Swedish results show that reduction in mortality from breast cancer can be achieved in women older than 50 by using mammography alone. However, they leave unanswered the question of the amount that mammography adds to the benefit of physical examination, and so far they provide no evidence of effectiveness in younger women. Whether this is a result of a relative lack of sensitivity of single-view mammography in younger women or just a function of a short follow-up period will eventually be determined by further follow-up.

United Kingdom Study

In the United Kingdom a geographically based quasi-experimental study is ongoing.[44] In two districts, population screening has been initiated; in two others, breast self-examination (BSE) teaching in clinics or groups is offered; and in four more, data are being gathered for comparative purposes, but no screening or BSE teaching offered. Women are recruited for screening by letters written to them from their family physicians after age-sex registers are created in the practices in the area. In both centers offering screening, mammography is done biennially, with one single-view and one two-view examination. Annual physical examinations are also offered. In one of the two screening districts, some of the practices have been randomized to a control group. Although response has approximated 70 percent in the screening centers, there was a lower response to invitations for breast self-examination teaching.[33] Mortality results have been reported.[44a] There is a significant reduction in breast cancer mortality in years 6 and 7 in the screening districts.

Canadian National Breast Screening Study

The Canadian National Breast Screening Study (NBSS) commenced in January, 1980,[34] with the following objectives:

1. To determine, in volunteers aged 40 to 49 on entry to the study, whether unselective annual screening by mammography and physical examination when used as an adjunct to the highest standard of care in the Canadian health care system reduces the mortality from breast cancer.

2. To determine, in volunteers aged 50 to 59 on entry to the study, the additional contribution of routine annual mammographic screening to screening by physical examination alone.

3. To assess whether an appropriate combination of risk factors for breast cancer can be derived to permit restricting screening to those at highest risk of the disease.

4. To provide the data necessary for an analysis of the cost effectiveness of breast cancer screening in Canada using current mammography techniques.

5. To provide data on the natural history of breast cancer for incorporation into computer simulation approaches to evaluate the optimum age at which screening should commence and its periodicity at different ages.

It was planned to recruit 90,000 women into the project, 50,000 aged 40 to 49 and 40,000 aged 50 to 59. This required 15 screening centers across the country with an individual recruitment target ranging from 1,000 to 15,000 women. Five screening examinations were originally planned to be conducted annually, but in order to set a termination date to the study, women recruited toward the end of the recruitment phase were offered only four annual screens, as in the HIP study. After cessation of screening, follow-up will be performed by computerized record linkage with the Canadian Cancer Incidence and Mortality files, and can therefore be continued indefinitely.[32]

Recruitment in the NBSS was completed in March, 1985, and screening was completed in May, 1988. A total of 89,968 women were allocated: 26,653 aged 40 to 44; 23,819 aged 45 to 49; 22,903 aged 50 to 54; and 16,593 aged 55 to 59. The detection rates by age on initial and repeat screening approximated those antici-

pated from other studies, though with slightly higher proportions of cancers detected on physical examination alone, possibly a reflection of more efficient physical examination.

DEMONSTRATION PROJECTS AND CASE-CONTROL STUDIES OF SCREENING

Breast Cancer Detection Demonstration Projects (BCDDP)

In 1973 the American Cancer Society initiated the concept of centers designed to assess the extent to which women would attend for breast cancer screening. This idea was taken up by the National Cancer Institute and eventually extended to include 28 centers in 27 cities throughout the United States. In each city 10,000 women between the ages of 35 and 74 were to be recruited. They were to provide information on risk factors for breast cancer and to be screened using physical examination, thermography, and mammography.

In their recruitment drives, the centers were eminently successful. Recruitment was facilitated by the publicity surrounding the development of breast cancer in the wives of the then president and vice president.

Unfortunately the program was not designed to evaluate the outcome in the women screened. Thus, in the absence of defined populations from which the women who volunteered for the projects were drawn and the lack of a suitable control group, it is not possible to determine effectiveness in terms of mortality reduction.[10]

An analysis of the cancers identified during the 5 years of the BCDDPs[9] confirmed that the detection ability of mammography in women younger than 50 was much improved over that in the HIP study, though it is possible that some of the apparent increased sensitivity of mammography compared to physical examination may have been a result of less efficient physical examinations.

The apparent improvement in the detection ability of mammography and the favorable stage distribution of the cancers detected led to the publication by the American Cancer Society of guidelines for mammography[1] that updated the Society's previous guidelines and those of the American College of Radiology.[4] These were again updated in 1983.[2] The difficulty with these guidelines is that they were based on assumptions about benefit using endpoints that are suggestive of but do not prove that mortality reduction can be attributed to mammography. This consideration led directly to the design of one of the components of the Canadian NBSS.

With hindsight, it seems clear that the BCDDP did not serve to advance the cause of breast cancer screening in the United States. This was largely caused by the concerns that arose from radiation risk from mammography,[6] concerns that with modern mammography now seem groundless.[15] Nevertheless, as a result of the controversy, many of the projects were terminated, and it required evidence from the continued follow-up of the

HIP study and the results from the trials in Europe to rectify the situation.

Five-year survival data have been published on all cancers detected in the BCDDP.[37] These show, both for women younger than 50 and for those older than 50, considerably better survival than for cancers diagnosed in the NCI Surveillance, Epidemiology, and End Results (SEER) program. The authors claimed that "there is no doubt of the very successful results of screening for breast cancer with mammography in younger as well as older woman."[37]

This claim can be criticized. First, although 1-year lead time was allowed for screen detected cancers, with modern mammography, lead times are much longer.[48] Second, and perhaps critically, no allowance was made for selection bias. The importance of this is shown by the fact that the survival of all breast cancers in the control groups in the NBSS (in women both older and younger than 50) is at least as good as that in the BCDDP. Even taking the BCDDP improved survival at face value, Eddy et al.[20] have concluded that screening women younger than 50 with mammography is not likely to be cost effective.

Studies in the Netherlands

Two screening projects were initiated in the Netherlands. In Utrecht, all women older than 50 on the population register were invited to attend a center at which they were offered mammography and physical examination. Mammography used the xeroradiographic process and was a standard two-view examination; physical examination was performed by the radiology technicians.[17] In Nijmegen, another city in the Netherlands, single-view (lateral) mammography was used alone in a similar population study. In this study women aged 35 and older were recruited. In both cities, approximately 70 percent of those invited attended, but after four screens, attendance fell to a little more than 50 percent.[33]

Initial results from both studies were derived using the case-control approach to analysis. In Utrecht, the breast cancer mortality among those presenting at least once for screening was 70 percent less than for those who refused (relative risk-0.30; 95 percent confidence interval 0.13–0.70).[13] In Nijmegen, a 52 percent reduction in risk of death was seen (relative risk = 0.48; 95 percent confidence interval 0.23–1.00).[46]

The case-control approach is a relatively new way of analyzing the results of screening[36] and is not as valid as a randomized controlled trial. Case-control studies essentially mimic the approach that would be taken in a cohort study, and questions have to be raised as to the comparability of the cases and controls. The analysis essentially compares the screening history in those who die of breast cancer with comparable people drawn from the source population who have not. In both cities, it was found that a higher proportion of those who died had not attended screening than had controls (i.e., more of the deaths included women who had refused to attend screening than controls).

In the Utrecht study, it was possible to show that the non-responders had similar breast cancer incidence and stage distribution to that seen immediately before screening started and in a control town,[13] so that little bias seemed to be operating in terms of incidence of breast cancer. Nevertheless, it is still possible that some selection bias in the factors that influence mortality from breast cancer may have been present. If unknown factors led to a higher probability of death from breast cancer in those who refused to enter the screening program than in those who accepted the invitation to be screened, then the result that was seen could have been anticipated.

Although the numbers of deaths were small when considered by age, both studies suggest different effects of screening by age. In Utrecht, a lower effect of screening was seen in women aged 50 to 59 than in older women, a reverse of the effect seen in the HIP study; so in practice, the Utrecht study provides most confirmation of the effectiveness of screening women aged 60 or more. In Nijmegen, in a further analysis using a different control group and including deaths up to 1982, those younger than 50 at first invitation to screening had no reduction in breast cancer mortality (relative risk-1.23; 95 percent confidence interval 0.31–4.81).[47]

Continued follow-up of mortality from breast cancer in the city of Utrecht among women in the birth cohorts invited for screening compared to similar women in 17 other cities in the Netherlands shows stability of breast cancer mortality in Utrecht, while in the 17 other cities, mortality is increasing (as would be expected as the cohorts age).[16] This is important confirmation of the validity of the conclusions derived from the case-control analysis.

Florence Study

Mass screening for breast cancer using conventional two-view mammography was started in Florence in 1970.[35] Women aged 40 to 70 years were invited by mail to attend. The average compliance on first invitation was 60 percent. The average interval between two consecutive screening rounds was 2.5 years. Results have now been assessed using the case-control approach. There were 57 deaths from breast cancer in women of eligible ages who were matched with 285 population controls. The ratio of death from breast cancer among screened women compared to that in women who had never been screened was 0.53 (95 percent confidence interval 0.29–0.95). The protective effect was almost completely restricted to women aged 50 and older.

THE WOMAN'S ROLE IN DETECTION/ DIAGNOSIS AND BREAST SELF-EXAMINATION

All the studies considered in the previous section (with the possible exception of that in Florence[35]) were either special research studies to determine the effectiveness of screening, or demonstration projects. If screening for breast cancer is going to make an important impact on prevention of mortality from breast cancer, the proportion of women receiving screening will have to increase substantially, as emphasized in the NCI's goals for the year 2000.[18]

To achieve this, a considerable investment in professional and public education will be required. Professional education is required because the Canadian National Breast Screening Study[7] and the American Cancer Society Surveys[3] have noted a reluctance of physicians either to perform breast physical examinations or to refer their patients for mammography. Public education (including women to request that their physicians refer them for screening) may help to overcome this, at least in part. Increased public education is, indeed, part of the program of both the American Cancer Society and the NCI and can be expected to increase substantially from now on.

In addition to compliance in screening, women have a potentially more direct role in detection and diagnosis through breast self-examination. As part of their educational approaches to the problem of cancer, the Cancer Societies of North America have provided information to the public on breast cancer in the hope that women will not delay seeing their physician if they find a lump in the breast. In addition, they have urged women to practice BSE on a regular basis in the hope that if a change does occur, the woman will detect it promptly. Neither the general public education messages nor BSE have ever been appropriately evaluated. Some investigators have evaluated the stage distribution of cases found on BSE,[23, 26] but for the reasons already discussed, it is impossible to equate these measures with eventual reduction in deaths from breast cancer. Cole and Austin[12] concluded that BSE may contribute more in situations in which women do not utilize other screening modalities, but this conclusion was based on a review of studies that used surrogate measures to assess outcome. On a worldwide basis, BSE may have more potential applicability than other screening tests for breast cancer, as it does not involve complex technology.[31] It is currently being evaluated in the study of breast screening in the United Kingdom,[44] in a randomized study based on cluster sampling in the USSR,[45] and in a cohort study of women enrolled in the MAMA program in Finland.[25] The Canadian Breast Screening Study has shown that reinforcement of training is necessary in order for an appreciable proportion of women to practice it well, even when initially taught on an individual basis.[8] Hence, costs associated with its use are not negligible, and it has been concluded that BSE cannot yet be advocated as public health policy until more information on its effectiveness is available.[31]

Nevertheless, all screening studies have shown that interval cancers occur between screens (approximately one per 1000 per year), and only BSE has the potential to reduce mortality from them. Studies in Vermont have produced suggestive evidence that women who perform BSE have lower mortality from breast cancer than those who do not,[22] and these studies also demonstrate that community-based BSE instruction programs are feasible. In the interim before the results of the BSE trials are available, it would seem appropriate to continue to advocate BSE, and for physicians to incorporate BSE instruction as a component of their clinical breast examination.

It is important to recognize that, even for women participating in a regular program of breast screening, BSE offers a potential advantage that may not be demonstrable, except in the context of a case-control study as planned for the Canadian NBSS. This advantage is the avoidance of false reassurance. It was partly for this reason that it was taught to all participants in the NBSS, and there is some evidence that this objective was secured.

CONCLUSION

There is clearly still some controversy as to whether breast cancer screening requires further evaluation or can be adopted as public policy. Many radiologists, especially in North America, are not prepared to abandon double-view mammography, and they are not able to offer the low-cost mass approach developed in Sweden or even in the NBSS in Canada. Perhaps the most important lesson to be derived from the experience of the past decade is that we are beyond the stage when large-scale population screening programs for cancer, or indeed any disease, can be introduced on the basis of assumed benefits. Benefits will have to be established in large-scale studies. The studies that are necessary to fully evaluate breast cancer screening are now in place, and the answers we need should be available by the end of the current decade.

In the meantime, it is clear that with consistent evidence of screening effectiveness in women older than 50, population policies for breast cancer screening can now be advocated. The project on screening of the International Union Against Cancer has concluded that "In countries where breast cancer is common and where the necessary resources are available, screening using mammography alone or mammography plus physical examination is applicable as public health policy."[15] However, we also noted that "The greatest initial benefit will occur in women age 50–69."

References

1. American Cancer Society: Mammography 1982. CA 32:226, 1982.
2. American Cancer Society: Mammography guidelines 1983: background statement and update of cancer-related check-up guidelines for breast cancer detection in asymptomatic women age 40 to 49. CA 33:255, 1983.
3. American Cancer Society: Survey of physicians' attitudes and practices in early cancer detection. CA 35:197, 1985.
4. American College of Radiology: Board approves mammography policy, summary of current opinion. Bull Am Coll Radiol 32:1, 1976.
5. Andersen I, Andren L, Hildell J, Linell F, Ljungqvist U, Pettersson H: Breast cancer screening with mammography. A popu-

lation-based, randomized trial with mammography as the only screening mode. Radiology 132:273, 1979.

5a. Andersson I, Aspegren K, Janzon L, Landberg T, Lindholm K, Linell F, Ljungberg O, Ranstam J, Sigfusson B: Mammographic screening and mortality from breast cancer: The Malmö mammographic screening trial. Br Med J 297:943, 1988.

6. Bailar JC: Mammography: a contrary view. Ann Intern Med 84:77, 1976.

7. Baines CJ: Impediments to recruitment in the Canadian National Breast Screening Study: response and resolution. Controlled Clin Trials 5:129, 1984.

8. Baines CJ, Wall C, Risch HA, Kuin JK, Fair IJ: Changes in breast self-examination behaviour in a cohort of 8214 women in the Canadian National Breast Screening Study. Cancer 57:1209–1216, 1986.

9. Baker LH: Breast cancer detection demonstration project: five-year summary report. CA 32:194, 1982.

10. Beahrs O, Shapiro S, Smart C: Report of the Working Group to Review the National Cancer Institute American Cancer Society Breast Cancer Detection Demonstration Projects. J Natl Cancer Inst 62:640, 1979.

11. Breslow L, Thomas LB, Upton AC: Final reports of the National Cancer Institute ad hoc working groups on mammography in screening for breast cancer and summary report of their joint findings and recommendations. J Natl Cancer Inst 59:467, 1977.

12. Cole P, Austin H: Breast self-examination: an adjuvant to early cancer detection. Am J Public Health 71:572, 1981.

13. Collette HJA, Day NE, Rombach JJ, et al: Evaluation of screening for breast cancer in a non-randomized study (the DOM project) by means of a case-control study. Lancet 1:1224, 1984.

14. Dales LG, Friedman GD, Collen MF: Evaluating periodic multiphasic health check-ups: a controlled trial. J Chronic Dis 32:385, 1979.

15. Day NE, Baines CJ, Chamberlain J, Hakama M, Miller AB, Prorok PC: UICC project on screening for cancer: report of the workshop on screening for breast cancer. Int J Cancer 38:303–308, 1986.

16. Day NE, Chamberlain J: Screening for breast cancer: workshop report. Eur J Cancer Clin Oncol 24:55, 1988.

17. de Waard F, Collette HJA, Rombach JJ, Baanders-van Halewijn EA and Honing C: The Dom project for the early detection of breast cancer, Utrecht, the Netherlands. J Chronic Dis 37:1, 1984.

18. Division of Cancer Prevention and Control: Cancer control objectives for the nation 1985–2000. NCI Monogr, number 2, 1986.

19. Eagan RL: Mammography. Springfield, IL, Charles C Thomas, 1964.

20. Eddy DM, Hasselblad V, McGivney W, Hendee W: The value of mammography screening in women under age 50 years. JAMA 259:1512, 1988.

21. Flay BR: Efficacy and effectiveness trials (and other phases of research) in the development of health promotion programs. Prevent Med 15:451–474, 1986.

22. Foster RS, Costanza MC: Breast self-examination practices and breast cancer survival. Cancer 53:999–1005, 1984.

23. Foster RS, Lang SP, Costanza MC, et al: Breast self-examination practices and breast cancer stage. New Engl J Med 299:265, 1978.

24. Friedman GD, Collen MF, Fireman BH: Multiphasic health check-up evaluation: a 16-year follow-up. J Chronic Dis 39:453, 1986.

25. Gastrin G: Breast Cancer Control. Stockholm, Almqvist and Wiksell International, 1981.

26. Greenwald P, Nasca PC, Lawrence CE, et al: Estimated effect of breast self-examination and routine physician examinations on breast-cancer mortality. New Engl J Med 299;271, 1978.

27. Habbema JDF, van Oortmarssen GJ, van Putten DJ, Lubbe JT, van der Maas PJ: Age specific reduction in breast cancer mortality by screening: an analysis of the results of the Health Insurance Plan of greater New York study. J National Cancer Inst 77:317–320, 1986.

28. Hutchison GB, Shapiro S: Lead time gained by diagnostic screening for breast cancer. J Natl Cancer Inst 41:665, 1968.

29. Lundgren B: Efficiency of single-view mammography: rate of interval cancer cases. J Natl Cancer Inst 62:799, 1979.

30. Miller AB: Approaches to the control of breast cancer. In Rich M, Hager JC, Furmanski P (eds): Understanding Breast Cancer: Clinical and Laboratory Concepts. New York, Marcel Dekker, 1983, pp 3–25.

31. Miller AB, Chamberlain J, Tschckovski M: Self-examination in the early detection of breast cancer. A review of the evidence, with recommendations for further research. J Chronic Dis 38:527, 1985.

32. Miller AB, Howe GR, Wall C: The national study of breast cancer screening. Clin Invest Med 4:227, 1981.

33. Miller AB, Van Slooten EA: Screening and diagnosis in breast cancer; workshop report. Eur J Cancer Clin Oncol 19:1711, 1983.

34. National Cancer Institute of Canada: National breast-cancer screening study gets underway. Can Med Assoc J 122:243, 1980.

35. Palli D, del Turco MR, Buiatti E, Carli S, Ciatto S, Toscani L, Maltoni G: A case control study of the efficacy of a non-randomized breast cancer screening program in Florence (Italy). Int J Cancer 38:501–504, 1986.

36. Prorok PC, Chamberlain J, Day NE, et al: UICC workshop on the evaluation of screening programmes for cancer. Int J Cancer 34:1, 1984.

37. Seidman H, Gelb SK, Silverberg E, LaVerda N, Lubera JA: Survival experience in the breast cancer detection demonstration project. CA 37:258, 1987.

38. Shapiro S: Evidence on screening for breast cancer from a randomized trial. Cancer 39:2772, 1977.

39. Shapiro S, Strax P, Venet L, et al: Changes in 5-year breast cancer mortality in a breast cancer screening program. Seventh National Cancer Conference Proceedings, American Cancer Society, January, 1974, pp 663–678.

40. Shapiro S, Venet W, Strax P, et al: Ten to fourteen-year effects of screening on breast cancer mortality. J Natl Cancer Inst 69:349, 1982.

41. Shapiro S, Venet W, Strax P, Venet L: Current results of the breast cancer screening randomized trial: the Health Insurance Plan (HIP) of greater New York study. In Day NE, Miller AB (eds): Screening for Breast Cancer. Toronto, Hans Huber, 1988, pp 3–15.

42. Tabar L, Fagerberg CJG, Gad A, et al. Reduction in mortality from breast cancer after mass screening with mammography. Randomized trial from the breast cancer screening working group of the Swedish National Board of Health and Welfare. Lancet 1:829, 1985.

43. Tabar L, Gad A: Screening for breast cancer: the Swedish trial. Radiology 138:219, 1981.

44. UK Trial of Early Detection of Breast Cancer Group: Trial of early detection of breast cancer: description of method. Br J Cancer 44:618, 1981.

44a. UK Trial of Early Detection of Breast Cancer Group: First results on mortality reduction in the UK trial of early detection of breast cancer. Lancet ii:441, 1988.

45. USSR/WHO study: Protocol of the study of the role of breast self-examination in reduction of mortality from breast cancer. In preparation, 1990.

46. Verbeek ALM, Hendriks JHCL, Holland R, et al: Reduction of breast cancer mortality through mass screening with modern mammography: first results of the Nijmegen project 1975–1981. Lancet 1:1222, 1984.

47. Verbeek ALM, Hendriks JHCL, Holland R, et al: Mammographic screening and breast cancer mortality age specific effects in Nijmegen project, 1975–1982. (Letter) Lancet 1:865, 1985.

48. Walter SD, Day NE: Estimation of the duration of a pre-clinical disease state using screening data. Am J Epidemiol 118:865, 1983.

Chapter 24

DIAGNOSTIC RADIOLOGICAL IMAGING FOR BREAST DISEASES

Joseph T. Ennis, M.D.

Cancer of the breast is the most common malignant disease in women in the western world, and certain "at risk" groups are associated with a three- to fourfold increase in eventual breast cancer development.[48] These include first degree female members (mothers and sisters who have breast cancer); patients with previous breast cancer; nulliparity; age greater than 30 years at the first pregnancy; and early menarche or late menopause. Women with fibrocystic disease have a higher risk of developing breast cancer only where hyperplastic changes are associated with atypical epithelial cells (see chapter 14).[77] Apocrine metaplasia, when extensive, carries an increased risk for breast cancer.[98] More recent studies suggest an increased risk for young women on long-term oral contraceptives.[95]

MINIMAL BREAST CANCER

Minimal breast cancer is defined as cancer less than 0.5 cm in diameter and can refer to lobular carcinoma in situ, intraductal cancer, and invasive cancers [Fig. 24–1(*A, B*)]. Other cancers exhibiting a favorable clinical potential, such as mucinous, colloid, and papillary cancers, can be considered as minimal, and present with a smooth palpable mass that on mammography and clinical examination can appear benign.

Most cancers that are clinically palpable measure 1 cm or greater in size, have gone through approximately 30 doubling times, and contain 1 billion cells. Even minimal breast cancers of 0.5 cm, regarded as clinically early, will already have passed through 27 doubling times and represent a biologically late tumor. The average size of cancers detected by self-examination is greater than 2 cms.[101] Where there are metastasizing phenotypes, breast cancer will metastasize early, even before it can be detected by modern diagnostic methods, and it therefore has been estimated that 50 percent of patients with diagnostically minimal breast cancer will have systemic disease.[8]

Breast cancer, however, behaves less predictably than other cancers, and while some patients with untreated disease can survive for long periods, other patients with minimal breast cancer can succumb very quickly.[62] The important features in predicting the severity of breast cancer include the magnitude of the host response and the tumor characteristics. Survival in breast cancer patients is directly related to the size of the tumor at initial diagnosis and to the presence or absence of positive axillary nodes.[39] Therefore, early diagnosis not only influences prognosis but encourages cosmetically more acceptable surgery that can yield relapse-free and survival rates comparable to more dramatic and aggressive surgical interventions.

While most breast cancers appear to evolve from a sequence of pathological change described as hyperplasia, atypical hyperplasia, and carcinoma in situ, such progression is nonobligate or discontinuous. However, the proliferative form of fibrocystic disease, characterized by ductal hyperplasia, papillomatosis, epitheliosis, and multiple papillomas, does represent one form of precancerous change, and there is compelling evidence that at least the proliferative form of fibrocystic disease is not just a precursor of breast cancer, but one of its earliest morphological expressions.[35] The early diagnosis of breast cancer would be enormously advanced if techniques could accurately and noninvasively detect these hyperplastic precancerous changes. Wolfe's[104] classification (Figs. 24–2 and 24–3), for all its limitations, has attempted to concentrate the diagnostic capability of mammography into defining structural alterations in the breast stroma. The progression of sclerosing lesions presents problems pathologically and radiologically, because the morphological and radiological changes mimic a scirrhous carcinoma, even in the precancerous stage.[74]

EARLY DIAGNOSIS OF BREAST CANCER

The critical importance of diagnostic mammography is the early detection of breast cancer [i.e., before the cancer has reached 5 mm (Fig. 24–4) in size], which can reduce mortality. This is of particular importance where screening programs are being implemented at considerable cost. With clinical diagnostic referrals in which an abnormality has been detected by either the patient or

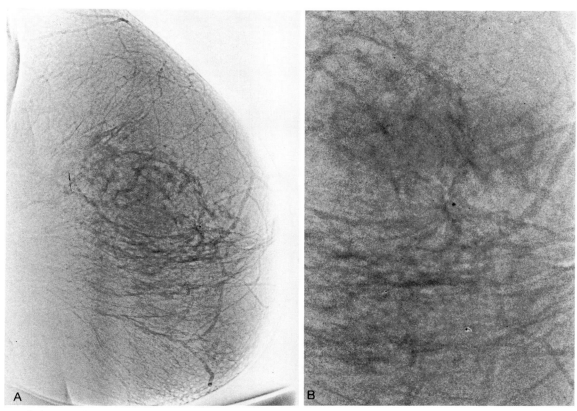

Figure 24–1. *A,* Slight parenchymal distortion in the retroareolar region with a single area of coarse calcification. *B,* Magnified view demonstrating spiculation characteristic of early breast cancer.

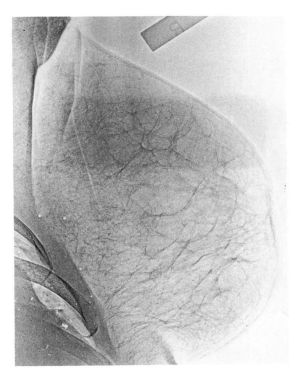

Figure 24–2. Xeromammography demonstrating predominantly fatty tissue with normal trabeculae.

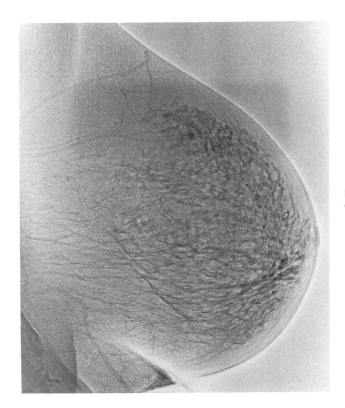

Figure 24–3. Prominent ductal pattern in a normal breast consistent with a P2 classification.

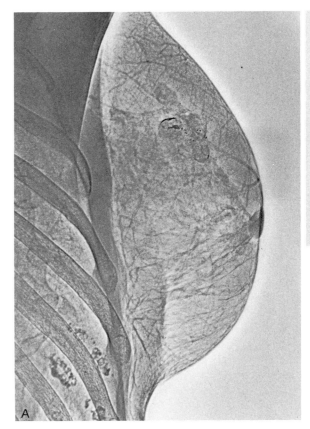

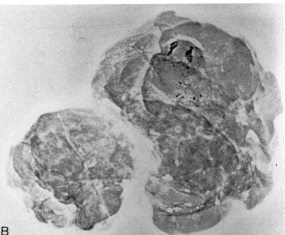

Figure 24–4. *A,* Mass lesion in the superior aspect with areas of coarse calcification. Anteriorly and inferiorly are several areas of microcalcification that are clustered. *B,* Resection specimen shows clearly the benign fibroadenoma with coarse calcification, and inferiorly, the typical microcalcification of intraductal carcinoma.

the referring clinician, or where there is a clinical suspicion of an abnormality, x-ray mammography can precisely define the abnormality, detect multicentric disease, and identify the presence of synchronous cancers. Ultrasound accurately excludes cystic disease, but palpable mass lesions that are solid, irrespective of the mammographic criteria in women older than 50 years, should be evaluated by biopsy.

While it is accepted that microcalcification plays a significant part in the early detection of breast cancer, calcification will occur in less than half of nonpalpable cancers.[84] Equally important is that less than half of these calcific foci will demonstrate the classic appearances suggestive of malignancy. Similarly, less than half of the dominant mass lesions may have spiculated or irregular margins, and 20 percent of the cancers will be discovered by secondary signs such as architectural distortion, asymmetry, duct dilatation, and developing densities. The accurate diagnosis of early breast cancer requires the radiologist to be familiar with subtle parenchymal alterations. Microcalcification, as a sign of malignancy, is of more importance in younger women, in whom it may be the sole mammographic feature.[43] The importance of calcification as a sign of breast cancer decreases with the age of the patient. Careful analysis of direct and indirect signs are essential to ensure that the benign-to-malignant biopsy ratio is surgically acceptable. The positive predictive value of certain mammographic signs increases dramatically when parenchymal distortion, poorly defined mass lesions, typical malignant-type calcifications, and stellate opacities, are present.[10]

The impetus gained from the Health Insurance Plan (HIP) study[81] which demonstrated conclusively a reduction of 33 percent in mortality in those patients who were screened by mammography, has been accentuated by the data from the Breast Cancer Detection Demonstration Project (BCDDP).[5] The significant findings of the BCDDP was that mammography conducted in optimal surroundings had a true-positive rate greater than 90 percent and was significantly more accurate than clinical examination in detecting small cancers.[5] In both the HIP and BCDDP studies, 80 percent of those patients who had carcinomas detectable only by mammogram had no axillary nodal disease. This contrasts with patients who have clinically detected breast cancer, in which more than 50 percent will have axillary node involvement. In addition, only one of the 44 patients whose cancer was detected by mammography alone in the HIP study had died in a 10-year follow-up. Mammography, which superficially appears to be a simple procedure, demands the most meticulous attention to detail and dedicated personnel to produce acceptable and reproducible results. Performed optimally, the sensitivity and specificity of mammographic investigations can be greater than 90 percent, but in inexperienced hands there can be disastrous results.

The introduction, therefore, of newer techniques that may have attractive features, such as being noninvasive and having no associated radiation risks, are only of importance in breast cancer analysis if they can (1)

detect lesions smaller than 5 mm in diameter, (2) help to accurately localize small abnormalities for surgical removal, (3) allow procurement of cytological or histological material for accurate preoperative assessment, and (4) provide some information relative to chemotherapeutic responses.

The radiation risks[4] associated with x-ray mammography are currently considered negligible. In the worst possible scenario, it has been suggested that if 1,000,000 women had two mammographic examinations per year, 7000 clinically unsuspected early breast cancers would be detected, at the theoretical cost of inducing six new cancers. The decreasing radiation dosages with film/screen and new xeroradiographic processes ensure that the benefit-to-risk ratio of x-ray mammography is enormous for the patient.

MORTALITY REDUCTION THROUGH SCREENING PROGRAMS

Most breast cancers, whether discovered by the patient or by a clinician as a palpable lump, will measure 1 to 1.5 cms in diameter, will have gone through approximately 30 doubling times and, in many cases, will have become a systemic disease. There is clinical evidence that the more extensive the tumor at the time of diagnosis and initial treatment, the worse the prognosis.

Lowering the diagnostic threshold for a particular tumor should, therefore, improve the clinical outcome.[92] In breast cancer, increasing the diagnostic accuracy is possible only through x-ray mammography, which when performed and interpreted optimally, can detect lesions smaller than 5 mm in diameter. Several controlled prospective clinical trials have established the benefits of early detection through mammography. The HIP study,[81] the first randomized controlled trial to investigate the possibility of reducing the mortality rate from breast cancer, was a prospective, scientifically designed study to determine the effectiveness of mammography and physical examination. The initial results demonstrating a 30 percent decrease in mortality have been sustained in an 18-year follow-up. The two county Swedish trials,[93] begun in October 1977, demonstrated a 25 percent reduction in the number of stage II or more advanced cancers, and a 31 percent reduction in mortality in the study group. Two nonrandomized studies reported from the Netherlands in 1984[15, 96] demonstrated a significant protection in patients who had been screened by mammography. The combined results of the HIP, BCDDP, Swedish, and Dutch trials clearly indicate that early detection may alter the natural history of breast cancer.

Few diagnostic methods for breast disease have been evaluated as thoroughly as mammography. This technique is simple, acceptable to patients, has a high sensitivity and specificity, is reproducible, cost effective, and has a low risk-to-benefit ratio. Properly performed and interpreted, mammography has a sensitivity greater than 90 percent, but poor mammographic technique can have disastrous consequences for the patient. Lowering the sensitivity and specificity will result in either many cancers being missed or in unnecessary surgical intervention through an increase in the false-positive rate.

The poorly understood biological behavior of breast cancer, the questionable importance of in situ carcinoma, the discrepancy in the malignant potential of different tumors, and the influence of lead-time bias on survival have all been used as potent arguments against screening to detect early malignancy. To accept that breast cancer mortality cannot be altered and that the depressing statistics that persisted for 100 years prior to 1971 will remain unchanged is untenable. In the absence of breast cancer screening, most cancers will be detected by either the patient or a clinician as a palpable lump, and in more than 50 percent of these patients, metastases to the axillary nodes will have occurred.[33, 34] The natural history of a disease can therefore be altered by early mammographic diagnosis, which greatly improves the survival and the quality of life. Minimal breast cancer is associated with a 93 percent 20-year survival compared with a 10 percent 5-year survival in patients with distant metastases.[34] The continuing improvement in mammographic technique and in interpretation over the past years can be gauged by comparing the HIP with the BCDDP studies. The cancer detection rate in the BCDDP study was twice as great as in the HIP study, most probably because of the increased sensitivity of the technique and the greater diagnostis acumen. It would appear that biannual screening for women aged 50 and older should now be the acceptable objective. The evidence that screening benefits younger women is accumulating, and this is significant in light of the findings that young women on contraceptive medication are more prone to develop breast cancer.[95] The effectiveness of the screening program will depend entirely on the sensitivity of the techniques. Where sensitivity is high, the objective (i.e., reducing mortality) will be met. This sensitivity will depend on state-of-the-art equipment, proper processing facilities, trained and motivated radiologists, and a population that has been properly informed regarding the risks and benefits of screening programs.

Promotion of an active health care program to reduce breast cancer mortality in women demands a multidisciplinary approach.[30] Diagnostic radiologists must be specifically trained in breast cancer screening techniques that differ considerably from routine clinical methods. Surgeons should have a particular interest in the latest developments in breast cancer surgery, be familiar with the problems involved in screening programs, and be prepared to initiate research into newer and more appropriate surgical techniques. Cytologists with a detailed knowledge of breast pathology and confident in handling small tissue samples play a crucial role in an effective screening program. Medical oncology has become increasingly important with the introduction of adjuvant chemotherapy. The involvement of general practitioners and community health care workers will determine how successful the program will be, both in educating the population and in maximizing participation.

Counseling is a necessary component in most success-ful programs in the continuous assessment of patients. The technique of mammography is absolutely critical to sustain acceptable results. The equipment must be state-of-the-art, and the radiographers must be full-time in the field of mammography, trained to the highest level, and specifically motivated.

While the use of stereotactic-guided biopsy for cytology and histology will significantly reduce the requirements for open breast biopsy,[3] any breast cancer screening program will undoubtedly increase the surgical workload. Any screening program that fails to give due consideration to the financial requirements of all of the involved departments will be an abysmal failure.

IMAGING TECHNIQUES FOR THE DIAGNOSIS OF BREAST CANCER

Reduction in mortality from breast cancer depends on detecting minimal disease before there has been systemic spread. In patients with clinically palpable abnormalities, demonstration of multicentric or bilateral carcinomas makes mammography a valuable preoperative technique, but the evidence that cancers smaller than 5 mm will have undergone at least 27 doubling times and, in many cases, have become a systemic disease makes it essential that imaging technology be able to detect evidence of systemic disease. The primary sites for systemic involvement are the bone, bone marrow, and lymph nodes. The value of contemporary imaging techniques in breast cancer detection, therefore, lies in the ability to detect small lesions and to accurately assess whether these lesions have become metastatic.

Xeromammography

Xeroradiography has considerably improved resolution, with reduced radiation and consistent image quality, with the development of new technology such as the 126 and 175 systems. Xeroradiography produces a dry image using a selenium-coated aluminium plate, a good conductor in the presence of x-rays, instead of a radiographic cassette. Prior to mammography, the plate is positively charged in a Xerox conditioning unit so that the selenium layer contains positive charges, while an equal number of negative electrons are attracted to the aluminium surface. This plate, enclosed in an airtight electrically insulated cassette, is positioned under the breast as with a radiographic plate and the mammographic examination conducted appropriately. The discharge of the x-rays dissipates the charge in inverse proportion to the density of the overlying tissue so that a high-resolution latent image of the breast is formed on the selenium-coated plate. In the Xerox processing unit, negatively charged blue toner powder, proportional to the positive charge, is concentrated on the xerographic plate. The image is then transferred onto a plastic-coated sheet of paper charged electrostatically so that the toner adheres and, after heating and cooling, is radiologically interpreted.

The new developments in Xerox processing afford greater control over the quality of the examination. The

175 system affords a combination of decreased radiation dosages with higher resolution and less image noise as a result of the smaller-sized toner particle, fewer charges per particle, and decreased turbulence of the liquid toner fountain.

Most xerographic plates are exposed using a positive imaging technique, but negative xeromammography is more effective in distinguishing subtle calcifications, reducing radiation dosage to the breast by about 35 percent. Both techniques are effective in detecting microcalcification, but the negative mode has a major advantage in that there is less toner deletion from areas such as those containing calcification or from the insertion of prostheses, which therefore makes it a very valuable technique in detecting subtle changes.

The unique characteristics of xeromammography compared with other imaging techniques are edge enhancement and wide recording latitude (Figs. 24–5, 24–6, and 24–7). The wide recording latitude allows detail of the soft tissues of the breast, the chest wall, and the thinner peripheral portions of the breast to be recorded on one exposure. Xeromammography presents a high-contrast image of the breast from the chest wall to the nipple and can be recorded on a single mediolateral view. Xerox's recent decision to cease development of xeromammography is regrettable.

Film/Screen Mammography

Recent developments in film/screen mammography have considerably improved the diagnostic accuracy and

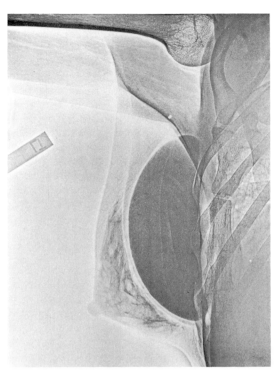

Figure 24–6. Xeromammography in a patient with subpectoral prosthesis.

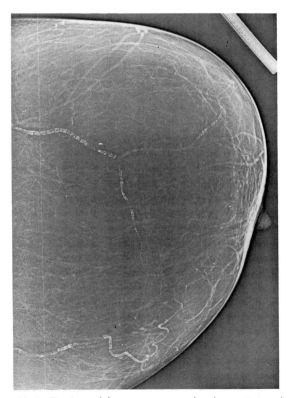

Figure 24–5. Craniocaudal xeromammography demonstrates characteristic vascular calcification.

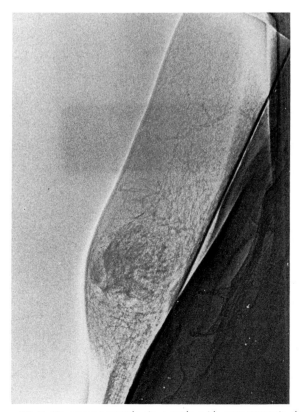

Figure 24–7. Xeromammography in a male with gynecomastia demonstrating the typical parenchymal pattern.

reduced the radiation dosages.[60] Dedicated mammographic equipment, vigorous breast compression, and soft x-ray beams to accentuate contrast are absolute requirements (Fig. 24–8). Film processing is an essential component of film/screen mammography, and poor processing will result in inappropriate examinations with many artifacts. Compression of the breast is of more significance with film/screen than with xeroradiographic mammography. Vigorous compression can increase geometric sharpness by reducing the object film distance, enhance contrast, reduce scatter, and minimize motion artifact. Further benefits from compression include reduced radiation dosages, more accurate assessment of densities, and better visualization of the borders of the lesion that can distinguish benign from malignant densities. The use of grids has been of particular importance in film/screen mammography by increasing the contrast resolution, but at a cost of slightly increased radiation dosages. Most of the films available for use in film/screen mammography have similar resolution characteristics.

Optimal technique demonstrates the breast parenchyma in two planes. Standard views, such as craniocaudal and upright or reclining mediolateral, are usually sufficient to demonstrate breast pathology. The mediolateral view demonstrates more of the breast, including the posterior wall, and should be the first view taken. Deep-seated lesions seen on the mediolateral projection may require extended craniocaudal views, either medial or lateral extension, to demonstrate the lesion adequately. The importance of biplane assessment is critical when needle localization is indicated. In addition, close apposition of the breast to the cassette and the elimination of skin fold are technical considerations. In film/screen mammography, the posterior wall cannot be demonstrated, because the thick posterior of the breast cannot be sufficiently compressed to allow adequate imaging with the lower kilovolts peak (kVp) technique. Supplementary views that give useful information include contact mediolateral, the lateromedial, and the oblique lateral. The value of the contact projection is that it eliminates magnification and therefore produces better resolution. Uniform compression of the breast is essential to reduce radiation, improve resolution, increase contrast, and decrease geometric un-sharpness.

Optimal mammographic images, with proper positioning and the use of dedicated mammographic equipment, greatly facilitate the diagnosis of breast pathology. Difficulty in interpretation results when the images are substandard, the position is inadequate, and the equipment inappropriate.

In a recent recommendation from the American College of Radiologists, accreditation is only given to those units that have state-of-the-art mammographic equipment, trained personnel (both radiographic and radiological), and quality control that ensures radiation dosage is minimal.

Magnification Mammography

Magnification radiography improves sharpness in detail and increases diagnostic accuracy in angiography, skeletal radiography, and breast cancer. Dedicated mammographic equipment is essential for good magnification mammography.

The optimal degree of magnification is 1.5 times life size. It has been shown both qualitatively and quantitatively that the improved sharpness of magnification mammography results from both increased resolution and reduced effective noise. The margins of breast masses and the degree and specificity of microcalcifications are more clearly defined.[76] The increased diagnostic accuracy of magnification readily translates into patient management, with many lesions that were regarded as equivocal or abnormal being reinterpreted positively. This technique can significantly reduce the number of patients referred for biopsy.

MAMMOGRAPHIC SIGNS OF BREAST CANCER

Performed and interpreted optimally, mammography will detect approximately 90 percent of all breast cancers and is the single most effective method for the detection of minimal breast cancer. The false-negative results occur most frequently in dense breasts in which the architectural changes are concealed by the overlying parenchyma (Fig. 24–9). Some carcinomas are difficult to visualize in the atrophic breast because of similar density attenuation properties of the surrounding tissue.

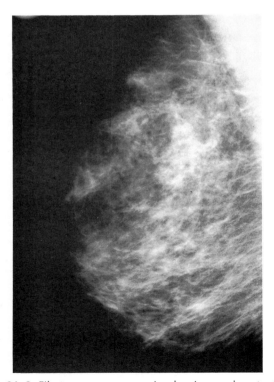

Figure 24–8. Film/screen mammography showing good contrast with normal parenchymal architecture.

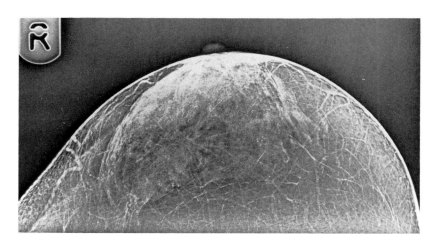

Figure 24–9. Marked parenchymal distortion in a dense breast, consistent with scirrhous carcinoma.

The mammographic features of breast cancer include primary and secondary signs. The presenting *primary signs* include a dominant mass, architectural distortion, and microcalcification, while the *secondary signs,* such as skin thickening, lymphatic permeation, increased vascularity, lymph node involvement, and ductal dilatation are much less specific.[103]

Dominant Mass

Although the presence of microcalcification plays a critical part in the diagnosis of early breast cancer, the most frequently observed abnormality representing carcinoma is a mass.[40] Most breast cancers measure at least 1 cm in diameter when they are discovered clinically and present mammographically as a mass lesion (Figs. 24–10 and 24–11). The shape of this mass can discriminate between benign and malignant lesions, as planar or rodlike structures are less likely to be malignant than more volumetric-shaped abnormalities. Tumor masses may have irregular contours or be well circumscribed (Figs. 24–12, 24–13, and 24–14). Those cancers with irregular margins present less difficulty with differential diagnosis than well circumscribed lesions. Careful analysis of the abnormality on the mammogram to localize suspicious areas of spiculation can enhance the diagnosis

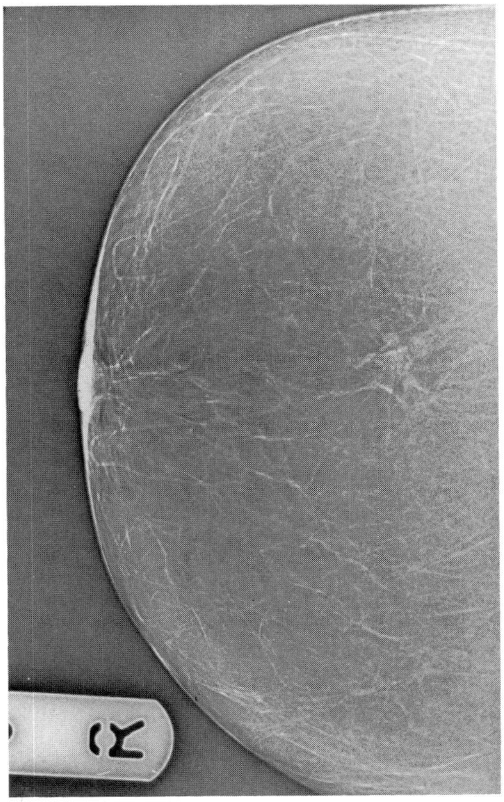

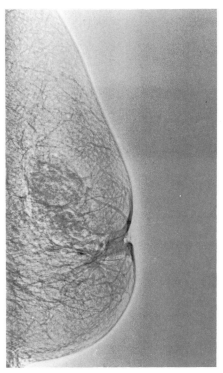

Figure 24–10. Irregular mass in the posterior aspect of the breast. Slight skin thickening. These appearances are consistent with an early tumor.

Figure 24–11. Ductal hypertrophy with nipple retraction, with a small area of desmoplasia in the retroareolar region due to intraductal cancer.

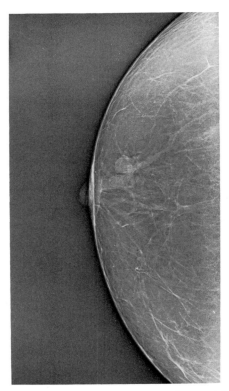

Figure 24–12. Marked ductal hypertrophy with a nodular irregular density in the outer aspect.

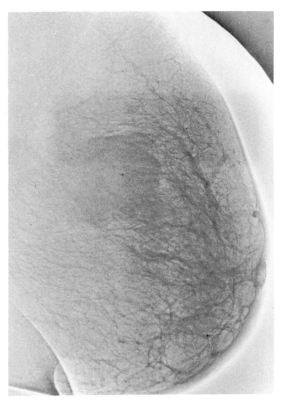

Figure 24–14. A large 3 cm mass with poorly defined margins and obscuration posteriorly. There is associated skin thickening and edema.

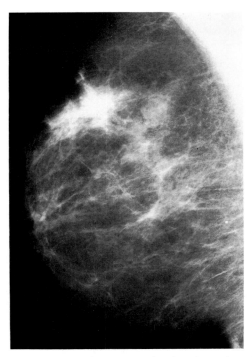

Figure 24–13. Mediolateral projection showing dense, irregular mass with superior spiculation, typical for a neoplasm.

of breast cancer. This may require supplementary views (Figs. 24–15 and 24–16), including magnification, for detection.[70] Spiculated masses can present typical appearances of scirrhous carcinoma (Figs. 24–17, 24–18, 24–19, and 24–20) resulting from the fingerlike extensions into the breast parenchyma representing desmoplastic reaction, retraction, and lymphatic engorgement, but frequently these signs are subtle and can be overlooked (Fig. 24–21). These cancers are characterized microscopically by extensive reactive fibrosis and are larger on palpation than on mammography because of extensive desmoplasia. The more aggressive breast cancers are associated with striking stellate appearance and are reported to have a higher hormonal receptor content than do circumscribed or nodular carcinomas, which may be less anaplastic.[9, 75] Stellate abnormalities demonstrated on high quality mammograms must be considered potentially malignant until proven otherwise by biopsy, and the addition of typical calcifications greatly increases the probability of cancer. The suggestion of parenchymal invasion is an important sign of malignancy and can be demonstrated mammographically by effacement of the contours in any part of any one projection. This is particularly important where adequate compression has been applied, and when present, must be considered as a malignant sign. Cancers tend to be more inhomogeneous than benign lesions, which on compression will present uniform homogeneity.[40]

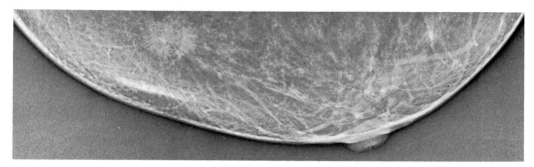

Figure 24–15. Extended craniocaudal view, better demonstrating a carcinoma.

Several benign entities can present with a stellate appearance mimicking carcinoma, resulting in diagnostic problems (Figs. 24–22 and 24–23). The postsurgical radial scar can present as a tumorlike mass lesion with tissue retraction and may simulate carcinoma. The history of previous surgery is critical in making the correct diagnosis. Serial examinations will show reduction in the size of the associated mass following surgery. Fat necrosis usually results from surgery and can present as a spiculated mass lesion or with typical tumorlike calcifications that make radiological differentiation difficult. Careful analysis of the mammogram will often demonstrate areas of reduced density representing fat in the region of the mass, which may give some indication of the benign etiology. Other entities that may sometimes simulate carcinoma are abscesses and hematomas. Abscesses are usually found peripherally in the subareolar region, and both the abscess and hematoma will show rapid resolution on serial mammography. Frequently there is extensive subareolar edema in association with abscess and hematoma, but these changes will again quickly resolve. A baseline mammogram (Fig. 24–24) following segmental removal of a carcinoma is essential for accurate follow-up. Serial mammographic examinations will demonstrate rapid reduction in the postsurgical changes, with a relative return to normality of the breast parenchymal tissue.

Circumscribed carcinomas include medullary carcinoma, mucinous carcinoma, and cystosarcoma phyllodes, which may have malignant potential. In older patients, masses that are solid on ultrasound should be surgically removed. Adequate radiographic projections, including supplementary views, optimal compression, and magnification, are necessary to ensure that the borders of the circumscribed mass are well defined (Figs. 24–25 and 24–26). With xeromammography, a halo sign, 1 mm thick, entirely surrounding the circumscribed lesion in both projections is necessary to suggest a benign etiology, such as fibroadenoma or cyst (Figs. 24–27 and 24–28). Cysts will change shape with compression, and ultrasound can determine the cystic nature. Aspiration of the cyst and the use of pneumocystography can be helpful in eliminating the presence of rare intracystic tumors[91] (Fig. 24–29). In cases in which masses are clinically palpable but indistinct on mammography, biopsy of these lesions is mandatory. Most peripherally located solid lesions are not malignant and represent lymph nodes, particularly when found in the upper outer

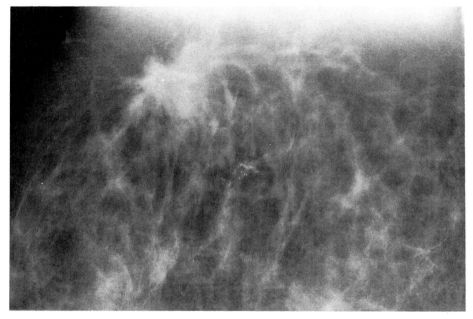

Figure 24–16. Magnified craniocaudal projection shows lobulated, irregular mass anteriorly and a cluster of microcalcification in patient with multicentric cancer.

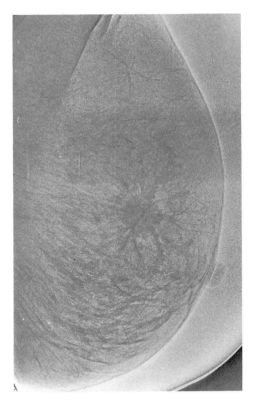

Figure 24–17. Spiculated scirrhous carcinoma.

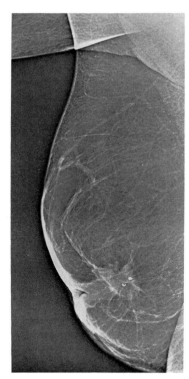

Figure 24–19. Marked skin thickening, nipple retraction, and ductal dilatation with a posterior spiculated mass containing coarse areas of calcification.

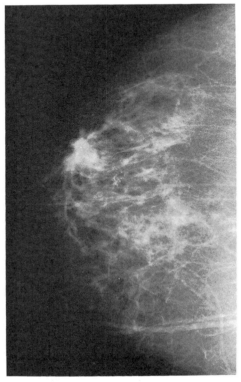

Figure 24–18. Irregularly contoured density in the superior aspect of the right breast with marked nodularity.

quadrant of the breast. Most lymph nodes measure less than 1 cm in length, have a characteristic bean-shaped appearance, sometimes with a fat sinus. Neoplastic lymph nodes are solid, round, and measure greater than 1.5 cm in diameter. It is unusual to find breast cancer in the periphery of the breast, and most abnormalities found in the subcutaneous fat have a benign etiology. Most cancers occur in the fibroglandular tissue and are therefore predominantly found in the subareolar region extending into the upper outer quadrant, where most of the fibroglandular tissue persists. Border effacement, asymmetry, and developing densities are important signs of cancer (Figs. 24–30, 24–31, and 24–32).

Calcification

Calcifications are frequently found in the breast; most of these are benign and may have typical presentations. Calcifications are the smallest structures seen on a mammogram and to be identified need high-resolution mammography, vigorous compression of the breast, elimination of geometric unsharpness, and magnification radiography. While it has been stated that xeroradiography is superior in detecting microcalcification, high-resolution film/screen mammography can be equally diagnostic.[82] The overlap between benign and malignant microcalcifications is considerably increased where technique and interpretative skills are poor, resulting in many unnecessary excision biopsies.

Text continued on page 442

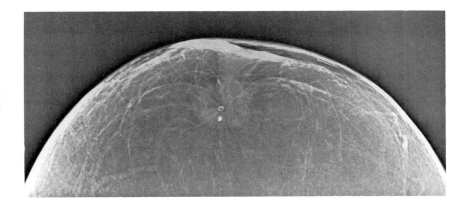

Figure 24–20. Same patient as in Figure 24–19. Craniocaudal projection demonstrates the typical features of a scirrhous carcinoma incorporating coarse, benign calcification.

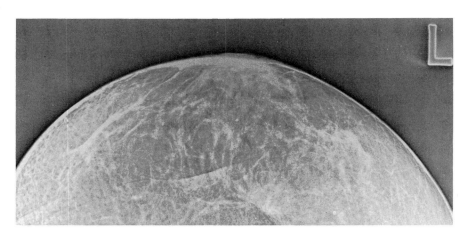

Figure 24–21. Craniocaudal view. Posteriorly there is a suggestion of parenchymal desmoplasia in a patient with no palpable mass and histologically confirmed carcinoma.

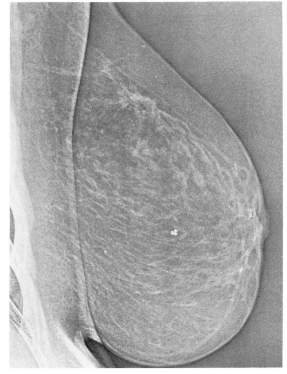

Figure 24–22. Superiorly irregular density in the postoperative breast, mimicking carcinoma. Benign calcification in the retroareolar region. Normal lymph nodes.

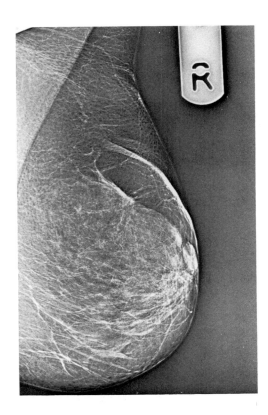

Figure 24–23. Postsurgical change showing parenchymal distortion with some spiculation.

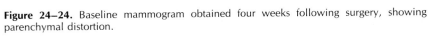

Figure 24–24. Baseline mammogram obtained four weeks following surgery, showing parenchymal distortion.

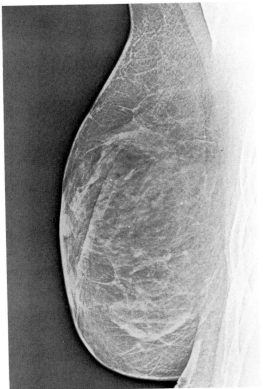

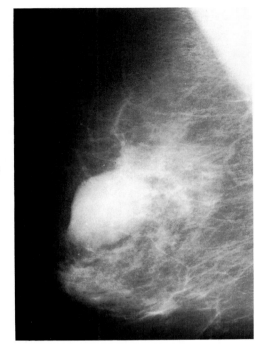

Figure 24–25. Mass lesion with well-defined margins superiorly but effacement posteriorly, representing carcinoma.

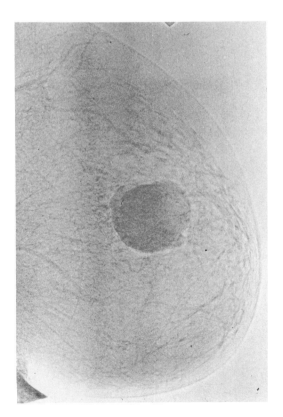

Figure 24–26. Reasonably well-defined mass lesion with partial "halo" sign, but the posterior irregularity and effacement of the interface is very suggestive of carcinoma.

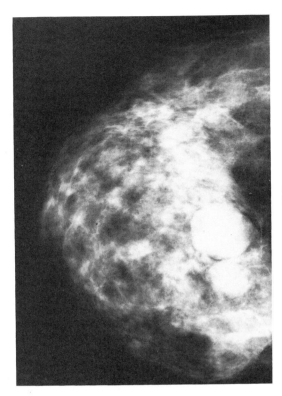

Figure 24–27. Two well-defined homogeneous densities in a breast with marked ductal hypertrophy. These represent cysts, confirmed on ultrasound.

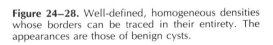

Figure 24–28. Well-defined, homogeneous densities whose borders can be traced in their entirety. The appearances are those of benign cysts.

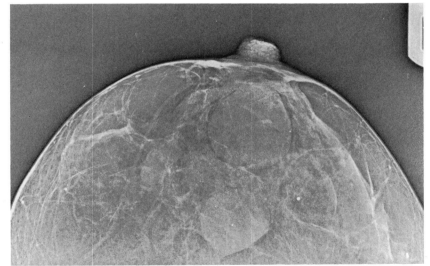

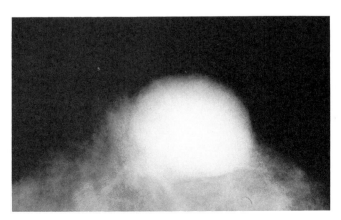

Figure 24–29. Homogeneous, well-circumscribed density that has the appearances of a cyst. However, on the lateral margins there is irregularity and a suggestion of spiculation. This represented an associated carcinoma. (Courtesy of Dr. G. Svane and Dr. E. Azavedo, Karolinska Hospital, Stockholm, Sweden.)

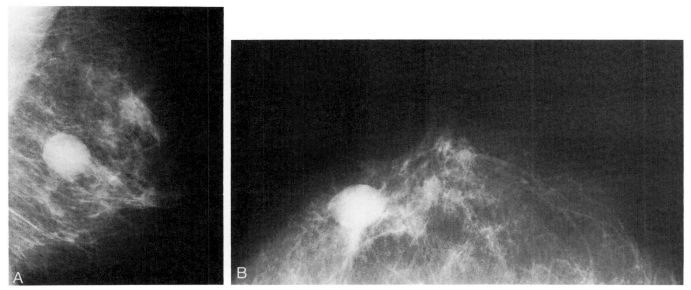

Figure 24–30. *A*, Reasonably well-defined density on the mediolateral projection with some ductal prominence. *B*, Posterior effacement of the parenchyma due to tumor infiltration in the same patient.

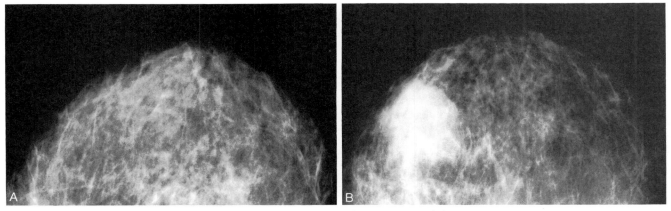

Figure 24–31. *A*, Normal breast with prominent ductal pattern. *B*, Marked asymmetrical density representing a tumor in same patient.

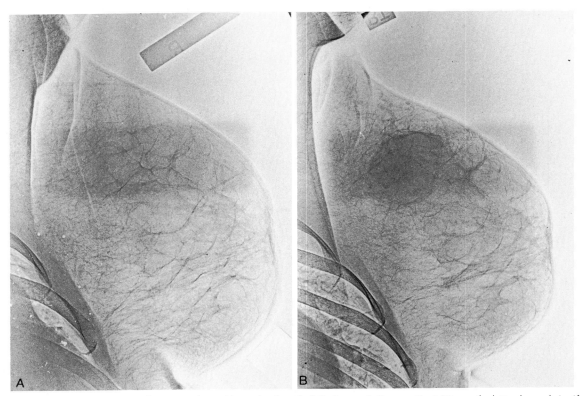

Figure 24–32. *A,* Normal xeromammography in a patient with predominantly fatty tissue. *B,* Same patient 18 months later showed significant density that developed in the upper quadrant. Histology confirmed this to be a tumor.

Obvious benign calcifications can be clearly identified. Arterial calcification can be seen as undulating parallel lines, usually bilateral, and presents diagnostic difficulties only in the early stages (see Fig. 24–5). Fibroadenomas will eventually produce the pathognomonic "popcorn" calcification appearances, but in the early stages some difficulty may exist. The calcific foci associated with fibroadenomas tend to be larger than calcification associated with malignancy (Fig. 24–33). In later stages, when the fibroadenomas have degenerated, calcific appearances may mimic other benign calcifications, such as microcysts. Calcifications with radiolucent centers are almost always benign. These calcifications can be seen as entirely circumscribed or partially complete. They are usually widely scattered, and although their etiology is not completely known, they may be associated with fat necrosis. The calcifications associated with secretory disease (Fig. 24–34), because of calcified inspissated secretions, are typically bilateral, widely spread throughout the breast, and larger in length and diameter than calcifications that are malignant. These calcifications are often associated with ductal dilatation and are orientated on the lines of the ducts toward the areola. Milk of calcium cysts characteristically show density differences on the craniocaudal and lateral oblique projections (Fig. 24–35). Milk cysts are usually manifested by small, widely scattered calcifications and may have incomplete contours.

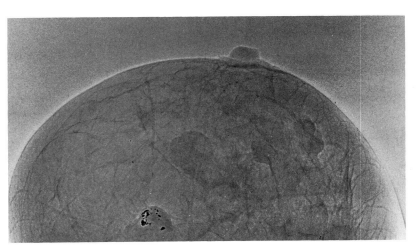

Figure 24–33. Multiple well-defined densities with typical "popcorn" calcification in the most posterior mass. This represents fibroadenoma.

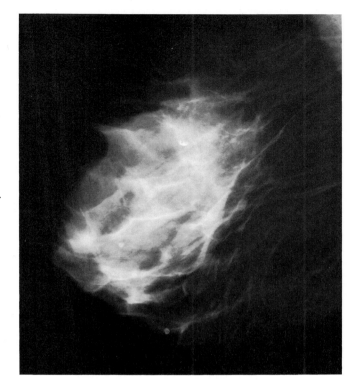

Figure 24–34. Curvilinear calcification consistent with microcysts.

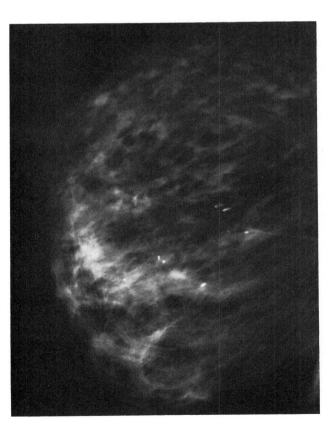

Figure 24–35. Elongated linear calcification with lucent centers.

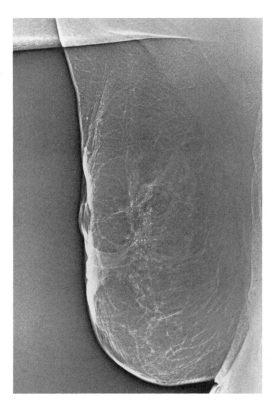

Figure 24–36. Marked skin thickening with nipple retraction. Punctate, irregularly contoured microcalcification extending toward the areola in a patient with intraductal carcinoma.

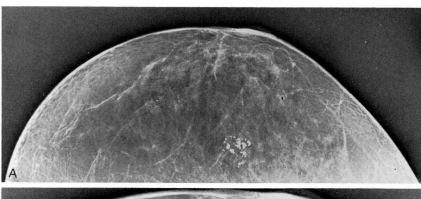

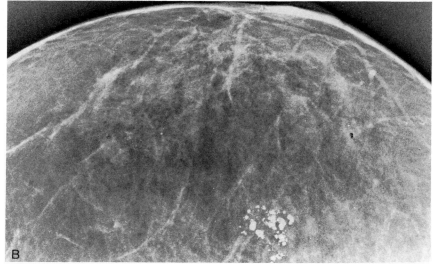

Figure 24–37. *A,* Tightly clustered linear microcalcification with irregular contours. *B,* Magnification demonstrating the classic appearances of malignant calcification.

The contours of the individual calcific foci and their distributive pattern can help to separate benign from malignant calcification on mammography. Calcifications that are well defined, widely scattered, and of reasonably uniform size are associated with benign fibrocystic disease. In secretory disease, calcifications are linear, produce ductal configurations with branching patterns, and may be associated with nipple discharge. Milk of calcium cysts are usually widespread, bilateral, and have a linear or curvilinear appearance on one of the two projections.

Microcalcifications are one of the most important mammographic signs of early breast cancer and can occur as the sole finding in 30 percent to 47 percent of early breast cancers. Since their discovery in breast cancer by Leborg,[58] they have been characterized in several ways (Fig. 24–36). Microcalcifications that have a high association with breast cancer are linear, branching, small, irregularly contoured, angular (Fig. 24–37), and localized or in separate groups.[24, 69] These calcifications may be the only evidence of malignancy on a mammogram and in occult cancer occur in 75 percent of cases. In the majority of tumor calcifications, the calcium is deposited within the ducts, and their ramifications can be curvilinear or branching, conforming to the lumen of the duct, and orientated toward the nipple in a discontinuous fashion. Most of the calcifications will be associated with a surrounding density, but between 10 percent and 20 percent will have no demonstrable architectural mass. The number of calcifications does not indicate whether the process is benign or malignant, and cancers can have as few as five calcifications and as many as hundreds.

A comprehensive analysis of the morphological features of microcalcification in malignant and benign disease, carried out by Lanyi in 1985, demonstrated certain useful findings that were not pathognomonic.[56] In malignant lesions, the calcium groups formed a triangular or trapezian configuration in 65 percent of patients and a square or rectangular configuration in 9.5 percent. Less frequently the groups had a club-shaped or stellate form. The shape of the single microcalcification in breast cancer fell into four readily defined forms: punctiform of varying size, bean-shaped, undulating lines of varying length not greater than 3 mms, and branching or Y-shaped patterns (Figs. 24–38, 24–39, and 24–40).

Magnification radiography is important in determining the number, size, shape, and configuration of the calcific foci. Calcifications that are irregular and asymmetrically distributed (although grouped) are potentially malignant and require surgical biopsy. Unfortunately, appearances similar to malignancy can occur in patients with fat necrosis and with sclerosing adenosis. Even in benign processes, such as early calcification in fibroadenoma and in ductal ectasia, the appearances can mimic carcinoma, and the exact procedure for management of these patients will depend on institutional policy.

One of the most difficult calcifications to distinguish is that associated with sclerosing adenosis.[74] The calcifi-

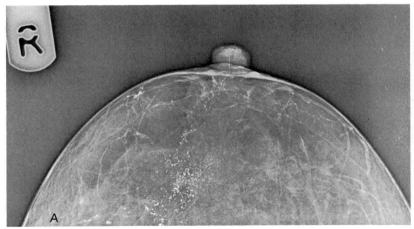

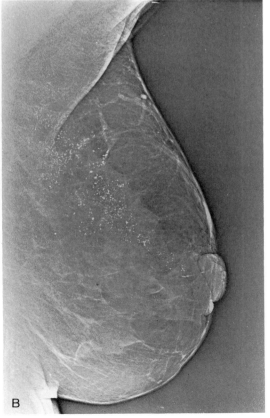

Figure 24–38. *A,* Intraductal carcinoma with typical microcalcifications extending toward the nipple. *B,* Craniocaudal projection of the same patient demonstrating the asymmetry, irregularity, and linearity.

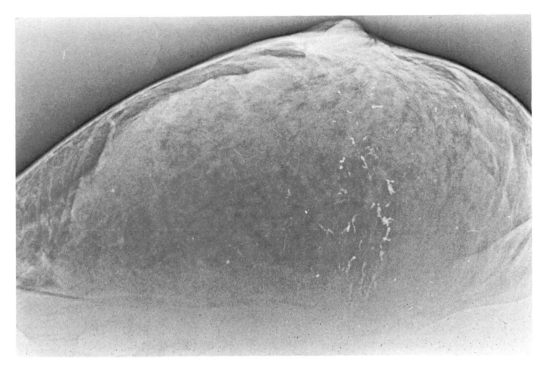

Figure 24–39. Intraductal carcinoma with linear branching, Y-shaped, irregularly contoured calcifications extending toward the nipple.

cations can mimic carcinoma, and parenchymal distortion can support the diagnosis of malignancy and very often will lead to a biopsy (Figs. 24–41, 24–42, and 24–43). Multicentric cancers can occur in approximately five percent of patients (Figs. 24–44 and 24–45). Bilateral cancers are often only detected through x-ray mammography, which must be performed when a clinical diagnosis of breast cancer has been made. Interval breast

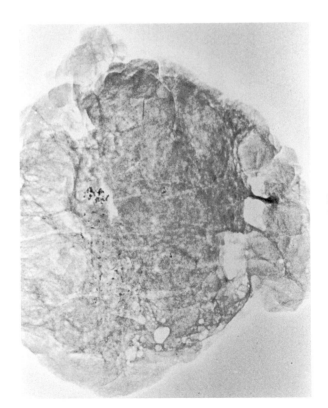

Figure 24–40. Resected specimen showing the irregularity and linearity of the intraductal calcifications.

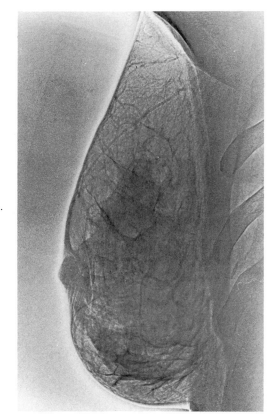

Figure 24–41. Microcalcific group in the retroareolar region, which appears punctate.

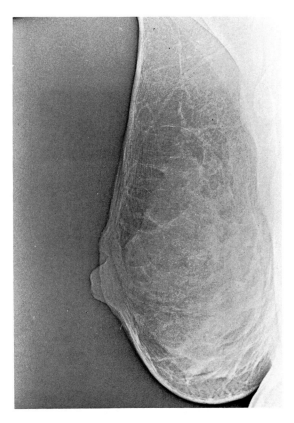

Figure 24–42. Same patient two years later. Calcifications again are grouped, are punctate, and appear to have increased in number.

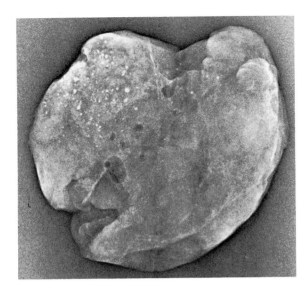

Figure 24–43. Same patient as Figures 24–41 and 24–42. Resected specimen demonstrating that the calcific foci are rounded and reasonably well contoured, but with no definite evidence of linearity. Histology confirmed the presence of sclerosing adenosis.

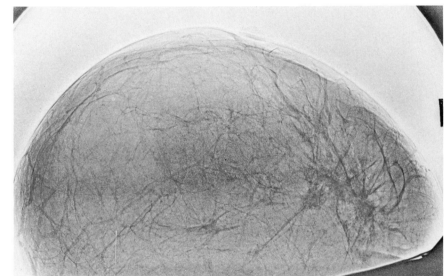

Figure 24–44. Multicentric carcinoma with three separate cancers.

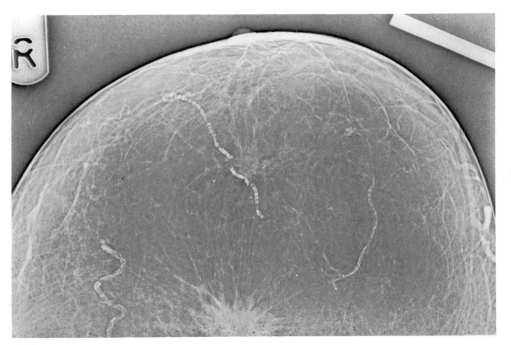

Figure 24–45. Multicentric cancer. The anterior section contains typical calcifications.

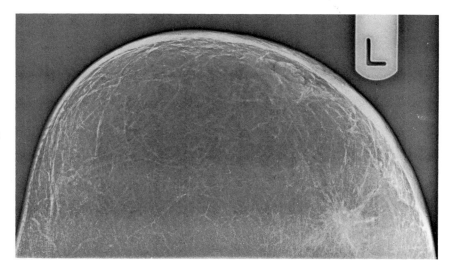

Figure 24-46. Spiculated scirrhous carcinoma with associated edema and marked skin thickening.

cancers can be either true or false. The incidence of false interval breast cancers is a measure of the sensitivity of diagnostic mammography.

Architectural Distortion

Architectural distortion presents one of the earliest and most challenging signs of breast cancer. The positive predictive value of architectural distortion is significantly less than signs such as stellate opacities or clustered microcalcifications. The associated fibrotic changes can give rise to the classic "purse-string" appearance consistent with a carcinoma. Thickening and straightening of the trabeculae can occur asymmetrically, and this spiculation may indicate an underlying neoplasm. In the absence of previous surgical biopsy, asymmetric density in one breast can also be indicative of an underlying carcinoma.

SECONDARY SIGNS OF BREAST CANCER

Edema of the breast is nonspecific and is caused primarily by benign diseases such as inflammation, lymphatic obstruction, cardiac failure, or (rarely) Mondor's disease. In some cases, however, edema may be the only sign of malignancy when the tumor is small, deep-seated, and produces extensive edema that masks the posteriorly positioned lesion (Fig. 24-46).

Thickening and tethering of the skin will occur when there is lymphatic permeation, and while this may be seen often following surgical intervention, its presence in the absence of surgery needs careful evaluation. Increased vascularity may occur in normal breasts and is of no significance, but asymmetry can be associated with neoplasia. Bilateral dilatation of the ducts is common in postmenopausal women, but unilateral dilatation may be associated with carcinoma and requires assessment. In some cases, ductography can be of value in demonstrating intraductal abnormalities such as papillomas and, rarely, tumors.

Normal lymph nodes measure less than 1.5 cms in diameter, are oval-shaped, and usually contain a lucent fat sinus. Intramammary lymph nodes are common and, while smaller than axillary nodes, will have a similar structural appearance (Fig. 24-47). Malignant lymph nodes are round, solid, and measure greater than 2 cms in diameter (Figs. 24-48, 24-49, and 24-50). Enlarged lymph nodes can be present because of local spread from breast carcinoma or represent metastatic disease from other primary malignancies.

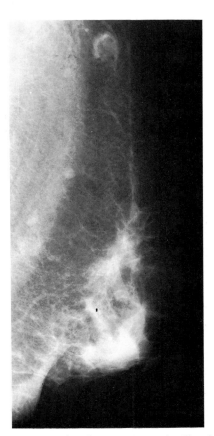

Figure 24-47. Prominent ductal pattern. Normal axillary lymph nodes. Intramammary lymph nodes are present.

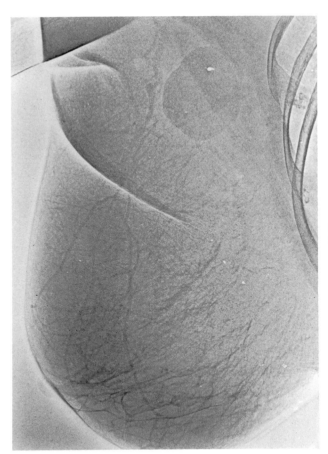

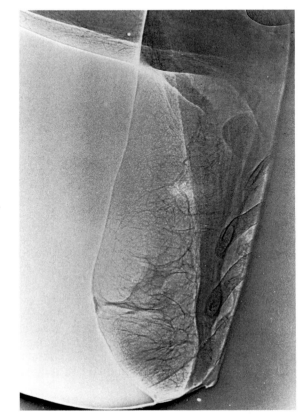

Figure 24–48. Large homogeneous lymph node in the axilla, the result of metastases.

Figure 24–49. Normal breast with secondary lymph node involvement in the axilla.

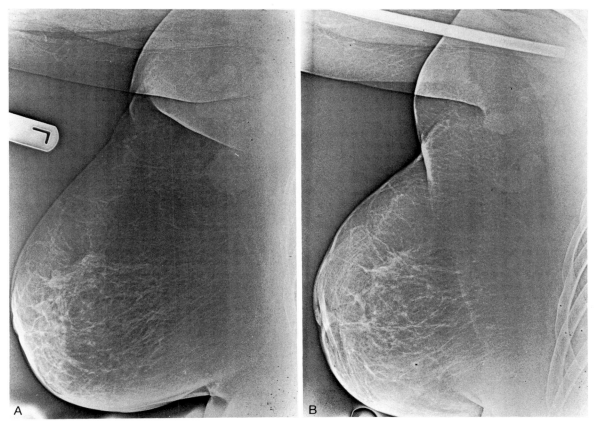

Figure 24–50. *A,* Breast cancer with involved enlarged nodes in the left axilla. *B,* Following chemotherapy. There has been a marked reduction in the lymph node size.

FALSE-NEGATIVE MAMMOGRAMS

False-negative mammography may lead to a delay in biopsy, and the prognosis may be adversely affected. The most important causes of false-negative mammograms are as follows:

1. Dense breast tissue. Where there is insufficient fat to separate the abnormality from the surrounding breast parenchyma, then mammography may fail to identify a palpable abnormality. If a lesion is clinically palpable but has negative findings on mammography, it must be investigated further. Ultrasound may be of value in demonstrating an abnormality that is clinically palpable but mammographically negative and in locating the lesion for aspiration biopsy. When the patient has mammary implants, xeromammography is superior to the film/screen technique in detecting subtle parenchymal changes indicative of carcinoma.

2. Technical factors. State-of-the-art dedicated x-ray equipment, well-trained mammographers, and radiologists who can interpret subtle signs of breast cancers are essential to limit false-negative results. Properly performed, good compression and demonstration of the posterior chest wall will contribute significantly to the overall accuracy. With inadequate technical factors, then the false-negative results will increase.

3. Errors in Interpretation. The primary errors in interpretation assume that well-circumscribed lesions are benign, that calcifications without the characteristic branching pattern cannot have a malignant basis, or failure to interpret the subtle indirect signs of parenchymal distortion. A greater awareness and a greater emphasis on training can make radiologists more adept at distinguishing early parenchymal changes indicative of breast cancer. The introduction of adjunctive techniques and the more reliable use of aspiration cytology, under stereotactically guided biopsy, can be of value.

OTHER IMAGING TECHNIQUES

Ultrasound

The uniquely attractive features of ultrasound as a diagnostic tool (i.e., no ionizing radiation, noninvasiveness, reproducibility, and high patient acceptability) have stimulated extensive investigations into its role for the detection of breast cancer. Despite rapid developments in technology from the prototype water-bath[100] to the automated immersion scanners,[49, 50, 54] the role of ultrasound in the diagnosis of minimal breast cancer remains equivocal.[7, 46]

The sole objective of breast cancer screening is to reduce mortality, which can be achieved by the diagnosis of minimal breast cancer (i.e., lesions smaller than 5 mm in diameter and before the disease has become

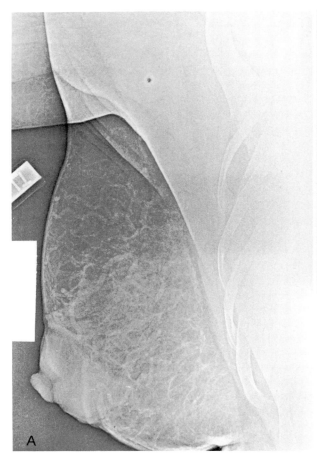

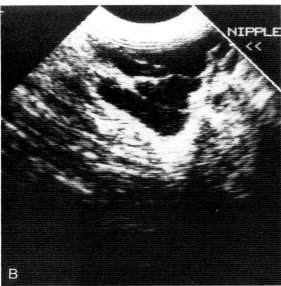

Figure 24–51. *A,* Asymmetrical density extending from the areola into the posterior aspect of the breast. *B,* Contact sonogram demonstrating the cystic multilocular components.

systemic). Diagnostic ultrasound in its present format is incapable of consistently diagnosing such lesions. Most series demonstrating high correlative accuracy with mammography have usually been obtained with the prior knowledge of mammographic findings. Ultrasound has consistently been inferior to mammography in detecting breast cancer.[13, 23] In one large series, ultrasound failed to demonstrate 92 percent of cancers smaller than 1 cm in diameter.[85]

The importance of diagnostic ultrasound in the management of breast cancer is in the resolution of equivocal mammography (Fig. 24–51), the diagnosis of cystic disease, and the demonstration of solid abnormalities with specific ultrasonographic features. The resolution of ultrasound is inferior to high-resolution mammography, and lesions smaller than 1 cm in diameter, unless cystic, will not be detected. Sonographically demonstrated abnormalities, when physical examination and x-ray mammography are normal, are in most cases not significant.[7, 52] Contact scanning of the breast, using real-time high-resolution ultrasound scanners, provides the most comprehensive information regarding palpable abnormalities, which may help specifically in the diagnosis or in location for biopsy.[53] Patients with multiple abnormalities or nonpalpable abnormalities with equivocal mammograms are best examined by automated waterbath scanning techniques. It is, however, questionable

whether the investment in expensive automated waterbath scanners as a method for breast cancer screening is justified.

Clinical Applications of Diagnostic Ultrasound

Ultrasound demonstrates cysts superbly, and lesions as small as 2 mm can be detected with the use of high-resolution transducers (7.5–10 MHz). Ultrasound has an accuracy greater than 95 percent in diagnosis of breast cysts.[47, 86] Ultrasonically guided aspiration can be extremely beneficial in both drainage of the cyst and in providing cytological specimens. Cysts on ultrasound are always well circumscribed with smooth margins and have an echo-free center, irrespective of the sensitivity setting (Figs. 24–52 and 24–53), with typical distal echogenic shadowing.[85] Cysts are thin-walled and may be round, oval, lobulated, or septated. An abscess or hematoma may also be fluid-filled but can be distinguished from cysts by the thickness of the walls and through altering central echo pattern with changing sensitivity, particularly in chronic abscesses (Fig. 24–54). Abscesses will demonstrate resolving patterns in response to therapy, with reduction in size associated with thickening and demonstrating bright echoes.

While certain criteria have been established to distin-

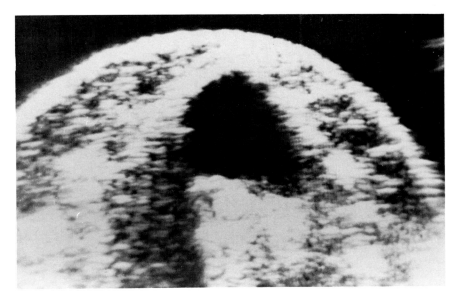

Figure 24–52. Breast cyst. Hypoechoic with acoustic shadowing.

guish benign from malignant lesions on sonography, these criteria lack specificity. Benign solid masses usually show smooth contours, round or oval shapes with weak internal echoes, and well-defined anterior and posterior margins. However, ultrasound is unable to distinguish solid benign from solid malignant lesions with consistent accuracy, and therefore all solid lesions detected on ultrasound should be evaluated by biopsy.[18, 86]

Malignant lesions have characteristically jagged, irregular walls (Fig. 24–55), compared with the usually smooth margin of benign masses. However, malignant lesions can have smooth margins with acoustic enhancement. Scirrhous carcinomas produce severe desmoplasia, have irregular margins of various shapes, and contain weak, nonuniform internal echoes with characteristic acoustic attenuation.[12] The internal echoes

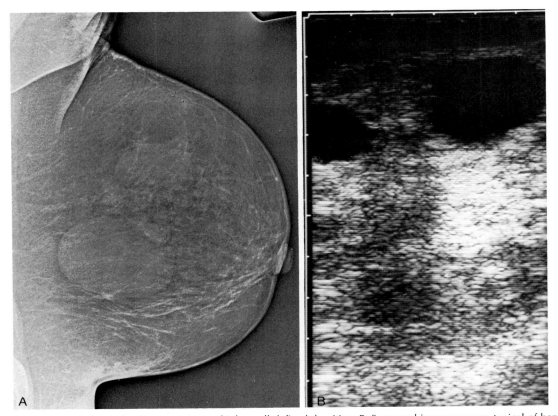

Figure 24–53. *A,* Xeromammography demonstrating multiple, well-defined densities. *B,* Sonographic appearances typical of benign cysts.

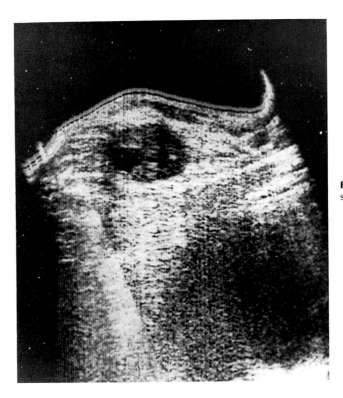

Figure 24–54. Irregular density with inhomogeneous echographic pattern and some posterior shadowing in a patient with a breast abscess.

in malignant lesions are inhomogeneous compared with the homogeneity demonstrated in most benign masses, but have considerable overlap that makes consistent distinction impossible. Attenuation shadowing is considered a prominent sonographic feature of malignant mass lesions in the breast, but attenuation shadowing can also occur in benign masses.

Blood flow in malignant breast lesions is considerably increased.[2] Doppler flow signals can detect the increased blood flow and distinguish benign from malignant lesions. Malignant lesions produce Doppler signals of higher frequency and amplitude with continuous flow through diastole.[99] Doppler flow analysis could play a role in distinguishing benign from malignant tissue but is not sensitive enough for screening.

The attractions of diagnostic ultrasound include the absence of radiation, its noninvasiveness, and the ability to repeat the examination without morbidity. It is therefore ideal for monitoring resolution of inflammatory and trauma changes.[36, 47] Breast masses can be conclusively demonstrated to be cystic or solid, and ultrasonic guidance can be particularly useful in obtaining biopsy

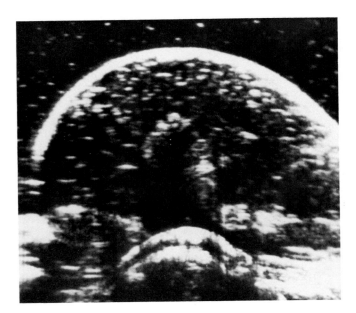

Figure 24–55. Thick, irregular walls, suggestive of a neoplasm.

material either for cytology or histology. While there has been a major improvement to the spatial resolution of ultrasound scanners with high-frequency transducer systems, large fatty breasts, which are the ones most easily examined by mammography, present difficulty for ultrasound, despite the advantages of breast compression.[79] Although ultrasound had been proposed as a screening method for breast cancer detection, neither automated ultrasonic scanning techniques nor high-resolution contact scanning[7] can reliably detect minimal breast cancer, and both significantly fail to detect microcalcification, the most significant marker for breast cancer in younger women.[43, 45, 85] The ultrasonic contribution to resolving equivocal areas is of some importance and, combined with high-resolution mammography, may increase the diagnostic yield.

Thermography

Thermography was first utilized for the diagnosis of breast disease in 1956,[57] when it was noted that breast cancers were associated with a rise in temperature of the overlying skin. However, this technique has always been a controversial means of investigation. Transmission of heat from the breast is nonspecific and in carcinoma probably results from the increased blood perfusion or hypervascularity that frequently accompanies carcinomas. There are three methods currently available for thermography: telethermography, contact thermography, and computerized thermography.[66] All examinations are performed in a draft-free room with controlled humidity and temperature regulated to 20°C. Cooling of the breast is essential. The principal advantage of computer thermography is that the analysis of data is objective; in both other methods, the interpretation of the thermographic scans is qualitative. The criteria for abnormal thermograms are abnormal vascular patterns with varying dynamic responses to cooling. With computerized methodology, diagnostic algorithms have been used for linear discriminant analysis of the temperature reading. The value of thermography has been and remains equivocal, and the results are so variable and inaccurate that it ceased to be part of the Breast Cancer Detection Demonstration Project. The sensitivity is less than 50 percent, and it is not now being advocated as a routine screening method.[73] Thermography is unable to detect minimal breast cancer and therefore cannot be used as a screening method. The suggestion that changing thermographic patterns of the breast could be used as a determinant for patients at risk for developing breast cancer has been refuted.[71, 72]

Light Scanning of the Breast

The technique of light scanning is noninvasive and relatively inexpensive, and therefore has attracted considerable attention as a method of diagnosing breast cancer. When an electromagnetic wave impinges on a transparent medium, the wave is scattered and absorbed; this light attenuation will vary depending on the biological tissue.[32] The attenuation is significantly influenced by the hemoglobin content of the tissue.[97] The transmission of light is inhibited by hemoglobin, and thus the neovascularity associated with many breast cancers will influence the transmission patterns in transillumination.

In the normal breast there should be symmetrical absorption of light, with the veins, because of their high hemoglobin content, appearing black on the monochrome scan and blue-black with color analysis.[20] However, venous patterns on breast tissue can be asymmetric, and so asymmetry of light transmission is an unreliable sign of abnormality.

The most important and consistent sign of breast cancer is increased light absorption as a result of the high hemoglobin content, with a decrease in luminence that can be displayed on the black-and-white mode as focal, regional, or total. Total light absorption is seen with large carcinomas, extensive intraductal carcinomas, diffuse carcinomatosis, or inflammatory cancers.[38] The indirect signs of breast cancer, such as focal or regional attenuation, vascular asymmetry, and skin retraction, are less reliably demonstrated by light scanning. In addition, a decrease in light transmission may occur following biopsy or hematoma, and this can mimic carcinoma. Attenuation patterns mimicking carcinoma may also occur in the subareolar region, which is frequently vascular. Papillomas may contain increased amounts of hemoglobin, and biopsy scars, as in mammography, are indistinguishable from cancer. The retromammary area close to the chest wall cannot be examined, and light scanning, like conventional mammography, cannot distinguish sclerosing adenosis from breast cancer.

Light scanning technique is the most operator-dependent of all techniques for breast cancer detection, and requires extensive physician-time. It is a technique that needs further evaluation, and its major role may be like that of Doppler ultrasound in demonstrating abnormal flow patterns resulting from the neovascularity associated with breast cancer that could help to determine the presence of minimal breast cancer. Currently, the sensitivity of light scanning in the determination of breast cancer is limited. With lesions smaller than 1 cm in diameter, the sensitivity varies from 19 percent[83] to 44 percent.[6] Size of the cancer is therefore critical in the diagnosis of breast cancer. The serious limitation of light scanning is in the detection of minimal breast cancer. Of 24 biopsy-proven carcinomas, 14 (58 percent) were detected with light scanning, compared with 21 (88 percent) detected by mammography. With nonpalpable breast lesions, light scanning demonstrated only five of 15 invasive cancers and two of eight intraductal cancers, so that 16 (70 percent) of 23 cancers were not visible with light scanning.[67, 68]

Of more significance are the findings with larger cancers,[21] where in 20 cancers smaller than 2 cm, light scanning detected 11, compared with 19 detected by conventional mammography. It is clear from the current data that light scanning is not a technique that can be reliably used in breast cancer screening.

Magnetic Resonance Imaging

While magnetic resonance imaging (MRI) has proven to be of great diagnostic value in the spine and the musculoskeletal system and in monitoring tumor responses,[78] its value as a potential screening method in breast cancer is equivocal. There is no ionizing radiation and no known radiobiological hazards, and MRI can produce high resolution images that have similar criteria for the diagnosis of benign and malignant disease as mammography. MRI of the breast is conducted using specially designed surface coils to give maximum resolution for breast images, and using this technique, it is possible to study details of the breast parenchyma, the axilla, and the posterior wall of the chest (Fig. 24–56), which makes MRI superior to either light scanning or ultrasound. The breast can be examined using conventional spin-echo T_1 and T_2 weighted sequences, preferably in the sagittal plane, but coronal and axial images can also be obtained. Gradient echo images will allow faster imaging sequences and help to separate small density differences.[88]

Conventional imaging sequences in magnetic resonance present excellent morphological data regarding breast tissue.[28] However, with conventional spin-echo imaging there is considerable overlap between benign and malignant tissue.[89] This overlap in signal intensity between benign and malignant tissue significantly reduces the potential of MRI to detect early breast cancer. In addition, the inability to detect microcalcification,

which is the single most important mammographic sign of early malignancy, is a significant limitation.

On T_1 weighted sequences, fat is seen as a high-intensity signal, and small infiltrating mass lesions can be clearly separated. Normal ductal tissue is an intermediate-intensity signal and cannot be separated from Cooper's ligaments or from normal vascular structures. The muscles posteriorly are well demonstrated, and tumor extension more effectively gauged. In addition, it is possible to image the axilla and to quantitate the number and size of lymph nodes. Breast cysts as small as 3 cm to 4 cm can be demonstrated as low signal intensity, well encapsulated on T_1, with bright signal intensity on all T_2 sequences (Fig. 24–57). Fibroadenomas are usually seen as a well-encapsulated low- to moderate-intensity signal on T_2 weighted sequences (Fig. 24–58). However, in some instances these signal intensities reflecting the composition of the fibroadenoma can be higher than those of fat, presenting diagnostic difficulties.[89] Calcified fibroadenomas produce inhomogeneity of signal intensity because of signal loss from the calcific foci. There are three patterns of abnormality in fibroadenoma: low signal intensity, high signal intensity with small areas of inhomogeneity, and gross inhomogeneity signal resulting from calcium deposition. These provide overlapping signals that cannot clearly separate fibroadenoma from carcinoma on low field-strength magnets.[17]

Malignant tissue may be discriminated on MRI using the same morphological criteria as mammography. Irregularly marginated spiculated masses, secondary skin changes, and enlarged glandular tissue are signs of malignancy. The hope that improvements in T_2 weighted sequences (Fig. 24–59) would distinguish benign from

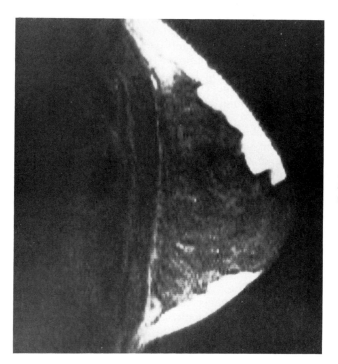

Figure 24–56. MR image. Sagittal section in a normal breast, T_1 weighted. Subcutaneous fat with high signal intensity. Normal breast parenchyma, posterior muscles well demonstrated.

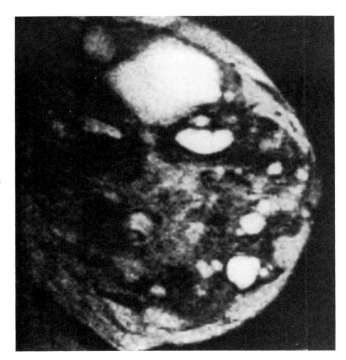

Figure 24–57. T$_2$ weighted image showing the high signal consistent with multiple, fluid-filled cysts.

malignant tissue more readily than would T$_1$ weighted images has not been realized.[29]

Imaging with gadolinium-DTPA has proved disappointing in that similar signal intensities can occur in malignant and nonmalignant tissue, particularly in inflammatory lesions and fibroadenomas,[44] using standard spin-echo techniques (Fig. 24–60). In addition, proliferative dysplastic lesions may enhance, resulting in false-positive diagnosis of carcinoma by MRI. Dynamic uptake of gadolinium-DTPA has proven to be more efficacious than other methods in distinguishing vascular from nonvascular tissue and separating benign from

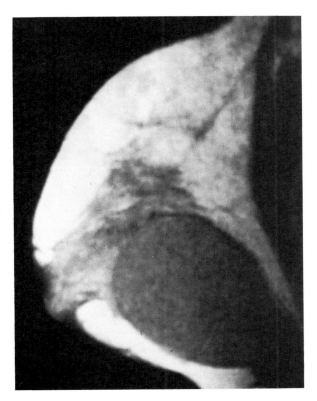

Figure 24–58. Well-encapsulated mass and intermediate signal of a fibroadenoma.

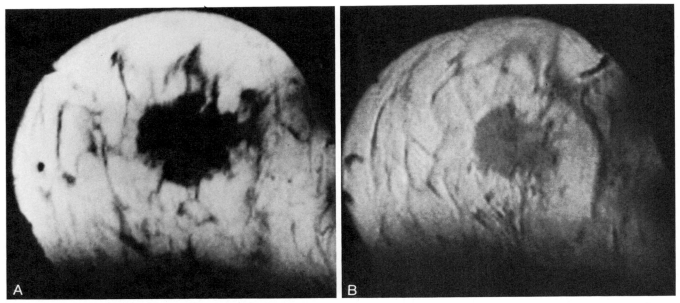

Figure 24–59. *A,* Irregular, jagged margins with low signal intensity of carcinoma on a T_1 weighted sequence. *B,* T_2 weighted sequence in the same patient demonstrates the changing signal intensity.

malignant tissue (Figs. 24–61 and 24–62). There is a clear demarcation (Fig. 24–63) between fibrocystic, fibroadenoma, and malignant tissue.[88] The rapid concentration of contrast medium in malignant tissue is based on the proliferative vascularity of the lesion, which distinguishes it from fibroadenoma and from other benign entities. The absence of high blood flow in benign tissue helps to separate these lesions from the malignant stroma. The neovascularity associated with most neoplasms can distinguish benign from malignant tissue and

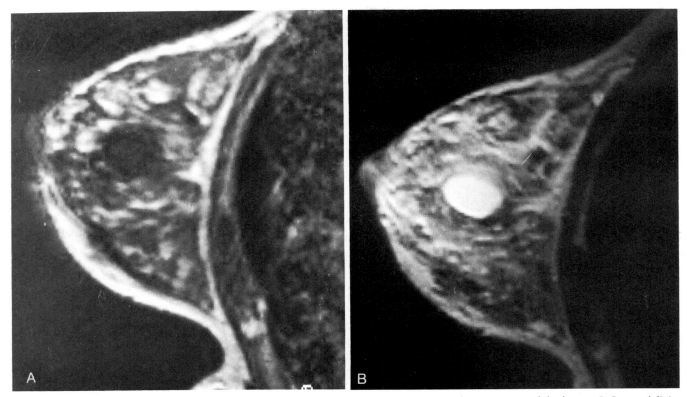

Figure 24–60. *A,* Precontrast scan demonstrates low intensity area with well-defined margins in the center part of the breast. *B,* Post gadolinium-DTPA injection showing significant enhancement.

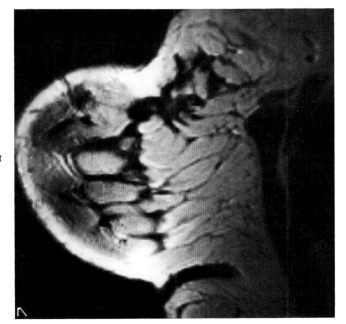

Figure 24–61. Irregular mass in the superior aspect, with enhancement following gadolinium-DTPA, in the central part of a scirrhous carcinoma.

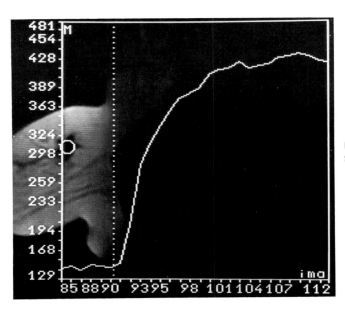

Figure 24–62. Profile scanning showing the rapid accumulation of the gadolinium-DTPA in the cancer.

Figure 24–63. Intensity profiles following dynamic gadolinium scanning can separate carcinoma from dysplastic breast tissue.

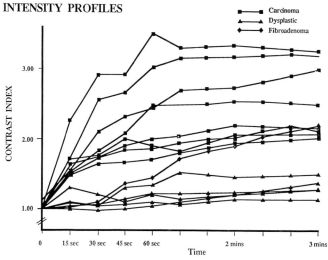

INTENSITY PROFILES

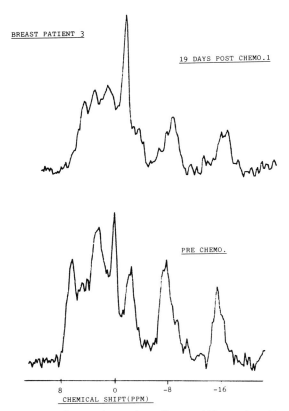

Figure 24–64. Pre- and postchemotherapy MR spectroscopy scans demonstrate the change in spectra represented by diminution in the phosphomono and phosphodiester peaks.

reduce the number of biopsies from equivocal mammograms through use of ferromagnetic contrast agents.[88]

An additional, more important role of MRI may develop in monitoring chemotherapeutic responses in breast cancer patients.[78] MRI spectroscopy, pre- and post-chemotherapy, may have a role in determining the treatment rationale of patients (Fig. 24–64). Spectral changes in malignant masses can be observed 1 hour following chemotherapy, and certain trends in spectral changes can be observed on a daily basis that can indicate the benefits of a particular therapeutic regimen.

INTERVENTIONAL TECHNIQUES

Ductography

Ductography is performed by injecting a radiopaque contrast into one of the mammary ducts with subsequent mammographic images.[94] The main indications are discharges from the nipple, particularly when these are serosanguinous or bloody. It has been established that carcinoma will be the cause of the discharge in only a small number of patients, but nevertheless, this is a very useful technique. Ductography is simple but can successfully be performed only in those patients in whom there is a discharge at the time of the examination and where the orifice can be visualized. The duct is gently

dilated using a Nettleship dilator. A small blunt cannula, under sterile conditions, is inserted into the orifice and, with the patient in the supine position, 0.1 to 0.2 ml of a dilute contrast medium is injected until the patient experiences fullness. Craniocaudal and mediolateral mammographic views are obtained, with no compression.

In the normal appearances the duct should measure no more than 2 mm in diameter and have a triangular branching pattern in the retroareolar region (Fig. 24–65). The walls of the normal duct are smooth and straight, with a gradually tapering caliber, until they join the acini. In patients who have secretory disease there may be dilatation of the duct to about 1 cm in diameter. Intraductal masses can be demonstrated as filling defects (Fig. 24–66) surrounded by the contrast medium. Filling defects are caused by either cysts or intraductal papillomas. Cysts may opacify if they are connected to the ducts when the contrast is injected. Carcinomas may be occasionally identified by ductography and may appear as irregular masses, but more frequently appear as multiple intraluminal filling defects.

Localization of Nonpalpable Breast Lesions

Localization of nonpalpable breast cancers has become an integral part of patient management (see chapter 28). Occult lesions can only be surgically removed if there is accurate preoperative localization. While surface localization and spot method identification are still currently in use, the mammographically controlled place-

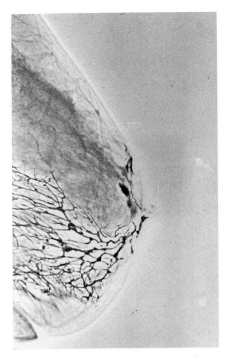

Figure 24–65. Normal ductogram demonstrates the normal-caliber distribution of the mammary ducts.

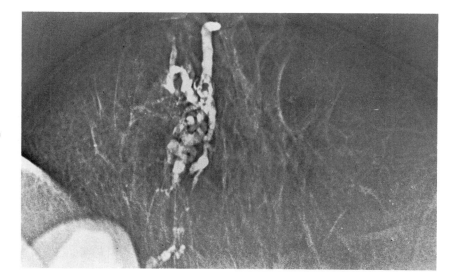

Figure 24–66. Marked ectasia of the ductal system with a solitary filling defect representing a papilloma.

ment of a hooked wire is considerably more accurate.[102] The stylet, under local anesthetic, is accurately placed parallel to the chest wall using an acrylic plastic compression plate containing multiple holds, all of which must be larger than the hub of the stylet needle. The needle is withdrawn when the lesion is accurately localized on mammography, and the tiny wire hook is left in position. The position of the needle must be carefully assessed before the stylet is removed and the hook left in position.[45, 51] However, the greatest advances in localization and diagnosis have been in the use of stereotactic needle placement (Figs. 24–67 and 24–68) with cytologic aspiration.[3, 37] With this technique occult breast cancers can be localized successfully in more than 90 percent of patients, and the sensitivity and specificity of the cytologic aspirate for occult breast cancers is greater than 95 percent. Fine needle aspiration has become one of the most impressive diagnostic tools in selecting patients for surgical excision (see chapter 26). While blind placement of fine needles can be successful, Goodson et al.[42] have shown that stereotactic controlled needle placement is impressively more accurate and leads to more finite results. The addition of immunohistochemistry, using monoclonal antibody, enhances the overall cytology diagnostic accuracy.[61]

Specimen Radiography

Needle localization and excision of the abnormal tissue must be evaluated by specimen radiography to ensure that the appropriate mammographically detected abnormality has been completely removed (Fig. 24–69) (see chapter 28). Before dissection, a radiograph of the intact specimen can be obtained using conventional mammographic equipment or, for better resolution, a dedicated specimen radiographic unit. Xeroradiography or film/screen techniques will provide excellent detail of the presence of microcalcification, architectural distortion, or subtle masses (Fig. 24–70).[90]

Radiological/pathological correlation is essential for accurate histopathological diagnosis. Specimen radiography directs the pathologist to the precise localization of an abnormality to ensure that appropriate tissue is obtained. Accurate radiological and pathological correlation greatly enhances conservative resection.[90] While most calcifications in resected specimens can be clearly identified, high-resolution specimen radiography can ac-

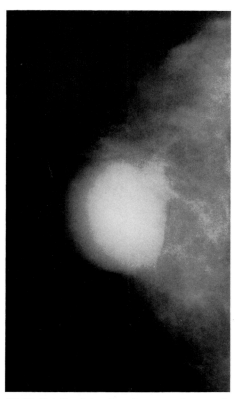

Figure 24–67. Well-defined density whose margins are obscured posteriorly by a malignant mass. (Courtesy of Dr. G. Svane and Dr. E. Azavedo, Karolinska Hospital, Stockholm, Sweden.)

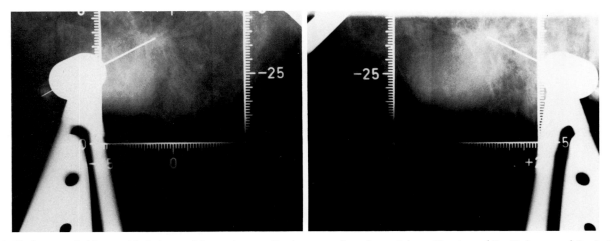

Figure 24–68. Stereotactic biopsy with drainage of the cystic area. Carcinoma confirmed on cytology. (Courtesy of Dr. G. Svane and Dr. E. Azavedo, Karolinska Hospital, Stockholm, Sweden.)

curately detect occult noncalcified abnormalities. This combined approach, involving surgeon, pathologist, and radiologist, has a significant impact on patient management.

IMAGING OF METASTATIC DISEASE

The rapid tumor doubling time of some breast cancers means that many of these cancers will have become systemic at the time of initial diagnosis. Cancers most frequently metastasize to the bone or to the lymph nodes.[16] The long-term survival of patients with breast cancer will depend on the stage of the disease at the time of initial diagnosis. In patients with minimal disease at initial diagnosis, 93 percent will be alive 20 years later, compared with none of the patients with extensive metastatic disease at the time of initial diagnosis.[34] This emphasizes the critical role of diagnostic imaging in establishing, at the time of diagnosis, the extent of disease.

While bone scintigraphy is superior to skeletal radiography in the detection of bony metastases (Fig. 24–71), there is considerable discrepancy between the frequency of metastatic bone disease at autopsy and that reported at the initial diagnosis of breast cancer and surgical treatment. This would suggest that many patients with breast cancer have occult bony metastases that are undetected by conventional methods.[1] This explains why some patients with minimal breast cancer (stage I disease) and an apparently good prognosis, have a short survival time. Bone pain is an unreliable indicator of

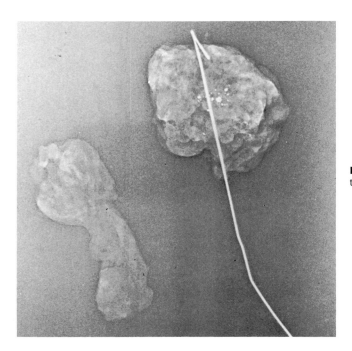

Figure 24–69. Specimen radiograph with the hooked stylet, demonstrating typical tumor calcifications.

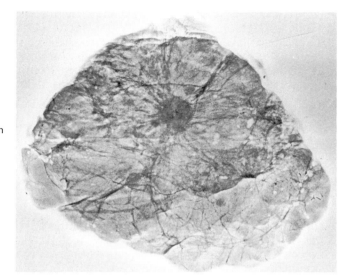

Figure 24–70. Specimen radiograph demonstrating architectural distortion of carcinoma.

the presence or absence of bone metastases, which can occur in 44 percent of patients with no pain.[63] The incidence of bone metastases detected on scintigraphy in stage I and stage II breast cancer varies between two percent and six percent increasing to 14 percent in stage III disease.[64] The sensitivity of the bone scan over skeletal radiography is such that the scan has a lead of 6 to 18 months over the radiograph in demonstrating abnormal results. While there is little uniform agreement about the appropriate protocol for scanning patients with breast cancer, McNeill et al. have argued that all patients with stage III disease should have preoperative

bone scans, while patients with stage I and stage II disease should have baseline scans at the time of diagnosis, with follow-up scans at varying intervals.[64] Coleman et al.[14] demonstrated the incidence of bone metastases to be zero percent for stage I, three percent for stage II, seven percent for stage III, and 47 percent for stage IV, to reinforce this concept. False-positive bone scans can occur and emphasize the need for radiological correlation. False-negative rates as low as 0.08 percent may be impressive,[14] but most probably underestimate the extent of systemic marrow disease. False-negative bone scans occur where the lesions are osteolytic with

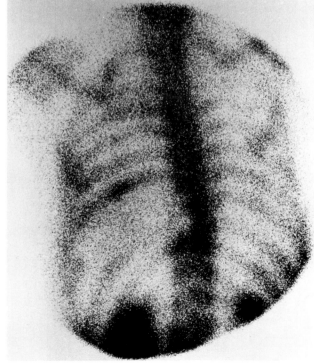

Figure 24–71. Bone scintigraphy. Multiple secondary infiltration of the spine and rib cage.

relatively little reactive osteogenesis. In these cases, skeletal radiography is essential. While most solitary bone lesions have a low association with malignant spread, solitary sternal lesions have a high correlation with metastases.[55] Patients relapsing with breast cancer may have solitary bone lesions as the sole manifestation of metastases in 21 percent of patients.

While bone scanning plays a fundamental role in acquiring baseline data for management,[11, 14, 59] the bone scan is unable to detect marrow infiltration that precedes involvement of the bony cortex. The infiltration of bone marrow and occult lymph node involvement explain why many patients with Stage 1 breast cancer may have a poor outcome. The objective of radiology is to detect metastases at the earliest stage. Conventional x-ray techniques are of little value in demonstrating lymph node involvement or marrow infiltration that produce no reactive bone changes. False-negative bone scans are common in patients who have positive marrow aspirations.[31] Although data suggest a low incidence of bone involvement,[41, 80] analysis with modern imaging techniques should be completed. Marrow imaging has assumed significance in baseline studies in patients who have minimal breast cancer. The techniques currently in use include marrow scanning with ^{99m}Tc-nanocolloid, which can demonstrate evidence of marrow infiltration as photon-deficient areas (Fig. 24–72). The addition of single-photon emission computed tomography (SPECT) can significantly enhance the pickup rate of radionuclide marrow imaging.

MRI of the marrow cavity to demonstrate local and diffuse marrow disease[31] is increasing in importance. MRI bone marrow scans performed in coronal and sagittal planes, with conventional spin-echo sequences, demonstrate marrow as uniform high signal intensity, while gradient echo sequences for rapid imaging produce a uniform low signal intensity (Fig. 24–73). Alteration in the marrow signals by infiltration with tumor can be solitary, multiple but well defined, or diffuse. Sequential marrow imaging is useful for demonstrating response to chemotherapy.[31] Bone metastases in breast cancer may appear between 20 months and 4 years after mastectomy, and although bone scintigraphy is the most effective method of detecting these metastases,[19] marrow imaging would provide a longer lead time.

The most frequent sites for breast cancer metastases are bone, lungs, mediastinum, and lymph nodes. Pulmonary involvement characteristically includes pulmonary effusions, most of which are unilateral, pulmonary nodules and, occasionally, lymphangitic carcinomatosis. These appearances can be assessed accurately through plain chest radiography (Fig. 24–74). Computerized tomography will give exquisite detail about the involvement of mediastinal lymphadenopathy and help to characterize nonspecific pulmonary nodules. Pulmonary metastases tend to occur at a very advanced stage of breast cancer, and conventional x-ray techniques provide adequate information for patient management.

CT can undoubtedly demonstrate the presence of mediastinal and retrosternal nodes, but both CT and chest radiography underestimate the involvement of internal mammary node chain with metastatic breast cancer. Mammary lymphoscintigraphy has been used to study the lymphatic drainage of the breast.[25, 26] Metastases to the internal mammary lymph nodes may be present in the absence of axillary node involvement, and the incidence may be as high as 18 percent for patients with negative axillary nodes.[27] Lymphoscintigraphy is performed by the subcostal injection of ^{99m}Tc-nanocolloid, followed by planar or single-photon emission tomographic images of the mediastinum, to include the axillae. Normal distribution shows symmetrical uptake by the internal mammary lymph chains bilaterally. Metastatic infiltration of the lymph nodes results in nonvi-

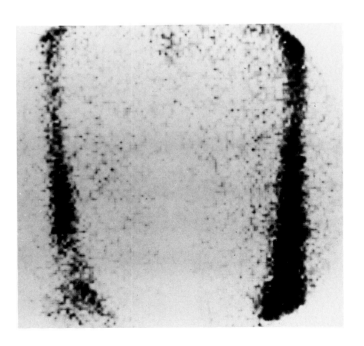

Figure 24–72. Marrow scanning with technetium^{99m} nanocolloid, demonstrating photon-deficient areas in the right femur.

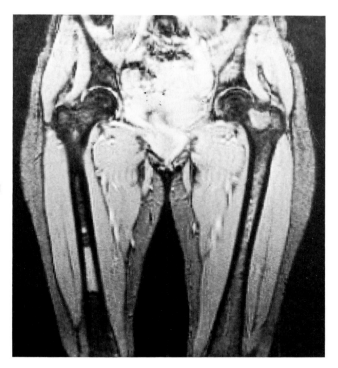

Figure 24–73. Gradient echo marrow MR image demonstrating bilateral marrow infiltration.

sualization or partial visualization of the affected nodal chain (Fig. 24–75). Single-photon emission tomography can provide three-dimensional information for therapeutic planning regarding the involved lymph nodes, and there is a high correlation between negative lymphoscintigraphy and the recurrence rate of the tumor (Fig. 24–75). The technique is simple to perform, has a high sensitivity and specificity, and is well tolerated by the patients.[65]

Radioimmunoscintigraphic detection of primary and metastatic cancer has made significant progress, both in diagnosis and treatment. This technology could provide

a simple test to demonstrate the presence of occult metastases throughout the body. Developments in antibody production, purification, fragmentation, and labeling, combined with improvements in instrumentation and knowledge of the clinical and technical factors associated with radioimmunoimaging, has improved the reliability and availability of these techniques.[22]

Monoclonal antibodies are now more specific and have less antigenicity to the patient. The development of newer isotope labeling techniques and the use of instrumentation provide better in-depth resolution.[105]

Response to chemotherapy can be monitored in sev-

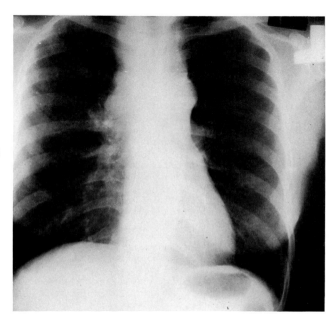

Figure 24–74. Chest x-ray of a patient with breast cancer, demonstrating bilateral hilar lymph node involvement.

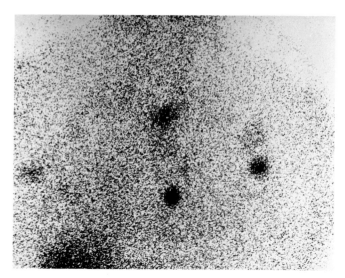

Figure 24–75. Lymphoscintigraphy demonstrating nonfilling of the right mammary chain and asymmetrical filling of the left mammary chain. These appearances are consistent with metastatic involvement of the mammary lymph nodes.

eral ways using imaging techniques. Plain radiography will demonstrate lytic lesions converting to sclerotic radiographic abnormalities. Sequential scintigraphy, using profile imaging techniques, can demonstrate diminution in activity levels in response to therapy. Computerized tomography is effective in demonstrating reduction in tumor bulk size. However, all these techniques are insensitive in detecting early changes in response to chemotherapeutic intervention. MR spectroscopy can effectively demonstrate chemotherapeutic responses within 24 hours of administration.[78] MR spectroscopy offers a unique diagnostic tool to monitor early responses and to demonstrate persistent changes before morphological alterations have occurred.

References

1. Alazraki N: In Resnick D, Niwayama G (eds): Diagnosis of Bone and Joint Disorders. Philadelphia, WB Saunders, 1988, pp 470–471.
2. Atkinson P, Woodcock JP: Döppler Ultrasound and Its Use in Clinical Measurement. New York, Academic Press, 1982, pp 228–236.
3. Azavedo E, Svane G, Auer G: Stereotactic fine needle biopsy in 2,594 mammographically detected non-palpable lesions. Lancet 1:1033–1035, 1989.
4. Bailar JC: Mammography—a contrary view. Ann Intern Med 84:77–84, 1976.
5. Baker LH: The Breast Cancer Demonstration Project: five-year summary report. CA 32(4):194–198, 1982.
6. Bartrum RJ, Crowe HC: Transillumination light scanning to diagnosis breast cancer: a feasibility study. AJR 142:409–414, 1984.
7. Basset LW, Kimme-Smith C, Sutherland LK, Gold RH, Sarti D, King W III: Automated and hand-held breast ultrasound. Radiology 165:103–108, 1987.
8. Bauer W, Igot JP, Le Gal Y: Chronologie du cancer mammaire utilisant un modele de croissance de Gompertz. Ann Anat Pathol 25:39–56, 1980.
9. Broberg A, Glas U, Gustafsson SA, Hellstrom L, Somell A: Relationship between mammographic pattern and estrogen receptor content in breast cancer. Breast Cancer Res 3:201–207, 1983.
10. Ciatto S, Cataliotti L, Distante V: Non-palpable lesions detected with mammography: review of 512 consecutive cases. Radiology 165:99–102, 1987.
11. Citrin DL, Hougen C, Zwiebel W, Schlise S, Pruitt B, Ershler W, Davis TE, Harberg J, Cohen AI: Use of serial bone scans in assessing response of bone metastases to systemic treatment. Cancer 47:680, 1981.
12. Cole-Beuglet C: Ultrasound: Breast Cancer Detection. New York, Grune and Stratton, 1987, pp 153–167.
13. Cole-Beuglet C, Goldberg BB, Kurtz AB, Rubin CS, Patchefsky AS, Shaber GS: Ultrasound mammography—a comparison with mammography. Radiology 139:693–698, 1981.
14. Coleman RE, Rubens RD, Fogelman I: Reappraisal of the baseline bone scan in breast cancer. J Nucl Med 29(6):1045–1049, 1988.
15. Collette HJA, Day NE, Rombach JJ, deWard F: Evaluation of screening for breast cancer in a non-randomised study by means of a case control study. Lancet 1:1224–1226, 1984.
16. Cutler SJ, Asire AJ, Taylor SG: Classification of patients with disseminated cancer of the breast. Cancer 34:861–869, 1969.
17. Dash N, Lupetin AR, Daffner RH, Deeb ZL, Sefczek RJ, Schapiro RL: Magnetic resonance imaging in the diagnosis of breast disease. AJR 146:119–125, 1986.
18. Dempsey PJ: Breast sonography: clinical applications in image interpretation. Breast Imag 99–104, 1986.
19. Derimanov SG: For or against bone scintigraphy in patients with breast cancer. Nucl Med Comm 8:79–86, 1987.
20. D'Orsi CJ, Bartrum RJ, Moskowitz MM: Light Scanning of the Breast in Breast Cancer Detection. New York, Grune & Stratton, 1987, pp 169–177.
21. Drexler B, David JL, Schofield G: Diaphanography in the diagnosis of breast cancer. Radiology 157:41–44, 1985.
22. Eary JF, Schroff RW, Abrams PG, Fritzberg AR, Morgan AC, Kasina S, Reno JM, Srinivasan A, Woodhouse CS, Wilbur DS, Natale RB, Collins C, Stehlin JS, Mitchell M, Nelp WB: Successful imaging of malignant melanoma with Tc99m labelled monoclonal antibodies. J Nucl Med 30:25–32, 1989.
23. Egan R, Egan KL: Detection of breast cancer: comparison of water-bath whole breast sonography, mammography and physical examination. AJR 145:1–8, 1985.
24. Egan RL, Sweeney MB, Sewell CW: Intramammary calcifications without an associate mass in benign or malignant diseases. Radiology 137:1, 1980.
25. Ege GN: Internal mammary lymphoscintigraphy: the rationale technique—interpretation in clinical application. Radiology 118:101–107, 1976.
26. Ege GN: Internal mammary lymphoscintigraphy in the conservative surgical management of breast carcinoma. Clin Radiol 31:559–563, 1980.
27. Ege GN, Elhakin T: The relevance of internal mammary lymphoscintigraphy in the management of breast carcinoma. J Clin Oncol 2:774–781, 1984.
28. El Yousef SJ, O'Connell DM: Magnetic resonance imaging of the breast. Mag Res Ann 177–195, 1986.

29. El Yousef SJ, O'Connell DM, Duchesneau RH, Smith MJ, Hubay CA, Guyton SP: Benign and malignant breast disease: magnetic resonance radiofrequency pulse sequences. AJR 145:1–8, 1985.
30. Ennis JT: Reducing mortality from breast cancer. IMJ 81:2, 1988.
31. Ennis JT, Stack JP, Redmond O, Kirby B, Scully M, Carney DN: MR imaging of bone marrow involvement in small cell lung cancer. Radiology (suppl)169:66, 1988.
32. Ertefai S, Profoio AE: Spectral transmission and contrast in breast diaphanography. Med Phys 4:393–400, 1985.
33. Feig SA: The role of new imaging modalities in staging and follow-up of breast cancer. Semin Oncol 13:402–414, 1986.
34. Feig SA: Decreased breast cancer mortality through mammographic screening: results of clinical trials. Radiology 167:659–665, 1988.
35. Fisher ER: Relationship of fibrocystic disease with cancer of the breast in breast cancer. Breast Cancer CRC 120–135, 1981.
36. Friedrich M: Recent Progress in the Ultrasonic Detection of Early Breast Cancer. New York, Springer-Verlag, 1984, pp 155–173.
37. Gent HJ, Sprenger E, Dowlatshahi K: Stereotactic needle localisation and cytological diagnosis of occult breast lesions. AJR 145:580, 1986.
38. Geslien GE, Fisher JR, De Laney C: Transillumination in breast cancer detection: screening failures and potential. AJR 144:619–622, 1985.
39. Getty DJ: Minimal breast cancer: a clinical meaningful term? Semin Oncol 4:384–392, 1986.
40. Getty DJ, Pickett RM, D'Orsi CJ, Swets JA: Enhanced interpretation of diagnostic images. Invest Radiol 23:240–252, 1988.
41. Gibbons J, Holleb A, Farrow JH: An evaluation of routine preoperative skeletal survey for the patient with operable breast cancer. NY J Med 61:4219–4220, 1961.
42. Goodson WH, Mailman R, Millar T: Three-year follow-up of benign fine needle aspiration biopsies of the breast. Am J Surg 154:58–60, 1987.
43. Hermann G, Janus C, Schwartz IS: Occult malignant breast lesions in 114 patients: relationship to age in the presence of microcalcifications. Radiology 169:321–324, 1988.
44. Heywang SH, Fenzl G, Eiermann W, Beck R, Hahn D, Permanetter W, Lissner J: Magnetic resonance imaging of the breast with Gd-DTPA: development of diagnostic criteria. San Diego, Proceedings of an International Workshop on Contrast Agents and Magnetic Resonance Imagings, 1986, pp 155–158.
45. Homer MJ: Non-palpable lesion localisation using curved end retractable wire. Radiology 157:259–260, 1985.
46. Jackson VP, Rothschild PA, Kreipke DL, Mail JT, Holden RW: Spectrum of sonographic findings of fibroadenoma of the breast. Invest Radiol 21:34–40, 1986.
47. Jellins J, Kossoff G, Reeve TS, et al: Detection and classification of liquid-filled masses in the breast by grey-scale echography. Radiology 125:205–212, 1977.
48. Kelsey JL: A review of the epidemiology of human breast cancer. Epidemiol Rev 1:49, 1979.
49. Kobayashi T: Grey-scale echography for breast cancer. Radiology 122:207–214, 1977.
50. Kobayashi T: Ultrasonic detection for breast cancer. Clin Obstet Gynaecol 25:409–423, 1982.
51. Kopans DB, de Luca S: A modified needle hooked wire technique to simplify pre-operative localisation of occult breast lesions. Radiology 134:781, 1980.
52. Kopans DB, Meyer JF, Lindfors KK, Bucchianeri SS: Breast sonography to guide cyst aspiration and wire localisation of occult solid lesions. AJR 143:489–492, 1984.
53. Kopans DB, Meyer JF, Lindfors KK: Whole breast ultrasound imaging: four year follow-up. Radiology 157:505–507, 1985.
54. Kossoff G, Carpenter DA, Robinson DE, et al: Octoson: a new, rapid and general purpose echoscope. In White D, Barnes R (eds): Ultrasound in Medicine, vol 2. New York, Plenum, 1976, pp 333–339.
55. Kwai AH, Stomper PC, Kaplan WD: Clinical significance of isolated scintigraphic sternal lesions with breast cancer. J Nucl Med 1988; 29:324–328, 1988.
56. Lanyi M: Morphologic analysis of microcalcifications in early breast cancer. In Zander J, Baltzer J (eds): Early Breast Cancer. New York, Springer-Verlag, 1985, pp 113–135.
57. Lawson R: Implications of surface temperatures in the diagnosis of breast cancer. Can Med Assoc J 75:309–310, 1956.
58. Leborg NER: Diagnosis of tumor to the breast by simple roentgenography: calcifications and carcinomas. AJR 65:1, 1951.
59. Lee Y: Bone scanning in patients with early breast carcinoma: should it be a routine staging procedure? Cancer 47:486, 1981.
60. Logan WW, Janus JA: Screen/film Mammography in Breast Cancer Detection. New York, Grune & Stratton, 1987, pp 75–87.
61. Lundy J, Lozowski M, Mishriki Y: Monoclonal antibody B72.3 as a diagnostic adjunct in fine needle aspirates of breast masses. Ann Surg 203:399–402, 1986.
62. McKay EN, Sellars AH: Breast cancer at the Ontario Cancer Clinic—a statistical review. Medical Statistics Branch, Ontario Department of Health, 1965, pp 1938–1956.
63. McNeill BJ: Value of bone scanning in neoplastic disease. Semin Nucl Med 14:277, 1984.
64. McNeill BJ, Pace PD, Gray EB, Adelstein SJ, Wilson RE: Preoperative and follow-up of bone scans in patients with primary carcinoma of the breast. Surg Gynecol Obstet 147:745, 1978.
65. Mazzeo F, Accurso A, Petrella G, Capuano S, Maurelli L, Celentano L, Squame G, Salvatore M: Preoperative axillary lymphoscintigraphy in breast cancer experienced with subareolar injection of Tc^{99m} nano colloidal albumin. Nucl Med Comm 7:5–16, 1986.
66. Milbrath JR: Thermography in Breast Cancer Detection. New York, Grune & Stratton, 1987, pp 145–152.
67. Monsees B, Destouet JM, Gersell D: Light scanning of non-palpable breast lesions: re-evaluation. Radiology 167:352, 1988.
68. Monsees B, Destouet JM, Totti WG: Light scanning vs. mammography in breast cancer detection. Radiology 163:463–465, 1987.
69. Moskowitz M: Screening is not diagnosis. Radiology 133:265–268, 1979.
70. Moskowitz M: Screening for breast cancer: how effective are our tests? A critical review. CA 33:26–27, 1983.
71. Moskowitz M: Thermography: a risk indicator for breast cancer. J Reprod Med 30(6):451–459, 1985.
72. Moskowitz M: Breast cancer screening: all's well that ends well or much ado about nothing? AJR 151:659–665, 1988.
73. Moskowitz M, Milbrath J, Garthside P, Zermeno A, Mandel D: Lack of efficacy in thermography as a screening tool for minimal and Stage 1 breast cancer. New Engl J Med 295:249–252, 1976.
74. Nielsen NS, Nielsen BB: Mammographic features of sclerosing adenosis presenting as a tumor. Clin Radiol 37:371–373, 1986.
75. Nielson NS, Poulsen H: Relation between mammographic findings and hormonal receptor content in breast cancer. AJR 145:501–504, 1985.
76. Oestmann JW, Kopans DB, Linetsky L, Hall DA, McCarthy KA, White G, Swann C, Kelley JE, Johnson LL: Comparison of two screen-film combinations in contact and magnification mammography. Radiology 168:657–659, 1988.
77. Page DL, Dupont WD, Rogers LW: Breast cancer risk of lobular-based hyperplasia after biopsy. Cancer Detect Prevent 9:441–448, 1986.
78. Redmond O, Stack JP, Ennis JT: Tumor response to therapy in breast carcinoma. Radiol (suppl)169:272, 1988.
79. Reilly M, Ennis JT: Ultrasound of the breast. Br J Radiol 54:642, 1981.
80. Roberts JG, Gravelle IH, Baum M, Bligh AS, Leach KG, Hughes LE: Evaluation of radiography in isotope scintigraphy detecting skeletal metastases in breast cancer. Lancet 1:237–239, 1976.
81. Shapiro S: Evidence for screening of breast cancer from a randomization trial. Cancer 39:2772–2782, 1977.
82. Sickles EA: Mammographic detectibility of breast microcalcifications. AJR 139:913–918, 1982.

83. Sickles EA: Breast cancer detection with transillumination in mammography. AJR 142:841–844, 1984.

84. Sickles EA: Mammographic features of 300 consecutive non-palpable breast cancers. AJR 146:661–663, 1986.

85. Sickles EA, Filly RA, Callen PW: Breast cancer detection with sonography and mammography: comparison using state-of-the-art equipment. AJR 140:843–845, 1983.

86. Sickles EA, Filly RA, Callen PW: Benign breast lesions: ultrasound detection and diagnosis. Radiology 151:467–470, 1984.

87. Silverberg E, Lubera J: Cancer Statistics 1987. CA 37:2–19.

88. Stack JP, Redmond O, Codd MB, Heffernan SJ, Dervan PA, Carney DN, Ennis JT: Tissue enhancement profiles with Gd-DTPA in breast carcinoma. Radiology 169 (suppl):22, 1988.

89. Stelling CB, Powell DE, Mattingly SS: Fibroadenomas: histopathological and MR imaging features. Radiology 162:399–407, 1987.

90. Stomper PC, Davis SP, Sonnenfeld MR, Meyer JE, Greenes RA, Eberlein TJ: Efficacy of specimen radiography of clinically occult non-calcified breast lesions. AJR 151:43–47, 1988.

91. Tabar L, Bentek Z, Dean PB: The diagnostic and therapeutic value of breast cyst puncture and pneumocystography. Radiology 14:659–663, 1981.

92. Tabar L, Dean PB: The control of breast cancer through mammography screening. Radiol Clin North Am 25:993–1005, 1987.

93. Tabar L, Fagerberg CJG, Gad A, Baldetorp L, Holmberg LH, Grontoft O, Ljungquist U, Lundstrom B, Manson JC, Eklund G, Day NE, Pettersson F: Reduction in mortality from breast cancer after mass screening with mammography. Lancet 1:829–832, 1985.

94. Threatt B: Ductography: Breast Cancer Detection. New York, Grune & Stratton, 1987, pp 119–129.

95. United Kingdom National Case Control Study Group: Oral contraceptive use and breast cancer risk in young women. Lancet 1:973–982, 1989.

96. Verbeek ALM, Holland R, Sturmans F, Hendriks JHCL, Mravunac M, Day NE: Reduction in breast cancer mortality through mass screening with modern mammography. Lancet 1:1222–1224, 1984.

97. Watmough DJ: Diaphanography: mechanism responsible for the images. Acta Radiol (Oncol) 21:11–15, 1982.

98. Wellings SR, Alpers CF: Apocrine cystic metaplasia. Hum Pathol 18:381–386, 1987.

99. Wells PNT: Döppler ultrasound in medical diagnosis. Br J Radiol 62:399–420, 1989.

100. Wells PNT, Evans KT: An immersion scanner for two-dimensional ultrasonic examination of the human breast. Ultrasonics 6:222–228, 1968.

101. Wertheimer MD, Castanza ME, Dodson TF, D'Orsi C, Pastides H, Zapka JG: Minimal breast cancer. JAMA 255:1311–1315, 1986.

102. Wilhelm C, Paredes ES, Pope T, Wanebo HJ: The changing mammogram. Arch Surg 121:1311–1313, 1986.

103. Winchester DP, Lasky HJ, Silvester J, Maher ML: Television promoted mammography screening pilot project in the Chicago Metropolitan Area. CA 38(5):291–309, 1988.

104. Wolfe JW: Risk for breast cancer determined by mammographic parenchymal pattern. Cancer 37:2486–2492, 1976.

105. Yokiama K, Kacarrasquillo JA, Chang AE: Differences in bio distribution of Indium-111 and Iodine-131 labelled B72.3 monoclonal antibodies in patients with colorectal cancer. J Nucl Med 30:320–327, 1989.

Chapter 25

INTERVAL BREAST CANCER AND THE KINETICS OF NEOPLASTIC GROWTH

John E. Niederhuber, M.D.

In the large population-based, randomized screening trials designed to evaluate the efficacy of mammography to detect early occult breast cancer, a subset of women had their cancers diagnosed after a negative mammogram but prior to the next scheduled screening examination.[2, 6, 14, 36, 45, 50] Fortunately, the incidence of these *interval* cancers in the screened population is low, which in itself is a measure of the effectiveness of mammography as a screening tool. Concern, however, has always existed that these interval breast cancers represent tumors with a shorter doubling time, and therefore a more aggressive metastatic potential.[3, 10, 16, 17, 31] The question of a biological difference between interval cancers and screen-detected cancers has been further confused by the possibility that there exists among screen-detected cancers an excess of slow-growing tumors.[24] These observations have led to the suggestion that interval cancers should be treated more aggressively.[10]

Recent reports, however, indicate that interval cancers have a similar prognosis to cancers diagnosed in an unscreened population (i.e., the control population).[18, 36] These observations would seem to be at odds with the frequently stated hypothesis that the more rapid growth rate of the interval cancer results in a greater metastatic potential. Obviously, the significance of interval cancers and the relationship of growth rate to prognosis relate directly to decisions regarding appropriate therapy. This chapter will attempt to review the available clinical trials data relevant to the natural history of interval cancers and the relationship among breast cancer doubling time, metastatic potential, and overall prognosis.

INTERVAL CANCERS

While a number of screening trials have provided data concerning the incidence of interval breast cancers, almost all of our information concerning interval breast cancers and their relative risk comes from two large randomized trials: the Health Insurance Plan (HIP) study of New York and the Swedish two-county study.[36, 45] The Swedish trial has contributed significantly to this subject because it was designed with longer inter-screen-ing intervals. The longer time between screens made it possible to study the effect of interval length on the incidence of interval cancers and their clinical stage. The proportion of cancers detected as interval cancers and the prognosis (i.e., stage) of the cancers diagnosed at the next screen are what determines an acceptable interval between screens. The design of the Swedish study with longer screen intervals provided an opportunity to look at these important factors in greater detail.

The first breast cancer screening trial to use randomization in its design was the HIP study, initiated in 1963. Two systematic random samples of 31,000 women aged 40 to 64 years were selected from HIP, a comprehensive prepaid group practice in New York. Following an initial screening examination, the study group women were offered three additional examinations on an annual basis. The control group was not screened and continued to receive their usual medical care. By the end of 10 years, the study group mortality resulting from breast cancer was approximately 30 percent lower than that in the control group.[45] Interestingly, the small number of interval cancers diagnosed in the HIP study group had the same case-fatality rate as the control group.[36]

The two-county Swedish study is even more enlightening because of its design and because it was able to make use of the many technical advances in mammography that have occurred since the 1960s. The Swedish trial began in 1977 and involved 162,981 women aged 40 or older.[45] The women were randomly assigned to study or control on a population-block basis drawn from small local administrative units or parishes in two counties. Between the first and second screenings, the average interval was 33 months for women 50 years of age and older, and 24 months for women younger than 50 years. The average interval between the second and third examinations was 24 months for all age groups. Compliance for the three screening examinations was quite good, being 89.2 percent, 83.3 percent, and 84.0 percent, respectively. This study had another interesting design feature that incorporated screening of the control population after the completion of the third round of screening for those aged 50 or older and after the fourth screen in those younger than 50 years. In 1986, the Swedish group reported that during the first 7 years of screening, 104 of 465 breast cancers presented as interval cancers.[18] Ten of the 104 were in situ and were excluded from analysis. In addition, a blinded radiological review of the cases revealed only six that were judged to be cancers missed on prior screen. These 94 interval cancers were compared to 178 breast cancers in the control group.

Overall, the survival rate was higher in the interval cancer group than in the control cancers, but this difference was not significant. A similar trend of even greater difference was observed when comparing the disease-free intervals. These observations remained true even with a proportional hazards analysis, which introduced age, tumor size, axillary nodal involvement, and TNM stage into the analysis. Furthermore, when the authors analyzed the time between last screen and diagnosis of the interval cancer by the proportional hazards model, they could not demonstrate that this time factor was related to prognosis. Thus these findings confirmed the observations in the earlier HIP project and were perhaps even more significant when considering that the equipment used in this more recent trial had greater sensitivity. Therefore, the Swedish series should be weighted for selection of interval cancers that were likely to be more rapid growing than those detected in the HIP study.

The Swedish trial also observed that the proportion of deaths among women who refused screening increased rapidly with age, reaching 50 percent in the 70- to 74-year-old age group, whereas the proportion of deaths found in the interval cancer group decreased rapidly with age.[43] In their analysis of the screened population, they observed that more than 50 percent of deaths from breast cancer in the 40- to 49-year-old age group were from interval cancers.

It is important to examine the incidence of interval cancers based on the length of time between screens and the age of the screening population. To do this, the Swedish group determined the incidence of breast cancers each year in the randomly selected control population. This provided the basis for estimating the number of cases that should be detected by screening each year. The ratio of the number of cases observed and the number expected (i.e., the number predicted from the control population) gives the *proportional incidence* of interval cancers.

The contrast between the proportional incidence of interval cancers in the 40- to 49-year-old and the 50- to 69-year-old age groups was quite significant. In the younger women, screening detected 62 percent of the cancers that would have surfaced in the first 12 months, and only 32 percent of the cancers predicted for the second 12 months. In contrast, the screening exam detected 87 percent for the first and 71 percent for the second 12 months in the 50- to 69-year-old group.[43] The Swedish trial also found that the proportion of Stage II cancers in the interval cases, 57.5 percent, was essentially the same as for the cancers diagnosed in the control group (59.2 percent). In this case, age had no effect on the percent of Stage II cases found in either group.[43]

The results of the HIP and Swedish randomized trials

support the conclusion that the prognosis of interval cancers is the same as that of similarly staged cancers diagnosed in a nonscreened population. Although interval cancers may be more rapidly growing tumors, no evidence can be found that patients with interval cancers are at greater risk for a more rapid course of systemic dissemination and death. Clearly, the value of screening is in the earlier stage of cancers detected at repeat screening, especially with increasing age (38 percent Stage II, age 40 to 49 years; 25 percent Stage II, age 50 to 59 years; and 17 percent Stage II, age 60 to 69 years). Although it is tempting to compare interval cancers with cancers detected at regularly scheduled screening examinations, this would be invalid because of the length bias sampling error in the screened population.[44, 51]

It should be recalled that the Swedish study consisted of only a single-film view of the breast. Therefore, the incidence of interval cancer can be expected to be even lower using annual two-view screening mammography combined with physical examination of the breast. In addition, shorter-interval follow-up is often indicated when uncertainties arise. Overall, even with an optimum screening program, the incidence of interval cancers can be expected to be about 12 percent.

KINETICS OF BREAST CANCER GROWTH

General Observations and the Cell Cycle

The rate of growth of the primary breast cancer and its metastases is a major determinant of the patient's ultimate survival. Breast cancer cells, like other tumor cells, undergo binary division, grow to a certain state, and then repeat the division—a process known as the *cell cycle*.[19] This cycle of cell division, as with normal cells, is divided into four stages: G_1, S (DNA synthesis), G_2, and M (mitosis) (Fig. 25–1).[30, 42, 53] G_1 is the "gap" between completion of cell division and the beginning

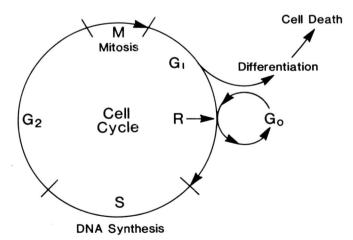

Figure 25–1. The cell cycle is divided into two phases: interphase and mitosis (M). Interphase has been subdivided into: gap 1 (G_1), a phase of DNA synthesis (S), and gap 2 (G_2). A restriction point (R) exists in G_1 and determines whether the cell can progress to S phase. If the cell is not triggered to DNA synthesis, it may be shunted to a resting state termed G_0.

of the next round of DNA synthesis in the S phase. The two daughter cells generated by mitosis reside in either G_1 or G_0 (the resting state) and retain a diploid set of chromosomes.

Cells in culture usually spend several hours in G_1; for example, NIH-3T3 cells generally have a G_1 of 6 hours, and L cells a G_1 of 12 hours. The G_1 transit time is, however, highly variable, even from one cell to another within the same culture, and it is during G_1 that the cell is most affected by external conditions. Studies of cell cycle kinetics suggest that a specific control event, called a *restriction point,* exists within the G_1 stage, and this control point determines whether the cell can progress to DNA synthesis.[32]

If the cell is not triggered to DNA synthesis, it may be shunted into a resting state termed G_0, from which the cell can reenter G_1 when conditions are appropriate. It appears to be rare for tumor cells to enter G_0. During the S phase, cells synthesize DNA, and chromosomal replication begins. The average duration of the S phase of NIH-3T3 cells in culture is 8 hours, and at the completion of DNA synthesis, the cell has replicated its entire complement of genetic material and thus has two diploid sets of chromosomes. The S phase is followed by a second gap termed G_2, averaging approximately 3 hours for NIH-3T3 cells in culture.

The daughter chromosomes generated during the S phase remain intimately associated with their partners until mitosis. During G_1, S, and G_2 (the *interphase* of the cell cycle), RNA and protein synthesis are steadily increasing with duplication of all organelles, including ribosomes and mitochondria. Mitosis, the shortest segment of the cycle, represents the culmination of cell growth that has occurred during G_1, S, and G_2 and is the process by which the cell distributes two sets of identical chromosomes to the two daughter cells. As noted, the most variable period of the cell cycle is the first gap, G_1. G_1 essentially determines the length of the cycle by responding or not responding to intrinsic or extrinsic signals that trigger entry into the S phase.[4, 32]

The best estimates for cell cycle time of human solid tumors (including breast cancer), obtained using the percentage-labeled mitosis method, indicate that 90 percent fall within 15 and 120 hours (median, 48 hours).[48] The duration of the S phase is less variable, with 90 percent being between 9.5 and 24 hours (median, 16 hours). While the duration of the cell cycle may vary significantly from one cell to another within a tumor, there appears to be less variation based on tumor histology. In fact, differences in cell cycle time cannot explain the much greater variation observed for actual tumor doubling time.

The growth rate of the primary breast cancer and its metastases is determined by a complex set of interrelated events that are a balance between cell gain (cell proliferation) and cell loss. Cell gain is determined by the fraction of tumor cell mass that is actively dividing and by the time each dividing cell spends completing the cell cycle. Some information exists to estimate the fraction of breast tumor cells actively dividing. The most recent is an analysis of 1000 breast tumors by Dressler et al.[11]

They found that the median proportion of cells in S phase was 2.6 percent if the tumors were diploid and 10.4 percent if they were aneuploid.

The tumor, while growing, is also losing cells through cell death and via the shedding of tumor cells into the circulation (vascular and lymphatic) or into an adjacent body cavity. Thus the actual measured tumor doubling time represents a net effect of all these concurrent processes. For various tumors, including breast, it has been possible to measure cell cycle time, and on occasion serial measurements of imaged tumor masses have given direct information about actual tumor doubling time.

Spratt and Spratt have described three patterns of tumor growth within a tumor.[41] The first, termed *linear growth,* describes a cancer that has its linear dimensions increased a specific amount each day—an increment that is not altered by tumor size. This pattern implies that the majority of cell proliferation is occurring only at the periphery of the mass. The second example is termed *exponential growth.* In this case, the tumor has a randomly steady increase in volume per unit of time. This model requires a uniform cell cycle and a uniform but random rate of cells entering cell division. In addition, cell loss must be minimal or at least constant. Both of these types of growth can be described by mathematical equations.[41]

A number of additional factors, however, impact on the growth rate of human tumors. For example, as size increases, parts of the tumor may outgrow the tumor blood supply and develop areas of necrosis or ischemia. Thus the rate of cell proliferation may vary even within the tumor. In the case of breast cancer, growth is also influenced considerably by hormonal mechanisms, namely estrogens and other growth factors, both stimulatory and inhibitory.

This example in which the growth rate decreases as size increases has been described mathematically as a *Gompertzian function.*[23, 33, 40, 41] A cancer following Gompertzian growth initially grows rapidly, but as its size increases, its growth curve is downwardly concave and approaches a horizontal asymptote. The potential slowing of growth as size increases makes it difficult to determine the date of tumor initiation by simply extrapolating from observed doubling time. Nevertheless, despite the Gompertzian growth curve, measuring tumor doubling time contributes valuable information. It is also important to note that while the same tumor type in different patients may have different doubling times, the various metastatic lesions in an individual patient tend to show a very uniform rate of growth—a rate that is generally more rapid than the original primary lesion.[48]

Direct Observations of Breast Cancer Growth

In 1963, Gershon-Cohen and colleagues reported on 18 patients who had not had immediate biopsy until two or more mammograms had been obtained.[15] An additional case from the Ellis Fisehel State Cancer Hospital in Missouri was added and used to calculate a median observed doubling time (DT) of 120 days (range, 23 to 209 days).[41] One study reported on 147 breast cancers that had 388 serial mammograms prior to definitive treatment. The observation time ranged from 2 months to 11 years and averaged 27 months.[5] Measured tumor volume DTs were 44 to 1869 days, with an average of 212 days. From these observations, the authors concluded that the smallest lesion detectable by mammography would be 1 to 2 mm in diameter, or about 20 doublings. Growth from this size to 10 mm required, on the average, 4 additional years, or a total of 20 years from initial transformed cell to a 2-cm tumor. No correlation was found between DT and tumor differentiation, and no relationship between DT and the incidence of axillary lymph node metastases was demonstrated.[5] Others, however, have found that the growth rate was higher in patients younger than 50 years with nodal involvement.[47] From these direct observations of early primary breast cancer growth using mammography, the average growth curve is more consistent with an exponential function than a Gompertzian curve.

Indirect Measurement of Tumor Growth

In the early 1970s, investigators introduced the technique of tritiated thymidine labeling of tumor cell DNA during S phase. This technique for identifying specific cells in the process of dividing is based on the fact that DNA is synthesized in the cell only during active division and in so doing will take up exogenous thymidine. Providing the dividing cells with a source of radiolabeled thymidine makes it possible to identify these cells. Labeled cells are exposed to a plate coated with a photographic emulsion, and the number of radioactive cell nuclei are counted. This ratio of labeled to unlabeled cells is termed the "labeling index" (LI) and provides an estimate in vitro of the potential tumor DT.[5, 26, 28, 47, 49] Of course, cell loss in growing tumors may be low or in excess of 90 percent of the rate of cell production[47] and therefore may make the actual DT longer than predicted by the measured LI. Nevertheless, LI correlates quite well with actual DT.

The Institute Gustave-Roussy has reported the measurement of the LI in 128 consecutive breast cancers. Their results, initially reported in 1975 and updated several times, have shown a higher LI in patients with relapse.[26, 47, 49] Other studies examining large numbers of patients have reached a similar conclusion.[27, 29, 38] Subjecting LI to multivariant analysis has shown that its prognostic impact on relapse and death is independent of stage, tumor size, and nodal involvement. The LI does, however, show a strong correlation with nuclear and histological grade.[26, 28, 38]

Silvestrini et al. determined the LI on fresh tumors of 258 node-negative patients (Stages T1, T2, and T3a) treated by radical mastectomy. In their study, the probability of a 6-year relapse-free survival was 80.5 percent for patients with a low LI and 59.6 percent for patients with a high LI ($p = 0.00004$).[39] Tubiana points out that the low incidence of relapse in the low LI patients cannot be solely the result of differences in growth rates but must be partly the result of differences in metastasizing potential.[47]

Recently, the application of DNA flow cytometry and image cytometry has provided a more accurate assessment of the number of tumor cells in S phase.[25] Furthermore, by substituting bromodeoxyuridine (BrdU) for tritiated thymidine, the labeled cells can be detected by an anti-BrdU antibody. Thus, it is possible to determine the proportion of cells engaged in a cell cycle, the duration of the cycle, and the DNA ploidy of the breast tumor.[9]

Preliminary data indicate that breast cancers with diploid DNA content tend to be of low histological grade and high ER content, while tumors with higher DNA ploidy are more anaplastic and low in receptor content.[7, 9] As a result, the simultaneous measurement of these prognostic indicators provides a useful method of identifying the subsets of patients at increased risk.

Natural History of Breast Cancer

As noted, it has been possible to use the large population-based randomized breast cancer screening trials to study a broader range of questions concerning the biology of breast cancer. The analysis of the observed prevalence of cancer detected at the time of a given screen and the incidence of cancers discovered during the intervals between screens has provided insight into the kinetics of breast cancer cell growth and the biological activity (metastatic potential) of the disease. During the asymptomatic preclinical phase of breast cancer growth, there is a time when the *prevalent cancer* has reached a size detectable by screening mammography. This time point is determined by a number of variables, including rate of tumor cell growth, the suitability of the breast for optimal imaging, the sensitivity of equipment used, and the skill of the physician(s) interpreting the results.

The interval between the time of detection by screening and the time when the cancer becomes clinically incident (*incident cancer*) is defined as the *lead time* (Fig. 25–2). Thus the longer the lead time the better the prognosis. Lead time, of course, depends directly on the length of time a breast cancer is in the preclinical (asymptomatic) phase, but is detectable by screening. The longer this preclinical phase of detectable cancer, the longer the lead time.

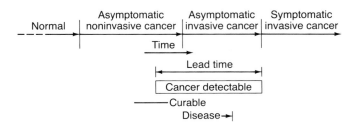

Figure 25–2. A model of breast cancer progression. Estimates suggest that mammography is capable of detecting tumors once they have reached 1 to 2 mm in diameter.

Table 25-1. ANALYSIS OF PRECLINICAL PHASE OF BREAST CANCER

Report	Data Base	Estimated Mean Pre-clinical Duration (years)	Estimated Mean Lead Time (years)
Hutchison and Shapiro[20]	HIP	1.7	0.85
Zelen and Feinleib[52]	HIP	2.4	2.4
Shapiro et al.[35]	HIP	1.3	0.65
Tallis and Sarfaty[46]	Melbourne Cancer Registry	1.8	—
Seidman[34]	BCDDP	—	1.4
Fox et al.[13]	BCDDP	—	3.0
Albert et al.[1]	HIP	1.8	—
Shwartz[37]	HIP, BCDDP	—	1.9
Dubin[12]	HIP	—	0.4
Walter and Day[8, 51]	HIP	1.7	1.7

Abbreviations: BCDDP = Breast Cancer Detection Demonstration Project study; HIP = Health Insurance Plan study.
(From Walter SD, Day NE: Am J Epidemiol 118:865, 1983. Reprinted by permission.)

If the breast cancer has developed to the point where it is no longer curable at the time of screening, the time between diagnosis and death is prolonged only by the lead time. Earlier detection, in this case, does not affect the time of death. It is also possible that screening may detect breast cancers with a long asymptomatic noninvasive phase; some of these might never have become clinically detectable (*length bias sampling*), and their detection by screening would have little impact on breast cancer mortality.

Using the HIP study, Walter and Day determined an estimated lead time of 1.387 years for breast cancer detected in the first year of screening.[8, 51] In subsequent years, the number of cases found at screening diminished, presumably as the number of prevalent cases in the screened population gradually decreased. Table 25-1 summarizes the results of a number of investigators who have determined the preclinical phase and the lead time. As can be seen, there is a large variation in estimates of lead time, ranging from 0.4 to 3.0 years. This large variation is undoubtedly the result of using numerous unverified assumptions in the calculations and a great diversity of mathematical approaches. In addition, some authors used data from the Breast Cancer Detection Demonstration Project (BCDDP), a nonrandomized screening study, for their calculation of lead time. The best estimate of lead time for cancers detected by mammography appears to be the one calculated by Walter and Day of 1.7 years for each screening period.[8, 51]

Recently, studies of a large group of breast cancer patients at the Institute Gustave-Roussy divided cancers according to their volume at surgical excision and plotted for each subset of volumes the actuarial cumulated proportion of patients with metastases as a function of time from treatment up to 25 years.[21] From their extensive analysis of these data, the investigators have concluded that the capacity for lymphatic spread is acquired much earlier than the capacity for hematogenous spread. In rapidly growing tumors, initial axillary node invasion was estimated in their model to have occurred when the primary tumor was 2 mm to 3 mm in diameter, and distant metastasis was estimated to have occurred with a tumor diameter of less than 1.5 cm.[21] This differed markedly from what was observed for tumors with a slow growth rate, where the predictions for axillary node invasion and distant metastasis were for tumors with a diameter of 4 cm and 6 cm, respectively.

The ability of screening mammography to diagnose breast cancer early during the lead time when it is either noninvasive or early in its invasive growth emphasizes the importance of assessing the biological parameters for each tumor. In the future, the patient's risk for occult metastases will be determined by assessing tumor growth rate, histological grade, receptor content, and DNA ploidy. From such a profile it will be possible to predict the patient's position on the risk curve and thereby select the appropriate surgical and adjuvant therapy.

References

1. Albert A, Gertman PM, Louis TA: Screening for the early detection of cancer. 1. The temporal natural history of a progressive disease state. Math Biosci 40:1–59, 1978.
2. Andersson I, Janzon L, Sigfirsson BF: Mammographic breast cancer screening—a randomized trial in Malmo, Sweden. Maturitas 7:21–29, 1985.
3. Bland KI, Buchanan JB, Mills DL, Kuhns JG, et al: Analysis of breast cancer screening in women younger than fifty years. JAMA 10:1037–42, 1981.
4. Brooks RF, Bennet DC, Smith JA: Mammalian cell cycles need two random transitions. Cell 19:493, 1980.
5. Chavaudra N, Richard JM, Malaise EP: Labelling index of human squamous cell carcinomas. Comparison of *in-vitro* and *in-vivo* labelling methods. Cell Tissue Kinet 12:145–152, 1979.
6. Collette HJA, Day NE, Rombach JJ, et al: Evaluation of screening for breast cancer in a non-randomized study (the DOM project) by means of a case-control study. Lancet i:1224–1226, 1984.
7. Coulson PB, Thornthwaite JT, Woolley TE, Sugarbaker EV, Seckinger D: Prognostic indicators including DNA histogram type, receptor content and staging related to human breast cancer survival. Cancer Res 44:4187–4196, 1984.
8. Day NE, Walter SD: Simplified models of screening for chronic disease: estimation procedures from mass screening programmes. Biometrics 40(1):1–14, 1984.
9. Dean PN, Dolbeare F, Gratzner H, Rice GC, Gray JW: Cell-cycle analysis using a monoclonal antibody to BrdUrd. Cell Tissue Kinet 17:427–436, 1984.
10. DeGroote R, Rush BF, Milazzo J, Warden MJ, Rocko JM: Interval breast cancer: a more aggressive subset of breast neoplasias. Surgery 94:543–547, 1983.
11. Dressler LG, Owens M, Seamer L, McGuire WL: Identifying breast cancer patients for adjuvant therapy by DNA flow

cytometry and steroid receptors; a 1000 patient study. (Abstract 238) Proceedings Twenty-second Annual Meeting of ASCO, May 4-6, 1986, Los Angeles, Calif.

12. Dubin N: Benefits of screening for breast cancer: application of a probabilistic model to a breast cancer detection project. J Chronic Dis 32:145–51, 1979.

13. Fox SH, Moskowitz M, Saenger EL, Keriakes JG, Milbrath J, Goodman MW: Benefit/risk analysis of aggressive mammographic screening. Radiology 128:359–365, 1978.

14. Frisell J, Glas U, Hellstrom L, et al: Randomized mammographic screening for breast cancer in Stockholm. Breast Cancer Res Treat 8:45–54, 1986.

15. Gershon-Cohen J, Berger SM, Klickstein HS: Roentgenography of breast cancer moderating concept of "biologic predeterminism." Cancer 16:961–964, 1963.

16. Heuser L, Spratt JS, Polk HC: Growth rates of primary breast cancer. Cancer 43:1888–1894, 1979.

17. Heuser LS, Spratt JS, Kuhns JG, Chang AF-C, Polk HC Jr, Buchanan JB: The association of pathologic and mammographic characteristics of primary human breast cancers with "slow" and "fast" growth rates and with axillary lymph node metastases. Cancer 53:96–98, 1984.

18. Holmberg LH, Adami HO, Tabar L, Bergstrom R: Survival in breast cancer diagnosed between mammographic screening examinations. Lancet ii:27–30, 1986.

19. Howard A, Pelc S: Nuclear incorporation of ^{32}P as demonstrated by autoradiographs. Exp Cell Res 2:178–187, 1951.

20. Hutchison GB, Shapiro S: Lead time gained by diagnostic screening for breast cancer. J Natl Cancer Inst 41:665–681, 1968.

21. Koscielny S, Tubiana M, Lee MG, et al: Breast cancer, relationship between the size of the primary tumor and the probability of metastatic dissemination. Br J Cancer 49:709–715, 1984.

22. Koscielny S, Tubiana M, Valleron AJ: A simulation model of the natural history of human breast cancer. Br J Cancer 52:515–524, 1985.

23. Laird AK: Dynamics of tumor growth: comparison of growth rates and extrapolation of growth curve to one cell. Br J Cancer 19:278–291, 1965.

24. Love RR, Camilli AE: The value of screening. Cancer 48:489–494, 1981.

25. McDivitt RW, Stone KR, Meyer JS: A method for dissociation of viable human breast cancer cells that produces flow cytometric kinetic information similar to that obtained by thymidine labeling. Cancer Res 44:2628–2633, 1984.

26. McGurrin JF, Doria MI, Dawson PJ, et al: Assessment of tumor cell kinetics by immunohistochemistry in carcinoma of breast. Cancer 59:1744–1750, 1987.

27. Meyer JS, Friedman E, McCrate MM, Bauer WC: Prediction of early course of breast carcinoma by thymidine labeling. Cancer 51:1879–1886, 1983.

28. Meyer JS, Hixon B: Advanced stage and early relapse of breast carcinomas associated with high thymidine labeling indices. Cancer Res 39:4042–4047, 1979.

29. Meyer JS, Prey MU, Babcock DS, McDivitt RW: Breast carcinoma cell kinetics, morphology, stage and host characteristics: a thymidine labeling study. Lab Invest 54:41–51, 1986.

30. Mitchison JM: The Biology of the Cell Cycle. London, Cambridge University Press, 1971.

31. Panoussopoulos D, Chang J, Humphrey LJ: Screening for breast cancer. Ann Surg 186:356–362, 1977.

32. Pardee AB: A restriction point for control of normal animal cell proliferation. Proc Natl Acad Sci USA 11:1286–1290, 1974.

33. Salmon SE, Smith BA: Immunoglobulin synthesis and total body tumor cell number in IgG multiple myeloma. J Clin Invest 49:1114–1121, 1970.

34. Seidman H: Screening for breast cancer in younger women: life expectancy gains and losses. CA 27:66–87, 1977.

35. Shapiro S, Goldberg JD, Hutchinson GB: Lead time in breast cancer detection and implications for periodicity of screening. Am J Epidemiol 100:357–366, 1974.

36. Shapiro S, Venet W, Strax P, Venet L, Roeser R: Ten to fourteen year effect of screening on breast cancer mortality. J Natl Cancer Inst 69:349–355, 1982.

37. Shwartz M: An analysis of the benefits of serial screening for breast cancer based upon a mathematical model of the disease. Cancer 41:1550–1564, 1978.

38. Silvestrini R, Daidone MG, Valagussa P, Salvadori B, Rovini D, Bonodonna G: Cell kinetics as a prognostic marker in locally advanced breast cancer. Cancer Treat Rep 71:375–379, 1987.

39. Silvestrini R, Daidone MG, Gasparini G: Cell kinetics as a prognostic marker in node negative breast cancer. Cancer 56:1982–1987, 1985.

40. Sommers SC: Growth Rates, Cell Kinetics and Mathematical Models of Human Cancers. Pathobiology Annual, vol 3. New York, Appleton-Century-Crofts, 1973, p 309.

41. Spratt JS, Spratt JA: Growth rates. In Donegan NL, Spratt JS (eds): Cancer of the Breast. Major Problems in Clinical Surgery, vol 5. Philadelphia, WB Saunders, 1979, pp 197–220.

42. Stanners CP, Till JE: DNA synthesis in individual L-strain mouse cells. Biochem Biophys Acta 37:406–419, 1960.

43. Tabár L, Faberberg G, Day NE, Holmberg L: What is the optimum interval between mammographic screening examinations? An analysis based on the latest results of the Swedish two-county breast cancer screening trial. Br J Cancer 55:547–551, 1987.

44. Tabàr L, Dean PB: The control of breast cancer through mammography screening. What is the evidence? Radiol Clin North Am 25:993–1005, 1987.

45. Tabár L, Faberberg CJG, Gad A, et al: Reduction in mortality from breast cancer after mass screening with mammography: randomized trial from the breast cancer screening working group of the Swedish National Board of Health and Welfare. Lancet i:829–832, 1985.

46. Tallis GM, Sarfaty G: On the distribution of the time to reporting cancers with application to breast cancer in women. Math Biosci 19:371–376, 1974.

47. Tubiana M, Koscielyn S: Cell kinetics, growth rate and the natural history of breast cancer. The Heuson Memorial Lecture. Eur J Cancer Clin Oncol 24:1879–1886, 1983.

48. Tubiana M, Malaise EP: Growth rate and cell kinetics in human tumors: some prognostic and therapeutic implications. In Symington T, Carter RL (eds): Scientific Foundations of Oncology. London, Heinemann, 1976, pp 126–136.

49. Tubiana M, Pejovie MH, Chavaudia N, Contesso G, Malaise EP: The long-term prognostic significance of the thymidine labelling index in breast cancer. Int J Cancer 33:441–445, 1987.

50. Verbeek ALM, Hendricks JHCL, Holland R, et al: Reduction of breast cancer mortality through mass screening with modern mammography: first results of the Nijmegen project, 1975–1981. Lancet i:1222–1224, 1984.

51. Walter SD, Day NE: Estimation of the duration of a preclinical disease state using screening data. Am J Epidemiol 118:865–886, 1983.

52. Zelen M, Feinleib M: On the theory of screening for chronic diseases. Biometrika 56:601–613, 1969.

53. Zetterberg A: Nuclear and cytoplasmic growth during interphase in mammalian cells. Adv Cell Biol 1:211–232, 1970.

Chapter 26

CYTOLOGICAL NEEDLE SAMPLING OF THE BREAST: TECHNIQUES AND END RESULTS

Edward J. Wilkinson, M.D., Daisy A. Franzini, M.D., and Shahla Masood, M.D.

HISTORY OF BREAST FINE NEEDLE ASPIRATION

The use of fine needle aspiration (FNA) for the diagnosis of tumor is attributed to Martin and Ellis, who in 1930 published their classic study on this procedure.[104] The work on FNA was prompted by Dr. James Ewing, who had objections to preliminary surgical excision of breast tumors because of concern regarding the dissemination of the tumor by biopsy.[160] It is of interest that the pathologist who interpreted these samples was Dr. Fred Stewart.[160] Stewart[173] in 1933, and Martin and Ellis[104] in 1934, published further studies on the use of FNA. The procedure, however, did not gain acceptance for a variety of reasons, one of which was concern regarding spreading of tumor as a result of needle puncture. Tumor growing out the needle tract had been reported in a few but highly influential cases. It required the careful and comprehensive work on FNA by Franzen and Zajicek to reintroduce the procedure. Their publications, from 1967 through 1974, were influential in renewing interest in FNA in the United States and elsewhere.[50, 199, 200] However, only in the past few years has concerted interest in breast FNA occurred. Cost and associated hospital utilization have been major factors stimulating interest in breast FNA. Breast FNA is rapid and cost effective when compared to breast biopsy.[150] Improved understanding of the biology of malignant tumors has also provided a rationale for the reintroduction of FNA. It is now understood that once an epithelial tumor is established and extends beyond its intra-epithelial site, it grows into the adjacent subepithelial tissue, gaining access to the extracellular space and vascular spaces. From there it has access to the peripheral circulation. This process, as well as it is understood, is not influenced by FNA. Follow-up studies comparing women who had FNA on their breast tumors to those who did not, reveal that there are no significant differences in the recurrence or survival in these two groups.[10, 81, 147]

A large number of terms have appeared in the literature referring to the FNA procedure. These terms are listed in Table 26–1. For the purpose of clarity, the acronym "FNA" or the term "fine needle aspiration" will be used throughout this text. This term has the advantage that it includes needle size (fine needle) and the technique (aspiration) to clearly delineate it from needle biopsy, with which it may be confused. It is generally the most common term used in referring to this procedure.

COMPARISON OF FNA TO LARGE NEEDLE BIOPSY

Fine needle aspiration results have been compared to biopsy results with a large needle such as the TruCut needle. In general the FNA is more accurate[67, 153] and has a lower false-negative rate than large needle biopsy, the latter having a false-negative rate as high as 20 percent.[56] Some reports identify no statistical difference in either sensitivity or specificity between the two procedures.[22] The results of large needle biopsies studied

Table 26–1. EQUIVALENT TERMS USED TO DESCRIBE FINE NEEDLE ASPIRATION FOR CYTOLOGIC STUDY

Fine needle aspiration (FNA)
Fine needle aspiration cytology
Fine needle aspiration biopsy
Fine needle biopsy
Needle aspiration biopsy (NAB)
Needle biopsy
Needle aspiration cytology
Aspiration biopsy
Aspiration cytology
Aspiration biopsy cytology
Thin needle aspiration biopsy

by frozen section are comparable in speed to FNA, but at considerably greater cost. Both procedures can be performed in the outpatient setting, thus reducing the cost by 90 percent when compared to hospitalization and excisional biopsy.[74]

The large needle biopsy is a more painful procedure than FNA. The specimen obtained, when submitted for frozen section, often reveals extensive crush artifact and accompanying fat. Most pathologists who are experienced with both breast FNA and large needle preparations prefer examination of the FNA sample for diagnosis. Currently, however, more pathologists are familiar with the interpretation of breast biopsies (including large needle biopsies) on frozen section than are familiar with breast FNA.[166] With the current interest in FNA by pathologists, it is anticipated that greater experience and skill with FNA of the breast is only a matter of training and time.

EVALUATION OF BREAST MASSES BY FINE NEEDLE ASPIRATION

General Principles

A basic principle of FNA is that it is not performed unless there is a palpable mass or a mass that has been identified by mammography or similar screening procedure. There is no reason to attempt needle aspiration of nonspecific changes in the breast or to use FNA as a screening technique on a breast that is clinically interpreted as negative. The combination of physical examination, mammography, and FNA will give a diagnostic accuracy approaching 100 percent.[63] A negative FNA finding in the presence of a palpable mass, however, does not exclude tumor when the mass is clinically suspicious, because the sensitivity of the test is approximately 80 percent.[169] The false-negative rate of breast FNA varies between approximately two percent and ten percent.[160, 190, 199]

Localization of the Breast Mass and Palpable Lymph Nodes

Following the identification of a palpable breast mass, FNA can be performed in an outpatient setting. The procedure usually does not require an anesthetic. If the mass is identified by mammography and is not palpable, then stereotactic, radiological, or some other guidance method is necessary to place the needle into the area being studied. The use of localizing needles to direct the biopsy has been reported.[12] A compression plate coordinating system[75, 187] and a stereotaxic technique[12, 75, 175, 187] have both been effectively employed. In one study[135] the use of ultrasound to localize the mass significantly reduced the unsatisfactory rate of FNA for inexperienced physicians performing the aspiration. Ultrasound localization was also found to be of value when the mass was less than 3 cm in diameter.[135] The sensitivity and specificity of FNA by these techniques approaches that of FNA on palpable masses.

Fine needle aspiration for the evaluation of lymph nodes or palpable masses outside the breast is approached essentially the same as for a breast mass. Pneumothorax following aspiration of axillary or supraclavicular lymph nodes is a recognized complication, and great care must be taken with insertion of the needle.[1] Follow-up chest radiographs to evaluate the chest for pneumothorax may be indicated depending on the physician's judgment of the procedure or if symptoms of pneumothorax are detected. In approaching enlarged lymph nodes, selection of a node that can be fixed between the palpating fingers is necessary so that the node can be held in place as the needle is inserted. Deep, freely moveable, barely palpable nodes are extremely difficult to aspirate, and generally FNA is best not attempted on such nodes. When lymph nodes are aspirated, we prefer to examine an air-dried Diff-Quik (American Scientific Products, McGaw Park, IL) smear at the bedside. If tumor is not identified or lymphoma or an inflammatory process is considered, additional cellular material is collected in Eagle's medium for flow cytometry and appropriate cell markers. In addition, cultures of the aspirate are performed if inflammation is considered clinically or suggested from evaluation of the aspirate.

Complications

The risk of tumor growing out the needle tract is real and has been described primarily in bone tumors. This risk is markedly influenced by two factors. The first is needle size. The needles used in the cases reported with tumor growing out the needle site were usually large, ranging from 12 gauge to 16 gauge. Needles of this size are commonly used for needle biopsy, and a wide variety are available for this purpose; however, needles of this size are unnecessary for FNA cytology. In evaluating tumors of the breast by FNA there is no reason to use a needle any larger than 20 gauge. Usually 22- or 20-gauge needles are very satisfactory. These smaller needles are not associated with tumor spread into the needle tract. Second, the risk of needle tract involvement by tumor following FNA is eliminated when the needle tract is excised at the time the tumor is surgically removed. The surgical approach to a breast mass, whether it be by lumpectomy or mastectomy, can usually readily encompass the skin puncture site and needle tract resulting from the breast FNA.

Both acute mastitis and pneumothorax can occur as complications of breast FNA, but these complications are rare.[1, 81] Hematomas may occur following FNA of the breast and can result in false-positive mammographic studies. An interval of 2 weeks is generally advised between FNA and mammography.[157]

Approach to the Patient

The approach to the patient with a palpable mass requires that the procedure be explained to the patient and that informed consent be obtained. For most women, breast FNA is less painful than venipuncture, a procedure with which women who have regular medical care are familiar. There is usually no need to use anesthesia, although some physicians prefer to use a small amount of local anesthetic (e.g., 1 cc of one percent lidocaine or equivalent) injected into the skin at the site of the subsequent needle puncture. Usually a 33- or 25-gauge needle is used for the local anesthetic procedure. This generally has more disadvantages than advantages. The major disadvantage is that if excessive amounts of anesthetic are injected, or if hematoma results, the mass may be obscured to palpation and thus reduce the probability of a successful FNA. Adverse effects, including anaphylaxis, may also occur from local anesthetic.

The skin is usually prepared with 70 percent alcohol or an iodine solution. The proposed needle site is air dried thoroughly before aspiration. Aseptic technique is necessary. Slides for the aspirate should be properly labeled with the patient's name, and an appropriate requisition form for the cytopathology laboratory should be completed. We prefer to have a cytotechnologist available at the bedside to prepare the slides and quick-stain representative air-dried slides to evaluate adequacy of the aspirate. We prefer a 20-cc syringe within a syringe holder to enable the physician performing the FNA to control the syringe and needle with one hand while positioning and holding the breast mass with the opposite hand. Smaller syringes, manipulated by hand without a syringe holder, can also be used.[81] There are a number of syringe holders available (Fig. 26–1). Some of these syringe holders can be sterilized, if desired, and some can be heat autoclaved. It is an uncommon practice to sterilize the syringe holder except within an operating

Table 26–2. CHECKLIST FOR THE PERFORMANCE OF BREAST FINE NEEDLE ASPIRATION

1. Identify breast mass
2. Review clinical history
3. Review allergy history (query allergy to local anesthetic if to be used)
4. Signed informed consent
5. Labeled glass slides (polylysine-treated slides if ER-PR receptors or other immunoperoxidase procedures are to be performed)
6. 20-cc disposable sterile syringe
7. Syringe holder
8. 22- and 20-gauge sterile needles for aspiration
9. 26- or 33-gauge sterile needles (if local anesthetic to be used)
10. One per cent lidocaine or equivalent (if local anesthetic to be used)
11. 95 per cent ethyl alcohol or spray fixative
12. Tissue culture media for transport of needle washing
13. Cytopathology requisition form
14. Sterile gloves
15. Povidone-iodine or alcohol for skin preparation

room setting. Usually only the syringe, needles, and local anesthetic are sterile. We do not recommend storing the syringe holders in detergent-antiseptic solutions if sterilization is desired, because some viruses can survive in such solutions. Submersion in a ten percent fresh bleach solution for 20 minutes may be acceptable for cleaning, but even this treatment would not meet the standards established in some states for medical instrument handling. Disposable syringe holders significantly add to the cost of the procedure but may be a practical solution in some circumstances.

Once the patient is informed, the consent is signed, the slides appropriately labeled, the syringe prepared by placing it into the syringe holder, and the ideal position in which to place the patient during the procedure in order to gain optimal access to the breast mass established, then the needle aspirate may be performed. Table 26–2 provides a checklist that may be used in preparation for breast FNA.

At the University of Florida, we have a prepared cart, which is taken to the patient's bedside or clinic station (Fig. 26–2). In addition to the materials listed in Table 26–2, the cart contains the following:
Microscope and power cord
Block (10" × 10" × 7") to elevate scope for ease of viewing
All frosted slides (one box at least three fourths full)
Clear glass slides with frosted labels—(one box at least three fourths full)
Sterile rubber gloves (two pair)
20-, 22-, and 19-gauge needles, especially 20-gauge
Centrifuge tubes (1 to 3 cc, 1 to 6 cc)
1 sterile syringe (20 cc)
20-cc syringes
Needle holder (autoclaved)
Two to three tubes of normal saline (NS) and 50 percent ethyl alcohol (ETOH); fill tubes with ¼ NS and ¼ 50 percent ETOH to equal ½ of the tube filled

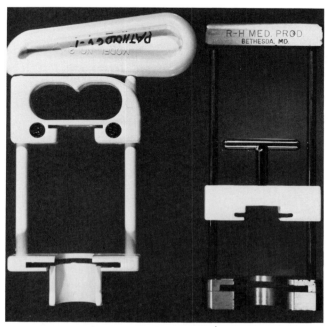
Figure 26–1. Two commonly used syringe holders for fine needle aspiration.

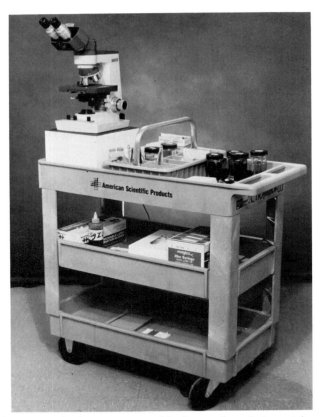

Figure 26–2. Cytology cart prepared for fine needle aspiration cytology.

Two tubes (6 cc) tissue culture media
Requisition forms
Paper towels
Black pen, pencil
Two Coplan jars of 95 percent ETOH
One Coplan jar of Carnoy's solution to lyse red blood
  cells (RBCs) before placing into 95 percent ETOH
1 Coplan jar of water to rinse slides after staining
Diff-Quik solutions I and II
Tweezers

Fine Needle Aspiration Technique

In most women a 1½-inch 22-gauge needle will be quite adequate for FNA of a breast mass. We prefer to withdraw 5 cc of air into the 20-cc syringe prior to attaching the needle to the syringe. The advantage of this is that following the procedure, there are 5 cc of air within the syringe that can be used to express the needle contents onto the slides without having to remove the syringe from the needle.

The performance of the aspirate is as follows. Holding the breast mass in a fixed position with one hand, advance the needle into the mass. Once the needle is in the mass, place full suction on the syringe (plunger to the 20-cc position) and move the needle slowly back and forth within the mass (Fig. 26–3). Moving the needle along a single needle tract will give a satisfactory cellular

yield in the majority of cases.[130] Keep the needle tip within the mass and full suction on the syringe until material can be seen coming into the *hub of the needle* (Fig. 26–4). The principle is to fill the needle, not the syringe, with cells. One needle can hold more than 100,000 cells, and this is usually adequate for cytologic diagnosis.[191] Once material is seen at the hub of the needle, release suction and return the plunger to the 5-cc mark. Withdraw the needle (still attached to the syringe) and express the needle contents onto the glass slides. To do this, the needle should touch the surface of the slide to avoid sample air drying. A small amount of material, usually a drop not exceeding 5 mm in diameter, should be expressed onto the slide (Fig. 26–5). It is usually preferable to place aliquots of the sample on several slides. The slides should lay flat on a towel placed on a firm surface such as a table top. Do not have a technologist or an assistant hold the slides. The risk of accidentally sticking the person holding the slide or spraying the assistant with the needle contents is real, and with the concerns of hepatitis and AIDS, this technique is best avoided. If all of the sample does not express from the needle, simply remove the needle from the syringe, withdraw the plunger to the 20-cc mark to fill the syringe with air, and reexpress the material by forcing air through the needle.

In our practice we use Eagle's tissue culture medium to rinse the needle and syringe and ensure that all of the cellular material is harvested. Within the cytopathology laboratory, cells are collected from the media using nucleopore filtration or cytocentrifugation, or are prepared for a cell block for paraffin embedding. Centrifugation depends on the amount of cellular material within the washings.

Preparation of Pathological Materials from FNA

There are several opinions on how to make preparations from the needle aspirate material.[48, 74, 81, 130] We

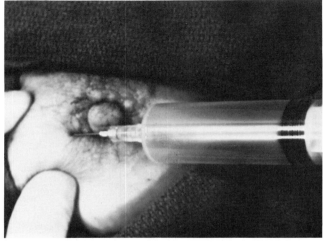

Figure 26–3. Needle in mass with full suction on the syringe.

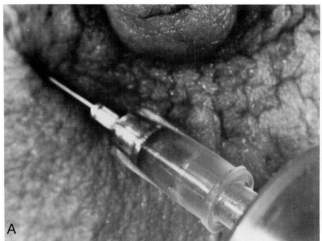
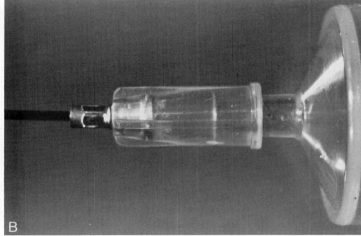

Figure 26–4. *A,* Breast aspirate material within the hub of the needle. *B,* Close view demonstrating cellular material within the needle hub.

prefer the "book opening" technique, which we find limits air drying and smear artifact and produces "mirror image" slides that are very useful when both air-dried and alcohol-fixed material is prepared. Once a drop of needle aspirate is placed on the slide, a second slide is laid on top of this slide, and gentle pressure is placed on the cover slide (Fig. 26–6). When this is done, the cellular sample will be seen to spread out between the two glass slides (Fig. 26–6). The slides are then turned apart, as in opening a book (Fig. 26–7). This technique preserves cell group orientation and avoids smear artifact, which makes interpretation difficult. In our laboratory we prepare both air-dried and 95 percent ethanol–fixed slides. There are differences of opinion as to the advantages or disadvantages of air-dried vs. alcohol-fixed material. Air-dried slides can be prepared and stained with Diff-Quik or a similar stain within a few minutes at the bedside. We use such preparations to evaluate adequacy of the smear. Air-dried slides give good cytoplasmic and cell orientation detail, but lack

the nuclear detail available with alcohol fixing. Unlike air-dried slides, alcohol-fixed slides can be used for immunoperoxidase procedures, such as the detection of cellular antigens [including carcinoembryonic antigen, cytokeratins, melanoma-associated antigens (e.g., HMB 45, S-100), and lymphoma-related antigens (e.g., T-200), which are all of value in dealing with tumors of the breast, including those that may be metastatic to the breast or of nonepithelial origin]. In our practice we use Poly-L-Lysine (Sigma, St. Louis) pretreated slides to improve cell-glass adherence. If immunoperoxidase, histochemical, or estrogen receptor procedures are to be performed on the cell sample, such slide pretreatment will reduce the loss of cells from the glass slide.

There is some debate as to who is best qualified to perform the actual fine needle aspiration of the breast. Some data indicate that when the pathologist is given full responsibility to both perform and interpret the FNA, the frequency of false-negative results is at a minimum (0.7 percent), whereas when surgeons perform

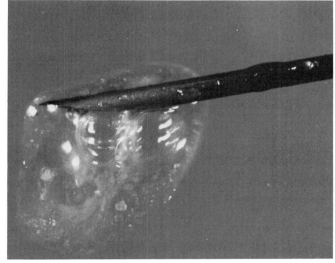

Figure 26–5. Aspirate material placed on the slide. Note that the needle touches the slide.

Figure 26–6. Book opening technique of cellular preparation of the fine needle aspiration sample. First, a second slide is placed over the slide containing the sample. The cellular material can be seen spread out between the two slides with slight pressure.

the FNA, the false-negative rate is 22.8 percent.[130] This is primarily because the needle aspiration technique and slide preparation are full of pitfalls that can result in unsatisfactory or false-negative reports. In our practice, although we offer FNA as part of our pathology service, the majority of breast FNAs are performed by the surgeon seeing the patient. The cytotechnologist prepares the smears following performance of the procedure and evaluates the cellular adequacy of the air-dried slides at the patient's bedside. In other hospitals and clinics the physician seeing the patient may prefer to have the pathologist do the FNA. The advantage of this is that a false-negative aspirate becomes the full responsibility of the pathologist and not of the physician seeing the patient. The availability of the pathologist to perform the FNA frees the surgeon to treat other clinic patients. A breast clinic's successful operation depends on the resources of the surgeon and cytopathologist and their respective services. The best care for the patient should be the determining factor in making these choices; this can only be achieved by thoughtful, cooperative interaction between the surgeon and cytopathologist in applying their combined resources in an optimum way.

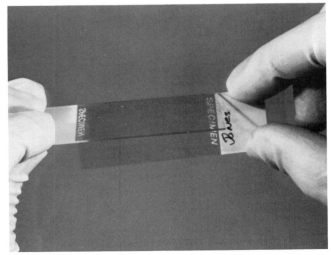

Figure 26–7. Book opening technique. The two slides are turned apart, as in opening a book.

INTERPRETATION OF CYTOPATHOLOGICAL FINDINGS OF BREAST FINE NEEDLE ASPIRATES

General Diagnostic Criteria

Benign breast disease

Normal structures of the breast include major lactiferous ducts, branched ducts, lobules, and connective tissue stroma. When normal breast tissue is aspirated, the cellular yield is quite low, with hypocellular or sometimes acellular smears. A few ductal cells may be present, arranged in sheets or in a monolayer-like pattern.[50] Benign processes generally are characterized by the common cellular features summarized in Table 26–3.

The specific cellular characteristics found in benign breast disease are summarized in Table 26–4 (Fig. 26–8). Although there are some rare exceptions, such as finding nucleoli in the cells of lactating adenoma, when these features are identified in an adequate and well-prepared sample, they are characteristic of the majority of benign processes within the breast.

Multiple needle aspiration passes may be necessary to increase the cellular yield when dealing with benign breast disease, because benign diseases usually produce hypocellular samples. The cellularity of the aspirate also depends on the quantitative proportion of cells and fibrous stroma. Occasionally, casts of large ducts or sheets of cells may be seen representing larger epithelial groups.

In addition to sheets of ductal cells, FNAs from benign breast disease also show variable numbers of single bare nuclei, (i.e., nuclei that are devoid of cytoplasm) (Fig.

Table 26–3. COMMON CELLULAR FEATURES OF BENIGN BREAST DISEASE

Low cell yield
Sheets or monolayers of ductal epithelial cells
Single, bare nuclei
Orderly cell arrangement
Uniformity in nuclear size
Absence of necrosis

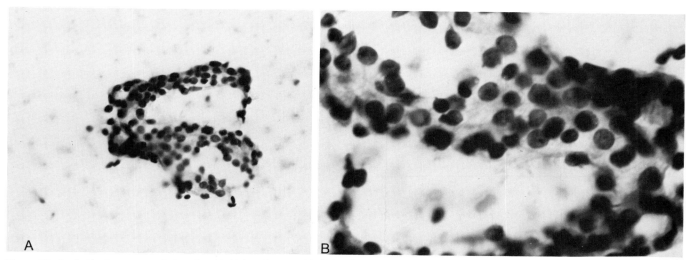

Figure 26–8. *A*, Benign group of ductal epithelial and myoepithelial cells (× 400). *B*, Benign ductal epithelial cells and benign myoepithelial elements (× 1000).

26–9). These have a bipolar shape, smooth and distinctive nuclear profile, compact chromatin, and indistinct nucleolus, and their size range is the same as that of benign ductal cell nuclei. The origin of the bare nuclei is unclear; myoepithelial, ductal, or stromal cells are all considered possible candidates.[178]

Malignant Breast Disease

Breast adenocarcinomas share some common cellular features, which are summarized in Table 26–5. Cellular groups are commonly found, and within these groups the nuclei are crowded together, often with nuclear molding. A marked variation in nuclear size (anisonucleosis) is also usually present (Fig. 26–10). The nuclear membranes show infolding, and the nuclear chromatin is usually coarse and radially dispersed against the nuclear membrane. There is cellular monomorphism where, in spite of the variations in size and shape, the cells appear similar to each other, whether occurring in groups or as single cells.[48, 199]

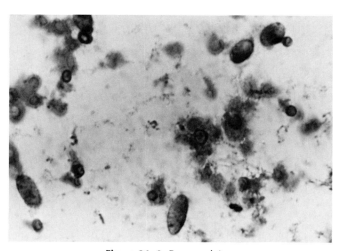

Figure 26–9. Bare nuclei.

Cytopathological Evidence of Benign Changes

Benign Mastopathies

Benign mastopathies are a heterogeneous group of benign diseases that include one or more of the features listed in Table 26–6. The histopathological heterogeneity of this diverse group of benign changes results in variable appearances on FNA. Lesions that are essentially fibrous or fatty will produce hypocellular smears. Epithelial hyperplasias will produce more cellular smears, with cellular groups bearing the benign characteristics described previously (Fig. 26–11). Depending on the degree of hyperplasia, nuclear crowding and overlapping may occur with irregular nuclear placement. The nuclei maintain relatively uniform size, and nuclear molding is not present.[50, 76, 85] There is no tendency for the cells to disassociate, and isolated intact single abnormal cells are absent. Bare nuclei vary from few to moderate numbers.

Apocrine Metaplasia

Apocrine metaplasia shows characteristic large cells of polygonal shape, large nucleus, and a single and

Table 26–4. CELLULAR CHARACTERISTICS OF BENIGN BREAST DISEASE

Nuclear size about 1 to 1.5 times that of RBCs
Uniformity of nuclear size
Regular nuclear placement in rows and columns
Smooth nuclear membranes
Absent nucleoli
Scanty cytoplasm and indistinct cell membranes
Cohesiveness of cell groups
Absence of single intact cells

Table 26–5. COMMON CELLULAR FEATURES OF BREAST CARCINOMA

High cellularity
Lack of cohesion of cellular groups
Presence of isolated intact single cells
Cellular monomorphism
Variation in nuclear size from cell to cell (anisonucleosis)
Nuclear membrane infolding
Chromatin clumping and radial dispersion of chromatin
Prominent nucleoli or macronucleoli

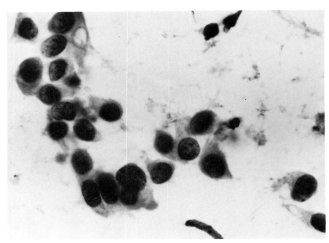

Figure 26–10. Cell groups and single cells with characteristic cellular features of adenocarcinoma of the breast.

prominent central nucleolus. Cytoplasm is prominent and often amphoteric (Fig. 26–12).

Apocrine cells often occur singly and are an exception to the cytologic criterion that a lack of cohesiveness on FNA is supporting evidence of malignancy. These findings are distinguishable from apocrine cell carcinoma of the breast, which can also be recognized on FNA.[48] Apocrine differentiation in lobular carcinoma has also been described in breast FNA.[43]

Fat Necrosis

In fat necrosis the aspirate usually consists of milky and/or oily fluid; fat is easily recognizable microscopically as macro- and microglobules, particularly on air-dried slides stained with Wright's stain. Ductal cells are few and cohesive. Macrophages may appear atypical with large nuclei, multinucleation, prominent nucleoli, and hyperchromasia; chronic inflammatory cells may also be present.

Mastitis

In mastitis, the usual bimodal benign cellular ductal epithelial components are present; acute and chronic inflammatory cells are seen. Some epithelial atypia, with nuclear enlargement and crowding, may be found. Single intact isolated cells are absent. Histocytes, multinucleated giant cells, and plasma cells are also present (Fig. 26–13).

Tuberculous mastitis may present as a breast mass and can be suggested by FNA findings from the breast. Acid-fast organisms are rarely identified. The cellular elements within the aspirate consist primarily of epithelioid-type histiocytes with Langhan's giant cells. Neutrophils are generally present.[122]

Pregnancy-Associated Changes

Pregnancy may be associated with benign breast adenomas (pregnancy adenomas that are characterized on FNA by hypercellular smears that may contain blood and amorphous debris that can be misinterpreted as necrotic material). Cell groupings lack cohesion, and individual intact cells may be present; nuclear enlargement is moderate (usually up to two times the size of RBCs), and nucleoli may be prominent. Differential

diagnosis is based on the presence of abundant fatty material in the background, uniformity of nuclear shape, and nuclear enlargement no more than two times the size of RBCs.[16] The cytoplasm is abundant and granular with distinct cell borders. On Papanicolaou's stain, the cytoplasm is blue-green and the granules are red; on Wright's stain, the cytoplasm is gray-blue with dark blue granules.

Cysts

Cysts usually produce fluid, which can be obvious at the time of aspiration. The fluid may be seen as finely granular background material on air-dried or alcohol-fixed slides. Cellular components include macrophages, hyperplastic ductal cells, and apocrine cells (Fig. 26–14).[176] In general, the fluid from benign cysts is clear to mildly cloudy and green to yellow in color. Fluid that is bloody, dark brown, opaque, or viscous is also supporting evidence for a benign lesion. Cytologic evaluation is often of value.[23] There is always the possibility of an associated carcinoma in the cyst wall, and if a cyst is aspirated, a follow-up mammogram may be of value to visualize the tissue surrounding the collapsed cyst.[170] Whenever a cystic lesion is aspirated, it is important to determine if a residual mass remains; in such event, it is advisable to obtain a repeat FNA or a surgical biopsy.

Table 26–6. CELLULAR FEATURES OF BENIGN MASTOPATHIES

Epithelial hyperplasia (also known as epitheliosus or papillomatosis)
Apocrine metaplasia
Duct ectasia
Cystic changes
Fibrosis
Fat infiltration
Adenosis

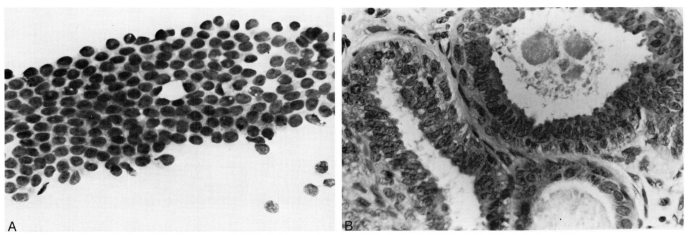

Figure 26–11. *A,* Ductal epithelial hyperplasia (× 400). *B,* Ductal epithelial hyperplasia (× 400).

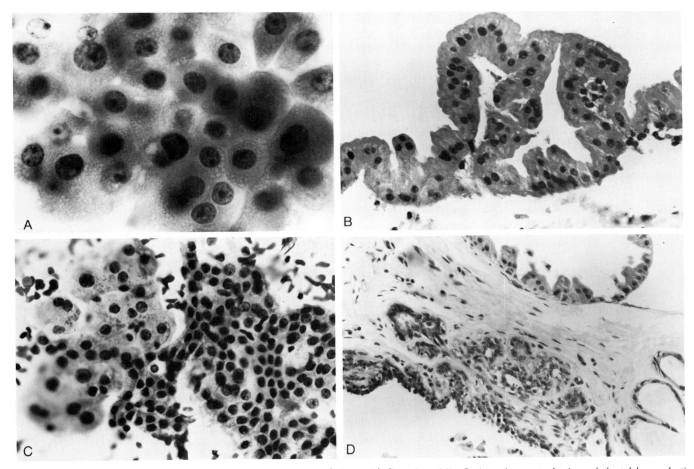

Figure 26–12. *A,* Apocrine metaplasia (× 1000). *B,* Apocrine cyst lining epithelium (× 400). *C,* Apocrine metaplastic and ductal hyperplastic cellular groups (× 400). *D,* Adjacent apocrine metaplasia with adjacent ductal epithelium from corresponding biopsy from C (× 200).

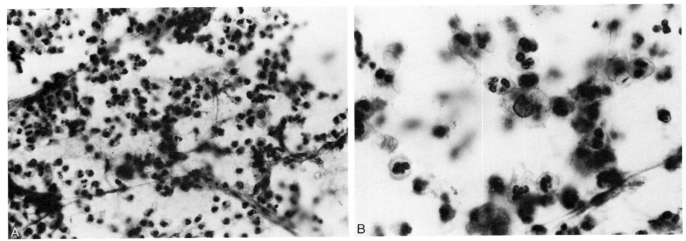

Figure 26–13. *A,* Acute mastitis (× 200). *B,* Acute mastitis (× 1000).

Benign Tumors

Fibroadenoma. Characteristically, the cellular yield from fibroadenomas on FNA is quite abundant, with numerous broad sheets of regularly arranged epithelial cells ("antler horns") identified (Fig. 26–15). The nuclei of the epithelial cells are slightly larger than those of normal ductal cells; they are uniform in size and shape, have finely granular chromatin, and one or two small nucleoli. Large numbers of bare nuclei are also present and are best appreciated at medium scanning power as abundant small dark dots.[50, 95, 192] The stroma is best seen on Wright's stain as metachromatic and fibrillar material. Stromal blood vessels appear as parallel rows of elongated endothelial nuclei. Giant fibroadenomas have a cytologic appearance similar to that of common fibroadenomas; in most cases, stromal elements predominate over epithelial elements. Bare nuclei, however, are even more numerous than they are in fibroadenomas. Carcinoma of the breast may rarely be found in a fibroadenoma.[164]

Intraductal Papilloma. Aspirates from intraductal papillomas can be similar to fibroadenomas. Clinical information such as nipple discharge or central subareolar lesion should alert the pathologist to the possibility of a papilloma when the smears resemble a fibroadenoma (Fig. 26–16).[48, 199]

Characteristic but inconsistent findings of a papilloma include the following:

1. Large numbers of foamy macrophages, indicating a cystic area where the papilloma protrudes.

2. Complex branching groups of hyperplastic ductal cells.

3. Tall columnar cells, probably representing hyperplastic epithelial cells of the cyst wall or of the papillary projections.

Nipple Adenoma (Periareolar Duct Hyperplasia). On FNA nipple adenoma present as cellular lesions, the

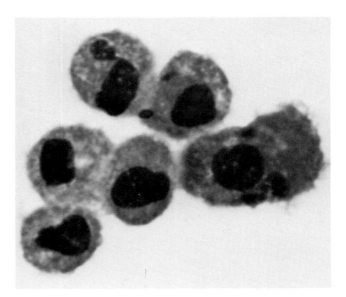

Figure 26–14. Cyst cellular contents (× 1000).

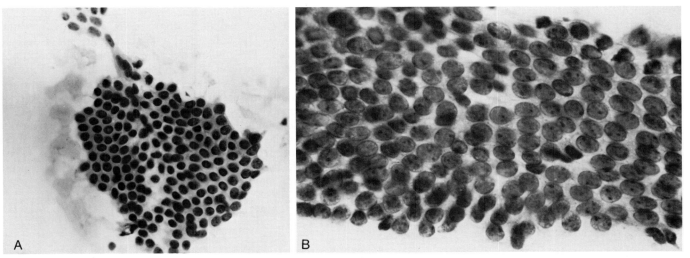

Figure 26–15. *A*, Fibroadenoma (× 400). *B*, Fibroadenoma (× 1000).

cells of which show some disassociation. The nuclei are uniform, but nucleoli may be prominent. Diagnosis of malignancy should only be made in the presence of many single cells with irregular nuclear profiles and marked anisocytosis.[174]

Granular Cell Tumor. Granular cell tumors may clinically simulate malignancy. Aspirates show syncytial clusters of cells with abundant, dense cytoplasm, prominent cytoplasmic granularity, and small round to oval central nuclei. Small nucleoli and bland nuclear chromatin pattern characterize this tumor.[96]

Cytopathological Evidence of Malignant Tumors of Epithelial Origin

In Situ Lobular Carcinoma and Intraductal Carcinoma

Generally, it is not possible to distinguish in situ and infiltrating carcinoma by FNA at an exclusively morpho-

logical level.[13] In situ lesions rarely form palpable masses, and when aspirated, the yield is frequently low; surgical biopsy is advised in such cases.

Invasive Carcinomas

There are two broad cytologic categories of invasive carcinomas: the usual adenocarcinoma of nonspecific type and histologically distinctive tumors.

Invasive Adenocarcinoma, Not Otherwise Specified (NOS). The usual invasive adenocarcinoma of the breast clinically presents as an ill-defined, hard nodule firmly attached to the adjacent breast tissue. The mammographic appearance of this tumor is characterized by infiltrative borders and typical calcifications.[14, 38, 86] Depending on the degree of fibrous response, aspirates can be quite hypocellular, and examiners must be very sensitive to the adequacy of the specimen. The diagnosis depends on finding the usual malignant criteria including hypercellularity, cellular lack of cohesion, characteristic cell groupings, monomorphism, anisonucleosis, nuclear

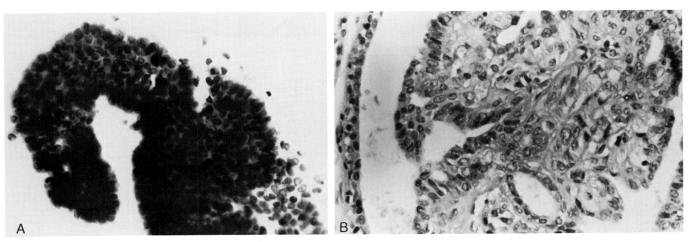

Figure 26–16. *A*, Intraductal papilloma (× 400). *B*, Intraductal papilloma. Biopsy corresponding to cytologic study *(A)* (× 400).

chromatin, and membrane changes; prominent nucleoli are frequently observed. Nuclear molding, overriding, and crowding are also commonly observed (Fig. 26–17).

Most of these tumors are readily diagnosed; however, the tumor cells may appear benign because of relative uniform size and bland appearance. Increased nuclear size, assessed by comparison with adjacent benign ductal cells and RBCs, usually indicates the true nature of the process. The presence of many intact single cells and cell groups with the absence of bare nuclei provides additional clues to the diagnosis.

Lobular Carcinoma. Invasive lobular carcinoma has characteristic cytological features including small- to medium-sized isolated single cells with few cellular groupings. The cells have a small amount of ill-defined cytoplasm. The nuclei have fine, uniform chromatin and prominent nucleoli. Anisonucleosis is minimal (Fig. 26–18).[48, 81] In cases where cellular groups predominate, differentiation from the usual adenocarcinoma cannot be made. Likewise, metastatic small-cell adenocarcinomas to the breast may appear lobular.[198] Argyrophilic small-cell carcinomas arising primary in the breast may also occur and have been reported in breast FNA samples.[145] The FNA diagnosis of lobular carcinoma

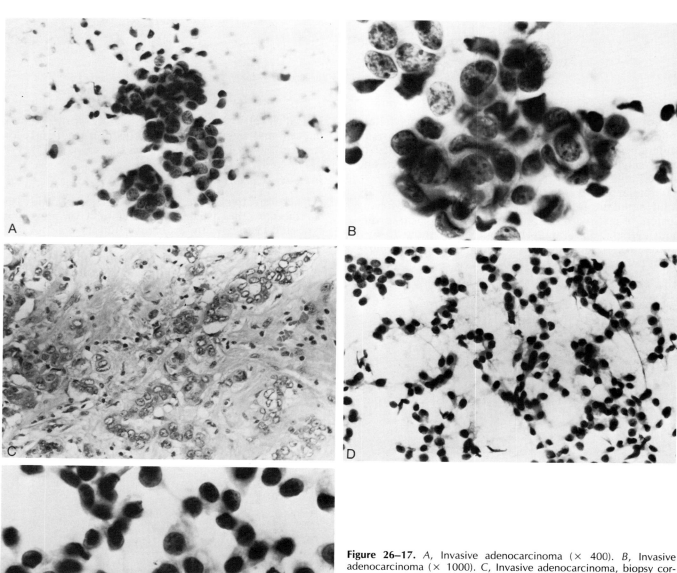

Figure 26–17. *A,* Invasive adenocarcinoma (× 400). *B,* Invasive adenocarcinoma (× 1000). *C,* Invasive adenocarcinoma, biopsy corresponding to *A* and *B* (× 400). *D,* Invasive adenocarcinoma (× 250). *E,* Invasive adenocarcinoma (× 400).

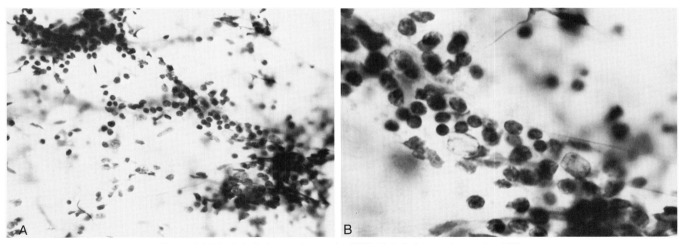

Figure 26–18. *A,* Lobular carcinoma (× 250). *B,* Lobular carcinoma (× 400).

may therefore be only presumptive, and the final histopathological tumor classification may require biopsy and permanent sections.

Medullary Carcinoma. Medullary carcinomas contain medium-to-large cells with little intracellular cohesion, abundant cytoplasm (sometimes resembling squamous carcinoma), and marked nuclear abnormalities including nucleoli and nuclear membrane folding.[48, 74] Necrotic material, lymphocytes, and plasma cells may be found within the background (Fig. 26–19). Mixed apocrine medullary carcinoma of the breast diagnosed by FNA has been reported.[17]

Mucinous (Colloid) Carcinoma. Well- or moderately differentiated adenocarcinomas are usually associated

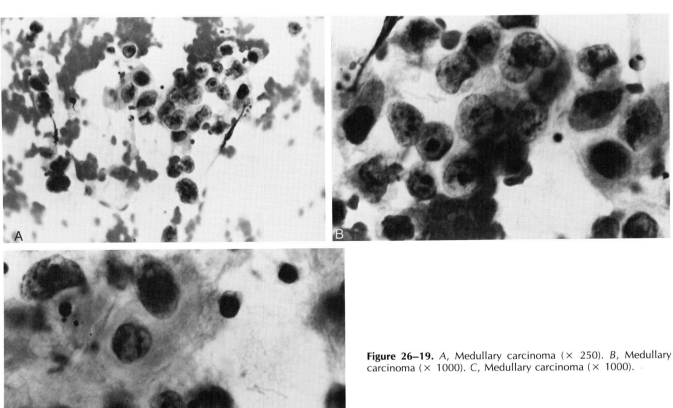

Figure 26–19. *A,* Medullary carcinoma (× 250). *B,* Medullary carcinoma (× 1000). *C,* Medullary carcinoma (× 1000).

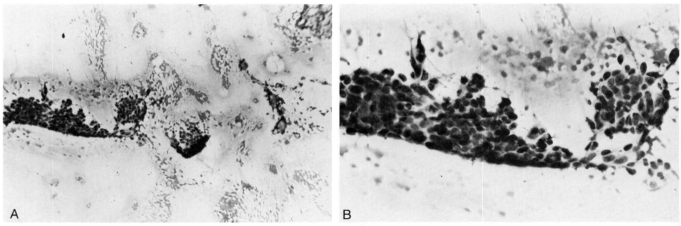

Figure 26–20. *A,* Mucinous (colloid) carcinoma (× 250). *B,* Mucinous (colloid) carcinoma (× 400).

with mucus secretion. On PAP stain, the mucin appears as a subtle light-blue to orange background; on Wright's stain, it appears purple and is easily recognized. The tumor cells are frequently arranged in compact groups ("balls") and demonstrate a moderate degree of nuclear pleomorphism (Fig. 26–20). The characteristic mucinous background may be lost if only filter material is available for cytologic review.[190] Mucinous carcinoma may be mixed with other adenocarcinoma cell types that may not be evident on FNA. Because this finding will influence prognosis and therapy, definitive diagnosis requires study of the excised tumor.[132]

Tubular Carcinoma. Tubular carcinomas are well differentiated, have minimal nuclear abnormalities, and maintain cell cohesion. Characteristic glandular (tubular) structures are usually found within the FNA smear appearing in groupings. Monolayers and sheets of cells may predominate. Nuclear enlargement, evident on comparison with benign ductal cells, is a consistent finding.[48, 81] Other features that may suggest the diagnosis of tubular carcinoma include extremely orderly nuclear placement, nuclear regularity, large but relatively uniform nucleoli, and focal areas showing a lack of cellular cohesion.

Inflammatory Carcinoma. Knowledge of the distinctive clinical presentation of inflammatory carcinoma is essential for appropriate diagnosis by FNA. Aspirates are usually cellular with all the malignant criteria (Fig. 26–21) usually found in breast adenocarcinoma.[48] Inflammatory carcinoma is not a specific tumor type, but rather a distinctive clinical presentation. The tumor type is typically invasive adenocarcinoma, NOS.

Mammary Paget's Disease. Smears prepared from scrapings from the nipple in Paget's disease will show a background of keratinous debris, inflammatory cells, and squamous cells. Large cells, singly or in groups, with obvious nuclear malignant features and abundant pale cytoplasm typify Paget's disease.[42, 199] The differential diagnosis includes subareolar duct papillomatosis and other periareolar duct hyperplasias; in these cases, cohesive aggregates of uniform cells without nuclear features of malignancy are present. Most patients with

Paget's disease of the breast have underlying intraductal or invasive adenocarcinoma of the breast, usually of nonspecific type. Needle aspiration of a palpable breast associated with Paget's disease is indicated.

Other Breast Carcinoma Types. Squamous carcinoma may arise as a primary tumor within the breast, and its diagnosis by FNA has been well described.[65, 89] Groups and sheets of cells are usually seen with keratin and/or dyskeratotic cells being important diagnostic features.

Secretory carcinoma of the breast is rare; however, the cytologic findings on FNA have been observed. Distinctive features include sheets of neoplastic cells with prominent intracellular spaces, cytoplasmic vacuolization, and signet ring cell formation.[34]

Carcinoma of the breast with osteoclast-like, stromal giant cells has been identified on breast FNA.[142] Characteristically, multinucleating giant cells mixed with neoplastic epithelial cell elements are identified on FNA. The giant cells have been identified as being of histiocytic origin.

Argyrophilic small-cell tumors, including primary carcinoid tumors, may arise in the breast and be diagnosed by FNA. The relatively small, uniform tumor cells may

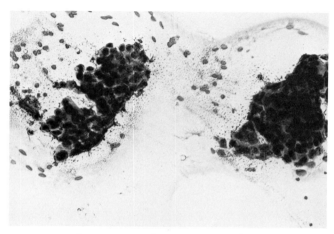

Figure 26–21. Inflammatory carcinoma.

be argyrophil-positive.[90, 145] These cells are characteristically immunoreactive for neuron-specific enolase and chromogranin, distinguishing them from typical lobular carcinoma.

Apocrine Carcinomas

Apocrine carcinoma, an unusual variant of ductal carcinoma, is composed of large apocrine cells with abundant granular eosinophilic cytoplasm and central large nuclei with prominent nucleoli.

On needle aspirates (Fig. 26–22) these tumors yield numerous cells with apocrine features, large size (15 μm to 20 μm), and abundant granular cytoplasm. The cytoplasm is typically well delineated in isolated cells, but rather indistinct in cell groupings. Nuclear anisocytosis and prominent nucleoli, often occupying half of the nuclear volume, are usually seen.[81]

Cytopathological Evidence of Sarcomas of the Breast

Cystosarcoma Phyllodes

The FNA characteristics of cytosarcoma phyllodes (CSP) are similar to those of fibroadenomas. The aspirate is usually cell rich, with cellular fronds and loosely cohesive clusters; bare nuclei are also evident. Occasional multinucleated giant cells, anisonucleosis, and macronucleoli may also be seen. The principal difference between CSP and fibroadenoma is the stromal connective tissue, which is more cellular and vascular and contains abundant fibroblasts with elongated nuclei in CSP. In most cases, the correct interpretation of the FNA requires clinical correlation.[172] Cystosarcoma phyllodes are considered malignant based on evaluation of margins of the tumor, lack of epithelial component, and high mitotic counts. Such findings cannot be evaluated on an aspirate alone. The suspicion of malignancy should be raised when abundant stromal nuclei, sparse epithelial groups, mitotic figures, and atypical nuclei are noted in smears with the general appearance of fibroadenomas.

Sarcomas of the breast arise from the mesenchymal component and are quite rare. The aspirate of a sarcoma of the breast, as reported by Kline,[81] contained large irregular and elongated cells with pleomorphic nuclei in abundant hemorrhagic material. Similar findings in breast sarcomas had been previously observed by Degrell.[35]

Fine needle aspiration samples from angiosarcomas of the breast have an abundant amount of blood and

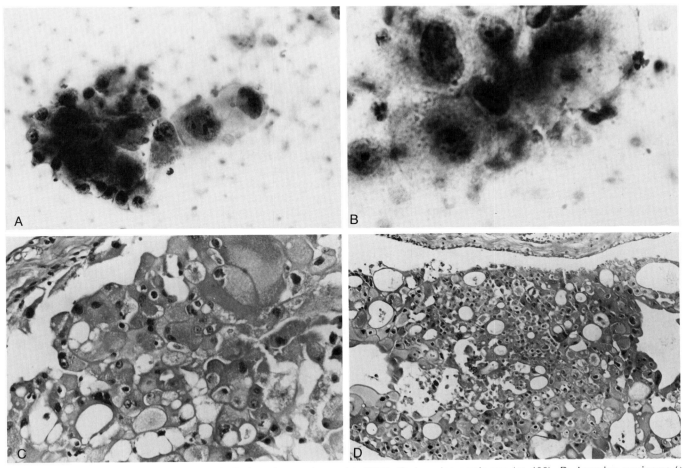

Figure 26–22. *A,* Apocrine carcinoma (× 400). *B,* Apocrine carcinoma (× 1000). *C,* Apocrine carcinoma (× 400). *D,* Apocrine carcinoma (× 250).

tumor cells that are sparse and difficult to identify. This is particularly true in low-grade angiosarcomas, in which the malignant endothelial cells have little tendency to proliferate in solid clusters.[102] These tumors are rich in factor VIII, which can be identified within the malignant endothelial cells by employing immunohistochemical techniques.

Primary rhabdomyosarcoma of the breast has been identified by FNA.[177] Large striated cells and rhabdomyoblasts may be seen. Immunohistochemical detection of desmin, actin, myosin, and myoglobin may assist in the identification of such tumors.

IMMUNOFLUORESCENCE, IMMUNOPEROXIDASE, AND ELECTRON MICROSCOPY PROCEDURES IN FNA

Hormone Receptor Studies

In most centers estrogen receptor (ER) and progesterone receptor (PR) analysis is performed on fresh, surgically excised specimens. There are clinical situations, however, such as breast tumor metastasis to deep nodes, organs, or bone in which tumor excision for ER or PR receptor analysis would be either impossible or compromising for the patient. In such cases, hormone receptor studies can be performed on the tumor cellular material obtained by fine needle aspiration. There are several potential advantages to using FNA rather than surgical biopsy for hormone receptor assays on the cellular material. First, fine needle aspiration is a relatively easy, cost-effective, and nontraumatic procedure compared with surgical biopsy. FNA can readily be employed in patients with inoperable, recurrent, or metastatic breast cancer in whom the tumor size or accessibility to conventional biopsy may present a problem. Second, in cases selected for preoperative irradiation, hormone receptor analysis on aspirates may be the only possible alternative, since the primary tumor undergoes severe degeneration or totally regresses after irradiation. Third, in patients with advanced breast cancer, hormone receptor status may be studied at intervals in cells obtained by fine needle aspiration. This may provide information regarding the effects of therapy and may improve understanding of the tumor biology of breast adenocarcinoma.[18] The detection of hormone receptors in cells aspirated from pleural effusion and ascitic fluid, as well as from visceral lesions, may help differentiate between a primary tumor and a metastatic lesion.[59]

An isoelectric focusing technique has been applied to the measurement of estrogen and progesterone receptors in fine needle aspirates by several investigators.[116, 144, 159] This procedure is based on the electrofocusing of 3H-estradiol–bound receptors in tumor cells within polyacrylamide gel. This method is cumbersome, requiring a highly cellular aspirate, and is not applicable for general cytologic use.[144]

Several biochemical methods have proven to be reliable in assaying cytosol steroid receptors in breast cancer homogenates, with the dextran-coated charcoal (DCC) technique being the most commonly used.[27, 193] These techniques are discussed in detail elsewhere in this book. Conventional biochemical methods for measuring steroid hormone receptors require from 0.5 gm to 1.0 gm of tissue. Thus cytologic material is not suitable for such analyses.

Cytochemical Techniques Using Fluorescent-Conjugated Estrogens and Progestins

Cytochemical techniques use steroid hormones that are directly or indirectly linked to trace molecules such as fluorescein or rhodamine to permit direct visualization of the hormone binding site by fluorescence microscopy.[124, 186] Cytochemical techniques offer significant technical and economical advantages when compared with existing isotope binding assays and are particularly adaptable to imprint preparation and fine needle aspirates of tumors.[6, 33, 111] Cytochemical tests also provide data regarding tumor heterogeneity.

Fluorescent cytochemical methods for detecting steroid hormone receptors in tissue prepared by using frozen section or imprint preparation have been described. This assay employs 17β-estradiol-6-carboxymethyloxime-bovine serum albumin-fluorescein isothiocyanate conjugated into a single agent for detection of estrogen receptor, and 11α-hydroxyprogesterone hemisuccinate-bovine serum albumin tetramethyrhodamine isothiocyanate congregate for detection of progesterone receptor.

The direct fluorescent technique may employ the Fluoro-cep method (Zeus Technologies, Raritan, NJ). Estrogen receptor-positive cells give a bright-yellowish fluorescence when examined using fluorescent microscopy. Progesterone receptor-positive cells luminesce with a brilliant cytoplasmic orange-red color under fluorescent microscopy. The results of such assays have shown a 78 percent to 90 percent correlation with conventional biochemical methods.[33, 106, 107] Most of the specimens examined in these studies were composed of varying populations of positive and negative tumor cells. Heterogeneity of staining was conspicuous. Intensity of staining was frequently variable among different positive cells of the same specimen. In most tumor cells, cytoplasmic staining was predominant. Nuclear staining was occasionally observed but was generally associated with cytoplasmic staining.

Comparing our cytochemical results with the conventional DCC biochemical method employing the Fluoro-cep assay for estrogen and progesterone receptors, an 80 percent correlation for estrogen receptors and an 85 percent correlation for progesterone receptors was observed. Sensitivity for ER was 82 percent, and specificity was 80 percent. The sensitivity and specificity for PR were 88 percent and 82 percent, respectively.[108] Curtin et al. reported 83 percent correlation for estrogen binding in 41 cases and 87 percent correlation for progesterone binding in 31 cases.[33] In none of the studies was any consistent correlation found between the percentage of fluorescent-positive tumor cells and the quantitative values of the biochemical tests. This finding may be a result of the effect of mixed stromal and benign epithelial components that are frequently included in the biochemical assay.

Further studies also suggest that cytochemistry has a potential similar to that of biochemical hormone receptor determination for predicting clinical response to endocrine therapy in stage IV breast carcinoma.[140, 141]

There are suggested limitations in the use of cytochemical techniques as a result of controversy regarding the exact receptors being recognized by the fluorescent technique.[124] The conjugate prepared against estrogen and progesterone receptors in this method seems to bind to a lower-affinity binding site common to multiple classes of steroid hormones.[68] The fluorescent cytochemical technique detects hormone-specific binding, the presence of which may correlate with the presence of estrogen and progesterone receptors,[115] and that may explain why the fluorescent cytochemical technique has generally compared favorably with the biochemical assay.

Immunoperoxidase Techniques Using Monoclonal Antibodies to Estrogen and Progesterone Receptors

The production by Greene and Hensen of monoclonal antibodies highly specific to ER has provided a new and perhaps improved approach to the study of ERs in hormone-responsive tumors.[58] An immunoperoxidase technique since developed has been repeatedly employed in immunocytochemical ER study of human breast tumor and has shown to be highly specific and sensitive.[78, 97, 113, 139, 189] This technique has only recently been utilized to study ERs in fine needle aspirates of patients with breast cancer.[46, 106–108, 146] Most commonly, the reagents used in estrogen receptor immunocytochemical assay have been obtained from commercially available kits. The technique is based on visualization of estrogen receptor–binding sites using monoclonal antibodies with specific affinity for these receptors. Cellular material obtained from fine needle aspirates is smeared and fixed on microscope slides and treated with a blocking reagent to prevent specific binding of successive reagents. Specimens are then incubated with monoclonal antibody against estrogen receptor (H222 Sp λ). Goat anti-rat IgG immunoglobulin is added to form a "bridge" between the primary antibody and a horseradish peroxidase-antiperoxidase (PAP) complex. The peroxidase portion of this complex uses a chromogen substrate to form a colored product. ER presence is identified with a light microscope as brown staining localized in cell nuclei. The percentage of tumor cells with detectable estrogen receptor and the intensity of nuclear staining are then recorded. This percentage may be used for semiquantitative evaluation of estrogen receptor contact in aspirated material.

Quantitative receptor assay methods are currently employed to evaluate positivity or negativity of tumor tissue for sex steroid receptors. Although many investigators believe that quantitation of hormone receptors may be of value in predicting the patient's prognosis,[36, 70, 134] it has not been shown that quantitative values beyond a defined minimum are helpful in selecting treatment options. It is therefore generally adequate to determine that receptors are either positive or negative within the assay limits of the test and to initiate or withhold hormonal therapy on this basis.[111] Fine needle aspiration cytologic material is usually adequate, in the presence of tumor, to depict the presence or absence of sex steroid receptors using the previously described methods.

Recent studies have shown significant correlation between the results of the monoclonal antibody technique in fine needle aspirates and the biochemical analysis of the excised malignant tumor.[46, 97, 106–108, 113, 189] In 41 fine needle aspiration biopsy specimens studied by Flowers et al., sensitivity and specificity of the monoclonal antibody technique was reported as 80 percent, with an 89 percent positive predictive value and 84 percent negative predictive value. We studied the usefulness of the monoclonal antibody technique in 62 cases of breast fine needle aspirates and compared the results to the biochemical method. The sensitivity was 93 percent and specificity 88 per cent.[106–108] These studies suggest that through the immunoperoxidase technique, a cytologic preparation of aspirated cells can be examined for presence of ERs, and a semiquantitative evaluation of estrogen receptor content may be possible.[106–108]

Substantial evidence indicates the clinical usefulness of determining both estrogen and progesterone receptor levels in breast carcinoma. Monoclonal antibodies suitable for determining progesterone receptors in a fashion similar to that presently described for recognition of cells containing estrogen receptor are available, and several of these monoclonal progesterone receptor antibodies are under investigation.[196]

Immunoperoxidase Techniques to Detect Tumor-associated Antigens

The application of fine needle aspiration for earlier detection of primary breast carcinoma requires development of confirmatory tests to increase the diagnostic accuracy of this procedure. The immunoperoxidase technique has become a powerful adjunctive diagnostic tool in surgical pathology and is now widely used in pathology practice. This method can provide information about the histogenesis of a variety of neoplasms using various tissue-specific markers. It also may be useful to distinguish between primary and metastatic tumor. The demonstration of different classes of intermediate cytoskeletal filaments helps in differentiating among carcinomas, lymphomas, and sarcomas.[57]

Various immunoperoxidase-coupled antigens have been employed in an attempt to define the immunoexpression of different breast lesions and to differentiate between benign and malignant lesions of the breast. The primary ones include epithelial membrane antigen, carcinoembryonic antigen, keratin, antitumor monoclonal antibody B72.3, α-lactalbumin, S-100 protein, human chorionic gonadotropin, ABH blood group isoantigens, neuron-specific enolase, gross cystic disease fluid protein, and actin.

Monoclonal antibody (MAb) B72.3 demonstrates selective reactivity for carcinoma cells over normal human adult tissue.[72] This is the basis of an immunocytochemical approach employing MAb B72.3 to stain fine needle aspirates of breast masses.[127] Monoclonal antibody B72.3 obtained by standard hybridoma technology is directed against a membrane protein of human breast cancer. Using this immunoperoxidase technique on 50 breast fine needle aspirates, Lundy et al. reported a ten percent increase in their diagnostic accuracy.[98] All of their cases considered cytologically malignant were confirmed by immunocytochemistry. They also suggested that MAb B72.3 may be used as a valuable diagnostic adjunct in atypical and suspicious cases, particularly those in which hypocellular or cellular monomorphism preclude a diagnosis of malignancy by routine cytologic examination. Monoclonal antibody B72.3 was also used in 52 of our breast fine needle aspirates. All of our 32 malignant cases and none of our 20 benign cases were immunoreactive. The overall diagnostic accuracy was 96 percent, sensitivity was 94 percent, and specificity was 100 percent.[109]

Actin is a contractile protein that is present in muscular and normovascular cells. Using the immunoperoxidase technique, Mukai et al.[119] demonstrated actin in smooth and striated muscle, in pericytes, and in myoepithelial cells of the salivary glands, breast, and sweat gland.[119] In the study by Papotti et al., actin was used to differentiate between benign and malignant papillary lesions of the breast.[133]

These studies have been performed primarily on surgically removed breast specimens. Further investigation is warranted on breast tumor–associated antigens, especially in consideration of the potential value for assessment of metastatic and atypical breast lesions in fine needle aspirates. Actin, S-100 protein, and epithelial membrane antigen immunoperoxidase studies may assist in differentiating between atypical ductal hyperplasia and carcinoma in situ in fine needle aspirates sampled from the breast.

Electron Microscopy

Electron microscopy study of fine needle aspiration material enhances the ability to recognize unusual breast lesions and assists in the characterization of metastatic tumors of the breast.[99] We prefer to fix separate fresh cellular specimens for possible electron microscopic studies. The aspirated material is then processed immediately, but sectioning for electron microscopy is deferred pending our decision on whether the ultrastructural study is required based on the FNA findings.

Several techniques have been described to process aspirated material for electron microscopy. The most commonly used method is to eject the aspirate into a small centrifuge tube containing the appropriate fixative.

The sample is then centrifuged, and the pellet is removed and processed in the conventional way (i.e., as a tissue fragment).

In our laboratory, the aspirated material is expressed directly into Trump's agarized fixative. The sample is then centrifuged several times, and the pellet is resuspended in buffer and agar, respectively. The agarized cell pellet then is cut into suitable slices and processed in the conventional way.

Fine needle aspirates are suitable for ultrastructural study provided they contain adequate representative cellular material and are handled appropriately.[99] The small yield of cells may lead to problems in localization and interpretation, and single cells are prone to artifactual distortion; therefore particular care should be exercised in preparing the specimen for electron microscopy.

INTERPRETING REPORTS ON FINE NEEDLE ASPIRATES FROM THE BREAST

Calculation of Sensitivity, Specificity, Predictive Value, and Efficiency (Diagnostic Accuracy)

Display of Results for Analysis

To calculate sensitivity, specificity, predictive value, and efficiency, it is necessary to know the total negative, total positive, total false-negative (FN), and total false-positive (FP) cases. From these data the total true-positive (TP) and total true-negative (TN) cases can be calculated once this data is collected. The calculations are best set up in a binomial 2 × 2 table (Table 26–7).

Definitions and Methods of Calculation

The definitions and methods of calculation for sensitivity, specificity, predictive value, and efficiency are summarized in Table 26–8.[52, 163] As a general rule, cases that are classified as atypical (benign atypia, class II) are included in the negative calculation number. Cases that are considered suspicious are not included in the calculation, because such cases are truly indeterminate. In most laboratories, 50 percent to 74 percent of suspicious findings on breast FNA will have malignant findings at biopsy. Unsatisfactory cases are also not included in the calculations. Because breast FNA cytology is not used as a screening procedure (i.e., where no mass is

Table 26–7. RESULTS TO CALCULATE SPECIFICITY, SENSITIVITY, PREDICTIVE VALUE, AND EFFICIENCY OF BREAST FNA

FNA Diagnosis	Breast Biopsy Diagnosis	
	Carcinoma Present	*Carcinoma Absent*
Malignant	True-positive	False-positive
Benign	False-negative	True-negative

Table 26–8. DEFINITIONS AND CALCULATIONS FOR SENSITIVITY, SPECIFICITY, PREDICTIVE VALUE AND EFFICIENCY

Definition	Calculation
Sensitivity (positivity in disease)	$\dfrac{TP}{TP + FN} \times 100$
Specificity (negativity in health)	$\dfrac{TN}{TN + FP} \times 100$
Efficiency of the test (diagnostic accuracy)	$\dfrac{TN + TP - FN}{TP + FP + TN} + FN$
Predictive value of a positive result	$\dfrac{TP}{TP + FP} \times 100$

palpable), the specificity of negative findings is not as meaningful as it would be in a setting in which cytology is used in screening (e.g., for cervial carcinoma).

The true usefulness of fine needle aspiration cytology in the evaluation of breast masses can be properly assessed by examining the sensitivity, i.e., "the incidence of the positive results obtained when a test is applied to patients known to have the disease."[52] The FN rate is the percentage of needle aspirates interpreted as negative (no tumor present) when tumor is present. The FP rate is the percentage of needle aspirates interpreted as containing tumor where no tumor is found. The specificity is " . . . the incidence of true-negative results obtained when a test is applied to subjects known to be free of the disease."[52] The predictive value of a positive test is defined as "the percentage of positive results that are true positives when the test is applied to a population containing both healthy and diseased subjects."[52]

Diagnostic Accuracy of Breast Fine Needle Aspiration

The sensitivity of breast FNA performed on palpable masses is reported as approximately 90 percent (80 percent to 98 percent). The sensitivity and efficiency are influenced primarily by false-negative FNA results, which are discussed in the following section.

The sensitivity, specificity, and predictive value have been studied in detail by several investigators.[82, 86] The specificity and the predictive value of breast FNA approach 100 percent because false-positive results are rare (see section on false-positive results). Efficiency of the test ranges from 84 percent to 99.5 percent in studies in which it has been calculated.[163, 190, 195]

False-Negative Results

A false-negative result is a negative result in the presence of tumor. In reviewing the published literature, the false-negative rate of FNA of the breast ranges from 0.7 percent to 22 percent.[62, 130, 190] This figure is quite variable, depending on whether the breast mass was significant enough to require biopsy in spite of the FNA findings. In our own experience, 3.3 percent of our total cases interpreted as negative were false-negative; however, when only biopsy cases were reviewed, the false-negative rate was 11.1 percent.[190] Fifty-seven percent of our false-negative cases resulted from a lack of diagnostic tumor cells on the needle aspirate (sample error). These cases were excluded from the unsatisfactory needle aspirates because they contained benign breast cellular elements. Aspirates that contain adequate appearing benign cell elements are usually interpreted as negative.

Steps that can be taken to reduce false-negative results include having assistance in performing the aspirate so that appropriate smears can be made and rapidly fixed in 95 percent ethanol or air-dried for optimum cytologic evaluation. When alcohol-fixed material is desired, rapid fixation after performing the smear is imperative to avoid air-drying artifact. When air-dried slides are made, the smear should also be made rapidly, because attempting to smear cells that have partially dried results in cellular disruption, which seriously interferes with appropriate evaluation. Immediate staining of the processed sample at the patient's bedside and microscopic evaluation for adequacy of the smear by an experienced cytotechnologist or pathologist are very useful in determining whether a repeat aspirate is necessary. Definitive interpretation at the bedside by the pathologist is not generally necessary, but this service is provided by us and by some other pathologists in hospital settings. When multiple slides are made, unless the findings obviously indicate a tumor, a final diagnosis of "negative" requires careful screening of all cytologic material available for study, and any initial negative diagnostic statement should imply that the final diagnosis is pending review of all of the cytologic material obtained. Some investigators believe that a negative FNA should be followed by an open biopsy.[2, 187] False-negative results also occur in frozen section evaluation of the breast at a rate of approximately four percent.[161, 162] Evaluations based on the combined findings of physical exam, mammography, and FNA may assist in avoiding unnecessary biopsies, especially in women younger than 40 years.[24, 37, 88] When there are suspicious clinical or radiological findings despite a negative FNA result, biopsy is indicated.[136]

The false-negative rate can be reduced by increasing the number of aspirates performed. In one study the sensitivity increased from 61 percent with one aspirate to 91 percent with three aspirates.[136] False-negative results are most significantly related to the skill and experience of the physician performing the aspiration.[8]

A false-negative diagnosis may be suspected when an adequate clinical history, including physical findings, strongly suggests that tumor is present, and the cellular sample is minimal. Some estimate of the expected cell sample size can be made from the initial clinical evaluation of the mass. When a negative diagnosis results from minimal cellular material, it may be prudent for the pathologist to instead render an "unsatisfactory" diagnosis, recognizing the limitations of the sample. This is especially true in postmenopausal women, in whom the incidence of breast carcinoma is higher. The tumor type itself may also be a factor; for example, lobular carcinoma has a generally higher false-negative rate than do other breast tumor types.[9, 73, 136] In the experience of Ortel, the lowest false-negative rate (0.7 percent) was observed when the pathologist performed the aspirate and was responsible for all phases of the FNA procedure. Certainly this approach has many advantages to the patient as well as to the pathologist and surgeon; however, this is possible only in a hospital-based system or one in which a pathologist is readily available.

False-Positive Results

A false-positive result is a positive diagnosis for tumor when no tumor is present. False-positive results are rare and among experienced cytopathologists occur at a rate of zero to 0.4 percent, with an approximate average rate of 0.17 percent.[44, 67] Many pathology services have reported sizeable series without any false-positive results.* Some pathology services have reported significantly higher false-positive rates, but in several of these services the false-positive results decreased with increased pathologist experience.[91, 143] Cytologic tests carried out by experienced pathologists have a higher level of sensitivity and specificity.[28] False-positive results are the responsibility of the pathologist, which is also the case with frozen section diagnosis of breast masses, in which the false-positive rate is very low (0.06 percent).[148] False-positive results can sometimes be avoided by being aware of the clinical history and physical findings. Breast carcinomas, for example, are rare in women younger than 30 years. Fine needle aspirate interpretative difficulties may occur in cell samples from hematomas, breast fat necrosis, and irradiated breasts; all of which have been misinterpreted as malignancy on FNA by experienced pathologists.[48, 84, 130, 137] Fulfillment of diagnostic cytologic criteria for malignancy is necessary to avoid false-positive results. If the FNA lacks adequate evidence for malignancy but reveals cellular findings such as single isolated cells suggestive of carcinoma, it is best to report the results as "suspicious", but not diagnostic, preferably adding a comment regarding the problem and discussing these findings with the surgeon when necessary. Between four percent and 18 percent of FNA performed on breasts bearing tumor are interpreted as suspicious, whereas 70 percent to 92 percent are correctly interpreted as positive for tumor. In evaluating FNA in benign breast disease, two percent or less of aspirates performed on breasts with benign changes are interpreted as suspicious.[81] Most of these occur in benign breast disease (fibrocystic disease); however, fibroadenomas, gynecomastia, papillomas, pregnancy-associated hyperplasia, and granulation tissue may all be associated with FNA findings interpreted as suspicious.[81]

---

*References 20, 38, 61, 66, 123, 165, 167, 190, and 195.

The risk of a false-positive result is very minimal, and a number of investigators employ definitive surgical therapy for the breast carcinoma based on the results of the FNA alone, thereby eliminating interval frozen sections or biopsy.[39, 84, 187, 188]

The false-positive rate of FNA is substantially lower than that of either mammography or physical examination. False-positive rates between 15 percent and 28 percent have been reported for mammography, with rates between 12 percent and 20 percent reported for physical exam.[7, 19, 165, 181]

References

1. Abele JS, Miller TR, Goodson WH III, Hunt TK, Hohn DC: Fine-needle aspiration of palpable breast masses. A program for staged implementation. Arch Surg 118:859–863, 1983.
2. Adye B, Jolly PC, Bauermeister DE: The role of fine-needle aspiration in the management of solid breast masses. Arch Surg 123(1):37–39, 1988.
3. Allegra JC, Lippman ME, Thompson EB, Simon R, Barlock A, Green L, Huff KK, Do HM, Aitken SC, Warren R: Estrogen receptor status: an important variable predicting response to endocrine therapy in metastatic breast cancer. Eur J Cancer 16:323–331, 1980.
4. American College of Physicians: The use of diagnostic tests for screening and evaluation of breast lesions. Ann Intern Med 103:147–151, 1985.
5. Aretz HT, Silverman, ML, Kolodziejski JL, Witherspoon BR: Fine needle aspiration. Why it deserves another look. Postgrad Med 75:49–56, 1984.
6. Azavedo E, Baral E, Skoog L: Immunohistochemical analysis of estrogen receptors in cells obtained by fine needle aspiration from human mammary carcinomas. Anticancer Res 6:263–266, 1986.
7. Azzarelli A, Guzzon A, Pilotti S, Quagliuolo V, Bono A, Di Pietro S: Accuracy of breast cancer diagnosis by physical, radiologic and cytologic combined examinations. Tumori 69(2):137–141, 1983.
8. Barrows GH, Anderson TJ, Lamb JL, Dixon JM: Fine-needle aspiration of breast cancer. Relationship of clinical factors to cytology results in 689 primary malignancies. Cancer 58(7):1493–1498, 1986.
9. Bell DA, Hajdu SI, Urban JA, Gaston JP: Role of aspiration cytology in the diagnosis and management of mammary lesions in office practice. Cancer 51:1182–1189, 1983.
10. Berg JW, Robbins GF: A late look at the safety of aspiration biopsy. Cancer 15:826–827, 1962.
11. Bhambhani S, Rajwanshi A, Pant L, Das DK, Luthra UK: Fine needle aspiration cytology of supernumerary breasts. Report of three cases. Acta Cytol 31(3):311–312, 1987.
12. Bibbo M, Scheiber M, Cajulis R, Keebler CM, Wied GL, Dowlatshahi K: Stereotaxic fine needle aspiration cytology of clinically occult malignant and premalignant breast lesions. Acta Cytol 32(2):193–201, 1988.
13. Bigelow R, Smith R, Goodman PA, Wilson GS: Needle localization of nonpalpable breast masses. Arch Surg 120:565–569, 1985.
14. Bjurstam N, Hedberg K, Hultborn KA, et al: Diagnosis of breast carcinoma: evaluation of clinical examination, mammography, thermography and aspiration biopsy in breast disease. Progr Surg 13:1–65, 1974.
15. Bondeson L: Aspiration cytology of radiation-induced changes of normal breast epithelium. Acta Cytol 31(3):309–310, 1987.
16. Bottles K, Taylor RN: Diagnosis of breast masses in pregnant and lactating women by aspiration cytology. Obstet Gynecol 66(Suppl 3):76S–78S, 1985.
17. Burt AD, Seywright MM, George WD: Mixed apocrine-medullary carcinoma of the breast. Report of a case with fine needle aspiration cytology. Acta Cytol 31(3):322–324, 1987.
18. Burton G, Flowers J, Cox E, Gersinger K, et al: Monoclonal

antiestrogen receptor antibody (H222) in fine needle aspiration cytologies of breast cancer. A predictive marker of response to hormonal therapy. Breast Cancer Res Treat 6:164, 1985.

19. Cardona G, Cataliotti L, Ciatto S, Rosselli-Del-Turco M: Reasons for failure of physical examination in breast cancer detection (analysis of 232 false-negative cases). Tumori 69(6):531–537, 1983.

20. Carlson GW, Ferguson CM: Needle aspiration cytology of breast masses. Am Surg 53(4):235–237, 1987.

21. Castro A, Buschbaum P, Nadji M, Voigt W, Taber S, Morales A: Immunochemical demonstration of human chronic gonadotropin (hc5) in tissue of breast carcinoma. Acta Endocrinol 94:511–516, 1980.

22. Cheung PS, Yan KW, Alagaratnam TT: The complementary role of fine needle aspiration cytology and Tru-cut needle biopsy in the management of breast masses. Aust NZ J Surg 57(9):615–620, 1987.

23. Ciatto S, Cariaggi P, Bulgaresi P: The value of routine cytologic examination of breast cyst fluids. Acta Cytol 31(3):301–304, 1987.

24. Ciatto S, Smith AH, DiMaggio C, Pescarini L, Lattanzio E, Ancona A, Punzo C, DeLeo G, Burke P, Bonomini MG, et al: Breast cancer diagnosis under the age of forty years. Tumori 73(5):457–461, 1987.

25. Clark CL, Zaino RJ, Feil PD, Miller JV, Steck ME, Ohlsson-Wilhelm BM, Satyaswaroop PG: Monoclonal antibodies to human progesterone receptor: characterization by biochemical and immunohistochemical techniques. Endocrinology 121:1213–1222, 1987.

26. Clark GM, McGuire WL, Hubay CA, Pearson OH, Marshall JS: Progesterone receptors as a prognostic factor in stage II breast cancer. N Engl J Med 309:1343–1347, 1983.

27. Clark JH, Peck EJ, Shraden WT, O'Malley BW: Estrogen and progesterone receptors: methods for characterization, quantification and purification. Methods Cancer Res 12:367–417, 1976.

28. Cohen MB, Rodgers RP, Hales MS, Gonzales JM, Ljung BM, Beckstead JH, Bottles K, Miller TR: Influence of training and experience in fine-needle aspiration biopsy of breast. Receiver operating characteristics curve analysis. Arch Pathol Lab Med 111(6):518–520, 1987.

29. Colcher D, Hand PH, Nuti M, Schlom J: A spectrum of monoclonal antibodies reactive with human mammary tumor cells. Proc Natl Acad Sci USA 78:3199–3203, 1981.

30. Cook SS, DeMay R: Adenocarcinoma of the breast with osseous metaplasia. Acta Cytol 28:317–320, 1984.

31. Craig JP: Secretory carcinoma of the breast in an adult. Acta Cytol 29:589–592, 1985.

32. Crone P, Hertz N, Nilsson T, Junze J, Hoier-Madsen K, Kennedy M, Bojsen-Moller J, Diepereen P, Hahn-Pedersen A, Jorgensen SJ: Predictive value of three diagnostic procedures in the evaluation of palpable breast tumors. Ann Chir Gynaecol 73:273–276, 1984.

33. Curtin CT, Pertschuk L, Mitchell V: Histochemical determination of estrogen and progesterone binding in fine needle aspirates of breast cancer. Correlation with conventional biochemical assays. Acta Cytol 26:841–846, 1982.

34. d'Amore ES, Maisto L, Gatteschi MB, Toma S, Canavese G: Secretory carcinoma of the breast. Report of a case with fine needle aspiration biopsy. Acta Cytol 30(3):309–312, 1986.

35. Degrell I: Fine needle biopsy of sarcomas of the breast. Acta Med Hung 37:73–81, 1980.

36. DeSombre ER, Jensen EV: Estrophilin assays in breast cancer. Quantitative features and application to the mastectomy specimen. Cancer 46:2783–2788, 1980.

37. Di Pietro S, Fariselli G, Bandieramonte G, Lepera P, Coopmans de Yoldi G, Viganotti G, Pilotti S: Diagnostic efficacy of the clinical-radiological-cytological triad in solid breast lumps: results of a second prospective study on 631 patients. Eur J Surg Oncol 13(4):335–340, 1987.

38. Dixon JM, Anderson TJ, Lamb J, Nixon SJ, Forrest APM: Fine needle aspiration cytology in relationship to clinical examination and mammography in the diagnosis of a solid breast mass. Br J Surg 71:593–596, 1984.

39. Dixon JM, Clarke PJ, Crucioli V, Dehn TC, Lee EC, Greenall MJ: Reduction of the surgical excision rate in benign breast disease using fine needle aspiration cytology with immediate reporting. Br J Surg 74(11):1014–1016, 1987.

40. Dwarakanath S, Lee AK, Delellis RA, Silverman ML, Frasca L, Wolfe HJ: S-100 protein positivity in breast carcinomas: a potential pitfall in diagnostic immunohistochemistry. Hum Pathol 18:1144–1148, 1987.

41. Egan MJ, Neuman J, Crocher J, Collard M: Immunohistochemical localization of S-100 protein in benign and malignant conditions of the breast. Arch Pathol Lab Med 111:28–31, 1987.

42. Eisen MJ, Taft RH: Cytologic diagnosis of mammary cancer associated with incipient Paget's disease of the nipple. Cancer 4:150–153, 1951.

43. Eusebi V, Betts C, Haagensen DE, Gugliotta P, Bussolati G, Azzopardi JG: Apocrine differentiation in lobular carcinoma of the breast: a morphologic immunocytologic and ultrastructural study. Hum Pathol 15:134–140, 1984.

44. Feldman PS, Covell JL: Breast and lung. In Fine Needle Aspiration Cytology and Its Clinical Application. Chicago, American Society of Clinical Pathologists Press, 1985, pp 27–43.

45. Fessia L, Ghiringhello B, Arisio R, Botta G, Aimone V: Accuracy of frozen section diagnosis in breast cancer detection. Pathol Res Pract 179:61–66, 1984.

46. Flowers JL, Burton GV, Cox EB, McCarty KS Sr, Dent GA, Geisinger RR, McCarty KS Jr: Use of monoclonal antiestrogen receptor antibody to evaluate estrogen receptor content in fine needle aspiration breast biopsies. Ann Surg 203:250–254, 1986.

47. Forsman LM, Karhi KK, Autero M, Gahmberg CG, Andersson LC: Antiserum against formalin-fixed human milk fat globule glycoprotein for immunohistochemistry of normal and malignant apocrine epithelium. Acta Pathol Microbiol Immunol Scand (A) 92:331–337, 1984.

48. Frable WJ: Thin Needle Aspiration Biopsy. Philadelphia, WB Saunders, 1983, pp 20–73.

49. Frable WJ: Needle aspiration of the breast. Cancer 53:671–676, 1984.

50. Franzen S, Zajicek J: Aspiration biopsy in diagnosis of palpable lesions of the breast. Critical review of 3479 consecutive biopsies. Acta Radiol 7:241–262, 1968.

51. Fritsches HG, Muller EA: Pseudosarcomatous fasciits of the breast. Cytologic and histologic features. Acta Cytol 27(1):73–75, 1983.

52. Galen RS, Gambino SR: The predictive value and efficiency of medical diagnosis. In Beyond Normality. New York, John Wiley and Sons, 1975.

53. Gardner DG, Wittliff JL: Specific estrogen receptors in the lactating mammary gland of the rat. Biochemistry 12:3090–3096, 1973.

54. Gent HJ, Sprenger E, Dowlatshahi K: Stereotaxic needle localization and cytological diagnosis of occult breast lesions. Ann Surg 204(5):580–584, 1986.

55. Gentling PA: Fine needle aspiration—an aid to breast diagnosis. NC Med J 46:481–482, 1985.

56. Gonzalez E, Grafton WD, Morris DM, Barr LH: Diagnosing breast cancer using frozen sections from Tru-Cut needle biopsies. Ann Surg 202:696–701, 1985.

57. Gown AM, Gabbiani G: Intermediate-sized (10 mm.) filaments in human tumors. In DeLellis RA (ed): Advances in Immunohistochemistry. New York, Masson Publishing USA, 1984, p 89.

58. Greene GL, Hensen EV: Monoclonal antibodies as probes for estrogen receptor detection and characterization. J Steroid Biochem 16:353–359, 1982.

59. Gunduz N, Zheng S, Fisher B: Fluoresceinated estrone binding by cells from human breast cancers obtained by needle aspiration. Cancer 52:1251–1256, 1983.

60. Haag D, Goerttler K, Tschahargane C: The proliferative index (pi) of human breast cancer as obtained by flow cytometry. Path Res Pract 178:315–322, 1984.

61. Halvey A, Reif R, Bogokovsky H, Orda R: Diagnosis of carcinoma of the breast by fine needle aspiration cytology. Surg Gynecol Obstet 164(6):506–508, 1987.

62. Hammond S, Keyhani-Rofagha S, O'Toole RV: Statistical analysis of fine needle aspiration cytology of the breast. A review

of 678 cases plus 4,265 cases from the literature. Acta Cytol 31(3):276–284, 1987.

63. Hermansen C, Poulsen HS, Jensen J, Langféldt B, Steenskov V, Frederiksen P, Jensen O: Palpable breast tumours: "triple diagnosis" and operative strategy. Acta Chir Scand 150:625–628, 1984.

64. Homer MJ, Smith TJ, Marchant DJ: Outpatient needle localization and biopsy of nonpalpable breast lesions. JAMA 252:2452–2454, 1984.

65. Hsiu JG, Hawkins AG, D'Amato NA, Mullen JT: A case of pure primary squamous cell carcinoma of the breast diagnosed by fine needle aspiration biopsy. (Letter) Acta Cytol 29:650–651, 1985.

66. Ingram DM, Sterrett GF, Sheiner HJ, Shilkin KB: Fine-needle aspiration cytology in the management of breast disease. Med J Aust 2(4):170–173, 1983.

67. Innes DJ Jr, Feldman PS: Comparison of diagnostic results obtained by fine needle aspiration cytology and Tru-cut or open biopsies. Acta Cytol 27(3):350–354, 1983.

68. Janssens JP, Pylyser K, Bekaert J, Roelens J, Stuyck J, DeKeyser LJ, Lasuneryns JM, De Loecker W: Biochemical and histochemical analysis of steroid hormone binding sites in human primary breast cancer. Cancer 55:2600–2611, 1985.

69. Jayaram G: Cytomorphology of tuberculous mastitis. A report of nine cases with fine needle aspiration cytology. Acta Cytol 29(6):974–978, 1985.

70. Jensen EV, DeSombre ER, Jungblut PW: Estrogen Receptors In Hormone Responsive Tissues and Tumors. Chicago, University of Chicago Press, 1967.

71. Jobis AC, DeVries GP, Meiyer AEFH, et al: The immunohistochemical detection of prostatic acid phosphatase, its possibilities and limitations in tumor histochemistry. Histochem J 13:961, 1981.

72. Johnston WW, Szpak CA, Thor A, Simpson JF, Schlom J: Applications of immunocytochemistry to clinical cytology. Cancer Invest 5(6):593–611, 1987.

73. Kambouris AA: The role of fine needle aspiration cytology in the management of solid breast tumors. Am Surg 49(6):310–313, 1983.

74. Kaminsky DB: Aspiration biopsy in the context of the new Medicare fiscal policy. Acta Cytol 28(3):333–336, 1984.

75. Kehler M, Albrechtsson U: Mammographic fine needle biopsy of non-palpable breast lesions. Acta Radiol (Diagn) 25:273–276, 1984.

76. Kern WH, Dermer GB: The cytopathology of hyperplastic and neoplastic mammary duct epithelium. Acta Cytol 16:120–129, 1972.

77. Keshgegian AA, Inverso K, Kline TS: Determination of estrogen receptor by monoclonal antireceptor antibody in aspiration biopsy cytology from breast carcinoma. Am J Clin Pathol 89(1):24–29, 1988.

78. King WJ, DeSombre ER, Jensen EV, Greene GL: Comparison of immunocytochemical and steroid binding assays for estrogen receptor in human breast tumor. Cancer Res 45:293–304, 1985.

79. Kiovuniemi AP: Fine needle aspiration of the breast. Ann Clin Res 8:272, 1976.

80. Kline TS: Maquerades of malignancy. A review of 4241 aspirates from the breast. Acta Cytol 25:263–266, 1981.

81. Kline TS: Breast. In Handbook of Fine Needle Aspiration Biopsy Cytology, ed 2. New York, Churchill Livingstone, 1988, pp 199–252.

82. Kline TS, Joshi LP, Neal HS: Fine needle aspiration of the breast: Diagnoses and pitfalls. A review of 3545 cases. Cancer 44:1458–1464, 1979.

83. Kline TS, Neal HS: Needle aspiration of the breast—why bother? Acta Cytol 20:327, 1976.

84. Knight DC, Lowell DM, Heimann A, Dunn E: Aspiration of the breast and nipple discharge cytology. Surg Gynecol Obstet 163(5):415–420, 1986.

85. Kreuzer G: Aspiration biopsy cytology in proliferative benign mammary dysplasia. Acta Cytol 22:128–132, 1978.

86. Kreuzer G, Boquoi E: Aspiration biopsy cytology, mammography and clinical exploration: a modern set-up in diagnosis of tumor of the breast. Acta Cytol 20:319, 1976.

87. Kreuzer G, Zajicek J: Cytologic diagnosis of mammary tumors from aspiration biopsy smears. III. Studies on 200 carcinomas with false negative or doubtful cytologic reports. Acta Cytol 16:249–252, 1972.

88. Lamb J, Anderson TJ, Dixon MJ, Levack PA: Role of fine needle aspiration cytology in breast cancer screening. J Clin Pathol 40(7):705–709, 1987.

89. Lazarevic B, Katatikarn V, Marks RA: Primary squamous cell carcinoma of the breast. Diagnosis by fine needle aspiration cytology. Acta Cytol 28(3):321–324, 1984.

90. Lazarevic B, Rodgers JB: Aspiration cytology of carcinoid tumor of the breast. A case report. Acta Cytol 27(3):329–333, 1983.

91. Learmonth GM, Hayes MM, Hacking A, Gudgeon A, Dent DM, Stander W, Slater P, Holden S: Fine-needle aspiration biopsy cytology of the breast. A review of the Groote Schuur Hospital experience. S Afr Med J 72(8):525–527, 1987.

92. Leclercq G, Heuson JC: Therapeutic significance of sex steroid hormone receptors in the treatment of breast cancer. Eur J Cancer 13:1205–1215, 1977.

93. Lee SH: Validity of a histochemical estrogen receptor assay. J Histochem Cytochem 32:305–310, 1984.

94. Lever JV, Trott PA, Webb AJ: Fine needle aspiration cytology. J Clin Pathol 38:1–11, 1985.

95. Linsk J, Kreuzer G, Zajicek J: Cytologic diagnosis of mammary tumors from aspiration biopsy smears. II. Studies on 210 fibroadenomas and 210 cases of benign dysplasia. Acta Cytol 16:130–138, 1972.

96. Lowhagen T, Rubio CA: The cytology of the granular cell myoblastoma of the breast. Acta Cytol 21:314–315, 1977.

97. Lozowski MS, Mishriki Y, Chao S, Grimson R, Pai P, Harris MA, Lundy J: Estrogen receptor determination in fine needle aspirates of the breast. Correlation with histologic grade and comparison with biochemical analysis. Acta Cytol 31:557–562, 1987.

98. Lundy J, Lozowski M, Mishiriki Y: Monoclonal antibody B72.3 as a diagnostic adjunct in fine needle aspiration of breast masses. Ann Surg 203:399–402, 1986.

99. MacKay B, Bruner J, Nelson G, et al: Electron microscopy in surgical pathology. Lab Med 19:13–17, 1988.

100. Magdelenat H: Estrogen and progestin receptors on drill biopsy samples of human mammary tumors. Recent Results Cancer Res 91:45–49, 1984.

101. Malberger E, Gutterman E, Bartfeld E, Zajicek G: Cellular changes in the mammary gland epithelium during the menstrual cycle. A computer image analysis study. Acta Cytol 31(3):305–308, 1987.

102. Mann M, Masin F: Cytology of angiosarcoma of the breast. Acta Cytol 22:162–164, 1978.

103. Marchetti E, Nenci I: Immunohistochemical demonstration of steroid receptors. Recent Results Cancer Res 91:61–67, 1984.

104. Martin HE, Ellis EB: Biopsy by needle procedure and aspiration. Ann Surg 92:169–181, 1930.

105. Martin HE, Ellis EB: Aspiration Biopsy. Surg Gynecol Obstet 59:578–589, 1934.

106. Masood S: Fluorescent cytochemical detection of estrogen and progesterone receptors in breast fine needle aspirates. (Abstract) Modern Pathology 2(1)59A, 1989.

107. Masood S: The potential value of imprint cytology in cytochemical localization of steroid hormone receptors in ovarian cancer. Diagn Cytopathol 4:42–47, 1988.

108. Masood S: Use of monoclonal antibody in assessment of estrogen receptor content in fine needle aspiration biopsy specimen from patients with breast cancer. Arch Pathol Lab Med 113:26–30, 1989.

109. Masood S: Use of monoclonal antibody B72.3 in breast fine needle aspirates. J Breast Cancer Treat 14:159, 1989.

110. Masood S, Frykberg ER, Mitchum DG, McLellan GL, Scalapino MC, Bullard JB: The potential value of mammographically guided fine needle aspiration biopsy of nonpalpable breast lesions. Am Surg 55:226–231, 1989.

111. Masood S, Johnson H: The value of imprint cytology in cytochemical detection of steroid hormone receptors in breast cancer. Am J Clin Pathol 87:30–36, 1987.

112. Mayar M, Saxena H: Tuberculosis of the breast. A cytomorphologic study of needle aspirates and nipple discharges. Acta Cytol 28:325–328, 1984.

113. McClelland RA, Berger O, Wilson P, Powless TJ, Trott PA, Easton D, Gazet JC, Combs RC: Presurgical determination of estrogen receptor status using immunocytochemically stained fine needle aspirate smears in patients with breast cancer. Cancer Res 15(47):6118–6122, 1987.

114. McGuire WL, Carbone PP, Volmer EP (eds): Estrogen Receptors. In Human Breast Cancer. New York, Raven Press, 1975.

115. Mercer WD, Lippman ME, Wahl TM, Carlson CA, Wahl DA, Lezotte D, Teague PO: The use of immunocytochemical techniques for the detection of steroid hormones in breast cancer cells. Cancer 46:2859–2868, 1980.

116. Merle S, Zajdela A, Magdelenat H: Progesterone receptor assay in fine needle aspirates of breast tumors. (Letter) Acta Cytol 29:496–497, 1985.

117. Millis RR: Needle biopsy of the breast. (Review) Monogr Pathol 25:186–203, 1984.

118. Mooler JC, et al: Fine needle aspiration of the breast. A five year series. Ugeskr Laeger 140:1847, 1978.

119. Mukai K, Schollmeyer JV, Rosai J: Immunohistochemical localization of actin. Am J Surg Pathol 5:91–97, 1981.

120. Mushlin AI: Diagnostic tests in breast cancer. Ann Int Med 103:79–85, 1985.

121. Mushlin AI: The use of diagnostic tests for screening and evaluating breast lesions. Ann Int Med 103:147–151, 1985.

122. Nayar M, Saxena H: Tuberculosis of the breast. A cytomorphologic study of needle aspirates and nipple discharges. Acta Cytol 28:325–328, 1984.

123. Naylor B: Fine needle aspiration cytology of the breast. An overview. Am J Surg Pathol 12(suppl 1):54–61, 1988.

124. Nenci I: Estrogen receptor cytochemistry in human breast cancer: Status and prospects. Cancer 48:2674–2686, 1981.

125. Norton LW, Davis JR, Wiens JL, Trego DC, Dunnington GL: Accuracy of aspiration cytology in detecting breast cancer. Surgery 96:806–814, 1984.

126. Nuti M, Mottolese M, Viora M, Donnorso RP, Schlom J, Natali PG: Use of monoclonal antibodies to human breast-tumor-associated antigens in fine-needle aspirate cytology. Int J Cancer 37(4):493–498, 1986.

127. Nuti M, Teramoto YA, Mariani-Constantini R, Hand PH, Colcher D, Schlom J: A monoclonal antibody (B72.3) defines patterns of distribution of a novel tumor-associated antigen in human mammary carcinoma cell populations. Int J Cancer 29:539–545, 1982.

128. Oatham SA, Randall KJ: Problems in the diagnosis of breast aspirates. Acta Cytol 21:711, 1977.

129. Orell SR, Sterrett GF, Walters M, Whitaker D: Fine Needle Aspiration Cytology. London, Churchill Livingstone, 1986.

130. Ortel YC: Fine Needle Aspiration of the Breast. Boston, Butterworths USA, 1987.

131. Osborne CK, McGuire WL: Current uses of steroid hormone receptor assays in the treatment of breast cancer. Surg Clin North Am 58:777–787, 1978.

132. Palombini L, Fulciniti F, Vetrani A, Galligioni A, Montaguti A, Pennelli N: Mucoid carcinoma of the breast on fine-needle aspiration biopsy sample: cytology and ultrastructure. Appl Pathol 2(2):70–75, 1984.

133. Papotti M, Eusebi V, Gugliotta P, Bussolati G: Immunohistochemical analysis of benign and malignant papillary lesions of the breast. Am J Surg Pathol 7:451–461, 1983.

134. Paridaens R, Sylvester RJ, Ferrazzi E, Legros N, Leclerq G, Henson JC: Clinical significance of the quantitative assessment of estrogen receptors in advanced breast cancer. Cancer 46:2889–2895, 1980.

135. Patel JJ, Gartell PC, Guyer PB, Herbert A, Taylor I: Use of ultrasound localization to improve results of fine needle aspiration cytology of breast masses. J R Soc Med 81(1):10–12, 1988.

136. Patel JJ, Gartell PC, Smallwood JA, Herbert A, Royle G, Buchanan R, Taylor I: Fine needle aspiration cytology of breast masses: an evaluation of its accuracy and reasons for diagnostic failure. Ann R Coll Surg Engl 69(4):156–159, 1987.

137. Pedio G, Landolt U, Zobeli L: Irradiated benign cells of the breast: a potential diagnostic pitfall in needle aspiration cytology. (Letter). Acta Cytol 32(1):127–128, 1988.

138. Perrot-Applanat M, Groyer-Picard M, Lorenzo F, Jolivet A, Hai MT, Pallud C, Spyratos F, Milgrom E: Immunocytochemical study with monoclonal antibodies to progesterone receptor in human breast tumors. Cancer Res 47:2652–2661, 1987.

139. Pertschuk LP, Eisenberger K, Carter AC, Feldman JG: Immunohistologic localization of estrogen receptors in breast cancer with monoclonal antibodies. Cancer 55:1513–1518, 1985.

140. Pertschuk LP, Tobin EH, Gaetjens E, Carter AC, Degeshein GA, Bloom ND, Brigati DJ: Histochemical assay of estrogen and progesterone receptors in breast cancer. Correlation with biochemical assays and patients' response to endocrine therapies. Cancer 46:2896–2901, 1980.

141. Pertschuk LP, Tobin EH, Tanapat P, Gaetjens E, Carter AC, Bloom ND, Macchia RJ, Eisenberg KB: Histochemical analyses of steroid hormone receptors in breast and prostate carcinoma. J Histochem Cytochem 28:779–810, 1980.

142. Pettinato G, Petrella G, Manco A, di Prisco B, Salvatore G, Angrisani P: Carcinoma of the breast with osteoclast-like giant cells. Fine-needle aspiration cytology, histology and electron microscopy of 5 cases. Appl Pathol 2(3):168–178, 1984.

143. Pilotti S, Rilke F, Delpiano C, Di Pietro S, Guzzon A: Problems in fine-needle aspiration biopsy cytology of clinically or mammographically uncertain breast tumors. Tumori 68(5):407–412, 1982.

144. Poulsen HS, Schulz H, Bichel P: Estrogen receptor determinations on fine needle aspirations from malignant tumours of the breast. Eur J Cancer 15:1431–1438, 1979.

145. Ravinsky E, Cavers DJ: Cytology of argyrophilic carcinoma of the breast. Acta Cytol 29:1–6, 1985.

146. Reiner A, Spona J, Reiner G, Schemper M, Kolb R, Kwasny W, Fugger R, Jakesz R, Holzner JH: Estrogen receptor analysis on biopsies and fine needle aspirates from human breast carcinoma. Am J Pathol 125:443–449, 1986.

147. Rosemond GP, Maier WP, Brobyn TJ: Needle aspiration of breast cysts. Surg Gynecol Obstet 128:351–354, 1969.

148. Rosen PP: Frozen section diagnosis of breast lesions. Recent experience with 556 consecutive biopsies. Ann Surg 187:17–19, 1978.

149. Rosen P, Hadju SJ, Robbins G, et al: Diagnosis of Carcinoma of the Breast by Aspiration Biopsy. Surg Gynecol Obstet 134:837–838, 1972.

150. Rosenthal DL: Breast lesions diagnosed by fine needle aspiration. Pathol Res Pract 181:645–656, 1986.

151. Russ JE, Winchester DP, Scanlon ET, Christ MA: Cytologic findings of aspiration of tumors of the breast. Surg Gynecol Obstet 146:407–411, 1978.

152. Sartorius OW, Morris PL, Benedict DF: Fine needle aspiration for the cytologic diagnosis of benign and malignant breast lesions. Proc Am Assoc Cancer Res 20:275, 1979.

153. Scanlon EF: The case for and against two-step procedure for the surgical treatment of breast cancer. Cancer 53(Suppl 3):677–680, 1984.

154. Schondorf H (translated by Schneider V): Aspiration Cytology of the Breast. Philadelphia, WB Saunders, 1978.

155. Schwartz GF, Feig SA, Rosenberg AL, Patchefsky AS, Schwartz AB: Localization and significance of clinically occult breast lesions: Experience with 469 needle guided biopsies. Recent Results Cancer Res 90:125–132, 1984.

156. Shousha S, Lyssiotis T, Godfrey VM, Scheuer PJ: Carcinoembryonic antigen in breast cancer tissue: a useful prognostic indicator. Br Med J 1:777–779, 1979.

157. Sickles EA, Klein DL, Goodson W III, Hunt TK: Mammography after needle aspiration of palpable breast masses. Radiology 145:395–397, 1983.

158. Silfversward C, Humla S: Estrogen receptor analysis on needle aspirates from human mammary carcinoma. Acta Cytol 24:54–57, 1980.

159. Silfversward C, Wallgren, Nordenskjold A, Humla S: Estrogen receptor analysis on fine needle aspirates from human breast carcinoma. Recent Results Cancer Res 91:41–44, 1984.

160. Silver CE, Koss LG, Brauer RJ, Kamholz SL, Pinsker KL, Rosenblatt R, Esposti PL: Needle aspiration cytology of tumors at various body sites. Curr Prob Surg 22:1–67, 1985.

161. Silverman JF, Feldman PS, Covell JL, Frable WJ: Fine needle aspiration cytology of neoplasms metastatic to the breast. Acta Cytol 31(3):291–300, 1987.

162. Silverman JF, Lannin DR, O'Brien K, Norris HT: The triage role of fine needle aspiration biopsy of palpable breast masses. Acta Cytol 31:731, 1987.

163. Silverman JF, Lannin DR, Unverferth M, Norris HT: Fine needle aspiration cytology of subareolar abscess of the breast. Spectrum of cytomorphologic findings and potential diagnostic pitfalls. Acta Cytol 30(4):413–419, 1986.

164. Simpson RHW, James KA, Holdstock JB, Kelly RM, Yankah DHT: Carcinoma in a breast fibroadenoma. Acta Cytol 31(3):313–316, 1987.

165. Smallwood J, Herbert A, Guyer P, Taylor I: Accuracy of aspiration cytology in the diagnosis of breast disease. Br J Surg 72(10):841–843, 1985.

166. Smeets HJ, Saltzstein SL, Meurer WT, Pilch YH: Needle biopsies in breast cancer diagnosis: techniques in search of an audience. J Surg Oncol 32(1):11–15, 1986.

167. Smith C, Butler J, Cobb C, State D: Fine-needle aspiration cytology in the diagnosis of primary breast cancer. Surgery 103(2):178–183, 1988.

168. Smith TJ, Safaii H, Foster EA, Reinhold RB: Accuracy and cost effectiveness of fine needle aspiration biopsy. Am J Surg 149:540–545, 1985.

169. Somers RG, Young GP, Kaplan MJ, Bernhard VM, Rosenberg M, Somers D: Fine needle aspiration biopsy in the management of solid breast tumors. Arch Surg 120:673–677, 1985.

170. Squires JE, Betsill WL: Intracystic carcinomas of the breast. Acta Cytol 25:267–271, 1981.

171. Stavric GD, Tercer DT, Kaftandjiev DR, et al: Aspiration biopsy cytologic method in diagnosis of breast lesions. A critical review of 250 cases. Acta Cytol 28:729–732, 1973.

172. Stawickl ME, Hsiu JG: Malignant cystosarcoma phyllodes. Report with cytologic presentation. Acta Cytol 23:61–64, 1979.

173. Stewart FW: The diagnosis of tumors by aspiration. Am J Pathol 9:801–812, 1933.

174. Stormby N, Bondenson L: Adenoma of the nipple. Acta Cytol 28:729–732, 1984.

175. Svane G, Silversward C: Sterotaxic needle biopsy of nonpalpable breast lesions: cytologic and histopathologic findings. Acta Radiol (Diagn) 24:283–288, 1983.

176. Takeda T, Suzuki M, Sato Y, Hase T, Yamada S: Aspiration cytology of breast cysts. Acta Cytol 26:37–38, 1982.

177. Torres V, Ferrer R: Cytology of fine needle aspiration biopsy of primary breast rhabdomyosarcoma in an adolescent girl. Acta Cytol 29(3):430–434, 1985.

178. Tsuchiya S, Maruyama Y, Koike Y, Yamada K, Kobayashi Y, Kagaya A: Cytologic characteristics and origin of naked nuclei in breast aspirate smears. Acta Cytol 31(3):285–290, 1987.

179. Tucker AK: Breast screening. Practitioner 229:217–223, 1985.

180. Ulanow RM, Galblum L, Canter JW: Fine needle aspiration in the diagnosis and management of solid breast lesions. Am J Surg 148:653–657, 1984.

181. Venet L, Strax P, Venet W, Shapiro S: Adequacies and inadequacies of breast examination by physicians. Cancer 24:1187–1191, 1969.

182. Vinores SA, Bonnin JM, Rubinstein LJ, Marangos PJ: Immunohistochemical demonstration of neuron-specific enolase in neoplasma of CNS and other tissues. Arch Pathol Lab Med 108:536–540, 1984.

183. Vorherr H: Breast aspiration biopsy. Am J Obstet Gynecol 148:127–133, 1984.

184. Walker HC, Delaney JP, Gedgaudas E: Locating nonpalpable breast lesions for the surgeon. Minn Med 68:437–439, 1985.

185. Walker RA: The binding of peroxidase labeled sections to human breast epithelium-normal, hyperplastic and lactating breast. J Pathol 142:279–291, 1984.

186. Walker RA, Cove DH, Howel A: Histological detection of oestrogen receptor in human breast carcinomas. Lancet 1:171–173, 1980.

187. Wanebo HJ, Feldman PS, Wilhelm MC, Covell JL, Binns RL: Fine needle aspiration cytology in lieu of open biopsy in management of primary breast cancer. Ann Surg 199(5):569–579, 1984.

188. Watson DP, McGuire M, Nicholson F, Given HF: Aspiration cytology and its relevance to the diagnosis of solid tumors of the breast. Surg Gynecol Obstet 165(5):435–441, 1987.

189. Weintraub J, Weintraub D, Redard M, Vassilakos P: Evaluation of estrogen receptors by immunocytochemistry on fine needle aspiration biopsy specimens from breast tumors. Cancer 15(60):1163–1172, 1987.

190. Wilkinson EJ, Schuettke CM, Ferrier CM, Franzini DA, Bland KI: Fine needle aspiration of breast masses: analysis of 276 aspirates. Acta Cytol 33:613–619, 1989.

191. Wilkinson EJ, Xiang J, Braylan RC, Benson NA, Spanier SS, Enneking WF, Springfield DS: Potential value of fine needle aspiration in the cytologic and cytometric analysis of bone and soft tissue tumors. Lab Invest 48(1):93A–94A, 1983.

192. Wilkinson S, Forrest APM: Fibroadenoma of the breast. Br J Surg 72(10):838–840, 1985.

193. Wittliff JL: Steroid binding proteins in benign and neoplastic mammary cells. Meth Cancer Res 11:293–354, 1975.

194. Wolberg WH, Tanner MA, Wei-Yin L, Janichsetakal N: Statistical approach to fine needle aspiration diagnosis of breast masses. Arch Surg 124(7):814–818, 1989.

195. Wollenberg NJ, Caya JG, Clowry SJ: Fine needle aspiration cytology of the breast. A review of 321 cases with statistical evaluation. Acta Cytol 29(3):425–429, 1985.

196. Zaino RJ, Clarke CL, Mortel R, Satyaswarrop PG: Heterogeneity of progesterone receptor distribution in human endometrial carcinoma. Cancer Res 48:1889–1895, 1988.

197. Zajdela A, Arsclain B, Ghossein NA: Comparison between the nuclear diameters of primary and metastatic breast cancer cells obtained by cytologic aspiration. Cancer 56:1605–1610, 1985.

198. Zajdela A, Ghossein NA, Pilleron JP, Ennuyer A: The experience of aspiration cytology in the diagnosis of breast cancer. Experience at the Foundation Curie. Cancer 35:499–506, 1975.

199. Zajicek J: Aspiration Biopsy Cytology, part I: cytology of supradephragmatic organs. Monogr Clin Cytol 4:1–211, 1974.

200. Zajicek J, Franzen S, Jakobson P, Rubio C, Unsgaard B: Aspiration of mammary tumors in diagnosis and research—a critical review of 2200 cases. Acta Cytol 11:169–175, 1967.

201. Zaloudek C, Oertel Y, Orenstein JM: Adenoid cystic carcinoma of the breast. Am J Clin Pathol 81:297–307, 1984.

Section IX

Clinical Trials: Biostatistical Applications

Chapter 27

DESIGN AND CONDUCT OF CLINICAL TRIALS FOR BREAST CANCER

Alfred A. Bartolucci, Ph.D., Marilyn Raney, M.A., and Robert Birch, Ph.D.

This chapter will outline the important principles for the design and conduct of therapeutic clinical trials in breast cancer. Such trials have become extremely sophisticated and complicated. We will not cover every single aspect of these types of trials but instead will highlight the major points.

This chapter will concentrate on prospective clinical trials and will not focus on retrospective trials (i.e., the after-the-fact abstracting of data and data interpretation by investigators) except to say that retrospective trials are often tainted by biases inherent in the data and biases inherent in the investigators. Well-planned prospective trials assure objectivity.

Spilker[28] indicated that biases, in general, occur as a consequence of the study design used, the tests used, the people involved in the study, the patients, and the analyses or perspectives used in interpreting the data. Sackett[22] attributes most biases to the investigator who designs, conducts, and analyzes the study. We will outline, in as much detail as possible, the various salient points of well-conducted breast cancer trials that avoid the problems of biases or other underlying shortcomings for which the trial can be criticized.

There are three types of clinical trials usually used: phase I, phase II, and phase III clinical trials. Each of these types of trials is geared to a specific patient population, and the objectives may vary according to the type of sample under study. If these trials are conducted according to good scientific practice, then they are said to be generalizable to the particular population for which they were designed. Phase IV studies, discussed later, are also sometimes used.

PHASE I STUDIES

Phase I studies usually involve the determination of a generally safe or well-tolerated dose of a new drug by the patient. This is often referred to as a "maximally tolerated dose" in patients. The objective is to seek dose-limiting toxicity. The end points usually involved are commonly noted adverse reactions, characteristics of the drug, and perhaps characteristics of the drug at different dose levels. This involves identifying laboratory parameters affected by the drug. Spilker[28] referred to this as seeking an initial pharmacokinetic profile. A second objective, which is often serendipitous, is usually a determination of efficacy of the drug in some situations. Again, this depends on the therapy under study and the parameters of efficacy that are being considered in the particular population under study.

PHASE II STUDIES

Phase II studies in breast cancer usually involve identifying tumor types for which the treatment appears promising. The major end point is generally the magnitude of efficacy (i.e., the level of response), which will be discussed later. Other end points may include the duration of the effects produced (often referred to as duration of response or survival), the doses of the drug that are effective, and additional information on suitable dose regimens or schedules of the drug. Toxicities are also measured.

499

PHASE III STUDIES

The purpose of phase III studies is to determine the effect of a new treatment relative to a standard therapy. These are often referred to as comparative trials. Another benefit of a phase III study is to determine the effect of a treatment relative to the natural history of the disease or to determine if a new treatment is relatively as effective as a standard therapy but is associated with less morbidity or toxicity. Many special studies are frequently associated with phase III trials; these may include studies of demographic or environmental characteristics, particular patient clinical values (laboratory values), or other characteristics that may be influential in terms of prognostic significance of a particular therapy or group of therapies.

End points of phase III studies may include the evaluation of chemotherapeutic, radiotherapeutic, or surgical procedures. Other considerations may involve the activity of immunostimulants, biotherapeutic agents, antiemetics, and pain control agents, and measurement of the quality of life during the conduct of the trial. It must also be remembered that the trials conducted are usually specific to a particular patient population. For example, phase I and II studies are sometimes conducted in refractory or relapsed types of patient populations. Phase III studies usually involve early stage disease or metastatic disease, depending on the end points of interest.

PHASE IV STUDIES

The phase IV study is less scientific than the phase III study and usually involves the safety, tolerance, and efficacy of the drug in the general population of patients for which the drug or therapy is intended. Once the therapy has become "standard" practice, early indications of unexpected or expected beneficial activities can be studied further in the general population. Phase IV studies usually involve post-marketing surveillance, epidemiology, and the marketing of therapeutic agents. Thus in these studies, the science is now extended to the general population for treatment of a specific disease, which in our case is breast cancer.

PROTOCOL DESIGN FROM THE STATISTICAL PERSPECTIVE

Content of Experimental Design

All well-planned strategies involve a protocol. In a breast cancer clinical trial, this is a written document detailing the scientific questions to be reviewed, giving a justification for the type and number of patients to be studied as well as a scientific basis for the study. The elements of a protocol typically include objectives, background and rationale, therapeutic agents, patient selection criteria, studies to be done, stratification and randomization procedures, treatment regimens, toxicity and dosage estimates, evaluation of response, reporting procedures, and statistical considerations.

Objectives

Objectives are well-stated hypotheses addressing the types of questions the protocol is designed to address. Usually just prior to the objectives or following the objectives, or sometimes in the appendices of a protocol, a schema, which is a schematic diagram showing an overview of the study design, may be included. It is very important to list these study objectives quite specifically in the protocol. This enables all concerned to clearly understand the research plan. As will be seen later, the objectives also help determine the size of the study (i.e., the numbers of patients and controls), depending on the type of study that is being conducted. Unfortunately, for a number of trials that are published, the stated sample size is never fully met, often because of extenuating circumstances. However, studies are often ended too early with inadequate numbers, and as a result, the conclusions can be questionable. The objectives of the study usually include the elements outlined in the phase I, II, and III trial descriptions. Thus in a phase I trial, the question is one of dose-limiting toxicity (i.e., the maximal dose to obtain a toxic effect). The objective then is to move on to a phase II study and to conduct a response or efficacy trial, in which the maximal tolerable dose is often indicated and the objective changes from determination of toxicity to evaluation of treatment efficacy. Once the phase II objective is met and it is found that the treatment in question does have satisfactory efficacy, the study will move on to a phase III trial, which involves a comparative study. Two or more treatments or therapeutic modalities are then tested against one another to determine which is the most efficacious in the patient population under study.

Background and Rationale

The background and rationale of a proposed protocol include previous studies that have attested to the therapeutic efficacy of a particular treatment or combination of treatments; as a result, these treatments or combinations have been given a "green light" to be studied further in a particular patient sample of interest. The background and rationale section of a protocol is often filled with many references, much past data, and good scientific indications for the proposed study. The background and rationale of a phase III study could, in fact, include data from phase I and phase II studies as a prelude to the present design.

Therapeutic Agents

Therapeutic agents are usually the agents or modalities (e.g., surgery, radiation, immunotherapy, chemotherapy) that will be used in the protocol. In chemotherapy, the section on therapeutic agents usually includes a description of the chemical aspects of the drugs under consideration, the routes of administration, and known side effects. The surgery section may include a detailed description of the type of surgery required. In the case of breast cancer this may include a description of a segmental, total, modified, or radical mastectomy, for example. The radiation therapy section usually includes the procedure for the type of radiation to be delivered and the sites, dosage, and timing as well as the toxicity that is expected to be encountered.

Criteria for Patient Selection

The patient eligibility criteria section is an extremely important section of the protocol, as it usually describes the types of patients who may benefit from the types of therapies under study. As a result, the protocol treatments, if successful, can then be extended to the general patient population with the characteristics of the patients in the particular sample under study in the protocol. The patients identified for a particular protocol should be those who would most likely benefit from the new therapy or therapies under study. The eligibility limitations can be altered as a result of phase I and phase II trials, in which the objectives may extend beyond a particular patient sample. For example, eligibility criteria may include the tumor type that is under study—in our case, breast cancers. Therefore the protocols would be targeted toward women with breast cancer. The eligibility criteria may further be refined to include a certain stage of breast cancer. The criteria may also restrict the type of past therapy that patients under study would be allowed to have had prior to coming into a particular protocol. There may be specifications as to the time limit in which a patient can be entered on protocol following certain procedures. For example, in adjuvant breast studies there may be limitations on the number of days a patient may enter a protocol for chemotherapy following surgery or radiation therapy. The eligibility criteria may extend to a patient's physiological function. This would include, for example, adequate absolute granulocyte count, adequate bilirubin and blood urea nitrogen (BUN), and absence of infection or septicemia.

The criteria for patient selection of the protocol or document may also list a number of reasons why patients would be ineligible for a study. For example, if a woman is coming into a breast cancer protocol, she may be ineligible if she has had a previous history of cancer other than breast cancer. Especially in the adjuvant setting, the objective of a protocol may be to determine the effect on prolongation of life with chemotherapy following surgery, and a woman may be ineligible if she has had any previous chemotherapy. The same may apply to those who have received previous radiation, especially if there is a radiotherapy question in the protocol. In the case of metastatic disease, sometimes the protocol is restricted to the sites of disease as well as to types of previous therapies the patient has received. Sometimes preexisting conditions will also disqualify a patient from a study.

It was previously stated that the eligibility criteria are set so that the results of the study under question may be generalized to a broader population of individuals. There are often problems with eligibility criteria. If the criteria are too narrow, then the study may yield results that are not generalizable beyond the patients of the restricted types that have been included. A balance must be struck between attaining a homogeneous group in order to answer the protocol question and having a general group so that the results of the study can be applied to a broad population base. This has political and ethical as well as scientific implications. Simon[24] gives a good discussion of this type of controversy.

Studies to be Done

The section on the studies to be done usually includes the clinical work-up and follow-up of patients during the course of the protocol. This may involve, for example, physical examinations, laboratory readings, or CT scans. Typically the timing and requirements of these are described. The statistical issues involved here are to ensure that all patients are supported and evaluated the same way on protocol, thus protecting the reliability of study results.

Stratification and Randomization Procedures

For phase I and phase II studies, stratification and randomization procedures are not usually important. The only criterion for stratification in a phase II study is usually the inclusion of several types of populations of patients to determine if a treatment is efficacious within these particular populations. For example, stratification might be done according to stage of disease in order to test a treatment within those subgroups for efficacy.

Randomization and stratification are most important in phase III randomized trials. Randomization is the "random" allocation of patients to the various treatments under study. The technique used in randomization may be simple or complex, depending on the protocol. The purpose is to ensure that all patients in a study have an equally likely chance to be allocated to the treatments under consideration. Patients are usually stratified according to specific criteria based on patient characteristics believed to be related to response to therapy. For example, in an adjuvant breast cancer study, patients may be stratified by the number of positive axillary lymph nodes. Some patients may present at surgery with limited metastatic disease in the axilla (one to three positive nodes). Others may present with more extensive axillary disease (four or more positive nodes). To ensure that patients allocated to the treatments under consideration are not allocated disproportionately, randomization within the nodal status is often done. Suppose treatments A and B were to be tested to determine which was more efficacious in prolonging disease-free survival or overall survival. Patients with one to three positive nodes would be randomized to A or B, and those presenting with four or more positive nodes would also be randomized to either A or B. The strategy is to ensure that approximately 50 percent of the patients with one to three positive nodes are allocated to A, and 50 percent are allocated to B, and likewise for patients with four or more positive nodes. This guards against the possibility of one of the treatments being applied to the majority of patients within either nodal status and thus possibly biasing the results of the study in favor of A or B.

Randomization and stratification are usually described in quite a bit of detail in the written protocol. Researchers may stratify by a number of factors, but it must be remembered that the subgroups created are the number of randomization arms multiplied by the number of possible combinations of stratification grouping. It is easily possible for this to become very complex. Randomization and stratifications as well as justifications for stratifications are usually written into a treatment protocol.

Treatment Regimens

The treatment regimen section of the protocol includes the timing and dosage of therapy to be given in a particular study. This will include the timing and dosage of chemotherapy and timing and dosage of radiation therapy. If surgery is involved, then the surgical procedures are often outlined or at least referenced for the respective surgeons who will participate in the study.

Toxicity and Dosage Estimates

The toxicity and dosage estimates part of the protocol will involve the expected toxicities and the types of treatments, adjustments, delays, and modifications required to accommodate these toxicities. This section of the protocol may also involve statements as to the notification of appropriate personnel should unexpected or life-threatening toxicities be encountered. This administrative procedure is necessary so that others who are writing similar protocols or wish to pursue similar studies will be aware of the types of problems they may encounter during the course of their particular study. Toxicities are usually graded as to severity according to specific criteria included either in this section of the protocol or in the appendices.

Evaluation of Response

The type of response that an investigator wishes to evaluate will depend on the type of trial being conducted and the type of question under study. For example, as discussed previously, a phase I trial measures responses to determine the correct dose to limit toxicity. A phase II trial usually measures tumor shrinkage, and appropriate types of procedures for measuring tumor response are often indicated in the protocol. In some circumstances phase II studies have measured disease-free intervals or prolonged survival. This is not really the purpose of a phase II study, but some trials have added these as secondary end points to determination of tumor response to treatment.

A phase III trial may study tumor shrinkage or disease-free interval. Metastatic disease protocols will often measure tumor response to treatment. Basically a tumor or group of tumors within an individual is sited for observation, and during the course of the therapy, whether the tumor has responded to therapy and the degree of response (i.e., the amount of shrinkage in the tumor) will be determined.

Phase III adjuvant studies, which, for example, determine the effect of chemotherapy on prolongation of disease-free survival after surgical removal of a tumor, often have the end point of disease-free interval or overall survival. The analysis section will consider both metastatic and adjuvant phase III studies. The disease-free interval in the adjuvant protocol is usually defined as beginning when the patient has either received surgery or has started on protocol and ending when the disease or tumor recurs, either during the progress of the adjuvant therapy or after therapy is completed. Evaluation of the response often coincides with the "Studies to be Done" section. For example, a chest radiogram, bone scan, or liver scan may be used to determine whether disease has recurred. In addition, these are used throughout the protocol to evaluate the progress of the patient. It is most important that the dates of evaluations and their results be recorded during the course of a study so that an accurate assessment can be made of the·relative efficacy of various treatments and their effect on the end points or the responses to be evaluated.

Reporting Procedures

The reporting procedures involve the timely notification of a central office or reviewing organization as to the progress of the patients on study. Usually summary results of a patient's progress are required within certain specified periods of time as the study progresses. Indications or provisions in the reporting procedures are usually made if a recurrence occurs prior to a scheduled reporting time. It is just as important for reporting procedures to be followed as it is for response criteria and timing to be followed so that fair comparisons can be made among therapeutic strategies in the evaluation of certain tumor types. It has become an extremely important and sensitive quality control issue to accurately maintain the files of patients both at the site of treatment and at some central location so that the integrity of all data received, reported, and analyzed can be ensured.

In both metastatic breast cancer studies and adjuvant breast cancer studies, all patients are usually followed at regular intervals until death, and all reporting procedures with all relevant details are expected to be carried out until that time or until the question in the protocol has been satisfactorily answered. In adjuvant trials, a median disease-free interval (i.e., the time at which approximately half the patients are still disease free) may be as long as 5 or 10 years, and the follow-up status and reporting procedures can go on for a very long time. The reporting of a study not only in publication form but also in case record form can involve much time and expense. The questions studied and the patient population considered must be of sufficient scientific as well as practical interest to justify undertaking such a commitment.

Statistical Considerations

Previous sections have dealt with specific statistical objectives and their impact on the other sections of the protocol. The statistical considerations section of the protocol basically outlines the experimental design in terms of the stratification and randomization of the patients. This section restates the objectives and the hypotheses of the protocol associated with the objectives.

Based on the objectives, the sample size requirements (i.e., number of patients needed for the study) are then derived and reviewed. Other topics in the statistical considerations include the expected time frames and the proposed analyses of the particular study.

The statistical considerations follow from the protocol document and should be consistent with the entire document. For example, if the objective is a phase III question, then the sample size as stated in the statistical section should not be that for a phase II study. The sample size usually follows very closely from the objectives of the study. In a phase III trial of adjuvant therapy, the objective may be to study the disease-free interval (DFI) and survival of patients who have undergone radical mastectomy for carcinoma of the breast with positive axilliary nodes; patients are randomized to one of three adjuvant therapies. The statistical consideration then assumes the null hypothesis that the three therapies (A, B, and C) are equally effective with respect to the length of DFI and overall survival. The null hypothesis is often stated:

H : The three therapies are equivalent.

The alternative is often stated:

H : The three therapies are not equivalent.

The alternative hypothesis can also be stated as A being better than B or C, or B being better than C or A, or C being better than A or B. A particular alternative or combination of alternatives may be appropriate for the therapeutic agents under the study.

The statistical literature contains several methodologies for determining the appropriate numbers of patients for each treatment group in order to have a valid clinical trial.* Sample size considerations will often take into account the duration or the expected duration of a study,[12] and also depend on the type of analysis that will be conducted in a particular study. For example, in a mestastatic disease protocol with a response objective,

the response can be defined in several ways. In measuring tumor response or tumor shrinkage, a complete response (CR) is considered to be complete disappearance of the tumor. A partial response (PR) is considered to be a shrinkage totaling at least 50 percent of the tumor diameter. Tumor shrinkage can be controversial, because it depends on the actual types of measurement and measurement instrumentations that are used in the study. A stable response (S) is usually considered to be either no change in the tumor or a tumor shrinkage of less than 50 percent. Tumor progression indicates that the tumor has not responded to therapy or has increased in size, or new tumors have been found. Sample size considerations become important when comparing the ability of two regimens to shrink a tumor in size. The null hypothesis for comparing two treatments with respect to their degree of efficacy is often stated

$$H : P_A = P_B$$

This is often used in a null hypothesis to state that the two treatments are equal with respect to the proportion of individuals in which a response will be achieved. The variable denotes the proportion of response and is often considered to be the combination of both the complete and partial responses. There are many techniques for comparing these proportions and for reaching conclusions as to the superiority of one treatment to another in its ability to shrink the tumor. A comprehensive outline of these techniques can be found in Bartolucci.[2]

The sample size in a clinical trial, depending on the end point or objective, is determined by the magnitude of the expected differences between A and B at the initiation of the clinical trial. Usually the greater the magnitude, the fewer the patients required in each of the two treatment arms. The sample size required in each treatment arm is also dependent on statistical issues such as the size and power of the statistical procedure used to test the null hypothesis. The size of the test or alpha level, sometimes denoted as p value, is usually set at 0.05. This is the probability of rejecting the null hypothesis when, in fact, it is true. This is also commonly called the type I error. The p value often quoted in the literature is analogous to this alpha level, which statisticians use to determine the sample size of the test.

The other statistical consideration in determining sample size, the power of the test, is the probability of rejecting the null hypothesis when, in fact, it is false. This is analogous to the probability of declaring the two treatments to be different at a given magnitude when in reality they are different. The complement of the power is called the type II error. This is the probability of accepting the null hypothesis when, in fact, it is false. When computing the sample size, both type I and type II errors should be minimized; by minimizing the type II error, the power of the test is maximized. The power is usually set to be at least 80 percent to 95 percent in most trials. The literature often indicates a p value or significance level associated with the results of a clinical trial, but the power of the test is also important. It is

---

*References 4, 8, 10, 12, 14, 21, 23, 24, and 29.

quite possible with inadequate sample size to get a significant *p* value yet achieve inadequate power.

End points such as survival and disease-free interval can also be considered in the conduct of statistical tests. The statistical procedures are different than those just considered with respect to their methodology of computation, but the underlying theory of limiting type I and type II errors holds throughout. Also it should be noted that a conventional type I error of 0.05 is not always appropriate. A statistician should be consulted to determine if the alpha level should be increased or decreased for the questions being asked.

The statistical considerations section should also contain a paragraph or two stating the types and timing of analyses according to the stated objectives of the protocol. Later sections in this chapter will discuss various types of analyses that are appropriate for either metastatic or adjuvant breast cancer protocols.

Other Protocol Sections

Other sections of a treatment protocol usually include a bibliography or references for the background of the protocol design, a list of investigators who are authoring the study, and an example of a consent form. The consent form usually seeks the patient's permission to participate in the study, summarizes the study's purpose, and outlines the risks and benefits of the therapeutic alternatives.

TOOLS FOR CONDUCTING BREAST CANCER TRIALS

The essence of a good clinical trial is a strong and knowledgeable team of individuals experienced in the procedures that have been discussed. These individuals also contribute to the development and implementation of the tools necessary to conduct a well-designed breast cancer clinical trial. This section will discuss the specific tools necessary for designing and implementing a clinical trial and the organization needed to put such a trial in place. One such tool is the data collection form on which information relevant to the clinical trial is transcribed. These data collection instruments must be designed once the study objectives have been defined. Again, we see the pivotal value of the study objectives. The types of forms follow the same sequence or order as that used for the collection of information as the patient progresses through the trial. The data collection and reporting schedules are summarized in the sections of the protocol entitled "Studies to be Done" and "Reporting Procedures." Everything done in a clinical trial, from data collection to analysis, depends on the written protocol.

Data Collection Forms

On-Study Form

Once a patient is randomized and registered in the trial, the on-study form is completed. It contains such patient information as basic demographics, past treatment history, initial laboratory work-up, tumor measurements, sites of disease, and clinical stage of disease. Sometimes, depending on the study, information particular to the eligibility or stratification criteria may be requested on this form. For example, for adjuvant breast studies, information about axillary staging is requested on the form as well as the date of primary surgery and type of surgery (radical mastectomy, modified radical mastectomy, or segmental mastectomy). Examples of all forms, which were obtained from the Southeastern Cancer Study Group (SEG), may be found in the appendix to this chapter. [All forms are reproduced at the end of this chapter, following the references.]

Flow Sheet

The information to be entered on the flow sheet depends on the study and usually includes dates and dosages of therapies given, basic patient clinical data, laboratory data, the tests or procedures to be done, and the results of those procedures. These tests and procedures are usually recorded on a periodic basis (i.e., weekly, bi-weekly, monthly, etc.), depending on the instructions given in the protocol and the timing of the treatment and suggested delays according to the toxicity criteria in the protocol. This is usually very detailed information during the course of the patient's treatment on study.

Response or Summary Form

The response form contains information summarizing the patient's progress on study with respect to the end points discussed in the protocol. Such information includes the disease-free status (usually disease-free or not disease-free), survival information (either dead or last known date alive), and response criteria if a tumor measurement is required (i.e., complete response, partial response, stable, or progression). For breast cancer clinical trials, specific information such as the sites of relapse may also be included on this form. As time progresses, the protocol may require that this form be updated occasionally should a patient's status change, usually to coincide with the completion of specific cycles of therapy. The reporting procedures of the protocol will dictate when and how often this particular form is to be completed and submitted for central review.

Follow-up Form

The follow-up form is normally completed and submitted every 6 months or yearly, depending on the protocol, and contains information concerning the patient's end-point status (i.e., recurrence date, death date, or last known date alive), and possible subsequent therapy. In some respects this form may overlap with the response form, and in some circumstances it may not be very detailed. Again, an example is given in the appendix.

Other Forms

This has been a brief overview of the major types of forms that may be required by the protocol document. There are, however, other specialized forms. For example, in an adjuvant breast study, a surgical report detailing the type of surgery and other relevant information may be required. A radiation summary form may also be required if radiation was part of the treatment plan. A pathology form may be necessary for documentation of the diagnosis. A pathology form and radiation summary may also be required for a metastatic breast disease protocol in certain circumstances.

Computerized Data Base

Patients are usually entered on study via a remote site (e.g., hospital, private practice, or university medical center). Eligibility or patient selection criteria are checked at these remote sites but are also checked at a central administrative and statistical organization experienced in study design, data collection, quality control, and data computerization. All the data relevant to a particular protocol are reported to this central organization for appropriate synthesis, checking, analysis, and reporting. All forms are entered centrally on a computer data base for report generation; the ultimate goal is publication of the trial.

The central collection of forms can become cumbersome and time consuming. Several investigators have been working on systems commonly called "distributed data base systems." This involves not only collection at a remote site, but also data entry directly into a personal computer or computer terminal with communication (e.g., diskette, or phone line) to the host computer (PC, minicomputer, or main frame) at the central location. With current software and technology, much of this is feasible and can be implemented. This type of a system allows for instant data checking, processing, and feedback queries regarding missing, inconsistent, or out-of-range data. Thus data are always available and can be checked much more rapidly than if handled through the postal service. Techniques have been developed to assist investigators with this type of data transmission and checking procedures. Bartolucci[1] described the application of these techniques to oncologic clinical trials. The technology is not only available but is also constantly being updated.

Computerization of any data base is a costly and time-consuming undertaking. Therefore these trials must always be approached with much caution and great organization. The protocol's importance to a well-organized clinical trial cannot be overemphasized. It affects every aspect of the trial (i.e., the general conduct and organization of the trial from start to finish, the results and reporting of the trial, and finally, the publication of the trial for public scrutiny and evaluation).

Quality Control Procedures

We have already established that patients entered on breast cancer clinical trials (as well as other types of trials) can be from multiple sites (e.g., hospitals, private practices, or university medical centers) and that the trial is centrally administered. Multiple-site participation is usually necessary because a clinical trial requires many more patients than can normally be obtained at a single site in a reasonable amount of time. A phase III trial should not take longer than 3 to 5 years for patient entry (with less time for phase I or II trials—usually 2 years or less).

The central organization that is responsible for the conduct of the trial (design, data collection, data base management, and analysis) is usually staffed by individuals who are an educational resource for quality control. Quality control is defined here as monitoring of the study to guarantee a number of assurances (e.g., that only eligible patients are entered; that forms are completed properly by the contributing investigator or by data personnel; that data are submitted in a timely manner; and that all data are accurate and complete). To achieve this high quality of data accuracy, the central staff publishes general data collection guidelines that may be amended to accommodate protocols asking for specialized data or end points. This is usually called a procedures document or manual and is made available to all study participants. Contents of the document usually include methods for manual data entry and checks. Usually additional computerized checks of the data are made centrally and are often referred to as "edit," "consistency," or "range" checks. Quality control in breast cancer trials also includes confirmation of correct treatment being delivered. Often the patient's case record and forms are further checked by a surgeon, chemotherapist, radiologist, and pathologist not treating the patient to ensure that the patient was followed with respect to the procedures of treatment delivery detailed for each modality in the protocol. Again, failure to comply with protocol guidelines with respect to these quality control procedures has serious implications for the interpretation of the outcome of any study.

ANALYSES OF CLINICAL BREAST STUDIES

Analyses examples will be confined to oncologic trials, although the techniques apply broadly. Two well-designed clinical trials, one a study of metastatic breast cancer and the other a study of adjuvant breast disease, will be examined.

Metastatic Breast Cancer Study

The Southeastern Cancer Study Group Protocol of metastatic breast cancer (a phase III trial) involved a randomized comparison between two chemotherapeutic combinations in women with metastatic breast cancer. The objective of the study was to determine the complete and partial response rates of metastatic breast carcinoma to the regimens listed in Table 27–1. The treatment plan is also given in Table 27–1. Treatment duration was approximately 25 weeks.

Table 27–1. COMBINATION CHEMOTHERAPY REGIMEN

Regimen	Dosage	
A (CAF)		
Cyclophosphamide	500 mg/m² i.v. (day 1)	
Adriamycin	50 mg/m² i.v. (day 1)	} q 3 weeks
Fluorouracil	500 mg/m² i.v. (day 1)	
B (CMFVP)		
Cyclophosphamide	400 mg/m² i.v. (day 1)	
Methotrexate	30 mg/m² i.v. (day 1,8)	
Fluorouracil	400 mg/m² i.v. (day 1,8)	} q 28 days
Vincristine	1 mg i.v. (day 1,8)	
Prednisone	20 mg q.i.d. p.o. (day 1–7)	

This was a multi-institutional study with 16 institutions participating. Patients were assigned to either regimen A or B (see Table 27–1) after eligibility was confirmed and the patient had signed an informed consent. Eligibility criteria included the following:

1. All patients with metastatic breast adenocarcinoma with at least one measurable tumor mass (excluding radiographic bone lesions, previously irradiated lesions, liver scan abnormalities, and pleural effusion) who had not received any of the six drugs (or other alkylating agents) in the trial were eligible provided symptoms were present or there had been a recent enlargement of a metastatic lesion. Patients with elevated bilirubin levels prior to study were not eligible.

Patients with radiographic bone lesions as their only manifestation were eligible for entry on regimen A. They were not randomized. Their survival was compared to that of the other patients entered on regimen A. They were evaluated for response at 6 weeks.

Patients with local recurrence at the mastectomy site, with or without ipsilateral supraclavicular or axillary nodes, with or without bone metastasis by bone scan or by x-ray and liver scan were eligible for entry on regimen A. They were not randomized. They were evaluated for response at 6 weeks.

2. Premenopausal patients, defined as women who were still menstruating, had been amenorrheic less than 1 year, or had had a hysterectomy but were still younger than 50 years, were not eligible unless there had been previous ovarian ablation by surgery or radiation.

3. Following oophorectomy, patients were eligible no sooner than 3 weeks postop with progressive disease and 10 weeks postop with unresponsive (i.e., stable) disease.

4. At least 3 weeks must have lapsed following discontinuation of any hormone therapy, and there had to be evidence of stable or progressive disease (e.g., patients with regressing disease following discontinuation were ineligible).

5. Patients with a bilirubin level >1.2 mg/dl, an absolute granulocyte count of <1500 mm³, or platelet count <100,000/mm³ were not eligible.

6. Patients with skeletal metastases must have undergone a bone marrow biopsy. If there was tumor involvement, the patient was treated with a 50 percent dose of all drugs except vincristine and prednisone. They were

analyzed separately, along with patients who had only bone disease and no other measurable lesions. Dose was escalated 25 percent with each subsequent course if grade I toxicity had not occurred.

The analysis of this study will involve only the randomized patients and not the nonrandomized bone lesion cases.

Table 27–2 lists the response status of the 306 eligible patients entered on study. The statistical considerations of the study as originally designed required approximately a 20 percent difference in complete plus partial response rates between the two combinations, with an alpha level of 0.05 and power of 80 percent. This required approximately 110 to 120 patients on each treatment arm. The study clearly met its objective.

There were 160 patients assigned to each arm, but response data were not available on four subjects on arm A and 10 subjects on arm B. The response rate of A was 74/156 (47.4 percent) and on B was 52/150 (34.7 percent), or approximately a 13 percent difference. This had a significance level of 0.025, denoted as $p = 0.025$, which meant that if the two regimens were equal in their ability to induce a response, then the chance of observing a difference was 2.5 percent. Thus they were not equivalent in their ability to induce a response. The power appears to be adequate (approximately 90 percent). Thus statistically we can say that A was superior to B. However, an important consideration is clinical significance. There was significantly more morbidity associated with regimen A than with regimen B. Future studies will have to consider the risk-benefit ratios of such therapies (see Spilker[28]).

End points such as survival time (time from entry in study to death) and duration of disease control (time from entry in study to observed progression) are given in Figures 27–1 and 27–2. There was no advantage with either regimen. The median survival (the point in time at which approximately 50 percent of the sample were still alive or free of progression) is equivalent on both regimens.

This is a general overview of a study from its stated objectives to the primary analysis. Often large phase III studies such as this one would probe the data further to impose a regression structure to determine, for example, which underlying variables (e.g., site of metastasis, patient demographics, or initial lab work-up) most influenced the response or survival outcome. Such was done with this study. Smalley et al.[26, 27] discuss in detail the clinical patterns of metastases found in this study; further detail can be found in Smalley and Bartolucci.[25]

The techniques used to analyze regression relationships are well established.[3, 5, 6, 9, 13] However, results

Table 27–2. RESPONSE STATUS OF 306 PATIENTS IN METASTATIC BREAST CANCER STUDY

Regimen	Eligible	Complete Response	Partial Response	Stable	Progression
A (CAF)	156	23	51	37	45
B (CMFVP)	150	7	45	40	58

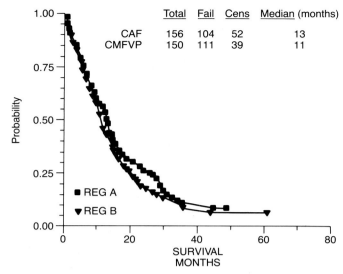

	Total	Fail	Cens	Median (months)
CAF	156	104	52	13
CMFVP	150	111	39	11

■ REG A
▼ REG B

Figure 27–1. Time from date on study: all induction entries.

should be interpreted with caution. One shortcoming in these types of analyses is that there may be insufficient numbers of observations compared with the variables considered in the regression equation.[16] One guideline is to have at least ten to 15 times as many observations as variables. A thorough statistical evaluation of all planned methodology is advised prior to any attempt to analyze the data base. The safest and most reliable analyses usually are those for which the study was originally designed.

Adjuvant Breast Disease Study

In 1976 the Southeastern Cancer Study Group initiated a trial to compare the disease-free interval (DFI) and survival of patients who had undergone radical or modified radical mastectomy for breast carcinoma with positive axillary nodes; patients were randomized to one of three adjuvant therapies:

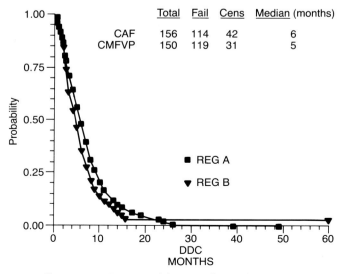

	Total	Fail	Cens	Median (months)
CAF	156	114	42	6
CMFVP	150	119	31	5

■ REG A
▼ REG B

Figure 27–2. Duration of disease: all induction entries.

1. Short-term chemotherapy: six cycles of cyclophosphamide, methotrexate, and 5-fluorouracil (CMF).
2. Long-term chemotherapy: 12 cycles of CMF.
3. Radiation therapy plus short-term chemotherapy: six cycles of CMF.

A secondary objective was to compare the tolerance of patients in each of the regimens. The objectives here were different than in the previous example, since a different population of women was involved. The eligibility criteria for patient selection for this study included the following:

1. Women of all ages with proven stage II carcinoma of the breast who had undergone radical or modified radical mastectomy and whose pathological specimens had shown one or more positive axillary nodes, regardless of level, were eligible. Stage II was defined as any combination of T1a, T1b, T2a, T2b, T3a, N, N1a, or N1b, according to the International Staging System. The staging was defined in the appendix of the protocol.
2. Patients were entered on study within 56 days of standard or modified radical mastectomy and after complete healing of the surgical wound.
3. Patients were eligible if they had adequate physiological function, defined as absolute granulocyte count of >1500/mm³ or platelets >100,000/mm³; bilirubin levels <1.2 mg/dl; BUN <25 percent or creatinine <1.2 mg/dl; and absence of infection or septicemia.

The following were ineligible for study:
1. Patients with previous history of cancer in the other breast.
2. Patients who had received prior chemotherapy or hormone therapy for breast cancer.
3. Patients who had received prior radiation therapy.
4. Patients with inflammatory carcinoma of the breast.
5. Patients with residual foci of metastatic disease as judged by careful physical examination and by appropriate studies (chest roentgenogram, liver scan, and bone scan).
6. Patients who did not meet listed criteria for adequate physiological function.
7. Patients whose personal circumstances did not permit adequate treatment and follow-up as outlined.
8. Patients with preexisting medical conditions that would make them poor candidates for adjuvant therapy.

The details of the treatment plan will not be discussed here, except to say that the timing of a cycle was approximately 1 month. The study was stratified by nodal status (one to three positive axillary nodes vs. four or more), pre- vs. postmenopausal status, interval after surgery (less than 28 days vs. 28 to 56 days), and type of mastectomy (radical vs. modified radical). The study initially included regimens A (short-term chemotherapy) and B (long-term chemotherapy) within the one-to-three–node women and regimens A, B, and C (radiation + short-term chemotherapy) within the four-or-more–node women. Later the study was revised to include only regimens A and C in the four-or-more–node women. Twenty-four institutions participated in this study.

The objectives of this study dictated that the sample size in each nodal stratum be between 200 and 240 patients. With an alpha level of 0.05 and power of 80 percent, the alternative hypothesis stated that the 12-month CMF regimen would reduce the relapse rate at 2 years from 30 percent to 10 percent in the one-to-three–node group. For the four-or-more–node group, the addition of radiotherapy was hypothesized to reduce the 2-year relapse rate by the same magnitude (30 percent to 10 percent).

Table 27–3 lists the patient characteristics by the strata set out in the protocol; clearly the accrual objectives were met. There were 301 eligible entries in the one-to-three–node group and 241 eligible entries in the four-or-more–node group. These numbers do not include the 55 patients on the long-term chemotherapy arm in the four-or-more–node group.

Figures 27–3 to 27–6 show no statistical advantage of any of the regimens with respect to DFI or survival. This was a case in which the null hypothesis was not rejected. Some may argue that further subsetting of the data is required to ferret out statistical differences among the strata of interest. This is precisely the situation to avoid, since the study was not designed to accommodate and the objectives did not hypothesize a subgrouping effect. At best, trends in the data can be investigated, as shown in Figure 27–7. Even if a statistical difference is seen in regimen A vs. regimen C in the DFI of premenopausal woman with four or more positive nodes there are only two avenues to take. One is to conclude that statistical significance has been reached by pure chance. This is the multiplicity issue in statistics, which says that if subsets of data continue to be analyzed then a significant result may be found by chance, and the conclusions are more superficial than real. In this study, the 95 percent confidence intervals around these curves overlapped; thus the difference was not as real as it appeared. This can be avoided by employing the regression techniques discussed previously with the appropriate cautions outlined. This way we can determine if treatment adjusted for menopausal status, nodal status, etc., was a determinant in the DFI. The problem of multiplicity in analyses has been discussed by Bartolucci.[2]

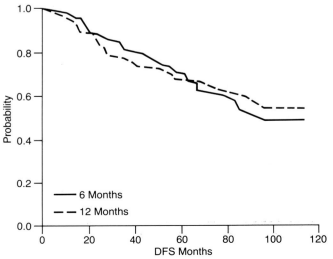

Figure 27–3. Disease-free survival time: one to three nodes.

The other avenue to pursue given such a finding is to investigate this phenomenon further in a clinical trial of premenopausal women with four or more positive nodes. If this result were real, it might be used to set up an entirely new clinical trial with precisely stated objectives, thus leading to adequate sample size. However, the narrowness of the eligibility criteria might preclude the feasibility of conducting such a trial.

As previously stated, a secondary objective of the study was to compare the tolerance of patients for each of the regimens. Table 27–4 summarizes these results. The following is an example of the type of toxicity report found in most such studies:

Of the 597 eligible cases, 548 have toxicity evaluations on file. Toxicities are reported as mild, severe, and life-threatening. No lethal toxicity has been reported during protocol therapy and no deaths secondary to therapy are known to have occurred in patients off study. Toxicities reported appear in Table 27–4. Other reported adverse events are at 6 mo.: chemo-weight, tearing of eyes, fatigue, hot flashes, conjunctivitis, anorexia, vaginal yeast infection, and tinnitus; 12 mo.: chemo-weight, folliculitis, conjunctivitis, fatigue, nasal mucositis, corneal ulcerations, and mucositis; RT + 6 mo.: chemo-anxiety, tearing of eyes, and fatigue.

In summary, studies must be designed and reported in such a way as to prevent reporting and publishing misleading anecdotes. This section has discussed two examples of studies generated from well-designed protocols, with significant results confirmed by a check on the power of the statistical procedures, and with results reported as stated in the objectives.

OVERVIEW OF PRESENT CONTROVERSIES

Randomization

The controversy over randomization concerns two types of randomization: conventional randomization and pre-randomization. Conventional randomization occurs when the patient has been demonstrated to be eligible, has had the details and purposes of the study explained, and has signed an informed consent document. Included in the explanation of the details of the study are the possible risks and benefits of the therapeutic alternatives. The patient can refuse to participate in the study at any time—even prior to signing the informed consent. Thus there may not be any record of the patient even being approached for the study, and most written protocols do not require investigators to keep an accounting of all eligible patients who were approached and subsequently refused to participate.

Pre-randomization occurs when the physician randomly assigns the patient to treatment after determining eligibility but before discussing the study and its implications with the patient and obtaining informed consent. This approach eliminates the uneasiness experienced by most physicians when they have to obtain the patient's consent to participate in the trial but are not able to tell the patient what treatment will be administered, something that makes many patients unwilling to participate

Table 27–3. CHARACTERISTICS OF PATIENTS IN ADJUVANT BREAST DISEASE STUDY

	1 to 3 Nodes				4+ Nodes					
	6 Mo.		12 Mo.		6 Mo.		12 Mo.		RT+6 Mo.	
	No.	*%*	*No.*	*%*	*No.*	*%*	*No.*	*%*	*No.*	*%*
Premenopausal										
Number of cases	70	100	70	100	49	100	22	100	48	100
Type of Surgery										
Radical	18	26	12	17	9	18	6	27	9	19
Modified radical	52	74	58	83	40	82	16	73	39	81
Time from Surgery										
<28 days	19	27	19	27	14	29	11	50	13	27
≥28 days	51	73	51	73	35	71	11	50	35	73
Age										
<40	31	44	24	34	24	49	9	41	21	44
≥40	39	56	46	66	25	51	13	59	27	56
TNM Stage										
T1+T2	58	82	53	76	40	82	15	68	31	65
T3	6	9	12	17	8	16	5	23	12	25
Unknown	6	9	5	7	1	2	2	9	5	10
Performance Status										
<70 percent	1	1	0	0	0	0	2	9	1	2
≥70 percent	69	99	67	96	48	98	19	86	46	96
Unknown	0	0	3	4	1	2	1	5	1	2
Estrogen Receptor Status										
Yes	24	34	27	39	20	47	4	18	13	27
No	15	21	10	14	8	19	2	9	8	17
Unknown	31	44	33	47	21	34	16	73	27	56
Number of Nodes+										
4–6					16	33	7	32	16	33
7–12					22	45	7	32	15	31
≥12					11	22	8	36	17	36
Postmenopausal										
Number of Cases	85	100	76	100	73	100	33	100	71	100
Type of Surgery										
Radical	11	13	12	16	15	21	11	33	11	15
Modified radical	74	87	64	84	58	79	22	67	60	85
Time from Surgery										
<28 days	27	32	21	28	25	34	13	39	20	28
≥28 days	58	68	55	72	48	66	20	61	51	72
Age										
<40	1	1	2	3	0	0	1	3	0	0
≥40	83	98	74	97	73	100	32	97	70	99
Unknown	1	1	0	0	0	0	0	0	1	1
TNM Stage										
T1+T2	72	85	66	87	50	69	24	73	47	66
T3	5	6	4	5	16	22	5	15	14	20
Unknown	8	9	6	8	7	9	4	12	10	14
Performance Status										
<70 percent	1	1	0	0	0	0	0	0	1	1
≥70 percent	79	93	74	97	71	97	31	94	66	93
Unknown	5	6	2	3	2	3	2	6	4	6
Estrogen Receptor Status										
Yes	34	40	27	36	24	33	11	33	24	34
No	7	8	14	18	7	10	2	6	13	18
Unknown	44	52	35	46	42	57	20	61	34	48
Number of Nodes+										
4–6					34	47	13	39	30	42
7–12					15	21	9	27	22	31
≥12					24	32	11	34	19	27

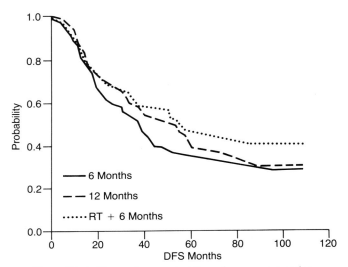

Figure 27–4. Disease-free survival time: four or more nodes.

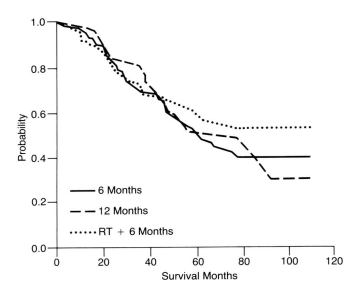

Figure 27–6. Survival time from date on study: four or more nodes.

in the trial. Many physicians argue that some clinical trials cannot be accomplished without the accrual enhancement technique of pre-randomization. A variation of this technique, called the "randomized-consent design" has been discussed by Zelen.[30] Both Zelen[30] and Ellenberg[7] have reported the negative implications of this procedure. A particular statistical concern is the refusal rate of patients with this type of design and the adverse impact it has on the overall efficiency of the study. To achieve a valid study, the accrual has to be inflated to accommodate the study efficiency lost by refusal to receive the assigned treatment. For example, if the refusal rate on a pre-randomized study is ten percent, the overall accrual has to be increased by almost 60 percent. This assumes an overall selection bias when, for example, patients on a two-arm study have a prognosis that prompts them to choose one treatment in favor of another.[7] The National Surgical Adjuvant Breast and Bowel Project (NSABP) used pre-randomization in its study comparing total mastectomy with

segmental mastectomy with or without radiation therapy.

Because of the statistical controversy associated with pre-randomization, many individuals advocate the use of conventional randomization. The critics of pre-randomization are often accused of not having had adequate experience with large-scale cooperative group trials and the problems associated with obtaining adequate accrual. Also, pre-randomization is a victim of its own technique. With pre-randomization, the rate of refusal for a study is known, since a random assignment is recorded and registered. However, with conventional randomization, the patient's refusal is never recorded. Therefore the refusal rate can be just as frequent and biased in a conventionally randomized study as in a pre-randomized study, and it may go undetected. Regardless of the randomization technique employed, the patient

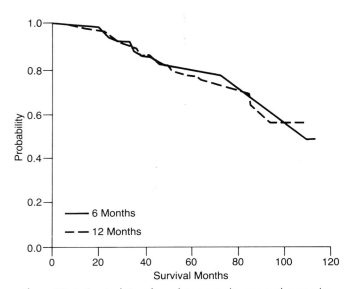

Figure 27–5. Survival time from date on study: one to three nodes.

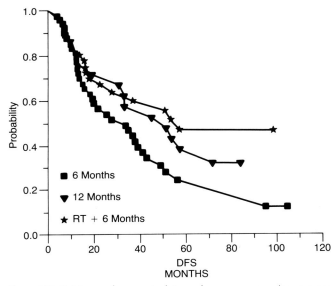

Figure 27–7. Disease-free survival time: four or more nodes: premenopausal patients.

Table 27–4. TOXICITIES IN ADJUVANT BREAST DISEASE STUDY

	Number of Patients								
	258			187			103		
	6 mo. (%)			12 mo. (%)			RT + 6 mo. (%)		
Toxicity	Mild	Severe	Low Tolerance	Mild	Severe	Low Tolerance	Mild	Severe	Low Tolerance
Hemoglobin	12	1	—	16	2	—	8	1	—
Granulocytes	39	21	2	43	19	2	34	11	—
Platelets	11	3	—	18	4	2	12	2	—
Cardiovascular	<1	—	—	1	—	—	—	—	—
Oral	9	4	1	3	6	1	4	2	2
Gastrointestinal	28	11	1	28	13	5	32	9	1
Genitourinary	2	1	—	6	1	1	1	4	—
Liver	2	2	—	2	4	—	2	1	—
CNS*	<1	<1	<1	1	—	—	2	1	—
Skin and hair	28	3	—	25	3	—	22	4	—

*Psychological

is of primary concern. Honest and open discussions of all options, risks, and benefits are necessary. If a patient's physician believes that a particular treatment option is best for a patient, then a randomized trial may not be appropriate.

Subset and Interim Analyses

A previous section discussed the problem of multiple testing (i.e., looking for significant comparisons in subsets of the data). The danger is that of achieving statistical significance purely by chance. For example, the chance of committing at least one type I error at alpha level ($\alpha = 0.05$) when c = 10 tests are conducted is

$$1 - (1 - \alpha) = 1 - (1 - 0.05)^{10} = 0.40.$$

The accommodation of the many factors in a patient sample and their associated influence on the major end points of the study can be best dealt with by using the appropriate analytic tools.[5, 6]

Another problem in the analysis of clinical trials is that of interim analysis. The generally accepted procedure is to fully analyze the study at its conclusion because type I error can be increased by repeated testing (i.e., interim analyses) throughout the course of the trial.[19, 20] Interim analyses can be misleading, because differences in treatment response could be noted for patients entered early on the trial who may be of a different prognostic characterization than those entered later on the trial. Interim analyses can cause unjustified early termination of a trial for the reasons stated. Also these misleading results can influence the rate of accrual to a study, cause individual physicians to adopt a particular treatment strategy prematurely, and influence the way particular study end points are evaluated. Only a selected subgroup of individuals (which should include a statistician) should review interim results and thoroughly investigate any striking differences in outcomes

and morbidity to date. If this review panel decides for ethical or scientific reasons that the study should be terminated, then this recommendation should be made to all participating physicians. Peto[17] has suggested techniques for terminating clinical studies early on the basis of highly statistically significant p values.

Nonrandomized Controls

The use of nonrandomized (historical) controls in clinical trials is primarily an economic move to expedite the initiation and completion of those trials. Gehan and Freireich[11] have discussed the rationale and conditions for the use of nonrandomized controls. The success of the technique depends on the success of matching concurrent and historical groups based on relevant prognostic variables. This can be tenuous, since archived prognostic data may not be available and certain underlying prognostic data influencing the results may be unknown to those analyzing the data. However, Makuch and Simon[14, 15] have discussed the sample size requirements for using this technique if the use of historical data is relevant.

Meta-Analysis

Meta-analysis, although not new, has recently been advocated by Peto[18] as a possible technique in analyzing results from many studies. One of the purposes of this technique is to decide the future direction in the study of a disease. The technique involves the continued analysis of past studies in the literature for a particular type and stage of cancer. By combining the results of many small trials using similar therapies for a particular disease, the past sample size and power of the studies can be increased. This may allow more definitive conclusions concerning the relative efficacy of past treatments. This technique suffers from many of the same pitfalls found in the technique using historical controls (i.e., possible prognostic incomparability of the samples and possible lack of relevant demographic or clinical information).

Quality of Life

Another issue not yet discussed is that of the quality of life. Many clinical groups are beginning to include this assessment as part of the clinical protocols. End points such as response and survival may be of primary clinical interest. However, other health-related professionals such as psychologists and nutritionists are now becoming important partners in the conduct of clinical trials. Methodological tools are constantly being developed and tested to assess the psychological well-being of patients on study. This is especially important in trials in which the overall mortality over time may be decreased, but the morbidity becomes a real detriment to the patient. Future reports of clinical studies are likely to incorporate an ever-increasing analysis of the quality of life.

References

1. Bartolucci AA: The role of microcomputers in clinical trials. The Southeastern Cancer Study Group experience. Community Clinical Oncology Program Workshop, Bethesda, MD, National Cancer Institute, 1983.
2. Bartolucci AA: Estimation and comparison of proportions. *In* Buyse M, Sylvester R, Staquet M (eds): Cancer Clinical Trials. Methods and Practice. Oxford, Oxford University Press, 1984, pp 337–360.
3. Bartolucci AA, Fraser MD: Comparative step up composite tests for selecting prognostic indicators associated with survival. Biomet J 19:437–448, 1977.
4. Cassagrande JT, Pike MC, Smith PG: An improved formula for calculating sample sizes for comparing two binomial distributions. Biometrics 34:483–486, 1978.
5. Cox DR: Analysis of Binary Data. Methuen Monograph Series. London, Methuen, 1970.
6. Cox DR: Regression models and life tables (with discussion). J R Statist Soc B 34:187–220, 1972.
7. Ellenberg SS: Randomization designs in comparative clinical trials. N Engl J Med 310:1404–1408, 1984.
8. Fleiss JL: Statistical Methods for Rates and Proportions. New York, John Wiley and Sons, 1973.
9. Fraser MD, Bartolucci AA, Smith WA: A Bayesian decision procedure for selecting prognostic variables associated with survival. (In press.)
10. Gehan EA: The determination of the number of patients required in a preliminary and followup trial of a new chemotherapeutic agent. J Chronic Dis 13:346–353, 1961.
11. Gehan EA, Freireich EJ: Non-randomized controls in cancer clinical trials. N Engl J Med 290:198–203, 1974.
12. George SL, Desu MM: Planning the size and duration of a clinical trial studying the time to some critical event. J Chronic Dis 27:15–24, 1974.
13. Lee ET: A computer program for linear logistic regression analysis. Comput Prog Biomed 4:80–92, 1974.
14. Makuch R, Simon R: Sample size requirements for evaluating a conservative therapy. Cancer Treat Rep 62:1037–1040, 1978.
15. Makuch RW, Simon R: A note on the design of multi-institution three treatment studies. Cancer Clin Trials 1:301–303, 1978.
16. Marascuilo LA, Levin JR: Multivariate Statistics in the Social Sciences—A Researchers Guide. Monterey, CA, Brooks Cole, 1983.
17. Peto R: Clinical trial methodology. Biomedicine 28:24–36, 1978.
18. Peto R: Yes or no adjuvant chemotherapy apart from trials? Which aspects need to be studied in trials? London, Fourth European Organization for the Research and Treatment of Cancer Breast Cancer Working Conference, July 1987.
19. Peto R, Pike MC, Armitage P, et al: Design and analysis of randomized clinical trials requiring prolonged observation of each patient. 1. Introduction and design. Br J Cancer 34:585–612, 1976.
20. Peto R, Pike MC, Armitage P, et al: Design and analysis of randomized clinical trials requiring prolonged observation of each patient. 2. Analysis and examples. Br J Cancer 35:1–39, 1977.
21. Pocock SJ: Size of cancer clinical trials and stopping rules. Br J Cancer 38:757–766, 1978.
22. Sackett DL: Biases in analytic research. J Chronic Dis 32:51–63, 1979.
23. Schoenfeld DA, Gelber RD: Designing and analyzing clinical trials which allow institutions to randomize patients to a subset of the treatments under study. Biometrics 35:825–830, 1979.
24. Simon R: Design and conduct of clinical trials. *In* DeVita VT Jr, Hellman S, Rosenberg SA (eds): Cancer—Principles and Practice of Oncology. Philadelphia, JB Lippincott, 1982, pp 198–225.
25. Smalley RV, Bartolucci AA: Variations in responsiveness and survival of clinical subsets of patients with metastatic breast cancer to two chemotherapy combinations. European J Cancer 16(suppl 1): 141–146, 1980.
26. Smalley RV, Lefante J, Bartolucci AA, Carpenter J, Vogel C, Krauss S: A comparison of cyclophosphamide, adriamycin and 5-fluorouracil (CAF) and cyclophosphamide, methotrexate, 5-fluorouracil, vincristine, prednisone (CMFVP) in patients with advanced breast cancer. A Southeastern Cancer Study Group project. Breast Cancer Res Treat 3:209–220, 1983.
27. Smalley RV, Bartolucci AA, Moore M, Vogel C, Carpenter J, Perez CA, Velez-Garcia E, Marcial V, Lefante J, Wittliff J, Ketcham A, Durant J: Southeastern Cancer Study Group—breast cancer studies 1972–1982. Int J Radiat Oncol 9:1867–1874, 1983.
28. Spilker B: Guide to Clinical Interpretation of Data. New York, Raven, 1986.
29. Zelen M: Aspects of the planning and analysis of clinical trials in cancer. A survey of statistical design and linear models. New York, North Holland, 1975, 629–645.
30. Zelen M: A new design for randomized clinical trials. N Engl J Med 300:1242–1245, 1979.

Appendices

Stat Off Only

	B	R	1

BREAST ON-STUDY

This form should be filled out at the Institution. Copy and return the original to the Statistical Center within two weeks of date on study.

Protocol _____   Institution _____

Accession # _____   Hospital or Soc. Sec. # _____

Patient Name _____
        Last   *First*

----

	mo	day	yr
Date On Study	☐☐	☐☐	☐☐
Date of Birth	☐☐	☐☐	☐☐

Sex (*1-Male; 2-Female*) .... ☐

Race (*1-Cauc.; 2-Black; 3-Other*) .... ☐

Weight (*kg*) .... ☐☐☐

Height (*cm*) .... ☐☐☐

Surface Area (M²) .... ☐☐

Karnofsky's Performance Status (%) .... ☐☐☐

	mo	day	yr
Date of Original Diagnosis Biopsy Proven	☐☐	☐☐	☐☐

Histology .... ☐☐

Stat Off Only

Surgery Performed By _____

M.D. Responsible for Chemotherapy _____

M.D. Responsible for Radiation _____

NARRATIVE ----   *Must include important history & physical data. Please type or print plainly.*

_____   _____
Investigator's Signature   Name of Person Completing Form

BREAST ON-STUDY

Patient Name _____

PRIOR TREATMENT

If patient is entering an adjuvant study, go to next page.

RESPONSE CODES (for ALL prior treatments)	
1-No	4-Stable
2-Yes, Complete	5-Adjuvant Treatment
3-Yes, Partial	6-Nonevaluable/Uk

PRIOR SURGICAL/HORMONE THERAPY (*1-No; 2-Yes*) .... ☐

	MO	YR	RESP
Oophorectomy			
Adrenalectomy			
Hypophysectomy			

PRIOR CHEMOTHERAPY/IMMUNOTHERAPY/HORMONAL THERAPY (*1-No; 2-Yes*) .... ☐

AGENT	STARTED		STOPPED		RESP	DRUG CODE Stat Off Only		
	MO	YR	MO	YR				
_____								
_____								
_____								
_____								
_____								
_____								
_____								
_____								

PRIOR RADIOTHERAPY (*1-No; 2-Yes*) .... ☐

For Primary Treatment (*1-None; 2-Preoperative; 3-Postoperative; 4-Definitive; 5-Other; 6-Xrt done, no details available*) ..... ☐

For Recurrent Disease (*1-No; 2-Yes*): Local recurrence .... ☐

Lymph nodes .... ☐

Brain .... ☐

Bone .... ☐

Other, specify _____ ☐

TYPE CODES: 1-Ortho; 2-CO^{60}; 3-Linac; 4-Beta; 5-Other

SPECIFY AREA	STARTED		RESP	TUMOR DOSE × 1000R	TYPE	AREA CODE Stat Off Only		
	MO	YR						
_____								
_____								
_____								
_____								
_____								

BREAST ON-STUDY

Patient Name _____

CLINICAL & ANATOMICAL DATA -

Menopausal Status . . . . ☐

    1-Premenopausal
    2-In menopause
    3-Postmenopausal, natural
    4-Postmenopausal, surgical WITH
      bilateral oophorectomy
    5-Postmenopausal, surgical WITHOUT
      bilateral oophorectomy
    6-Postmenopausal, radiation induced

Date of Last   MO   DAY   YR
Menstrual Period   ☐☐   ☐☐   ☐☐

ORIGINAL TUMOR INVOLVEMENT & STAGING

Type of Initial Surgery . . . . ☐

    1-None or biopsy only
    2-Local excision
    3-Total (simple) mastectomy
    4-Modified radical
    5-Radical mastectomy
    6-Segmental or partial mastectomy
    7-Surgery done, no details avail.
    8-Other,
       specify _____

Right   Left

Site of Primary
(Code in site of right and/or left by number)

Right . . . . ☐

Left . . . . ☐

    1-Upper lateral
    2-Lower lateral
    3-Upper medial
    4-Lower medial
    5-Subareola
    6-Axillary

Axillary Node Staging at Initial Surgery
    (1-Not Done; 2-Dissection; 3-Sampling) . . . . ☐

Initial Axillary Node Involvement

                    # Positive   # Removed

Right . . . .   ☐☐   . . . .   ☐☐

Left . . . .   ☐☐   . . . .   ☐☐

TNM Staging

    Tumor . . . . T   ☐☐

    Nodes . . . . N   ☐☐

    Metastases . . . . M   ☐

Date of Diagnosis of   MO   DAY   YR
Recurrence or Progression   ☐☐   ☐☐   ☐☐

Estrogen Receptor Status
(1-Negative; 2-Positive; 3-Equivocal; 4-Not obtained)

    At initial surgery . . . . ☐

    Site taken from _____

    fmoles . . . . ☐☐☐

    At relapse . . . . ☐

    Site taken from _____

    fmoles . . . . ☐☐☐

Progesterone Receptor Status
(1-Negative; 2-Positive; 3-Equivocal; 4-Not obtained)

    At initial surgery . . . . ☐

    Site taken from _____

    fmoles . . . . ☐☐☐

    At relapse . . . . ☐

    Site taken from _____

    fmoles . . . . ☐☐☐

BREAST ON-STUDY

Patient Name _____

AREA(S) OF TUMOR INVOLVEMENT

    1-Negative
    2-Positive, cytology &/or biopsy
    3-Positive, clinical incl. radiographic
    4-Positive, clinical only
    5-Positive, other (specify) _____
    6-Questionable
    7-Not examined

How was diagnosis established in patient whose primary lesion was not treated with surgical procedure? .... ☐

Local Recurrence .... ☐

LYMPH NODES:

Axillary ipsilateral .... ☐

Axillary contralateral .... ☐

Supraclavicular ipsilateral .... ☐

Supraclavicular contralateral .... ☐

Internal mammary (on CXR) .... ☐

Mediastinal (on CXR) .... ☐

DISTANT METASTASIS:

Liver .... ☐

Meninges or CSF .... ☐

Brain .... ☐

Subcutaneous .... ☐

Opposite breast .... ☐

CHEST X-RAYS:

Lung nodular .... ☐

Lung lymphangitic .... ☐

Pleural lesion .... ☐

Pleural effusion .... ☐

BONE:

Lytic .... ☐

Blastic .... ☐

Marrow .... ☐

Other (specify) _____ ☐

FLOW SHEET

SOLID TUMOR

DIAGNOSIS _____ M² _____ NAME _____ Pg# _____

Protocol/Access #

_____

Date on Study
REMARKS
(Date Each)

		Phase/Course#								
		Date Yr 19 (Mo/Day)								
		Day or Week on Study								
THERAPY	1	SURGERY								
	2	RADIATION								
	3	DRUGS								
	4									
	5									
	6									
	7									
	8									
	9									
	10	ANTIBIOTICS								
	11	TRANSFUSION (RBC/PLAT)								
Measurable Disease (in 2 diam.)	12	LIST SITE & IF ON PE, SCAN, XR								
	13									
	14									
	15									
SUM	16	PRODUCTS OF DIAMETERS								
NEW LESIONS	17									
	18									
P.E.	19	LIVER								
	20	SPLEEN								
	21	TEMPERATURE								
SUBJECTIVE FINDINGS	22	PERFORMANCE STATUS								
	23	WEIGHT								
	24	PAIN								
	25	NAUSEA/VOMITING								
	26	RESPIRATORY DIFFICULTY								
	27									
	28									
BLOOD COUNTS	29	HEMOGLOBIN/HEMATOCRIT								
	30	WBC ($\times 1000$)								
	31	SEGS + BANDS (%)								
	32	ABSOLUTE GRANULOCYTE CT								
	33	EOS/BASOS (%)								
	34	LYMPHOCYTES (%)								
	35	MONOCYTES (%)								
	36	(%)								
	37	PLATELETS ($\times 1000$)								
BLOOD CHEMISTRIES	38	BUN/CREATININE								
	39	BILIRUBIN								
	40	ALKALINE PHOSPHATASE								
	41	SGOT								
	42	LDH								
	43									
	44									
OTHER	45	CREATININE CLEARANCE								
	46	URINALYSIS								
	47	EKG								
	48									
Marker	49	MARKERS								
	50									
	51									
TOXICITY	52									
	53									
	54									
	55									
	56									

RESPONSE FORM

Instructions: This form should be completed at the end
of each phase of treatment as specified by protocol.

☐ Induction   ☐ Consolidation   ☐ Crossover   ☐ Maintenance
☐ Reinduction   ☐ Induction-Revis   ☐ Continuation   ☐ Off-study

Protocol _____   Institution _____

Accession # _____   Hospital or
Soc. Sec. # _____

Patient Name _____
           Last   *First*

	MO	DAY	YR			MO	DAY	YR

Date on Study ....   Date Patient Evaluated ....
(for this phase)

Investigator _____

NARRATIVE ---
                                        (Please type or print plainly)

_____   _____
Investigator's Signature   Name of person completing this form

RESPONSE FORM

NAME _____

ACCESSION # _____

TOXICITIES:
(for phase being evaluated)

Instructions: Box A—use grading 0–4 as outlined in Toxicity Criteria, code 9 for toxicities not assessed.
Box B—grade clinical significance of each grade 4 toxicity reported.
0—Not Life Threatening or Not Applicable
1—Life Threatening complication occurred, but not causing death
2—Fatal

Box C—grade D for protocol therapy related, Q for questionably protocol related, N for definitely not protocol related.

	(A) GR	(B) SIGN	(C) DRUG R.		(A) GR	(B) SDIGN	(C) DRUG R.
HEMATOLGIC				**PULMONARY**			
WBC/mm^3	☐	☐	☐	PFT	☐	☐	☐
Absolute Granulocyte Count/mm^3	☐	☐	☐	Clinical	☐	☐	☐
Platelets/mm^3	☐	☐	☐	**CARDIAC**			
Hgb/dl or HCT %	☐	☐	☐	EKG: A. Rate, Rhythm	☐	☐	☐
Clinical Anemia	☐	☐	☐	B. QRS Voltage decrease	☐	☐	☐
Hemorrhage: 2 to thrombocytopenia	☐	☐	☐	Ejection Fraction	☐	☐	☐
INFECTION	☐	☐	☐	Clinical	☐	☐	☐
GENITOURINARY				**NEUROLOGIC**			
BUN (mg%)	☐	☐	☐	Peripheral Nerves	☐	☐	☐
Creatinine (mg%)	☐	☐	☐	Central Neurologic	☐	☐	☐
Creatinine Clearance (% change)	☐	☐	☐	Mental Status (Circle O)	☐	☐	☐
Hematuria (unrelated to thrombocytopenia	☐	☐	☐	(Circle one if >0) State of Consciousness Mood Ideation Memory			
Proteinuria	☐	☐	☐	Headache	☐	☐	☐
HEPATIC				Seizure Disorder (Motor Act)	☐	☐	☐
SGOT (IU)	☐	☐	☐	Cerebellar	☐	☐	☐
Alkaline Phosphatase	☐	☐	☐	**CUTANEOUS**			
Bilirubin (mg%)	☐	☐	☐	Skin (Local Reaction)	☐	☐	☐
Clinical	☐	☐	☐	Hair	☐	☐	☐
GASTROINTESTINAL				**ALLERGY**			
Nausea & Vomiting	☐	☐	☐	Dermatological (Rash)	☐	☐	☐
Abdominal Cramps/Diarrhea	☐	☐	☐	Pulmonary	☐	☐	☐
Mucositis	☐	☐	☐	**FEVER** (No other cause)	☐	☐	☐
				OTHER, specify _____	☐	☐	☐

Note: Please report severe toxicities to NCI and the Operations Office by phone and complete a Drug Experience Report, FDA 1639. Attach a copy of this form to the case.

RESPONSE FORM

Patient's Name _____ Accession # _____

Response

CATEGORIES OF DISEASE (CLASSES I–IV)

I—Bidimensional Measurable Disease

	At time on-study this phase		At time of this evaluation	

Stat Off. Only

I—(rows)

_____ □□□ cm X □□□ cm   □□□ cm X □□□ cm

_____ □□□ cm X □□□ cm   □□□ cm X □□□ cm

_____ □□□ cm X □□□ cm   □□□ cm X □□□ cm

_____ □□□ cm X □□□ cm   □□□ cm X □□□ cm

CT Scan or Ultrasound
Volume Measurements:

At time on-study this phase   At time of this evaluation

_____ □□□ X □□□ X □□□   □□□ X □□□ X □□□

_____ □□□ X □□□ X □□□   □□□ X □□□ X □□□

_____ □□□ X □□□ X □□□   □□□ X □□□ X □□□

II—Unidimensional Measurable Disease (e.g., Mediastinal mass on CXR/CT, intraabdominal mass, liver enlargement)

Parameter	At time on-study this phase	At time of this evaluation
_____	_____	_____
_____	_____	_____
_____	_____	_____

III—Nonmeasurable Disease (e.g., bone scan, lymphangitic, pulmonary)

Parameter	At time on-study this phase	At time of this evaluation
_____	_____	_____
_____	_____	_____
_____	_____	_____

IV—Indirect Parameters of Disease Activity (hepatic enzymes, tumor markers, serum calcium, serum & urinary abnormal proteins)

Parameter	At time on-study this phase	At time of this evaluation
_____	_____	_____
_____	_____	_____
_____	_____	_____

MO DAY YR

Date any response as defined by protocol was FIRST observed
  (if during this period) .... □□ □□ □□

Date of BEST OBTAINED response (if during this period) .... □□ □□ □□

Response to this Phase, 1 = CR, 2 = PR, 3 = Fair PR, 4 = ?Improvement, 5 = Stable, 6 = Worse, 7 = Dead .... □

RESPONSE FORM

Patient Name _____   Accession # _____

If the patient has completed all required treatment for this phase, which of the following apply (circle one):

Patient has completed all phases of protocol **0.0**

Patient is being observed on study until change of status **0.1**

Patient is continuing on study **0.2**

Patient is going off study because ineligible for next phase **0.3**

Patient would be eligible for next phase but is going off study early (circle reason under Treatment Complication) **0.4**

Patient would be eligible for next phase but is going off study early to receive another modality (circle which one(s)) **0.5**

    Surgery   Radiotherapy   Immunotherapy   Chemotherapy

    Antiemetics   BMT   Other, specify _____

Stat Off only [|]

If the patient has been removed from study before completing all required treatment for this phase OR 0.3 is circled for the question above, circle the number of the most appropriate reason below:

TREATMENT COMPLICATION:

Toxicity

Not cause of early death **1.1**

Cause of early death **1.2**

Circle the modality (or modalities) that caused the toxicity

    Surgery   Radiotherapy   Immunotherapy   Chemotherapy

    Antiemetics   BMT   Other, specify _____

Stat Off only [|]

Rapid Progression of Disease

Not cause of early death **2.1**

Cause of early death **2.2**

Intercurrent Disease

Not cause of early death **3.1**

Cause of early death **3.2**

Removal by Investigator

for other reasons than 1.1–3.2 (Explain in narrative on page 1) **4.0**

Patient Non-Compliance

Lost to Follow-up **5.1**

Refused to begin therapy **5.2**

Refused further therapy **5.3**

Schedule not followed by patient **5.4**

Early death without follow-up studies **5.5**

Change in initial disease status preventing beginning of treatment **5.6**

Other, specify _____ **9.5**

RESPONSE FORM—REVIEW PAGE
PROJECT CHAIRMAN/STAT OFFICE DATA COORDINATOR

Page 5

Patient Name _____   Accession # _____

DATA COORDINATOR ONLY

Drugs Received	Code	# of Courses	Total Dosage Patient Actually Received
_____	☐☐☐	☐☐	☐☐☐☐☐☐
_____	☐☐☐	☐☐	☐☐☐☐☐☐
_____	☐☐☐	☐☐	☐☐☐☐☐☐
_____	☐☐☐	☐☐	☐☐☐☐☐☐
_____	☐☐☐	☐☐	☐☐☐☐☐☐
_____	☐☐☐	☐☐	☐☐☐☐☐☐

Status . . . . ☐☐

Evaluability . . . . ☐

Response . . . . ☐

Date Review Received . . . .   MO ☐☐ DAY ☐☐ YR ☐☐

Reviewing Investigator . . . .   ☐☐☐☐

	Data Coordinator		Project Chairman	
	No	Yes	No	Yes
Is the patient eligible?				
Reason why ineligible				
Incorrect Disease	6.1		6.1	
Incorrect Staging	6.2		6.2	
Incorrect Lab Values	6.3		6.3	
Incorrect Prior Therapy	6.4		6.4	
Incorrect Performance Status	6.5		6.5	
Incorrect Response/Recovery to Previous Phase . . .	6.6		6.6	
No Measurable Disease or No Elevated Markers . . .	6.7		6.7	
Previous Phase Not Fully Evaluable	6.8		6.8	
Concurrent Malignancy or Prior Cancer . . .	6.9		6.9	
Improper Evaluation of Patient for Treatment . . .	7.0		7.0	
Other, specify _____	9.6		9.6	
Is the patient evaluable for:				
Survival	No	Yes	No	Yes
Toxicity	No	Yes	No	Yes
Response	No	Yes	No	Yes
Please give response as follows:				
1 = CR, 2 = PR, 3 = Fair PR, 4 = ? Improvement, 5 = Stable, 6 = Worse 7 = Dead	1 2 3 4 5 6 7		1 2 3 4 5 6 7	

Overall Assessment of Protocol Compliance . . . . ☐

RESPONSE FORM—REVIEW PAGE (Continued)   Page 6

Patient Name _____ Accession # _____

	Data Coordinator	Project Chairman
Reason why patient not fully evaluable or went off study:		
Non-Compliance due to Investigator error		
Over dosage of major significance (% deviation _____)	4.1	4.1
Under dosage of major significance (% deviation _____)	4.2	4.2
Incorrect timing of major significance		
Specify _____	4.3	4.3
Incorrect adjustments of major significance		
Specify _____	4.4	4.4
Insufficient data	4.5	4.5
Unjustified early removal from study by Investigator	4.6	4.6
Incorrect protocol therapy	4.7	4.7
Required follow-up studies not done	4.8	4.8
Other, specify _____	9.4	9.4
Non-Compliance (not due to Investigator error)		
Lost to follow-up	5.1	5.1
Refused to begin therapy	5.2	5.2
Refused further therapy	5.3	5.3
Schedule not followed by patient	5.4	5.4
Early death without follow-up studies	5.5	5.5
Change in initial disease status preventing beginning of treatment	5.6	5.6
Other, specify _____	9.5	9.5
Treatment Complication:		
Toxicity		
Not cause of early death	1.1	1.1
Cause of early death	1.2	1.2

Circle the modality (or modalities) that caused the toxicity:

Stat Off
only
[|]

    Surgery   Radiotherapy   Immunotherapy   Chemotherapy

    Antiemetics   BMT   Other, specify _____

	Data Coordinator	Project Chairman
Rapid Progression of Disease		
Not cause of early death	2.1	2.1
Cause of early death	2.2	2.2
Intercurrent Disease		
Not cause of early death	3.1	3.1
Cause of early death	3.2	3.2

FOLLOW-UP

INSTRUCTIONS: Complete this form at time of each Response Form
and every 6 months after study ended until death.

Protocol _____   Institution _____
                                             Hospital or
Accession # _____   Soc. Sec. # _____

Patient Name _____
            Last   First
Investigator _____

                                                              MO   DAY   YR
Date of Last Evaluation . . . . □ □ □   Date of this Evaluation . . . . □□ □□ □□

ADJUVANT PATIENTS . . . . □

                                                              MO   DAY   YR
Status: 1—No Evidence of Disease; 2-Recurrence . . . . □□ □□ □□

Last Known Date NED or Date of Recurrence . . . .

Give Sites	**Date Diagnosed**			**Sites of Recurrence:**
	MO	DAY	YR	

Give Sites	MO	DAY	YR
_____	□□	□□	□□
_____	□□	□□	□□
_____	□□	□□	□□
_____	□□	□□	□□

Sites of Recurrence:
- Area Code □□□
- Stat. Office Only □□□ □□□ □□□

METASTATIC PATIENTS

Has the patient experienced a stable or better response because of protocol therapy?
(1-No, 2-Yes) . . . . □

Note: If a Response improves from one type to another, list all dates.
(Status code: 1-Ongoing, 2-Relapsed)

STATUS		**STARTED**			**ENDED**		
		MO	DAY	YR	MO	DAY	YR
Complete Response	□	□□	□□	□□	□□	□□	□□
Partial Response	□	□□	□□	□□	□□	□□	□□
Stable	□				□□	□□	□□

Sites of Progression:

Give Sites	**Date Diagnosed**			
	MO	DAY	YR	
_____	□□	□□	□□	Area Code □□□
_____	□□	□□	□□	
_____	□□	□□	□□	Stat. Office Only □□□
_____	□□	□□	□□	□□□

Continued, Next Page

FOLLOW-UP FORM

Page 2

Patient's Name _____ Accession # _____

Has the patient experienced a second response (stable or better) because of therapy?
(i.e., crossover or reinduction) (1-No, 2-Yes) . . . . ☐

Record Second Response Below

	STATUS	STARTED			ENDED		
		MO	DAY	YR	MO	DAY	YR
Complete Response	☐	☐	☐	☐	☐	☐	☐
Partial Response	☐	☐	☐	☐	☐	☐	☐
Stable	☐				☐	☐	☐

Sites of Progression:

Give Sites	**Date Diagnosed**	Area Code Stat. Office Only
_____	☐☐☐☐	☐☐☐☐
_____	☐☐☐☐	☐☐☐☐
_____	☐☐☐☐	☐☐☐☐
_____	☐☐☐☐	☐☐☐☐

CURRENT RESPONSE STATUS (All Patients)

Current Response Status: (Metastatic: Code 1-5, Adjuvant: Code 1, 3, or 5) . . . . ☐

1-Remission NED   2-Stable Disease   3-Progression Recurrence   4-Dead   5-Lost to Follow-Up

Has the patient developed a new primary cancer? (1-No, 2-Yes) . . . . ☐

If YES, Give Site _____   Stat. Off. Only ☐☐☐

Cell Type _____   ☐☐☐

Date of Diagnosis . . . . ☐☐ ☐☐ ☐☐

Has the patient received subsequent therapy? (1-No, 2-Yes, 3-Yes, details unknown) . . . . . . ☐

Date of death or Last Known Alive . . . .   MO ☐☐ DAY ☐☐ YR ☐☐

Cause of Death . . . . ☐
1-Disease Primary Cause   4-Unrelated to Disease or Therapy
2-Disease Contributing Cause   5-Unknown
3-Due to Toxicity   Stat. Off. Only ☐

IF SUBSEQUENT THERAPY RECEIVED, COMPLETE NEXT PAGE

FOLLOW-UP FORM

Patient's Name _____   Accession # _____

SUBSEQUENT THERAPY --

INSTRUCTIONS	CODES FOR ALL TREATMENTS

INSTRUCTIONS

If subsequent information has previously been completed on this patient, enter only additional information below.

CODES FOR ALL TREATMENTS

RESPONSE CODES	TYPE CODES
1-Yes, Complete	1-Ortho
2-Yes, Partial	2-CO^{60}
3-Yes, Fair Partial	3-Linac
5-Stable	4-Beta
6-Worse	5-Other
7-Inevaluable	

SUBSEQUENT SYSTEMIC THERAPY: (CHEMOTHERAPY, IMMUNOTHERAPY, HORMONE THERAPY):

Has the patient received SUBSEQUENT SYSTEMIC THERAPY? (1-No, 2-Yes) . . . .

	THERAPY				DURATION OF RESPONSE				R E S P	STAT OFFICE ONLY
	STARTED		STOPPED		STARTED		STOPPED			
	MO	YR	MO	YR	MO	YR	MO	YR		

SUBSEQUENT RADIOTHERAPY: Has the patient received SUBSEQUENT RADIOTHERAPY?

(1-No, 2-Yes, 3-Yes, palliative). . . . .

	THERAPY				DURATION OF RESPONSE				R E S P	TUMOR DOSE × 1000R	T Y P	STAT OFFICE ONLY
	STARTED		STOPPED		STARTED		STOPPED					
	MO	YR	MO	YR	MO	YR	MO	YR				

SUBSEQUENT SURGERY: Has the patient received SUBSEQUENT SURGERY? (1-No, 2-Yes) . . . .

INTENT OF SURGERY: 1-Palliative, 2-Curative, 3-Diagnostic

Type of Surgery	Date of Surgery			Inten
	MO	DAY	YR	

Surgery for Benign and Malignant Disease of the Breast: Techniques and Complications

Chapter 28

INDICATIONS AND TECHNIQUES FOR BIOPSY

Wiley W. Souba, M.D., Sc.D. and Kirby I. Bland, M.D.

Even though a presumptive diagnosis of breast cancer can be made from a patient's history and physical examination or from radiological studies, the actual removal of tissue from the breast or from a metastatic site, followed by microscopic examination, is essential to confirm the diagnosis. Unfortunately most breast masses that appear to be benign have a real, although relatively small, probability of malignancy that cannot be ruled out until a biopsy is performed.[8, 35, 45] The morbidity and mortality associated with breast biopsy is acceptably low, primarily because of adherence to careful surgical technique and to the frequency with which local anesthesia can be utilized. A 1980 study[6] on the cost-effectiveness of breast cancer management demonstrated that screening costs are very high and that the most effective means of containing the economic cost of this illness is through the targeted selection of high-risk patients for breast biopsy using local anesthesia. However, given the emotional impact of the possibility of a breast mass being cancerous and the traditional teaching that all breast masses in women older than 35 years should be removed, can the need for breast biopsy be questioned? Open biopsy of a breast mass under general or local anesthesia remains relatively low in morbidity with essentially no mortality. Although most biopsies of "suspicious" breast lesions prove to be benign, certain clinical and mammographic features are associated with a high probability of malignancy.[9, 10, 15, 16, 27, 31, 32] The history, physical examination, and preoperative staging will all influence the timing and the type of breast biopsy performed. Should the patient have cancer confirmed by biopsy, the information gained from the specimen is crucial to staging, assessment of prognosis, and selection of the appropriate therapy. Properly done, the biopsy

findings will be of great assistance in planning the workup and definitive treatment of the patient. On the other hand, inconclusive data derived from insufficient tissue or a biopsy incision placed in the wrong position may limit therapeutic options or make definitive treatment difficult or inconsequential.

The decision to perform a breast biopsy requires thorough assessment of the individual patient and her radiographic and clinical presentation. Breast masses in adolescent and young adult women are often benign lesions that can generally be followed at specified intervals unless an indication for biopsy is apparent (e.g., positive family history or suspicious mammogram). In women older than 35 years, there are several clinical situations in which a biopsy is generally indicated without reservation. The first is the presence of a previously unrecognized three-dimensional mass that is anatomically distinct from the remainder of the breast tissue. Even though the mammogram is entirely normal, the presence of a new mass is usually an indication for biopsy. Criteria that should influence the surgeon's decision to perform the biopsy include mammographic findings that are suspicious for carcinoma,[13] the presence of a positive family history for breast cancer or a previous history of breast cancer,[24] and physical findings (e.g., skin dimpling, peau d'orange, or clinically positive axillary nodes) indicative of neoplastic disease.[8] The second indication for breast biopsy is the presence of xeromammographic findings that are suggestive of carcinoma.[4, 13, 27, 28, 37, 38] These radiographic features include architectural distortion of the surrounding breast tissue that may be suggestive of carcinoma or clustered microcalcifications (see section 8, chapter 24). In the absence of any physical abnormality, these findings are generally an indication to perform an excisional biopsy of the nonpalpable lesion.

NONPALPABLE LESIONS

A "normal" breast may not present any apparent physical signs of an underlying breast cancer but may harbor a neoplasm in the noninfiltrating (in situ) stage or, less often, as an occult infiltrating breast carcinoma.[16] Nonpalpable breast lesions are generally discovered on routine screening mammogram,[27] although incidental breast masses have been found on chest computed tomography (CT) scans. In the past decade, the widespread application of high-quality xeromammography has resulted in the detection of increasing numbers of nonpalpable breast lesions. The xeroradiographic criteria on which the decision to perform a biopsy is based include (1) a localized soft tissue mass within the breast parenchyma; (2) architectural distortion, including contracture of trabeculae producing stellate alterations, with severe asymmetric periductal and lobular thickening; and (3) cluttered microcalcifications with or without the aforementioned features.[8, 10, 13]

Preoperative Localization of Nonpalpable Breast Lesions

As previously stated, the widespread use of mammography has resulted in the detection of increasing numbers of suspicious but nonpalpable lesions of the breast.[13] Such lesions may represent up to one half of the detected cancers in screening clinics and account for a substantial proportion of breast tumors that undergo biopsy. Despite the frequency and simplicity of xeroradiographic or film/screen mammographic identification of suspicious lesions, intraoperative localization with subsequent adequate excision presents challenging technical problems. This is because of the shape and position of the breast during compression mammography, which is often quite different from that seen by the surgeon in the operating room. This has led to the development of several methods for preoperative localization of nonpalpable lesions.* The aim of these methods is to facilitate complete removal of the tumor with the first attempt at excision, while simultaneously minimizing the size of the resected specimen and shortening the duration of anesthesia. Radiologically guided, invasive, preoperative localization of nonpalpable breast lesions is a safe, simple, and established procedure that allows for accurate and expeditious biopsy that can often be performed under local anesthesia. It should be uniformly available wherever mammography and breast biopsies are performed. Since nonpalpable breast masses are often discovered as clustered microcalcifications or architectural distortions, they may remain nonpalpable even on examination of the resected specimen. Thus specimen radiography (mammography) is mandatory to document removal of

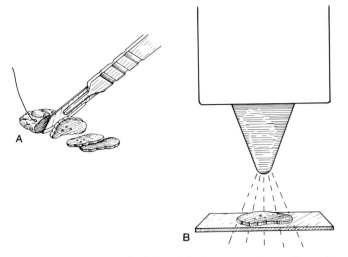

Figure 28–1. *A,* "Bread loafing" of the biopsy specimen allows the exact site of the lesion to be determined and submitted for pathological evaluation. *B,* Following excision of the suspicious lesion, specimen radiography is completed to confirm the presence of the suspect lesion in the excised tissue.

the suspicious area and to facilitate histological examination.*

Noninvasive Localization Techniques

Noninvasive techniques for localization of mammographically suspicious breast lesions include visual estimation, external breast markers,[3] coordinates plotted on a diagram of the breast,[44] stereomammograms,[2] and grid compression devices.[44] Although superficial lesions of the mamma or lesions adjacent to the nipple may be adequately localized preoperatively by visual estimation, deeper suspect areas cannot be accurately localized by noninvasive localization techniques.[3] Extrapolation of the depth and surface distances of the lesion obtained during compression mammography in the supine position introduces unacceptable error.

External breast markers such as indelible ink or the needle-scratch technique were introduced more than 25 years ago; Stevens and Jamplis[44] were among the first investigators to describe preoperative localization of nonpalpable breast lesions with use of a "mammographic map" that established the relative position for the suspicious area within the breast using coordinates. With the use of this localization technique, a wedge biopsy with adequate margins could be obtained. The authors emphasized the need for roentgenographic confirmation of removal of the suspicious lesion. Following "bread loafing" of the specimen and repeat roentgenography, the exact site of the suspicious lesion may be localized and submitted for pathological evaluation (Fig. 28–1). Although this technique for localization of nonpalpable lesions was an improvement over "blind" biopsy methods, it was fraught with error and inaccurate sampling of the suspicious breast lesion.

---

*References 2, 3, 5, 14, 17, 19, 20, 21, 25, 26, 36, 40, 43, and 44.

*References 1, 23, 29, 33, 34, 40, 41, and 46.

Invasive Localization Procedures

Localization of occult breast masses has markedly improved with the use of small radiopaque needles that may be radiographically guided into the breast.[18, 20, 21, 25, 30] These needles are inserted by the radiologist in the radiology suite; subsequent mammography demonstrates the relationship of the needle to the suspect lesion. The success of breast localization procedures requires patient cooperation and communication between the radiologist and surgeon; when specimen radiography is necessary, communication among the radiologist, surgeon, and the pathologist is of utmost importance. Failure of these individuals to communicate at preoperative planning of the procedure is a common cause of unsuccessful localization and excision of the nonpalpable breast lesion following needle localization.[3]

Injection (Spot) Localization

In 1972, Simon et al.[39] first described the technique of spot localization of nonpalpable breast lesions using a percutaneously inserted needle. The site for insertion of the localizing needle is selected by using coordinate measurements taken from the craniocaudal and mediolateral mammograms in relation to the nipple. Following local anesthesia of skin and subcutaneous tissues, the needle is inserted through the skin in the direction and depth determined by the biplanar radiological measurements. Repeat craniocaudal and mediolateral radiograms are obtained with the needle in position to confirm its relationship to the suspect lesion and to indicate any necessary changes in needle position. Once the needle has been satisfactorily positioned, a 0.1-ml solution of equal parts of Evans blue dye and radiopaque contrast is injected. Thereafter a small amount of air is flushed through the needle to ensure that all of the dye has been delivered into the breast. The needle is withdrawn, and repeat craniocaudal and mediolateral radiographic views are taken to determine the distance and direction of the lesion relative to the radiopaque contrast. This information is communicated to the surgeon, and the final set of radiographs are sent with the patient to the operating room. The surgeon performs the biopsy using the dyed outline of breast tissue and its relationship to the area of suspicion on mammogram as a guide. The spot method of localization overcame the disadvantage of localization that was based on coordinates alone (i.e., these coordinates tended to shift substantially when the patient was placed in the supine position on the operating table). Unfortunately this technique was limited by rapid absorption of the biodegradable dye from the vicinity of the tumor and the needle tract, and by dissemination of the dye well beyond the anatomical location of the tumor.

Needle Localization

Needle localization methods that utilized percutaneously placed needles in the vicinity of the suspect mass as a biopsy guide were first described by Dodd.[7] This technique, however, did not gain widespread acceptance until screening mammography achieved universal application. Variations of this technique have been reported by many radiologists[20, 21] and became popular and routinely accepted in the late 1970s. Thereafter Libshitz et al.[25] reported complete success in the removal of 83 suspicious breast lesions. Unfortunately the authors did not state how often more than one biopsy was required to remove the suspicious area, or the frequency of lesions that were palpable during the surgical procedure. Common technical problems with this method of localization include (1) movement of the nonmalleable needle during the time between placement and operation, even when the needle hub is taped or secured in place; (2) compression of the breast during mammography and localization, creating tissue stress that may alter the position of the needle even when it is sutured in place; and (3) unavoidable dislodgement of the needle during the procedure, with operator manipulation often leading to inadequate tissue sampling (false-negative results) or inadvertent transection of the tumor with incomplete removal of the suspect mass.

Self-Retaining Wire Localization

The two principal problems with needle localization of breast lesions are the nonpliability of the stainless steel needle and the unreliability of the position of the needle following breast compression, patient movement, and surgical manipulation.[14] These problems have been overcome, for the most part, by placing a flexible hooked wire within the localizing needle, a technique first described by Frank et al.[11] The hook ideally lodges within the suspicious breast lesion and prevents dislodgement from the specimen (Fig. 28–2). Local anesthesia is utilized, and a small puncture wound is made in the skin that directly overlies the lesion using a no. 11 scalpel blade. The rigid introducer needle with the hooked wire within it is directed into the breast using biplane mammographic guidance. The rigid needle is then removed, leaving the hooked wire in place. Because of its self-retaining feature, the wire is not easily withdrawn, advanced, or redirected. The operative approach is directed parallel and deep to the axis of the wire; the hooked tip of the wire is excised with contiguous tissues that surround the suspect lesion (Fig. 28–3). Although wire localization has gained widespread acceptance, several technical problems have been reported. The surgeon may have difficulty locating the flexible localization wire, especially if the lesion is approached via a circumareolar incision remote from the suspicious mass. To help eliminate this problem, Homer et al.[18] advocate the use of a post-localization needle. This needle is guided percutaneously by the surgeon over the flexible hooked wire, which has been previously placed by the radiologist. The rigidity of the needle allows easy palpation of its course during the operative procedure.

Methods for preoperative localization represent a

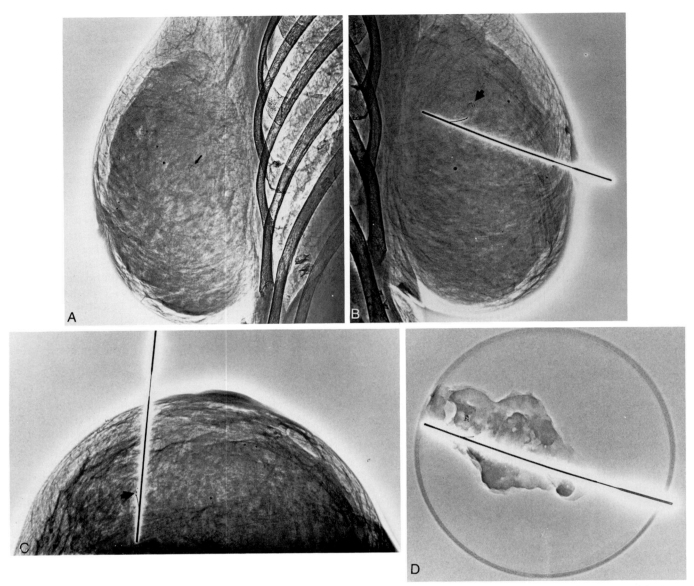

Figure 28–2. Preoperative needle localization of a nonpalpable breast lesion *(A)* requires mediolateral *(B)* and craniocaudal *(C)* views of the breast. It is mandatory to obtain specimen mammography of the excised tissue *(D)*, preferably with the localization wire in place to confirm extirpation of the suspect lesion.

major contribution to the operative treatment of suspicious occult (nonpalpable) lesions of the breast. The success and effectiveness of any invasive breast localization procedure to facilitate specimen removal, decrease operating time, and reduce biopsy size is enhanced by an experienced surgeon working in close cooperation with the radiologist.

PALPABLE LESIONS

While nonpalpable breast lesions require needle localization prior to definitive biopsy, palpable lesions may undergo biopsy by one of several techniques. The choice of the biopsy technique will be influenced by the physical characteristics and size of the breast mass, the location of the suspicious lesion in the breast, the use of local or general anesthesia, and the method of treatment decided on should a malignancy be confirmed. For example, an incisional biopsy of a large breast tumor performed under local anesthesia in a woman who presents with bony metastases provides histological confirmation of the malignancy and adequate tissue for hormone receptor analysis prior to the initiation of preoperative chemotherapy. On the other hand, fine needle aspiration biopsy of a suspicious mass done in an outpatient setting in a woman with clinical stage I breast cancer provides a diagnosis and allows the surgeon and patient to discuss treatment strategies and options prior to the definitive surgical procedure. It is critical that the biopsy specimen be handled appropriately in both clinical situations, as failure or delay in transport to the

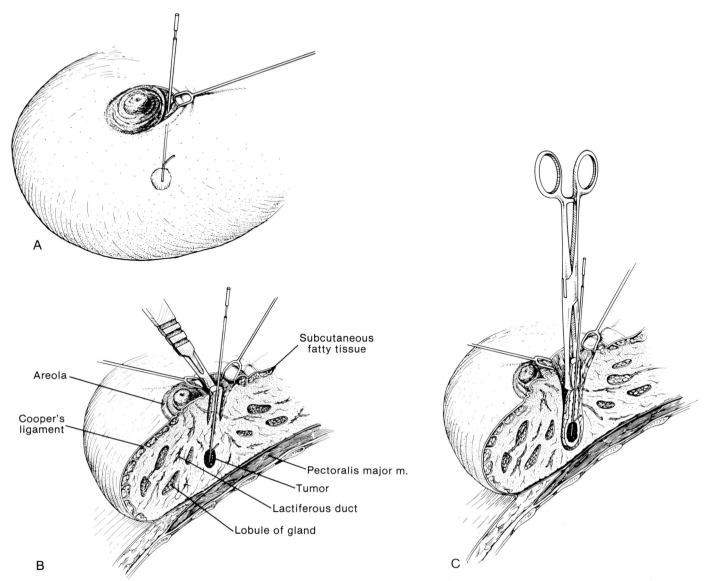

Figure 28–3. Operative technique for needle localization biopsy: The suspicious lesion is "localized" on the mammogram immediately prior to surgery. *A,* At operation the needle serves as a guide for the surgeon to perform the biopsy. *B,* Development of tissue planes circumferential and parallel to the localization wire. *C,* Controlled dissection of the wire, which is purchased with tissues using an Allis clamp. The suspicious lesion is incorporated in the dissection, which is inclusive of tissue beyond the tip of the hooked wire. Specimen radiography confirms excision of the suspicious, nonpalpable mammographically identified lesion.

surgical pathology laboratory may render a specimen invalid for histological or hormone receptor analysis (see chapter 43).

Collection of Specimens for Cytological Examination

Direct Smear

Specimens for exfoliative cytology in the patient with suspected Paget's disease of the breast may be obtained with direct smear of the weeping eczematoid lesion of the nipple. If the aroela and surrounding skin is scaly

and encrusted, a sterile glass slide can be used to gently scrape this area. The direct smear technique is simple and can be performed in the surgeon's office. Although it may be possible to differentiate invasive cancer from carcinoma in situ with this technique, the treatment of choice in Paget's disease is modified radical mastectomy following confirmed diagnosis.

Fluid Aspiration

Fluid from breast cysts is simple to aspirate with a needle and syringe (Fig. 28–4). If the cyst is not palpable, ultrasound may confirm its presence and can be used as a guide to direct the depth and location of the

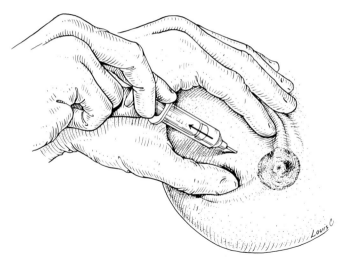

Figure 28–4. Technique for aspiration of fluid from a breast cyst.

biopsy needle. The return of greenish-brown fluid virtually confirms the diagnosis of benign (nonproliferative) cystic disease and, unless otherwise indicated, should not be submitted for cytologic examination. Bloody cystic fluid, on the other hand, is more likely to be indicative of malignancy and therefore should *always* be examined histologically, either following direct smear or after centrifugation of the aspirated contents. Palpable breast cysts should no longer be detectable after aspiration of their contents, since the walls of the cyst should subsequently collapse and conform to the configuration of contiguous breast tissues. Clinical and mammographic follow-up of patients who undergo fluid aspiration is mandatory, since excisional biopsy of the suspicious mass is indicated, in most patients, should the mass recur within 6 weeks of aspiration.

Fine Needle Aspiration Biopsy

Fine needle aspiration (FNA) biopsy of breast masses is a safe and reliable diagnostic technique that can be performed in the office using local anesthesia.[12] The skin overlying the palpable lesion is infiltrated with one percent plain lidocaine. The breast lump is held relatively immobile, using one hand to gently, but firmly, stabilize the quadrant containing the mass. Using a special cytology aspiration gun (Cameco, Enebyberg, Sweden) that activates the plunger of a disposable 10-cc or 20-cc syringe attached to a 22-gauge needle, the biopsy can be effectively performed using this technique (Fig. 28–5). (See section VIII, chapter 26.) The needle is inserted into the mass through the anesthetized skin, and maximum suction is applied to the syringe. On moving the needle into the suspect lesion at variable angles over an area of no more than 1 cm, clumps of cells may be dislodged from the tumor, aspirated into the syringe, and submitted for cytologic examination. FNA is quite safe, although the individual performing the procedure must be cognizant at all times of the relationship of the aspiration needle to the chest wall, as entry of the parietal pleura with iatrogenic pneumo-

thorax is a potentially dangerous, although rare, complication. Following aspiration needle biopsy of any breast mass, local pressure should be applied to the skin puncture site to prevent dispersion of cells and ecchymosis.

The diagnostic accuracy of fine needle aspiration biopsy of breast masses approximates 80 percent.[22] False-positive results are unusual when the aspirated specimen is properly prepared and reviewed by a qualified cytopathologist. False-negative results are much more common, and it must be emphasized that *the absence of malignant cells in the aspirate does not exclude the diagnosis of cancer. Hence, any clinical or mammographically suspicious breast mass that undergoes fine needle aspiration biopsy and does not yield a diagnosis of malignancy must be subjected to an incisional or excisional biopsy.* For patients who undergo fine needle aspiration of the breast to confirm the diagnosis of metastatic cancer prior to the institution of preoperative chemotherapy, quantitative hormonal (estrogen and progesterone) receptor assays cannot be performed, because the tissue sample is of inadequate volume. Newer qualitative immunofluorescent monoclonal antibody techniques can be applied to the cytology specimen and may aid in eliminating the problem of insufficient tissue to provide accurate hormone receptor data.

Cutting Needle Biopsy

The technique of biopsy with a needle that incises a core of tissue from the breast is termed "cutting-needle biopsy." The standard Tru-Cut (Travenol, Deerfield, IL) needle (Fig. 28–6) is the most commonly utilized cutting needle for breast biopsy. The false-positive diagnostic rate is lower with tissue procured by cutting needles than with fine needle aspiration biopsy specimens, because more tissue is retained and can be submitted for analysis. However, a core biopsy that yields no malignant cells cannot conclusively be considered benign, since only a portion of the mass that did not contain cancer may have been sampled (sampling error). Thus, like FNA biopsy, the cutting needle biopsy is only useful when the results are positive for malignancy. Cutting needles are 12 gauge or larger in size and thus require local anesthesia prior to use. Since the biopsy yields a core of solid tissue, rather than clumps of cells, the potential risk for hemorrhage and tissue disturbance is higher than with needle aspiration methods. Care must be taken not to advance the cutting needle beyond the suspect mass, since the contiguous normal breast or the chest wall could be implanted with malignant cells. Such complications can be reduced with operator experience. The site of the puncture and the biopsy tract should always be planned so that these areas can be excised en bloc with the neoplasm at the time of the definitive surgical treatment.

Incisional Biopsy

An incisional biopsy of a suspicious breast mass involves removal of a portion of the lesion, which is then submitted for pathological examination. This type of

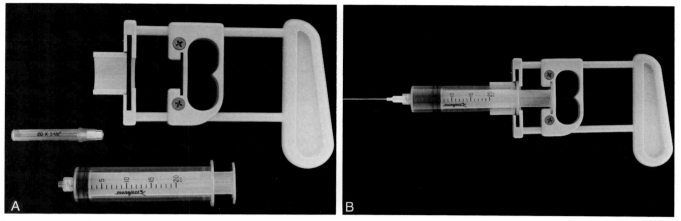

Figure 28–5. *A* and *B*, Aspiration of a solid breast mass is best performed using a cytology fine needle "aspiration gun" (Cameco, Enebyberg, Sweden).

biopsy is indicated in patients with large (≥4 cm) primary breast lesions and who will undergo preoperative chemotherapy or radiotherapy. The incisional biopsy should only excise the amount of tissue necessary for histological confirmation of the diagnosis and for hormone receptor studies.

Technique. The biopsy site should be marked on the breast, typically in curvilinear fashion paralleling Langer's lines, to enable the surgeon to excise the entire scar and the primary neoplasm at the time of definitive surgical therapy (see section X, chapter 29). Meticulous attention to hemostasis is mandatory to prevent the spread of potentially malignant cells. The technical aspects of incisional biopsy of breast masses are relatively simple and straightforward. Local anesthesia of one percent plain lidocaine is infiltrated into the dermis of the planned skin incision directly over the tumor. The actual biopsy of tumor is best performed using the scalpel, since electrocautery may distort the histological features of the tissue and possibly invalidate accurate tissue levels (mg/cytosol protein) of hormonal receptors.

Biopsy of a portion of the mass is followed by closure with absorbable 2–0 or 3–0 sutures.

Excisional Biopsy

As the terminology implies, excisional biopsy of a breast mass removes the entire lesion and generally includes a margin of normal breast tissue that surrounds the suspicious mass. It should be considered an error in surgical technique if the tumor is transected during the excisional biopsy. Such technical errors virtually guarantee the contamination of adjacent tissues with malignant cells. Occult suspicious breast lesions that are apparent only on mammogram should undergo excisional biopsy using preoperative needle localization. If the volume of tissue removed is small (≤1 cm³), only permanent histological sections of the lesion should be planned, as the pathologist may not be able to distinguish between severe atypia and carcinoma on frozen section specimens. On rare occasion, excisional biopsy

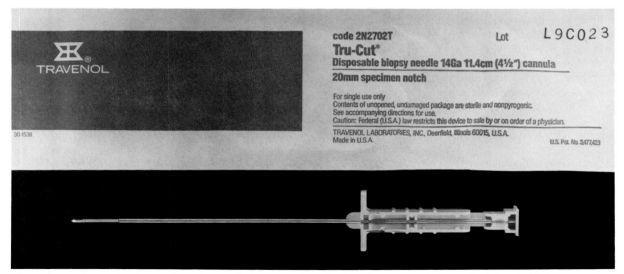

Figure 28–6. The TruCut (Travenol) cutting needle is commonly utilized to obtain a core biopsy of solid, palpable breast masses.

of a large breast mass (e.g., giant fibroadenomas), is indicated to provide definitive therapy for breast disease.

Lumpectomy (Segmental Mastectomy)

When the National Surgical Adjunctive Breast Project (NSABP) was implemented in the 1950s, the standard surgical treatment for carcinoma of the breast was modified radical or radical mastectomy. Surgeons had essentially no familiarity with "breast conservation surgery" or terms such as tylectomy, lumpectomy, segmental mastectomy, and quadrantectomy. Through a series of workshops and other educational tools, the participating NSABP surgeons were instructed in the methods mandated by the protocol. Lumpectomy with axillary dissection (Levels I and II) followed by radiation therapy to the breast is now an acceptable surgical treatment for certain carcinomas of the breast. A detailed review of the indications and techniques for conservation surgery advocated by Fisher and other investigators of the NSABP is provided in Section X, Chapter 29.

Curvilinear incisions are recommended for the majority of lumpectomies regardless of the location of the primary breast lesion. Although radial incisions are preferred by some surgeons for lesions in the lower half of the breast, we use nonradical incisions in the majority of patients, as cosmetic results are equivalent or superior with curvilinear incisions that follow the breast contour parallel to Langer's lines. Chapter 29 reviews the placement of incisions in various quadrants of the breast for suspect breast masses. The surgeon must always be cognizant of the occasional necessity to convert a planned segmental mastectomy into a total mastectomy. Thus placement of breast incisions that are readily incorporated into cosmetically acceptable incisions for total mastectomy is essential to planning the operative procedure.

It is helpful if the preoperative diagnosis of cancer has been established by needle aspiration biopsy or core biopsy. Breast lesions suggestive of carcinoma that require needle localization should have the needle directed into the lesion perpendicular to the skin and as close to the planned curvilinear incision as possible to avoid extensive flap elevation with subsequent wound hemorrhage and skin slough. The incision for lumpectomy should be placed directly over the lesion. Tunneling through and elevation of contiguous breast tissue at an angle is not recommended, as tumor-free margins are invariably difficult to obtain. In patients referred with biopsy-proven carcinoma, reexcision of the old scar and the entire biopsy site is essential to diminish the probability of tumor implantation and local recurrence in the scar and skin flaps.

It is imperative to excise a margin of "normal" breast tissue contiguous with the suspicious mass. Careful palpation of margins of the tumor by the operating surgeon during excision provides a three-dimensional perspective of the lesion that is essential to ensure that the tumor is not violated and is excised within the sphere of extirpated breast tissue. This technique does not necessitate removal of a predetermined volume of normal tissue;

the goal of the operative procedure is to obtain margins that are grossly free of tumor. Skin edges need not be undermined, and the pectoralis major fascia is not included in the resected margin unless the lesion is contiguous with or is fixed to the fascia. The specimen should be oriented in all dimensions, using suture for tags. The designations "cranial-caudal," "medial-lateral," and "superficial-deep" allow the surgeon to appropriately designate the varying margins of the excised specimen for the pathologist. Such margins may be dyed with indelible vital stains (e.g., india ink) to verify areas of concern and ensure histological extirpation of the cancer. Thereafter, the pathologist completes the frozen section analysis of the margins of all biopsy specimens to ensure histologically clear margins (see chapter 29). The pathologist's role is most important in confirming the diagnosis, establishing the presence of tumor-free margins, and submitting tissue for estrogen and progesterone receptor analyses. The surgeon must be cognizant of tumor orientation with respect to the wound and chest wall during resection of the breast mass; the presence of a positive margin will require reexcision of any area in which the frozen section was histologically positive. For instances in which lumpectomy cannot assure tumor-free margins (e.g., multifocality, multicentricity, multiple histological types, diffuse microcalcifications, etc.), a total mastectomy is performed.

Following confirmation of tumor-free margins by the pathologist, meticulous hemostasis is achieved and wound closure is begun. Special attention is paid to closure of the wound, since tissue defects created with lumpectomy may result in cosmetically unacceptable scars that may be further exaggerated on completion of breast irradiation. Care must be taken with closure of the wound, as unacceptable cosmetic results occur when superficial or deep tissues are approximated under tension. Large defects are preferably closed in multiple layers with interrupted 2–0 or 3–0 absorbable chromic gut or synthetic sutures. Some surgeons make no attempt to obliterate dead space, and others make no effort to drain this space. Interrupted absorbable sutures are placed in the subcutaneous tissues, and the skin is closed using a running subcuticular absorbable 4–0 or 5–0 synthetic suture.

Surgical Biopsy of the Breast

Only by removing a sample of breast tissue sufficient for histological preparation can a diagnosis be made with ultimate confidence. The accuracy of pathological information obtained is limited only by the accuracy of sampling and morphological interpretation. Because a negative biopsy result can be caused by sampling error, cancer cannot be excluded unless representative pathological tissue is removed and examined thoroughly. This principle is most important, as therapy for cancer can only be predicated on histological verification of its presence.

Breast biopsy is best performed in a surgical suite, under sterile conditions and with techniques using local or general anesthesia. This may be done on an outpatient basis, but the setting is dependent on patient and physician preference. It is essential that incisions be cosmetically designed, since approximately 70 percent of breast biopsies confirm benign (proliferative and nonproliferative) disease. Since the lines of tension in the skin of the breast are generally concentric with the nipple (Fig. 28–7), incisions that parallel these lines (Langer's lines) generally result in thin and cosmetically acceptable scars.[42] It is best to keep these incisions within the boundaries of potential incisions for future mastectomy or wide local excision should those therapies be required for definitive treatment (Fig. 28–8). Principles for planning breast biopsy are further reviewed in Section X, Chapter 29, and Section XIV, Chapter 36. The most cosmetically acceptable scars result from circumareolar (curvilinear) incisions. Most centrally located subareolar lesions can be approached in this manner.

Once the patient is comfortably positioned on the operating table, the thorax is slightly elevated ipsilaterally on the side of the suspect lesion (using folded sheets), and the arm is placed in a relaxed position on an arm board. Commonly used incisions for all quadrants are depicted in Figure 28–5. In general, dermal tension is concentric, with the nipple becoming transverse over the sternum and diagonal toward the extreme upper lateral anterior chest. Periareolar and concentric lesions follow these lines of tension and therefore are optimally cosmetic. The proposed incision is marked on the skin after the dimensions of the tumor are estimated, and local anesthesia (one percent plain lidocaine) is infiltrated into the dermis (cutis vera). The surgeon is admonished to avoid lidocaine injections with epinephrine for fear of epidermolysis of the injection site with subsequent slough of the epidermis. It is not necessary to fill subcutaneous tissues with the local anesthetic, as this may make it difficult to palpate margins of the suspicious mass. This principle is most important if excisional biopsy is planned. Injection of the tumor with anesthetics is also contraindicated, as this adds nothing

to patient comfort but creates the potential to disseminate neoplastic cells into contiguous tissues. Biopsy should be performed with the scalpel rather than electrocautery, as the latter can devitalize tissue and invalidate detectable hormone receptor values. We prefer to obtain estrogen and progesterone receptor data from tissue removed at biopsy rather than from residual tumor that is present in the mastectomy specimen, particularly because warm ischemia time during mastectomy may alter the estrogen and progesterone content (see Section XVII, Chapter 43).

Once the incision is completed and dermal and subcutaneous bleeding is controlled, the incision is carried through the subcutaneous fat with sharp (scalpel) dissection to expose the tumor mass. Unless incisional biopsy is planned because of the size (≥4 cm) of the neoplasm, every effort is made technically to avoid incision of the tumor. Using sharp dissection guided by careful and gentle digital palpation by the operating surgeon, the mass is excised with a small rim of normal breast parenchyma. If the tumor is large (≥4 cm), only an incisional biopsy should be performed to confirm the diagnosis of cancer. If the diagnosis of cancer is not determined at histological review of permanent sections, the entire mass should be removed and the specimen immediately placed in a saline-soaked sponge for transport to the pathologist. Should prolonged transport of the tumor be anticipated with warm ischemia time that exceeds 20 minutes, the specimen should be packed on ice and delivered expeditiously to the pathology department.

During excisional biopsy, retractors can be utilized to facilitate exposure for dissection of the mass, but care must be taken not to violate the area that is undergoing biopsy. Once the specimen is removed, attention to meticulous hemostasis with electrocautery or suture ligatures is mandatory. Wound drainage with soft rubber Penrose drain (¼-inch) is optional. Closure of the breast tissue defect is not mandatory, although we recommend closure with interrupted 2-0 or 3-0 absorbable chromic

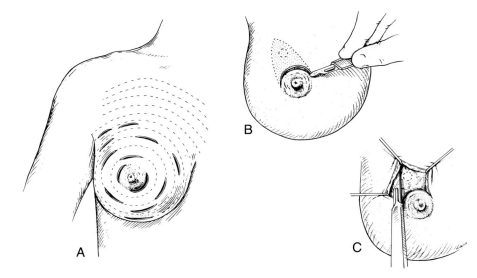

Figure 28–7. Recommended locations of incisions for performing breast biopsy. *A,* The most cosmetically acceptable scars result from circumareolar incisions that follow the contour of Langer's lines. *B* and *C,* Technique for dissection of breast masses within 3 cm of the areolar margin. Thin skin flaps must be avoided to ensure cosmetically contoured and viable tissues about the areola.

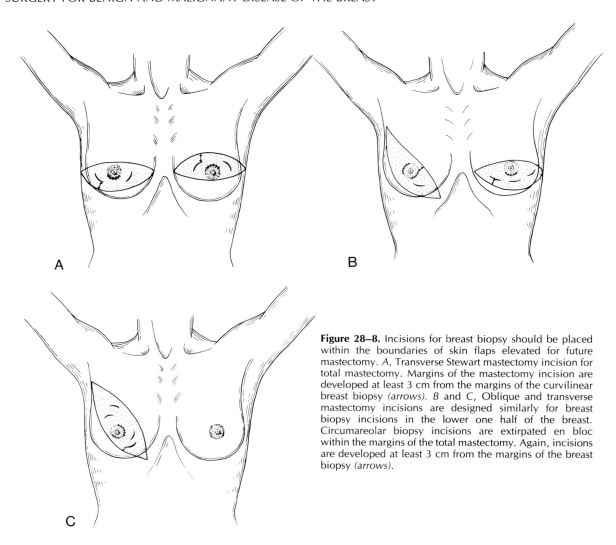

Figure 28–8. Incisions for breast biopsy should be placed within the boundaries of skin flaps elevated for future mastectomy. *A,* Transverse Stewart mastectomy incision for total mastectomy. Margins of the mastectomy incision are developed at least 3 cm from the margins of the curvilinear breast biopsy *(arrows). B* and *C,* Oblique and transverse mastectomy incisions are designed similarly for breast biopsy incisions in the lower one half of the breast. Circumareolar biopsy incisions are extirpated en bloc within the margins of the total mastectomy. Again, incisions are developed at least 3 cm from the margins of the breast biopsy *(arrows).*

gut or synthetic sutures. The subcutaneous tissues are closed with 3-0 or 4-0 interrupted, absorbable sutures. A running subcuticular closure of the skin using 5-0 synthetic suture is performed, followed by Steri-Strip approximation of the skin edges. A light occlusive dressing is applied.

CHOICE OF ANESTHESIA IN ONE- AND TWO-STAGE PROCEDURES

The choice of anesthesia (local or general) for breast biopsy depends on the following factors:

1. The presence of a lesion that is palpable or non-palpable
2. The age and general medical condition of the patient
3. The presumptive diagnosis
4. The necessity to procure adequate amounts of tissue for hormone receptor analysis prior to the initiation of anticancer therapy
5. The type of biopsy (incisional/excisional/FNA) that the physician plans to perform
6. The location of the mass within the breast

7. The personal preference of the physician and the patient.

In general, efforts should be made to avoid sequential general anesthesia when treating patients with a potentially malignant breast mass. This is not always feasible or possible. For example, nonpalpable lesions that are located deep in the breast may be best excised under general anesthesia. In addition, an anxious patient who is apprehensive of the biopsy under local anesthesia may elect a general anesthetic if her medical condition is conducive to this technique.

Biopsy as a separate procedure under general anesthesia should be avoided when needle biopsy, cutting needle biopsy, or biopsy under local anesthesia can be safely and comfortably accomplished with supplemental anesthesia (sedation with amnesia). The great majority of palpable and nonpalpable breast masses can be excised with local anesthesia and sedation incurring minimal morbidity and no mortality. Local agents such as lidocaine are safe and effective and initiate minimal discomfort following injection of the dermis and surrounding breast tissues. Contraindications to local anesthesia for breast biopsy generally include (1) a palpable or nonpalpable lesion that is located deep within the breast parenchyma in which significant manipulation of tissue near the fascia is anticipated; (2) an anxious, apprehensive patient or a patient who prefers to have the biopsy done under general anesthesia; and (3) a patient with a breast mass suggestive of carcinoma who agrees to undergo biopsy, frozen section, and definite operative therapy all during one procedure under general anesthetic. When it is anticipated that general anesthesia will be required for biopsy of a suspicious breast mass, a full work-up, including staging (see section VI, chapter 17), with plans to implement comprehensive operative therapy should be completed *prior* to the procedure to avoid a second operation. Therefore informed consent for definitive therapy should be obtained prior to any procedure in the patient with a suspicious breast mass. Additionally, the surgeon and operating room personnel must arrange preoperatively for specimen mammography to be performed (if needle localization is required) as soon as the biopsy is completed to allow analyses of the freshly procured tissue. Such arrangements with the radiologist and pathologist will minimize the duration of the general anesthetic with its inherent morbidity.

In the patient with a highly suspicious lesion, a two-stage procedure under general anesthesia is not recommended if frozen section evaluation at the time of the biopsy could provide the diagnosis and allow the surgeon to proceed with definite therapy as a one-stage procedure. General anesthesia for biopsy should not be used solely because the clinic or hospital lacks the facilities for needle biopsy or frozen section analysis.

References

1. Bauermeister DE, Hall MH: Specimen radiography—a mandatory adjunct to mammography. Am J Clin Pathol 59(6):782–789, 1973.
2. Becker W: Stereotactic localization of breast lesions. Radiology 133:240–241, 1979.
3. Bigongiari LR, Fidler W, Skerker LB, Comstock C, Threatt B: Percutaneous localization of breast lesions prior to biopsy: analysis of failures. Clin Radiol 28:419–425, 1977.
4. Block MA, Reynolds W: How vital is mammography in the diagnosis and management of breast carcinoma. Arch Surg 108:588–591, 1974.
5. Dietler PC, Wineland RE, Marolo NM: Localization of nonpalpable breast lesions detected by xeromammography. Ann Surg 42(11):810–811, 1976.
6. Doberneck RC: Breast biopsy, a study of cost-effectiveness. Ann Surg 192:152–156, 1980.
7. Dodd GD: Pre-operative radiographic localization of non-palpable lesions. *In* Gallagher HS (ed): Early Breast Cancer—Detection and Treatment. New York, John Wiley and Sons, 1975, pp 151–152.
8. Egan RL: Breast biopsy priority: cancer versus benign preoperative masses. Cancer 35(3):612–617, 1975.
9. Eagan RL, McSweeney MB, Sewell CW: Intramammary calcifications without an associated mass in benign and malignant diseases. Radiology 137:1–7, 1980.
10. Egeli RA, Urban JA: Mammography in symptomatic women 50 years of age and under, and those over 50. Cancer 43:878–882, 1979.
11. Frank HA, Hall FM, Steer ML: Preoperative localization of nonpalpable breast lesions demonstrated by mammography. N Engl J Med 295:259, 1976.
12. Frazier TG, Rowland CW, Murphy JT, Woolery CT, Ryan SM: The value of aspiration cytology in the evaluation of dysplastic breasts. Cancer 45:2878–2879, 1980.
13. Gallager HS: Breast specimen radiography: obligatory, adjuvant and investigative. Am J Clin Pathol 64:749–755, 1975.
14. Hall FM, Frank HA: Preoperative localization of nonpalpable breast lesions. AJR 132(1):101–105, 1979.
15. Hassler O: Microradiographic investigations of calcifications of the female breast. Cancer 23:1103–1109, 1969.
16. Hickey RC, Gallager HS, Dodd GD, Samuels BI, Paulus DD, Moore DI: The detection and diagnosis of early, occult and minimal breast cancer. Adv Surg 10:287–312, 1976.
17. Homer MJ, Rangel DM, Miller HH: Pre- and transoperative localization of nonpalpable breast lesions. Am J Surg 139:889–891, 1980.
18. Homer MJ, Fisher DM, Sugarman HJ: Post-localization needle for breast biopsy of nonpalpable lesions. Radiology 140(1):241–242, 1981.
19. Horns JW, Arndt RD: Percutaneous spot localization of nonpalpable breast lesions. Am J Roentgenol 127:253–256, 1976.
20. Jensen SR, Luttenegger TJ: Wire localization of nonpalpable breast lesions. Radiology 132:484–485, 1979.
21. Kalisher L: An improved needle for localization of nonpalpable breast lesions. Radiology 128:815–817, 1978.
22. Kline TS, Neal HS: Role of needle aspiration biopsy in diagnosis of carcinoma of the breast. Obstet Gynecol 46(1):89–92, 1975.
23. Koehl RH, Synder RE, Hutter RVP: The use of specimen roentgenography to detect small carcinomas not found by routine pathologic examination. Cancer 21(1):2–10, 1971.
24. Kolbenstvedt A, Heldaas O: Value of radiography of the remaining breast following mastectomy for carcinoma. Acta Radiol Diagn 14(4):435–441, 1973.
25. Libshitz HI, Feig SA, Fetouh S: Needle localization of nonpalpable breast lesions. Radiology 121:557–560, 1976.
26. Loh CK, Perlman H, Harris JH, Rotz CT, Royal DR: An improved method for localization of nonpalpable breast lesions. Radiology 130:244–245, 1979.
27. McLelland R: Mammography in the detection, diagnosis and management of carcinoma of the breast. Surg Gynecol Obstet 146(5):735–740, 1978.
28. Millis RR, McKinna JA, Hamlin IME, Greening WP: Biopsy of the impalpable breast lesion detected by mammography. Br J Surg 63:346–348, 1976.
29. Moss JP, Voyles RG: Operative localization of the suspicious lesion on mammography. J Ky Med Assoc 76(7):324–326, 1978.
30. Muhlow A: A device for precision needle biopsy of the breast at mammography. Am J Roentgenol Radium Ther Nucl Med 121(4):843–845, 1974.
31. Pollei SR, Mettler FA, Bartow SA, Moradian G, Moskowitz M: Occult breast cancer: prevalence and radiographic detectability. Radiology 163:459–462, 1987.
32. Rogers JV, Powell RW: Mammographic indications for biopsy of clinically normal breasts: correlation with pathologic findings in 72 cases. Am J Roentgenol Radium 115:794–780, 1972.
33. Rosen PP, Snyder RE, Robbins G: Specimen radiography for nonpalpable breast lesions found by mammography: procedures and results. Cancer 34:2028–2033, 1974.
34. Rosen P, Snyder RE, Foote FW, Wallace T: Detection of occult carcinoma in the apparently benign breast biopsy through specimen radiography. Cancer 26(4):944–952, 1970.
35. Roses DF, Harris MN, Gorstein F, Gumport SL: Biopsy for microcalcification detected by mammography. Surgery 87(3):248–252, 1980.
36. Schwartz AM, Siegelman S: A technique for biopsy of nonpalpable breast tumors. Surg Gynecol Obstet 23(6):1321–1322, 1966.
37. Seidman H, Gelb SK, Silverberg E, LaVerda N, Lubera JA: Survival experience in the breast cancer detection demonstration project. CA 37(5):258–290, 1987.
38. Sickles EA, Herzog KA: Mammography of the postsurgical breast. AJR 136(3):585–588, 1981.
39. Simon N, Lesnick GJ, Lerer WN, Bachman AL: Roentgenographic localization of small lesions of the breast by the spot method. Surg Gynecol Obstet 134:572–574, 1972.

40. Synder RE: Specimen radiography and preoperative localization of nonpalpable breast cancer. Cancer 46(4)(suppl):950–956, 1980.
41. Synder RE, Rosen P: Radiography of breast specimens. Cancer 28(6):1608–1611, 1971.
42. Spratt JS, Donegan WL: Surgical management. *In* Donegan WL, Spratt JS (eds): Cancer of the Breast, ed 3. Philadelphia, WB Saunders, 1988, pp 403–416.
43. Stephenson TF: Chilba needle-barbed wire technique for breast biopsy localization. AJR 135:184–186, 1980.
44. Stevens GM, Jamplis RW: Mammographically directed biopsy of nonpalpable breast lesions. Arch Surg 102:292–295, 1971.
45. Urban JA: Biopsy of the "normal" breast in treating breast cancer. Surg Clin North Am 49(2):291–301, 1969.
46. Wallace TI: Radiographic identification of calcifications in breast specimens. Cancer 21(1):11–12, 1971.

Chapter 29

PRIMARY THERAPY FOR BREAST CANCER: SURGICAL PRINCIPLES AND TECHNIQUES

Kirby I. Bland, M.D., Edward M. Copeland, III, M.D., Bernard Fisher, M.D., Eric R. Frykberg, M.D., Scott A. Hundahl, M.D., Jerome A. Urban, M.D., Umberto Veronesi, M.D.

Evolution of Surgical Principles for the Management of Breast Cancer

Eric R. Frykberg, M.D. and Kirby I. Bland, M.D.

> To understand a science it is necessary to know its history
>
> Auguste Comte (1798–1857)

> Let us not lightly cast aside things that belong to the past, for only with the past can we weave the fabric of the future.
>
> Anatole France (1844–1924)

> Those who cannot remember the past are condemned to repeat it.
>
> George Santayana (1863–1952)

> We see so far, because we stand on the shoulders of giants.
>
> Sir Isaac Newton (1643–1727)

ANCIENT RECORDS

Most of the recorded history of carcinoma of the breast has involved the development of thought regarding its biology and pathophysiology and the application of these concepts to a rational treatment. Its description in the earliest medical literature indicates that this disease has always been the relatively common and virulent entity that we know today.

The Edwin Smith Papyrus, discovered at Thebes, Egypt, in 1862, is the oldest known medical document, thought to date from between 3000 B.C. and 2500 B.C. It contains the oldest reference to tumors or ulcers of the breast.[16, 20, 109, 153] Believed to have been written by the first known physician, Imhotep, it describes "bulging tumors" of the breast that were cool, spreading, and hard; had no granulation; formed no fluid; and generated no secretion. These tumors were probably malignant lesions, and it was asserted that "there is no treatment" for them, even though cauterization with a "fire-drill" was used for lesions thought to represent benign cysts or breast abscesses.[32, 109] Writings from India and Assyria that date from this same period also mention breast malignancy.[32] There is no evidence of the application of an operative procedure for breast carcinoma in these ancient records.

The earliest reference to breast carcinoma found in the ancient Greek civilization was made by the historian Herodotus (ca. 484–425 B.C.). He credited the Persian physician Democedes (ca. 525 B.C.) with the successful treatment of a breast tumor that had already ulcerated and spread in Atossa, daughter of Cyrus and wife of Darius.[20, 32, 85, 109] This may represent the first description of local and metastatic spread of cancer, although the fact that it was apparently cured raises doubt that it was a true malignancy.[20, 187] The hindrance of early diagnosis by a woman's fear and cosmetic considerations, a problem that persists to the present day, is also well demonstrated by this anecdote.[109]

Hippocrates, the "Father of Medicine" (ca. 460–370 B.C.), devoted little attention to breast "Karkinoma" in his vast collection of works. His diligent observations of disease processes did include two references to apparently advanced cases of breast malignancy:[20, 29, 109]

"The whole body becomes emaciated . . . When they have gone as far as this, they do not recover, but die of this disease."

This probably also represents an early reference to metastatic breast carcinoma. Hippocrates was the first to distinguish benign from malignant breast neoplasms, applying the latter term to any growth that spread and caused death.[187] He advocated withholding any treatment for "hidden" or deep-seated breast tumors (presumably referring to those that had not yet involved the overlying skin) in view of his observations that medical therapy caused a "speedy death, but to omit treatment is to prolong life." Some have interpreted these hidden cancers to mean those occurring within the body (i.e., metastatic lesions), for which this caution is logical.[29] There is no evidence that surgery was then applied to this disease.

Aulus Cornelius Celsus (ca. 30 B.C.–38 A.D.) was a Roman scholar and encyclopedist who, although not a physician, wrote one of the most extensive surveys of the practice of medicine of that era. This work, *De Medicina*, demonstrated a remarkable insight into the natural history of cancer, particularly as it applied to the breast.[17, 109] He provided one of the first descriptions of the "dilated tortuous veins" that typically surround a tumor,[20] which later led Galen to liken to a crab and apply the label of "cancer."[32] Celsus described four stages in the clinical evolution of breast cancer, the first of which ("cacoethes") represented either an early malignancy or a benign premalignant lesion. He advised treatment only at this stage, first with caustics, followed by surgical excision and cauterization if symptoms improved. In keeping with his Egyptian and Greek predecessors, he advised against any treatment for the three more advanced stages of malignancy, since any surgery seemed to "irritate" the process and hasten the demise of the patient. Despite this cautious approach, it is evident that extensive surgery was commonly carried out for breast carcinoma in this ancient Roman period. Celsus advised against removal of the pectoral muscles if breast amputation were done. He thus indicated the benefits of early detection and treatment and the dangers of surgery for locally advanced disease that were ultimately confirmed some 2000 years later.[20, 29, 109, 187]

Galen (ca. 131–203 A.D.) was a Greek physician whose abundant works on medicine centered around the humoral principle of disease that was first elaborated by Hippocrates. He asserted that cancer was a local manifestation of "melancholia" caused by an excess of black bile in the body. This was the rationale behind his recommendation that all treatment should include purgatives, bleeding, proper nutrition, and a restarting of menstruation (he noted that most cases of breast carcinoma occurred in postmenopausal females). Such a concept represents perhaps one of the earliest views of breast malignancy as a systemic disease requiring systemic treatment and served to explain its poor prognosis at that time.[32, 53] After such treatment, Galen recommended surgical excision of the diseased breast if it was amenable to removal. In what may be the first description of an operation for cancer of any kind, he advised incising the breast through healthy, uninvolved tissue so as to widely encompass the whole tumor without leaving behind "a single root" that would allow recurrence. He

also advised against the use of both ligatures and cautery, since a free flow of blood was thought to maximize the drainage of black bile and thus minimize the chance of local recurrence and spread.[20, 29, 109]

The Greek physician and surgeon Leonides, who worked in the great school of Alexandria around 180 A.D., provided the first detailed factual description of a mastectomy as it was widely practiced during that time. He, like Galen, advocated wide excision of the tumor through normal tissues, but he used cautery to both stem the bleeding and eradicate the disease. The common association of enlarged axillary nodules with breast malignancy was noted in his writings.[20, 32, 153] He was the first to describe nipple retraction as a clinical sign of breast cancer. He advised against surgical intervention in cases of locally advanced disease and also advocated a systemic "detoxification of the body" in both the preoperative and postoperative phases of treatment.[29, 109, 146] His practice of performing mastectomy by alternate incision and cautery persisted largely unchanged for at least the next 1500 years.

Substantial progress was made in these ancient years in understanding the pathophysiology of breast carcinoma and in developing some of the basic surgical principles of its treatment that we still follow today. In the next several centuries further progress was scant, and some concepts were even forgotten.

MEDIEVAL AND RENAISSANCE PERIODS

The humoral theory of disease prevailed throughout the Dark Ages, and a rigid adherence to Galen as the ultimate authority in medical matters prevented any further evolution in the treatment of breast carcinoma. A conservative and nihilistic view of this disease process was held by virtually all medical practitioners. The influence of the Church on all scholarly matters in this era is suggested by the fact that the Council of Tours in 1162 banned the "barbarous practice" of surgery for breast tumors.[20, 32] Cautery, purgatives, and caustic agents served as the mainstays of treatment, as they largely had in the ancient Greek and Roman cultures. The treatises of the Spanish-Arabian surgeon Albucasis (ca. 1013–1106 A.D.) and the French surgeons Henri de Mondeville (ca. 1260–1320 A.D.) and his pupil Guy de Chauliac (ca. 1300–1367 A.D.) reflected Galen's approach to breast malignancy in advocating only a limited role for surgery in those tumors able to be completely removed.[124] De Chauliac emphasized the need for wide excision of these tumors to include all the "rests" of the disease when surgery was indicated. Lanfranc (ca. 1296), the "Father of French Surgery," practiced the same technique for mastectomy that Leonides had described 1100 years before and was largely responsible for this operation becoming the standard treatment for breast cancer in the larger schools of medicine in Europe.[20, 109, 153]

As the Renaissance philosophy of enlightenment and learning spread throughout Europe in the fifteenth and sixteenth centuries, many of the principles that eventually led to the modern era of breast cancer treatment were developed or rediscovered. At the same time, however, several extreme and irrational modes of treatment persisted. The Spanish surgeon Francisco Araceo (1493–1571) cut directly into breast tumors to place a large ligature in an attempt to "dissolve" the disease. Some physicians applied frogs and bisected chickens or puppies to breast tumors. William Clowes (1560–1634), physician to Queen Elizabeth, advocated the laying on of hands by the monarch to cure this disease. Peter Lowe (ca. 1597) applied goat's dung, and James Cooke (1614–1688) advised bleeding from the basilic vein.[20, 32, 109] Incising into a diseased breast and through tumor in a piecemeal approach to removing the malignancy appears to have been commonly practiced during this period. The poor results of this practice, in terms of the rapid recurrence of ulcerating tumors, led Fabricius ab Aquapendente (1537–1619), the famed Italian surgeon and anatomist who was William Harvey's teacher, to condemn partial excisions as worthless. He performed radical excisions of the entire breast, but only when the patient requested it.[20, 109, 190] This idea recalled the advice of Galen and Leonides that breast tumors be widely excised through normal tissue and represented an important conceptual basis for the ultimate evolution of the modern mastectomy.

One of the first scholars of this period to reject the entrenched doctrines of Galen and thus pave the way for a new era of medical progress was Andreas Vesalius (1514–1574), the "Father of Modern Anatomy." He also advocated wide surgical excision of breast tumors but substituted the use of ligatures for cautery in the control of hemorrhage. Ambrose Pare (1510–1590), the French military surgeon and "Father of Modern Surgery," treated large and advanced breast malignancies with milk, vinegar, and ointments in the galenic tradition. He also widely excised smaller tumors, using sulfuric acid instead of hot cautery to control bleeding. He attempted a less mutilating procedure originally introduced by Lenard Fuchs (1501–1566) involving crushing the diseased breast between lead plates.[153] The observation of the probable relationship between breast carcinoma and swelling of the axillary glands was an important advance credited to Pare. His pupil, Bartholemy Cabrol, took a more radical approach to breast cancer by advocating mastectomy and removal of the underlying pectoral muscles, as did Jacques Guillemeau (1550–1601) and Michael Servetus (1509–1553). Servetus, a Spanish surgeon who was burned at the stake by Calvinists, was also perhaps the first to recommend that axillary lymph nodes be removed along with the radical excision of the breast in the treatment of breast carcinoma.[153, 190] This latter idea was also advanced by the Italian surgeon Marcus Aurelius Severinus (1580–1659), who was perhaps the first author since Hippocrates to emphasize the distinction between benign and malignant breast tumors. He also recommended excision of benign lesions to prevent their development into cancers.[27, 32, 109]

The sixteenth and seventeenth centuries were marked by a variety of innovations in the technique of mastectomy for breast cancer that led to a more efficient, thorough, and swift operation in this preanesthetic age.

Wilhelm Fabry von Hilden, also known as Fabricius Hildanus (1560–1624), a German surgeon taught by Vesalius, invented a surgical instrument that compressed the base of the breast to allow easy amputation with a knife. He emphasized the need for tumors to be mobile in order to be candidates for surgery and to avoid leaving behind "sprouts," asserting:[9]

"But before everything we must carefully make out whether the tumour can be shifted and moved from one point to another, and whether it can be radically excised. For the operation will be fruitless if any part of the tumour, however minute—nay, even the membranes in which tumours of this sort are usually enveloped—be left behind. For the disease sprouts up again, and becomes more malignant than ever, while there is no hope that we can remove what remains behind by cauterising."

Fabry also removed axillary lymph nodes as a part of his procedure.[20, 36, 97, 153]

Johannes Scultetus (1595–1645) was another German surgeon whose method of treatment for breast carcinoma involved traction on the diseased breast with cords placed through the base with large needles,[160] allowing complete amputation with a knife (see Figs. 1–7 and 1–8). Bidloo (1708) and Tabor (1721) described similar instruments and methods. In all cases the large open wounds were cauterized, which generally led to a high incidence of infection and death.[29, 32]

The Reverend John Ward described in 1666 a mastectomy performed on a Mrs. Townsend, in which two surgeons bluntly separated a breast tumor from surrounding tissues by hand, after the skin incision. The skin was apparently closed back over the wound temporarily and in the succeeding 2 days reopened several times to allow further removal of more tumor. Several months later the patient died with malignancy still present in the breast, confirming the admonition against piecemeal removal of breast tumors given a century earlier by Fabricius ab Aquapendente.[29, 109, 146] Attempts at this more limited form of operation may have been initiated by a desire to be kinder to the patient by lessening the degree of mutilation and perhaps also to avoid the catastrophic complications from the large cauterized open wounds that took several months to heal if the patient survived. The flaw in these attempts, as noted by Moore two centuries later,[127] became obvious when these tumors quickly recurred and hastened the patient's death, presumably from residual tumor left behind.[20] This observation had been made by Celsus 1600 years earlier. One of the first surgical attempts to allow healing by direct union of the incised skin edges following mastectomy was recorded by Van der Mullen in 1698. The fact that this patient also died contributed to the controversy over the safety of primary wound closure.[29]

THRESHOLD OF THE MODERN PERIOD

One of the greatest impediments to the advancement of knowledge of the treatment of breast carcinoma through these years was in the failure of physicians to keep comprehensive records of their results, the absence of scientific analysis of such results, and the poor communication of ideas among physicians. With the advent of the Age of Enlightenment in the eighteenth century, this situation began to change. The great hospitals of Paris and London became centers of scholarly study in both theoretical and practical aspects of medicine. Formal lectures in anatomy and surgery were instituted, prizes were awarded for scientific research, and in 1731 one of the first surgical societies was founded in France, the Academie de Chirurgie.[29] Its publication, *The Memoires*, was the first journal devoted entirely to surgery, and it pioneered the spread of surgical knowledge throughout Europe.

The systemic theory of origin of breast carcinoma persisted during this period, although derangements of the newly discovered and described lymphatic system replaced Galen's black bile as the stimulating agent.[32, 109, 187] John Hunter (1728–1793) was a proponent of this idea, believing that cancer made its appearance wherever lymph coagulated. He also believed, however, that a local component of disease origin was important in the treatment of breast carcinoma, which required wide excision beyond the grossly visible disease if recurrences were to be avoided.[30] This typified the views of many surgeons of this period, and such views marked the beginning of a trend toward more aggressive and thorough local treatments that ultimately led to greatly improved results for women afflicted with breast cancer. The report of Guillaume de Houpeville in 1693 describing his removal of a breast with surrounding healthy tissue as well as the underlying pectoral muscle, indicated a revival of the radical operation first advocated 150 years before by Cabrol, Guillemeau, and Servetus.[153] Such an operation was not commonly performed at that time, but de Houpeville's report did illustrate the beginning of the idea that breast cancer may initially develop as a localized disease.

One of the greatest contributions to this changing attitude was made by the French surgeon Henri Francois LeDran (1685–1770), who practiced at the Hôpital St. Come. He courageously repudiated the classic humoral theory of Galen, which was still firmly entrenched in the contemporary teachings of medical schools, by asserting in 1757 that breast cancer began in its earliest stages as a local process within the breast proper. As it grew, he believed it spread initially to the regional axillary lymphatics and then to distant sites through the general circulation.[107] He thus claimed that "we may hope for a perfect cure" by an aggressive surgical ablation in its earliest stages. This presaged the benefits of early detection of this disease that were to be well demonstrated more than 200 years later,[161, 162, 170] as well as the benefits of a wide surgical resection of disease that were to be so famously demonstrated by Halsted 150 years later.[68] LeDran's operation included the dissection of enlarged axillary lymph nodes, as previously advocated by Servetus, Severinus, and Fabry. He also recognized the dismal prognostic implications of axillary lymph node involvement by the malignant process.[29, 109, 153, 187] The results of these efforts can only be surmised

by LeDran's statement, characteristic of this period, that he carried out "a great number" of such operations, "many" with success.

Jean Louis Petit (1674–1750) was LeDran's contemporary and was a prominent French surgeon and the first Director of the Academie Francoise de Chirurgie (Fig. 29–1). He is credited by many as being the first to introduce an improved operation for breast carcinoma with the goal of curing the malignancy rather than simply removing an inevitably fatal tumor.[20, 32, 109, 141, 146, 153] His book, *Traites des Operations*, was not published until 24 years after his death. In it he recommended total removal of the breast and of any enlarged axillary lymph nodes as well as the pectoralis major muscle if it was involved by tumor. It is not clear whether the lymph nodes were removed in continuity, but he did begin the operation with their removal.[29] He discouraged the practice of partial and piecemeal removal of tumor and breast tissue that was so prevalent at the time and asserted that "the roots of a cancer (of the breast) were the enlarged lymphatic glands." This principle of wide excision without incising or even viewing the tumor itself recalls the original philosophy set forth by Galen.

Although Petit's operation may be considered the direct forerunner of the modern radical mastectomy in both principle and technique, it did differ primarily in the amount of skin removed. He advised leaving the greater portion of overlying skin, and even the nipple, and dissecting breast tissue out from beneath it. His pupil and colleague, Rene Garangeot (1688–1760), was largely responsible for preserving and spreading the

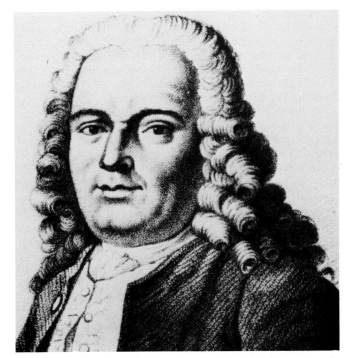

Figure 29–1. Jean Louis Petit (1674–1750), the French surgeon who was the first to apply surgical intervention as a curative modality for breast carcinoma. (From Robinson JO: Am J Surg 151:317–333, 1986. Reprinted by permission.)

teachings of this eminent surgeon who was so far ahead of his time. Garangeot explained the rationale for skin preservation in mastectomy in his own book, *Traite des Operations de Chirurgie* (1720):

"sewing up the lips of the wound immediately after operation, as was practiced by J. L. Petit, is not only the safest method of arresting hemorrhage but is also the quickest way of healing the wound and preventing the return of the cancer."

It probably also served to reduce the considerable number of infectious complications derived from the typically large and open wounds that most surgeons of that era left, although no definitive results were ever published.[146] Petit did recognize the necessity of removing any skin directly involved by the cancer, asserting:[141]

"Where the integuments are also affected and strictly joined to the cancer there is little hope to expect a perfect cure if they are not both cleanly extirpated together."

This further reinforced the principle of wide excision of all clinically evident malignancy. He also recognized the poor prognosis of cervical and supraclavicular lymph node involvement.[109, 153]

These principles of breast carcinoma beginning as a localized disease process and necessitating wide excision of the entire breast and surrounding tissues if cure was to be achieved gained momentum during this period. Lorenz Heister (1683–1758), a famous German surgeon, used a guillotine device to amputate the entire breast. He was also aware of the morbid implications of axillary lymph node involvement. Removal of axillary contents, the pectoralis major muscle, and even portions of the chest wall if necessary for excision of the gross tumor were recommended by him in conjunction with mastectomy.[32, 82, 153] Bernard Peyrilhe (1735–1804) also embraced the concept that breast cancer begins as a local disease in the breast and later spreads by way of the lymphatics.[142] Like Heister and Petit, he advocated the total removal of a cancerous breast along with the axillary contents and pectoralis major muscle.[29, 32, 187]

Samuel Sharpe, an English surgeon, advocated a similarly aggressive approach in his *Treatise on the Operations of Surgery*, published in 1735. He recommended removal of the entire breast through a longitudinal incision for small tumors, although an oval segment of skin was taken for larger tumors in order to facilitate the dissection. He claimed that the breast should be cleaned away from the pectoral fascia and that this operation was impractical if the tumor involved the pectoral muscles. The necessity of removing any "knobs" in the armpit was also asserted by Sharpe, who wrote:[9, 97, 153]

"The possibility of extirpating these knobs without wounding the great vessels is very much questioned by surgeons, but I have done it when they have not laid backwards and deep."

Benjamin Bell (1749–1806), surgeon to the Edinburgh Royal Infirmary, not only advocated a radical operation for all breast tumors but also emphasized the importance of early diagnosis.[28, 109, 146, 153] He echoed Petit's views in his book, *A System of Surgery* (1784), in which he wrote:[12]

"When practitioners have an opportunity of removing a cancerous breast early they should always embrace it, that as little skin as possible should be removed, and that the breast should be dissected off the pectoral muscle, which ought to be preserved. If any indurated glands be observed, they should be removed and particular care should be given to this part of the operation. For unless all the diseased glands be taken away, no advantage whatever will be derived from it."

These principles of treatment of breast carcinoma remained the standard in Scotland for the next century.

Henry Fearon (1750–1825) was a British surgeon of this period who also recognized the importance of early detection of breast carcinoma as well as the unlikely probability of achieving this goal. In 1784 he asserted:[30]

"The early period of the complaint is beyond all doubt the most favorable period for extirpating it, however patients can seldom be convinced that there is any necessity for an operation while the disease continues in a mild state."

In the latter years of the eighteenth century and the first half of the nineteenth century, a greater degree of conservatism and pessimism toward breast carcinoma pervaded the medical literature and the practice of many surgeons. This arose primarily from the poor results of the bold operations described above. William Hunter stated in 1778:[9]

"Amputation of the breast is an easy operation but a doubtful remedy. The little success attending it deters the patient, wherefore it ought not to be undertaken without great probability of cure, as we run the risque of a general prejudice against the operation, which may so affright others that they will not run the hazard, tho' their disease may be really curable."

Thus, although many agreed that the goal of surgery should be the complete removal of the disease, the consensus was that no operation should be performed at all if this goal was not feasible.

The Dutch surgeon Hendrik Ulhoorn asserted in 1747 that even small breast cancers had already spread throughout the body, and there was thus no point in operating on this disease.[29] Such a belief was remarkably similar to the theories of breast carcinoma held more than 200 years later. His contemporary, Petrus Camper, indicated the reluctance of most surgeons at that time to perform mastectomy for breast carcinoma; he reported in 1757 that "not six times a year a breast was amputated with reasonable chance of cure" in Amsterdam, which had a population of 200,000.[29, 31, 153]

The first efforts to record and analyze the results of treatment of breast carcinoma occurred in this period and reinforced these pessimistic attitudes. Most of the literature consisted of case reports of mastectomies. Alexander Monro Senior (1697–1767) reviewed the cases of 60 patients with this disease who had been treated by contemporary methods and found only four patients free of disease after 2 years.[125] He noted that the disease almost always returned either locally or in distant sites soon after operation. Operative mortality alone was reported to be as high as 20 percent, predominantly from sepsis.[32]

The Scottish surgeon James Syme (1799–1870) wrote in 1842 in his *Principles of Surgery* that palliative procedures for carcinoma of the breast should be abandoned when axillary glands are involved or the tumor is too extensive or fixed to allow complete removal.[109, 153, 169] He found that surgery is more likely to "excite greater activity" of the tumor left behind, thus echoing the observations of Celsus nearly 1900 years earlier.

A. Velpeau reviewed this subject in 1856 and listed several authors who had reported dismal results following the treatment of breast carcinoma.[178] According to him, Boyer found four cases of cure out of 100 operations,[29] and Mayo reported only a five percent cure rate. MacFarlane had not seen a single cure after 118 operations. Although Velpeau did not attach great importance to these observations because of their lack of scientific foundation, his own experience led him to believe that a true breast malignancy could not be cured.[28, 153]

Sir James Paget (1814–1899) wrote in 1856 that breast carcinoma was such a hopeless disease that he doubted the substantial mortality and morbidity of its treatment could be justified.[135] He found that women with "scirrhous" carcinoma of the breast actually lived longer without surgical intervention than those who underwent attempts at surgical excision.[29] In 235 cases he had an operative mortality of ten percent and had never seen a cure or a case in which recurrence was delayed beyond 8 years.[109, 153]

Robert Liston (1794–1847) wrote in 1840 that only under the most favorable circumstances should a woman be subjected to operation for breast carcinoma and that it was rash and cruel to remove axillary lymph glands involved with tumor.[111, 153]

The first hospital ward for indigent cancer patients was opened in Middlesex Hospital in London in 1792.[29] The surgeon John Howard provided the major initiative in this effort by arguing that such a ward would not only benefit the patients themselves but would also provide an opportunity to study the natural history of this disease, which could lead to improvements in treatment. Private endowments eventually allowed this goal to be realized by contributing to its development into perhaps the first modern cancer institute. From this establishment came some of the most important advances in our knowledge and experience with carcinoma of the breast in the ensuing years.

By the middle of the nineteenth century, the basic principles for the surgical treatment of carcinoma of the breast had been laid down. Several surgeons had already performed what would later be called the standard radical mastectomy. However, there was no consistency among various surgeons or between different geographic regions in the overall management of this disease or in the specific operations performed. This can be attributed to a less-than-optimal mechanism for widespread communication and dissemination of ideas, a lack of understanding of the basic pathology and pathophysiology of the malignant process, and the poor results of treatment evident in the few scientific analyses available. Advances in these areas were necessary for the evolution of a truly

effective and widely accepted treatment for breast carcinoma.

THE MODERN ERA

Two major advances that paved the way for an effective operation for carcinoma of the breast were the discovery and development of general anesthesia and the dissemination of the germ theory of disease and the principles of antisepsis.[29] These both occurred in the mid to late 1800s. One other series of scientific advances occurred during this same period that led to a basic understanding of tumor biology that many consider the most important contribution to the ultimate development of a rational treatment for breast carcinoma. The widespread use of the microscope led to the birth of cellular pathology, and such scientists as Raspail (1826), Schleiden (1838), Schwann (1838), Muller (1838), and Remak (1852) established the cell as the basic structural and functional unit of normal tissue as well as neoplasms.[109] The growth and behavior of malignancies were found by (among others) Virchow and Leydig to be primarily caused by cell division, thus removing cancer from the realm of body humors. Recamier first used the term "metastasis" in 1829 and also described local tumor infiltration and venous invasion.[187] Rene Laennec (1781–1826) was the first to devise a classification of tumors based on scientific principles. Hannover (1843) and Lebert (1845) first described a "cancer cell," which identified a malignancy and distinguished it from benign growths. Hannover also asserted that these cells could be found circulating in the blood and were responsible for distant metastases.[29, 187]

Virchow believed that these malignant cells originated from connective tissue. The meticulous and extensive studies of Thiersch (1822–1895) and Waldeyer (1872), however, established the epithelial origin of all carcinomas. These investigators also supported the mechanical theory of metastasis, asserting that emboli of cancer cells through the lymphatics and blood stream are responsible for the spread of disease.[187]

These scientific advances fostered an enlightened atmosphere in the second half of the nineteenth century, which led to the reemergence of radical surgery for breast carcinoma. The increasing acceptance of the local theory of origin of this disease and the desire to eliminate its local recurrence further contributed to a decline in pessimistic and fatalistic attitudes and to the establishment of a more rational approach to management. Joseph Pancoast (1805–1882) was a professor of surgical anatomy at Jefferson Medical College in Philadelphia (Fig. 29–2). He revived the teachings of Petit and Bell advocating routine removal of the entire breast for tumors of any size as well as removal of axillary lymph nodes if they were clinically involved. His assertion that the axillary contents should be removed in continuity with the breast represented the first description of an en bloc resection.[28, 29, 136, 146] This was not then a widely held view, as suggested by the fact that Pancoast's successor,

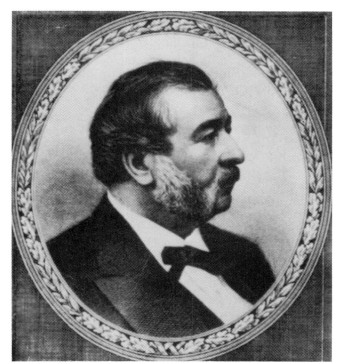

Figure 29–2. Joseph Pancoast (1805–1882), the American surgeon who supported wide breast excision and first described en bloc axillary lymph node dissection. (From Robinson JO: Am J Surg 151:317–333, 1986. Reprinted by permission.)

Samuel D. Gross (1805–1884), felt that "the proper operation is amputation, not excision."[146] Gross taught that as much skin as possible should be preserved and that axillary lymph nodes should not be removed in view of the hopelessness of cure if they were involved.

Thomas Bryant, an assistant surgeon at Guy's Hospital in London, echoed Pancoast's views in 1864.[146] He believed that local recurrence of breast carcinoma was caused by inadequate surgical resection and thus taught that the entire breast along with a wide margin of overlying skin should be removed in all cases of breast carcinoma.

A landmark paper by Charles Hewitt Moore (1821–1870) was presented before the Royal Medical and Surgical Society in London in 1867.[127] Moore was surgeon to the Middlesex Hospital, where he observed several breast cancer patients who had been subjected to the various operations then being practiced for this disease and who had subsequently developed local recurrences. He postulated that since these recurrences were virtually always near the surgical scar, they probably represented direct extension of the primary disease rather than new foci of malignancy. They thus appeared to result from incomplete removal of the disease at the original operation rather than from a systemic predisposition or diathesis. He advocated removal of the entire breast for any breast carcinoma along with a wide margin of overlying skin, especially if there was any doubt as to skin involvement by the tumor. Another principle set

forth in this paper was to avoid cutting into the tumor or even seeing it in the course of its resection so as to prevent any of its cells from lodging in the wound. He also recommended removing "diseased axillary glands" en bloc with the breast, although he later stated that even normal-appearing axillary lymph nodes can never be assumed to be healthy, suggesting that axillary dissection should be a routine part of the operation.[20, 29, 146, 153] He did not recommend removal of the pectoral muscles. It is interesting to note that he reported the placement of a "drainage tube" through the armpit as early as 1858.[146] Moore gave new impetus to the theory of local origin of breast carcinoma with this report, and his remarkable clinical insight into the underlying pathophysiology of this disease served as the foundation on which a standard and widely accepted operation would later be developed.

Richard Sweeting, a British surgeon from Stratford, advocated the same principles of wide excision but extended Moore's operation to include "the lower two-thirds" of the pectoralis major muscle.[168] He did not mention removal of the axillary contents but stated the concept of the local origin of disease by saying:

"For if a purely localized cancer is to be cured by incisions, and is sure to return if not completely removed, then we are more likely to succeed in proportion as our incisions are as deep and as extensive as is consistent with the patient's safety."

He reported three patients who were "cured" by this operation on follow-up of 7 months, 25 months, and 31 months.

Joseph Lister (1827–1912) of Edinburgh, Scotland, revolutionized the surgical approach toward breast carcinoma with his introduction of antiseptic techniques; he also supported the principles laid down by Moore. In 1870 he reported removing the entire breast in continuity with the axillary glands and was the first to describe division of the origins of both pectoral muscles to facilitate the axillary dissection.[110]

In 1877 William Mitchell Banks, surgeon to the Liverpool Royal Infirmary, read a paper before the British Medical Association supporting the principles of Moore and emphasizing the merits of routine axillary dissection in continuity with wide excision of the entire breast.[8, 146] Banks' views were supported by his own clinical experience and that of his contemporaries in attempting to avoid the axillary recurrence that was often noted when the axillary lymph nodes were left in situ. He reiterated Moore's observation that it was impossible to clinically judge axillary node involvement. Also described in his paper was the technique of first removing the breast until it was attached only to the axillary pedicle, which could then be meticulously dissected free of the axillary vein as far as the clavicle (thus recalling the advice of Sharpe more than a century before). He employed "undercutting" of the remaining skin to facilitate primary closure of the wound. He did not find it necessary to divide the pectoral muscles as Lister had but did subscribe to Lister's antiseptic techniques. By 1902, he had performed this operation 300 times and documented the course of 175 patients. In his last 80 consecutive cases he reported only one operative mortality and several ancedotal reports of cure. He also expressed an opinion that was to be increasingly shared by others in subsequent years concerning the desirability to achieve earlier detection of breast carcinoma in order to improve its cure:[9]

"Have you ever imagined what the results would be if all cancers were thoroughly excised when they were no bigger than peas? But if this happy consummation is to be reached, it will not be by performing tremendous operations upon practically hopeless cases."

A German surgeon from Berlin, Ernst Küster (1839–1922), had practiced routine clearance of the axilla in conjunction with mastectomy since 1871.[102] A review of 95 recurrences in his series demonstrated only one in the axilla.[158] Halsted later credited Küster with being the first to advocate routine systematic axillary dissection.[32]

Theodor Billroth (1824–1887), the famous professor of surgery in Vienna, elevated the practice of surgery to a scientific discipline. He related the clinical manifestations of breast carcinoma to its underlying pathophysiology and in this way developed a rational mode of treatment. Although he generally removed the entire breast with the underlying pectoral fascia, he felt that wide local excision of smaller tumors might be just as effective. After removal of the breast he lengthened the incision into the axilla, where he digitally removed any enlarged nodes and the axillary fat pad. He also removed a portion of the pectoral muscle if involved by the tumor.[13] The overall mortality of this operation was 15.7 percent, and it was 21.3 percent in those cases involving axillary dissection. With the introduction of antiseptic wound techniques, these rates were reduced to 5.8 percent and 10.5 percent, respectively. As was characteristic of most mastectomies of this period, 82 percent of Billroth's patients developed local recurrence, and only 4.7 percent had survived by the end of 3 years.[63]

Richard von Volkmann (1830–1889), a German professor of surgery from Halle, was among the first to apply histological observations to the treatment of breast carcinoma. He reported several cases in which the pectoral fascia was involved with tumor that was clinically evident, but microscopic foci were not. This led him to routinely supplement mastectomy and axillary dissection with removal of the pectoral fascia.[181] He also advocated removal of a wide margin of skin as well as a generous portion of underlying muscle if the tumor were fixed to it. In 38 cases of greatly advanced disease, he reported a 14 percent 3-year survival rate and no local recurrence.[109] It was Volkmann's belief that survival without disease for 3 years was a firm indication of cure, an idea that pervaded virtually all studies of this period.[29]

Lothar Heidenhain (1860–1940), an assistant to Küster, reported the histological observation of metastases in lymphatic channels running between the breast and pectoral muscle in two thirds of the cases of breast carcinoma.[81] He believed that contraction of the muscle

was a major route of disease spread. Based on these observations, Heidenhain extended the surgical treatment of this disease to routinely include a superficial layer of the muscle for movable tumors and complete removal of the entire pectoralis major muscle and its underlying connective tissue if the tumor were fixed to it.

Samuel Weissel Gross (1837–1889) was a lecturer in clinical surgery at the Jefferson Medical College in Philadelphia where his father, Samuel D. Gross, had succeeded Pancoast as professor of surgery. Unlike his father, he endorsed the tenets of Pancoast and Moore in advocating total mastectomy, including all skin covering the breast, routine axillary dissection, and excision of the pectoral fascia. This became known as the "dinner plate operation" because of the shape of the wound it left.[109, 146, 153] In his report of 207 patients, he demonstrated a 19.4 percent 3-year survival rate and 53 percent rate of local recurrence, with only a 4.6 percent operative mortality.[58] He also showed that 87.5 percent of all nonpalpable axillary lymph nodes were actually involved with tumor, reinforcing his belief in the necessity of routine axillary dissection.

Sir Henry Butlin provided figures at about this same period from his own experience with carcinoma of the breast that supported a conservative and more selective approach toward axillary dissection.[97, 153] He recommended this procedure only in those cases in which enlarged axillary glands could be palpated. His operative mortality rate (20 percent) and 3-year survival rate (five percent) among 209 women whose axillae were opened were substantially worse than those rates (ten percent and 18 percent, respectively) among 101 women who did not undergo axillary dissection as a part of their operation. He interpreted these figures as indicating that axillary dissection was dangerous, although in retrospect it can be seen that he was describing the more favorable prognosis associated with earlier lesions in which axillary lymph nodes would not be clinically evident. The high operative mortality was typical of that period and was primarily a result of infection.

Johannes Adrianus Korteweg (1851–1930) was a Dutch professor of surgery whose critical approach toward evaluating his operative experience was typical of European surgeons at the end of the nineteenth century.[98, 99] He reviewed the operative mortality and cure rates of surgery for breast carcinoma from several European clinics and made several observations. The widely differing operative procedures and degree of adherence to antiseptic techniques between various surgeons made comparison difficult and largely explained the range of differences in their results.[20] Korteweg noted a lower level of local recurrence before the introduction of listerian antisepsis than after, presumably because of an increasing preference to preserve more skin for primary wound closure once infection became less of a threat. He postulated that some forms of breast carcinoma are more malignant than others, thus foreshadowing our present knowledge of the differences in tumor biology and growth characteristics among different individuals with this disease. He noted the substantially higher 3-year survival rates in patients without axillary nodal involvement than in those with axillary involvement. He also shared a misconception common in the history of medicine, believing that no further improvement could be expected in the cure rates following the treatment of this disease.

Development of the Standard Radical Mastectomy

The evolution of a standardized, effective, and widely accepted operation for the treatment of carcinoma of the breast culminated primarily with the efforts of William Stewart Halsted (1852–1922). Completing his undergraduate education at Yale in 1874 and his medical education at Columbia in 1877, Halsted then spent 2 years (1878–1880) in Europe observing the practice of the noted surgeons of that era (Fig. 29–3). For much of this period he worked in Vienna under Billroth, whose experience he later reviewed along with that of many other European surgeons. He developed a working knowledge of the state of the art of that period in the surgical treatment of breast carcinoma, which predominantly involved Volkmann's operation. He returned to New York with a firm idea, based on his observations and analyses of the results of others, of what the appropriate surgical attack on this disease should encompass.[63] The high rates of local recurrence and low rates of survival of the operations performed by the prominent European surgeons led him to extend the concept of wide excision, based on the theory of local origin of breast carcinoma. Halsted believed these poor results must be caused by an inadequate and inconsistent re-

moval of tissue surrounding the tumor, thus failing to give the malignancy a wide enough berth to avoid leaving any cancer cells behind. He pronounced Volkmann's operation "a manifestly imperfect one."[66] Although Halsted's philosophy toward breast carcinoma was very much like that of Moore and Banks, he never referred to the work of these surgeons in his early reports. This was probably a result of the small circulation of the British journals in which they were published.[146]

The major contribution that Halsted made in this area was his advocacy of the routine removal of the pectoralis major muscle in addition to removal of the entire breast and meticulous clearing of the axillary tissue. He performed all of these maneuvers as an en bloc resection so as to avoid cutting across any cancer-containing tissues. He firmly believed that the spread of cancer was entirely through the lymphatics and not through the blood stream, having been influenced by Heidenhain's studies that showed a high incidence of microscopic involvement of the pectoral muscles with tumor cells. He later asserted:[65]

"From the careful microscopical examination of many very small cancers of the breast I am convinced that the pectoralis major muscle is usually at the time the operation involved in the new growth. Strange to say, no authority so far as I know suggests the advisability of always removing the pectoralis muscle or a portion of it in operations for the cure of cancer of the breast; and still stranger there are many surgeons of the first rank—surgeons in favor of methodically clearing out the axilla—who instead of recommending the excision of the muscle advise the removal of the fascia only from the pectoral muscle . . . Surely it is absurd not to remove the muscle when its fascia is, even to the naked eye, diseased."

Halsted first performed his "complete operation" at the Roosevelt Hospital in New York City in 1882. In 1883 it was used by him in "almost every case" of breast carcinoma, ultimately becoming known as the "radical mastectomy."[32, 63] His first 13 cases were summarized in an article he published on wound healing in 1891.[65] In 1894 he published his landmark study that described in detail both the operation he developed and the follow-up results from his first 50 patients.[66] There were no operative deaths in this series. The local recurrence rate of 6 percent (3 of 50 patients) and the 3-year survival (cure) rate of 45 percent stood in stark contrast to all of Halsted's contemporaries, whose results he meticulously analyzed in this same report (Table 29–1). These results were in spite of his findings that 27 of these 50 patients had been labeled as "hopeless or unfavorable" on presentation, that all had axillary node metastases, and that 10 percent had supraclavicular node metastases. By modern standards, his actual local recurrence rate was 18 percent. A follow-up study of this population by Lewis and Rienhoff in 1932[108] reported this local recurrence rate to have increased to 31.5 percent, which still represented a substantial improvement at that time. Another perspective was provided in 1980 by Henderson and Canellos,[32, 84] whose analysis of Halsted's data showed only an 8 percent disease-free survival at 4 years and no more than a 12 percent overall improvement in

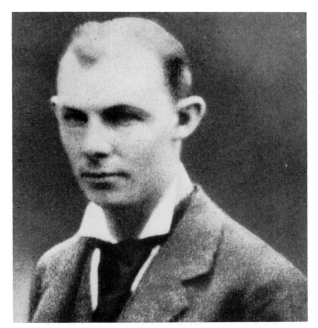

Figure 29–3. William Stewart Halsted (1852–1922) at age 25 upon completion of medical education at Columbia University and internship at Bellevue Hospital in 1877. (Courtesy of Johns Hopkins Hospital.)

Table 29–1. RESULTS OF SURGICAL TREATMENT OF BREAST CARCINOMA UP TO 1894

Surgeon	Time	No. Cases	Local Recurrence (%)	Three Year Cure (%)
Banks	1877	46	—	20
Bergmann	1882–1887	114	51–60	20
Billroth	1867–1876	170	82	4.7
Czerny	1877–1886	102	62	18.8
Fischer	1871–1878	147	75	—
Gussenbauer	1878–1886	151	64	—
Konig	1875–1885	152	58–62	—
Küster	1871–1885	228	59.6	21.5
Lucke	1881–1890	110	66	16.2
Volkmann	1874–1878	131	60	11
Halsted	1889–1894	50	6	45

Compiled from Halsted WS: Johns Hopkins Hosp Rep 4:297–350, 1894–1895; and Cooper WA: Ann Med Hist 3:36–54, 1941.

survival. Halsted himself continued to update his results,[67, 68] which he perceived as vindicating his original premise and reinforcing the then-prevalent concept of breast carcinoma as a disease that arises locally and spreads exclusively via the lymphatics.

Halsted's radical mastectomy involved a wide excision of skin through a teardrop incision extending across the deltopectoral groove onto the arm, excision of the entire pectoralis major muscle, and simple division of the pectoralis minor muscle to expose the axillary contents for dissection (Fig. 29–4). By the time of his follow-up report in 1898,[67] he had extended the operation to routinely include excision of the supraclavicular lymph nodes and pectoralis minor muscle and immediate skin graft of all wounds. He learned this latter technique from Thiersch in Germany and was one of the few in this country at that time to have mastered it. Halsted also described the dissection of mediastinal nodes by his house surgeon, Harvey Cushing, in three cases of recurrent breast carcinoma, prompting his prediction that this would probably be a routine part of the primary operation in the future. Halsted also favored stripping the

fascial sheaths of the rectus, serratus anterior, subscapularis, and latissimus dorsi muscles in locally advanced cases and even indicated that "a part of the chest wall should, I believe, be excised in certain cases."[68]

In 1907, Halsted reported before the American Surgical Association an update of his results on 232 patients who underwent his complete operation at Johns Hopkins,[68] where he had served as professor of surgery since 1891. All patients in this series had been subjected to at least 3 years of follow-up. His operative mortality was 1.7 percent (four patients), and only 18 patients had been lost to follow-up. No axillary lymph node metastasis was found in 64 of these 232 patients, (27.6 percent) and in this group there was a 70 percent overall cure rate (45 of 64 patients) and an 80 percent (51 of 64 patients) 3-year disease-free survival rate. In 15 of these node-negative patients (23.4 percent), metastasis or local recurrence ultimately occurred; six developed such recurrence more than 3 years after treatment. This contrasted with the 24.5 percent cure rate found in those 110 patients with axillary lymph node involvement but negative supraclavicular nodes, and the 7.5 percent cure

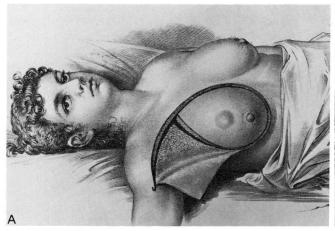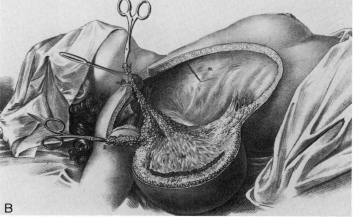

Figure 29–4. A and B, Plates X and XI from Halsted's landmark 1894 paper (Johns Hopkins Hospital Reports, 4:297–350, 1894–1895) showing his incision and dissection for the radical mastectomy. (Courtesy of Johns Hopkins Hospital.)

rate in 40 patients with both axillary and supraclavicular lymph node involvement.

Halsted was pessimistic in this paper about the efficacy of routine supraclavicular node dissection and had abandoned this practice in those cases with no clinical evidence of axillary or neck disease. He stated[68]:

"Before accepting the statement of anyone that he has cured a case of breast cancer with neck involvement, incontrovertible proof should be demanded . . . We should demand as further proof of cure in these positive neck cases that the patient live at least five years after the operation . . . With these stipulations fulfilled I should still be sceptical (sic) as to the cure."

This remarkable 1907 paper contained many of the fundamental precepts that are currently taken for granted. It was evident that the natural history of this disease was more protracted than previously thought. The number of recurrences found more than 3 years after primary treatment led Halsted to first advance the idea that perhaps at least 5 years of survival was a more appropriate measure of "cure." His data also clearly demonstrated the importance of axillary lymph node involvement as a prognostic factor and that the prognosis of breast carcinoma is related to its stage, or level of advancement at the time of diagnosis and treatment. This reinforced the findings of Butlin from several years before. The poor outcome of those patients with supraclavicular node involvement, regardless of the extent of surgery, suggested systemic dissemination, which led Halsted to eventually abandon supraclavicular dissection. By 1910 Halsted made his final modification to the operation, which was the elimination of the upper extension of the incision onto the arm. Instead, he carried his incision straight upward from the circular incision around the breast to the midclavicle.

All these observations emphasized the advantage of early detection of breast carcinoma, a principle strongly advocated by Halsted and one of the most vigorous thrusts of current research. Both the importance and the difficulty of such efforts was accurately described by Halsted:[68]

"But women are now presenting themselves more promptly for examination, realizing that a cure of breast cancer is not only possible, but, if operated upon early, quite probable. Hence the surgeon is seeing smaller and still smaller tumors, cancers which give not one of the cardinal signs . . . It would undoubtedly be possible for the expert to discover of the scirrhous growth earlier stages than he encounters, but unfortunately the tumor must first be recognized by the patient, and a scirrhous cancer large enough to attract her attention has quite surely already gone afield. Our problem, therefore, is to discover these tumors before the afflicted one can do so."

Halsted's operation resulted in the most significant improvement in survival and overall control of breast carcinoma that had occurred up to that time, which was reflected in its rapid and widespread adoption by the turn of the century as the standard treatment for this disease.[153] This was the first time in the long history of treatment of breast carcinoma that any single procedure was uniformly embraced. Halsted's 1907 paper, however, also contained the seeds of the eventual demise of

the radical mastectomy some 70 years later. The fact that 23.4 percent of node-negative patients died of disseminated disease, despite having undergone the complete operation, provided the first indication that the theory of local origin does not adequately explain the underlying biology of this disease. Halsted was troubled by this observation but simply concluded that a more diligent and comprehensive surgical attack and an effort to diagnose the disease at an earlier stage would lead to an improved rate of cure in this group. Further studies in subsequent years were to confirm that metastasis must occur earlier than originally thought (i.e., while the disease is still at a microscopic stage) and that more extensive local excision does not, in fact, improve the approximately 20 percent rate of relapse in stage I patients.[37, 43] This aspect of breast cancer biology led eventually to a diminished emphasis on ever wider and more extensive surgical excision in the initial treatment of primary disease.

The end of the nineteenth century provided an atmosphere of enlightenment and scientific approaches to disease that allowed the principles of breast cancer surgery to take root and flourish. In fact, in 1894 a professor of surgery at the New York Postgraduate Medical School, Willy Meyer (1858–1932), reported the details of an operation very similar to Halsted's radical mastectomy before the Section on Surgery of the New York Academy of Medicine.[122] Meyer (Fig. 29–5), born and educated in Germany, had independently conceived this operation based on the observations of Heidenhain

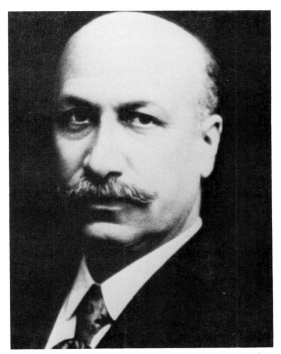

Figure 29–5. Willy Meyer (1858–1932), German-born New York surgeon who conceived of and performed radical mastectomy independently of Halsted in 1894. (From Ravitch MM: A Century of Surgery, Vol 1. Philadelphia, JB Lippincott, 1980, p 612. Reprinted by permission.)

and many of the other European surgeons who had also influenced Halsted.[2] Meyer's report was given only 10 days after the publication of Halsted's landmark paper on the "complete operation," although Meyer had performed his first fully developed operation only 2 months before and had performed only six other similar operations since 1891. The basis of Meyer's operation, like Halsted's, was the en bloc removal of the entire breast, pectoralis muscles, and axillary contents. Meyer advocated the routine removal of the pectoralis minor muscle, a modification later adopted by Halsted,[67] and began his operation with the axillary dissection so as to minimize tumor manipulation and lymphatic dissemination. Although he did not excise the supraclavicular lymph nodes at that time, he did add that to his procedure after reading Halsted's paper. He left more skin than did Halsted and sutured as much of the skin together as possible (Fig. 29–6). He grafted skin to any remaining defect only after 8 to 10 days in order to allow a bed of granulation tissue to develop. Drainage tubes were routinely placed in the axilla. Overall he preferred his method to that of Halsted since it seemed to be "more anatomical," although he recognized "Halsted's unprecedented percentage of cures." Meyer concluded:[122]

"That this kind of radical operation will be 'the' operation for the extirpation of carcinoma of the breast, there can be no doubt . . . I venture to hope that, by absolutely and continuously working everywhere around the seat of disease, by never trespassing on the belly of the muscles, and always removing the latter completely, this extremely gratifying result might also be secured by others.

"Thus will then, at last, it is to be hoped, also this terrible foe of suffering mankind, this dread especially of the female sex, become oftener silenced and made more submissive to the surgeon's knife, provided the operation is done early, before remote parts of the system have become infected."

Here is still another independent observation recognizing the value of early detection and treatment of breast carcinoma.

Meyer published an update of the results of his operation after a 10-year experience with 72 procedures in 70 patients.[123] His only modifications included supraclavicular dissection in those cases of upper quadrant tumors and preservation of a portion of the pectoralis minor muscle to facilitate skin grafting. The operation took an average of 30 minutes to perform, with one case being done in 12 minutes. He reported a 1.4 percent operative mortality (one patient who had died of diabetic coma). Follow-up results were available for 67 patients, 30 (44.8 percent) of whom were alive at the time of his report. Twenty-four (35.8 percent) of these survivors were disease free, and six had developed local, regional, or distant recurrence. Of the 30 study patients with a 5- to 10-year follow-up, eight (26.7 percent) were still alive, of whom seven (23.3 percent) were disease free, and one had developed a regional recurrence 8 years after surgery. There was a 50 percent disease-free survival (14 of 28 patients) among those patients followed for 1 to 3 years. Thirty-five patients (52.3 percent) had died of their disease. Twenty-seven of those who died had distant metastases, accounting for 40.3 percent of all 67 traceable patients, while four died with regional recurrence, and the remaining four died with both local recurrence and distant metastasis. Meyer concluded this paper, as he did his original report, with an observation on the value of early detection:[123]

"I am convinced that final results could be further improved only, if we could get patients to come earlier for operation. The important task before us, therefore, is that of educating the public. . . . In view of the excellent results that can be obtained by radical operation . . . physicians, too, should advise early operation, not only in the plainly recognizable cases, but also in the doubtful ones, rather than keep such patients under observation until the disease has become manifest beyond question, and, perhaps, developed to a stage where it is beyond surgical reach."

Meyer was perhaps the first to believe in an immunological basis for cancer, an idea that developed from

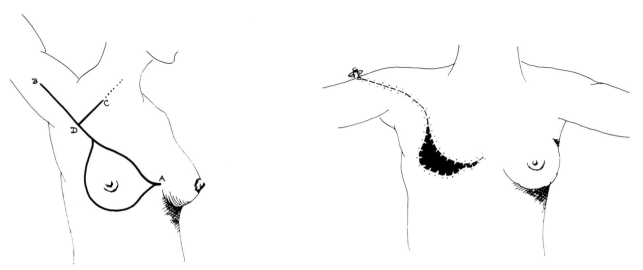

Figure 29–6. Meyer's incision and closure for his radical mastectomy. (From Meyer W: JAMA 45:297–313, 1905. Copyright, 1905, American Medical Association. Reprinted by permission.)

his observation of the regression of a case of ulcerating breast carcinoma after the patient had developed and recovered from erysipelas.[2] He developed this thesis in his book, *Cancer,* published in 1931, and came to regard this disease as a systemic process, thus reviving a theory found in ancient writings that had not been prevalent for more than 200 years.

An obscure report in *The Lancet* of February 4, 1893, is cited by Donegan[32] as evidence that other surgeons were performing similar radical breast excision at the time of both Halsted's and Meyer's papers, perhaps even predating them. This report related a presentation by the British surgeon Arbuthnot Lane before the Clinical Society of London in 1893,[104] which described his operation as involving en bloc excision of the breast, underlying pectoral muscles, and complete clearance of axillary contents:

"By these means not only were the primary growth and the cancerous glands removed, but, also, all the lymphatic channels along which infection had extended."

Halsted has nevertheless been accorded the primary credit for the radical mastectomy in view of his meticulous and diligent correlation of the pathophysiology of breast carcinoma with an appropriate surgical attack as well as the esteem he engendered in his surgical pupils, who then became effective disciples of his technique.[29, 109, 153] Matas explained Halsted's prominence in this field by stating:[118]

"Though old the thought and oft expressed, 'tis his at last who says it best."

In the first decade of the twentieth century, several surgeons published their experiences with the radical mastectomy, indicating again how rapidly and widely it was accepted (Table 29–2). One of the most comprehensive such reports was published by J. Collins Warren of Boston in 1904,[185] describing the results of 100 consecutive cases of breast carcinoma accumulated during a 20-year period in which at least a 3-year follow-up was available. There was only a 2 percent operative mortality among these patients, a 6 percent rate of local or regional recurrence, and a 30 percent rate of cure at 3 years. In following patients beyond 3 years, Warren found only a 12 percent rate of cure at 5 years and 5 percent at 10 years, leading him to assert that "the three year limit does not by any means constitute an infallible test of cure." He found that 56 percent of all locoregional recurrences that occurred did so within 5 years of surgery, and 37 percent occurred within 2 years. At the time of his report, nine patients treated for local recurrence were still alive and well, two of them living for 10 and 16 years, respectively, after resection of these recurrences. This was perhaps the first indication that local recurrence is not necessarily the inevitable death knell that past authors had suggested. Skin involvement by the primary tumor had been noted in 17 percent of patients. Among 17 patients who had no axillary lymph node involvement, a 64 percent rate of cure was observed. An 8 percent rate of bilateral breast malignancy was also observed in this population. Another important observation made by Warren in this series was that the preoperative duration of symptoms did not appear to influence the prognosis.

Warren's first 50 cases had involved only total mastectomy with excision of the pectoral fascia and axillary lymph nodes, while his last 50 patients were subjected to the "Halstedian operation." Interestingly, there was no difference in the overall survival of these two groups. In actuality, Warren's procedure more closely approximated that of Meyer in that the axillary dissection was carried out first. He also added a hook-shaped lateral extension onto Halsted's classic racket-shaped (teardrop) incision (Fig. 29–7) and extended an incision onto the neck of several patients for supraclavicular node excision. This latter portion of the procedure was eventually abandoned by him, as it was by Halsted about this same time. Although Warren believed, as did Halsted, that "any method which permits of an easy approximation of the edges of the wound is out of date," he was nevertheless able to close most of his wounds

Table 29–2. RESULTS OF RADICAL OPERATION FOR THE TREATMENT OF BREAST CARCINOMA SINCE 1904

Author	Date	No. Cases	Operative Mortality (%)	Loco-regional Recurrence (%)	Five Year Survival (%)
Warren[185]*	1904	100	2	6	12
Meyer[123]	1905	72	1.4	9	26.7
Greenough[56]*	1907	376	3.6	47.7	11.2
Halsted[68]	1907	232	1.7	19.5	30.9
Ochsner[133]*	1907	98	3	—	18.4
Lee[150]	1924	75	—	—	15
White[186]	1927	157	—	22.6	36
Harrington[78]	1929	2083	0.76	—	34
Jessop[91]	1936	217	3.2	—	48
Rodman[154]	1943	132	—	2.2	46
Taylor[172]	1950	2000	0.65	—	51
Haagensen[62]	1951	495	1.8	22.8	58.2

*Includes a mixture of cases, some of which were subjected to "complete" operations, others to lesser procedures.

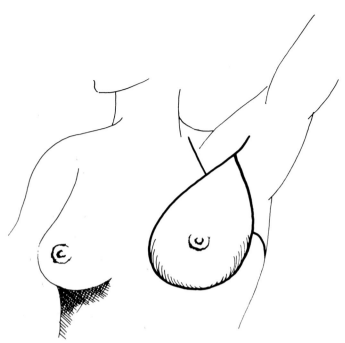

Figure 29–7. Incision used by J. C. Warren of Boston for radical mastectomy. (From Warren JC: Ann Surg 40:805–833, 1904. Reprinted by permission.)

primarily by extensive mobilization of flaps and the opposite breast (Fig. 29–8). He thus made use of those same "plastic procedures" decried by Halsted,[68] yet increasingly utilized by most other surgeons for primary wound closure. A unique addition introduced by Warren was his insistence that a pathologist be present in the operating room throughout the procedure to confirm that all margins were free of tumor before completion of the dissection.

In 1906 Jabez N. Jackson of Kansas City, Missouri, published a detailed description of his own modification of the radical mastectomy, which he had performed on eight patients.[89] His operation involved a circular incision encompassing most of the breast skin and extending into the axilla and superiorly toward the supraclavicular area (Fig. 29–9). He also began his dissection at the axilla. This incision allowed a ready mobilization of flaps for primary closure of the wound as well as elimination of dead space in the axilla (Fig. 29–10).

Albert J. Ochsner of Chicago published in 1907 the results of his surgical treatment of breast carcinoma in 98 patients who were able to be followed out of a total of 164 patients treated.[133] He reported 54 patients (55 percent) still alive at intervals ranging from 1 to 13 years after surgery, with 36 of these being within 5 years of operation. Only five patients were alive 10 or more years after surgery. There was only a 3 percent (five of 164) operative mortality in this population. This paper typified the problems with many reports of this period in that it included patients of differing stages of disease and subjected to different operative procedures. Ochsner's results dated back to 1887, and he did not perform his first radical mastectomy until 1896. Almost one third of his patients, therefore, underwent lesser procedures,

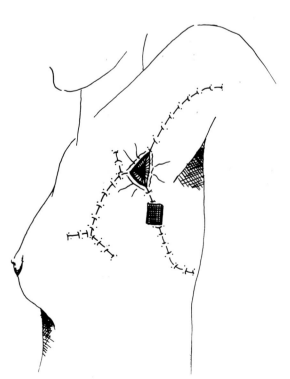

Figure 29–8. Warren's closure following radical mastectomy. (From Warren JC: Ann Surg 40:805–833, 1904. Reprinted by permission.)

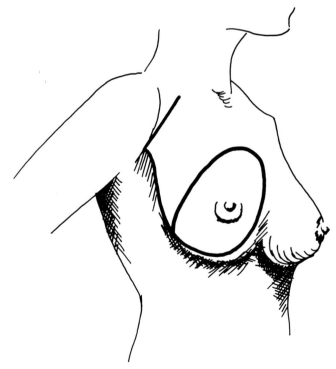

Figure 29–9. Jabez Jackson's incision for radical mastectomy. (From Jackson JN: JAMA 46:627–633, 1906. Copyright 1906, American Medical Association. Reprinted by permission.)

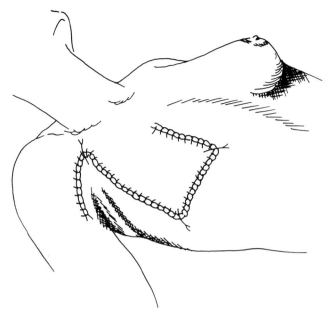

Figure 29–10. Jackson's closure following radical mastectomy. (From Jackson JN: JAMA 46:627–633, 1906. Copyright 1906. American Medical Association. Reprinted by permission.)

usually involving only total mastectomy and axillary dissection.

Robert B. Greenough, a Boston surgeon on the faculty of Harvard Medical School, presented "The Results of Operations for Cancer of the Breast at the Massachusetts General Hospital from 1894 to 1904" before the American Surgical Association in 1907.[56] There were 416 primary operations for breast cancer during this period, of which 376 patients (90 percent) could be adequately traced for long-term follow-up. These operations were performed by 20 different surgeons (one of whom was J. C. Warren). Only 160 patients had undergone a "complete operation," while a "semi-complete" procedure (differing only in that the pectoralis minor muscle was left in place) was performed in 75 patients. "Incomplete" procedures, which lacked any one of the essential elements of a radical mastectomy, were performed in 85 patients, and 56 patients with hopelessly advanced disease underwent palliative procedures that probably left tumor behind. The 3-year survival rate in this last category was, predictably, only 7 percent. Paradoxically, though, a 25 percent 3-year disease-free survival rate was found in the "incomplete" and "semi-complete" groups, while the "complete" group showed only a 16 percent rate. The authors attributed this difference to selection bias, again indicating the problem with failing to stratify a study population according to stage of disease. The overall operative mortality was 3.6 percent, dropping from 5.1 percent in the first 5 years to only 2 percent in the last 5 years. The overall disease-free survival rate at 3 years, excluding the palliative group, was 21 percent and in the last 5 years of the study was 26 percent. Of the 64 patients alive and well 3 or more years after operation,

42 (65.6 percent) had survived 5 or more years, and 17 (26.6 percent) had survived 10 or more years. Almost 50 percent of the patients evaluable for recurrence (126 of 264) developed local chest wall recurrence, and the authors noted that local recurrence was least likely to be found in those having the widest and most complete primary resections. Seventeen (19 percent) of the 88 patients free of disease at 3 years developed recurrence later; in four cases recurrence occurred more than 6 years after operation. This led to speculation that 3-year disease-free survival was probably not an adequate measure of cure.

Greenough et al.'s paper documented several clinical features associated with a poor prognosis, all of which were later recognized to be ominous signs.[60, 61] These included skin involvement, ulceration, axillary gland involvement, supraclavicular gland involvement (in which group there was not a single cure), bilateral cancer, and chest wall or axillary vein attachment. Also, like Warren, these authors found that preoperative duration of disease did not seem to influence prognosis.

In 1950 Taylor and Wallace updated this experience at the Massachusetts General Hospital.[172] They analyzed 2500 cases of women with primary breast carcinoma, 2000 of whom had undergone radical mastectomy. A greater degree of uniformity was apparent in this study population, since patients with Greenough's unfavorable factors were eliminated from study. The operative mortality decreased to 0.65 percent. They reported a 51 percent overall 5-year "cure" rate. Those without axillary nodal involvement had a 77 percent rate of cure, while axillary involvement resulted in a 33 percent cure rate. Again, axillary node status was shown to be a significant prognostic factor. There was still a 76 percent cure rate if only one or two axillary nodes were involved.

These survival figures for breast cancer must be viewed within the context of what is known of the natural history of this disease. Bloom et al. in 1962[14] reviewed the clinical courses of 250 women with a confirmed diagnosis of breast carcinoma who had been admitted to the Middlesex Hospital Cancer Ward between 1805 and 1933 and were not treated. He found a median survival of 2.7 years from the onset of symptoms, with 20 percent alive at 5 years, 5 percent alive at 10 years, and approximately 1 percent still alive at the end of 15 years (Fig. 29–11). Thus radical mastectomy in some series at the turn of this century did not appear to influence survival at all.

Theories of Metastatic Dissemination

The perceived means by which carcinoma of the breast spreads throughout the body has, appropriately, always influenced its primary surgical treatment. The ancient belief that malignancy represented a systemic affliction mediated through bodily humors[53] persisted into the nineteenth century, when it was reinforced by Virchow's assertion that cancer was disseminated by a toxic fluid from the primary neoplasm.[180] This philosophy led to a pessimistic attitude toward the local surgical ablation of

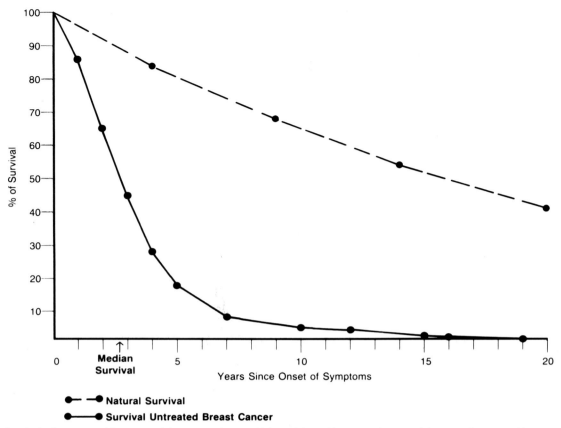

Figure 29–11. Survival of women with untreated breast carcinoma. (Adapted from Bloom et al: Natural history of untreated breast cancer (1805–1933). Br Med J 2:213–221, 1962.)

breast carcinoma. In the late nineteenth century, Thiersch and Waldeyer demonstrated that metastasis occurred through a seeding of distant organs with cells of the primary tumor by way of embolization through the lymphatics and blood stream.[187] This formed the basis of the "mechanical theory" of tumor dissemination that was widely accepted at the beginning of the twentieth century.

William Sampson Handley (1872–1962) was a British surgeon at London's Middlesex Hospital who made a meticulous study of the pathological anatomy of the lymphatic circulation and cancer dissemination and applied his observations to the clinical management of carcinoma of the breast (Fig. 29–12). He extended the principle first espoused by his predecessor, Charles H. Moore, asserting that cancer cells spread centrifugally from the primary tumor, but more through continuous permeation of the lymph vessels rather than through episodic embolization. He believed that the lymphatics were the sole route by which this dissemination occurred, referring to earlier studies that indicated that blood-borne tumor cells are routinely destroyed by their stimulation of a thrombotic process.[32, 97, 187] According to Handley's theory, regional lymph nodes act as filters for these permeating cancer cells, and only after the cells are able to grow beyond them are they capable of reaching the blood stream for embolic spread. These

principles contributed to the idea that breast cancer begins as a local process within the breast proper and then spreads in an orderly, stepwise fashion first to the regional lymphatics and then to distant sites. This formed the conceptual basis for radical mastectomy, because according to this theory, complete ablation of all tissues through which the lymphatics travel provided the only chance of curing the disease as long as it is not so advanced as to already have reached distant sites through the blood stream. It also supported the practice of excising all tissues in continuity, so as not to cut across and disperse the tumor-filled regional lymphatics. Not surprisingly, Halsted embraced and endorsed Handley's theory,[68] and its publication in Handley's first book on breast cancer in 1906[75] represented a significant contribution to the management of this disease that affected surgical practices throughout the world.[153] Handley recommended the modification of Halsted's operation to include lesser areas of skin and greater portions of the deep fascia in order to more fully encompass the offending lymphatics.[20]

One of Halsted's major concerns, derived from the mechanical theory of tumor dissemination, was the danger of manipulating a breast malignancy, especially for purposes of diagnosis. Moore had voiced these same concerns some 30 years earlier. Halsted asserted:[67]

"Tumors should never be harpooned, nor should pieces

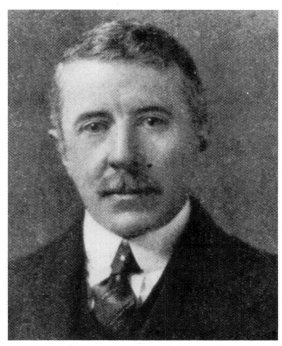

Figure 29–12. William Sampson Handley (1872–1962), surgeon to Middlesex Hospital, whose permeation theory of breast cancer dissemination was embraced by Halsted. (Courtesy of Middlesex Hospital, London.)

even be excised from malignant tumors for diagnostic purposes. Think of the danger of rapid dissemination of the growth from . . . snipping off a piece of the tumor with scissors.

"In studying the published histories of cases of malignant tumors, particularly sarcoma, I have been impressed with the great number of cases in which general dissemination of the neoplasm has seemed to follow swiftly upon exploratory incisions.

"Breast tumors should not be incised on the operating table prior to their removal. The surgeon must learn to recognize malignant tumors not only with the microscope, but also with his naked eye and fingers.

". . . If the surgeon cannot, in a given case, make a diagnosis prior to operation . . . he should excise the breast or, at least, give the tumor a wide berth. If then, on incision, the tumor proved to be malignant, the complete operation should be performed immediately."

These concerns were supported by experimental evidence, published in 1913, of tumor dissemination after manipulation of breast tumors in the Japanese waltzing mouse,[173] although this was never corroborated in humans.

The perceived necessity for a one-stage operation that encompassed both the diagnostic biopsy and definitive procedure led to the development at Johns Hopkins of the frozen section examination. William H. Welch is credited with first using this technique in 1891 on a patient operated on by Halsted for a benign breast tumor.[153] In 1895 a detailed description of this technique was published.[23] The one-stage procedure was to remain the standard approach to diagnosis and surgical man-

agement of primary breast carcinoma for the next 80 years.

Handley's permeation theory eventually was discredited in favor of the original theory of tumor cell embolization.[97] J. H. Gray[55] showed in an extensive series of observations that cancer cells can only rarely be found along the entire course of a lymphatic channel, a well-known observation that Handley explained by postulating that an obliterative lymphangitis obscured cancer cells.[76] He also found that the deep fascia was virtually devoid of lymphatics, contrary to Handley's assertion. Abundant evidence also accumulated of the existence of cancer cells in the circulating blood,[6, 33] which is now felt to be the primary route of metastatic dissemination. These changing attitudes toward the underlying biology of breast carcinoma were among many that led in ensuing years to changing attitudes toward the extent of surgery necessary to control the disease.

Results and Modifications of Radical Mastectomy

Halsted made very little modification to his procedure during the 40 years that he performed it. Supraclavicular dissection, mediastinal dissection, and stripping of the fascia of the rectus and serratus muscles were all temporary additions that he eventually abandoned. In 1913 he published a fourth paper on breast cancer that summarized the technique and advantages of skin grafting in radical mastectomy, a part of the procedure to which he remained firmly committed.[63, 69] His last paper, published in 1921, dealt with lymphedema of the arm following radical mastectomy.[70] He emphasized the meticulous attention that must be paid to suturing the flaps and grafts without tension and to avoiding infection, both of which he believed to be major factors in the development of arm edema. As mentioned earlier, he had already abandoned the extension of his incision onto the arm in an effort to avoid arm edema.

Most of the modifications made by other surgeons to Halsted's procedure were relatively minor and unimportant but served to reinforce the essential principles he espoused,[20] which remained widely accepted and practiced well beyond his death in 1922 (Fig. 29–13). In fact, the operation done by most surgeons during the next several decades resembled Meyer's procedure more than Halsted's, especially in the sacrifice of lesser areas of skin to usually allow primary closure. F. T. Stewart[164] introduced the transverse incision in 1915.

In 1924 Burton J. Lee, a surgeon at the Cornell Medical School in New York, presented before the American Surgical Association the first survival curve for treated breast carcinoma.[150] Seventy-five of 87 cases were available for a long-term follow-up, which showed a 15 percent 5-year recurrence-free survival. Like many other surgeons of this period, he advocated abandoning the 3-year standard for defining "cure."

In 1929 Stuart W. Harrington of the Mayo Clinic (Fig. 29–14) updated the results of operation for primary

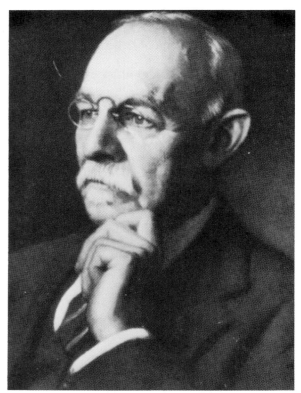

Figure 29–13. William Stewart Halsted shortly before his death at age 70. (From Robinson JO: Am J Surg 151:317–333, 1986. Reprinted by permission.)

breast carcinoma[78] that had originally been reported by Judd and Sistrunk in 1914.[92] In 2083 operations, he reported an operative mortality of only 0.76 percent. Axillary lymph node involvement was clearly demonstrated in this series to be "the most important factor in the prognosis" of breast carcinoma, a principle that has remained valid up to the present.[39, 167, 177] Those without lymphatic involvement had an overall 3-year survival rate of 74.7 percent and a 10-year survival rate of a 44.1 percent, while those patients with regional lymph node involvement had a 39 percent 3-year survival rate and a 13.4 percent 10-year survival rate. Harrington's skin incision was not uniform but was tailored to the extent of disease in each individual case. He made a vertical incision for upper or lower quadrant lesions (Fig. 29–15) and a transverse incision for lateral or medial lesions, approaching this part of the procedure with the following philosophy:

"I believe it important to make a wide excision of the skin, and, if the margins cannot be approximated, I graft skin. This, however, is not often necessary if the incision is properly planned, except in extensive cases."

Harrington found a gradual improvement in survival from this operation up to 1915, which he attributed to "improvement and standardization of technic and the gradual increase of the operative procedure." After 1915 these results reached a plateau, indicating the limits of surgery for this disease. There was an 80 percent 3-year

survival rate and 53 percent 10-year survival rate among those undergoing primary radical operation without axillary nodal involvement, representing the best results obtained up to that time. He also observed the failure of various extensions to the operation, such as supraclavicular dissection, excision of the contralateral axillary nodes, and removal of the opposite breast, to improve results.

Harrington made several observations in this paper that were to become important issues in the future. Five patients who were pregnant at the time of operation had poor outcomes, leading him to an ultimately misguided conclusion that pregnancy represents a poor prognostic factor. A group of 112 patients who had undergone inadequate forms of treatment before having a radical operation at the Mayo Clinic had substantially lower survival rates than those undergoing radical operation initially, demonstrating the validity of Moore's original thesis published more than 60 years earlier. There were 51 patients with bilateral malignancy, in whom it was found that the second malignancy did not have any additional adverse effect on survival. In 1092 cases "roentgen ray" treatment was used in addition to radical operation without any demonstrable benefit on survival, which was to be expected with the state of knowledge at that time as indicated by Harrington's statement:

"If the radical operation is performed, it should accomplish what the term implies, complete removal of the diseased tissue, and should not depend on the roentgen ray to destroy remaining malignant tissue. . . . The best opportunity of eradicating the malignant disease is at the first operation and the magni-

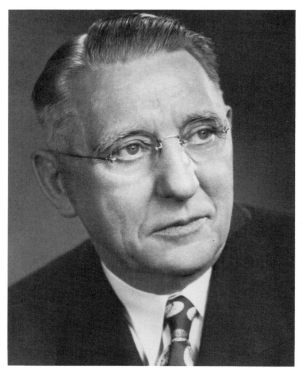

Figure 29–14. Stuart W. Harrington of the Mayo Clinic. (Courtesy of Mayo Clinic, Rochester, MI.)

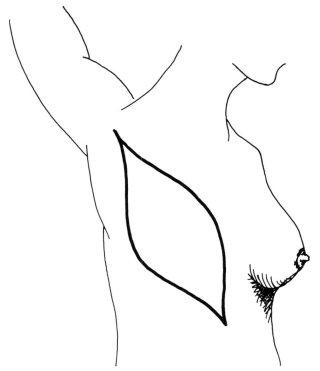

Figure 29–15. The vertical skin incision of S. W. Harrington of the Mayo Clinic. (From Harrington SW: JAMA 92:208–213, 1929. Copyright 1929, American Medical Association. Reprinted by permission.)

tude of this operation must be sufficient to remove all of the diseased tissue. The prognosis depends on the possibility of accomplishing this."

Thus Harrington understood the fact that radiation therapy was strictly a modality for local control of disease that should not substitute for an incomplete or poorly done operation. Since breast cancer is a systemic illness that ultimately kills the patient, radiation treatment should have no effect on survival.

Harrington also emphasized the benefits of early detection of disease, which were evident in his statistics relating survival to lymph node involvement. He was concerned that the incidence of lymph node involvement had actually increased from 59 percent before 1915 to 67 percent since then, suggesting that patients were presenting at later stages of disease. He stated:

"The results in these cases can be greatly improved if operation is performed early in the course of the disease. If operation is delayed until the signs of malignancy are obvious, it is too late to expect much more than a palliative result. There are few if any single tumors of the breast in which delay in the institution of treatment is safe for the patient, and few physicians care to assume the responsibility of determining the presence or absence of malignancy by the physical characteristics of the tumor."

He also supported Halsted's belief that in doubtful cases a definite diagnosis must be made by wide excision of the tumor, microscopic examination, and immediate radical operation in one stage if the lesion is malignant.

J. Stewart Rodman of Philadelphia published in 1943 the results of 132 women who had undergone a modification of the Halsted radical mastectomy first proposed in 1908 by William L. Rodman.[154] This procedure combined a wide removal of skin with the ability to close the wound in virtually every case and resulted in a negligible incidence of arm edema or limitation of arm function. Rodman reported a 2.2 percent incidence of local recurrence, among the lowest reported in the literature, and a 46 percent disease-free 5-year survival (63.5 percent in those without axillary metastasis).

In 1927 William Sampson Handley (see Fig. 29–12), still devoting his career at London's Middlesex Hospital to the investigation of breast carcinoma, published a report that revived an awareness of the internal mammary and mediastinal lymph node chains as a route of metastatic dissemination.[77] He observed that despite the lower incidence of local recurrence (especially in the axilla) following radical mastectomy, involvement of axillary lymph nodes with tumor was still predictive of death from disseminated disease. Most of the recurrences in his patients occurred along the sternal border of the excised breast, from which he concluded that these lymph nodes must be seeded with microscopic deposits of tumor quite early in the course of the disease. The extent of surgical treatment would have no influence on outcome in these patients unless these nodes were also treated. Handley did not believe that surgical excision was appropriate in view of the time and morbidity it added to the radical mastectomy, but he did advocate the routine placement of radium tubes along the sternal border as an adjunct to mastectomy. This practice resulted in a 56.5 percent disease-free survival at 3 years, which he considered to be a significant improvement over the 47 percent 3-year survival in his patients not subjected to this treatment. He also noted that local recurrences only rarely occurred in the sites where radium had been inserted.

Following World War II, Handley's son, Richard S. Handley (1909–1984), published the results of his practice of routine biopsy of the internal mammary lymph nodes in all cases of carcinoma of the breast.[71, 72] In 119 patients, these nodes were involved with metastases in 34 percent of patients overall and in 48 percent of those with axillary lymph node metastasis. He felt this explained both the recurrence of disease when radical mastectomy is performed for "early" lesions and the fact that the lungs and pleura are the most common sites of distant metastasis. However, Handley seemed skeptical about the possibility of surgically eradicating these nodes, much as his father had been.[73]

The implications of Handley's observations, that one third of all mastectomies are doomed to failure from the start, led some surgeons to advocate treatment of breast carcinoma with an "extended" radical mastectomy, which included an en bloc resection of the internal mammary lymph nodes. The first to do this routinely was the Italian surgeon Margottini in 1948,[32, 116] although Halsted had described this being done in three cases by his house surgeon, Harvey Cushing, in 1898.[67].

In 1952 Jerome Urban published his initial experience

with radical mastectomy in continuity with en bloc internal mammary dissection at Memorial Hospital in New York.[175] He developed this procedure after observing that more than 70 percent of chest wall recurrences following radical mastectomy occurred in the medial parasternal area.[174] There was one operative mortality among 57 patients who underwent this procedure and no local recurrences, with 28 patients (49 percent) having internal mammary node metastasis. Like Handley, he found that medial quadrant lesions had the greatest risk of internal mammary involvement. Although the short follow-up period did not allow any assessment of survival, Urban postulated a significant improvement and even considered the following:

"The next step to be considered is the further extension of this procedure to include en bloc dissection of the lymphatic-bearing tissues at the base of the neck."

Wangensteen and associates had already been performing a "super-radical" mastectomy including supraclavicular, internal mammary, and mediastinal lymph node dissection.[183, 184] They found that 58 percent of their cases of operable breast carcinoma had internal mammary node involvement, but they were unable to demonstrate any significant improvement in survival with this procedure. Because of a 12.5 percent operative mortality, they abandoned the procedure in treating breast carcinoma.

Dahl-Iversen published several reports from Denmark detailing an operation that also combined radical mastectomy with supraclavicular and internal mammary dissection, although these extensions were not performed in continuity.[24-26] Prudente[149] described upper extremity amputation en bloc with radical mastectomy for locally advanced disease.

In 1964, E. D. Sugarbaker published a retrospective review of 156 extended radical mastectomies with internal mammary node dissection and compared them to 97 historical controls who were very comparable in stage and demographic features and who had undergone conventional radical mastectomies.[165] The 5-year survival rate in the former group was 70 percent, compared to 57 percent in the latter group, prompting the conclusion that operable breast carcinoma should be treated by extended radical mastectomy. Other series, though, demonstrated either no difference in overall results between simple mastectomy plus postoperative irradiation and extended radical mastectomy[93] or simply inefficacy of the internal mammary node dissection in improving survival.[179] These extended procedures never became widely accepted because of the absence of any clear benefit despite the substantial added risk; however, they are still used selectively in some centers.[27]

During these same years the bilaterality of carcinoma of the breast became evident in a small percentage of cases, with victims of this disease showing an increased risk of a second malignancy developing metachronously in the contralateral breast. In 1951 Pack[134] advocated bilateral mastectomy for any unilateral breast malignancy, an idea that has continued to be sporadically advocated. Urban,[176] Fracchia et al.,[49] and Pressman,[147]

among others, have suggested routine contralateral blind biopsy in conjunction with ipsilateral mastectomy and excision of the contralateral breast in those 10 percent to 20 percent of patients showing any microscopic finding of malignancy. Robbins and Berg[152] demonstrated that the cumulative risk of developing clinically evident contralateral breast carcinoma following ipsilateral disease was less than 1 percent per year, which is less than the incidence of clinically occult carcinoma in the opposite breast detected by routine blind biopsy. Because of the doubts this raises of the clinical significance of occult contralateral malignancy, most surgeons do not intervene in the opposite breast unless there is some clinical indication.

Emergence of Lesser Operative Procedures

Halsted's major contributions to the treatment of breast carcinoma include (1) substantial reduction in operative mortality rates through adherence to the surgical principles of sharp dissection, meticulous hemostasis, elimination of dead space, wound closure using skin grafts, and antiseptic techniques; (2) the demonstration of the importance of wide surgical excision in preventing loco-regional recurrence of disease; and (3) the value of applying scientific principles of anatomy, physiology, and analysis of results to the development of a rational and effective treatment for this disease.

The basic flaw in the theory of local disease origin was quickly manifest by the fact that surgery alone did not consistently yield high rates of cure, regardless of how extensive the procedure or early the diagnosis. Although survival at 3 years appeared to show an improvement over earlier procedures, longer follow-up revealed steadily diminishing rates. The efforts of many surgeons to extend the scope of the radical mastectomy indicated their recognition of its inadequacy as the sole form of treatment for breast carcinoma. The abandonment of these extensive procedures by most surgeons, including Halsted himself, further testifies to the failure of surgery alone to eradicate most cases of this disease.

Rudolf Matas (1860–1957) of Tulane University asserted in 1898 that Halsted's operation could never be considered "complete" because of all the lymphatic channels left behind.[117] Lane-Claypon published the first epidemiological analysis of the results of surgical treatment of breast carcinoma in 1924[105] and concluded in this and a follow-up report in 1928[106] that whatever improvement in survival may exist was primarily attributable to earlier diagnosis rather than to the radical mastectomy itself. In a retrospective review of 20,000 operations for breast carcinoma in the medical literature, she showed a 43 percent 3-year survival and a 33 percent 5-year survival for those subjected to radical mastectomy. Those treated with lesser operations had a 3-year survival of only 29 percent. Also shown was a twofold increase in survival in the absence of lymph node involvement.[29]

William Crawford White, a surgeon at New York's Roosevelt Hospital, reported survival data on 157 radical mastectomies in 1927.[186] He typified the tendency to extend the reporting interval to 5 years or more, showing a 36 percent 5-year survival and only a 24 percent survival at 10 years. This study also demonstrated the impact of disease stage as determined by axillary node status on prognosis.

The noted New York pathologist, James Ewing, was also pessimistic about the true value of the radical mastectomy during this period, agreeing that the relatively good survival in most reports was more appropriately attributed to early detection than to the surgery. He was concerned that this operation was being performed too often on relatively harmless and sometimes benign lesions, while it seemed to make little difference on ultimate mortality in those with highly malignant and advanced lesions.[34, 153] In 1928 he stated[35]:

"I have drawn the impression that in dealing with mammary cancer surgery meets with more peculiar difficulties and uncertainties than with almost any other form of the disease. The anatomical types are so numerous, the variations in clinical course so wide, the paths of dissemination so free and diverse, the difficulties of determining the actual conditions so complex, and the sacrifice of tissues so great, as to render impossible in the majority of cases a reasonably accurate adjustment of a means to an end."

The pessimistic extreme was represented by Park and Lees, who in 1950[137] published an extensive and elegant analysis of treatment results for breast carcinoma. They cautioned that the variability of individual tumor growth rates may render survival rates meaningless, and that the available forms of treatment were unlikely to alter mortality rates, since these rates were largely caused by distant metastases. They concluded that there was no firm evidence that treatment had any effect on survival whatsoever.

The evident shortcomings of the surgical treatment of breast carcinoma led some to consider using lesser procedures in conjunction with other modalities in order to spare patients an unnecessary degree of tissue loss. Radiation therapy was one of the first adjunctive modalities applied to breast carcinoma for this purpose, first being used in this way by Emile Grubbe in Chicago within 2 months of the discovery of x-rays by Wilhelm Roentgen in 1895.[59] In 1917 Janeway described the use of interstitial irradiation of operable breast carcinoma instead of mastectomy, finding it an acceptable alternative for those patients who refused surgery or for those tumors that were not amenable to surgical ablation.[90]

Geoffrey Keynes, a surgeon at St. Bartholomew's Hospital in London, began applying radium needles to the treatment of breast carcinoma in 1922 under the direction of his superior, George Gask.[97, 153] They treated only advanced, inoperable cases at first but extended the use of the procedure as their success became evident. In their first 42 patients treated by radium implantation alone without surgery, 13 (31 percent) were "apparently cured,"[94] of whom six had been judged to have inoperable cancers. The follow-up in this series ranged from 8 months to 4 years, with only four patients having more than a 2-year follow-up. In 1932 Keynes reported similar

results for 171 cases treated during a 7-year period,[95] pointing out some of the harmful effects of this method on both patient and physician. In this report he also first speculated that radium may be more efficacious if the bulk of the tumor were first surgically removed. Several patients had been subjected to this combination of surgery and radiotherapy by 1937, when Keynes published his results from 250 patients in whom at least a 3-year follow-up was available.[96] He stratified these patients according to disease stage, with 85 patients being clinically stage I. Pathological staging was not possible, since axillary dissections were not performed. There was a 71.4 percent 5-year survival in these patients, and a 29 percent 5-year survival in those patients clinically judged to be stage II at presentation. This compared to 69 percent stage I and 30.5 percent stage II 5-year survivals among patients subjected to surgery alone as reported in a contemporary series by Jessop.[91] Assuming a 27 percent error rate in the clinical assessment of axillary nodes, Keynes speculated that the actual 5-year survival rate among his stage I patients might be as high as 86 percent. Since it is now known such an error may be as high as 40 percent to 50 percent,[3, 145] Keynes' results appear to be remarkable. They demonstrated for the first time the possibility that a lesser degree of surgical ablation of breast carcinoma may provide acceptable results.

George E. Pfahler, a Philadelphia radiologist, analyzed in 1932[143, 144] a series of 1022 cases in which radiation therapy was applied to breast carcinoma. In those patients in whom radiation followed surgery, a 90 percent increase in 5-year survival was found over the use of surgery alone. By 1939, Keynes was also convinced of the necessity to routinely remove the gross bulk of tumor prior to irradiation because of an otherwise high local recurrence rate.[97, 153] This was the first assertion of the principle that is now widely accepted, that surgery should be most effectively and appropriately applied to the removal of clinically evident disease, while radiation is best applied to ablation of the subclinical disease that is virtually always left behind after surgery. In other words, these modalities are complementary rather than competing forms of local treatment for breast carcinoma, though neither one can effectively treat the distant metastases that are largely responsible for mortality from this disease.

Haagensen and Stout in 1943[60, 61] defined those clinical features of breast carcinoma that predicted a poor outcome following radical mastectomy in terms of a prohibitively high rate of local recurrence and poor overall survival rate (Table 29–3). Such cases were considered "inoperable." This report recognizes the same limitations of surgery, especially for locally advanced disease, that such authorities as Banks, Moore, Petit, LeDran, and Hippocrates had espoused in centuries past.

In 1951, Haagensen and Stout reviewed, according to their strict and specific criteria of operability,[62] a series of 495 radical mastectomies performed at Columbia Presbyterian Hospital in New York between 1935 and 1942. They reported a 1.8 percent operative mortality,

Table 29–3. GRAVE SIGNS OF INOPERABILITY IN PATIENTS WITH BREAST CARCINOMA*

Skin edema
Skin ulceration
Chest wall fixation
Matted, enlarged, or fixed axillary nodes
Satellite skin nodules
Supraclavicular node enlargement
Arm edema
Inflammatory carcinoma

*Compiled from Greenough et al: Surg Gynecol Obstet 3:39–50, 1907; and Haagensen and Stout: Ann Surg 118:859–876, 1032–1051, 1943.

a relative 5-year survival rate of 58.2 percent and relative 5-year clinical "cure" rate of 48.7 percent, which were among the best results ever achieved following radical mastectomy. These results represented a 10 percent to 75 percent improvement over earlier rates from that hospital,[109] although the obvious selection bias contributing to these results cannot be overlooked.

Following World War II, efforts to investigate the feasibility of lesser operative procedures for breast carcinoma continued. High-voltage external beam radiation was developed, allowing more effective and safer delivery of radiation to the breast with better cosmetic results. In 1948 Robert McWhirter, a surgeon at the Royal Infirmary in Edinburgh, Scotland, published the results of treatment of 1345 patients who presented with breast carcinoma between 1941 and 1945.[120] Simple mastectomy and radiotherapy were carried out in 757 patients in whom the disease appeared to be clinically localized to the breast. The surgery involved only limited skin excision and limited undermining of flaps, with no axillary dissection in the absence of clinically palpable nodes. Radiation was applied to the chest wall, axilla, and supraclavicular fields in a minimum dose of 3750 rad during 3 weeks. The 5-year survival rate of these patients was 62.1 percent, which was substantially better than those cases undergoing radical mastectomy alone in most series.

McWhirter emphasized the validity of study techniques that are necessary to clarify optimal treatment regimens. Exclusion of untreated patients (selection bias), use of historical or noncomparable controls, lack of comprehensive follow-up, short follow-up intervals, incomplete histological confirmation, and failure to consistently stratify cases according to stage of disease at presentation were all flaws in study design that he identified in many published series that contributed to confusion and misconceptions of the appropriate treatment of breast carcinoma. He asserted that if these factors were taken into account and radical mastectomy was the only form of treatment available, then the 5-year survival rate of all patients with breast carcinoma was no more than 25 percent.[153] The overall survival rate of all 1345 cases of breast carcinoma referred to McWhirter's institution during the study period of 1941 to 1945 was 43.7 percent. In those 389 patients with only locally advanced but inoperable disease subjected

only to radiotherapy, there was a 29 percent 5-year survival. In those 1146 cases with no evidence of distant metastasis, the 5-year survival rate was 50.5 percent. These results were interpreted as demonstrating the efficacy of radiation as the sole treatment of the axilla, although future investigators, like Keynes in prior years,[96] were not to find this true. In 1964 McWhirter emphasized the need to address flaws in study design in order to scientifically determine the optimal treatment for breast carcinoma.[121] He advised that multicenter prospective clinical trials should be organized for this purpose, something that was to actually occur in the near future.

Two surgeons from London's Middlesex Hospital, D. H. Patey (1889-1977) (Fig. 29–16) and W. H. Dyson, initiated a revolutionary change in the surgical management of breast carcinoma with the publication in 1948 of their technique of modified radical mastectomy.[139] There appeared to these authors to be no valid reason for routine removal of the pectoralis major muscle in conjunction with mastectomy, except in those rare cases in which it was actually invaded by tumor. The work of Gray[55] supported this contention in showing an absence of lymphatics in the muscle and its fascia, which was contrary to the observations of Heidenhain in the nineteenth century. The primary conceptual basis of Halsted's removal of the muscle was the belief that it served as a route of lymphatic dissemination of tumor. The steadily decreasing rates of survival following radical mastectomy with lengthening follow-up intervals also raised the question of the importance of the extent of local treatment. Mr. Patey did believe in the necessity

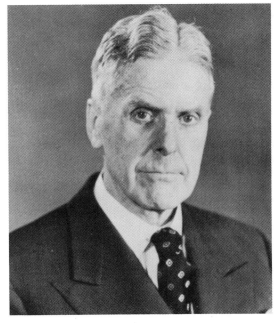

Figure 29–16. D. H. Patey (1889–1977), surgeon to London's Middlesex Hospital, who demonstrated the benefits of the modified radical mastectomy in 1948 with complete dissection of Levels I to III nodes following removal of the pectoralis minor. (Courtesy of Middlesex Hospital, London.)

for wide skin excision and thorough axillary dissection, with the latter including excision of the pectoralis minor muscle to ensure completeness. He also emphasized preservation of the lateral pectoral nerve. The advantages of leaving the pectoralis major muscle included the improved cosmetic result, less operative blood loss, and it provided "a more suitable bed for skin grafting than ribs and costal cartilages." This plea to preserve the pectoralis major muscle echoed the similar advice given by Celsus almost 2000 years ago.

Patey had first performed this modified radical mastectomy in 1932 and began using it routinely in 1936. The results on his first 118 patients, stratified according to axillary lymph node involvement and types of operative procedures, showed equivalent outcomes between modified radical mastectomy and standard radical mastectomy (83 percent vs. 78 percent 3-year survival in node-negative patients). The influence of postoperative irradiation could not be assessed, since it was applied inconsistently in both groups. This similarity of results, in terms of both survival and local recurrence rates, was confirmed in an updated review by Patey in 1967[138] of 146 patients, 69 of whom underwent modified radical mastectomy. "Good" results were achieved in 38 patients, all with follow-ups of at least 8 years.

In his 1948 report, Mr. Patey described ten cases in which a partial mastectomy and axillary dissection were performed. Interestingly enough, the survival rate of these patients did not appear to be significantly different from that of those who underwent total mastectomy, although the high rate of local recurrence led Patey to abandon this breast-sparing approach. Had he used radiation therapy on these patients, he could have been far ahead of his time in establishing an even more radical departure from the standard radical mastectomy.

Handley and Thackray of the Middlesex Hospital reported in 1969 their 10-year results of 143 patients who underwent Patey's modified radical mastectomy, in whom it was specified that no adjuvant hormonal manipulation or chemotherapy was used.[74] They included in this procedure the biopsy of the medial ends of the upper three intercostal spaces. Their adherence to Patey's philosophy of wide skin removal was reflected in the fact that 50 percent of their patients required skin grafting. Fifty-four percent of these patients were stage A of the Columbia Clinical Classification, and this group showed a 61 percent 10-year survival and 16 percent rate of local recurrence. In no case was there noted to be a local recurrence arising from the pectoralis major muscle. This was felt to be equivalent to results following standard radical mastectomy.

Williams et al. published in 1953 a retrospective review of 1044 cases of breast carcinoma treated by various methods at St. Bartholomew's Hospital in London between 1930 and 1939 in an effort to assess any difference in outcome according to the treatment methods.[188] The results indicated that there was no difference in 10-year survival rates between radical mastectomy, modified radical mastectomy, or simple mastectomy, whether or not radiation therapy was used. Local recurrence rates appeared to be significantly diminished only

in the radical mastectomy group and did not appear to be influenced by the use of radiation therapy. The conclusion of these authors was "that where efficient radiotherapy is available radical mastectomy should be abandoned in favor of conservative surgery." This supported the efforts of such contemporary investigators as McWhirter and Patey to explore the efficacy and safety of lesser procedures and presaged the eventual widespread acceptance of these procedures.

Hugh Auchincloss, a surgeon at the Columbia Presbyterian Hospital, advanced the cause of the modified radical mastectomy using many of the same arguments as Patey to conceptually justify its use.[7] He analyzed a series of 107 radical mastectomies for breast carcinoma associated with axillary metastases. Of 31 of these patients who were clinically free of disease 8 to 10 years following surgery, 27 had involvement of four or fewer nodes, all of which had been situated in the lower two axillary levels. This suggested that all disease could just as effectively have been removed by the modified procedure, with the same chance of cure. Auchincloss's procedure used a transverse elliptical incision but differed from that of Patey in leaving the pectoralis minor muscle in place and only dissecting the lower two thirds of the axilla to avoid the morbidity of arm edema. Postoperative irradiation to the chest wall and upper axilla was given only to those patients with axillary nodal involvement, thus achieving the best aspects of both radical surgery and radiation with the least morbidity.

John L. Madden of New York began in 1958 to routinely perform modified radical mastectomy on his patients with carcinoma of the breast, removing the chest wall musculature only when direct invasion occurred, and using neither routine radiotherapy nor chemotherapy.[113] He used a vertical elliptical skin incision similar to that described by Harrington in 1929[78] and extensive subcutaneous dissection of the skin flaps that rarely required skin graft closure. The pectoralis fascia was removed. The en bloc axillary dissection included all three levels, being more extensive than Auchincloss's procedure, and both pectoralis muscles were left in situ. Although, like Patey and Auchincloss, Madden made a point of removing the intermuscular nodes of Rotter, he did not believe these were clinically important because of their rare involvement by tumor. Drains were routinely placed under the skin flaps postoperatively. In subsequent reports, Madden's results were also compatible with those of the more extensive radical mastectomy. An important finding in his series was the absence of any local recurrences at 10 years in the pectoral muscles.[114]

Roses et al. reported in 1981 another variation of the modified radical mastectomy and advocated abandoning this term in favor of a more accurately descriptive name, since there are so many "modifications" of the radical mastectomy.[157] Their procedure involved a transverse or oblique skin incision and division of the humeral insertion of the pectoralis major muscle, with medial reflection of the sternal portion of this muscle to allow complete axillary dissection up to the apex. The pectoralis minor muscle is excised in continuity with the breast and axillary contents, preserving the lateral pectoral and long thoracic nerves, usually preserving the thoracodorsal nerve and sacrificing the intercostobrachial nerve and thoracodorsal vessels. The pectoralis major muscle is then resutured to its insertion on the humerus prior to skin closure and drain placement underneath the flaps. They called this procedure a "total mastectomy with complete axillary lymph node dissection" and asserted that a similar procedure leaving the pectoralis minor muscle in place (i.e., that of Auchincloss or Madden) should be called a "total mastectomy with lateral axillary dissection." "Total mastectomy" is a term they reserved for procedures that only sample low-level axillary nodes. Roses' procedure is reminiscent of that originally described by Lister more than 110 years earlier.

The modified radical mastectomy is essentially the same operation described by Moore in 1867, although it was another century before this procedure became the standard surgical treatment for breast carcinoma. A report by the American College of Surgeons Commission on Cancer demonstrated a dramatic decline in the use of the radical mastectomy, from 47.9 percent of cases in 1972 to 3.4 percent in 1981 (Fig. 29–17). The modified radical mastectomy was increasingly utilized during this same period, making up 27.7 percent of cases in 1972 and 72.3 percent in 1981.[4, 27, 131] An NIH Consensus Development Conference in 1980 concluded that the modified radical mastectomy is a satisfactory alternative to the Halsted radical mastectomy for stage I or stage II breast carcinoma.[128] This was further supported by a randomized prospective clinical trial published in 1983[115] showing no significant difference in disease-free or overall survival or in local recurrence rates at 5 years between radical mastectomy and modified radical mastectomy. What differences that existed in this study were attributable to a small number of stage III patients, indicating that locally advanced disease is not amenable to surgery alone and should probably not be included in these trials. The routine use of chemotherapy in those patients with involved axillary lymph nodes also distinguished this trial from prior studies.

As the validity of lesser local treatment for breast carcinoma became established through the 1950s and 1960s, it seemed reasonable to postulate that tumor extirpation alone may be as effective as mastectomy. Keynes had approached this goal with the addition of radiotherapy,[97] but Patey's small experience with a high local recurrence rate among patients undergoing only partial mastectomy[139] lent a pessimistic outlook to this procedure. The reluctance of surgeons to attempt anything less than a total mastectomy for this disease can be understood in the context of history, since such authorities as LeDran, Petit, Moore, and Halsted, among others, had all demonstrated the dangers of "inadequate operation" in terms of a prohibitive rate of local recurrence and death from disease.[127] Of course

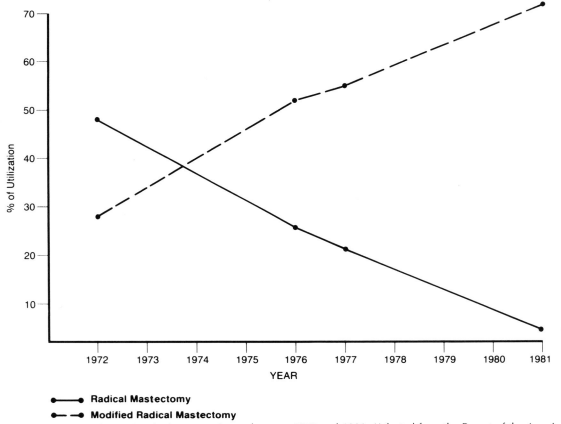

Figure 29–17. Changing patterns of operation for breast carcinoma between 1972 and 1981. (Adapted from the Report of the American College of Surgeons Commission on Cancer, October 22, 1982.)

the nature and extent of the disease being treated in the mid twentieth century was quite different from the locally advanced disease most commonly treated by the foregoing authorities, and the understanding of tumor biology and surgical principles had advanced to a remarkable degree during the intervening years.

Adair[1] in 1943 reported a small series of patients with breast carcinoma who had undergone local excision only; they actually had a better 5-year survival (88 percent) than a larger group of patients who had undergone radical mastectomy, simple mastectomy, or local excision plus radiotherapy during the same time period. The failure to stratify these patients according to variables, such as stage (known to influence survival) and the degree of selection bias, made these results inconclusive. Stimulated by these results, though, Crile and colleagues analyzed several series of patients during a 25-year period.[21, 22, 86] Their results suggested that partial mastectomy resulted in rates of local recurrence and overall survival that were statistically similar to the results of radical mastectomy. This similarity was most prominent when partial mastectomy was applied to patients with small tumors and no involvement of axillary lymph nodes and persisted up to 15 years of follow-up.[86] The retrospective and uncontrolled study design, the failure to microscopically confirm clear margins, and the involvement of selection bias in these studies, though, cast some uncertainty on these findings. Tagart in 1981[171] added to this uncertainty with his finding of a prohibitively high rate of local recurrence (37 percent) at only 3 years following wide local excision of operable (stage I or II) breast carcinoma in 44 patients, in whom a 2-cm margin of grossly normal tissue was obtained around all tumors. Montgomery et al. followed a group of 31 patients with small (T1 or T2) breast carcinomas treated only with a "wide biopsy excision."[126] At 5 years the overall loco-regional recurrence rate was 33 percent. They stated the basic concerns that must be addressed in the treatment of breast carcinoma in the light of our current knowledge of tumor biology:

"Treatment of breast cancer by radical surgery with or without radiotherapy has as its objective cure of the patient,

or at least the prevention of distressing local recurrence. It is widely believed that recurrence in the operation area predisposes to early dissemination and, since we now realize that the curative role of mastectomy is at least debatable, treatment is directed to preventing local tumor recurrence."

Lagios et al. in 1983 prospectively studied 43 patients who underwent segmental mastectomy alone for primary operable breast carcinoma, comparing their outcomes with those of a similar group of patients who underwent total mastectomy.[103] A significantly greater incidence of local recurrence was found in the former group after an average follow-up of 24 months (28 percent vs. 7.5 percent). A major factor related to this incidence of local recurrence was the unsuspected involvement of the resection margin by carcinoma in several cases. This emphasized the importance of assuring an adequate resection of tumor, preferably by microscopic confirmation, if segmental mastectomy is to be at all successful. If the dangers of local recurrence are to be avoided, whether they be a persistent potential for distant dissemination or simply the morbidity associated with salvage mastectomy, these authors feel that any involvement of resection margins by tumor mandates either further surgery or the addition of postoperative radiotherapy.

Several studies have confirmed the original observations of Keynes and McWhirter regarding the efficacy and safety of limited surgery followed by postoperative radiotherapy.* These studies demonstrate no differences in ultimate outcome of segmental mastectomy plus postoperative radiation when compared with more extensive surgery alone (Table 29–4). The addition of radiotherapy appears to control those multicentric or residual foci of subclinical disease in the breast that presumably give rise to the high rates of local recurrence observed following segmental mastectomy alone.

A small number of studies have explored the value of radiation therapy as the sole treatment for carcinoma of the breast. Although the results have been quite comparable with those of surgery at follow-up of 5 and 10 years, longer follow-up has revealed increased levels of

---

*References 19, 50, 79, 121, 129, 140, 145, 148. 155, 163, and 189.

Table 29–4. RESULTS OF PARTIAL MASTECTOMY AND POSTOPERATIVE IRRADIATION FOR OPERABLE STAGE I AND STAGE II BREAST CARCINOMA

Author	No. Patients	Follow-up Interval (yrs)	Local Recurrence (%)	Overall Survival (%)
Mustakallio[129]*	127	10	26	71
Porritt[145]†	263	10	—	70
Peters[140]*	124	10	5	45
Wise[189]†	49	10	8	62
Prosnitz[148]†	49	5	2	97
Freeman[50]*	115	5	15.6	80
Clark[19]*	680	10	16.3	62
Romsdahl[155]†	103	10	6.8	78
Fisher[38]*	566	5	7.7	91

*Stage I and stage II cases combined
†Stage I cases only

local recurrence and distant metastases as well as severe late radiation damage of the treated breast. Radiation therapy is therefore generally applied as the sole form of treatment only to inoperable forms of breast carcinoma, in which its role is strictly one of palliation rather than cure.[37, 87]

The appropriate roles of breast-sparing surgery and radiation therapy in the treatment of breast carcinoma appeared to be definitively established by the results of the National Surgical Adjuvant Breast and Bowel Project (NSABP) B-06 protocol.[38] This study improved on the design flaws of prior reports in its prospective controlled design, its uniform assurance of complete tumor excision in those undergoing segmental mastectomy through microscopic confirmation of clear margins, the use of pathological staging through the performance of axillary dissection in all patients, and the treatment of all node-positive patients with chemotherapy. One finding at 39 months of mean follow-up was a significantly higher local recurrence rate in patients subjected to segmental mastectomy alone (28 percent) compared to those subjected to either total mastectomy or segmental mastectomy plus postoperative irradiation (8 percent). Also found was an absence of any significant difference in overall survival between the three treatment modalities.

It thus seems that surgery is best applied to controlling grossly evident disease, and any extension of its application to attempt eradication of subclinical or microscopic disease increases its morbidity with no compensatory gain in survival. Conversely, it is this subclinical disease that is best controlled by radiation therapy, the morbidity of which becomes prohibitive when it is extended to the treatment of gross disease.[83] It has been demonstrated that a postoperative radiation dose of 5000 rad to a breast free of clinically detectable disease should provide control in 100 percent of cases.[48, 50]

It could be argued that segmental mastectomy alone is also justified by the results of the B-06 protocol if a predictably high rate of local recurrence is acceptable (i.e., approximately 30 percent, and perhaps higher for those lesions such as invasive lobular carcinoma or ductal carcinoma in situ known to be associated with high rates of multicentricity). The prognostic implications of local recurrence in the breast remain unresolved. Although many authors view local recurrence as a strong indicator, and perhaps instigator, of distant disease,[11, 18, 50, 54, 126, 159, 171] many reports demonstrate that when it follows segmental mastectomy, it can be effectively treated by reexcision or salvage mastectomy without any apparent adverse effects on ultimate survival.[19, 100, 101, 163] In the B-04 protocol of the NSABP,[42, 44] 88 percent of the local recurrences in the group undergoing radical mastectomy were ultimately associated with distant metastasis, while only 58 percent of local recurrences in the group undergoing total mastectomy developed distant disease. Fisher has postulated from this observation that local recurrence following more radical surgical procedures may be caused by tumor cells that are already systemically disseminated lodging in the operative site; following lesser procedures, especially segmen-

tal mastectomy, it may result from residual or incompletely excised tumor in the absence of distant disease.[43] This may justify a less pessimistic attitude toward local recurrences following breast-sparing procedures and may explain their apparent lack of impact on survival in many series when appropriately treated.

Another perspective on this issue of local recurrence was provided by the results of the NSABP B-06 trial summarized previously.[38] In node-positive patients, local recurrence had no effect on survival. In node-negative patients, however, local recurrence was associated with a significant reduction in disease-free survival ($p = 0.005$) and distant disease–free survival ($p = 0.02$). This suggests that local recurrence should be vigorously prevented in order to optimize the chance of cure in those patients most capable of being cured. This provides the stongest argument against treating breast carcinoma with segmental mastectomy alone and tends to vindicate the basic beliefs of Petit, Moore, and Banks.

REFLECTIONS AND PREDICTIONS

The one common thread found in virtually all recent studies concerning the surgical treatment of breast carcinoma is that the type and extent of local and regional treatment does not substantially affect survival. This concept represents a major change in thinking regarding the biology of breast carcinoma from the Halstedian beliefs that predominated at the turn of the twentieth century. This change has at least partially resulted from scientific observations of the results of treatment that was predicated on the belief that this disease is local in origin. For several decades it has been apparent that breast carcinoma must in fact be a systemic disease at its earliest stages, with the actual development of distant metastases dependent on a number of factors relating to tumor cell kinetics, tumor growth rate, and complex host-tumor interactions, perhaps mediated through hormonal and immunological mechanisms that are unique to each afflicted individual.[37, 43, 83, 145]

Experimental studies have further shown that breast carcinoma does not evolve in the orderly, stepwise fashion envisioned by Halsted and his contemporaries. Fisher and Fisher demonstrated that lymph nodes do not act as barriers to tumor cell dissemination[40] and also that there is an extensive and complex intercommunication between the lymphatics and blood stream that contradicts the premise of the mechanical theory of tumor extension elaborated by Thiersch, Waldeyer, Handley, and Gray.[41] These observations suggest that the status of regional lymph nodes in the patient with breast carcinoma should be viewed as a "marker" of the particular host-tumor relationship that exists, which is either conducive to (i.e., positive nodes) or prohibitive of (i.e., negative nodes) the development of distant metastasis. This concept assumes that all patients have some potential for systemic dissemination from the earliest phases of disease development.[43]

The greatest promise for an effective cure must therefore lie in systemic treatment. Patey's understanding of this concept is reflected in the following assertion[139]:

"Until an effective general agent for the treatment of carcinoma of the breast is developed, a high proportion of cases are doomed to die of the disease whatever combination of local treatment by surgery and irradiation is used, because in such a high proportion of cases the disease has passed outside the field of local attack when the patient first comes for treatment."

The abundant experimental and clinical evidence that has emerged in support of this hypothesis has led to the current acceptance of a dimished emphasis on locoregional treatment of this disease, as discussed in the previous section, while systemically oriented modalities have been increasingly emphasized. Hormonal manipulation was the first systemic therapy applied to breast carcinoma when Sir George Beatson of Glasgow performed oophorectomy for an advanced case in 1896.[10] Since then hormonal therapies of various types have continued to be used, showing promising though less than optimal results.[88, 112, 119, 130, 166] Cytotoxic chemotherapy became popular in the late 1950s[80] and has since become a mainstay of adjuvant systemic therapy following surgical treatment and as such has demonstrated improved survival over surgery alone.[15, 43, 57] Advances in molecular biology have led to the discovery of oncogenes, which offer the opportunity of perhaps manipulating the process of malignancy to prevent its occurrence altogether.[132] Adoptive immunotherapy is another form of systemic treatment involving the application of the lymphokine interleukin-2 to activate "killer" lymphocytes with antitumor activity; this is currently being investigated for clinical use and may represent the next generation of treatment for breast carcinoma.[156]

The surgeon has thus become an integral part of a multidisciplinary team that manages the patient with breast carcinoma. This team includes the diagnostic radiologist, radiation oncologist, medical oncologist, and pathologist. The surgeon's role has evolved to diagnosing and assuring the removal of all clinically evident disease so as to maximize the efficacy of radiation and systemic therapy.[37] All members of this team must be committed to the total patient and to a thorough understanding of the disease process and management options. Mastectomy is still a valid and sometimes preferable option in cases of operable (stage I and II) breast carcinoma as well as in all cases of locally advanced disease judged to be amenable to operation.

Axillary dissection may assume a diminished importance in the future treatment of breast carcinoma. Recent studies have demonstrated that there is no survival advantage to the routine removal of axillary lymph nodes[3, 37, 42, 44-46] and that the only therapeutic advantage of this practice is a substantial reduction in the rate of regional axillary recurrence. The clinical significance of axillary lymph node involvement, beyond its prognostic implications, has also been questioned.[46] In the past, the status of axillary lymph nodes has been the primary determinant of the need for systemic adjuvant chemotherapy. However, the National Cancer Institute now recommends routine systemic therapy even in the absence of axillary metastases.[5] It would therefore seem reasonable, because of the absence of data to suggest

any detriment to survival, to perform axillary dissection only in those patients who present with palpable adenopathy or who develop such adenopathy following primary treatment. This approach is currently practiced by some in the treatment of malignant melanoma.

The therapeutic challenge posed by noninvasive breast carcinoma will be increasingly faced in the future because of the more frequent detection of these lesions resulting from the current emphasis on early detection of breast carcinoma and the use of mammography. In situ breast malignancies may be the one form of this disease that may still be governed by the precepts of the local origin theory, since by definition systemic dissemination should not yet have occurred at this stage. Aggressive local treatment alone may thus be curative, as has been demonstrated in a number of studies.[51, 161, 182] The currently available evidence of the natural history of lobular carcinoma in situ suggests that it may best be managed expectantly, and may be more of a marker of increased risk for the future development of invasive carcinoma than an actual precursor of such.[52] Ductal carcinoma in situ appears to be a more ominous lesion that requires definitive surgery, although breast-sparing procedures with postoperative irradiation result in survival rates comparable to those of total mastectomy, which, as would be predicted at this stage of disease, approach 100 percent.[47, 151, 161] Further advances in hormonal manipulation and molecular biology may halt the progression of these lesions to invasive carcinoma.

As we come to the end of the twentieth century, breast carcinoma is increasingly seen as a systemic disease. This same philosophy was held by Imhotep, Hippocrates, Galen, and Hunter at the crest of many other cycles of belief and practice. Although these swings in philosophy during the past several centuries may appear arbitrary, they have actually occurred in response to advances in clinical experience and scientific knowledge. It is likely that the remarkable rate of scientific advances currently being made in this field will result in further shifts in conceptual and practical approaches to breast carcinoma in the future. Hopefully this cycle will end with an ideal management regimen for this complex disease process. This sentiment was expressed by Lewison in 1953[109]:

"The soundest predication of future progress must come from a realistic view of the past. Only by carefully examining our present precepts and practice can we intelligently plan for the future. Our resolute purpose must always be to promote the best interest of each individual patient, and not those of surgery, radiotherapy or chemotherapy."

Bernard Fisher, among others, has greatly contributed to achieving this purpose by developing and establishing the clinical trial, as McWhirter had recommended.[121] This has become the primary tool for testing hypotheses and determining optimal treatment for breast carcinoma. He has asserted the following[43]:

"Therapeutic strategies for breast cancer have evolved over time in step-wise fashion and are the result of biological information, which has led to a better understanding of this disease. It is logical to anticipate that this course will continue and that future gains will occur as a result of the testing of new biological hypotheses. Breast cancer management has been, is, and will be related to science and not to populism!"

Interestingly enough, Fisher's sentiment on this issue closely echoes one of Virchow's many dictums, stated in 1896, as cited by DeMoulin[29]:

"Indeed, a great deal of industrious work is being done and the microscope is extensively used, but someone should have another bright idea!"

This impatience with the status quo and commitment to shed light on the unknown will continue to advance the frontiers of our knowledge of breast carcinoma.

References

1. Adair FE: Role of surgery and irradiation in cancer of the breast. JAMA 121:553–558, 1943.
2. Anonymous: Dr. Willy Meyer. Am J Surg 17:287–292, 1932.
3. Anonymous: Cancer research campaign working party: Cancer research campaign (King's/Cambridge) trial for early breast cancer. Lancet 2:55–60, 1980.
4. Anonymous: Report by the American College of Surgeons Commission on Cancer. Chicago, October 22, 1982.
5. Anonymous: Clinical alert from the National Cancer Institute, Department of Health and Human Services. Betheseda, MD, May 16, 1988.
6. Ashworth TR: A case of cancer in which cells similar to those in the tumours were seen in the blood after death. Med J Aust 14:146–148, 1869.
7. Auchincloss H: Significance of location and number of axillary metastases in carcinoma of the breast: a justification for a conservative operation. Ann Surg 158:37–46, 1963.
8. Banks WM: A plea for the more free removal of cancerous growths. Liverpool and Manchester Surgical Reports, 192–206, 1878.
9. Banks WM: A brief history of the operations practised for cancer of the breast. Br Med J 1:5–10, 1902.
10. Beatson GT: On the treatment of inoperable cases of carcinoma of the mamma: suggestions for a new method of treatment, with illustrative cases. Lancet 2:104–107, 1896.
11. Bedwinek JM, Lee J, Fineberg B, Ocwieza M: Prognostic indicators in patients with isolated local-regional recurrence of breast cancer. Cancer 47:2232–2235, 1981.
12. Bell B: A System of Surgery, vol 5. Edinburgh, Bell, Bradfute, 1791, pp 436–460.
13. Billroth T: Die krankheiten der brust drusen. Stuttgart, F Enke, 1880.
14. Bloom HJG, Richardson WW, Harries EJ: Natural history of untreated breast cancer (1805–1933). Br Med J 2:213–221, 1962.
15. Bonadonna G, Valagussa P: Dose-response effect of adjuvant chemotherapy in breast cancer. N Engl J Med 304:10–15, 1981.
16. Breasted JH: The Edwin Smith Surgical Papyrus, vol 1. Chicago, University of Chicago Press, 1930, pp 363, 463.
17. Celsus AM: De Medicina, vol 2. Translated by Spencer WG. Cambridge, MA, Harvard University Press, 1953, p 129.
18. Chu FCH, Lin F-J, Kim JH, et al: Locally recurrent carcinoma of the breast. Cancer 37:2677–2681, 1976.
19. Clark RM, Wilkinson RH, Mahoney LJ, Reid JG, MacDonald WD: Breast cancer: a 21 year experience with conservative surgery and radiation. Int J Radiol Oncol Biol Phys 8:967–975, 1982.
20. Cooper WA: The history of the radical mastectomy. Ann Med Hist 3:36–54, 1941.
21. Crile G: Treatment of breast cancer by local excision. Am J Surg 109:400–403, 1965.
22. Crile G, Hoerr SO: Results of treatment of carcinoma of the breast by local excision. Surg Gynecol Obstet 132:780–782, 1971.
23. Cullen TS: A rapid method of making permanent specimens from frozen sections by the use of formalin. Bull Johns Hopkins Hosp 6:67–73, 1895.
24. Dahl-Iversen E, Soerener B: Recherches sue les metastases microscopiques des ganglions lymphatiques parasterneaux dans le cancer du sein. J Int Chir 11:492–509, 1951.
25. Dahl-Iversen E, Tobiassen T: Radical mastectomy with parasternal and supraclavicular dissection for mammary carcinoma. Ann Surg 157:170–176, 1963.
26. Dahl-Iversen E, Tobiassen T: Radical mastectomy with parasternal and supraclavicular dissection for mammary carcinoma. Ann Surg 170:889–894, 1969.
27. Danforth DN, Lippman ME: Surgical treatment of breast cancer. In Lippman ME, Lichter AS, Danforth DN (eds): Diagnosis and Management of Breast Cancer. Philadelphia, WB Saunders Company, 1988, pp 95–154.
28. Degenshein GA, Ceccarelli F: The history of breast cancer surgery, part 1: early beginnings to Halsted. Breast 3:28–36, 1977.
29. De Moulin D: A Short History of Breast Cancer. Boston, Martinus Nijhoff, 1983.
30. Dobson J: John Hunter's views on cancer. Ann R Coll Surg Engl 1:176–181, 1959.
31. Doets CJ: De heelkunde van Petrus Camper 1722–1789. Thesis. Leiden, 1948, p 25.
32. Donegan WL: Introduction to the history of breast cancer. In Donegan WL, Spratt JS (eds): Cancer of the Breast, ed 3. Philadelphia, WB Saunders, 1988, pp 1–15.
33. Engell HC: Cancer cells in the circulating blood. Acta Chir Scand 201(suppl):1–70, 1955.
34. Ewing J: Neoplastic Diseases, ed 2. Philadelphia, WB Saunders, 1922.
35. Ewing J: Neoplastic Diseases, ed 3. Philadelphia, WB Saunders, 1928, p 582.
36. Fabry W: Observationum et curationum chirurgicarum centuriae, cent. II. Lugduni, IA Huguetan, 1641, pp 267–269.
37. Fisher B: A commentary on the role of the surgeon in primary breast cancer. Breast Cancer Res Treat 1:17–26, 1981.
38. Fisher B, Bauer M, Margolese R, et al: Five year results of a randomized clinical trial: comparing total mastectomy and segmental mastectomy with or without radiation in the treatment of breast cancer. N Engl J Med 312:665–673, 1985.
39. Fisher B, Bauer M, Wickerham DL, et al: Relationship of number of positive axillary nodes to the prognosis of patients with primary breast cancer—an NSABP update. Cancer 52:1551–1557, 1983.
40. Fisher B, Fisher ER: Transmigration of lymph nodes by tumor cells. Science 152:1397–1398, 1966.
41. Fisher B, Fisher ER: The interrelationship of hematogenous and lymphatic tumor cell dissemination. Surg Gynecol Obstet 122:791–798, 1966.
42. Fisher B, Montague ED, Redmond C, et al: Comparison of radical mastectomy with alternative treatments for primary breast cancer: a first report of results from a prospective randomized clinical trial. Cancer 39:2827–2839, 1977.
43. Fisher B, Redmond C, Fisher ER, et al: The contribution of recent NSABP clinical trials of primary breast cancer therapy to an understanding of tumor biology—an overview of findings. Cancer 46:1009–1025, 1980.
44. Fisher B, Redmond C, Fisher ER, et al: Ten-year results of a randomized clinical trial comparing radical mastectomy and total mastectomy with or without radiation. N Engl J Med 312:674–682, 1985.
45. Fisher B, Wolmark N, Bauer M, et al: The accuracy of clinical nodal staging and of limited axillary dissection as a determinant of histological nodal status in carcinoma of the breast. Surg Gynecol Obstet 152:765–772, 1981.
46. Fisher ER, Sass R, Fisher B: Biologic considerations regarding the one and two step procedures in the management of patients with invasive carcinoma of the breast. Surg Gynecol Obstet 161:245–249, 1985.
47. Fisher ER, Sass R, Fisher B, et al: Pathologic findings from the National Surgical Adjuvant Breast Project (protocol 6). I. Intraductal carcinoma (DCIS). Cancer 57:197–208, 1986.

48. Fletcher GH: Clinical dose-response curves of human malignant epithelial tumors. Br J Radiol 46:1–12, 1973.
49. Fracchia AA, Robinson D, Legaspi A, et al: Survival in bilateral breast cancer. Cancer 55:1414–1421, 1985.
50. Freeman CR, Belliveau MD, Kim TH, Boivin J-F: Limited surgery with or without radiotherapy for early breast carcinoma. J Can Assoc Radiol 32:125–128, 1981.
51. Frykberg ER, Bland KI, Copeland EM: The detection and treatment of early breast cancer. In Tompkins RK (ed): Advances in Surgery, vol 23. Chicago, Yearbook Medical Publishers, 1990, pp 119–194.
52. Frykberg ER, Santiago F, Betsill WL, O'Brien PH: Lobular carcinoma in situ of the breast. Surg Gynecol Obstet 164:285–301, 1987.
53. Galen: De tumoribus praeter naturam. In Kuhn CG (ed): Opera Omnia, vol 7. Lipsiae, C Knobloch, 1821, pp 726–728.
54. Gilliland MD, Barton RM, Copeland EM: The implications of local recurrence of breast cancer as the first site of therapeutic failure. Ann Surg 197:284–287, 1983.
55. Gray JH: The relation of lymphatic vessels to the spread of cancer. Br J Surg 26:462–495, 1938.
56. Greenough RB, Simmons CC, Barney JD: The results of operations for cancer of the breast at the Massachusetts General Hospital from 1894–1904. Surg Gynecol Obstet 3:39–50, 1907.
57. Greenspan EM, Fisher M, Lesnick G, Edelman S: Response of advanced breast carcinoma to the combination of the antimetabolic methotrexate and the alkylating agent Thio-Tepa. Mt Sinai J Med 33:1–26, 1963.
58. Gross SW: An analysis of two hundred and seven cases of carcinoma of the breast. Med News 51:613–617, 1887.
59. Grubbe EH: X-ray treatment: its origin, birth and early history. St Paul, MN, Bruce Publishing, 1949.
60. Haagensen CD, Stout AP: Carcinoma of the breast, I. Criteria of operability. Ann Surg 118:859–876, 1943.
61. Haagensen CD, Stout AP: Carcinoma of the breast, II. Criteria of operability. Ann Surg 118:1032–1051, 1943.
62. Haagensen CD, Stout AP: Carcinoma of the breast: results of treatment 1935–1942. Ann Surg 134:151–172, 1951.
63. Haagensen CD: The history of the surgical treatment of breast carcinoma from 1863–1921. In Haagensen CD (ed): Diseases of the Breast, ed 3. Philadelphia, WB Saunders, 1986, pp 864–871.
64. Haddow A, Watkinson JM, Paterson E: Influence of synthetic oestrogens upon advanced malignant disease. Br Med J 2:393–398, 1944.
65. Halsted WS: The treatment of wounds with especial reference to the value of the blood clot in the management of dead spaces. Johns Hopkins Hosp Rep 2:255–314, 1890–1891.
66. Halsted WS: The results of operations for the cure of cancer of the breast performed at the Johns Hopkins Hospital from June 1889 to January 1894. Johns Hopkins Hosp Rep 4:297–350, 1894–1895.
67. Halsted WS: A clinical and histological study of certain adenocarcinomata of the breast: and a brief consideration of the supraclavicular operation and of the results of operations for cancer of the breast from 1889 to 1898 at the Johns Hopkins Hospital. Ann Surg 28:557–576, 1898.
68. Halsted WS: The results of radical operations for the cure of carcinoma of the breast. Ann Surg 46:1–19, 1907.
69. Halsted WS: Developments in the skin grafting operation for cancer of the breast. JAMA 60:416–435, 1913.
70. Halsted WS: The swelling of the arm after operations for cancer of the breast—elephantiasis chirurgica—its cause and prevention. Bull Johns Hopkins Hosp 32:309–313, 1921.
71. Handley RS, Thackray AC: Invasion of the internal mammary lymph glands in carcinoma of the breast. Br J Cancer 1:15–20, 1947.
72. Handley RS, Thackray AC: Internal mammary lymph chain in carcinoma of the breast: Study of 50 cases. Lancet 2:276–278, 1949.
73. Handley RS: Further observations on the internal mammary lymph chain in carcinoma of the breast. Proc R Soc Med 45:565–566, 1952.
74. Handley RS, Thackray AC: Conservative radical mastectomy (Patey's operation). Ann Surg 170:880–882, 1969.
75. Handley WS: Cancer of the Breast, ed 2. New York, Paul B Hoeber, 1906.
76. Handley WS: Cancer of the Breast and Its Operative Treatment. London, John Murray, 1922.
77. Handley WS: Parasternal invasion of the thorax in breast cancer and its suppression by the use of radium tubes as an operative precaution. Surg Gynecol Obstet 45:721–728, 1927.
78. Harrington SW: Carcinoma of the breast: surgical treatment and results. JAMA 92:208–213, 1929.
79. Harris JR, Connolly JL, Schnitt SJ, et al: The use of pathologic features in selecting the extent of surgical resection necessary for breast cancer patients treated by primary radiation therapy. Ann Surg 201:164–167, 1985.
80. Heidelberger C, Chaudhuri NK, Danneburg P, et al: Fluorinated pyrimidines, a new class of tumour—inhibitory compounds. Nature 179:663–666, 1957.
81. Heidenhain L: Ueber die ursachen der localen krebsrecidive nach amputation mammae. Arch Klin Chir 39:97–166, 1889.
82. Heister L: General System of Surgery, part II, section 4. London, Innys, 1745, p 13.
83. Hellman S, Harris JR: The appropriate breast cancer paradigm. Cancer Res 47:339–342, 1987.
84. Henderson IC, Canellos GP: Cancer of the breast: the past decade. N Engl J Med 302:17–20, 787–800, 1980.
85. Herodotus: The Histories. New York, Penguin, 1967.
86. Hermann RE, Esselstyn CB, Crile G, Cooperman AM, Antunez AR, Hoerr SO: Results of conservative operations for breast cancer. Arch Surg 120:746–751, 1985.
87. Hochman A, Robinson E: Eighty-two cases of mammary cancer treated exclusively with roentgen therapy. Cancer 15:670–673, 1960.
88. Huggins C, Bergenstal DM: Inhibition of human mammary and prostatic cancers by adrenalectomy. Cancer Res 12:134–141, 1952.
89. Jackson JN: A new technic for breast amputation. JAMA 46:627–633, 1906.
90. Janeway HH: Radium Therapy in Cancer at Memorial Hospital. New York, Hober, 1917, pp 184–190.
91. Jessop WHG: Results of operative treatment in carcinoma of the breast. Lancet 2:424–426, 1936.
92. Judd ES, Sistrunk WE: End-results in operation for cancer of the breast. Surg Gynecol Obstet 28:289–294, 1914.
93. Kaae S, Johansen H: Breast cancer: five year results: two random series of simple mastectomy with postoperative irradiation versus extended radical mastectomy. AJR 87:82–88, 1962.
94. Keynes G: Radium treatment of primary carcinoma of the breast. Lancet 2:108–111, 1928.
95. Keynes G: The radium treatment of carcinoma of the breast. Br J Surg 19:415–480, 1932.
96. Keynes G: Conservative treatment of cancer of the breast. Br Med J 2:643–647, 1937.
97. Keynes G: Carcinoma of the breast: a brief historical survey of the treatment. St. Bartholomew's Hosp J 56:462–466, 1952.
98. Korteweg JA: Die statistischen resultate der amputation des brustkrebses. Arch Klin Chir 38:679–685, 1889.
99. Korteweg JA: Carcinoom en statistiek. Ned Tijdschr Geneeskd 39:1054–1068, 1903.
100. Kurtz JM, Amalric R, Brandone H, Ayme Y, Spitalier J-M: Results of salvage surgery for mammary recurrence following breast-conserving therapy. Ann Surg 207:347–351, 1988.
101. Kurtz JM, Amalric R, Brandone H, Ayme Y, Spitalier J-M: Results of wide excision for mammary recurrence after breast-conserving therapy. Cancer 61:1969–1972, 1988.
102. Küster E: Zur behandlung des brustkrebses. Arch Klin Chir 29:723–735, 1883.
103. Lagios MD, Richards VE, Rose MR, Yee E: Segmental mastectomy without radiotherapy: short-term followup. Cancer 52:2173–2179, 1983.
104. Lane WA: A case illustrating a more effectual method of removing a cancerous breast, lymphatics and glands. Trans Clin Soc London 26:85–87, 1893.
105. Lane-Claypon JE: Cancer of the breast and its surgical treatment. Reports on public health and medical subjects No. 28. London, Ministry of Health, 1924.
106. Lane-Claypon JE: Report on the late results of operation for

cancer of the breast. Reports on public health and medical subjects No. 51. London, Ministry of Health, 1928.

107. LeDran F: Memoire avec une precis de plusiers observations sur le cancer. Mem Acad R Chir Paris 3:1–56, 1757.

108. Lewis D, Rienhoff WF: A study of the results of operations for the cure of cancer of the breast performed at the Johns Hopkins Hospital from 1889–1931. Ann Surg 95:336–400, 1932.

109. Lewison EF: The surgical treatment of breast cancer: an historical and collective review. Surgery 34:904–953, 1953.

110. Lister J: Collected Papers, vol 2. Oxford, Clarendon Press, 1909.

111. Liston R: Practical Surgery. London, J Churchill, 1837.

112. MacMahon CE, Cahill JL: The evolution of the concept of the use of surgical castration in the palliation of breast cancer in pre-menopausal females. Ann Surg 184:713–716, 1976.

113. Madden JL: Modified radical mastectomy. Surg Gynecol Obstet 121:1221–1230, 1965.

114. Madden JL, Kasndalaft S, Bourque R: Modified radical mastectomy. Ann Surg 175:624–633, 1972.

115. Maddox WA, Carpenter JT, Laws HL, et al: A randomized prospective trial of radical (Halsted) mastectomy versus modified radical mastectomy in 311 breast cancer patients. Ann Surg 198:207–212, 1983.

116. Margottini M: Recent developments in the surgical treatment of breast cancer. Acta Unio Int Contra Cancrum 8:176–190, 1952.

117. Matas R: In discussion of WS Halsted. Trans Am Surg Assoc 16:165–178, 1898.

118. Matas R: William Stewart Halsted, 1852–1922: an appreciation. Bull Johns Hopkins Hosp 36:2–7, 1925.

119. McGuire WL, DeLaGarza M: Similarity of the estrogen receptor in human and rat mammary carcinoma. J Clin Endocrinol Metab 36:548–552, 1973.

120. McWhirter R: The value of simple mastectomy and radiotherapy in the treatment of cancer of the breast. Br J Radiol 21:599–610, 1948.

121. McWhirter R: Should more radical treatment be attempted in breast cancer? AJR 92:3–13, 1964.

122. Meyer W: An improved method of the radical operation for carcinoma of the breast. Med Rec 46:746–749, 1894.

123. Meyer W: Carcinoma of the breast: ten years' experience with my method of radical operation. JAMA 45:297–313, 1905.

124. deMondeville H: Die chirurgie des Heinrich deMondeville. Berlin, A. Hirschwald, 1892.

125. Monro A: Collections of blood in cancerous breasts. In The Works of Alexander Monro: Published by His Son Alexander Monro. Edinburgh, Ch. Elliot, 1781, pp 484–491.

126. Montgomery ACV, Greening WP, Levene AL: Clinical study of recurrence rate and survival time of patients with carcinoma of the breast treated by biopsy excision without any other therapy. J R Soc Med 71:339–342, 1978.

127. Moore CH: On the influence of inadequate operations on the theory of cancer. R Med Chir Soc London 1:244–280, 1867.

128. Moxley JH, Allegra JC, Henney J, et al: Treatment of primary breast cancer: summary of the National Institutes of Health Consensus Development Conference. JAMA 244:797–799, 1980.

129. Mustakallio S: Treatment of breast cancer by tumor extirpation and roentgen therapy instead of radical operation. J Fac Radiol 6:23–26, 1954.

130. Nathanson IT: The effect of stilbestrol on advanced cancer of the breast. (Abstract) Cancer Res 6:484, 1946.

131. Nemoto T, Vana J, Bedwani RN, et al: Management and survival of female breast cancer: results of a national survey by the American College of Surgeons. Cancer 45:2917–2924, 1980.

132. Nowell PC: Molecular events in tumor development. N Engl J Med 319:575–577, 1988.

133. Ochsner AJ: Final results in 164 cases of carcinoma of the breast operated upon during the past fourteen years at the Augustana Hospital. Ann Surg 46:28–42, 1907.

134. Pack GT: Argument for bilateral mastectomy. Surgery 29:929–931, 1951.

135. Paget J: On the average duration of life in patients with scirrhous cancer of the breast. Lancet 1:62–63, 1856.

136. Pancoast J: A treatise on operative surgery. Philadelphia, R Hart, 1852, pp 269–271.

137. Park WW, Lees JC: The absolute curability of cancer of the breast. Surg Gynecol Obstet 93:129–152, 1951.

138. Patey DH: A review of 146 cases of carcinoma of the breast operated on between 1930 and 1943. Br J Cancer 21:260–269, 1967.

139. Patey DH, Dyson WH: The prognosis of carcinoma of the breast in relation to the type of operation performed. Br J Cancer 2:7–13, 1948.

140. Peters MV: wedge resection and irradiation: an effective treatment in early breast cancer. JAMA 200:144–145, 1967.

141. Petit JL: Oeuvres Completes, section VII. Limoges, R Chapoulard, 1837, pp 438–445.

142. Peyrilhe B: Dissertatio Academia de Cancro. Paris, De Hansy Jeune, 1774.

143. Pfahler GE: Results of radiation therapy in 1,022 private cases of carcinoma of the breast from 1902 to 1928. AJR 27:497–508, 1932.

144. Pfahler GE, Parry LD: Roentgen therapy in carcinoma of the breast: a statistical study of 977 private cases. Ann Surg 93:412–427, 1931.

145. Porritt A: Early carcinoma of the breast. Br J Surg 51:214–216, 1964.

146. Power D: The history of the amputation of the breast to 1904. Liverpool Med Chir J 42:29–56, 1934.

147. Pressman PI: Selective biopsy of the opposite breast. Cancer 57:577–580, 1986.

148. Prosnitz LR, Goldenberg IS, Packard RA, et al: Radiation therapy as initial treatment for early stage cancer of the breast without mastectomy. Cancer 39:917–923, 1977.

149. Prudente A: L'amputation inter-scapulo-mammothoracique (technique et resultats). J Chir 65:729–735, 1949.

150. Ravitch MM: A Century of Surgery, vol I. Philadelphia, JB Lippincott, 1980, p 612.

151. Recht A, Danoff BS, Solin LJ, et al: Intraductal carcinoma of the breast: results of treatment with excisional biopsy and radiation. J Clin Oncol 3:1339–1343, 1985.

152. Robbins GF, Berg JW: Bilateral primary breast cancers: a prospective clinicopathological study. Cancer 17:1501–1527, 1964.

153. Robinson JO: Treatment of breast cancer through the ages. Am J Surg 151:317–333, 1986.

154. Rodman JS: Skin removal in radical breast amputation. Ann Surg 118:694–705, 1943.

155. Romsdahl MM, Montague ED, Ames FC, Richards PC, Schell SR: Conservation surgery and irradiation as treatment for early breast cancer. Arch Surg 118:521–528, 1983.

156. Rosenberg SA, Lotze MT, Muul LM, et al: Observations on the systemic administration of autologous lymphokine-activated killer cells and recombinant interleukin-2 to patients with metastatic cancer. N Engl J Med 313:1485–1492, 1985.

157. Roses DF, Harris MN, Potter DA, Gumport SL: Total mastectomy with complete axillary dissection. Ann Surg 194:4–8, 1981.

158. Schmid H: Zur statisk der mammacarcinome und der heitung. Dtsch Z Chir 26:139–145, 1887.

159. Schnitt SJ, Connolly JL, Khettry V, et al: Pathologic findings on re-excision of the primary site in breast cancer patients considered for treatment by primary radiation therapy. Cancer 59:675–681, 1987.

160. Scultetus J: Armamentarium Chirurgicum. Ulm, B Kuhnen, 1653, pp 50–51.

161. Seidman H, Gelb SK, Silverberg E, et al: Survival experience in the Breast Cancer Detection Demonstration Project. CA 37:258–290, 1987.

162. Shapiro S, Venet W, Strax P, et al: Ten-to-fourteen year effect of screening on breast cancer mortality. J Natl Cancer Inst 69:349–355, 1982.

163. Stehlin JS, Ipolyi PD, Greeff PJ, Gutierrez AE, Hardy RJ, Dahiya SL: A ten year study of partial mastectomy for carcinoma of the breast. Surg Gynecol Obstet 165:191–198, 1987.

164. Stewart FT: Amputation of the breast by a transverse incision. Ann Surg 62:250–251, 1915.

165. Sugarbaker ED: Extended radical mastectomy: its superiority in the treatment of breast cancer. JAMA 187:96–99, 1964.

166. Suntzeff V, Burns EL, Moskop M, Loeb L: The effect of

injections of estrin on the incidence of mammary cancer in various strains of mice. Am J Cancer 27:229–245, 1936.

167. Sutherland CM, Mather FJ: Long-term survival and prognostic factors in breast cancer patients with localized (no skin, muscle, or chest wall attachment) disease with and without positive lymph nodes. Cancer 57:622–629, 1986.

168. Sweeting R: A new operation for cancer of the breast. Lancet 1:323, 1869.

169. Syme J: Principles of Surgery. London, H Balliere, 1842, p 73.

170. Tabar L, Fagerberg CJG, Gad A, et al: Reduction in mortality from breast cancer after mass screening with mammography. Lancet 1:829–832, 1985.

171. Tagart REB: Partial mastectomy for breast cancer. Br Med J 2:1268, 1978.

172. Taylor GW, Wallace RH: Carcinoma of the breast: fifty years experience at the Massachusetts General Hospital. Ann Surg 132:833–843, 1950.

173. Tyzzer EE: Factors in the production and growth of tumor metastases. J Med Res 28:309–333, 1913.

174. Urban JA: Radical excision of the chest wall for mammary cancer. Cancer 4:1263–1285, 1951.

175. Urban JA, Baker HW: Radical mastectomy in continuity with en bloc resection of the internal mammary lymph-node chain: a new procedure for primary operable cancer of the breast. Cancer 5:992–1008, 1952.

176. Urban JA: Bilaterality of cancer of the breast. Cancer 20:1867–1870, 1967.

177. Valagussa P, Bonadonna G, Veronesi U: Patterns of relapse and survival following radical mastectomy. Cancer 41:1170–1178, 1978.

178. Velpeau A: A Treatise on the Diseases of the Breast and Mammary Regions. Translated by Henry M. London, The Sydenham Society, 1856.

179. Veronesi U, Valagussa P: Inefficacy of internal mammary node dissection in breast cancer surgery. Cancer 47:170–178, 1981.

180. Virchow R: Cellular Pathology. Translated by Chance F. Philadelphia, JB Lippincott, 1863.

181. Volkmann R: Beitrage zur Chirurgie. Leipzig, Breitkoff und Hartel, 1875, pp 329–338.

182. Von Rueden DG, Wilson RE: Intraductal carcinoma of the breast. Surg Gynecol Obstet 158:105–111, 1984.

183. Wangensteen OH: Carcinoma of the breast. Ann Surg 132:833–843, 1950.

184. Wangensteen OH, Lewis FJ, Arhelger SW: The extended or super-radical mastectomy for carcinoma of the breast. Surg Clin North Am 36:1051–1062, 1956.

185. Warren JC: The operative treatment of cancer of the breast: with an analysis of a series of one hundred consecutive cases. Ann Surg 40:805–833, 1904.

186. White WC: Late results of operations for carcinoma of the breast. Ann Surg 86:695–701, 1927.

187. Wilder RJ: The historical development of the concept of metastasis. J Mt Sinai Hosp 23:728–734, 1954.

188. Williams IG, Murley RS, Curwen MP: Carcinoma of the female breast: conservative and radical surgery. Br Med J 2:787–796, 1953.

189. Wise L, Mason AY, Ackerman LV: Local excision and irradiation: an alternative method for the treatment of early mammary cancer. Ann Surg 174:392–401, 1971.

190. Wolff J: Die lehre von der krebskrankenheit, vol 1. Jena, G Fischer, 1907.

General Principles of Mastectomy

Kirby I. Bland, M.D. and Edward M. Copeland III, M.D.

Following an established diagnosis of invasive carcinoma of the breast, a complete history, physical examination, and an accurate clinical staging evaluation are required before treatment of the primary lesion. Mammary adenocarcinoma that is smaller than 5 cm in transverse diameter and limited to the central or lateral aspect of the breast with the absence of pectoral fascia, skin fixation, and axillary lymphadenopathy can usually be treated by surgery alone. Lesions that are smaller than 4 cm in diameter may be optionally treated by segmental mastectomy (partial mastectomy, lumpectomy, or tylectomy) and postoperative irradiation, with results comparable to radical surgical techniques; this is discussed in a subsequent section of this chapter. For cancers larger than 5 cm in transverse diameter (stage IIIA or IIIB), a combination of radical surgery and radiation therapy is often essential to achieve local and regional control of the breast, axilla, and chest wall (see section XV, chapter 40).

For stage I and II breast cancers, the type of surgical procedure and the sites that should receive irradiation depend on the location of the primary tumor in the breast and the presence or absence of axillary metastases. Lesions in the *lateral aspect of the breast* drain principally via axillary lymphatic channels (see section II, chapter 2). Disease in this location can be eradicated from the chest wall by employing the modified radical mastectomy. This procedure is defined as a total mastectomy with en bloc removal of the pectoralis minor muscle and Levels I to III axillary lymph nodes. These laterally placed neoplasms, with axillary lymph node metastases, may be associated with internal mammary or supraclavicular lymph node metastases in as much as 25 percent to 30 percent of patients; thus irradiation therapy has been utilized to treat the peripheral lymphatic areas (internal mammary chain, supraclavicular sites).[4a] *Centrally located lesions* that are attached to the pectoralis major fascia or high-lying (superiorly located) fixed lesions to this fascia may be treated by radical mastectomy or by a combination of radical mastectomy and peripheral lymphatic and chest wall irradiation when palpable axillary lymph node metastases smaller than 2 cm are evident. These centrally placed lesions commonly metastasize via lymphatics that parallel the course of the neurovascular bundle medial to the pectoralis minor muscle. This medial neurovascular bundle that contains the lateral pectoral nerve and innervates the pectoralis major muscle is preserved in the modified radical mastectomy to ensure function of the pectoralis major muscle after mastectomy. In the radical mastectomy procedure, this neurovascular bundle, associated lymphatics, and areolar tissue are resected en bloc with the specimen to accomplish adequate surgical extirpation of regional disease.

The principal lymphatic drainage of *medially located cancers* is via routes that course to lymph nodes near the ipsilateral internal mammary vessels. These medial lesions may be associated with metastasis to the internal mammary lymphatics in 10 percent to 30 percent of patients, as previously confirmed by Handley.[13] The presence of pathologically-positive axillary metastasis with an associated medial lesion escalates this incidence of internal mammary metastasis to as much as 50 percent. In the absence of clinically positive axillary metastases, medially located cancers may be adequately treated by modified radical mastectomy and peripheral lymphatic irradiation. It is common to include chest wall irradiation when axillary metastases are identified pathologically in more than 20 percent of the removed axillary lymphatics. This principle was originally established because of the high incidence of skin flap recurrence evident with metastatic disease that courses to the axilla via the subdermal lymphatics from medially located primary lesions.

The *pathological stage* of the primary lesion is the main determinant of actuarial survival of the treated breast primary lesion. It is the responsibility of the surgeon and the radiation therapist to plan an operative procedure that encompasses, en bloc, the extent of the disease and provides the maximum probability for local and regional chest wall control of the tumor. It is also their responsibility to achieve this end result with minimal morbidity and mortality. These principles are best served by the avoidance of axillary irradiation following the Patey (complete) surgical dissection of Levels I to III axillary lymphatics; otherwise, the incidence of lymphedema of the ipsilaterally irradiated extremity will be increased some seven- to tenfold. Following radical resection of lymphatic channels with en bloc dissection of Levels I to III, the remaining lymphatics are destroyed by radiation therapy, thus increasing the incidence of lymphedema. In principle, operable breast cancer (stages I and II) treated by total mastectomy and axillary node removal with the radical or modified radical mastectomy should not require postoperative irradiation. In contradistinction, for the treatment of stage III disease with axillary metastases that clinically present with large, matted, or multiple nodes, the radiation therapist should plan the application of tangential fields to the apex of the axilla with inclusion of the peripheral lymphatics and chest wall after the extended simple (total) mastectomy is performed. This therapeutic regimen is essential, because Level III (apical) lymphatics remain intact after a resection that includes lymphatics lateral to the border of the pectoralis major

and minor muscles. With the extended simple mastectomy performed for stage III breast cancer, the primary cancer and/or lymphatics that are larger than 1 cm in diameter are unlikely to be sterilized by irradiation and are thus surgically removed. Extension of the primary neoplasm into the axillary space with invasion of the axillary artery, vein, or brachial plexus does not technically allow surgical removal and is best treated with ionizing irradiation to the area. Radiotherapy should be added to low or central axillary nodes that are determined pathologically to have *extranodal extension,* because local and regional control rates are enhanced with this modality, despite the increased risk of lymphedema to the ipsilateral arm. In the absence of clinically palpable nodes with primary neoplasms that exceed 5 cm in diameter, preoperative radiation therapy or combination chemotherapy may induce regression of the primary lesion. Thereafter surgical treatment of the breast is dependent on the extent (volume) of regression of the primary tumor, the presence or absence of fixation to pectoralis major fascia, location, and the presence or absence of local grave signs (ulceration, skin edema and fixation, satellitosis, etc.).

Surgeons should plan the operation with the objective of achieving, at minimum, 3- to 5-cm skin margins in all directions from the tumor, which can be accomplished with a radical, modified radical, or extended simple mastectomy. Patients who present with distant metastases, including supraclavicular lymph node metastases, are best treated with systemic chemotherapy. Again, it is the responsibility of the surgeon and the radiotherapist to achieve local and regional control except when adequate surgical margins are unobtainable without regression of the tumor, thereby reducing the probability of radiotherapeutic responses. The choice of these operative procedures must be individualized for the patient following determination of the site, clinical stage, and histological type of the primary neoplasm. Similar principles guide the management of inflammatory breast cancers, which may be large, fixed, or ulcerated (see section XV, chapter 40).

As indicated in section IV, chapter 9, and section XVII, chapter 43, estrogen and progesterone receptor activity should be obtained on all pathological breast cancer specimens to aid the therapeutic planning of endocrine replacement therapy should metastatic disease occur. The prospective data available for analysis suggest that mean survival rates for patients receiving either chemotherapy or hormonal manipulation are higher for patients who have positive estrogen and progesterone receptor activity than for those who do not. Regardless of the pathological stage of the tumor or the receptor activity, the optimal chemotherapeutic regimen for patients with metastatic breast cancer is still evolving. Nonetheless, both the quantitative and qualitative values for receptor activity of the primary neoplasm are of significant value to the oncologist and should be obtained from the primary lesion and metastatic sites to prospectively guide subsequent therapy.

Because proper processing of tissues that contain estrogen receptor (ER) and progesterone receptor (PR)

Table 29–5. STEROID HORMONE RECEPTOR VS. ISCHEMIA TIME*[6, 7]

Receptor (n = 11)	Ischemic Time (min)†				
	0	*30*	*60*	*90*	*150*
ER	100	79 ± 10‡	67 ± 11‡	54 ± 11‡	56 ± 13‡
PR	100	101 ± 21	101 ± 26	94 ± 14	84 ± 27
AR	100	57 ± 12‡	53 ± 15‡	28 ± 9†	42 ± 12‡

*Ischemia significantly decreased ER levels within the first 30 minutes ($p = 0.05$). ER values had sustained decrease throughout 150 minutes of ischemia. Similarly, AR levels were significantly lower by 30 minutes of ischemia ($p = 0.002$) and remained so throughout 150 minutes of ischemia. The largest decrease in ER and AR levels occurred within the first 30 minutes of ischemia. In contrast, PR levels were unchanged throughout 150 minutes of ischemia.

†Values are mean ± SEM, expressed as percent of control at baseline. AR = androgen receptor; ER = estrogen receptor; PR = progesterone receptor.

‡$p < 0.05$ compared with baseline by analysis of variance.

activity is essential to the design and implementation of future chemotherapy protocols for specific patients, the surgeon's attention to the preservation and processing of biopsy tissues is mandatory. Despite the importance of the ER and PR activity in guiding future therapies, processing of neoplastic tissue for pathology, in all cases, must take precedence over determination of steroid receptor activity. The surgeon should also be aware of the potential for the electrocautery to diminish steroid receptor activity. This has been confirmed by Ellis and associates[6, 7] and by Bland et al.[3] to be dependent on heat inactivation by the ambient temperature and by devascularization (Table 29–5). The procurement of primary breast cancer tissue for pathological diagnosis and for determination of quantitative and qualitative steroid receptor activity is best accomplished with the cold scalpel. This technique avoids the possibility of heat-induction artifact, tissue necrosis, cellular death, and temperature-dependent inactivation of steroid receptor activity in the procured tissues. The indications and techniques for biopsy of suspicious breast masses are comprehensively reviewed in section X, chapter 28.

TOPOGRAPHIC SURGICAL ANATOMY

Section II, chapter 2 contains a detailed review of the anatomy of the breast, including discussions of regional vasculature, neurological structures, and lymphatics. Hollingshead[14] observed that the fibrous and fatty components of breast tissue occupied that interval between the second or third rib superiorly with extension to the sixth or seventh ribs inferiorly. The breadth of extension includes the parasternal to the midaxillary lines. The glandular portion of the breast rests largely on the pectoral fascia and the serratus anterior musculature; however, mammary tissue extends typically into the anterior axillary fold (tail of Spence) and may be visible as a well-defined superolateral extension from the upper outer quadrant of breast tissue. Extent of the mammary tissue is ill defined and varies considerably with patient habitus and lean muscle mass.

Breast volume, with anterior and lateral projections, is variable and is dependent on lean body mass, habitus, age, and ovarian functional status. Because the ductal and lobular components are almost exclusively sensitive to the trophic effects of secretory estrogen and progestational compounds, the breast remains underdeveloped and rudimentary in the male. In men, short ducts with poorly developed acini are evident. Thus a deficiency of parenchymal fat and nipple-areola development are apparent and contribute to the nonspheroidal or flat appearance of the male breast.

In contradistinction to the male breast, the virginal breast is hemispheric and somewhat flattened above the nipple. The multiparous breast, on the other hand, is large and replaced in part with fat, which accounts for its lax, soft appearance; it rarely regains its initial configuration until menopause, when atrophy of glandular tissue is initiated. The breast is circumscribed anteriorly by a superficial layer and posteriorly by a deep layer of the superficial investing fascia of the chest wall. The superficial layer of the superficial fascia of the chest wall derives its anterior boundaries from the fibrous tissue of the tela subcutanea. Haagensen[11] observed the deep layer of the superficial fascia to be contiguous with the pectoral fascia.

With the loss of estrogen influence on breast parenchyma and ductal structures, the postmenopausal breast is consistently noted to lack parenchymal fat and active (proliferative) glandular components. Spratt and Donegan[23] note the nonlactating breast to weigh between 150 g and 225 g, whereas the lactating organ may weigh as great as 500 g.

Neural Supply to Pectoral Muscles

In major surgical texts, the surgical anatomy of the pectoral nerves and the innervation of the pectoral muscles has evoked only minimal interest. Major textbooks of anatomy have long considered the names of the medial pectoral and lateral pectoral nerves on the basis of origin from the *brachial plexus*. Therefore the

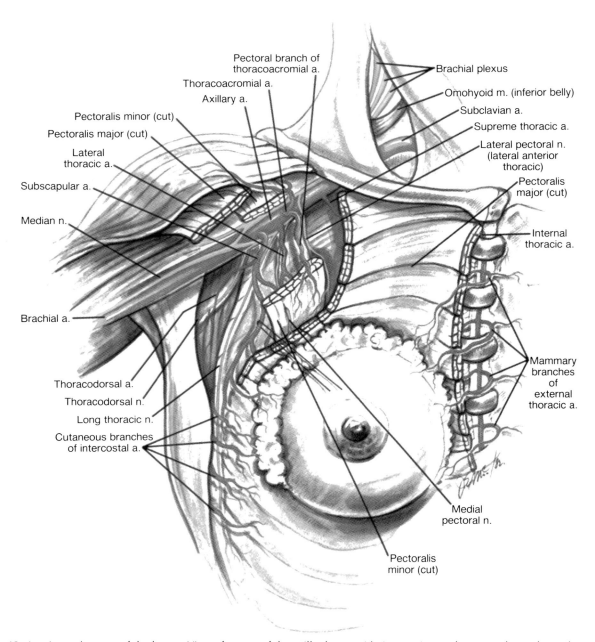

Figure 29–18. Arteries and nerves of the breast. View of nerves of the axilla that provide innervation to the pectoral muscles and muscles of the chest wall and posterior axillary space. The *long thoracic nerve* is identified and protected at the juncture where the axillary vein passes over the second rib. Injury or division of this nerve will result in "winged scapula" due to paralysis of the serratus anterior. The *thoracodorsal nerve* is found in the posterior axillary space with origin medial to the thoracodorsal vessels. This nerve may accompany the thoracodorsal artery and vein en route to its innervation of the latissimus dorsi. Injury results in weakness of abduction; internal rotation of the shoulder will result. The medial (anterior thoracic) pectoral nerve is superficial to the axillary vein and lateral to the pectoralis minor muscle, which it variably penetrates en route to its innervation of the pectoralis major muscle. The lateral (anterior thoracic) pectoral nerve lies at the medial edge of the pectoralis minor muscle and superficial to the axillary vein. With origin from the lateral cord of the brachial plexus, this nerve supplies major motor innervation to the pectoralis major. (From Gray SW, Skandalakis JE, McClusky DA: Atlas of Surgical Anatomy for General Surgeons. Baltimore MD, Williams & Wilkins, 1985. Reprinted by permission.)

names in classic anatomical teaching are *not* correlated with the anatomical position found at operation (Fig. 29–18). Moosman,[19] however, completed a detailed study of the pectoral nerves by dissection of 100 adult fixed and fresh cadaver pectoral regions (56 male and 44 female) and transposed the names of the medial and lateral pectoral nerves according to their anatomical relationship to the pectoral muscles and to the anterior chest wall. These nerves, sometimes referred to as the *anterior thoracic nerves,* originate cephalad and posterior to the axillary vein from an anastomotic nerve loop of variable size between the medial and lateral brachial plexus cords.

In his anatomical dissections, Moosman[19] noted the *lateral pectoral nerve* to arise anatomically *medial* to the pectoralis minor and, in its course, to divide into two to four branches that pass downward and medial to supply the clavicular, manubrial, and sternal components of the pectoralis major muscle. Thereafter the nerve passes through the costocoracoid foramen with the thoracoacromial vessels and enters the interpectoral space to mix with tributaries of vascular origin to the muscle. Moosman observed that this nerve is larger than the medial pectoral nerve because of the greater volume of muscle it innervates.

The smaller *medial pectoral nerve* was observed to be approximately 1 mm to 2 mm in diameter and 10 cm to 15 cm in length, with origin medial or posterior to the pectoralis minor. This nerve sends branches to the pectoralis minor and descends on its dorsal surface. Typically this nerve crosses the axillary vein and is accompanied by small tributaries from the axillary or thoracoacromial vessels. It enters the interpectoral space and supplies the lower third of the costoabdominal portion of the pectoralis major muscle. In this extensive review of the anatomy of the medial and pectoral nerve, Moosman[19] observed the relationship of the medial pectoral nerve to the pectoralis minor to be one of several variants: (1) descension as a single branch around the lateral border of the lower half of the muscle (38 percent); (2) division into two branches with one branch passing *through* the muscle and the other *around* its lateral margin (32 percent); (3) descension as a single branch that passed *through* the muscle (22 percent); and (4) descension as two or three branches of varying size, each of which passed through the muscle often at different levels (8 percent). He observed motor branches to the pectoralis major coursing through the pectoralis minor in 62 percent of cases.

In rare circumstances, the medial pectoral nerve may pass through the medial muscular components of the pectoralis minor or in other cases may remain entirely on its medial surface. When numerous branches arise from the major trunks, a more diminutive size can be expected for branches that innervate the pectoralis major. The nerve is observed to remain relatively large when it is a single branch, while multiple branches passing through the muscle may be of thread size.[19]

Regardless of the anatomical nomenclature utilized, the surgeon must be cognizant of the potential for damage to the nerve supply to the pectoralis muscles at all levels of dissection. Manipulation, traction, electrocautery, or removal may destroy the lateral or medial pectoral nerves unless they are carefully separated from nerve branches of variable size.

For purposes of clarity and consistency, the editors have retained the classic anatomical description and nomenclature for the pectoral (anterior thoracic) nerves and the accompanying neurovascular bundles (see section II, chapter 2). The name of the neurovascular bundle (lateral or medial) is synonymous with its course (position) in the axilla. Classic anatomy teaches that the pectoral nerves take the name of the brachial cord (medial or lateral) from which they originate. In the technical description of operative procedures within this chapter and in anatomical descriptions in other sections of this text, we have retained the classic nomenclature.

Vascular Supply

Nutrient arterial supply to the skin and breast is via branches of the *lateral thoracic arteries,* the *acromiothoracic branch of the axillary artery,* and the *internal mammary artery.*[1] The venous drainage system includes the intercostal veins, which traverse the posterior aspect of the breast from the second or third through the sixth or seventh intercostal spaces to terminate and enter posteriorly into the vertebral veins. The intercostal veins may arborize centrally with the azygos system to terminate in the superior vena cava. The deep venous drainage of the breast in large part parallels the pectoral branches of the acromiothoracic artery and the lateral thoracic artery.

Much of the surface area of the superior, central, and lateral aspects of the breast is drained by tributaries that enter the *axillary vein.* Venous supply from the pectoralis major and minor muscles also drain into tributaries that enter the axillary vein. Perforating veins of the *internal mammary venous system* drain the medial aspect of the breast and the pectoralis major muscle. This large venous plexus can be observed to traverse the intercostal musculature and terminate in the innominate vein, providing a direct embolic route to the venous capillary network of the lungs. Each plexus of veins in the lateral and medial aspects of the breast is observed to have multiple, racemose anastomotic channels.

Lymphatic Drainage and Routes for Metastases

Lymphatic drainage generally parallels the arterial and venous supply of the breast. This lymphatic flow is primarily unidirectional except in subareolar and central aspects of the breast or in circumstances in which physiological lymphatic obstruction occurs as a consequence of neoplastic, inflammatory, or developmental processes that initiate a reversal of flow with bidirectional egress of lymph.[9] This bidirectional lymphatic flow (see Figs. 2–12 and 2–14) may account for metastatic proliferation in sites remote from the primary neoplasm (i.e., the opposite breast and axilla). The delicate lymph vessels of the corium are valveless and encircle the lobular parenchyma to enter each echelon of the regional lymphatic nodes in a progressive and orderly fashion (e.g., Level I → Level II → Level III). As indicated in chapter 2 (Figs. 2–14, 2–15, and 2–16), multiple lymphatic capillaries anastomose and fuse to form fewer lymph channels that subsequently terminate in the large left thoracic duct or the smaller right lymphatic duct (chapter 2, Figs. 2–6 and 2–16). As a consequence of the predominant unidirectional flow of lymph, two accessory drainage routes exist for lymph en route to nodes of the apex of the axilla and include the *transpectoral* and the *retropectoral* routes as defined by Anson and McVay.[1] Lymphatics of the *transpectoral* or *interpectoral* routes that occupy the position between the pectoralis major and minor muscles were described by Rotter, a German pathologist, and bear his name: Rotter's nodes. Cody et al.[4] and Netter[20] observed Rotter's nodes to be present in up to 75 percent of individuals, with an average of two to three nodes per patient. Cody et al.[4] observed that 0.5 percent of node-negative patients and 8.2 percent of patients who were axillary node positive had evidence of Rotter lymph node metastases. This observation was rarely reported by Haagensen.[11] Therefore although the Patey axillary dissection, included in the Halsted radical[12] and in the modified radical mastectomy, removes the interpectoral Rotter group en bloc, this nodal group plays only a diminutive role in the diagnosis and therapy of breast cancer. The retropectoral lymphatics, however, may play a more important physiological role in drainage of the breast, because they are exposed to the superior and internal portions of the mammary glands. These lym-

phatics arborize lateral and posterior to the surface of the pectoralis major muscle and terminate at the apex of the axilla. To achieve an adequate en bloc resection of major axillary nodal groups, a thorough conceptualization of breast lymphatic drainage is essential to the surgeon. Familiarization with the anatomy of this area is essential for staging and for curative resection.

Section II, chapter 2 deals with the *principal axillary nodal groups* as described by Anson and McVay.[1] Figure 29–19 topographically depicts anatomical Levels I to III of the axillary contents with the relations to the neurovascular bundle, the pectoralis minor, the latissimus dorsi, and the chest wall. The following principal axillary nodal groups are included in *Level I*:

1. The *external mammary group,* which parallels the course of the lateral thoracic artery from the sixth or seventh rib to the axillary vein. This group occupies the loose areola tissue inferior and lateral to the pectoralis major muscle in the medial distal axillary space.

2. The *subscapular group,* which is contiguous with thoracodorsal branches of the subscapular vessels. This group extends from the ventral surface of the axillary vein to the lateral thoracic chest wall and includes loose areola tissue on the serratus anterior and subscapularis musculature.

3. The *axillary vein group,* which is the most laterally placed nodal group of the axillary space. This group also contains the largest group of nodes in the axilla and is observed to be caudal and ventral to the surface of the axillary vein.

Level II, or the *central nodal group,* is immediately beneath the pectoralis minor muscle and is the most centrally located of the axillary lymphatic groups. This nodal group is located between the anterior and poste-

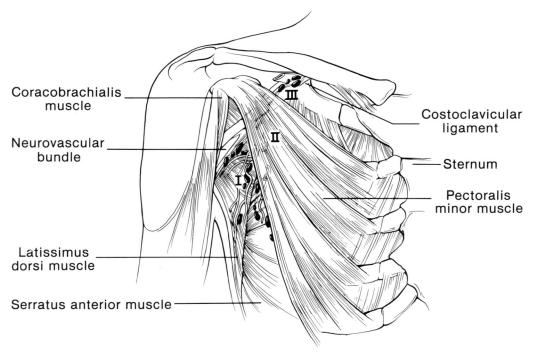

Coracobrachialis muscle

Neurovascular bundle

Latissimus dorsi muscle

Serratus anterior muscle

Costoclavicular ligament

Sternum

Pectoralis minor muscle

Figure 29–19. Topographical anatomical depiction of Levels I, II, and III of the axillary contents with relation to the neurovascular bundle, pectoralis minor, latissimus dorsi, posterior axillary space, and chest wall. Level 1 comprises three principal axillary nodal groups, including the external mammary group, the subscapular group, and the axillary vein (lateral) group. Level II, the central nodal group, is centrally placed immediately beneath the pectoralis minor muscle. The subclavicular (apical) group is designated Level III nodes and is superomedial to the pectoralis minor muscle.

rior axillary fold and occupies a superficial position beneath the skin and fascia of the midaxilla. The highest and most medially placed of the lymph node groups is the *subclavicular (apical group),* designated as *Level III.* This is the cephalomedial lymph node group that is located just proximal to the termination of the axillary vein at its confluence with the subclavian vein at the level of *Halsted's (costoclavicular) ligament* (condensation of the clavipectoral fascia). Figure 29–19 illustrates the position of the nodes relative to the pectoralis minor muscle and the posterior axillary space. These nodal groups are described relative to topographic anatomical relationships with the pectoralis minor muscle and the medial, lateral, and posterior axillary space. These lymphatics may be different from the nodal groups described by pathologists to indicate the area of metastic involvement within the axilla.

EVOLUTION OF SURGICAL TECHNIQUES FOR MASTECTOMY

In 1894, Halsted[12] and Meyer[18] simultaneously reported their operations for treatment of cancer of the breast. By demonstrating superior local and regional control rates using en bloc radical resection techniques, these eminent surgeons established the radical mastectomy as the "state-of-the-art" modality of that era to control cancer of the breast. Subsequently, many modifications of the original incision developed by Halsted have been reported and include those of Meyer, Kocher, Rodman, Stewart, Warren, Greenough, Orr, and MacFee, to mention only a few variations of the incision.[8] Many of the original incisions were developed to permit multiple approaches for extirpation of the mamma and to allow access to the axillary contents.

The Halsted and Meyer radical mastectomies differed technically in the sequence in which the breast and nodes were removed. Halsted insisted on primary resection of the breast and pectoral muscles prior to dissection of the axillary contents. In contrast, the Meyer technique (modified Halsted incision) completed the axillary dissection first, which was followed in sequence by breast and pectoral muscle resections, respectively. As indicated in Figure 29–20, the result achieved and the final cosmetic appearance for the Halsted and Meyer mastectomies are similar. Both procedures use a vertical incision to facilitate detachment of the pectoralis major from the clavicle and humerus and removal of the pectoralis minor from the coracoid process of the scapula. The incisions that have been subsequently adopted by various European and American surgeons are indicated in Figure 29–20 and represent incision modifications for operable breast cancer that presents in each quadrant of the organ. It should be noted that Halsted[12] and Meyer[18] strongly advocated the necessity of en bloc resections for extirpation of the breast and the contents of the axilla but had little appreciation for clinical staging and the ultimate consequences of systemic disease. At that time, no modalities existed to provide effective cytoreduction of the advanced primary lesion; thus ad-

vanced stages of disease were extirpated with the use of wider skin margins and larger flaps. For this reason, incision modifications that incorporate breast resection and wound closure were developed.

As appreciated by eminent breast surgeons of the late nineteenth and early twentieth centuries, the total mastectomy incision should incorporate both the nipple and the biopsy site to reduce the possibility of tumor implantation in the wound. In original dissections of the axilla, both Halsted[12] and Meyer[18] advocated complete axillary dissection of *all* nodal levels from the latissimus dorsi muscle laterally to the thoracic outlet medially. Both surgeons routinely resected the long thoracic nerve and the thoracodorsal neurovascular bundle en bloc with the axillary contents. Therefore it is not surprising that much of the initial criticism levied upon the radical mastectomy in the treatment of breast carcinoma concerned itself with the limitation of motion in the shoulder and the ipsilateral lymphedema that followed the surgery. It may also be argued that the survival rates for these patients, especially those with advanced local and regional disease, were not increased in proportion to the resultant disabilities (e.g., the "winged scapula" and shoulder fixation) evident with the procedures. Subsequently, Haagensen[11] advocated preservation of the long thoracic nerve to avoid the winged scapula disability and motor apraxia evident with loss of innervation to the serratus anterior. Additionally, Haagensen[11] commonly advocated removal of the thoracodorsal neurovascular bundle (with neural innervation to the latissimus dorsi muscle) to allow clearance of the subscapular and external mammary lymphatics that may follow the course of this neurovascular structure. However, most breast surgeons currently make an attempt to preserve *both* the long thoracic and the thoracodorsal nerves in the absence of gross invasion by the neoplasm or nodal fixation to these nerves. These principles are maintained to ensure function of the scapula and to preserve viability and function of the latissimus dorsi such that myocutaneous breast reconstruction may be considered at a future date.

It should be noted that contemporary modifications of the Halsted or Meyer radical mastectomy, with preservation of the long thoracic nerve, can be performed with little or no increase in morbidity when compared with the simple mastectomy.[8, 9] Additionally, any argument based on the value of the simple versus the radical procedure should be concerned with the long-term survival of the patient, which is the ultimate goal of therapy. To deny the patient the benefit of an adequate operative procedure on the basis of difficulty in placing cosmetic incisions or difficulty with wound closure is tantamount to admitting that the surgeon should not be treating the cancer.

The important contributions of D. H. Patey[21, 22] of the Institute of Clinical Research, Middlesex Hospital, London should be recognized. His careful clinical development and scientific demonstration of the worth of the "modified radical mastectomy" technique are quite laudable. In Britain in the 1930s, only a small minority of physicians questioned the absolute necessity of the rad-

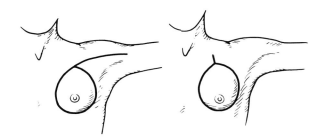

Original Halsted Incision   Modified Halsted Incision

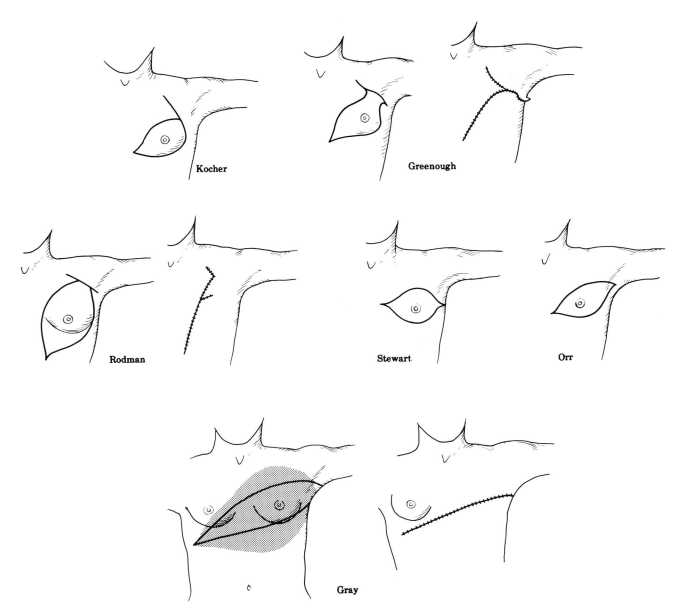

Figure 29–20. Variants of the radical mastectomy incision utilized in the therapy of primary carcinoma of the breast by various surgeons. The original Halsted incision was revised to avoid encroachment on the cephalic vein, which was preserved in subsequent procedures.

ical mastectomy for carcinoma of lesser size with absence of fixation to the pectoral muscles (stage I or II). Three major influences led Patey to consider alternatives and design the modified radical mastectomy technique. The first and most important consideration was the development and organization of radiation therapy. The second influence was the growing feeling of dissatisfaction with Sampson Handley's theory of "lymphatic permeation" as the primary process for the dissemination of carcinoma of the breast—a theory that, in its day, provided a logical pathological basis for some of the technical details of the radical mastectomy.[21] Lastly, with newer techniques for the study of lymphatic anatomy, Patey was able to refute the unproven postulates on which the original radical operations were based.[9, 22] Thereafter, Mr. Patey and his colleagues developed the technique for incontinuity removal of the breast and axillary contents with preservation of the pectoralis major muscle. This technique removed the pectoralis minor, like the standard radical operation, as an essential step to provide complete clearance of the axillary contents. Thereafter, objective demonstration of the efficacy for removal of axillary lymphatics with the technique was proven with lymphangiography by Kendall et al.[15] in 1963. Although this operation was performed by Patey for the first time in 1932, it was not adopted as a routine alternative to the standard radical mastectomy until late 1936.[22]

Although Patey is responsible for the application of the modified radical mastectomy as a standard approach for operable breast cancer, Auchincloss[2] and Madden[17] also developed modified radical mastectomy approaches. As indicated above, the Patey mastectomy differs from the Halsted mastectomy in that the pectoralis major muscle is preserved. Patey acknowledged the importance of the complete axillary dissection and appreciated the anatomical necessity for preservation of the medial and lateral pectoral (anterior thoracic) nerves, which may serve as dual innervation to the pectoralis major. In contrast, the Madden[17] and Auchincloss[2] modified radical mastectomies advocated preservation of *both* the pectoralis major and minor muscles. The similarities of the approaches were that these techniques required total mastectomy with at least partial axillary lymph node dissection. Because these approaches preserved the pectoralis minor, dissection of the apical (subclavicular, Level III) nodes was restricted, and in all cases, nodal recovery was less than with the Patey modified technique. The advantage of the Auchincloss[2] and Madden[17] procedures may be the higher probability for preservation of the medial pectoral nerve, which runs in the lateral neurovascular bundle of the axilla and may course through the pectoralis minor to supply the lateral border of the pectoralis major muscle. Expectantly, the Madden and Auchincloss techniques dissect only Levels I and II nodes and leave Level III lymphatics intact. Some surgeons advocate preservation of the pectoralis minor and simply detach the tendinous portion of the muscle from the coracoid process of the scapula to allow complete dissection of Level III nodes to Halsted's ligament. On completion of the nodal dissection, the tendon of the pectoralis minor was reapproximated to the coracoid with stainless steel wire or nonabsorbable suture.

The student of breast surgery should recognize that incisions for the modified radical mastectomy are narrow, and wounds are usually closed primarily. In contrast, radical procedures utilize wide incision margins, and skin is routinely grafted to wound defects. Because of modern radiobiological techniques and cytoreductive chemotherapy, skin incisions designed to totally ablate the skin of the breast (Fig. 29–20) are rarely utilized. Prior to the application of modern adjuvant techniques, incisions for large tumors that were considered to be locally advanced (because of ulceration, edema, and other grave signs) were designed to encompass these lesions with wide margins.

All skin flaps should be designed so that the incision incorporates skin at least 3 cm from the periphery of the tumor in three dimensions. In principle, less skin is excised when lesions are located deep within the breast and are small in transverse diameter (T1 < 2 cm). As indicated in chapter 2, viable breast tissue is anatomically distributed on the chest wall from the sternum to the axilla and from the clavicle to the aponeurosis of the rectus abdominis tendon. Haagensen[11] demonstrated that small foci of glandular tissue can be histologically identified in close proximity to the dermis just beneath the superficial fascia. Halsted[12] and Haagensen[11] each considered that wide skin excision of at least 5 cm in all directions from the tumor was essential because of the rich superficial lymphatic channels of the central subareolar tissue and subcutaneous dermal lymphatic plexuses of the breast. The anatomical and pathological rationale of the classic radical mastectomy is increasingly being challenged because of the availability of adjuvant modalities that enhance local and regional control with potential lengthening of disease-free and overall survival rates.

Questions have also been raised with regard to the *thickness* of skin flaps that should be elevated in the planning of the total mastectomy as part of the radical or modified radical procedure. Krohn et al.[16] recently completed a two-arm study to evaluate the necessity of the ultrathin skin flap and the autogenous skin graft as methods to enhance local wound control and 5- and 10-year survival. A similar group of women who underwent radical mastectomy with narrow margins of skin excision, with primary wound closure and without ultrathin flaps, had comparable 5- and 10-year survival and local recurrence rates. Wound complications, hospital stay, and subsequent lymphedema, however, were significantly greater in the patients with thinner skin flaps. Most surgeons acknowledge that superior cosmetic results are achievable with well-vascularized flaps and the avoidance of split-thickness skin grafting. We maintain these basic tenets and avoid ultrathin flaps. Flaps developed at the plane of insertion of Cooper's ligament in the cutis with subcutaneous fat assure extirpation of the underlying breast parenchyma. In general, flaps of 7 to 8 mm thickness usually ensure generous vascularity to the skin. As much subcutaneous fat is preserved as is consistent with complete breast resection. Although the deep layer of the superficial investing fascia that intervenes between the subcutaneous fat and the breast tissue is easily identified, the thickness of this well-vascularized flap varies considerably with the patient's habitus and lean body mass.

The design of operations intended for total mastectomy of operable breast cancer not amenable to conservation surgical techniques has been previously addressed. In general, advanced primary lesions (T2 or T3), with pectoralis major fixation, high-lying lesions, and perhaps some lesions with grave signs should be treated by radical or modified radical techniques. As previously discussed, the operations designed by Halsted, his predecessors, and his students reflect the necessity of designing wider flaps with large incisions that encompass the primary lesion by at least 5 cm. When considering the advanced primary lesions that were treated in that era without adjuvant techniques, the necessity of larger resections can be rationalized, because surgery was the only option for treatment.

Incisions designed for removal of the entire mammary gland (total or simple mastectomy) must incorporate the nipple-areola complex with the primary tumor in a three-dimensional aspect such that margins are free of disease. Donegan et al.[5] previously determined that incisions that resect skin and breast parenchyma at a distance of more than 4 cm from any margin of the palpable tumor achieve nothing therapeutically. The majority of surgeons consider a 3- to 4-cm margin adequate to achieve local control without tumor implantation. As discussed in chapter 28, incisions placed in the breast for suspicious breast masses must be planned with consideration for the subsequent need for total mastectomy. Incisions should incorporate the primary biopsy scar, which should be well planned at the time of biopsy to allow complete extirpation of the neoplasm with the definitive mastectomy. When the primary breast lesion has been totally removed with the original biopsy as an excisional technique, incisions at the time of total mastectomy should incorporate the skin and scar of the biopsy site by a 3-cm margin in all directions. We prefer incisions that are slightly oblique from the transverse line and that extend cephalad toward the axilla. Under no circumstances should the design of a cosmetic scar in any way compromise the successful extirpation of the primary neoplasm. Split-thickness skin grafting becomes necessary when wider margins and larger flaps are required to achieve the 3- to 4-cm free margin.

Figures 29–21 through 29–26 depict the various locations of breast primaries in which adequate therapy, with or without irradiation and chemotherapy, necessitates the total mastectomy.

DESIGN OF INCISIONS FOR MASTECTOMY IN THE TREATMENT OF BREAST CANCER

Central and Subareolar Primary Lesions

Figure 29–21 depicts the design of the classic Stewart elliptical skin incision (Fig. 29–20) that is utilized for mastectomy of subareolar or central breast primaries. The original biopsy is preferably done via a periareolar incision for lesions in this location. The residual scar should have measurements for the cephalad and caudad extents of the incision to include at least a 3-cm margin. Availability of adequate skin to complete a primary closure is rarely difficult in the pendulous or large breast. For the majority of patients with small breasts, the Stewart incision will allow primary closure of skin except when more than 4 to 5 cm of skin are encompassed in the primary resection or if evidence of skin devascularization is apparent following completion of the procedure. Loss of skin secondary to ultrathin dissection planes or trauma to the flaps may necessitate even wider resections of skin margins.

Figure 29–22 shows an optional elliptical incision in the contour of the breast for an inner quadrant primary lesion. This incision would perhaps best be described as the *modified Stewart incision,* which has a predominant extension in a more oblique and cephalad direction toward the ipsilateral axilla. The Stewart incision is commonly preferred by plastic surgeons anticipating reconstruction with myocutaneous flaps, especially when a contralateral simple mastectomy is planned for treatment of benign or potentially malignant disease or as a prophylactic procedure.

Lesions of the Upper Outer or Lower Inner Quadrants

Figures 29–23 and 29–24 denote the incision design for operable breast cancer in the upper outer or lower inner quadrants. Minimal skin margins of 3 cm from the primary neoplasm are incorporated in a *modified Orr incision* that is slightly oblique from the transverse line with cephalad extension toward the axilla. Similar to the Orr and Stewart incisions, although somewhat more oblique, these incisions lend themselves to cosmetically satisfactory breast reconstruction using myocutaneous or subpectoral augmentation breast implants.

Lesions of the Upper Inner Quadrants

Lesions of the upper inner quadrants of the breast are often difficult to manage because of their anatomical location. The surgeon should recognize the inherent problems encountered with elevation of skin flaps that allow adequate surgical margins while providing cosmesis for wound closure and potential reconstruction. On occasion, the surgeon is able to develop a 3-cm margin for lesions that are in this quadrant, providing the lesion is not cephalad (infraclavicular). These lesions may be operated via the modified Stewart incision. Commonly the surgeon encounters the dilemma of designing an elliptical incision that is widely based near the cephalomedial aspect of the breast to incorporate a 3-cm margin of the tumor with extension laterally and inferiorly such that the incision terminates at the anterior axillary line (Fig. 29–25). The surgeon should plan the cephalic portion of the incision for the superior flap such

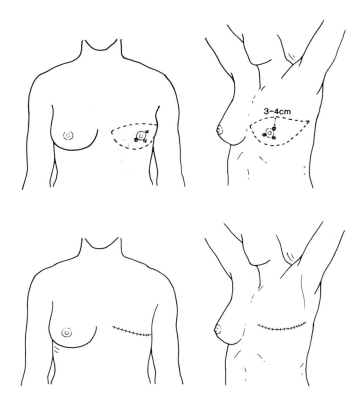

Figure 29–21. Design of the *classic Stewart* elliptical incision for central and subareolar primary lesions of the breast. The *medial* extent of the incision ends at the margin of the sternum. The *lateral* extent of the skin incision should overlie the anterior margin of the latissimus dorsi. The design of the skin incision should incorporate the primary neoplasm en bloc with margins that are 3 to 4 cm from the cranial and caudal edges of the tumor.

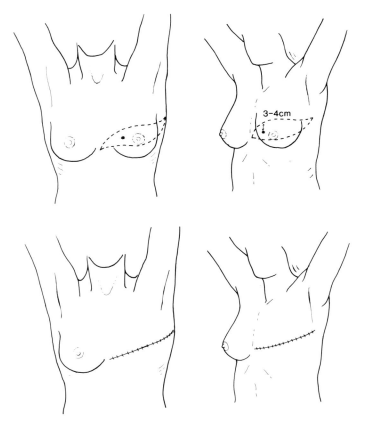

Figure 29–22. Design of the obliquely placed *modified Stewart* incision for cancer of the inner quadrant of the breast. The medial extent of the incision often must incorporate skin to the midsternum to allow a 3 to 4-cm margin in all directions from the edge of the tumor. Lateral extent of the incision ends at the anterior margin of the latissimus.

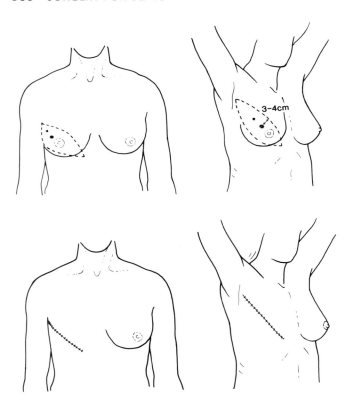

Figure 29–23. Design of the *classic Orr* oblique incision for carcinoma of the upper outer quadrants of the breast. The skin incision is placed 3 to 4 cm from the margin of the tumor in an oblique plane that is directed cephalad towards the ipsilateral axilla. This incision is a variant of the original Greenough, Kocher, and Rodman techniques for flap development.

Figure 29–24. Variation of the *Orr* incision for lower inner and vertically placed (6 o'clock) lesions of the breast. The design of the skin incision is identical to that of Figure 29–22, with attention directed to margins of 3 to 4 cm.

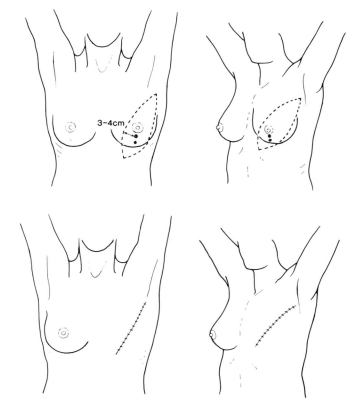

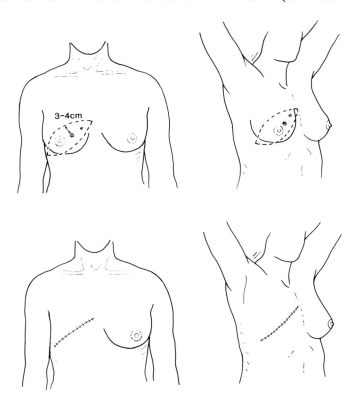

Figure 29–25. Design of skin flaps for upper inner quadrant primary tumors of the breast. The cephalad margin of the flap must be designed to allow access for dissection of the axilla. With flap margins 3 to 4 cm from the tumor, variation in the medial extent of the incision is expectant and may extend beyond the edge of the sternum.

On occasion, the modified Stewart incision can incorporate the tumor en bloc, provided that the cancer is not too high on the breast and craniad from the nipple-areola complex. All incision designs must be inclusive of the nipple-areola when total mastectomy is planned with primary therapy.

that adequate access to the pectoralis major and to the axillary contents is assured.

Lesions of the Lower Outer Quadrants

Lesions of the lower outer quadrants of the breast should have an incision design similar to those of the upper inner quadrant, with margins of 3 to 4 cm around the primary lesion (Fig. 29–26) and with maximum extension of the cephalad margin to provide access to flaps for dissection of the pectoralis major and the axillary contents.

High-lying (Infraclavicular) Lesions

With large lesions (T2, T3, T4) that are high lying, infraclavicular, or fixed to the pectoralis major, incisions designed to provide a 3- to 4-cm margin will necessitate

Figure 29–26. Incisions for cancer of the lower outer quadrants of the breast. The surgeon should design incisions that achieve margins of 3 to 4 cm from the tumor with cephalad margins that allow access for dissection of the axilla. The medial extent is the margin of the sternum. Laterally, the inferior extent of the incision is the latissimus.

skin grafting of the defect. The original Halstedian and Meyer incisions, with subsequent modifications by Greenough, Rodman, and Gray (see Fig. 29–20), are used for treatment of these primary lesions of T2, T3, and T4 size.[8] For T1 lesions in this position, design of an elliptical incision placed in a vertical dimension from the clavicle provides adequate access for axillary dissection and clearing of the pectoralis major muscle when indicated. Figure 29–27 depicts the design of the vertical, elliptical incision for these high-lying lesions and the vertical closure. As these incisions are placed perpendicular to Langer's lines, cosmesis is minimized and the planes of cleavage for the medial breast are lost.

Incisions for Axillary Dissection

Figure 29–28 depicts the preferred incision and the optional incisions for axillary dissections performed syn-

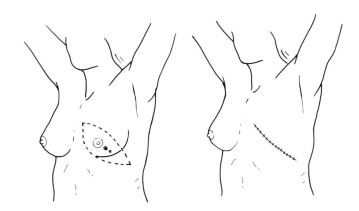

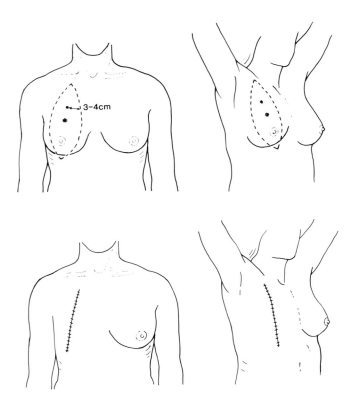

Figure 29–27. Depiction of skin flaps for lesions of the breast that are high lying, infraclavicular, or fixed to the pectoralis major muscle. Fixation to the muscle necessitates Halsted radical mastectomy with skin margins of a minimal 3 cm. Skin grafting is necessary when large margins of skin are resected for T3 and T4 cancers. Primary closure for T1 and some T2 tumors is often possible.

chronously with lumpectomy (segmental mastectomy, tylectomy). We prefer incisions placed parallel with Langer's lines and designed in a curvilinear fashion just caudal to the axillary hairline. Preferably axillary incisions are made separately from incisions of the segmental mastectomy. Optional incisions indicated in Figure 29–28 obliquely cross Langer's lines and are not positioned in axillary skin folds. It is perhaps for this latter reason that delay in primary healing and inferior cosmetic results are obtained. Adequate skin exposure should be provided so that dissection of Level I and Level II nodes beneath the pectoralis minor is possible without undue traction on the pectoralis major or minor muscles. This principle prevents damage to the medial and lateral (anterior thoracic) pectoral nerves located in the lateral and medial neurovascular bundles, respectively. Incisions placed in a curvilinear transverse, oblique, or vertical fashion all allow adequate access to the axillary vein, the medial border of the pectoralis minor muscle, and the lateral aspect of the latissimus dorsi muscle. This exposure should permit visualization of the long thoracic nerve to the serratus anterior and the thoracodorsal nerve to the latissimus dorsi.

References

1. Anson BJ, McVay CB: Breast or mammary region. *In* Anson BJ, McVay CB (eds): Surgical Anatomy, vol 1. Philadelphia, WB Saunders, 1971, pp 339–356.
2. Auchincloss H: Significance of location and number of axillary metastases in carcinoma of the breast: a justification for a conservative operation. Ann Surg 158:37–46, 1963.
3. Bland KI, Freedman BE, Harris PL, Yun-Jo H, Wittliff JL: The effects of ischemia on estrogen and progesterone receptor profiles in the rodent uterus. J Surg Res 42(6):653–660, 1987.
4. Cody HS, Egeli RA, Urban JA: Rotter's node metastases. Ann Surg 199:266–270, 1984.
4a. Copeland EM III: Carcinoma of the breast. *In* Copeland EM III (ed): Surgical Oncology. New York, John Wiley & Sons, 1983, pp 43–58.
5. Donegan WL, Perez-Mesa CM, Watson FR: A biostatistical study of locally recurrent breast carcinoma. Surg Gynecol Obstet 122:529–540, 1966.
6. Ellis LM, Wittliff JL, Bryant ML, Hogancamp WE, Sitren HS, Bland KI: Correlation of estrogen, progesterone and androgen receptors in breast cancer; significance of the androgen receptor. Am J Surg 157(6):577–581, 1989.

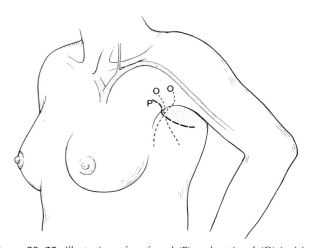

Figure 29–28. Illustration of preferred (P) and optional (O) incisions utilized in axillary dissection. Ideally, incisions are placed in skin folds that parallel Langer's lines. Incisions are preferably curvilinear with placement just caudal to the hairline of the axilla.

Optional incisions depicted are oblique or vertically placed with the chest wall. As these optional incisions cross the lines of tension (Langer's lines), delay in wound repair and inferior cosmetic results may be observed.

7. Ellis LM, Wittliff JL, Bryant MS, Sitren HS, Hogancamp WE, Souba WW, Bland KI: Lability of steroid hormone receptors following devascularization of breast tumors. Arch Surg 124:39–42, 1989.
8. Gray DB: The radical mastectomy incision. Am Surg 35(10):750–755, 1969.
9. Gray JH: The relation of lymphatic vessels to the spread of cancer. Br J Surg 26:462–495, 1939.
10. Gray SW, Skandalakis JE: Atlas of Surgical Anatomy for General Surgeons. Baltimore, MD, Williams and Wilkins, 1985.
11. Haagensen CD: Anatomy of the mammary gland. *In* Haagensen CD (ed): Diseases of the Breast, ed 2. Philadelphia, WB Saunders, 1971, pp 1–28.
12. Halsted WS: Results of operation for cure of cancer of breast performed at Johns Hopkins Hospital from June 1889 to January 1894. Ann Surg 20:497–555, 1894.
13. Handley RS: The conservative radical mastectomy of Patey: ten year results in 425 patients breasts. Dis Breast 2:16, 1976.
14. Hollingshead WH: The breast. *In* Hollingshead WH (ed): Anatomy for Surgeons: Vol 2. Thorax, Abdomen, and Pelvis, ed 2. New York, Harper & Row, 1971, pp 11–17.
15. Kendall BE, Arthur JF, Patey DH: Lymphangiography in carci-

noma of the breast: a comparison of clinical, radiological, and pathological findings in axillary lymph nodes. Cancer 16:1233–1242, 1963.
16. Krohn IT, Cooper DR, Bassett JG: Radical mastectomy. Arch Surg 227:760–763, 1982.
17. Madden JL: Modified radical mastectomy. Surg Gynecol Obstet 121:1221–1230, 1965.
18. Meyer W: An improved method of the radical operation for carcinoma of the breast. Med Rec NY 46:746–749, 1894.
19. Moosman DA: Anatomy of the pectoral nerves and their preservation in modified mastectomy. Am J Surg 139:883–886, 1980.
20. Netter FH: CIBA collection of medical illustrations, 7:6, Summit NJ, CIBA Pharmaceutical, 1979.
21. Patey DH: A review of 146 cases of carcinoma of the breast operated upon between 1930–1946. Br J Cancer 21:260–269, 1967.
22. Patey DH, Dyson WH: Prognosis of carcinoma of the breast in relation to type of operation performed. Br J Cancer 2:7–13, 1948.
23. Spratt JS Jr, Donegan WL: Anatomy of the breast. *In* Donegan WL, Spratt JS Jr (eds): Cancer of the Breast, ed 3. Philadelphia, WB Saunders, 1979.

HALSTED RADICAL MASTECTOMY

Kirby I. Bland, M.D. and Edward M. Copeland III, M.D.

"With the exception of perhaps Billroth, Volkmann is the only one of the surgeons quoted who occasionally removed the pectoral muscles. But his operation is an imperfect one. It admits of the frequent division of tissues which are cancerous and it does not give the disease a sufficiently wide berth. Why should we shave the under-surfaces of the cancer so narrowly if the pectoralis major muscle or a part of it can be removed without danger, and without causing subsequent disability, and if there are positive indications for its removal? The pectoralis major muscle, entire, all except its clavicular portion, should be excised in every case of cancer of the breast because the operator is enabled thereby to remove in one piece all of the suspected tissues. The suspected tissues should be removed in one piece lest the wound become infected by the division of tissue invaded by the disease, or by division of the lymphatic vessels containing cancer cells, and because shreds or pieces of cancerous tissue might readily be overlooked in a piecemeal extirpation."

William Stewart Halsted (1894)

HISTORY

The student of surgery of the breast will immediately recognize that the Halsted radical mastectomy, begun in 1882 by Halsted at the Johns Hopkins Hospital in Baltimore, embodied the concept of routine complete en bloc resection of the breast with the pectoralis major muscle and the regional lymphatics.[9, 10] Indeed, the rationale of the Halstedian approach was largely directed at the proposition of preventing local or regional recurrences. Halsted's synthesis of the techniques of his predecessors in surgery and pathology allowed him to achieve local and regional recurrent rates of 6 percent and 22 percent, respectively.[4, 9, 10] The en bloc technique described by Halsted, although published simultaneously by Willy Meyer,[18] allowed a reduction in the local recurrence rate to 6 percent from rates of 51 percent to 82 percent for contemporary European surgeons. Table 29–6 compares the operations available to European surgeons during the Halstedian era with the accompanying 3-year estimated cure rates for breast carcinoma.

Halsted was not the first surgeon to resect the pectoralis major muscle in the course of a radical mastectomy. Wolff[32] documents that Barthélemy Cabrol of Montpellier, France, reported the cure of a mammary carcinoma in a 35-year-old woman in whom the pectoralis major muscle was excised and the wound sprinkled with vitriol.[4] The patient survived 12 years, only to succumb to cancer of the lower lip. Great European surgeons such as Petit, Billroth, Volkmann, and others of that period not infrequently removed portions of the pectoral muscles in resection of certain malignancies of the breast.[31] Joerss[14] has attributed the modern operation to Heidenhein. Nonetheless it was Halsted who advocated routine resection of the pectoralis muscles en bloc with breast tissues and axillary nodes. In its final form, the technique of the radical mastectomy espoused by Halsted embodied the following principles:

1. Wide excision of the skin, covering the defect with Thiersch grafts.

Table 29–6. CHRONOLOGY OF THE MASTECTOMY FOR TREATMENT OF BREAST CANCER WITH EXPECTANT (AVERAGE) 3-YEAR "CURE RATES"

Type of Operation	Author	Year	No. Cases	Percent 3-Year Cures
Simple mastectomy	V. Winiwarter (Billroth)[30]	1867–1875		4.7
Average				4.7
Complete mastectomy and	Oldekop[21]	1850–1878	229	11.7
axillary dissection in	Dietrich (Lucke)[6]	1872–1890	148	16.2
majority of cases	Horner[12]	1881–1893	144	19.4
	Poulsen[24]	1870–1888	110	20
	Banks[3]	1877	46	20
	Schmid (Kuster)[26]	1871–1885		21.5
Average				18.1
Complete (total) mastectomy,	Sprengel (Volkmann)[28]	1874–1878	200	11
axillary dissection, removal	Schmidt[27]	1877–1886	112	18.8
of pectoral fascia and	Rotter[25]		30	20
greater or lesser amounts of	Mahler[17]	1887–1897	150	21
pectoral muscle	Joerss[14]	1885–1893	98	28.5
Average				19.9
Modern radical mastectomy	Halsted[9]	1889–1894	76	45
	Halsted[10]	1907	232	38.3
	Hutchinson's collected figures[13]	1910–1933		39.4

From Cooper WA: The History of the Radical Mastectomy. *In* Annals of Medical History, Vol III. New York, Paul B. Hoeber, 1941, pp 36–54.

2. Routine removal of *both* pectoral muscles.
3. Routine axillary dissection (Levels I to III).
4. Removal of all tissues in one block, cutting as wide as possible on all sides of the growth.

The evolution of the modern radical mastectomy was a tedious and laborious process that began with Cabrol in 1570 and terminated with Halsted in 1890.[4] The evolution of the operation is one of discordant retrogressions. The wide acceptance of the incurability of carcinoma, the consequences of sepsis, and the necessity for anesthesia played prominent roles in delay of the development for surgery of the breast. To attribute the development of the modern operation to a single individual would discredit the remarkable contributions of Halsted's predecessors. The early surgery and pathology pioneers extended the operation because of the clinical observations for the natural history of breast cancer. These leaders of medical science lacked the salient background in pathology, anatomy, and statistics that was to enable Halsted to complete the evolution of the radical mastectomy in the late nineteenth century.

BREAST CANCER TREATMENT IN THE UNITED STATES

The American College of Surgeons conducted two surveys for the treatment of breast carcinoma in the United States: a long-term survey in 1976 and a short-term survey in 1982.[30] Table 29–7 shows that in the short-term survey, more than twice the percentage of patients were treated by partial mastectomy (7.2 percent) compared with the long-term survey, which re-

ported that 2.8 percent of surgeons utilized this technique in the primary therapy of breast cancer ($p < 0.0001$). The most significant changes in this survey were in the type of operations used for treatment of operable breast cancer. There is an increased use of modified radical mastectomy (55.6 percent in the long-term survey compared with 78.2 percent in the short-term survey) and a marked decline in the reported use of the Halsted radical mastectomy (27.5 percent of the patients in the long-term survey compared with 3.4 percent in the 1981 data) (Fig. 29–29). For each stage of disease, there was a greater reported use of the modified radical procedure in the more recent short-term survey data compared with that for patients operated on 5 years earlier. Interestingly, no significant changes were observed in the other types of surgical procedures between 1976 and 1981.

When treatment modalities were evaluated according to clinical stage in the American College Survey, 95 percent of the patients were treated in the long- and short-term survey by surgical treatment alone or in combination with other modalities. Table 29–8 shows that in the long-term survey, 60.6 percent of patients were treated by operation alone compared with 58.8 percent in the short-term analysis. Additionally, the use of surgical therapy plus irradiation (with or without chemotherapy) was observed to decrease from 19.8 percent to 16.6 percent, and the use of chemotherapy (with or without irradiation) with operation was noted to increase from 16.4 percent to 22.7 percent over this 5-year period. The change was limited to patients with regional and distant disease, and there was no significant change in the use of other treatment modalities between

Table 29–7. TYPE OF OPERATION AND STAGE DISTRIBUTION OF PATIENTS WITH CARCINOMA OF THE BREAST

| | Clinical Stage Regional To: | | | | | | | | | |
| Operation | Localized | | Axillary Nodes With or Without Adjacent Tissue | | Adjacent Tissue Only | | Distant | | Total | |
	No.	Percent	No.	Percent	No.	Percent	No.	Percent	No.	Percent
Long-Term Survey (1976)										
Partial mastectomy	408	3.0	74	0.8	58	8.1	153	14.3	693	2.8
Total mastectomy only	1,261	9.3	203	2.2	178	24.7	278	26.0	1,920	7.8
Total mastectomy with low axillary dissection	632	4.6	509	5.5	35	4.9	98	9.2	1,274	5.2
Modified radical mastectomy	7,584	55.7	5,481	59.1	295	41.0	361	33.7	13,721	55.6
Radical (Halsted) mastectomy	3,571	26.2	2,909	31.4	144	20.0	169	15.8	6,793	27.5
Extended radical mastectomy	152	1.1	99	1.1	9	1.2	11	1.0	271	1.1
Total	13,608	100.0	9,275	100.0	719	100.0	1,070	100.0	24,672	100.0
Short-Term Survey (1981)										
Partial mastectomy	819	8.5	236	3.4	58	12.1	170	22.1	1,283	7.2
Total mastectomy only	530	5.5	129	1.9	73	15.2	184	23.9	916	5.2
Total mastectomy with low axillary dissection	511	5.3	340	5.0	26	5.4	83	10.8	960	5.4
Modified radical mastectomy	7,436	77.1	5,777	85.0	302	62.9	312	40.6	13,827	78.2
Radical (Halsted) mastectomy	295	3.0	272	4.0	17	3.5	19	2.5	603	3.4
Extended radical mastectomy	57	0.6	41	0.6	4	0.8	1	0.1	103	0.6
Total	9,648	100.0	6,795	100.0	480	100.0	769	100.0	17,692	100.0

From Wilson RE et al: Surg Gynecol Obstet 159:309–318, 1984.

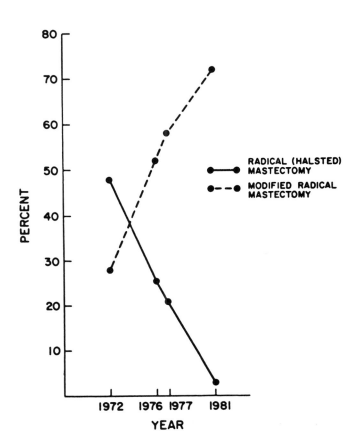

Figure 29–29. Trends in the type of operation performed from 1972 to 1981 in the 1982 National Survey of Carcinoma of the Breast in the United States by the American College of Surgeons Survey. (From Wilson RE et al: Surg Gynecol Obstet 159:309–318, 1984.)

the long- and short-term surveys. For both the long- and short-term analyses, 82 percent of the patients in the localized disease stage were treated by surgery alone. For both surveys, the use of operative therapy as a sole modality decreased with advancing stage of disease, and the proportion of patients treated by operation alone was similar in both surveys (Table 29–8). Further, operation plus irradiation was used more often than operation plus chemotherapy in treatment of patients having cancer diagnosed as localized or regional to adjacent tissue. For the long-term study, operation plus irradiation and operation plus chemotherapy were used equally (24.2 percent vs. 24.1 percent) for treatment of patients with axillary node involvement. The short-term study confirmed that operation plus chemotherapy was 3.5 times more likely to be utilized than operation plus radiation (35 percent vs. 10.4 percent) for treatment of patients with positive axillary nodes. Wilson et al.[30] noted that in both surveys, similar proportions of patients with regional disease underwent operation followed by both radiation and chemotherapy. For patients observed to have disease in the advanced stage, irradiation, chemotherapy, or hormone therapy, alone or in combination, were used more often (42.1 percent long-term and 38.7 percent in the short-term surveys).

Trends and Patterns of Care, 1971–1981

Figures 29–17 and 29–29 confirm that the majority of surgeons used the modified radical mastectomy on patients reported in 1971, 1976, 1977, and 1981. In 1972, 48 percent of patients were reported to have had a Halsted-type radical mastectomy, whereas only 3 percent of patients underwent this procedure in 1981. Trends in the use of radiation therapy and chemotherapy also showed dramatic alterations in application from 1972 through 1981. The trends for the use of radiation therapy in these years are depicted in Figure 29–30. The proportion of patients at all stages reported to have received irradiation decreased from 33 percent in 1972 to 18 percent in 1981. This trend is most apparent for regional stage disease. In contrast, the introduction of effective adjuvant and systemic chemotherapy and the emerging principles of pharmacotherapeutics caused a dramatic increase in the application of chemotherapy.

Table 29–8. TYPE OF TREATMENT AND STAGE DISTRIBUTION OF PATIENTS WITH CARCINOMA OF THE BREAST

	Localized		Clinical Stage Regional To: Axillary Nodes With or Without Adjacent Tissue		Adjacent Tissue Only		Distant		Total	
Operation	*No.*	*Percent*	*No.*	*Percent*	*No.*	*Percent*	*No.*	*Percent*	*No.*	*Percent*
Long-Term Survey (1976)										
Surgical treatment only	11,592	84.4	3,395	35.8	454	53.9	261	14.1	15,702	60.6
Surgical treatment and radiation	1,275	9.3	2,289	24.2	148	17.6	165	8.9	3,877	15.0
Surgical treatment and chemotherapy	460	3.4	2,284	24.1	57	6.8	215	11.6	3,016	11.6
Surgical treatment and hormone therapy	75	0.5	132	1.4	12	1.4	103	5.6	322	1.2
Surgical treatment, radiation, and chemotherapy	154	1.1	911	9.6	34	4.0	142	7.7	1,241	4.8
Surgical treatment and others*	52	0.4	264	2.8	14	1.7	184	10.0	514	2.0
Others*	120	0.9	198	2.1	123	14.6	778	42.1	1,219	4.7
Total	13,728	100.0	9,473	100.0	842	100.0	1,848	100.0	25,891	100.0
Short-Term Survey (1981)										
Surgical treatment only	8,065	82.2	2,444	35.0	285	53.5	140	11.2	10,934	58.8
Surgical treatment and radiation	1,035	10.6	731	10.4	94	17.6	56	4.5	1,916	10.3
Surgical treatment and chemotherapy	355	3.6	2,444	35.0	44	8.3	209	16.7	3,052	16.4
Surgical treatment and hormone therapy	78	0.8	179	2.6	8	1.5	96	7.7	361	1.9
Surgical treatment, radiation and chemotherapy	88	0.9	857	12.3	37	6.9	181	14.4	1,163	6.3
Surgical treatment and others*	27	0.3	140	2.0	12	2.3	87	6.9	266	1.4
Others*	162	1.6	192	2.7	53	9.9	485	38.7	892	4.8
Total	9,810	100.0	6,987	100.0	533	100.0	1,254	100.0	18,584	100.0

*Radiation, chemotherapy, or both, and radiation, hormone therapy, or both.
From Wilson RE et al: Surg Gynecol Obstet 159:309–318, 1984.

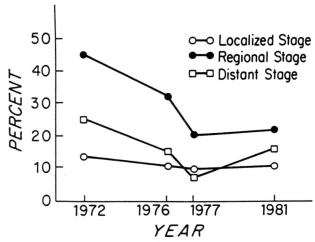

Figure 29–30. Trends in the use of radiotherapy from 1972 to 1981 as reported in the 1982 National Survey of Carcinoma of the Breast in the United States by the American College of Surgeons Survey. (From Wilson RE et al: Surg Gynecol Obstet 159:309–318, 1984.)

Chemotherapy increased from 7 percent of patients treated in 1972 to 22.7 in 1981. As depicted in Figure 29–31, this exponential increase in the use of chemotherapy was limited to patients with regional and distant stages of disease. Currently the use of adjuvant chemotherapy for treatment of localized disease (stages O and I) has seen a renaissance. A discussion of the application of adjuvant chemotherapy and hormonal therapy for breast cancer is presented in section XIV, chapter 39.

The 1982 National Survey evaluated 5-year survival rates by stage, type of treatment, and type of adjuvant therapy. Table 29–9 depicts survival rates for patients treated in 1976 by type of operation, with or without adjuvant irradiation and chemotherapy. Similar survival rates for patients with localized disease were observed for treatment by partial mastectomy alone and by partial mastectomy plus irradiation to either the breast, the

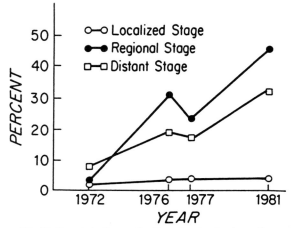

Figure 29–31. Trends in the application of systemic chemotherapy from 1972 to 1981 as reported in the 1982 National Surgery of Cancer of the Breast in the United States reported by the American College of Surgeons Survey. (From Wilson RE et al: Surg Gynecol Obstet 159:309–318, 1984.)

axilla, or both. Additionally, 5-year survival rates for patients treated by the modified radical mastectomy technique were similar to 5-year survival rates for those treated by the Halsted radical mastectomy. Wilson et al.[30] noted that survival rates were also similar for those who received additional irradiation therapy or chemotherapy with one of the two surgical procedures.

It must be emphasized that these short- and long-term surveys are not prospective trials, and bias in treatment selection cannot be eliminated. In addition, follow-up studies are short, and data represent only trends. Nonetheless there has been an important transition in curative surgical procedures utilized by American surgeons from the Halsted radical to the modified radical mastectomy techniques.[29] This transition was apparent at the time of the 1977 survey reported by Nemoto et al.,[19, 20] and the 1981 survey[20] confirmed that the vast majority of patients treated had had a modified radical rather than a radical mastectomy (77 percent vs. 3 percent). The results of the short-term survey also confirmed an increase in the proportion of patients being treated by partial mastectomy, largely because of the convincing results of recent clinical trials conducted by Fisher et al.[7, 8] in association with the National Surgical Adjuvant Breast Project (NSABP). These data will almost certainly undergo rapid change with the next American College of Surgeons' survey. Survival rates of patients treated by the various procedures are *not* comparable in the absence of more detailed data, because of confounding biological and patient-related factors that may affect prognosis. Clearly, prospective follow-up studies using equivalent disease staging are needed to make long-term comparisons for the value of the various operative approaches.

INDICATIONS FOR THE RADICAL MASTECTOMY

Despite the application of modern radiobiology and chemotherapy as modalities to allow cytoreduction of the primary breast neoplasm, radical mastectomy is occasionally necessary to achieve local and regional control of disease in the breast, axilla, and chest wall. Breast cancer mortality rates before and after the introduction of the Halsted mastectomy attest to the effectiveness of this treatment as the most definitive step in the management of breast cancer.[1] Until the advent of adjuvant chemotherapy and modern irradiation, little improvement in survival data for patients with breast cancer was documented. In the past two decades, a growing body of data confirm that the extent of the procedure can be lessened while maintaining survival rates equivalent to that of the radical approach for the treatment of breast cancer.*

The major consideration for less extensive operations than the classic Halsted mastectomy is based on tissue preservation to enhance the cosmetic result. Nevertheless, with presentation of gross involvement of the pectoralis major muscle, whether fixed to the pectoralis

---

*References 2, 5, 7, 8, 11, 15, 16, 19, 20, 22, and 23.

Table 29–9. FIVE-YEAR SURVIVAL RATE IN PERCENT BY STAGE, TYPE OF OPERATION, AND TYPE OF ADJUVANT THERAPY

| | Type of Adjuvant Therapy by Stage | | | | | | | | |
| | Localized | | | Regional | | | Distant | | |
Type of Operation	*None*	*Radiation*	*Chemotherapy*	*None*	*Radiation*	*Chemotherapy*	*None*	*Radiation*	*Chemotherapy*
Partial mastectomy									
Five-year survival (%)	82.6	83.9	100.0	64.4	56.9	81.0	29.0	9.5	20.4
No. of patients	301	81	7	54	45	8	32	18	37
Total mastectomy only									
Five-year survival (%)	86.8	81.0	80.1	66.0	51.3	55.9	30.2	23.4	19.7
No. of patients	1,034	154	37	183	116	32	72	44	43
Total mastectomy with low axillary dissection									
Five-year survival (%)	92.6	88.0	82.7	75.0	64.7	74.0	24.8	19.0	36.4
No. of patients	540	55	24	242	159	77	15	17	13
Modified radical mastectomy									
Five-year survival (%)	92.4	89.2	84.3	80.2	72.3	71.6	46.1	29.4	32.4
No. of patients	6,537	630	280	2,131	1,292	1,553	85	55	85
Radical (Halsted) mastectomy									
Five-year survival (%)	92.8	89.4	88.7	78.0	73.1	71.1	52.5	51.4	51.5
No. of patients	3,058	335	104	1,190	795	640	50	29	37

Adapted from Wilson RE et al: Surg Gynecol Obstet 159:309–318, 1984.

minor or not, any operation less than the Halsted mastectomy will be insufficient to achieve en bloc extirpation of the neoplasm. In addition, high-lying peripheral lesions near the clavicle or sternum, with deep fixation, commonly necessitate the radical mastectomy with combination irradiation to control the neoplasm. Consideration must also be given the radical procedure for deep or central tumors of the breast with fixation to the pectoral fascia in solitary or multicentric sites. Many surgeons advocate the Halsted radical procedure for lesions that exceed 4 cm in transverse diameter, as the advantage of total mastectomy with wide margins (minimal 4 cm) is best achieved with this procedure.

TECHNIQUE OF RADICAL MASTECTOMY

Following induction of general anesthesia, the patient is positioned supine on the operative table with a sheet roll that allows slight elevation of the ipsilateral shoulder and hemithorax. The ipsilateral hemithorax should be positioned at the margin of the operative table. The operator must be cognizant of the potential for subsequent subluxation and abduction of the shoulder on the arm board to prevent stretch of the brachial plexus with potential injury by motor denervation of the shoulder and arm. This complication is best avoided by padding the arm board to allow elevation of the forearm and hand in a relaxed position (Fig. 29–32). The operator should confirm that the ipsilateral arm and shoulder have free mobility for adduction across the chest wall; the elbow should be easily flexed and extended without tension.

The involved breast with the ipsilateral neck and hemithorax is prepped to the table margin inclusive of the shoulder, axilla, arm, and hand. Towels may be

stapled or secured with towel clips to the skin with draping of the shoulder, lower neck, sternum, and upper rectus abdominus musculature within the planned operative field (Fig. 29–32). The authors prefer to isolate the hand and forearm with an occlusive Stockinette (DeRoyal Industries, Powell, TN) cotton dressing and secure same with a Kerlex or Kling (Johnson and Johnson, New Brunswick, NJ) cotton roll that is carefully tied below the elbow. Thereafter, sterile sheets isolate the anesthesiologist from the operating site. We prefer to position the first assistant over the shoulder

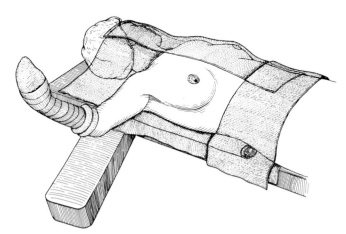

Figure 29–32. Typical position for draping patient for operations of cancer of the right breast. The ipsilateral hemithorax is positioned at the margin of the operative table with a sheet roll that provides slight elevation to the ipsilateral shoulder and hemithorax. This position potentially prevents subluxation and abduction of the shoulder with stretch of the brachial plexus. Draping of the periphery of the breast is inclusive of the supraclavicular fossa and the entire shoulder to allow adequate mobility for adduction of the shoulder and arm across the chest wall. The elbow should be easily flexed and extended without undue tension.

(cephalad to the arm board) on the ipsilateral side of the procedure (Fig. 29–33) such that the muscular retraction with extension and abduction of the arm and shoulder that is necessary for dissection of the axilla can be accomplished without undue stretch on the brachial plexus.

The operation is initiated with the ipsilateral arm in a relaxed, extended position on the arm board. Incisions are made following the planned guidelines discussed in the subsection of this chapter entitled, "General Principles of Mastectomy."

The Halsted radical mastectomy is utilized for larger breast lesions (T2, T3, T4) that present with gross involvement (fixation) of the skin or pectoralis major (Fig. 29–34, inset) and for peripheral (high-lying) lesions near the clavicle in patients who are otherwise not candidates for radiation therapy. The skin flaps are designed to encompass wider margins than those for modified radical techniques. To obtain adequate surgical margins that encompass the primary neoplasm and involved skin, the operator may need to elevate skin flaps at the periphery of the breast (Fig. 29–34). This procedure necessitates an en bloc resection of the breast and the skin overlying the tumor as well as the pectoralis major and minor muscles, with a complete axillary dissection of Levels I to III nodes. The limits of the dissection are delineated *superiorly* by the inferior border of the clavicle at the subclavius muscle, *laterally* by the anterior margin of the latissimus dorsi muscle, *medially* at the midline of the sternum, and *inferiorly* at the inframammary fold with extension to the aponeurosis of the rectus abdominus tendon, some 3 to 4 cm inferior to the caudal extent of the breast. As described previously, cutaneous flaps should be elevated with a thickness of 7 to 8 mm; however, flap thickness is invariably dependent on the patient's habitus and lean body mass. The interface for elevation of this flap is the plane deep to the cutaneous vasculature, which can be accentuated with tension on the flaps by towel clips placed in the margins of the incision or by retraction hooks. This technique of retraction is essential to allow exposure of the subcutaneous component of the flap as it overlies the breast parenchyma. Flap elevation may be accomplished with electrocautery or cold scalpel dissection. Constant tension on the periphery of the elevated flaps at right angles to the chest wall exposes the superficial and deep layers of the superficial fascia to allow the operator to dissect to the anatomical boundaries previously delineated. With dissection, the surgeon must ensure that flap thickness is consistent with elevation to avoid devascularization of the skin or the creation of "buttonholes" that contribute to skin necrosis and wound seroma.

Typically, exposure of the superolateral aspect of the wound allows identification of the humeral insertion of the pectoralis major muscle and then continuation of the dissection in a central and superomedial direction with muscular elevation to allow exposure of the pectoralis minor. The insertion of the pectoralis major on the humerus is transected and rotated medially. The operator must be cognizant of the anatomical position of the cephalic vein and its relationship to the deltopectoral triangle. The dissection commences medially with resection of the pectoralis major at its craniad clavicular attachments. This maneuver allows the surgeon direct access to the axilla; thereafter the tendinuous portion of the pectoralis minor muscle is divided at its insertion on the coracoid process of the scapula (Fig. 29–35). This muscle is likewise elevated from the axilla with careful ligature and division of perforating musculature branches from the thoracoacromial artery and vein. The *medial (anterior thoracic) pectoral nerve,* which commonly penetrates the pectoralis minor before innervation of the pectoralis major, is ligated and divided at its origin from the medial cord of the brachial plexus. As the surgeon continues the medial resection of the pectoralis major, the *lateral (anterior thoracic) pectoral nerve* (which originates from the lateral cord and runs in the medial neurovascular bundle) should be identified, ligated, and divided. We prefer to continue the dissection in the superomedial-most aspect of the elevated flap such that the pectoralis major is divided from its medial origin at the costosternal junction of ribs 2, 3, 4, 5, and 6 (Fig. 29–36). The resection of the pectoralis musculature invariably allows the operator to encounter multiple perforator vessels (lateral thoracic and anterior intercostal arteries) at its periphery that are end arteries to the pectoralis major and minor. Perforator branches from the intercostal muscles that take origin from the intercostal arteries and veins are also encountered. All divided tributaries should be individually clamped, ligated, and tied with nonabsorbable 2-0 or 3-0 suture. With division of the pectoral muscles and inferomedial traction of the specimen, the axillary contents are fully exposed, and origin of the pectoralis minor on ribs 2 to 5 can be visualized and divided at this level. With this maneuver, *Rotter's interpectoral nodes* are swept en bloc into the specimen to allow full visualization of the axillary vein to the level of Halsted's (costoclavicular) ligament, which is recognized as condensation of the clavipectoral fascia. *Level III (apical, subclavicular) nodes* can be dissected at this level.

Thereafter we prefer to work lateral to medial to allow en bloc dissection of the axillary contents. The reader is referred to the subsection of this chapter entitled, "Modified Radical Mastectomy" for figures that illustrate the techniques for axillary dissection. The axillary vein is identified, and the investing deep layer of superficial fascia of the axillary space is incised sharply with the scalpel on the ventral and anterior surface of the vein, with dissection and exposure of all venous tributaries. It is inadvisable to dissect the axilla with electrocautery for fear of thermal damage to the axillary vein and electrostimulation of the brachial plexus or its motor branches. As the medial and lateral (anterior thoracic) pectoral nerves have previously been sacrificed with elevation of the pectoralis major and minor muscles, the entire extent of dissection along the anterior axillary vein allows ligation and division of venous tributaries coursing inferiorly and anteriorly without fear of neural injury.

All loose areolar tissues at the juncture of the axillary

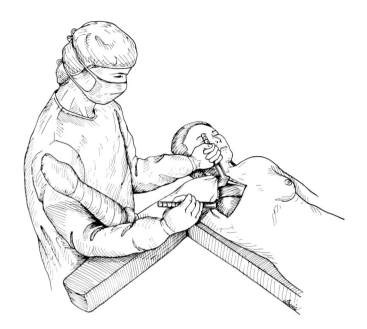

Figure 29–33. Position of the first assistant for right radical mastectomy. The surgical assistant, positioned cephalad to the armboard and shoulder, is able to provide traction, control, and protection of the arm and shoulder. Undue traction of chest wall musculature with potential damage to the brachial plexus can be avoided by ensuring free mobility of the shoulder and elbow that is being controlled by the first assistant.

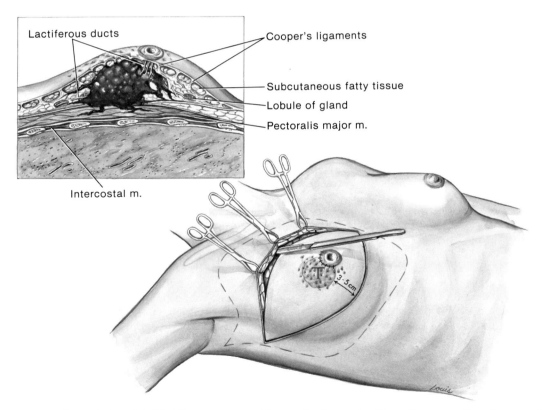

Figure 29–34. *Inset,* Large breast lesions (T2, T3, T4) may present with gross fixation to the skin and/or pectoralis major musculature. The radical mastectomy is designed to encompass wider skin flaps than does the modified technique. The margins designed and developed should encompass normal skin and breast parenchyma 3 to 5 cm from the periphery of the tumor.

The design of elevated flaps is inclusive of skin margins at the periphery of the breast on the chest wall. The broken line indicates the limits of the dissection and includes the following: *superior,* the inferior border of the clavicle at the subclavius muscle; *lateral,* the anterior margin of the latissimus dorsi muscle; *medial,* midline of the sternum; and *inferior,* the inframammary fold with extension of dissection to the cephalic extension of the aponeurosis of the rectus abdominis tendon.

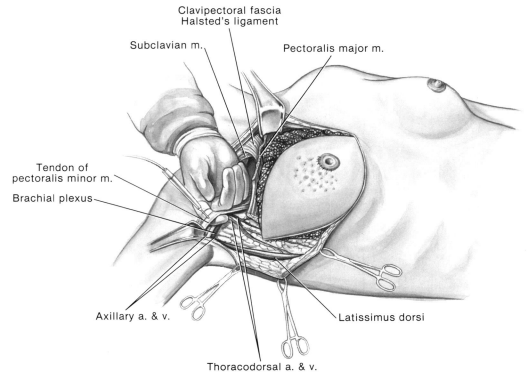

Figure 29–35. Exposure of the superiolateral aspect of the mastectomy wound following division of the humeral insertion of the pectoralis major muscle. The insertion of the pectoralis minor on the coracoid process of the scapula is transected and rotated medially with en bloc dissection of Rotter's interpectoral nodes. Technically, the dissection commences on the anterior and ventral aspects of the axillary vein to incorporate Levels I to III nodes. Division of the pectoralis major and minor tendons allows the surgeon direct access to the floor of the axilla.

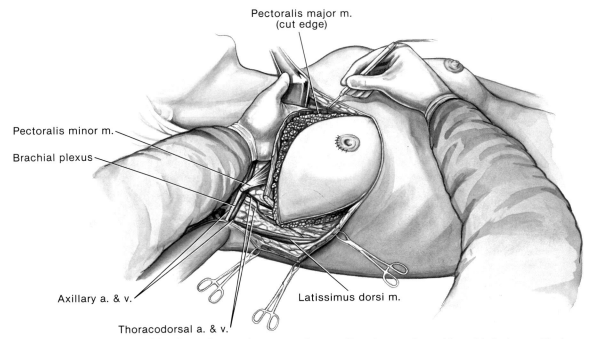

Figure 29–36. Superomedial dissection of the elevated pectoralis minor and pectoralis major muscles en bloc with the breast. The breast parenchyma remains intact with the pectoralis major fascia. Illustrated is the medial extent of the dissection along the costoclavicular margin with division of insertion of the pectoralis major on ribs 2 through 6 and the pectoralis minor on ribs 2 through 5. Multiple perforator branches from the intercostal muscles are encountered at the origin of the intercostal arteries and veins. Following superomedial and inferomedial dissection, the axillary contents are fully exposed to allow completion of the Patey axillary dissection of Levels I to III nodes.

vein with the anterior margin of the latissimus dorsi are swept inferomedially to be inclusive of the *lateral (axillary) nodal group (Level I)*. Care is taken to preserve the thoracodorsal artery and vein, and the operator should be cognizant of the origin of the *thoracodorsal nerve*, which is medial to this vascular structure. This nerve originates from the posterior cord and may run a variable course in the central axillary space as it courses inferolaterally to innervate the latissimus dorsi muscle. As dissection in the axilla commences, the major branch of the *intercostobrachial nerve*, which transverses the axillary spaces at right angles to the latissimus medial to lateral, will be identified. This nerve, which is sensory to the medial arm and axilla with fibers from lateral cutaneous branches of the second and third intercostal nerves, is sacrificed without prolonged morbidity.

Typically the *lateral (axillary) nodal group* is swept anteriorly or posteriorly about the thoracodorsal neurovascular bundle to be incorporated en bloc with the *subscapular group of nodes (Level I)*, which are medially placed between the thoracodorsal nerve and the lateral chest wall. With dissection of these two nodal groups and the investing areolar tissues, the posterior boundary of the axillary space with exposure of the teres major muscle is evident. Medial dissection with clearing of the ventral surface of the axillary vein allows direct visualization of the subscapularis muscle. Inferior dissection of the *external mammary nodes of Level I* is deferred. Preferably dissections of the *central nodal group (Level II)* and the *apical or subclavicular (Level III) nodes* are completed *prior to* removal of the external mammary level. We favor this technique with clearing of the superomedial areolar and nodal contents to the costoclavicular (Halsted's) ligament. Thereafter the Level III group can be labeled with a metallic marker or suture to provide the pathologist precise identification of this nodal group, which may have therapeutic and prognostic value. These two nodal groups are subsequently retracted inferiorly with the partially dissected components of Level I groups. Nodal dissection commences with en bloc removal of the external mammary group that is medial and contiguous with the breast. The operator is admonished to dissect from a cephalad to caudad direction *parallel with* the thoracodorsal neurovascular bundle. This maneuver is important in dissection to prevent neural injury and allows direct access to venous tributaries posterior to the axillary vein. Thereafter the surgeon will encounter the chest wall, and dissection is continued in a cephalocaudal direction to allow identification of the *long thoracic nerve (respiratory nerve of Bell)* that provides motor innervation to the serratus anterior muscle. After incision of the serratus fascia, this nerve is dissected throughout its course in the medial axillary space from its superior-most origin near the chest wall to the innervation of the serratus anterior.

On occasion, extranodal extension of metastatic disease with nodal involvement of the external mammary, subscapular, or lateral (axillary) nodal groups of Level I initiates tumor fixation and invasion of the thoracodorsal neurovascular bundle. When such pathology is encountered, the surgeon should advisedly sacrifice this

neurovascular structure at the ventral surface of the axillary vein. Both artery and vein should be ligated separately with nonabsorbable 2-0 sutures to avoid subsequent hematoma formation. Relatively little disability is evident with denervation of the latissimus dorsi muscle; however, myocutaneous flaps that utilize the latissimus dorsi must be excluded for reconstruction purposes. Every attempt should be made to preserve the long thoracic nerve for fear of permanent disability with the "winged scapula" and shoulder apraxia that follow denervation of the serratus anterior.

Thereafter the axillary contents anterior and medial to the long thoracic nerve are swept inferomedially with the specimen, and the operator should ensure that division of the inferior-most boundaries of the axillary contents is deferred until preserved innervations of the long thoracic and thoracodorsal nerves are visualized. Any point of origin of the pectoralis major muscle from the second through the sixth rib left intact with the medial dissection is divided such that en bloc resection of the pectoralis major is accomplished over the retromammary bursa. The surgeon continues the dissection in this avascular plane to sweep the breast and axillary contents toward the aponeurosis of the rectus abdominus tendon to complete extirpation of the specimen as an en bloc procedure (Fig. 29–37).

The surgeon and assistants as well as the scrub nurse should reglove (and optionally regown). Clean instruments for flap closure are preferred to avoid the potential for wound implantation of tumor. Thereafter the wound is copiously irrigated with distilled water or saline to evacuate residual tissue and clots. Points of bleeding from intercostal perforators are identified, clamped, and ligated to diminish hematoma and seroma accumulation. Closed-suction catheters (18–20 French) are placed via separate stab-type incisions that enter the inferior margin of the flap at approximately the anterior axillary line (Fig. 29–37, inset). These Silastic catheters are positioned with the lateral catheter in the axillary space just medial to or on the surface of the latissimus dorsi to provide drainage of the axilla. The second, longer catheter is placed via the anterior-most skin incision superomedially to evacuate serum and blood of the large surface area dissected from the chest wall. The drains are secured at skin level with 2-0 nonabsorbable sutures. Suction catheters should not be secured to the chest wall with sutures because of the potential for causing muscle injury and hemorrhage with removal.

Skin margins should be carefully inspected to evaluate devascularization that results with the trauma of dissection or tangential incisions that contribute to subsequent skin necrosis and wound dehiscence. We prefer closure with interrupted 2-0 absorbable synthetic sutures placed in the subcutaneous tissues without tension. The skin may be closed optionally with subcuticular 4-0 synthetic absorbable sutures or stainless-steel staples. Steri Strips are applied across (vertical to) the incision when subcuticular sutures are utilized in the closure. Following irrigation, the closed-suction catheters are connected and maintained on continuous low to moderate suction with large reservoir vacuum bottles. Light, bulky dress-

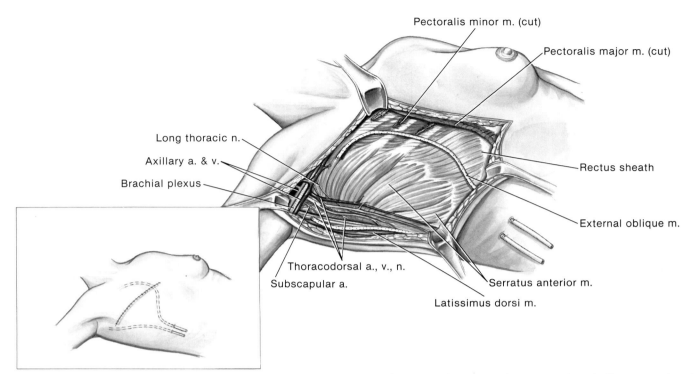

Pectoralis minor m. (cut)

Pectoralis major m. (cut)

Long thoracic n.

Axillary a. & v.

Brachial plexus

Rectus sheath

External oblique m.

Thoracodorsal a., v., n.

Subscapular a.

Serratus anterior m.

Latissimus dorsi m.

Figure 29–37. The completed Halsted radical mastectomy with residual margins of the pectoralis major and minor muscles. Ideally, preservation of the long thoracic nerve ensures innervation of the serratus anterior. Innervation of the latissimus dorsi muscle is ensured with preservation of the thoracodorsal nerve that accompanies the neurovascular bundle of the posterior axillary space. Inset depicts position of closed-suction catheters (18–20 French) placed via separate stab wounds that enter the inferior margin of the flap at approximately the anterior axillary lines.

ings are applied to the entire area of dissection and are taped securely in place, although some surgeons prefer compression dressings over flaps inclusive of the margins of dissection. This practice may initiate central damage to the flap and potential skin necrosis if undue pressure is applied with taping. The dressing should remain intact until the third or fourth postoperative day. Wound

catheters may be removed when drainage becomes predominantly serous and has decreased to a maximum of 20 to 25 ml during a 24-hour interval. Shoulder exercises are initiated on the day following removal of the drainage catheters.

Often the defect created with the Halsted mastectomy is too great to allow primary wound closure. Thus the

Figure 29–38. Large defect that is expectant with creation of large skin flaps inclusive of the periphery of the breast for T3 and T4 lesions with fixation to the pectoralis major. Such large defects must be grafted with split-thickness skin (0.018–0.020 inch) that is preferably obtained via a dermatome from skin of the anterior/lateral thigh or buttock. An additional option for closure is the myocutaneous latissimus dorsi flap. *Bottom,* The partial-thickness skin graft held in position with a compression stent created with cotton gauze mesh. These large skin defects do not require catheter drainage. Alternatively, compression foam-mesh as the stent may be applied over the split-thickness skin graft. Foam mesh may be stapled in place at the margin of the skin defect.

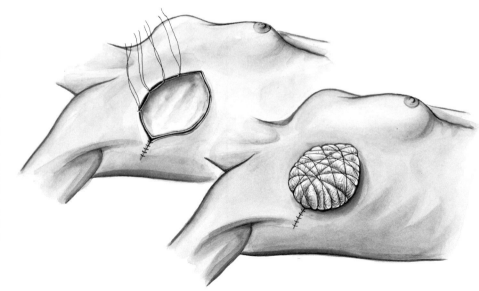

defect must be grafted with split-thickness skin (0.018 to 0.020 in) obtained with a dermatome from the anterolateral thigh or buttock (Fig. 29–38). To immobilize the skin graft and enhance the probability of adherence ("graft-take") to the chest wall, the partial-thickness skin is stented with bolsters (Fig. 29–38) or compression foam mesh. Catheters are not usually necessary when skin grafts are applied to the defect. The stents placed over the split-thickness skin grafts are not removed until the fifth or sixth postoperative day, unless undue drainage (serum, blood, or suppuration) from beneath the grafts is evident. This practice increases the probability of graft adherence, which is further enhanced with postoperative shoulder immobilization for large defects.

For patients who have protracted serosanguineous or serous drainage, the catheters may be shortened and the portable suction device secured in the most comfortable position for ambulation. This practice requires the patient to pay strict attention to hygienic care of the catheters and the sites of skin entry and necessitates frequent dressing changes. In addition, the patient should be instructed to temporarily limit the range of motion of the shoulder and arm to augment flap adherence to the chest wall. The physician should periodically inspect the volume and composition of fluid emanating from the catheter and should be cognizant of the potential for retrograde infection of the axillary space. Wound care and complications following mastectomy are reviewed more comprehensively in chapter 31.

References

1. Anglem TJ, Leber RE: Characteristics of survivors after radical mastectomy. Am J Surg 121:363–367, 1971.
2. Baker RR, Montague ACW, Childs JN: A comparison of modified radical mastectomy to radical mastectomy in the treatment of operable breast cancer. Am Surg 189(5):553–559, 1979.
3. Banks M: A plea for the more free removal of cancerous growths. *In* Liverpool and Manchester Surgical Reports. 1878, pp 192–206.
4. Cooper WA: The history of the radical mastectomy. *In* Annals of Medical History, vol 3. New York, Paul B. Hoeber, 1941, pp 36–54.
5. Dahl-Iversen E, Tobiassen T: Radical mastectomy with parasternal and supraclavicular dissection for mammary carcinoma. Am Surg 157:170–173, 1963.
6. Dietrich G (Lucke): Beitrag zur Statisik des Mammacarcinom. Dtsch Z F Chir 33:471–516, 1892.
7. Fisher B, Bauer M, Margolese R, Posson R, Pilch Y, Redmond C, Fisher ER, Wolmark N, Deutsch M, Montague E, Saffer E, Wickerham L, Lerner H, Glass A, Shibata H, Deckers P, Ketcham A, Oishi R, Russell I: Five-year results of a randomized trial comparing total mastectomy and segmental mastectomy with or without radiation in the treatment of breast cancer. N Engl J Med 312:665–673, 1985.
8. Fisher B, Redmond C, Poisson R, Margolese R, Wolmark N, Wickerham L, Fisher E, Deutsch M, Caplan R, Pilch Y, Glass A, Shibata H, Lerner H, Terz J, Sidorovich L: Eight-year results of a randomized clinical trial comparing total mastectomy and lumpectomy with or without irradiation in the treatment of breast cancer. N Engl J Med 320(13):822–828, 1989.
9. Halsted WS: The results of operations for the cure of cancer of the breast performed at the Johns Hopkins Hospital from June, 1889, to January, 1894. Ann Surg 20:497–555, 1894.
10. Halsted WS: The results of radical operations for the cure of cancer of the breast. Tr Am S A 25:61–79, 1907.
11. Handley RS: The conservative radical mastectomy of Patey: ten year results in 425 patient's breasts. Dis Breast 2:16, 1976.
12. Horner F: Uebr die Endresultate von 172 operierten Fällen maligner Tumoren der weiblichen Brust. Beitr Z Klin Chir 12:619–703, 1894.
13. Hutchison RG: Radiation therapy in carcinoma of the breast. Surg Gynecol Obstet 62:653–664, 1936.
14. Joerss J: Ueber die heutige Prognose der Exstirpatio mammae carcinomatosae. Dtsche Z F Chir 44:101–130, 1897.
15. Madden JL: Modified radical mastectomy. Surg Gynecol Obstet 121(6):1221–1230, 1965.
16. Maddox WA, Carpenter JT, Laws HL, Soong SJ, Cloud G, Urist MM, Balch CM: A randomized prospective trial of radical (Halsted) mastectomy vs modified radical mastectomy in 311 breast cancer patients. Ann Surg 198(2):207–212, 1983.
17. Mahler F: Ueber die in der Heidelberger Klinik 1887–1897 behandelten Fälle von Carcinoma Mammae. Beitr Z Klin Chir 26:681–714, 1900.
18. Meyer W: An improved method of the radical operation for carcinoma of the breast. Med Rec NY 46:746–749, 1894.
19. Nemoto T, Vana J, Bedwanni RN, Baker HW, McGregor FH, Murphy GP: Management and survival of female breast cancer; results of a national survey by the American College of Surgeons. Cancer 45:2917–2924, 1980.
20. Nemoto T, Vana J, Nararajan N, et al: Observations on short-term and long-term surveys of breast cancer by the American College of Surgeons. *In* Murphy GP (ed): International Advances in Surgical Oncology, Vol IV. New York, Alan R Liss, 1981, pp 209–239.
21. Oldekop J: Statische Zusammenstellung von 250 Fällen von Mamma-Carcinom. Arch F Klin Chir 24:536–581, 1879.
22. Patey DH: A review of 146 cases of carcinoma of the breast operated on between 1930 and 1943. Br J Cancer 21:260–269, 1967.
23. Patey DH, Dyson WH: Prognosis of carcinoma of the breast in relation to type of operation performed. Br J Surg 2:7, 1948.
24. Poulsen K: Die Geschwülste der Mamma. Arch F Klin Chir 42:593–644, 1891.
25. Rotter J: Günstigere Dauererfolge durch eine verbesserte operative Behandlung der Mammakarzinome. Berl Klin Wochenschr 33:69–72, 1896.
26. Schmid H (Kuster): Zur statistik der mammacarcinome und deren heilung. Dtsche Z F Chir 26:139, 1887.
27. Schmidt GB: Die Geschwülste der Brustdrüse. Beitr Z Klin Chir 4:40–136, 1889.
28. Sprengel O (Volkmann): 131 Fälle von Brust-Carcinom. Arch F Klin Chir 27:805–892, 1882.
29. Vana J, Bedwani R, Nemoto T, Murphy GP: Long-term patient care evaluation study for carcinoma of the female breast. American College of Surgeons Commission on Cancer Final Report, Chicago, 1979.
30. Wilson RE, Donegan WL, Mettlin C, Natarajan N, Smart CR, Murphy GP: The 1982 national survey of carcinoma of the breast in the United States by the American College of Surgeons. Surg Gynecol Obstet 159:309–318, 1984.
31. Winiwarter V (Billroth): Beiträge zur statisik d. carcinome. Stuttgart, 1878.
32. Wolff J: Die Lehre von der Krebskrankheit, vol 1. Jena, G Fischer, 1907, p 43.

MODIFIED RADICAL MASTECTOMY AND TOTAL (SIMPLE) MASTECTOMY

Kirby I. Bland, M.D. and Edward M. Copeland III, M.D.

"Sometimes the tumor only is removed; sometimes the segment of the breast (where the tumor lies) is taken away . . .; sometimes . . . the entire mamma. Mammary cancer requires the careful extirpation of the entire organ."

C. H. Moore (1867)

MODIFIED RADICAL MASTECTOMY

The rationale for the Halsted radical mastectomy was largely the prevention of local and regional recurrence on the chest wall and axilla. The synthesis of mastectomy techniques by Halsted's predecessors in surgery and pathology allowed him to achieve unprecedented success in obtaining this objective without the availability of irradiation and/or chemotherapy. From a historical perspective, C. H. Moore[49] was the first to introduce the concept of the modified radical mastectomy with *segmental resection* of the breast in which the tumor was located and *selective* axillary dissections for clinically positive nodal disease. He stated that "diseased axillary glands should be taken away by the same dissection as the breast itself, without dividing the intervening lymphatics."[49] Careful review of Moore's literature suggests that he performed axillary dissection *selectively* rather than as a routine procedure. Volkmann,[63] in 1875, followed the postulates espoused by Moore but was opposed to the performance of partial amputation of breast tissue. Regardless of the small size of the breast primary on initial evaluation, he advised total extirpation of the gland. He preserved the pectoralis major as the "floor" of the dissection, but stressed the necessity for resection of the pectoralis major fascia. When axillary lymphatics were observed to be "diseased," they were removed—a "cleaning of the axilla." Volkmann was also convinced of the inadvisability of supraclavicular node dissection when clinically involved and considered operation inappropriate with this presentation.

Like Volkmann, the American surgeon Samuel Gross,[26] in 1880, strongly advocated the principles and concepts developed by Moore.[49] Gross utilized total mastectomy and concomitant "cleaning out" of the axilla for the primary treatment of cancer in 19 of 48 patients (39.6 percent) treated for mammary carcinoma.[26] Gross allowed wounds to heal by secondary intention without skin grafting.

In 1882, Banks[3] of England reported a British series with use of the modified radical mastectomy in 46 patients. With regard to the axillary dissection, Banks stated: "As you cannot tell whether these glands are infected or not, remove them and dissipate the doubt." Banks indicated that Level III axillary lymphatics could be readily resected en bloc; he found no indication "for dividing the pectoral muscles." In this same year, Sprengel,[58] of Germany, reported the results of operations performed in 131 patients treated in the Volkmann Clinic between 1874 and 1878. He stressed the importance of the total mastectomy and "cleaned out" clinically involved axillary nodes as a staging and potentially therapeutic procedure. When disease was not palpable in the axilla, the "axilla was opened in order to ascertain the true diagnosis" (operative staging). Sprengel[58] treated 29 patients (22.1 percent) with total mastectomy, and the remaining 102 patients (77.9 percent) were treated with total mastectomy and concomitant dissection of varying levels of the axilla.

Soon after, in 1883, Küster[36] emphasized the importance of the total mastectomy performed in conjunction with routine dissection of the axillary nodes for the treatment of breast carcinoma. He advised axillary dissection despite node-negative clinical findings. Of 132 patients with carcinoma in Küster's series, 117 (88.6 percent) were so treated.[36] In the discussion of Küster's original presentation, Gussenbauer, von Langenbeck, and von Winiwater agreed that routine axillary dissection was an essential part of the therapy of breast carcinoma, despite the clinical negativity of the axilla with initial clinical staging.[36] Gussenbauer further advised the routine "extirpation of supraclavicular nodes . . . when the condition demanded it."[36]

In 1894, Halsted[27] and Meyer[48] independently reported their individual techniques for the successful therapy of breast carcinoma with radical mastectomy. The initial clinical experience by Halsted suggested that he removed only the pectoralis major concomitant with the axillary node dissection, which presumably included Levels I to III nodes. The pectoralis minor muscle was transected only for technical expediency in the conduct of the axillary dissection and was thereafter resutured to close the posterior superior axillary space. Soon after, Halsted advocated and was in complete agreement with Meyer's concept of the *routine* resection of *both* muscles. This concept espoused by Meyer and Halsted soon became the state-of-the-art operative procedure for cancer of the breast until challenged by American and British clinics on the basis of the worth of conservative methods for surgical management of the organ.

In 1912, J. B. Murphy[50] acknowledged that he had abandoned the Halsted radical mastectomy and did not remove either pectoral muscle. Murphy's practice for preservation of these muscles was based on the original report by Bryant of London, who acknowledged only one case of recurrent carcinoma of the breast in the pectoral muscles in patients followed during a 40-year clinical experience.[50] The recommendation by Grace,[25] in 1937, for use of the total (simple) mastectomy alone for the treatment of certain invasive carcinomas was unchallenged until the widely acclaimed report by McWhirter[46] in 1948 served to renew enthusiasm for the modified radical technique.

The notable and widely regarded contribution of Mr. D. H. Patey[53, 54] of the Middlesex Hospital, London, served to establish the modified radical mastectomy in its deserving place as appropriate therapy for select T1 and T2 lesions that were positioned in the breast and were not fixed to the pectoralis major to allow curative en bloc resection without pectoralis major muscle removal.

RETROSPECTIVE STUDIES OF MODIFIED RADICAL MASTECTOMY

Table 29–10 provides the results from various clinics and study groups for retrospective clinical trials conducted for the modified radical mastectomy. Inclusive are the absolute 5- and 10-year survival rates available from the various studies of these series between 1969 and 1985. In these series, completed in the United Kingdom, Canada, and the United States, it is evident that dramatic reductions in survival are expected with advancing stage of disease at operation. Handley and Thackray,[30] Baker et al.,[2] and Leis[39] employed the classic Patey mastectomy with resection of the pectoralis minor and all three levels of axillary nodes. In contrast, the series reported by Madden,[42, 43] Meyer et al.,[47] DeLarue et al.,[9] Hermann et al.,[33, 34] and Robinson et al.[55] utilized the Auchincloss-Madden technique for the modified radical mastectomy with preservation of the pectoralis minor to complement regional control with the total mastectomy. Nemoto et al.[51,] in reporting the American College of Surgeons Survey of 1978, expectantly analyzed a mixed series of patients having both the Patey and Auchincloss-Madden techniques performed in this large series of stage I and II (TNM classification) patients. As a consequence of the various classifications for staging utilized in the series reported in Table 29–10, a variance in the absolute survivals at 5 and 10 years is evident.

Attempts to make comparisons with statistical and reproducible validity among retrospective series with varied reported stages are virtually impossible. Therefore the series reported in Table 29–10 reflects a variance in the absolute survival at 5 years for stage I patients of 61.8 percent to 90 percent on the basis of these biological and anatomical differences in the tumor. However, the series clearly reflects the difference in survivorship at 5 and 10 years for stages I and II disease. Furthermore, with comparisons to Table 29–9 for the Halsted radical mastectomy and with consideration of stage classification, the results of the two procedures are comparable.

Table 29–10. RESULTS OF RETROSPECTIVE CLINICAL TRIALS OF PATIENTS TREATED BY MODIFIED RADICAL MASTECTOMY ALONE*

Author and Year	Clinic or Study Group	Number of Patients	Disease Stage	Absolute-Survival (%) 5-yr	Absolute-Survival (%) 10-yr
Handley et al, 1969[30]	UK	77	I	75	61
		58	II	57	25
DeLarue et al, 1969[9]‡	Toronto	75	I	61.8	—
		25	II	51.4	—
Madden, 1972[43]†	NYC	94	I	81.6	63
			II	32.4	17
Robinson et al, 1976[55]	Mayo Clinic	280	I	81	—
			II	54	—
Meyer et al, 1978[47]	Rockford, IL	175	I–III	74	43
Baker et al, 1979[2]‡	Johns Hopkins University	91	I	90	—
		22	II	72	—
		31	III	45	—
Leis, 1980[39]§	NY Medical College	397	I	—	72.2
		333	II	—	40.2
Nemoto et al, 1980[51]‡	American College of Surgeons	8,906	I	65.1	—
		7,832	II	35.1	—
Hermann et al, 1985[34]†	Cleveland Clinic	358	I	73	56
		211	II	55	28

*Includes some patients treated with radical mastectomy with equivalent therapy results.
†Manchester classification.
‡TNM classification.
§Columbia Clinical Classification.

Table 29–11. 5- AND 10-YEAR SURVIVAL RATES AS A FUNCTION OFAXILLARY NODAL STATUS FOLLOWING MODIFIED RADICAL MASTECTOMY

Author and Year	Clinic or Study Group	Number of Patients	Survival Rate for Patients with Negative Nodes		Survival Rate by Number of Positive Nodes					
					Any		1–3		≥4	
			5-yr	10-yr	5-yr	10-yr	5-yr	10-yr	5-yr	10-yr
Handley and Thackray, 1969[30]	UK	135	75	57	61	25	NA	NA	NA	NA
Madden et al, 1972[43]	NYC	94	82	63	32	17	NA	NA	NA	NA
Robinson et al, 1976[53]	Mayo Clinic	339	80† (93)		48† (55)		61† (72)		37† (42)	
Nemoto et al, 1980[51]	American College of Surgeons	24,136	71.8		40.4		63.1–58.8*		51.9–22.2*	
Hermann et al, 1985[34]	Cleveland Clinic	564	78	62	55	28	66	41	47	25

*Range inclusive of number of positive nodes.
† = Determinate survival.
NA = Not available.

With extensive analyses that allow comparisons of the Patey and the Auchincloss-Madden mastectomy techniques, the results of these two procedures would also appear to be similar with regard to survival. The retrospective analyses by Hermann et al.,[34] Robinson et al.,[55] DeLarue et al,[9] and Madden et al.[43] suggest that no benefit in survival is obtained with completion of the axillary dissection inclusive of Level III nodes following removal of the pectoralis minor.

Table 29–11 further analyzes the 5- and 10-year survival rates as a function of the status of the axillary nodes at the time of modified radical mastectomy for operable cancer. In five series reported between 1969 and 1985, survivorship directly correlated with the presence or absence of nodes containing tumor metastasis. Table 29–11 also reflects a diminishing survival with any positive node and a decreasing survival rate with the number of positive nodes (1–3, ≥4) reported in the operative series. These five series confirm for node-negative patients a 5-year survival rate of 71.8 percent to 82 percent and a 10-year survival rate of 57 percent to 63 percent. The presence of *any* positive node statistically diminished the probability of 5- and 10-year survival for all series. In this retrospective analysis, patients with any positive nodes had an expectant 5-year survival that varied from 32 percent to 61 percent and a 10-year survival of 17 percent to 28 percent. Robinson et al.,[55] Nemoto et al.,[51] and Hermann et al.[34] further confirm the statistically significant effect of reduction in 5-year survival as the number of nodes increases. Robinson et al.,[55] in the Mayo Clinic series of 339 patients, observed a 61 percent absolute (72 percent determinate) survival rate at 5 years for one to three nodes. Absolute 5-year survival data for four or more positive nodes was 37 percent (42 percent determinate). In the large series reported by Nemoto et al.[51] of the American College of Surgeons Survey of more than 24,000 patients, any positive node had the effect of reducing 5-year survivorship by greater than 30 percent. Vana et al.,[61] Nemoto et al.,[51] and Hermann et al.[34] further confirm that the number of positive nodes

recovered at axillary dissection for operable breast cancer has a reciprocal effect on 5- and 10-year survivorship.

The 5- and 10-year local and regional recurrence rates for chest wall, scar, operative field, and axilla are analyzed from five series in Table 29–12. The series by Madden et al.,[43] Handley and Thackray,[30] and Leis[39] reported 10-year recurrence rates, whereas the series by DeLarue et al.[9] and Baker et al.[2] indicated 5-year relapse rates. Adjunctive irradiation was utilized in the series reported by Baker et al.[2] but was excluded for patients in the Leis, Handley and Thackray, DeLarue et al., and Madden et al. analyses. Interestingly, DeLarue et al.[9] observed no recurrence at any site for stage I disease (n = 43) at 5-year follow-up. Leis[39] observed no recurrence in any site for stage 0 (minimally invasive ductal carcinoma ≤ 1 cm; in situ ductal and lobular carcinoma); for stage I disease, Leis noted a 5 percent recurrence rate at 10 years for chest wall, scar, and operative field, with a low axillary recurrence rate of 0.8 percent when using the classic Patey mastectomy technique. This low axillary recurrence rate was similarly observed by Handley and Thackray[30] for Columbia Clinical Classification Stage A and B lesions of 1.8 percent and 0.1 percent, respectively.

Madden et al.[43] extol the virtues of the Auchincloss technique and stress the necessity to dissect completely the axillary contents. Auchincloss[1] originally questioned the value of removal of the apical (Level III) nodes if they were invaded. In 38 patients who had metastases to apical nodes, only four (10.5 percent) remained free of disease in follow-up 8 to 10 years subsequently. Conversely, when apical nodes were clinically negative, Auchincloss considered completion of the axillary dissection unnecessary, as results equivalent to excision of the lower nodes (Level I/II) alone with removal of the breast and preservation of the pectoral muscles had control and survival rates identical to the more radical approaches. Furthermore, Crile[5-7] has previously presented inconclusive but intriguing data that supported the concept that node-negative cancer of the breast should have delayed axillary node dissection, performed

Table 29–12. LOCAL AND REGIONAL 5- AND 10-YEAR RECURRENCE RATES OF VARIOUS SITES IN RETROSPECTIVE STUDIES FOLLOWING MODIFIED RADICAL MASTECTOMY

Author and Year	Clinic or Study Group	Number of Patients	Disease Stage	Site (%)	
				Chest Wall, Scar, or Operative Field	Axilla
DeLarue, 1969[9]	Toronto General* (Canada)	43	I	0	0
		32	II	12.5	—
		25	III	15.0	—
Madden, 1972[43]	NYC†	94	I–III	10	0
Handley, 1976[29]	UK†	77	A‡	10.0	1.8
		58	B	22.6	0.1
		8	C	63.6	9.1
Baker, 1979[2]	Johns Hopkins*	91	I	13.2	1.1
		22	II	9.1	4.5
		31	III	22.6	22.6
Leis, 1980[39]	NY Medical College†	116	0	0	0
		397	I	5.0	0.08
		333	II	13.8	0.08

*5-year recurrence rates.
†10-year recurrence rates.
‡Columbia Clinical Classification.
Staging is TNM unless otherwise noted.

only if nodal metastases became clinically evident. Crile[5–7] used experimental data to confirm the concept that excision of normal regional lymph nodes may remove a natural protective immunological barrier to the systemic dissemination of primary breast tumors.

In the series reported by Madden et al.,[43] the local recurrence rate using the Auchincloss-Madden technique was ten percent. None of the patients in this series received prophylactic irradiation to the chest wall or peripheral lymphatics. Madden and associates considered removal of the pectoralis minor unnecessary on the basis of the experimental data noted previously by Crile and the lack of evidence to suggest a reduction in survival or control rates when delayed metastases were evident. Furthermore, in this series of 93 patients, Madden et al.[42, 43] noted no involvement of Rotter's nodes and considered the clearance of this group of interpectoral lymphatics unnecessary. These authors considered preservation of both pectoral muscles to be equivalent to standard or extended radical procedures for the treatment of breast cancers when axillary nodes were clinically negative. The superior control rates for the axilla obtained by these authors justify this technique's application in the treatment of stage I patients.

Baker et al.[2] of Johns Hopkins University compared the results of modified radical mastectomy (n = 144) to radical mastectomy (n = 188) in the treatment of operable cancer of the breast. For 205 patients with stage I cancer, 60 with stage II disease, and 67 with stage III disease (TNM system), there were no statistically significant differences in 5-year survival when the results of the radical mastectomy were compared to those of the modified radical mastectomy. Furthermore, no statistically significant differences in incidence of local/regional recurrence were evident in patients with

stage I and II disease when the results of the two surgical procedures were compared. In contrast, individuals with stage III disease treated by modified radical mastectomy had a statistically significant ($p = 0.002$) higher incidence of local recurrence (chest wall and axilla) when compared with patients treated with the radical mastectomy. Baker et al.[2] concluded that the modified radical mastectomy is the treatment of choice in patients with TNM stage I and II disease. For patients with stage III disease, the radical mastectomy provided a greater probability of local/regional control of disease but did not enhance survival.

These and other observations support the conclusion that extirpation of the pectoralis major muscle is not essential to provide local/regional control of stage I and stage II disease (Columbia Clinical Classification A and B). It must be noted that either the modified radical mastectomy or the Halsted procedure *alone* would be inadequate procedures for achieving local/regional control of TNM stage III and Columbia Clinical Classification C and D tumors (see discussion of stage III and IV disease, chapters 40, 41, and 42). In properly selected patients with stage I and II disease, these retrospective analyses for the modified radical procedure show survival and control rates comparable to the more radical procedure. Chapter 31 contains a comprehensive discussion of local, regional, and systemic complications that may ensue with the modified radical mastectomy.

PROSPECTIVE TRIALS FOR MODIFIED RADICAL MASTECTOMY

In contrast to the Halsted radical mastectomy, the modified radical mastectomy implies a total mastectomy with removal of the tumor, overlying skin, and axillary lymphatics with preservation of the pectoralis major muscle. Thus the modified radical technique has the established precedent for preservation of the major muscle group, which preserves cosmesis of the chest wall. Retrospective analyses by Handley[29] and Dahl-Iversen and Tobiassen[8] confirm survival results similar to those of the classic radical mastectomy. Subsequently, Nemoto and Dao[52] reported that the modified radical mastectomy, which uses the Patey approach, can recover as many axillary lymphatic nodes as possible with the radical mastectomy. Similarly, the report by Fisher et al.[17] of the National Surgical Adjuvant Breast Project (NSABP) confirmed the modified technique to be equivalent to the radical mastectomy in disease-free and overall survival in a carefully-controlled prospectively randomized trial.

Manchester Trial

Between 1969 and 1976, Turner et al.[60] in Manchester, England, prospectively randomized and treated TNM T1 or T2 (N0 or N1) carcinomas of the breast with either Halsted radical mastectomy or modified radical mastectomy. Neither adjuvant chemotherapy nor irradiation were given following the operative procedure performed by six surgeons participating in the trial. In this series, Halsted radical mastectomy was performed in 278 patients, and modified radical mastectomy was performed in 256 patients.

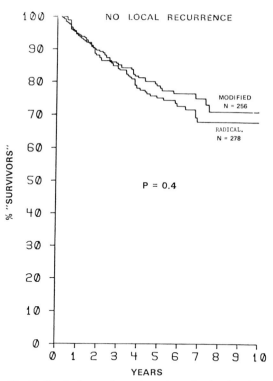

Figure 29–40. Survival rates for patients free of either local recurrence or distant metastasis. (From Turner L, et al: Ann R Coll Surg Engl 63:241, 1981. Reprinted by permission.)

At a median follow-up period of 5 years, Turner et al.[60] found no statistical differences with regard to disease-free or overall survival between the two surgical treatment groups. This was also true for local recurrence and distant metastases for stage I and stage II tumors (Figs. 29–39 to 29–42). Table 29–13 confirms that for clinical and pathological stage I and stage II patients, the 5-year local/regional recurrence rates for the chest wall, axilla, and skin were equivalent. Indeed, a trend favoring the modified radical technique was evident for all cases (25 percent local recurrence rate for radical versus 21 percent for modified radical). This clinical trial suggested that the modified radical mastectomy provided overall and disease-free survival rates similar to those of the Halsted radical technique and the incidence of local recurrence and distant metastases was not significantly different between the two operations.

Investigators of the Manchester trial acknowledge the violation of protocol stipulations in eight patients who received surgical procedures other than those assigned to the study. In addition, the number of positive nodes recovered per patient is not reported, and the precise axillary dissection (Patey versus Auchincloss) methodology with which Levels II and III nodes were recovered is not specified for either surgical procedure. Despite these variances in reporting, staging classifications are equivalent. With regard to randomization, the only variance is that patients in the Halsted radical group were, on average, 3 years older than those in the modified radical group. Despite the minor infractions of

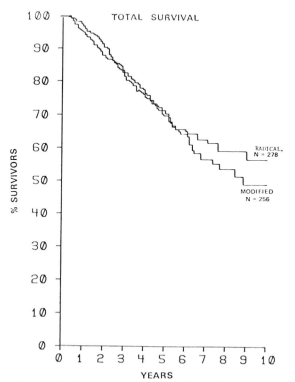

Figure 29–39. Total survival rates for each of the two operations, including disease-free, locally recurrent disease, and metastatic disease. (From Turner L, et al: Ann R Coll Surg Engl 63:241, 1981. Reprinted by permission.)

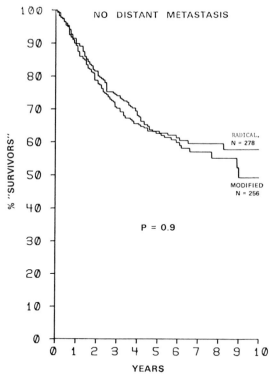

Figure 29–41. Local recurrence rates following each of the two operations regardless of any other outcome. (From Turner L et al: Ann R Coll Surg Engl 63:241, 1981. Reprinted by permission.)

protocol variation, the Manchester trial supports the comparability of the two surgical techniques with regard to overall survival, disease-free survival, and recurrence.

University of Alabama Trial, 1975–1978

In the absence of any clear consensus about the appropriate standard for surgical therapy of primary breast cancer, a controlled-network cancer demonstration project was initiated between 1975 and 1978 by Maddox and associates[44, 45] of the University of Alabama in Birmingham (UAB). This study was approved and supported by the Alabama Chapter of the American College of Surgeons with the primary goal of establishing a prospective randomized trial to compare alternative forms of surgical therapy and adjuvant chemotherapy. Patients with operable breast cancer were prerandomized to receive either a Halsted radical mastectomy or a modified radical mastectomy. Three hundred and eleven patients with primary operable cancer were entered into this surgical and adjuvant chemotherapy trial. Although conducted and controlled by a single institution, a total of 91 surgeons participated (all Diplomates of the American Board of Surgery and Fellows of the American College of Surgeons). Patients with histologically positive metastatic axillary lymph nodes were randomized further to receive one of two forms of adjuvant chemotherapy (a combination of cyclophosphamide, methotrexate, and fluorouracil or the single agent melphalan).

At the median follow-up of 5.5 years, Maddox et al.[44] found no statistically significant difference in disease-free survival between the two operative groups. However, at this early operative follow-up interval, a trend toward improvement in the 5-year survival rate was evident for the Halsted mastectomy group when compared to the modified radical group (84 percent versus 76 percent, respectively; $p = 0.14$). This trend became more evident when analysis was completed at 10 years[45] (Fig. 29–43). Figure 29–44 shows an improvement in survival rates for patients treated with the Halsted radical technique for T2 tumors with clinically positive axillary nodes and for T3 tumors. Maddox et al.[45] confirmed a statistically significant reduction in the local/regional recurrence rate ($p = 0.04$) following treatment with the radical mastectomy technique when compared with the modified technique (Fig. 29–45). Table 29–14 depicts the comparison of 5- and 10-year recurrence rates between the two techniques according to stage of disease. At the 5-year analysis, patients treated with the modified radical mastectomy technique (n = 175) had a local recurrence rate of 9.1 percent compared to 4.4 percent for 136 patients treated with Halsted mastectomy ($p = 0.09$). At 10-year follow-up, these investigators confirmed an increase in local recurrence rate for the modified radical technique that was twice that of the radical mastectomy technique ($p = 0.04$). This increase in recurrence was evident with subset analysis of the more advanced stage lesions and, as expected, was greatest for stage III disease. This subset of patients

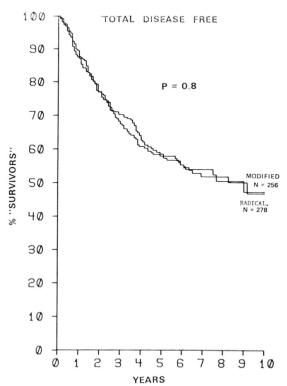

Figure 29–42. Distant metastasis rates regardless of any other outcome. (From Turner L, et al: Ann R Coll Surg Engl 63:241, 1981. Reprinted by permission.)

Table 29–13. MANCHESTER TRIAL RESULTS: OVERALL SURVIVAL, DISEASE-FREE SURVIVAL, AND LOCAL AND DISTANT DISEASE–FREE SURVIVAL RATES (%) FOR RADICAL AND MODIFIED RADICAL MASTECTOMY ACCORDING TO CLINICAL AND PATHOLOGICAL STAGE AT ENTRY

	Number of Patients Followed Up	Overall Survival, 5 yrs	Disease-Free Local Recurrence,* 5 yrs	Disease-Free of Distant Metastases,* 5 yrs	Overall Disease-Free Survival,* 5 yrs
All cases					
Radical	278	70	75	63	58
Modified	256	70	79	63	58
Clinical stage I					
Pathological stage I					
Radical	119	80	85	79	69
Modified	108	79	90	79	71
Pathological stage II					
Radical	52	57	57	52	39
Modified	49	62	74	62	57
Clinical stage II					
Pathological stage I					
Radical	41	85	91	79	79
Modified	38	78	88	71	70
Pathological stage II					
Radical	64	55	59	47	38
Modified	59	55	56	45	30

*Figures indicate the percentages of patients not experiencing each event regardless of any other outcome.
From Turner L, et al: Ann R Coll Surg Engl 63:240–243, 1981. Reprinted by permission.

with more advanced cancers (T2 and T3 with clinically positive axillary nodes) experienced significantly better survival at 10 years following the radical mastectomy compared with the modified radical mastectomy (59 percent versus 38 percent, respectively).

The results of this prospective randomized UAB study demonstrated no significant difference in the overall survival rates for the two techniques. However, there was a trend of increased survival rates for those having the radical mastectomy. These results are virtually identical to those reported by Turner et al.[60] in the Man-

chester trial (Table 29–13 and Figs. 29–39 and 29–40) for overall survival between the two surgical treatment groups. However, disease-free survival was different at 10 years in the analysis by Maddox and associates.[45] Furthermore, this well-controlled and monitored study produced remarkable concurrence between the community pathologists and referees. Despite the large number of qualified surgeons who participated in the trial, recurrence rates among stages I and II patients were comparable at 5 years. The higher local/regional recurrence rate experienced using the lesser technique

Table 29–14. UNIVERSITY OF ALABAMA PROSPECTIVE RANDOMIZED TRIAL TO COMPARE THE HALSTED RADICAL MASTECTOMY TO THE MODIFIED RADICAL MASTECTOMY: LOCAL RECURRENCE RATES OF THE TWO TECHNIQUES

Disease Stage	Modified Radical Mastectomy						Halsted Radical Mastectomy					
	No. of Patients	%	Local Recurrence				*No. of Patients*	%	Local Recurrence			
			5-year		10-year				5-year		10-year	
			No.	%	*No.*	%			*No.*	%	*No.*	%
I	43	13.8	4	9.3	NA	NA	37	11.9	2	5.4	NA	NA
II	112	36.0	8	7.1	NA	NA	83	26.7	3	3.6	NA	NA
III	20	6.4	4	20.0†	NA	NA	16	5.0	1	6.3†	NA	NA
Total	175	56.2	16	9.1*	20	11.4‡	136	43.7	6	4.4*	8	5.8‡

*p = 0.09.
†p = NS.
‡p = 0.04.
NA = Not Available.
Modified from Maddox WA et al: Ann Surg 198:207–212, 1983, and Arch Surg 122:1317–1320, 1987.

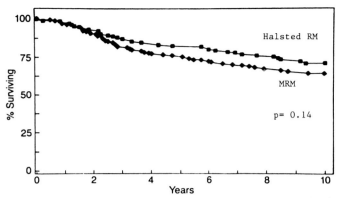

Figure 29–43. Overall survival of patients who underwent radical (squares, n = 136) and modified radical (diamonds, n = 175) mastectomy (*p* = 0.14). (From Maddox WA, et al: Arch Surg 122:1319, 1987. Reprinted by permission.)

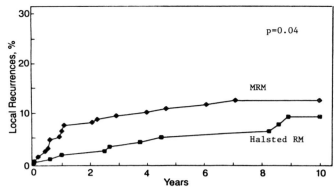

Figure 29–45. Overall local recurrence rates in patients who underwent radical (squares, n = 136) and modified radical (diamonds, n = 175) mastectomy. Local recurrence rate was significantly higher after modified radical mastectomy (*p* = 0.04). (From Maddox WA, et al: Arch Surg 122:1319, 1987. Reprinted by permission.)

suggests that more advanced local disease (T2, T3 with clinically positive nodes) substantially benefited from the more comprehensive operation. This study further demonstrated the importance of conducting long-term follow-up analysis to confirm the results of a trial in which trends are evident in the earlier stages of the analysis. The results of this study indicate that although overall survival was similar for patients treated with the two techniques, patients with more advanced disease had better ultimate survival when treated by the radical mastectomy.

TOTAL MASTECTOMY (WITH AND WITHOUT IRRADIATION)

The term "total mastectomy" should be considered synonymous with "simple mastectomy." This technique represents a further modification of the modified and Halsted radical mastectomies in that the total mastectomy preserves *both* pectoral muscles and does not utilize any variant of the axillary dissection in the

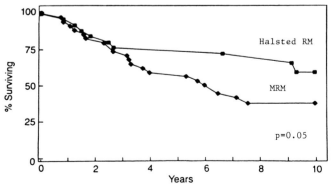

Figure 29–44. Survival curves comparing radical (squares, n = 25) and modified radical (diamonds, n = 36) mastectomy for patients with T2 tumors with clinically positive axillary nodes and T3 tumors. There was significantly better survival after radical mastectomy (*p* = 0.05). (From Maddox WA, et al: Arch Surg 122:1319, 1987. Reprinted by permission.)

treatment of breast cancer. As discussed in a subsequent section of this chapter, the rationale for the procedure developed from the alternative hypothesis concept, which, in the most simplistic terms, considers breast cancer to be a biologically heterogeneous, systemic disease involving a complexity of host-tumor interrelationships. Furthermore, this alternative hypothesis suggests that variations in local/regional therapy are unlikely to substantially affect survival. Fisher and colleagues[20] of the NSABP have contributed significantly to this hypothesis.

It has previously been determined that regional lymph nodes have greater biological than anatomical importance and do not provide a barrier to tumor dissemination as considered by Halsted,[27] Meyer,[48] and others during the late nineteenth and early twentieth centuries. These original concepts of the "orderliness" about tumor dissemination and the probability that clinically recognizable cancer was in many circumstances a local/regional disease have been essentially dispelled by the recognition of systemic disease in the presence of early stages of breast cancer. In that era, surgeons considered cancers of the breast to be more curable if the surgeon designed a more expansive operation to extirpate wider margins that encompassed the locally confined disease process. In this earlier era of breast cancer therapy, local/regional recurrences were considered to be the result of inadequate applications of surgical skill rather than a manifestation of systemic dissemination.

Fisher, Saffer, and Fisher[22] confirmed that biological rather than anatomical factors are responsible for metastatic dissemination. The findings of these investigators confirmed that hematogenously-located tumor cells enter the lymph nodes and concluded that the hematopoietic and lymphatic systems are unified inasfar as tumor cell dissemination. Furthermore, there appeared to be no orderly pattern of tumor cell dissemination based upon the primitive concepts of mechanical considerations and orderly permeation of lymphatics prior to systemic disease.[16] These investigators conducted important experiments in the 1950s to determine host factors for development of metastases and established that the tumor is not autonomous of its host.[15] Evidence for a "dormant" tumor cell was confirmed experimentally, and Fisher and Fisher[15] identified host perturbations that could produce lethal metastasis from these dormant cells. Other experiments support divergent hypotheses regarding the biology of breast cancer, with particular reference to the mechanism for tumor dissemination, and provide the major rationale for disagreement as to the surgical management for cancer of this organ. However, *these experiments support the concept that cancer of the breast is a systemic disease, perhaps from its inception.*[20] In contradistinction, this premise and its biological rationale do not suggest that every patient will develop overt metastasis (stage IV disease). It is this rationale that led Fisher and Fisher[18, 19] to formulate the thesis that the regional lymph node basin represents an *indicator* of the "existent host-tumor relationship." These and many other investigators consider the positive regional lymph node to be a reflection of the interrelationship that permits development of metastases rather than maintains the role as the instigator of distant disease. These principles[159, 160] and the evolution of scientific debate led to the establishment of the use of the total mastectomy alone or in combination with irradiation for the treatment of breast cancer. Data for the effectiveness of the total mastectomy with or without irradiation or chemotherapy for treatment of disease are derived from both retrospective and prospective randomized trials.

Because the total (simple) mastectomy is designed to treat local or regional recurrence, some authors have postulated that the addition of the regional node dissection should not influence survival. This premise maintains that the total mastectomy provides overall survival rates equivalent to those of the modified radical and radical mastectomy without incurring an additional op-erative risk or unnecessary cosmetic deformity. It has also been postulated that the intact axillary nodal basin may enhance immune competency and inherent tumor-icidal activities. Should this be confirmed, we would expect a reduction in the local/regional recurrence rate reflected in an increased disease-free survival.

RETROSPECTIVE AND PROSPECTIVE STUDIES OF TOTAL MASTECTOMY

The previously cited data demonstrate the biological and anatomical considerations for use of the total mastectomy in the treatment of operable breast cancer. These data are derived from both retrospective studies and prospective randomized clinical trials. These series make comparisons of the total mastectomy with and without radiation therapy; other studies make comparisons with radical surgical procedures.

Table 29–15 documents the survival results for nine retrospective clinical trials performed by seven institutions or study groups utilizing total mastectomy with and without irradiation of the peripheral lymph nodes and chest wall. The Manchester and TNM classification systems were used in these trials, which varied in homogeneity and patient accrual size. Expectantly, 3-, 5- and 10-year survival rates show a progressive attrition over time for patients who underwent irradiation of the peripheral lymphatics or for those in whom this modality was not used in postoperative therapy. Turnbull et al.[59] reported from Southamptom (United Kingdom) the 3-year follow-up results of patients treated by simple mastectomy alone or by simple mastectomy with radical irradiation. There were no statistically significant differences in survival of patients in the two groups at 3 years, but local recurrence was significantly more frequent (28

Table 29–15. SURVIVAL RESULTS OF RETROSPECTIVE CLINICAL TRIALS FOR TOTAL MASTECTOMY ± RADIOTHERAPY (RT)

| Author and Year | Clinic or Study Group | No. of Patients | Disease Stage | Absolute Survival (%) | | | |
| | | | | 5-year | | 10-yr | |
				−RT	+RT	−RT	+RT
Williams, 1953[64]	St. Bartholomew (UK)	110	I	77	67	33	40
		45	II	—	35	—	21
Smith, 1959[57]	Rockford, IL	97	I & II	54	—	32	—
Shimkin, 1961[56]	Rockford, IL	103	I & II	51	—	31	—
Devitt, 1962[11]	Ottawa (Canada)	119	I	—	68	—	45
		30	II	—	56	—	47
Den Besten, 1965[10]	University of Iowa	133	I	55.7	—	—	—
		95	II	33.7	—	—	—
Kyle, 1976[37]	Cancer Research Campaign (UK)	1152	I*	78	79	—	—
		1116	II	71	76	—	—
Turnbull, 1978[59]	Southampton (UK)	96	I	84†	85†	—	—
		54	II	72†	81†	—	—
Meyer, 1978[47]	Rockford, IL	252	I & II	69	—	40	—
Hermann, 1985[34]	Cleveland Clinic	355	I	78	—	60	—
		47	II	53	—	37	—

*Manchester Staging Classification.
†3-year survival.

percent) in the mastectomy-alone group. Early survival was not adversely affected by irradiation.

For these various trials, the 5-year survival rate for clinical TNM stage I tumors ranged from 51 percent to 78 percent; for clinical TNM stage II cancers, the range was 33.7 percent to 71 percent. Radical radiotherapy administered to the peripheral lymphatics in these nine series appears to have had little overall benefit in the groups compared by Williams et al.[64] at 5 years. However, at 10 years, absolute survival appeared to be improved in patients who had undergone radical irradiation of the peripheral lymphatics. Hermann et al.[34] reported a 10-year absolute survival of 60 percent for stage I and 37 percent for stage II, respectively. No comparisons were made at 10 years for usage of radical irradiation in this series. These data must be viewed with the knowledge that these trials span three decades and use diverse techniques by varying physicians in retrospective reports. However, it seems evident that the survival rates achieved with total mastectomy (both with and without radiation therapy) are comparable to those obtained with radical mastectomy.

Table 29–16 catalogues local/regional recurrence rates following total mastectomy with and without irradiation in nine retrospective and prospective clinical trials conducted in the United Kingdom, South Africa, and the United States. The series by Williams et al.[64] of St. Bartholomews-St. Albans Hospitals (UK) represents a 10-year study of patients with stage I, II, or III cancer. With comparable matching of patients in these stages, the authors used total mastectomy with and without

irradiation or total mastectomy with radium implants. No differences were observed between the treatment groups utilizing external beam irradiation or radium implants versus the surgery only group. Recurrences at the chest wall, scar, or supraclavicular sites are not documented in this series.[64]

Crile[6] of the Cleveland Clinic treated operable stage I and II breast cancer with simple mastectomy alone (stage I) and occasionally used radical irradiation of the peripheral lymphatics for stage II disease. In 69 reported cases at this institution, five patients (7.2 percent) treated by simple mastectomy had local recurrence in the chest wall or the axilla; in a comparable group of 62 patients treated by radical operation, five (8.1 percent) had similar recurrence. Crile does not document recurrence rates in chest wall, scar, operative field, or supraclavicular sites.

Helman and associates[31] reported on a controlled trial to investigate the efficacy of simple mastectomy versus radical mastectomy in the treatment of TNM stage I and II operable breast cancer at the Groote Schuur Hospital in Capetown, South Africa. This interim study was rapidly terminated as follow-up analysis at the time of the report confirmed that five of 51 patients (9.8 percent) having simple mastectomy developed lymph node recurrence in the axilla, and seven (13.7 percent) developed skin flap recurrence. Recurrence rates in the operative scar, chest wall, or supraclavicular sites are not reported. In contrast, Helman and associates[31] confirmed that of 44 patients undergoing radical mastectomy, only one (2.3 percent) developed skin flap recurrence, and none

Table 29–16. LOCAL AND REGIONAL RECURRENCE RATES FOLLOWING TOTAL MASTECTOMY ± RADIOTHERAPY

Author and Year	Clinic or Study Group	No. of Patients	Disease Stage	Follow-up (yrs)	Chest Wall	Scar	Operative Field	Supra-clavicular
Williams, 1953[64]	St. Bartholomew	55*	I–III	10	—	—	16	—
	St. Albans (UK)	63†	I–III	10	—	—	14	—
		98§	I–III	10	—	—	13	—
Crile, 1964[7]	Cleveland Clinic*†	69	I + II	5	7.2	—	—	—
Helman, 1972[31]	Groote Schuur (Capetown, S. Afr.)	51	I + II	2–5	—	—	13.7	—
Kyle, 1976[37]	Cancer Research Campaign (UK)	1152*	I + II	5	3.2	—	4.9	2.2
	King's College	1116†	I + II	5	0.8	—	1.5	0.7
Turnbull, 1978[58]	Holt Radium Inst.	76*	I + II	1–4	—	—	27.6	—
	Southampton, (UK)	74†	I + II	1–4	—	—	10.8	—
Langlands, 1980[38]	Southeast Scotland	131†	I	12	—	—	8.4	3.1
		64†	II	12	—	—	12.5	6.3
		47†	III	12	—	—	12.8	4.3
Forrest, 1974, 1982[23, 24]	Edinburgh (Cardiff/St. Mary's)	75*	I	5	—	5.3	2.7	—
		49†	II	5	—	8.0	4.0	—
		39‡	II	10	25.6	—	—	—
Berstock, 1985[4]	Cancer Research Campaign (UK)	1121*	I + II	14	12.4	—	—	3.9
	King's College	1122	I + II	14	6.5	—	—	3.4
Fisher, 1985[17]	NASBP (B-04)*	365	I	10	5.2	1.6	0.8	3.0
	NSABP (B-04)†	352	I	10	0.9	0.3	0.0	0.3
	NSABP (B-04)†	294	II	10	0.7	0.3	0.7	0.0

*Total mastectomy alone.
†Total mastectomy with radical irradiation.
‡Total mastectomy with axillary irradiation only.
§Total mastectomy + radium implant.

developed axillary nodal recurrence at the time of this brief follow-up of 2 to 5 years. This high rate of local/regional recurrence for the simple mastectomy persuaded the authors to recommend techniques that include axillary node dissection or postoperative irradiation therapy for treatment of operable breast cancer.

In the original report of the Cancer Research Campaign of the United Kingdom, Kyle and associates[37] compared the results of a radical therapeutic regimen (total mastectomy and radiotherapy) to those of a conservative policy (total mastectomy alone) in a prospective controlled clinical study. The study included 2268 patients to ensure that small but significant differences between the two treatments would be evident. Within a 5-year follow-up interval, there was no evidence that routine postoperative radiation therapy was detrimental to wound repair; however, this modality also conferred no additional benefit as to survival or distant recurrence. Irradiation did, however, significantly reduce the incidence of local/regional recurrence, as indicated in Table 29–16. Almost a fourfold reduction in chest wall recurrence and a threefold reduction in supraclavicular recurrence was evident at 5-year follow-up with the addition of irradiation. Similar trends were observed in recurrence at the operative site. Berstock and associates[4] continued this trial, with follow-up ranging from 9 to 14 years (median, 11.4 years). Again, updated analyses showed no significant differences in survival and distant recurrence between the two treatment groups. Conversely, patients who received prophylactic irradiation postoperatively continued to have a reduced risk for development of local recurrence as the first sign of treatment failure ($p < 0.001$). A twofold reduction was evident in chest wall recurrence at the median follow-up of 11.4 years. Specifics with regard to site and operative field recurrence were not reported. Interestingly, at the median follow-up of 11.4 years, prophylactic irradiation appeared to confer minimal benefit for control of the supraclavicular site.

A prospective randomized trial was conducted by Turnbull et al.[59] in Southampton, UK, for treatment of early breast cancer with total mastectomy alone versus total mastectomy with radical radiotherapy. These investigators matched groups for age, menopausal status, duration of symptoms, size of tumor, and nodal involvement. In stage I and II patients (n = 76) treated with total mastectomy alone and followed for 1 to 4 years, operative field recurrence was 27.6 percent. Seventy-four patients with TNM stages I and II disease who were followed concurrently at the same interval but were treated with postoperative irradiation showed a reduction in operative field recurrence to 10.8 percent. Early survival was not adversely affected by radiation therapy.

In the randomized trial conducted by Langlands et al.[38] in southeast Scotland, the overall survival rate with use of radical mastectomy was equivalent to that for patients treated by simple mastectomy and radical irradiation. At 12 years follow-up, these authors confirmed that survival in the radical mastectomy treatment group

was significantly better ($p < 0.05$), but only for those with clinical stage I disease. The pattern of survival after recurrence was detected confirmed interesting differences between the two treatment modalities. Overall there was a significantly prolonged survival following detection of recurrence in the radical mastectomy group ($p < 0.05$); this was greatest when local recurrence and distant metastases coincided ($p < 0.01$). Forrest and associates[23, 24] of the University Department of Clinical Surgery, Royal Infirmary, Edinburgh, confirmed scar recurrence rates of 5.3 percent and 8.0 percent for TNM stages I and II, respectively. Recurrence rates in the operative field were 2.7 percent and 4.0 percent at 5-year follow-up for stages I and II, respectively.

In the National Surgical Adjuvant Breast Project (NSABP) B-04 trial, Fisher et al.[17] conducted a randomized study to compare alternative local and regional treatments of breast cancer. Life table estimates were obtained for 1665 women enrolled for a mean of 126 months (see critique in this chapter). For patients treated by total (simple) mastectomy without axillary irradiation but with regional irradiation versus those treated by total mastectomy alone, no differences were observed between patients with clinically positive nodes or clinically negative nodes with respect to disease-free survival, distant disease–free survival, or overall survival at 10 years follow-up. Ten-year survival was approximately 57 percent for node-negative patients and 38 percent for node-positive patients. These investigators concluded that variations of local and regional treatment were not important in determining survival of patients with breast cancer. Results obtained at 5 years accurately predicted outcome at 10 years. Despite these similarities in survival, chest wall recurrence was significantly greater at 10-year follow-up for stage I patients treated with mastectomy alone (5.2 percent) versus patients treated with total mastectomy and radical irradiation (0.9 percent). Table 29–16 further documents the reduction in scar, operative field, and supraclavicular recurrence for stage I and stage II disease in patients treated with adjunctive radiotherapy.

The axillary recurrence rates for node-negative and node-positive patients treated with total mastectomy with and without radiation are depicted in Table 29–17. The series by Kyle et al.[37] and Berstock et al.[4] represent trials of the Cancer Research Campaign of the United Kingdom. The series reported by Langlands et al.[38] was updated at 10 years in the Cardiff-St. Mary's study by Forrest and associates.[23, 24] In the report by Crile[6] of 103 node-negative and 35 node-positive patients, the axillary recurrence rate for node-negative patients was 30.0 percent at 6-year follow-up. The recurrence rate for node-positive patients was not reported in this series.

In the Cancer Research Campaign of the UK initially reported by Kyle et al.,[37] with detailed follow-up at 14 years by Berstock and associates,[4] the benefit of radiotherapy was evident in the node-negative group. At 5 years, a reduction in axillary recurrence rate for stage I disease from 9.5 percent to 1.7 percent was attributed to the use of prophylactic radiotherapy. At 14 years

Table 29–17. AXILLARY RECURRENCE RATES FOR PATIENTS TREATED WITH TOTAL MASTECTOMY ± RADIOTHERAPY

Author and Year	Clinic or Study Group	No. of Patients Neg./Pos.	Follow-up Interval (yrs)	Recurrence Rates (%) Node-negative	Node-positive
Crile, 1964[7]	Cleveland Clinic	103/35	6	30.0	NA
Kyle, 1976[37]	Cancer Research Campaign (UK)‡	877/275	5	9.5*	—
		843/273	5	1.7†	—
Langlands, 1980[38]	Southeast Scotland	131/111	5	13.7	10.8 +
Forrest, 1982[24]	Edinburgh (Cardiff)§	64/39	10	15.6	25 +
Berstock, 1985[4]	Cancer Research Campaign (UK)‡	877/275	14	23.8*	—
		843/273	14	6.4†	—
Fisher et al, 1985[17]	NSABP (B-04)	365/294	10	1.1§	—
		352/294	10	3.1†	11.9†

*Overall axillary recurrence for node-positive + node-negative without radiation therapy.
†Overall axillary recurrence for node-positive + node-negative with radiation therapy.
‡No axillary node histology available at therapy.
§Treated with axillary radiotherapy if nodes positive clinically.
NA-Not available.

follow-up, Berstock et al.[4] documented an axillary recurrence rate of 23.8 percent for stage I disease. A reduction of the relapse rate to 6.4 percent was evident in patients who had undergone radical radiotherapy to the chest wall and regional lymphatics. In the Scottish trial initially reported by Langlands et al.[38] with follow-up by Forrest et al.,[23, 24] 5-year axillary recurrence rate for node-negative and node-positive patients was 13.7 percent and 10.8 percent, respectively. The recurrence rate at 10 years was 15.6 percent for node-negative and 25 percent for node-positive patients. In the Cardiff-St. Mary's trial, patients were treated with axillary radiotherapy only if nodes were clinically positive.

Fisher and associates[17] of the NSABP B-04 cooperative trial reported a 10-year axillary recurrence rate of 1.1 percent in stage I node-negative patients treated by total mastectomy alone, which was equivalent to the relapse rate for radical mastectomy (1.4 percent) for this site. The addition of irradiation therapy to the total mastectomy group conferred no benefit in this subset of patients with clinically negative nodes. For patients with clinically positive nodes, the axillary recurrence rate was 11.9 percent in the group treated with irradiation and total mastectomy, which was significantly higher than that in the group treated by radical mastectomy alone (1.0 percent). These analyses note minimal enhancement of absolute survival at 5 and 10 years; some studies confirm that peripheral irradiation in the clinically node-positive group reduced local/regional relapse rates. These data further indicate the necessity of histological sampling of the axillary lymphatics for invasive ductal and lobular carcinoma to guide future therapy strategies. Unless axillary lymphatics are sampled at the time of total mastectomy, this information will not be available for the planning of peripheral irradiation and/or subsequent systemic chemotherapy. The advantages of adding systemic chemo- and/or hormonal therapy to the pre- and postmenopausal patient will be subsequently discussed in chapters 39, 42, and 44.

PROSPECTIVE TRIALS FOR TOTAL MASTECTOMY WITH AND WITHOUT IRRADIATION

A previous section in this chapter gave the history of the development of the Halsted radical mastectomy and its necessity in the absence of effective adjuvant therapy to control local and regional disease. This section has defined the rationale for the modified radical mastectomy as a more conservative approach than the Halsted procedure that can achieve similar local/regional and survival benefit. The evolution toward more conservative approaches with effective adjuvant therapy has led to prospective randomized clinical trials for the treatment of breast cancer with total mastectomy both with and without irradiation.

Groote Schuur Trial, 1968–1971

A prospective controlled trial was conducted in the breast clinic of the Groote Schuur Hospital in Cape Town, South Africa, to evaluate the efficacy of simple mastectomy versus radical mastectomy in the treatment of stage I (T1N0, T2N0) and stage II (T1N1, T2N1) carcinoma of the breast. Helman and associates,[31] in an interim report, felt that conservative approaches for the treatment of operable breast cancer should be investigated. The authors did not utilize routine postoperative radiotherapy or chemotherapy in the treatment of 51 patients undergoing simple mastectomy and 44 patients undergoing radical mastectomy. The median follow-up was not determined.

At the time of analysis, the authors confirmed that five of the 51 patients (9.8 percent) having simple mastectomy developed lymph node recurrences in the axilla; seven (13.7 percent) developed skin flap recurrence. In contrast, for the 44 patients undergoing radical mastectomy, only one (2.3 percent) developed skin flap recurrence, and none developed axillary node recurrence. After reviewing these results and the apparent discrepancy between the local recurrence rates after simple and radical mastectomy, the Groote Schuur Breast Clinic terminated the trial because of the high rate of axillary node recurrence in patients undergoing simple mastectomy.

Helman and associates[31] admitted that they had no justifiable predictions of prognosis for patients in the simple mastectomy trial. The authors concluded that simple mastectomy, in the absence of routine postoperative irradiation, should not be used for operable breast cancer. Because of the satisfactory survival data obtained with the radical mastectomy, the authors suggest that this operation or any other form of mastectomy that includes axillary node dissection with postoperative irradiation is an effective therapy for breast cancer.

It is unfortunate that this trial was terminated after only 3.25 years. The small number of patients in each arm of the study and the short duration of the trial make ultimate conclusions difficult to formulate. Furthermore, the authors do not state in the study design the mechanism for allocating patients to each of the randomization arms with regard to stage of disease. Without knowledge of the number of positive nodes and tumor size allocated into each arm, firm conclusions cannot be drawn. Despite these factors, the disturbingly high incidence of progression of disease in the axillary lymphatics (9.8 percent) of the simple mastectomy only group is significant. The low local/regional recurrence rate (2.2 percent) and the absence of failure of the axilla in the Halsted radical group confirms the efficacy of the radical mastectomy to control axillary recurrence.

Edinburgh Trial, 1964–1971

Between 1964 and 1971, Hamilton et al.[28] and Langlands et al.[38] conducted a study for the treatment of operable cancer of the breast in the southeast region of Scotland. In this controlled clinical trial, 490 women aged 35 to 69 years were randomized to treatment by

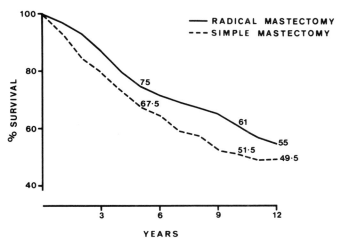

Figure 29–46. Crude survival rates for 256 radical mastectomies and 242 simple mastectomies plus radiotherapy. Percentage survivals are indicated for 5, 10, and 12 years. (From Langlands AO, et al: Br J Surg 67:171, 1980. Reprinted by permission.)

either radical mastectomy (n = 256) or by simple mastectomy and postoperative radiotherapy (n = 242). Figure 29–46 confirms crude survival rates for the radical and simple mastectomy groups. Follow-up data for the first 12 years indicated that survival in the radical mastectomy group was significantly better ($p < 0.05$); however, the benefit accrued only to patients with clinical stage I disease (Fig. 29–47).

Table 29–18 demonstrates the pattern of survival once recurrence has been detected, confirming survival differences between the two treatment groups. Overall there was a significant prolongation of survival following detection of recurrence in the radical mastectomy group ($p < 0.05$), which was greatest when local recurrence and distant metastases were observed ($p < 0.01$). At 12 years on study, Langlands et al.[38] confirmed that duration of survival was independent of clinical stage of disease, tumor size, or menstrual status at diagnosis of recurrent disease. However, the duration of survival was observed to be directly proportional to the duration of the disease-free interval ($p < 0.01$) (Fig. 29–48 and Table 29–19).

Figure 29–47. Crude survival rates for cases according to international stage of the disease and treatment option (RM I = radical mastectomy for Stage I, SM III = simple mastectomy plus radiotherapy for Stage III, and so forth). (From Langlands AO, et al: Br J Surg 67:172, 1980. Reprinted by permission.)

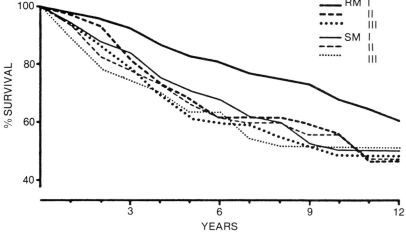

Table 29–18. EDINBURGH TRIAL (1964–1971): SURVIVAL ACCORDING TO TYPE OF RECURRENCE

Type of Recurrence	Treatment	Observed No. of Patients	Expected No. of Deaths	No. of Deaths	X^2
Local only	RM	35	27	28.45	0.20
	SM	28	19	17.55	
Distant only	RM	58	45	51.26	1.56
	SM	69	62	55.74	
Local and distant	RM	12	9	13.88	7.32 ($p<0.01$)
	SM	10	10	5.12	
Combination	RM	105	81	93.59	4.09 ($p<0.05$)
	SM	107	91	78.41	
All recurrences without stratification	RM	105	81	96.43	5.90 ($p<0.05$)
	SM	107	91	75.57	

RM = Radical mastectomy; SM = simple mastectomy.
From Langlands AO et al: Br J Surg 67:170–174, 1980. Reprinted by permission.

In summary, the enhanced survival determined in the Edinburgh trial is seen exclusively in the radical mastectomy group but is accounted for entirely by the use of this technique for the treatment of stage I disease. This well-controlled prospective study further demonstrated an excess number of deaths in the simple mastectomy plus irradiation group that were attributed to causes other than cancer. However, the difference in the pattern of local recurrence, which appears to be excessive in the simple mastectomy plus irradiation group, is almost entirely accounted for by recurrence in the axilla, which occurred in 12 percent of the simple mastectomy group compared with three percent in the radical mastectomy group. This recurrence appeared to be unaffected by stage of disease at the time of presentation. Recurrence in skin flaps was more commonly observed in stage III disease; paradoxically, such recurrences were greater in the radical mastectomy group and are perhaps accounted for by the advantage of postoperative irradiation. Distant disease–free survival was equivalent for the two treatment groups.

Edinburgh Royal Infirmary–Cardiff Trial, 1967–1973

To determine if simple mastectomy combined with lower axillary node sampling (Level I/II node biopsy) was a safe therapeutic option for conservation of the breast, Forrest and associates[23, 24] of the Royal Infirmary, Edinburgh, Scotland, initiated the Cardiff trial. Two hundred patients were included in the study, all with tumors of TNM classification T1, T2, N0N1M0. Patients were randomized according to the site of tumor, clinical stage, and menopausal status and were randomly selected within subgroups for conservative (n = 103) or radical (n = 97) therapy. Patients treated by the conservative approach (simple mastectomy and axillary node sampling) received postoperative irradiation only if the node sample proved to be positive. Radiation therapy was restricted to the axilla and was given in ten fractions (40 Gy) over 3 weeks. The protocol also

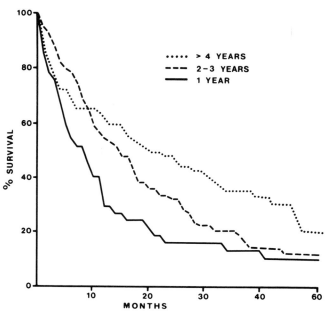

Figure 29–48. Subsequent survival of patients according to the length of the disease-free interval. (From Langlands AO, et al: Br J Surg 67:174, 1980. Reprinted by permission.)

Table 29–19. EDINBURGH TRIAL (1964–1971): DISEASE-FREE INTERVAL ACCORDING TO TYPE OF RECURRENCE*

Stratum	RM Group	SM Group
Local recurrence only	33.5 (+ 4.8)	34.9 (+ 5.2)
Distant metastases only	45.8 (+ 4.4)	38.4 (+ 3.4)
Synchronous local and distant	41.4 (+ 7.4)	31.0 (+ 6.8)

*Mean times in months (+ standard errors) from initial treatment until the first detection of recurrent disease according to the three strata defined in the text.
RM = Radical mastectomy; SM = simple mastectomy.
From Langlands AO et al: Br J Surg 67:170–174, 1980. Reprinted by permission.

required that a biopsy sample be taken from the edge of the removed skin in proximity to the tumor; if biopsy results were positive, radiation therapy was also given to the chest wall. Patients randomized to the radical policy (Halsted radical mastectomy) also received irradiation when positive nodes were identified in the axillary specimen.

As of 1981 (14 years on study), the major revelation of this Scottish study was in the success of the two policies of treatment to achieve local control.[24] There was an increased incidence of recurrent disease affecting the axilla in patients who, on the basis of clinically negative nodes, were treated by simple mastectomy alone compared to those treated by radical mastectomy (Table 29–20). With simple mastectomy alone, axillary recurrence was noted in ten of 64 patients (15.6 percent); only one of 66 patients (1.5 percent) treated with radical mastectomy had axillary recurrence. For patients having simple mastectomy and axillary radiotherapy for positive nodes, the observed chest wall recurrence rate was 25.6 percent (ten of 39 patients); only two of 31 patients (6.5 percent) with positive nodes having radical mastectomy and radical irradiation had chest wall recurrence (Table 29–21). Despite these differences in local/regional control and axillary recurrence rates, the overall survival rates with the two therapies proved to be identical ($p = 0.4147$) (Fig. 29–49). Results from the Edinburgh trial shown in Table 29–22 suggest that radical irradiation may benefit patients with histologically negative or unidentified pectoral nodes recovered at mastectomy; this benefit is greater for patients with unidentified nodes (i.e., unstaged pathologically).

Manchester Regional Breast Study, 1970–1975

Lythgoe and associates[40, 41] reported a prospective clinical trial for treatment of operable breast cancer initiated by the Manchester Regional Association of Surgeons. Patients with TNM clinical stage I cancer (T1, T2, N0M0) were randomly allocated to be treated by total mastectomy and postoperative radiotherapy (TM

Table 29–21. EDINBURGH ROYAL INFIRMARY—CARDIFF TRIAL (1967–1973): CHEST WALL TUMOR RECURRENCE*

| Treatment | Number of Patients | |
	Total	With Chest Wall Recurrence (%)
Simple mastectomy and axillary radiotherapy	39	10 (25.6)
Radical mastectomy and radical radiotherapy	31	2 (6.5)

*Patients had positive nodes at the time of mastectomy.
From Forrest APM et al: Ann Surg 196(3):371–378, 1982. Reprinted by permission.

+ RT) or by total mastectomy (TM) alone. Patients with clinical stage II cancers (T1, T2, N1M0) were randomly allocated to treatment by TM + RT or by radical mastectomy (RM) alone.

Between March, 1970, and October, 1975, 1022 patients (714 stage I and 308 stage II) were admitted to this prospective trial. At a follow-up of 5 to 10 years, no statistically significant differences in overall survival were evident between clinical stage I cancers treated by TM + RT versus those treated by TM alone (Fig. 29–50). Local recurrence (defined as recurrence at the chest wall, axilla, or supraclavicular fossa) was observed twice as frequently in the group treated with TM alone, and this difference was statistically significant ($p < 0.0001$) (Fig. 29–51). Of clinical stage II breast cancers randomly allocated to either TM + RT or RM alone (n = 308), no statistically significant differences in survival or in the frequency of local/regional recurrence were observed between the two treatment groups. Table 29–23 depicts

Table 29–20. EDINBURGH ROYAL INFIRMARY—CARDIFF TRIAL (1967–1973): AXILLARY RECURRENCE IN PATIENTS WITH NEGATIVE AND NONIDENTIFIED NODES TREATED BY SIMPLE AND RADICAL MASTECTOMY

| Treatment | Number of Patients | |
	Total	With Axillary Recurrent (%)
Mastectomy alone (simple mastectomy)	64	10 (15.6)
Mastectomy with axillary clearance (radical mastectomy)	66	1 (1.5)

From Forrest APM et al: Ann Surg 196(3):371–378, 1982. Reprinted by permission.

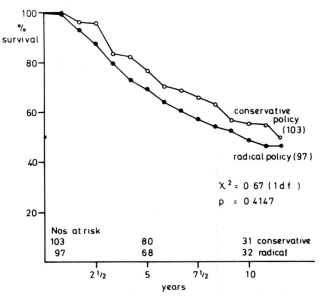

Figure 29–49. Survival of all patients included in the Cardiff trial in April 1981. (From Forrest APM, et al: Ann Surg 196:371, 1982. Reprinted by permission.)

Table 29–22. EDINBURGH TRIAL: LOCAL/REGIONAL RECURRENCE ACCORDING TO WHETHER NODES WERE IDENTIFIED OR NONIDENTIFIED FOR HISTOLOGICAL EXAMINATION AT MASTECTOMY

Treatment	Number of Patients, Nodes Identified and Histologically Negative		Number of Patients, Nodes Not Identified	
	Total	*With Recurrence (%)*	*Total*	*With Recurrence (%)*
Mastectomy alone	114	18 (16)	59	24 (41)
Mastectomy with radiotherapy	112	6 (5)	57	11 (19)

From Forrest APM et al: Ann Surg 196(3):371–378, 1982. Reprinted by permission.

the primary control rates related to the clinical stage of disease and the treatment allocated for the Manchester study. For clinical stage II disease, postoperative irradiation therapy utilized with total mastectomy appears to have a 10-year survival rate equivalent to that of radical mastectomy. In addition, primary control rates of the chest wall, axilla, and supraclavicular fossa appear to be equivalent with the two modalities for this more advanced stage.

Cancer Research Campaign Clinical Trial, 1970–1975

Berstock and colleagues[4] of the King's College/Cambridge School of Medicine, United Kingdom, reported on the Cancer Research Campaign Multicenter Trial for the management of operable breast cancer. Patients were managed with two treatment policies, a total mastectomy alone ("watch policy") and a total mastectomy plus radiotherapy given as a four-field technique employing a recommended dose of 1320 to 1510 ret (radiation equivalent therapy) during a 6-week period. Of 2800 patients randomized, 2243 were deemed fully evaluable in these groups in which no formal axillary dissection was performed. Follow-up ranged from 9 to

14 years (median, 11.4 years). As seen in Figure 29–52, these data confirm no significant differences in terms of survival ($p = 0.37$) for the "watch policy" versus irradiated patients following total mastectomy. However, the incidence of local recurrence in the two treatment groups (Fig. 29–53) shows a marked and significant difference favoring the radiotherapy group and represents a hazard ratio of observed-to-expected events in the "watch policy" group of 2.69 compared with the irradiated group ($p < 0.001$). The effect of radiotherapy on the distribution of local recurrence as reported by the authors of this trial is interesting, because irradiation tended to protect most effectively against axillary recurrence (hazard ratio = 3.95) and less effectively against chest wall recurrence (hazard ratio = 2.03). Furthermore, the use of irradiation appeared to have no protection whatsoever against supraclavicular recurrence, in spite of the supraclavicular field being included in the recommended protocol and employed in 92 percent of the patients studied. The most significant variable that determined the future development of local recurrence was the histological grade of the primary tumor. As reported by Elston and associates[14] of this study, high-grade tumors had a significantly higher incidence of local recurrence than did histologically low-grade tumors (Fig.

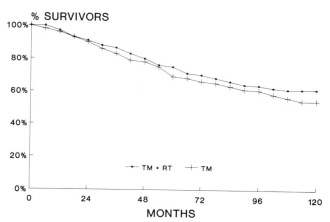

Figure 29–50. Survival curves for all surgical cases entered as stage I. TM = Total (simple) mastectomy; TM + RT = total (simple) mastectomy and postoperative radiation therapy. (From Lythgoe JP, Palmer MK: Br J Surg 69:693, 1982. Reprinted by permission.)

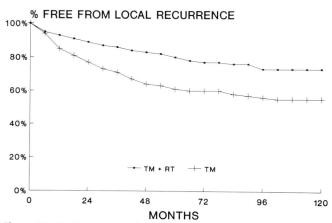

Figure 29–51. Percentage of stage I patients free of local recurrence. TM + RT = Total mastectomy plus postoperative irradiation; TM = total mastectomy alone. The differences observed for local recurrence of the chest wall, axilla, and supraclavicular fossa were statistically significant ($p < 0.0001$). (From Lythgoe JP, Palmer MK: Br J Surg 69:693, 1982. Reprinted by permission.)

Table 29–23. MANCHESTER REGIONAL BREAST STUDY (1970–1975): PRIMARY CONTROL RELATED TO CLINICAL STAGE AND TREATMENT FOR STAGE I AND II DISEASE

| Clinical Stage | Treatment | No. of Patients | % Free from Recurrence ||||||
| | | | Chest Wall || Axilla || Supraclavicular Fossa ||
			5 yr	10 yr	5 yr	10 yr	5 yr	10 yr
I	Simple mastectomy	359	84	80	67	63	89	85
	Simple mastectomy + radiotherapy	355	94	91	84	81	92	89
			$p = 0.0002$		$p = 0.0001$		$p = 0.20$	
II	Radical mastectomy	149	66	64	76	71	80	77
	Simple mastectomy + radiotherapy	159	77	63	75	72	87	86
			$p = 0.22$		$p = 0.95$		$p = 0.15$	

From Lythgoe JP, Palmer MK: Br J Surg 69:693–696, 1982. Reprinted by permission.

29–54). The site of the primary tumor within the breast, dose of radiation therapy received, and menstrual status had little bearing on the subsequent development of local recurrence.

Of interest in the study is the finding that survival following development of local recurrence was different between the two treatment groups. Paradoxically, the radiotherapy arm did worse than the "watch policy" group ($p = 0.05$). The 5-year survival rate following any local/regional recurrence was 35.6 percent for the "watch policy" group and 30.6 percent for the total mastectomy plus irradiation group. Mean survival time was 3.3 years for the "watch policy" group and 2.7 years for the total mastectomy plus irradiation group (Table 29–24).

In conclusion, this study confirms that patients at high risk of local recurrence are those with high histological grade tumors, those with clinically or pathologically positive axillary nodes, and those with cancers that had diameters greater than 2 cm. Of patients who subse-quently developed local/regional recurrence and died, 67 percent in the total mastectomy plus irradiation group and 56 percent in the "watch policy" group did so with evidence of uncontrolled local/regional disease; the incidence of uncontrolled local disease at death was greater in the "watch policy" group (13.2 percent versus 6.8 percent, $p < 0.001$). While much of the local/regional recurrence can be controlled by surgery, radiation therapy, chemotherapy, or adjunctive endocrine measures, this study indicated that a percentage of patients will remain uncontrolled with the disease until death. Importantly, this prospective study establishes the rationale for use of prophylactic irradiation for patients considered at high risk for recurrence to reduce the unfortunate sequelae of uncontrolled disease.

National Surgical Adjuvant Breast Project (B-04), 1971–1974

Fisher and other investigators[17] at 34 American and Canadian institutions participated in B-04 of the

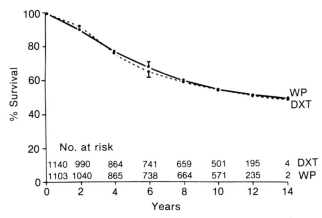

Figure 29–52. All evaluable patients. Survival in watch policy and radiotherapy groups [$\chi^2 = 0.02$, $p = 0.88$, hazard ratio (HR) = 1.0]. "No. at risk" represents the number of patients alive at entry and biennially thereafter. This number decreases in the later years, since there are fewer patients with relevant trial times. Vertical bars indicate the 95 percent confidence intervals. (From Berstock DA, et al: World J Surg 9:667, 1985. Reprinted by permission.)

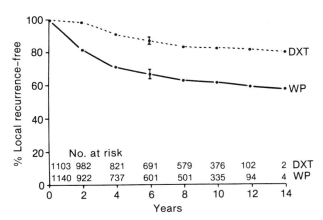

Figure 29–53. All evaluable patients: local recurrence–free in watch policy and radiotherapy groups ($\chi^2 = 120.93$, $p < 0.001$, HR = 2.69). "No. at risk" represents the number of patients alive at entry and biennially thereafter. This number decreases in the later years, since there are fewer patients with relevant trial times. Vertical bars indicate the 95 percent confidence intervals. (From Berstock DA, et al: World J Surg 9:667, 1985. Reprinted by permission.)

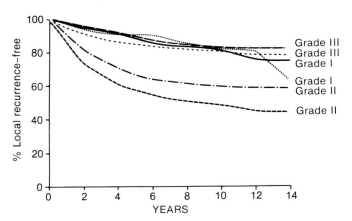

Figure 29–54. Patients with histologically graded tumors subdivided by treatment policy: Grade I (n = 180) $- \chi^2$ = 0.01 ns, HR = 1.04; Grade II (n = 903)χ^2 = 59.79, p < 0.001, HR = 2.98; Grade III (n = 456) $- \chi^2$ = 42.21, p < 0.001, HR = 3.28. (From Berstock DA, et al: World J Surg 9:667, 1985. Reprinted by permission.)

NSABP, a prospectively randomized trial to compare alternative local and regional treatments of breast cancer, all of which employed breast removal. The findings presented by these investigators are drawn from 1655 eligible patients who were enrolled on study for 108 to 145 months (average, 126 months). One hundred patients (5.7 percent) were considered ineligible for analysis. Women who had clinically negative axillary nodes and met rigid protocol requirements (T1, T2N0, N1; or T3N0 tumors) were randomized to receive one of three distinctly different local/regional treatment regimens: a conventional radical mastectomy (RM); a total (simple) mastectomy followed by local/regional irradiation (TM + RT); or a total mastectomy alone (TM). Removal of axillary regional lymphatics was to be completed only when nodes became clinically positive. Similarly, clinically node-positive patients were treated with RM or TM + RT. No adjunctive chemotherapy was given to patients in any of the three randomization arms. Patients considered to have clinically negative nodes were randomly assigned so that one third were treated by RM, one third by TM + RT, and one third by TM alone.

Table 29–24. CANCER RESEARCH CAMPAIGN TRIAL (1970–1975): SURVIVAL FOLLOWING THE DEVELOPMENT OF LOCAL RECURRENCE

Site	5-Yr Survival, % (± SE)		Median Survival (yr)	
	WP	DXT	WP	DXT
Chest wall	33.9 (4.2)	32.2 (5.9)	3.1	2.8
Axilla	33.7 (3.0)	26.7 (5.4)	3.2	2.6
Supraclavicular fossa	16.9 (5.8)	7.9 (4.4)	1.6	1.1
Overall	31.6 (2.5)	30.6 (3.9)	3.3	2.7

WP = Watch policy group; DXT = irradiated group.
From Berstock DA et al: World J Surg 9:667–670, 1985. Reprinted by permission.

Patients with clinically positive axillary nodes were randomized such that one half were treated by RM and one half by TM + RT. A node biopsy was performed in patients with clinically negative axillary nodes who had undergone a total mastectomy without irradiation and subsequently had clinical evidence of axillary node involvement in the absence of other disease manifestations. When regional lymphatics were pathologically reported as positive, a delayed axillary dissection was completed. Patients whose disease progressed with positive axillary nodes following TM + RT were considered treatment failures.

Irradiation was administered using supervoltage techniques; radiation dosages of 4500 rads over 25 fractions were administered to both the internal mammary and supraclavicular nodes at a depth of 3 cm. For patients with clinically negative axillary nodes, a dose of 5000 rads in 25 fractions was delivered to the midaxilla. Most of the dosage was delivered from the anterior supraclavicular portal, and the remainder from the posterior axillary portal. Patients with clinically positive nodes received a boost of 1000 to 2000 rads via a direct appositional portal.[17]

Figure 29–55 shows that there was no significant difference (p = 0.2) in disease-free survival during the entire period of follow-up among groups of patients with *clinically negative nodes* treated by RM, TM + RT, or TM (panel A). When disease-free survival was evaluated in the first and second 5-year periods of follow-up, Fisher and colleagues observed no differences among groups within the first 5 years following surgery

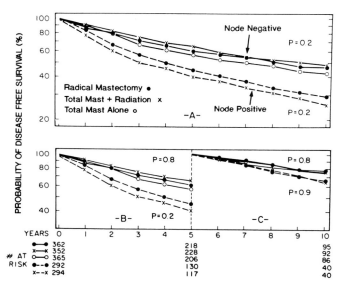

Survival Free of Disease through 10 Years (A), during the First 5 Years (B), and during the Second 5 Years for Patients Free of Disease at the End of the 5th Year (C).

Figure 29–55. Disease-free survival for patients treated by radical mastectomy (solid circle), total mastectomy plus radiation (x), or total mastectomy alone (open circle). There were no significant differences among the three groups of patients with clinically negative nodes (solid line) or between the two groups with clinically positive nodes (broken line). (From Fisher B, et al: N Engl J Med 312(11):674, 1985. Reprinted by permission.)

(p = 0.08) (panel B). Interestingly, an additional 15 percent of patients in all three groups had a treatment failure between the fifth and tenth year. There were no statistical differences in the probability of failure among the three groups during the second 5 years of follow-up (p = 0.8) (panel C). For each group, approximately 75 percent of patients who were free of disease at the end of 5 years remained so at the end of the tenth year. It is apparent that differences observed in the initial 5 years occurred secondary to the higher incidence of local/regional disease and occurred as the first evidence of disease in the total mastectomy group. The differences were not related to an increase in distant disease occurring as a first treatment failure (Fig. 29–56, upper panel). These investigators noted that patients undergoing TM + RT had a lower incidence of local and regional recurrence than did those in the other two groups.

This study showed no significant differences in disease-free survival among patients in the two groups (see Fig. 29–55) treated with RM or TM + RT who presented with *clinically positive nodes* (p = 0.2). These data held for the first and second 5-year intervals of follow-up. Almost two thirds of patients who were free of disease at the end of the fifth year remained so within the next 5-year interval of follow-up. Additionally, this

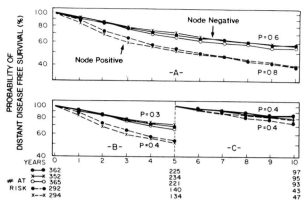

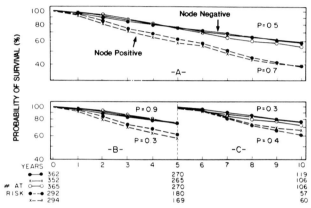

Survival Free of Distant Disease through 10 Years (A), during the First 5 Years (B), and during the Second 5 Years for Patients Free of Distant Disease at the End of the 5th Year (C).

Survival through 10 Years (A), during the First 5 Years (B), and during the Second 5 Years for Patients Alive at the End of the 5th Year (C).

Figure 29–57. Distant disease–free survival and overall survival for patients treated by radical mastectomy (solid circle), total mastectomy and radiation (x), or total mastectomy alone (open circle). There were no significant differences among the three groups of patients with clinically negative nodes (solid line) or between the two groups with positive nodes (broken line). (From Fisher B, et al: N Engl J Med 312(11):674, 1985. Reprinted by permission.)

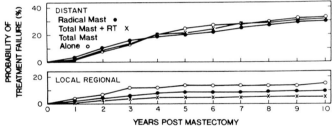

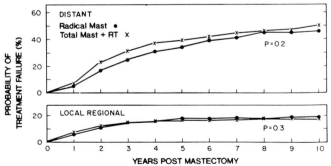

Figure 29–56. Local or regional and distant treatment failures as the first evidence of disease in patients with clinically negative and positive nodes who were treated by radical mastectomy (solid circle), total mastectomy and radiation (x), or total mastectomy alone (open circle). For node-negative patients there were no significant differences in distant disease occurring as a first treatment failure among the three groups, whereas local and regional disease was best controlled in the group receiving radiation. For node-positive patients there was no significant difference in distant or local and regional disease between the two groups. (From Fisher B, et al: N Engl J Med 312(11):674, 1985. Reprinted by permission.)

NSABP study[17] observed little difference between the two groups with respect to the occurrence of distant, local, or regional disease (Fig. 29–56, lower panel).

Fisher et al.[17] observed no significant differences in the probability of survival free of any distant disease, whether occurring as a first treatment failure or after local or regional disease, among patients in the three randomized arms who had *clinically negative nodes* (p = 0.6) (Fig. 29–57, upper panel A). In addition, no significant differences were observed when groups were examined according to the first and second 5-year postoperative intervals for patterns of recurrence (p = 0.3 and 0.4, respectively) (Fig. 29–57, upper panels B and C).

A similar trend was also observed for patients with *clinically positive nodes,* with no significant differences in distant disease–free survival between those undergoing RM and those treated with TM + RT (p = 0.8) (Fig. 29–57, lower panel A). At 5 years follow-up, the distant disease–free survival for patients with clinically positive nodes was 53 ± 3.0 percent for patients treated by RM and 51 ± 3.0 percent for those treated by TM + RT ($p = 0.4$) (Fig. 29–57, upper panel B). At 10 years, the NSABP investigators noted the corresponding figures were 39 ± 3.1 percent and 40 ± 3.1 percent. Thus the probability of distant disease occurring in the second 5-year interval was identical for the two treatment arms ($p = 0.4$) (Fig. 29–57, upper panel C). The occurrence of distant treatment failures reported by the NSABP suggests that the first evidence of recurrent disease does not differ significantly among node-negative (Fig. 29–56, upper panel) and node-positive (Fig. 29–56, lower panel) treatment subgroups.

It is no surprise that overall survival was not significantly different ($p = 0.5$) among the three *node-negative groups* (Fig. 29–57, lower panel A). Overall survival at mean follow-up of 126 months for the three arms were: 58 ± 2.6 percent for the RM group, 59 ± 2.7 percent for the TM + RT group, and 54 ± 2.7 percent for the TM group. The probability of survival during the first and second 5-year follow-up intervals was not significantly different ($p = 0.9$ and 0.3, respectively) (Fig. 29–57, lower panels B and C). Approximately 75 percent of patients with negative nodes who were alive in the first 5 years of follow-up remained alive at 10 years.

No statistical differences were observed in the *node-positive group* with respect to survival at 10 years follow-up ($p = 0.7$) (Fig. 29–57, lower panel A). The probability of survival in the first 5 years and second 5 years of follow-up were not statistically different ($p = 0.3$ and 0.4, respectively) (Fig. 29–57, lower panels B and C). At the end of the tenth year of follow-up, only 38 ± 2.9 percent of the RM group and 39 ± 2.9 percent of the TM + RT group were alive. The authors observed that approximately 65 percent of patients with positive nodes who lived 5 years survived an additional 5 years.

Tumor Location and Survival

Figure 29–58 indicates the relationship of treatment to survival according to tumor location in the NSABP study. Adjustments were made for intralymphatic extension, cell reaction, histological grade, and clinical tumor size.[17] For patients with clinically negative nodes and medial-central or laterally located tumors, no statistical differences ($p = 0.6$) were observed in outcome among the three treatment groups. For patients with clinically positive nodes, treatment was not observed to affect survival in those with lateral ($p = 0.8$) or medial-central tumors ($p = 0.3$).

Axillary Recurrence Following Total Mastectomy

Among 365 patients with clinically negative axillary nodes who had total mastectomy without irradiation, Fisher et al.[17] observed that 17.8 percent subsequently developed histologically confirmed ipsilateral adenopa-

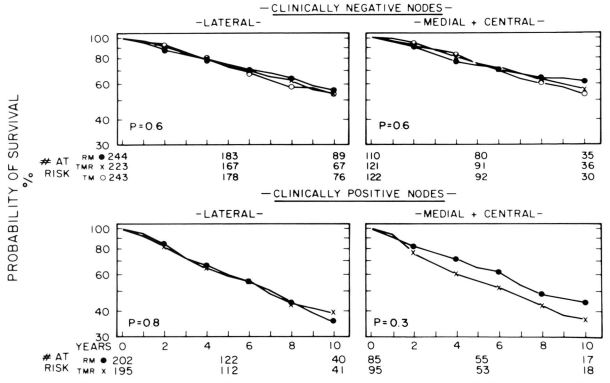

Figure 29–58. Relation of treatment to survival according to tumor location. Patients were treated by radical mastectomy (solid circle), total mastectomy and radiation (x), or total mastectomy alone (open circle). The outcome for patients with clinically negative or positive nodes and lateral tumors or medial and central tumors was not affected by the treatment. (From Fisher B, et al: N Engl J Med 312(11):674, 1985. Reprinted by permission.)

thy. These patients were treated by delayed axillary dissection. Median time from TM to axillary dissection for recurrent disease was 14.7 months (range, 3 to 112.6 months). The majority of delayed axillary dissections (78.5 percent) were completed within 24 months of the original mastectomy. Only 4.6 percent of delayed dissections were completed in the second 5-year follow-up interval.

Summary

This well-controlled prospective study used patients who were meticulously analyzed for treatment results and follow-up. The findings of the NSABP group[17] indicate that location of the breast tumor does not influence prognosis and that irradiation of the internal mammary chain in patients with inner quadrant lesions does not improve survival. This clinical trial demonstrated that results obtained at 5 years accurately predict the outcome to be expected at 10 years. It would appear from this important study that variations of local and regional treatment parameters have less importance in determining survival of the patient with breast cancer than originally considered.

MODIFIED RADICAL MASTECTOMY TECHNIQUE

For the planning of mastectomy incisions, the reader is referred to the section entitled "General Principles of Mastectomy," which describes the techniques for elevation of flaps for tumors of central-subareolar sites and each quadrant of the breast. The initial steps of the operation are conducted with the ipsilateral arm and shoulder in a relaxed, extended position on the arm board (see Fig. 29–32).

As indicated previously, the modified radical mastectomy, with removal of the pectoralis minor muscle (Patey dissection), allows access to Level III nodes such that all nodal levels can be extirpated. The Patey modified radical mastectomy is intended for lesions that cannot be extirpated with clear margins at the time of tylectomy and for lesions of so large a size (>T2, >5 cm) that cosmetic reconstruction and regional control cannot be accomplished with confidence. It is not intended for large tumors (T2, T3, T4) with evidence of skin or pectoralis major fixation for which major resection of this muscle is necessary to achieve adequate surgical margins. Therefore patients with high-lying (peripheral) lesions near the clavicle are not considered candidates for the Patey,[52, 53] Auchincloss,[1] or Madden[42] techniques.

The modified radical mastectomy necessitates en bloc resection of the breast, the axillary lymphatics, and overlying skin near the tumor with a 3- to 5-cm margin to ensure marginal clearance of the tumor. The names "Auchincloss"[1] and "Madden"[42] (and occasionally "Handley"[29]) are used synonymously as modified radical techniques. The Patey mastectomy acknowledges the importance of the complete axillary dissection and the

anatomical necessity for preservation of the medial and lateral pectoral (anterior thoracic) nerves, which may serve as dual innervation to the pectoralis major. Both the Madden and Auchincloss mastectomies advocate preservation of both the pectoralis major and minor muscles, thus allowing adequate access to Level II lymphatics with incomplete dissection (or preservation) of Level III. These approaches are similar in that both require total mastectomy with at least partial axillary lymph node dissection. With the limitation for dissection of the apical (subclavicular) nodal group, the Auchincloss[1] and Madden[42] procedures allow for higher probability of preservation of the *medial (anterior thoracic) pectoral nerve*, which courses in the *lateral neurovascular bundle* of the axilla and commonly penetrates the pectoralis minor to supply the lateral border of the pectoralis major muscle.

The patient is positioned supine for induction with general anesthesia. A roll sheet allows modest elevation of the ipsilateral hemithorax and shoulder such that there is no limitation of range of motion of the shoulder and arm with abduction and adduction. The positioning of the patient at the margin of the operative table is important to allow the operator and assistant simple access without undue retraction on the major muscle groups or brachial plexus (Fig. 29–59).[101] With positioning, the operator should be cognizant of potential subluxation and abduction of the shoulder. This complication is best prevented with padding of the armboard to avoid stretch of the brachial plexus and denervation of major muscle groups of the shoulder and arm. The surgeon must confirm adequate mobility of the ipsilateral arm for adduction and extension during operation.

The ipsilateral breast, neck, shoulder, and hemithorax are prepped with povidone iodine to the table margin and well beyond the midline (see Fig. 29–32). Additionally, the axilla, arm, and hand are fully prepped within the operative field. Towels are secured with clips or stainless steel staples to the skin within the operative field, which includes the shoulder, lower neck, sternum, and upper abdominal musculature. Alternative methods exist to include the arm and hand in the operative field. Our preference is to isolate the hand and forearm with an occlusive Stockinette (DeRoyal Industries, Powell, TN) cotton dressing that is further secured with Kling or Kerlex cotton roll (Johnson and Johnson, New Brunswick, NJ) distal to the elbow. Free mobility of the elbow, arm, and shoulder must be ensured with isolation of the forearm and hand. As in the Halsted radical mastectomy, we position the first assistant over the shoulder (craniad to the armboard) of the ipsilateral breast such that appropriate muscle retraction at the time of axillary dissection can be accomplished with free mobility of the shoulder to allow extension, abduction, and adduction without undue stretch of neurovascular structures of the axilla (see Fig. 29–33).

The limits of the modified radical mastectomy, regardless of the skin incisions utilized, are delineated *laterally* by the anterior margin of the latissimus dorsi muscle, *medially* by the midline of the sternum, *superiorly* by the subclavius muscle, and *inferiorly* by the

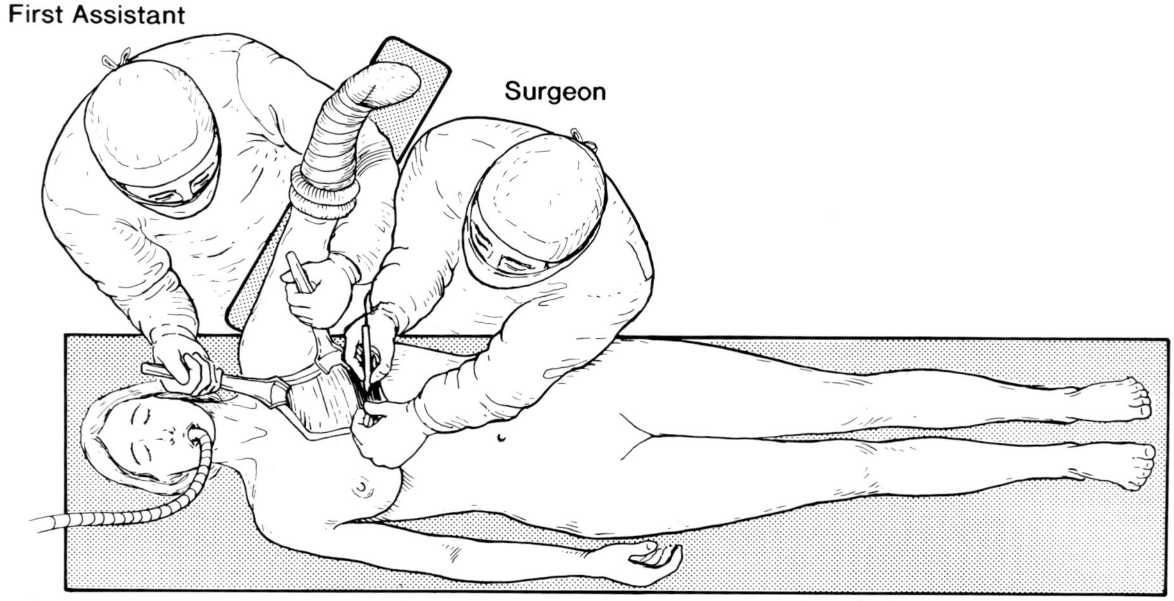

First Assistant

Surgeon

Figure 29–59. Position of patient for left modified radical mastectomy at margin of operative table. The first assistant is cephalad to the armboard and shoulder of the patient to allow access to the axillary contents without undue traction on major muscle groups. Depicted is the preferential isolation of the hand and forearm with an occlusive Stockinette cotton dressing secured distal to the elbow. This technique allows free mobility of the elbow, arm, and shoulder to avoid undue stretch of the brachial plexus with muscle retraction.

caudal extension of the breast some 3 to 4 cm inferior to the inframammary fold (Fig. 29–60, inset).

The design of skin flaps is carefully planned with relation to the quadrant in which the primary neoplasm is located so that adequate margins can be ensured. In the majority of cases, primary closure should be possible unless undue tension or flap devascularization and the necessity of margin debridement is evident. Incisions and skin flaps should be developed perpendicular to the subcutaneous plane. Thereafter retraction hooks or

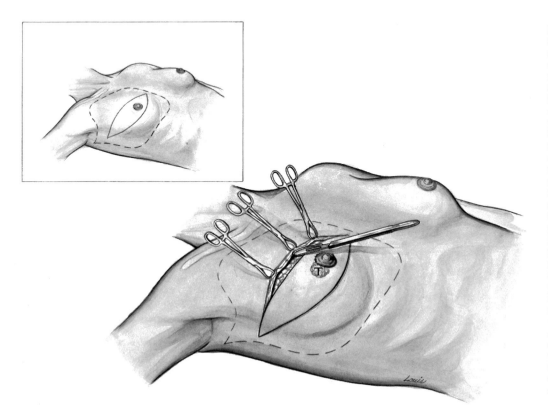

Figure 29–60. *Inset,* Limits of the modified radical mastectomy are delineated *superiorly* by the subclavius muscle, *laterally* by the anterior margin of the latissimus dorsi muscle, *medially* by the midline of the sternum, and *inferiorly* by the caudal extension of the breast approximately 3 to 4 cm inferior to the inframammary fold. Skin flaps for the modified radical technique are planned with relation to the quadrant in which the primary neoplasm is located. Adequate margins are ensured by developing skin edges 3 to 5 cm from the tumor margin. Incisions are planned so that they are developed perpendicular to the subcutaneous plane and are inclusive of skin and parenchymal tissue 3 to 5 cm around the neoplasm. Flap thickness is dependent on patient habitus and proportional lean body mass. Flaps should be 7 to 8 mm in thickness inclusive of the skin and tela subcutanea. Flap tension should be perpendicular to the chest wall with flap elevation deep to the cutaneous vasculature, which is accentuated by flap retraction.

towel clips are placed on skin margins for appropriate elevation. Flaps are retracted with constant tension on the periphery of the elevated margin at right angles to the chest wall to expose the superficial and deep layers of superficial fascia. This maneuver allows the operator access to the anatomical boundaries described previously. Flap thickness varies with patient habitus and proportional lean body mass. Ideally, flap thickness should be 7 to 8 mm, inclusive of skin and tela subcutanea. The interface for flap elevation is developed deep to the cutaneous vasculature, which is accentuated by flap traction as previously described. The surgeon must be cognizant of the necessity for flap elevation with consistent thickness to avoid creating devascularized subcutaneous tissue that contributes to wound seroma, skin necrosis, or flap retraction.

We prefer to elevate the cephalad skin flap with constant thickness to the level of the subclavius muscle. Dissection commences from lateral to medial with the optional use of the cold scalpel or electrocautery. Thereafter the pectoralis major fascia is dissected from the pectoralis musculature in a plane that is parallel with the course of the muscle bundle from the origin of ribs two to six to its insertion on the humerus (Fig. 29–61). The operator places inferior traction (perpendicular to the clavicle) on the breast and fascia; this traction is maintained constantly with elevation of the fascia from the muscle. Multiple perforator vessels from the lateral

thoracic or anterior intercostal arteries are invariably encountered in moving from lateral to medial with the dissection. These vessels represent end-arteries that supply the pectoralis major and minor and should be carefully identified, clamped, and ligated with 2-0 or 3-0 nonabsorbable suture. The breast and skin, inclusive of the elevated pectoralis fascia from the lateral humeral extension to the medial costochondral junction, is elevated en bloc to approximately the fifth or sixth rib, leaving the inferiormost portion of the breast intact. Depending on location of the lesion, if access to the central and lower aspect of the breast is not possible, the inferior flap should then be elevated as delineated previously. Preferably the lateral margin of the flap is then elevated to the anterior margin of the latissimus dorsi with exposure from inferior to superior directions (Fig. 29–62). The loose areolar tissue of the lateral axillary space is elevated with identification of the lateral most extent of the axillary vein in its course anterior and caudal to the brachial plexus and axillary artery. Dissection craniad to the axillary vein is inadvisable for fear of damage to the brachial plexus and the infrequent observation of nodal tissues cephalad to the vein. The axillary vein should be sharply exposed with cold scalpel dissection on its anterior and ventral surfaces following division of the investing deep layer of superficial fascia of the axillary space. Dissection with electrocautery may cause thermal damage to the surface of the anterior or

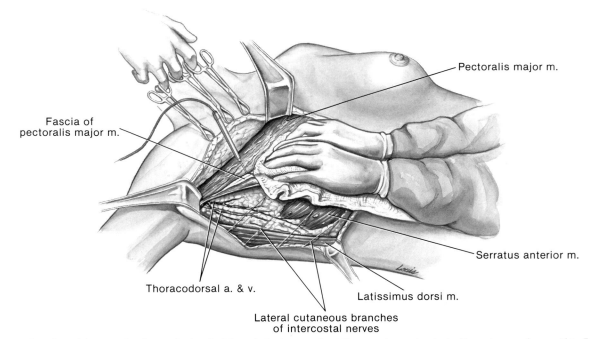

Fascia of pectoralis major m.

Pectoralis major m.

Serratus anterior m.

Thoracodorsal a. & v.

Latissimus dorsi m.

Lateral cutaneous branches of intercostal nerves

Figure 29–61. Elevation of the superior flap to the level of the subclavius muscle at the superiormost extent of breast parenchyma. Skin flap thickness is constant at 7 to 8 mm from lateral to medial. Thereafter, dissection of the pectoralis major fascia from the pectoralis musculature may be completed with cold scalpel or electrocautery. Dissection commences lateral to medial in a plane that parallels the muscle bundles of the pectoralis major muscle from origin of ribs 2–6 to insertion on the humerus. Countertraction in a caudal direction allows tension on the fascia to facilitate its removal from the pectoralis major. Perforator vessels from the lateral thoracic or anterior intercostal arteries are encountered as end-arteries that supply the pectoralis major and minor muscles. Thereafter, the inferior flap is elevated medially in similar fashion to the midline, inferiorly to the aponeurosis of the rectus abdominis tendon, and laterally to the anterior margin of the latissimus. The inferiormost portion of the breast is left intact following clearing of the superolateral margin of the pectoralis major. This maneuver ensures an en bloc resection of the axillary contents with the breast, leaving the axillary tail of Spence intact.

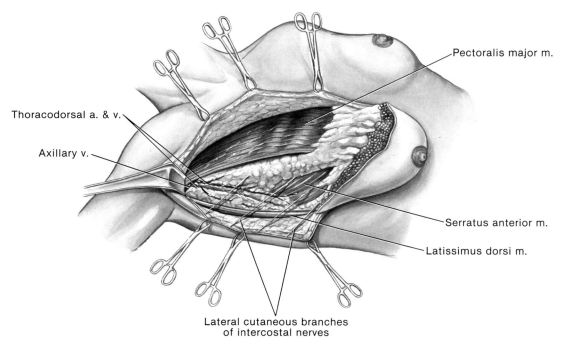

Figure 29–62. The completed superior and inferior flap with breast parenchyma intact with the axillary tail of Spence and the axillary contents. The pectoralis major is completely cleared of its fascia en bloc with the breast parenchyma. At this juncture, the pectoralis minor has not been exposed to allow access to the axilla (Level II and III nodes). The latissimus dorsi muscle has been dissected on its anterior surface to delineate the lateral boundary of dissection. Illustrated in this view is the cutaneous innervation of skin of the lateral chest, axilla, and medial arm by intercostobrachial sensory nerves. These nerves are commonly divided in the course of dissection of the axilla and lateral skin flap following identification of the latissimus dorsi.

inferior vein wall. Electrical stimulation with electrocautery of the brachial plexus or its motor branches to muscles of the arm and shoulder is an additional technical problem.

As the operator proceeds medially to complete dissection of the lateralmost margin of the pectoralis major, abduction of the shoulder and extension of the arm with finger dissection of the lateral and inferior margin of the pectoralis major allow visualization of the insertion of the pectoralis minor on the coracoid process of the scapula. The tendinous portion of the pectoralis minor is divided near its insertion on the coracoid process (Fig. 29–63, inset). The surgeon must be cognizant of the anatomical location of the lateral neurovascular bundle in which the medial pectoral nerve courses to its innervation of the pectoralis minor and major. If possible, this nerve should be preserved to abrogate the probability of atrophy of the lateral head of the pectoralis major. Should the entire nerve trunk penetrate the pectoralis minor, sacrifice may be necessary. It may also be necessary to sacrifice penetrating *branches* of the medial pectoral nerve with elevation and medial retraction of the pectoralis minor to its origin on ribs two through five. With this maneuver, the *interpectoral nodes (Rotter's nodes)* are included en bloc with the operative specimen. Furthermore, resection of the pectoralis minor allows full visualization of the extent of the axillary vein in its course beneath the pectoralis minor and its entry into the chest wall at its confluence with the subclavian vein beneath the costoclavicular (Halsted's)

ligament. With resection of the pectoralis minor muscle, exposure of Level II and III nodes is possible.

The operator should continue to work lateral to medial with complete visualization of the anterior and ventral surfaces of the axillary vein. The investing fascia of the axillary vein is dissected with elevation of the deep layer of superficial fascia and cold scalpel division following exposure, ligation, and division of all venous tributaries. With identification and retraction of the superomedial aspect of the pectoralis major, the lateral pectoral (anterior thoracic) nerve with origin from the lateral cord is exposed with the medial neurovascular bundle. This neurovascular structure should likewise be protected to ensure innervation to the medial heads of the pectoralis major (Fig 29–64). Dissection is continued medially on the anterior/ventral surface of the axillary vein to the costoclavicular ligament, which represents the condensation of the clavipectoral fascia.

Caudal to the vein, the loose areolar tissue at the juncture of the axillary vein with the anterior margin of the latissimus dorsi is swept inferomedially to include the *lateral (axillary) nodal group (Level I)*. The operator should take care to preserve the thoracodorsal artery and vein, which are deep in the axillary space and fully invested with loose areolar tissue and nodes of the lateral group. The operator should also be cognizant of the origin of the *thoracodorsal nerve* from the posterior cord, whose origin is medial to the thoracodorsal artery and vein. This nerve has a variable inferolateral course en route to its innervation of the latissimus dorsi muscle

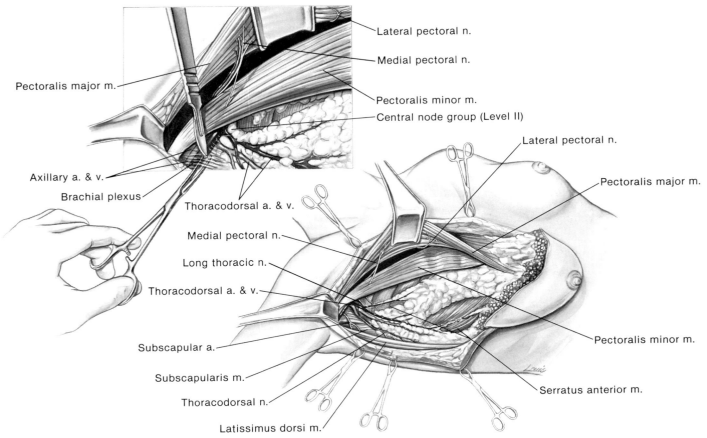

Pectoralis major m.

Lateral pectoral n.

Medial pectoral n.

Pectoralis minor m.

Central node group (Level II)

Lateral pectoral n.

Pectoralis major m.

Axillary a. & v.

Brachial plexus

Thoracodorsal a. & v.

Medial pectoral n.

Long thoracic n.

Thoracodorsal a. & v.

Pectoralis minor m.

Subscapular a.

Subscapularis m.

Thoracodorsal n.

Serratus anterior m.

Latissimus dorsi m.

Figure 29–63. *Inset,* Juncture of the latissimus (unexposed) with the ventral surface of the axillary vein. Sharp division with scalpel to incise the investing fascia of the axillary space. Following isolation of the tendinous portion of the pectoralis minor muscle with finger dissection, the insertion of this tendon on the coracoid process of the scapula can be readily identified. The surgeon must be cognizant of the anatomical location of the lateral neurovascular bundle and the laterally placed medial pectoral nerve, which takes origin from the medial cord. (See section entitled "General Principles of Mastectomy" for variance of this nerve.) Every attempt should be made to preserve the medial pectoral nerve, as sacrifice of the main trunk may allow atrophy of the lateral head of the pectoralis major. Further, the lateral pectoral nerve, which takes origin from the lateral cord and is medially placed, should also be preserved.

and must be visualized and protected throughout its course if subsequent reconstruction using myocutaneous flaps that incorporate the latissimus is planned. Thereafter the lateral axillary nodal group is retracted inferomedially and anterior to the *thoracodorsal neurovascular bundle* to be dissected en bloc with the *subscapular group of nodes (Level I)*, which are medially located between the thoracodorsal nerve and the lateral chest wall. Dissection of the posterior contents of the axillary space and division of multiple tributaries from the thoracoacromial artery and vein allow free access to exposure of the posterior boundary of the axilla. With this dissection, the heads of the teres major laterally and the subscapularis muscle medially are visualized.

The dissection commences medially with extirpation of the *central nodal groups (Level II)* and *apical (subclavicular) (Level III)* nodes. The superomedial-most aspect of the dissection at the level of the costoclavicular ligament represents the point of termination of the dissection; this nodal group should be identified with a metallic marker or suture. This practice avails the pathologist the opportunity to examine for extension of

nodal disease, which may have subsequent therapeutic and prognostic significance.

It is essential that the operator continue this dissection en bloc to avoid the separation of nodal groups and disruption of lymphatic vessels in the axilla. Inferomedial retraction of Level II and III nodes en bloc with the specimen, which is inclusive of the *external mammary group (Level I)*, is conducted in a cephalad to caudad direction in parallel with the thoracodorsal neurovascular bundle. This dissection maneuver incorporates nodal groups en bloc and avoids neural injury while providing direct access and exposure of venous tributaries posterior to the axillary vein. With medial dissection, the operator encounters the chest wall deep in the medial axillary space and is able to identify the *long thoracic nerve (respiratory nerve of Bell)* applied in the deep investing (serratus) fascia of the axillary space. This nerve is constant in its location anterior to the subscapularis muscle and is closely applied to the investing fascial compartment of the chest wall. Every effort should be made to preserve the long thoracic nerve; otherwise, permanent disability with a winged scapula and shoulder apraxia will follow denervation of the serratus anterior. This nerve is dissected throughout its course to innervation of the serratus anterior (Fig. 29–63 and Fig. 29–64). The axillary contents anterior and medial to the nerve are swept inferomedially with this specimen, and the operator should ensure that innervations of the long thoracic and thoracodorsal nerves are visualized prior to division of the inferiormost extent of the axillary contents. Incompletely divided origins of the pectoralis minor from ribs two through five are resected with electrocautery, and the remaining portions of the muscle are swept en bloc with the axillary contents to be inclusive of Rotter's interpectoral and the retropectoral groups. The dissection continues in a

caudal direction such that the entire breast and fascia are cleared medially and inferiorly from the aponeurosis of the rectus abdominis muscle (see Fig. 29–64). The specimen is immediately sent to the pathology department for examination of the fresh specimen and to procure steroid hormone receptors of the tumor if this procedure was not completed at the initial biopsy. It is essential that tissue be forwarded promptly to the laboratory for tissue preservation, as hormone receptor analyses are thermo- and ischemia-labile within the ambient temperature of the operating room environment.[12, 13]

Points of bleeding are inspected, clamped, and ligated individually with nonabsorbable 2-0 and 3-0 sutures.

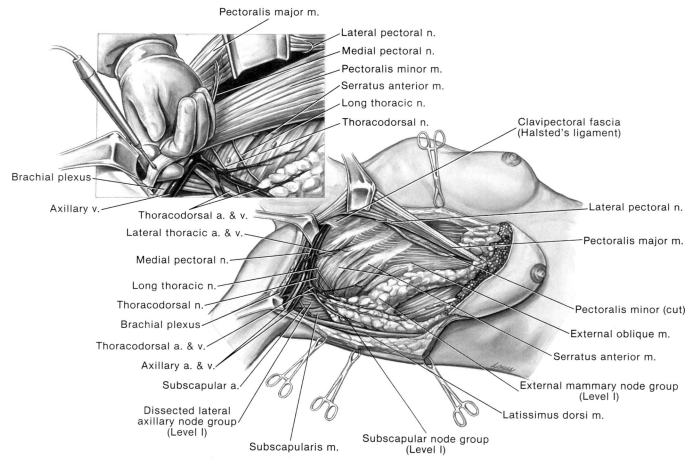

Figure 29–64. *Inset,* Digital protection of the brachial plexus for division of the insertion of the pectoralis minor muscle on the coracoid process. All loose areolar and lymphatic tissues are swept en bloc with the axillary contents to insure resection of the interpectoral (Rotter's) nodes.

Dissection commences lateral to medial with complete visualization of the anterior and ventral aspects of the axillary vein. Dissection craniad to the axillary vein is inadvisable, for fear of damage to the brachial plexus and the infrequent observation of gross nodal tissue cephalic to the vein. Investing fascial dissection of the vein is best completed with the cold scalpel following exposure, ligation, and division of all venous tributaries on the anterior and ventral surfaces. Caudal to the vein, loose areolar tissue at the junction of the vein with the anterior margin of latissimus is swept inferomedially inclusive of the lateral (axillary) nodal group (Level I). Care is taken to preserve the neurovascular thoracodorsal artery, vein, and nerve in the deep axillary space. The thoracodorsal nerve is traced to its innervation of the latissimus dorsi muscle laterally. Lateral axillary nodal groups are retracted inferomedially and anterior to this bundle for dissection en bloc with the subscapular (Level I) nodal group. Preferentially, dissection commences superomedially before completion of dissection of the external mammary (Level I) nodal group. Superomedial dissection over the axillary vein allows extirpation of the central nodal group (Level II) and apical (subclavicular) Level III group. The superomedialmost extent of the dissection is the clavipectoral fascia (Halsted's ligament). This level of dissection with the Patey technique allows the surgeon to mark, with metallic clip or suture, the superiormost extent of dissection. All loose areolar tissue just inferior to the apical nodal group is swept off the chest wall, leaving the fascia of the serratus anterior intact. With dissection parallel to the long thoracic nerve (respiratory nerve of Bell), the deep investing serratus fascia is incised. This nerve is closely applied to the investing fascial compartment of the chest wall and must be dissected in its entirety, cephalic to caudal to ensure innervation of the serratus anterior and avoidance of the "winged scapula" disability.

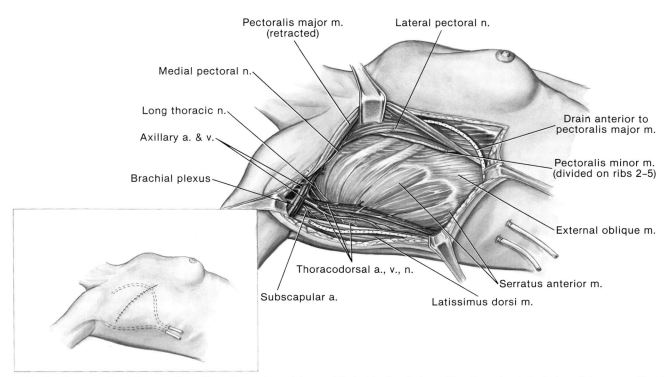

Figure 29–65. The completed Patey axillary dissection variant of the modified radical technique. The dissection is inclusive of the pectoralis minor muscle from origin to insertion on ribs 2–5. Both medial and lateral pectoral nerves are preserved to ensure innervation of the lateral and medial heads, respectively, of the pectoralis major. With completion of the procedure, remaining portions of this muscle are swept en bloc with the axillary contents to be inclusive of Rotter's interpectoral and the retropectoral groups.

Inset, Following copious irrigation with distilled water and saline, closed-suction Silastic catheters (18–20 French) are positioned via stab incisions placed in the inferior flap at the anterior axillary line. The lateral catheter is placed approximately 2 cm inferior to the axillary vein. The superior, longer catheter placed via the medial stab wound is positioned in the superomedial aspect of the defect anterior the pectoralis major muscle beneath the skin flap. The wound is closed in two layers with 2-0 absorbable synthetic sutures placed in subcutaneous planes. Undue tension on margins of the flap must be avoided; it may necessitate undermining of tissues to reduce mechanical forces. The skin is optionally closed with subcuticular 4-0 synthetic absorbable sutures or stainless steel staples.

Following completion of wound closure, both catheters are irrigated copiously with saline to ensure patency and are connected and maintained on low to moderate continuous suction provided by reservoir portable vacuum bottles. Light, bulky dressings of gauze are placed over the dissection site and taped securely in place with occlusive dressings. The surgeon may elect to place the ipsilateral arm in a sling to provide immobilization.

Prior to wound closure, the margins of the wound are carefully inspected for devascularization initiated by the trauma of flap retraction or by tissue dissection of thin, poorly-vascularized skin. Obvious sites of devascularization are debrided back from the skin margin parallel with the original skin incision such that adequate closure without tension is possible. For equivocal areas of devascularized tissue, systemic intravenous injection of 4 to 5 cc of fluoroscein will allow the operator to visualize viable skin margins with a Wood's light.

It is advisable for the surgeon and all assistants, inclusive of the scrub nurse, to reglove and optionally regown. Additionally, sterile instruments are utilized for wound closure to avoid the potential for implantation of exfoliated tumor cells in the wound. Thereafter the wound may be closed following copious irrigation with distilled water or saline, which augments evacuation of residual tissue, clots, and serum. The wound is again inspected for bleeding sites, and if none are found, closed-suction Silastic catheters (18–20 Fr) are positioned via separate stab incisions that enter the inferior flap at approximately the anterior axillary line (Fig. 29–

65). The lateral Silastic catheter is positioned in the axillary space approximately 2 cm inferior to the axillary vein on the ventral surface area of the latissimus dorsi muscle to provide drainage of the axilla. A longer, second catheter placed via the medial stab incision is positioned in the superomedial aspect of the defect (Fig. 29–65, inset) to provide continual evacuation of serum and blood that may accumulate within the large surface area of the dissected pectoralis major muscle. Both catheters are secured at skin level with a 2-0 nonabsorbable suture. We prefer not to secure the catheters to pectoral muscles or to the latissimus for fear of initiating bleeding at the time of catheter removal.

The flap margins are again inspected to evaluate sites of devascularization or "buttonhole" defects that result from tangential incisions or the trauma of dissection with flap elevation. The wound is closed in two layers with 2-0 absorbable synthetic sutures placed in the subcutaneous tissues. Undue tension on margins of the flap may necessitate extensive undermining of these tissues to reduce mechanical forces and maximize adherence to the underlying pectoralis major. The skin is optionally closed with subcuticular 4-0 synthetic absorbable sutures or stainless steel staples. Wounds closed with subcuticular sutures should have Steri-strips applied perpendicular to the incision to enhance wound repair. Thereafter both catheters are irrigated copiously with saline to ensure patency and are then connected and maintained on continuous low-to-moderate suction by large reservoir portable vacuum bottles. Light bulky dressings of cotton are applied to the dissection site and are taped securely in place. Optionally, the surgeon may immobilize the ipsilateral arm in an arm sling.

The dressings should remain intact on the operative wound until the third or fourth postoperative day, unless the surgeon is concerned about the viability of the dissected flap. Wound catheters should remain in the site of dissection until the drainage becomes predominantly serous and diminishes to 20 to 25 ml during a 24-hour interval. Most surgeons initiate shoulder and arm exercises on the day following removal of the drainage catheters.

We follow the same recommendations previously given for the Halsted radical mastectomy for patients with protracted serosanguinous or serous drainage. This is evident in approximately 20 percent of operative wounds and may be managed by continued suction using the lateralmost (dependent) Silastic drain. However, long-term catheter preservation requires the patient to be cognizant of hygienic care of the catheters and of the sites of skin entry and necessitates frequent changes of dressings. It is our practice to limit the range of motion of the arm and shoulder for patients with protracted drainage, as shoulder immobilization augments flap adherence to the chest wall. The surgeon must periodically inspect wound discharge from the catheters to evaluate the potential for retrograde bacterial infection of the axillary space, particularly when drainage catheters remain in place longer than seven days.

References

1. Auchincloss H: Significance of location and number of axillary metastases in carcinoma of the breast. Ann Surg 158:37–46, 1963.
2. Baker RR, Montague ACW, Childs JN: A comparison of modified radical mastectomy to radical mastectomy in the treatment of operable breast cancer. Ann Surg 189(5):553–557, 1979.
3. Banks WM: On free removal of mammary cancer with extirpation of the axillary glands as a necessary accompaniment. Br Med J 2:1138, 1882.
4. Berstock DA, Houghton B, Haybittle J, Baum M: The role of radiotherapy following total mastectomy for patients with early breast cancer. World J Surg 9:667–670, 1985.
5. Crile GC Jr: Results of simple mastectomy without irradiation in the treatment of operative stage I cancer of the breast. Ann Surg 168:330–336, 1968.
6. Crile GC Jr: Results of conservative treatment of breast cancer at ten and 15 years. Ann Surg 181:26–30, 1975.
7. Crile GC Jr: Results of simplified treatment of breast cancer. Surg Gynecol Obstet 517–523, 1964.
8. Dahl-Iversen E, Tobiassen T: Radical mastectomy with peristernal and supraclavicular dissection for mammary carcinoma. Am Surg 157:170–173, 1963.
9. DeLarue NC, Anderson WD, Starr J: Modified radical mastectomy in the individualized treatment of breast carcinoma. Surg Gynecol Obstet 129:79–88, 1969.
10. Den Besten L, Ziffren SE: Simple and radical mastectomy: a comparison of survival. Arch Surg 90:755–759, 1965.
11. Devitt JE: The influence of conservative and radical surgery on the survival of patients with breast cancer. Can Med Assoc J 87:906–910, 1962.
12. Ellis LM, Wittliff JL, Bryant MS, Sitren HS, Hogancamp WE, Souba WW, Bland KI: Effects of ischemia on breast tumor steroid hormone-receptor levels. Curr Surg 45(4):312–314, 1988.
13. Ellis LM, Wittliff JL, Bryant MS, Sitren HS, Hogancamp WE, Souba WW, Bland KI: Lability of steroid hormone receptors following devascularization of breast tumors. Arch Surg 124:39–42, 1989.
14. Elston CW, Gresham GA, Rao GS, Zebro T, Haybittle JL, Houghton J, Kerney G: The Cancer Research Campaign (King's/Cambridge) Trial for early breast cancer: clinical pathological aspects. Br J Cancer 45:655, 1982.
15. Fisher B, Fisher ER: Experimental evidence in support of the dormant tumor cell. Science 130:918–919, 1959.
16. Fisher B, Fisher ER: Transmigration of lymph nodes by tumor cells. Science 152:1397–1398, 1966.
17. Fisher B, Redmond C, Fisher ER, Bauer M, Wolmark N, Wickerham L, Deutsch M, Montague E, Margolese R, Foster R: Ten-year results of a randomized clinical trial comparing radical mastectomy and total mastectomy with or without radiation. N Engl J Med 312(11):674–681, 1985.
18. Fisher ER, Fisher B: Host influence on tumor growth and dissemination. In Schwartz E (ed): The Biological Basis of Radiation Therapy. Philadelphia, JB Lippincott, 1966, pp 484–517.
19. Fisher B, Fisher ER: The interrelationship of hematogenous and lymphatic tumor cell dissemination. Surg Gynecol Obstet 122:791–798, 1966.
20. Fisher B, Redmond C, Fisher ER, et al: The contribution of recent NSABP clinical trials of primary breast cancer therapy to an understanding of tumor biology—an overview of findings. Cancer 46:1009–1025, 1980.
21. Fisher B, Redmond C, Poisson R, Margolese R, Wolmark N, Wickerham L, Fisher E, Deutsch M, Caplan R, Pilch Y, Glass A, Shibata H, Lerner H, Terz J, Sidorovich L: Eight-year results of a randomized clinical trial comparing total mastectomy and lumpectomy with or without irradiation in the treatment of breast cancer. N Engl J Med 320(13):822–828, 1989.
22. Fisher B, Saffer EA, Fisher ER: Studies concerning the regional lymph node in cancer. VII. Thymidine uptake by cells from nodes of breast cancer patients relative to axillary location and histopathologic discriminants. Cancer 33:271–279, 1974.
23. Forrest APM, Roberts MM, Preece P, Henk JM, Campbell H, Hughes LE, Desai S, Hulbert M: The Cardiff-St. Mary's trial. Br J Surg 61:766–769, 1974.
24. Forrest APM, Stewart HJ, Roberts MM, Steele RJC: Simple mastectomy and axillary node sampling (pectoral node biopsy) in the management of primary breast cancer. Ann Surg 196(3):371–378, 1982.
25. Grace E: Simple mastectomy in cancer of the breast. Am J Surg 35:512, 1937.
26. Gross SW: A Practical Treatment of Tumors of the Mammary Gland Embracing Their Histology, Pathology, Diagnosis and Treatment. New York, D Appleton & Co, 1880, pp 222–227.
27. Halsted WS: The results of operations for the cure of cancer of the breast performed at the Johns Hopkins Hospital from June 1889 to January 1894. Arch Surg 20:497–544, 1894.
28. Hamilton T, Langlands AO, Prescott RJ: The treatment of operable cancer of the breast: a clinical trial in the South-East region of Scotland. Br J Surg 61:758–761, 1974.
29. Handley RS: The conservative radical mastectomy of Patey: 10-year results in 425 patients' breasts. Dis Breast 2:16, 1976.
30. Handley RS, Thackray AC: Conservative radical mastectomy (Patey's operation). Ann Surg 170(6):880–882, 1969.
31. Helman P, Bennett MB, Louw JH, Wilkie W, Madden P, Silber W, Sealy R, Heselson J: Interim report on trial of treatment for operable breast cancer. South Afr Med J 46:1374–1375, 1972.
32. Henderson IC, Mourisden H, et al: Effects of adjuvant tamoxifen and of cytotoxic therapy on mortality in early breast cancer: an

overview of 61 randomized trials among 28,896 women. N Engl J Med 319(26):1681–1692, 1988.

33. Hermann RE, Steiger E: Modified radical mastectomy. Surg Clin North Am 58(4):743–754, 1978.

34. Hermann RE, Esselstyn CB Jr, Crile G Jr, Cooperman AM, Antunez AR, Hoerr SO: Results of conservative operations for breast cancer. Arch Surg 120:746–751, 1985.

35. Hoffman GW, Elliott LF: The anatomy of the pectoral nerves and its significance to the general and plastic surgeon.

36. Küster E: Zur behandlung des brustkrebses verhandlungen der deutschen gesellschaft für Chirurgie. Leipsiz 12:288, 1883.

37. Kyle J, et al: Management of early cancer of the breast: report on an international multicentre trial supported by the Cancer Research Campaign. Br Med J 1:1035–1038, 1976.

38. Langlands AO, Prescott RJ, Hamilton T: A clinical trial in the management of operable cancer of the breast. Br J Surg 67:170–174, 1980.

39. Leis HP Jr: Modified radical mastectomy: definition and role in breast cancer surgery. Int Surg 65(3):211–217, 1980.

40. Lythgoe JP, Leck I, Swindell R: Manchester regional breast study: preliminary results. Lancet 1:744–747, 1978.

41. Lythgoe JP, Palmer MK: Manchester regional breast study—5 and 10 year results. Br J Surg 69:693–696, 1982.

42. Madden JL: Modified radical mastectomy. Surg Gynecol Obstet 121(6):1221–1230, 1965.

43. Madden JL, Kandalaft S, Bourque RA: Modified radical mastectomy. Ann Surg 175(5):624–634, 1972.

44. Maddox WA, Carpenter JT Jr, Laws HL, Soong SJ, Cloud G, Urist MM, Balch CM: A randomized prospective trial of radical (Halsted) mastectomy versus modified radical mastectomy in 311 breast cancer patients. Ann Surg 198(2):207–212, 1983.

45. Maddox WA, Carpenter JT Jr, Laws HT, Soong S-J, Cloud G, Balch CM, Urist MM: Does radical mastectomy still have a place in the treatment of primary operable breast cancer? Arch Surg 122:1317–1320, 1987.

46. McWhirter R: The value of simple mastectomy and radiotherapy in the treatment of cancer of the breast. Br J Radiol 21:599–610, 1948.

47. Meyer AC, Smith SS, Potter M: Carcinoma of the breast. A clinical study. Arch Surg 113:364–367, 1978.

48. Meyer W: An improved method for the radical operation for carcinoma of the breast. Med Rec NY 46:746–749, 1894.

49. Moore CH: On the influence of inadequate operations on the theory of cancer. Roy Med Chir Soc London 1:244–280, 1867.

50. Murphy JB: Carcinoma of breast. Surg Clin JB Murphy I(6): 779, 1912.

51. Nemoto T, Vana J, Bedwani RN, Baker HW, McGregor FH, Murphy GP: Management and survival of female breast cancer: results of a national survey by the American College of Surgeons. Cancer 45(12):2917–2924, 1980.

52. Nemoto T, Dao TL: Is modified mastectomy adequate for axillary lymph node dissection? Ann Surg 182:722–723, 1975.

53. Patey DH, Dyson WH: The prognosis of carcinoma of the breast in relation to the type of operation performed. Br J Cancer 2:7–13, 1948.

54. Patey DH: A review of 146 cases of carcinoma of the breast operated on between 1930 and 1943. Br J Cancer 21:260–269, 1967.

55. Robinson GN, Van Heerden JA, Payne WS, Taylor W, Gaffey TA: The primary surgical treatment of carcinoma of the breast: a changing trend toward modified radical mastectomy. Mayo Clin Proc 51:433–442, 1976.

56. Shimkin MB, Koppel M, Connelly RR, Cutler SJ: Simple and radical mastectomy for breast cancer: a re-analysis of Smith and Meyer's report from Rockford, Illinois. J Natl Cancer Inst 27:1197–1215, 1961.

57. Smith SS, Meyer AC: Cancer of the breast in Rockford, Illinois. Am J Surg 98:653–656, 1959.

58. Sprengel O: Mittheilungen über die in den Jahren 1874 bis 1878 aur der *Volkmann'schen Klinik operativ behandelten 131 Falle von Brust-carcinom. Archir F Klin Chir 27:805, 1882.

59. Turnbull AR, Chant ADB, Buchanan RB, Turner DTL, Shepherd JM, Fraser JD: Treatment of early breast cancer. Lancet 2:7–9, 1978.

60. Turner L, Swindell R, Bell WGT, Hartley RC, Tasker JH, Wilson WW, Alderson MR, Leck IM: Radical vs modified radical mastectomy for breast cancer. Ann R Coll Surg Engl 63:239–243, 1981.

61. Vana J, Bedwani R, Nemoto T, Murphy GP: American College of Surgeons Commission on Cancer Final Report on Long-Term Patient Care Evaluation Study for Carcinoma of the Female Breast. Chicago, American College of Surgeons, 1979.

62. Veronesi U, Valagussa P: Inefficacy of internal mammary nodes dissection in breast cancer surgery. Cancer 47:170–175, 1981.

63. Volkmann R: Geschwülste der mamma (36 Fälle) Beitrage zur Chirurgie. Leipzig, 1895, pp 310–334.

64. Williams IG, Murley RS, Curwen MP: Carcinoma of the female breast: conservative and radical surgery. Br Med J 2:787–796, 1953.

65. Wilson RE, Donegan WL, Mettlin C, Smart CR, Murphy GP: The 1982 National Survey of Carcinoma of the Breast in the United States by the American College of Surgeons. Surg Gynecol Obstet 159:309–318, 1984.

EXTENDED RADICAL MASTECTOMY

Jerome A. Urban, M.D., D.Sci. (Hon) and Scott A. Hundahl, M.D.

RATIONALE FOR THE EXTENDED RADICAL MASTECTOMY

The internal mammary lymphatics constitute an important route of spread for breast cancers, particularly those located centrally or medially. Hidden beneath the medial chest wall, internal mammary nodes elude palpation and, unless specifically subjected to a biopsy, histological examination. Despite the independent prognostic significance of internal mammary metastases[17] (particularly if such metastases are not adequately treated[2]), staging systems have, until recently,[8] disregarded such involvement. The possibility that even carefully controlled, prospective, randomized trials of therapy have been confounded by failure to stratify for internal mammary metastases should not be dismissed.

Before succumbing to the popular neglect of the internal mammary lymphatics, the following conditions should be considered:

I. No internal mammary metastases
   A. No systemic dissemination
   B. Systemic dissemination

II. Internal mammary metastases
   A. No systemic dissemination
   B. Systemic dissemination

Patients in category I, who have no internal mammary metastases, will not benefit from internal mammary treatment, although prognostic information can be gleaned from internal mammary node biopsy samples. Similarly, patients in category IIB, who have involved internal mammary nodes and systemic dissemination, will not benefit from internal mammary treatment but may benefit from histological confirmation of nodal metastases if this alters adjuvant therapy decisions. It is the patients in subgroup IIA, who have internal mammary metastases but no systemic dissemination who will benefit from internal mammary treatment—ideally, en bloc resection of the internal mammary lymphatics through a properly performed extended radical mastectomy. What proportion of breast cancer patients fit into this subgroup? Is it a significant proportion? Are there selection criteria by which this subgroup may be identified? Is measurable survival benefit associated with internal mammary nodal treatment?

We believe that the subgroup of breast cancer patients at high risk for internal mammary metastases are identifiable and that they indeed do benefit from surgical removal of the internal mammary lymphatics by a properly performed extended radical mastectomy. This view has now been confirmed by both large retrospective studies and prospective randomized trials.

RISK FACTORS FOR INTERNAL MAMMARY METASTASES

Which patients harbor internal mammary metastases? In an effort to answer this question, R. S. Handley,[4] continuing the pioneering work of his father,[6] took biopsy specimens from the internal mammary nodes of 1000 patients with primary breast cancer. Handley reported his results according to location of the primary tumor and axillary nodal status. He found that patients with central or medial tumors, as well as patients with involved axillary nodes, exhibited internal mammary nodal metastases more frequently. Handley's data are presented in Table 29–25.

Handley's technique of sampling the internal mammary nodes through intercostal space incisions precluded a complete analysis of the internal mammary nodes, suggesting the possibility that internal mammary metastases were underestimated. In 1984, Li and Shen reported a large series of consecutive, unselected cases of primary breast cancer treated by extended radical mastectomy.[12] In this series, because all internal mammary lymph nodes were removed and available for histological analysis, sampling error was eliminated. Li and Shen's findings, shown in Table 29–26, are similar to Handley's; both centromedial location of the primary tumor and axillary metastases were associated with internal mammary metastases.

Other possible risk factors for internal mammary involvement, gleaned from a retrospective review of

Table 29–25. RESULTS OF 1000 INTERNAL MAMMARY NODE BIOPSIES

Axillary Nodal Status	Location of Breast Cancer	
	Outer (% positive)	Central or Medial (% positive)
Negative (N = 465)	4	10
Positive (N = 535)	21	48
Total (N = 1000)	14	30

From Handley RS: Ann R Coll Surg Engl 57:59–66, 1975. Reprinted by permission.

1119 patients treated by extended radical mastectomy at the National Cancer Institute of Milan, are size of the primary tumor (diameter $\leq$ 2 cm, 16 percent; diameter > 2 cm, 24 percent; p = 0.007) and age of the patient (age $\leq$ 40 years, 27.6 percent; age 41 to 50 years, 19.7 percent; age > 50 years, 15.6 percent; p = 0.01). Although this study confirmed axillary metastases as a risk factor (negative axillary nodes, 9.1 percent; positive axillary nodes, 29.1 percent; $p < 10^{-6}$), location of the primary tumor was not shown to be a statistically significant risk factor (p = 0.07).[17] This finding differs from the findings of virtually all other studies of internal mammary metastases.

PROGNOSIS OF TREATED AND UNTREATED PATIENTS WITH INTERNAL MAMMARY METASTASES

Donegan[2] has reported a series of 113 patients treated by radical mastectomy who underwent simultaneous internal mammary node biopsy. Twenty-five patients (22 percent) had histologically documented internal mammary metastases, and of these, 20 received no further treatment and five received adjuvant chest wall (but not internal mammary) irradiation. Only one of these 25

Table 29–26. INTERNAL MAMMARY METASTASES IN 1242 CONSECUTIVE UNSELECTED CASES TREATED BY EXTENDED RADICAL MASTECTOMY

Axillary Nodal Status	Location of Breast Cancer	
	Outer (% positive)	Central or Medial (% positive)
Negative (N = 607)	2	9
Positive (N = 635)	25	35
Total (N = 1242)	14	22

From Li KY, Shen ZZ: Breast 10:10–19, 1984. Reprinted by permission.

Table 29–27. REPORTED 10-YEAR SURVIVAL RATES ACCORDING TO STATUS OF AXILLARY AND INTERNAL MAMMARY NODES

Reference	Surgical Treatment	Adjuvant Radiotherapy	Adjuvant Chemotherapy	Nodal Status (%)			
				Ax − *IM −*	*Ax +* *IM −*	*Ax −* *IM +*	*Ax +* *IM +*
Donegan[2] (113 cases)	RM	5/113	—	40	21	0	6
Handley[5] (425 cases)	MRM	Yes	—	69	44	40	20
Veronesi and Valagussa[18] (342 cases)	ERM	—	—	79.5	Not Given	45.8	20
Urban[16] (815 cases)	ERM	Yes	—	82	63	56	38
Li & Shen[12] (1242 cases)	ERM	—	—	84.5	44	61	27
Deemarski and Seleznev[1] (325 cases)	ERM	—	Yes	77.4	57	46	39

Abbreviations: Ax = Axillary nodes; ERM = extended radical mastectomy; IM = internal mammary nodes; MRM = modified radical mastectomy; RM = radical mastectomy; + = positive; − = negative.

patients with untreated internal mammary metastases survived 10 years (4 percent 10-year survival), and even this patient subsequently died of disseminated cancer.[2]

In Table 29–27, Donegan's results with untreated internal mammary metastases are compared to results obtained when such metastases are treated by internal mammary radiotherapy[5] or by extended radical mastectomy.[1, 12, 16, 18] When only internal mammary metastases are present, 10-year survival rates for treated patients range from 40 percent to 61 percent. When both axillary and internal mammary metastases are present, 10-year survivals of 20 percent to 38 percent are obtained.

This investigator[2] confirmed internal mammary metastases to be most frequent in the presence of axillary nodal spread, medial primaries, and clinically advanced lesions. Axillary metastases were evident in 58 percent of the patients and were accompanied by internal mammary nodal involvement in 34 percent. Only 6 percent of patients without axillary disease had metastases confirmed by internal mammary node biopsies. The majority of patients (88 percent) with internal mammary nodal disease also had axillary metastases.

INTERNAL MAMMARY IRRADIATION VERSUS EXTENDED RADICAL MASTECTOMY

Comparison of Handley's results with those of investigators treating internal mammary metastases by extended radical mastectomy (see Table 29–27) suggests that surgical resection of the internal mammary nodes may be superior to internal mammary irradiation.

Ten-year survival of patients with both axillary and internal mammary metastases may be further improved if adjuvant treatment follows extended radical mastectomy. Urban and Egli's 38 percent 10-year survival rate for this subgroup, obtained when adjuvant base of neck

and supraclavicular irradiation* was utilized,[16] is similar to the 39 percent 10-year survival reported by Deemarski and Seleznev when adjuvant chemotherapy was employed.[1] Combined adjuvant irradiation and adjuvant chemotherapy for patients with internal mammary metastases treated by extended radical mastectomy awaits investigation.

Ignoring, for the moment, the possible survival advantage associated with extended radical mastectomy, an additional argument against internal mammary irradiation relates to the increased incidence of myocardial infarction among patients receiving internal mammary irradiation. In a trial of postoperative radiotherapy conducted at the Norwegian Radium Hospital in Oslo, there was a significant increase in deaths from myocardial infarction in the group treated with cobalt 60 for internal mammary irradiation.[7] Although the technique used for internal mammary irradiation in this study may be criticized, this study demonstrates the distinct possibility that internal mammary irradiation carries a treatment-related cardiac mortality that may partially offset the advantages of irradiating internal mammary metastases.

COMPARISON OF EXTENDED RADICAL MASTECTOMY WITH RADICAL MASTECTOMY IN HIGH-RISK PATIENTS

Risk factors for internal mammary metastases that are identifiable preoperatively include central or medial location of the breast tumor,[4, 9, 12, 16] size > 2 cm,[17] presence of axillary lymph node metastases,[4, 9, 12, 16, 17] and age ≤ 40 years.[17] While it is not possible to stratify the data from available studies according to all these

---

*Within this series, however, no statistically significant survival advantage for adjuvant radiotherapy was demonstrable.

Table 29–28. RESULTS OF NONRANDOMIZED STUDIES OF EXTENDED RADICAL MASTECTOMY VS. RADICAL MASTECTOMY IN PATIENTS WITH CENTRAL OR MEDIAL TUMORS

Reference	Tumor Size or Stage	No. of Patients with Central or Medial Tumor	Adjuvant Treatment		Axillary Node Status	Follow-up Interval (yrs)	Percent Survival		p value*
			Radio-therapy	Chemo-therapy			ERM	RM	
Li and Shen[12]	Stage I	161	No	No	−	10	83.1	79.8	NS
						20	78.6	79.8	NS
	Stage II	354	No	No	±	10	66	51.8	<0.02
						20	63	46	<0.01
	Stage III	429	No	No	±	10	45	27	<0.001
						20	42	24	<0.001
Deemarski and Seleznev[1]	T1	119	For RM pts. only	Yes	±	10	72	62	NS
	T1 + T2 combined	311	For RM pts. only	Yes	−	10	77	60	0.001
		233	For RM pts. only	Yes	+	10	58	29	<0.001

*P values, not included in the original reports, were calculated by the chi-squared test.
Abbreviations: ERM = Extended radical mastectomy; NS = not significant; RM = radical mastectomy; + positive; − = negative.

risk factors, detailed analysis of the patients with central or medial tumors is possible.

Ten-year and 20-year data from nonrandomized, large series comparing the survival of patients treated by extended radical mastectomy with that of concurrently treated patients who underwent radical mastectomy are available.[1, 12] Because extended radical mastectomy is likely to benefit only those patients with internal mammary metastases but no systemic dissemination, no study, except the extremely large series by Li and Shen,[12] has documented a statistically significant improvement in the overall survival of unselected patients undergoing extended radical mastectomy versus radical mastectomy. When analysis is restricted to the subgroup of patients with central or medial tumors greater than 2 cm in size, however, significant differences are apparent (Table 29–28). Data from Deemarski and Seleznev[1] as well as from the trials summarized in Table 29–29, suggest that such differences are even more pronounced in the subgroup of patients who also have axillary metastases.

In the prospective randomized trials listed in Table 29–29, a similar analysis of the subgroup of patients with central or medial tumors confirms significant differences in survival following extended radical mastectomy versus radical mastectomy. If a subgroup of patients with all of the identified risk factors for internal mammary metastases could be compared, the results could be even more striking.

RECOMMENDATIONS

Patients who are at risk for internal mammary metastases (i.e., those with central or medial tumors greater than 2 cm in diameter or with axillary metastases) are candidates for resection of the internal mammary lymphatics by extended radical mastectomy.[15] Adjuvant treatment may further enhance the survival benefit of extended radical mastectomy in patients with internal mammary metastases.

For patients who are not at high risk for internal mammary metastases, radical mastectomy or modified

Table 29–29. RESULTS OF PROSPECTIVE, RANDOMIZED TRIALS OF EXTENDED RADICAL MASTECTOMY VS. RADICAL MASTECTOMY IN PATIENTS WITH CENTRAL OR MEDIAL TUMORS

Trial	Tumor Size	No. of Patients with Central or Medial Tumor	Adjuvant Treatment		Axillary Node Status	Follow-up Interval (yrs)	Percent Survival		p Value
			Radio-therapy	Chemo-therapy			ERM	RM	
Chicago Trial[3, 13]	T1–T2	70	No	Yes	±	10	85.7	59.7	0.028
International Cooperative Trial[9, 13]	T1–T2	192	No	No	+	5	71	52	0.01
						10	Subgroup not analyzed		
Milan[18]*	T1–T3a	286	No	No	±	10	62	56	NS
Inst. Gustave Roussy[10]*	T1–T2	70	No	No	+	15	53	28	0.05

*Data from centers participating in International Cooperative Trial.
Abbreviations: ERM = Extended radical mastectomy; NS = not significant; RM = radical mastectomy; + = positive; − = negative.

radical mastectomy or wide excision with axillary dissection and radical radiotherapy are reasonable treatments, depending on the clinicopathological setting. Extrapleural biopsy of the internal mammary lymph nodes in the second intercostal space should be performed, however. If these biopsy results are positive, treatment should be altered accordingly (i.e., extended radical mastectomy or at least internal mammary radiotherapy).

The choice of the most appropriate treatment for the patient with breast cancer should not be made according to a dogmatic algorithm, but instead should be individualized. Factors such as poor medical condition must also be considered. The preceding recommendations are intended to aid rather than replace careful clinical judgment.

OPERATIVE PROCEDURE

Histological confirmation of malignancy is mandatory prior to any surgical therapy. If immediate treatment is undertaken, gloves, instruments, and drapes should be changed following the biopsy.

A wide skin incision should be made extending at least 4 cm from the nearest palpable margin of the tumor and encompassing the areola. A transverse incision extending from just below the axillary hairline to the parasternal area is cosmetically more acceptable but less convenient than the more vertical incision indicated in Figure 29–66. Skin flaps are developed outside the superficial fascia, which separates the subcutaneous fat from the underlying breast parenchyma. This fascia is transected at the base of the flap, and the incision is beveled off to the underlying muscle fascia (Fig. 29–

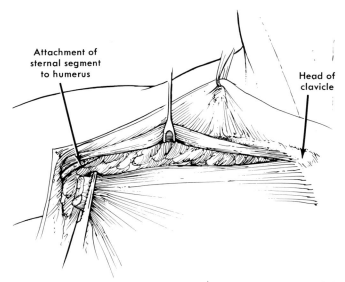

Figure 29–67. Separation of the clavicular and sternal heads of the pectoralis major muscle.

66). Flaps are developed to the clavicle above, to the sternum medially, to the anterior margin of the latissimus laterally, and inferiorly to the sixth rib.

The fascia overlying the clavicular head of the pectoralis major muscle is dissected from this muscle downward to the plane that separates the sternal and clavicular heads. The pectoralis major muscle is separated in this plane (Fig. 29–67). Tissues overlying the first rib and the arch of the manubrium are dissected down to the bony structures and reflected inferiorly, exposing the lower margin of the first rib and the arch of the manubrium.

Inferiorly, the rectus sheath is cleared to the level of the sixth rib, where it is incised, or to the level of the fifth rib and reflected superiorly, exposing the lower portion of the fourth or fifth interspace (Fig. 29–68). The pectoralis muscle is freed from the underlying chest wall by inserting a finger beneath this muscle just lateral to the second costochondral junction and elevating the muscle from the level of the first interspace above to the fifth interspace below. Inferiorly, the pectoralis major muscle is transected at its attachment to the costochondral junction of the fifth rib, and the tunnel beneath the muscle is completed (Fig. 29–69).

The chest is entered through the first interspace just outside the costochondral junctions of the first and second ribs. The internal mammary artery, lying just beneath the first rib, can now be palpated from within the chest. The artery usually extends upward and laterally, whereas the vein extends upward and medially at this level. The base of the neck can be explored by palpation from within the chest, and the deeper mediastinal structures can also be examined before committing to resection of the internal mammary area. If no gross evidence of metastatic disease is noted in these areas, the procedure is continued.

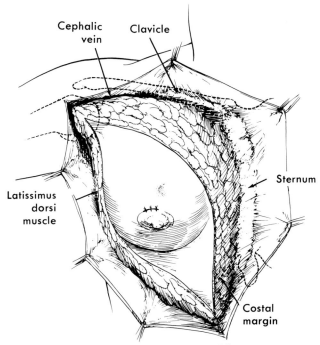

Figure 29–66. Development of flaps.

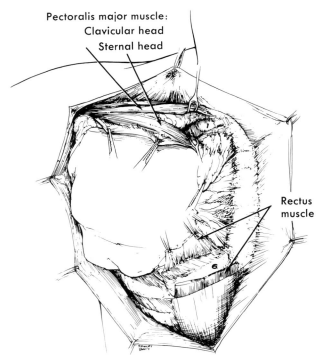

Figure 29–68. The first and fifth interspaces are exposed (label identifies the sixth rib).

The intercostal muscles of the first interspace are cut from the lower margin of the first rib and the arch of the manubrium, exposing the areolar tissue (between the parietal pleura and the intercostal muscle) that contains the internal mammary vessels and nodes. This is reflected downward toward the operative specimen, the internal mammary vessels are doubly tied and cut, and the parietal pleura is transected just below the lower margin of the first rib.

In a similar fashion, dissection is carried through the lowermost portion of the fourth or fifth interspace, depending on the location of the primary tumor in the breast. With an upper inner quadrant lesion, dissection is usually carried down to the fourth interspace. If disease is found in the lower portion of the breast, dissection is usually carried down to the upper margin of the sixth rib to include this drainage area more thoroughly. Inferiorly, the internal mammary vessels lie between the intercostal muscles anteriorly and the anterior transverse thoracic muscle posteriorly. Dissection is carried through the entire thickness of the chest wall, and the vessels are isolated, tied off, and cut just above the lower rib.

The sternum is split vertically just inside its ipsilateral margin, developing a trap door in the chest wall (Fig. 29–70). This portion of the chest wall, which contains the internal mammary vessels and lymph nodes, is then resected from the chest wall by cutting through the ribs and soft parts at the level of the costochondral junctions of the second and third ribs with scissors. The chest wall area containing the internal mammary lymph node complex is now reflected laterally, still in continuity with the overlying breast and pectoralis major muscle (Fig. 29–71). The intercostal bleeders are tied off with 3-0 silk

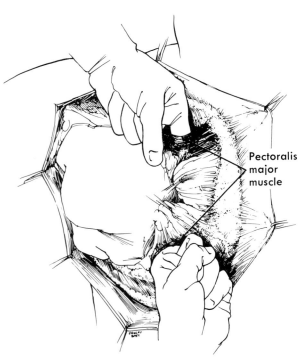

Figure 29–69. A tunnel is developed beneath the pectoralis major muscle.

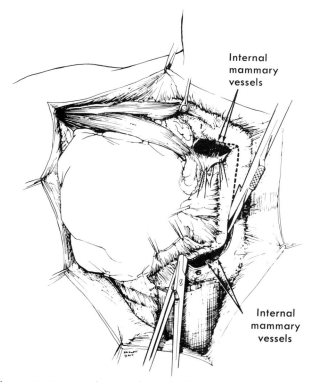

Figure 29–70. Near the sternal margin, the sternum is split vertically with a Lebsche sternal knife.

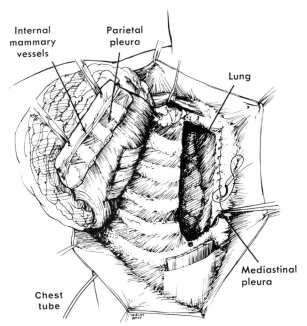

Figure 29–71. A "trap door" excision of the parasternal chest wall, pleura, and internal mammary lymphatics is performed. The mediastinal pleura is sewn to the sternal periosteum. A chest tube is inserted.

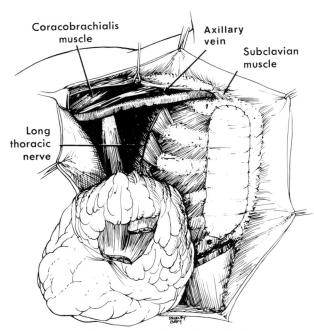

Figure 29–73. The breast, pectoral muscles, and axillary contents are excised as indicated.

sutures, and bone wax is used to control oozing from the sternal marrow cavity.

The pectoralis major and minor muscles are then reflected from the chest wall laterally. A no. 28 French chest tube, connected to water seal drainage, is inserted into the chest cavity through a separate inferolateral skin incision in the midaxillary line and secured with a stout dermal suture (Fig. 29–71).

Reconstruction of the chest wall defect is then begun by suturing the free margin of the mediastinal pleura to the fascia overlying the sternum with a running suture of fine catgut. The cut rib margins are then approximated to the sternal margin with four separate, parallel, heavy, stay sutures of no. 2 nylon (Fig. 29–72). These are applied through the anterior margin of the sternum

first, carried across the space through the rib, over the rib, back through the rib, and back through the anterior margin of the sternum. The sutures are all put in place and then snubbed up tightly to minimize the chest wall defect and also to stabilize the chest wall. The defect in the chest wall is usually diminished by approximately one third by this maneuver, and the tense sutures serve as a stabilizing support (Fig. 29–72). Finally, sterile ox fascia, autologous fascia lata, or synthetic Gore-Tex is applied over the stabilized chest wall and anchored under tension to the margins of the defect with inter-

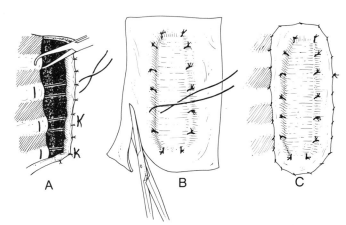

Figure 29–72. Reconstruction of the chest wall defect.

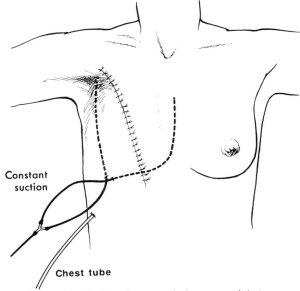

Figure 29–74. Skin closure and placement of drains.

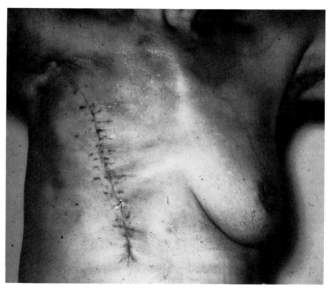

Figure 29–75. Typical result following healing.

rupted double 0 nylon. Excess fascia is trimmed off, and the margins are approximated to the underlying chest wall with a running atraumatic 00 chronic catgut suture. This type of closure results in a flexible support of the chest wall that greatly prevents paradoxical motion.

Radical mastectomy is then completed in the usual fashion (Fig. 29–73). Two Reliavac catheters are placed through the lower skin flap, and the skin margins are closed. The chest tube is attached to a Pleurovac underwater drainage system, and the Reliavac drains are connected to a suitable container (Figs. 29–74 and 29–75).

POSTOPERATIVE CARE AND COMPLICATIONS

Patients undergoing the extended radical mastectomy are usually hospitalized for 8 days. The chest tube (usually left in place for 2 days) and the Reliavac catheters (usually left in place for 5 to 7 days) are not removed until total drainage is less than 150 cc and 50 cc, respectively, for a 24-hour period.

One of the authors (JAU) has performed 1000 extended radical procedures with only three postoperative deaths within 1 month of surgery. One death occurred from a coronary infarction, another from a cerebrovascular accident, and a third from an uncontrolled perforated peptic ulcer. This minimal mortality is only possible through careful postoperative care of the patients, with particular attention to pulmonary ventilation and pleural drainage. The incidence of nonpulmonary postoperative complications is similar to that seen following radical mastectomy.

References

1. Deemarski LY, Seleznev IK: Extended radical operations on breast cancer of medial or central location. Surgery 96:73–77, 1984.
2. Donegan WL: The influence of untreated internal mammary metastases upon the course of mammary cancer. Cancer 39:533–538, 1977.
3. Ferguson DJ: Personal communication concerning 10-year results of Chicago Trial (manuscript in preparation).
4. Handley RS: Carcinoma of the breast. Ann Coll Surg Engl 57:59–66, 1975.
5. Handley RS: The conservative radical mastectomy of Patey: 10-year results in 425 patients. Breast 2(3):16–19, 1976.
6. Handley WS: Parasternal invasion of the thorax in breast cancer and its suppression by the use of radium tubes as an operative precaution. Surg Gynecol Obstet 45:721–782, 1927.
7. Host H, Brennhoud IO, Loeb M: Post-operative radiotherapy in the treatment of breast cancer—long-term results from the Oslo study. Int J Radiol Oncol Biol Phys 12:727–732, 1986.
8. Hutter RVP: At last—worldwide agreement on the staging of cancer. Arch Surg 122:1235–1239, 1987.
9. Lacour J, Bucalossi P, Caceres E, et al: Radical mastectomy versus radical mastectomy plus internal mammary dissection. Cancer 37:206–214, 1976.
10. Lacour J, Lé MG, Hill C, et al: Is it useful to remove internal mammary nodes in operable breast cancer? Eur J Surg Oncol 13:309–314, 1987.
11. Lacour J, Moniqué L, Caceres E, et al: Radical mastectomy versus radical mastectomy plus internal mammary dissection. Cancer 51:1941–1943, 1983.
12. Li KY, Shen ZZ: An analysis of 1,242 cases of extended radical mastectomy. Breast 10:10–19, 1984.
13. Meier P, Ferguson DJ, Karrison T: A controlled trial of extended radical mastectomy. Cancer 55:880–891, 1985.
14. Urban JA, Baker HW: Radical mastectomy in continuity with en bloc resection of the internal mammary lymph node chain. Cancer 5:992–1008, 1952.
15. Urban JA, Castro EB: Selecting variations in extent of surgical procedure for breast cancer. Cancer 28:1615–1623, 1971.
16. Urban JA, Egeli RA: Extended radical mastectomy. In Strombeck JO, Rosato FE (eds.): Surgery Of The Breast. New York, Thieme, 1986, pp 138–147.
17. Veronesi U, Cascinelli N, Greco M, et al: Prognosis of breast cancer patients after mastectomy and dissection of internal mammary nodes. Ann Surg 202:702–707, 1985.
18. Veronesi U, Valagussa P: Inefficacy of internal mammary node dissection in breast cancer surgery. Cancer 47:170–175, 1981.

QUADRANTECTOMY

Umberto Veronesi, M.D.

GENERAL PRINCIPLES

A quadrantectomy is an operation that removes the quadrant of the breast where the primary carcinoma is located. For small tumors, the classic concepts of good oncological surgical practice (i.e., removal of an extensive portion of normal tissue around the primary, en bloc removal of overlying skin and underlying muscular fascia) may be maintained without performing a total mastectomy. This concept follows a similar evolution of thought in other fields of surgical oncology (e.g., lobectomy instead of total thyroidectomy; lung lobectomy or removal of a lung segment instead of pneumonectomy; partial resection of the bladder instead of a total cystectomy) when small tumors are found.

These concepts have evolved primarily because of the great change in the characteristics of the patient population that has occurred in the past 20 years. Better education, more extensive information, more refined diagnostic tools, and diffuse screening campaigns all contribute to earlier detection of cancer, particularly breast carcinoma in women. It would be unwise to perform the classic surgical procedures that were introduced at the beginning of the century to treat patients with tumors that were totally different in character and more often than not were locally advanced. Many current patients bear breast tumors of very limited dimensions, sometimes not even palpable. We have to consider that the feeling of women toward breast cancer and breast cancer surgery has also greatly changed; women today are aware that if the primary tumour is small, most of the breast may be spared with adequate surgical and radiotherapeutic procedures. This new optimistic view of breast cancer treatment has also stimulated women to participate more actively in detection programs and in breast self-examination, knowing that if a small cancer is found, treatment can preserve the breast rather than produce the scarring mutilation prevalent in previous eras.

Certainly, the quadrantectomy poses some cosmetic problems. In a breast of normal size, it produces acceptable results, but in small breasts the cosmetic results may be unsatisfactory. Therefore in selected cases the option of total mastectomy and immediate reconstruction may be considered. However, surgeons must be trained to reshape the breast after quadrantectomy, possibly with the help of a plastic surgeon, who may in the future become a component of the modern breast surgery team.

What must be emphasized is that the quadrantectomy is a surgical procedure that may be defined as "radical," in the sense that it aims at removal of all the tumor cells of the primary carcinoma. Other procedures, such as the lumpectomy, tylectomy, or tumorectomy, are just "debulking" operations whose objective is to reduce the mass of cancer tissue in order to improve the efficacy of postsurgical radiotherapy.

Quadrantectomy followed by radiotherapy has had excellent results, not only in the overall survival but also in the incidence of local recurrences, with rates ranging from three to five percent, which is comparable to the rate of recurrence following the Halsted mastectomy and probably lower than the rate of local recurrence after modified radical mastectomy.[2, 4] Results of the QUART protocol (quadrantectomy, axillary dissection, radiotherapy) are reviewed comprehensively in chapter 38.

SURGICAL TECHNIQUE

Biopsy

In principle no definitive treatment for suspicious breast cancer should be adopted until diagnosis is established by a satisfactory pathological examination. If a fine needle biopsy has previously unequivocally proven the diagnosis of malignancy and there are clear clinical and mammographic findings of invasive carcinoma, an open biopsy may be avoided and the quadrantectomy performed directly.

Obtaining an adequate biopsy specimen has the following objectives:

1. To remove an adequate quantity of cancer tissue for an accurate pathological diagnosis and to allow an accurate measurement of the lesion.

2. To limit the disruption of the anatomical integrity of the breast to a minimum.

3. To avoid implantation of cancer cells.

As regards the last point, since cancer cells are easily transplantable, the surgeon must take special care not to implant them in the operative field. Therefore in the removal of the involved quadrant, the surgeon should avoid reentering the biopsy site.

The incision must be made just over the site of the lesion in a radial direction. The tumor nodule must be carefully dissected and totally removed with a very limited margin of normal tissue in all directions. The surgeon should then cut the tumour in two parts and observe the cutting surface. In most cases the diagnosis is easy to assess with this macroscopic examination. If the mass is less than 2 to 3 cm in maximum diameter, the patient is considered to be a candidate for quadrantectomy. In the case of an extemporary biopsy, while the specimen is being processed in the pathology department to obtain the final histological diagnosis by frozen section examination, the mammary gland is carefully reconstructed with one layer of interrupted suture with 0 silk. Because the wound may contain free-floating cancer cells, it is filled with a gauze soaked in a solution (i.e., hypotonic saline or distilled water) apt to destroy free cancer cells. The skin is closed with a continuous or interrupted suture. This suture must be tight, and no fluid should spill from the wound. If this should happen, there is a risk of implantation of cancer cells during the subsequent quadrantectomy. If final surgery is delayed, some time (7 to 10 days) should elapse between the biopsy and the quadrantectomy, as this is much more easily performed if the area of the biopsy has undergone a reparative fibrotic process.

Removal of the Quadrant

The quadrantectomy technique aims to remove an entire quadrant of the breast, including the skin and the superficial pectoralis fascia.[3] The objective is to obtain a radical removal of the primary tumor and its potential surrounding infiltrations through an excision of one fourth of the entire breast. To perform such an operation, it is necessary that the primary cancer be of limited size; it is difficult to do an appropriate quadrantectomy for tumors whose diameter is larger than 2 to 3 cm, unless the breast is large.

After the biopsy has been terminated and the malignant nature of the lesion confirmed, all the instruments, gloves, and drapes must be changed, and the skin resterilized.

The incision in the skin is first outlined with a sterile marking pencil. The shape of the incision is elliptical, with the major axis radial from the nipple. There must be a margin of at least 2 cm from the biopsy incision (Fig. 29–76).

Should the axillary dissection be performed in continuity, a peripheral extension of the incision is made to

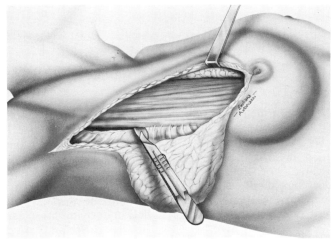

Figure 29–77. Removal of the quadrant. Two to 3 cm of normal mammary tissue around the primary carcinoma is removed.

give adequate exposure of the axilla. The en bloc operation is generally done when the primary tumor is situated in the upper external quadrants close to the axilla. In all other situations, the quadrantectomy must be carried out separately from the axillary dissection. The skin flaps are prepared with great accuracy to expose a portion of the mammary gland and allow an incision in the mammary gland at least 2 cm from the border of the tumor or the biopsy incision. The deep plane of the excision is the superficial fascia of the pectoralis major muscle (Fig. 29–77). This plane of dissection may be many centimeters from the primary cancer if the tumor is superficial, but when the cancer is deeply situated, only a few millimeters may separate the border of the tumor from the pectoralis muscle; thus the plane of dissection is very close to the edge of the tumor. In this case the corresponding superficial portion of the pectoralis major muscle may be dissected en bloc with the breast quadrant.

Because a good cosmetic result is one of the major objectives of the quadrantectomy, it is important that the breast and the nipple be reconstructed with great care. This step will require time and often the collaboration of a plastic surgeon. The edges of the mammary gland must be sutured along one or two planes according to the thickness of the breast. However, the extent of reconstruction of the mammary tissue must be carefully evaluated in each case, since it is sometimes advisable to limit reconstruction to a minimum to avoid possible subsequent skin retraction or a bulky and excessively prominent breast.

Special care is needed for the good appearance of the nipple. One of the consequences of the quadrantectomy may be the excessive protusion of the nipple and sometimes its distortion. The protruded nipple tends in fact to bend in the direction of the removed quadrant. To avoid nipple distortion, it is advisable to free it from the mammary gland through an extensive dissection of the skin and by cutting the major ducts.

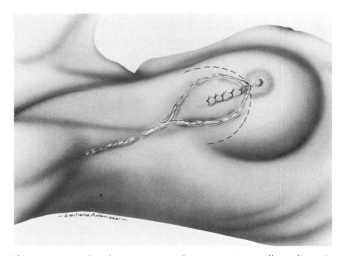

Figure 29–76. Quadrantectomy and in-continuity axillary dissection lines of skin incision.

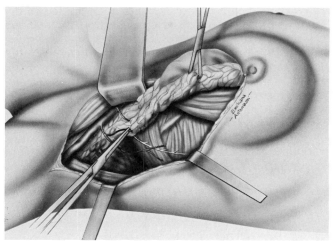

Figure 29–78. Dissection of axillary nodes, with preservation of the major pectoralis muscle.

Axillary Dissection

The axillary dissection may sometimes be performed in continuity with the quadrantectomy. In the majority of cases it is done in discontinuity through a separate incision, preferably a posteroanterior one that crosses the axillary fossa in an upward direction. The incision follows the cutaneous lines of Langer, 3 to 4 cm down the axillary fold, and has a length of 12 to 15 cm. It gives excellent access to the axillary vein but should be retracted downward to obtain access to the thoracodorsal vessels and nodes (Fig. 29–78).

The first step of the axillary dissection, after the preparation of the skin flaps, is the exposure of the latissimus dorsi muscle. This muscle is a key part of the technique and, once identified, must be carefully followed upward to its white tendinous portion. After the latissimus dorsi muscle has been isolated, the axillary vein, which lies on the white tendon of the latissimus dorsi, is easily identified.

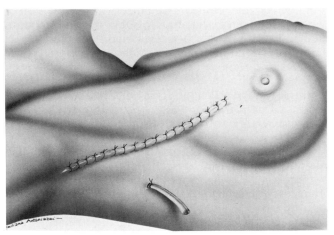

Figure 29–80. The breast is reconstructed and the wound closed.

When the vein has been isolated in its lateral portion, the thoracodorsal vessels and nerve are exposed (Fig. 29–79). This may be done by cutting the deep pectoralis fascia. At this point the surgeon should free the lateral margin of the pectoralis major muscle from its fascial connections. The muscle is then retracted upward to give access to the structures situated deep in the axilla. Great care must be taken not to injure the thoracoacromial vessels and the nerves to the pectoralis major. The pectoralis minor muscle is then freed from its connections and isolated, keeping its nerves and vessels intact.

The next step is the dissection of the apex of the

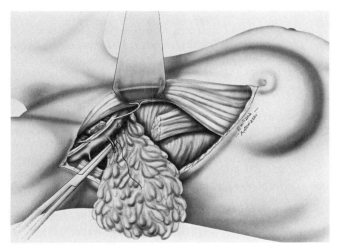

Figure 29–79. The axillary dissection is completed.

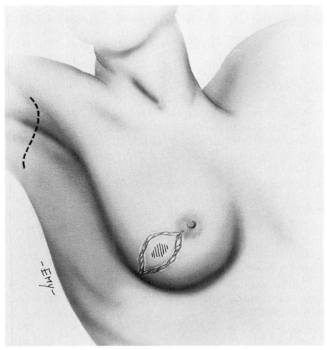

Figure 29–81. Quadrantectomy and axillary dissection with separate incision.

axilla, which may easily be obtained with the incision of the costocoracoid fascia at the point of its reflection into the chest wall. To improve the visibility of the apex of the axilla, the minor pectoralis muscle is retracted laterally. The fat and areolar tissues in the area between the chest wall and the medial aspect of the minor pectoralis muscle contain the highest axillary lymph nodes. To help the pathologist orient the specimen, it is advisable to put a metal disc on the tissue excised from the apex of the axilla.

Once the apex of the axilla has been cleared, the operation continues by dissecting the entire axillary vein and artery, with isolation and ligation of all their branches directed toward the breast. After the long thoracic nerve is identified and isolated, all the axillary fatty and areolar tissues containing the axillary lymph nodes and vessels are set free and removed (Fig. 29–80). A suction drain is employed, and then the wound is closed (Fig. 29–81).

SUMMARY

Quadrantectomy has as its objective the removal of all the cancer tissue in the breast. In principle, therefore, it might not need to be followed by radiotherapy; in Europe clinical trials are in progress to evaluate this.[1]

However, experience until now has been limited to the QUART protocol, which involves postquadrantectomy radiotherapy and axillary dissection. With this technique the results are equal, if not superior, to the Halsted mastectomy. The significance of the QUART protocol is its extremely low rate of local recurrence of disease, which approximates three to five percent in large series of cases.[1] A high rate of local recurrences often implies a second operation, which, in many cases, is a mastectomy, thus frustrating the objectives of the conservative procedure and creating serious psychological distress to the patient.

References

1. Veronesi U: Rationale and indications for limited surgery in breast cancer: current data. World J Surg 11:493–498, 1987.
2. Veronesi U, Banfi A, Del Vecchio M, et al: Comparison of Halsted mastectomy with quadrantectomy, axillary dissection, and radiotherapy in early breast cancer: long-term results. Eur J Cancer Clin Oncol 22:1085–1089, 1986.
3. Veronesi U, Costa A, Saccozzi R: Surgical technique of breast quadrantectomy and axillary dissection. *In* Stömbeck JO, Rosato FE (eds): Surgery of the Breast. Diagnosis and Treatment of Breast Disease. Stuttgart, Thieme Verlag, 127–131, 1986.
4. Veronesi U, Saccozzi R, Del Vecchio M, et al: Comparing radical mastectomy with quadrantectomy, axillary dissection, and radiotherapy in patients with small cancers of the breast. N Engl J Med 305:6–11, 1981.

LUMPECTOMY (SEGMENTAL MASTECTOMY) AND AXILLARY DISSECTION

Bernard Fisher, M.D.

In less than two decades, revolutionary changes in the local/regional management of primary breast cancer have taken place. During that time, radical and extended radical mastectomy have become historic "milestones" against which progress can be measured. Total mastectomy (modified radical mastectomy) and axillary dissection can be considered the "radical" surgery of the present era. It is likely that in the foreseeable future, these procedures will likewise be relegated to a position of historic significance. Breast-conserving procedures are being employed with ever-increasing frequency. How strong is the justification for the changes that have occurred? Why have they come about? Has science played a role? Have these changes resulted because of anecdotal reporting of the experiences of a few who dared to tamper with tradition, or are there nebulous reasons, such as "consumer" pressure, that some would suggest are the cause?

For more than a quarter of a century I have reported the results of laboratory and clinical investigations that have had an impact on the primary treatment of breast cancer, and I have repeatedly presented my perception of the reasons for the change in the surgical management of cancer.[12–17, 19, 20, 30, 36] The altered comprehension of cancer biology acquired over the past two decades is primarily responsible for the formulation of a new basis for cancer surgery, and any contribution from "nonscience" (anecdotage) has been entirely fortuitous.

On numerous occasions I have chronicled the pathway of change from Halsted's time to the present and have emphasized laboratory and clinical research conducted by me and my associates that led to the formulation of a hypothesis alternative to that of Halsted. I have also repeatedly reported the results of clinical trials carried out to test the new paradigm. Space prohibits more than a brief presentation of the highlights of those efforts, and the reader is referred to the original publications and a complete bibliography for greater detail. This chapter will provide information obtained from the only randomized trial in America carried out to determine the efficacy of breast conservation for the treatment of primary breast cancer. That study (protocol B-06) was begun in 1976 by the National Surgical Adjuvant Breast and Bowel Project (NSABP). This chapter will present findings through 8 years of follow-up and will also provide commentary regarding those major issues that have arisen as a result of the use of breast conservation and that have not been previously addressed in the literature. The original study reports used the term "segmental mastectomy" to identify the operative procedure employed for breast preservation. The term was intended to indicate that the operation removed only enough breast tissue to ensure that margins of the resected surgical specimen were free of tumor. The term "segmental mastectomy," however, failed to convey the image of the operation employed and was judged inappropriate since there are no true segments of breast as in other anatomical structures (e.g., the lung). Consequently, we have resorted to the use of the term "lumpectomy," which, although inelegant and equally imprecise, better conveys the intent of the operation. Other terms, such as "tylectomy," "local excision," or "tumorectomy," are also imprecise and fail to indicate whether the primary tumor is completely or partially removed and whether an attempt is made to remove the tumor so that the specimen margins are tumor free. In this chapter the terms "lumpectomy" and "segmental mastectomy" are, on occasion, used interchangeably. In no circumstances was a quadrantectomy employed.

FROM HALSTED'S RADICAL MASTECTOMY TO LUMPECTOMY: A HISTORICAL OVERVIEW

The Anecdotal Period

There must be a firm rationale for the surgical management of cancer. In tracing the evolution of cancer surgery, it is important to know how those who formulated and influenced treatment at a particular time in history conceived of the disease, for it was their conception of the disease process that provided the rationale for the therapy they employed.

The first true paradigm for cancer management was formulated in the late nineteenth century by William S. Halsted. To understand the rationale for the type of surgery he advocated, it is important to appreciate Halsted's concept of the biology of cancer, particularly his perception of the phenomenon of metastases. Halsted formulated a hypothesis based on a diverse group of findings that had been obtained by others around 1880. This hypothesis ultimately had its expression in the radical mastectomy. Of particular importance were the findings of Goldman and Schmidt that cancer cells in blood excited thrombosis and that the thrombosis destroyed or rendered cancer cells harmless.[43] The report by Handley that tumor cells spread along lymphatic pathways by direct extension rather than by embolization had a seminal effect on Halsted's thinking.[41] The investigations of Virchow indicating that regional lymph nodes were effective filters also influenced the evolution of Halstedian concepts.[71] Another precept in harmony with Halsted's hypothesis was that a growing tumor remains localized at its site of origin for a period of time, but at some instant during its growth, tumor cell invasion of lymphatics and dissemination to regional nodes takes place. After a further interval, during which the tumor is local/regional only, systemic dissemination occurs as the tumor increases in size.

As a consequence of these precepts and the understanding of the mechanism of cancer metastases at the time, there arose an "anatomic" basis for cancer surgery. The "proper" cancer operation consisted of removal of the primary tumor together with regional lymphatics and lymph nodes by en bloc dissection. Because there was deemed to be a certain orderliness about tumor spread and because clinically recognizable cancer was considered in many instances to be a local/regional disease, it was considered that tumors would be more curable if surgeons would only be more expansive in their interpretation of what constituted the "region" and if, above all, they utilized better technique so that they could eradicate every cancer cell. Local/regional reoccurrences were more often than not considered to be the result of inadequate application of surgical skill rather than a manifestation of systemic disease. There was hope that one more lymph node dissection would cure more cancers. Radical cancer surgery based on those anatomical considerations persisted for 75 years and still endures to varying degrees. The Halstedian paradigm remained intact because of few substantive challenges to it arising from the results of laboratory and clinical investigation. Findings from studies that were carried out could not be unified to produce a competing hypothesis.

The efficacy of performing the radical mastectomy to fulfill the tenets of the Halstedian hypothesis began to be seriously challenged during the 1950s and 1960s. The challenge was not to the principles on which the hypothesis was based, but rather to whether the radical mastectomy adequately embodied those principles. If the removal of the entire lymphatic drainage area was of paramount importance, then the radical operation for breast cancer was inadequate since lymph nodes other than those in the axilla were frequently involved with tumor. A flurry of anecdotal reports by such leaders in surgery as Wangensteen,[73] Margottini,[55] Urban,[69] Dahl-Iversen,[2] Lacour,[51] Veronesi,[70] Caceres,[4] and Sugarbaker[68] appeared that recorded their personal experiences with the *extended* radical mastectomy. In 1970, after an extensive evaluation of these reports, I concluded that the information presented by those investigators had not demonstrated that the extended radical procedure was more efficacious than the conventional radical mastectomy.[12] Despite the large number of patients used in many of the studies, the evaluations were inadequate to test the worth of the extended radical operation. Nothing came from those reports that could provide a basis for challenging Halstedian principles and nothing arose from them that added to comprehension of the disease.

At the same time that more encompassing operations were being carried out, other investigators were reporting their experience with operations less extensive than the radical mastectomy. The deviation from radical mastectomy was not a result of the Halstedian hypothesis being displaced by new facts or concepts, but of a dissatisfaction with the results of the operation. The considerations of McWhirter, who in 1948 reported his results with simple mastectomy combined with postoperative radiotherapy, best exemplify that attitude.[56] McWhirter adopted his "new" therapeutic regimen because of his concern that radical operations were not "radical" enough, in that they failed to get rid of all tumor tissue in the operative area, and "at the time of operation tissues actually invaded by tumor must often be divided." It was McWhirter's opinion that, as a result of this trauma, malignant cells would have an increased tendency to disseminate to other sites. Although he appreciated the possibility that such cells could still be liberated from the area of operation when a simple mastectomy was performed, McWhirter was of the opinion that these cells would be trapped by the intact barrier of the axilla. Moreover, since wound healing was likely to take place more rapidly after simple rather than radical mastectomy, radiotherapy could be applied with less delay, thus reducing the interval during which cells could be disseminated to distant sites. McWhirter's views were in keeping with the mechanistic approach to both tumor dissemination and eradication; they did not challenge the prevailing paradigm. As with extended radical mastectomy, aside from a demonstration of personal conviction, the data regarding operations less extensive than radical mastectomy were nondefinitive. The data failed to demonstrate unequivocally whether simple mastectomy was a procedure that should supplant the radical operation. While clinicians were debating the relative merits of radical, extended radical, and simple mastectomy, a few were reporting their experiences with modified radical mastectomy or local excision and radiation. The most ardent of the few supporters of the modified radical mastectomy (Patey operation) was Handley.[42] Handley's rationale for that operation was based on his conviction that the radical mastectomy was inadequate because it left behind internal mammary nodes. It was his view that the use of radiation following modified radical mastectomy would be more beneficial, since the internal mammary nodes would be treated by employing this procedure.

The results of local excision of breast tumors followed by breast radiation were reported by Mustakallio[58] in 1954 and by Porritt,[64] Peters,[59] and Crile[11] in the 1960s. While these studies failed to clearly determine the relative merits of that regimen, they did demonstrate that patients could survive free of disease for many years following such treatment. The more recent reports by Calle et al.,[5] Hellman et al.,[48] Prosnitz et al.,[65] Montague et al.,[57] and Pierquin et al.[63] continue to attest to that fact. It is difficult to determine the rationale employed by the early advocates of breast conservation. What seems most certain is that there was no clear biological principle that directed their approach. In many instances, as noted by Mustakallio, the procedure was initially performed because patients refused to have a radical mastectomy.

Despite the fact that clinical efforts from 1950 to 1970

failed to determine with certainty the relative merits of the various methods for the local/regional treatment of breast cancer, failed to evolve new biological principles, and failed to test the Halstedian hypothesis (allowing it to remain the paradigm for breast cancer management), operations of lesser extent were becoming accepted in clinical practice and in some places were considered "standard." Thus, as previously mentioned, the retreat from radical mastectomy was more the result of frustration with its inability to fulfill the tenets of the hypothesis than because there were new principles attracting attention.

Laboratory and Clinical Research in the 1960s

During the time that anecdotal clinical information was accumulating, a series of laboratory and clinical investigations directed toward obtaining a better comprehension of the biology of metastases was being conducted by ourselves and others. These studies (1958–1970) influenced our thinking relative to metastatic mechanisms and revealed that the blood and lymphatic vascular systems are so interrelated that it is impractical to consider them as independent routes of tumor cell dissemination.[28] The studies also revealed that the residence of a vast majority of tumor cells gaining access to an organ via the blood stream was transient.[26] As a consequence, we concluded that patterns of tumor spread are not solely dictated by anatomical considerations but are also influenced by intrinsic factors in tumor cells and in the organs to which they gain access. The thesis was accepted that there is no orderly pattern of tumor cell dissemination that could be based on mechanical and temporal factors.

Results from other experiments indicated that regional lymph nodes are not, as Virchow proposed, effective barriers to tumor spread.[8] Tumor cells traverse lymph nodes and gain access to the blood vascular system by lymphatic-venous communications in nodes. Additional studies indicated the biological importance of regional nodes, which were found to have a role in both initiation and maintenance of tumor immunity.[27] It was demonstrated that regional node cells are capable of destroying tumor cells; therefore, the presence of negative nodes may be a result of such a circumstance (because tumor cells traverse nodes) rather than the result of removal of a tumor prior to its dissemination.[33] Our findings indicated that biological rather than anatomical factors may be the reason that certain nodes contain metastases and others do not. Thus we concluded that consideration of regional nodes as mechanical receptors for tumor cells and way stations for tumor dissemination is an anachronism. The findings also indicated that host factors are important in the development of metastases and that a tumor is not autonomous from its host, as was believed in Halsted's time. The existence of dormant tumor cells was demonstrated for the first time, and it was shown that perturbation of a host by a variety of means could produce lethal metastases from those cells.[25] Our findings led us to consider that local reoccurrences following operation were apt to be the result of systemically disseminated cells lodging and growing at a site of trauma rather than because of inadequate surgical technique.[29] We proposed that a tumor is a systemic disease, probably from its inception. That premise does not imply that all patients will at some time develop overt metastases, nor does it imply that only patients with metastases have disseminated disease. We theorized in the 1960s that the regional node is an indicator of host-tumor relations. The lymph node that contains tumor cells reflects an interrelation between host and tumor that permits the development of metastases; it does not reflect a situation in which the lymph node is an instigator of distant disease.

Concurrent with the laboratory studies, a series of clinical trials carried out by us provided new information that raised questions regarding concepts on which treatment was based. Tumor recurrence and survival of breast cancer patients were found to be independent of the number of axillary nodes removed and examined,[34] and tumor location failed to influence prognosis.[35]

Regardless of whether the results of all of the laboratory studies and clinical observations were interpreted correctly, whether they resulted from the methodologies and models employed rather than from biological circumstances, whether they could or could not be confirmed in every setting and in every detail, or whether they were obtained from simplistic experiments that did not really provide positive proof for any of our assumptions, they all had the same characteristic: they did not conform to the concepts that provided the principles for the Halstedian hypothesis. They provided a matrix within which an alternative thesis could be formulated. That hypothesis, synthesized by us in 1968, is biological in concept, rather than anatomical and mechanistic. Its components are completely antithetical to those in the Halstedian hypothesis (Table 29–30).

Clinical Trials Testing the Alternative Hypothesis and Providing Justification for Evaluating Lumpectomy

During the time that laboratory investigations were reshaping thinking regarding the biology of metastases and anecdotal reporting was flourishing, one of the great advances of our time was taking place. The prospective, randomized, controlled trial was being introduced into clinical medicine as a mechanism for testing hypotheses, obtaining natural history information, and evaluating the worth of a particular therapy. The use of that highly sophisticated methodology instead of anecdotal reports represents a major step toward transforming medicine from an art to a science.

In August, 1971, a clinical trial (NSABP B-04) was begun, not only to test the validity of the principles on which our alternative hypothesis was based but also to simultaneously evaluate, in an unbiased fashion, different regimens of surgical management for primary breast

Table 29–30. TWO DIVERGENT HYPOTHESES OF TUMOR BIOLOGY

Halstedian	Alternative
Tumors spread in an orderly defined manner based on mechanical considerations.	There is no orderly pattern of tumor cell dissemination.
Tumor cells traverse lymphatics to lymph nodes by direct extension, supporting en bloc dissection.	Tumor cells traverse lymphatics by embolization, challenging the merit of en bloc dissection.
The positive lymph node is an indicator of tumor spread and is the instigator of disease.	The positive lymph node is an indicator of a host-tumor relationship that permits development of metastases rather than the instigator of distant disease.
Regional lymph nodes are barriers to the passage of tumor cells.	Regional lymph nodes are ineffective as barriers to tumor cell spread.
Nodes are of anatomical importance.	Nodes are of biological importance.
The blood stream is of little significance as a route of tumor dissemination.	The blood stream is of considerable importance in tumor dissemination.
A tumor is autonomous of its host.	Complex host-tumor interrelationships affect every facet of the disease.
Operable breast cancer is a local/regional disease.	Operable breast cancer is a systemic disease.
The extent and nuances of operation are the dominant factors influencing patient outcome.	Variations in local/regional therapy are unlikely to substantially affect survival.
No consideration is given to tumor multicentricity.	Multicentric foci of tumor are not necessarily a precursor of clinically overt cancer.

cancer. The results of that trial, obtained from information on more than 1500 women, indicate that in patients without clinical evidence of axillary node involvement (40 percent of whom had histologically positive nodes), three distinctly different treatment regimens [radical mastectomy, total (simple) mastectomy with local/regional irradiation, or total mastectomy and removal of nodes that later became clinically positive] yielded no significant difference in overall treatment failure, distant metastases (Fig. 29–82), or survival through more than 14 years of follow-up.[31] When patients free of disease at the end of 5 years were evaluated between 5 and 10 years, not only was there no difference among the treatment groups, but the positive-node patients had results similar to those in patients with negative nodes. The same findings were observed between 10 and 14 years. Thus the 5-year results were indicative of future findings. In patients with clinical evidence of node involvement, there was no significant difference between the group treated by radical mastectomy and the group treated by total mastectomy and local/regional irradiation. The findings also indicated that radiation of internal mammary nodes in patients with inner quadrant lesions did not improve survival and

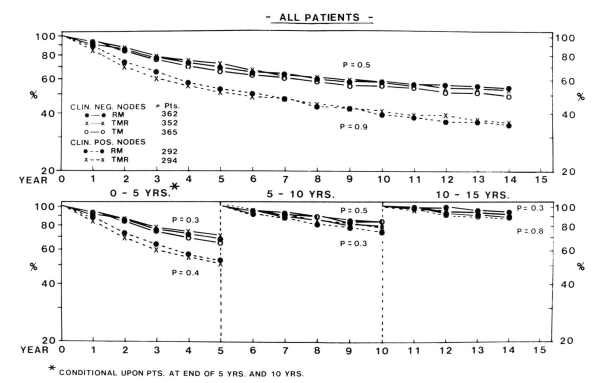

Figure 29–82. Distant disease–free survival at intervals following mastectomy.

that results obtained at 5 years accurately predicted the outcome through 10 years.

It was concluded that variations of local/regional treatment used in the study were not important in determining survival of breast cancer patients. The multiple findings from this study support and confirm the validity of the various components of the alternative hypothesis.

During the 1970s, other trials were unwittingly putting the alternative hypothesis to further test. A major trial in the United Kingdom employed women with clinical stage I or stage II carcinoma of the breast.[7] A simple mastectomy was performed in all patients without surgical attention to the axillary nodes. Patients received either a course of regional radiotherapy or no further primary treatment (the "watch policy" group). Ten years later, no differences were found between the two groups, findings that lend support to the alternative hypothesis.

When early findings from the NSABP B-04 study indicated that patients treated by total mastectomy without axillary node dissection and pectoral muscle removal were at no higher risk for distant disease or death than were those undergoing a Halsted radical mastectomy, we considered it clinically and scientifically justifiable to begin a new study (B-06) to evaluate the worth of breast conservation by local tumor excision with or without radiation therapy. The rest of this chapter provides an overview of findings obtained from the NSABP study, which is the only randomized trial in America to evaluate the worth of lumpectomy with and without breast radiation.

DESIGN OF THE NSABP LUMPECTOMY TRIAL

To ensure credibility of the findings from the NSABP lumpectomy trial, a sophisticated experimental design was necessary (Fig. 29–83). Beginning in 1976, patients were randomly assigned to one of three treatment groups: total mastectomy, lumpectomy, or lumpectomy followed by breast irradiation. Women in all the treatment groups had an axillary dissection, and those with positive nodes received chemotherapy. The lumpectomy operation completely abandoned conventional concepts of cancer surgery by removing only enough breast tissue to ensure that the margins of the resected surgical specimens were free of tumor. All resected lumpectomy specimens were examined pathologically to ensure that the margins were free of tumor. The study was designed to determine (1) the effectiveness of lumpectomy for breast preservation, (2) whether radiation therapy reduces the incidence of tumor in the ipsilateral breast after segmental mastectomy, (3) whether breast conservation results in a higher risk of distant disease and death than does mastectomy, and (4) the clinical significance of multicentricity.

The protocol required that a subsequent mastectomy be performed if the margins of specimens removed by lumpectomy were not tumor free. It also mandated that a total mastectomy be carried out should tumor occur in the operated breast subsequent to lumpectomy. Such a tumor occurring following a previous lumpectomy was designated a tumor "reoccurrence" and was not consid-

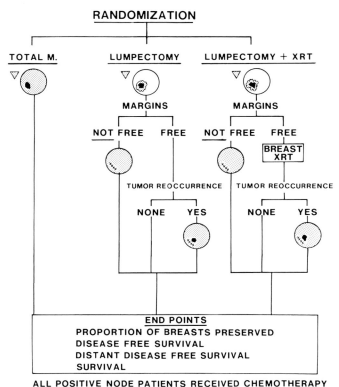

ALL POSITIVE NODE PATIENTS RECEIVED CHEMOTHERAPY
SHADED AREA INDICATES REMOVAL
Figure 29–83. Treatment strategy NSABP B-06.

ered to be a "treatment failure" unless the tumor was so extensive that it could not be completely removed by mastectomy. However, because the breast was removed, the patient was regarded as having a "cosmetic failure." It must also be emphasized that when determining disease-free survival (DFS), distant disease–free survival (DDFS), and survival (S) in the three treatment groups, it was necessary that all patients in each group be included—even those in the two lumpectomy groups who had margins involved and consequently had a mastectomy. Margin involvement was found to be associated with tumors having a poorer patient prognosis than tumors associated with free margins. Consequently, elimination of those patients from the segmental mastectomy groups would have created a bias, because patients with a similarly poor prognosis existed in the total mastectomy group. Elimination would have resulted in segmental mastectomy patients appearing to have a much more favorable outcome than those who had total mastectomy.

Recurrences of tumor in the chest wall and operative scar, but not in the ipsilateral breast, were classified as local treatment failures. Tumors in the internal mammary, supraclavicular, or ipsilateral axillary nodes were classified as regional treatment failures. Tumors in all other locations were considered distant treatment failures. Patients classified as having any distant disease included those with a distant metastasis as a first treatment failure, a distant metastasis after a local or regional

reoccurrence, or a second cancer (including tumor in the other breast). Overall survival refers to survival with or without recurrent disease.

OPERATIVE TECHNIQUE FOR LUMPECTOMY

When the NSABP study to evaluate the worth of local tumor excision was implemented in 1976, American surgeons had little familiarity with breast-conserving procedures. Through a series of workshops and other educational mechanisms, those NSABP surgeons participating in the trial were apprised of the methodologies mandated by the protocol. With only minor variations, those procedures have been used in several thousand lumpectomies in patients entered into the initial and subsequent NSABP trials evaluating local/regional and systemic therapy for breast cancer. The following descriptions highlight the operative procedures employed; these procedures have previously been described in detail.[38, 54]

Incisions and Skin Removal

Curvilinear incisions are employed by us no matter where in the breast a lesion occurs (Fig. 29–84). Such incisions should be used even when tumors are in the upper outer quadrant of the breast near the axilla. A separate incision for the axillary dissection is almost always made when a tumor is in that portion of the breast. To achieve the best cosmetic results, radial incisions are *not* recommended (Fig. 29–85). Some NSABP surgeons, however, prefer radial incisions for lesions at the "6 o'clock" position in the breast. Our own preference is for curvilinear incisions even when tumors are in that location. To perform a satisfactory lumpectomy, it is essential that the incision be placed directly over the tumor [Fig. 29–86(A)]. The use of a circumareolar incision for removal of a lesion that is not in proximity to the areola is inappropriate. Tunneling through breast tissue to remove a lesion that is not

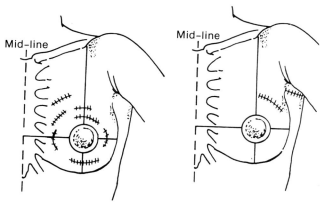

Figure 29–84. Recommended incisions.

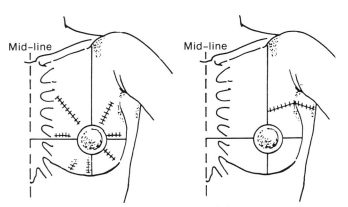

Mid-line   Mid-line

Figure 29–85. Nonrecommended incisions.

beneath the incision is to be condemned. Tumor-free specimen margins are difficult and often impossible to obtain when such an incision is made. Reexcision of the tumor site to obtain free margins is equally difficult. Whether the patient is a candidate for lumpectomy should be determined prior to operation, and the incision should not be made with concern as to how it might relate to skin removal if a conventional mastectomy is required. In those rare instances in which it is found at operation that a planned lumpectomy cannot be carried out because of the inability to obtain tumor-free margins, the mastectomy incisions are tailored to accommodate the lumpectomy incision.

Because lumpectomy is not a Halstedian operation and patients with tumor involving the overlying skin are not apt to be candidates for the operation, skin removal is not a requisite of the operation. A small ellipse of skin may be removed with the underlying lesion to orient the pathologist as to the anterior or superficial border of the specimen, but its removal does not enhance the effectiveness of the operation. We do not ordinarily remove any skin, because in our experience, the quality of cosmesis is inversely related to the amount of skin removed. If a prior biopsy has been performed, skin encompassing the biopsy site is removed when lumpectomy is done.

Tumor Removal and Examination of Specimen Margins

The tumor is removed so that it is completely enveloped in normal fat or breast tissue. This does not necessitate removal of a predefined amount of normal tissue around the lesion. The aim is to remove an amount that is adequate to achieve specimen margins grossly free of tumor [Fig. 29–86(B)]. A special point to be emphasized is that when the excision is being carried out, skin edges are not undermined (i.e., thin skin flaps are not desirable) [Fig. 29–86(C)]. Undermining of skin, like skin removal, results in an unfavorable cosmetic result. No special effort is made to include pectoral fascia in the specimen unless the lesion lies in close proximity to it.

Our practice is to tag the specimen before it leaves the operating field [Fig. 29–86(B)]. Any system for doing this may be employed. A long silk suture is used to mark the lateral surface, a short suture to identify the medial aspect of the specimen, and two short tags close together to identify the "top" of the specimen (i.e., the anterior or superficial margin). If so desired, additional tags may be placed to designate the superior, or cephalic, margin and the inferior, or caudal, border. The specimen is immediately delivered to the pathologist, or ideally, he or she is present in the operating room to receive it. The pathologist's role is to confirm or establish the diagnosis of cancer, to aid the surgeon in deciding intraoperatively whether the specimen margins are *grossly* free of tumor, and to take an aliquot of tumor for estrogen and progesterone receptor analyses. Our procedure is to not close the operative incision until the pathologist reports on the status of the specimen margins.

When the pathologist receives the specimen, he or she carefully orients it by means of the suture tags that the surgeon has placed (Fig. 29–87). After measurement, the uncut specimen is inspected for gross margin involvement. If there is evidence that the tumor has been transected, the surgeon is immediately apprised of the precise location of the margin involvement so that additional tissue can be removed from that area while

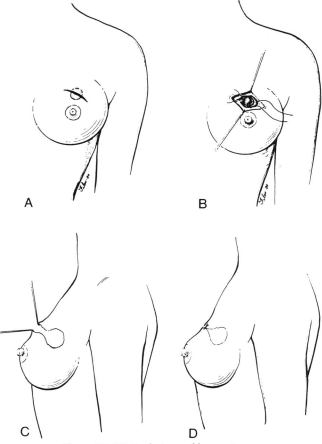

A   B

C   D

Figure 29–86. Technique of lumpectomy.

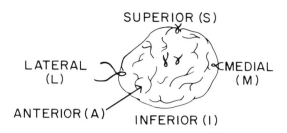

- ORIENT AND MEASURE SPECIMEN

- INSPECT FOR GROSS MARGIN INVOLVEMENT.

Figure 29–87. Orientation of the lumpectomy specimen.

the pathologist is completing inspection of the specimen. The pathologist then coats the entire surface of the specimen with india ink [Fig. 29–88(A)], blots it dry, and then bisects the tumor and specimen transversely. The anteroposterior and mediolateral diameters of the tumor are then measured, and the specimen is further examined to determine if the tumor is grossly "close" to any margin of the specimen. If there is concern about any border, the pathologist may do a frozen section to determine margin involvement. Our preference is to remove additional breast tissue in the area to obtain a new true margin any time that it is considered advisable

that frozen section be done to check margin involvement. Rarely will there be a subsequent report of microscopic tumor at margins that have been reported to be grossly free. A multiplicity of frozen sections is *not* carried out to determine if the margins are free of tumor. Rarely is a frozen section done for that purpose. If tumor is found on gross examination to be "close" to a portion of the resected tissue margin, the resection in that area is extended by removal of an additional rim of breast tissue and fat. The new true margin of the area that was considered to be "close" is identified for the pathologist by placing methylene blue on the surface of the re-resected portion of tissue that is farthest from the initial resection site.

Aliquots of tumor are taken for receptor studies and for the preparation of blocks from which permanent sections are made [Fig. 29–88(B)]. While the technique for examining the specimen for margin involvement may vary among pathologists, the following approach established by the NSABP project pathologist[40] is provided as a guideline that may be varied with circumstances. Blocks of the lateral, medial, anterior, and posterior margins are prepared from the original transverse block. The remaining hemispheres are fixed for 1 to 2 hours to facilitate subsequent blocking [Fig. 29–88(C)]. These remnants are then blocked sagittally, with the cut surfaces placed down [Fig. 29–88(D)]. This procedure provides for measurement of the superior-inferior diameter of the tumor and for the preparation of blocks

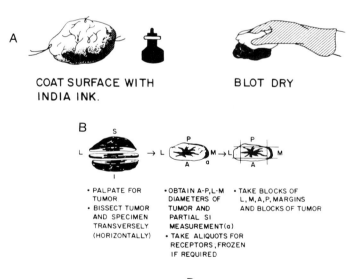

Figure 29–88. Preparation of specimen for determination of margin involvement. *A,* Application of India ink. *B,* Taking of blocks. *C,* Fixing tissue for additional blocks. *D,* Taking further blocks.

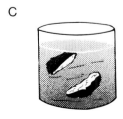

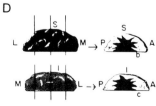

that provide sections for additional examination of margins. At least 12 to 20 blocks are made from each specimen, depending on its size. Although there have been, and will continue to be, variations of this scheme by hospital pathologists, at least five lines of resection were available for review in patients having lumpectomy in the NSABP study.

Pathological assessment of lines of resection in a lumpectomy specimen is admittedly difficult because of the large surface area. This assessment is confounded by vague pathological criteria utilized for making a decision relative to whether tumor involves specimen margins. Many pathologists have the tendency to infer margin involvement by such subjective designations as tumor "too" or "very" close to it. When hospital pathologists resorted to these subjective criteria, there was residual cancer in only 12 percent of total mastectomy specimens removed because of presumed margin involvement. Thus it is most appropriate to regard lines of resection as involved only when cancer is transected.

Closure of the Lumpectomy Wound

After a decision has been made concerning the status of the specimen margins and meticulous hemostasis of the lumpectomy site has been achieved, closure of the wound is carried out [Fig. 29–86(D)]. Because lumpectomy is a cosmetic procedure, meticulous attention must be given to this part of the operation. Attempts at breast reconstruction by approximating breast tissue and deep fat can lead to unfavorable cosmesis, particularly following removal of tumors in the upper half of the breast. For optimal cosmesis, our approach is to make no attempt to obliterate the "dead space" in the breast by approximating breast tissue or fat, and no drain of any type is ever placed in the wound [Fig. 29–86(C)]. In recent years we have found it desirable to use interrupted Dexon (5-0) sutures to approximate the subcutaneous fat. The skin is then carefully approximated by the use of a continuous subcuticular suture of the same material [Fig. 29–86(D)].

Subareolar Tumors or Tumors >4 cm

The aim of the NSABP lumpectomy protocol was to carry out the operation so that a normal appearing breast resulted in all patients. Because subareolar tumors or those close to that position might require removal of the nipple and areola to ensure tumor-free specimen margins, with a resultant cosmetic defect, lesions in such a location were not considered to be amenable to lumpectomy. Patients with subareolar or periareolar lesions were considered candidates for lumpectomy when tumor-free margins could be obtained without removal of the nipple and areola and when a satisfactory cosmetic result could be achieved. This was particularly the case in women with large breasts and posteriorly located tumors. Recent experience has indi-

cated that the removal of subareolar lesions with the nipple and areola can be carried out with a satisfactory cosmetic result. The resulting breast mound is more normal than that achieved by breast reconstruction following total mastectomy.

Following publication of the results of our trial, the impression was erroneously created that lumpectomy was appropriate only for those patients with very small tumors. This misconception occurred despite the fact that it had clearly been stated that women with tumors ≤4 cm were eligible. That tumor size was originally selected because it had been demonstrated by us that the incidence of multicentricity was apt to be greater in tumors larger than 4 cm. We have recently liberalized the tumor size requirement so that patients with tumors ≤5 cm are eligible for our present protocols, providing they have an ample-sized breast so that a favorable cosmetic result can be obtained. Thus patients with clinical stage I and II tumors are eligible for lumpectomy regardless of tumor location. It is our opinion that, when technically feasible, women with larger tumors and/or clinically positive nodes are better served by lumpectomy, because they are at great risk for the development of distant metastases and death regardless of the operation performed.

AXILLARY DISSECTION

We do not recommend axillary "sampling" as a substitute for axillary dissection. The purpose of an axillary dissection is to use the information obtained relative to lymph node involvement with tumor (1) for determining patient prognosis, (2) for staging relative to the use of adjuvant chemotherapy, and (3) for local/regional disease control. Axillary dissection is not employed with the intent of enhancing curability, since it is our contention that regional lymph nodes serve as indicators of distant metastatic disease rather than as instigators of significance for such tumor. Although we have demonstrated that the qualitative status of axillary lymph node involvement (i.e., either positive or negative) may be accurately determined by examining relatively few nodes, a more complete dissection is required for accurately determining the number of nodes involved.[37] Because patient prognosis is significantly related to the number of positive nodes present (i.e., 1–3, 4–9, ≥10), a sufficient number must be obtained to quantitate patient prognosis more accurately.[24]

As previously mentioned, the incision used for axillary dissections is separate from that used for removal of the tumor in the breast. We prefer a curvilinear transverse incision just below the axillary hairline. Some surgeons favor a longitudinal incision placed along the posterolateral margin of the pectoralis major muscle; either incision is appropriate. In all NSABP breast protocols, an axillary dissection includes all nodes from at least axillary levels I and II. The anatomical delineation of this dissection is the latissimus dorsi muscle laterally, the axillary vein superiorly, and the medial border of the pectoralis minor muscle medially. Removal of the pectoralis minor muscle is not required. The nerves to the serratus anterior and latissimus dorsi muscles should be identified and preserved. The axillary vein should be visualized and followed under the pectoralis minor muscle to the medial border. These are the minimal limits for the dissection. The average number of nodes removed compares favorably with the number obtained following a radical mastectomy or a modified radical mastectomy in previous NSABP trials. In all NSABP studies since 1971, the number of axillary nodes removed (a mean number of 15) has remained remarkably constant. Although the surgical site in the breast is not drained, a suction drain in the axilla is present for several postoperative days.

When a lumpectomy is carried out for lesions in the upper outer quadrant of the breast, even when separate incisions are used for removal of the tumor and for the axillary dissection, the two cavities (i.e., those in the breast and in the axilla) may sometimes become confluent. In such a situation, we omit the use of any drain in the axilla or the breast. An axillary drain in such a circumstance will prevent the accumulation of serum at the lumpectomy site, resulting in an unfavorable cosmetic result. The omission of such a drain has produced no undesirable effect, and a seroma of the axilla has not been observed.

A question asked with increasing frequency is whether all patients having a lumpectomy require an axillary dissection. The question arises most often regarding patients with small tumors (≤ 1 cm), particularly patients whose lesions were detected by mammography and who have clinically negative axillary nodes. We demonstrated in a prior NSABP study (B-04) that patients who were treated by simple mastectomy and an axillary dissection when nodes became clinically positive had an outcome similar to that for those who were treated by total mastectomy and an initial axillary dissection. Those findings indicate that such a dissection does not enhance curability. Moreover, if all negative- and positive-node patients are given the same systemic adjuvant therapy, there is no reason to know the nodal status except for predicting patient prognosis. That is not yet entirely the case. Consequently I currently recommend that all patients receiving lumpectomy have an axillary dissection. NSABP studies currently being carried out may provide reason to alter that view.

RADIATION THERAPY FOLLOWING LUMPECTOMY

In 1924, an English surgeon, Geoffrey Keynes, of St. Bartholomeus Hospital, London, began to treat breast carcinoma by implantation of radium needles, often resulting in good local control of cancer.[50] For the next half century, although a few surgeons such as Mustakallio of Finland; Porritt in England; and Adair, Crile, and Cope in the United States were attracting attention with their writings, much of the impetus for breast

conservation in the management of mammary cancer came from radiation therapists. The French were particularly influential.[1, 3, 6, 10, 62, 72] Reports by Peters,[59–61] Prosnitz et al.,[65] Montague et al.,[57] and Hellman et al.[44, 46, 47, 52, 74] are representative of the activities of American radiation therapists who were early advocates of breast preservation. Some of these investigators promulgated the thesis of "primary treatment of breast cancer by radiation"—a misleading description of therapy, because the radiation was administered following tumor excision. Essentially, it was only Baclesse, from the Institute Curie of Paris, who in 1965 reported his experience with the treatment of breast cancer exclusively by radiation.[3]

Reports in the 1960s were anecdotal and related to findings from heterogeneous groups of patients varying in stage of disease, operation employed, techniques of radiation, and other patient and tumor characteristics. While failing to provide definitive information regarding the worth of breast radiation, these reports, together with evolving biological information, provided justification for evaluating the worth of breast irradiation in conjunction with breast conservation surgery by means of a proper clinical trial such as was conducted by the NSABP.

Radiation used by the NSABP in protocol B-06 was aimed at eliminating occult tumor foci remaining in the ipsilateral breast. The dose level used in the NSABP trial was a level that was considered to be cancericidal and not likely to produce distortion and fibrosis of the breast or other undesirable sequelae. The dose used to meet those requirements was efficacious, as indicated by the findings from the study. The marked reduction in breast tumor reoccurrence following radiation, the failure to observe undesirable cosmetic sequelae, and the absence of complications such as rib fractures and pneumonitis that have been reported by others attest to the propriety of the techniques and the amount of radiation administered.

The intent of the radiation therapy was to treat the skin, breast tissue, muscle, lymphatics, and entire scar of the breast. No attempt was made to include axillary, supraclavicular, interpectoral, and internal mammary lymph nodes. Because the internal mammary nodes, however, lie at the medial edge of the treatment field, they were sometimes either partially or wholly included. No special attempt was made to exclude them, because that would have interfered with irradiation of the entirety of the breast. Our findings over the years indicate no advantage for axillary radiation when an axillary dissection has been carried out, and radiation of the internal mammary nodes has resulted in no survival benefit in any of the NSABP trials.

When segmental mastectomy and axillary dissection were performed through separate incisions, if the scar of the axillary dissection was extrinsic to the breast, no radiation was directed to that scar. If the axillary dissection scar was in continuity with that of the segmental mastectomy, no special attempt was made to irradiate the portion of the scar that was beyond the breast tissue.

Radiation therapy was initiated no later than 6 weeks after lumpectomy in patients with negative nodes and no later than 8 weeks after surgery in those with positive nodes. In patients with positive nodes, radiation therapy was delayed to permit completion of the first course of adjuvant chemotherapy. A minimum dose of 5000 rad was administered. This dose was calculated at a depth of two thirds distance between the skin overlying the breast and the base of the tangential fields at midseparation. This depth generally ranged from 3 cm to 7 cm. The maximum dose to the point of calculation did not exceed 5300 rad. The dose was given at a rate of 1000 rad per week (200 rad per day, 5 days per week), calculated at the minimum dose point. Both tangential fields were treated daily, with 100 rad T.D. given to each. Dry desquamation with pigmentation and/or erythema at the end of treatment were considered desirable; limited patches of moist desquamation were acceptable. Extensive areas of moist desquamation were avoided.

Because the proper administration of radiation is as important as the surgical technique for obtaining a good cosmetic result and for preventing ipsilateral breast tumor reoccurrence, it is appropriate to present a detailed account of the method of irradiation employed in all lumpectomy patients entered into NSABP studies.

Patients lie supine, head straight (no pillows are used unless dorsal convexity of the patient is extreme), and the upper arm abducted 90°, with the forearm supported in an upright position by a vertical armboard. The breast (and the chest wall) are treated through opposing tangential fields to avoid direct irradiation of the lung.

The field boundaries employed are as follows. The medial border lies along the midsternal line and the lateral border lies along the midaxillary line. If the scar extends beyond this line, the lateral border may, within limits, be moved posteriorly to include the entire scar. The extent to which this line may be moved posteriorly should be guided by the amount of lung tissue that would be irradiated if this border is parallel-opposed to the medial border. If the irradiated slice of lung tissue exceeds a width of 5 cm, the lateral portal should be left along the midaxillary line and the end of the surgical scar treated by superficial irradiation. The inferior border of the tangential field is drawn horizontally across the hemithorax at a level about 2 cm below the inframammary fold. This line can be drawn by extension from the contralateral fold if the ipsilateral breast is distorted. The superior border is located along a horizontal line that bisects the sternomanubrial junction (angle of Louis). If necessary, this border may be moved superiorly to be sure that the entire breast and the tail of the breast are included. If the scar extends above this boundary, the line should be moved superiorly to include the entire scar. The central axes of the medial and lateral fields lie on the same line. The angle of treatment ($\pm 180°$) can be determined with a rolling ball or an inclinometer bridge or by rotating the head of the machine until the back pointer and the front pointer lie on the lateral and medial field boundaries, respectively.

Cobalt 60 or a linear accelerator x-ray machine is employed. Superficial irradiation may be used only to treat or boost portions of the surgical scar as described. The use of a beam-blocking device ("breast gadget") greatly facilitates treatment of the breast. Because the lower half of the beam is blocked near its central axis, the tangential fields do not diverge into the lung.

The extent to which bolus should be used depends greatly on the details of the treatment situation at each institution. Bolus is added to reach the desired skin reaction (i.e., dry desquamation and erythema). Any accessories that enhance secondary electron scatter will increase the dose to the skin and thus limit the need for buildup. Plastic blocking trays or shields may enhance the skin dose to the extent that the use of additional bolus is neither necessary nor desirable. In general, bolus may safely be used two to four times with each tangential field when no intervening tray is used.

The worth of radiation therapy following lumpectomy has been demonstrated by our findings. Of greatest importance is the fact that those results were achieved using radiation therapy that did not include the use of radiation boosts or external beam or interstitial implants; radiation of regional nodes was not employed. Our incidence of breast tumor reoccurrence approximated that observed by proponents of such additive therapy, so it would seem that the need for a radiation boost to the excision site is not necessary when proper attention is paid to specimen margins. A clinical trial to evaluate the effectiveness of radiation with and without boosts or to evaluate external beam boosts versus boosts by interstitial implant would be nearly impossible to undertake because of the size of the patient population that would be required. Moreover, considering such a trial a high priority could be questionable. We are currently evaluating our data with respect to patient and tumor characteristics associated with tumor reoccurrence following radiation in an attempt to indicate which patients might benefit from a boost. Despite our findings indicating the lack of need for a boost, if there are circumstances in which the radiation therapist feels more benefit would accrue by using a boost, an external beam boost is more appropriate than interstitial implants because of the need for additional hospitalization, higher morbidity, imprecision of the radiation dose delivered, and the lack of data demonstrating the superiority of interstitial implants.

It is frequently asked whether all patients who have a lumpectomy need to have breast irradiation. For example, do women with small tumors (≤ 1 cm) and negative axillary nodes require such therapy? Data from the NSABP trial continue to indicate that even in such patients the use of radiation reduces the incidence of ipsilateral breast tumor reoccurrence. Whether radiation is required for patients who have microinvasive tumors treated by lumpectomy is uncertain, particularly if these patients receive systemic therapy such as tamoxifen. There are no data to clarify this issue. Consequently we currently advocate the use of breast radiation even for this subset of patients.

RESULTS FROM THE NSABP B-06 TRIAL EVALUATING LUMPECTOMY

Tumor Involvement of Specimen Margins

In our initial report we indicated that of the 1257 patients who were initially treated by lumpectomy, 10 percent were found to have tumor at the margins of resected specimens and subsequently had a total mastectomy.[23] The incidence of positive specimen margins was related to certain patient and tumor characteristics. Evaluation according to patient age showed that about 10 percent of patients ≤49 years of age and 10 percent of those ≥50 years of age had positive margins. A higher percentage of patients with positive nodes (15 percent) than with negative nodes (7 percent) had positive margins after segmental mastectomy, and the larger the number of positive axillary nodes, the higher the incidence of positive specimen margins; 33 percent of patients with ≥10 positive nodes had margins containing tumor. Women with larger tumors (2.1 cm to 4 cm) had a higher percentage of positive margins (13 percent) than did those with tumors between 0 and 2 cm (7 percent). Women with centrally located tumors were the most apt to have margin involvement.

Central review of material obtained from hospital pathologists relative to specimen margin involvement with tumor disclosed a disagreement in interpretation of the findings in some instances. This discrepancy was clearly related to hospital pathologists' statements indicating that tumor was "too" or "very" close to a line of resection, whereas it has been our practice to regard only transected invasive or noninvasive cancer as evidence of such involvement. Residual cancer was noted in 67 percent of the mastectomy specimens available for review when there was agreement as to line of involvement; however, it was noted in only 12 percent of the mastectomy specimens in which hospital, but not headquarters, pathologists had considered margins to be involved. This study did not allow for a direct evaluation of the contribution of inadequate assessment of the lines of excision to the incidence of breast tumor reoccurrence, since total mastectomy was performed when involvement was considered to have been present.

When the specimen margin contains an amount of tumor that indicates that the tumor has been transected, there is little problem deciding the future surgical management of the patient. Either a reexcision (lumpectomy) of the area should be done to obtain free margins, or a mastectomy should be performed, if it is deemed that clear margins cannot be obtained by lumpectomy. If, however, the margin is involved with only a few cells, the question arises as to whether reexcision is necessary or whether radiation, perhaps with an external beam boost, will eliminate the minimal tumor that may or may not be present. No clear information exists to supply an answer, because in our study, either reexcision or mastectomy was performed in such patients. Radiation with an external beam boost may be adequate, particularly since all primary breast cancer patients receive systemic therapy that may, in conjunction with the radiation, be adequate for preventing breast tumor reoccurrence.

Tumor Reoccurrence

Findings demonstrating the probability of patients remaining free of tumor in the ipsilateral breast after 8 years support the worth of radiation (Fig. 29–89).[32] Whereas 90 percent of those treated by lumpectomy and radiation were free of tumor, only 61 percent of those having a lumpectomy and no radiation were tumor free. The finding that a higher percentage of positive-node patients treated by segmental mastectomy and radiation (94 percent) remained free of tumor than did similarly treated negative-node patients (88 percent) is of special interest, because those with positive nodes received adjuvant chemotherapy in addition to radiation therapy.

Shortly after the initial report of our findings with lumpectomy,[23] we provided information regarding our pathological experience with this procedure, particularly as it related to ipsilateral breast tumor reoccurrence.[37] Eighty-six percent of all breast tumor reoccurrences were noted within 4 years following lumpectomy, and 95 percent had occurred within 5 postoperative years. A review of the location of reoccurrences indicated that 95 percent involved the mammary parenchyma, and the

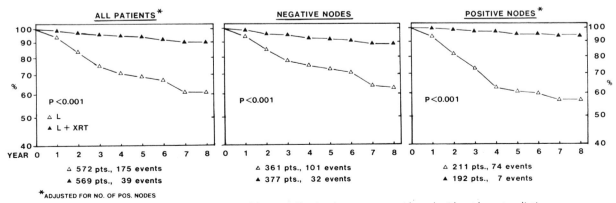

Figure 29–89. Tumor free in ipsilateral breast following lumpectomy with and without breast radiation.

remaining 5 percent involved the skin and/or nipple only. Ten percent of those in the breast parenchyma were noninvasive. The most common presentation of the reoccurrence (86 percent) was as a localized mass within or close to the quadrant of the cancer removed by lumpectomy. Fourteen percent of the reoccurrences within the breast were not only in the same quadrant as the primary cancer but were also diffusely extended into other quadrants as well. Pathologically, intralymphatic extension in this type was pronounced, being evident in remote quadrants and not infrequently in overlying skin and/or nipple as in so-called inflammatory or occult inflammatory breast cancer.[53] The extraparenchymal local breast tumor reoccurrences appeared to involve only the lymphatics (71 percent), the dermis of the skin or lymphatics, or the ducts or epidermis (Paget's disease) of the nipple. There were no significant differences in the time of appearance of the invasive and noninvasive breast tumor reoccurrences or those invasive forms appearing locally or more diffusely in the breast. Too few examples of reoccurrences involving only the skin and/or nipple were available for this determination.

The histological types and grades of 93 recurrent, invasive cancers of breast parenchyma were identical to those of the original tumor in 86 percent of cancers, whereas in 14 percent the histological type differed from that of the initial lesion (Table 29–31); however, in eight (nine percent) of these, the recurrent cancer could have represented one portion of a combination tumor type. The histological grade of these 13 cancers was similar to that of the initial cancer in seven, better differentiated in four, and less differentiated only in two.

When the probability of developing a breast tumor reoccurrence was related to the pathological features of tumors (Table 29–32), there was a significantly greater ($p \leq 0.05$) incidence in patients whose tumors were ≥ 2 cm, of high nuclear and histological grades, or revealed intralymphatic extension. Reoccurrences were less frequent with tubular type primary cancers or with types 1 and 4 scar cancers. The majority of the latter cancers were tubular. Except for intralymphatic extension, the

Table 29–31. INCIDENCE OF HISTOLOGICAL TYPES OF INITIAL AND RECURRENT INVASIVE CANCERS INVOLVING BREAST PARENCHYMA ONLY

Same Types		
Type	No.	%
NOS	40	50
Medullary	13	16
NOS + tubular	13	16
Papillary	6	8
Tubular	4	5
NOS + lobular invasive	4	5
Total	80	100

Different Types		
Initial	Recurrence	No.
Mucoid	Mucoid + papillary*	1
Mucoid	NOS	2
NOS	NOS + tubular*	1
NOS	NOS + lobular invasive*	1
NOS	Lobular invasive + tubular	1
NOS + tubular	NOS*	2
NOS + tubular	Lobular invasive	1
NOS + lobular invasive	NOS*	1
NOS + lobular invasive	Lobular invasive*	1
Lobular invasive	NOS + lobular invasive*	1
Medullary	NOS + tubular	1
Total		13

*Could represent portion of combination tumor.
NOS = Not otherwise specified.

magnitude of difference noted with these discriminants was not great. For instance, 12 percent of patients with tumors ≥ 2 cm had reoccurrences, whereas 7 percent with tumors <2 cm had such an event. Reoccurrences in the lumpectomy and irradiation group were related only to intralymphatic extension in the primary cancer ($p = 0.07$).

There was no relationship between reoccurrences in the breast and the level of estrogen and progesterone receptors of the primary cancer. The mean largest

Table 29–32. PATHOLOGICAL FEATURES RELATED TO LOCAL BREAST TUMOR REOCCURRENCE

Feature	After All Lumpectomies		After Lumpectomy + Radiation	
	%	p	%	p
Tumor size ≥ 2 cm	12 vs 7*	0.02	5 vs. 2	0.16
Nuclear grade		0.002		0.42
Grade 1	4		5	
Grade 2	8		3	
Grade 3	13		5	
Histological grade		0.01		0.11
Grade 1	2		0	
Grade 2	9		3	
Grade 3	12		6	
Intralymphatic extension		0.0004		0.07
Yes	41†		8	
No	12		3	

*12% of patients with tumors ≥ 2 cm had reoccurrence, whereas 7% with tumors <2 cm had reoccurrence.
†41% of patients with intralymphatic extension had reoccurrence, whereas 12% without intralymphatic extension had reoccurrence.

diameters of the initial and recurrent cancers were 2.5 ± 1.3 and 2.4 ± 1.4, respectively.

These findings indicate that the majority of breast tumor reoccurrences are a result of residual tumor. Whether those reoccurrences that exhibited a different histological appearance represent de novo cancers or are a portion of a combination tumor cannot be stated with certainty. Nevertheless, at the time of these analyses, the findings minimize the clinical significance of multicentric foci of cancer within the breast as a deterrent to performing lumpectomy.

This study has revealed three presentations of local tumor reoccurrence. In the most common presentation, the recurring lesion appears localized. In the second, more diffuse breast involvement is apparent, both clinically and pathologically. This presentation simulates inflammatory breast cancer or its occult form[53] and is often associated with skin and/or nipple involvement. The tumor is exceedingly multifocal or infiltrative or reflects the phenomenon of intramammary metastases. Intralymphatic extension is conspicuous, not only locally but in other quadrants and often in the skin of the breast as well. The third form of reoccurrence may represent a variant of the second and is characterized by intralymphatic extension to dermal or nipple lymphatics.

The second and third forms of reoccurrence appear to be local phenomena of highly aggressive cancers rather than an induced biological change attendant with lumpectomy. In support of this view is the failure to recognize any significant difference in the histological grades of all except two of the primary cancers and their local reoccurrences. In neither of these two with differing grades was the reoccurrence of the diffuse type. This information also suggests that, once established, it is highly unlikely that the histological grade vis-à-vis differentiation of breast cancer changes. This interpretation coincides with our previous assessment of the nuclear grades of primary breast cancer and their nodal metastases.[39]

Several pathological discriminants were recognized that appear to be statistically related to reoccurrence following lumpectomy. The magnitude of their significance, however, does not appear to be great. The only feature suggestively found to be related to reoccurrence in the lumpectomy and irradiation group was intralymphatic extension. Our experience differs from that of Schnitt, Harris, Connolly and associates,[9, 45, 66] who related reoccurrence following biopsy and irradiation of breast cancer to anaplasia and a marked or moderate intraductal component of the initial cancer. One reason for the failure to recognize the latter component as significant may well be the relatively frequent (44 percent) presence of an intraductal component at the periphery of all invasive breast cancers. The failure to discern any adverse effect of local reoccurrence on the ultimate survival of patients indicates to us that some of these events, particularly those mimicking occult inflammatory cancer, represent local manifestations of highly aggressive cancers that would not be influenced by any form of local control. This, as well as the relative infrequency of local breast tumor reoccurrence following lumpectomy and irradiation, indicates to us that there are no pathological discriminants that would appear to contraindicate lumpectomy and irradiation.

Disease-Free Survival, Distant Disease–Free Survival, and Overall Survival

Life table estimates at the end of 8 years of follow-up indicate no significant difference in disease-free survival, distant disease–free survival, or overall survival between patients treated by total mastectomy and axillary dissection and those treated by lumpectomy and axillary dissection without breast radiation (Table 29–33). Similarly, there was no significant difference when the patients treated by total mastectomy were compared with those managed by lumpectomy, axillary dissection, and breast radiation. The means $\pm$ S.E. for the three treatments are remarkably similar when examined relative to each of the outcome determinants. Life table plots through the entire 8 years of follow-up further emphasize the lack of difference between the groups (Figs. 29–90 and 29–91).

When negative-node patients treated by total mastectomy were compared with those managed by lumpectomy and breast radiation, there was no significant difference at 8 years after operation between the two groups relative to the three end points of outcome

Table 29–33. COMPARISON OF TOTAL MASTECTOMY (TM) WITH LUMPECTOMY AND WITH LUMPECTOMY PLUS RADIATION (XRT): LIFE TABLE ESTIMATES 8 YEARS AFTER OPERATION

	TM (590 pts.), %	Lumpectomy (636 pts.), %	Lumpectomy + XRT (629 pts.), %
Disease–free survival	58 ± 2.6*	54 ± 2.4 ($p = 0.3$)	59 ± 2.5 ($p = 0.2$)
Distant disease–free survival	65 ± 2.6	62 ± 2.3 ($p = 0.4$)	64 ± 2.5 ($p = 1.0$)
Survival	71 ± 2.6	71 ± 2.4 ($p = 0.8$)	65 ± 2.1 ($p = 0.3$)

*Mean $\pm$ S.E.

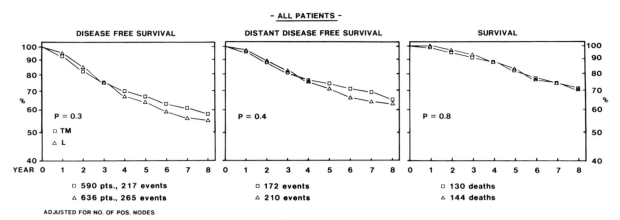

Figure 29–90. Total mastectomy vs. lumpectomy.

(Table 29–34). A comparison of negative-node patients managed by total mastectomy with those treated by lumpectomy without irradiation also indicated no significant survival difference after 8 years. There was a 5 percent greater disease-free survival and a 4 percent greater distant disease–free survival for those in the total mastectomy group. There was no significant difference in any of the three end points of outcome when positive-node patients treated by total mastectomy were compared with similar patients in either of the lumpectomy groups.

When a comparison was made between the two lumpectomy groups, (i.e., those with and without breast radiation), there was a 5 percent greater disease-free survival for all patients receiving breast radiation ($p = 0.01$; Fig. 29–92). There was, however, no significant difference between the two groups with respect to distant disease–free survival ($p = 0.2$) or overall survival ($p = 0.3$). In negative-node patients, there was a 5 percent greater disease-free survival after 8 years of follow-up for those undergoing lumpectomy and radiation therapy, but there was no significant difference in distant disease–free survival (1.8 percent; $p = 0.1$) or overall survival (5.3 percent; $p = 0.5$). In patients with positive nodes, there was no significant difference between the two groups for each of the three end points.

COMMENTS

The increasing use of lumpectomy has given rise to several issues that require attention. The following paragraphs present personal views regarding those issues that I deem to be important.

Reappraisal of Breast Biopsy. Paradoxically, just at the time when the two-stage biopsy procedure has gained acceptance, not only is there a need to reassess the merit of that approach, but it is also necessary to reappraise and modify the entire method for breast cancer biopsy. With the increasing use of breast-conserving operations and evidence supporting their credibility, there is a need to reevaluate the surgical strategy employed in breast cancer management. I recently described how my experience acquired with lumpectomy altered not only my views and policies relative to breast biopsy, but also my entire approach to breast cancer surgery.[18] A detailed algorithm describing an optimal surgical strategy for the management of primary breast cancer was presented (Fig. 29–93). It was pointed out that as a result of the increasing acceptance of lumpectomy, arguments for use of the two-stage procedure are in many, if not most, instances nullified and obsolete. As in the Halstedian era (but now for different reasons), there is justification for performing more, rather than

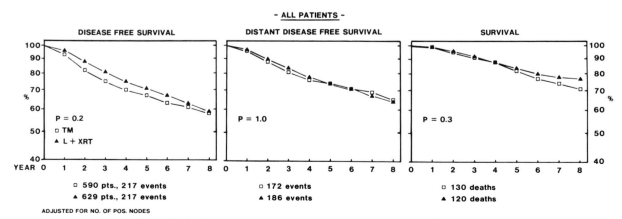

Figure 29–91. Total mastectomy vs. lumpectomy plus breast radiation.

Table 29–34. COMPARISON OF TOTAL MASTECTOMY WITH LUMPECTOMY AND WITH LUMPECTOMY PLUS RADIATION THERAPY ACCORDING TO NODAL STATUS: LIFE TABLE ESTIMATES 8 YEARS AFTER SURGERY

Treatment Group	Disease–Free Survival (%)	Distant Disease–Free Survival (%)	Survival (%)
NEGATIVE-NODE PTS.			
Total Mastectomy (N = 366)	65.5 ± 3.3*	73.8 ± 3.2	78.7 ± 3.2
Lumpectomy (N = 392)	60.7 ± 2.8	69.6 ± 2.6	76.6 ± 2.8
Lumpectomy and Irradiation (N = 399)	65.6 ± 3.3	70.7 ± 3.2	82.9 ± 2.3
POSITIVE-NODE PTS.†			
Total Mastectomy (N = 224)	44.5 ± 4.0	50.7 ± 4.2	59.9 ± 4.1
Lumpectomy (N = 244)	41.6 ± 4.1	49.1 ± 4.6	60.3 ± 4.5
Lumpectomy and Irradiation (N = 230)	46.6 ± 4.1	53.1 ± 3.9	68.3 ± 3.9

*Mean ± S.E.
†Values are adjusted for the number of positive nodes (1 to 3, 4 to 9, or ≥10).

fewer, biopsies with general anesthesia and for carrying out biopsy and the definitive operation more frequently in one stage. It is an absolute dictum that all open breast biopsies be carried out as if a lumpectomy were being performed. Attention must be given to ensuring that specimen margins are likely to be free of tumor should a tumor be encountered. Today, biopsy done without attention to specimen margins is inappropriate. In all circumstances where breast conservation is feasible, the operation carried out to establish the definitive *diagnosis* of a breast lesion becomes the definitive *treatment* along with axillary dissection.

Lumpectomy in Conjunction with Systemic Therapy. It is becoming increasingly meaningless to discuss the surgical management of breast cancer without considering how other therapeutic modalities might influence the surgeon's operative approach. It is highly likely that with the use of more effective systemic therapy following operation, the incidence of breast tumor reoccurrence will be lower than has been observed as a result of lumpectomy and breast radiation alone. This finding is already evident in more recent NSABP studies. The NSABP B-06 study, which provided data for this chapter, was almost entirely concerned with assessing local/regional disease control by lumpectomy and radiation without serious regard for how systemic therapy might affect patient outcome as influenced by the surgery. The study has, however, provided evidence to indicate the value of chemotherapy in enhancing the benefit from lumpectomy and radiation. In the B-06 trial, only positive-node patients received systemic chemotherapy (melphalan + 5-fluorouracil), which had been demonstrated in a prior NSABP study to modestly improve disease-free survival and survival of positive-node patients following total mastectomy and axillary dissection. It has been observed that the incidence of breast tumor reoccurrence in the B-06 trial was lower in positive-node lumpectomy patients who received breast irradiation than in negative-node lumpectomy patients who received breast irradiation but no chemotherapy.

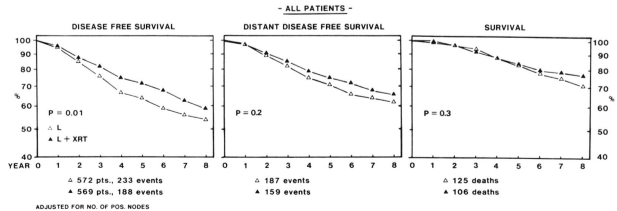

Figure 29–92. Lumpectomy vs. lumpectomy plus breast radiation.

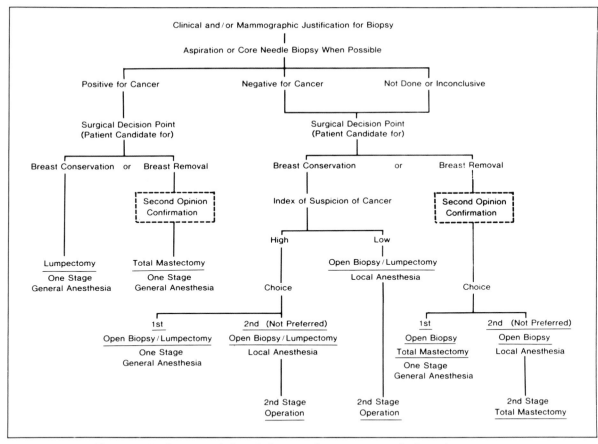

Figure 29–93. Recommended surgical strategy for management of primary breast cancer.

In two recent NSABP studies evaluating the use of adjuvant chemotherapy in node-negative breast cancer patients, evidence has indicated that effective systemic therapy reduces the incidence of breast tumor reoccurrence following lumpectomy and radiation.[21, 22] Those patients with estrogen receptor–(ER-) negative tumors received either no systemic therapy or methotrexate followed by 5-fluorouracil and leucovorin calcium. The patients with ER-positive tumors were randomized between placebo and tamoxifen. After 4 years of follow-up in both studies, the lumpectomy-treated, breast-irradiated patients who received either methotrexate and fluorouracil or tamoxifen had fewer breast tumor reoccurrences than did the untreated or placebo-treated control groups. In regard to the incidence of breast tumor reoccurrence, we are awaiting findings from ongoing NSABP trials evaluating more aggressive chemotherapy regimens in stage II lumpectomy-treated patients.

Systemic therapy may also influence breast-conserving procedures by its use prior to operation. Recently the NSABP judged that there is sufficient biological and clinical information available to justify the conduct of a randomized clinical trial to determine whether preoperative chemotherapy will more effectively prolong the disease-free survival and overall survival of patients with stages I and II breast cancer than will the same therapy given postoperatively. That study (B-18), which has already been implemented, will also evaluate the response of the primary tumor to preoperative chemotherapy and will correlate the response to the ultimate disease-free survival and survival of the patient. That study is of particular importance to the surgeon. It will determine whether preoperative chemotherapy can reduce the size of a large primary tumor sufficiently to permit a breast-conserving operation with a low incidence of ipsilateral breast tumor reoccurrence.

It is likely that a reduction in the extent of surgery may indeed result, since it has been demonstrated by other investigators that there was a 90 percent objective response following the use of primary chemotherapy for stage III disease.[67] A complete response was observed in 50 percent of these patients. Others have reported a similar experience with locally advanced disease.[49] Thus it is reasonable to speculate that the present paradigm used for the management of breast cancer—operation followed by systemic therapy—may be replaced by another that makes current management anachronistic. With the advent of increasingly better diagnostic procedures and the availability of better regimens of therapy, this outcome is almost inevitable.

SUMMARY

This chapter provides results obtained from patients who were entered into the NSABP clinical trial evaluating breast conservation. Eight years following operation, the findings continue to justify the use of lumpectomy followed by breast irradiation for patients with stages I and II breast cancer ≤4 cm, provided that resected specimen margins are free of tumor and that systemic adjuvant therapy is administered to those with pathologically positive axillary lymph nodes. The findings continue to support the validity of the alternative paradigm for breast cancer management that I proposed in the 1960s.

ACKNOWLEDGMENTS

Most of the information presented was obtained as a result of support by a Public Health Service grant from the National Cancer Institute (NCI-U10-CA-12027) and by a grant from the American Cancer Society (ACS-RC-13).

References

1. Amalric R, Santamaria F, Robert F, Seigle J, Altshuler C, Pietra JC, Amalric F, Kurtz JM, Spitalier JM, Brandone H, Ayme Y, Pollet JF, Bressac C, Fondarai J: Conservative therapy in operable breast cancer—results at five, ten and fifteen years in 2216 consecutive cases. *In* Harris JR, Hellman S, Silen W (eds): Conservative Management of Breast Cancer. Philadelphia, JB Lippincott, 1983, pp 15–21.
2. Andreassen M, Dahl-Iversen E, Sorensen B: Extended exeresis of regional lymph nodes at operation for carcinoma of the breast and result of 5-year follow-up of first 98 cases with removal of axillary as well as supraclavicular gland. Acta Chir Scand 107:206–213, 1954.
3. Baclesse F: Five year results in 431 breast cancers treated solely by roentgentherapy. Ann Surg 161:103–104, 1965.
4. Caceres E: An evaluation of radical mastectomy and extended radical mastectomy for cancer of the breast. Surg Gynecol Obstet 125:337–341, 1967.
5. Calle R, Pilleron JP, Schlienger P, Vilcoq JR: Conservative management of operable breast cancer: ten years experience at the Foundation Curie. Cancer 42:2045–2053, 1978.
6. Calle R, Vilcoq JR, Pilleron JP, Schlienger P, Durand JC: Conservative treatment of operable breast carcinoma by irradiation with or without limited surgery—ten-year results. *In* Harris JR, Hellman S, Silen W (eds): Conservative Management of Breast Cancer. Philadelphia, JB Lippincott, 1983, pp 3–9.
7. Cancer Research Campaign Working Party: Cancer research campaign (King's/Cambridge) trial for early breast cancer. Lancet 2:55–60, 1980.
8. Coman DR: Mechanisms responsible for the origin and distribution of blood-borne tumor metastases: a review. Cancer Res 13:397–404, 1953.
9. Connolly JL, Schnitt SJ, Harris JR, Hellman S, Cohen RB: Pathologic correlates of local tumor control following primary radiation therapy in patients with early breast cancer. *In* Harris JR, Hellman S, Silen W (eds): Conservative Management of Breast Cancer. Philadelphia, JB Lippincott, 1983, pp 123–136.
10. Cope O, Wang CA, Chu A, Wang CC, Schulz M, Castleman B, Long J, Sohier WD: Limited surgical excision as the basis of a comprehensive therapy for cancer of the breast. Am J Surg 131:400–406, 1976.
11. Crile G Jr: Treatment of breast cancer by local excision. Am J Surg 109:400, 1965.
12. Fisher B: The surgical dilemma in the primary therapy of invasive breast cancer: a critical appraisal. Curr Probl Surg, October: 3–53, 1970.
13. Fisher B: Cancer: A Comprehensive Treatise, vol 6. New York, Plenum, 1977, pp 401–421.
14. Fisher B: Breast cancer management: alternatives to radical mastectomy. N Engl J Med 301:326–328, 1979.
15. Fisher B: Laboratory and clinical research in breast cancer—a personal adventure: the David A Karnofsky Memorial Lecture. Cancer Res 40:3863–3874, 1980.
16. Fisher B: The interdependence of laboratory and clinical research in the study of metastases. *In* Nicolson GL and Miles L (eds): Cancer Invasion and Metastasis: Biologic and Therapeutic Aspects. New York, Raven Press, 1984, pp 27–46.
17. Fisher B: The Role of Science in the Evolution of Breast Cancer Management. Austin, TX, University of Texas Press, 1984, pp 1–21.
18. Fisher B: Reappraisal of breast biopsy prompted by the use of lumpectomy. JAMA 253:3585–3588, 1985.
19. Fisher B: The revolution in breast cancer surgery: science or anecdotalism? World J Surg 9:655–666, 1985.
20. Fisher B: Conservative surgery: the American experience. Semin Oncol 13:425–433, 1986.
21. Fisher B: Sequential methotrexate and 5-fluorouracil for the treatment of node negative breast cancer patients with estrogen receptor negative tumors: results from NSABP protocol B-13. N Engl J Med 320:473–478, 1989.
22. Fisher B: Tamoxifen for the treatment of node negative breast cancer patients with estrogen receptor positive tumors: results from NSABP protocol B-14. N Engl J Med 320:479–484, 1989.
23. Fisher B, Bauer M, Margolese R, Poisson R, Pilch Y, Redmond C, Fisher ER, Wolmark N, Deutsch M, Montague E, Saffer E, Wickerham L, Lerner H, Glass A, Shibata H, Deckers P, Ketcham A, Oishi R, Russell I: Five-year results of a randomized clinical trial comparing total mastectomy and segmental mastectomy with or without radiation in the treatment of breast cancer. N Engl J Med 312:665–673, 1985.
24. Fisher B, Bauer M, Wickerham L, Redmond CK, Fisher ER: Relation of number of positive axillary nodes to the prognosis of patients with primary breast cancer—an NSABP update. (With the contribution of Anatolio Cruz, Roger Foster, Bernard Gardener, Lerner Harvey, Margolese R, Poisson R, Shibata H, Volk H, and other NSABP Investigators) Cancer 52:1551–1557, 1983.
25. Fisher B, Fisher ER: Experimental evidence in support of the dormant tumor cell. Science 130:918, 1959.
26. Fisher B, Fisher ER: The organ distribution of disseminated ^{51}Cr-labeled tumor cells. Cancer Res 27:412, 1967.
27. Fisher B, Fisher ER: Studies concerning the regional lymph node in cancer I. Initiation of immunity. Cancer 27:1001, 1971.
28. Fisher B, Fisher ER: The interrelationship of hematogenous and lymphatic tumor cell dissemination. Surg Gynecol Obstet 122:791, 1976.
29. Fisher B, Fisher ER, Feduska N: Trauma and the localization of tumor cells. Cancer 20:23–30, 1967.
30. Fisher B, Gebhardt MC: The evolution of breast cancer surgery: past, present and future. Semin Oncol 5:385–394, 1978.
31. Fisher B, Redmond C, Fisher ER, Bauer M, Wolmark N, Wickerham L, Deutsch M, Montague E, Margolese R, Foster R: Ten year results of a randomized clinical trial comparing radical mastectomy and total mastectomy with or without radiation. N Engl J Med 312:674–681, 1985.
32. Fisher B, Redmond C, Poisson R, Caplan R, Wickerham L, Wolmark N, Fisher E, Deutsch M, Margolese R, Pilch Y, Glass A, Shibata H, Lerner H, Terz J, Sidorovich L. Eight year results of the NSABP randomized clinical trial comparing total mastectomy and lumpectomy with or without radiation in the treatment of breast cancer. N Engl J Med 320(13):822–828, 1989.
33. Fisher B, Saffer E, Fisher ER: Studies concerning the regional lymph nodes in cancer. IV. Tumor inhibition by regional lymph node cells. Cancer 33:631–636, 1974.
34. Fisher B, Slack NH: Number of lymph nodes examined and the prognosis of breast carcinoma. Surg Gynecol Obstet 131:79, 1970.

35. Fisher B, Slack NH, Ausman RK, Bross IDJ: Location of breast carcinoma and prognosis. Surg Gynecol Obstet 129:705–716, 1969.
36. Fisher B, Wolmark N: New concepts in the management of primary breast cancer. Cancer 36:627–632, 1975.
37. Fisher B, Wolmark N, Bauer M, Redmond C, Gebhardt M: The accuracy of clinical nodal staging and of limited axillary dissection as a determinant of histologic nodal status in carcinoma of the breast. Surg Gynecol Obstet 152:765–772, 1981.
38. Fisher B, Wolmark N, Fisher ER, Deutsch M: Lumpectomy and axillary dissection for breast cancer: surgical, pathological, and radiation consideration. World J Surg 9:692–698, 1985.
39. Fisher ER, Palekar AS, Sass R, Fisher B: Pathologic findings from the National Surgical Adjuvant Breast Project (protocol 4): IX. Scar cancers. Breast Cancer Res Treat 3:39–59, 1983.
40. Fisher ER, Sass R, Fisher B, Gregorio R, Brown R, Wickerham L, and collaborating NSABP investigators: Pathologic findings from the National Surgical Adjuvant Breast Project (protocol 6). II. Relation of local breast recurrence to multicentricity. Cancer 57:1717–1724, 1986.
41. Halsted WS: The results of radical operations for the cure of carcinoma of the breast. Ann Surg 46:1–19, 1907.
42. Handley RD: The technic and results of conservative radical mastectomy (Patey's operation). Prog Clin Cancer 1:462, 1965.
43. Handley WS: *In* Murray A (ed): Cancer of the Breast and Its Operative Treatment. London, Hoeber Publishing, 1922.
44. Harris JR, Botnick L, Bloomer WD, Chaffey JT, Hellman S: Primary radiation therapy for early breast cancer: the experience at the joint center for radiation therapy. Int J Radiat Oncol Biol Phys 7:1549–1552, 1981.
45. Harris JR, Connolly JL, Schnitt SJ, Cohen RB, Hellman S: Clinical pathologic study of early breast cancer treated by primary radiation therapy. J Clin Oncol 1:184–189, 1983.
46. Harris JR, Hellman S: Primary radiation therapy for early breast cancer. Cancer 52:2547–2552, 1983.
47. Harris JR, Levine MB, Hellman S: Results of treating stage I and II carcinoma of the breast with primary radiation therapy. Cancer Treat Rep 62:985–991, 1978.
48. Hellman S, Harris JR, Levene MB: Radiation therapy of early carcinoma of the breast without mastectomy. Cancer 46:988–994, 1980.
49. Jacquillat C, Baillet F, Blondon J, Auclerc G, Lefranc JP, Maylin CI, Weil M: Preliminary results of "neoadjuvant" chemotherapy in initial management of breast cancer (BC). Proc Am Soc Clin Oncol 2:C-437, 112, 1983.
50. Keynes G: Radium treatment of primary carcinoma of the breast. Lancet 2:108, 1928.
51. Lacour J: The place of the Halsted operation in treatment of breast cancer. Int Surg 47:282, 1967.
52. Levene MBF, Harris JR, Hellman S: Treatment of carcinoma of the breast by radiation therapy. Cancer 39:2840–2845, 1977.
53. Lucas FV, Perez-Mesa C: Inflammatory carcinoma of the breast. Cancer 41:1595–1605, 1978.
54. Margolese R, et al: The technique of segmental mastectomy (lumpectomy) and axillary dissection: a syllabus from the National Surgical Adjuvant Breast Project workshops. Surgery 102:828–834, 1987.
55. Margottini M, Bucalossi P: El metastasi lymphoghiandolari mammario interne nel cancro delia mammella. Boll Oncol 23:2, 1949.
56. McWhirter R: The value of simple mastectomy and radiotherapy in the treatment of cancer of the breast. Br J Radiol 21:599–610, 1948.
57. Montague ED, Gutierrez AE, Barker JL, Tapley N, Fletcher GH: Conservative surgery and irradiation for the treatment of favorable breast cancer. Cancer 43:1058–1061, 1979.
58. Mustakallio S: Treatment of breast cancer by tumor extirpation and roentgen therapy instead of radical operation. J Fac Radiol 6:23, 1954.
59. Peters MV: Wedge resection and irradiation, and effective treatment in early breast cancer. JAMA 200:134–135, 1967.
60. Peters MV: Cutting the "Gordian Knot" in early breast cancer. Ann R Coll Phys Surg Can 8:186–192, 1975.
61. Peters MV: Wedge resection with or without radiation in early breast cancer. Int J Radiat Oncol 2:1151–1156, 1977.
62. Pierquin B: Conservative treatment for carcinoma of the breast: experience of Creteil—ten year results. *In* Harris JR, Hellman S, Silen W (eds): Conservative Management of Breast Cancer. Philadelphia, JB Lippincott, 1983, pp 11–14.
63. Pierquin B, et al: Radical radiation therapy of breast cancer. Int J Radiat Oncol Biol Phys 6:17, 1980.
64. Porritt A: Early carcinoma of the breast. Br J Surg 51:214, 1964.
65. Prosnitz LR, Goldenberg IS, Packard RA, Levene MB, Harris J, Hellman S, Wallner PE, Brady LW, Mansfield CM, Kramer S: Radiation therapy as initial treatment for early stage cancer of the breast without mastectomy. Cancer 39:917–923, 1977.
66. Schnitt SJ, Connolly JL, Harris JR, Hellman S, Cohen RB: Pathologic predictors of early local recurrence in stage I and II breast cancer treated by primary radiation therapy. Cancer 53:1049–1057, 1984.
67. Sorace RA, Bagley CS, Lichter AS, Danforth DN, Wesley MW, Young RC, Lippman ME: The management of nonmetastatic locally advanced breast cancer using primary induction chemotherapy with hormonal synchronization followed by radiation therapy with or without debulking surgery. World J Surg 9:775–785, 1985.
68. Sugarbaker ED: Extended radical mastectomy. Its superiority in the treatment of breast cancer. JAMA 187:96–99, 1964.
69. Urban JA: Discussion on radical mastectomy in breast cancer with supraclavicular and/or internal mammary node dissection. Proc Natl Cancer Conf 2:243, 1952.
70. Veronesi U, Zingo L: Extended mastectomy for cancer of the breast. Cancer 20:677–680, 1967.
71. Virchow R: Cellular Pathology. Translated by Frank Chase. Philadelphia, JB Lippincott, 1863.
72. Volcoq JR, et al: The outcome of treatment of tumorectomy and radiotherapy of patients with operable breast cancer. Radiat Oncol Biol Phys 7:1327, 1981.
73. Wangensteen OH: Super-radical operation for breast cancer in the patient with lymph node involvement. Proc Natl Cancer Conf 2:230, 1952.
74. Weber E, Hellman S: Radiation as primary treatment for local control of breast carcinoma. A progress report. JAMA 234:608–611, 1975.

EXTENDED SIMPLE MASTECTOMY

Edward M. Copeland III, M.D. and Kirby I. Bland, M.D.

The surgical definition of extended simple mastectomy is removal of the breast in continuity with Level I lymph nodes. In the procedure, the surgeon deliberately leaves intact Levels II and III lymph nodes of the axilla. The need for such an operation arises when radiation therapy to the apical axilla and supraclavicular region is indicated in conjunction with an axillary dissection or when an axillary lymph node sampling is required at the time of an indicated total mastectomy.

In 1972, Charles McBride[4] of the M.D. Anderson Hospital popularized the operation, although a look at the specimen photographed in Halsted's initial description of the radical mastectomy indicates the contents of the procedure may have been only the breast and Level I lymph nodes.[2] No chest wall muscles are visible.

Radiation therapy to the axilla should not be used in conjunction with complete surgical dissection (Patey operation) of the axilla. Major lymphatic channels are removed surgically, and collateral channels draining the arm are damaged by radiation therapy. The result is symptomatic lymphedema of the ipsilateral extremity. When the surgeon determines that all disease cannot be removed from the axilla by any surgical procedure and that radiation therapy to this area is inevitable, then only the bulky metastatic disease in Level I and Level II lymph nodes should be removed surgically. As a rule, moderate doses of radiation therapy will sterilize lymph nodes 1 cm or smaller in size; therefore metastatic cancer in smaller, centrally located axillary lymph nodes (high Level II and Level III), often attached to or invasive of axillary structures and not adequately removed surgically, is sterilized by radiation therapy. By such a combination of therapeutic modalities, the entire axilla is treated with minimal overlap of radiation portals with the surgically dissected portion of the axilla. The entire axilla is irradiated with less chance of resultant symptomatic lymphedema.

The operation is ideally suited to the treatment of advanced stage III and inflammatory breast cancer. Preoperative chemotherapy will reduce the size of axillary metastases and will often reduce the size of the primary lesion, making operation possible. Even if a complete response to chemotherapy is obtained, extended simple mastectomy is still recommended, since the majority of patients will have microscopic residual breast cancer.[1, 3] Radiation therapy to the chest wall, apical axilla, and internal mammary and supraclavicular lymph nodes is used postoperatively to decrease the incidence of chest wall recurrence. Radiation therapy should be started as soon as adequate wound healing has occurred. Consequently, thick skin flaps should be elevated, using the plane of the retinaculae cutis. All attempts to prevent skin slough should be employed. Because radiation therapy will be used, the skin incision to initiate the skin flaps can be relatively close to the tumor mass, since any residual disease remaining after the dissection will be in the radiation treatment field.

Extended simple mastectomy is also indicated when preoperative radiation therapy (with or without chemotherapy) is employed with treatment fields that cover the apical axilla or the supraclavicular region. A therapeutic dose of radiation should sterilize these areas. Surgical dissection of high Level II and Level III lymph nodes adds minimal therapeutic benefit and dramatically increases (seven- to tenfold) the incidence of symptomatic lymphedema of the ipsilateral arm.

The need for sampling of lymph nodes and the need for mastectomy when treating carcinoma *in situ* is controversial. Certainly, when intraductal carcinoma is multifocal, knowledge of axillary nodal status is important, since microscopic foci of invasive breast cancer may coexist and have the potential to metastasize to axillary lymph nodes. If total mastectomy is the treatment selected for the breast, the en bloc Level I axillary lymph node dissection adds minimum morbidity, gives adequate information as to the pathological status of the axilla, and allows easy access to the subpectoral area for breast reconstruction.

TECHNIQUE

The arm is draped free so that the elbow may be flexed or extended and the arm adducted across the chest wall. A roll is placed parallel to the thoracic spine beneath the ipsilateral scapula.

The orientation of the skin incision is somewhat dictated by the location of the tumor mass. To minimize bleeding of the inferior incision while the superior flap is developed, the superior flap is elevated first, before beginning the incision that outlines the inferior flap. Medially, the upper margin of the superior flap is the medial half of the clavicle; laterally, it is the deltopectoral triangle and cephalic vein. The lateral portion of the superior flap is developed until the anterior edge of the latissimus dorsi muscle is identified, at which point the superior flap is developed laterally and superiorly following the anterior edge of the latissimus dorsi muscle cephalad (Fig. 29–94). As the dissection continues toward the axilla, the major branch of the intercostobrachial nerve is identified and sacrificed. This nerve is

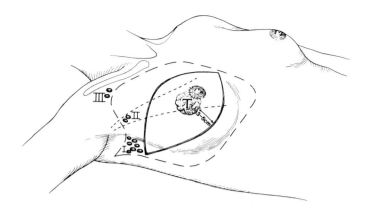

Figure 29–94. Limits of dissection for the extended simple mastectomy (dotted line). The dissection is inclusive of tumor and overlying skin, with an adequate skin margin to allow primary wound closure. Only Level I and lower Level II nodes are dissected en bloc with the breast.

composed of fibers from the lateral cutaneous branches of the second and third intercostal nerves and runs at right angles and anterior to the latissimus dorsi muscle. It should not be confused with either the thoracodorsal or long thoracic nerve. The dissection is continued cephalad following the anterior border of latissimus dorsi muscles until the white tendon of the latissimus dorsi muscle is identified. Immediately superior and anterior to this tendon, the axillary vein is identified and exposed.

Attention is then turned to dissection of the inferior flap, a portion of the operation that should proceed expeditiously, since the investing fascia of the breast is usually easy to identify inferiorly, and the position of the anterior border of the latissimus dorsi muscle is known laterally. In raising the skin flaps medially, the plane of penetration of the pectoralis major fascia by the perforating branches of the internal mammary vessel should be used as a guide for the medial extension of the dissection. Several of these branches often can be preserved, and the dissection should not need to extend to the middle of the sternum to remove all breast tissue.

The breast is dissected free from the pectoralis major muscle, beginning superomedially and progressing inferolaterally until the lateral border of the muscle is identified almost in its entirety (except for the superiormost portion, which crosses anterior and lateral to the latissimus dorsi muscle to insert on the humerus).

Allis clamps are placed on the lateral border of the pectoralis major muscle, and the muscle is retracted anteriorly and medially. Dissection is continued lateral and posterior to the pectoralis major muscle to identify the lateral border of the pectoralis minor muscle. The entire innervation of the pectoralis major and minor muscles can be preserved in this operation. The medial pectoral nerve is identified coursing lateral to (or penetrating) the pectoralis minor muscle at approximately the juncture of the superior two thirds of the muscle with the lateral one third. Only rarely will the medially placed lateral pectoral nerve be visualized in this procedure, as Level II and Level III nodes are incompletely exposed. The (lateral) neurovascular bundle that contains the medial pectoral nerve can be easily severed inadvertently. It represents an important landmark as it courses posterior to the pectoralis minor muscle with

vascular and neural origin from the thoracoacromial trunk of the axillary artery, the axillary vein, and the medial cord of the brachial plexus.

The clavipectoral fascia lateral to the pectoralis minor muscle is opened, and the axillary vein is again identified.

Working laterally along the axillary vein, the venous tributaries coursing inferiorly are divided and ligated. Laterally, the neurovascular bundle to the latissimus dorsi muscle is identified; this bundle contains the thoracodorsal nerve and major branches of the subscapular artery and vein. The lateral thoracic artery is usually identified just medial to it. The full extent of the thoracodorsal neurovascular bundle is often best demonstrated by dissecting the fibrofatty tissue from the anterior border of the latissimus dorsi muscle and retracting it laterally and inferiorly. At the site of confluence of the thoracodorsal neurovascular trunk with the latissimus dorsi muscle, a venous tributary courses medially to join the chest wall. At this site, with meticulous dissection in a plane parallel with the long axis of the patient, the long thoracic nerve to the serratus anterior muscle (respiratory nerve of Bell) is best identified. The long thoracic nerve is traced superiorly until it exits the operative field posterior to the axillary vein.

The axillary contents are removed from the serratus anterior muscle anterior and medial to the long thoracic nerve. The superior extent of the axillary dissection was defined previously by the axillary vein, and the medial extent of the dissection is represented by the lateral borders of the pectoralis major and minor muscles as well as the medial pectoral nerve and accompanying vascular structures. Any lymph nodes that are clinically positive and larger than 1 cm in size should be removed from beneath the pectoralis minor muscle (within Level II lymph nodes). As the Level I axillary contents are removed from the serratus anterior muscle, the lateral cutaneous branches of the second and third intercostal nerves and accompanying vascular structures are identified, severed, and ligated.

The specimen is removed from the operative field, and the wound is irrigated copiously with warm saline. Instruments and gloves are discarded for clean ones. Two large-bore suction catheters are inserted, one anterior to the pectoralis major muscle and the other posterior to it within the dissected axilla. The drains are sutured in place at the skin entrance site. The wound is closed with interrupted absorbable sutures in the subcutaneous tissue, and the skin is closed with staples or optional subcuticular absorbable sutures. Continuous suction is maintained on the drains by attachment to a suction apparatus that generates approximately 60 cm of water-negative pressure, and a pressure dressing is applied to be removed within 48 hours. The drains are removed when their output falls below 20 ml per 24 hours. Following drain removal, shoulder exercises are begun.

References

1. Bonadonna G, Valagussa P, Zambetti M, Zucali R: Locally advanced breast cancer: 10-year results after combined treatment. Proc Am Soc Clin Oncol 7:9, 1988.
2. Halsted WS: The results of operations for the cure of cancer of the breast performed at the Johns Hopkins Hospital from June 1889, to January 1894. Ann Surg 20:497–555, 1894.
3. Manji M, Ragaz J, Worth A, Plenderleith IH, Harman J, Knowling M, Olivotto I, Basco V: Is mastectomy indicated in patients with stage III breast cancer treated with preoperative (neoadjuvant) therapy? Proc Am Soc Clin Oncol 7:36, 1988.
4. McBride CM: Extended simple mastectomy: anatomic definition and uses. South Med J 65:1427–1431, 1972.

Chapter 30

BREAST RECONSTRUCTION FOLLOWING MASTECTOMY

John B. McCraw, M.D., Anne R. Cramer, M.D., and Charles E. Horton, M.D.

FUNCTIONAL ASPECTS OF BREAST RECONSTRUCTION

We usually think of a *functional* replacement as one in which bodily functions, strength, or range of motion are enhanced or replaced, but this definition is not applicable to the breast. After the age of lactation has been passed, the only purpose or function of the mature adult breast is the part it plays in the body form (i.e., its appearance). In this case, the replacement of the breast *form* constitutes the replacement of the breast *function*. Although the adult breast has been described as an unnecessary appendage, an absent breast has the same functional significance as an absent nose or ear. It is certainly possible to live without these visible structures, but their absence materially diminishes the quality of life.

It is only within the past 10 years that reconstructive procedures on the breast following mastectomy have been considered "functional" rather than "cosmetic" in nature. A cosmetic procedure is one that improves the appearance of a feature that would be considered to be within the broad range of normal to the average observer. For instance, a large nose might be unattractive, but it could be perceived as "normal." Alternatively, it is not "normal" for a nose or a breast to be absent, even though neither causes any functional problem. Although a person's appearance may be improved by replacing the nose or the breast, such replacement is not a cosmetic procedure.

There are five essential elements of any reconstructive procedure that also apply to the extirpation and reconstruction of the breast:

1. *Survival* of the extirpation (e.g., coverage of major vessels or a chest wall defect).

2. Facilitation of an *adequate extirpation* so that coverage will be assured no matter what the extent of the surgery (e.g., mastectomy).

3. Correction of an *irradiated or scarred* operative site through the introduction of new (flap) blood supply into the injured area.

4. Recreation of the *form* of the lost part.

5. Replacement of *function* of the lost part.

The first three elements relate to soft tissue coverage and are done for reasons of safety rather than for reasons of appearance. These flap closures would be applicable to any extended type of mastectomy, such as a neglected tumor or failure of a lumpectomy-irradiation procedure. No justification is needed for these procedures other than the achievement of a healed wound.

Women are no different from men in their desire to correct a physical deformity, yet the only cancer patients who are not routinely considered for some form of reconstructive surgery are breast cancer patients. Many procedures in other areas of the body are done purely to improve form, such as the correction of a bulging but otherwise asymptomatic ventral hernia, excision of gynecomastia in the male, placement of a scrotal prosthesis, or removal of an unsightly skin graft on the arm. For some reason, it is not necessary to justify these procedures to third party carriers, but it is *always* necessary to justify any contour change or improvement of the female breast. Following a mastectomy, it must be established that the planned reconstructive procedure is not "cosmetic" (i.e., improvement of a normal breast), even though the mastectomy deformity by definition is not "normal."

It is fair to say that the eventual goal of virtually every mastectomy patient is to dress in normal clothes. To achieve this, women will go to great lengths to obtain sufficient breast symmetry to enable them to dress in sundresses and bathing suits, whether this is accomplished through the use of an external prosthesis or a reconstructive operation. Now that breast reconstruction is a reasonable surgical option in most patients, it has become the patient's choice as to what procedure will be done. It is important that the patient understand her responsibility in personally influencing the course of her future care, because these are sophisticated surgical choices. Most patients possess only selected information and have no surgical background with which to make a reasonable judgment without guidance.

For these reasons, every effort should be made to assist the patient so that sound choices will be made by all parties. It is also necessary for the oncologic surgeon to recognize the context of each type of reconstructive breast procedure to both guide the patient and develop a comprehensive treatment plan.

HISTORICAL EVOLUTION OF BREAST RECONSTRUCTION

The history of breast reconstruction primarily involves the development of silicone implants, myocutaneous flaps, and autogenous tissue transfers. These clinical applications have all occurred within the past 20 years, but their general acceptance has been realized only in the past 5 years. The clinical applicability of these new modalities has radically altered the surgical approach to the absent breast.

Silicone Implants

Silicone implants were first introduced in 1964 by Cronin and Gerow.[11] This pioneering surgical work was done in collaboration with Silas Braley of the Dow Chemical Company. Silicones are polymers that are constructed from silicon, an elemental metal adjacent to carbon on the periodic table. Silicone was chosen as the implant material because of its nonreactive implantation potential. Even today, the U.S. Pharmacopeia uses medical grade silicone as its standard for biocompatibility against which all other compounds are compared. The second reason for choosing silicone was its physiochemical characteristics, which allow a broad range of design capabilities. Linear, short-chain, lightweight silicon polymers form oils. The viscosity of silicone increases with increasing molecular weight, and heat or catalysts cause branching of the chains to form gels. With side branching of the linear chains, the oils are vulcanized into elastomers, which can be used as adhesives, sealants, and rubbers. The initial silicone implant design, a silicone gel contained within a thin, solid silicone envelope sealed with silicone adhesive, is basically unchanged to the present time.

Compared with the previously available implants made of steel, polyurethane foam, or paraffin, as well as cadaveric and autologous free fat grafts, all of which were capable of disastrous complications, the silicone gel implants represented an historic medical breakthrough. This was also the foundation for the future development of a number of new medical products from silicone, including silicone tubes, lubricants, and linings, which were similarly biologically inert.

From the outset it was presumed that these new silicone implants would contribute to some breast "firmness" through the body's normal defenses to a foreign object (i.e., scar isolation and encapsulation). The implant itself does not become firm, but the scar surrounding the implant contracts, tightens the silicone gel envelope, and converts the "teardrop" contour of the implant into a round shape. This is analogous to squeezing a balloon in your hands and causing "firmness" of the balloon. Removing your hands then causes "softness" of the balloon, even though the balloon itself is unchanged. With improvements in silicone gel during the early 1970s, it was recognized that at least some implants remained soft and barely palpable, so that naturally soft breast implantation seemed to be an achievable goal. This led to the hope that silicone breast implantation might be a reasonable method of breast enlargement for any woman with small breasts.[6, 12] A vast array of "new" implants were produced, including saline-filled implants, double-lumen implants of saline and silicone, and even an acceptable implant made of polyurethane foam, in an effort to achieve a predictably "soft" implant.[19, 37, 39–41] By the mid 1970s "Mother Nature" was the recognized winner in the determination of which breast implants would remain "soft," no matter what type of implant was used.[7, 8]

Reconstructive surgeons then attempted to favorably affect this biological balance by using pectoralis and latissimus muscle flap coverage of the implants to enhance the softness of the implants. This maneuver was helpful, but it was not the final answer hoped for. Any number of ancillary techniques were also used, including irrigation of the pocket with antibiotics, instillation of corticosteroids, and perfect hemostasis; still, a significant number of implants eventually developed "firmness."[9] The biological determination of softness or firmness of breast implants was confirmed by the unilaterality of the event. Empirical observation revealed that the usual conclusion of bilateral breast implantation was a soft implant in one breast and a firm implant in the other breast, rather than a soft or firm implant in both breasts. It was then recognized that the relative probability of bilateral versus unilateral capsular contracture followed mathematical projections for a random phenomenon. This suggests that somehow the breast itself is the determining factor, rather than any specific characteristic of the implant or some general physiological mechanism. Surgeons are always loathe to ascribe an outcome to random probabilities, particularly when it is an event they want to control, but capsular contracture around a simple implant proved to be beyond surgical control.

The incidence of capsular contracture is directly related to the quality of the soft tissue covering the implant. For instance, larger breasts are less likely to develop capsules than small breasts, and muscular coverage of the implant further reduces the incidence of this problem. When standard implants are used in normal breasts, the rate of contracture is 35 percent to 55 percent.[7] The more difficult situation of an implant placed beneath mastectomy flaps results in a contracture rate of virtually 100 percent.

This clinical problem led to the development of externally inflatable tissue expansion devices, which were introduced as a physical method of manipulating the scar around the breast implant. Tissue expanders were designed to stretch skin through a mechanism that is probably similar to the stretching of abdominal skin during pregnancy. Overexpansion of the device (and the implant capsule) for a prolonged period of 3 to 12 months creates a "larger" pocket for the implant and better soft tissue cover. The theory is that the expanded and stable capsular scar, like postpartum abdominal skin, will not return to its original size and will therefore preserve the space around the implant. Because it does not conform to the margins of the implant, this permanent enlargement of the implant pocket allows the implant to remain soft.

It is now clear that tissue expansion offers major advantages over simple implants in terms of softness. As is usually the case, Mother Nature extracts a price for this from both the patient and the surgeon. Completion of the tissue expansion generally requires 30 to 40 office visits and three or more operations. For some reason, perhaps mechanical ischemia of the skin flaps, tissue expansion is also associated with a high incidence of both early and late hematomas and infections, and the overall complication rate is thought to range from 30 percent to 40 percent. Once the process is completed, the long-term benefits of softness and shape are maintained with time.

Myocutaneous Flaps

Professor Iginio Tanzini of Padua, Italy, described the use of the latissimus dorsi myocutaneous flap to close the radical mastectomy defect in 1896; this was a popular method in both Europe and North America until about 1920. Tanzini introduced this method as a way of obtaining a primarily healed radical mastectomy, since partial loss of the mastectomy flaps was nearly a universal event at that time. It was never intended as a method of breast reconstruction but was proposed specifically for the purpose of wound closure. Halsted is known to have considered this an unnecessary procedure, as the mastectomy flaps were not a problem when *he* performed his operation. Halsted's role in the demise of the latissimus myocutaneous flap is not known, but the procedure did fall into disuse shortly after his Grand European Tour in 1920, and it is clear that Halsted said, "Beware of the man with the plastic operation." The myocutaneous flap method was then completely lost until it was repopularized by McCraw, Dibbell, Carraway, and others in the late 1970s.[26-28, 35] Since that time, the use of myocutaneous flaps has been integral to almost all aspects of breast reconstruction.

Subpectoral Breast Reconstruction

Horton first suggested the subpectoral implant reconstruction of the breast following a total mastectomy in 1974.[20, 21] This placement of the implant beneath the pectoralis major muscle reduced the incidence of capsular contracture from nearly 100 percent to less than 30 percent and was the first biological attempt to correct the capsular contracture problem in the reconstructed breast. The effectiveness of the method is well recognized, and it is still commonly used in favorable candidates.[34, 38, 45, 51, 53] When used in combination with the polyurethane-covered implant, the softness of the reconstruction is quite acceptable. Although this reconstruction is not as soft as an autologous reconstruction, it is a dramatic improvement over the standard implant placed beneath mastectomy skin.

Latissimus Dorsi–Implant Reconstruction

The latissimus dorsi breast reconstruction was introduced in 1977 by Schneider, Hill, and Brown and popularized by Bostwick and others.* Two new concepts of breast reconstruction were represented by this dramatic development: immediate replacement of the lost mastectomy skin and complete muscular coverage of the silicone implant. The muscular coverage of the implant was expected to reduce the rate of capsular contracture to a minimal level, which it did for a period of 1 to 2 years. However, a study of the 5-year results of the standard latissimus reconstruction by McCraw and Maxwell shows a "normal" incidence of capsule formation with time.[30] Significant capsules, causing either firmness or contour deformities, developed in 39 percent of the modified mastectomy patients and 75 percent of the radical mastectomy patients. As an isolated problem, firmness could be accepted, and approximately half of the patients eventually developed a "soft" breast. Late deformation of the breast contour by the capsular contracture proved to be a more intractable problem that resulted in two to three additional operations in the average patient. The expected three-dimensional expansion of the mastectomy defect by the latissimus reconstruction was not realized because of this capsular contracture problem. Mechanical overexpansion of the capsule with a tissue expander during the first year may alleviate a part of the capsular "deformation" that is the source of the multiple reoperations.

From the time of its description in 1977 to the height of its popularity in 1982, the latissimus breast reconstruction was recognized as the standard by which all other methods of breast reconstruction should be measured. By 1985, however, the standard latissimus reconstruction was all but abandoned in most major breast centers in favor of tissue expansion or the more complex autogenous transverse rectus abdominis myocutaneous (TRAM) flap reconstruction. The intention of tissue expansion is to avoid a complex flap transfer whereas the intention of the TRAM flap is to avoid the problems of implants altogether. These two schools of thought are still the major influences of current breast reconstruction.

Tissue Expansion

The fundamental choice that must be made in any patient is the choice between tissue expansion and autologous tissue transfers. Simple implantation alone is now considered to be an "antique" method, and the latissimus dorsi–implant procedure offers few advantages over tissue expansion. Because each operative stage is brief and straightforward, tissue expansion is the most popular method in use today. The primary disadvantage of the method is that it requires a major investment of time and energy by the patient, because between three and five operations are usually required

---

*References 2–4, 10, 13, 22–25, 31, 33, 35, 36, 46, and 52.

for completion of the reconstruction. Insurance carriers became justifiably concerned about what they perceived to be an inordinate number of "revisions" of tissue expansion procedures, and they suspected that some of these operations were the result of either "makework" or "perfectionism." However, it is now recognized that the evolutionary changes in the implant capsule are the primary cause for the multiple revisions of the implants.

Tissue expansion is also a common addition to the closure of the mastectomy defect as an immediate reconstruction, since it adds very little time to the closure, even when it does not turn out to be the definitive method of reconstruction (i.e., when the implant is subsequently replaced with autogenous tissue). It is also a simple choice for the expectant mastectomy patient to make at a time when the patient is asked to decide among several methods for treatment of the tumor as well as between adjuvant chemotherapy and radiation therapy. One definite benefit of immediate expansion is that the results of immediate tissue expansion are much better than those of "delayed" (e.g., 3 months later) expansion. Immediate tissue expansion adds almost no wound healing complications, so if tissue expansion is a serious option, it is probably best employed at the time of the mastectomy.

Delayed tissue expansion at 3 months following the mastectomy is the most commonly used method of breast reconstruction today. The "delay" is employed because (1) it does not encumber the original extirpative procedure with reconstructive considerations, and (2) it allows definitive planning of the adjuvant therapy based on the pathological findings. When either chemotherapy or radiation therapy is anticipated, tissue expansion is usually deferred until therapy has been completed or is ruled unnecessary. However, tissue expansion is commonly used in patients with less than favorable disease, since the permanent implant does not interfere with later radiation therapy or chemotherapy for chest wall recurrences.

The "ideal" candidate for delayed tissue expansion has (1) a unilateral mastectomy, (2) an innervated pectoralis major muscle, (3) thick and redundant mastectomy skin flaps with an intact inframammary fold, and (4) less than 20 percent obesity. The absence of even one of these factors can be expected to lead to a below-average result. For instance, the large opposite breast or the obese patient requires a large reconstructive breast implant to match the size of the opposite breast. This can only be achieved by using a broad-based and round implant, which seldom provides adequate symmetry with a normal teardrop shape. Symmetry is *the* criteria of success in any breast reconstruction. It is even harder to obtain in the bilateral mastectomy patient, because every problem associated with single implants is doubled in the bilateral condition. For instance, one implant may be soft, ptotic, and low, whereas the other implant, placed in precisely the same fashion, may be firm, round, and high. The capsule formation around any implant is, for the most part, beyond the control of the surgeon, and although this capsule may not cause a problem in the unilateral case, it can make symmetry almost unobtainable in bilateral cases. These problems with bilateral reconstructions, however, should not detract from the value of tissue expanders in general. In the "ideal" candidate, tissue expansion is safe and effective and should be an option for most mastectomy patients.

Autogenous Tissue Transfers

The current alternative choice to tissue expansion is an autogenous tissue transfer. This is criticized as the "Rolls Royce" method, because it is elegant as well as unnecessarily complex, (i.e., like the car). These critics admit, however, that the most natural results, as far as softness and symmetry, are achieved with autogenous tissue. Autogenous tissue transfers follow the basic principle of "replacing lost tissue with like tissue," so objections to the principle must consist of reasoned objections. The real question is whether the results are worth the risk and expense of a very sophisticated procedure. This deliberation is unnecessary if a sophisticated replacement is not sought by the patient and a simpler procedure will achieve the desired goals.

Choosing among the various autogenous myocutaneous flaps is not easy, because there are several good options. The TRAM flap, which was described by Hartrampf in 1982, is the forerunner of all the autogenous flaps that have been suggested for breast reconstruction.[5, 14–18, 32, 42–44, 49, 50] The other "local" myocutaneous flap, the latissimus dorsi "J" reconstruction, was recently described by McCraw et al.[29] The final option is provided by free microvascular myocutaneous flap transfers, including the "free" TRAM flap, the superior gluteal flap, the inferior gluteal flap, and the tensor fascia lata flap. Undoubtedly, other options will follow. The primary indication for this type of reconstruction is the need for massive replacements of soft tissue in the breast area, found in the following:

1. The radical mastectomy with loss of skin, pectoralis major muscle, and breast volume.

2. The modified radical mastectomy with tight chest wall skin or heavy irradiation, a failed previous reconstruction, or the need to match a large and ptotic opposite breast.

3. The subcutaneous mastectomy "cripple."

4. The major congenital chest wall and breast defect.

TRAM Flap. The TRAM flap employs the rectus abdominis muscles to "carry" the redundant lower abdominal skin and fat to the area of the breast. This procedure, like any autogenous myocutaneous flap transfer, constitutes a major operation, and the candidates must be carefully chosen. Obesity (over 20 percent) and smoking are relative contraindications because of the increased risk of abdominal hernia formation and flap loss, respectively. The most common criticism of the TRAM procedure is the closure of the abdominal wall defect. Unless this can be safely performed, this operation should not be seriously considered. The keys to postoperative abdominal wall competence are (1) patient selection (i.e., avoiding the obese patient) and (2) proper surgical closure. The largest experience has been reported by Hartrampf, who noted a single hernia in one early, obese patient (patient number 26) out of 400 total patients, for an incidence of 0.3 percent. Hartrampf now has more than 400 consecutive patients who have not developed a hernia, and this establishes the benchmark. This favorable experience with the abdominal wall closure should be expected, since the width of the anterior fascial sheath removal is usually limited to 3 to 4 cm, and this can be primarily closed without any difficulty. The functional loss of a single rectus abdominis muscle is seldom noticed, and 95 percent of Hartrampf's patients felt that their work performance and sports activities were unchanged or improved following surgery.

Whether the surgical effort of the TRAM flap reconstruction is worthwhile can best be answered by the patients who have experienced it. Hartrampf asked the first 300 patients these questions:

"Was the operation worth the time and effort you invested in it?"

"Would you recommend this method of breast reconstruction to other patients?"

Both questions were answered affirmatively by 98 percent of the patients. The TRAM flap, as performed by Hartrampf, should be considered the "gold standard," and all other methods must be compared with it because of the known excellent results as well as its low recorded complication rate and donor site morbidity.

Latissimus Dorsi "J" Reconstruction. The latissimus dorsi myocutaneous flap is presently the only "local" autogenous flap other than the TRAM that is accessible to the breast area. The large latissimus muscle can be used to carry sufficient fat and skin from the back so that an implant is not necessary. Unlike the standard latissimus dorsi–implant reconstruction, the "J" reconstruction includes a horizontal ellipse of skin along the "fat roll" of the back, as well as a vertical ellipse of the redundant axillary fat that is left after a mastectomy. This method is particularly applicable to the moderately obese patient or the smoker who may not be a candidate for the TRAM procedure.

The latissimus flap can be raised at the time of mastectomy if the patient is placed in a lateral decubitus position, and an immediate reconstruction can be performed with only a moderate increase in operative time. It is more definitive than any type of implant procedure and is significantly less complex than any of the other autogenous tissue transfers. This, and the favorable donor site of the back, should make the "J" latissimus flap reconstruction a reasonable routine consideration at the time of mastectomy.

In the future, the "J" latissimus reconstruction will be a necessary consideration for the lumpectomy-irradiation "failure" patient with a tumor-filled breast. Some of these patients will require a massive mastectomy, either because of the failure to control the local disease or because of the ravages of irradiation. In either case, the only plausible replacement of the damaged breast tissue is with autogenous tissue. Since this replacement will need to be carried out immediately, if only to obtain a healed wound, the "J" latissimus reconstruction will be an important cancer tool to provide a healed wound in these patients.

Microvascular Tissue Transfers. Free tissue transfers have recently become reasonable methods of breast reconstruction with the advent of "large vessel" myocutaneous flaps.[5, 47–50] Some of these donor site flap vessels, including the deep inferior epigastric (used for the TRAM procedure), the inferior gluteal (gluteus maximus), and the lateral circumflex femoral (tensor fascia lata, TFL), are nearly as large as the radial artery. These myocutaneous flaps have "high flow" vascular trees in which the extensive runoff helps prevent venous clotting of the vascular anastomosis. The development of the end-to-side anastomosis into the axillary vessels further promotes high flow and should make total loss of the flap a rarity.

Free tissue transfers have traditionally been criticized for their excessive operative time and their unreliability. Those criticisms were previously justified, but the predictability of "large vessel" myocutaneous flaps has made it necessary to reconsider this procedure. Several microvascular surgeons have experience with more than 100 consecutive free muscle flaps without a failure. In fact, many of these free flaps were placed in the lower extremity, which is a much more difficult transfer than that to the axillary vessels. The operative time is still long, but this is related more to the complex dissection of the flap than to the vascular anastomosis, which can usually be completed in less than an hour.

The technical advances in breast reconstruction in the past 10 years have eclipsed all previous surgical history of this area. Breast reconstruction is now accepted by the surgical community, even though the rapidly changing scope and rationale of various methods are less than well understood. It is important for the oncologic surgeon to recognize the context of these methods in the overall treatment plan, not because breast reconstruction should be considered a routine matter, but because certain types of breast reconstruction may be more appropriate for some patients. For example, the "J" latissimus reconstruction adds little time to the mastectomy, is totally reliable, and adequately replaces the breast in a single stage. This will become an important future consideration in management of the patient with failure of the lumpectomy-irradiation method.

RECOVERY PROCESS

The physical and mental adjustment to both the diagnosis of breast cancer and the removal of the breast is, by definition, a recovery process. In its simplest conceptual form, this is seen as an adjustment of the focus of life's purpose away from a "preparation for dying" to a "preparation for living." Reconstruction of the breast is an important aspect of the recovery process, but a number of issues must be resolved before surgical intervention can be considered.

Preparation for dying is also described by the "grief reaction," which is an emotional response that is experienced with any loss. This grief reaction occurs in sequential stages and includes the following feelings:

1. *Disbelief.* "This can't be happening to me. The biopsy must be wrong."

2. *Denial.* "This is not cancer, after all. My surgeon is not even sure what kind of mastectomy I should have."

3. *Anger.* "I wish I had found this sooner. My surgeon has absolutely no bedside manner, because he told me that the tumor had been there for several years."

4. *Depression.* "I hate having cancer. The surgeon did more surgery than was needed. Look at how terrible I look."

5. *Acceptance.* "I do have cancer, but I am doing my best to survive. My surgeon has been so caring and nice to me. I really like him."

It is essential that the patient obtain a satisfactory resolution of these negative feelings prior to the consideration of an elective reconstruction. Some patients deny these feelings completely and never reach the acceptance stage. These patients should not be considered for a breast reconstruction, because an "external" solution to these profound emotional concerns cannot bring happiness any more than buying a new dress can bring happiness.

Preparation for living follows the grief reaction temporarily and is also called "acceptance." This includes the following stages:

1. *Acceptance of death.* "I may die, but I have had a full life."

2. *Acceptance of survival.* "I can survive, and I am going to do everything in my power to make that happen."

3. *Hope.* "I have good doctors, and they have given me the best chance of a cure."

4. *Life is worth living.* "Life is really good, whether I live for a day, a year, or a very long time."

These feelings are universally experienced by breast cancer patients to some degree, whether they undergo a mastectomy or a lumpectomy followed by irradiation. In fact, the lumpectomy patient may have more difficulty working through the grief reaction than the mastectomy patient. It is easier for lumpectomy patients to end the emotional progression of the grief reaction at the denial phase, since they have experienced very little "loss" from the experience of the lumpectomy and irradiation. Following their cancer treatment, the breast is still present, and it does not *appear* that they have had a breast cancer; as a result, this group of patients may not have experienced the deep negative feelings related to loss of the breast. Furthermore, the form of treatment chosen by the patient was selected because it is less deforming, not because it is more effective. This makes it particularly difficult for them to cope with a recurrence, because emotionally, survival was *expected* rather than hoped for. It was their choice to have a form of breast "conservation" treatment, and they may feel guilty that the recurrence is the result of their personal choice of treatment rather than the biological behavior of the disease.

With the proper emotional support, a progression of positive feelings evolves. Survival becomes a reasonable possibility, and eventually the feeling arises that life is good and should be approached positively. Only after a favorable attitude and a positive self-esteem are reestablished does the patient usually become concerned with the correction of the mastectomy deformity and the mastectomy stigma. Reconstruction of the breast should be reserved for the time when the patient's feelings about the breast cancer and the mastectomy are completely stabilized. Offering an immediate reconstruction as a way of preventing negative feelings is just as bad as offering tranquilizers to obliterate unpleasant feelings related to any loss. Both of these methods merely defer the time when these feelings must be faced, since the eventual experience of these feelings is unavoidable.

The psychological aspects of the recovery process are not well understood by some surgeons, because the emotional healing has been traditionally left to outside groups (e.g., Reach to Recovery) that function independently of the surgeon. These groups are effective primarily because their members have actually lived through the disease themselves. Psychiatrists, no matter how well they understand this process from a learned and theoretical standpoint, may not be as effective in their counseling as other mastectomy patients, because they haven't lived through the pain of a lost breast. The surgeon can get involved in this healing process at any point by simply asking the patient about her feelings. Questions directed toward feelings (e.g., "You look sad; are you sad?" and "You look angry; are you angry?") can open the door for the patient who is not doing well coping by herself. At least it can help point out her need to seek help with her feelings from others.

Generally, breast reconstruction is an appropriate addition to the late recovery process, at a time when self-esteem is high and life is viewed as "worth living." At this point doing "something for yourself" is seen as healthy rather than as a way of denying or rationalizing unpleasant truths. It is clearly a mistake to proceed with plans for a breast reconstruction before these issues have been resolved by the patient.

REASONS FOR CONSIDERATION OF BREAST RECONSTRUCTION

Patients have become increasingly sophisticated in their expectations of breast reconstruction. They generally seek consultation 2 or more years following the mastectomy after a great deal of introspective thought and self-education on the subject. They are usually exceedingly well informed and capable of understanding the differences among the various methods of reconstruction, and they frequently come with a number of personal prejudices for or against certain methods. Our ability to achieve a result that satisfies their expectations is a subject of vital interest, and the number of cases in our experience is an expected question that should not be offensive. Postmastectomy patients are uniform in their initial complaints of their inability to wear clothes, their dislike of the external prosthesis, and their weariness of the mastectomy deformity and the postmastectomy stigma.

Inability to Wear Normal Clothes

"Normal" clothes are generally defined as what other people wear and what the patient wore prior to the mastectomy. This euphemism of "normal" really implies sundresses and bathing suits, because these garments present a special problem to the mastectomy patient, and so they are carefully avoided. For example, the loss of upper breast "fill" is obvious in anything other than a high-necked blouse or sweater, and this is accentuated by bending over. External prostheses, helpful as they may be, cannot camouflage the mastectomy deformity in these revealing clothes.

Dislike of the External Prosthesis

The external prosthesis camouflages the breast deformity very well in certain clothes, but it has the disadvantages of being hot and heavy and also serves as a constant reminder of the breast abnormality. A conscious decision is required to wear it, and this is not always easy to make. For instance, it is difficult for the patient to know whether to wear the prosthesis beneath a nightgown when answering the door or beneath a bathing suit outdoors. Because the external prosthesis is vulnerable to accidents of dislodgement (e.g., popping out of the bathing suit), this dreaded embarrassment precludes its use in many situations. Although many patients are served very well by the external prosthesis, it is seen as an unnatural attachment after a few years of use.

Weariness of the Mastectomy Deformity

"Weariness" of the mastectomy deformity is something that takes months to years to develop, but it is a uniform finding. Mastectomy patients may accept the mastectomy and the cancer without question, but they still dislike their appearance in the mirror. Whether the problem is perceived to be the anatomical deformity, the asymmetry of the breasts, or something that can be translated into a loss of femininity, the mirror is a constant reminder. To avoid the unpleasant fact of the mastectomy, many patients treat the mastectomy deformity as a "secret" that can be covered up by conscious decision. The secret is protected by not being seen naked and even by wearing a bra and an external prosthesis to bed.

Postmastectomy Stigma

Mastectomy patients tire of being grouped as a special social class of "abnormals" who are somehow different from other women. This is termed the postmastectomy stigma, in which well-intentioned nonmastectomy women ascribe great strength and character to the mere survival of a mastectomy, and others feel obligated to tell these patients how they should feel. It is particularly common for female parents and friends to say seemingly helpful things such as, "You are so strong," "You should be stronger," "You shouldn't feel that way," and "All mastectomy patients need to . . ." These stigmatized patients long for the time when they will be allowed to think, feel, and express themselves as "whole" persons rather than as people who are perceived to be different. This usually begins to occur at about 2 years following the mastectomy, as soon as the doctors give the impression that survival is a definite possibility and the family has accepted the mastectomy as a remote event.

RECONSTRUCTIVE GOALS OF THE PATIENT

When the recovery process has advanced to the point of "acceptance," the following reconstructive goals of the patient can be addressed:

1. *Symmetry.* No matter what type of reconstruction is proposed, symmetry with the opposite breast is the paramount goal. This is seldom obtainable without the use of an autogenous reconstruction, and it must be the active choice of the patient to decide on a method that provides acceptable symmetry.

2. *Lasting result.* A lasting result is expected as an implied warranty, even though this can only be assured with autogenous tissue transfers, which are not expected to change with time.

3. *Aesthetic factors of form, consistency, and size.* Patients are generally undefinitive about these considerations initially, but only because of their inability to express themselves. Once the postoperative result is visible, no patient has a problem describing her preferences for the desired softness, size, and ptosis.

4. *Forgetting about the mastectomy.* This is the "ultimate" goal of any breast reconstruction. One would hope that the trauma of both the mastectomy and the reconstruction would be lost to memory at some future point. As ambitious as it sounds, it does occur.

The patient's expectations of the breast reconstruction must be determined at the outset, since all of the subsequent decisions are predicated on one of the following surgical goals:

A *limited surgical goal* of replacing the external prosthesis with an internal prosthetic mound can be accomplished in one or two procedures using a simple silicone prosthesis. This is applicable in the situation in which there is adequate skin cover, an innervated pectoralis major muscle, and a small and nonptotic opposite breast.

A *moderate surgical goal* of reasonable breast softness and symmetry can be accomplished with a tissue expander followed by a subsequent custom-designed permanent implant. This usually requires two to four operative procedures, but the initial tissue expansion of the existing skin generally provides a mound which is softer, more ptotic, and less round than the simple implant.

An *ambitious surgical goal* is to create a breast that mimics the opposite normal breast in contour, form, and consistency. An ambitious goal may also be necessitated by a condition that can only be corrected by a major tissue replacement. Tissue expanders are not effective in some extensive mastectomies (e.g., in failed lumpectomy-irradiation patients), because the tissue deficit of muscle, skin, and breast volume cannot be overcome without adding new flap tissue. The transfer of autogenous tissue from the abdomen or another distant site is almost always necessary to accomplish such a sophisticated restoration.

METHODS

Simple Implantation

The basic mound of a reconstructed breast can be formed with a simple implant. This was previously done beneath the mastectomy flaps alone, but the provided "cover" proved inadequate to prevent the routine formation of a fibrous capsule. Placement of the implant beneath the pectoralis major muscle gives a much more satisfactory result in both softness and shape. When the mastectomy skin is "tight," it is frequently necessary to augment the soft tissue cover with a myocutaneous flap. Even though the initial implant procedure is successful, reoperation for asymmetry and scar encapsulation is common with simple implantation (Figs. 30–1 to 30–6).

Tissue Expansion

A tissue expander is a saline-filled implant with a valve that can be used to inflate the implant in the physician's office. The tissue expander is primarily used to stretch the mastectomy skin flaps, but it is also a mechanical method of controlling the scar capsule. Although it is not understood exactly why pressure "softens" scars, the internal pressure exerted by the tissue expander has the same positive effect that external pressure has on a burn scar. The expander is progressively inflated over a period of several months until the scar capsule is soft and the overlying skin is redundant. When this is successful, it provides a ptotic skin envelop that allows the implant to mimic the normal droop of the opposite breast. True ptosis is seldom achieved, but acceptable softness is obtained in approximately 70 percent of the cases. Occasionally, an immediate capsule develops around the tissue expander and precludes permanent implantation. In this event, tissue expansion is abandoned, and an autogenous tissue transfer is done to replace the breast volume. Overall, tissue expansion is a great improvement over simple implantation in every respect, and it is less complex than most flap reconstructions. The complication rate has been high, but it is apparently improving with experience (Figs. 30–7 to 30–30).

Autogenous Tissue Transfer

Autogenous tissue transfers offer the only method that can be expected to mimic the form, shape, and consistency of the opposite breast. A number of myocu-

Text continued on page 675

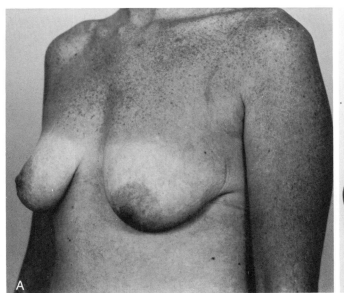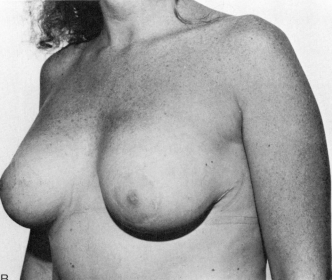

Figure 30–1. *A,* Simple subpectoral implantation and mastopexy in a young patient. *B,* An acceptable aesthetic result is expected when a silicone implant is placed beneath a moderate-sized breast.

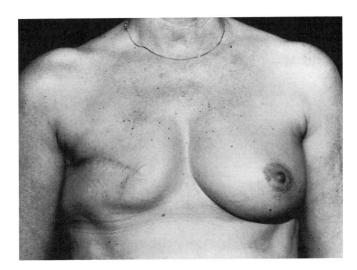

Figure 30–2. Fifty-year-old patient who is an ideal candidate for a simple implant reconstruction following a right modified mastectomy. The pectoralis major muscle is intact, the mastectomy flaps are thick, and the inframammary fold is present. The opposite breast is also favorable in terms of obtaining symmetry, since there is no ptosis.

Figure 30–3. Even in a favorable candidate, the simple implant usually gives a round appearance and does not mimic the "teardrop" shape of the normal breast. The implant is soft, but it is high and nonptotic.

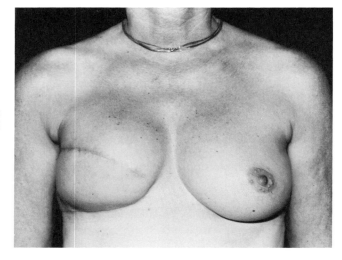

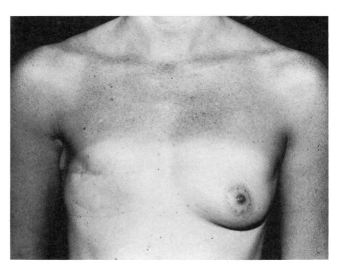

Figure 30–4. Less favorable candidate for a simple implantation. The mastectomy flaps are thin, and the pectoralis major muscle is not large enough to provide good coverage of the implant.

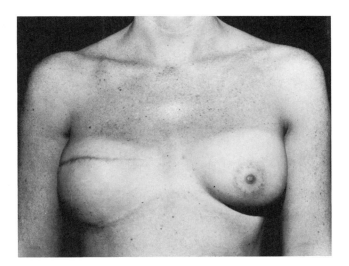

Figure 30–5. Although the initial result was reasonably symmetrical, the implant beneath the normal breast has migrated superiorly, and the reconstructive implant has been pushed laterally by the scar capsule. This type of capsule can usually be prevented by the use of a tissue expander.

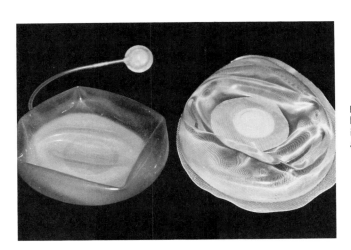

Figure 30–6. Saline inflatable tissue expansion devices. The right implant has a remote filling valve that is attached by a silicone tube. The right implant valve is contained within the implant. The valves are self-sealing, and can be punctured multiple times with No. 23 needles.

Figure 30–7. Thirty-two-year-old female following a left modified mastectomy. The skin envelope of the ptotic right breast will be tightened with a mastopexy. The patient is an excellent candidate for skin expansion, because of the low and oblique mastectomy scar and the lax, ptotic skin of the left breast.

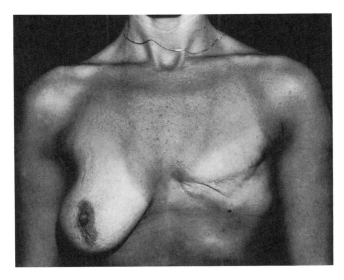

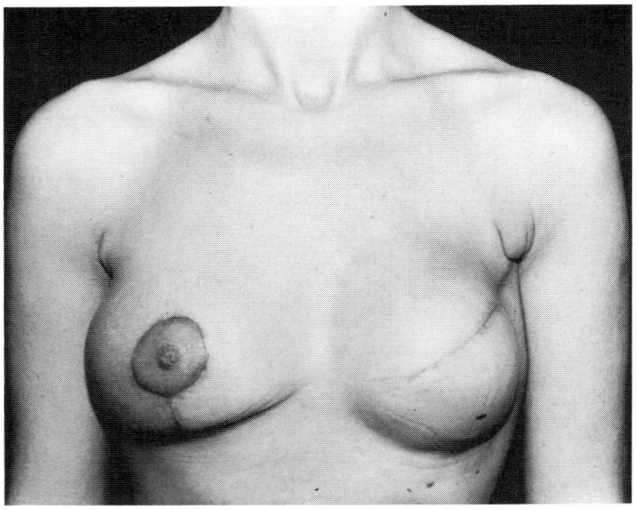

Figure 30–8. Result 3 months following a right mastopexy and skin expansion of the left breast. The patient is ready for a nipple-areolar reconstruction and recreation of the left inframammary fold.

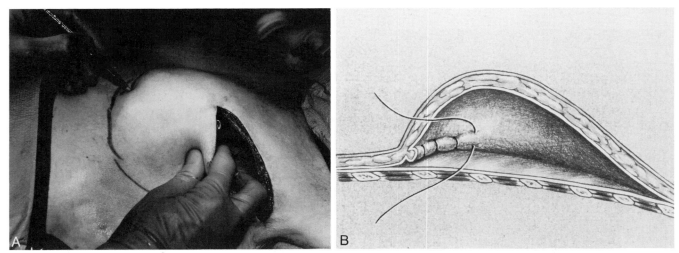

Figure 30–9. A, The inframammary fold is formed by suture plication of the internal capsule under direct vision, as shown on the cutaway diagram (B).

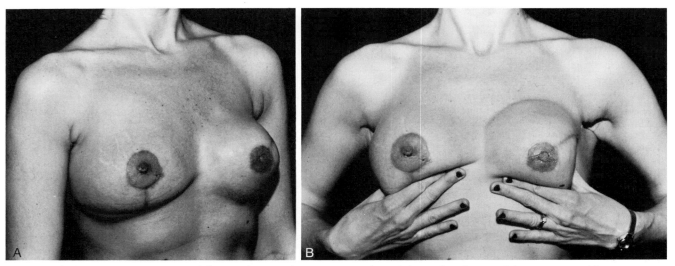

Figure 30–10. A, Appearance following the second stage. B, Note the mobility and "softness" of the reconstructed breast.

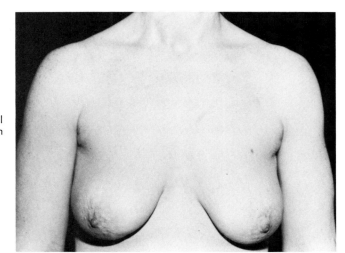

Figure 30–11. Thirty-six-year-old surgical nurse with bilateral intraductal carcinomas of the breasts. The patient refused the mastectomies unless an "immediate" reconstruction could be done.

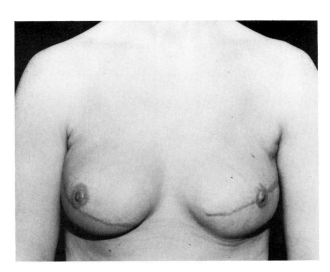

Figure 30–12. Six months following "immediate" breast reconstructions with tissue expansion devices. The nipple-areolar reconstructions were done in a separate stage under local anesthesia. The implants are completely "soft," and remarkably good ptosis was achieved with the tissue expanders.

Figure 30–13. Forty-year-old female with a biopsy-proven adenocarcinoma of the right breast. A modified left mastectomy had been done 3 years earlier. A bilateral reconstruction will be done at the time of the right mastectomy, using tissue expanders.

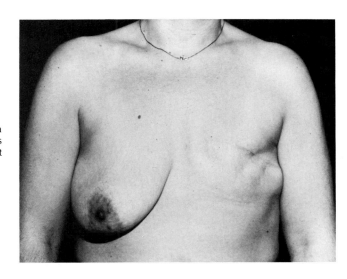

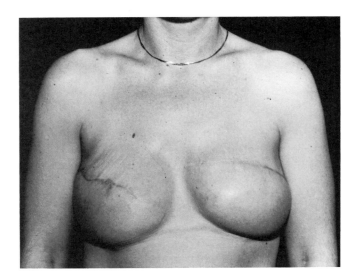

Figure 30–14. Inflated tissue expanders 6 months following the mastectomy. Note the excellent ptosis.

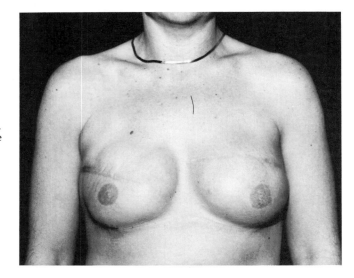

Figure 30–15. Four years following the placement of permanent implants. Late elevation of the implants by the scar capsule has resulted in some loss of the ptosis, even though the implants are still "soft."

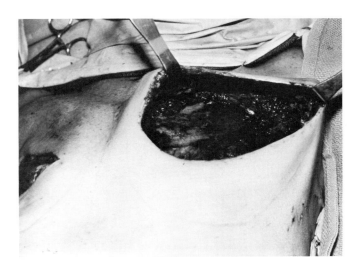

Figure 30–16. "Immediate" reconstruction with tissue expanders at the time of bilateral mastectomies. Note the thin mastectomy flaps.

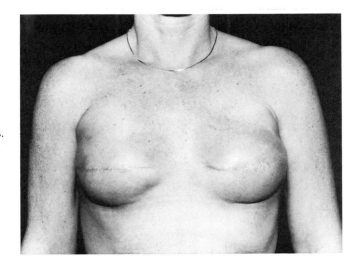

Figure 30–17. The early result of the tissue expansion is good at 3 months.

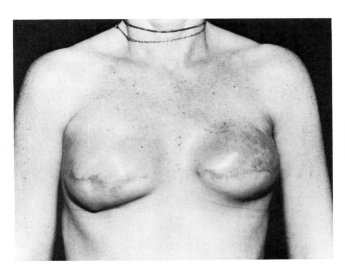

Figure 30–18. The later result at 6 months is poor because of scar encapsulation around the tissue expanders. This is a common problem when the tissue expanders are covered only by thin mastectomy flaps.

Figure 30–19. The result was salvaged by open capsulotomies and placement of Becker implants.

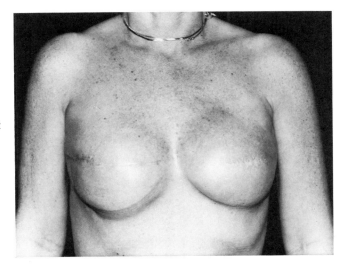

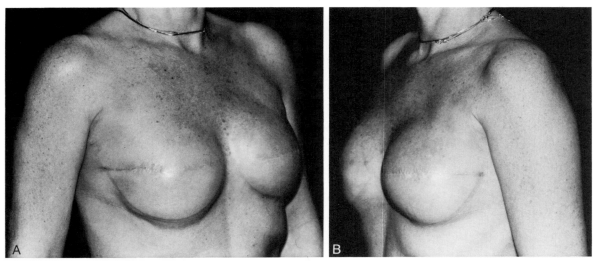

Figure 30–20. *A* and *B*, Oblique views of the Becker tissue expanders. This is an unusually good result in view of the deficient cover for the implant.

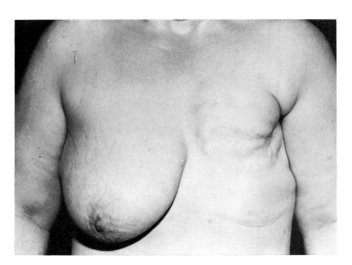

Figure 30–21. Forty-six-year-old female 6 years following an extensive left mastectomy and postoperative irradiation for an advanced adenocarcinoma. The patient is a poor candidate for tissue expansion, because the densely scarred mastectomy flaps cannot be expected to stretch adequately.

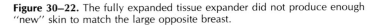

Figure 30–22. The fully expanded tissue expander did not produce enough "new" skin to match the large opposite breast.

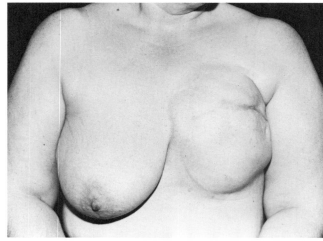

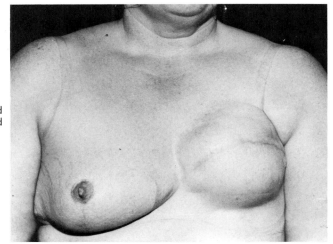

Figure 30–23. Two years following placement of the permanent implant and a reduction mammoplasty of the right breast. The implant is firm, high, and asymmetrical, even though two open capsulotomies had been done.

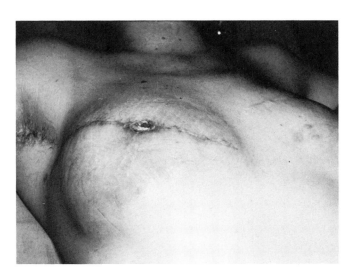

Figure 30–24. Example of a late infection and erosion of a tissue expander at 6 weeks. The implant is visible in the line of the scar and will have to be removed. These late infections appear to be related to small seromas, but they can also be caused by the repeated injections of the implant.

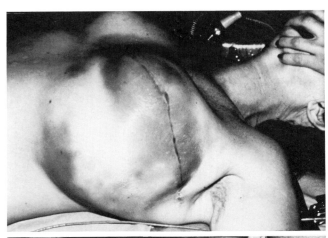

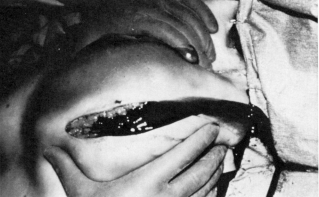

Figure 30–25. Example of a late hematoma around a tissue expander at 7 weeks. The cause of the hematoma is usually a mystery.

Figure 30–26. Leakage from a tissue expander is rare, even though the implant has been punctured repeatedly.

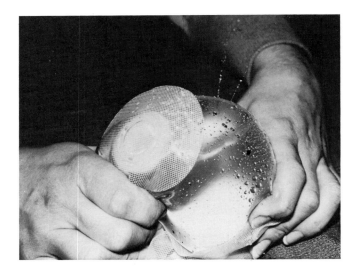

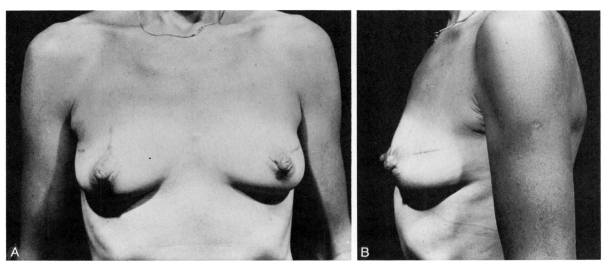

Figure 30–27. *A* and *B,* Forty-one-year-old female with bilateral lobular carcinoma of the breasts. An ''immediate'' bilateral latissimus dorsi muscle flap and implant reconstruction are planned.

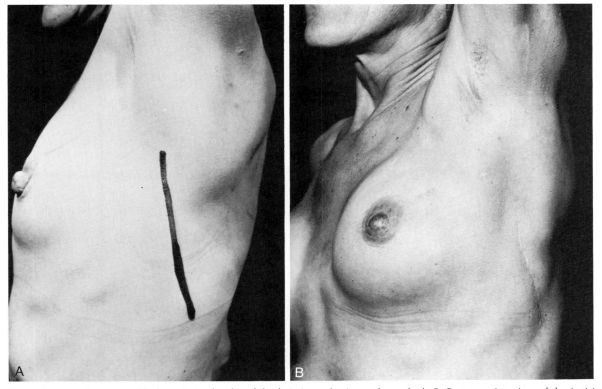

Figure 30–28. *A,* Preoperative view with the anterior border of the latissimus dorsi muscle marked. *B,* Postoperative view of the incision used to retrieve the latissimus muscle.

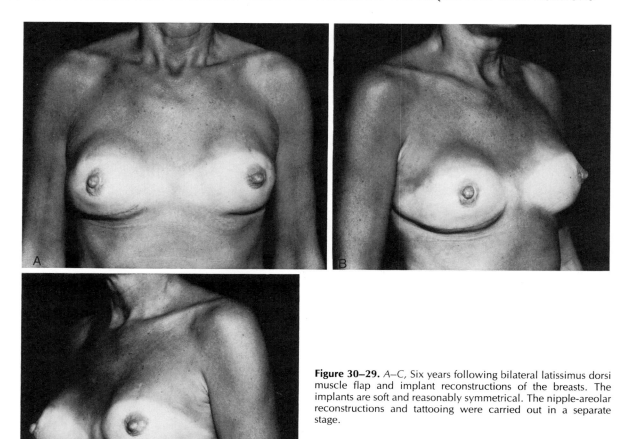

Figure 30–29. A–C, Six years following bilateral latissimus dorsi muscle flap and implant reconstructions of the breasts. The implants are soft and reasonably symmetrical. The nipple-areolar reconstructions and tattooing were carried out in a separate stage.

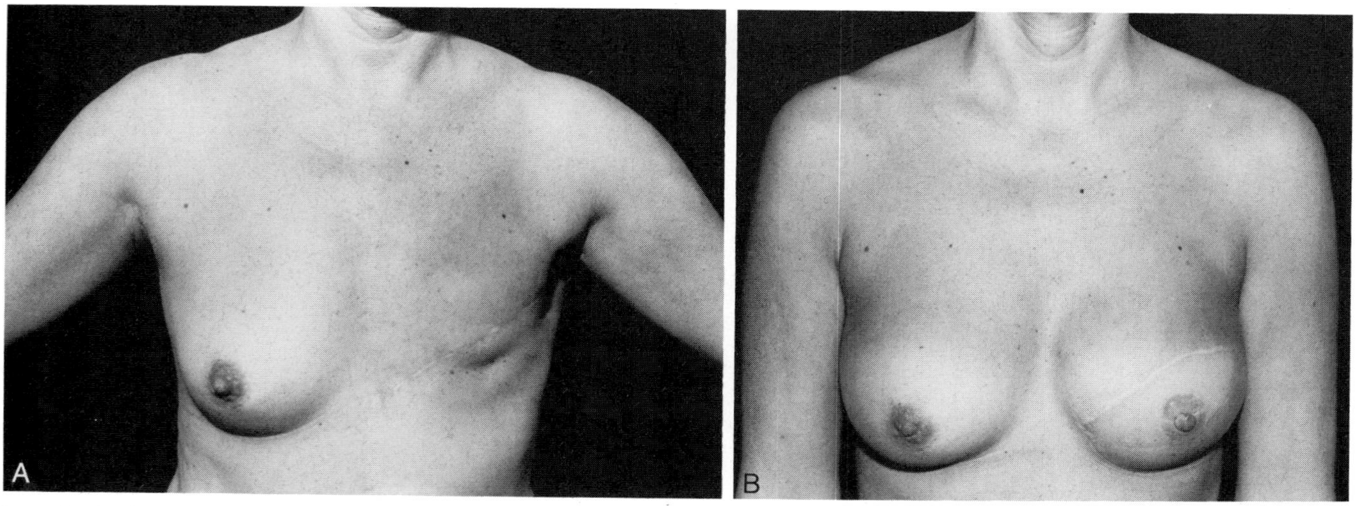

Figure 30–30. Preoperative (A) and postoperative (B) views of an ideal result from using a latissimus dorsi myocutaneous flap and an implant. A subpectoral implant was used in the right breast for symmetry.

taneous flaps are available for transfer to the breast area, and each offers a definitive and lasting result. The recent refinements in myocutaneous flaps make flap loss highly unlikely, and even the microvascular transfers are nearly 100 percent reliable. The donor site is the usual reason for choosing a particular flap procedure, since an acceptable contour can be created from any of the properly chosen flaps. The functional loss from the use of a myocutaneous flap is seldom a consideration, and the donor site pain is brief and manageable. Although highly sophisticated anesthetic management is a necessity for these lengthy procedures, anesthetic complications should become infrequent when these procedures become routine. Usually fewer operations are required than with the implantation methods, because the final shaping is definitive at the initial operation in more than half of the cases.

Latissimus Dorsi "J" Reconstruction

The standard latissimus myocutaneous flap reconstruction requires an implant, because the flap itself does not provide enough bulk to recreate the breast mound. The alternative "J" latissimus reconstruction does not require an implant and is an alternative autogenous transfer in the moderately obese patient or the smoker who would otherwise not be a good candidate for a more extensive procedure. The "J" design of the latissimus reconstruction includes a long horizontal ellipse of skin with a vertical extension into the redundant fatty tissue of the posterior axillary fold. The entire width of the latissimus muscle is elevated along with the fat on the surface of the muscle. This provides a breast volume of 300 gm in thin patients and as much as 2000 gm in obese patients.

The "J" latissimus reconstruction is also an excellent method of immediate breast reconstruction because of the favorable donor site. An immediate reconstruction

adds approximately 1 hour and 30 minutes to the time of a mastectomy and should not necessitate additional transfusion. The softness of the reconstruction facilitates the follow-up examination of the mastectomy site, and postoperative irradiation and chemotherapy can usually be started within 10 days of the surgery. Since the latissimus flap has even more predictable healing than the mastectomy flaps, an immediate reconstruction is a reasonable consideration in many patients (Figs. 30–31 to 30–58).

Vertical Rectus Abdominis Flap

The skin "island" of the rectus abdominis flap can be oriented either vertically or horizontally. The vertical orientation carries the skin directly over the muscle and is primarily used for surface coverage of major mastectomy defects rather than for breast reconstruction. The flap elevation can be done at the same time as the mastectomy, and the anterior fascia can usually be primarily closed. If two surgical teams are used, the mastectomy and the flap reconstruction can both be completed within a 1½- to 2-hour operative session. Because of the reliability of this flap, there should almost never be any reason for a skin graft of the mastectomy site. The coverage provided by this flap is better than a skin graft, healing is more predictable, and the difference in operative time is negligible (Figs. 30–59 to 30–68).

Horizontal Rectus Abdominis Flap

The horizontal design of the rectus abdominis flap provides the most ideal replacement tissue for the breast and can be used to reconstruct virtually any defect. It is a technically demanding procedure, but it offers the most elegant contour restoration of the breast. It is not recommended in obese patients (weight 20 percent more

Text continued on page 689

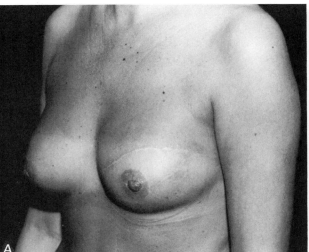
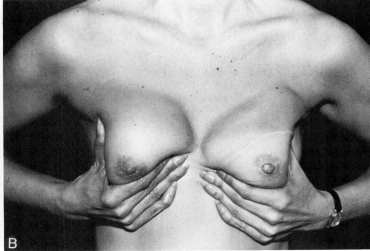

Figure 30–31. Oblique (*A*) and "squeeze" (*B*) postoperative views. The patient was 26 years old at the time of the mastectomy, and 12 lymph nodes were positive. An early reconstruction was recommended by the patient's oncologist *because* of the unfavorable prognosis. The patient was free of disease for seven years.

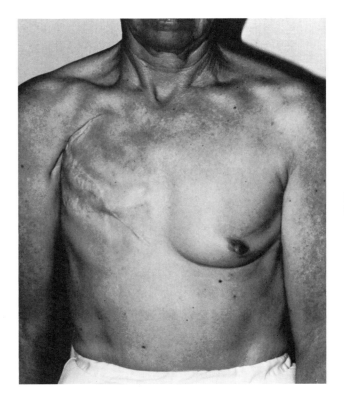

Figure 30–32. Fifty-six-year-old woman who had undergone a radical mastectomy and skin graft closure 15 years earlier.

Figure 30–33. A latissimus dorsi myocutaneous flap and implant reconstruction was initially acceptable but became painful, firm, and elevated with time. In retrospect, it is unreasonable to attempt the correction of such a large defect without autogenous tissue.

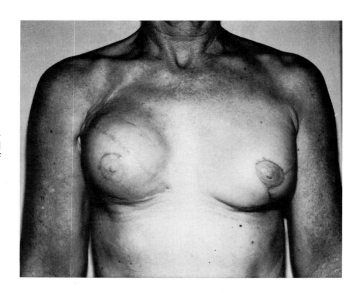

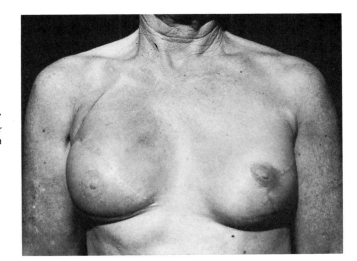

Figure 30–34. The implant was removed and replaced with a "buried" TRAM flap. Note the complete replacement of the contour of the anterior axillary fold and the upper breast, which is not possible to do with an implant.

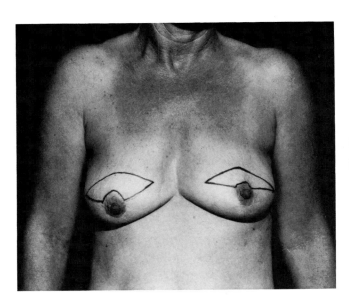

Figure 30–35. Bilateral siliconomas of the breast in a 49-year-old woman. The breasts were painful and impossible to evaluate. Because of the previous problem with silicone, the patient is not a good candidate for implants.

Figure 30–36. Outline of the planned "J" latissimus dorsi reconstruction, which will not use an implant.

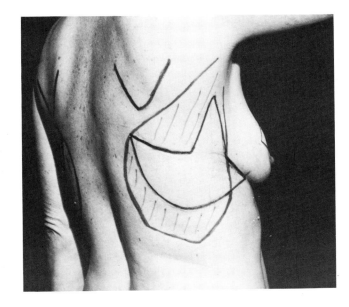

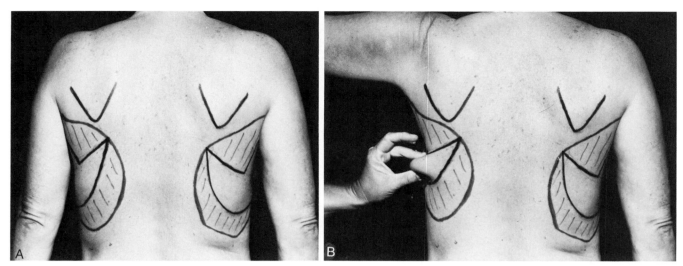

Figure 30–37. *A* and *B,* Adequate volume for reconstruction of the breasts can be obtained from the ''J'' latissimus reconstruction even in a thin patient.

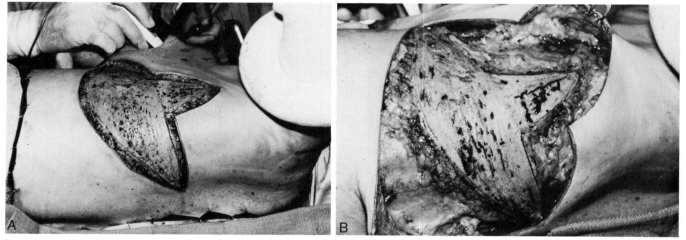

Figure 30–38. *A* and *B,* Intraoperative view of the de-epithelialized latissimus flap. Note the fat that is ''carried'' on the surface of the latissimus muscle.

Figure 30–39. Intraoperative view of the total replacement of the breast volume with the de-epithelialized latissimus flap.

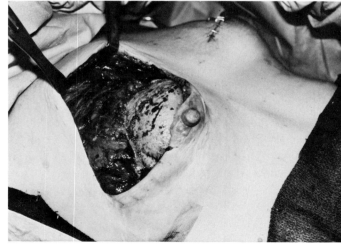

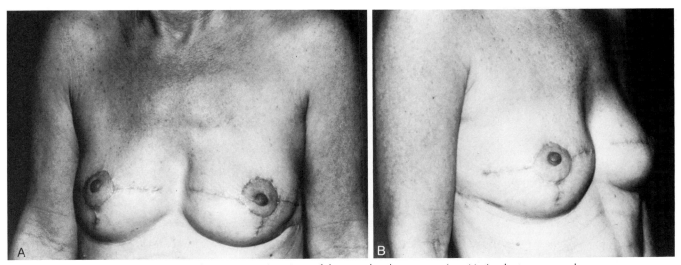

Figure 30–40. *A* and *B,* Postoperative views of the completed reconstruction. No implants were used.

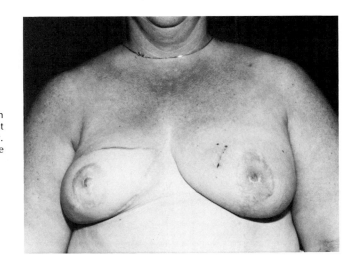

Figure 30–41. Obese 42-year-old surgical nurse with a biopsy-proven adenocarcinoma in the medial aspect of the left breast. A modified right mastectomy and TRAM flap reconstruction had been done 7 years earlier. An immediate "J" latissimus reconstruction was chosen because of the planned postoperative irradiation.

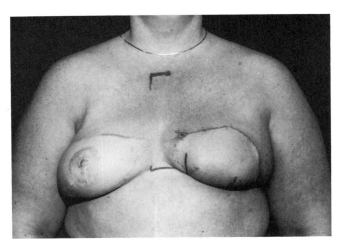

Figure 30–42. Two weeks following the immediate reconstruction without an implant. Note the parasternal irradiation markings.

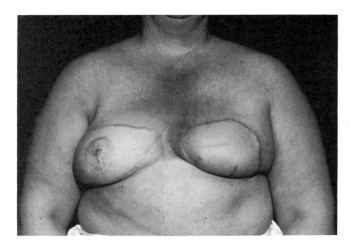

Figure 30–43. Appearance 6 months after the irradiation treatments.

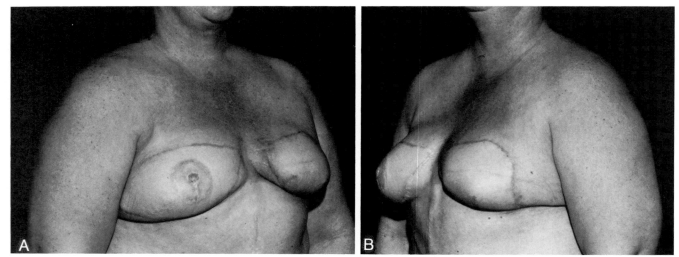

Figure 30–44. *A* and *B*, Oblique views of the ptosis at 6 months. The volume replacement in the left breast exceeded 1500 gm.

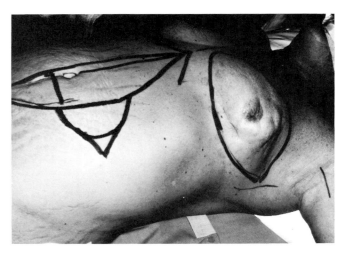

Figure 30–45. Elderly patient with a tumor-filled right breast from a neglected primary. A radical mastectomy is planned and will be followed by irradiation. An L-shaped vertical rectus abdominis myocutaneous flap is outlined on the abdomen. A flap was chosen instead of a skin graft in order to facilitate early adjunctive therapy.

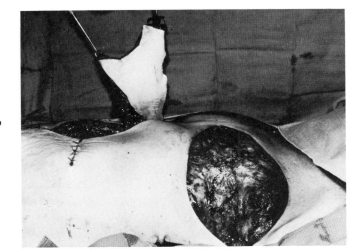

Figure 30–46. Completed radical mastectomy and myocutaneous flap elevation.

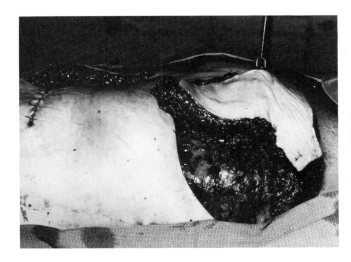

Figure 30–47. Transfer of the flap for the mastectomy closure. Both the mastectomy and the flap closure were completed within 2 hours by using two surgical teams.

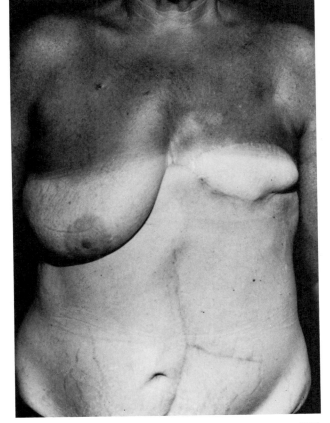

Figure 30–48. Healed flap reconstruction at 6 months. The patient was free of disease for 4 years.

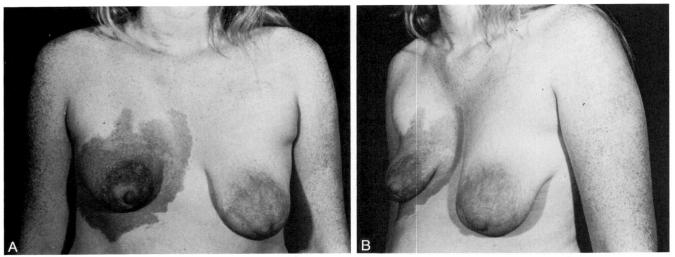

Figure 30–49. *A* and *B*, Twenty-four-year-old female with a malignant tumor of the right breast that did not involve the congenital hemangioma. An "immediate" reconstruction with a vertical rectus abdominis flap is planned.

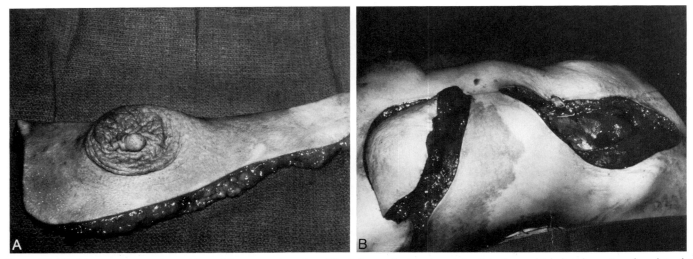

Figure 30–50. Mastectomy specimen (*A*) and intraoperative view (*B*) of the vertical rectus abdominis flap, which has been transferred to the mastectomy site. The entire procedure was completed in less than 2 hours using two surgical teams.

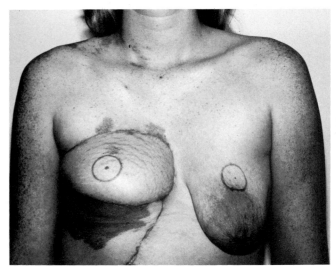

Figure 30–51. Six weeks following the immediate reconstruction. A right nipple-areolar reconstruction and a left mastopexy are planned.

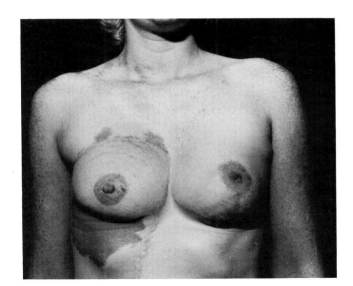

Figure 30–52. One year following the left mastopexy and the nipple reconstruction. The rectus abdominis flap did not interfere with the patient's vigorous outdoor hobbies.

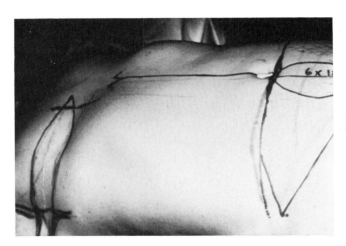

Figure 30–53. Intraoperative view of a lower abdominal TRAM flap, which will be used to reconstruct a modified mastectomy of the right breast.

Figure 30–54. The breast volume was totally replaced by the TRAM flap, which provides excellent symmetry of the upper breast and the axillary tail. No implant was used.

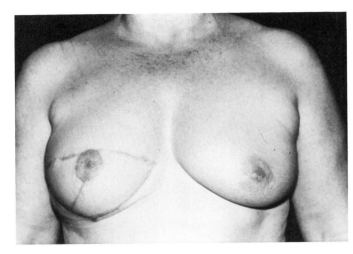

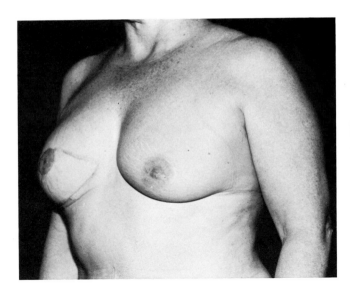

Figure 30–55. The visible portion of the TRAM flap is seen in the area between the inframammary fold and the previous transverse mastectomy scar.

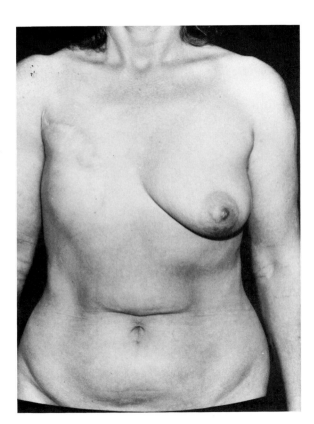

Figure 30–56. Thirty-five-year-old patient following a right radical mastectomy through a high, vertical incision.

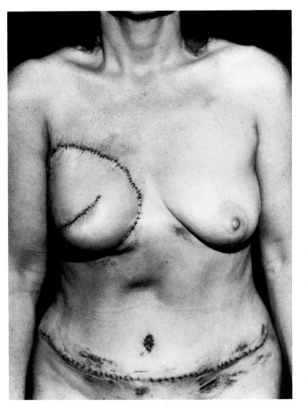

Figure 30–57. Appearance one week following the TRAM flap reconstruction of the right breast. Note the massive amount of skin replacement that was required.

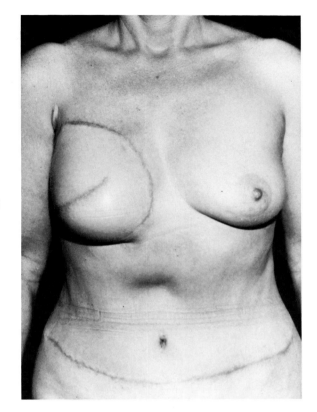

Figure 30–58. Appearance at 6 weeks. A minor revision of the inframammary fold and a nipple reconstruction will complete the reconstruction.

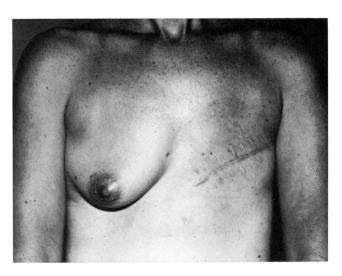

Figure 30–59. Tight left radical mastectomy closure and a partially denervated pectoralis major muscle in a young female. The patient would not be a good candidate for a tissue expander.

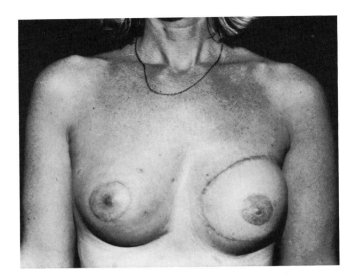

Figure 30–60. A TRAM flap was used to replace the missing breast skin and volume. A large defect such as this cannot be satisfactorily reconstructed without using autogenous tissue. A right augmentation-mastopexy was done for purposes of symmetry.

Figure 30–61. Thirty-four-year-old patient with premalignant disease of the breasts. The redundant abdominal pannus offers the ideal replacement tissue for the bilateral mastectomy defect.

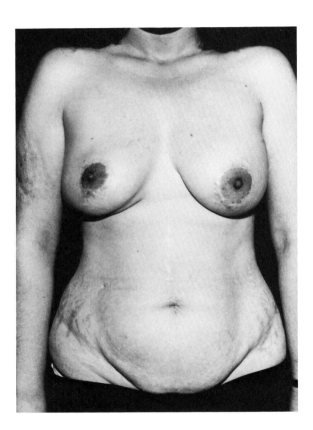

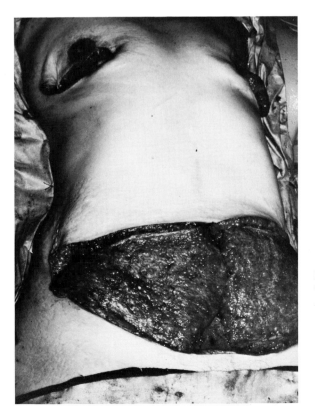

Figure 30–62. An "immediate" bilateral reconstruction was carried out using a completely de-epithelialized and buried TRAM flap. The nipple was discarded.

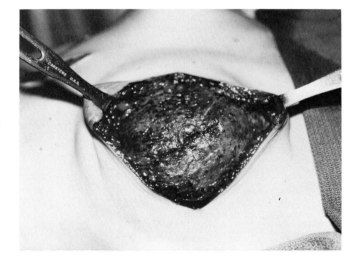

Figure 30–63. Inset of the "buried" TRAM flap beneath the retracted left breast skin.

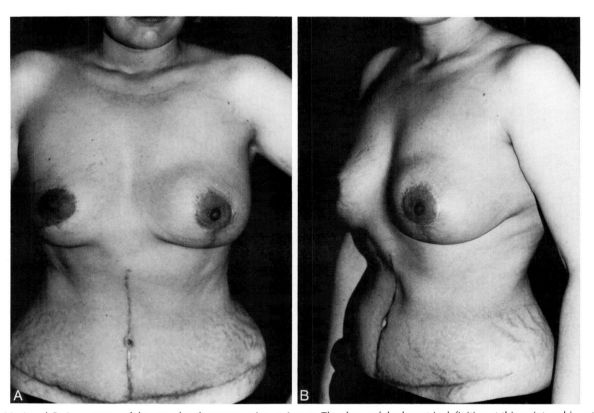

Figure 30–64. *A* and *B,* Appearance of the completed reconstruction at 1 year. The shape of the breast is definitive at this point and is not expected to change. The previous midline abdominal scar was revised at the time of the original procedure.

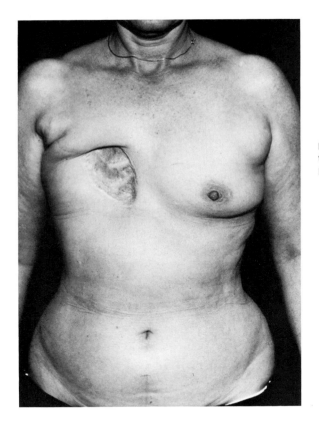

Figure 30–65. Fifty-six-year-old female who had undergone a right radical mastectomy with a skin graft closure *17 years* earlier. A left modified mastectomy is planned for biopsy-proven disease.

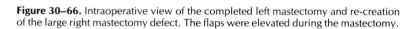

Figure 30–66. Intraoperative view of the completed left mastectomy and re-creation of the large right mastectomy defect. The flaps were elevated during the mastectomy.

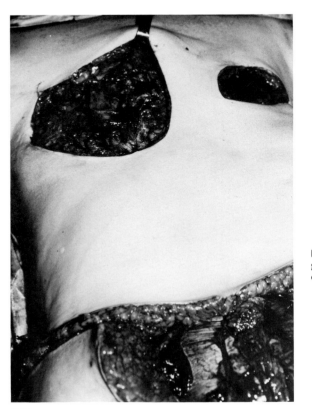

Figure 30–67. A white patch of "scar" was biopsied on the surface of the skin grafted sixth rib and proved to be *persistent* tumor. An unplanned full-thickness chest wall resection was then done.

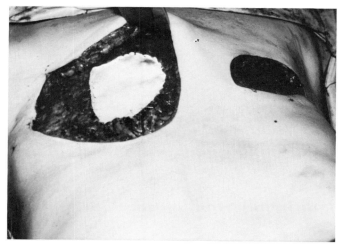

Figure 30–68. A Gore-Tex patch was used to repair the chest wall defect, and the planned procedure was completed.

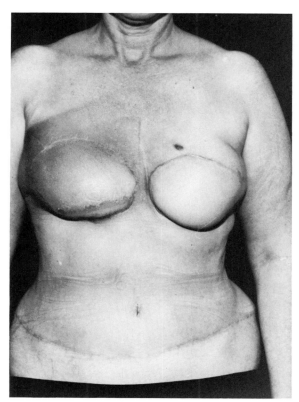

Figure 30–70. Appearance at 6 months. The postoperative irradiation was facilitated by the excellent blood supply of the TRAM flap.

than ideal) or in smokers, because of the healing problems in the flap and the donor site. The donor site is the subject of the most debate, because of the 0.3 percent incidence of hernia formation. A competent abdominal wall should be expected if only a single rectus abdominis muscle is elevated, and this seldom affects the muscular function of the abdominal wall. Approximately one third of the patients surveyed felt that the abdominal contour was unimproved following the removal of the abdominal pannus, even though this was the case from a photographic standpoint.[18] The postoperative donor site pain is significant and is usually compared to the discomfort of a Kocher incision. It is interesting to note that the postoperative pain is related to the dissection of the abdominal flap away from the lower ribcage rather than from the closure of the abdominal fascial defect (Figs. 30–69 to 30–74).

"Free" Microvascular Transfers

Microvascular transfers of myocutaneous flaps to the breast area can now be performed with essentially 100 percent reliability because of three factors that mitigate vascular thrombosis: (1) large flap vessels of 3 to 4 mm, (2) "high flow" myocutaneous flaps, and (3) "end-to-side" vascular anastomosis into the axillary vessels. Even

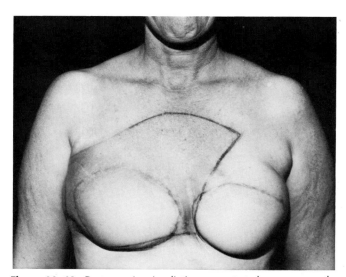

Figure 30–69. Postoperative irradiation was started as soon as the sutures were removed. The irradiation discoloration of the skin is visible at 6 weeks.

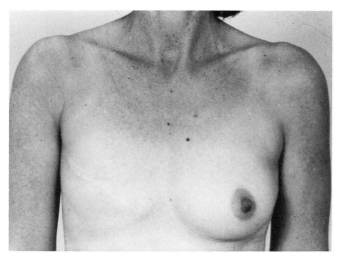

Figure 30–71. Modified mastectomy in a thin patient. The mastectomy flaps are thin, and the pectoralis major muscle is partially denervated.

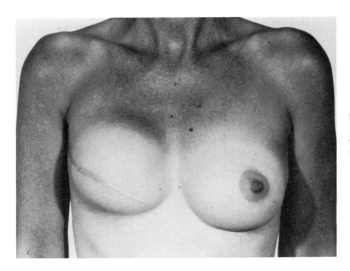

Figure 30–72. The mastectomy was reconstructed with a simple subpectoral implant, which became firm and painful. Multiple attempts with open capsulotomies were not successful in correcting the scar encapsulation. The subpectoral implant in the left breast remained soft.

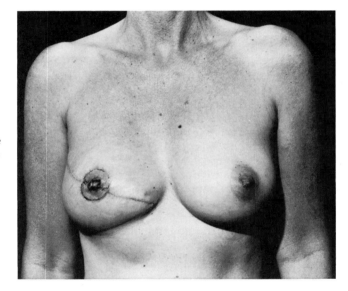

Figure 30–73. A "buried" TRAM flap was used to completely replace the right breast volume. The nipple reconstruction was done at a separate stage.

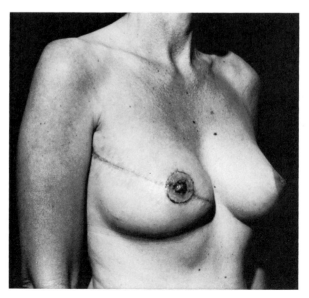

Figure 30–74. Oblique view of the excellent symmetry and ptosis.

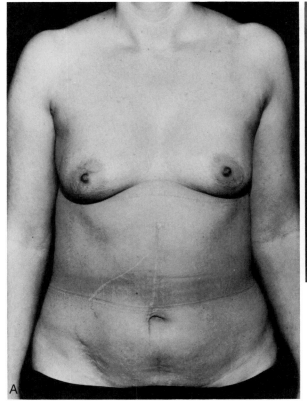

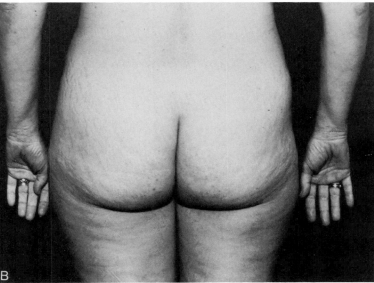

Figure 30–75. Fifty-two-year-old patient with bilateral lobular carcinoma in situ. *A,* Bilateral TRAM flap reconstructions could not be done because of the previous abdominal scars. *B,* A superior gluteus maximus myocutaneous "free" flap reconstruction was chosen as an autogenous replacement.

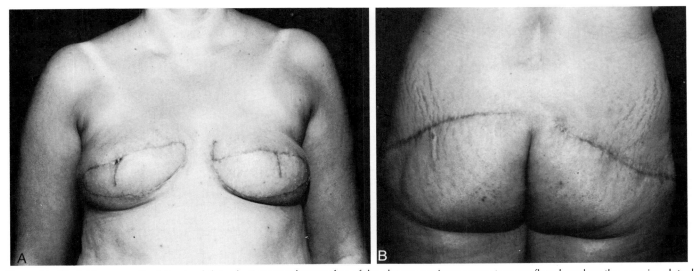

Figure 30–76. *A,* Three months following bilateral microvascular transfers of the gluteus maximus myocutaneous flaps based on the superior gluteal vessels. *B,* The contour of the buttocks is essentially unchanged.

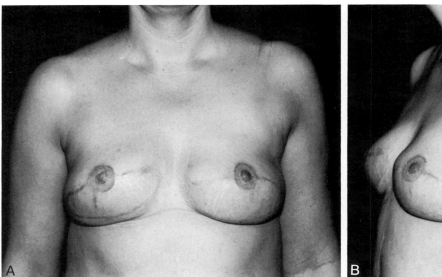
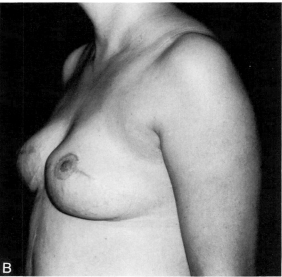

Figure 30–77. *A* and *B,* Appearance of the completed reconstruction at 1 year. The contour of the autogenous reconstruction is definitive at this point.

though the vascular anastomosis can be completed within an hour, the more tedious flap dissection extends the operative time of the "free" flap reconstruction. Two surgical teams are required to complete the procedure in a timely fashion, because the recipient vessels should be prepared while the flap is being elevated. Although the initial operative time is longer for the "free" flap procedure, the reconstruction usually can be completed in a single stage and is cost effective for this reason. The "free" flap donor site discomfort is significantly less than that of other myocutaneous flaps because of the smaller muscular dissection (Figs. 30–75 to 30–77).

SUMMARY

The role of breast reconstruction in the care of the mastectomy patient is expanding now that reliable methods of tissue expansion and myocutaneous flap transfer are available. Definitive and lasting results can be expected, and the replication of the form and consistency of the normal breast should be the desired goal. Flap reconstructions also offer a safer method for closure of difficult wounds of the chest wall and breast and should be routinely considered for major mastectomy and post-irradiation defects.

REFERENCES

1. Becker H: Breast augmentation using the expander mammary prosthesis. Plast Reconstr Surg 79:192–199, 1987.
2. Bostwick J III, Vasconez LO, Jurkiewicz MJ: Breast reconstruction after a radical mastectomy. Plast Reconstr Surg 61(5):682–693, 1978.
3. Bostwick J III, Scheflan M: Latissimus dorsi musculocutaneous flap: a one-stage breast reconstruction. Clin Plast Surg 7:71–78, 1980.
4. Bostwick J III: Latissimus dorsi flap: current applications. Ann Plast Surg 9(5):377–380, 1982.
5. Boyd JB, Taylor GI, Corlett R: The vascular territories of the superior epigastric systems. Plast Reconstr Surg 73:1–16, 1984.
6. Broadbent TR, Woolf RM: Augmentation mammaplasty. Plast Reconstr Surg 40:517–523, 1967.
7. Burkhardt BR: Capsular contracture: hard breasts, soft data. Clin Plast Surg 15:521–532, 1988.
8. Burkhardt BR: Comparing contracture rates: probability theory and the unilateral contracture. Plast Reconstr Surg 74:527–529, 1984.
9. Burkhardt BR, Fried M, Schnur PL, Tofield JJ: Capsules, infection, and intraluminal antibiotics. Plast Reconstr Surg 68:43–49,1981.
10. Cohen BE, Cronin ED: Breast reconstruction with the latissimus dorsi musculocutaneous flap. Clin Plast Surg 11:287–302, 1984.
11. Cronin TD, Gerow F: Augmentation mammaplasty: A new "natural feel" prosthesis. *In* Transactions of the Third International Congress of Plastic Surgeons. Amsterdam, Exerpta Medica, 1964.
12. Dempsey WC, Latham WD: Subpectoral implants in augmentation mammaplasty. Plast Reconstr Surg 42:515–521, 1968.
13. Dowden RV, Horton CE, Rosato FE, McCraw JB: Reconstruction of the breast after mastectomy for cancer. Surg Gynecol Obstet 149:109–115, 1979.
14. Drever JM: The lower abdominal transverse rectus abdominis myocutaneous flap for breast reconstruction. Ann Plast Surg 10(3):179–185, 1983.
15. Hartrampf CR Jr, Scheflan M, Black PW: Breast reconstruction with a transverse abdominal island flap. Plast Reconstr Surg 69(2):216–225, 1982.
16. Hartrampf CR Jr: Transverse Abdominal Island Flap Technique for Breast Reconstruction after Mastectomy. Baltimore, University Park Press, 1984.
17. Hartrampf CR Jr: Abdominal wall competence in transverse abdominal island flap operations. Ann Plast Surg 12(2):139–146, 1984.
18. Hartrampf CR, Bennet GK: Autogenous tissue reconstruction in the mastectomy patient: a critical review of 300 patients. Ann Surg 105(5):508–519, 1987.
19. Hester TR: The polyurethane-covered mammary prosthesis: facts and fiction. Perspect Plast Surg 2:135, 1988.
20. Horton CE, Adamson JE, Mladick RA, Carraway JH: Simple mastectomy with immediate reconstruction. Plast Reconstr Surg 53:42–47, 1974.

21. Horton CE, Carraway JH: Total mastectomy with immediate reconstruction for premalignant disease. *In* Goldwyn RM (ed): Plastic and Reconstructive Surgery of the Breast. Boston, Little, Brown & Co, 1976, p 459.
22. Lejour M, De Mey A, Mattheiem W: Local recurrences and metastases of breast cancer after 194 reconstructions. Chir Plast 7:131–134, 1983.
23. Lejour M, Alemanno P, De Mey A: Analysis of 56 breast reconstructions using the latissimus dorsi flap. Ann Chir Plast Esthet 30:7, 1985.
24. Marshall DR, Anstee EJ, Stapleton MJ: Immediate reconstruction of the breast following modified radical mastectomy for carcinoma. Br J Plast Surg 35:438–442, 1982.
25. Maxwell GP: Latissimus dorsi breast reconstruction: an aesthetic assessment. Clin Plast Surg 8:373–387, 1981.
26. McCraw JB, Dibbell DG: Experimental definition of independent myocutaneous vascular territories. Plast Reconstr Surg 60:212–227, 1977.
27. McCraw JB, Dibbell DG, Carraway JH: Clinical definition of independent myocutaneous vascular territories. Plast Reconstr Surg 60:341–352, 1977.
28. McCraw JB, Massey FM, Shanklin KD, Horton CE: Vaginal reconstruction with gracilis myocutaneous flaps. Plast Reconstr Surg 58(2):176–183, 1976.
29. McCraw J, Papp C, Zanon E: Breast volume replacement using the de-epithialized latissimus dorsi myocutaneous flap. Eur J Plast Surg 11(3):120–125, 1988.
30. McCraw JB, Maxwell GP: Early and late capsular "deformation" as a cause of unsatisfactory results in the latissimus dorsi breast reconstruction. Clin Plast Surg 15:717–726, 1988.
31. Millard DR Jr: Breast aesthetics when reconstructing with the latissimus dorsi musculocutaneous flap. Plast Reconstr Surg 70:161–172, 1982.
32. Milloy FG, Anson BJ, McAfee DK: The rectus abdominis muscle and the epigastric arteries. Surg Gynecol Obstet 110:293–302, 1960.
33. Muhlbauer W, Olbrisch R: The latissimus dorsi myocutaneous flap for breast reconstruction. Chir Plast 4:27, 1977.
34. Noone RB, Murphy JR, Spear SL, Little JW III: A 6 year experience with immediate reconstruction after mastectomy for cancer. Plast Reconstr Surg 76:258–269, 1985.
35. Olivari N: The latissimus flap. Br J Plast Surg 29:126–128, 1976.
36. Olivari N: Use of thirty latissimus dorsi flaps. Plast Reconstr Surg 64:654–661, 1979.
37. Peters W, Smith D: Ivalon breast prostheses: evaluation 19 years after implantation. Plast Reconstr Surg 67(4):514–518, 1981.
38. Pickrell KL, Puckett CL, Given KS: Subpectoral augmentation mammaplasty. Plast Reconstr Surg 60:325–336, 1977.
39. Pollock H: Polyurethane-covered breast implant. Plast Reconstr Surg 74:729, 1984.
40. Rees T, Guy C, Coburn J: The use of inflatable breast implants. Plast Reconstr Surg 52:609–615, 1973.
41. Reiffel RS, Rees TD, Guy CL, Aston SJ: A comparison of capsule formation following breast augmentation by saline-filled or gel-filled implants. Aesthetic Plast Surg 7:113–116, 1983.
42. Robbins TH: Rectus abdominis myocutaneous flap for breast reconstruction. Aust NZ J Surg 49(5):527–530, 1979.
43. Robbins TH: Post-mastectomy breast reconstruction using a rectus abdominis musculocutaneous island flap. Br J Plast Surg 34:286–290, 1981.
44. Robbins TH: Breast reconstruction using a rectus abdominis musculocutaneous flap: 5 year follow-up. Aust NZ J Surg 55(1):65, 1985.
45. Rosato FE, Fink PJ, Horton CE, Payne RL: Immediate post-mastectomy reconstruction. J Surg Oncol 8:277–280, 1976.
46. Schneider WJ, Hill HL Jr, Brown RG: Latissimus dorsi myocutaneous flap for breast reconstruction. Br J Plast Surg 30:277–281, 1977.
47. Shaw WW: Breast reconstruction by superior gluteal microvascular free flaps without silicone implants. Plast Reconstr Surg 72(4):490–501, 1983.
48. Shaw W, Feng L: A comparison of the superior vs. inferior pedicles of the transverse rectus abdominis myocutaneous flap: implications in breast reconstruction. Plast Reconstr Surg (in press).
49. Taylor GI, Corlett RJ, Boyd JB: The extended deep inferior epigastric flap: a clinical technique. Plast Reconstr Surg 72(6):751–765, 1983.
50. Taylor GI, Corlett RJ, Boyd JB: The versatile deep inferior epigastric (inferior rectus abdominis) flap. Br J Plast Surg 37(3):330–350, 1984.
51. Tebbetts JB: Transaxillary subpectoral augmentation mammaplasty: long-term follow-up and refinements. Plast Reconstr Surg 74:636–647, 1984.
52. Wolf LE, Biggs TM: Aesthetic refinements in the use of the latissimus dorsi flap in breast reconstruction. Plast Reconstr Surg 69:788–793, 1982.
53. Woods JE, Irons GB, Arnold PG: The case for submuscular implantation of prostheses in reconstructive breast surgery. Ann Plast Surg 5:115–122, 1980.

Chapter 31

WOUND CARE AND COMPLICATIONS OF MASTECTOMY

Kirby I. Bland, M.D.

Rehabilitation of the postmastectomy patient produces problems of varying complexity. This chapter reviews commonly utilized approaches for the care of the postmastectomy wound and addresses the complications encountered in these patients.

WOUND CARE

The various operative techniques employed in the treatment for breast carcinoma are described in detail in chapters 28, 29, and 30. The surgeon should recognize that the essential parts of optimal wound repair are the application of meticulous technique, hemostasis, and wound closure at operation. We prefer closed-suction catheter drainage of the mastectomy wound, commercially available as Hemovac, Davol, or Jackson-Pratt tubing, and each system should be appropriately placed at operation to allow superomedial and inferolateral positioning of these apparati to ensure thorough, dependent aspiration. After the wound is closed, the tubing is connected to ensure removal of all wound contents (e.g., clots, serum). An optional technique includes wound irrigation with saline via the closed flaps to flush the drainage system and provide patency of the suction catheters. Thereafter the skin margins may be covered with strips of nonadherent, nonporous dressing (Telfa) or a porous dressing (Adaptic). The application of the operative dressing is an essential part of the operative procedure and should not be delegated to surgical assistants or nurses unfamiliar with this detail. Optionally, surgeons may apply fluffs of 4 × 4 dressings of cotton gauze, inclusive of the entire operative site, to provide uniform gentle compression within the limits of flap dissection. These compression dressings are then taped with Elastoplast or an equivalent elastic adherent dressing that is further secured by the application of benzoine over the periphery of the dissected operative sites. This technique affords optimal coverage of the axilla with uniform gentle compression, yet leaves the upper arm and forearm free of dressing application. Other surgeons criticize the application of pressure dressings over the dissected skin flaps and prefer occlusive dressings alone (e.g., light dressing, Opsite). This technique is inadvisable when suction drainage methods are not used, as flap adherence is reduced with subsequent seroma formation. Suction catheter drainage, as a rule, is necessary for 4 to 7 days postoperatively. Premature removal of the catheters is only allowed when the function of this closed-system technique is compromised. Routinely, catheters are removed only when less than 20 ml of serous or serosanguinous drainage is evident during a 24-hour interval. Thereafter the wound is carefully inspected with regard to flap adherence, and the patient is encouraged to begin graded, active range of motion of the ipsilateral arm and shoulder.

The patient usually experiences moderate pain in the operative site, shoulder, and arm in the immediate postoperative period. Because of the necessity of extensive flap development, the patient may note hypesthesia and paresthesia as well as occasional "phantom" hyperesthesia. Hypesthesia is a common postmastectomy complaint and results from denervation of one or more of the intercostobrachial nerves traversing the axillary space that are sectioned in the conduct of the axillary dissection. These sensations disappear gradually with wound healing.[25] The patient should be assured that abnormal sensations will usually subside within 3 to 8 months postoperatively. However, normal sensation may never return to the denervated axilla, medial arm, and hemithorax.

In the immediate postoperative period, the patient is encouraged to resume activity on the evening following her operative procedure. We regularly prescribe fluids by mouth within 2 to 4 hours postoperatively, and often the patient is able to eat a normal or light meal before retiring. Early ambulation is encouraged. Use of portable suction units allows the patient to be up and about her room early postoperatively. We routinely encourage the patient to continue immobilization of the ipsilateral shoulder and upper arm, while mobility is permitted below the elbow in the forearm and hand. Application of closed-suction catheter techniques ensures wound evacuation in this circumstance. Isometric exercises, such as squeezing a ball, increase blood and lymph volume but do not facilitate lymph flow. Initial exercises should include graded, active shoulder exercises.

Although a moderate degree of bacterial contamination can be demonstrated in mastectomy procedures, we do not routinely administer preoperative, perioperative, or postoperative antibiotics unless other medical conditions (e.g., cardiac valvular disease, prosthetic appliances, or skin ulceration) are present. If postoperative erythema and cellulitis are evident, treatment with topical antibacterial creams such as Silvadene are of particular value to prevent progressive epidermolysis and invasive soft tissue infections. Early debridement of obviously devascularized tissue is an important prophylactic adjunct to prevent progressive invasive infection.

Skin grafting following radical mastectomy as originally proposed by Halsted[11] continues to hold a prominent role in the management of the mastectomy wound. Stents applied over split-thickness skin grafts, which are necessary for large tissue defects, should be removed on the fifth or sixth postoperative day. Early and periodic wound care, including debridement with wet-to-dry saline dressings, affords optimal wound management to ensure adequate "take" of the graft application.

COMPLICATIONS OF MASTECTOMY

The operative therapy of breast carcinoma can produce a variety of physical problems with regard to patient care. Rehabilitation for the postmastectomy patient has been greatly facilitated by the Reach to Recovery programs sponsored by the American Cancer Society and similar patient/family rehabilitation agencies. In most circumstances, the breast cancer patient is allowed to begin the gradual resumption of presurgical activities within 2 weeks after surgery. Younger women usually regain full range of motion of the arm and the shoulder before leaving the hospital, whereas older patients may require intense (supervised) exercise for several months before attaining their former levels of activity. Visits from volunteers of the American Cancer Society or the Visiting Nurse Association are of particular value for psychosocial and physical recovery of the postmastectomy patient.

Lymphedema

The pathogenesis of ipsilateral arm lymphedema following radical, modified, and segmental mastectomy is comprehensively reviewed in chapter 32. Lymphedema results as a consequence of the en bloc ablation of lymphatic routes (nodes and channels) within the field of resection of the primary mammary tumor. The subsequent increase in plasma hydrostatic pressure that results with removal of these conduits may follow the surgical procedure, irradiation, or uncontrolled progression of neoplasm. Injury, capillary disruption, infection, obstruction to lymphatic or venous outflow, hyperthermia, or exercise will accelerate protein leakage into these tissues. Previous attempts to evaluate the degree of arm lymphedema have been classified by Stillwell[27] according to the percentage of volume increase. We

grade an increase of less than 10 percent in arm volume as insignificant, whereas an increase of greater than 80 percent is classified as severe. Lymphedema affects some 50 percent to 70 percent of all radical mastectomy patients but is severe and incapacitating in only approximately 10 percent.[26] Gilchrist[10] stresses the importance of free and complete active range of motion of the arm and shoulder in the early postoperative period. Patient education emphasizing the avoidance of excessive sun exposure, injections, infections, or other potentially active or passive injury to the ipsilateral extremity is paramount to avoid lymphedema. Further, early recognition of incipient edema by the patient and immediate therapy with compression massage of the area by the patient or nursing personnel may abrogate the ensuing morbidity of lymphedema. Early application of compression massage with the thumb, including stroking of the edematous extremity, will often alleviate and augment the prophylaxis of further edema. When lymphedema is severe, hospitalization for mechanical expression of tissue fluid, with application of an intermittent pneumatic compression device (Jobst pump), may be of value. The Jobst compression pump allows sequential, uniform, and progressive compression of the involved extremity in a proximal direction, thus allowing egress to the obstructed flow of lymph. The physician may wish to prescribe antibiotics, especially if there is evidence of supervening cellulitis. Additionally, it is advisable to prescribe diuretic therapy concomitant with a low salt diet. An elastic Ace bandage is applied when the patient is not treating herself with the pump, and the arm should be elevated above heart level when the patient is inactive. We recommend daily measurements at a fixed point on the extremity before and after Jobst therapy is initiated. The arm circumference is measured daily at positions above and below the elbow. These measurements should be recorded prior to and following therapy. This method is completed in a repetitious cycle when progressive resolution of the edema is evident. When optimal improvement is apparent, the patient is measured for a Jobst Venous Pressure sleeve, which is custom-tailored with specific circumferential compression pressure (30 to 40 mm Hg). Daily application of compression treatments are necessary until the sleeve is received and the results of therapy are realized.

Wound Infection

Although wound infection occurs infrequently, infection and cellulitis of the mastectomy wound or ipsilateral arm may represent serious morbidity in the postoperative patient (see chapter 5). The majority of reported wound infections occur as a result of the primary tissue ischemia resulting from extensive tissue dissection that creates thin, devascularized skin flaps. Thereafter progressive tissue necrosis provides a medium that supports bacterial proliferation with invasive tissue infection. The 18.9 percent infection rate reported for radical mastectomy by the National Research Council is exorbitantly high for a clean operation. In contrast, the 4.3 percent rate identified in the modified radical mastectomy series by Cruse[7] may be lower because the operation is of lesser magnitude, but more likely it is less because of the efficient evacuation of hematoma and serum with closed wound suction drainage.

Except in patients with preexisting medical diseases (e.g., prosthetic devices, cardiac valvular disease, or ulcerative carcinoma), we do not administer prophylactic antibiotics routinely; however, irrigation of the wound with antibiotics at operation is desirable for reduction of the bacterial flora.

Wound infection or cellulitis produces an immediate disability that may progress to late postoperative lymphedema of the arm. The compromised lymphatic flow, with resultant stasis produced by the standard technique of developing thin skin flaps, predisposes the wound to resultant infection. Early attempts should be made to culture the wound for aerobic and anaerobic organisms with immediate Gram stain of identifiable strains in order to document the bacterial contaminant. In the absence of lymphedema, wound cellulitis uniformly responds to appropriate antibiotic therapy and elevation of the extremity.

Seroma

Seromas occur in the axillary dead space beneath the elevated skin flaps and represent the most frequent complication of mastectomy. In the reports by Say and Donegan[24] and Budd et al.,[6] the incidence of seroma formation varied from 24.6 percent to 52.0 percent through the past two decades. In a retrospective analysis of 87 axillary regional lymph node (Patey) dissections performed as isolated procedures discrete from en bloc breast resections, Bland et al.[3] observed seromas in 26 percent of patients.

With surgical ablation of the breast, the intervening lymphatics and fatty tissues are resected en bloc; thus the vasculature and lymphatics of the gland are transected. Thereafter transudation of lymph and the accumulation of blood in the operative field are expected. Further, extensive dissection of the mastectomy flaps results in a large potential dead space beneath the flaps, as does the irregularity of the chest wall, especially in the deep axillary fossa. Continual chest wall respiratory excursions and motion in the shoulder initiate shearing forces that further delay flap adherence and wound repair. Operative technique should minimize lymphatic spillage and transudation of serum to allow rapid adherence of the skin flaps to deep structures without compromise of blood flow to skin flaps or the axilla. Various techniques for flap fixation and wound drainage have been utilized to enhance primary wound repair and to minimize seroma accumulation. Two types of external suture fixation have been advocated. In the study by Orr,[22] tension sutures tied over a rubber tubing bolster to fixate the flaps to underlying intercostal muscles and the latissimus dorsi muscle were used. In the report by Keyes et al.,[14] through-and-through flap sutures were tied directly to the skin surface to secure the breast flap

to the chest wall. Penrose drains were utilized to drain excessive accumulation of lymph and blood. Thereafter Larsen and Hugan[15] recommended the application of buried fixation sutures of silk or absorbable material to secure the flaps. These authors secured skin flaps with 30 to 50 subcutaneous cotton sutures and avoided the insertion of any type of drain when possible.

Removal of serum accumulation was first accomplished by the use of static drains, such as Paul's tubing, and the insertion of various soft Penrose drains. Both Paul's tubing and Penrose drains required bulky gauze dressings and multiple dressing changes for the continuous serous soilage expected with wound discharge. Murphy,[21] in 1947, and Morris,[20] in 1973, proposed continuous closed-suction drainage methods to prevent serum collection beneath extensive flaps. Presently, the majority of surgeons utilize this technique of closed-suction drainage to aspirate excessive collections of serum, lymph, and blood from the mastectomy wound.

In the classic report by Maitland and Mathieson,[16] in 1970, 1193 wounds were drained during a 5-year period. Of 153 mastectomies, 72 underwent traditional drainage (i.e., wicks, Penrose), whereas 81 had suction drainage. For operations at various sites, including the genitourinary, alimentary, and biliary tract and soft tissue areas (e.g., breast, thyroid), significant differences were not evident for the two techniques. However, in evaluation of the breast as a subset of the overall analysis, the incidence of wound infection with suction drainage (4.9 percent) versus traditional drainage (12.50 percent) was 1.7 times less frequent ($p = 0.045$). For this subset of the patient population, the authors noted a diminished wound infection rate and increased primary healing with the application of closed-suction drainage techniques. These results were confirmed by Morris[20] following a controlled clinical trial performed to compare the effectiveness of suction drainage with that of static drainage. For radical mastectomy wounds, this trial established that the rate of wound repair was superior with suction drainage technique. Furthermore, the volume of aspirated drainage was greater with the closed-suction method, which also afforded a reduction in the infection, tissue necrosis, and wound disruption frequency.

Thereafter Bourke and associates[5] conducted a randomized, prospective trial of closed-suction wound drainage compared with corrugated wound drainage following simple mastectomy for early breast cancer (lesion confined to the breast and without skin ulceration). In 51 patients admitted to the study, there were no statistically significant differences between the two groups with respect to local complications such as infection, serum collection beneath the flaps, skin necrosis, and wound repair. However, as shown in Table 31–1, the number of dressing changes required were significantly reduced with suction catheters as opposed to corrugated drainage, and suction drains could be removed significantly sooner than corrugated drains. In today's cost-conscious medical environment, the reduction in dressing changes per day and the morbidity related to prolonged *in situ* drainage clearly favors the usage of closed-suction drainage methods.

Table 31–1. FREQUENCY OF DRESSINGS, LENGTH OF DRAINAGE, AND TIME OF SUTURE REMOVAL

	Suction Drains ($n = 24$)	Corrugated Drains ($n = 27$)	t	p
Number of dressings/day	0.071 ± 0.19	1.02 ± 0.30	3.88	0.001
Drains *in situ* (days)	4.79 ± 1.66	6.55 ± 1.33	4.18	0.001
Sutures removed (days)	9.91 ± 0.65	10.28 ± 0.93	1.15	NS

NS = Not significant.
From Bourke JB, et al: Br J Surg 63:67–69, 1976. Reprinted by permission.

Aitken et al.[1] evaluated 204 consecutive mastectomies in which the techniques used for flap closure and wound management were identical. All potential dead space was obliterated with absorbable sutures that incorporated the pectoralis major, serratus anterior, and latissimus dorsi muscles as well as the subdermal skin of the axillary flap. Two closed-suction Hemovac drains, one placed in the axillary apex along the lateral part of the chest wall and the other placed over the anterior portion of the chest, were inserted via a separate lower flap stab incision. The average initial volume and total volume of the fluid aspirated from the wounds were similar in both radical and modified radical mastectomy groups (91.1 ml vs. 91.7 ml). Table 31–2 summarizes the wound complications observed in this series. Postoperative fluid accumulation occurred in 9.31 percent, with greater frequency in the radical mastectomy group. Infected seroma was identified only in the radical mastectomy group, with an overall frequency of 0.98 percent. The magnitude of the radical mastectomy procedure perhaps also accounted for the frequency of superficial wound infections, which were more than four times as frequent in this group as in the modified radical mastectomy group. Aitken and Minton[2] identified a decreased incidence of seroma accumulation in these less extensive operations on the breast (simple mastectomy had less incidence than modified radical, which in turn had less incidence than radical mastectomy). These results agree with the results of other reports.[24] In addition, the wound infection rate of 3.4 percent compares most favorably with those in other series,[6, 24] which ranged from 8.4 percent to 14.2 percent.

Tadych and Donegan[28] determined the daily wound drainage and total hospital drainage (THD) for 49 consecutive patients undergoing mastectomy to evaluate the frequency of seroma and lymphedema formation. Of this series of patients undergoing modified radical mastectomies and who did not receive irradiation, all had wound closure with suction drainage and none had flap necrosis or infection. THD varied from 227 to 3607 ml and did not correlate with body weight. Twenty-six patients had wound seromas requiring drainage for periods of as much as 7 months, most often requiring repeated aspirations and, more infrequently ($n = 4$), open drainage. No patient with less than 20 ml of drainage in the 24 hours prior to catheter removal developed a seroma. Ipsilateral edema of the arm directly correlated with THD. No patient with less than 500 ml of THD had edema, whereas the frequency rate was 75 percent in patients with THD that exceeded 900 ml. These authors concluded that THD likely reflects the magnitude of lymphatic interruption after mastectomy and thus the probability of lymphatic insufficiency and the development of lymphedema.

The utilization of closed-system suction catheter drainage during the past decade has greatly facilitated the reduction in protracted serum collections. Seromas of the axillary dead space and the anterior chest wall are manifested in the first week postoperatively. Therapy consists of retention of the suction apparatus until drainage diminishes to <20 ml per day. Thereafter compression dressings are applied following catheter removal in anticipation of protracted wound discharge.

McCarthy et al.[17] reported on attempts at management of the chronic serous discharge from mastectomy wounds that were observed in approximately 25 percent of their patients. In this prospective, randomized controlled trial, the effect of tetracycline as a sclerotherapy agent for flap adherence was evaluated. Six patients in the control group and eight patients in the treated group were evaluated. One patient in the control group developed a seroma following drain removal. In contrast, one half of the patients treated with tetracycline therapy developed seromas following removal of drains. Because of the severe pain associated with tetracycline sclerotherapy treatment and the lack of demonstrable benefit to those treated, the study was aborted by the investigators.

The effect of shoulder mobility restriction in diminishing serous wound discharge following radical mastec-

Table 31–2. SUMMARY OF WOUND COMPLICATIONS

Complication	Type of Mastectomy			
	Radical ($n = 72$)	Modified Radical ($n = 117$)	Simple ($n = 15$)	Total ($n = 204$)
Hematoma or seroma	14 (19.44)	5 (4.27)	—	19 (9.31)
Infected seroma	2 (2.78)	—	—	2 (0.98)
Superficial wound infection	5 (6.94)	2 (1.71)	—	7 (3.43)

Numbers in parentheses are percentages.
From Aitken DR, et al: Surg Gynecol Obstet 158:327–350, 1984. Reprinted by permission.

tomy was evaluated in a randomized prospective clinical trial by Flew.[9] Of 64 consecutive patients nursed in the wards of the Guy's Breast Unit in London, shoulder movement restriction reduced the mean volume of drainage by 40 percent in those who had immobility for the first 7 postoperative days when compared with the group in whom early arm exercises were encouraged (Table 31–3). This study confirmed a reduction in drainage duration (days) by 29 percent. Both the number of patients and the need for multiple aspirations were reduced in the shoulder-restricted group; however, differences were not statistically significant between the two subgroups in duration of hospital stay. Shoulder mobilization did not result in increased shoulder stiffness, although the author confirmed an increased incidence of mild, but transient, lymphedema of the arm when the technique was utilized. It may be concluded from this study that active shoulder movement immediately following mastectomy is not advisable. Furthermore, there is evidence that immobilization significantly decreased drainage in volume ($p < 0.01$) and duration ($p < 0.05$) without affecting eventual shoulder mobility, as shown in Table 31–3. It appears that the liability of lymphedema is enhanced with use of the restriction technique but can be limited in extent when the complication is recognized.

Pneumothorax

Pneumothorax, a rare complication, develops when the surgeon perforates the parietal pleura with extended tissue dissection or with attempts at hemostasis for perforators of the intercostal musculature. Pneumothorax is more commonly seen in patients undergoing a radical mastectomy following removal of the pectoralis major musculature. Respiratory distress is recognized in the operative or the immediate postoperative periods, and pneumothorax is confirmed by chest roentgenogram. Immediate therapy with closed thoracostomy drainage of the pleural space is essential as soon as pneumothorax is verified.

Tissue Necrosis

A commonly recognized complication of breast surgery is necrosis of the developed skin flaps or skin margins. Zintel and Nay[29] observed major skin necrosis in four percent of their patients, a rate similar to that observed by other series. Bland et al.[3, 4] observed an incidence of 21 percent for minor and major necrosis of skin flaps with associated wound infection for this operative site. Fitts et al.[8] noted an incidence of marginal necrosis for 39 percent of patients in their series and demonstrated that patients with skin edge necrosis were observed to have an increased incidence of postoperative arm edema.

Local debridement is usually not necessary in minor areas of necrosis (i.e., ≤ 2 cm² area). Larger areas of partial or full-thickness skin loss require debridement and, on occasion, the application of split-thickness skin grafts. Rotational composite skin flaps and subcutaneous skin tissue can be utilized from the lateral chest wall or the contralateral breast to cover the defect.

Hemorrhage

The utilization of closed-suction catheter drainage allows early recognition of hemorrhage, an infrequent complication of mastectomy. Hemorrhage is reported as a postoperative complication in one to four percent of patients and is manifested by undue swelling of flaps of the operative site.[3, 4, 29] Early recognition of this complication is imperative. Hemorrhage may be treated by aspiration of the liquefied hematoma and the establishment of patency of the suction catheters. The application of a light compression dressing reinforced with Elastoplast tape should diminish the recurrence of this adverse event. Moderate to severe hemorrhage in the immediate postoperative course is rare and is best managed with wound reexploration. Early, severe hemorrhage is most often related to arterial perforators of the thoracoacromial vessels or internal mammary arteries. Direct suture ligature is advisable. Thereafter closed drainage systems are replaced, and tubing patency is ensured prior to wound closure.

Surgeons hold varying opinions as to the best technique to elevate skin flaps for performance of total mastectomy. Electrocautery, cold scalpel, Shaw hot knife, and, more recently, the laser have been utilized to create skin flaps for modified radical and radical

Table 31–3. WOUND DRAINAGE FOLLOWING MODIFIED RADICAL MASTECTOMY: EFFECT OF RESTRICTION OF SHOULDER MOVEMENT

	Fixed (*n = 29*)		Free (*n = 35*)	
Drainage volume (ml, mean ± S.E.)		725.4 ± 77.3		1203.1 ± 137.7†
Total drainage time* in days (range and mean)	4–21	11.69 ± 0.93	6–60	16.40 ± 1.79‡
Time until removal of all drains (range and mean)	4–21	11.17 ± 0.92	6–31	13.66 ± 0.93§
Aspirations				
No. patients		2		7§
No. aspirations		4		33 ‖
Hospital stay (days, mean ± S.E.)		14.66 ± 0.66		16.03 ± 0.75§

*Including aspirations.
†$t = 2.862$; $p < 0.01$.
‡$t = 2.195$; $p < 0.05$.
§N.S.
‖ $t = 1.791$; $p < 0.1$.

Group	Shoulder Abduction at 4 Months	
	Limitation > 30° (No. of Patients)	*Mean Limitation* (Degrees ± S.E.)
Fixed (*n = 29*)	8	19.8 ± 3.3
Free (*n = 34*)	13	21.2 ± 3.6

The differences are not significant.
From Flew TJ: Br J Surg 66:302–305, 1979. Reprinted by permission.

mastectomies. The cold scalpel has the advantage of minimal tissue injury but may present formidable bleeding problems unless used concomitantly with direct suture ligature or electrocoagulation. Excessive bleeding may obscure the operative field with blood, and the extensive dissection may leave the hematologically compromised patient anemic at termination of the procedure. In contrast, electrocoagulation minimizes blood loss.[2, 12] However, the experimental studies by Keenan et al.[13] suggest that the tissue damage initiated with cautery injury may diminish the autoimmune response of host tissues to infection.

In Osborne and coinvestigators'[23] prospective, nonrandomized study of 60 patients undergoing total mastectomy, no statistical differences for infection rate, operating time, wound discharge, or hospital stay were noted with use of the cold scalpel compared with the electrocautery. These authors determined that use of the electrocautery allowed significantly greater blood loss, estimating that blood loss was 440 versus 651 ml for the scalpel and electrocautery, respectively. Kakos and James[12] completed a similar prospective analysis for comparison of blood loss with the electrocautery versus the scalpel in 50 mastectomy patients. Average blood loss in this series was 960 ml in the scalpel group vs. 160 ml in the electrocautery group. Twenty-four of 25 scalpel patients (96 percent) received transfusions, compared with only six of 25 (24 percent) in the electrocautery group. Wound necrosis was not different in the two groups.

More recently, Miller and associates[19] conducted a randomized prospective study to investigate differences in blood loss and postoperative complications in patients undergoing modified radical mastectomy with use of the electrocautery and scalpel. Table 31–4 demonstrates the demographic features identifiable with use of electrocoagulation versus the scalpel in mastectomies. Twenty-

four patients had skin flaps created with the cold scalpel, and 25 had skin flaps created with the electrocautery. The two groups were similar with respect to age, stage of disease, size of tumor, and body weight. Use of the electrocautery allowed patients to have significantly reduced operative blood loss when compared with scalpel patients (352 vs. 507 ml, respectively; $p < 0.05$). No electrocautery patient required transfusion. The primary advantage of the electrocautery was the reduction in blood loss; surprisingly, operating time was not significantly shortened with use of the electrocautery technique. These authors acknowledge that the axillary dissection is the time-limiting factor of the procedure, and, because of neurological injury induced with use of electrocoagulation, axillary dissection techniques utilized by the surgeons were identical in both subgroups. Total postoperative Hemovac drainage and hospital stay were not significantly different between the two groups. Although the number of fever days and wound complications were slightly higher in the electrocoagulation group, this difference was not statistically significant. Miller and coinvestigators[19] concluded that use of the electrocautery for development of skin flaps in the performance of a mastectomy reduces blood loss without incurring a greater incidence of wound complications. Cautery appears to be the most suitable surgical instrument for tissue plane dissection in the procedure. However, it has the expectant limitation of neurostimulation and heat injury with dissection around motor nerves, such as the brachial plexus, and of motor innervation to muscles of the axillary space, including the medial/lateral pectoral, long thoracic, and thoracodorsal nerves to the pectoralis major/minor, serratus anterior, and latissimus dorsi muscles, respectively. For these reasons, the combination of both techniques is utilized by the majority of surgeons.

As indicated by Miller et al.,[18] the known risk for blood transfusions include hepatitis (0.26 to one percent), transfusion allergic reactions (one to 19 percent), and a lower, but fatal, risk for acquisition of the acquired immunodeficiency syndrome (AIDS). Each of these transfusion-related complications necessitate constant reexamination of the indications for transfusion with deliberate attempts to reduce transfusion requirements at mastectomy in the nonanemic patient.

Injury to Neurovascular Structures of the Axilla

Injury to the brachial plexus is also a rare complication of mastectomy. This is most commonly avoided by meticulous (cold scalpel) sharp dissection in and about the neurovascular bundle and by development of tissue planes that parallel the neurilemma and the wall of the axillary vein to allow en bloc resection of lymphatic structures and fatty tissues. More common are injuries to the thoracodorsal nerve and the long thoracic nerve (respiratory) of Bell in the postoperative period. The thoracodorsal, or subscapular, nerve innervates the latissimus dorsi muscle in its course with the thoracodorsal

Table 31–4. BLOOD LOSS, HEMATOCRIT CHANGE, TRANSFUSION, LENGTH OF OPERATION, DRAINAGE, STAY, AND INFECTIONS IN SCALPEL AND ELECTROCAUTERY MASTECTOMY PATIENTS

	Scalpel Patients	Electrocautery Patients	p Value
Estimated blood loss (ml)	507 ± 122	352 ± 106	<0.05
Decrease in hematocrit	8.2 ± 2.2	5.9 ± 1.6	<0.05
Number transfused	3	0	<0.005
Length of operation (minutes)	120 ± 19	117 ± 20	NS
Postoperative drainage (ml)	208 ± 56	256 ± 66	NS
Stay (days)	5.8 ± 0.1	5.9 ± 0.6	NS
Number fever days	6	9	NS
Wound complications	3	6	NS
Cellulitis	2	5	NS
Flap necrosis	1	1	NS

NS = Not significant.
From Miller E, et al: Am Surg 54:284–286, 1988. Reprinted by permission.

(subscapular) vessels and is commonly sacrificed when lymphatics are discovered to be involved with metastases at axillary dissection. Sacrifice of this nerve allows minimal physical disability; the patient observes weakness of internal rotation and abduction of the shoulder following denervation and paralysis of the latissimus dorsi muscle.

Conversely, injury or transsection of the long thoracic nerve of Bell, which innervates the serratus anterior muscle, produces instability and unsightly prominence of the scapula ("winged scapula"). The patient sustaining such an injury will often complain of shoulder pain at rest and with motion for many months following the procedure. All attempts should be made to preserve this nerve, yet its involvement with invasive neoplasm or nodal extension may require that it be sacrificed to ensure adequate en bloc resection.

The lateral and medial pectoral nerves to the pectoralis major muscles and the motor innervation to the pectoralis minor exit the brachial plexus to enter the posterior aspects of these muscles in the proximal axilla. Preservation of the pectoralis major and its function is the objective of the modified radical mastectomy. Thus maintenance of the integrity of the medial and lateral pectoral nerves is paramount to ensure subsequent function of the pectoralis major. Section of the medial pectoral nerve with motor denervation of the pectoralis musculature allows progressive atrophy of these muscle groups with resultant cosmetic and neurological morbidity.

Technical precision must be exercised in dissection of the axillary vein and its tributaries. The surgeon should dissect in a plane that is parallel, anterior, and ventral to the vein surface with inclusion of perivascular fat and lymphatics (see section X, chapter 29). The rare complication of injury to the vein with dissection is immediately controlled by use of compression and vascular clamps and by suture repair with fine cardiovascular nylon suture. Tumor invasion of the axillary vein is best managed by vein resection and subsequent ligation of the proximal and distal ends. Ligation of the axillary vein for preexisting venous tumor invasion has not been associated with an increased incidence of postoperative edema of the extremity.[29]

Injuries to the axillary artery likewise must be carefully repaired with cardiovascular suture; however, such injuries are less likely to occur than are venous injuries, as the axillary artery is located posterior and superior to the axillary vein. The axillary vein must be "skeletonized" when performing the axillary dissection, but there is no need to dissect the axillary artery. Lymphatics about the axillary artery serve an important physiological purpose in preventing postoperative arm edema. These perivascular lymphatics are involved with metastatic disease only in advanced stages of regional disease in which locally invasive tumor or extranodal involvement extends into the axilla space.

REFERENCES

1. Aitken DR, Hunsaker R, James AG: Prevention of seromas following mastectomy and axillary dissection. Surg Gynecol Obstet 158:327–330, 1984.
2. Aitken DR, Minton JP: Complications associated with mastectomy. Surg Clin North Am 63:1331–1351, 1983.
3. Bland KI, Klamer TW, Polk HC Jr, Knutson CO: Isolated regional lymph node dissection: morbidity, mortality, and economic considerations. Ann Surg 193:372–376, 1981.
4. Bland KI, Heuser LS, Spratt JS Jr, Polk HC Jr: The postmastectomy patient: wound care, complications, and follow-up. *In* Strombeck JO, Rosato FE (eds): Surgery of the Breast. Stuttgart, Thieme Verlag, 1986, pp 158–173.
5. Bourke JB, Balfour TW, Hardcastle JD, Wilkins JL: A comparison between suction and corrugated drainage after simple mastectomy: a report of a controlled trial. Br J Surg 63:67–69, 1976.
6. Budd DC, Cochran RC, Sturtz DL, Fouty WJ Jr: Surgical morbidity after mastectomy operations. Am J Surg 135:218–220, 1978.
7. Cruse P: Infection surveillance: identifying the problems and the high-risk patient. South Med J 70(1):408, 1977.
8. Fitts WT, Keuhnelain JG, Ravdin IS, Schor S: Swelling of the arm after radical mastectomy. A clinical study of its cause. Surgery 35:460, 1954.
9. Flew TJ: Wound drainage following radical mastectomy: the effect of restriction of shoulder movement. Br J Surg 66:302–305, 1979.
10. Gilchrist RK: The postmastectomy massive arm. A usually preventable catastrophe. Am J Surg 122:363, 1971.
11. Halsted WS: Developments in the skin-grafting operation for cancer of the breast. JAMA 60:416–418, 1913.
12. Kakos GS, James AG: The use of cautery in "bloodless" radical mastectomy. Cancer 26:666–668, 1970.
13. Keenan KM, Rodeheaver GT, Kenney JG, Edlich RF: Surgical cautery revisited. Am J Surg 147:818–821, 1984.
14. Keyes IW, Hawk BO, Sherwin CS: Basting the axillary flap for wounds of radical mastectomy. Arch Surg 66:446–451, 1953.
15. Larsen BB, Hugan C: Fixation of skin flaps in radical mastectomy by subcutaneous sutures. Arch Surg 71:419–423, 1955.
16. Maitland IL, Mathieson AJM: Suction drainage: a study in wound healing. Br J Surg 57(3):193–197, 1970.
17. McCarthy PM, Martin JK, Wells DC, Welch JS, Ilstrup DM: An aborted, prospective, randomized trial of sclerotherapy for prolonged drainage after mastectomy. Surg Gynecol Obstet 162:418–420, 1986.
18. Miller PJ, O'Connell J, Leipold A, Wenzel RP: Potential liability for transfusion associated AIDS. JAMA 253:3419–3423, 1985.
19. Miller E, Paull DE, Morrissey K, Cortese A, Novak E: Scalpel versus electrocautery in modified radical mastectomy. Am Surg 54:284–286, 1988.
20. Morris AM: A controlled trial of closed wound suction drainage in radical mastectomy. Br J Surg 60:357–359, 1973.
21. Murphy DR: The use of atmospheric pressure in obliterating axillary dead space following radical mastectomy. South Surg 13:372–375, 1947.
22. Orr TG: An incision and method of wound closure for radical mastectomy. Ann Surg 133:565–566, 1951.
23. Osborne MP, Andrakis C, Rankin RA: The thermal scalpel: comparative study with conventional scalpel and electrocautery. Contemp Surg 29:51–54, 1986.
24. Say CC, Donegan WL: A biostatistical evaluation of complications from mastectomy. Surg Gynecol Obstet 138:370–376, 1974.
25. Schoenberg B, Carr AC: Loss of external organs: limb amputation, mastectomy, and disfiguration. *In* Schoenberg B, Carr, AC, Peretz D, Kutscher AH (eds): Loss and Grief: Psychological Management in Medical Practice. New York, Columbia University Press, 1970.
26. Schottenfeld D, Robbins GF: Quality of survival among patients who have had radical mastectomy. Cancer 26:650, 1970.
27. Stillwell GK: Treatment of postmastectomy lymphedema. *In* Modern Treatment. New York, Harper and Row, Hoeber Medical Division, 1969.
28. Tadych K, Donegan WL: Postmastectomy seromas and wound drainage. Surg Gynecol Obstet 165:483–487, 1987.
29. Zintel HA, Nay HR: Postoperative complications of radical mastectomy. Surg Clin North Am 44:313, 1964.

Chapter 32

LYMPHEDEMA IN THE POSTMASTECTOMY PATIENT

J. Shelton Horsley, III, M.D. and Toncred Styblo, M.D.

Lymphedema is the accumulation of lymph in the interstitial spaces, principally in the subcutaneous fat, caused by a defect in the lymphatic system. In the patient who has undergone treatment for primary breast cancer, a swollen arm is a worrisome complication. It may vary from a slight measurable enlargement of the arm, not noticeable to the patient or the physician, to a grotesquely enlarged, heavy, impaired upper extremity.

In 1921, Halsted[11] suggested the term "elephantiasis chirurgica" for the swollen arm following radical mastectomy. He referred rather extensively to an article by Matas[22] published in 1913 that stated "by elephantiasis we mean a progressive histopathologic state or condition which is characterized by a chronic inflammatory fibromatosis or hypertrophy of the hypodermal and dermal connective tissue which is preceded by and associated with lymphatic and venous stasis, and may be caused by any obstruction or mechanical interference with the return flow of the lymphatic and venous currents. . . ."

Swelling of the arm may occur in the immediate postoperative period as a complication secondary to the operative trauma. This is usually transitory and will respond to restoration of normal arm and shoulder function. The baggy enlargement of the ventral aspect of the upper arm in the obese woman is localized. It is probably caused by dividing and removing the axillary fascia and is limited in extent. Lymphedema that occurs on a chronic basis, often delayed in onset, is the subject of this chapter.

INCIDENCE

For many years, the accepted treatment for potentially curable breast cancer was the radical mastectomy with removal of the breast and both pectoral muscles and complete axillary dissection as described by Halsted[12] and further defined by Haagensen.[8] The reported incidence of lymphedema was highly variable depending on the criteria employed. Arm circumference measurement is the most common method used, but arm volume measurement is the most accurate. Despite the great range of incidence, 40 percent is a reasonable average.[36]

With the advent of more conservative surgical procedures in the past few years, the incidence has decreased. Lymphedema is found in 15.4 percent of patients follow-ing modified radical mastectomy[21] and in only two to three percent after both local removal of the cancer plus axillary dissection[14] and local excision plus radiation therapy.[29]

ETIOLOGY

The mammalian lymphatic system is thought to evolve from the fusion of clefts in perivenous mesoderm. The more superficial or primary lymphatics form a complex dermal network of capillary-like channels and have no valves. These drain into larger secondary channels or lymphatics containing valves located in the subdermal space. Both of these systems parallel the course of superficial veins and drain into a third deeper layer in the subcutaneous fat adjacent to the fascia. Active and unidirectional lymphatic flow is aided by a muscular wall and numerous valves in these subcutaneous lymphatics. An intramuscular system of lymphatics also exists, paralleling the deep arteries and draining the muscular compartment, joints, and synovium. There is lymphangiographic evidence that this intramuscular system communicates with the superficial system near regional lymph nodes. However, these two systems probably function independently except in abnormal states.[5, 30]

The main function of the lymphatic system is to return fluid and protein that have accumulated in the interstitial spaces back to the blood vascular system. Lymphatic vessels, unlike blood vessels, have an absent or poorly developed basement membrane. This facilitates intercellular movement of plasma proteins and lipids that are too large for venous reabsorption. Normally, lymphatic pressure is negative or zero mm H_2O. Intralymphatic pressure becomes positive and lymphatic flow can be 10 times slower than normal following destruction of the normal lymphatic architecture.[3]

Capillary fluid filtration is promoted by capillary hydrostatic pressure and the colloid osmotic pressure of the interstitial fluid; it is impeded by interstitial hydrostatic pressure and the osmotic pressure of plasma proteins. Under normal conditions, the capillary wall is permeable to water and electrolytes, and filtration exceeds resorption, resulting in a net fluid flow from the capillaries to the interstitial spaces. This fluid is removed from the tissues by the lymphatic vessels. Abnormal interstitial fluid accumulation, or edema, occurs when there is a disequilibrium in this balanced fluid exchange. This can be classified by the principal causes leading to its development.

There are two primary mechanisms responsible for clinical edema: increased filtration and reduced absorption. Causes of increased filtration include increased capillary hydrostatic pressure, decreased tissue pressure, and increased membrane permeability. Reduced absorption can be caused by decreased plasma oncotic pressure, increased oncotic pressure of tissue fluid, and lymphatic obstruction.

Lymphedema of the upper extremity is usually divided into primary and secondary types. *Primary lymphedema* is defined as a primary abnormality or disease of the lymph-conducting elements or lymph nodes. *Secondary lymphedema* includes all forms of lymphedema caused by disease not originating in the lymph-conducting elements and nodes. Various preoperative, operative, and postoperative factors may contribute to lymphatic insufficiency. These include extended surgical removal and destruction of lymphatic channels, fibrosis, venous obstruction, radiation of the axilla, infection, and neoplastic replacement.

In 1938, Veal[37] performed venography in postmastectomy arm edema and attributed swelling to axillary vein obstruction in most cases. His belief was not supported by subsequent investigators. By 1955, Kinmouth et al.[18] were studying postmastectomy lymphedema with venography and lymphography. They published conclusive evidence of lymphatic obstruction without axillary vein obstruction and concluded that postmastectomy lymphedema was a result of lymphatic rather than venous obstruction. Axillary vein obstruction has been documented in association with postmastectomy lymphedema in about 20 percent of patients.[24] Although chronic axillary vein thrombosis and venous hypertension rarely result in arm swelling, when mastectomy includes axillary dissection, many of the venous tributaries capable of forming collateral circulation are removed, making the consequences of axillary vein obstruction more serious than simple ligation. Important venous tributaries participating in the development of collaterals include the superficial system over the anterior shoulder and chest, the subscapular vein, the cephalic vein, and the recanalized axillary vein.

Fibrosis of the axilla is an almost universal phenomenon following mastectomy and has been implicated as a cause of venous and lymphatic obstruction. Hughes and Patel[16] suggested that postmastectomy fibrous tissue formation not only compresses the main lymphatic trunks and axillary vein, but also acts as a sclerotic barrier to regeneration of lymphatic and venous collateral channels. Mustard and Murillo[28] reported decreased lymphedema if the areola tissue around the axillary vein was preserved. They reported no decrease in 5-year survival with this operative technique.

Many authors[19, 36] agree that radiation therapy to the axilla following axillary node dissection greatly increases the incidence of lymphedema. Treves[36] reported a 52 percent incidence of lymphedema among patients undergoing radiation after radical mastectomy, whereas the incidence in groups treated without radiation was 25 percent.

Radiation therapy causes fibrosis of lymph nodes and may cause radiodermatitis. Acute obstruction of the dilated, tortuous network of collateral dermal lymphatics may precipitate overt lymphedema. Similarly, minor skin trauma or secondary streptococcal invasion as a result of radiodermatitis-induced infection may precipitate dermal lymphatic occlusion and cause lymphedema. Several authors[10, 27] suggest that infection was the single most important etiological factor in the appearance of secondary lymphedema, once attendant dermal lymphatic collaterals developed.

Although rare, recurrent breast cancer as a cause of lymphedema should always be considered. Usually this is easy to detect because of the presence of obvious recurrent or metastatic disease.

All of these factors may play an important role in the development of lymphedema, either by promoting a vulnerable, functional adaptation or by triggering malfunction leading to irreparable damage and overt lymphedema. It does appear that lymphedema is most often the result of a combination of several factors. Certainly the most common cause is the interference and obstruction of the lymph flow from the arm by the division and removal of the lymphatic channels and the lymph nodes of the axilla.

DIAGNOSIS

The wide variation in the reported incidence of lymphedema is largely a result of the lack of uniform diagnostic criteria. Subjective criteria include size, heaviness, functional activity, and appearance (Fig. 32–1). The objective criteria are based on measurement (circumferential or volumetric). Lymphangiograms, venograms, injection of patent blue dye, and radioisotopic studies have all been done, but these have been employed to better delineate the etiology rather than to diagnose clinical lymphedema. There is no uniform agreement on the criteria for lymphedema. Kissen et al.[19] found that water displacement measurement 15 cm above the epicondyle was the most sensitive index. A value of 200 ml included 96.4 percent of patients with subjective lymphedema. This would appear to be the best objective criterion with which to judge lymphedema.

PREVENTION

What can we do to prevent lymphedema? The radical mastectomy has been almost totally replaced by the modified radical mastectomy or local resection (lumpectomy or segmental resection) with axillary node dissection and radiation of the breast tissue. All of these surgical procedures involve an axillary node dissection. Nevertheless, the incidence of lymphedema decreases significantly with the more conservative procedures.[19] Mustard and Murillo[28] advocated leaving the areolar

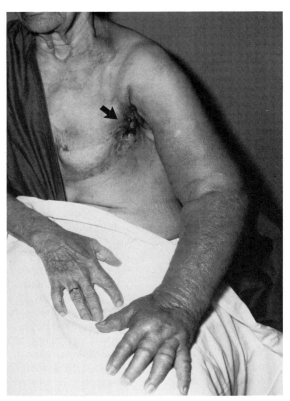

Figure 32–1. Eighty-year-old female with onset of lymphedema in left arm and hand two years post modified radical mastectomy for high-grade carcinoma of upper outer quadrant of breast. Progressive lymphedema was evident with the appearance of recurrent carcinoma (*arrow*) in left axilla and a 3 cm mass in left supraclavicular region. Patient was treated with chest wall and axillary irradiation and thereafter placed on a cytotoxic chemotherapy regimen. Lymphedema was managed with the Jobst pneumatic compression pump and sleeve, with partial resolution, until her death, which was related to pulmonary metastases.

deep margins on the pectoral muscle, should not include the axilla. Even with metastases in the axillary nodes, the recurrence rate in the axilla is extremely low following dissection.[9] As has been pointed out previously, radiation of the dissected axilla has a high rate of lymphedema and should be avoided (see chapters 37 and 41).[19, 36]

The long-term care of the arm on the side of the axillary node dissection is important. A list of "do's" and "don'ts" for the patient should be helpful. Resumption of normal shoulder and arm function is beneficial. Proper exercises and the assistance and encouragement of an American Cancer Society Reach to Recovery Volunteer are of real benefit. Any trauma or infection, should receive special attention, as cellulitis of the arm can lead to lymphedema. The patient should be made aware of this possibility and counseled to be alert. Once cellulitis has occurred, prompt treatment with antibiotics and immobilization and elevation are mandatory. Severe cases may require hospitalization with bed rest, elevation of the arm, and intravenous antibiotics. Fortunately, most cases are secondary to a streptococcus infection and respond promptly to oral antibiotics such as penicillin. Rarely, because of recurrent infections, prophylactic antibiotics are used, but the real efficacy of this approach is unproven.

TREATMENT

The management of *postmastectomy lymphedema* is divided into nonsurgical and surgical therapy. Most patients are satisfactorily treated by conservative means. Surgical intervention should be utilized only after an unsuccessful trial of medical management.[31] The majority of patients with lymphedema never require surgical intervention.

There are two broad categories of conservative therapy: mechanical and pharmacological. Important mechanical modalities include elevation of the arm, custom-fitted graded pressure garments, meticulous skin hygiene to prevent infection, weight control, elimination of injections, and avoidance of blood pressure cuffs on the involved arm. Extremity pumps utilizing intermittent pneumatic compression as demonstrated in Figure 32–2 are extremely helpful in the management of the edematous arm. The cuff is alternately inflated and deflated according to a controlled time cycle prescribed for each patient. This increases fluid flow in veins and lymphatics and prevents accumulation of residual fluid in the arm. Pharmacological therapy utilizes antibiotics for treatment and prevention of bacterial cellulitis and lymphangitis. A variety of different drugs have been used, including diuretics, anticoagulants, pantothenic acid, pyridoxine, and hylauronidase. These drugs have no proven therapeutic value and may cause adverse reactions. The patient should be educated about the possibilities of lymphedema, and attention to details of prevention should be stressed.

Surgical therapy is indicated in those patients who fail nonoperative therapy. There are a variety of reasons

tissue around the axillary vein, which lessened the incidence of edema of the arm following radical mastectomy with no adverse effect on survival. However, no one else has reported similar results. Current findings of more limited surgical procedures demonstrate a very low incidence of lymphedema (see chapter 29, Extended Simple Mastectomy).

Primary healing creates less fibrosis than does the scarring of healing by secondary intention. Attention to sound surgical principles of sharp dissection, meticulous hemostasis, closure without tension that may occasionally require split-thickness skin grafting, and suction drainage to remove serous fluid are all important details. Sepsis following mastectomy is often more frequent than originally thought, particularly when an excisional biopsy has been performed several days before the definitive mastectomy.[2] Infection should, of course, be avoided. However, precise attention to surgical technique, not antibiotic therapy, is the best prevention of infection.

Postoperative radiation therapy, when employed as part of the definitive initial therapy with lumpectomy and axillary node dissection or because of inadequate

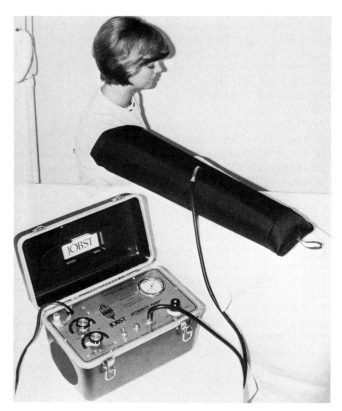

Figure 32–2. Jobst pneumatic compression pump and compression sleeve for the therapy of the lymphedematous arm. The cuff pressures actuated are inflated and deflated in a rhythmic time cycle prescribed for each patient. After each course of daily therapy, the patient is instructed to wear a custom-fitted compression sleeve from fingers to shoulder.

for failure including impairment of function as a result of excess weight and size leading to recurrent episodes of lymphangitis and cellulitis; aesthetic considerations; and, rarely, lymphangiosarcoma.

Many operations have been devised for the treatment of lymphedema, and these can be classified into two broad categories: physiological and excisional. The first surgical procedure attempted for lymphedema was done by Lis Franc in 1841.[26] In 1908, Handley[13] attempted the first physiological operation to improve lymphatic drainage by implanting silk threads subcutaneously and creating an ascending lymph flow utilizing capillary action. The relatively high rates of infection and extrusion, coupled with only transient improvement, resulted in the rejection of this particular operation. Replacement of the silk threads by nylon threads,[40] fine polyethylene tubes,[15] and multifilament Teflon[35] have prolonged the improvement and minimized complications.

An omental transposition flap for treatment of chronic lymphedema was introduced in 1966.[7] Unfortunately, initial successes were diminished by major complications such as intestinal obstruction, wound hernias, and wound infections. Histological encapsulation of the omental flap, preventing lymphatic absorption, and the inability to demonstrate long-term lymphatic connections from the extremity to the omentum were found.

Pedicle flaps were introduced by Gillies and Frazer in 1935[6] as bridging procedures to transpose normal tissue across an area of interrupted lymphatic drainage. There are several prerequisites for a successful pedicle flap; the flap must contain lymphatics, the valves must be oriented to ensure lymphatic drainage in the direction of transposition, and competent draining lymphatics in the arm must be directed away from the functional blockade.[17] Axial pattern myocutaneous and intestinal flaps have also been applied in the treatment of chronic lymphedema.[23]

A variety of lymphatic anastomotic techniques have been developed, including buried dermis flap,[15] lymph node–to-venous anastomosis,[17] lymph vessel–to-vein anastomosis,[20] and lymphaticolymphatic anastomosis.[1] These techniques are theoretically attractive, but additional experimental and clinical evaluation is needed to determine long-term results.

Excisional techniques were first employed by Charles in 1912.[4] All involved skin and subcutaneous tissue were removed, followed by split-thickness and full-thickness skin grafts to cover deep fascia or muscle. Variations of his procedure, including staged excisions of subcutaneous tissue and skin, are still in use. However, complications (which include hypertrophic scarring, sensory loss of the skin, graft loss, scar contracture, and ulceration) may restrict its use to patients with severe lymphedema with chronic, massive subcutaneous fibrosis.

The satisfactory management of postmastectomy lymphedema rarely requires surgical intervention, and it should never be considered without a serious trial of conservative management. The staged excision of skin and subcutaneous tissue, the *Charles procedure,* and the dermal flap are the most popular operations in the United States. The number of surgical procedures advocated demonstrates the lack of satisfactory results with any one operation. Continued investigations emphasizing long-term follow-up, with objective radiological documentation of lymphatic continuity and function, will provide better surgical therapy for lymphedema. An algorithm outlining the management of the patient with lymphedema of the arm is presented in Figure 32–3.

LYMPHANGIOSARCOMA

Lymphangiosarcoma is a rare but lethal complication of chronic lymphedema. Since it was first described 30 years ago by Stewart and Treves,[34] approximately 300 cases have been described in the literature. Of all patients surviving 5 or more years following mastectomy, 0.07 to 0.45 percent of them will develop lymphangiosarcoma. The mean time between mastectomy and lymphangiosarcoma is 10.25 years, and the median survival is 1.33 years.

The cause of lymphangiosarcoma is unknown. The presence of chronic lymphedema appears to be the most important factor. Most often, it involves the upper extremity after radical mastectomy with or without radiation therapy. Lymphangiosarcoma has also been reported in different locations. Several mechanisms have been suggested to explain its development in the chron-

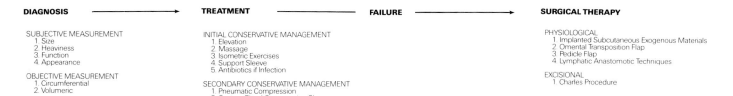

Figure 32–3. Algorithm for management of the lymphedematous arm.

ically lymphedematous extremity. The protein-rich edema apparently causes degeneration of collagen and fat in the dermal and subdermal tissues and stimulates fibroblastic proliferation. In addition, the long-standing lymphedema may be a "relatively immunologically privileged site" allowing sarcomatous degeneration to go unnoticed by the immune system.[32] The development of immunohistochemical markers enabled Miettinen et al.[25] to demonstrate conclusively the endothelial origin of postmastectomy lymphangiosarcoma and to rule out its derivation from the primary mammary cancer.

Clinically, lymphangiosarcoma presents as single or multiple bluish-red hemorrhagic nodules on the edematous limb with proximal and distal progression. Initially, there is a solitary, purple-red focus in the skin of the arm, slightly raised, macular or nodular type, and usually described by the patient as a "bruise." Later, satellite tumors arise, and the nodules grow. Death usually results from metastatic (usually pulmonary) and residual growths.

There is no established method of treatment of lymphangiosarcoma in chronic lymphedema. Modalities include amputation, local excision, radiation therapy, and chemotherapy, separately or in combination. The reported series by Woodward et al.[38] and Sordillo et al.[33] concluded that initial radical amputation of the affected limb offers the best hope of cure. Recurrence almost always follows local excision and radiation. Once recurrent lesions appear, no therapeutic regimen seems to be able to prevent further progression and death from pulmonary metastasis within a short time. There have been rare long-term survivals following treatment with chemotherapy including 5-fluorouracil, methotrexate, and combinations of adriamycin and dacarbazine with or without vincristine.[39]

Overall prognosis is poor. Fifty percent of patients died within 19 months of the appearance of lesions. Lymphangiosarcoma in nonpostmastectomy lymphedema has a somewhat better prognosis. Only a few patients survive for 5 or more years. The patient's prognosis is not influenced by age or duration of lymphedema before diagnosis. Early diagnosis increases survival and therapeutic efficacy and is the key to survival. All postmastectomy lymphedematous extremities should be followed carefully with life-long examinations. Biopsy is indicated if there is increased pain, swelling, ecchymosis, or purple-red nodules. Cutaneous angiosarcoma arising at the site of therapeutic radiation exposure has been observed in a few instances. This diagnostic consideration may become particularly important as radiation therapy for the treatment of breast cancer becomes more popular.

SUMMARY

Lymphedema of the arm, occurring after mastectomy or a breast-conserving procedure such as lumpectomy or segmental resection, is initiated by axillary node dissection, which disrupts the lymphatic drainage. The incidence is decreasing with less radical surgical procedures and the abandonment of postoperative radiation therapy to the surgically dissected axilla. Circumferential measurements are most frequently employed, but volumetric determination appears to be more accurate. Prevention by employing precise surgical technique and good postoperative care and rehabilitation is essential. The treatment is basically conservative, and only when a serious medical management effort fails is surgical therapy contemplated. No operative technique can cure this problem, but significant improvement may be obtained with surgery.

REFERENCES

1. Baumeister RG, Seifert J: Microsurgical lymph vessel transplantation for the treatment of lymphedema: experimental and first clinical experiences. Lymphology 14:90, 1981.
2. Beatty JD, Robinson GV, Zaia JA, Benfield JR, Kemeny MM, Meguid MM, Riihimaki DU, Terz JJ, Lemmelin ME: A prospective analysis of nosocomial wound infection after mastectomy. Arch Surg 118:1421–1424, 1983.
3. Blocker TG Jr, Lewis SR, Smith JR, Dunton EF, Kirby EJ, Meyer JV: Lymphodynamics. Plast Reconstr Surg 25:337–348, 1960.
4. Charles RH: A System of Treatment, vol III. London, J & A Churchill, 1912, p 504.
5. Crockett DJ: Lymphatic anatomy and lymphedema. Br J Plast Surg 18:12–25, 1965.
6. Gillies H, Frazer FR: The treatment of lymphedema by plastic operation: a preliminary report. Br Med J 1:96–98, 1935.
7. Goldsmith HS, De Los Santos R, Beattie EJ: Relief of chronic lymphedema by omental transposition. Ann Surg 166:572–585, 1966.
8. Haagensen CD: A technique for radical mastectomy. Surgery 19:100–131, 1946.
9. Haagensen CD: Disease of the Breast, ed 3. Philadelphia, WB Saunders, 1986, pp 911–912.
10. Haagensen CD: Diseases of the Breast, ed 3. Philadelphia, WB Saunders, 1986, pp 915–919.
11. Halsted WS: Swelling of the arm after operation for cancer of the breast—elephantiasis chirurgica—its cause and prevention. Bull Johns Hopkins Hosp 32:309–313, 1921.
12. Halsted WS: The results of operations for the cure of cancer of the breast performed at the Johns Hopkins Hospital from June 1889 to January 1894. Ann Surg 20:497–555, 1894.
13. Handley WS: Lymphangioplasty: a new method for the relief of the brawny arm of breast cancer and for similar conditions of lymphatic oedema. Lancet 1:783–785, 1908.
14. Hayward JL, Winter PJ, Tong D, Rubens RD, Payne JG, Chaudary MA, Habibollahi F: A new approach to the conservative treatment of early breast cancer. Surgery 95:270–274, 1984.

15. Hogeman K: Artificial subcutaneous channels in draining lymphedema. Acta Chir Scand 110:154–156, 1955.
16. Hughes JH, Patel AR: Swelling of the arm following mastectomy. Br J Surg 53:4–14, 1966.
17. Kerstein MD, Licalzi L: Microvascular procedures in the management of lymphedema. Vasc Surg 11:188–195, 1977.
18. Kinmouth JB, Harper RA, Taylor GW: Lymphangiography. A technique for its clinical use in the lower limb. Br Med J 1:940–942, 1955.
19. Kissin MW, Querci Della Rovere G, Easton D, Westbury G: Risk of lymphedema following the treatment of breast cancer. Br J Surg 73:580–584, 1986.
20. Laine JB, Howard JM: Experimental lymphatico-venous anastomosis. Surg Forum 14:111–112, 1963.
21. Leis HP: Selective moderate surgical approach for potentially curable breast cancer. *In* Gallagher HS, Leis HP, Snyderman RK, Urban JA (eds): The Breast. ed 1. St Louis, CV Mosby, 1978, p 232.
22. Matas R: Surgical treatment of elephantiasis and elephantoid states dependent upon chronic obstruction of lymphatic and venous channels. Am J Trop Dis 1:60–85, 1913.
23. Mathes SJ, Nahai F: Clinical Atlas of Muscle and Musculocutaneous Flaps. St Louis, CV Mosby, 1979.
24. McIvor J, O'Connell D: The investigation of postmastectomy edema of the arm by lymphography and venography. Clin Radiol 29:457–462, 1978.
25. Miettinen M, Lehto V-P, Virtanen I: Postmastectomy angiosarcoma (Stewart-Treves syndrome). Light microscopic immunohistological and ultrastructural characteristics of two cases. Am J Surg Pathol 7:329–339, 1983.
26. Miller TA, Harper J, Longmire WP: The management of lymphedema by staged subcutaneous excision. Surg Gynecol Obstet 136:586–592, 1973.
27. Mozes M, Papa MZ, Karasik A, Reshef A, Adar R: The role of infection in postmastectomy lymphedema. Surg Ann 14:73–83, 1982.
28. Mustard RL, Murillo C: Prevention of arm lymphedema following radical mastectomy. Ann Surg 154(suppl):282–285, 1961.
29. Osborne MP, Ormiston N, Harmer CL, McKinna JA, Baker J, Greening WP: Breast conservation in the treatment of early breast cancer. A 20-year follow-up. Cancer 53:349–355, 1984.
30. Puckett CL: Microlymphatic surgery for lymphedema. Clin Plast Surg 10:133–138, 1983.
31. Savage RC: The surgical management of lymphedema. Surg Gynecol Obstet 160:283–290, 1985.
32. Schreiber H, Barry FM, Russell WC, Macon WL IV, Ponsky JL, Pories WJ: Stewart-Treves syndrome: a lethal complication of postmastectomy lymphedema and regional immune deficiency. Arch Surg 114:82–85, 1979.
33. Sordillo PP, Chapman R, Hajdu SI, Magill GB, Golbey RB: Lymphangiosarcoma. Cancer 48:1674–1679, 1981.
34. Stewart FW, Treves N: Lymphangiosarcoma in postmastectomy lymphedema: a report of six cases of elephantiasis chirurgica. Cancer 1:64–81, 1948.
35. Thompson N: The surgical treatment of chronic lymphedema of the extremities. Surg Clin North Am 47:445–503, 1967.
36. Treves N: An evaluation of the etiological factors of lymphedema following radical mastectomy: an analysis of 1,007 cases. Cancer 10:444–459, 1957.
37. Veal JR: Pathologic basis for swelling of the arm following radical amputation of the breast. Surg Gynecol Obstet 67:752–760, 1938.
38. Woodward AH, Ivins JC, Soule EH: Lymphangiosarcoma arising in chronic lymphedematous extremities. Cancer 30:562–572, 1972.
39. Yap B-S, Yap H-Y, McBride CM, Bodey GP: Chemotherapy for postmastectomy lymphangiosarcoma. Cancer 47:853–856, 1981.
40. Zieman SA: Re-establishing lymph drainage for lymphedema of the extremities. J Int Coll Surgeons 15:328–331, 1951.

Radiation Therapy for Breast Cancer: History, Techniques, and Complications

HISTORY OF IRRADIATION IN THE PRIMARY MANAGEMENT OF APPARENTLY REGIONALLY CONFINED BREAST CANCER

Gilbert H. Fletcher, M.D.

EVOLUTION OF CLINICAL DATA

Two sets of clinical data had a profound impact on the management of apparently confined breast cancer: prognostic factors based on the clinical features of the disease both in the breast and the axilla, and the demonstration that the internal mammary chain nodes are a primary route of spread. These data forced clinicians to consider radiotherapy as an effective complement or option to surgery, which had once been the universal treatment of choice for breast cancer.

Criteria of Clinical Operability

The Halsted operation extended the mastectomy by removing the whole of the sternal head of the pectoralis major muscle with division of the clavicular head and the pectoralis minor muscle, thus giving better access to the lymph nodes in the infraclavicular fossa. In his first 50 cases, Halsted also dissected the supraclavicular nodes, a procedure he later abandoned as a routine but continued to practice in many cases. All of Halsted's first 50 patients were found to have invasion of the axillary lymph nodes.

Until World War II, the radical mastectomy was regarded as the routine treatment in most cases of cancer confined to the breast and the axillary nodes on the same side. The first critical appraisal of the radical mastectomy was done by Haagensen and Stout. Their paper, published in 1943, is a milestone in the evaluation of the effectiveness of the surgical procedure.[19] It demonstrated that in patients with criteria of clinical inoperability, the radical mastectomy was not only futile but also possibly harmful, since almost all patients died within 5 years and the incidence of local/regional failures was 47 percent. Haagensen and Stout[19] noted the following:

"From these correlations we have drawn up rules for judging operability in breast carcinoma as follows: women of all age-groups, who are in good enough general condition to run the risk of major surgery, should be treated by radical mastectomy, except as follows:

1. When the carcinoma is one which developed during pregnancy or lactation.
2. When extensive edema of the skin over the breast is present.
3. When satellite nodules are present in the skin over the breast.
4. When intercostal or parasternal tumor nodules are present.
5. When there is edema of the arm.
6. When proved supraclavicular metastases are present.
7. When the carcinoma is the inflammatory type.
8. When distant metastases are demonstrated.
9. When any two, or more, of the following signs of locally advanced carcinoma are present:
   a. Ulceration of the skin.

b. Edema of the skin of limited extent (less than one-third of the skin over the breast involved).
c. Fixation of the tumor to the chest wall.
d. Axillary lymph nodes measuring 2.5 cm or more in transverse diameter, and proved to contain metastases by biopsy.
e. Fixation of axillary lymph nodes to the skin or the deep structures of the axilla, and proved to contain metastases by biopsy.

If these criteria had actually been followed in judging operability in the series of 640 radical mastectomies which we have reported, the fate of 109 of the patients would not have been affected." (See Table 33-1.)

In his book, *Diseases of the Breast,* Haagensen elaborated on the clinical features of the primary tumor and the axillary status as prognostic factors, particularly in local/regional failures.[18] A high incidence of local/regional recurrences was also reported in another series.[36] These two analyses prompted us to combine the surgical procedure with pre- or postoperative irradiation or to use irradiation alone to cut down on this high recurrence rate (Table 33-2).[14]

Internal Mammary Chain Nodes

The invasion of the internal mammary chain nodes was recorded for the first time in an autopsy report from Middlesex Hospital Cancer Ward on October 22, 1806. Halsted was probably the first to attempt to excise the internal mammary nodes as part of the surgical attack on breast cancer. In 1922, Sampson Handley, a surgeon at Middlesex Hospital, explored the mediastinum in six patients and found involvement of the chain in two. In 1927, Handley again documented his belief in the importance of the internal mammary chain route of metastases:

"It is the fact that in more than half of my recurrent cases, before I began the prophylactic use of radium, the return of the disease manifested itself either by an enlargement of the gland of the lower and inner angle of the posterior triangle, or by the appearance of nodules, later merging in sternal recurrence, upon the deep fascia at the inner end of the first, second, or third intercostal spaces. The position of these recurrences accurately along the line of the internal mammary artery shows, I think, beyond doubt that they are due to invasion of the lymphatic glands which lie along its course."[20]

Richard Handley, son of Sampson Handley, began in 1946 to excise the nodes at the first three intercostal spaces at the completion of the radical mastectomy. In 1949, he reported his findings in 50 patients, correlating the involvement of the chain with the histological status of the axilla and the location of the tumor in the breast.[22] He later published graphs of that correlation (Fig. 33-1).[21]

Treatment of the internal mammary chain nodes by dissecting them became very popular in conjunction with conventional radical mastectomy (extended radical mastectomy). The survival benefits of the treatment were controversial, and so an intercontinental randomized trial of radical mastectomy versus radical mastectomy plus dissection of the chain nodes was structured. Initially it seemed to show survival benefits in patients with histologically positive axillary nodes and the tumor located in the inner quadrants. With longer follow-up, the statistical difference disappeared in most patients, but was maintained in the patients treated at the Institut Gustave Roussy.[25] The results of irradiation of the internal mammary nodes have also not been consistent. A review of the irradiation techniques showed that in several techniques, the coverage of the nodes was inadequate.[16]

HISTORY OF BREAST IRRADIATION

Pioneer Era (1896–1930)

After the discovery of x-rays by Roentgen in 1895, Emil Grubbe, a Chicago medical student, developed a severe dermatitis of the skin of his hand while testing Crookes' tubes with that hand. A physician who had seen Grubbe's lesion referred a patient with breast cancer to him for irradiation, because of the apparent biological damaging effect of the recently discovered x-rays.

From 1900 until the 1920s, the practice was to give one treatment that produced a brisk skin erythema. The dose was called Haut (skin) Erythema Dosis or HED. Later, the HED was measured to be approximately 1000 roentgen. It was believed that the dose killing the epithelium of the skin would kill cancer. In the 1920s, after the Coolidge tube was invented, somewhat more

Table 33–1. HAAGENSEN-STOUT CRITERIA OF OPERABILITY APPLIED TO PRESBYTERIAN HOSPITAL SERIES OF RADICAL MASTECTOMIES, 1915–1934

Group	No. of Cases	5-Year Local Recurrence		5-Year Clinical Cures		Permanent Cures
		No.	*%*	*No.*	*%*	
Cases in which radical mastectomy was actually performed (1914–1934)	640	161	25.2	231	36.1	Many still well
Cases that would now be classified as inoperable	109	52	47.7	3	2.8	None
Cases that would now be classified as operable	531	109	20.5	228	42.9	Many still well

From Haagensen CD, Stout AP: Ann Surg 118:859–870; 1032–1051, 1943. Reprinted by permission.

Table 33–2. IRRADIATION IN THE PRIMARY TREATMENT OF NONDISSEMINATED BREAST CANCER AT M. D. ANDERSON CANCER CENTER (1948–1975)

Modality of Treatment	No. of Patients
Radical or modified radical mastectomy + postoperative irradiation	1250
Preoperative irradiation + radical mastectomy	677
Simple mastectomy + postoperative irradiation	720
Irradiation alone	711
Tumorectomy + postoperative irradiation	84
Total	3442

From Fletcher GF: Int J Radiat Oncol Biol Phys 11:2133–2142, 1985. Reprinted by permission.

systematic treatments of breast cancer were done with external irradiation. Technical advances were made in external irradiation treatment planning, such as the introduction of tangential fields for irradiating the breast. Inoperable lesions were irradiated and some regression resulted, a phenomenon that was noticed with interest. Also at this time, irradiation began to be used pre- or postoperatively. The rationale for preoperative irradiation was the same as it is today, that by diminishing the tumor cell population, the spread of cancer would be less likely during the surgical procedure.

In the early 1920s, radium needles were made available in the Surgical Department of St. Bartholomew's Hospital in England. Geoffrey Keynes, a surgeon, began in 1922 to treat patients who had recurrent disease and found that the tumor in nearly every instance disappeared. The method was extended to treatment of primary disease in 1924, initially for very advanced or inoperable tumors and later for operable lesions (Fig. 33–2).[23] In 1937, Keynes reported that long-term, disease-free survival rates were comparable to those obtained with radical mastectomy and considered this method an alternative to radical mastectomy. He also carefully mentioned the disadvantages, specifically the development of fibrosis and neuropathies.[24]

Preoperative Irradiation Followed by Radical Mastectomy

In the 1930s, Baclesse gave, at best estimate, a radiation dose to 21 patients of at least 5000 roentgen over an 8- to 13-week period. The surgery was performed 4 to 8 weeks after irradiation. In one third of the surgical specimens, no tumor at all could be detected, and only two specimens had cancer cells with no marked morphological changes.[5] As a result, preoperative irradiation had some popularity in the 1930s and 1940s, but since 1950, the interest in preoperative irradiation has been limited, and few series of patients have been available for analysis. At the University of Texas M. D. Anderson Cancer Center, patients with lesions of borderline clin-

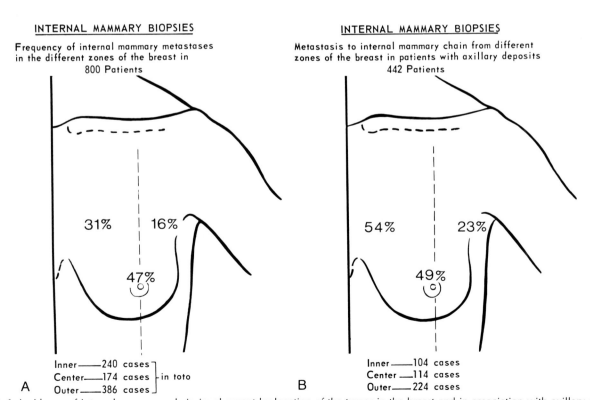

Figure 33–1. Incidence of internal mammary chain involvement by location of the tumor in the breast and in association with axillary deposits. *A,* All patients. *B,* Patients with histologically positive axillary nodes. (From Handley RS: A surgeon's view of the spread of breast cancer. Cancer 24:1232, 1969. Reprinted by permission.)

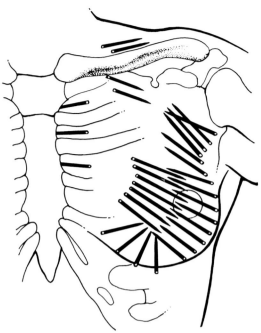

Figure 33–2. Diagram showing usual distribution of needles. (From Keynes G: The radium treatment of breast cancer. Br J Surg. 19:415, 1932. Reprinted by permission.)

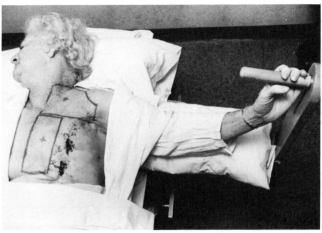

Figure 33–3. Peripheral lymphatics irradiation technique with en face portals, since two portals had to be used with 250 kV irradiation. Only the apex of the axilla is covered. The internal mammary chain field is 6 cm wide with the medial margin on the midline. A skin dose of 4000 rad was delivered in four weeks at the central axis of the supraclavicular portal. (From Fletcher GH: Textbook of Radiotherapy, 1st ed. Philadelphia, Lea & Febiger, 1966, p. 344. Reprinted by permission.)

ical operability or with large ecchymoses after an outside biopsy were treated with preoperative irradiation, first with 250 kV and later with cobalt 60. An analysis of the long-term results showed a lower percentage than expected of patients with histologically positive axillary nodes and a low incidence of local/regional failures. Survival rates were similar to those in patients given postoperative irradiation.[33]

Irradiation After Radical Mastectomy

In 1949 in Manchester, England, a randomized trial comparing the results of radical mastectomy with and without postoperative irradiation was started using two different techniques. The quadrate technique essentially irradiated the chest wall, and the other technique irradiated the peripheral lymphatics but did not irradiate the chest wall. No survival benefits were seen with either technique, although there was a diminution of local/regional failure rates with both techniques. Paterson and Russell concluded that one could wait for failures to appear before treating them.[31]

Since 1948 at M. D. Anderson Cancer Center, postoperative irradiation has been given to the lymphatics of the apex of the axilla, supraclavicular area, and internal mammary chain with an en face L-shaped portal (Fig. 33–3).[11] Because of the variable location of the nodes, they may be only marginally covered unless an en face portal or sophisticated techniques are used to identify their location. Kilovoltage was first used, then cesium 137, cobalt 60, and finally, since 1963, electron beam. An analysis of the incidence of failures in the supraclavicular area in patients with initially clinically negative supraclavicular nodes showed that approxi-

mately 5000 rad in 4 weeks reduced the incidence of failures at this site to almost zero (Table 33–3),[12] compared with 25 percent rates at Manchester and Memorial Hospital, New York, where no postoperative irradiation was given. Since 1963, the chest wall has been irradiated with an electron beam if there was a heavy involvement of the axilla in the surgical specimen, aggressive features of the disease in the breast, or both (Fig. 33–4). An analysis of the disease-free survival rates and the local/regional failures was done in 1982.[37]

Simple Mastectomy and Postoperative Irradiation

In 1941 in Edinburgh, McWhirter initiated the use of simple mastectomy followed by postoperative irradiation for operable breast cancer instead of a radical mastectomy. In 1948, he reported 5-year survival rates comparable to the ones obtained with radical mastectomy.[26] The so-called McWhirter technique was the first chal-

Table 33–3. INCIDENCE OF DISEASE DEVELOPING IN THE SUPRACLAVICULAR AREA AFTER RADICAL MASTECTOMY* AT M. D. ANDERSON CANCER CENTER, JANUARY 1955–DECEMBER 1967

Treatment	No.	%
Postoperative irradiation		
250 kV: 4000 rad skin dose in 4 weeks (<3500 rad node dose)	6/89	7
Cesium 137, cobalt 60, electron beam: 5000 to 5500 rad given in 4 weeks	4/273	1.5
Preoperative irradiation		
Cobalt 60: 4000 rad given in 4 weeks	4/121	3

*When axillary nodes are positive in the surgical specimen.
Modified from Fletcher GH: Cancer 29:545–551, 1972.

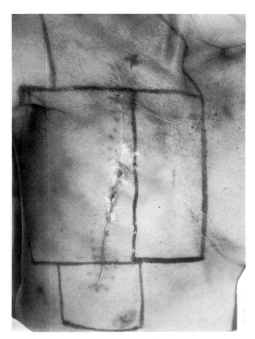

Figure 33–4. A 60-year-old woman with a T4 upper outer quadrant breast cancer. A radical mastectomy was performed on June 25, 1970; 14 axillary nodes were positive out of 28 recovered. Postoperative irradiation to the chest wall (5000 cGy with 7 MeV electron beam), internal mammary chain (5000 cGy with 15 MeV electron beam), and supraclavicular area (5000 cGy with 11 MeV electron beam) was completed in September 1970. The patient remained disease free until January 1989. (From Tapley N duV, et al: Cancer 49:1316–1319, 1982. Reprinted by permission.)

lenge to the radical mastectomy, which had been considered the only curative procedure. The historical importance of the Edinburgh experiment cannot be overemphasized, because it justified the use of surgical procedures less extensive than the classical radical procedures.

At the M. D. Anderson Cancer Center, simple mastectomy followed by irradiation has been used since 1948 in patients with stage III and stage IV disease. Later, dissection of the lateral axilla was added. The results showed approximately ten percent local/regional failures and disease-free survival rates of 35 percent in patients without clinically positive supraclavicular nodes.[27]

Irradiation Alone

Baclesse was the first to explore the use of external irradiation alone for the curative treatment of breast cancer. Between 1936 and 1945, 145 patients, some with operable and some with inoperable lesions, were treated with irradiation alone. Only ten of the patients had had the tumor removed by an excisional biopsy. Baclesse reported on this series in 1948, including detailed sketches of the treatment portals.[3] It can be estimated that doses of 7000–9000 roentgen were given to a large mass in the breast in 16 weeks. The supraclavicular area received a 5000 roentgen skin dose in 12 weeks if there

were no palpable nodes; in-between doses were given to the intermediately sized axillary nodes. A correlation was made between the size of the tumor mass and the amount of irradiation necessary to control it. For instance, doses as low as 4100 rad produced control in relatively small tumors, whereas in large tumors higher doses and a minimum of 3 months of treatment time were necessary. It is of interest that nine of the ten patients whose tumor had been removed by excisional biopsy were alive, disease free, 5 years or more following removal. Baclesse concluded in 1959 that in properly selected patients, the percentage of cures was not significantly different from that obtained by more conventional methods, and although it was not a method to replace all others, radiotherapy was an alternative to consider for those patients who refused mutilating surgery.[4]

At M. D. Anderson Cancer Center, patients with unresectable lesions or who met Haagensen's criteria of clinical inoperability were treated with irradiation alone by the Baclesse technique, initially with 250 kV and later with cobalt 60. The total dose in some patients was as high as 10,000 rad. In 1965, an analysis confirmed that gross masses can be controlled with very large doses, with significant survival rates.[15] A later analysis showed that fibrosis and sometimes ulceration developed in all patients.[35]

Tumorectomy Followed by Irradiation

In 1945, Mustakallio initiated careful dissection of early tumors, leaving only sound tissue, followed with 2100 rad (6 × 350) to the breast through tangential portals.[28] The axilla was treated through front and back portals and the supraclavicular area through a direct portal. In 1969, an analysis of long-term results showed survival rates comparable to those obtained with radical mastectomy, but with a 20 percent recurrence rate in the breast.[32]

In 1955, at Guys Hospital in London, a randomized clinical trial of radical mastectomy versus wide excision (extended tylectomy) followed by postoperative irradiation was initiated.[2] The doses were inadequate by present standards. Fifteen local/regional failures occurred in 112 patients with clinical stage I disease (clinically negative axilla) and 30 failures occurred in 70 patients with clinical stage II disease (clinically positive axilla). The incidence of failures in the axilla in patients with clinically positive nodes corresponds with the expected percentage of patients who would have had histologically positive axillary nodes had a radical mastectomy been performed.

Evolution of the Concept of Radiosensitivity of Breast Cancer

Until relatively recently, the concept of radiosensitivity had been based on histology; within the same histology, there were subsets of tumors that, for no obvious

Table 33–4. PERCENTAGE CONTROL IN ADENOCARCINOMA OF THE BREAST CORRELATED WITH DOSE AND VOLUME OF CANCER

	Radiation Dose		Volume of Cancer (cm)	Control (%)
	Rad	*Weeks*		
Clinically negative lymphatic areas (elective irradiation)	5000	5	Subclinical	>90
Clinically positive axillary nodes	7000	7	2.5–3	90
Gross disease in the breast (biopsy only)	7000–8000	8–9	2–5	65
			>5	30
	8000–9000	8–10	>5	56
	8000–10,000	10–12	5–15	75

Modified from Fletcher GF: Textbook of Radiotherapy, ed 2. Philadelphia, Lea & Febiger, 1973.

reasons, were radiosensitive or radioresistant. This was best expressed by the following quotation from Paterson on the radiosensitivity of breast cancer[30]:

"A few fall into the highly radiosensitive group already discussed; the majority seem to respond in a surprising way to doses at the 4/5000 r level. But on the other hand, there are cases which definitely do not respond to even 7000 r. The breast group of tumors, as a whole, lacks the interesting consistency of the true squamous epitheliomata, and promises to present an interesting research problem for the pathologist and therapist jointly."

Baclesse must be credited with demonstrating that breast cancer can be eradicated by irradiation only. His work on breast cancer has great significance, because it established the correlation among dose, control, and size of the tumor. The fact that he gave much smaller doses to clinically negative lymphatic areas is important, but the effectiveness of these doses on subclinical disease cannot be assessed, since he did not report the incidence of failures in electively irradiated areas: at that time, the 5-year survival rate was the only analyzed end point.

Elective irradiation of the supraclavicular areas has shown that 4500–5000 rad given in 5 weeks eradicates more than 90 percent of occult deposits (Table 33–3). These data are the basis of the regimen in which 5000 rad is given to the breast after a segmental resection of the tumor. A boost is given if the margins are poor. Table 33–4 summarizes the relationships of control, dose, and tumor volume.[13]

Curability of Breast Cancer

At the middle of this century, after investigating breast cancer mortality since 1900, some epidemiologists concluded that survival rates of patients with breast cancer were not at all affected by any treatment.[29] In their study, the 5-year survival rate was used as an index. Other authors have constructed mathematical models of the behavior of breast cancer and have concluded that at any one time the same proportion of patients experience failure, so that eventually all patients die from breast cancer.[9, 10] Other studies have indicated that less than 15 percent of breast cancer patients with positive axillary lymph nodes will be free of disseminated disease.[8] However, some models of breast cancer survival suggest that a fraction of patients are cured by

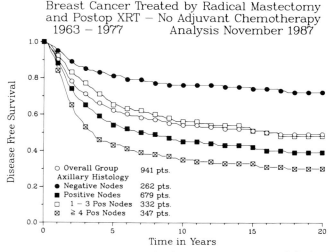

Figure 33–5. Proportion disease free by years post treatment. Calculated by the life-table method,[6] death was considered a censoring event, not a failure in this calculation. (From Fletcher GH, McNeese MD, Oswald MJ: Int J Radiol Oncol Biol Phys. 17:11–14,1989. Reprinted by permission.)

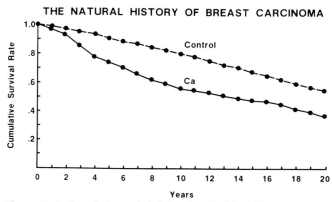

Figure 33–6. Cumulative probabilities of survival for 662 women treated by radical mastectomy for carcinoma of the breast are compared with age-adjusted survival rates for women in the general population of New York State. (From Haagensen CD: Diseases of the Breast, 2nd ed. Philadelphia, WB Saunders, 1971. Reprinted by permission.)

therapy.[34] There are data in the literature showing that patients with histologically positive axillary nodes can survive a long time. For instance, of 1958 breast cancer patients treated at Memorial Hospital in New York City in the years 1940–1943, 184 were known to be alive for an average of 30.6 years; 60 of them had had positive axillary nodes.[1] At M. D. Anderson Cancer Center, an analysis done in 1987 of the results in patients who had received postoperative irradiation between 1963 and 1977 showed that 40 percent of the patients with histologically positive axillary nodes are alive and free of disease after 20 years (Fig. 33–5).[17]

A graph in Haagensen's second edition of his book, *Diseases of the Breast,* compares the mortality of breast cancer patients 10 years after treatment with the mortality of the general population (Fig. 33–6).[18] After 15 years, the curves are parallel, indicating that a certain proportion of patients is cured. In another series comparing the mortality of breast cancer patients with the mortality of the general population, some patients were also shown to be cured.[7]

ACKNOWLEDGMENTS

This investigation was supported in part by grants CA06294 and CA16672 awarded by the National Cancer Institute, U.S. Department of Health and Human Services.

References

1. Adair F, Berg J, Joubert L, Robbins GF: Long-term follow-up of breast cancer patients: the 30-year report. Cancer 33:1145–1150, 1974.
2. Atkins H, Hayward JL, Klugman DJ, Wayte AB: Treatment of early breast cancer: a report after ten years of clinical trial. Br Med J 20:423–429, 1972.
3. Baclesse F: La roentgentherapie seule dans le traitement des cancers du sein operables et inoperables. Troisieme rapport. Presented at the Association francaise de Chirurgie, 51st Congress francais de Chirurgie, Paris, 1948.
4. Baclesse F: Roentgen therapy alone in cancer of the breast. Acta Un Int Cancer 15:1023, 1959.
5. Baclesse F, Gricouroff G, Tailhefer A: Essai de roentgentherapie du cancer du sein suivie d'operation large. Resultat histologiques. Bull Cancer 28:729–743, 1939.
6. Berkson J, Gage RP: Calculation of survival rates for cancer. Mayo Clin Proc 25:270–286, 1950.
7. Brinkley D, Haybittle JL: The curability of breast cancer. Lancet 2:95–97, 1975.
8. Bross IDJ, Blumenson LE: Predictive design of experiments using deep mathematical models. Cancer 28:1637–1646, 1971.
9. Cutler SJ, Axtell SJ: Partitioning of a patient population with respect to different mortality risks. Am Stat Assoc J 6:701–712, 1963.
10. Ederer F, Cutler SJ, Goldberg IS, Eisenberg H: Causes of death among long-term survivors from breast cancer in Connecticut. J Natl Cancer Inst 30:933–947, 1963.
11. Fletcher GH: Textbook of Radiotherapy, ed 1. Philadelphia, Lea and Febiger, 1966.
12. Fletcher GH: Local results of irradiation in the primary management of localized breast cancer. Cancer 29:545–551, 1972.
13. Fletcher GH: Textbook of Radiotherapy, ed 2. Philadelphia, Lea and Febiger, 1973.
14. Fletcher GH: History of irradiation in the primary management of apparently regionally confined breast cancer. Int J Radiat Oncol Biol Phys 11:2133–2141, 1985.
15. Fletcher GH, Montague ED: Radical irradiation of advanced breast cancer. Am J Roentgenol 93:573–584, 1965.
16. Fletcher GH, Montague ED: Does adequate irradiation of the internal mammary chain and supraclavicular nodes improve survival rates? Int J Radiat Oncol Biol Phys 4:481–492, 1978.
17. Fletcher GH, McNeese MD, Oswald MJ: Long-range results for breast cancer patients treated by radical mastectomy and postoperative radiation without adjuvant chemotherapy: an update. Int J Radiat Oncol Biol Phys 17:11–14, 1989.
18. Haagensen CD: Diseases of the Breast, ed 2. Philadelphia, WB Saunders, 1971.
19. Haagensen CD, Stout AP: Carcinoma of the breast. II. Criteria of operability. Ann Surg 118:859–870; 1032–1051, 1943.
20. Handley WS: Parasternal invasion of the thorax in breast cancer and its suppression by the use of radium tubes as an operative precaution. Surg Gynecol Obstet 45:721, 1927.
21. Handley RS: A surgeon's view of the spread of breast cancer. Cancer 24:1231, 1969.
22. Handley RS, Thackray AC: The internal mammary lymph chains in carcinoma of the breast. Lancet 2:276–278, 1949.
23. Keynes G: The radium treatment of carcinoma of the breast. Br J Surg 19:415–480, 1932.
24. Keynes G: Conservative treatment of cancer of the breast. Br Med J 2:643–647, 1937.
25. Lacour J, Le M, Caceres E, Koszarowski T, Veronesi U, Hill C: Radical mastectomy versus radical mastectomy plus internal mammary dissection. Ten year results of an international cooperative trial in breast cancer. Cancer 51:1941–1943, 1983.
26. McWhirter R: The value of simple mastectomy and radiotherapy in the treatment of cancer of the breast. Br J Radiol 21:599–610, 1948.
27. Montague ED, Spanos WJ Jr, Fletcher GH: Die Entwicklung der Behandlungsmethoden bei der Primartherapie des nichtmetastasierten Mammakarzinoma. *In* Frischbier HJ (ed): Die Erkrankungen den weiblichen Brustdruse. Stuttgart, Georg Thieme Verlag, 1982, pp 201–208.
28. Mustakallio S: Uber die Moeglichkeiten der roentgentherapie bei der Behandlung des Brustkrebses. Acta Radiol (Stockh) 26:503–511, 1945.
29. Park WW, Lees JC: The absolute curability of cancer of the breast. Surg Gynecol Obstet 93:129–152, 1951.
30. Paterson R: The radical x-ray treatment of the carcinomata. Br J Radiol 9:671–679, 1936.
31. Paterson R, Russell M: Clinical trials in malignant disease, part III. Breast cancer: evaluation of postoperative radiotherapy. J Fac Radiologist 10:175–180, 1959.
32. Rissanen PM: A comparison of conservative and radical surgery combined with radiotherapy in the treatment of stage I carcinoma of the breast. Br J Radiol 42:423–426, 1969.
33. Rodger A, Montague ED, Fletcher GH: Preoperative or postoperative irradiation as adjuvant treatment with radical mastectomy in breast cancer. Cancer 51:1388–1392, 1983.
34. Rutqvist LE, Wallgren A, Nilsson B: Is breast cancer a curable disease? A study of 14,731 women with breast cancer from the cancer registry of Norway. Cancer 53:1793–1800, 1984.
35. Spanos WJ, Montague ED, Fletcher GH: Late complications of radiation only for advanced breast cancer. Int J Radiat Oncol Biol Phys 6:1473–1476, 1980.
36. Spratt JS: Locally recurrent cancer after radical mastectomy. Cancer 20:1051, 1967.
37. Tapley N duV, Spanos WJ, Fletcher GH, Montague ED, Schell S, Oswald MJ: Results in patients with breast cancer treated by radical mastectomy and postoperative irradiation with no adjuvant chemotherapy. Cancer 49:1316–1319, 1982.

Management of Benign Breast Disease

Chapter 34

EVALUATION AND TREATMENT OF BENIGN BREAST DISORDERS

Wiley W. Souba, M.D., Sc. D.

Benign lesions of the breast are common. However, benign pathological states have always been neglected in comparison to cancer even though they account for as much as 90 percent of the clinical presentations related to the breast.[40] The term "benign," when applied to a biopsy sample of a breast mass, is nonspecific and may be misleading (Table 34–1). Substantial variations for designation of specific disease processes, in conjunction with the observation that many women with "lumpy breasts" never have breast biopsy, have resulted in inaccurate estimates of the true clinical incidence of benign disorders of this organ.

Table 34–1. SYNONYMS FOR COMMON BENIGN BREAST DISORDERS

Cyclical nodularity
　Fibrocystic disease
　Fibroadenosis
　Schimmelbusch's disease
　Chronic cystic mastitis
　Cystic mastopathy

Duct ectasia/periductal mastitis
　Plasma cell mastitis
　Comedo mastitis
　Mastitis obliterans
　Secretory disease

Giant fibroadenomatous tumor
　Giant fibroadenoma
　Cystosarcoma phyllodes
　Phyllodes tumor
　Juvenile fibroadenoma

Modified from Hughes LE, et al: Benign Disorders and Diseases of the Breast. Concepts and Clinical Management. London, Bailliere Tindall, 1989, pp 1–4.

There has been the tendency in many international clinics to include all benign breast disorders and pathology under the designation of "fibrocystic disease."[8, 34, 55, 93, 94] This nomenclature confuses normal physiological and morphological transformations in the breast with specific disease processes and is based on the assumption that all nonmalignant breast symptoms are etiologically derived from similar pathophysiological processes. The result is often one of increased confusion, both clinically and pathologically, and this approach has prevented the systematic study of benign breast disease.

This chapter will review the treatment of benign breast diseases, with the exception of infectious and inflammatory disorders of the breast, which have been previously discussed in section III, chapter 5. Emphasis will be placed on the application of appropriate terminology and on management strategies, as the epidemiology and histopathology of these lesions are described elsewhere (section III, chapter 6 and section IV, chapter 12).

CLINICAL FEATURES OF BENIGN BREAST DISORDERS

A useful classification system for benign breast disease has been described by Love and colleagues[55, 56] and is based on symptoms and physical findings. Six general categories have been identified (Table 34–2), which include physiological swelling and tenderness, nodularity, mastalgia, dominant lumps, nipple discharge, and inflammation. This classification emphasizes the variety of benign breast disorders seen by clinicians. It is important to consider that many women develop premenstrual breast swelling and tenderness that is mild and

Table 34–2. CLASSIFICATION OF BENIGN BREAST DISEASE BASED ON CLINICAL FEATURES

I. Physiological swelling and tenderness
II. Nodularity
III. Mastalgia (breast pain)
IV. Dominant lumps
    A. Gross cysts
    B. Galactoceles
    C. Fibroadenoma
V. Nipple discharge
    A. Galactorrhea
    B. Abnormal nipple discharge
VI. Breast infections
    A. Intrinsic mastitis
        1. Postpartum engorgement
        2. Lactational mastitis
        3. Lactational breast abscess
    B. Chronic recurrent subareolar abscess
    C. Acute mastitis associated with macrocystic breasts
    D. Extrinsic infections

Modified from Love SM, et al: N Engl J Med 307:1010–1014, 1982; Love SM, et al: Benign Breast Disorders. Philadelphia, J. B. Lippincott Company, 1987.

physiological and therefore should *not* be termed a disease or even a symptom requiring therapy. In addition, it should be emphasized that pain, nodularity, or lumps may occur synchronously, metachronously, unilaterally, or bilaterally. When communicating to his or her peers, the physician should make every effort to apply pathophysiological descriptive nomenclature and avoid usage of the nondescriptive term "fibrocystic disease."

Physiological Swelling and Tenderness

At recurrent intervals premenopausally, most women clinically experience premenstrual tenderness, which is often associated with mild breast swelling. These changes are physiological, expectant, and limited to the reproductive years, since they are hormonally regulated (see section II, chapter 3). Cyclic physiological swelling and tenderness should not be labeled as a breast disorder and generally does not require therapy. These cyclic alterations in breast structure, contour, and size result from variations in plasma concentrations of gonadotrophic and ovarian hormones.[41] Further, these concentrations may fluctuate significantly with each menstrual cycle. Prior to onset of menses, mammary lobules, stroma, and ducts become engorged; thereafter, ducts shrink with the onset of menses, and epithelial cells desquamate and are maintained to initiate proliferation by the second week of the cycle.[41] The connective stroma and ductal epithelial cells increase in size and number. These remarkable variations and alterations of the hormonal milieu are clinically evident with resultant effects of hypoplastic and hyperplastic dilation of all mammary components (e.g., connective tissue stroma, ducts, and lobules). With menopause, there is regression to an atropic or hypoplastic epithelium of the lobules and ducts, while periductal fibrous tissue becomes more

dense and is recognizable to the clinician as cords of homogenous tissue. The senile or postmenopausal breast transforms to progressive involution as a result of cessation of parenchymal and ductal stimulation by ovarian estrogens and progesterones. The clinician may observe dilation of the lactiferous duct network in isolated lobules. Macrocystic formation occurs following enlargement of the lobular acini depleted of their columnar epithelium. Thus on examination the postmenopausal breast is commonly asymmetric, with lobular irregularity and variation of cyst size. With progressive diminution in total fat content of the organ, the senescent breast will shrink in volume and the parenchyma and stroma will blend into a more spherical or pendulous mass.

Nodularity

A pattern of diffuse lumpiness or nodularity is generally not abnormal and represents the responsiveness of breast parenchyma and stroma to circulating estrogenic and progestational hormones.[15, 42] The nodularity may be finely granular or grossly lumpy and may involve the entire breast or a specific focus of the mamma. Patey[82, 83] coined the term "pseudolump" to describe a dominant area of lumpiness that coalesces into the surrounding breast tissue. Although many surgeons today would designate such areas as "fibrocystic disease," most histological entities grouped broadly in this nondescriptive category do not form gross nodules or lumps. Hence the term "fibrocystic disease" should be abandoned, and clinicians must be educated as to the often poor correlation between clinical nodularity and significant pathological entities.

Mastalgia

Mastalgia, or pain in the mammary gland, is common and is of concern to the patient, as evidenced by the large number of women who present to their doctor with such complaints.[45] These individuals are generally seeking reassurance that they do not have cancer or another serious breast disorder. A careful history and physical examination and mammogram will help the physician to rule out this possibility. With such patients an explanation of the hormonal nature of the breast pain is helpful in alleviating anxiety, and generally no other treatment is necessary. Mastalgia and nodularity are discussed in greater depth in a subsequent section of this chapter.

Dominant Lumps

A dominant lump in the breast must be clinically differentiated from carcinoma. Dominant lumps that are benign include macroscopic cysts, galactoceles, and fibroadenomas.[10] As a general rule discrete lumps may be aspirated with a needle (section X, chapter 28) to determine if they are cystic or solid. The physical and radiographic features of these lesions are important for accurate clinical assessment. Differentiation of solid and cystic characteristics is aided with use of mammography and ultrasonography (section VIII, chapter 24). If the lesion is cystic, the wall will collapse with needle aspiration, and the cyst will no longer be palpable. If the lesion is solid, further evaluation with biopsy to rule out cancer is advisable.

Nipple Discharge

Nipple discharge can be classified as galactorrhea or abnormal nipple discharge.[48, 56] Galactorrhea is the spontaneous nipple discharge of milklike fluid as a result of stimulation of the breast by elevated prolactin secretion from the pituitary. Prolactin levels may be elevated in patients who use oral contraceptives, in thyroid disease, and as a result of a functional pituitary adenoma. Appropriate management includes thyroid tests and determination of the serum prolactin level.

Abnormal nipple discharge is bloody or blood-tinged or is sticky and clear. Takeda et al.[91] noted that the presence of red blood cells and clusters of more than 30 ductal cells are suggestive of malignancy. The most common causes of bloody discharge from the nipple are intraductal papilloma, duct ectasia, and carcinoma (see section II, chapter 3).

Breast Infections

Infections of the female breast are rare excluding the postpartum period. These inflammatory states may be classified as intrinsic infections of the breast (secondary to abnormalities in breast architecture or function) or extrinsic (secondary to an infection in an adjacent organ or structure that involves the breast).[56] Intrinsic mastitis includes postpartum engorgement, lactational mastitis, and lactational breast abscess. Chronic recurrent subareolar abscess occurs primarily in women in the reproductive years and has a high incidence of squamous metaplasia of involved ducts.[21] Antibiotics are generally not of therapeutic benefit, and resolution of the infection depends on excision of the chronically involved site. Acute mastitis associated with gross cysts may be observed in the patient with macrocystic breasts who develops a localized area of redness, pain, edema, and fever. The entity can mimic inflammatory cancer; therefore the involved lesion should be aspirated or sampled by biopsy for culture and histology. Rupture of a gross cyst within the breast parenchyma that elicits an inflammatory response may result in acute mastitis and systemic sepsis.

Extrinsic infections may develop secondary to an infectious process in the skin overlying the breast or within the thoracic cavity. A complete review of the pathology, clinical presentation, and management of infectious and inflammatory diseases of the breast is provided in section III, chapter 5.

PATHOLOGY OF NONPROLIFERATIVE AND PROLIFERATIVE BENIGN BREAST DISORDERS

Although there has been a tendency to classify all benign breast diseases under the global category of "fibrocystic disease," from a pathological viewpoint this term is nondescriptive for any specific entity.[55] Histologically, the term encompasses a broad spectrum of pathological abnormalities and physiological variations and hence is imprecise and inaccurate. For example, biopsy of a nodular (lumpy) area of the breast may demonstrate fibroglandular tissue and mammary epithelium. Although these are considered to be normal tissues of breast stroma and parenchyma, they often are reported in many institutions as "consistent with fibrocystic disease, mammary dysplasia, or chronic cystic mastitis."

Of paramount clinical significance is the histopathological differentiation of benign and atypical changes of ductal and lobular components of the breast from frank neoplasia.[68, 69] The histopathological evaluation of the biopsy specimen will also help determine the subsequent risk of developing carcinoma if the lesion represents atypia of lobules or ductal epithelium. This information, together with the surgeon's knowledge of other risk factors, will greatly influence the frequency of follow-up and future mammography as well as the timing and necessity for additional biopsies. Determining the clinical significance of pathological characteristics of the biopsy specimen in the absence of carcinoma is a difficult problem that has been compounded by the lack of consistent nomenclature. This problem has been addressed by Page and coworkers[26, 67–70] and has led to a classification system adopted by the American College of Pathologists.[20] This system emphasizes the uselessness of the terms "fibrocystic disease" and "chronic cystic mastitis" and provides a practical classification of benign breast pathology that is clinically relevant. With use of this classification, the relative risk for developing invasive breast carcinoma, based on the pathological evaluation of benign breast tissue, is provided. The classification system developed by Page separates the various types of benign breast lesions into three clinically relevant groups: nonproliferative lesions, proliferative lesions without atypia, and proliferative lesions with atypia (Table 34–3). This classification completely eliminates potentially confusing terminology and incorporates histopathological criteria that may be associated with an increased risk for development of breast cancer.[50] Provision of essential pathology features of the biopsy to allow precise classification, together with the clinician's knowledge of the family history, establishes the relative risk for cancer. These data, together with the mammographic and physical examination findings, will determine the management strategy and follow-up for the patient. A review of the classification system introduced by Page is essential to define neoplastic risk for benign breast disease and to objectively provide recommendations for management.

Table 34–3. PATHOLOGICAL CLASSIFICATION OF BENIGN BREAST DISORDERS

I. Nonproliferative lesions of the breast
  A. Cysts and apocrine metaplasia
  B. Duct ectasia
  C. Mild ductal epithelial hyperplasia
  D. Calcifications
  E. Fibroadenoma and related lesions
II. Proliferative breast disorders without atypia
  A. Sclerosing adenosis
  B. Radial and complexing sclerosing lesions
  C. Moderate and florid ductal epithelial hyperplasia
  D. Ductal involvement by cells of atypical lobular hyperplasia
  E. Intraductal papillomas
III. Atypical proliferative lesions
  A. Atypical lobular hyperplasia (ALH)
  B. Atypical ductal hyperplasia (ADH)

Modified from Consensus Meeting: Arch Pathol Lab Med 110:171–173, 1986; Dupont WD, Page DL: N Engl J Med 312:146–151, 1985.

Pathological Classification of Benign Breast Disorders

The pathology classification system proposed by Page for benign diseases of the breast is outlined in Table 34–3. A more detailed review of the histological features associated with each specific entity is provided in section III, chapter 6. This brief pathology review is intended for the practitioner. Clinicians involved in breast diagnosis and surgeons who operate on the breast should become familiar with this classification system and its implications to ensure effective communication with the pathologist and to appropriately determine subsequent risk for developing carcinoma once the histological features of the biopsy specimen are determined. This level of familiarization with the system is essential, as only microscopic evaluation of the examined specimen can provide this information.

Nonproliferative Lesions of the Breast

Nonproliferative lesions of the breast account for approximately 70 percent of benign lesions and carry no increased risk for the development of carcinoma.[67, 96] Cysts and apocrine metaplasia, duct ectasia, mild ductal epithelial hyperplasia, calcifications, and fibroadenomas and related lesions are included in this category.

Cysts and Apocrine Metaplasia. Cysts are defined by the presence of fluid-filled walled spaces.[46, 72] Cysts in the breast may vary tremendously in size and number and may be microscopic or macroscopic. These lesions are almost always multifocal and bilateral and almost never malignant.[37, 39, 51, 78] Cysts originate from the terminal duct lobular unit, probably from hormonally regulated dilatation of the lobule and failure to shrink after the onset of menses. Cysts may also arise from an obstructed ectatic duct. The typical macroscopic cyst is round and bluish in color (blue-domed cyst) and usually contains dark fluid ranging in color from green-gray to brown. Often the epithelium of the cyst is flattened or even absent. Apocrine metaplasia of epithelium lining

the wall of the cyst is not infrequently present (Table 34–4). This term denotes histological similarities to apocrine epithelium, which is composed of large columnar cells.[1] The apical aspect of these cells frequently has a rounded protrusion into the cyst space that has been termed an "apocrine snout." The stroma surrounding these cysts is generally fibrotic and is often infiltrated with numerous lymphocytes, plasma cells, and histiocytes (see section III, chapter 6).

Duct Ectasia. Duct ectasia is a disease complex that involves the large and intermediate ductules of the breast.[11] It is most often recognized clinically by the presence of palpable dilated ducts filled with sticky grumous debris of desquamated ductal epithelium and secretory proteinaceous contents. Duct ectasia is common; autopsies have shown it to be present in nearly one half of women older than 60 years.[30] Periductal inflammation is a distinguishing histological characteristic in this condition. It is generally accepted that duct ectasia is preceded by destruction of the elastic periductal tissues, thus initiating ectasia and periductal fibrosis. The greatest clinical significance of duct ectasia lies in its mimicry of invasive ductal carcinoma when the duct ectasia is extreme.[36, 74] There is no demonstrated relationship to cancer risk.

Mild Ductal Epithelial Hyperplasia. The fundamental feature of epithelial hyperplasia is an increased number of cells relative to that normally observed above the basement membrane (Table 34–4).[77] Normally two cell layers are evident; therefore three or more cells above the basement membrane is pathognomonic of hyperplasia of the duct epithelium. Epithelial hyperplasia does not include conditions in which glandular (stromal) cells are increased in number relative to the basement membrane, a condition known as adenosis.[73]

Mild hyperplasia of the usual (ductal) type is defined as an increase in the number of epithelial cells to more than two to three layers above the basement membrane without crossing the lumen.[56, 77] Cells may vary in size and are often elliptical but are not atypical. Other than cyst formation, lobular hyperplasia of the usual type is the most frequent alteration in the breast recognized as abnormal. Despite its frequency, this diagnosis is often made by exclusion, representing any epithelial hyperplasia that lacks lobular, apocrine, or atypical features.

Table 34–4. EPITHELIAL HYPERPLASIA OF THE BREAST

I. Apocrine type
  A. Apocrine metaplasia (most commonly seen in the lining of cysts)
II. Ductal type
  A. Mild ductal hyperplasia
  B. Moderate ductal hyperplasia
  C. Florid ductal hyperplasia
  D. Atypical ductal hyperplasia (ADH)
III. Lobular type
  A. Atypical lobular hyperplasia (ALH)
  B. Ductal involvement by cells of ALH

Compiled from Consensus Meeting: Arch Pathol Lab Med 110:171–173, 1986; Dupont WD, Page DL: N Engl J Med 312:146–151, 1985.

This type of epithelial hyperplasia is recognized primarily to distinguish it from the more marked changes characteristic of moderate to florid epithelial hyperplasia, which have been demonstrated to indicate an increased risk of breast cancer[26, 77] (Tables 34–4 and 34–5). Thus a pathology report revealing foci of mild hyperplasia does not imply any clinically significant risk of carcinoma.

Calcifications. Calcifications are quite common in ductal, lobular, and stromal tissues of the breast. They may be macroscopic or microscopic and may be seen in blood vessels or lobules, free in the stroma, or associated with epithelium. Diffuse microcalcifications are most commonly seen in sclerosing adenosis.[56, 73] In the absence of other risk factors, calcifications do not increase the probability for development of breast cancer.

Fibroadenoma and Related Lesions. Fibroadenoma is a benign tumor of fibrous and epithelial elements.[28] The gross appearance of the typical fibroadenoma is usually diagnostic. It is a sharply circumscribed, spherical mass that may be unilobular or multilobular. The cut surface is white or yellow, and on gross examination the fibroadenoma is pseudoencapsulated and sharply delineated from the surrounding breast tissue.[56] These tumors originate from the breast lobule.[95] Microscopically, fibroadenomas have both an epithelial and stromal component. The histological pattern depends on which of these components is predominant. In general, the epithelial component consists of well-defined glandlike and ductlike spaces with varying degrees of epithelial hyperplasia. The stromal elements consist of connective tissue with variable collagen content and, rarely, mature adipose tissue[11] or smooth muscle.[31] In the elderly, fibroadenomas may become quite dense as a result of calcification and the lack of epithelial elements.

Autopsy studies demonstrate that fibroadenomas are present in approximately ten percent of women.[44] The peak incidence occurs between the second and third decades of life, but fibroadenomas are not uncommon in the elderly. Fibroadenomas that are allowed to enlarge after initial detection have a doubling time of approximately 1 year and generally cease growing once they reach 3 cm in diameter. The tumor is usually painless, spherical, smoothly marginated, and mobile within the breast.

Approximately five to ten percent of fibroadenomas that occur in teenagers are designated as *juvenile fibroadenomas*. This term is applied when the tumor (1) occurs in an adolescent, (2) rapidly enlarges, (3) reaches a size that is two to four times that of the opposite breast, (4) stretches the skin, and (5) displaces the nipple.[44] The juvenile fibroadenoma is not a specific histological entity in and of itself, although it tends to have an abundant cellular stroma compared to the typical fibroadenoma. Approximately 100 cases of either noninvasive or invasive carcinoma arising within fibroadenomas have been reported.[29, 66] Almost one half of these tumors have been lobular carcinoma, while another one third demonstrate features of invasive ductal carcinoma. The phyllodes tumor is the only entity that combines both epithelial and fibrous components into a pattern that resembles the fibroadenoma. The presence of these pathological features may result in difficulty distinguishing between certain low-grade cystosarcomas and fibroadenomas (section IV, chapter 10). These pathological cellular features are essential to differentiate benign from malignant lesions and will influence the clinician's management and follow-up of the patient. Should a presumed fibroadenoma recur, wide local excision rather than enucleation is appropriate therapy. Fibroadenomas and phyllodes tumors are reviewed in further detail later in this chapter when management of benign breast disorders is discussed.

Adenomas of the breast are well-circumscribed tumors composed of benign epithelial elements with sparse stroma.[56, 63] This latter histopathological feature differentiates these lesions from fibroadenomas, in which the stroma is abundant as an intrical part of the tumor. Adenomas may be divided into tubular adenomas and lactating adenomas.[28] Tubular adenomas present in young women as well-defined freely mobile lesions that clinically resemble fibroadenomas. Lactation adenomas present during pregnancy or during the postpartum period. On microscopic examination, these lesions have lobulated borders and are composed of glands lined by cuboidal cells with secretory activity identical to the lactational changes normally observed in breast tissue during pregnancy and lactation.

Hamartomas are discrete breast lesions that are most commonly 2 to 4 cm in diameter and are firm and sharply circumscribed.[5, 28] Microscopically, numerous lobules are present that may be discrete or may coalesce to form a homogeneous mass. Hamartomas and fibroadenomas share the features of gross circumscription and the presence of lobules, but the lobules in hamartomas are a major component except for fatty areas. The stroma of a fibroadenoma is usually more cellular than the stroma of a hamartoma; hamartomas have areas of fat replacement, a rare observation in fibroadenomas.

Adenolipomas consist of sharply circumscribed nodules of fatty elemets that have normal lobules and ducts interspersed.[90] Microscopically, the fat is normal, and the lobules and ducts are fairly evenly distributed throughout the tumor. Most of the lobules, however, are set in the fat without any fibrous stroma.

Table 34–5. RISK FOR DEVELOPMENT OF INVASIVE CARCINOMA AFTER BREAST BIOPSY

Lesion	Approximate Relative Risk
Nonproliferative lesions of the breast	No increased risk
Sclerosing adenosis	No increased risk
Intraductal papilloma	No increased risk
Moderate and florid hyperplasia (of usual type)	1.5- to twofold
Atypical lobular hyperplasia	Fourfold
Atypical ductal hyperplasia	Fourfold
Ductal involvement by cells of atypical ductal hyperplasia	Sevenfold
Lobular carcinoma *in situ*	Tenfold
Ductal carcinoma *in situ*	Tenfold

Compiled from Dupont WD, Page DL: N Engl J Med 312:146–151, 1985; Page DL, et al: J Natl Cancer Inst 61:1055–1063, 1978.

Proliferative Breast Disorders Without Atypia

Proliferative breast disorders without atypia include sclerosing adenosis, intraductal papillomas, and moderate and florid ductal epithelial hyperplasia, among others.[9] There is a slightly increased risk for the development of invasive breast cancer (approximately 1.5 to 2 times normal) when the biopsy specimen demonstrates moderate or florid ductal epithelial hyperplasia (Table 34–5). It is therefore imperative that the surgeon be knowledgeable of the implications of these diagnoses, since they will influence the future management of the patient.

Sclerosing Adenosis. Sclerosing adenosis is a lobular change involving an enlargement and distortion of lobular units (Table 34–3).[47] Sclerosing adenosis is formed following proliferation of both stromal and epithelial units of the terminal duct lobular unit.[73] Microscopically, the disease is characterized by an increased number of acinar structures and fibrosis of the lobular stroma, but the normal two-cell population central to the enveloping basement membrane is maintained. Sclerosing adenosis most commonly occurs in multiple microscopic cysts and occasionally presents as a palpable mass.[32] Diffuse microcalcifications are most commonly seen in sclerosing adenosis, and the most significant clinical aspect of sclerosing adenosis is its mimicry of carcinoma.

Sclerosing adenosis may be confused with carcinoma at physical examination, mammography, and at gross examination in the surgical pathology laboratory. The borders of the lesion are irregular. Maintenance of the lobular architecture, determined by low-power evaluation under the light microscope, allows sclerosing adenosis to be identified as a benign lesion.

Sclerosing adenosis is confined for the most part to the child-bearing and perimenopausal years. It has no proven premalignant implications. The importance of sclerosing adenosis for practicing physicians is its macroscopic and microscopic resemblance to carcinoma.[57] Only excisional biopsy and histopathological study of the lesion can differentiate these entities.

Radial Scars and Complex Sclerosing Lesions. Radial scars and complex sclerosing lesions of the mamma are characterized by central sclerosis and varying degrees of epithelial proliferation, apocrine metaplasia, and papilloma formation (Table 34–3).[75] (This is reviewed in chapter 6.) However, their gross and microscopic mimicry of cancer has rendered these lesions most important to diagnostic histopathology. The term "radial scar" is reserved for the smaller lesions (up to 1 cm in diameter), whereas the diagnostic terminology "complex sclerosing lesion" is appropriate for the larger masses. The possibility that the epithelial elements of some of these lesions represent an early stage of breast evolution, as suggested by Linell,[53] remains to be proved.

Radial scars originate at the point of terminal duct branching.[4] With the naked eye the appearance is often unremarkable, but with slight magnification the radiality is evidenced around a central white area of fibrosis flecked by elastic streaks. The *complex sclerosing lesion* measures more than 10 mm and has essentially the same characteristics of the radial scar but on a greater scale. A stellate appearance best describes the lesion that is usually seen around the firm fibrous center. All of the histological features of the radial scar are seen in these larger lesions, but the involved elements show a greater disturbance of structure with papilloma formation, apocrine metaplasia, and occasionally sclerosing adenosis.[3]

Moderate and Florid Ductal Epithelial Hyperplasia. Moderate and florid hyperplasia of the usual type are found in more than 20 percent of biopsy samples and thus are the most common variants of proliferative lesions of the breast.[77] These entities are characterized by an increase in cell number within the ducts. *Moderate hyperplasia* is defined arbitrarily as having more than three cells in height above the basement membrane.[77] *Florid hyperplasia* consists of a proliferation of cells that occupy at least 70 percent of the duct lumen and often distend the involved spaces. With florid hyperplasia, the combined histological and pattern features of atypical hyperplasia and carcinoma *in situ* are absent. Architecturally, epithelial hyperplasia is either solid or papillary and may be characterized by intracellular spaces that are irregular, slitlike, and variably shaped.

Ductal Involvement by Cells of Atypical Lobular Hyperplasia. Ductal involvement with cells characteristic of atypical lobular hyperplasia is an unusual phenomenon (Tables 34–3 and 34–4). Small irregular lobular cells usually spread beneath the ductal epithelium. When the ductal involvement with cells typical of lobular proliferative regions is extensive, it is usually seen in conjunction with an invasive lobular cancer or lobular carcinoma *in situ*.

Intraductal Papillomas. *Solitary intraductal papillomas* are tumors of the major lactiferous ducts and are most commonly observed in premenopausal women (Table 34–3).[56, 76] The most common presenting symptom is nipple discharge, which may be serous or bloody. Intraductal papillomas are generally less than 0.5 cm in diameter but may be as large as 4 or 5 cm.[18] Grossly, these lesions are tannish-pink, friable lesions within a duct or cyst. The tumor is usually attached to the wall of the duct by a stalk. Microscopically, these tumors are composed of multiple branching papillae within a central fibrous vascular core and a superficial layer of epithelial cells. Variable amounts of fibrosis may be present between the epithelial elements. It is often difficult to differentiate between benign papilloma and papillary carcinoma on frozen section. Moreover, there has been considerable debate regarding the malignant potential for solitary intraductal papillomas. It is rare for these lesions to undergo malignant transformation. In addition, the risk of developing carcinoma for a woman with an intraductal papilloma appears to be no greater than that of the general population.

Multiple intraductal papillomas tend to occur in younger patients and are associated with nipple discharge less often than are solitary intraductal papillomas.[56] These lesions are more often peripheral and bilateral, and most importantly, the pathological entity appears to be susceptible to the development of carcinoma. In Haagensen's series[34] of 39 patients with multiple papillomas, the simultaneous presence of carcinoma was observed in 38 percent of patients. Peripheral papillomas, in contrast to solitary central papillomas, seem to be highly susceptible to malignant transformation.

Atypical Proliferative Lesions

The category of atypical proliferative lesions includes both ductal and lobular lesions. These are lesions with some but not all of the features of carcinoma *in situ*. Even the most experienced pathologists may disagree as to whether to classify a given lesion as atypical hyperplasia or carcinoma *in situ*.

Atypical Lobular Hyperplasia. Atypical lobular hyperplasia fulfills some but not all of the criteria of lobular carcinoma *in situ*.[6, 14, 67–70, 77] The cytology of atypical lobular hyperplasia is usually quite bland with round, somewhat lightly stained eosinophilic cytoplasm. The uniformity and roundness of the cell population is pathognomonic to the diagnosis of atypical lobular hyperplasia. The lobular unit must be less than half filled with these cells, and no significant distortion of the lobular unit should be present.[77] If any lobular unit fulfills the criteria for lobular carcinoma *in situ* thereafter (section IV, chapter 8), this diagnosis overrides the presence of atypical lobular hyperplasia from a prognostic and therapeutic perspective. Cells of atypical lobular hyperplasia may involve the ducts, with pathological features identical to lobular carcinoma *in situ*.[71, 88] The solid pattern of lobular carcinoma *in situ* involvement of ducts is not seen with atypical lobular hyperplasia.

This spectrum from lesser examples of atypical lobular hyperplasia up to and including lobular carcinoma *in situ* may best be termed "lobular neoplasia," as suggested by Haagensen et al. in 1978.[35] Adoption of the degree of filling, distortion, and distension of the lobular acini as the determinant criteria for separation of atypical lobular hyperplasia from lobular carcinoma *in situ* has revealed a relative risk of subsequent invasive carcinoma for atypical lobular hyperplasia that is four times that of the general population in two separate studies.[25, 26, 69, 70] This risk is approximately tenfold when lobular carcinoma is not further treated after biopsy. Other than the magnitude for subsequent risk of carcinoma, atypical lobular hyperplasia does not differ from analogous carcinoma *in situ* lesions in clinical correlates and implications. The incidence of atypical lobular hyperplasia present in benign biopsies is slightly greater than one percent; the great majority of cases occur in the perimenopausal era. As with atypical ductal hyperplasia, there appears to be an increased risk in patients with a strong family history of breast cancer. Women with atypical lobular hyperplasia at biopsy and a family history of breast cancer in a first degree relative have a risk of invasive carcinoma twice that of the patient who presents with atypical lobular hyperplasia alone.[26]

Atypical Ductal Hyperplasia. Atypical ductal hyperplasia of no special variant (usual type) is diagnosed when either the cytological or pattern criteria of ductal carcinoma *in situ* (DCIS) are present histologically but are not both evident at pathological review. Page et al.[69] have emphasized the following criteria as most indicative of DCIS: (1) a uniform population of cells, (2) smooth geometric spaces between cells or micropapillary formations with uniform cellular placement, and (3) hyperchromatic nuclei. Atypical ductal hyperplasia has some of these features but lacks the complete histological criteria for DCIS. Any biopsy specimen with one of the first two major criteria will be diagnostic of atypical ductal hyperplasia. In this presentation, the secondary pathological criteria are evident as a noncomplete (suggestive) variant. The third criteria will be viewed as contributory, but neither specific nor sufficient for the diagnosis of atypical ductal hyperplasia. This pathological entity is appropriately placed in an intermediate position as a cancer risk between proliferative breast disease without atypia and ductal carcinoma *in situ*. The natural history of atypical ductal hyperplasia[69] suggests an intermediate risk (approximately fourfold) for invasive cancer development (Table 34–5; see also chapter 14).

The clinical importance of diagnosing atypical ductal hyperplasia in the breast biopsy specimen resides in its prognostic significance for breast cancer risk. Women followed for 15 years after biopsy alone develop invasive breast cancer about four times as frequently as women in the general population. This relative risk translates into an absolute risk that indicates that about ten percent of women with atypical ductal hyperplasia will develop invasive carcinoma within 10 to 15 years of biopsy.[69, 70]

OVERALL MANAGEMENT OF BENIGN DISORDERS OF THE BREAST

A variety of therapeutic modalities have been proposed in the treatment of the patient with benign lesions of the breast.[7, 12, 13, 16, 23, 38] The results have been variable. It should be emphasized that, in general, any dominant mass that does not yield fluid on aspiration should undergo biopsy to histologically exclude cancer of the organ.[49] Moreover, the majority of breast lumps should be aspirated in order to assess the consistency of the mass, obtain fluid that may be diagnostic of a cyst, and obtain a cytological specimen if the lesion is solid or yields bloody fluid. Furthermore, any solid or cystic breast mass in which the histopathology on fine needle aspiration (FNA) is equivocal should undergo incisional or, preferably, excisional biopsy (section X, chapter 28). Similarly, any nonpalpable mammographic abnormality that is suspicious for carcinoma (i.e., a stellate lesion with diffuse microcalcifications) should be excised by needle localization technique (section X, chapter 28). The histopathology of the specimen will be of great value to the surgeon in determining future treatment strategies.

The majority of patients with benign breast disease present to their physician with complaints of physiological swelling, nodularity, or mastalgia. The management of these patients (assuming the physical examination

Table 34–6. CANCER WITH BREAST PAIN

Author	Percentage of Cancers With Breast Pain
Haagenson[34]	5
Preece[85a]	7
Smallwood[89a]	18
River[87a]	24

and mammogram are normal) primarily consists of re-assurance. The importance of breast self-examination should be emphasized, and the hormone-related perturbations of breast tenderness can be explained.

Breast Pain and Nodularity

Breast pain (mastalgia) is the most common complaint associated with disorders of the breast.[45] Mastalgia denotes the symptom of pain in the breast parenchyma or stroma in the absence of any specific physical or pathological abnormality. The frequency of breast pain as a presenting breast symptom ranges from 45 percent to 84 percent. It is important to emphasize that although breast pain is an uncommon complaint in breast cancer, this presentation does not exclude the diagnosis (Table 34–6). Although mastalgia associated with cancer has no specific features, it differs from cyclical premenstrual mastalgia in that its persentation is unilateral, intense, and constant in nature. Haagensen[33] noted that only five percent of patients with breast cancer presented with pain, whereas others have noted an incidence as great as 24 percent (see Table 34–6).

Preece et al.[86] studied the pattern and natural history of mastalgia in patients who presented with complaints of breast pain and nodularity (Table 34–7). The most common type, cyclical pronounced pattern, was so named because it identifies a definite relationship to hormonal perturbations of the menstrual cycle. Patients with this pattern of mastalgia (mean age, 34 years) almost invariably have nodularity in the breast and have mastalgia for at least the week preceding the menstrual cycle. Careful studies using pain charts document that the discomfort is significant; when interviewed, women apply terms such as "heaviness" and "tenderness" to

Table 34–7. PATTERNS OF MASTALGIA

Pattern/Diagnosis	No. (%)
Cyclical pronounced	93 (40.1)
Noncyclical	62 (26.7)
Tietze's syndrome	25 (10.8)
Trauma (postbiopsy)	19 (8.2)
Sclerosing adenosis	11 (4.7)
Cancer	1 (0.4)
Miscellaneous/nonbreast	21 (9.1)
Total	232 (100)

Compiled from Hughes LE, et al: Benign Disorders and Diseases of the Breast. Concepts and Clinical Management. London, Bailliere Tindell, 1986, pp 75–92; Preece PE, et al: Lancet 2:670–673, 1976.

describe their discomfort. The mastalgia is premenopausal, and the pain is invariably relieved by menstruation; resolution in the perimenopausal or menopausal eras is typical.

The second most common pattern of breast pain identified by Preece et al.[86] was the noncyclical pattern, which accounted for slightly more than one fourth of women presenting with breast pain. Noncyclical mastalgia (patient mean age, 43 years) is distinguished from the cyclical pattern principally by its lack of relationship with events in the menstrual cycle. The cyclical pronounced pattern occurs exclusively in premenopausal women. In contradistinction, the noncyclical pattern occurs in pre- and postmenopausal women. Women use terms such as "drawing" and "burning" to describe their discomfort, which is not relieved with the onset of menses. In this entity, nodularity is much less prominent than in the cyclical pattern type, and there may be no palpable abnormality at the site of pain, which is typically subareolar or in the medial quadrants of the breasts. Mammography has been of some interest in the noncyclical type, since radiological abnormalities consistent with coarse calcifications and ductal dilatation are commonly seen. In the study by Preece et al.,[86] more than two thirds of women with noncyclical mastalgia had radiological evidence of duct ectasia, and one half of these patients had identifiable calcifications at the site of the complaint. However, it should be emphasized that there is no histological evidence that noncyclical pain results from the pathological changes of duct ectasia.

Tietze's syndrome, or painful costochondral junction syndrome, is not true mastalgia, but the pain is often considered to emanate from the region of the breast that overlies the tender costocartilage.[45] There is no palpable abnormality, but the pain is typically identified in the medial quadrants of the breast. Tietze's syndrome is often unilateral and may occur in any age group. The disease generally runs a chronic course. A smaller group of patients with postbiopsy mastalgia (trauma related) complain of a persistent, noncyclical variant of pain that is localized to the breast biopsy scar. Although some women in this group may have had a biopsy complicated by wound infection or hematoma that required evacuation, this is not a universal finding. Nearly five percent of patients with mastalgia have pain in a focal area of the breast that is replaced by sclerosing adenosis.[45] Cancer represents an uncommon cause of breast pain (less than one percent); the pain is generally noncyclical in nature. About ten percent of patients presenting with breast pain will be found to have a cause remote from the breast (Table 34–7).

The etiology of mastalgia and nodularity has been a source of debate for many years. The notable physical symptoms and emotional concern with cancer phobia experienced by many women with mastalgia and nodularity have been documented. Haagensen[45] observed that women with severe breast pain were "in general, unstable and hypochondriacal although they were not frankly psychotic." Edema caused by water and salt retention secondary to fluctuating estrogen and progesterone levels in the blood and their steroidal effects has been suggested as the cause of both mastalgia and nodularity. However, Preece et al.[86] demonstrated that there were no significant differences in water retention between the fifth and twenty-fifth days of the menstrual cycle when mastalgia patients were compared with normal controls. This was equally true for patients in the cyclical group, who displayed a typical premenstrual increase in breast pain. In the nineteenth century, Sir Astley Cooper suggested that mastalgia patients were "of a nervous disposition," but Preece and colleagues tested the psychoneurotic profiles of 300 patients who presented with cyclical and noncyclical mastalgia. These investigators demonstrated conclusively that there was no scientific basis for the hypothesis that mastalgia patients were psychoneurotic.

The introduction of accurate hormonal assays into clinical medicine has led to the development of three theories of the cause of the painful nodular breast: increased estrogen production by the ovary, diminished progesterone production, and hyperprolactinemia. Despite one report[89] that confirmed a significantly depressed level of luteal progesterone, additional studies have failed to show a defect in luteal phase progesterone values between mastalgia patients and controls. Moreover, a recent review[95] concludes that there are no significant differences in basal levels of sex steroids and gonadotropins in women with benign breast diseases compared with control patients. Pituitary regulation of prolactin release may be abnormal in patients with cyclic and noncyclic mastalgia.[60] Peters et al.[85] examined the stimulated prolactin response to thyrotropin releasing hormone (TRH) in a group of patients with benign disorders of the breast. These authors noted that patients with mastalgia had a significantly greater rise in TRH-induced prolactin release compared to controls. Additional studies[45] suggest that there is a disturbance in hypothalamic feedback control of prolactin secretion in patients with cyclic mastalgia and that this defect may contribute to the development of painful nodular breasts.

Management

The first step in the management of patients with mastalgia and nodularity is a thorough history and physical examination.[43] If a dominant or discrete lump is present, it should be aspirated to determine if the lesion is cystic. Solid lumps should undergo biopsy (see section X, chapter 28). However, the vast majority of patients seen in breast clinics will present with mastalgia and nodularity without a dominant lump or with diffusely nodular breasts that are painless. This latter group requires no active treatment and may be followed with interval physical examinations and mammography. For patients with mastalgia, regardless of the variant, the best overall management is reassurance that the pain is expectant and physiological.[84] The physician should allay the cancerophobic concerns of most of these patients following examination and review of mammographic findings. Billroth emphasized the importance of

"friendly advice and assurance and the banishment of suspicion of the dread disease."[45] Reassurance does not provide resolution of the patient's breast pain; however, professional advice from a concerned physician who offers a thorough, clear explanation of breast physiology will abrogate the perception of mastalgia and nodularity as serious problems. It has been demonstrated that approximately 85 percent of patients with mastalgia can be successfully treated with reassurance alone.[16, 45]

In a small percentage of patients, mastalgia interferes considerably with daily activity.[79] The pain, and its psychological and emotional impact, may be severe enough to initiate marital discord. In such patients, a variety of available psychiatric and medical therapies may be useful.[64] Medical management is reviewed in the following sections.

Hormonal Therapy

Progesterone. Conceptually, the use of progesterone in the treatment of cyclic mastalgia is based on the physiological and bioassay analyses that confirm a deficiency of circulating progesterone relative to estrogen during the luteal phase of ovarian secretion.[61] Several studies have demonstrated a significant improvement in breast pain and nodularity with intramuscular and oral progesterone derivatives.[19, 22] Other studies have not shown a benefit.[52] Animal studies that have examined the use of progestin on the development of premalignant breast lesions are controversial.[65]

Bromocriptine. Bromocriptine (Parlodel) is a prolactin antagonist that may enhance luteal function in patients with luteal insufficiency and hyperprolactinemia. Several double-blind studies have demonstrated a significant improvement in breast pain, tenderness, and nodularity with bromocriptine therapy.[2, 17, 24, 97] These encouraging results were confirmed in the Cardiff Mastalgia Clinic in a prospective, controlled, double-blind trial conducted for 53 patients using a bromocriptine dosage of 2.5 mg twice a day.[45] The results of this trial showed that breast pain in women with cyclical mastalgia was significantly reduced by the prolactin antagonist compared to placebo, whereas those with the noncyclical pattern of pain failed to respond. Blood sampling during the study confirmed the reduction of serum prolactin levels in patients taking bromocriptine. It is not currently understood how the lowering of prolactin levels improves mastalgia symptoms, but the mechanism is presumed to be a decreased hormone-related stimulation of breast stroma and parenchyma by prolactin. These results have been corroborated in other control trials,[17, 58] and it is evident that this drug is consistently effective in reducing breast pain. The potential side effects with use of bromocriptine are nausea, vomiting, and dizziness. Additionally, the drug is expensive.

Tamoxifen. Tamoxifen (Nolvadex), an estrogen analog and antagonist, may also alleviate mastalgia. In one study, more than two thirds of women with severe breast pain who were treated with tamoxifen had a complete remission of symptoms as well as disappearance of nodularity as assessed by physical examination and ultrasonography.[87] The side effects associated with tamoxifen therapy are minimal, but the drug is expensive.

Danocrine. Danocrine (Danazol) is a synthetic derivative of testosterone that has been shown to be effective in treating patients with severe mastalgia.[32, 92] Danocrine may have significant side effects because of its mild androgenic properties and its direct effects on hypothalamic-pituitary function. Side effects include menstrual irregularities, growth of facial hair, voice changes, water retention, and gastrointestinal complaints.

Danocrine, like bromocriptine, is unique on its action on the pituitary-ovarian axis.[59] A double-blind placebo study at the Cardiff Mastalgia Clinic confirmed that danocrine given to women with cyclic mastalgia provided symptomatic relief and reduction of nodularity with doses as low as 200 mg per day.[45] This low dose was associated with an acceptable rate of side effects, and only a ten percent noncompliance rate was recorded in the trial. The notable side effect of amenorrhea was observed in all patients treated at doses of 600 to 800 mg per day. Side effects such as weight gain, acne, and hirsuitism may also develop. Currently, danocrine appears to be an excellent drug for the treatment of breast pain and nodularity, with an overall improvement rate of approximately 70 per cent.

Thyroid Hormones. It has been suggested that there may be a relationship between hypothyroidism and benign breast disorders. Several studies have demonstrated improvement of pain and nodularity in patients with clinical hypothyroidism who were treated with thyroxine.[56] A study of Peters and associates[85] demonstrated that an 8-week course of thyroxine diminished thyrotrophin-releasing hormone (TRH)–induced hyperprolactinemia. Thyroid hormone supplementation did not affect luteal function, but mastalgia was significantly improved in the treatment group.

Evening Primrose Oil. A recent hypothesis proposes that mastalgia occurs as an abnormality of prostaglandin synthesis secondary to inadequate essential fatty acid (EFA) intake in the diet. This hypothesis has led to treatment of mastalgia by supplementing the diet with EFAs. One potential therapy includes the oil of the evening primrose flower, which is unique in that it contains seven percent linolenic acid and 72 percent linoleic acid. The oil of this flower represents the richest source of essential fatty acids known. A recent trial has suggested that this compound may be useful in treating mild cases of cystic mastalgia.[81] This agent is ingested orally and is potentially useful in mild-to-moderate cases of mastalgia, as it has no known side effects. Patient compliance is generally good, since evening primrose oil is viewed as a "naturally occurring substance" rather than a drug.

Methylxanthine Restriction. The relationship between methylxanthine intake and "fibrocystic disease" was first reported in 1979.[62] Although several studies suggest that abstinence from caffeine may aid in resolution of mastalgia and nodularity symptoms, the design of these studies has been subject to criticism. The randomized, controlled study by Parazzini et al.[80] demonstrated no relationship between caffeine intake and fibrocystic disease when patients were evaluated by physical examination, symptoms, and thermography. Thus the data demonstrating an association between methylxanthine consumption and benign breast disease have not been substantiated.

Vitamin E. There is also controversy in the literature regarding the efficacy of alpha-tocopherol (vitamin E) supplementation and benign breast disease. Two randomized, double-blind, controlled trials from separate investigators demonstrated no significant difference between vitamin E and placebo in resolution of the symptoms of benign breast disease when evaluated radiographically and clinically.[27, 54]

Diuretics. The use of diuretics in the management of benign breast diseases is based on the premise that cyclic mastalgia and nodularity may be related to fluid and salt retention and subsequent breast engorgement. The only study that has examined this hypothesis confirmed no statistical changes in total body water in the premenstrual period following the usage of diuretics.[86a]

Other Therapies. Several other management strategies have been proposed for the treatment of benign breast disease, but the majority of such therapies are based on anecdotal reports. These treatments include the use of a well-fitted brassiere providing ample support, injection of steroids into painful breasts, and deletion of ginseng tea from the diet. Expectantly, variable response rates with usage of these regimens are recorded for symptomatic benign disease.

FIBROADENOMA AND RELATED TUMORS

There are three tumors of the breast that have conspicuous stromal elements: fibroadenoma, benign phyllodes tumors, and phyllodes sarcomas.[44] Phyllodes tumors are benign, whereas phyllodes sarcoma is malignant. Differentiation of these entities is made on the degree of cytologic aberration. Both tumors are composed of variable combinations of stromal and epithelial elements. Pure sarcoma of the breast is a tumor solely of connective (mesenchymal) tissue origin that behaves clinically and biologically in a more malignant fashion than phyllodes sarcoma (see section IV, chapter 10). The group of tumors with stroma of markedly increased cellularity and atypia, but without malignant features, is termed "phyllodes tumor" (see chapter 10).

Fibroadenomas

Fibroadenomas are discrete, benign tumors of the breast showing evidence of connective tissue, and epithelial proliferation.[44] The typical fibroadenoma is easy to recognize and manage; atypical variants of fibroadenomas that exhibit rapid growth and hypercellularity may create substantial clinical and pathological confusion. The key to the classification of fibroadenomas is the fibrous stromal element; any epithelial variant should be treated secondarily. Thus the term "fibroadenoma" is used for any tumor in which the fibrous stroma is of low cellularity without cytologic atypia.

Clinical Features

Fibroadenomas generally appear in young women and present as rubbery, firm, discrete, mobile masses. When left untreated, these tumors will gradually increase in size to 2 to 3 cm; this growth process may take as long as 5 years. During the growth phase, the tumor doubles in size in 6 to 12 months and then stabilizes or even decreases in size. The infrequency of fibroadenomas after menopause suggests the hormonal dependency of the lesion; they may regress in the postmenopausal woman.

Fibroadenomas can be classified into four main categories: (1) the small fibroadenoma (3 to 4 mm), which is palpable in the superficial breast; (2) the most common variant, which reaches a diameter of 1 to 3 cm (80 percent of fibroadenomas); (3) intermediate fibroadenomas (4 to 5 cm); and (4) giant fibroadenomas of adolescence and the perimenopausal age groups.

Approximately 55 per cent of fibroadenomas are found in the left breast.[44] They are most commonly located in the upper outer quadrant. The tumors probably develop from the breast lobule. Although the cause of fibroadenomas is unclear, they may develop as a result of lobular stimulation by estrogen. Macroscopically, these tumors are characterized by a marginated surface that is somewhat irregular, white, glistening, and bulging. This appearance differs from that of phyllodes tumors, which characteristically have a brown surface. In young women, the diagnosis can be made with confidence, as the fibroadenoma is generally smooth, round (sometimes lobulated), firm, and discrete. These fibroadenomas are very mobile. The incidence of multiple fibroadenomas in the breast has been reported to be 10 to 20 percent, and these lesions may be synchronous or metachronous.[28]

Although some physicians recommend removal of all fibroadenomas, it is our policy to adapt a flexible approach, particularly in those patients younger than 25 years. In these women, the incidence of cancer is rare enough that the typical fibroadenoma can be observed through several menstrual cycles. The use of fine needle aspiration (FNA) can help make the diagnosis of fibroadenoma certain. Some of these tumors will regress, but most remain stable. Should the lesion increase in size, excision is advised.

Giant Fibroadenoma

Giant fibroadenomas are rare and biphasic in occurrence: peak incidence is in the 15- to 20-year age group and the 50- to 60-year age group. The lesions are designated as "giant" primarily on the basis of their clinical size. Sudden, rapid growth is a prominent feature of adolescent giant fibroadenomas. The giant fibroadenoma of adolescence is more than 5 cm in diameter and usually presents in patients between the ages of 11 and 20 years. Onset at or soon after puberty, short doubling time, prominent veins overlying the tumor, and occasional skin ulceration resulting from pressure are common features. From a pathological standpoint, a wide spectrum of changes in both epithelial and connective tissue elements may be found in these tumors, but it is important to emphasize that significant cellular atypia is not a feature.

From a practical perspective, giant fibroadenomas of adolescence are benign lesions. They can therefore be excised by enucleation and with minimal risk of local recurrence. These lesions may best be approached by a submammary incision, since they tend to be deep in the breast parenchyma. Simple mastectomy is *not* recommended. Flap rotations and prosthesis are also inappropriate. The breast remnant generally returns to a normal configuration and contour following removal of the fibroadenoma, a process that would be inhibited by an implant.

Phyllodes Tumors

Phyllodes tumors are usually large, benign tumors of epithelial and mesenchymal origin that occur primarily in the perimenopausal era. However, the tumors may be small and may be observed in any age group. Phyllodes tumors have a fairly dramatic clinical presentation and an aggressive histological pattern, although they usually exhibit benign clinical behavior.[44] This tumor is neither cystic nor sarcomatous, and thus the designation "cystosarcoma phyllodes" should be abandoned in favor of the term "phyllodes tumor" or, in the case of malignant transformation, "phyllodes sarcoma" (see section IV, chapter 10).

Although phyllodes tumors are microscopically and macroscopically distinct from giant fibroadenomas, it is important to emphasize that the diagnosis is a histopathological one. The pathologist should decide, based on histological findings, whether the term "sarcoma" is justified. To diagnose the malignant counterpart, both epithelial and fibrous stromal elements must be present, with the stroma demonstrating marked pleomorphism, hypercellularity, irregularity, and significant numbers of mitotic figures.[44] Although giant fibroadenomas and phyllodes tumors can behave similarly, there are certain clinical features that help distinguish these entities. The giant phyllodes tumor is macroscopically brown, irregular, and cellular. The peripheral configuration of the gross tumor resembles a leaflike mass, thus the designation phyllodes (Greek: *phyllon*, leaf, and *eidos*, form). These tumors often exhibit central necrosis and hemorrhage. The giant fibroadenoma, on the other hand, is macroscopically uniform with a whitish, fibrous appearance. Microscopically, the giant fibroadenoma shows hypocellular stroma, whereas the phyllodes tumor shows hypercellular stroma with pleomorphism.

The majority of phyllodes tumors occur in women between the ages of 35 and 55 years. They are far less common than fibroadenomas (occurring approximately 1/40 as frequently). Bilateral tumors are rare. Most lesions grow rapidly and become massive before the patient presents to the physician. Unlike large carcinomas, these tumors are characteristically noninvasive. Even though the lesion may virtually occupy the entire breast and produce evidence of skin ulceration, phyllodes tumors are almost invariably mobile on the chest wall. The axillary lymph nodes are infrequently involved with metastases; phyllodes sarcoma has approximately a ten percent incidence of positive lymph nodes.

On sectioning, phyllodes tumors are well demarcated by may invade the pseudocapsule. This histological finding explains the tendency for local recurrence following simple enucleation. The brown color of the phyllodes tumor is characteristic and may alert the pathologist and surgeon to the diagnosis. Although these tumors have a tendency to recur locally, distant metastases are uncommon. Hence phyllodes tumors (excluding phyllodes sarcomas) have an excellent prognosis. The principal determinants of prognosis for the malignant variant are the size and number of mitoses per high-powered field.

Proper management of these lesions is not entirely clear, but wide local excision is probably the best treatment of benign phyllodes tumors. Haagensen[34] noted a recurrence rate of 28 percent in patients treated by local excision. If the lesion is large and replaces most of the breast tissue, a simple mastectomy is recommended. For small lesions, an excisional biopsy that includes a rim of normal breast tissue is usually adequate therapy. If the diagnosis is established histologically by fine needle aspiration or needle core biopsy prior to definitive therapy, wide local excision of the scar with normal adjacent surrounding tissue is the procedure of choice.

In summary, phyllodes tumors are uncommon breast masses. They are generally large and are usually benign. Clinically, these lesions cannot be distinguished from the giant fibroadenoma and must be differentiated histologically to formulate a treatment plan. Distinction of the two phyllodes tumors is essential to the planning of appropriate therapy and to providing prognostic information.

CASE EXAMPLES OF BENIGN BREAST DISEASE

For the practicing general surgeon who operates on patients with diseases of the breast, the following case examples may be useful in illustrating the management of benign disorders of the breast.

CASE 1. A 38-year-old woman presents to her physician with a lump in the superior aspect of the right breast. She has no family history of breast cancer, no history of previous breast disease, and has had no previous mammogram. Physical examination demonstrates diffuse nodularity of both breasts with a 1-cm dominant mass in the upper outer quadrant of the right breast. The axillae and supraclavicular fossae are without palpable adenopathy. An initial bilateral xeromammogram reveals a normal parenchymal pattern without microcalcifications. Aspiration of the lump is performed in the office and returns 10 ml of greenish-brown fluid. The fluid is discarded, and the lump is noted to disappear. The patient is scheduled to return to the office for a follow-up visit in 6 weeks.

Clinical Impression: Diffuse bilateral nodularity
Gross cyst of the right breast, upper outer quadrant

Comment: The diagnosis should be made clinically based on the classification system outlined in Table 34–1. The term "fibrocystic disease" should be avoided. If the cyst is again palpable in 6 weeks, the area should undergo biopsy. If the cyst does not recur, the patient can be seen again in 1 year, at which time the mammogram is repeated.

CASE 2. A 47-year-old female is noted to have an area of clustered microcalcifications with irregular nodules in the upper outer quadrant of the left breast on routine follow-up (annual) mammography. These calcifications were not present on mammogram 1 year earlier. Physical examination of the breasts reveals minimal nodularity without a dominant lump or axillary adenopathy. The surgeon elects to perform needle localization biopsy of this area. Microscopically, the lesion demonstrates proliferation of both the stroma and epithelium of several terminal duct-lobular units. Diffuse microcalcifications are present, and a histological diagnosis of sclerosing adenosis is confirmed.

Comment: Diffuse microcalcifications are commonly seen in sclerosing adenosis. It has no proven premalignant implications. The importance of sclerosing adenosis for the surgeon is its macroscopic and microscopic resemblance to carcinoma. The patient described should be taught breast self-examination and scheduled to return for a follow-up office visit with mammography in 6 to 12 months (see chapter 53).

CASE 3. A 50-year-old woman is referred with a 2 × 2–cm mass in the upper inner quadrant of the left breast. The lesion is discrete on mammography, and there are no microcalcifications present. Physical examination confirms the presence of the mass. The remainder of the breast and peripheral lymphatic examination is normal. The lesion is excised under local anesthesia. Microscopic examination reveals cystic lesions and apocrine metaplasia with moderate and florid hyperplasia of the usual ("ductal") type.

Comment: Moderate and florid hyperplasia of the usual type are present in more than one fifth of breast biopsies. These pathological entities are characterized by an increase in cell number within the ducts. In florid hyperplasia, the proliferating ductal cells fill at least 70 percent of the lumen of the duct, which may lead to distention of the involved spaces. The combined histological and pattern features of atypical hyperplasia and carcinoma *in situ* are absent. Moderate and florid epithelial hyperplasia are classified as proliferative disorders without atypia (PDWA) and are associated with as much as a 1.5 to twofold risk for developing invasive carcinoma in the future. The patient discussed in this case should continue breast self-examination with a repeat mammogram and clinical examination in 6 months.

CASE 4. A 44-year-old woman is referred to a surgeon following a breast biopsy in which the specimen was diagnosed by an outside pathologist as lobular carcinoma *in situ* (LCIS). On examination, the biopsy incision is well healed, and the breast and lymphatic examinations are within normal limits. The patient has an older sister who was diagnosed with breast cancer 3 years earlier. Review of the slides by the pathologist reveals atypical, round, uniform cells that fill less than one half of the involved lobules. There is no lobular distortion. The official pathology report reads: "lobular neoplasia most consistent with atypical lobular hyperplasia."

Comment: The uniformity, roundness, and lack of lobular distortion is key to the diagnosis of atypical lobular hyperplasia (ALH). Adoption of the degree of filling and distortion of the lobular acini as a determinant criterion to distinguish ALH from LCIS in biopsy specimens has revealed a relative risk of subsequent invasive carcinoma development for ALH that is four times that of the general population. Women with a family history of cancer in a first degree relative as well as ALH at biopsy have a risk of developing invasive carcinoma that is twice that of women who have ALH alone. Thus the patient discussed in this case example has an absolute risk of approximately 15 percent to 20 percent of developing an invasive breast cancer during the next 20 years. She should be followed closely by a physician for the remainder of her life with regularly scheduled office visits and mammography. Breast self-examination is essential to early detection, and its importance must be emphasized to the patient.

SUMMARY

The proper approach to the management of benign breast diseases requires the clinician to be familiar with the clinical and pathological classifications discussed in this chapter. The term "fibrocystic disease" should be excluded when these disorders are being discussed by the pathologist and the clinician. Appropriate treatment strategies can thereafter be most effectively implemented when relative risk of the pathological variants is thoroughly established.

References

1. Ahmed A: Apocrine metaplasia in cystic hyperplastic mastopathy. Histochemical and ultrastructural observations. J Pathol 115:211–214, 1975.
2. Andersen AN, Larsen JF, Steenstrup OR, Svendstrup B, Nielsen J: Effect of bromocriptine on the premenstrual syndrome. A double-blind clinical trial. Br J Obstet Gynaecol 84:370–374, 1977.
3. Andersen JA, Gram JB: Radial scar in the female breast: a long term follow-up study of 32 cases. Cancer 53:2557–2560, 1984.
4. Anderson JA, Battersby S: Radial scars of benign and malignant breast: comparative features and significance. J Pathol 147:23–32, 1985.
5. Arrigoni MG, Dockerty MB, Judd ES: The identification and treatment of mammary hamartoma. Surg Gynecol Obstet 133:577–582, 1971.
6. Ashikari R, Huvos AG, Synder RE, Lucas JC, Hutter RVP, McDivitt RW, Schottenfeld D: A clinicopathological study of atypical lesions of the breast. Cancer 33:310–317, 1974.
7. Atkins HJB: Treatment of chronic mastitis. Lancet 1:707–712, 1938.
8. Azzopardi JG: Problems in Breast Pathology. Philadelphia, WB Saunders, 1979, pp 213–223.
9. Azzopardi JG: Benign and malignant proliferative epithelial lesions of the breast: A review. Eur J Cancer Clin Oncol 19:1717–1720, 1983.
10. Azzopardi JG: Problems in Breast Pathology. Philadelphia, WB Saunders, 1979, pp 29–56.
11. Azzopardi JG: Problems in Breast Pathology. Philadelphia, WB Saunders, 1979, pp 59–71.
12. Barnes WC: Management of cystic disease of the breast. Am J Surg 129:324–325, 1975.
13. Bischoff VJ, Wenderlein JM: Die bedeutung der mastalgie in der mammadiagnostik. Fortschr Geb Rontgenstr 130:706–710, 1979.
14. Black MM, Barclay THC, Cutler SJ, Hankey BF, Asire AJ: Association of atypical characteristics of benign breast lesions with subsequent risk of breast cancer. Cancer 29:338–343, 1972.
15. Bland KI, Copeland EM: Breast disease: physiologic considerations in normal benign and malignant states. *In* Miller T, Rowlands B (eds): The Physiologic Basis of Modern Surgical Care. St Louis, CV Mosby, 1988, pp 1019–1056.
16. Blichert-Toft M, Watt-Boolsen S: Clinical approach to women with severe mastalgia and the therapeutic possibilities. Acta Obstet Gynecol Scand 123(suppl):185–188, 1984.
17. Blichert-Toft M, Anderson AN, Henriksen OB, Mygind T: Treatment of mastalgia with bromocriptine: a double-blind crossover study. Br Med J 1:237–238, 1979.
18. Carter D: Intraductal papillary tumors of the breast: a study of 78 cases. Cancer 39:1689–1692, 1977.
19. Colin C, Gasparou, Lambotte R: Relationship of mastodynia with its endocrine environment and treatment in a double blind trial with lynestrenol. Arch Gynakol 225(I):7–13, 1978.
20. Consensus Meeting: Is "fibrocystic disease" of the breast precancerous? Arch Pathol Lab Med 110:171–173, 1986.
21. Crile G, Chatty EM: Squamous metaplasia of lactiferous ducts. Arch Surg 102:533–534, 1971.
22. Dennerstein L, Spencer-Gardiner C, Gotts G, Brown JB, Smith MA, Burrows GD: Progesterone and the premenstrual syndrome; a double blind crossover trial. Br Med J 290:1617–1621, 1985.
23. Doberl A, Tobiassen T, Rasmussen T: Treatment of recurrent cyclical mastodynia in patients with fibrocystic disease. Acta Obstet Gynecol Scand 123(suppl):177–184, 1984.
24. Dogliotti L, Mussa A, Sandrucci S: Prolactin and benign breast disease with special emphasis on bromocriptine therapy. *In* Angeli A, et al (eds): Endocrinology of Cystic Breast Disease. New York, Raven Press, 1983.
25. Donnelly PK, Baker KW, Carney JA, O'Fallon WM: Benign breast lesions and subsequent breast carcinoma in Rochester, Minnesota, Mayo Clinic Proc 50:650–656, 1975.
26. Dupont WD, Page DL: Risk factors for breast cancer in women with proliferative breast disease. N Engl J Med 312:146–151, 1985.
27. Ernster VL, Goodson WH, Hunt TK, Petroakis NL, Sickles EA, Miike R: Vitamin E and benign breast "disease": a double-blind, randomized clinical trial. Surgery 97:490–494, 1985.
28. Fechner RE: Fibroadenoma and related lesions. *In* Page DL, Anderson TJ (eds): Diagnostic Histopathology of the Breast. New York, Churchill Livingstone, 1987.
29. Fondo EY, Rosen PP, Fracchia AA, Urban JA: The problem of carcinoma developing in a fibroadenoma. Recent experience at Memorial Hospital. Cancer 43:563–567, 1979.
30. Frantz VK, Pickren JW, Melcher GW, Auchincloss H: Incidence of chronic cystic disease in so-called "normal breasts," a study based on 225 postmortem examinations. Cancer 4:762–783, 1951.
31. Goodman ZD, Taxy JB: Fibroadenomas of the breast with prominent smooth muscle. Am J Surg Pathol 5:99–101, 1981.
32. Greenblatt RB, Nazhat C, Ben-Nun I: The treatment of benign breast disease with danazol. Fertil Steril 34:242–245, 1980.
33. Haagensen CD: Diseases of the Breast. Philadelphia, WB Saunders, 1971.
34. Haagensen CD: Diseases of the Breast, ed. 3. Philadelphia, WB Saunders, 1986.
35. Haagensen CD, Lane N, Lattes R, Bodian C: Lobular neoplasia (so-called lobular carcinoma in situ) of the breast. Cancer 42:737–769, 1978.
36. Haagensen CD: Mammary-duct ectasia: a disease that may stimulate carcinoma. Cancer 4:749–761, 1951.
37. Harrington E, Lesnick G: The association between gross cysts of the breast and breast cancer. Breast 7:13–19, 1981.
38. Hendrick JW: Results of treatment of cystic disease of the breast. Surgery 44:457–482, 1958.
39. Herrman JB: Mammary cancer subsequent to aspiration of cysts in the breast. Ann Surg 173:40–43, 1971.
40. Hughes LE, Mansel RE, Webster DJT: Problems of concept and nomenclature of benign disorder of the breast. *In* Benign Disorders and Diseases of the Breast. Concepts and Clinical Management. London, Bailliere Tindall, 1989, pp 1–4.
41. Hughes LE, Mansel RE, Webster DJT: Breast anatomy and physiology. *In* Benign Disorders and Diseases of the Breast. Concepts and Clinical Management. London, Bailliere Tindall, 1989, pp 5–13.
42. Hughes LE, Mansel RE, Webster DJT: Aberrations of normal

development and involution (ANDI): a concept of benign breast disorders based on pathogenesis. *In* Benign Disorders and Diseases of the Breast. Concepts and Clinical Management. London, Bailliere Tindall, 1989, pp 15–26.

43. Hughes LE, Mansel RE, Webster DJT: The approach to assessment and management of breast lumps. *In* Benign Disorders and Diseases of the Breast. Concepts and Clinical Management. London, Bailliere Tindall, 1989, pp 41–48.

44. Hughes LE, Mansel RE, Webster DJT: Fibroadenoma and related tumors. *In* Benign Disorders and Diseases of the Breast. Concepts and Clinical Management. London, Bailliere Tindall, 1989, pp 59–74.

45. Hughes LE, Mansel RE, Webster DJT: Breast pain and nodularity. *In* Benign Disorders and Diseases of the Breast. Concepts and Clinical Management. London, Bailliere Tindall, 1989, pp 75–92.

46. Hughes LE, Mansel RE, Webster DJT: Cysts of the breast. *In* Benign Disorders and Diseases of the Breast. Concepts and Clinical Management. London, Bailliere Tindall, 1989, pp 93–102.

47. Hughes LE, Mansel RE, Webster DJT: Sclerosing adenosis. *In* Benign Disorders and Diseases of the Breast. Concepts and Clinical Management. London, Baillere Tindall, 1989, pp 103–106.

48. Hughes LE, Mansel RE, Webster DJT: Nipple discharge. *In* Benign Disorders and Diseases of the Breast. Concepts and Clinical Management. London, Bailliere Tindall, 1989, pp 133–142.

49. Hughes LE, Mansel RE, Webster DJT: Operations. *In* Benign Disorders and Diseases of the Breast. Concepts and Clinical Management. London, Bailliere Tindall, 1989, pp 187–206.

50. Hutchinson WB, Thomas DB, Hamlin WB, Roth GJ, Peterson AV, Williams B: Risk of breast cancer in women with benign breast disease. J Natl Cancer Inst 65:13–20, 1980.

51. Kodlin D, Winger EE, Morgenstern NL, Chen U: Chronic cystic mastopathy and breast cancer: a follow-up study. Cancer 39:2603–2607, 1977.

52. Lafaye C, Aubert B: Action de la progesterone locale dans les mastopathies benignes. J Gynecol Obstet Biol Reprod 7:1123–1139, 1978a.

53. Linell F, Ljungberg O, Andersson I: Breast carcinoma. Aspects of early stages, progression and related problems. Acta Pathol Microbiol Scand (A) 272(suppl):1–233, 1980.

54. London RS, Sundaram GS, Murphy L, Manimekalai S, Reynolds M, Goldstein PJ: The effect of vitamin E on mammary dysplasia: a double-blind study. Obstet Gynecol 65:104–106, 1985.

55. Love SM, Gelman RS, Silen WS: Fibrocystic "disease" of the breast: a non-disease. N Engl J Med 307:1010–1014, 1982.

56. Love SM, Schmitt SJ, Connolly JL, Shirley RL: Benign Breast Disorders. Philadelphia, J. B. Lippincott Company, 1987, pp. 15–53.

57. MacErlean DP, Nathan BE: Calcification in sclerosing adenosis simulating malignant breast calcification. Br J Radiol 45:944–945, 1972.

58. Mansel RE, Preece PE, Hughes LE: A double blind trial of the prolactin inhibitor bromocriptine in painful benign breast disease. Br J Surg 65:724–727, 1978.

59. Mansel RE, Hughes LE: The clinical and hormonal effects of treating mastalgia with danazol. *In* Angeli A, et al (eds): Endocrinology of Cystic Breast Disease. New York, Raven Press, 1983.

60. Marzetti L, Framarino dei Malatesta ML, Aaragona C: Prolactin and benign breast diseases. *In* Angeli A, et al (eds): Endocrinology of Cystic Breast Disease. New York, Raven Press, 1983.

61. Mauvais-Jarvis P, Sterkers N, Kuttenn F, Beauvais J: Traitement des mastopathies benignes par la progesterone, et les progestatifs. J Gynecol Obstet Biol Reprod 7:477–484, 1978.

62. Minton JP, Foecking MK, Webster DJT, Matthews RH: Caffeine, cyclic nucleotides and breast disease. Surgery 86:105–109, 1979.

63. Moross T, Land AP, Mahoney L: Tubular adenoma of breast. Arch Pathol Lab Med 107:84–86, 1983.

64. Murley RS: Treatment of benign breast disease. Ann Coll Surg Engl 58:385–387, 1976.

65. Nagasawa H, Fujii M, Hagiwara K: Inhibition by medroxyprogesterone acetate of precancerous mammary hyperplastic alveolar nodule formation in mice. Breast Cancer Res Treat 5:31–36, 1985.

66. Ozzello L, Gump FE: The management of patients with carcinomas in fibroadenomatous tumors of the breast. Surg Gynecol Obstet 160:99–104, 1985.

67. Page DL, Vanderzwaag R, Rogers LW, Williams LT, Walker WE, Hartmann WH: Relation between the component parts of fibrocystic disease complex and breast cancer. J Natl Cancer Inst 61:1055–1063, 1978.

68. Page DL: Cancer risk assessment in benign biopsies. Hum Pathol 17:871–874, 1986.

69. Page DL, Dupont WD, Rogers LW, Rados MS: Atypical hyperplastic lesions of the female breast. A long-term follow-up study. Cancer 55:2698–2708, 1985.

70. Page DL, Dupont WD, Rogers LW: Breast cancer risk of lobular-based hyperplasia after biopsy: "ductal" pattern lesions. Cancer Detect Prevent 9:441–448, 1986.

71. Page DL, Dupont WD, Rogers LW: Ductal involvement by cells of atypical lobular hyperplasia in the breast. Hum Pathol 19:201–207, 1988.

72. Page DL, Anderson TJ: Cysts and apocrine change. *In* Diagnostic Histopathology of the Breast. New York, Churchill Livingstone, 1987.

73. Page DL, Anderson TJ: Adenosis. *In* Diagnostic Histopathology of the Breast. New York, Churchill Livingstone, 1987.

74. Page DL, Anderson TJ: Miscellaneous non-neoplastic conditions. *In* Diagnostic Histopathology of the Breast. New York, Churchill Livingstone, 1987.

75. Page DL, Anderson TJ: Radial scars and complex sclerosing lesions. *In* Diagnostic Histopathology of the Breast. New York, Churchill Livingstone, 1987.

76. Page DL, Anderson TJ: Papilloma and related lesions. *In* Diagnostic Histopathology of the Breast. New York, Churchill Livingstone, 1987.

77. Page DL, Vander Zwaag R, Rogers LW, Williams LT, Walker WE, Hartmann WH: Relation between component parts of fibrocystic disease complex and breast cancer. J Natl Cancer Inst 61:1055–1063, 1978.

78. Page DL, Dupont WD: Are breast cysts a premalignant marker? Eur J Cancer Clin Oncol 22:635–636, 1986.

79. Page DL, Mansel RE, Hughes SE: Clinical experience of drug treatments for mastalgia. Lancet 2:373–377, 1985.

80. Parazzini F, La Vecchia C, Riundi R, Pampallona S, Regallo M, Scanni A: Methylxanthine, alcohol-free diet and fibrocystic breast disease. A factorial clinical trial. Surgery 99:576–581, 1986.

81. Pashby NL, Mansel RE, Hughes LE, Hanslip J, Preece PE: A clinical trial of evening primrose oil in mastalgia. Br J Surg 68:801–805, 1981.

82. Patey DH: Two common non-malignant conditions of the breast. Br Med J 1:96–99, 1949.

83. Patey DH, Nurck AW: Natural history of cystic disease of breast treated conservatively. Br Med J 1:15–17, 1953.

84. Peacock EE: Biological basis for management of benign disease of the breast. Plast Reconstr Surg 55:14–20, 1975.

85. Peters F, Pickardt CR, Zimmerman G, Breckwoldt M: PRL, TSH and thyroid hormones in benign breast disease. Klin Wochenschr 59:403–407, 1981.

85a. Preece PE, Baum M, Mansel RE, Webster DJT, Fortt RW, Gravelle IH, Hughes LE: The importance of mastalgia in operable breast cancer. Br Med J 284:1299–1300, 1982.

86. Preece PE, Hughes LE, Mansel RE, Baum M, Bolton PM, Gravelle IH: Clinical syndromes of mastalgia. Lancet 2:670–673, 1976.

86a. Preece PE, Richards AR, Owen GM, Hughes LE: Mastalgia and total body water. Br Med J 4:498–500, 1975.

87. Ricciardi I, Ianniruberto A: Tamoxifen-induced regression of benign breast lesions. Obstet Gynecol 54:80–84, 1979.

87a. River L, Silverstein J, Grout J, Nicholar E, Schairer A, Carlson B, Tanoue R, Tope J: Carcinoma of the breast: the diagnostic significance of pain. Am J Surg 82:733–735, 1951.

88. Rosen PP, Kosloff C, Adair F, Lieberman PH, Braum DW: Lobular carcinoma in situ of the breast: detailed analysis of 99 patients with average follow-up of 24 years. Am J Surg Pathol 2:225–251, 1978.

89. Sitruk-Ware R, Sterkers N, Mauvais-Jarvis P: Benign breast disease I: hormonal investigation. Obstet Gynecol 53:457–560, 1979.

89a. Smallwood JA, Kye DA, Taylor I: Mastalgia: is this commonly associated with operable breast cancer? Ann R Coll Surg 68:262–263, 1986.

90. Spalding JE: Adenolipoma and lipoma of the breast. Guy's Hosp Rep 94:80–84, 1945.

91. Takeda T, Suzuki M, Sato Y, Hase T: Cytologic studies of nipple discharges. Acta Cytol 26:35–36, 1982.

92. Tobiassen T, Rasmussen T, Doberl A, Rannevik G: Danazol treatment of severely symptomatic fibrocystic breast disease and long-term follow-up—the Hjorring project. Acta Obstet Gynecol Scand 123(suppl):159–176, 1984.

93. Veronesi U, Pizzocaro G: Breast cancer in women subsequent to cystic disease of the breast. Surg Gynecol Obstet 126:529–532, 1968.

94. Vorherr H: Fibrocystic breast disease: pathophysiology, pathomorphology, clinical picture and management. Am J Obstet Gynecol 154:161–179, 1986.

95. Wang DY, Fentiman IS: Epidemiology and endocrinology of benign breast disease. Breast Cancer Res Treat 6:5–36, 1985.

96. Wellings SR, Jensen HM, Marcum RG: An atlas of subgross pathology of the human breast with special reference to possible precancerous lesions. J Natl Cancer Inst 55:231–273, 1975.

97. Ylostalo P: Cycle of continuous treatment of the premenstrual syndrome (PMS) with bromocriptine. Eur J Obstet Gynecol Reprod Biol 17:337–343, 1984.

Section XIII

Current Concepts and Management of Early Breast Carcinoma

CURRENT CONCEPTS FOR MANAGEMENT OF EARLY (*IN SITU* AND OCCULT INVASIVE) BREAST CARCINOMA

Eric R. Frykberg, M.D., Frederick C. Ames, M.D., and Kirby I. Bland, M.D.

The prognosis of a patient with breast carcinoma depends to a significant extent on the stage of disease at the time of diagnosis,[41, 51, 94, 122, 231] a principle that has led to a major emphasis on early detection. Mammographic screening has been the most effective modality allowing this goal to be achieved.[59, 131, 176, 201, 204, 216] Evidence accumulated during the past century has demonstrated some relation between tumor size, axillary lymph node involvement, and curability of breast carcinoma, thus leading many to equate small size with an "early" stage of disease that is associated with improved survival.[44, 51, 178] This is consistent with the standard concept of earlier years that breast cancer develops in an orderly and progressive pattern from normal cells through phases of epithelial hyperplasia, cellular atypia, intraepithelial carcinoma, and finally invasive carcinoma.[79, 171] This "transition theory" of disease evolution also holds that invasive malignancy begins as a localized lesion and progressively spreads first to regional axillary lymph nodes and finally to distant metastatic sites by way of the lymphatics and blood stream.[86, 87, 92] The rationale behind the radical mastectomy, as developed by Halsted and Meyer in the late nineteenth century, derived largely from this principle.[103, 140] The significant reduction in local recurrence and mortality rates from breast cancer resulting from this procedure lent considerable support to the validity of the transition theory.

This concept of orderly transition in the evolution of breast carcinoma has been shown to be somewhat simplistic as more knowledge of tumor biology and the natural history of this disease has become available. A substantial percentage of small, nonpalpable breast tumors manifest evidence of systemic spread in the form of regional lymph node involvement.[1, 95, 219] Patients with such small malignancies have a lower survival rate following treatment than would be expected from purely localized disease, supporting the current consensus that carcinoma of the breast may be a systemic disease from its origin.[3, 107, 231] This has led to a shift in therapeutic direction away from local treatment and toward systemic treatment, although definite survival benefits have nevertheless continued to be demonstrated for early detection and treatment.

The potential for improved survival from early breast cancer detection has been appreciated for hundreds of years. Henry Fearon, a British surgeon of the eighteenth century, claimed that "The early period of the complaint is beyond all doubt the most favorable period for extirpating it."[50] Cheatle showed remarkable insight into this issue with the following assertion in 1906:

"A small cancer need not necessarily be an early one; and if one considers upon what the clinical signs of cancer of the breast depend, one must at once realize that the definite and classical clinical signs—even the earliest of them—owe their existence to a degree of spread of the disease which must reach certain stages before the signs for which we so anxiously search are recognizable . . . during the watching period cases must frequently pass from the curable into the incurable stages, and in the early treatment of cancer the saving of time means the saving of life."[38]

Although early detection and treatment of breast carcinoma have resulted in a significant reduction in mortality from this disease in select populations, the overall mortality has not changed appreciably during the past 50 years in the United States.[99, 201, 211, 231] Both the complexity and the promise of this aspect of carcinoma of the breast warrant an analysis of its epidemiology, natural history, and management options. The major categories of early breast cancer that will be dealt with in this chapter include lobular carcinoma *in situ* (LCIS), ductal carcinoma *in situ* (DCIS), and clinically occult invasive carcinoma.

EARLIEST FORMS OF BREAST MALIGNANCY

The key to many of the persistent questions and controversial issues surrounding the natural history and appropriate management of carcinoma of the breast may lie in its earliest stages, where the origins of the malignant process are harbored. The actual point at which benign tissue becomes malignant and those criteria that most accurately define "malignancy" have long been debated. Those benign proliferative forms of breast disease that most likely give rise to carcinoma have been reviewed in section III, chapter 6.[15, 53, 162, 164, 165] Atypical hyperplasia is thought to represent a borderline stage of evolution between benign and malignant disease. The evidence supporting this concept has prompted Fisher[68] to assert "that at least the proliferative form of fibrocystic disease represents not only a precursor of mammary carcinoma, but perhaps one of its earliest morphologic expressions."

Most investigators agree that all breast carcinomas pass through a stage of intraepithelial confinement in the course of their evolution from benign to malignant disease, in accordance with the transition theory. The duration of such a premalignant phase remains open to question.[79, 181] Studies of carcinoma of the uterine cervix have most conclusively documented such a systematically progressive evolution, and a great deal of evidence supports this pattern in carcinoma of the breast.[41]

Evolution of the "*In Situ*" Concept

Shield[56, 205] provided one of the first illustrations of what was later recognized as intraepithelial carcinoma, describing this lesion as "the earliest change usually observable by the microscope in carcinoma of the mamma." In 1908 Cornil described the morphological similarity between the cells of invasive breast carcinoma and those still confined to the epithelium of origin in cases of such early malignancy.[43] Ewing labeled such lesions as "precancerous changes," not considering them malignant unless there was invasion into the surrounding

stroma.[54] This view was also held by others.[31, 94] Bloodgood noted in 1916 that an increased proportion of such "borderline" breast lesions were detected among the increased number of breast biopsy samples that resulted from public education campaigns.[29] This presaged the currently accepted benefits of diagnostic screening and cancer education. Cheatle and Cutler[40] were among the first to consider these intraepithelial lesions as a form of carcinoma, also emphasizing the malignant characteristics of the cells and the process by which these cells extruded beyond their basement membrane to become invasive.

Broders[34] coined the term "in situ carcinoma" for these intraepithelial malignancies and established this as a distinct pathological entity with the following definition: "Carcinoma in situ is a condition in which malignant epithelial cells and their progeny are found in or near positions occupied by their ancestors before the ancestors underwent malignant transformation." Broders also noted the essential importance of this pathological entity and stated in 1932:

"If carcinoma in situ appears alone, its recognition is necessary, for failure to recognize it may constitute an error of omission fraught with grave danger to the patient; if it goes unrecognized, carcinoma is allowed to masquerade as a benign or not more than a precarcinomatous process, with the possibility of its becoming too far advanced to be amenable to treatment."[34]

The two recognized histological categories of *in situ* carcinoma of the breast correspond to those of invasive breast carcinoma: ductal carcinoma *in situ*, otherwise known as intraductal carcinoma, and lobular carcinoma *in situ*. These forms differ in their presumed sites of origin (i.e., the major lactiferous ducts and the terminal duct-lobular units, respectively) as well as in natural history and histological characteristics.

Lobular Carcinoma *In Situ*

Epidemiology

The distinctive histopathological features of lobular carcinoma *in situ* (LCIS) are well established[75, 82, 137] and have been described in section IV, chapter 8. LCIS occurs almost exclusively in females and is diagnosed at an average age of 44 to 47 years. The fact that this age range is 5 to 15 years younger than that of women most commonly diagnosed with invasive breast carcinoma tends to support the transition theory of disease development.[82, 152, 179] This theory is further supported by the coexistence of LCIS and invasive breast carcinoma at an average age of 54 years, which is between the average ages at which each are diagnosed individually.[48, 181]

LCIS itself never manifests any clinical indications of its presence. It is a microscopic entity that is always found incidentally in biopsy specimens that were obtained for clinically suspicious lesions (usually a lump) or for mammographic lesions (most commonly microcalcifications).[8, 82, 96, 191] For this reason, its true incidence in the general population cannot be accurately determined. It has been reported to occur in 0.8 percent to 8 percent of breast biopsy specimens,[91, 197, 235] although its incidence in more recent series of nonpalpable, mammographically detected breast lesions is much higher.[126] Autopsy studies of its incidence should provide the most accurate figures, but very few have been done, and their results are conflicting.[4, 154] It is certainly evident that LCIS is not the "rare form of mammary carcinoma" originally described.[75]

The important role that hormonal influence must play in the etiology and natural history of this entity is indicated by the fact that two thirds of all women with LCIS are premenopausal, unlike the pattern found in women with invasive breast carcinoma.[55, 102, 180, 188] Lobular carcinoma in general also has a significantly higher rate of estrogen receptor activity than does ductal carcinoma.[8, 49, 127, 185, 188] The specific estrogen receptor activity of LCIS has not been accurately established because it is not clinically detectable in the tissue in which it exists, leading to biochemical assay results that are probably contaminated by surrounding benign tissue.[185] Currently available immunocytochemical assay techniques that utilize monoclonal antibodies against hormone receptors now allow this evaluation to be performed directly on histological or cytological sections of confirmed disease.[134, 166]

Natural History

Abundant evidence indicates that the presence of LCIS imparts one of the greatest risks of the development of subsequent invasive carcinoma. The probability of future malignancy in a number of reports ranges from ten percent to 37 percent (Table 35–1). A single percentage, though, is not considered the most accurate expression of this risk in view of its cumulative effect during a lifetime as well as the differences in length of follow-up, patient selection criteria, and forms of treatment that are found in these studies.[96, 99, 169] Relative risk figures tend to be more informative and correct for differences in age and follow-up found in individual series. These are derived from the ratio of observed cancers to expected cancers in a large and stable population. For LCIS this risk ranges from six to 12 times the

risk for developing invasive carcinoma of the breast in the general population. A unique aspect of LCIS is that this risk applies equally to both breasts regardless of which breast harbors the focus of disease.[7, 20, 102, 115, 116, 136, 230]

A literature review of 515 patients with LCIS treated only by biopsy shows that the risk of subsequent development of invasive carcinoma was 15 percent in the ipsilateral breast and 11 percent in the contralateral breast (Table 35–2). This risk pattern has important therapeutic implications in that both breasts should be treated equally and should be considered a single organ.[169] In this collective review, 37 of the 515 patients (seven percent) died of carcinoma, with ranges from four percent to 19 percent in individual series. Rosen et al. have cautioned that these subsequent invasive carcinomas may be expected to have at least a 20 percent risk of regional lymph node metastasis,[178, 185] with rates ranging as high as 35 percent to 50 percent in published series.[7, 185] Mortality has been reported to be as high as 24 percent among these patients. In contrast to these observations are those of Haagensen, who reported no mortality among all patients with LCIS who subsequently developed invasive carcinoma, with a follow-up of 1 to 16 years.[102, 127] This good prognosis is most likely related to increased surveillance and earlier detection as a result of the diagnosis of LCIS. It is reasonable to postulate that these subsequent carcinomas are not intrinsically more or less aggressive simply because of their temporal relation to LCIS.[82]

Rosen[181] has shown that the incidence of simultaneous foci of invasive carcinoma in either breast at the time of diagnosis of LCIS was four percent in his own series and averaged seven percent in those series he reviewed.[37, 203] Although other authors have reported finding simultaneous invasive carcinoma in 11 percent to 13 percent of patients with LCIS,[220, 223] the usually reported rate for either breast is five percent.[115, 183, 189] These observations indicate the importance of a diligent and thorough pathological sectioning and review of biopsy specimens to ensure the correct diagnosis. The incidence of axillary nodal metastasis in patients with only LCIS found in mastectomy specimens appears to be very low, between one percent and two percent.[37, 178] Such metastases are presumably a result of either overlooked foci

Table 35–1. INCIDENCE OF BREAST CARCINOMA SUBSEQUENT TO A BIOPSY SHOWING LOBULAR CARCINOMA *IN SITU* OF THE BREAST

Author	No. Patients	No. Lost to Follow-up	Years Follow-up Mean	Years Follow-up Range	Subsequent Cancers No.	Subsequent Cancers %	Relative Risk*
Andersen[7]	52	0	15.0	2–28	15	29	12
Curletti and Giordano[46]	19	0	11.7	7–21	2	11	—
Giordano and Klopp[91]	19	—	—	—	2	10.5	—
Haagensen[99]	285	2	16.3	1–47	53	18.5	6
Hutter and Foote[116]	52	3		4–27	14	28.6	—
McDivitt et al.[136]	42	8		2–23	9	22.5	10
Rosen et al.[185]	99	15	24.0	1–35	31	37	9
Wheeler et al.[235]	35	0	15.7	1–24	6	17	18

*Compared to women from Denmark (Andersen[7]), Connecticut (Haagensen,[99] McDivitt et al.,[136] and Rosen et al.[185]), and historical controls from literature (Wheeler et al.[235]).

Table 35–2. LATERALITY OF RISK AND MORTALITY OF SUBSEQUENT INVASIVE BREAST CARCINOMA FOLLOWING A BIOPSY DIAGNOSIS OF LOBULAR CARCINOMA *IN SITU*

Author	Years Follow-up		No. Ipsilateral Breasts/ Carcinoma	No. Contralateral Breasts/Carcinoma	Mortality (No.)
	Mean	*Range*			
Andersen[7]	15	2–28	46/9	52/9	6
Haagensen et al.[102]	16.3	1–47	281/33	286/37	11
Hutter and Foote[116]		4–27	40/10	49/7	2
Rosen et al.[185]	24	1–35	83/18*	83/17*	16
Wheeler et al.[235]	15.7	1–24	25/1	34/5	2
Total (N = 515)			475/71 (15%)	504/75 (15%)†	37 (7%)

*One patient excluded, side not known.
†11 per cent if prior carcinoma excluded.
Adapted from Haagensen CD: Diseases of the Breast, ed 3. Philadelphia, WB Saunders, 1986, p 209.

of occult invasive disease in the breast or regression of an invasive focus.

The pattern of subsequent development of invasive carcinoma in women with LCIS provides an interesting perspective on this disease. Most of these women will never develop a future malignancy. The majority of those malignancies that do develop occur more than 15 years after the diagnosis of LCIS, and 38 percent occur more than 20 years later.[115] Rosen et al.[185] documented that the "hazard rate" of development of future invasive carcinoma in this setting actually increases with time. This risk pattern differs from that of other forms of breast carcinoma in which recurrences generally occur within 5 years of diagnosis and then taper off in frequency.[26, 57, 74, 191] The histology of 50 percent to 65 percent of these invasive malignancies is a form of ductal carcinoma. This is contrary to the predominance of invasive lobular carcinoma that would be expected according to the transition theory, which specifies that LCIS is a precursor lesion that directly evolves into invasive carcinoma.[47, 48, 69, 181, 185, 234] Although invasive lobular carcinoma does in fact occur in this setting at 18 times its expected rate,[235] these observations raise some doubt as to the validity of the transition theory and suggest a more complex mechanism governing cancer development. The known high rate of coexistence of lobular and ductal carcinoma *in situ* in breast tissue has provided one explanation for this phenomenon.[69, 177, 185] The differential growth rates of these two entities could then explain the predominance of subsequent ductal carcinomas, since DCIS tends to give rise to a higher rate of invasive carcinoma during a shorter period of time than does LCIS.[26, 163, 185] A recent study supports this idea in showing a significantly greater proportion of ductal histology among all invasive breast carcinomas than among all noninvasive carcinomas in a population of women who underwent mammographic screening.[202] In past years patients with the earlier appearing ductal invasive carcinomas uniformly underwent mastectomy, which served to prevent the appearance of the more slowly growing lobular carcinomas. The current trend toward breast-sparing procedures for invasive carcinoma may change this pattern.

These unique biological features of LCIS have led many authors to view it as a "marker" lesion that indicates an increased risk of future invasive disease in all genetically identical breast tissue, without the anatomical lesion itself necessarily being the actual focus that becomes invasive.[1, 82, 96, 102, 115, 127, 169] LCIS may thus be considered a risk factor viewed in much the same way as family history, contralateral breast cancer, and atypical hyperplasia, all of which are also bilateral in their risk and associated with no clinically detectable manifestations. This concept contrasts somewhat with the transition theory, but currently available evidence can support both theories of natural history to some extent. The fact that neither can completely explain the behavior of LCIS is a reflection of how much more we have yet to learn about this disease.[82]

Haagensen has applied the term "lobular neoplasia" to this disease to emphasize its clinically benign behavior and to discourage physicians from inappropriately aggressive treatment.[96, 99, 102, 127] The original term, "lobular carcinoma *in situ*," still prevails in current usage because of the "morphologic identity" of its cells with those of invasive lobular carcinoma as well as their similarity to cells of DCIS[177, 234]; it does not imply an inevitable progression to invasive carcinoma.[10, 16, 46, 179, 234]

Ductal Carcinoma *In Situ*

Ductal carcinoma *in situ* (DCIS), a noninvasive carcinoma of the breast, appears to have a higher incidence than its lobular counterpart, and its status as a direct precursor of subsequent invasive carcinoma is more certain. Although DCIS has long been described pathologically, it has been recognized as a distinct entity for a shorter period of time than has LCIS and has also been subject to less comprehensive investigation.[125, 238] Several aspects of its biology are still unclear and continue to raise questions as to its implications.[81, 181, 193, 208, 215]

Historical Overview

One of the first investigators to recognize a "transition stage" of ductal epithelium between benign forms and obvious malignancy was J. C. Warren of Boston, who termed this pathological entity "abnormal involution."[229] Illustrations of what would later be known as ductal carcinoma *in situ* were published by both Cheatle[38-40] and Bloodgood[30-32] in the early years of the twentieth century and were collectively termed by Bloodgood "borderline breast tumors."[31] He specifically named this lesion "comedo-carcinoma" on the basis of its characteristic gross and histological pattern of necrotic debris in the center of ductal lumens filled with proliferating epithelium.[32] Retrospective analysis of Bloodgood's series indicates that no distinction was made between invasive and noninvasive forms of this lesion, although it was noted that women with a "pure comedo tumor," analogous to DCIS, did not show axillary nodal metastasis and did not die of breast carcinoma. This favorable prognosis was confirmed by the 85 percent 5-year "cure" rate reported by Lewis and Geschickter,[130] who, along with Muir[145] stressed the importance of distinguishing Bloodgood's pure comedo tumor from the less favorable forms that showed microscopic invasion beyond the investing basement membrane. Although Bloodgood considered this entity a benign precancerous lesion, Lewis and Geschickter interpreted it as an indolent and slowly growing carcinoma with a favorable prognosis. This latter perspective can still be supported by current available evidence.[96, 233] Gillis et al. were probably the first to apply the term "*in situ*" to this ductal form of noninvasive carcinoma[90] but attributed the first recognition of this lesion as a noninvasive carcinoma to Foote and Stewart.[76] This established it as an analogous entity to the already well-defined lobular carcinoma *in situ*.

The distinctive histopathological characteristics of DCIS have been described in section IV, chapter 8. As is true of any *in situ* carcinoma,[34] its cells are completely contained within the investing borders of the duct with no infiltration into surrounding tissues. This has led to the application of the term "intraductal" carcinoma to DCIS, although this term tends to be frequently confused with invasive forms of disease. Another term used in this context is "comedocarcinoma," which has also encompassed both invasive and noninvasive lesions.[32, 130] It is derived from that specific gross and histological feature first described by Bloodgood, which does not necessarily correlate with the presence or absence of invasion. Many of the disparate and surprisingly low survival statistics reported for this entity[130, 191] probably stem from imprecise and misleading terms leading to imprecision in pathological diagnosis and staging. Some have thus recommended that these terms no longer be used[74] and that an accurately descriptive name such as "ductal carcinoma *in situ*" be uniformly applied to this lesion.

Epidemiology

DCIS occurs predominantly in females, and makes up approximately five percent of all male breast carcinomas.[111] The average age at diagnosis is 54 years to 56 years, ranging from 48 years to 63 years.* Westbrook

*References 14, 35, 125, 142, 163, 191, 194, 228, 233, and 238.

Table 35–3. PUBLISHED RATES OF DIAGNOSIS OF DUCTAL CARCINOMA *IN SITU* (DCIS)

Author	No. Breasts	Incidence DCIS No.	%
Brown et al.[35]*	1,300	40	3.0
Gillis et al.[90]*	603	36	6.0
Kramer and Rush[123]†	140	4	2.9
Nielsen et al.[154]†	83	9	13.3
Page et al.[163]*	2,404	52	2.2
Rosner et al.[191]*	23,972	202	0.8
Schwartz et al.[196]*	1,132	81	7.2
Total	29,634	424	1.4

*Clinical series.
†Autopsy series.

and Gallager[233] found no statistically significant difference in age at diagnosis between women with DCIS and women with invasive breast carcinoma, suggesting a "closer" relationship to a true malignancy than LCIS. The reported incidence of DCIS in various series is in the same range as that for LCIS (Table 35–3). The current widespread use of mammography for the detection of nonpalpable breast lesions has led to a predominance of DCIS among all *in situ* lesions diagnosed (Table 35–4), although in earlier years LCIS tended to predominate.[10, 56] The presentation of a substantial proportion of cases of DCIS as clinically palpable masses may also explain its greater incidence when compared with the wholly microscopic presentation of LCIS.[14, 228, 233]

Natural History

There is much uncertainty as to the biological behavior of DCIS, because most patients with this diagnosis in the past underwent mastectomy.[193, 238] Those few long-term follow-up studies that are available (Table 35–5), although flawed by selection bias, small numbers, and uncertain diagnostic criteria, report the probability of subsequent invasive carcinoma following a biopsy diagnosis of DCIS to be in the range of 25 percent to 50 percent. A relative risk of 11-fold has been computed,[163] and approximately ten percent of patients who develop subsequent invasive carcinoma have died of the disease.[163, 181] Virtually all malignancies that follow DCIS

Table 35–4. PROPORTIONS OF DCIS AND LCIS DETECTED BY BREAST BIOPSY

Author	No. *In Situ* Carcinomas	DCIS No.	%	LCIS No.	%
Farrow[56]	385	149	38.7	236	61.3
Frazier et al.[79]	155	138	89.0	17	11.0
Rosen et al.[189]	122	64	52.5	58	47.5
Rosner et al.[191]	323	202	62.5	121	37.5
Schwartz et al.[196]	101	81	80.0	20	20.0
Sunshine et al.[212]	106	70	66.0	36	34.0
Total	1192	704	59.0	488	41.0

Table 35–5. INCIDENCE OF BREAST CARCINOMA SUBSEQUENT TO BIOPSY RESULT SHOWING DUCTAL CARCINOMA *IN SITU* OF THE BREAST

Author	No. Patients	Years Follow-up Mean	Years Follow-up Range	Subsequent Cancers No.	Subsequent Cancers %	Years to Subsequent Cancer Mean	Years to Subsequent Cancer Range
Betsill et al.[26]	10	21.6	7–30	7	70	9.7	0.8–24.0
Farrow[56]	25	?		5	20		1.0–8.0
Lagios et al.[125]	20	7.25		3	15	1.5	0.75–3.0
Lewis and Geschickter[130]	8		1–11	6	75	1.6	1.0–4.0
Mills and Thynne[142]	8		5–20	2	25	3.8	0.5 and 7.0
Page et al.[163]	25	16.25	8–27	7	28	6.1	3.0–10.0
Total	96			30	31.25		

are histologically ductal forms that occur within 10 years of diagnosis, and they not only predominantly occur in the same breast but also in the same quadrant as the initial biopsy.[26, 125, 163, 193, 194] Thus despite the similarity of overall risk between DCIS and LCIS, there are many significant differences between these two entities in biology and prognostic implications (Table 35–6). These characteristics have led many to consider DCIS as a more ominous lesion that behaves as a more direct precursor to invasive carcinoma.[238]

Another factor that lends uncertainty to the natural history of DCIS is that most published reports involve patients treated in earlier years, before the widespread use of mammography, in whom DCIS was usually clinically palpable and amenable to detection only by physical examination. It is unknown whether a lesion that presents as a mass, pain, or nipple discharge will display the same biological behavior as a clinically occult microscopic lesion more commonly detected in recent years by mammography. The degree to which the treatment rendered to the patients in a study affects the natural history of DCIS is also uncertain. Most studies involve follow-up of DCIS that was only diagnosed by biopsy and treated no further. We can only speculate whether

the subsequent clinical course in these patients would be the same as that in patients whose disease was deliberately treated with wide surgical excision with or without radiation therapy.[97, 125]

Recent evidence indicates that the size or extent of DCIS is directly related to the incidence of multicentricity and synchronous invasive foci as well as to the risk of future malignancy.[125] This may explain some of the differences between data reported in various series from earlier years[14, 90, 142, 233] and those from more recent studies.[125, 163, 196] These observations support the emphasis of Gump et al.[96, 97] on distinguishing between the gross and microscopic presentations of DCIS in making a therapeutic decision.

Following biopsy of a lesion that proves to be DCIS, residual foci of disease have been found in 60 to 66 percent of cases, most commonly in the area of the biopsy site.[37, 189] This has led to an estimate of a 50 percent overall risk of DCIS developing into invasive carcinoma[163, 199] and also suggests that a more complete excision may reduce this risk.[74] The true risk of invasive carcinoma subsequent to DCIS may never be known, since it could be argued that removal of the lesion for diagnosis either ablates or reduces this risk. This may be the reason that all women with a diagnosis of DCIS do not develop invasive carcinoma on long-term follow-up after biopsy only, as would be expected if this were an obligate precursor (see Table 35–5).

A review of 694 axillary dissections in 754 patients with DCIS from the literature showed a rate of axillary metastasis of less than two percent (Table 35–7). Many series have documented no axillary lymph node involvement in these patients.[74, 206, 212, 228]

In the past DCIS has been viewed as an aggressive disease process on the basis of its rarity as an isolated entity and its frequent association with invasive disease, suggesting that the *in situ* phase is transient and its progression is rapid.[90, 209] More recent information on age distribution, the long duration of symptoms in many women prior to diagnosis, and the large size that these lesions may attain supports a more indolent disease process with a long preinvasive phase.[233] Whether DCIS is considered a benign process, as earlier reports maintained,[31, 94] or an already malignant lesion with a favorable prognosis,[159] it is generally agreed that if DCIS is left alone long enough, invasive carcinoma will develop,

Table 35–6. SALIENT CHARACTERISTICS OF DCIS AND LCIS OF THE BREAST

Characteristic	LCIS	DCIS
Age (yrs)	44–47	54–58
Incidence (%)	2.5	2–3
Clinical signs	None	Mass, pain, nipple discharge
Mammographic signs	None	Microcalcifications
Premenopausal	2/3	1/3
Incidence of synchronous invasive carcinoma (%)	5	18
Multicentricity (%)	60–90	40–80
Bilaterality (%)	50–70	10–20
Axillary metastasis (%)	1	2
Subsequent carcinomas		
Incidence (%)	25–35	25–70
Laterality	Bilateral	Ipsilateral
Interval to diagnosis (yrs)	15–20	5–10
Histology	Ductal	Ductal

Table 35–7. INCIDENCE OF AXILLARY METASTASIS IN PATIENTS WITH DCIS

Author	No. Patients	No. Axillary Dissections	No. Positive Nodes
Ashikari et al.[14]	112	113	1
Brown et al.[35]	40	21	1
Carter and Smith[37]	38	26	1
Fisher et al.[74]	78	78	0
Lagios et al.[125]	53	53	1
Rosner et al.[191]	210	210	8
Silverstein et al.[206]	100	100	0
Sunshine et al.[212]	70	61	0
Von Rueden and Wilson[228]	53	32	0
Total	754	694	12 (1.7%)

Modified from Swain SM, Lippman ME: *In* Lippman ME, Lichter AS, Danforth DN Jr (eds): Diagnosis and Management of Breast Cancer. Philadelphia, WB Saunders, 1988, pp 296–325.

and the opportunity to alter this progression will be lost. The wide variation in its presentation and behavior probably reflects each individual patient's own host resistance as well as differences in the biology of individual tumors in terms of growth rates and metastatic potential.[68, 233]

Clinically Occult Invasive Carcinoma

Any invasive carcinoma of small size without clinical evidence of distant spread is presumed to be "early" in its development and to thus have a more favorable prognosis than "later" larger lesions. Some have defined clinically occult invasive carcinoma, also known as microinvasive carcinoma, as any neoplasm in which as little as ten percent of its mass consists of invasive carcinoma.[198] Gallager and Martin[87] defined it as any invasive tumor 0.5 cm or less in diameter and included it, along with LCIS and DCIS, in the category of "minimal breast cancer." It was predicted that patients with this form of breast carcinoma would have less than a five percent incidence of axillary lymph node metastasis and at least a 90 percent 10-year survival rate. Subsequent reviews confirmed this good prognosis,[79, 83, 110] although at that time there were few implications for treatment, since most patients underwent mastectomy for any form of carcinoma.

Although this concept of minimal breast cancer emphasized the importance and the benefits of early breast cancer detection, many currently object to using the term,[1, 68, 186, 197, 198] in view of increasing evidence of a more complex tumor biology than originally postulated.[86] The three components of this category have also been found to have very different biological behaviors, as has already been shown (see Table 35–6). Thus the category of minimal breast cancer includes a diverse group of clinicopathological entities that should be analyzed separately in therapeutic considerations.[238]

Natural History and Risk Factors

Any microscopic evidence of invasion beyond the investing basement membrane into surrounding tissues significantly alters the prognosis of breast carcinoma. The mere presence of invasive disease diminishes the 10-year survival rate to 65 percent from the 96 percent 10-year survival rate expected for women with *in situ* breast carcinoma.[2, 3, 66, 149, 197] Even the smallest invasive tumors of up to 1 cm in size may show axillary nodal involvement in as many as 45 percent of cases.[23, 150, 198, 208] Although tumor size does correlate with prognosis to some degree, this correlation is not accurate enough to predict survival in and of itself.[108, 203, 233] Studies analyzing breast tumor doubling times[95] estimate that a tumor of 0.1 cm in size may have already been present for about 7 years. A 0.5-cm breast carcinoma has already undergone approximately 27 doublings, with evidence now suggesting that metastases probably occur within the first 10 to 20 doublings.[68] Thus a clinically early lesion (i.e., small) may actually be biologically late, so it is not surprising that perhaps as many as 45 percent of women with a carcinoma of the breast 1.0 cm in size may already have systemic disease.[3, 23, 68, 219]

The fallacy of assuming a linear relationship between tumor size and prognosis has been demonstrated in two studies. A review of more than 8500 cases of breast cancer from the Surveillance, Epidemiology and End Results (SEER) Project of the National Cancer Institute[208] showed that 17.2 percent of patients with invasive carcinomas smaller than 0.5 cm had positive axillary lymph node involvement, and 20.2 percent of patients with tumors 0.5 to 0.9 cm in size had disease-positive regional lymph nodes. In a long-term survey of breast cancer patients conducted by the American College of Surgeons, the incidence of regional lymph node metastasis was 23 percent for patients with invasive carcinomas measuring up to 0.5 cm and 20.9 percent for patients whose tumors were 0.6 to 1.0 cm in size.[23, 150, 191] With this degree of metastatic potential, invasive tumors up to 1 cm in size are not profoundly different from any other T1 (i.e., up to 2.0 cm) breast carcinoma and may not represent any distinct biological subgroup, as has been suggested.[21] In addition, since noninvasive breast cancers metastasize to lymph nodes in only about one percent of patients, their significant biological difference from any invasive cancer is further reinforced.[181, 215]

The most accurate single parameter that correlates with overall survival in women with invasive breast carcinoma is the status of axillary lymph nodes.[68, 108, 213, 238] A reduction in 10-year survival from 80 percent to 38 percent has been demonstrated between women without nodal involvement and those with involved axillary lymph nodes, as has an inverse correlation between survival and the number of lymph nodes harboring metastatic disease.[62, 66, 68, 98, 213, 224] The relatively greater prognostic importance of axillary node metastasis as compared with tumor size is also suggested by the fact that node-negative women with tumors larger than 2.0 cm (T2) have a 10-year survival rate equivalent to those with smaller T1 lesions.[187, 201] Stratification of lymph node involvement according to tumor size provides a highly accurate means of assessing prognosis.[66, 108, 150, 224]

Most women with clinically occult invasive breast

carcinoma have no axillary lymph node involvement, but several factors have been recognized that influence their prognosis (Table 35–8). The presence of tumor emboli in lymphatic channels and high nuclear or histological grade have been shown to correlate with poor outcome in this population.[9, 27, 68, 149, 186] Lymphocytic infiltration in the stroma surrounding a neoplasm has been correlated with a poor prognosis in stage I patients,[42] as has neoplastic invasion of blood vessels.[190] A significantly lower survival rate has been demonstrated in breast cancer patients older than 75 years and younger than 34 years.[113] DNA ploidy distributions and S-phase fractions in breast carcinoma specimens, as measured by flow cytometry, have shown some correlation with estrogen receptor status and survival.[22, 52, 65, 71, 214] Further research into tumor growth determinants promises to expand our understanding of these influences on prognosis and the effect of various treatments on the natural history of these early invasive malignancies.[77, 139]

Pathological Considerations

The accurate determination of invasion in borderline forms of breast malignancy is of critical importance, because the management may be entirely different from that of *in situ* disease. The pathologist carries the ultimate responsibility for this decision, which can be difficult and requires strict attention to a variety of histological and cytological factors that have been discussed in section IV, chapters 8 and 9 and section VIII, chapter 26. Subjective judgment may be necessary in some difficult cases, because there are no rigid or uniformly established morphological criteria by which invasion can be always determined.[82, 87, 114, 160]

Broders[34] established the essential role of the epithelial basement membrane surrounding mammary ducts and lobules in distinguishing between invasive and noninvasive breast carcinoma. A thorough examination of several histological sections of tissue is required to assure a diagnosis of *in situ* disease and to exclude any occult area of invasion as determined by neoplastic cells in the surrounding stroma. It is unusual to find a section that actually shows the extrusion of neoplastic cells through a basement membrane.[6, 81, 86] The earliest changes that may be associated with the transition from *in situ* to invasive breast carcinoma have been documented by Ozzello,[159–161] who showed that basement membranes are virtually always altered in some way in specimens of DCIS and may be attenuated, poorly defined, or

---

Table 35–8. FACTORS RELATED TO A POOR PROGNOSIS IN NODE-NEGATIVE CLINICALLY OCCULT INVASIVE BREAST CARCINOMA

Age
Negative estrogen receptor activity
Vascular invasion
Lymphatic invasion
High histological or nuclear grade
Aneuploid DNA patterns
Lymphocytic reaction

---

occasionally absent. Benign mammary tumors always had intact basement membranes, whereas those of frankly invasive carcinoma were always obliterated. Ultrastructural studies of the basal laminae showed these structures to be frequently disrupted in LCIS and DCIS, and a complex relationship was suggested between neoplastic epithelial cells and the "epithelial-stromal junction."[160, 161] This investigator found that the earliest stage of invasion appeared to be represented by neoplastic cytoplasmic protrusions through gaps in the basal lamina that could not be detected by light microscopy. This could explain the small incidence of axillary nodal metastasis seen in cases of *in situ* breast carcinoma as well as some of the unexpectedly high rates of recurrence and mortality following treatment of *in situ* disease.[130, 191] These observations support the idea that perhaps a truly noninvasive phase of breast carcinoma does not exist, but that these lesions simply represent an indolent and favorable form of an already invasive tumor.[82, 90, 160, 161]

Basement membrane appearance by light microscopy remains the standard determinant of diagnosis of the presence or absence of invasion.[90, 102, 137, 194] Fisher et al. have even claimed that they do not use the status of the basement membrane in their diagnosis of DCIS because of the wide disparities they find in this structure with various staining methods.[74] However, the distinction of DCIS from invasive carcinoma was the major source of disagreement among pathologists in that study, indicating how much more remains to be learned in this area.

The mechanism by which neoplastic cells manage to "escape" the confines of the basement membrane in the development of invasive carcinoma has been attributed to a number of possibilities. Pressure necrosis from a crushing effect of the proliferating epithelial cells on the peripheral myoepithelial cells has been postulated,[161, 218] as have a lytic action of the neoplastic cells[75] and enzymatic degeneration of the fibronectin that makes up basement membranes.[13, 210] The malignant process that governs tumor invasion appears to depend more on an interaction between the neoplastic cells and surrounding stroma than on any single element.[8, 10, 13]

Multicentricity and Bilaterality

Substantial evidence indicates that mammary carcinoma is a diffuse disease process involving all breast tissue.[79, 85, 86, 97, 171, 181, 198, 203] Evidence suggests that primary breast tumors represent a coalescence of neoplasms from multiple sites of origin within the breast.[86, 171] This may explain the substantial incidence of multiple foci of malignancy found in breasts with noninvasive carcinoma that do not appear to be influenced by histology (Table 35–9). These foci consist predominantly of the same *in situ* lesions as the primary neoplasm diagnosed.[37, 68, 189, 203] The fact that the size of the primary tumor has been shown to correlate with the extent of these multiple foci of occult malignancy[97, 112, 125] has led to the theory that this phenomenon represents spread of tumor cells from the primary lesion, most likely through the ductal system.[39] The diminishing fre-

Table 35–9. INCIDENCE OF MULTIPLE SITES OF INVASIVE AND NONINVASIVE CARCINOMA IN BREASTS WITH DCIS AND LCIS

	DCIS			LCIS		
		Malignant Foci			Malignant Foci	
Author	No. Patients	No.	%	No. Patients	No.	%
Carter and Smith[37]	38	25	66	49	34	69
Rosen et al.[189]	50	34	68	50	30	60
Schwartz et al.[196]	42	17	40.5	6	4	67
Shah et al.[203]	45	29	64	40	28	70
Total	175	105	60	145	96	66

quency of these foci with increasing distance from the tumor also supports this concept.[97, 112]

The wide variations in the frequency of multicentricity reported in the literature are partly a result of differences in the types of lesions and locations in the breast that are being included as well as of how thoroughly these foci are sought.[84, 86, 97, 217] It has been well demonstrated that the more histological sections are analyzed, the greater the yield of occult breast neoplasms.[10] Conversely, those series in which only a token effort is made to find multicentric foci of malignancy typically report low yields.[74] Confusion also exists in the definition of terms. Multicentricity should refer to malignancy found in sites outside the quadrant of the primary breast tumor, whereas multifocality and residual disease refer to sites within the same quadrant as the primary tumor.[68, 74] These terms are often used interchangeably in various studies,[35, 37, 217] which makes comparisons and conclusions difficult. Analysis of those particular studies that carefully adhere to the true definition of multicentricity shows that this phenomenon occurs in approximately one third of patients with DCIS (Table 35–10). Similar difficulties are encountered in studies dealing with LCIS, although this entity appears to have a higher rate of true multicentricity, one that is at least 50 percent and approaches 100 percent if diligently sought.[10, 56, 181]

The incidence of multicentricity in invasive breast carcinoma has been demonstrated to be lower than that in noninvasive disease. This may have some bearing on the good results of breast-sparing surgery accompanied by radiation therapy, since these results derive predom-

inantly from patients with invasive carcinoma.[61, 97] Further study of the clinical significance of multicentricity and its impact on conservative management of in situ breast carcinoma is warranted. The reader is referred to section XIX, chapter 48 for further discussion of the clinical management of bilateral breast cancer.

Bilaterality of in situ and clinically occult invasive breast carcinoma is probably a manifestation of the same etiological processes that give rise to multicentricity, and it also has an impact on therapeutic decisions.[129, 181] Shah et al.[203] reported a 22 percent incidence of bilaterality in 449 patients with a variety of breast carcinomas; 74 percent of these also demonstrated multicentricity in the ipsilateral breast. The rate of simultaneous bilaterality, like that of multicentricity, is also dependent on the extent to which it is sought, suggesting that most published rates probably underestimate the actual incidence.[112, 181] Unlike multicentricity, though, histology appears to significantly influence the probability of contralateral disease. As many as 90 percent of cases of LCIS have been found to have concurrent bilateral foci of disease,[101, 102, 173, 181, 220] which is consistent with the concept that this entity diffusely involves all breast tissue when it occurs.[10] LCIS was the only form of in situ carcinoma found to show a statistically significant rate of bilaterality.[230] Invasive lobular carcinoma has a similarly high bilaterality. Invasive ductal carcinoma, however, is generally associated with occult simultaneous contralateral carcinoma in ten percent to 15 percent of cases, and these foci are most commonly in situ lesions.[173, 194, 222] DCIS is also associated with a ten percent to 15 percent incidence of concurrent bilaterality,[14, 35, 228, 233] although some authors have reported much lower rates,[181, 223, 230] whereas others have reported rates as high as 30 percent.[79, 212]

Many of these studies provide conflicting data that are difficult to interpret in terms of how thoroughly these other foci of disease were sought, the reasons for contralateral biopsy, and what other risk factors were present in these patients. The clinical significance of multicentricity and bilaterality can also be appropriately questioned, because many of these studies do not correlate these phenomena with ultimate outcome in terms of recurrence and mortality.[125, 189, 198, 203] Available evidence indicates that the actual development of either ipsilateral or contralateral clinically evident breast carcinoma falls far short of the rates mentioned previ-

Table 35–10. INCIDENCE OF TRUE MULTICENTRICITY* IN PATIENTS WITH DUCTAL CARCINOMA *IN SITU* OF THE BREAST

		Multicentricity*	
Author	No. Patients	No.	%
Brown et al.[35]	40	13	32.5
Lagios et al.[125]	53	17	32.1
Nielsen et al.[154]	11	4	36.4
Rosen et al.[189]	53	10	18.9
Schwartz et al.[197]	11	4	36.4
Von Rueden and Wilson[228]	47	18	38.3
Total	215	66	31.0

*Malignant foci outside of quadrant of primary lesion.

ously.[78, 170, 174, 185, 230] Those cases that do develop most commonly occur within 5 years after diagnosis of the primary tumor, suggesting that they were probably present synchronously in a clinically occult form. It is also not specified in many studies whether these subsequent carcinomas occurred at the primary biopsy site, which would implicate incomplete excision of the primary tumor rather than a new malignancy.[68] Despite the high rates of multiple foci of malignancy reported for all forms of early breast carcinoma (see Table 35–9), the actual incidence of two or more malignancies detectable by physical examination in the same breast is rare (approximately 0.1 percent).[70] Autopsy studies have typically shown much higher rates of occult *in situ* breast carcinoma than clinically evident malignancy.[123] These considerations are important in assessing the appropriate treatment of *in situ* and clinically occult invasive carcinoma of the breast.

TREATMENT

The natural history of any disease must be understood before a rational treatment can be administered. In the case of breast carcinoma, Bloom et al.[33] have documented a comprehensive long-term follow-up of untreated women with this disease and have shown that 20 percent were alive 5 years after diagnosis, five percent at 10 years, and less than one percent at 15 years. Other studies have shown a 5-year survival rate for untreated disease as high as 68 percent.[68, 133] These data provide an important perspective from which to judge the results of published studies dealing with various treatment regimens. The controversies that still surround the many therapeutic options available for early breast carcinoma indicate that our knowledge of this disease is incomplete. It is thus important that the patient take an active role in the therapeutic decision.[82] The choice between the many therapeutic options available for early breast carcinoma (Table 35–11) must ultimately depend on the specific preferences and priorities of the individual patient, who should be thoroughly informed as to the potential risks and benefits of each option and included as an equal member of the medical team.

Until recently mastectomy was carried out for virtually all breast malignancies regardless of stage. This treatment was seldom modified for patients with the early forms of breast carcinoma discussed in this chapter, except perhaps for preserving the pectoral muscles in what is commonly called the modified radical mastectomy[64] or for limiting the extent of axillary dissection.[79] During the course of this century, however, advances in our understanding of the underlying biology and natural history of breast carcinoma have led to a diminished emphasis on local surgical treatment of the primary disease and a heightened awareness of the need to apply systemic treatment to an ever-broadening segment of the diseased population. These changing therapeutic approaches have resulted from evidence that systemic spread of disease has already occurred in many cases before the neoplasm becomes clinically manifest. Axillary nodal metastases and distant metastases may occur simultaneously rather than sequentially. Most deaths from carcinoma of the breast result from this systemic disease. Furthermore, many studies indicate that the extent of local treatment has little effect on mortality, although it may influence the incidence of local chest wall recurrence. The increasing acceptance of segmental mastectomy plus irradiation as an alternative to mastectomy for many patients with invasive breast carcinoma[61] is predicated on these observations. It is thus logical that patients with *in situ* and clinically occult invasive breast carcinoma should also be reassessed with regard to their suitability for breast conservation procedures.[238] A review of the current therapeutic options for these specific forms of disease follows.

Lobular Carcinoma *In Situ*

Ipsilateral radical mastectomy was the treatment originally recommended for LCIS because of the high rate of multicentricity and subsequent carcinoma with which it was associated.[75, 92, 141, 151] During the 1960s and 1970s, evidence accumulated as to its relatively benign course, its predominance among young females, the bilaterality of its risk of subsequent carcinoma in a minority of patients, and its unique pattern of increasing hazard rate after 15 years. These findings, which implicated LCIS as a marker of risk rather than an actual premalignant lesion, led to the current standard practice of nonoperative observation with lifelong surveillance as originally

Table 35–11. CURRENT THERAPEUTIC OPTIONS FOR DCIS, LCIS, AND CLINICALLY OCCULT INVASIVE CARCINOMA (COIC) OF THE BREAST

	LCIS	DCIS	COIC
1.	Nonoperative observation, lifelong follow-up of both breasts with mammography and physical examination	Total ipsilateral mastectomy, low-level axillary dissection ± breast reconstruction	Total ipsilateral mastectomy, level I or level II axillary dissection ± breast reconstruction
2.	Bilateral total mastectomy with low-level axillary dissection ± breast reconstruction	Wide local excision plus breast irradiation ± low-level ipsilateral axillary dissection	Wide local excision, ipsilateral level I or level II axillary dissection plus breast irradiation
3.	—	Wide local excision only (?)	—

advocated by Haagensen.[10, 91, 101, 115, 127, 169, 235] The goal of such surveillance is to detect any subsequent invasive carcinomas at an early enough stage to have a high likelihood of cure. The reasonableness of this practice is suggested by the results of many mammographic screening trials[201, 204, 216] and by Haagensen's own results.[102, 127] The predominance of the view that this lesion is a marker of risk rather than a preinvasive malignancy is indicated by a recent series that does not even include LCIS as a malignancy.[97]

The rationale behind nonoperative observation of LCIS raises an intriguing question as to the validity of the rigid distinction that is currently maintained between atypical lobular hyperplasia and LCIS.[1, 15, 102, 115, 137, 235] Both entities carry approximately the same bilateral risk for the development of invasive carcinoma,[15] both are most appropriately viewed as risk factors rather than actual precursors of malignancy, and both are so morphologically similar that a histological or cytological distinction is very difficult and many times subjective and arbitrary.[114, 132, 137, 234] Some have suggested abolishing the concept of *in situ* carcinoma based on these considerations and simply categorizing these forms as "precancerous mastopathy."[28, 94] This concept is probably more applicable to LCIS than to DCIS because of the more ominous malignant potential of the latter.

The major deterrents to the use of nonoperative observation following a biopsy diagnosis of LCIS are its known association with synchronous invasive carcinoma in approximately five percent of cases[183, 189] and its association with as much as a 90 percent rate of multicentricity.[115] However, the published long-term follow-up data indicate that the actual development of clinically apparent invasive carcinoma falls well below these levels (see Table 35–1). Also, at least 80 percent of the multicentric lesions are other foci of LCIS that do not necessarily require any more treatment than the primary lesion.[189] This suggests that LCIS is a diffuse disease process throughout all genetically identical breast tissue and is simply one manifestation of an underlying biological stimulus that also gives rise to separate foci of invasive carcinoma.[82] The doubtful clinical significance of synchronous invasive foci was suggested by Tulusan et al.,[220] who found a 16 percent rate of microscopic, clinically occult invasive carcinoma in subcutaneous mastectomy specimens from women who had had diagnosis of LCIS within 2 years prior to surgery. This represents more than 50 percent of the incidence expected after 24 years[185] and indicates that either most of these lesions may never become clinically evident or that they are very indolent in their growth. Although contralateral breast biopsy has been advocated for a diagnosis of LCIS,[99, 136, 223] such a practice may be considered unjustified on the basis of these considerations. The likelihood of finding a lesion that should be definitively treated (i.e., invasive carcinoma or DCIS) is small, and the clinical significance of such a lesion may be negligible. Also a negative contralateral biopsy cannot reliably exclude the presence of synchronous occult disease and cannot ensure that invasive carcinoma will not subsequently develop.

Bilateral mastectomy is a valid therapeutic option for LCIS that is consistent with the necessity to treat both breasts equally. Although few authors have advocated this as the primary management of choice,[25, 212] it remains the only rational alternative if surgical treatment is desired by the patient. The association of LCIS with invasive carcinoma in either breast poses a fourfold greater bilateral risk of future carcinoma than either entity alone and may be an indication for bilateral mastectomy.[48, 58] This procedure can be considered a prophylactic mastectomy, in this clinical setting, and considerations as to indications and patient preference, discussed in section IV, chapter 8 and section V, chapters 14 and 15, should apply. There is no evidence that radiation therapy has any benefit or role in the treatment of LCIS.

Wide excision of the biopsy site following a diagnosis of LCIS has been recommended.[82, 144] This idea derives from a standard practice currently used in breast-sparing procedures for invasive carcinoma,[61] the rationale for which is the removal of any residual foci of disease that may surround the primary lesion. However, this concept should not apply to LCIS because of its entirely microscopic status and diffuse involvement throughout the entire breast. Such clearance of margins has also not been shown to have any beneficial effect on ultimate outcome.[180, 185]

Subcutaneous mastectomy with preservation of the nipple-areola complex has been advocated as an appropriate surgical option for the treatment of LCIS.[24, 49, 220] Currently available evidence does *not* support this option, because of the increased amount of breast tissue left behind in comparison to a total mastectomy and the numerous reports of invasive carcinoma developing after subcutaneous mastectomy.[93, 115] There is also no evidence to suggest that any significant reduction in risk is brought about by reducing the amount of breast tissue present, short of total mastectomy.[82] The excellent cosmetic results that are currently achieved with reconstructive procedures should make total mastectomy a more acceptable surgical alternative to women with LCIS.

Opinion regarding the role of axillary dissection in the surgical management of LCIS is diverse and flexible. The incidence of axillary metastases is very low, as discussed previously. On the other hand, there is essentially no added morbidity to performing a low or level I axillary dissection in conjunction with a total mastectomy. Any diligent effort to remove all breast tissue from the axillary tail of Spence will, in fact, involve a removal of the low axillary lymph nodes. This will also occasionally uncover an unsuspected instance of synchronous invasion, which may alter the management. The small incidence of axillary metastasis associated with LCIS does not justify axillary dissection alone if nonoperative observation is chosen as the management option.

Ductal Carcinoma *In Situ*

For several decades mastectomy has generally been advocated as the appropriate treatment of DCIS because

Table 35–12. TREATMENT FAILURE AFTER MASTECTOMY FOR DUCTAL CARCINOMA *IN SITU*

Author	No. Patients	No. with Recurrence	No. Dead of Disease
Ashikari et al.[14]	112	1	1
Brown et al.[35]	40	0	0
Carter and Smith[37]	38	3	3
Fisher et al.[74]	27	1	1
Lagios et al.[125]	53	3	1
Sunshine et al.[212]	70	3	3
Von Rueden and Wilson[228]	47	1	0
Total	387	12 (3.1%)	9 (2.3%)

Modified from Swain SM, Lippman ME: *In* Lippman ME, Lichter AS, Danforth DN Jr (eds): Diagnosis and Management of Breast Cancer. Philadelphia, WB Saunders, 1988, pp 296–325.

of the same perceived hazards of multicentricity and subsequent risk of invasive carcinoma that characterized the initial observations of LCIS. Bloodgood viewed DCIS, or a "pure comedo tumor," as being essentially benign.[31, 32] He suggested that simple mastectomy with preoperative radiation for large tumors was adequate treatment. Lewis and Geschickter[130] also noted the excellent results of mastectomy even when axillary lymph nodes were involved, although simple excision of the tumor in their series led to a 75 percent recurrence rate within 4 years. They attributed this to an inability to reliably ascertain the "malignant potential" of this lesion (i.e., distinguish invasive from noninvasive forms; the former was apparently included in their population). Gillis et al.[90] also recommended radical mastectomy for DCIS because of the difficulties of identifying areas of microinvasion as well as their belief that this is a rapidly growing and aggressive tumor. Most investigators have since agreed with at least a total mastectomy as the appropriate treatment for DCIS.*

Total mastectomy cures virtually all patients with DCIS (Table 35–12) and currently remains the standard treatment. Ipsilateral mastectomy has generally been considered adequate, since the overall incidence of contralateral occult disease appears to be about the same as that for invasive carcinoma. The value of axillary dissection is debatable. Although axillary dissection was previously thought to improve survival in patients with invasive carcinoma, the results of the B-04 clinical trial of the National Surgical Adjuvant Breast Project (NSABP) suggest otherwise.[64] Therefore the major indication for axillary dissection is pathological staging to identify patients who may be candidates for systemic adjuvant therapy. Since only one percent to two percent of patients with DCIS have nodal metastases (see Table 35–7), the only potential benefit from any degree of axillary dissection is to ensure the completeness of the mastectomy, not to improve the reliability of pathological staging.[206] The low morbidity of axillary dissection and the small chance of uncovering unexpected invasive disease make this a reasonable

*References 1, 14, 35, 142, 182, 189, 194, 198, and 228

procedure to perform in conjunction with total mastectomy.

Segmental Mastectomy

The recurrences that develop in patients who have previously undergone biopsy or wide excision for a diagnosis of DCIS are most commonly found in the region of the biopsy site.[26, 74, 125, 194] Residual DCIS in biopsy sites in as many as 66 percent of cases[37, 189] may account for this pattern of recurrence and support the argument that a major reason for the high recurrence rate following biopsy is incomplete excision. Compelling support for this thesis was provided by Holland et al.,[112] who showed a substantial reduction in residual foci of DCIS by increasing the margin of resection from 2 cm to 5 cm. In many studies that evaluated recurrence subsequent to a diagnosis of DCIS, no attempt was made to widely excise this lesion or to microscopically confirm clear margins.[26, 163, 172, 182] Lagios et al.[125] prospectively treated 20 patients with small foci of DCIS by "tylectomy" but did not specify the extent of excision or how the margins of resection were confirmed. A substantial 15 percent recurrence rate resulted after a mean follow-up of 44 months. Fisher et al.[74] reported a recurrence rate of 23 percent after a mean follow-up of only 39 months among 22 women with DCIS who underwent "lumpectomy" alone with stringent measures documented to assure wide excision with microscopically clear margins. Rosner et al.[191] reported equivalent rates of both 5-year survival and recurrence for DCIS treated by either "wedge excision" or mastectomy. However, the surprisingly low 5-year survival reported (70 percent) suggests that invasive lesions were included in this series, which brings its results into question. Approximately 50 percent of all recurrences in these reports were invasive carcinoma.

The available evidence, although difficult to evaluate and compare, suggests that wide local excision alone is probably not adequate treatment for DCIS.[239]

Segmental Mastectomy Plus Radiotherapy

The application of radiation therapy to DCIS following excision was first reported in 1983[60] and resulted in two recurrences in 14 patients (14.3 percent) after 3 years. Recht et al.[172] reported 40 women who underwent excisional biopsy without any attempt to obtain a microscopically clear margin, followed by radiation to the breast of from 5000 rad to more than 6000 rad. Four recurrences (10 percent) occurred during 63 months of follow-up; one of these was invasive carcinoma, and all were in the primary excision site. All patients remained alive and well. However, the fact that 40 percent of the original lesions in the study were smaller than 1 cm and no patient who had an axillary dissection showed nodal metastasis suggests a significant selection bias.[89, 125] The contribution of radiation therapy to this lower recurrence rate is thus difficult to ascertain.

Fisher et al.[74] reported a substantially lower incidence of local recurrence (seven percent) in women with only

DCIS who were treated with wide local excision, microscopic clearance of margins, and postoperative breast irradiation, when compared with the group mentioned previously who had wide local excision only and experienced a 23 percent rate of recurrence. The average size of these tumors was 2.2 cm, and no patient had axillary nodal metastasis. Although this study was not specifically designed to assess the effects of radiation therapy on DCIS and follow-up averaged only 39 months, its results do suggest that this regimen may have substantial benefit in these women as long as they are appropriately selected and undergo wide excision with microscopically clear margins.

Montague[143] treated 34 patients who had a biopsy diagnosis of DCIS by excision followed by irradiation of at least 5000 rad to the breast during 5 weeks, and a boost to the tumor bed of 1000 to 2000 rad. At 44 months minimum follow-up there was one recurrence that involved the axillary lymph nodes (which had not been initially treated), but there were no failures involving the treated breasts.

Zafrani et al.[239] reported the results of treatment of 55 patients with DCIS who were treated at the Marie Curie Institute in Paris, France. All patients were treated with "wide excision," although there is no documentation of how this was assured, and 5000 rad to the breast, with a boost of between 1000 and 1500 rad to the tumor bed. Additional radiation to regional lymph nodes was given to 34 patients. After 55 months median follow-up, three recurrences had occurred, and one patient died of her disease.

These four series represent the results of treatment of 158 patients with a biopsy diagnosis of DCIS by tumor excision and radiation (Table 35–13). In this entire group, only nine patients (5.7 percent) experienced a failure in the treated breast, three of which (two percent) were invasive carcinoma, and one patient died of known disease. Although the average follow-up was relatively short, the addition of radiotherapy to excision appears to have reduced the incidence of treatment failure. Almost all patients with recurrences were successfully salvaged, even though 33 percent of these recurrences were invasive disease.

In contrast to these data are reports by Harris et al.[105, 106, 192] indicating that concomitant DCIS and invasive carcinoma treated by excisional biopsy and radiation

therapy has a substantially higher rate of local recurrence than does invasive carcinoma without DCIS. The retrospective study design and failure to control prognostic variables such as axillary nodal status, tumor size, and adequacy of excision make the significance of this apparent radiation resistance of DCIS uncertain. Others have found no such adverse effects from irradiation of DCIS.[73, 135]

Other Considerations

Lagios et al.[125] and Gump et al.[96, 97] have reported data suggesting that the size of the tumor significantly affects its degree of multicentricity and occult invasion and, ultimately, its recurrence and survival rates. A 44 percent rate of associated invasive carcinoma in lesions of DCIS larger than 2.5 cm[125] reinforces other studies that have shown similarly high rates[35, 37, 203] and lends credence to those who view DCIS as an indolent form of invasive carcinoma.[90, 130] The distinction between the gross and microscopic forms of DCIS has been advocated as a basis for deciding on the appropriate therapeutic regimen (i.e., mastectomy, breast conservation with radiation therapy, or wide excision only). A failure to make this distinction in many series accounts for the wide variation in results reported in the literature.[97] There is also a need to further study those microscopic lesions presenting as microcalcifications on mammography.

Further prospective randomized trials are necessary to assess the relative merits of observation, wide local excision, breast conservation with radiation therapy, and mastectomy as treatments of DCIS and to stratify these regimens according to prognostic variables. One such trial currently under way is the NSABP B-17 Protocol, which compares segmental mastectomy for this lesion with segmental mastectomy plus radiation. This directly addresses the issues of the natural history of DCIS and its radiosensitivity.[193, 238]

For those patients not able to enter into such a clinical trial, alternatives to total mastectomy may still be considered for DCIS, although there are no well-defined criteria for patient selection. It currently appears reasonable to treat small lesions that have no radiographic or microscopic evidence of extensive disease with wide excision and radiation therapy to the breast. The appro-

Table 35–13. BREAST CANCER RECURRENCE AND SURVIVAL OF PATIENTS WITH DCIS TREATED BY EXCISION PLUS RADIATION

Author	No. Patients	Follow-up (Mean Months)	Breast Recurrence Total/Invasive	Survival
Fisher et al.[74]	29	39	2/1	29
Montague[143]	34	44	0/0*	34
Recht et al.[172]	40	63	4/1	40
Zafrani et al.[239]	55	55	3/1	54
Total	158		9/3 (5.7%)	157 (99%)

*One axillary nodal recurrence.

priate radiation dose and the efficacy of irradiation to the regional lymph node basin have not been established by any substantial evidence. The short follow-up of less than 5 years in most studies of radiation therapy for DCIS should mandate caution in the interpretation of their results. The current data relating to wide local excision alone suggest that this treatment should probably not be applied to DCIS until more information is available. There appears to be little reason to perform axillary dissection if breast conservation is carried out. The therapeutic decision for DCIS should not be based on a frozen section diagnosis, because of the substantial rate of associated invasive carcinoma, the previously mentioned difficulties in histological analysis, and the absence of any demonstrated benefit of rapid diagnosis.[68]

If breast conservation is carried out, close clinical follow-up is mandatory, and a mammogram would seem prudent every 6 months for at least the first 3 years. Annual mammograms should be carried out indefinitely. Since the evolution of invasive carcinoma in these patients is poorly understood but may well take from 5 to 10 years, the optimal follow-up regimen remains to be defined.

Total mastectomy with low-level axillary sampling remains the standard treatment for DCIS and has excellent results. This should be applied to large and radiographically or histologically extensive manifestations of DCIS and to any case in which there is doubt as to the adequacy of lesser procedures. The contralateral breast should be managed with diligent surveillance, as is generally done for invasive carcinoma. There is no apparent reason to perform a biopsy or definitively treat the opposite breast in the absence of any established indications. Total mastectomy for such noninvasive lesions may be difficult to accept at a time when breast conservation is widely accepted for invasive lesions. However, DCIS may represent the most obvious circumstance in which aggressive local therapy can favorably affect overall survival, since theoretically there is no systemic disease present.

Clinically Occult Invasive Carcinoma

Treatment of the Breast

The abundant volumes of literature dealing with current treatment options for invasive breast carcinoma may appear confusing, but there are some basic points on which all therapeutic decisions should be based. First and foremost is that complete surgical ablation of the primary lesion is the sine qua non of maximal disease-free interval, optimal local control and palliation, as well as cure. Any compromise of the completeness with which clinically, histologically, or radiographically identifiable tumor is excised will compromise local control and perhaps survival.[156, 194] Adjuvant therapy is directed against carcinoma that is presumed to be present after removal of the primary tumor but cannot be identified. Any residual identifiable tumor will diminish the effectiveness of adjuvant therapy. The major objective and

efficacy of adjuvant radiation therapy is local control, whereas that of adjuvant chemotherapy is control of systemic disease. These modalities are used in those clinical settings in which known risk determinants suggest a high probability of local or systemic recurrence.

There is no convincing evidence that clinically occult invasive carcinoma of the breast that is smaller than 1 cm should be treated any differently than larger invasive lesions, as mentioned previously. These smaller tumors have been shown to be associated with rates of axillary metastasis exceeding 40 percent,[23, 208] which is little different from the 50 percent rate attributed to clinically palpable breast malignancies.[231] Estimates of prognosis and therapeutic decisions should take into account all factors of known prognostic importance, such as nodal status, hormone receptor activity, histological grade, and flow cytometry characteristics.[52, 65, 71] It would be helpful if large prospective trials involving patients with small breast malignancies were stratified according to tumor size to determine any prognostic or therapeutic differences based on this parameter.

The large amount of evidence suggesting that invasive breast carcinoma has a metastatic potential at a microscopic stage[1, 95, 219, 231] and the apparent absence of any association between the extent of surgical treatment of the primary lesion and rates of local recurrence or overall survival[44, 61, 63, 138, 146, 147, 237] have led to an increasing acceptance of breast-sparing procedures. The success of breast preservation depends to some extent on a small tumor size, since small lesions are more easily and reliably excised with histologically clear margins. This is therefore an option that should be seriously considered in cases of clinically occult invasive breast carcinoma.[36]

Wide local excision alone has been shown to result in a prohibitively high rate of local recurrence (28 percent), even with microscopic confirmation of clear margins and after a mean follow-up of only 39 months.[61] This suggests that something more must be done if breast conservation is to be safe and effective for these lesions. Radiation therapy has proven effective in the role of supplementing surgical excision, presumably by destruction of the substantial number of multicentric foci of occult malignancy that probably lead to clinical recurrence.[167]

The first application of radiation therapy to carcinoma of the breast has been attributed to Emile Grubbe in 1895, within only 2 months of Roentgen's discovery of x-rays.[175] Sir Geoffrey Keynes was one of the first to demonstrate that this modality was equivalent to mastectomy in terms of patient survival from breast carcinoma.[121] In succeeding years several nonrandomized trials as well as two well-controlled prospective randomized trials reported similarly optimistic results from wide local excision and breast irradiation for small invasive breast carcinomas. Veronesi et al.[226] compared radical mastectomy with quadrantectomy and radiotherapy for these tumors, and Fisher et al.[61] compared total mastectomy with both wide local excision alone and wide local excision followed by radiation. In both trials, survival rates of the control and experimental groups were equivalent. The latter trial demonstrated a significantly reduced rate of local breast recurrence (7.7 percent) among women undergoing wide local excision and radiotherapy as compared to those who had only wide local excision of the tumor (27.9 percent). All women in this study underwent axillary dissection and received chemotherapy if any nodal metastases were present.

These studies have established a definite benefit for wide local excision and radiation in the treatment of invasive breast carcinoma, but such success depends on patient selection. Any factors that have been shown to increase the probability of local recurrence or that adversely affect the cosmetic result will tend to diminish the safety and efficacy of breast-sparing therapy. Thus tumor size (less than 2 cm in the study by Veronesi et al. and less than 4 cm in the study by Fisher et al.), breast size, the size of the tumor relative to that of the breast, the extent to which the tumor is completely excised, and the method and dose of radiation therapy may all have a significant impact on the ultimate outcome.[36, 156, 186] The adverse influence that an extensive component of DCIS or high nuclear grade may exert on the results of radiation has been discussed previously.[105, 106] It would be prudent to offer total mastectomy and axillary dissection to any patient with clinically occult invasive breast carcinoma who has an elevated risk for local recurrence. At the University of Florida we also recommend mastectomy to any patient undergoing breast conservation in whom microscopic examination of the widely excised tumor specimen shows substantial tumor involvement of the margins, a practice also reported by Fisher et al.[61] The substantially increased costs to the patient of breast conservation as compared with mastectomy is another factor that may influence the treatment decision.[146]

Any diagnostic biopsy of the breast should be planned around the possibility of malignancy and should not interfere with the patient's therapeutic options. It would generally be prudent to perform all biopsies as wide local excisions and assure histologically clear margins at that time. The benefit of this approach lies in the avoidance of reexcising an already disturbed and potentially contaminated area if breast conservation is chosen by the patient in the event the biopsy sample is malignant.[19] Fine needle aspiration biopsy offers a similar opportunity to minimize the surgical disturbance of the breast and thus maximize the options and planning of definitive treatment.[36]

Some authors favor proceeding with breast conservation surgery despite the presence of elevated risks of local recurrence, because there is evidence that such recurrences can be successfully treated with either further local excision or "salvage mastectomy."[89, 109, 124] Others have documented a poor outcome in this situation.[18, 240] Local recurrences most commonly accompany distant metastases, a finding that has led many to view such recurrences as markers of systemic disease that are not affected by the extent of local treatment. Amalric[5] reported good results from salvage mastectomy, but these results appeared to be biased, because cases with no malignancy in the specimen were included. The implications of local recurrence that develops in the absence of distant metastases are unknown. Some evidence suggests that many cases of local recurrence are potentially preventable by more complete surgical excision.[89, 156] Compromising surgical treatment with the idea that local recurrence can be safely managed if it occurs may, in fact, adversely affect ultimate survival.[156] Proponents of Halsted's original view of the therapeutic value of wide en bloc local excision continue to report evidence of the efficacy of radical mastectomy.[100, 168] The relatively short follow-up interval of recent studies that show a benefit for breast conservation, the patterns of rising mortality in these patients after 10 years,[157, 186] and the uncertain long-term effects of the doses of radiation used in this clinical setting[80] are further indications that total mastectomy still remains an important part of the therapeutic regimen for clinically occult invasive breast carcinoma.

Treatment of the Axilla

Axillary lymph node dissection in patients with invasive breast carcinoma is currently felt to be primarily a staging procedure. Recent advances in our understanding of tumor biology have indicated that axillary lymph node metastasis probably occurs simultaneously with distant metastasis rather than preceding it. Regional node involvement thus probably reflects a particular host-tumor relationship that is conducive to distant metastasis.[67, 68, 225] Recent evidence has also suggested that axillary node metastasis has uncertain clinical significance and that axillary dissection may have no therapeutic benefit.[64, 72] Others perceive some therapeutic value to removing metastatic disease from the axilla, if only to prevent regional recurrence there. Radiation therapy is generally applied to the axilla by proponents of this latter view if there is any evidence of residual axillary disease following surgery.[195, 225]

Many believe that the disease status of level I axillary lymph nodes is reliably predictive of the status of higher levels and that complete axillary dissection is therefore seldom necessary.[68, 195, 200, 225] The number of lymph nodes involved with tumor has been shown to correlate with prognosis.[67] Although evidence suggests that the total number of lymph nodes sampled has no impact on prognosis, too limited an axillary dissection may increase the probability of sampling error and thus result in inaccurate staging.[88, 200] Axillary dissection of both level I and level II lymph nodes should provide an adequate specimen for prognostic and therapeutic purposes with a minimum of morbidity.[184] In cases of breast-sparing surgery, axillary dissection should generally be deferred until pathological examination of the widely excised breast tumor confirms clear margins. For this reason, some perform breast conservation surgery in two stages.[148]

Isolated axillary node involvement with metastatic adenocarcinoma in the absence of an identifiable primary lesion represents an unusual and challenging manifestation of clinically occult invasive breast carcinoma.[158] Ipsilateral mastectomy has been recommended in this setting if no extramammary foci of malignancy are found, even in the absence of any clinical or mammographic findings in the breast.[17, 117] Recently it has been found that a substantial number of such breasts do not harbor any malignancy, which may account for the good results of mastectomy in the past.[120] Axillary dissection and breast irradiation have thus been suggested as an alternative option, although a thorough physical examination and mammography are still important in order to exclude an identifiable primary lesion.[120, 232]

Implications of Time and Interval Between Diagnosis and Treatment

It was once theorized that the manipulation of a breast carcinoma during the diagnostic biopsy resulted in the distant spread of tumor cells and that this was a major contributor to metastasis. This belief led to the practice of immediate definitive mastectomy following diagnostic biopsy,[103] a practice that persisted through the 1970s. Some surgeons in the early part of this century based their diagnosis and therapeutic decision on the gross inspection of the tumor, partly to minimize the time interval to definitive treatment.[31] Others in these early years advocated careful diagnostic evaluation of permanent sections prior to embarking on surgery.[38] The development of the frozen section examination[236] provided the opportunity to make a rapid microscopic diagnosis, which facilitated the performance of immediate definitive surgery.[94] Tyzzer's experimental work reinforced this philosophy by demonstrating the development of metastatic disease in mice following tumor manipulation,[221] though evidence to support this observation in humans has never been reported.[68] Accurate and thorough pathological analysis is especially important for the early, borderline breast lesions discussed in this chapter and is currently felt to outweigh any need for rapid diagnosis by frozen section, which is suboptimal in its accuracy when compared to permanent paraffin sections.[68]

Therefore the two-stage procedure, in which diagnosis is temporally dissociated from definitive treatment, is currently the standard practice for small, early breast carcinomas. Evidence now indicates that there is no difference in survival between the one-stage and two-stage procedures.[72] However, the one-stage procedure carries the risk of diagnostic error inherent in the limitations of frozen section examination for *in situ* and clinically occult invasive malignancies.[119]

Role of Adjuvant Therapy

The role and importance of adjuvant radiation therapy in breast-sparing treatment for early breast carcinoma has already been discussed. Chemotherapy may be used in the treatment of clinically occult invasive breast carcinoma, with the purpose of diminishing the numbers of tumor cells that have spread systemically to a point that would allow the body's own host defense mechanisms to prevent their growth into a clinically evident tumor. In view of the known toxicity of these agents, their use has been recommended only in circumstances in which reliable clinical indications of systemic disease

are present (such as axillary nodal metastasis) and in which there is solid evidence of efficacy, such as in premenopausal females.[12] Some[149, 186] have also advocated the use of chemotherapy in patients with small tumors and no axillary lymph node involvement who manifest any of the risk factors for recurrence mentioned previously (see Table 35–8), although no benefit has yet been conclusively shown for these patients. A clinical alert from the National Cancer Institute has recently summarized the findings of three as-yet-unpublished studies purporting to show a significant survival advantage among women with node-negative clinically occult invasive breast carcinoma receiving adjuvant chemotherapy.[11] On the other hand, a recent overview of the results of adjuvant chemotherapy for breast carcinoma during the past 25 years indicated that no clear improvement in overall survival could be demonstrated and that the improvements that have been reported in disease-free survival appear to diminish with time.[118] There is no evidence that chemotherapy has any benefit for patients with *in situ* breast carcinoma.

Hormonal manipulation has shown some benefit in patients with breast carcinoma who relapse after primary treatment. This benefit tends to be more closely associated with the presence of estrogen receptor activity in the metastatic lesions rather than in the primary tumor.[107] Surgical oophorectomy has resulted in significant response rates in premenopausal females with recurrent disease but has been supplanted by the antiestrogen drug tamoxifen. Evidence exists that some metastatic lesions respond to tamoxifen even in the absence of estrogen receptor activity.[227] Current research efforts are directed at the use of hormonal therapy as a primary treatment for breast carcinoma, although results have not yet shown any distinct benefit in this setting.[107]

Management of the Contralateral Breast

The nature, extent, and uncertain clinical significance of occult foci of malignancy in the contralateral breast in patients with a primary breast carcinoma has already been discussed. Random contralateral biopsy samples yield malignancies in as many as 15 percent to 20 percent of these breasts.[78, 170, 173, 222] Most current evidence indicates that contralateral breast carcinoma has at least as favorable a prognosis as the ipsilateral carcinoma and thus should generally not influence the overall survival.[128, 207] Clinically evident malignancy develops in the contralateral breasts of only a small minority of women with primary breast carcinoma.[153, 174] This suggests that routine contralateral mastectomy or even blind contralateral biopsy would represent an unnecessary degree of overtreatment in these women. In view of these considerations, most surgeons manage the opposite breast with diligent lifelong surveillance, and biopsy or treatment is carried out only on the basis of clinically evident indications of malignancy.

SUMMARY

Research in the field of *in situ* and clinically occult invasive breast carcinoma has led to advances in our understanding of the physiology and epidemiology of these diseases, which has resulted in some of the most significant reductions in mortality from cancer in this century. Current investigations of the genetic patterns of breast carcinoma through flow cytometry and onco-gene analysis may significantly expand our diagnostic and prognostic capabilities. Treatment may also be improved with these modalities, which may allow an alteration of the earliest phases of the development of breast carcinoma through molecular biology.[155] The current trend toward a multidisciplinary management of the disease promises to optimize treatment results by providing early diagnosis and efficient, comprehensive follow-up.[104] Certainly an understanding of these earliest phases of breast malignancy may help to answer the many persistent questions concerning the biology of this disease. The physician involved in the management of these patients must be committed to such an understanding and able to rationally integrate what is known about this disease with the specific psychological and emotional patterns of the patient in order to maximize the success of treatment.

References

1. Ackerman LV, Katzenstein AL: The concept of minimal breast cancer and the pathologist's role in the diagnosis of "early carcinoma." Cancer 39:2755–2763, 1977.
2. Adair F, Berg J, Jonbert L, et al: Long term followup of breast cancer patients: One 30 year report. Cancer 33:1145–1152, 1974.
3. Albano WA, Hanf CD, Organ CH: Natural history of lymph node-negative breast cancer. Surgery 86:574–577, 1979.
4. Alpers CE, Wellings SR: The prevalence of carcinoma in situ in normal and cancer-associated breasts. Human Pathol 16:796–807, 1985.
5. Amalric R, Santamaria F, Robert F, et al: Conservation therapy of operable breast cancer—results at five, ten and fifteen years in 2216 consecutive cases. *In* Harris JR, Hellman S, Silen W (eds): Conservative Management of Breast Cancer. Philadelphia, JB Lippincott, 1983, pp 15–21.
6. Andersen JA: The basement membrane and lobular carcinoma in situ of the breast: a light microscopic study. Acta Pathol Microbiol Scand 83:245–250, 1975.
7. Andersen JA: Lobular carcinoma in situ of the breast: an approach to rational treatment. Cancer 39:2597–2602, 1977.
8. Andersen JA, Fechner RE, Lattes R, et al: Lobular carcinoma in situ (lobular neoplasia) of the breast (a symposium). Pathol Ann 15:193–223, 1980.
9. Andersen JA, Fischermann K, Hou-Jensen K, et al: Selection of high risk groups among prognostically favorable patients with breast cancer: an analysis of the value of prospective grading of tumor anaplasia in 1048 patients. Ann Surg 194:1–3, 1981.
10. Andersen JA, Schiodt T: On the concept of carcinoma in situ of the breast. Pathol Res Pract 166:407–414, 1980.
11. Anonymous: Clinical alert from the National Cancer Institute. Bethesda, MD, Department of Health and Human Services, May 16, 1988.
12. Anonymous: Consensus conference: adjuvant chemotherapy for breast cancer. JAMA 254:3461–3463, 1985.
13. Anonymous: Intraduct carcinoma of the breast (editorial). Lancet 2:24, 1984.
14. Ashikari R, Hajdu SI, Robbins GF: Intraductal carcinoma of the breast (1960–1969). Cancer 28:1182–1187, 1971.
15. Ashikari R, Huvos AG, Snyder RE, et al: A clinicopathologic study of atypical lesions of the breast. Cancer 33:310–317, 1974.
16. Ashikari R, Huvos AG, Urban JA, et al: Infiltrating lobular carcinoma of the breast. Cancer 31:110–116, 1973.
17. Ashikari R, Rosen PP, Urban JA, et al: Breast cancer presenting as an axillary mass. Ann Surg 183:415–417, 1976.
18. Auchincloss H: The nature of local recurrence following radical mastectomy. Cancer 11:611–619, 1958.
19. Auchincloss H: Conservative surgery. *In* Nealon TF (ed): Problems in General Surgery, vol 2(2). Philadelphia, JB Lippincott, 1985, pp 172–174.
20. Barnes JP: Bilateral lobular carcinoma in situ of the breast. Tex Med 55:581–584, 1959.
21. Beahrs O, Shapiro S, Smart C.: Report of the working group to review the National Cancer Institute/American Cancer Society breast cancer detection demonstration projects. J Natl Cancer Inst 62:639–710, 1979.
22. Bedrossian CWM, Raber M, Barlogie B: Flow cytometry and cytomorphology in primary resectable breast carcinomas. Anal Quant Cytol 3:112–116, 1981.
23. Bedwani R, Vana J, Rosner D, et al: Management and survival of female patients with "minimal" breast cancer: as observed in the long-term and short-term surveys of the American College of Surgeons. Cancer 47:2769–2778, 1981.
24. Benfield JR, Fingerhut AG, Warner NE: Lobular carcinoma of the breast 1969: a therapeutic proposal. Arch Surg 99:129–131, 1969.
25. Benfield JR, Jacobson M, Warner NE: In situ lobular carcinoma of the breast. Arch Surg 91:130–135, 1965.
26. Betsill WL, Rosen PP, Lieberman PH, et al: Intraductal carcinoma: long term follow-up after treatment by biopsy alone. JAMA 239:1863–1867, 1978.
27. Bilik R, Mor C, Wolloch Y, et al: Histopathologic high risk factors influencing the prognosis of patients with early breast cancer ($T_1N_0M_0$). Am J Surg 151:460–464, 1986.
28. Black MM, Barclay THC, Cutler SJ, et al: Association of atypical characteristics of benign breast lesions with subsequent risk of breast cancer. Cancer 29:338–343, 1972.
29. Bloodgood JC: Cancer of the breast: figures which show that education can increase the number of cures. JAMA 66:552–553, 1916.
30. Bloodgood JC: The pathology of chronic cystic mastitis of the female breast. Arch Surg 3:445–542, 1921.
31. Bloodgood JC: Borderline breast tumors. Ann Surg 93:235–249, 1931.
32. Bloodgood JC: Comedo carcinoma (or comedo-adenoma) of the female breast. Am J Cancer 22:842–853, 1934.
33. Bloom HJG, Richardson WW, Harries EJ: Natural history of untreated breast cancer (1805–1933): comparison of untreated and treated cases according to histological grade of malignancy. Br Med J 2:213–221, 1962.
34. Broders AC: Carcinoma in situ contrasted with benign penetrating epithelium. JAMA 99:1670–1674, 1932.
35. Brown PW, Silverman J, Owens E, et al: Intraductal "noninfiltrating" carcinoma of the breast. Arch Surg 111:1063–1067, 1976.
36. Cady B: Local excision and radiation therapy for early carcinoma of the breast. *In* Nealon TF (ed): Problems in General Surgery, vol 2(2). Philadelphia, JB Lippincott, 1985, pp 167–171.
37. Carter D, Smith RL: Carcinoma in situ of the breast. Cancer 40:1189–1193, 1977.
38. Cheatle GL: Early recognition of cancer of the breast. Br Med J 1:1205–1210, 1906.
39. Cheatle GL: Cysts, and primary cancer in cysts of the breast. Br J Surg 8:149–166; 1920–1921.
40. Cheatle GL, Cutler M: Tumors of the Breast. Philadelphia, JB Lippincott, 1931.
41. Christopherson WM: The changing concepts of early cancer. J Med Assoc Alabama 35:261–266, 1965.
42. Contesso JC, Delarue J, Mouriesse H, et al: Correlation between hormone receptors and histological characters in human breast tumors. Pathol Biol 31:747–754, 1983.
43. Cornil A-V: Les Tumeurs du Sein. Paris, Libraire Germer Bailliere and Company, 1908.
44. Crile G Jr: Treatment of breast cancer by local excision. Am J Surg 109:400–403, 1965.
45. Crile G Jr: Relationship of the size of the tumor and the size of involved nodes to survival. Am J Surg 124:35–38, 1972.

46. Curletti E, Giordano J: In situ lobular carcinoma of the breast. Arch Surg 116:309–310, 1981.
47. Dall'Olmo CA, Ponka JL, Horn RC, et al: Lobular carcinoma of the breast in situ. Arch Surg 110:537–542, 1975.
48. Davis N, Baird RM: Breast cancer in association with lobular carcinoma in situ: clinicopathologic review and treatment recommendation. Am J Surg 147:641–645, 1984.
49. Davis RP, Nora PF, Kooy RG, et al: Experience with lobular carcinoma of the breast: emphasis on recent aspects of management. Arch Surg 114:485–488, 1979.
50. Dobson J: John Hunter's views on cancer. Ann R Coll Surg Engl 1:176–181, 1959.
51. Donegan WL, Say CG: Invasive carcinoma of the breast: prognostic significance of tumor size and involved axillary lymph nodes. Cancer 34:468–471, 1974.
52. Dressler LG, Seamer LC, Owen SMA, et al: DNA flow cytometry and prognostic factors in 1331 frozen breast specimens. Cancer 61:420–427, 1988.
53. Dupont WD, Page DL: Risk factors in women with proliferative breast disease. N Engl J Med 312:146–151, 1985.
54. Ewing J: Neoplastic Diseases, ed 1. Philadelphia, WB Saunders, 1919.
55. Farrow JH: Clinical considerations and treatment of in situ lobular breast cancer. Am J Roentgenol 102:652–656, 1968.
56. Farrow JH: Current concepts in the detection and treatment of the earliest of early breast cancers. Cancer 25:468–477, 1970.
57. Fechner RE: Ductal carcinoma involving the lobule of the breast: a source of confusion with lobular carcinoma in situ. Cancer 28:274–281, 1971.
58. Fechner RE: Infiltrating lobular carcinoma without lobular carcinoma in situ. Cancer 29:1539–1545, 1972.
59. Feig SA, Schwartz GF, Nerlinger R, et al: Prognostic factors of breast neoplasms detected on screening by mammography and physical examination. Radiology 133:577–582, 1979.
60. Findlay P, Goodman R: Radiation therapy for treatment of intraductal carcinoma of the breast. Am J Clin Oncol 6:281–285, 1983.
61. Fisher B, Bauer M, Margolese R, et al: Five year results of a randomized clinical trial: comparing total mastectomy and segmental mastectomy with or without radiation in the treatment of breast cancer. N Engl J Med 312:665–673, 1985.
62. Fisher B, Bauer M, Wickerham DL, et al: Relationship of number of positive axillary nodes to the prognosis of patients with primary breast cancer—an NSABP update. Cancer 52:1551–1557, 1983.
63. Fisher B, Montague E, Redmond C, et al: Comparison of radical mastectomy with alternative treatments for primary breast cancer: a first report of results from a prospective randomized clinical trial. Cancer 39:2827–2839, 1977.
64. Fisher B, Redmond C, Fisher ER, et al: Ten-year results of a randomized clinical trial comparing radical mastectomy and total mastectomy with and without radiation. N Engl J Med 312:674–681, 1985.
65. Fisher B, Redmond C, Fisher ER, et al: Relative worth of estrogen or progesterone receptor and pathologic characteristics of differentiation as indicators of prognosis in node-negative breast cancer patients: findings from National Surgical Adjuvant Breast and Bowel Project B-06. J Clin Oncol 6:1076–1087, 1988.
66. Fisher B, Slack NH, Katrych D, et al: Ten-year followup results of patients with carcinoma of the breast in a cooperative clinical trial evaluating surgical adjuvant chemotherapy. Surg Gynecol Obstet 140:528–534, 1975.
67. Fisher B, Wolmark N, Bauer M, et al: The accuracy of clinical nodal staging and of limited axillary dissection as a determinant of histological node status in carcinoma of the breast. Surg Gynecol Obstet 152:765–772, 1981.
68. Fisher ER: The impact of pathology on the biologic, diagnostic, prognostic and therapeutic considerations in breast cancer. Surg Clin North Am 64:1073–1093, 1984.
69. Fisher ER, Fisher B: Lobular carcinoma of the breast: an overview. Ann Surg 195:377–385, 1977.
70. Fisher ER, Gregorio R, Fisher B: The pathology of invasive cancer: a syllabus derived from the findings of the National Surgical Adjuvant Breast Project (protocol 4). Cancer 36:1–85, 1975.
71. Fisher ER, Sass R, Fisher B: Pathologic findings from the National Surgical Adjuvant Project for Breast Cancers (protocol 4), X. Discriminants for tenth year treatment failure. Cancer 53:712–723, 1984.
72. Fisher ER, Sass R, Fisher B: Biologic considerations regarding the one and two step procedures in the management of patients with invasive carcinoma of the breast. Surg Gynecol Obstet 161:245–249, 1985.
73. Fisher ER, Sass R, Fisher B, et al: Pathologic findings from the National Surgical Adjuvant Breast Project (protocol 6), II. Relation of local breast recurrence to multicentricity. Cancer 57:1717–1724, 1986.
74. Fisher ER, Sass R, Fisher B, et al: Pathologic findings from the National Surgical Adjuvant Breast Project (protocol 6), I. Intraductal carcinoma (DCIS). Cancer 57:197–208, 1986.
75. Foote FW, Stewart FW: Lobular carcinoma in situ: a rare form of mammary carcinoma. Am J Pathol 17:491–495, 1941.
76. Foote FW Jr, Stewart FW: A histologic classification of carcinoma of the breast. Surgery 19:74–99, 1946.
77. Fossa SD, Thorud E, Vaage S, et al: DNA cytometry of primary breast cancer: a comparison of microspectrophotometry and flow cytometry and different preparation methods for flow cytometric measurements. Acta Pathol Microbiol Immunol Scand 91:235–247, 1983.
78. Fracchia AA, Robinson D, Legaspi A, et al: Survival in bilateral breast cancer. Cancer 55:1414–1421, 1985.
79. Frazier TG, Copeland EM, Gallager HS, et al: Prognosis and treatment in minimal breast cancer. Am J Surg 133:697–701, 1977.
80. Friedman N: The effects of irradiation on breast cancer and the breast. CA 38:368–371, 1988.
81. Frykberg ER, Bland KI, Copeland EM: The detection and treatment of early breast cancer. In Tompkins RK (ed): Advances in Surgery, vol 23. Chicago, Year Book Medical Publishers, 1990.
82. Frykberg ER, Santiago F, Betsill WL Jr, et al: Lobular carcinoma in situ of the breast. Surg Gynecol Obstet 164:285–301, 1987.
83. Gallager HS: Minimal breast cancer: results of treatment and long-term follow-up. In Feig SA, McLelland R (eds): Breast Carcinoma: Current Diagnosis and Treatment. New York, Masson Publishing USA, 1983, pp 291–294.
84. Gallager HS: Multicentricity in breast cancer. In Harris JR, Hellman S, Silen W (eds): Conservative Management of Breast Cancer. Philadelphia, JB Lippincott, 1983.
85. Gallager HS, Martin JE: The study of mammary carcinoma by mammography and whole organ sectioning. Cancer 23:855–873, 1969.
86. Gallager HS, Martin JE: Early phases in the development of breast cancer. Cancer 24:1170–1178, 1969.
87. Gallager HS, Martin JE: An orientation to the concept of minimal breast cancer. Cancer 28:1505–1507, 1971.
88. Gemsenjager E, Gyr K: Letter. Surg Gynecol Obstet 157:367–368, 1983.
89. Gilliland MD, Barton RM, Copeland EM III: The implications of local recurrence of breast cancer as the first site of therapeutic failure. Ann Surg 197:284–287, 1983.
90. Gillis DA, Dockerty MB, Clagett OT: Preinvasive intraductal carcinoma of the breast. Surg Gynecol Obstet 110:555–562, 1960.
91. Giordano JM, Klopp CT: Lobular carcinoma in situ: incidence and treatment. Cancer 31:105–109, 1973.
92. Godwin JT: Chronology of lobular carcinoma of the breast: report of a case. Cancer 5:229–266, 1952.
93. Goodnight JE, Quagliana JM, Morton DL: Failure of subcutaneous mastectomy to prevent the development of breast cancer. J Surg Oncol 26:198–201, 1984.
94. Greenough RB: Early diagnosis of cancer of the breast. Ann Surg 102:233–238, 1935.
95. Gullino PM: Natural history of breast cancer: progression from hyperplasia to neoplasia as predicted by angiogenesis. Cancer 39:2697–2703, 1977.
96. Gump FE: In situ cancers. In Harris JR, Hellman S, Henderson IC, et al (eds): Breast Diseases. Philadelphia, JB Lippincott, 1987.
97. Gump FE, Shikora S, Habif DV, et al: The extent and distri-

bution of cancer in breasts with palpable primary tumors. Ann Surg 204:384–390, 1986.

98. Haagensen CD: Treatment of curable carcinoma of the breast. Int J Radiat Oncol Biol Phys 2:975–980, 1977.

99. Haagensen CD: Diseases of the Breast, ed 3. Philadelphia, WB Saunders, 1986.

100. Haagensen CD, Bodian C: A personal experience with Halsted's radical mastectomy. Ann Surg 199:143–150, 1984.

101. Haagensen CD, Lane N, Lattes R: Neoplastic proliferation of the epithelium of the mammary lobules: adenosis, lobular neoplasia, and small cell carcinoma. Surg Clin North Am 52:497–524, 1972.

102. Haagensen CD, Lane N, Lattes R, et al: Lobular neoplasia (so-called lobular carcinoma in situ) of the breast. Cancer 42:737–769, 1978.

103. Halsted WS: The results of radical operations for the cure of carcinoma of the breast. Ann Surg 46:1–19, 1907.

104. Harness JK, Bartlett RH, Saran PA, et al: Developing a comprehensive breast center. Am Surg 53:419–423, 1987.

105. Harris JR, Connolly JL, Schnitt SJ, et al: Clinical-pathologic study of early breast cancer treated by primary radiation therapy. J Clin Oncol 1:184–189, 1983.

106. Harris JR, Hellman S: The results of primary radiation therapy for early breast cancer at the Joint Center for Radiation Therapy. In Harris JR, Hellman S, Silen W (eds): Conservative Management of Breast Cancer. Philadelphia, JB Lippincott, 1983, pp 47–52.

107. Harris JR, Hellman S, Canellos GP, et al: Cancer of the breast. In Devita VT, Hellman S, Rosenberg SA (eds): Cancer: Principles and Practice of Oncology, ed 2. Philadelphia, JB Lippincott, 1985, pp 1119–1177.

108. Harris JR, Henderson IC: Natural history and staging of breast cancer. In Harris JR, Hellman S, Henderson IC, et al (eds): Breast Diseases. Philadelphia, JB Lippincott, 1987, pp 233–258.

109. Harris JR, Recht A, Amalric R, et al: Time course and prognosis of local recurrence following primary radiation therapy for early breast cancer. J Clin Oncol 2:37–41, 1984.

110. Hartmann WJ: Minimal breast cancer: an update. Cancer 53:681–684, 1984.

111. Heller KS, Rosen PP, Schottenfeld D, et al: Male breast cancer: a clinicopathologic study of 97 cases. Ann Surg 188:60–68, 1978.

112. Holland R, Veling SHJ, Mravunac M, et al: Histologic multifocality of T_{1s}, T_{1-2} breast carcinoma. Cancer 56:979–990, 1985.

113. Host H, Lund E: Age as a prognostic factor in breast cancer. Cancer 57:2217–2221, 1986.

114. Hutter RVP: The pathologist's role in minimal breast cancer. Cancer 28:1527–1536, 1971.

115. Hutter RVP: The management of patients with lobular carcinoma in situ of the breast. Cancer 53:798–802, 1984.

116. Hutter RVP, Foote FW: Lobular carcinoma in situ. Cancer 24:1081–1085, 1969.

117. Iglehart JD, Ferguson BJ, Shingleton WW, et al: An ultrastructural analysis of breast carcinoma presenting as isolated axillary adenopathy. Ann Surg 196:8–13, 1982.

118. James AG: How effective is adjuvant cancer chemotherapy? Arch Surg 121:1233–1236, 1986.

119. Kagali VA: The role and limitations of frozen section diagnosis of a palpable mass in the breast. Surg Gynecol Obstet 156:168–170, 1983.

120. Kemeny MM, Rivera DE, Terz JJ, et al: Occult primary adenocarcinoma with axillary metastases. Am J Surg 152:43–47, 1986.

121. Keynes G: Radium treatment of primary carcinoma of the breast. Lancet 2:108–111, 1928.

122. Koscielny S, Tubiana M, Le MG, et al: Breast cancer: relationship between the size of the primary tumour and the probability of metastatic dissemination. Br J Cancer 49:709–715, 1984.

123. Kramer WM, Rush BF Jr: Mammary duct proliferation in the elderly. Cancer 31:130–137, 1973.

124. Kurtz JM, Amalric R, Brandone H, et al: Results of salvage surgery for mammary recurrence following breast-conserving therapy. Ann Surg 207:347–351, 1988.

125. Lagios MD, Westdahl PR, Margolin FR, et al: Duct carcinoma in situ: relationship of extent of noninvasive disease to the frequency of occult invasion, multicentricity, lymph node metastases and short-term treatment failures. Cancer 50:1309–1314, 1982.

126. Landercasper J, Gundersen SB, Gundersen AL, et al: Needle localization and biopsy of nonpalpable lesions of the breast. Surg Gynecol Obstet 164:399–403, 1987.

127. Lattes R: Lobular neoplasia (lobular carcinoma in situ) of the breast—a histological entity of controversial clinical significance. Pathol Res Pract 166:415–429, 1980.

128. Leis HP: Selective, elective, prophylactic contralateral mastectomy. Cancer 28:956–961, 1971.

129. Lesser ML, Rosen PP, Kinne DW: Multicentricity and bilaterality in invasive breast carcinoma. Surgery 91:234–240, 1982.

130. Lewis D, Geschickter CF: Comedo carcinoma of the breast. Arch Surg 36:225–244, 1938.

131. Lewis JD, Milbrath JR, Shaffer KA, et al: Implications of suspicious findings in breast cancer screening. Arch Surg 110:903–906, 1975.

132. Lewison EF: Lobular carcinoma in situ of the breast. Am Surg 31:787–789, 1965.

133. Mackay EN, Sellars AH: Breast cancer at the Ontario clinics: a statistical review. Ottawa, Ontario Department of Health, Medical Statistics Branch, 1938–1956, 1965.

134. Masood S: Use of monoclonal antibody for assessment of estrogen receptor content in fine needle aspiration biopsy specimens from patients with breast carcinoma. Arch Pathol Lab Med 113:26–30, 1989.

135. Mate TP, Carter D, Fischer DB, et al: A clinical and histopathologic analysis of the results of conservation surgery and radiation therapy in stage I and II breast carcinoma. Cancer 58:1995–2002, 1986.

136. McDivitt RW, Hutter RVP, Foote FW, et al: In situ lobular carcinoma: a prospective follow-up study indicating cumulative patient risks. JAMA 201:96–100, 1967.

137. McDivitt RW, Stewart FW, Berg JW: Tumors of the breast. Washington, DC, Armed Forces Institute of Pathology, 1968, pp 63–85.

138. McWhirter R: The value of simple mastectomy and radiotherapy in the treatment of cancer of the breast. Br J Radiol 21:599–604, 1948.

139. Meyer JS, Hixon B: Advanced stage and early relapse of breast carcinomas associated with high thymidine labelling indices. Cancer Res 39:4042–4047, 1979.

140. Meyer W: An improved method of the radical operation for carcinoma of the breast. Med Rec 46:746–749, 1894.

141. Miller HW, Kay S: Infiltrating lobular carcinoma of the female mammary gland. Surg Gynecol Obstet 102:661–667, 1956.

142. Millis RR, Thynne GSJ: In situ intraduct carcinoma of the breast: a long term follow-up study. Br J Surg 62:957–962, 1975.

143. Montague ED: Conservative surgery and radiation therapy in the treatment of operable breast cancer. Cancer 53:700–704, 1984.

144. Morris DM, Walker AP, Coker DC: Lack of efficacy of xeromammography in preoperatively detecting lobular carcinoma in situ of the breast. Breast Cancer Res Treat 1:365–367, 1982.

145. Muir R: Evolution of carcinoma of the mamma. J Pathol Bact 52:155–172, 1941.

146. Munoz E, Shamash F, Friedman M, et al: Lumpectomy vs. mastectomy: the costs of breast preservation for cancer. Arch Surg 121:1297–1301, 1986.

147. Mustakallio S: Treatment of breast cancer by tumor extirpation and roentgen therapy instead of radical operation. J Fac Radiol 6:23–26, 1954.

148. Nealon TF: Choice of operation based on histology of the tumor. In Nealon TF (ed): Problems in General Surgery, vol 2(2). Philadelphia, JB Lippincott, 1985, pp 175–184.

149. Nealon TF, Nkongho A, Grossi C, et al: Pathologic identification of poor prognosis stage I ($T_1N_0M_0$) cancer of the breast. Ann Surg 190:129–132, 1979.

150. Nemoto T, Vana J, Bedwani RN, et al: Management and survival of female breast cancer: results of a national survey by the American College of Surgeons. Cancer 45:2917–2924, 1980.

151. Newman W: In situ lobular carcinoma of the breast: report of 26 women with 32 cancers. Ann Surg 157:591–599, 1963.

152. Newman W: Lobular carcinoma of the female breast: report of 73 cases. Ann Surg 164:305–314, 1966.
153. Nielsen M, Chritensen L, Andersen JA: Contralateral cancerous breast lesions in women with clinical invasive breast carcinoma. Cancer 57:897–903, 1986.
154. Nielsen M, Jensen J, Andersen JA: Precancerous and cancerous breast lesions during lifetime and at autopsy. Cancer 54:612–615, 1984.
155. Nowell PC: Molecular events in tumor development. N Engl J Med 319:575–577, 1988.
156. Osborne MP: Limited resection and radical radiation therapy in the treatment of early stage breast cancer. In Nealon TF (ed): Problems in General Surgery, vol 2(2). Philadelphia, JB Lippincott, 1985, pp 159–166.
157. Osborne MP, Ormiston M, Harmer CC, et al: Breast conservation in the treatment of early breast cancer. Cancer 53:349–355, 1984.
158. Owen HW, Dockery MB, Gray HK: Occult carcinoma of the breast. Surg Gynecol Obstet 58:302–308, 1954.
159. Ozzello L: The behavior of basement membranes in intraductal carcinoma of the breast. Am J Pathol 35:887–899, 1959.
160. Ozzello L: Ultrastructure of intra-epithelial carcinomas of the breast. Cancer 28:1508–1515, 1971.
161. Ozzello L, Sanpitak P: Epithelial-stromal junction of intraductal carcinoma of the breast. Cancer 26:1186–1198, 1970.
162. Page DL: Cancer risk assessment in benign breast biopsies. Human Pathol 9:871–874, 1986.
163. Page DL, Dupont WD, Rogers LW, et al: Intraductal carcinoma of the breast. Cancer 49:751–758, 1982.
164. Page DL, Dupont WD, Rogers LW, et al: Atypical hyperplastic lesions of the female breast: a long-term follow-up study. Cancer 55:2698–2708, 1985.
165. Page DL, VanderZwaag R, Rogers LW, et al: Relation between component parts of fibrocystic disease complex and breast cancer. J Natl Cancer Inst 61:1055–1063, 1978.
166. Pertschuk LP, Eisenberg KB, Carter AC, et al: Immunohistologic localization of estrogen receptors in breast cancer with monoclonal antibodies: correlation with biochemistry and clinical endocrine response. Cancer 55:1513–1518, 1985.
167. Peters MV: Wedge resection and irradiation: an effective treatment in early breast cancer. JAMA 200:144–145, 1967.
168. Peterson CG: The treatment of breast cancer: II. A 20-year follow-up and reappraisal of the en bloc principle. Arch Surg 123:1059–1062, 1988.
169. Powers RW, O'Brien PH, Kreutner A: Lobular carcinoma in situ. J Surg Oncol 13:269–273, 1980.
170. Pressman PI: Selective biopsy of the opposite breast. Cancer 57:577–580, 1986.
171. Qualheim RE, Gall EA: Breast carcinoma with multiple sites of origin. Cancer 10:460–468, 1957.
172. Recht A, Danoff BS, Solin LJ, et al: Intraductal carcinoma of the breast: results of treatment with excisional biopsy and radiation. J Clin Oncol 3:1339–1343, 1985.
173. Ringberg A, Palmer B, Linell F: The contralateral breast at reconstructive surgery after breast cancer operation—a histological study. Breast Cancer Res Treat 2:151–161, 1982.
174. Robbins GF, Berg JW: Bilateral primary breast cancers: a prospective clinicopathological study. Cancer 17:1501–1527, 1964.
175. Robinson JO: Treatment of breast cancer through the ages. Am J Surg 151:317–333, 1986.
176. Rodes ND, Lopez MJ, Pearson DK, et al: The impact of breast cancer screening on survival: a 5 to 10 year follow-up study. Cancer 57:581–585, 1986.
177. Rosen PP: Coexistent lobular carcinoma in situ and intraductal carcinoma in a single lobular-duct unit. Am J Surg Pathol 4:241–246, 1980.
178. Rosen PP: Axillary lymph node metastases in patients with occult noninvasive breast carcinoma. Cancer 46:1298–1306, 1980.
179. Rosen PP: Lobular carcinoma in situ: recent clinicopathologic studies at Memorial Hospital. Pathol Res Pract 166:430–455, 1980.
180. Rosen PP: Clinical implications of preinvasive and small invasive breast carcinomas. Pathol Ann 16:337–356, 1981.
181. Rosen PP: Lobular carcinoma in situ and intraductal carcinoma of the breast. Monogr Pathol 25:59–105, 1984.
182. Rosen PP, Braun DW, Kinne DE: The clinical significance of preinvasive breast carcinoma. Cancer 46:919–925, 1980.
183. Rosen PP, Braun DW, Lyngholm B, et al: Lobular carcinoma in situ of the breast: preliminary results of treatment by ipsilateral mastectomy and contralateral breast biopsy. Cancer 47:813–819, 1981.
184. Rosen PP, Lesser ML, Kinne DW, et al: Discontinuous or "skip" metastases in breast carcinoma: Analysis of 1228 axillary dissections. Ann Surg 197:276–283, 1983.
185. Rosen PP, Lieberman PH, Braun DW, et al: Lobular carcinoma in situ of the breast: detailed analysis of 99 patients with average follow-up of 24 years. Am J Surg Pathol 3:225–251, 1978.
186. Rosen PP, Saigo PE, Braun DW, et al: Predictors of recurrence in stage I ($T_1N_0M_0$) breast carcinoma. Ann Surg 193:15–25, 1981.
187. Rosen PP, Saigo PE, Braun DW, et al: Axillary micro- and macrometastases in breast cancer: prognostic significance of tumor size. Ann Surg 194:585–591, 1981.
188. Rosen PP, Senie RT, Farr GH, et al: Epidemiology of breast carcinoma: age, menstrual status, and exogenous hormone usage in patients with lobular carcinoma in situ. Surgery 85:219–224, 1979.
189. Rosen PP, Senie RT, Schottenfeld D, et al: Noninvasive breast carcinoma: frequency of unsuspected invasion and implications for treatment. Ann Surg 189:377–382, 1979.
190. Roses DF, Bell DA, Flotte TJ, et al: Pathologic predictors of recurrence in stage I ($T_1N_0M_0$) breast cancer. Am J Clin Pathol 78:817–822, 1982.
191. Rosner D, Bedwani RN, Vana J, et al: Noninvasive breast carcinoma: results of a national survey by the American College of Surgeons. Ann Surg 192:139–147, 1980.
192. Schnitt SJ, Connolly JL, Harris JR, et al: Pathologic predictors of early local recurrence in stage I and II breast cancer treated by primary radiation therapy. Cancer 53:1049–1057, 1984.
193. Schnitt SJ, Silen W, Sadowsky NL, et al: Ductal carcinoma in situ (intraductal carcinoma) of the breast. N Engl J Med 318:898–903, 1988.
194. Schuh ME, Nemoto T, Penetrante RB, et al: Intraductal carcinoma: analysis of presentation, pathologic findings, and outcome of disease. Arch Surg 121:1303–1307, 1986.
195. Schwartz GF, D'Ugo M, Rosenberg AL: Extent of axillary dissection preceding irradiation for carcinoma of the breast. Arch Surg 121:1395–1398, 1986.
196. Schwartz GF, Feig SA, Patchefsky AS: Significance and staging of nonpalpable carcinomas of the breast. Surg Gynecol Obstet 166:6–10, 1988.
197. Schwartz GF, Feig SA, Rosenberg AL, et al: Staging and treatment of clinically occult breast cancer. Cancer 53:1379–1384, 1984.
198. Schwartz GF, Patchefsky AS, Feig SA, et al: Clinically occult breast cancer: multicentricity and implications for treatment. Ann Surg 191:8–12, 1980.
199. Schwartz GF, Patchefsky AS, Feig SA, et al: Multicentricity of nonpalpable breast cancer. Cancer 45:2913–2916, 1980.
200. Schwartz GF, Rosenberg AL, Danoff BF, et al: Lumpectomy and level I axillary dissection prior to irradiation for "operable" breast cancer. Ann Surg 200:554–560, 1984.
201. Seidman H, Gelb SK, Silverberg E, et al: Survival experience in the Breast Cancer Detection Demonstration Project. CA 37:258–290, 1987.
202. Sener SF, Candela FC, Paige ML, et al: Limitations of mammography in the identification of noninfiltrating carcinoma of the breast. Surg Gynecol Obstet 167:135–140, 1988.
203. Shah JP, Rosen PP, Robbins GF: Pitfalls of local excision in the treatment of carcinoma of the breast. Surg Gynecol Obstet 136:721–725, 1973.
204. Shapiro S, Venet W, Strax P, et al: Ten-to-fourteen year effect of screening on breast cancer mortality. J Natl Cancer Inst 69:349–355, 1982.
205. Shield AM: A Clinical Treatise on Diseases of the Breast. London, Macmillan, 1898.
206. Silverstein MJ, Rosser RJ, Gierson ED, et al: Axillary lymph node dissection for intraductal breast carcinoma—is it indicated? Cancer 59:1819–1824, 1987.

207. Slack NH, Bross IDJ, Nemoto T, et al: Experiences with bilateral primary carcinoma of the breast. Surg Gynecol Obstet 136:433–440, 1973.
208. Smart CR, Myers MH, Glockler LA: Implications from SEER data on breast cancer management. Cancer 41:787–789, 1978.
209. Somers SC: Histologic changes in incipient carcinoma of the breast. Cancer 23:822–825, 1969.
210. Stampfer MR, Viodavsky I, Smith HS, et al: Fibronectin production by human mammary cells. J Natl Cancer Inst 67:253–261, 1981.
211. Strax P: Mass screening for control of breast cancer. Cancer 53:665–670, 1984.
212. Sunshine JA, Moseley HS, Fletcher WS, et al: Breast carcinoma in situ: a retrospective review of 112 cases with a minimum of 10 year follow-up. Am J Surg 150:44–51, 1985.
213. Sutherland CM, Mather JF: Long-term survival and prognostic factors in breast cancer patients with localized (no skin, muscle or chest wall attachment) disease with and without positive lymph nodes. Cancer 57:622–629, 1986.
214. Sven-Borje E, Langstrom E, Baldetorp B, et al: Flow-cytometric DNA analysis in primary breast carcinomas and clinicopathologic correlations. Cytometry 5:408–415, 1984.
215. Swain SM, Lippman ME: Intraepithelial carcinoma of the breast: lobular carcinoma in situ and ductal carcinoma in situ. *In* Lippman ME, Lichter AS, Danforth DN Jr (eds): Diagnosis and Management of Breast Cancer. Philadelphia, WB Saunders, 1988, pp 296–325.
216. Tabar L, Fagerberg CJG, Gad A, et al: Reduction in mortality from breast cancer after mass screening with mammography. Lancet 1:829–832, 1985.
217. Tinnemans JGM, Wobbes T, Van der Sluis RF, et al: Multicentricity in nonpalpable breast carcinoma and its implications for treatment. Am J Surg 151:334–338, 1986.
218. Tobon H, Price HM: Lobular carcinoma in situ: some ultrastructural observations. Cancer 30:1082–1091, 1972.
219. Tubiana M, Chauvel P, Renaud A, et al: Growth rate and natural history of human breast cancers. Bull Cancer 62:341–358, 1975.
220. Tulusan AA, Egger H, Schneider ML, et al: A contribution to the natural history of breast cancer: lobular carcinoma in situ and its relation to breast cancer. Arch Gynecol 231:219–226, 1982.
221. Tyzzer EE: Factors in the production and growth of tumor metastases. J Med Res 28:309–333, 1913.
222. Urban JA: Bilaterality of cancer of the breast. Cancer 20:1867–1870, 1967.
223. Urban JA: Biopsy of the "normal" breast in treating breast cancer. Surg Clin North Am 49:291–301, 1969.
224. Valagussa P, Bonadonna G, Veronesi U: Patterns of relapse and survival following radical mastectomy. Cancer 41:1170–1178, 1978.
225. Veronesi U, Rilke F, Luini A, et al: Distribution of axillary node metastases by level of invasion: an analysis of 539 cases. Cancer 59:682–687, 1987.
226. Veronesi U, Saccozzi R, Del Vecchio M, et al: Comparing radical mastectomy with quadrantectomy, axillary dissection and radiotherapy in patients with small cancers of the breast. N Engl J Med 305:6–11, 1981.
227. Vogel CL, East DR, Voigt W, et al: Response to tamoxifen in estrogen receptor–poor metastatic breast cancer. Cancer 60:1184–1189, 1987.
228. Von Rueden DG, Wilson RE: Intraductal carcinoma of the breast. Surg Gynecol Obstet 158:105–111, 1984.
229. Warren JC: Abnormal involution of the mammary gland with its treatment by operation. Am J Med Sci 134:521–535, 1907.
230. Webber BL, Heise H, Neifeld JP, et al: Risk of subsequent contralateral breast carcinoma in a population of patients with in situ breast carcinoma. Cancer 47:2928–2932, 1981.
231. Wertheimer MD, Costanza ME, Dodson TF, et al: Increasing the effort toward breast cancer detection. JAMA 255:1311–1315, 1986.
232. Westbrook KC, Gallager HS: Breast carcinoma presenting as an axillary mass. Am J Surg 122:607–611, 1971.
233. Westbrook KC, Gallager HS: Intraductal carcinoma of the breast: a comparative study. Am J Surg 130:667–670, 1975.
234. Wheeler JE, Enterline HT: Lobular carcinoma of the breast in situ and infiltrating. Pathol Ann 11:161–188, 1976.
235. Wheeler JE, Enterline HT, Roseman JM, et al: Lobular carcinoma in situ of the breast: long-term follow-up. Cancer 34:554–563, 1974.
236. Wilson LB: A method for the rapid preparation of fresh tissue for the microscope. JAMA 45:1737, 1905.
237. Wise L, Mason AY, Ackerman LV: Local excision and irradiation: an alternative method for the treatment of early mammary cancer. Ann Surg 174:392–401, 1971.
238. Wolmark N: Minimal breast cancer: advance or anachronism? Can J Surg 28:252–255, 1985.
239. Zafrani B, Fourquet A, Vilcoq JR, et al: Conservative management of intraductal breast carcinoma with tumorectomy and radiation therapy. Cancer 57:1299–1301, 1986.
240. Zimmerman KW, Montague ED, Fletcher GH: Frequency, anatomical distribution and management of local recurrences after definitive therapy for breast cancer. Cancer 19:67–74, 1966.

Section XIV

Management of Stages I and II Breast Cancer

Chapter 36

CHOICE OF OPERATIONS FOR BREAST CANCER: CONSERVATIVE SURGERY VERSUS RADICAL PROCEDURES

Blake Cady, M.D.

SELECTION OF THERAPY IN EARLY BREAST CANCER

The definition of early breast cancer has been controversial and is not completely agreed on[61, 69]; for this chapter it will include breast cancers that could be expected to have better than a 75 percent disease-free survival rate at 10 years. Thus this would include cases that are noninvasive (T0) and all patients in stage I and stage IIa (Table 36–1).[2, 61] This arbitrary definition is chosen deliberately to highlight the surgeon's role in handling the increasing proportion of such patients and to emphasize the choice of decisions and the decision process regarding the management of the breast cancer itself, the breast as the host organ, and the patient, rather than the roles of adjuvant chemotherapy and hormone therapy, which are exhaustively presented in other chapters.

A few general comments should be made at the outset concerning general philosophy of treatment, approach to patients, use of early detection techniques, assessment of risk, and handling of the tissue specimens.

Primary breast cancer management is becoming increasingly complex, with rapid changes in management policy based on maturing clinical trials, new data, and the exploration of cellular prognostic indicators that may enable better treatment selection in more specific ways in the future. Because of the management complexity,

patient involvement in decision making is critical. Surgeons should accept the fact that this patient involvement requires a great deal of time in explanation and presentation of data as well as empathy and understanding about the complexity and anxiety the patients face. As long as surgeons are informed and willing to address the patients as individuals and include them in management decisions, and treatment facilities such as adequate pathology sophistication and radiotherapy units are available, modern breast cancer management can be conducted in any setting. Many patients are quite well informed through the public media about the turmoil in opinions and options in breast cancer management, and thus surgeons who do not explicitly recognize these aspects in dealing with their patients invite loss of confidence and a search for second opinions and consultations. Doctrinaire approaches to the management of early primary breast cancer ought to be avoided and programs that only recommend local excision are as improper as programs that only suggest mastectomy. Because the details of local breast cancer removal and management of the tissue specimen are critical to the conduct of contemporary breast cancer therapy, it is urged that surgeons seek special training and skill development in this area to develop confidence in breast-preserving therapy. The purpose of breast preservation therapy is cosmetic appearance, and it is vital that the details of the local breast cancer removal be well thought

753

Table 36–1. TNM BREAST CANCER CLASSIFICATION SYSTEM

Primary Tumor

TX		Primary tumor cannot be assessed
T0		No evidence of primary tumor
Tis		Carcinoma *in situ:* intraductal carcinoma, lobular carcinoma *in situ,* or Paget's disease of the nipple with no tumor
T1		Tumor 2 cm or less in greatest dimension
	T1a	0.5 cm or less in greatest dimension
	T1b	More than 0.5 cm but not more than 1 cm in greatest dimension
	T1c	More than 1 cm but not more than 2 cm in greatest dimension
T2		Tumor more than 2 cm but not more than 5 cm in greatest dimension
T3		Tumor more than 5 cm in greatest dimension
T4		Tumor of any size with direct extension to chest wall or skin
	T4a	Extension to chest wall
	T4b	Edema (including peau d'orange) or ulceration of the skin of the breast or satellite skin nodules confined to the same breast
	T4c	Both (T4a and T4b)

Regional Lymph Node

NX	Regional lymph nodes cannot be assessed (e.g., previously removed)
N0	No regional lymph node metastasis
N1	Metastasis to moveable ipsilateral axillary lymph nodes
N2	Metastasis to ipsilateral axillary lymph nodes fixed to one another or to other structures
N3	Metastasis to ipsilateral internal mammary lymph nodes

Pathological Classification (pN)

pNX		Regional lymph nodes cannot be assessed (e.g., previously removed or not removed for pathological study)
pN0		No regional lymph node metastasis
pN1		Metastasis to moveable ipsilateral axillary lymph nodes
	pN1a	Only micrometastasis (none larger than 0.2 cm)
	pN1b	Metastasis to lymph nodes, any larger than 0.2 cm
	pN1bi	Metastasis in 1 to 3 lymph nodes, any more than 0.2 cm, and all less than 2 cm in greatest dimension
	pN1bii	Metastasis to 4 or more lymph nodes, any more than 0.2 cm, and all less than 2 cm in greatest dimension
	pN1biii	Extension of tumor beyond the capsule of a lymph node metastasis less than 2 cm in greatest dimension
	pN1biv	Metastasis to a lymph node 2 cm or more in greatest dimension
pN2		Metastasis to ipsilateral axillary lymph nodes that are fixed to one another or to other structures
pN3		Metastasis to ipsilateral internal mammary lymph nodes

Distant Metastasis

MX	Presence of distant metastasis cannot be assessed
M0	No distant metastasis
M1	Distant metastasis (includes metastasis to ipsilateral supraclavicular lymph nodes)

Stage Grouping

Stage 0	Tis	N0	M0
Stage I	T1	N0	M0
Stage IIA	T0	N1	M0
	T1	N1	M0
	T2	N0	M0S
Stage IIB	T2	N1	M0
	T3	N0	M0
Stage IIIA	T0	N2	M0
	T1	N2	M0
	T2	N2	M0
	T3	N1, N2	M0
Stage IIIB	T4	Any N	M0
	Any T	N3	M0
Stage IV	Any T	Any N	M1

out and precise. Careful handling of the tissue specimen and a careful and collegial relationship with the pathologist are essential to achieve the data base for decision making.

Part of the contemporary approach of therapy selection in breast cancer involves having the patient make some of the ultimate decisions and consequently assume some of the associated risks and responsibilities. A thoughtful, open, and empathetic approach to patients yields enormous benefits in patient satisfaction, loyalty, and the personal gratification of guiding them through one of the most difficult experiences in their lives with implicit threats of mortality and physical disfigurement. This patient involvement should continue through the entire therapeutic process; patients frequently will want guidance from the surgeon regarding the use of radiation therapy and adjuvant therapy, and the surgeon should indeed be knowledgeable and involved in these decisions and in the careful, detailed follow-up important to the proper handling of patients selecting breast preservation therapy.

NONINVASIVE AND MARKER LESIONS

It must be emphasized that the increasing incidence of breast pathology that defines a high risk of associated or later breast cancer in and of itself carries no connotations of reduced survival. There are four histological entities that must be addressed separately and distinctly in this area: ductal carcinoma *in situ* (DCIS), lobular carcinoma *in situ* (LCIS), and atypical hyperplasia, both atypical ductal hyperplasia (ADH) and atypical lobular hyperplasia (ALH).

Ductal Carcinoma *In Situ*

Ductal carcinoma *in situ* is a lesion being encountered with increasing frequency as a result of the expanding use of screening mammography. In the premammography era, these lesions made up only one to two percent of palpable breast cancer.[60, 61] In more recent studies, DCIS may make up almost ten percent of all breast cancers and more than 20 percent of all breast cancers detected by mammography.[40, 63, 67, 71] With continued rapid expansion of mammographic screening programs, this will become an even more frequent entity that the patient will conceive of as cancer but the physician will recognize as a lesion that carries virtually a 100 percent cure. Prior to mammography, the DCIS lesions seen were either comedocarcinoma or incidental lesions discovered in the process of biopsy for other reasons. The vast majority were not only palpable but also frequently several centimeters in diameter. Even at that relatively advanced stage of intraductal carcinoma, if no invasive component was found, the prognosis for the patient undergoing mastectomy was virtually 100 percent freedom from disease. Now that small nonpalpable DCIS lesions are being found frequently, reevaluation of our traditional approach of mastectomy for noninvasive ductal carcinoma is necessary. At a time when mastectomy is routinely not required for invasive cancers, it is increasingly illogical to insist on mastectomy for noninvasive cancers. Important work is being done on the biological behavior, pathology, and outcome of conservative management of DCIS by Lagios et al.[40] In a series of papers culminating in a summary report in 1989,[40] Lagios et al. have empirically divided DCIS into lesions 25 mm or less and 26 mm or more in diameter. The median diameter of the small lesions was 8 mm, whereas the median diameter of the larger lesions was 50 mm. In 115 patients, there were no areas of microinvasion in the small lesions, but there was a 29 percent incidence of microinvasion in the larger lesions when the breasts were studied by whole organ sectioning after mastectomy for the original biopsy diagnosis of DCIS. Only two patients had positive nodes in these mastectomy specimens, and they were both patients with occult invasion and DCIS lesions of more than 68 mm in diameter. Both patients had micrometastases in a single lymph node. Almost half of the larger DCIS lesions had multifocal disease, whereas only a few of the smaller lesions were thus classified. Building on the basis of that extensive pathological survey involving whole organ sectioning of mastectomies, Lagios and colleagues treated a series of 79 patients[38, 40] with local excision only for DCIS lesions smaller than 25 mm that were detected mammographically by microcalcifications. In a recent presentation not published,[37] Lagios has cited 11 recurrences in these 79 patients (14 percent). Six of these recurrences (55 percent) were also DCIS and occurred a median of 13 months (range, 9 to 25 months) after the local excision; none of these six recurrences exceeded 23 mm in diameter. All these patients are living, and only one patient had a mastectomy for treatment of the recurrent DCIS. Five patients (45 percent) had recurrence in the form of invasive carcinoma a median of 36 months (range, 18 to 87 months) after the initial DCIS excision, and all of these lesions were 13 mm or less in diameter. These patients for the most part underwent mastectomy, but all are living free of disease at the present time.

Among the initial 20 patients in this series who were followed for a minimum of 80 months and a median of 118 months, there have been four recurrences (20 percent), whereas for the last 59 patients, there have been seven recurrences (12 percent) during a median 4-year follow-up, with a range from 1 to 80 months. Thus, based on this initial therapeutic trial by Lagios et al.,[40] it would appear that the local recurrence rate in the breasts of women treated by local excision for small DCIS may not exceed 20 percent even in long-term follow-up, although a number of these initial lesions were palpable. The later 59 patients constitute the only long-term prospective study of DCIS deliberately selected for local excision only of nonpalpable, mammographically detected lesions. There are numerous other retrospective reports of local excision for palpable or incidental lesions prior to the use of mammography that indicate higher recurrence rates. These recurrence rates range from 20 percent to more than 50 percent.[12, 17, 21, 33, 42, 45, 48, 58] It appears in other retrospective surveys that radiation therapy of DCIS lesions locally excised for clinically manifest tumors may reduce that recurrence rate considerably, at least by one half.[9, 17, 18, 46, 52, 65, 78] Tables 36–2 and 36–3 summarize the published literature for DCIS treated by local excision with or without radiation therapy. These reports demonstrate higher recurrence rates with longer follow-up periods.

Thus for women who want to preserve their breasts, it seems reasonable to treat small (<2.5 cm), mammographically discovered DCIS by local excision only. However, the patient must understand the risks of recurrence, and the various criteria suggested by Schnitt et al.[62] should be followed. These criteria are presented

Table 36–2. DCIS TREATED BY LOCAL EXCISION ONLY

Reference	Years	No.	Detection	Size	Local Recurrence (%)
42	1918–1936	8	Palpable	5–9 cm	75
33	Before 1961	4	Palpable	—	50
58	1940–1950	15	Incidental	Microscopic	67
12	1949–1967	25	—	—	20
45	1948–1968	8	Palpable	1–5 cm	25
48	1952–1968	28	Incidental	Microscopic	25
17	1976–1984	22	Mass	<4 cm	23
21	1944–1981	17	Mass 50%	1 cm median (0.4–7.0)	29
37, 38	1972–1980	20	Mass 25%	<2.5 cm	20
37, 38	1980–1988	59	Mammogram 100%	<2.5 cm	12

in Table 36–4 and indicate a reasonable and cautious approach to the management of small DCIS lesions. Of utmost importance are clear margins in the inked specimen, complete calcium removal as demonstrated by a postexcision mammogram, and extremely careful follow-up. Another important element of breast-preserving surgery is careful explanation of all the risks, benefits, and potential problems to the patient. It is essential that patients participate in decisions of nonstandard therapy as a way of ensuring mature judgment and protecting the surgeon from later recrimination if recurrences appear. Discussions with patients and families require presentation of data, consideration of alternatives, an empathetic attitude, and a great deal of time. Repeated discussion sessions are frequently required, but a rapid resolution of the clinical situation is not important, as the lesions are noninvasive and tiny.

For lesions between 2.5 cm (25 mm) and 5 cm (50 mm) in diameter, local excision only with or without radiation therapy may be considered, although the risk of a recurrence is higher than with the very small lesions, and the long-term results are less certain. In such patients, if margins are negative on the final inked specimen, radiotherapy may be considered, with a significant boost dose so the final local radiation exceeds 6000 cGy in order to minimize the risk of local recurrence.[52] However, the success of radiation therapy in reducing local recurrence rates in such patients is not completely known or well established. In a series of reports, the breast recurrence rate does seem somewhat

less (see Table 36–3) when comparing excision plus radiation with local excision only. The only prospective randomized trial to test such a thesis, however, did so indirectly, since the patients in the NSABP protocol B-06 were originally considered to have an invasive cancer, usually palpable, and only in retrospective review of the pathology slides were a small number of cases found to be noninvasive.[17] Twenty-nine cases were treated by excision and radiation therapy, 22 were treated by local excision alone, and 28 patients had mastectomy by random assignment. These patients had palpable masses smaller than 4 cm on presentation, with few exceptions. In those cases randomly allocated between radiation or no radiation after local excision, two (seven percent) of the 29 radiated patients and five (23 percent) of the 22 nonradiated patients had local recurrence. Roughly 50 percent of the recurrences were invasive carcinoma, as in most of the reports cited previously (see Tables 36–2 and 36–3). Current proto-

Table 36–4. GUIDELINES FOR THE EVALUATION OF PATIENTS BEING CONSIDERED FOR BREAST-CONSERVING TREATMENT WITH MAMMOGRAPHICALLY DETECTED NONPALPABLE LESIONS WITH MICROCALCIFICATIONS

1. Careful mammographic evaluation of the breast before biopsy, including magnification views, to delineate the extent of the microcalcifications.
2. Needle localization for the biopsy.
3. Specimen radiography, preferably with magnification views as well as contact views, to confirm that the lesion has been excised and to direct pathological sampling.
4. Careful gross description of the excised specimen by the pathologist.
5. Inking of the specimen margins by the pathologist before sectioning to facilitate evaluation of margins on permanent sections.
6. On microscopic examination, description of the relation of the calcifications to the lesion and the distance of the tumor from the inked margins of resection.
7. Postbiopsy mammography with magnification views to confirm that all suspicious microcalcifications have been removed.
8. Repeat excision of the primary site if residual microcalcifications are seen on postbiopsy mammography or if tumor involves margins of resection microscopically.

From Schnitt SJ, et al: N Engl J Med 318(14):898–903, 1988. Reprinted by permission.

Table 36–3. DCIS TREATED BY LOCAL EXCISION PLUS RADIOTHERAPY

Reference	Years	No.	Detection	Local Recurrence (%)
52	1976–1983	40	Mass 68%	10
17	1976–1984	29	Mass 100%	7
78	1967–1983	54	Mass 65%	5
18	1978–1985	46	Mass 48%	4
34	1975–1985	47	—	4
9	1956–1979	18	—	5
46	—	72	—	3
65	1980–1986	51	Mass 41%	2

cols further investigating the value of radiation therapy in the treatment of deliberately selected DCIS treated by local excision only are under way (NSABP-B-17), but results will not be available for several years.

For DCIS lesions of larger size (>5 cm in diameter) or when clear margins cannot be obtained in smaller lesions (2.5 to 5 cm), even after reexcision, or when a reasonable cosmetic result cannot be obtained, mastectomy should be performed. Axillary dissection may also be considered for such patients, since the incidence of occult invasion may exceed 50 percent,[40] and the incidence of lymph node metastases may be as high as five percent, although Lagios et al.[40] have reported that such positive axillary nodes are usually only micrometastases. For the most part, axillary dissection should be avoided, since the yield of positive lymph nodes is low and the morbidity of axillary dissection significant.

"Standard" therapy for DCIS of any size at this time, however, is total mastectomy, but axillary dissection is not required.

It should be emphasized in this discussion of DCIS that data are scant; patients are from earlier time periods and usually had palpable masses, and prospective trials are almost nonexistent. However, the clinical management trial of Lagios et al.[40] gives reasonable data indicating that local excision can be considered as an option in highly selective situations. The addition of radiotherapy may reduce the risk of local breast recurrence, but the extent, value, morbidity, and cost of this reduction is unclear. Patients will need thorough explanation and comprehension of the situation if they are to participate in informed decisions.

Lagios et al.[40] have reported that there are correlations between the particular pathological type and nuclear grade of DCIS and the recurrence rate after local excision only for limited DCIS. In patients with high nuclear grade and comedocarcinoma, the recurrence rate was 26 percent. In the intermediate nuclear grade, the recurrence rate was ten percent, and in the micropapillary pathology form of low nuclear grade, the recurrence rate was only three percent. Other authors have also correlated pathological variants and outcome.[51] Such data indicate the direction of future studies in analyzing particular features associated with recurrence and therefore perhaps with the more aggressive or progressive forms of DCIS. *Neu* oncogene overexpression has been reported by a group from Holland[72] as being associated with comedo-type DCIS, which, by implication, is the form of DCIS more likely to have microinvasion,[51] to recur following local excision,[40] and to exhibit progressive growth. Such specific prognostic indicators are vitally important in understanding the biology and progress of DCIS, particularly when of limited extent, and in selecting therapy. It seems clear that the larger DCIS lesions are slated to progress (i.e., develop the clinical course of invasive ductal carcinoma) in the majority of cases. However, many of the small DCIS lesions currently detected by mammography may well be pathological curiosities, since they are found with great frequency on routine autopsy studies of patients dying from other causes.[47] Since these lesions are all categorized as breast cancer in tumor registries, the detection by mammography of large numbers of such tiny focus DCIS (as well as LCIS) lesions may alter the incidence rates and survival rates of carcinoma of the breast; these changes may not be accurately assessed without a sophisticated analysis of cancer registry data. As in other hormone organ cancers, microscopic foci of noninvasive carcinoma may be frequent and in many cases of no biological significance. However, in the past it has been impossible to predict which tiny DCIS lesions might have the potential for progressive growth and which were clinically unimportant, a situation similar to that in prostate or thyroid cancer.

The most important consideration for local excision of small DCIS lesions has been to address the biological issue of whether extensive (large-sized) DCIS is the result of multifocal origin within the breast or of progressive intraductal growth without breaching of the basement membrane of a single initial focus of abnormal cells. The model of Paget's disease with progressive intraductal spread of cells even onto the surface of the nipple may illustrate the biological growth pattern of a significant proportion of DCIS.

Long-term follow-up results from the series reported by Lagios et al.[40] seem to indicate the absence of "multifocal" or "multicentric" DCIS in the breasts of people treated by local excision only and the fact that a significant proportion of the advanced comedo type of DCIS may arise as a single intraductal focus and spread only intraductally. If DCIS were truly a multifocal lesion, the low recurrence rates reported by Lagios et al. would not be possible, and recurrences would be multifocal and in other areas of the breast. In Lagios et al.'s series, the recurrences apparently are all in the same quadrant of the same breast as the original local excision, and lesions in other parts of the same breast have not been reported.[40] One patient had a primary invasive cancer develop in a different part of the ipsilateral breast, but it proved to be an invasive lobular carcinoma and thus apparently did not represent the late progression of multicentric DCIS. This hypothesis of ductal spread from a single focus has been explicitly proposed by Gump et al.[26] Clearly the most interesting biological information that will result from future trials of local excision of DCIS will be an answer to this question of the origin of extensive DCIS lesions and later comedocarcinoma.

Follow-up data are consistent with the assumption that DCIS is a true precursor or preinvasive lesion in a large proportion of patients; when later invasive disease occurs, it appears in the same breast and in the same quadrant. The risk of later invasive cancer occurring in the ipsilateral breast after local excision can be estimated and is presented in Table 36–5.[4] This continuing risk is probably at least two percent per year and may not abate with time. It undoubtedly is increased by the presence of a family history of premenopausal breast cancer. A specific pathological subtype may add to the predictability of invasive cancer recurrence, as suggested by the data of Lagios[8] and van de Vijver.[72] However, of most concern and importance is not the risk of later

Table 36–5. ESTIMATED OUTCOME IN PATIENTS WITH HIGH-RISK, NONINVASIVE BREAST PATHOLOGY TREATED BY LOCAL EXCISION

| Histology | Family History | Incidence of Invasive Cancer (%) | | Maximum Estimated 20-Year Mortality if Breast Preserved |
		Annually	*At 20 Years*	
ADH	No	0.5	10	1
ALH	Yes	1	20	2
LCIS	No	1	20	2
	Yes	2	40	4
DCIS	No	2	40	4
	Yes	(4)	(60 at 15 yrs)	(6)

Abbreviations: ADH = atypical ductal hyperplasia; ALH = atypical lobular hyperplasia; DCIS = ductal carcinoma *in situ;* LCIS = lobular carcinoma *in situ;* ( ) = no data available—author's estimate.

invasive breast cancer, but the risk of dying from a later cancer that would not have occurred if the breast had been sacrificed. Clearly this is only a small fraction of the invasive cancer incidence.

Estimates of death risk are extrapolated from survival rates achieved by screening programs such as Breast Cancer Detection Demonstration Project (BCDDP),[3] Health Insurance Plan of Greater New York (HIP),[64] and more contemporary trials of mammographic screening[64, 68, 69] and are less than five percent. In addition it was assumed that ten percent of new breast cancers will not be detected by screening programs and that these interval cancers may well carry a worse prognosis (50 percent survival).[29, 31] Thus at most, five percent of patients having cancers detected by screening will die, as will one half of those not detected (five percent), so that total risk of death will be no more than ten percent in the patients who actually develop invasive cancer.

Lobular Carcinoma *In Situ*

The other noninvasive breast cancer lesion of importance is lobular carcinoma *in situ*. In a series of reports in the literature[1, 3, 23, 27, 28, 56, 60, 76] and a collective review,[20] it seems clear that such lesions are *marker lesions* for patients at high risk of developing breast cancer and not explicit *precursor lesions* for the later local development of invasive carcinoma. This can be appreciated by the fact that later breast cancers that appear are as likely to be in the contralateral breast as in the ipsilateral breast and are as likely as not to be in a different quadrant of the ipsilateral breast from the original biopsy that revealed LCIS. Table 36–6 summarizes data from Haagensen et al.[28] illustrating this generalized risk. He prefers the term "lobular neoplasia" to LCIS to emphasize its risk effects rather than its precursor status. This is in marked contrast to the data reported in DCIS, where recurrences appear almost exclusively in the ipsilateral breast and in the same quadrant of the ipsilateral breast as the original biopsy when local excision only is performed. The risk of later invasive carcinoma developing in patients with LCIS treated by local excision seems to be roughly one percent per year (see Tables 36–5 and 36–6). This risk is probably doubled if there is an associated family history of premenopausal

breast cancer or a previous personal breast cancer.[27] Thus patients with LCIS need careful analysis of other risk factors, including family history, before making a decision regarding treatment.

Two aspects of LCIS that reemphasize the concept of its being a marker rather than a precursor lesion are the pathological types of invasive cancers that later develop and the age range at which LCIS occurs. In follow-up of patients with LCIS, invasive lobular carcinoma is not the predominant later cancer. Invasive ductal carcinoma is the most common subsequent cancer, which suggests that the lobular carcinoma *in situ* is not itself developing invasion. In addition, LCIS is found predominantly in premenopausal women. The incidence of LCIS in biopsy samples taken from postmenopausal women is not as high as in biopsy samples taken from premenopausal women. Autopsy studies also indicate a reduced incidence of LCIS with age.[47] Thus the implication of the high risk associated with LCIS is manifest even after the apparent regression of the LCIS lesion itself, probably because of the influence of declining estrogen levels. More specific prognostic aspects of LCIS have not been reported thus far, but clearly gene expression, DNA ploidy, histological subtypes, and patterns of growth need to be analyzed so that more specific individual prognostication can be made for patients with LCIS.

It seems illogical on the basis of the reports published thus far to treat LCIS by ipsilateral mastectomy, since risk is distributed apparently throughout all breast tis-

Table 36–6. INCIDENCE OF INVASIVE CANCER WHEN ORIGINAL LCIS WAS TREATED BY BIOPSY

Years After LCIS Diagnosis	No. at Risk	Cumulative Probability of Ipsilateral Breast Cancer (%)	Cumulative Probability of Contralateral Breast Cancer (%)
5	236	4	5
10	224	7	8
15	135	11	9
20	94	18	12
25	42	21	15

From Haagensen CD, et al (eds): Breast Carcinoma Risk and Detection. Philadelphia, WB Saunders, 1981, p 267. Reprinted by permission.

sue. The most logical therapeutic options seem to be bilateral mastectomy, a preventive attempt to remove the vast majority of breast tissue at risk, and local excision only with meticulous follow-up. Patients who have a diagnosis of LCIS with a strong family history, particularly of a premenopausal breast cancer in a first degree relative, may opt for bilateral mastectomy with or without reconstruction with the assumption that the marker lesion of LCIS indicates a genetic pattern with a high probability of invasive breast cancer.

In patients with repeated episodes of LCIS treated by biopsy only, even those without a family history, it would seem prudent to discuss the option of mastectomy; whether such multifocal LCIS or recurrent LCIS portends a higher risk of later development of invasive carcinoma in the absence of a strong family history or other risk factors is unknown. It is apparent that if local excision only is performed for LCIS, the follow-up of such patients must be continued permanently. Although data have only been reported for 20 years of follow-up, the risk seems to continue unabated at similar rates. Thus with the 40-year life expectancy of a woman who first underwent biopsy in her forties, it would appear that the risk of later invasive cancer might approach 40 percent in the absence of a family history and be even higher if a positive family history is present. The data presented indicate the need to discuss at great length the available therapeutic options, and the risks involved when patients who have LCIS are treated by biopsy. The long-term management of patients with LCIS treated by biopsy clearly requires involvement by the patient and implies that the patient understands and assumes the risks involved and will adhere to careful follow-up screening. This should include at least annual mammography and physical examination and careful breast self-examination to detect any abnormalities that may occur.

Table 36–5 indicates my interpretation of the risk of later invasive breast cancer and the probable maximum risk of dying of a breast cancer that would not have occurred if bilateral mastectomy had initially been elected.

Atypical Ductal Hyperplasia and Atypical Lobular Hyperplasia

Atypical ductal hyperplasia and atypical lobular hyperplasia have been shown by Page et al.[49] and Dupont and Page[11] to also be indicators of risk for the later development of invasive carcinoma of the breast. This risk is apparently doubled by the addition of a first-degree relative with breast cancer, although in their articles, the details of the family history were not recorded, and thus premenopausal or postmenopausal relatives were not distinguished. Interpretation of their articles and data indicates that the level of risk following biopsy only of atypical ductal or lobular hyperplasia is roughly ten percent at 20 years, or 0.5 percent per year cumulative, and roughly 20 percent at 20 years, or one percent per year cumulative, if there is a family history

of breast cancer. The location of the later carcinomas that develop in such patients is ipsilateral in 56 percent of ADH patients and 69 percent of ALH patients. Thus whether ADH and ALH represent precursor lesions or marker lesions is not known at the present time, but there is clearly a substantial risk in the contralateral breast.[49]

ADH and ALH make up less than five percent of benign breast lesions[11, 49] but may mark a significant proportion of patients at risk for later development of invasive breast cancer. Thus ductal hyperplasia without atypia and stromal changes in breast samples with non-proliferative ductal lesions were not associated with increased risks of invasive breast cancer during the 20-year follow-up period in the reports by Page et al.[48, 49] and Dupont and Page.[11] These studies cannot be over-emphasized, since they now provide clear-cut evidence that certain benign lesions serve as indicators for patients at higher risk of later invasive breast cancer. These patients might particularly benefit from screening, which would include at least yearly mammography and physical examination. Although these reports have not yet been confirmed by others, their comprehensive nature seems to secure this viewpoint and interpretation. A previous review by Love[43] pointed out the lack of a risk factor associated with "fibrocystic disease" generally and brought into focus the epithelial component of breast changes that might be associated with increased breast cancer risk.

Therapeutic recommendations in ADH and ALH consist of local excision and careful follow-up, since mastectomy or bilateral mastectomy would be unjustified except in patients with a strong family history. Whether the lesions of ADH and ALH are multifocal or ipsilateral or bilateral in nature remains to be elucidated. The majority of subsequent cancers are ductal, with a smaller number of other types. Only three of 16 cancers (19 percent) occurring after ALH were lobular carcinomas.

Table 36–5 summarizes my interpretation of the risks involved for later development of invasive carcinoma in the four lesions described (DCIS, LCIS, ADH, ALH) if treated by breast preservation.[4] However, in discussion with patients it is important to emphasize that the mere occurrence of invasive cancer after local excision only for these lesions is not the critically important feature by which to evaluate breast conservation therapy. The risk of death from cancer following breast preservation in contrast to the negligible risk after sacrifice of the breast or breasts should be the criterion for the acceptability of the limited surgical approach to these lesions and the basis on which discussion with patients should be undertaken. It should also be mentioned when discussing options with patients that unilateral or bilateral mastectomy used to treat LCIS or DCIS lesions and to prevent later invasive carcinoma is not uniformly successful, and cases of breast cancer developing after "preventive" mastectomy do occur, as every bit of breast tissue cannot be removed even by radical mastectomy.

In summary, recommendations to patients for management of ADH, ALH, LCIS, and DCIS are currently uncertain and will need refinement during coming years. Surgical therapy can be selected by addressing particular attention to the details of the histology of the lesion removed, the family history and other risk factors of the patient (i.e., previous invasive breast cancer or noninvasive disease), the patient's desire to retain the breast, and the patient's comprehension of and willingness to assume risks associated with what is currently nonstandard therapy. Careful detailed follow-up by the responsible surgeon with a willingness to perform a biopsy on any suspicious lesion that develops in breast tissue is required for such a program.

INVASIVE BREAST CANCER OF LIMITED EXTENT

The new staging criteria of carcinoma of the breast that have been adopted by the American Joint Committee on Cancer (AJCC) and the Union Internationale Contre le Cancer (UICC) suggest the importance of size in analysis of very early breast cancer.[4] In this new staging system (Table 36–1), T1 lesions are separated into those 0.5 cm or less in diameter (T1a), those between 0.5 and 1 cm in diameter (T1b), and those between 1 and 2 cm in diameter (T1c). Because size is the most important prognostic indicator in breast cancer, it is vital that future studies be more sophisticated in analyzing cancer size to be able to address new therapeutic issues such as local excision only. These small primary cancers will be increasing in incidence with widespread adoption of breast screening programs. The use of mammogram screening has not only reduced the percentage of advanced stage cases by 25 percent to 50 percent but has also significantly increased the number of very small invasive breast cancers.[29, 63, 68] In the BCDDP study, 27 percent of patients displayed invasive breast cancers of less than 1 cm in diameter. In a randomized clinical study, 36 percent of repeatedly screened patients had cancers of 1 cm or less in diameter, in contrast to ten percent of the control group.[29, 31]

Thus in the not too distant future it can be expected that close to 50 percent of breast cancers will be at an early stage, either noninvasive or invasive and less than 1 cm in diameter. In addition, nearly 50 percent of breast cancers in the future will be between 1 cm and 2 cm in diameter with either negative nodes or with only a few nodes involved. More than 60 percent of patients entering treatment facilities in the past decade had negative axillary lymph nodes, whereas in screening programs, 20 percent or less had positive nodes. Controlled trials of mammography screening in Sweden[68] and Holland[73] have indicated a significant reduction in the stage of presentation (i.e., smaller size and fewer lymph node metastases) of breast cancers that were detected as part of the screening program. Between 1981 and 1985, 75 percent of all patients with cancers detected by repeated screening were stage I.[29] All of these trends indicate that the majority of patients in the future will be classified as having early breast cancer.

Clear treatment guidelines for management of these patients is critical during this time of rapidly changing attitudes and procedures regarding breast cancer treatment.

The most informative current analysis of the results that might be achieved in patients with early breast cancer has been published by Rosen et al.[59] These patients originally had T1 primary cancers and either N0 or N1 and have been followed for 20 years. Patients with cancers 1 cm or less in diameter have a better than 80 percent disease-free survival rate at 20 years, and patients with cancers between 1 and 2 cm in diameter survive disease-free in 70 percent of cases. It is wise to keep in mind that these patients were first treated in the years 1964 to 1970, prior to mammography, and thus represent an historical analysis of patients from a different era. It could certainly be expected that patients encountered in the 1990s will have far earlier breast cancers and better results stage for stage, since even within overall stage categories there will be a shift toward earlier and smaller cancers as a result of early detection techniques. Rosen et al.'s analysis included *no* patients who were detected by mammographic screening,[59] but in recent years, the number of cancer patients detected by mammography is increasing, and these patients have a very early presentation. Of all patients encountered in one series between 1977 and 1987, lymph node metastasis was present in only five percent if the invasive cancer was less than 0.5 cm in diameter and in only ten percent if the invasive cancer was 1 cm in diameter or less.[54] As an indication of the continued improvement in clinical presentation, Rosen's patients treated in the late 1960s had an overall node-positive rate in all T1 lesions of 27 percent,[44] whereas the report of Reger et al.[54] of patients seen from 1977 to 1987 indicated a 23 percent overall incidence of positive nodes in T1 cancers. Thus for similarly staged cancers, clinical and pathological presentations will continue to improve as the overall incidence of lymph node metastases within each T category decreases as a result of the decreasing median diameter within each T category.

There may well be differences in outcome based on the detection methods even within limited cancer stage categories. In BCDDP patients, in whom 36 percent were detected by mammogram only, T1 node-negative primary cancers had a 10-year survival rate of 92 percent, whereas for Rosen's T1N0 patients, who were detected by physical examination, survival at the end of 10 years was 86 percent.[59] Thus we can expect that therapeutic results will continue to improve with the increasing use of mammography and screening.

It has been amply demonstrated in a variety of studies carried out throughout the world that the survival results after prolonged follow-up are essentially identical between lumpectomy plus radiation therapy and mastectomy.[6, 13, 15, 74] These results can be achieved regardless of the histological subtype.[36] In addition, patients who are at risk of failure after breast-preserving therapy have been well defined so that treatment selection can be relatively accurate.[35, 53] There is every expectation that local breast recurrence after breast preservation therapy can be reduced to three percent in the majority of patients who do not have an extensive intraductal component (EIC) and are older than 35 years[53] (Fig. 36–1). The increasing proportion of patients detected by mammography, the decreasing size of the primary invasive cancer, the improving overall prognosis, and the development of more precise prognostic studies such as flow cytometry, S-phase study, and oncogene analysis indicate that breast conservation can be done in the future with increasing confidence.

Several overall comments can be made regarding treatment selection for patients with early primary breast cancer. The essential decision in the selection of therapy for early breast cancer is the patient's desire about breast preservation. Even though breast preservation in the large majority of people has been found to be extremely satisfactory,[53] there are women who for a variety of reasons wish to have mastectomy. Perhaps this proportion will decrease in the future as breast preservation becomes more widely known, publicized, and accepted by the public and physicians. Nevertheless elderly patients who do not wish to travel extensively and repeatedly for radiation therapy and for whom the breast is of less cosmetic and functional importance may well choose mastectomy as the most expeditious therapy. In addition, of course, women who have an EIC within and around the primary cancer should continue to select mastectomy for treatment because of the extremely high local failure rate in the radiated breast despite extensive lumpectomy and even pathologically negative margins in the inked specimen.[53]

Another small proportion of women have cancers that are large in proportion to the breast size or have a centrally placed cancer that may require sacrifice of the nipple, areola, or more central breast tissue in the process of achieving adequate local excision; a more satisfactory long-term cosmetic result may be achieved

Table 36–7. RISK OF LOCAL BREAST RECURRENCE RELATED TO EXTENSIVE INTRADUCTAL COMPONENT (EIC) AFTER LOCAL EXCISION AND RADIOTHERAPY

EIC	Age (Years)	No.	Incidence (%)	5-Year Actuarial Risk of Local Recurrence (%)
Present	<35	18	4	38
Absent	<35	23	5	22
Present	35+	124	28	23
Absent	35+	279	63	3
Total		444	100	

From Recht A, et al: Int J Radiat Oncol Biol Phys 14:3–10, 1988. Reprinted by permission.

by mastectomy and reconstruction. Patients with two or more primary lesions in the same breast who are treated by local excision and radiation therapy have a very high likelihood of breast recurrence, a poor chance of retaining the breast, and a poor cosmetic outcome because of the need to radiate the entire breast at a high dose and the higher likelihood of EIC.[41] Very young age may also predispose to breast recurrence (Table 36–7).[53]

There is an increasing realization that lumpectomy without radiation therapy may be suitable for an as-yet-undefined proportion of patients with early breast cancer.[25, 39] The NSABP B-06 protocol at 8 years[15] demonstrates no statistically significant reduction in survival (distant disease–free or overall) in patients who had local excision only compared with those who had local excision plus radiation therapy for all cancers 4 cm or less in diameter. Since the entire trend of management of breast cancer during the past several decades has been toward more selective use of breast sparing, more restrictive use of radiation therapy (i.e., elimination of supraclavicular, axillary, and internal mammary node basin radiation), and more widely defined use of systemic adjuvant treatment, one can expect that the subset of patients who can be treated by local excision and careful follow-up without radiation therapy will increase. This will be the result of earlier detection, better definition of the risk of local recurrence in the breast, more widespread utilization of margin analysis pathologically, and the use of adjuvant tamoxifen, which may reduce the incidence of local recurrence and new primary cancers in other breast tissue (both ipsilateral and contralateral). It is difficult to predict what the standards of therapy will be for early breast cancer 10 or even 5 years in the future. However, expanded therapy selections will evolve from sophisticated subset analyses of patients in current trials, more careful individualization of therapy based on patient wishes, improved stage of disease, use of more sophisticated and individual prognostic indicators in primary breast cancer, and the expectation of excellent salvage that can occur even if locally excised breast cancers recur in the ipsilateral breast.

Therapy Selection

Therapy selection for patients with breast cancer can best be achieved by establishing the diagnosis, discussing

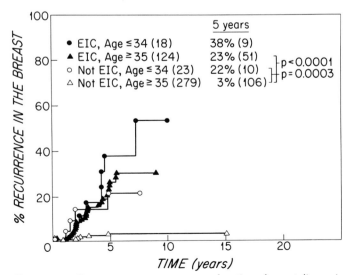

Figure 36–1. Breast cancer recurrence as a function of age at diagnosis and presence of an extensive intraductal component (EIC). (Excisional biopsy and dose to primary site ≥ 60 Gy, infiltrating ductal histology, with evaluable specimen.) (From Recht A, et al: Int J Radiat Oncol Biol Phys 14:3, 1988. Reprinted by permission.)

available options with patients during this critical initial phase of management, and then selecting the most appropriate therapy for the individual patient.

Mammographically Detected Invasive Breast Cancer

For those patients whose primary invasive cancer is detected by mammography as part of a screening program, the therapeutic selection process begins with wire (needle) localization of the mammographically identified calcification or mass and adequate local excision of this radiographic lesion. Careful discussion and a close working relationship with the radiologist who performs the mammography and wire localization are essential to achieve the best results. This and the subsequent biopsy can almost always be performed under local anesthesia. In general the incisions for removing mammographically detected breast cancer should be circular in the lateral three quarters of the breast but are better managed by a radial incision in the lower medial portion of the breast (Fig. 36–2). Breast biopsy incisions placed along Langer's lines give a superior cosmetic result and allow adequate excision of the breast lesions; they should be placed more centrally, however, to allow a subsequent mastectomy (if required) to be achieved without unusual length or arrangement of skin flaps or difficulty in approximation of the postmastectomy skin (Figs. 36–3 and 36–4). Slight tunnelling peripherally is acceptable to keep the incision as central as possible, but circumareolar incisions usually should be avoided except for very central masses.

After exposing the localization wire within the breast and pulling the wire into the excision site, the presumed area of the mammographic lesion surrounding the tip of the hooked wire should be widely circumscribed by the breast incision (performed either with electrocautery or knife) to completely encompass the suspected area (Fig.

36–5). Paradoxically the biopsy resection for nonpalpable lesions needs to be larger than the local excision of a palpable lesion of similar size, since it is unclear to the surgeon exactly where the lesion may be in relationship to the wire or within the excised tissue. The handling of the excised tissue specimen after wire localization and biopsy of a mammographically detected lesion is critical and is just as important as the sympathetic management of the patient herself during these biopsies.

Following removal of the specimen, the tissue must be carefully covered with india ink to mark the margins of excision for the pathologist. Sutures should be placed to orient the specimen also. This enables the surgeon and the pathologist to evaluate the margin and the adequacy of the removal of the primary cancer, but this is only possible if the tissue is removed as a single coherent piece and not excised in fragments or with a markedly irregular margin. In most situations (but always if calcifications were the reason for the biopsy), the specimen should be examined radiologically and compared with the mammogram to ensure adequacy of removal. Whether a frozen section is obtained of the tissue removed after the margins are inked and the mammographic examination of the specimen performed is a judgment of the surgeon. If the area of calcification or lesion is extremely small in size (less than 5 mm), it is probably better to avoid a frozen section and have the entire tissue analyzed carefully histologically by permanent sections. The histological definition of the cellular details are critical for very small lesions, and the destruction of even a portion of the tissue sample by frozen section analysis required for hormonal assay should be avoided. Patients with invasive cancers of such small size have outstandingly good prognoses that estrogen and progesterone receptor determinations are of minimal value in planning therapy. Furthermore, histochemical staining for estrogen receptor activity may

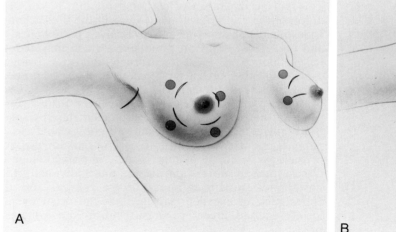
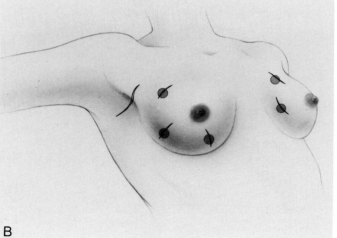

Figure 36–2. *A,* The preferred incisions: circular, except in the extreme medial aspect, and more centrally placed. The extent of peripheral dissection to excise the primary lesion should not be excessive, and circumareolar incisions are generally avoided. *B,* Commonly advocated incisions that are less suitable. Radial incisions inferiorly cross Langer's lines of skin tension. Incisions placed directly over peripheral cancers are cosmetically more difficult to hide under clothing and mandate more difficult mastectomy incisions. Radial incisions in the upper medial area are to be condemned, as they are difficult to conceal or incorporate within mastectomy incisions.

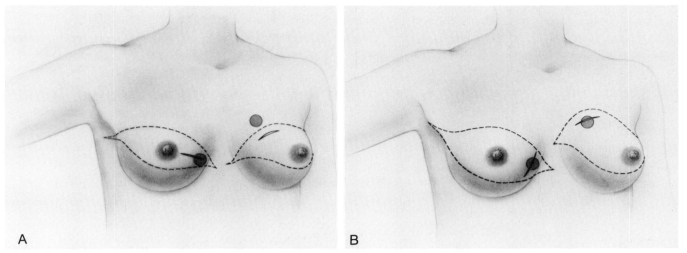

Figure 36–3. *A*, Mastectomy, if required, can be performed with minimal skin sacrifice if biopsy incisions are more centrally placed and if medial incisions are radial. *B*, With the biopsy incision placed directly over peripheral cancers, the later mastectomy incision may have to be contorted to achieve inclusion within the skin ellipse. If medial biopsies are circular, wide skin sacrifice is required in a location where excess skin is not available. Since 30 percent of patients may require mastectomy, careful biopsy incision placement is critical. Furthermore, with immediate reconstruction, minimal skin sacrifice is desirable.

be done later if necessary.[10] This is yet another reason that almost all breast cancer treatments should be performed in a two-step process, with the biopsy/lumpectomy performed as a completely separate procedure from axillary dissection or mastectomy. If the mass is of significant size or is palpable within the tissue removed at local excision and confirmed by postlumpectomy mammogram of the specimen, then the tissue block may be incised after inking, the gross lesion inspected visually for size and margin, and an appropriate tissue sample obtained for estrogen and progesterone receptors. The pathologist should be in attendance. Frozen section to evaluate margins may be undertaken if desired at this point, but frozen section analysis of margins is not highly accurate. Every biopsy of an early breast cancer should fulfill the requirements of a lumpectomy to minimize the need for later reexcision.

To reemphasize, with few exceptions this biopsy/lumpectomy should be the only step undertaken at the first operation; the concept of a two-step treatment program (first biopsy/lumpectomy, and then axillary dissection or mastectomy) is essential in the modern treatment of breast cancer. *A single-step process under general anesthesia is to be condemned.* Only after careful histological analysis of the removed specimen can final decisions be made about the adequacy of local excision, the suitability for conservative therapy as a result of extent in the intraductal component (EIC), the need for axillary dissection, the need for radiation therapy, and the specific prognostic aspects of the pathology. In addition, patients require prolonged discussion and presentation of data before they can make informed and adequate decisions. For simplicity and psychological comfort, patients should go into the operating room initially only for biopsy under local anesthesia and should not have a comprehensive discussion of therapeutic options until after it has been proven that they actually have cancer, and the full details of the histology have been carefully explored. This discussion can only occur in detail after the preliminary biopsy/lumpectomy. In some situations the cosmetic result can only be predicted after lumpectomy, particularly when a large cancer requiring major tissue loss or a reexcision needs to be performed. Since the majority of patients in premenopausal age groups do not have cancer as the cause of the mammographic changes, enormous savings in time and effort by both the surgeon and patient can be achieved by performing only the biopsy/lumpectomy at the first step. In postmenopausal patients with screening detected lesions, the extra discussion and time are

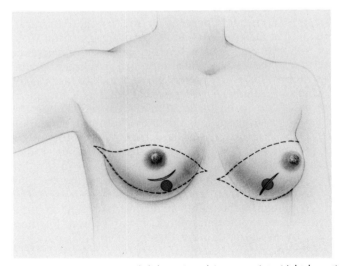

Figure 36–4. Appropriate (left breast) and inappropriate (right breast) biopsy incision placements are demonstrated with the resulting mastectomy incisions.

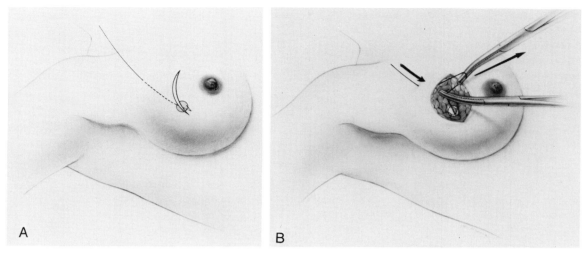

Figure 36–5. *A,* Central circular incisions are also used for lesions removed after mammographic wire localization. *B,* The wire is grasped beneath the skin by a Kelly clamp, and then the exterior portion is flipped into the wound. The wire, now completely within the biopsy incision, can be used for more accurate localization by gentle traction to demonstrate the area of the engaged hooked end near the lesion to be removed.

extremely helpful in achieving accommodation to the diagnosis by the patient, as the majority of suspicious lesions will be cancer.

Following the results of the biopsy report and careful analysis by the surgeon of the histology with the pathologist, the patient can be apprised of the size of the primary cancer, the extent of the surrounding intraductal carcinoma, the adequacy of the margins, the likelihood of a cure based on size, and the suitability of various therapeutic options. Since most of these mammographically detected breast cancers will be of small size with excellent prognosis, it is possible from the very first patient contact to provide a positive prognosis and a supportive environment for the patient when discussing outcome and therapeutic management.

If the excised specimen has negative margins of at least 1 cm and there is no extensive intraductal component (EIC), the first local excision is adequate for therapeutic purposes. If EIC is present and margins of the tissue sample are positive for intraductal or invasive cancer or are negative but less than 1 cm, a reexcision will be required of the biopsy/lumpectomy area in order to make a final decision about suitability for lumpectomy as a treatment of the mammographically discovered cancer. If EIC is present but of limited overall extent, reexcision will enable more complete evaluation of suitability for breast conserving therapy. Reexcisions are required in our referral center in at least ten percent to 20 percent of cases, reflecting the inability of frozen sections to detect accurately the presence and extent of EIC and the unsuspected involvement of margins by either invasive or intraductal carcinoma. These evaluations are much less satisfactorily obtained at frozen section and are unnecessary in the two-step process we advocate. Reexcisions should be kept to a minimum, as the cosmetic result may be adversely affected by reexcision and large volumes of biopsy specimens.

If the mammographically detected carcinoma is less than 5 mm in diameter (T1a) or even 6 to 10 mm in

diameter (T1b), the margins adequate, EIC not present, and the prognosis excellent, it may well be that no further therapy is required. Discussion about therapy selection in such patients should center on the usefulness of adding radiation therapy to reduce local recurrence rates in a tiny primary breast cancer, the projected incidence of lymph node metastases, the risk-benefit ratio of axillary dissection, and the risk-benefit ratio of adjuvant systemic therapy. Because of the near-perfect prognosis, therapy can frequently be markedly simplified. The use of radiation therapy to reduce local recurrence in such extremely small primary cancers has not been extensively studied, but in unpublished information from the B-06 study of the NSABP,[16] it appears that in lesions of 1 cm or less in size, the addition of radiation therapy (5000 rads to entire breast without a local boost) may only contribute a small reduction in local breast recurrence from about 20 percent in the nonirradiated breast to about ten percent in the irradiated breast. Greening et al.'s patients, after quadrant resection without radiotherapy, had a ten percent local recurrence rate if selected by age and tumor size.[25] Whether radiation therapy in every patient with a tiny breast cancer is worth the financial and physical costs is a judgment that will need to be made after discussions among the patient, the surgeon, and the radiotherapist. Radiation therapy is the current standard therapy, but for only a ten percent reduction in local breast recurrence, radiotherapy can be avoided with significant gains in simplicity of management. Clear cosmetic advantages may accrue to patients not requiring radiation therapy. For the 20 percent of patients recurring, subsequent local reexcision and radiotherapy become an option. Furthermore, by avoiding axillary dissection in such patients, the risks of general anesthesia and arm and breast edema (at least 15 percent incidence) can be avoided and shoulder function maintained.

It should be recognized that radiotherapy is *not* utilized after mastectomy. There is ample evidence that survival is not increased by postoperative radiation therapy after mastectomy. Postmastectomy radiation may, however, be used in a small, very select group of patients who have a small cancer very close to or involving the posterior margin and negative nodes. In such patients a local recurrence might not be associated with systemic disease but might instead be an isolated event because of the peculiar deep location of the cancer, and for these patients, extra protection from such a local recurrence might be justified. In this case the mastectomy bed is radiated, but the lymph node drainage basins are not.

Radiation therapy of the primary intact breast following breast preservation techniques is not extended to include regional lymphatic drainage basins. Breast tangents alone are utilized for the breast. The supraclavicular space, axillary apex, and internal mammary nodes are not radiated except as they occur within the field of the tangent radiation ports for the breast itself. This policy of limited radiation again reflects the fact that lymph node metastases are indicators but not governors of survival[5] and do not require separate therapy, since only half of positive nodes will ever become clinical problems if not treated; later treatment does not necessarily warrant radiation therapy, as hormone therapy and chemotherapy can be effective when used systemically. Because significant morbidity in terms of arm and breast edema does occur with extensive adjuvant radiation therapy to the lymphatics of the supraclavicular space and axillary apex, these complications can be avoided by limiting radiotherapy to the breast itself.

In a recent study,[54] the incidence of axillary lymph node metastases in all patients with cancers 1 cm or less in diameter was less than ten percent;[56] many of these patients have only micrometastasis, and the majority have minimal axillary involvement if nodes are positive.[14, 50] Of Rosen et al.'s patients with palpable cancers, two thirds had only one to three positive lymph nodes when axillas were involved (27 percent).[59] Thus whether axillary dissection is justified in screening-detected patients with very small cancers (T1a and T1b) is an open question. For T1c, lesions (1.1 to 2 cm in diameter), the incidence of lymph node metastases is approximately 20 percent, even when such cancers are discovered by mammography, and the risk of local recurrence in the breast is substantial after local excision. In the NSABP B-06 study, breast recurrence was more than 25 percent if axillary nodes were negative and more than 35 percent if nodes were positive. Local breast recurrences in such patients were reduced substantially by radiation therapy. If nodes were positive, these patients also received adjuvant systemic therapy; the reduction in local breast recurrence was quite dramatic, from about 35 percent to about five percent. Thus for patients with primary invasive cancers between 1.1 and 2 cm in diameter (T1c), whether detected by mammography or palpation, standard therapy should probably include radiation therapy to the breast even if there is an absence of EIC. However, if the cancer is of low grade or the patient is anxious to avoid radiation at the risk of a somewhat higher local recurrence rate in the breast and the axillary nodes are negative, avoiding radiation therapy should

at least be considered as an option.[25] Axillary dissection should be performed in T1c patients because of the much higher likelihood of positive axillary nodes and the subsequent benefit of adjuvant therapy. However, if adjuvant therapy is to be utilized, axillary dissection is optional in such patients regardless of axillary lymph node status, since the discovery of metastatic nodes will not alter the selection of therapy.

The entire thrust of sophisticated breast cancer management during the past decades has emphasized accurate staging. This has been stimulated by the need for accurate separation by stage to select the appropriate therapy, particularly systemic therapy. If such adjuvant therapy is to be administered regardless of stage, then accurate axillary staging operations are not necessarily required. Thus if prognostic features of the primary cancer itself (such as large size, estrogen receptor negativity, extremely poor histology, lymphatic permeation, flow cytometry indications, thymidine labeling index, oncogene expression, or other features) indicate that adjuvant systemic therapy will be selected, then avoidance of axillary dissection for staging is justified.[8] This simplifies breast cancer management considerably, as adequate axillary staging operations to obtain 10 nodes can only be performed under general anesthesia and require hospitalization and wound drainage and result in considerable (though temporary) shoulder stiffness. The numbness and disability from sacrifice of the brachiocutaneous nerve usually performed as part of the axillary dissection can also be avoided.

Sophisticated analysis of bone marrow with monoclonal antibodies[44] may also provide more accurate staging of systemic disease, encourage the use of breast conservation procedures, and decrease the number of axillary lymph node dissections.

The traditional staging of breast cancer (i.e., including axillary lymph node analysis) may have to be altered in the near future to reduce the morbidity of the treatment, expedite decision making, and reduce unnecessary costs. Although this suggestion defies traditional wisdom, it nevertheless reflects the inevitable result of current prognostic indicator development and more widespread use of adjuvant therapy in breast cancer management of node-negative patients.

Clinically Detected Invasive Breast Cancer

For palpable T1 or T2 breast cancers, and even for those lesions more than 5 cm in diameter but with negative axillary nodes (T3N0), decision algorithms similar to those for mammographically detected cancers are appropriate. For palpable breast cancers, histological confirmation can usually be obtained by needle aspiration or core cutting biopsy of the mass in the physician's office on the first patient visit. However, although the diagnosis of breast cancer in such situations can frequently be obtained in the office, the details of the local pathology cannot be determined without adequate total removal of the breast cancer itself. Thus lumpectomy should be carried out promptly under local anesthesia to assess the features of the primary cancer. Although there is usually a correlation between the palpable size of the cancer and the pathological measurement of the invasive component of the cancer, in some situations a small sclerosing invasive breast cancer can present with a mass apparently considerably larger by palpation and even by mammography than the actual invasive cancer itself. Thus even the exact size of the primary cancer cannot be determined until after the lumpectomy. Clearly the biopsy procedure should satisfy all of the previously described requirements of a lumpectomy: at least a 1-cm clear margin surrounding the palpable cancer, attention to cosmetically appropriate incisions (see Figs. 36–2, 36–3, and 36–4), inking of the specimen for margin analysis, careful control of bleeding in the residual biopsy cavity, avoidance of drains, and the performance of the usual two-step procedure. Exceptions to the two-step procedure may occur in elderly patients in whom office needle biopsy and cytologic proof of breast cancer are possible and the preliminary discussions regarding therapy indicate that mastectomy is desired. Thus mastectomy can be performed forthwith, since details of the local breast cancer excision margin, histology, and prognostic indicators will not alter the selection of treatment. However, for any patient who wishes to explore the option of breast preservation, the lumpectomy/biopsy should be performed as a separate procedure so that features of the primary cancer can be completely documented before discussion with the patient about options for therapy. In at least one third of such patients, local excision and radiation therapy may not be suitable because of extensive intraductal cancer surrounding the primary cancer, inability to obtain tumor-free margins, distortion and poor cosmetic outcome in a small breast by the removal of a relatively large carcinoma, or occurrence of multiple primary cancers. In these situations requiring mastectomy, immediate reconstruction of the breast can be offered, but the preliminary consultation and coordination of operative schedules with the plastic surgeon may require some period of delay. A considerable body of literature currently exists about the suitability of breast reconstruction and the lack of danger or adverse consequences of immediate reconstruction at the time of mastectomy.[22, 32, 77] Most reconstructions at the present time utilize a subpectoral implant that thrusts the entire operative field forward just under the skin so that local recurrences are not hidden from examination but can be readily detected.

Although axillary dissection should be considered standard therapy in patients with larger primary breast cancers, nevertheless, since the majority of these patients will be administered adjuvant chemotherapy (polychemotherapy if premenopausal or tamoxifen if postmenopausal), the relative value and usefulness of axillary dissection is virtually eliminated. Axillary lymph node metastases are "indicators but not governors of survival,"[5] and therefore axillary dissection is primarily a staging and not a therapeutic procedure. Thus in the absence of palpable axillary lymphadenopathy, and perhaps even with palpable lymph node metastases, a patient undergoing lumpectomy, radiation therapy, and adjuvant systemic therapy may choose to avoid axillary dissection after being given proper advice and explanation of risks and benefits. If the case is such that adjuvant therapy would not be given if axillary nodes are negative but would be given if nodes are positive, axillary dissection is clearly indicated. For clinical research trials in which detailed staging is critical for evaluation, axillary dissections should be performed.

Data indicate better disease-free survival rates after use of adjuvant therapy in node-negative patients (both premenopausal and postmenopausal) and mortality reduction in node-positive patients of approximately 20 percent (for postmenopausal patients administered tamoxifen) to 33 percent (for premenopausal patients given polychemotherapy).[30] When overall survival expectations at 10 years are no better than 75 percent, it seems clear that the benefits outweigh the risks for adjuvant therapy.[24, 77] Therefore patients with larger primary invasive breast cancer (T2 or T3) generally should receive adjuvant therapy.

In this time of rapidly evolving management changes in primary breast cancer, it is critical that patients be informed of the various options, risks, and benefits so they can make suitable judgments regarding appropriate therapy. Although some patients will choose standard therapy from a desire to conform and achieve maximal benefit from conventional wisdom, many patients are willing to explore variations in management and therapy with proper guidance, empathy, and information provided by the surgeon and medical oncologist. It is important to involve patients in therapeutic decisions, particularly in early breast cancer, since such a wide variety of options are currently available and more may be developed in the next decade. Because the word "cancer" terrifies most patients, careful detailed explanation of the realistic prognostic figures and outcomes are particularly important in patients with very early disease, since their outlook may be very favorable but their assumptions about outcome very gloomy. Patients may be frightened of a diagnosis of DCIS discovered mammographically, yet they may be heavy cigarette smokers incurring more risk to their life from that habit than from their innocuous focal DCIS. While it is vitally important to point out to patients the risks and benefits of their management decisions, it is also important to have them recognize and act on the basis of their personal philosophy regarding their physical body as well as their approach to life. (Are they risk takers? Are they body conscious? Are their breasts of major sexual or psychological importance?) Discussions about their breast cancer and the selection of variations in therapy have to be conducted at great length and, if at all possible, with other people present. Despite careful detailed explanation, emotion-laden material may not be properly comprehended by the anxious patient or family, and repeated discussions may need to occur. Unsophisticated, angry, or ignorant patients require great sensitivity and considerable time to resolve therapy selections.

Patients may urge the surgeon to make decisions to do what is "best." These pleas should resolutely be

Table 36–8. AUTHOR'S ESTIMATE OF DISEASE-FREE SURVIVAL AT 10 YEARS

T Category	Lesion Size (cm)	N Category	Disease-Free Survival at 10 Years (%)
Tis		N0	100
T1a	0–0.5	N0	99
		pN1ai + micrometastasis	95
		pN1bi + macrometastasis	80
T1b	0.6–1.0	N0	95
		pN1ai + micrometastasis	90
		pN1bi + macrometastasis	75
T1c	1.1–2	N0	90
		pN1bii + 1–3 macrometastases	70
		pN1biii + >3 macrometastases	<50
T2	2.1–3	N0	80
		N1	<50

Compiled from Rosen PP, et al: J Clin Oncol 7:355–366, 1989; Seidman H, et al: CA 5(37):258–290, 1987; Wilkinson LH, et al: Arch Surg 117:579–582, 1982.

deflected, since the "best" therapy is a completely relative term. What is "best" for one patient is hardly "best" for someone else, and the fact that true options exist in terms of equivalent survival means the patient must make the ultimate selection with guidance. This patient-based decision is required both for ultimate patient satisfaction and for physician protection and to avoid even the suggestion that the physician is autocratically dictating therapy for the uninformed patient. Such dictation of therapy by surgeons or physicians is inappropriate in the realm of contemporary breast cancer management, in which much publicity in the press has occurred and many therapeutic options are available. In 1950 or even 1960, there was only one realistic therapeutic alternative available for patients with breast cancer, but currently there are innumerable variations in treatment, perhaps totaling 50 or more. For each individual patient the therapeutic options may be numerous, and arbitrary imposition of a therapeutic pathway by the physicians and surgeons should be avoided. Such an approach, however, places a larger burden on patients and families.

Follow-Up

Follow-up of breast cancer patients is increasingly complicated when breast preservation is selected. For patients with mastectomy, routine subsequent physical examination can be performed at 6-month intervals initially and, after a few years, at yearly intervals. Examination should focus on the mastectomy area and regional nodes. Ample evidence exists that detailed laboratory-based follow-up is costly and of no help in improving prognosis.[66, 70] Symptom-based management is highly satisfactory and conserves patient and system resources. Thus routine blood studies, chest radiographs, and bone scans are not performed, but management utilizing specific symptomatic or physical examination indicators (backache, cough, fatigue, etc.) is used instead. If metastatic or recurrent disease is discovered,

a complete work-up is undertaken before therapy selection.

For patients with breast-preserving local therapy, however, follow-up of the breast must be more detailed, frequent, and careful, since local recurrence is not infrequent, and cure is often by mastectomy or by repeated local excision and radiation therapy if not previously utilized. Breast physical examination is performed every 3 months, perhaps alternating between surgeon and radiotherapist. Mammography is performed every 6 months for the first 2 years, with the understanding that prominent postlumpectomy scar can exactly mimic recurrent cancer. Suspicious thickening may occur because of radiation fibrosis, particularly if implantation techniques were used. A high index of suspicion must be maintained, and any worrisome mass or thickening of breast tissue should undergo needle aspiration or core cutting biopsy. Open biopsy is utilized cautiously, since late surgical incisions in the radiated breast exacerbate scar formation and mass development that continue the diagnostic problem. Mammographic changes that suggest recurrent or new cancer (i.e., clustered calcification or later mass) require localization and biopsy. The time sequence for locally recurrent disease is prolonged, although after 10 years, most cancers that arise are new primary cancers and not true recurrences.[70]

A summary of expected disease-free survival at 10 years from the various entities discussed in this chapter is given in Table 36–8.

References

1. Anderson J: Lobular carcinoma in situ: an approach to rational treatment. Cancer 39:2587–2602, 1977.
2. Beahrs OH, Henson DE, Hutter RVP, Myers MH (eds): Manual for Staging of Cancer, ed 3. American Joint Committee on Cancer. Philadelphia, JB Lippincott, 1988, p 147.
3. Bedwant R, Vana J, Rosner D, et al: Management and survival of female patients with "minimal" breast cancer: as observed in the long-term and short-term surveys of the American College of Surgeons. Cancer 47:2769–2778, 1981.
4. Cady B: New diagnostic, staging, and therapeutic aspects of early breast cancer. Cancer 65:634–647, 1990.

5. Cady B: Lymph node metastases: indicators but not governors of survival. Arch Surg 119:1067–1072, 1984.

6. Calle R, Vilcoq JR, Pilleron JP: Conservative treatment of operable breast cancer by irradiation with or without limited surgery: ten year results. *In* Harris JR, Hellman S, Silen W (eds): Conservative Management of Breast Cancer. Philadelphia, JB Lippincott, 1985, pp 3–9.

7. Carter CL, Allen C, Henson DE: Relation of tumor size, lymph node status, and survival in 24,740 breast cancer cases. Cancer 63:181–187, 1989.

8. Clark GM, Dressler LG, Owens MA, Pounds G, Ildaker T, McGuire WL: Prediction of relapse or survival in patients with node-negative breast cancer by DNA flow cytometry. N Engl J Med 320:627–633, 1989.

9. Delouche G, Bachelot F, Premont M, Kurtz JM: Conservation treatment of early breast cancer: long term results and complications. Int J Radiat Oncol Biol Phys 13:29–34, 1987.

10. DeRosa CM, Ozzello L, Habif DV, Konrath JG, Greene GL: Immunohistochemical assessment of estrogen and progesterone receptors in stored imprints and cryostat sections of breast carcinomas. Ann Surg 2:210:224–228, 1989.

11. Dupont WD, Page DL: Risk factors for breast cancer in women with proliferative breast disease. N Engl J Med 312:146–151, 1985.

12. Farrow JH: Current concepts in the detection and treatment of the earliest of the breast cancers. Cancer 25:468–477, 1970.

13. Findlay P, Lippman M, Danforth D, et al: A randomized trial comparing mastectomy to radiotherapy in the treatment of stage I–II breast cancer: a preliminary report. Proc Am Soc Clin Oncol 5:246–263, 1986.

14. Fisher B, Bauer M, Wickerham L, et al: Relation of number of positive axillary nodes to the prognosis of patients with primary breast cancer—an NSABP update. Cancer 52:1551, 1983.

15. Fisher B, Redmond C, Poisson R, Margolese R, Wolmark N, Wickerman L, Fisher E, et al: Eight-year results of a randomized clinical trial comparing total mastectomy and lumpectomy with or without irradiation in the treatment of breast cancer. N Engl J Med 320:822–828, 1989.

16. Fisher B: Presentation in Milan, Italy, 1989.

17. Fisher ER, Sass R, Fisher B, Wickerham C, Paik SM: Pathologic findings from the National Surgical Adjuvant Breast Project (protocol 6). I. Intraductal carcinoma (DCIS). Cancer 57:197–208, 1986.

18. Fowble BL, Solin LJ, Goodman RL: Results of conservative surgery and radiation for intraductal non-invasive breast cancer. (Abstract) Am J Clin Oncol (CCT) 10:110–111, 1987.

19. Frazier TG, Noone RB: Immediate reconstruction in the treatment of primary carcinoma of the breast. Surg Gynecol Obstet 157:413–414, 1983.

20. Frykberg E, Santiago F, Betsill WL, O'Brien PH: Lobular carcinoma in situ of the breast. Surg Gynecol Obstet 164:285–301, 1987.

21. Gallagher WJ, Koerner FC, Wood WC: Treatment of intraductal carcinoma with limited surgery: long-term follow-up. J Clin Oncol 7:373–380, 1989.

22. Georgiade GS, Georgiade NG, McCarty KS, Ferguson BJ, Seigler HF: Modified radical mastectomy with immediate reconstruction for carcinoma of the breast. Ann Surg 193:565–573, 1981.

23. Giordano JM, Klopp CT: Lobular carcinima in situ: incidence and treatment. Cancer 31:105–109, 1973.

24. Goldhirsch A, Gelber RD, Simes RJ, Glasziou P, Coates AS: Costs and benefits of adjuvant therapy in breast cancer: a quality-adjusted survival analysis. J Clin Oncol 7:36–44, 1989.

25. Greening WP, Montgomery CV, Gordon AB, Gowing NFC: Quadrantic excision and axillary node dissection without radiation therapy: the long-term results of a selective policy in the treatment of Stage I breast cancer. Eur J Surg Oncol 14:221–225, 1988.

26. Gump F, Jica DL, Ozzella L: Ductal carcinoma in situ (DCIS): a revised concept. Surgery 102:190–195, 1987.

27. Haagensen CD, Lane N, Lattes R, Bodian C: Lobular neoplasia (so-called lobular carcinoma in situ) of the breast. Cancer 42:737–769, 1978.

28. Haagensen CD, Bodian C, Haagensen D (eds): Breast Carcinoma Risk and Detection. Philadelphia, WB Saunders, 1981, p 267.

29. Hatschek T, Fagerberg G, Stal O, Sullivan S, Carstensen J, Grontoft O, Nordenskjolk B: Cytometric characterization and clinical course of breast cancer diagnosed in a population-based screening program. Cancer 64:1074–1081, 1989.

30. Henderson IC, Mouridsen H: Effects of adjuvant tamoxifen and of cytotoxic therapy on mortality in early breast cancer. An overview of 61 randomized trials among 28,896 women. N Engl J Med 319:1681–1692, 1988.

31. Holland R, Mravunac M, Hendriks JHCL, Bekker BV: So-called interval cancers of the breast. Pathologic and radiologic analysis of sixty-four cases. Cancer 49:2527–2533, 1982.

32. Johnson CH, van Heerden JA, Donohue JH, Martin JK, Jackson IT, Ilstrup DM: Oncological aspects of immediate breast reconstruction following mastectomy for malignancy. Arch Surg 124:819–824, 1989.

33. Kraus FT, Neubecker RD: The differential diagnosis of papillary tumors of the breast. Cancer 15:444–455, 1962.

34. Kurtz JM, Jacquemier J, Torhorst J, et al: Conservation therapy for breast cancers other than infiltrating ductal ca. (Abstract) Int J Radiat Oncol Biol Phys 15:194, 1988.

35. Kurtz JM, Amalric R, Brandone H, Ayme Y, Jacquemier J, Pietra JC, Hans D, Pollet JF, Bressac C, Spitalier JM: Local recurrence after breast-conserving surgery and radiotherapy. Frequency, time course, and prognosis. Cancer 63:1912–1917, 1989.

36. Kurtz JM, Jacquemier J, Torhorst J, Spitalier JM, Amalric R, Reinhard H, Walther E, Harder F, et al: Conservation therapy for breast cancers other than infiltrating ductal carcinoma. Cancer 63:1630–1635, 1989.

37. Lagios MD. Ductal Carcinoma *in Situ*. Presentation at Annual Meeting of Society of Surgical Oncology, San Francisco, May, 1989.

38. Lagios MD, Westdahl PR, Margolin FR, Rose MR: Duct carcinoma in situ: relationship of extent of noninvasive disease to the frequency of occult invasion, multicentricity, lymph node metastases, and short-term treatment failures. Cancer 50:1309–1314, 1982.

39. Lagios MD, Richards VE, Rose MR, Yee E: Segmental mastectomy without radiotherapy. Short-term follow up. Cancer 52:2173–2179, 1983.

40. Lagios MD, Margolin R, Westdahl PR, Rose MR: Mammographically detected duct carcinoma in situ. Cancer 63:618–624, 1989.

41. Leopold KA, Recht A, Schnitt SJ, Connolly JL, Rose MA, Silver B, Harris JR: Results of conservative surgery and radiation therapy for multiple synchronous cancers of one breast. Int J Radiat Oncol Biol Phys 16:11–16, 1989.

42. Lewis D, Geshickter CF: Comedo carcinoma of the breast. Arch Surg 36:225–234, 1938.

43. Love SM, Gelman RS, Silen W: Fibrocystic "disease" of the breast—a nondisease? N Engl J Med 307:1010–1014, 1982.

44. Mansi JL, Berger U, McDonnell T, Pople A, Rayter Z, Gazet JC, Coombes RD: The fate of bone marrow micrometastases in patients with primary breast cancer. J Clin Oncol 7:445–449, 1989.

45. Millis RR, Thynne GSJ: In-situ intraduct ca of the breast: a long term follow-up study. Br J Surg 62:957–962, 1975.

46. Montague E: Data presented at NSABP Intraductal Cancer Protocol Design Committee Symposium, November 29, 1984.

47. Neilsen M, Jensen J, Anderson J: Precancerous and cancerous breast lesions during lifetime and at autopsy. Cancer 54:612–615, 1984.

48. Page DL, Dupont WD, Rogers LW, Landenberger, M: Intraductal carcinoma of the breast: follow-up after biopsy only. Cancer 49:751–758, 1982.

49. Page DL, Dupont WD, Rogers LW, Rados MS: Atypical hyperplastic lesions of the female breast. A long-term follow-up study. Cancer 55:2698–2708, 1985.

50. Patchefsky AS, Shaber GS, Schwartz GF, Feig SA, Nerlinger RD: The pathology of breast cancer detected by mass population screening. Cancer 40:1659–1670, 1977.

51. Patchefsky AS, Gordon FS, Finkelstein SD, Prestipino A, Sohn SE, Singer JS, Feig SA: Heterogeneity of intraductal carcinoma of the breast. Cancer 63:731–741, 1989.

52. Recht A, Danoff BF, Solin LJ, et al: Intraductal carcinoma of the breast: results of treatment with excisional biopsy and irradiation. J Clin Oncol 3:1339–1343, 1985.

53. Recht A, Connolly JC, Schnitt SJ, et al: The effect of young age on tumor recurrence in the treated breast after conservative surgery and radiotherapy. Int J Radiat Oncol Biol Phys 14:3–10, 1988.
54. Reger V, Beito G, Jolly PC: Factors affecting the incidence of lymph node metastases in small cancers of the breast. Am J Surg 157:501–502, 1989.
55. Rose MA, Olivotto I, Cady B, Koufman C, Osteen R, Silver B, Recht A, Harris JR: Conservative surgery and radiation therapy for early breast cancer. Long-term cosmetic results. Arch Surg 124:153–156, 1989.
56. Rosen PP, Lieberman PH, Braun DW, et al: Lobular carcinoma in situ of the breast: detailed analysis of 99 patients with average follow-up of 24 years. Am J Surg Pathol 2:225–251, 1978.
57. Rosen PP, Saigo PE, Braun DW, Weathers E, Fracchia AA, Kinne DW: Axillary micro- and macrometastases in breast cancer, prognostic significance of tumor size. Ann Surg 5;194:585–591, 1981.
58. Rosen PP, Braun DW, Kinne DE: The clinical significance of pre-invasive breast carcinoma. Cancer 46:919–925, 1980.
59. Rosen PP, Groshen S, Saigo PE, Kinne DW, Hellman S: A long-term follow-up study of survival in stage I ($T_1N_0M_0$) and stage II ($T_1N_1M_0$) breast carcinoma. J Clin Oncol 7:355–366, 1989.
60. Rosner D, Bedwant RN, Vana J, et al: Noninvasive breast carcinoma: results of a national survey by the American College of Surgeons. Ann Surg 192:139–147, 1980.
61. Saccani Jotti, G, Petit JY, Contesso G: Minimal breast cancer: a clinically meaningful term? Semin Oncol 4(13):384–392, 1986.
62. Schnitt SJ, Silen W, Sadowsky NL, Connolly JL, Harris JR: Ductal carcinoma in situ (intraductal carcinoma) of the breast. N Engl J Med 318:898–903, 1988.
63. Seidman H, Gelb SK, Silverberg E, Laverda N, Lubera JA: Survival experience in the breast cancer detection demonstration project end results. CA 5:258–290, 1987.
64. Shapiro S: Determining the efficacy of breast cancer screening. Cancer 63:1873–1880, 1989.
65. Silverstein MJ, Rosser RJ, Gierson ED, et al: Axillary lymph node dissection for intraductal breast carcinoma—is it indicated? Cancer 59:1819—1824, 1987.
66. Stierer M, Rosen HR: Influence of early diagnosis on prognosis of recurrent breast cancer. Cancer 64:1128–1131, 1989.
67. Swain SM: Ductal carcinoma in situ-incidence, presentation, guidelines to treatment. Oncology March:25–31, 1989.
68. Tabar L, Dean PB: The control of breast cancer through mammography screening. What is the evidence? Radiol Clin North Am 25:993–1005, 1987.
69. Tinnemans JGM, Wobbes T, Holland R, Hendriks JHCL, et al: Treatment and survival of female patients with nonpalpable breast carcinoma. Ann Surg Feb:249–253, 1989.
70. Tomlin R, Donegan WL: Screening for recurrent breast cancer—its effectiveness and prognostic value. J Clin Oncol 5:62–67, 1987.
71. Unzeitig GW, Frankl G, Ackerman M, O'Connell TX: Analysis of the prognosis of minimal and occult breast cancers. Arch Surg 118:1403–1404, 1983.
72. van de Vijver MJ, Peterse JL, Mooi WJ, Wisman P, Lomans J, Dalesio O, Nusse R: Neu-protein overexpression in breast cancer: association with comedo-type ductal carcinoma in situ and limited prognostic value in stage II breast cancer. N Engl J Med 319:1239–1282, 1988.
73. Verbeek A, Hendricks J, Holland R, et al: Reduction of breast cancer mortality through mass screening with modern mammography. First results of the Nijmegen Project, 1975–1981. Lancet 1:1222, 1984.
74. Veronesi U: Rationale and indications for limited surgery in breast cancer: current data. World J Surg 11:493–498, 1987.
75. Webster DJT, Mansel RE, Hughes LE: Immediate reconstruction of the breast after mastectomy. Is it safe? Cancer 53:1416–1419, 1984.
76. Wheeler JE, Enterline HT, Roseman JM, et al: Lobular carcinoma in situ of the breast: long-term follow-up. Cancer 34:554–563, 1974.
77. Wilkinson LH, Peloso OA, Dail WG: Modified radical mastectomy with immediate breast reconstruction. Arch Surg 117:579–582, 1982.
78. Zafrani B, Fourquet A, Vilcoq JR, Legal M, Calle R: Conservative management of intraductal breast carcinoma with tumorectomy and radiation therapy. Cancer 57:1299–1301, 1986.

Chapter 37

ADJUVANT RADIATION THERAPY FOLLOWING MODIFIED RADICAL OR RADICAL MASTECTOMY

Nancy Price Mendenhall, M.D., Gilbert H. Fletcher, M.D., and Rodney R. Million, M.D.

INDICATIONS

Based on the incidence and pattern of local/regional recurrences following radical or modified radical mastectomy for operable breast cancer in historical series,[24, 29] Fletcher identified subsets of patients with a significant risk of local/regional recurrence and established the following indications for elective radiation following radical or modified radical mastectomy (see Table 37–1):[7]

1. Patients with outer quadrant lesions <5 cm and no involvement of axillary nodes do not receive postoperative irradiation.

2. Patients with histologically negative axillary nodes and central or medial breast cancers <2 cm receive irradiation to the internal mammary nodes only.

3. Patients with positive axillary nodes (but less than 20 percent of nodes involved) or patients with central or medial tumors >2 cm receive peripheral lymphatic irradiation (i.e., the internal mammary nodes and the supraclavicular and axillary apex nodes).

4. Patients with more than 20 percent of nodes involved receive not only peripheral lymphatic irradiation but also chest wall irradiation regardless of the size of the primary lesion or the location in the breast.
The whole axilla is never irradiated unless the dissection is incomplete, large (>2.5 cm) axillary nodes are present, or extranodal disease is histologically verified or clinically suspected because of matted adenopathy prior to surgery. The chest wall is also irradiated if the primary tumor is large (>5 cm), grave signs are present, the surgical margins are close or involved, or the primary tumor has extensive perineural or vascular space invasion.

TREATMENT

With the exception of posterior axillary fields, all standard radiation fields are treated with the patient supine on the treatment table. The patient is positioned on one of several prefabricated wedges [Fig. 37–1(A)] so that the chest wall from the suprasternal notch to the xiphoid is level. The patient's head is turned sharply to the contralateral side, and the ipsilateral arm is abducted to 90°. To ensure reproducibility of the patient's position each day of therapy, a customized polyurethane upper torso mold that fits over the wedge is then fashioned for each patient [Fig. 37–1(B)]. The patient's ipsilateral hand grasps a handle attached to the mold. The borders of anterior treatment fields are determined by anatomical landmarks. The posterior axillary field is simulated. Details of the design of the treatment portals are given in the following sections.

Internal Mammary Chain Field

The internal mammary chain nodes most at risk lie in a parasternal position within the first three rib interspaces. Approximately 85 percent of these nodes lie within a volume 1 to 4 cm lateral to midline and 4 cm deep to the skin surface.[25] Chest wall thickness may be determined from a cross-table lateral roentgenogram obtained at simulation [Fig. 37–2(A)], a CT scan,[19] or an ultrasound scan of the chest wall.[1, 6] Knowledge of the thickness of the chest wall provides a maximum potential depth for the internal mammary chain nodes so that an appropriate electron beam energy may be chosen.

The internal mammary chain nodes are treated with an en face field [Fig. 37–2(B)]. The lateral border is placed 6 cm from midline, and the medial border slopes from midline at the inferior border of the field to 1 cm contralateral to midline at the superior border of the field [Figs. 37–2(B), 37–3, and 37–4(C)]. The inferior border covers the third interspace. The superior border covers the first interspace or matches the inferior border of the supraclavicular field. With inferior medial or

Table 37–1. RADIATION THERAPY TREATMENT VOLUME GUIDELINES FOR OPERABLE (STAGES I AND II) BREAST CANCER FOLLOWING MODIFIED RADICAL OR RADICAL MASTECTOMY WITH PATEY OR FULL AXILLARY DISSECTION

Extent of Axillary Disease	Location of Primary	
	Medial	*Lateral*
Axilla negative, primary <2 cm	IMC	—
Axilla negative, primary ≥2 cm and ≤5 cm	PL	—
Axilla positive with ≤20 percent nodes positive	PL	PL
Axilla positive with >20 percent nodes positive	PL + CW*	PL + CW
Extranodal or large volume (≥2.5 cm) disease in axilla	PL + CW + AX	PL + CW + AX

*The chest wall is also treated whenever there are grave signs (skin edema, erythema, ulceration or fixation, pectoral fascia or chest wall fixation, axillary node matting, or fixation to the skin), a primary >5 cm, extensive perineural or vascular space invasion, multiple foci of invasive tumor, or close or positive margins on the primary tumor.

Abbreviations: AX = axilla; CW = chest wall; IMC = internal mammary chain nodes; PL = IMC + SC + axillary apex; SC = supraclavicular area.

central quadrant primaries, the fourth through sixth interspaces may be included. The internal mammary chain can be treated together with the chest wall within opposed tangential fields. However, it is necessary to extend the tangential fields across the midline to secure coverage of the internal mammary nodes. The volume of lung that is treated (as well as the heart in left-sided lesions) increases, and management of subsequent contralateral breast carcinomas is complicated (see Figs. 38–5 and 38–6, chapter 38).

The en face internal mammary chain field is treated preferably with electrons or with a combination of

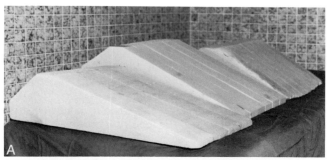

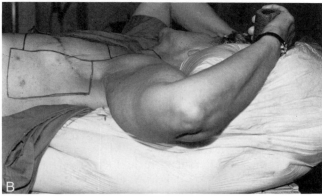

Figure 37–1. *A*, Patients are positioned on a Styrofoam wedge of appropriate size and shape so that the chest wall from the sternal notch to the xiphoid is level. *B*, After the appropriate wedge is selected, a customized polyurethane mold that fits over the wedge is made. The mold assures reproducible head and arm position and prevents torso rotation.

electrons and photons when the patient is very large or partial skin sparing is desired. An electron beam energy (usually 12 or 14 MeV electrons) or a combination of energies is selected so that the lymph nodes are contained within the 90 percent isodose volume. A given dose of 5000 cGy is delivered. For patients who were or will be exposed to doxorubicin HCl, it is essential to limit the dose to the heart from the internal mammary chain field by covering only the first three interspaces whenever possible [Fig. 37–4(D)] and by using an electron beam rather than photons.

Axillary Apex and Supraclavicular Node Field

The axillary apical-supraclavicular portal covers the lymph nodes in the axillary apex, which lie inferior to the clavicle just beneath the pectoral muscle, and the lymph nodes in the supraclavicular fossa, which are superficial laterally but deep to the insertion of the sternocleidomastoid muscle medially.

When peripheral lymphatic irradiation is indicated, the internal mammary chain and axillary apical-supraclavicular volumes may be treated separately or combined in a single hockey stick–shaped portal (Fig. 37–3). Two advantages of separate fields are the possibility of using different energies for separate fields and the ability to angle the supraclavicular portal 15° off the midline. The medial border of the supraclavicular field is 1 cm across the midline at the level of the sternal notch, extending superiorly to the thyrocricoid groove, laterally to include the supraclavicular fossa and axillary apex to the superior limits of surgical dissection in the axilla, and inferiorly to the first costal cartilage. If a full axillary dissection has been performed with removal of level I, II, and III nodes or if a level I and II dissection has revealed no tumor, the lateral border of the field can be placed at approximately the coracoid process, where the pectoralis minor muscle inserts. Clips placed in the axilla at the upper level of axillary dissection are also useful in setting the lateral border. When photons are used, the axillary apical-supraclavicular portal is

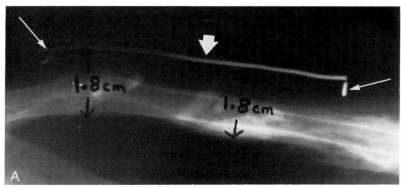

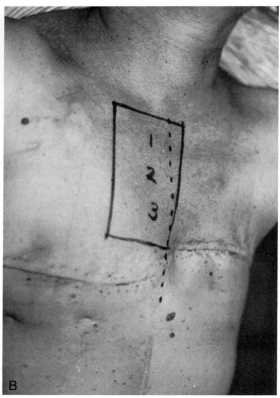

Figure 37–2. *A,* After field lines are drawn on the patient, a cross-table x-ray film is taken with solder placed on the skin at midline *(arrowhead)* and at the superior and inferior borders of the internal mammary field *(arrows).* The distance between the skin surface and posterior surface of the sternum is calculated and used to select an appropriate electron energy for the internal mammary field. *B,* Field for internal mammary chain treatment. The superior border is at the level of the suprasternal notch, and the inferior border is below the third intercostal space. The lateral border is 6 cm from midline (indicated by dotted line). The medial border is at midline inferiorly but slopes laterally to 1 cm across midline at the superior border of the field.

angled 15° laterally to avoid irradiation of the spinal cord. When electrons are used, the field is not angled.

Because of the varying target depths, high-energy photons are used for this field; cobalt 60 is ideal because of its maximum dose at 0.5 cm. Twenty percent to 40 percent of the dose may be delivered with electrons, which effectively decreases the dose to the lung and the incidence of acute symptomatic pneumonitis.[18] In elective irradiation of subclinical disease, the axillary apical-supraclavicular portal receives 200 cGy given dose a day to 5000 cGy; the superficial nodes therefore receive approximately 5000 cGy, and the deeper nodes at 3 cm receive approximately 4500 cGy.

Whole Axilla and Supraclavicular Node Field

The commonly involved axillary lymph nodes lie in the anterior half of the axilla. The most inferior axillary nodes lie at the midaxillary line [Fig. 37–4(A, B)]. The superior axillary nodes wrap anteriorly around the chest wall to drain into the apex of the axilla and the supraclavicular fossa. The target depth from the anterior skin surface ranges from 5 to 8 cm in the low to central axilla to 0.5 to 1 cm in the supraclavicular area and 1 to 4 cm beneath the sternocleidomastoid muscle insertion. In the apex of the axilla, the nodes lie beneath the pectoralis muscle, which varies considerably in thickness among patients.

When there are indications for treatment of the whole

axilla, the standard axillary apex and supraclavicular field may be extended laterally and inferiorly to incorporate the entire axilla. The medial and superior field borders are the same, but the lateral border crosses the acromioclavicular joint to cover the soft tissues of the axilla, and the inferior border of the field is extended to the second costal cartilage. Because the whole axilla-supraclavicular field is angled 15°, coverage in the lateral soft tissues of the axilla is increased, so it is not necessary for the beam to fall off the pectoral muscle [Fig. 37–4(C, D)].[7] The entire dose to the whole axilla-supraclavicular field is delivered with photons. When the whole axilla is treated, the skin of the superior chest wall flap is included in the treatment portal. To achieve an adequate skin dose, bolus material is applied to the skin below the clavicle, which is part of the superior chest wall flap. A posterior field is added to increase the dose to the mid and low axilla, which may be underdosed from the anterior supraclavicular field because of its relative depth in comparison to the more superficial axillary apex and supraclavicular fossa.

When a posterior axillary field is needed, a separate customized upper torso body mold is made with the patient prone and her head turned sharply to the contralateral side [Fig. 37–5(A)]. At simulation, a customized block is designed for treatment of the posterior axillary field. The medial border of the field shows a 1-cm rim of lung, the superior border splits the clavicle and the humerus, the lateral border includes the soft tissues of the axilla, and the inferior border coincides with the superior edge of the anterior chest wall fields

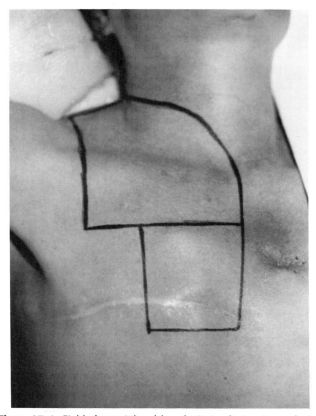

Figure 37–3. Fields for peripheral lymphatic irradiation (supraclavicular, axillary apical, and internal mammary nodes). This treatment volume may be treated in a single hockey stick–shaped field or in separate internal mammary and supraclavicular-axillary apical fields, as shown. When there are no indications for axillary irradiation, the lateral border of the supraclavicular-axillary apical field may be set over the coracoid process or, if clips placed at axillary dissection are visible, the border may be set to just overlap the medial extent of the surgical clips marking the proximal extent of the axillary dissection. The inferior border of the field is at the first costal cartilage. The beam for the field includes the first intercostal space or abuts an internal mammary field, which includes the first interspace as shown in Figure 37–4C. The medial border covers the insertion of the sternocleidomastoid muscle and joins the medial border of the internal mammary field. Superiorly, the field either falls off the skin edge or is blocked. This field is angled 15° laterally to avoid irradiation of the spine and esophagus and to increase lateral coverage. The supraclavicular-axillary apical field is treated with a combination of photons (usually cobalt 60 for 4000 cGy) and electrons (usually 10 to 14 MeV for 1000 cGy).

The internal mammary field may cover the nodes in the first three interspaces or abut the supraclavicular-axillary apical field to cover the second and third interspaces, as here. In patients with inferior-medial quadrant tumors, the internal mammary field extends caudad to cover the fourth through sixth interspaces. The medial field border is set 1 cm across the midline superiorly and at midline inferiorly. Superiorly, the field is 7 cm wide and inferiorly, 6 cm wide. The internal mammary field may be treated entirely with an appropriate energy of electrons (usually 12 or 14 MeV) or, if the patient is very large or skin sparing is desired, with photons alone or a combination of electrons and photons.

or approximately the lateral fourth rib [Fig. 37–5(B)]. The posterior axillary field is treated with high-energy photons. The total dose is 4500 cGy for subclinical disease and 5000 cGy for extensive extranodal disease. If gross residual disease is left in the axilla, the dose may be boosted through a reduced anterior or appositional field with an appropriate energy to 6000 cGy.

When the posterior axillary field is used, care is taken to ensure that the added dose contributions from the posterior and anterior portals throughout the treatment volume do not exceed a daily dose of 200 cGy. This may require treatment of the posterior axillary field on all or most treatment days.

Chest Wall Field

The main site of recurrence following mastectomy is in the skin of the chest wall flap. With standard modified radical and radical mastectomies, the chest wall flaps are quite thin, so that only a superficial volume of skin and subcutaneous tissue is at risk. With simple mastectomies, the chest wall flaps may be thicker.

In general, the superior and inferior chest wall flaps are included with at least a 5-cm margin beyond the mastectomy scar except at the extreme lateral and medial borders, where 2- to 3-cm margins are acceptable [Fig. 37–4(C)]. Chest wall irradiation may be delivered through en face electron-beam fields or opposed tangential photon fields.

The electron beam technique is chosen for the majority of patients because matching of abutting fields is easier to control, the dose to the lung is less, and a separate portal with higher energy electrons may be used for better coverage of the internal mammary nodes. Five MeV to 8 MeV electrons are chosen, and 0.5 cm of tissue-equivalent bolus material is applied to the skin during treatment to increase the skin dose to ≥90 percent of the specified dose; this approach produces a brisk erythema after delivery of 5000 cGy without concomitant chemotherapy in the majority of patients. If opposed tangential photon fields are used, bolus material should be applied as needed to achieve a brisk erythema by the end of treatment; with cobalt 60, bolus application every other day produces an appropriate skin reaction. With either technique, the matchlines for abutting fields are changed at least once during treatment to "feather" the dose inhomogeneity at the junction line.

For patients judged to be at a particularly high risk for chest wall recurrence because of extensive axillary node involvement or close surgical margins, the dose to a 2-cm strip of skin along the mastectomy scar is boosted with 5 MeV to 8 MeV electrons for an additional 1000 cGy in four to five fractions.

RESULTS OF TREATMENT

The goal of adjuvant irradiation following radical or modified radical mastectomy is prevention of local and regional recurrences. The primary end point by which the efficacy of this treatment must be measured then is local regional disease control. It was hoped when the indications for this treatment were defined that increased local/regional control rates would produce increased survival through prevention of distant metastases that occur as the result of seeding from uncontrolled lo-

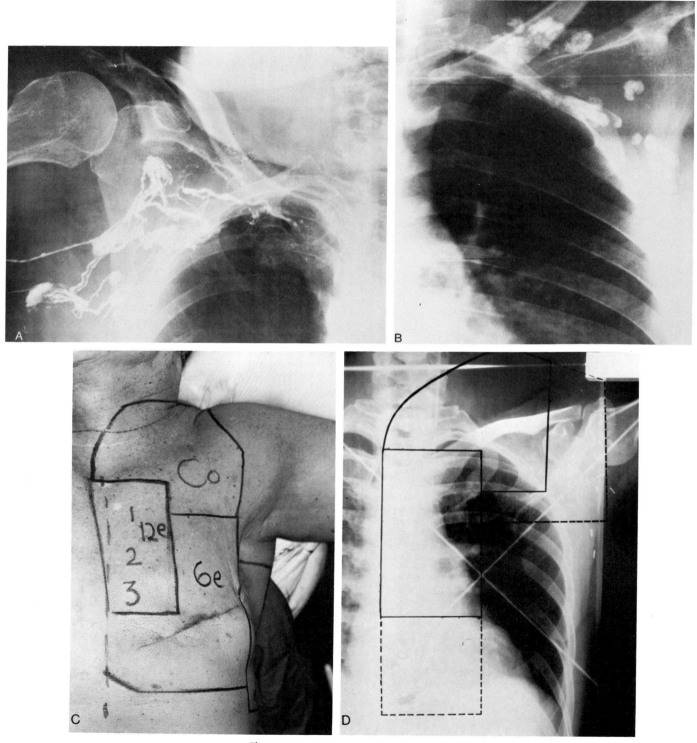

Figure 37–4. *See legend on opposite page*

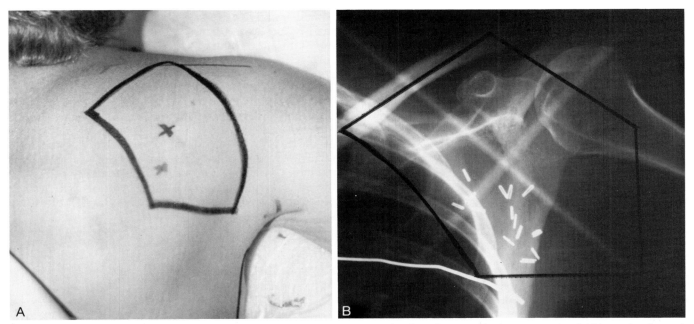

Figure 37–5. *A,* Posterior axilla field. The patient is treated prone in a customized polyurethane mold when a posterior field is used to boost the dose to the axilla. *B,* Simulation film of field. The field is simulated with the superior border along the clavicle, the medial border showing a 1-cm rim of lung, and the lateral border covering the soft tissues of the axilla and splitting the humerus. The inferior border matches the inferior border of the anterior supraclavicular-axillary portal (marked at simulation by a wire placed at the skin junction of the tangential or electron beam chest wall fields with the anterior supraclavicular-axillary field).

cal/regional disease. The secondary end points for evaluation of the efficacy of adjuvant irradiation, therefore, are survival and freedom from distant metastases.

Nonrandomized Studies of Postoperative Irradiation Without Adjuvant Chemotherapy

The results of postoperative irradiation after radical or modified radical mastectomy for 920 patients with operable breast cancer at the M. D. Anderson Hospital from 1963 to 1977 were reported in 1982.[35] Patients were electively irradiated postoperatively according to the indications listed previously. None of the patients received adjuvant chemotherapy. In 523 patients with

positive nodes who were observed for 10 years, the 10-year disease-free survival rate was 54 percent. Ten-year survival for patients with one to three positive lymph nodes was 56 percent, and for patients with four or more positive nodes, it was 33 percent. When compared with patients treated with radical mastectomy only in the placebo arm of NSABP trials from 1958–1963 (see Table 37–2), treatment failures were significantly fewer in the patients with both one to three and four or more positive nodes treated with postoperative irradiation at M. D. Anderson Hospital. Table 37–3 shows the site of local/regional recurrence according to histological status of the axilla and the area irradiated. Of interest were the low incidence (two percent) of supraclavicular failure and the increasing risk of failure in the chest wall

---

Figure 37–4. Axillary lymph nodes opacified by hand lymphangiogram *(A)* and reflux from foot lymphangiogram *(B).* The low axillary nodes lie at the midaxillary line. The apical nodes lie just beneath the pectoralis muscle. The nodes in the lateral supraclavicular fossa lie just beneath the skin. The depth of the medial supraclavicular nodes, which lie beneath the insertion of the sternocleidomastoid muscle, varies. (From Fletcher GH: Textbook of Radiotherapy. 3rd ed. Philadelphia, Lea and Febiger, 1983. Reprinted by permission.) *(C),* Anterior fields for a patient receiving chest wall, peripheral lymphatic, and axillary irradiation. The internal mammary node field is the same as in Figure 37–2B; it covers only the first three interspaces and is treated with 12 to 14 MeV electrons or photons. If the risk of disease in the internal mammary nodes in the fourth to the sixth interspace is judged to be high, the field may be extended caudally, but cardiac irradiation *(D),* which occurs when the fourth through the sixth interspaces are treated with high-energy electrons or photons, should always be avoided if possible (particularly when the patient has received or will receive doxorubicin). When axillary irradiation is indicated, the standard supraclavicular-axillary apical field is extended laterally to cross the acromioclavicular joint and inferiorly to the second costal cartilage for coverage of the axillary soft tissues. When axillary irradiation is indicated, the entire dose to the supraclavicular-axillary portal is delivered with photons, preferably cobalt 60, and the dose to the low and central axilla is boosted with a posterior portal. The chest wall fields cover the entire chest wall flaps, usually with at least a 5-cm margin on the mastectomy incision except at the medial and lateral ends of the incisions, where a 2-cm margin is acceptable. The chest wall fields are treated with 5 to 8 MeV electrons in most cases. *D,* Approximate volume of tissue irradiated with peripheral lymphatic irradiation *(solid lines)* covering only the internal mammary nodes in the first three interspaces and the supraclavicular and axillary apex nodes. The dotted lines indicate the extra volume of heart irradiated when the internal mammary field covers the fourth through the sixth interspaces and the extra lung and axillary soft tissue volume treated when there are indications for treatment of the whole axilla. This is an en face anteroposterior projection; sparing of the spine and some additional coverage of the axillary apex *(solid lines)* or whole axilla *(dotted lines)* is actually achieved when the beam for the supraclavicular-axillary field is angled 15° laterally. (The inferiormost portion of the axillary dissection bed is covered either in the en face electron fields or in tangential fields for the chest wall.)

Table 37–2. COMPARISON OF TREATMENT FAILURE RATES BETWEEN UTMDAH PATIENTS WITH RADICAL MASTECTOMY PLUS POSTOPERATIVE IRRADIATION AND NSABP PATIENTS WITH RADICAL MASTECTOMY WITHOUT IRRADIATION—NO ADJUVANT CHEMOTHERAPY IN BOTH GROUPS (10-YEAR MINIMUM FOLLOW-UP)

	Treatment Failures at 10 Yrs*			
	UTMDAH		**NSABP**	
Node Status	%	*No. Pts.*	%	*No. Pts.*
Negative	22.1	131	24.1	170
Positive	57.7†	392	76.1†	163
1–3 nodes	48.0‡	173	64.5‡	76
≥4 nodes	65.3§	219	86.2§	87

*Local/regional or at distant sites.
†*p* < 0.005
‡*p* < 0.02
§*p* < 0.005
Abbreviations: NSABP = National Surgical Adjuvant Breast and Bowel Project; UTMDAH = University of Texas M.D. Anderson Hospital.
From Tapley ND, et al: Cancer 49:1318, 1982. Reprinted by permission.

according to extent of axillary nodal involvement, which was significantly diminished by the addition of chest wall irradiation. The experience from M. D. Anderson Hospital therefore suggests that adjuvant irradiation following mastectomy not only improves local/regional control rates but also significantly decreases treatment failure rates.

Tubiana and coworkers[37] have compared four groups of patients treated at the Institut Gustave Roussy (IGR) in Villejuif between 1958 and 1967 for T0–T3 histologically node-positive breast cancers. Two groups were part of a multi-institutional cooperative study randomizing between radical mastectomy and extended radical mastectomy in which the internal mammary nodes were dissected. The other two groups of patients treated at the IGR during the same time period for breast cancers

of similar extent were ineligible for that study for various reasons and were treated with postoperative irradiation after either radical or extended radical mastectomy. The relapse-free and absolute survival rates for these four groups of patients are shown in Figures 37–6 and 37–7.[37] The data suggest not only a relapse-free survival benefit but also a survival benefit for patients with inner quadrant tumors whose internal mammary chain nodes were treated with surgery, irradiation, or a combination of the two. An analysis of the relative risks of local recurrence or distant metastasis in these four groups of patients (Fig. 37–8) suggests that elective treatment of the internal mammary nodes reduced not only the risk of local/regional recurrences but also the risk of distant metastases.

Prospective Randomized Trials of Postoperative Irradiation Without Adjuvant Chemotherapy

Five prospective randomized trials of adjuvant irradiation following radical mastectomy or modified radical mastectomy have been conducted. The first three studies, Manchester P, Manchester Q, and Oslo I, are not discussed here because they employed either radiotherapy doses that were unlikely to control subclinical disease or radiotherapy techniques that were unlikely to cover the volume at risk for subclinical disease.[11, 21–24] Results for the last two studies, Oslo II[11] and Stockholm I,[28, 38] are summarized in Table 37–4, which presents the results for rates of local/regional recurrence, distant metastases, and survival at 10 years for patients with histologically positive axillary nodes randomized to receive either modified or radical mastectomy with or without postoperative irradiation. Local/regional recurrence rates reported include all such events, not only those occurring in the absence of other disease, as the first sign of treatment failure is reported in other studies.[3] In both studies, there was a highly significant improvement in local/regional disease control in the

Table 37–3. LOCAL/REGIONAL RECURRENCE SITES IN PATIENTS TREATED WITH RADICAL MASTECTOMY AND POSTOPERATIVE IRRADIATION (NO ADJUVANT CHEMOTHERAPY): 1963–1977 (ANALYSIS, 1981)

Area Irradiated	Mean No. Pos. Nodes Per Pt. With Pos. Nodes	Axillary Node Status	Total No. Pts.	Chest Wall Only	Nodes Only		Chest Wall + Node*	Recurrence Rates	
					SC	Axilla		SC (%)	CW (%)
Peripheral lymphatics	3.5	0	207†	9	0	0	2 (2)	1	5
		1–3	221	15	1	0	4 (1)	2	9
		≥4	79	16	1	1	0	1	20
Peripheral lymphatics and chest wall	9.0	0	53	0	0	1	1	2	2
		1–3	102	8	0	1	0	1	8
		≥4	257	25	5	2 (1)	4	3	11

*All node recurrences were supraclavicular except one patient with an axillary recurrence and one patient with both.
†Includes 27 patients treated with internal mammary chain irradiation only.
( ) Indicates number of patients with node recurrence outside of treated field.
Abbreviations: CW = chest wall; SC = supraclavicular area.
From Tapley ND, et al: Cancer 49:1318, 1982. Reprinted by permission.

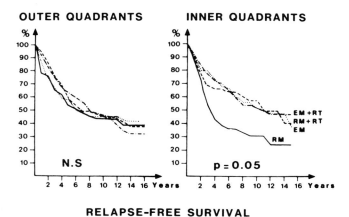

RELAPSE-FREE SURVIVAL

Figure 37–6. Relapse-free survival (RFS) in four groups of patients with breast tumors of the outer or inner quadrants treated at Villejuif by radical mastectomy (RM); radical mastectomy with postoperative radiotherapy (RM + RT); extended radical mastectomy with internal mammary chain dissection (EM); or extended radical mastectomy with internal mammary chain dissection and postoperative radiotherapy (EM + RT). No difference is observed between the four groups for tumors of the outer quadrants. For tumors of the inner quadrants, the RFS is significantly lower in patients treated by radical mastectomy alone. (From Tubiana M, Arriagada R, Sarrazin D: Int J Radiat Oncol Biol Phys 12:477, 1986. Reprinted by permission.)

irradiated patients. Both studies showed a decrease in the incidence of distant metastases in irradiated patients, which was statistically significant in the Stockholm study. In each study, there was a persistent but nonsignificant survival benefit of six to eight percentage points at 10 years in the irradiated patients. In the Oslo II study, patients with medial or central tumors and positive axillary nodes treated with irradiation showed a persistent 20 percent improvement in survival. The number of patients with medial or central tumors and positive axillary nodes treated with radical mastectomy (34 patients) or radical mastectomy and irradiation (38 patients) was so small that this substantial difference in survival only approached statistical significance ($p = 0.08$).

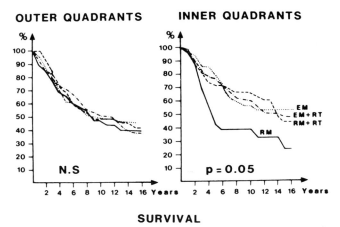

SURVIVAL

Figure 37–7. Absolute survival in patients with breast tumors. The groups of patients are the same as in Figure 37–6. (From Tubiana M, Arriagada R, Sarrazin D: Int J Radiat Oncol Biol Phys 12:477, 1986. Reprinted by permission.)

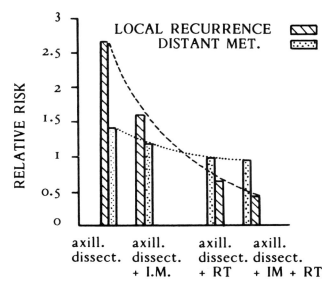

Figure 37–8. Relative risk of local regional recurrence and of distant metastases in four groups of patients with breast cancers treated at Villejuif by radical mastectomy (axillary dissection); radical mastectomy plus internal mammary chain dissection (axillary dissection + IM); radical mastectomy plus postoperative radiotherapy (axillary dissection + RT); and radical mastectomy plus internal mammary chain dissection plus postoperative radiotherapy (axillary dissection + IM + RT). Adjuvant chemotherapy was not used in any of the patients. The marked decrease in the incidence of local recurrence is associated with a slight decrease in the incidence of distant metastases. (From Tubiana M, Arriagada R, Sarrazin D: Int J Radiat Oncol Biol Phys 12:477, 1986. Reprinted by permission.)

Effect of Adjuvant Chemotherapy on Local/Regional Control

Several studies suggest that adjuvant chemotherapy, although effective for nondetectable distant disease, does little to reduce the risk of local/regional recurrence. Bonadonna and coworkers[3] have reported the prospective randomized 10-year experience in Milan with radical mastectomy followed by cyclophosphamide, methotrexate, and 5-fluorouracil (CMF)–based adjuvant chemotherapy or observation. Isolated local/regional recurrences as the first site of treatment failure occurred in 12 percent of patients who received 12 months of CMF chemotherapy versus 15 percent of patients treated with radical mastectomy alone. Stefanik and coworkers[30] reviewed the records of a series of 117 patients at Georgetown University treated with radical or modified radical mastectomy and adjuvant CMF chemotherapy only. An actuarial local/regional recurrence rate of 19 percent was found, similar to that in historical series using mastectomy alone. This study showed that primary tumor size (>5 cm), tumor site (central was more significant than lateral or medial), and extent of axillary nodal involvement (>4 nodes) were the most significant risk factors for local/regional recurrence following mastectomy and adjuvant chemotherapy. Finally, Fowble and coworkers reviewed a series of 627 patients entered into Eastern Cooperative Oncology Group protocols between 1978 and 1982.[8] At 3 years, 11 percent of patients had developed an isolated local/regional recurrence. Isolated local/regional recurrences represented 31 percent of all

Table 37–4. PROSPECTIVE RANDOMIZED TRIALS OF POSTOPERATIVE IRRADIATION (RT) FOLLOWING RADICAL MASTECTOMY (RM) OR MODIFIED RADICAL MASTECTOMY (MRM) IN PATIENTS WITH HISTOLOGICALLY POSITIVE AXILLARY LYMPH NODES

Trial	No. Pts.	LRR (%)		DM (%)		10-Year Survival (%)	
Stockholm I[28, 38]*							
MRM	120	45	} p = 0.001	60	} p = 0.01	42	} p = 0.21
MRM + RT	118	13		47		48	
Oslo II[11, 36]							
RM	91	32	} p < 0.01	~49		52†	} p = 0.15
RM + RT	95	10		~33		60†	

*Personal communication, L. Rutqvist, 1989.
†In patients with medial or central tumors and positive axillary nodes, an improvement in survival of 20 percentage points was noted in irradiated patients; the number of patients treated with radical mastectomy (34) and radical mastectomy plus radiation therapy (38) was small, so the difference only approached statistical significance ($p = 0.08$).
Abbreviations: DM = distant metastases; LRR = local/regional recurrence.

treatment failures, and the risk was related to the number of positive axillary nodes (>4 nodes), the primary tumor size (>5 cm), and the presence of tumor necrosis. Patients with four to seven positive axillary nodes had nearly as high a risk for isolated local/regional recurrence as for distant metastases. In fact, patients with four to seven involved nodes and a primary tumor size >5 cm had a 31 percent incidence of isolated local/regional recurrence at 3 years, which constituted almost two thirds of all recurrences seen in this subset of patients. A small subset of postmenopausal patients received no adjuvant chemotherapy; however, whether or not chemotherapy was given, there was no difference in either the rate of isolated local/regional recurrence or the rate of distant metastases.

Effectiveness of Postoperative Irradiation Following Mastectomy and Adjuvant Chemotherapy

Little information is available to assess the effectiveness of postoperative irradiation following radical mastectomy or modified radical mastectomy and adjuvant chemotherapy. In a prospective trial of radical mastectomy plus postoperative radiation therapy, radical mastectomy plus chemotherapy, and radical mastectomy plus postoperative radiation therapy and chemotherapy for stage III (locally advanced) breast carcinoma, Grohn and coworkers[10] showed enhanced local/regional disease control in the treatment arms receiving postoperative irradiation, and the best 3-year survival rate occurred when both adjuvant chemotherapy and postoperative irradiation were given. This study suggests that adjuvant chemotherapy does not negate the effectiveness of irradiation.

COMPLICATIONS OF RADIATION THERAPY

Visceral

The lung is the most sensitive tissue incidentally irradiated in the treatment of breast cancer. Depending on patient anatomy and treatment technique, a variable amount of lung is always irradiated when either the chest wall or regional lymphatics are treated. Acute pneumonitis is more likely when larger volumes of lung are irradiated.[26] Acute pneumonitis can be observed following elective chest wall irradiation when the electron beam energy selected is too high or when opposed tangential fields are too deep. The incidence of acute pneumonitis may be reduced by delivering a part of the dose to the supraclavicular fossa with electrons instead of photons.[18] Acute pneumonitis is characterized by a dry, hacking cough and occasionally fever and shortness of breath. Although it may last 2 to 3 weeks or longer, the pneumonitis is usually self-limited. In severe cases, steroids may be given; the steroid dosage must be tapered very gradually. Following radiation therapy, permanent fibrosis limited to the treatment volume is usually seen on chest roentgenograms. Although minor declines in pulmonary function parameters have been observed within the early follow-up period, there is rarely symptomatic compromise of pulmonary function.[12] Pleural effusion rarely occurs.

In patients with left-sided breast cancer, the anterior left ventricle is frequently included in tangential chest wall fields and in en face fields treating the internal mammary nodes. Host and coworkers[11] reported the results of a large prospective randomized trial evaluating the role of radiation therapy following radical mastectomy in 1115 patients who were observed for more than 10 years; an excess of nine cardiac deaths has been observed in stage I patients treated with postoperative irradiation over those not receiving irradiation. In the group showing an excess of cardiac deaths, treatment consisted of 5000 cGy delivered in 20 fractions of 250 cGy over 4 weeks to the peripheral lymphatics with an en face cobalt 60 field. No excess of cardiac deaths was observed in stage II patients, and no mention was made of any other potential factors affecting the risk of cardiac disease. Strender and coworkers[15, 32] prospectively studied 197 patients before, 6 months after, and 10 years after primary or adjuvant radiation therapy for breast cancer using exercise tests, heart volume determinations, and pulmonary function tests. Transient EKG changes were noted following irradiation, particularly in patients with left-sided cancers, but no functional impairment was noted, and no increase in the incidence of heart disease was found when the study group was compared with general population statistics. In this study, the daily dose per fraction was 200 cGy. Treatment techniques employed in the two studies differed and may account for the difference in late complications. Billingham and coworkers[2] reported a high proportion of endomyocardial damage when patients receiving doxorubicin HCl were also irradiated.

Musculoskeletal and Neurological

Mild atrophic and telangiectatic skin changes may occur following adjuvant irradiation of the chest wall after mastectomy, but severe fibrosis, necrosis, and soft tissue ulceration do not occur at doses of ≤5000 cGy with standard fractionation.

Arm edema is primarily related to the degree of axillary dissection and whether radiation therapy was delivered to the whole axilla. If only the apex of the axilla is irradiated, the risk of arm edema is less than when the whole axilla is treated. If whole axillary irradiation is used, the dose and fractionation scheme affect the risk of arm edema. Brismar and Ljungdahl[4] reported a prospective study of the development of arm edema in two patient populations receiving either radical or modified radical mastectomy with or without postoperative irradiation. Although no patients were judged to have severe (>6-cm difference in circumference) arm edema, the incidence was higher in irradiated patients. Among nonirradiated patients, the risk was higher with radical than with modified radical mastectomy. Swedborg and Wallgren[34] retrospectively studied the effects of radiation therapy in terms of arm edema, shoulder mobility, and gripping force in patients who had participated in a large prospective trial conducted by the Radiumhemmet. Patients with operable breast cancer had been randomized to receive modified radical mastectomy with or without preoperative or postoperative radiation therapy. Significant increases in arm edema and decreases in shoulder mobility were noted in patients receiving radiation therapy compared with those managed only with surgery. The degree of edema ranges from mild, when the patient is asymptomatic, to severe, when not only cosmesis but also function is compromised. Management (which includes elevation, elastic sleeves, pneumatic pumps, hand care, physical therapy with emphasis on strengthening the shoulder girdle, and prompt attention to cutaneous infections) is helpful but is usually ameliorative at best and does not fully eliminate the problem.[5] A rare complication of long-standing severe edema is lymphangiosarcoma.[31]

Spontaneous rib fractures occur in approximately ten percent of patients receiving radiation to the chest wall following mastectomy. The fractures may be asymptomatic and noticed only on routine chest roentgenogram or bone scan or they may be moderately painful. Typically, the fractures heal spontaneously within 6 to 8 weeks. Osteoradionecrosis occurs rarely, usually in the head of the clavicle or sternum, and is usually related to poor technique with overlap of treatment portals.

Brachial plexopathy secondary to radiation is a rare complication usually related to high total doses of radiation[13, 33] or nonstandard fractionation schemes.[16, 33] Whereas patients with brachial plexopathy secondary to tumor involvement often present with pain, Horner's syndrome, and neurological deficits involving the lower brachial trunks (C-8 and T-1), patients with radiation-induced plexopathy frequently present without pain but with edema[36] and signs of upper trunk (C-5 through C-7) dysfunction.[13] When brachial plexus symptoms are associated with lymphedema, management of lymphedema may ameliorate the brachial plexus symptoms.[9] Other therapeutic efforts such as nerve blocks, cordotomy, rhizotomy, and amputation have been disappointing. Most patients can be managed conservatively, but narcotics may be needed if pain becomes severe.

The incidence of subacute and late complications (including telangiectasia, fibrosis, rib fractures, osteoradionecrosis, arm edema, impairment of shoulder mobility, brachial plexopathy, acute pneumonitis, and pulmonary fibrosis) was significantly increased with the use of hypofractionation schemes[16, 20] in which large doses of irradiation were delivered to a treatment volume in a daily fraction; usually not all fields were treated each day. Such fractionation schemes are avoided in modern radiation therapy facilities, where all treatment fields are treated each day, and the daily dose is limited to 200 cGy.

Immune System

Multiple studies have demonstrated the transient or longstanding absence of certain subsets of T lymphocytes following local/regional irradiation for breast cancer.[27] The presence of such cell populations prior to irradiation is not always documented, and the clinical significance of such findings is unknown. Specifically, there has been no increased risk for infectious disease, distant metastases from breast cancer, or second malignancies observed in the radiotherapy arms of randomized trials that have long-term follow-up.[11, 28, 38]

Second Malignancies

Soft tissue sarcomas of the shoulder girdle and osteosarcomas of the rib cage are rarely seen after adjuvant irradiation following mastectomy. However, no increase in second thoracic malignancies, contralateral breast cancers, or leukemias has yet been reported in patients receiving adjuvant radiation therapy for breast cancer.[11, 14, 17] An increased risk may be observed when more patients have had longer follow-up, as the latency periods for radiation-induced neoplasms may be quite long.

References

1. Bernardino ME, Spanos W Jr: A simple technique for determining internal mammary chain depth by sonography. Int J Radiat Oncol Biol Phys 7:671–673, 1981.
2. Billingham ME, Bristow MR, Glatstein E, Mason JW, Masek MA, Daniels JR: Adriamycin cardiotoxicity: endomyocardial biopsy evidence of enhancement by irradiation. Am J Surg Pathol 1:17–23, 1977.
3. Bonadonna G, Valagussa BS, Rossi A, Tancini G, Brambilla C, Zambetti M, Veronesi U: Ten-year experience with CMF-based adjuvant chemotherapy in resectable breast cancer. Breast Cancer Res Treat 5:95–115, 1985.
4. Brismar B, Ljungdahl I: Postoperative lymphoedema after treatment of breast cancer. Acta Chir Scand 149:687–689, 1983.
5. Britton RC, Nelson PA: Causes and treatment of postmastectomy lymphedema of the arm: report of 114 cases. JAMA 180:95–102, 1962.
6. Cheung AYC, Chang KS: Effects of a sonographic technique for determining chest wall thickness in treatment planning for breast carcinoma. Int J Radiat Oncol Biol Phys 15:223–225, 1988.
7. Fletcher GH: Textbook of Radiotherapy, ed 3. Philadelphia, Lea and Febiger, 1980.
8. Fowble B, Gray R, Gilchrist K, Goodman RL, Taylor S, Tormey DC: Identification of a subgroup of patients with breast cancer and histologically positive axillary nodes receiving adjuvant chemotherapy who may benefit from postoperative radiotherapy. J Clin Oncol 6:1107–1117, 1988.
9. Ganel A, Engel J, Sela M, Brooks M: Nerve entrapments associated with postmastectomy lymphedema. Cancer 44:2254–2259, 1979.
10. Grohn P, Heinonen E, Klefstrom P, Tarkkanen J: Adjuvant postoperative radiotherapy, chemotherapy, and immunotherapy in stage III breast cancer. Cancer 54:670–674, 1984.
11. Host H, Brennhovd IO, Loeb M: Postoperative radiotherapy in breast cancer: long-term results from the Oslo Study. Int J Radiat Oncol Biol Phys 12:727–732, 1986.
12. Kaufman J, Gunn W, Hartz AJ, Fischer M, Hoffman RG, Schlueter DP, Komanduri A: The pathophysiologic and roentgenologic effects of chest irradiation in breast carcinoma. Int J Radiat Oncol Biol Phys 12:887–893, 1986.
13. Kori SH, Foley KM, Posner JB: Brachial plexus lesions in patients with cancer: 100 cases. Neurology 31:45–50, 1981.
14. Lavey RS, Prosnitz LR: Impact of radiation therapy (RT) and/or chemotherapy (CT) on the risk for a second malignancy following breast cancer. (Abstract) Den Haag, the Netherlands, 7th Annual Meeting of the European Society for Therapeutic Radiology and Oncology, September 5–8, 1988.
15. Lindahl J, Strender LE, Larsson LE, Unsgaard A: Electrocardiographic changes after radiation therapy for carcinoma of the breast: incidence and functional significance. Acta Radiol Oncol 22:433–440, 1983.
16. Montague ED: Experience with altered fractionation in radiation therapy of breast cancer. Radiology 90:962–966, 1968.
17. Montague ED, Ames FC, Schell SR, Romsdahl MM: Conservation surgery and irradiation as an alternative to mastectomy in the treatment of clinically favorable breast cancer. Cancer 54:2668–2672, 1984.
18. Montague ED, Schell SR, Romsdahl MM, Ames FC: Conservation surgery and irradiation in the treatment of breast cancer. Front Radiat Ther Onc 17:76–83, 1983.
19. Munzenrider JE, Tchakarova I, Castro M, Carter B: Computerized body tomography in breast cancer: I. Internal mammary nodes and radiation treatment planning. Cancer 43:137–150, 1979.
20. Overgaard M, Bentzen SM, Christensen JJ, Madsen EH: The value of the NSD formula in equation of acute and late radiation complications in normal tissue following 2 and 5 fractions per week in breast cancer patients treated with postmastectomy irradiation. Radiother Oncol 9:1–12, 1987.
21. Palmer MK, Ribeiro GG: Thirty-four year follow up of patients with breast cancer in clinical trial of postoperative radiotherapy. Br Med J 291:1088–1091, 1985.
22. Patterson R: Clinical trials in malignant disease: principles of random selection. J Fac Radiol 9:80–83, 1958.
23. Patterson R, Russell MH: Clinical trials in malignant disease: breast cancer: value of irradiation of the ovaries. J Fac Radiol 9:130–133, 1958.
24. Patterson R, Russell MH: Clinical trials in malignant disease: breast cancer: evaluation of postoperative radiotherapy. J Fac Radiol 10(4):175–180, 1959.
25. Recht A, Siddon RL, Kaplan WD, Andersen JW, Harris JR: Three-dimensional internal mammary lymphoscintigraphy: implications for radiation therapy treatment planning for breast carcinoma. Int J Radiat Oncol Biol Phys 14:477–481, 1988.
26. Rothwell RI, Kelly SA, Joslin CAF: Radiation pneumonitis in patients treated for breast cancer. Radiother Oncol 4:9–14, 1985.
27. Rotstein S, Blomgren H, Petrini B, Wasserman J, Baral E: Long term effects on the immune system following local radiation therapy for breast cancer. I. Cellular composition of the peripheral blood lymphocyte population. Int J Radiat Oncol Biol Phys 11:921–925, 1985.
28. Rutqvist LE, Cedermark B, Glas U, Johansson H, Rotstein S, Skoog L, Somell A, Theve T, Askergren J, Friberg S, Bergstrom J, Blomstedt B, Raf L, Silfversward C, Einhorn J: Radiotherapy, chemotherapy, and tamoxifen as adjuncts to surgery in early breast cancer: a summary of three randomized trials. Int J Radiat Oncol Biol Phys 16:629–639, 1989.
29. Spratt JS: Locally recurrent cancer after radical mastectomy. Cancer 20:1051–1053, 1967.
30. Stefanik D, Goldberg R, Byrne P, Smith F, Ueno W, Smith L, Harter K, Bachenheimer L, Beiser C, Dritschilo A: Local-regional failure in patients treated with adjuvant chemotherapy for breast cancer. J Clin Oncol 3:660–665, 1985.
31. Stewart FW, Treves N: Lymphangiosarcoma in postmastectomy lymphedema: a report of six cases in elephantiasis chirurgica. Cancer 1:64–81, 1948.
32. Strender LE, Lindahl J, Larsson LE: Incidence of heart disease and functional significance of changes in the electrocardiogram 10 years after radiotherapy for breast cancer. Cancer 57:929–934, 1986.
33. Svensson H, Westling P, Larsson LG: Radiation-induced lesions of the brachial plexus correlated to the time-dose-fraction schedule. Acta Radiol Ther Phys Biol 14:228–238, 1975.
34. Swedborg I, Wallgren A: The effect of pre- and postmastectomy radiotherapy on the degree of edema, shoulder-joint mobility, and gripping force. Cancer 47:877–881, 1981.
35. Tapley ND, Spanos WJ Jr, Fletcher GH, Montague ED, Schell S, Oswald MJ: Results in patients with breast cancer treated by radical mastectomy and postoperative irradiation with no adjuvant chemotherapy. Cancer 49:1316–1319, 1982.
36. Thomas JE, Colby MY Jr: Radiation-induced or metastatic brachial plexopathy? A diagnostic dilemma. JAMA 222:1392–1395, 1972.
37. Tubiana M, Arriagada R, Sarrazin D: Human cancer natural history, radiation induced immunodepression and postoperative radiation therapy. Int J Radiat Oncol Biol Phys 12:477–485, 1986.
38. Wallgren A, Arner O, Bergstrom J, Blomstedt B, Granberg P-O, Raf L, Silfversward C, Einhorn J: Radiation therapy in operable breast cancer: results from the Stockholm trial on adjuvant radiotherapy. Int J Radiat Oncol Biol Phys 12:533–537, 1986.

Chapter 38

POSTOPERATIVE IRRADIATION FOLLOWING BREAST-CONSERVING SURGICAL PROCEDURES

Nancy Price Mendenhall, M.D., Frederick C. Ames, M.D., Danièle Sarrazin, M.D., and Umberto Veronesi, M.D.

Overview

Nancy Price Mendenhall, M.D.

The use of postoperative irradiation to the breast following a breast-conserving surgical procedure for removal of the gross tumor is one of many examples of combined surgical and radiotherapeutic management of local and regional disease. Surgery is used for removal of clinically evident tumor, and moderate-dose irradiation is used for eradication of subclinical disease. Breast-conserving surgical procedures have been used extensively in Europe and Canada in lieu of mastectomy for patients with early breast cancer for many years.

TREATMENT

Selection

Selection of patients is based on clinical and radiographic criteria and patient preference. The relationship between tumor size and breast size must be such that there will be a reasonable cosmetic result after removal of the tumor and a margin of normal tissue. Therefore, patients with small tumors (T1–T2) and moderate-sized breasts are usually chosen [Fig. 38–1(A, B)]. In patients with T3 tumors, there is rarely adequate breast tissue remaining to assure a reasonable cosmetic result. Large breast size is *not* an absolute contraindication to conservative treatment, although large breasts are technically more difficult to irradiate, and dose homogeneity within the breast is more difficult to achieve. Cosmetic results in patients with large breasts are often not as good as in patients with moderate-sized breasts, but may be

quite satisfactory [Fig. 38–2(A, B)]. Alternatively, patients with large breasts who have undergone mastectomy without reconstruction often elect to undergo reconstruction later because of the unequal weight distribution in the upper torso. When reconstruction is performed in large-breasted women, reduction mammaplasty of the contralateral breast is frequently required to achieve symmetry. For women with breasts of all sizes, the advantages of irradiation over mastectomy and reconstruction are a more natural cosmetic appearance and the avoidance of extensive surgery, which often involves the contralateral breast or transposition of tissue flaps. The disadvantages of irradiation are the time required for a protracted course of treatment (usually 4.5 to 6 weeks) and the radiation exposure. In reconstructive procedures requiring transposition of tissue flaps, the recuperative time is actually similar to the time required for irradiation. Bilateral breast cancer, either synchronous or metachronous, is not a contraindication to breast-conserving surgery and irradiation, although technical care must be taken to avoid overlap of treatment fields or treatment of too much lung [Fig. 38–3(A, B)].

On mammography, the tumor must be solitary and discrete. Diffuse clustered microcalcifications suggest the possibility of extensive disease that would not be adequately removed by a breast-conserving surgical procedure.

Once a breast-conserving surgical procedure is performed, the margins of the surgical specimen are grossly and microscopically examined. In approximately ten

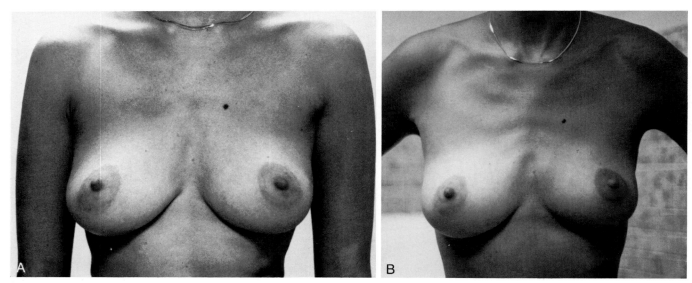

Figure 38–1. An excellent cosmetic result can be achieved with conservative surgery and postoperative irradiation in patients with small tumors and moderate-sized breasts. *A*, A 33-year-old patient following conservative surgery and axillary dissection for a T1, N0 carcinoma of the upper outer quadrant of the left breast, prior to irradiation. *B*, Five years after treatment. The planning CT scan and dosimetry for the external beam treatment in this patient are shown in Figure 38–4*(C and D)*, and the electron beam boost irradiation to the tumor bed is shown in Figure 38–7*(C)*.

percent of cases, margins that are grossly normal are extensively involved with tumor.[16] Patients in whom negative surgical margins cannot be achieved even with a reexcision are better served with mastectomy.

Technique

Recommended treatment volumes as a function of extent of disease and location of primary are shown in Table 38–1. The total dose to the breast (and peripheral lymphatics when indicated) ranges from 4600 cGy at 200 cGy per treatment to 5000 cGy at 180 to 200 cGy per treatment. One treatment is given each day. All fields are treated each day. In patients with large or pendulous breasts, the dose to the entire breast is often limited to 4500 cGy at 180 cGy per treatment because of dose inhomogeneities within the breast and increased acute skin reactions.

At simulation, the chest wall is leveled by placing the patient on a prefabricated wedge [Fig. 38–4*(A)*; also see Fig. 37–1*(A)*]. The patient's head is turned sharply to the contralateral side, and the ipsilateral arm is abducted. More than 90° of abduction is often required to allow for subsequent CT scanning with the patient in treatment position. To increase reproducibility of the patient's position each day, a customized polyurethane upper torso mold, which fits over the wedge, is then fashioned for each patient [Fig. 38–4*(A, B)*]. The ipsilateral hand is secured either behind the head or onto a handle attached to the polyurethane mold. The patient is then aligned on the simulator table with a laser beam marking the midline. Marks corresponding to the midline laser, to be used later in daily treatments, are placed at the suprasternal notch and xiphoid.

The medial border of the breast field is set at midline when only the breast is to be treated. The superior border is placed as high as is feasible with abduction of the arm. The lateral and inferior borders are placed approximately 2 cm posterior and inferior to palpable breast tissue. If the peripheral lymphatics are to be treated also, the superior border will match the inferior border of the supraclavicular-axillary field, and the medial border will either match the lateral border of the internal mammary chain field or be placed approximately 3 cm contralateral to the midline to encompass the internal mammary chain nodes within the tangential fields.

Appropriate opposing angles are chosen for entry of the medial and lateral tangential breast fields. The simulator is set at the correct angle, and the light fields

Table 38–1. TREATMENT VOLUME RECOMMENDATIONS AS A FUNCTION OF LOCATION OF PRIMARY TUMOR AND EXTENT OF DISEASE

| | **Histological Status of the Axilla** | | |
Primary Location	*Negative*	*Positive*	*Extensively Involved**
Lateral	B	B + PL	B + PL + AX
Medial T1	B + IMC†	B + PL	B + PL + AX
Medial T2	B + PL	B + PL	B + PL + AX

*Indications for treatment of the whole axilla and axillary soft tissues include extranodal axillary disease histologically verified or clinically suspected because of matted palpable nodes, axillary nodes greater than 2.5 cm, or an axilla not dissected or incomplete dissected.

†See text for discussion.

Abbreviations: AX = whole axilla; B = breast; IMC = internal mammary chain; PL = peripheral lymphatics (internal mammary nodes, supraclavicular fossa, and axillary apex).

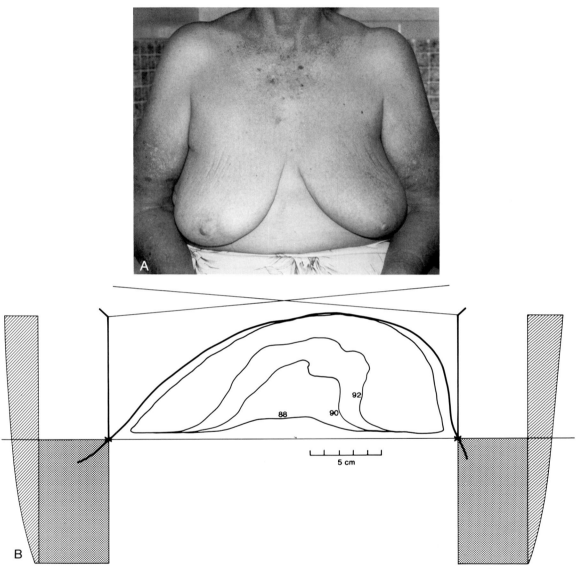

Figure 38–2. Large breast size is not an absolute contraindication to conservative treatment. *A,* A 59-year-old patient two years after treatment for a T1, N0 lesion of the upper central left breast. *B,* The dosimetry for her tangential photon treatment was achieved with a combination of medial and lateral cobalt 60 fields without a wedge block and medial and lateral 8 mV x-ray fields with a 45° wedge block. A dose of 5000 cGy in 28 fractions was specified to the 88 percent isodose line at the central axis. Because the tumor bed was contained in the 90 percent isodose line, it received 5100 cGy through the tangential breast fields. The 8 mV electron boost dose to the tumor bed was limited to 900 cGy.

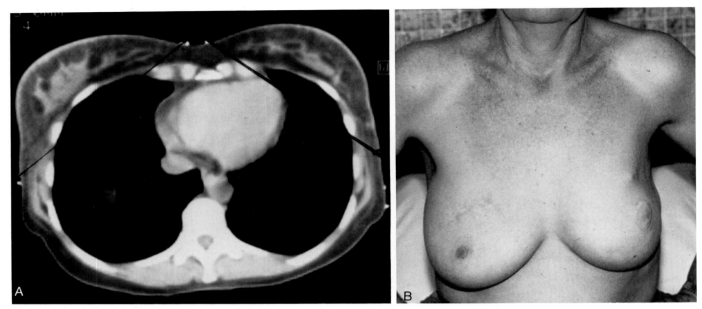

Figure 38–3. Bilateral concomitant or sequential breast carcinoma is not necessarily a contraindication to conservative treatment, as in this 53-year-old woman. *A*, If there is indication for treatment of the breasts only and not the peripheral lymphatics, the amount of lung treated is often minimal, as shown in the treatment-planning CT scan. *B*, Four years after treatment, the cosmetic result is good, and there are no signs or symptoms of acute or late pulmonary damage.

are marked on the patient. Half-beam blocks are used to eliminate field divergence with either an isocentric or fixed source-to-skin–distance technique. If regional lymphatic irradiation is also indicated (see chapter 37 for technique), appropriate couch rotation is chosen at this time for proper matching of the tangential and supraclavicular-axillary fields. After simulation, the patient undergoes a CT scan in the treatment position with all field lines marked with radiopaque catheters. From the CT scan, adequate coverage of the breast (and internal mammary nodes when indicated) may be verified, and the amount of lung and heart in the treatment field may be estimated [Figs. 38–4(C, D, E, F), 38–5(A, B), and 38–6(A, B)].

When the internal mammary nodes must be treated, coverage of the medial breast tissue and internal mammary nodes without undue heart and lung exposure may be difficult. In patients with medial tumors, it is often preferable to treat the internal mammary chain with the tangential fields (Fig. 38–5). In some cases, treatment of the internal mammary nodes is simply not feasible. In patients with lateral tumors or protuberant breasts, it is often preferable to treat the internal mammary chain with a separate field (Fig. 38–6).

Cobalt 60 or 4 MV, 6 MV, or 8 MV photons may be used. In small-breasted women, cobalt 60 or 4 MV photons may be preferable, whereas in large-breasted women, the higher energies are preferable. Wedge filters of 15° to 60° are used to decrease dose inhomogeneity in the conical treatment volume [Figs. 38–2(B), 38–4(D), 38–5(C), and 38–6(D)]. The dose may be specified to an arbitrary point or to an isodose volume, as shown in Figures 38–2(B), 38–4(D), 38–5(C), and 38–6(D). It is preferable to limit the dose inhomogeneity to ten

percent by choosing an isodose line of 90 percent or greater for dose specification.

It is unclear whether all patients require additional irradiation to boost the dose to the tumor bed for optimal local control. Centers that routinely deliver boost doses to the tumor bed following whole-breast irradiation with an interstitial implant,[20] electron beam,[33, 34, 49] or reduced photon fields report higher local control rates (>95 percent) than did the National Surgical Adjuvant Breast and Bowel Project (NSABP) study in which boosts were not routinely given.[15*]

The guidelines used at the University of Florida for boost irradiation following completion of whole-breast treatment are given in Table 38–2. An electron beam is used to boost the dose to the tumor bed when invasive disease is present and margins of the conservative tumor resection are negative. It may be used when margins are positive or unknown if neither reexcision nor interstitial implantation is feasible. The tumor bed is identified by palpation for postsurgical induration or the borders of nonapproximated normal tissue. The tumor bed may not always be located precisely beneath the incision scar in the treatment position. In most cases, a 3-cm margin is taken around the incision and the tumor

Text continued on page 789

---

*For more information on study results, the reader is referred to the following sections of this chapter: "Conservation Surgery and Radiation: The M. D. Anderson Cancer Center Experience," "Retrospective Study of Small Breast Cancers Treated by Conservative Surgery and Radiotherapy at the Institut Gustave-Roussy," "Conservation Surgery and Irradiation in Stages I and II Disease at the Istituto Nazionale Tumori (Milan)," and "Randomized Trial Comparing Conservative Treatment of Early Breast Cancers to Mastectomy at the Institut Gustave-Roussy."

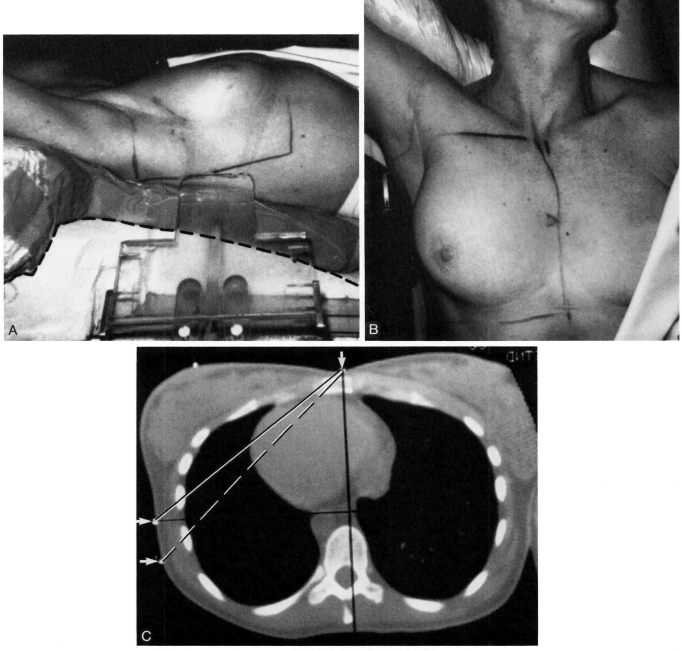

Figure 38–4. *A,* At treatment simulation, the patient's chest wall is leveled by placing a prefabricated wedge of Styrofoam (beneath the dashed line) of appropriate size and shape beneath her shoulders (see also Fig. 37–1A). The patient's arm is abducted to a position that will admit the head of the machine for tangential treatment and will also allow for patient entry into a CT scanner gantry in treatment position; this usually results in more than 90° of abduction. A customized polyurethane mold (above the dashed line) with a hand grip is then made to secure daily positioning of the arms, neck, and torso (see also Fig. 37–1B). *B,* Midline marks are placed in the center of the patient's suprasternal notch and xiphoid, and the patient is aligned on the simulation and treatment tables by laser beam. For patients with indications for breast irradiation only, the medial border of the field is at midline. A 2-cm margin beyond palpable breast tissue is taken for the inferior and posterior margins. The superior margin is placed as high as feasible after arm abduction. *C,* The field borders are then outlined with radiopaque catheters, and a CT scan is performed with the patient in treatment position. The CT scan is useful not only for verification of adequate coverage and sparing of critical tissues but also for an accurate contour of the treatment volume for computer-generated dosimetry through the central axis of the field as well as the plane of the tumor bed and high-risk internal mammary node interspaces. In this case, two angles *(solid and dotted lines)* for the tangential fields were marked with catheters *(arrows),* and the more shallow angle *(solid line)* was chosen for significant reduction of the heart and lung volume treated.

Illustration continued on following page

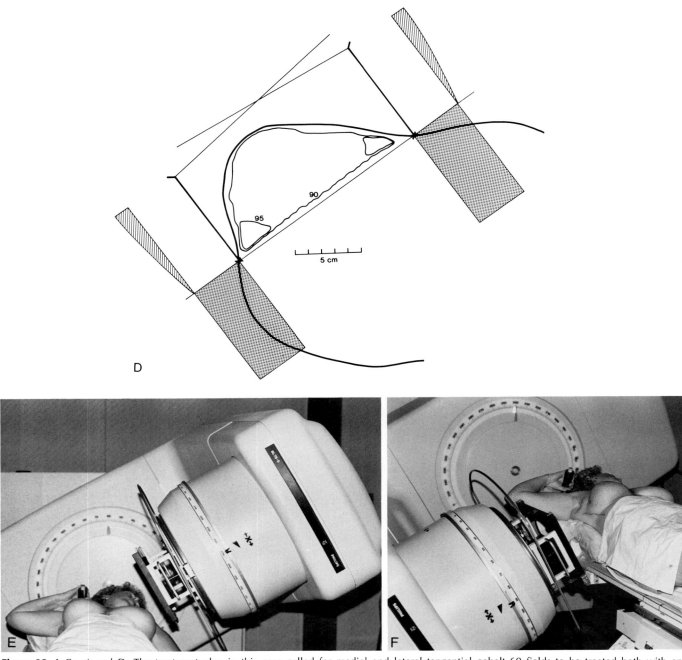

Figure 38–4 *Continued D,* The treatment plan in this case called for medial and lateral tangential cobalt 60 fields to be treated both with and without a 45° wedge filter (hatched area). The dose was specified to the 90 percent isodose line. A half-beam block was placed at the central axis to eliminate divergence of the beam (stippled area). Treatment to the breast is delivered through medial *(E)* and lateral *(F)* tangential fields.

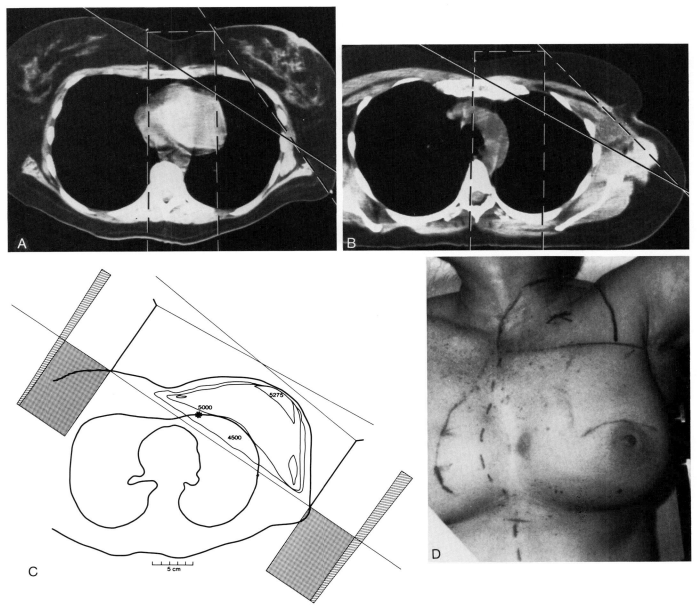

Figure 38–5. This 48-year-old premenopausal patient had a 2-cm supra-areolar carcinoma; she underwent conservative resection and Levels I and II axillary dissection. Microscopic examination of the breast specimen showed a mixed intraductal and infiltrating ductal tumor with negative surgical margins. Examination of the axillary specimen showed involvement confined to two of the 27 nodes retrieved. Because of the central location of the primary tumor and the contour of the breast and chest wall at the level of the central axis *(A)* and at the first interspace *(B)* (the most likely location of internal mammary nodes), the internal mammary nodes were best treated through the tangential breast fields *(solid lines).* A separate en face internal mammary field matched to more shallow breast tangents *(dotted lines)* would have resulted in an underdosed wedge of breast parenchyma in the vicinity of the tumor bed. *C,* As shown in the treatment plan, a dose of 5000 cGy was delivered to the breast with 8 mV x-rays. The supraclavicular field also received 5000 cGy. The area at highest risk for internal mammary nodes *(asterisk)* was contained within the 4500 cGy isodose line. *D,* The patient was positioned for treatment according to the solid lines drawn on the skin (which were generated at simulation and verified by planning CT scan). The medial contralateral breast tissue was then taped out of the field so that the beam actually entered and exited at the dotted line. This step reduced the volume of contralateral breast irradiated. An electron beam boost dose was subsequently delivered to the tumor bed to bring its dose to 6000 cGy.

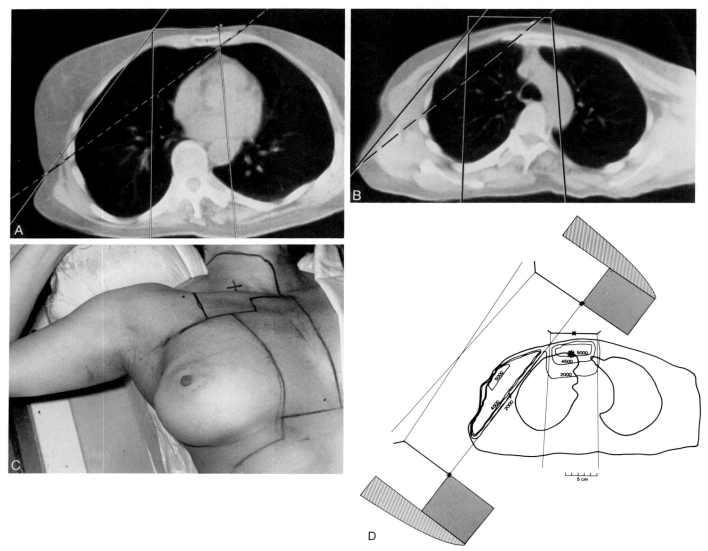

Figure 38–6. This 59-year-old postmenopausal woman underwent a conservative resection of a small lateral inframammary fold tumor and Level I dissection of the axilla. Microscopic examination of the breast specimen showed a 0.8-cm primary lesion with negative surgical margins. Examination of the axillary specimen showed that two of seven lymph nodes retrieved were totally replaced with tumor. Because of the contour of the breast and chest wall (shown on treatment-planning CT cuts through the central axis *(A)* and the first rib interspace *(B)*) and the lateral position of the tumor bed, better coverage of the internal mammary nodes with less lung irradiation was achieved by using separate en face electron fields *(solid lines)*. Inclusion of the internal mammary nodes within the tangential breast fields *(dotted lines)* would have increased the volume of lung irradiated substantially, in contrast to the situation illustrated in Figure 38–5. No attempt was made to cover the axillary hematoma apparent in *B*, as there were no indications for full axillary irradiation. *C*, The supraclavicular and internal mammary fields were matched to the tangential breast fields, and the field junction lines were changed at least once during the course of treatment. *D*, Computer-generated dosimetry demonstrates adequate doses in the area of the junction and the area at highest risk for internal mammary nodes *(asterisk)*. Because qualitative assays for estrogen and progesterone receptors on the primary tumor were strongly positive, the patient was also treated with adjuvant tamoxifen.

Table 38-2. GUIDELINES FOR BOOST TREATMENT OF THE TUMOR BED FOLLOWING BREAST-CONSERVING SURGERY AND POSTOPERATIVE IRRADIATION OF THE WHOLE BREAST

Surgical Procedure	Surgical Margin	Technique	Dosage
First excision	Unknown	Interstitial implant†	1500–2000 cGy
	Negative	Electron beam or photons	1000 cGy/4–5 fractions
	Positive	Interstitial implant†	1500–2000 cGy
Reexcision	No residual tumor	No boost	—
	Residual tumor with margins of reexcision negative	Electron beam or photons	1000 cGy/4–5 fractions
	Residual tumor with margins of reexcision positive	Interstitial implant‡	1500–2000 cGy

*The total dose to the tumor bed, including the dose given to the whole breast, is 6000 cGy when margins are negative, 6500 cGy when margins are close, and 7000 cGy to 7500 cGy when margins are positive. If the whole breast receives only 4500 cGy, then the boost dose is 1500 cGy in seven to eight fractions.
†Reexcision is preferred.
‡Mastectomy is preferred.

bed. The patient is positioned on the treatment table with pillows and wedges so that the volume to be treated is perpendicular to the electron beam. An electron beam energy is chosen based on information obtained from the preoperative mammogram and physical examination, the treatment-planning CT scan, and an estimation by physical examination of the thickness of breast tissue between skin and chest wall in the treatment position. If the depth of the tumor cannot be judged from preoperative studies and the treatment-planning CT, then an electron beam energy that will adequately cover the full thickness of the breast tissue from skin to chest wall is chosen. The energy most often chosen is 10 MeV, but 8, 12, and 14 MeV are frequently used. If the depth of the treatment volume is more than 4 cm, an interstitial implant or photon boost may be used to avoid the substantial skin and subcutaneous dose obtained with higher energy electrons. Interstitial implantation is used to boost the dose to the tumor bed when margins of conservative tumor resection are involved or are close to the tumor and reexcision is not feasible. The techniques used for electron beam and interstitial boosts are shown in Figures 38–7 and 38–8.

Sequencing of Irradiation and Chemotherapy

Irradiation and cyclophosphamide, methotrexate, and 5-fluorouracil (CMF) chemotherapy were delivered concomitantly in the Milan trial[51, 52] with no reported compromise of chemotherapy doses or schedules. Others using a doxorubicin-containing chemotherapy regimen have delayed the irradiation until after delivery of 2 or 3 months of chemotherapy without a noted increased

risk of recurrence. At the University of Florida, we have delivered irradiation concomitantly with CMF chemotherapy, with the only noticeable effect being a slight increase in the rate of pneumonitis. There is little experience with delay of irradiation in this setting more than 2 or 3 months after surgery.

RESULTS

Retrospective Experience

In 1949, Baclesse reported ten stage I patients treated with irradiation following excisional biopsy of their tumors.[3] Although one patient died early of distant metastases, the other nine remained free of disease. Other pioneers of the breast-conserving approach include Mustakallio in Finland,[35, 36] Porritt in England,[43] Peters in Canada,[38–41] and Adair,[1] Crile,[12] Cope,[11] and Rigby-Jones[47] in the United States. No detrimental effect on survival was observed when breast-conserving operations rather than radical mastectomy were employed for tumor removal. Peters performed a retrospective study of patients treated for breast cancer at the Princess Margaret Hospital with a variety of surgical and radiotherapeutic approaches.[41] The cases comprised T1–T2, N0, M0 lesions, had been followed for as long as 30 years, and were matched for primary size, patient age, and year of treatment. A total of 203 patients were treated with local excision with or without postoperative irradiation, and 609 patients had mastectomy with or without irradiation. Interestingly, the method of treatment had no effect on survival. Conservatively treated patients, in fact, developed fewer distant metastases (particularly to lung and bone) during the first 2 years after treatment. The local recurrence rate was eight

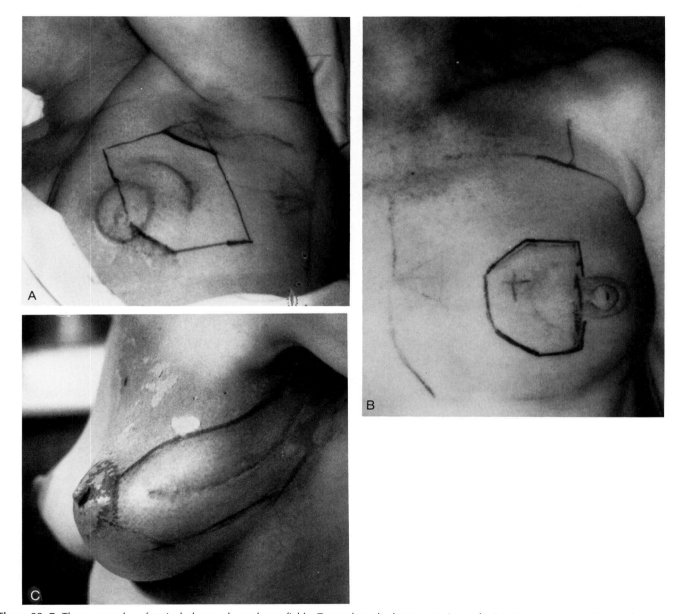

Figure 38–7. Three examples of typical electron beam boost fields. To produce the best cosmetic result, it is important to position each patient in such a way as to flatten the tumor bed. This minimizes the electron energy required and reduces the skin dose. *A,* Patient on her side with the ipsilateral arm elevated over her head so that the treatment volume is perpendicular to the electron beam. In this case, a 12 MeV electron beam was used. *B,* Patient supine with arms resting on the table to place the medial treatment volume in a position perpendicular to the electron beam. In this case, an 8 MeV electron beam was chosen. *C,* Because a single incision was used for the axillary dissection and breast resection, the electron beam treatment field covered the entire incision.

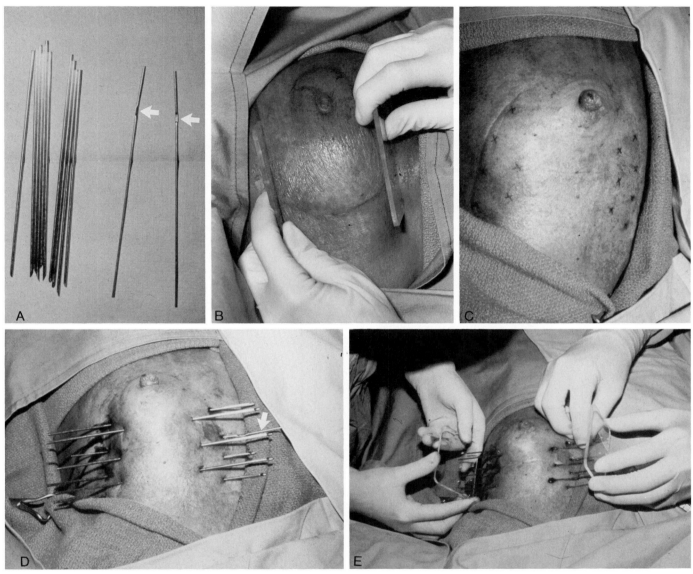

Figure 38–8. Interstitial implantation is performed when conservative surgical margins are close or involved by tumor. *A,* The beveled cutting trocars (left) used to penetrate the breast tissue and the stainless steel tubes (right) used to hold the ribbons of iridium seeds. The stainless steel tubes have 0.5 cm crimps *(arrows)* at one end to facilitate afterloading the iridium seed ribbons. *B,* With the patient under general anesthesia, the tumor bed is identified and the volume of tissue to be implanted is compressed between two lucite plates that contain complementary holes spaced 2 cm apart in staggered rows. The desired number and planar arrangement of the stainless steel tubes are then determined. Entrance and exit points through the compressed tissue are marked through the holes in the lucite plate with a 21-gauge needle and a marking pen. *C,* The lucite plates are removed. *D,* The beveled cutting trocars are forced from entry to exit point for each of the selected trocar tracks. The stainless steel tubes are then guided into place through the trocars, which are then withdrawn *(arrow).* *E,* The crimps in the stainless steel tubes are placed on the exit side of the implant volume just inside the skin surface. The lucite plates are then reapplied, to maintain spacing of the tubes.

Illustration continued on following page

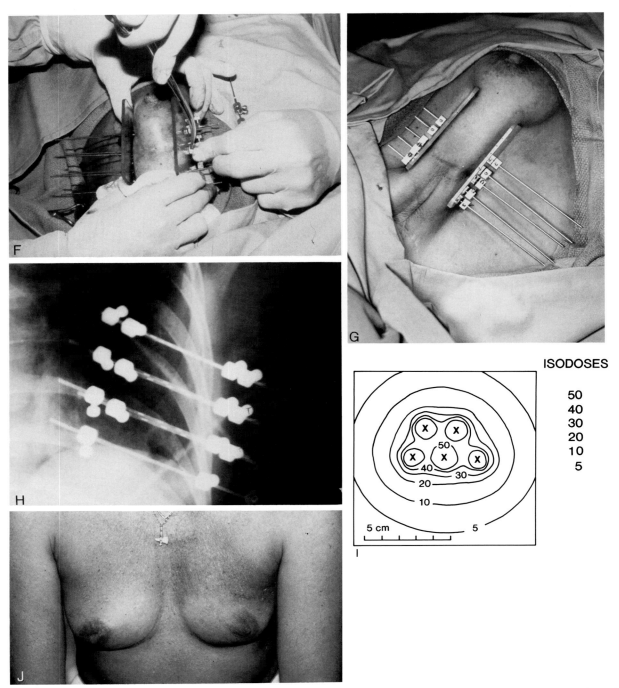

ISODOSES

50
40
30
20
10
5

Figure 38–8 *Continued F,* The plates are secured in parallel position by tightening socket-head setscrews placed just outside each plate. The plate on the exit side fits flush to the crimps just inside the skin and is tightened first. When tightening the screws, care must be taken not to crimp the stainless steel tubes on the entry side, which could complicate afterloading of the iridium seeds. *G,* The ribbons of iridium seeds are then loaded into the tubes through the uncrimped end. In afterloading the ribbons of iridium seeds into the stainless steel tubes, care must also be taken to place the end seeds no less than 0.5 cm from the skin surface. After the tubes are loaded, the position of the seeds is checked fluoroscopically *(H),* and computer-generated dosimetry is performed *(I).* The dose is specified to an isodose line encompassing all sources in a central plane perpendicular to the axis of the sources. In this case, the 30 cGy per hour line was selected. Alternatively, the Paris system may be used for dose specification.[42] *J,* A patient is shown five years after treatment for a T2 carcinoma of the upper outer quadrant on the left. She received 5000 cGy external-beam irradiation to the breast and peripheral lymphatics, followed by a two-plane implant to the tumor bed, indicated because surgical margins were positive after reexcision of the tumor bed and she refused a mastectomy. The only visible sequelae of the implant are tiny hypopigmented areas marking the entrance and exit points of the implant trocars.

percent, but only half of the local recurrences were associated with concurrent or subsequent distant metastases.

A large body of data concerning local control rates and survival rates has been accumulated by the many centers now experienced in the use of conservation surgery and postoperative irradiation for breast cancer (Table 38–3). Following complete excision of the tumor and moderate-dose irradiation to the breast (4500–5000 cGy) plus a boost dose (1000–2500 cGy) given just to the tumor bed, most institutions report local recurrence rates of five percent to ten percent at 5 years and ten percent to 25 percent at 10 years.* Five-year survival rates in most series range from 85 percent to 90 percent for clinical stage I patients and from 70 percent to 80 percent for clinical stage II patients.[6, 8, 10, 19, 20, 23, 33, 34, 37, 44, 49] Ten-year survival rates are 70 percent to 80 percent for stage I patients and 60 percent to 65 percent for stage II patients.[37] Detailed descriptions of the experience at two major institutions, the M. D. Anderson Hospital and the Institut Gustave-Roussy, are provided in chapter sections that follow.

Prospective Experience

Rarely in medicine have two forms of therapy been so thoroughly compared in prospective randomized trials

---

*References 6, 8, 10, 19, 20, 23, 31, 33, 34, 37, 44, and 49.

with such consistent results as have conservation surgery plus postoperative irradiation versus radical or modified radical mastectomy for early stage breast cancer. The results of four prospective trials have been reported. Detailed descriptions of trials from the Institut Gustave-Roussy in Villejuif, France, and the Istituto Nazionale in Milan, Italy, are provided in chapter sections that follow. The comprehensive NSABP trial for conservation surgery ± irradiation vs. total mastectomy and axillary dissection (protocol 13–06) is discussed in Fisher's section of chapter 29.

In these three trials, almost 3000 patients were studied, irradiation and surgical techniques were judged to have been adequate, and results (summarized in Table 38–4) were consistent. Conservative surgery (quadrantectomy, segmental mastectomy, or lumpectomy) with negative gross and microscopic surgical margins followed by irradiation in early stage breast cancer (T1–T2, N0–N1) produced local control and survival rates at least equal to those achieved with modified radical or radical mastectomy in all patient subsets. In both the Milan and NSABP studies, patients with histologically positive axillary nodes had a better disease-free survival rate if treated with the breast-conserving approach. An earlier prospective trial from Guy's Hospital in London[2] has been criticized for using irradiation techniques and doses that are considered significantly suboptimal.[34] The Guy's Hospital study, in contrast to the three studies described here, showed higher local/regional recurrence and death rates associated with the conservative surgery and irradiation approach.

Table 38–3. RETROSPECTIVE STUDIES OF LOCAL CONTROL AND SURVIVAL RATES FOR EARLY BREAST CANCER TREATED BY COMPLETE EXCISION AND POSTOPERATIVE IRRADIATION

Institution	No. of Pts.	Stage	5-Yr Rate of Local Recurrence (%)	5-Yr Rate of Survival (%)	10-Yr Rate of Survival (%)
Leon Berard[19]	195	CT1–2, N0*	4	87	n.d.
Curie[6]	324	CT1–2, N0*	8	90†	n.d.
A. Lacassagne[23]	108	CT1–2, N0–1*	6	90	n.d.
Gustave-Roussy[10]	592	CT0–2, N0*	6	92	80
Royal Marsden[37]	211	CT1, N0–1A	26‡	81	68
		CT2, N0–1A	18‡	76	61
Leuven[31]	168	1	10	n.d.	94
		II	n.d.	n.d.	58
M.D. Anderson[33, 34]	345	CT1–2, N0–1	5	78†	73†
Mass. General[8]	146	CI	8	93	—
		CII	17	73	—
Joint Center for Radiation Therapy[20]	255	CI	3	93	—
		CII	13	84	—
Univ. of Pennsylvania[49]	552	PI	6	97	—
		PII	n.d.	89	—
Yale[44]	179	CI	5	98	—
		CII	14	66	—

*<3 cm or <3.5 cm.
†Disease-free survival (alive and free of disease).
‡10-year results.
Abbreviations: C = clinical stage; n.d. = no data; P = pathological stage.

Table 38–4. PROSPECTIVE RANDOMIZED TRIALS COMPARING BREAST-CONSERVING SURGICAL PROCEDURES FOLLOWED BY BREAST IRRADIATION WITH MASTECTOMY

Institution*	No. of Pts Evaluated	Treatments Compared	Local Recurrence in Breast or Chest Wall (%)	% Distant Metastases	Disease-Free Survival (%)	Overall Survival (%)	Survival Interval (yr)
Gustave-Roussy, 1972–1979, stage T1, N0–1	179	Modified radical mastectomy	9	27	—	80	10
		Tumorectomy, axillary dissection, and breast irradiation	7	26	—	79	
Istituto Nazionale de Milan,† 1973–1980, stage C T1, N0	701	Halsted radical mastectomy	2	—	—	~75	15
		Quadrantectomy, axillary dissection, and breast irradiation	3	—	—	~75	
National Surgical Adjuvant Breast Project,† 1976–1984, stage C T1–2 (<4 mo), N0–1	1843	Total mastectomy and axillary dissection	5‡	35	58	71	8
		Segmental mastectomy and axillary dissection	4‡	38	54	71	
		Segmental mastectomy, axillary dissection, and breast irradiation	<1‡	36	59	65	

*Data from later sections of this chapter.
†All patients with histologically positive nodes received adjuvant chemotherapy.
‡5-yr cumulative (not actuarial) results; recurrences after segmental mastectomy alone not counted if salvage mastectomy was performed.
Abbreviation: C = clinical stage.

LOCAL RECURRENCE

Natural History

Approximately 75 percent of recurrences in the breast after a breast-conserving surgical procedure and postoperative irradiation occur in or marginal to the tumor bed or skin incision.[10, 33, 46] Although most recurrences in the breast occur within 5 years of treatment,[10, 33, 34] recurrences are often noted after that time.[37] In the series from the Joint Center for Radiation Therapy,[46] the hazard rate for local failure was fairly constant at approximately 2.5 percent per year from 2 to 6 years after treatment, dropping to one percent per year after 8 years. In a study by three institutes in France of patients alive and apparently cured 10 years after conservative treatment, Kurtz et al.[26] found that breast recurrences continued at a rate of approximately one percent per year during the second decade of follow-up. Montague[33, 34] noted that a high proportion of recurrences in the M. D. Anderson Hospital series after 6 years were in quadrants of the breast different from the location of the primary tumor. Recht et al.[46] showed that the hazard rate for marginal or tumor bed recurrences was approximately two percent per year until 5 years, then dropped to 0.5 percent per year after 8 years. In contrast, the hazard rate for a recurrence in the breast at a distance from the original primary remained constant at approximately one percent per year after 5 years. It is possible, therefore, that some of the "late" recurrences actually represented second primary cancers.

Prognostic Factors

An increased risk of local recurrence has been reported in patients whose tumors have extensive intraductal involvement.[4, 48] However, in institutions where wide gross margins are achieved initially or where reexcision is performed when the surgical margins are positive or unknown, an increased risk of local recurrence in tumors with an intraductal component has not been noted.[6, 17, 33, 34, 49] Patients in whom surgical margins are positive or unknown prior to irradiation are clearly at a higher risk for local recurrence.[8, 20, 31, 33, 34] In the NSABP B-06 trial, the most significant risk factor for local recurrence was extensive intralymphatic involvement within the primary tumor, which was associated with an inflammatory type of local recurrence.[16] Of interest is the finding of an increased risk of inoperable recurrences with chest wall or skin involvement in patients with stage II disease in the M. D. Anderson series (G. H. Fletcher, personal communication, 1989). It is probable that these same patients would be at high risk for local chest wall recurrence had mastectomy been the initial treatment. Young patients have a higher rate of local recurrence in most series.[4, 6, 28, 31, 45] Solin et al.[50] have found that young patients have an earlier pattern of failure but ultimately carry a prognosis similar to that of older patients for local, regional, and distant tumor control.

Salvage After Local/Regional Recurrence

Although reported results of management of limited recurrences in the breast after conservation surgery and postoperative irradiation with a second breast-conserving surgical procedure are good,[25] the standard salvage treatment in the United States is total mastectomy. Any chemotherapy or further irradiation must be tailored to the individual situation.

The results of treatment for isolated local/regional

recurrence following conservation surgery and postoperative irradiation obtained at various institutions are depicted in Table 38–5.[6, 10, 13, 27, 30, 33, 34, 37] Five-year disease-free survival rates range from 35 percent to 76 percent following salvage therapy. Kurtz et al.[27] reported the results of salvage surgery for local/regional recurrence in a series of patients treated with primary irradiation or limited surgery and postoperative irradiation to the intact breast. The 5-year survival rates after salvage surgery were 51 percent for the whole population, 71 percent for patients who originally had stage I tumors with no evidence of axillary disease at salvage surgery, and 36 percent to 37 percent for patients with histological evidence of axillary lymph node involvement either initially or at salvage surgery. The 10-year disease-free survival rates related to the original stage of disease were 70 percent, 55 percent, and 39 percent, respectively, for the stage I, II, and III patients not developing local/regional recurrence, and 70 percent, 49 percent, and 30 percent, respectively, for the stage I, II, and III patients who were able to undergo salvage surgery for local/regional recurrence.

As in local/regional recurrence following radical and modified radical mastectomy, several studies suggest that parameters of tumor burden and biology are prognostically significant. Kurtz et al.[27] identified original stage of disease and status of the axilla at the time of recurrence as the most important prognostic factors. Patients originally classified as T1–T2, N0 with negative nodes again at recurrence had a 71 percent 5-year survival rate compared with a 24 percent rate for patients originally classified as T3, N0–N1 with positive axillary nodes at recurrence. Clarke and coworkers[10] noted that size of recurrence in the breast was important in that no second local/regional recurrences were observed when the recurrence was ≤2 cm in diameter, whereas patients with larger tumors at recurrence developed second local/regional recurrences and were more likely to develop distant metastases. In the series from the Institut Gustave-Roussy[10] and from Marseilles,[27] the prognosis for patients with inoperable local/regional recurrence was dismal. Disease-free interval, an important prognostic factor for patients with local/regional recurrences following radical and modified radical mastectomies, has not been shown to be significant.[22]

COMPLICATIONS

Expected side effects of postoperative irradiation of the breast following a conservative surgical procedure are limited to a mild skin reaction. In patients with large or pendulous breasts, there is often mild moist desquamation of the inframammary area. Skin reactions heal within 1 or 2 weeks following treatment. Hyperpigmentation may remain for several months, particularly in patients who are also receiving chemotherapy. Transient breast edema is observed in practically all patients who have undergone axillary dissection and usually resolves within several months following treatment. When only tangential irradiation of the breast is given, pneumonitis is rare. If regional lymphatic irradiation is delivered, additional side effects may include pneumonitis and esophagitis. Transient ECG changes have been noted in patients treated for left-sided breast cancers, but no permanent cardiac damage has been identified.[32] Occasionally a patient reports easy fatigability.

Significant complications are rare,[8, 33, 34, 37, 49] but they include a low rate of severe breast fibrosis (one percent to two percent), ulceration (<1 percent), brachial plexopathy related to regional lymphatic irradiation (<1 percent), and spontaneous rib fracture (<1 percent).

Table 38–5. RESULTS OF TREATMENT FOR ISOLATED LOCAL/REGIONAL RECURRENCE FOLLOWING CONSERVATION SURGERY AND POSTOPERATIVE IRRADIATION FOR OPERABLE BREAST CANCER

Author (Institution)	Accrual Dates	No. of Pts.	5-Yr Rate of Survival (%)
Montague et al., 1984[33, 34] (M.D. Anderson, Houston)	1955–1980	16	67*
Osborne et al., 1984[37] (Royal Marsden, London)	1954–1969	12	42†
Delouche et al., 1987[13] (Centre de Charlebourg, Paris)	1956–1979	30	14/30
Kurtz et al., 1983[27] (Cancer Institute, Marseilles)	1960–1971	147‡	51*
Calle et al., 1986[6] (Institut Curie, Paris)	1960–1978	25	76†
Leung et al., 1986[30] (Hôpital H. Mondor, Créteil)	1961–1979	45	35†
Clarke et al., 1985[10] (Inst. G.-Roussy, Villejuif)	1970–1981	11	81§

*Overall survival calculated from time of recurrence.
†Disease-free survival or survival with no evidence of disease calculated from time of relapse.
‡This series includes some patients treated with radiation alone without surgical removal of tumor, although the majority had tumor excision.
§Disease-free survival calculated from time of primary treatment.

Significant pulmonary fibrosis and cardiac dysfunction have not generally been reported with this treatment. The risk of arm edema varies considerably with the extent of surgery[29] and the radiotherapy techniques employed,[14] but edema usually occurs only in patients who have undergone full axillary dissections with removal of level I, II, and III nodes. The risk of contralateral breast malignancies following irradiation appears to be similar to the risk following surgery alone.[33, 34] In a study of 2850 patients treated with radiation therapy alone or irradiation following breast-conserving surgery between 1960 and 1981, Kurtz and coworkers found the cumulative probability of contralateral breast cancer to be 4.5 percent at 5 years, 7.9 percent at 10 years, and 11 percent at 15 and 20 years.[24]

COSMETIC RESULTS

The majority of patients treated conservatively attain good or excellent cosmetic results.[5] In general, patients are less critical of the cosmetic result than is the treating physician.[7] Cosmetic results are judged on the basis of discrepancy in size, distortion, fibrosis, and skin changes. Discrepancy in size and distortion are often the result of the surgical procedure rather than the postoperative irradiation. Fibrosis and skin changes are related to the dose of irradiation and irradiation technique.[21] Cosmetic results are also related to both tumor size and breast size,[9] and patients with small tumors and small- to moderate-sized breasts generally have the best results.

FOLLOW-UP CARE

The overall follow-up evaluation for all patients with breast cancer discussed in chapters 46 and 47 is applicable to patients undergoing conservative surgery and postoperative irradiation for early breast cancer. In addition, lifelong surveillance of the irradiated breast is necessary because of the long-term risk of both local tumor recurrence and a second primary ipsilateral breast cancer. Recommended surveillance includes monthly breast self-examinations, regular physical examinations by a radiation oncologist experienced in this treatment, and bilateral mammograms.

The signs of recurrent tumor are the same as those of primary tumor. The most common finding is a painless lump in or near the primary tumor bed or incision. Fibrosis in the area of the tumor bed boost irradiation may be mistaken for recurrence; however, the fibrosis usually conforms to the borders of the boost field if an electron beam was used, to the needle tracks if an interstitial implant was used, or to a linear ridge in the upper part of the breast at the matchline of the tangential and supraclavicular fields. Occasionally the tumor bed is palpable as a tissue defect, particularly if the borders of the resection were not reapproximated at surgery. The borders of normal breast parenchyma may then be confused with a lump adjacent to the tumor

bed. Normal postirradiation skin erythema, hyperpigmentation, and edema or the occasional case of erysipelas may be distinguished from signs of an advanced or inflammatory recurrence in the skin by the time course or response to antibiotics. At the University of Florida, physical examinations are performed at 1 and 3 months after treatment, by which time most acute sequelae of irradiation are resolved. During the remainder of the first year, the patient is examined at 3-month intervals, then at 4-month intervals until 5 years, when follow-up intervals are extended to 6 months (or 1 year, if another physician is available for interval examinations). After 10 years, the patient is examined once a year. Follow-up examinations are performed more frequently if there are any equivocal or suspicious findings.

Mammographic signs of recurrent tumor are also similar to signs of primary tumor. These include mass density, parenchymal distortion, calcifications, and asymmetry in comparison with the uninvolved breast. After irradiation, there are often benign calcifications that are usually large and round compared with the suspicious clustered or linear microcalcifications that may reflect intraductal or invasive carcinoma. Suspicious microcalcifications present prior to treatment may or may not resolve after irradiation and are not necessarily a cause for concern. Increased density or distortion may be present after biopsy or after any surgical procedure in the breast. Skin edema is frequently present after breast irradiation and almost always present after axillary dissections. We recommend obtaining a mammogram between 3 and 6 months after treatment to be used in conjunction with the pretherapy mammogram as a baseline for evaluation of future mammograms, since interval change in distortion, density, or calcifications may be the best indication of recurrent tumor. For patients with equivocal or suspicious findings, the mammograms are repeated at 3- or 6-month intervals. Otherwise, mammograms are routinely performed at yearly intervals.

Any patient with a suspicious or persistently equivocal clinical or radiographic finding should have a biopsy performed, preferably with needle aspiration or needle localization technique. Biopsy should not be performed unless clearly indicated, however, as irradiated tissue may not heal quickly after trauma, and subsequent clinical or radiographic evaluation may be compromised by further fibrosis or distortion.

FUTURE DIRECTIONS

Because of the success of conservative surgical procedures with postoperative irradiation of the breast in selected early stage breast cancers (T1–T2, N0–N1), there is much interest in extending this approach to other presentations of breast cancer. In light of multiple reports of successful management of noninvasive disease with this approach,[17, 33, 34, 53] the NSABP has undertaken a prospective randomized trial to evaluate the role of postoperative irradiation after conservative surgical removal in patients with noninvasive disease (protocol B-

17). The Institut Gustave-Roussy has undertaken a trial of preoperative chemotherapy followed by a conservative surgical procedure and irradiation for patients with large T2 and T3 tumors. Preliminary reports of the conservative approach for Paget's disease are also promising.[18]

References

1. Adair FE: Role of surgery and irradiation in cancer of the breast. JAMA 121:553, 1943.
2. Atkins H, Hayward JL, Klugman DJ, Wayte AB: Treatment of early breast cancer: a report after ten years of a clinical trial. Br Med J 2:423–529, 1972.
3. Baclesse F: Roentgen therapy as the sole method of treatment of cancer of the breast. Am J Roentgenol Radium Thera 62:311–319, 1949.
4. Bartelink H, Borger JH, van Dongen JA, Peterse JL: The impact of tumor size and histology on local control after breast-conserving therapy. Radiother Oncol 11:297–303, 1988.
5. Beadle GF, Silver B, Botnick L, Hellman S, Harris JR: Cosmetic results following primary radiation therapy for early breast cancer. Cancer 54:2911–2918, 1984.
6. Calle R, Vilcoq JR, Zafrani B, Vielh P, Fourquet A: Local control and survival of breast cancer treated by limited surgery followed by irradiation. Int J Radiat Oncol Biol Phys 12:873–878, 1986.
7. Cedermark B, Askergren J, Alveryd A, Glas U, Karnstrom L, Somell A, Theve N-O, Wallgren A: Breast-conserving treatment for breast cancer in Stockholm, Sweden, 1977 to 1981. Cancer 53:1253–1255, 1984.
8. Chu AM, Cope O, Russo R, Lew R: Patterns of local-regional recurrence and results in stages I and II breast cancer treated by irradiation following limited surgery: an update. Am J Clin Oncol 7:221–229, 1984.
9. Clarke D, Martinez A, Cox RS: Analysis of cosmetic results and complications in patient with stages I and II breast cancer treated by biopsy and irradiation. Int J Radiat Oncol Biol Phys 9:1807–1813, 1983.
10. Clarke DH, Le MG, Sarrazin D, Lacombe M-J, Fontaine F, Travagli J-P, May-Levin F, Contesso G, Arriagada R: Analysis of local-regional relapses in patients with early breast cancers treated by excision and radiotherapy: experience of the Institut Gustave-Roussy. Int J Radiat Oncol Biol Phys 11:137–145, 1985.
11. Cope O: Breast cancer: has the time come for a less mutilating treatment? Psychiatry Med 2:263–269, 1971.
12. Crile G Jr: Treatment of breast cancer by local excision. Am J Surg 109:400–403, 1965.
13. Delouche G, Bachelot F, Premont M, Kurtz JM: Conservation treatment of early breast cancer: long-term results and complications. Int J Radiat Oncol Biol Phys 13:29–34, 1987.
14. Dewar JA, Sarrazin D, Benhamou E, Petit J-Y, Benhamou S, Arriagada R, Fontaine F, Costaigne D, Contesso G: Management of the axilla in conservatively treated breast cancer: 592 patients treated at Institut Gustave-Roussy. Int J Radiat Oncol Biol Phys 13:475–481, 1987.
15. Fisher B, Bauer M, Margolese R, Poisson R, Pilch Y, Redmond C, Fisher E, Wolmark N, Deutsch M, Montague E, Saffer E, Wickerham L, Lerner H, Glass A, Shibata H, Deckers P, Ketcham A, Oishi R, Russell I: Five-year results of a randomized clinical trial comparing total mastectomy and segmental mastectomy with or without radiation in the treatment of breast cancer. N Engl J Med 312:665–673, 1985.
16. Fisher ER, Sass R, Fisher B, Gregorio R, Brown R, Wickerham L: Pathologic findings from the National Surgical Adjuvant Breast Project (protocol 6) II. Relation of local breast recurrence to multicentricity. Cancer 57:1717–1724, 1986.
17. Fisher ER, Sass R, Fisher B, Wickerham L, Paik SM: Pathologic findings from the National Surgical Adjuvant Breast Project (protocol 6) I. Intraductal carcinoma (DCIS). Cancer 57:197–208, 1986.
18. Fourquet A, Campana F, Vielh P, Schlienger P, Jullien D, Vilcoq JR: Paget's disease of the nipple without detectable breast tumor: conservative management with radiation therapy. Int J Radiat Oncol Biol Phys 13:1463–1465, 1987.
19. Gerard JP, Montbarbon JF, Chassard JL, Romestaing P, Ardiet JM, Delaroche G, Talon B, Papillon J: Conservative treatment of early carcinoma of the breast: significance of axillary dissection and iridium implant. Radiother Oncol 3:17–22, 1985.
20. Harris JR, Hellman S: The results of primary radiation therapy for early breast cancer at the Joint Center for Radiation Therapy. In Harris JR, Hellman S, Silen W (eds): Conservative Management of Breast Cancer. Philadelphia, JB Lippincott, 1983, pp 47–52.
21. Harris JR, Levene MB, Svensson G, Hellman S: Analysis of cosmetic results following primary radiation therapy for stages I and II carcinoma of the breast. Int J Radiat Oncol Biol Phys 5:257–261, 1979.
22. Harris JR, Recht A, Amalric R, Calle R, Clark RM, Reid JG, Spitalier JM, Vilcoq JR, Hellman S: Time course and prognosis of local recurrence following primary radiation therapy for early breast cancer. J Clin Oncol 2:37–41, 1984.
23. Hery M, Namer M, Berschoore J, Monticelli J, Boublil J-L, Lalanne CM: Conservative treatment of breast cancer: a report on 108 patients. Int J Radiat Oncol Biol Phys 10:2185–2190, 1984.
24. Kurtz JM, Amalric R, Brandone H, Ayme Y, Spitalier J-M: Contralateral breast cancer and other second malignancies in patients treated by breast-conserving therapy with radiation. Int J Radiat Oncol Biol Phys 15:277–284, 1988.
25. Kurtz JM, Amalric R, Brandone H, Ayme Y, Spitalier J-M: Results of wide excision for mammary recurrence after breast-conserving therapy. Cancer 61:1969–1972, 1988.
26. Kurtz JM, Amalric R, Delouche G, Pierquin B, Roth J, Spitalier J-M: The second ten years: long-term risks of breast conservation in early breast cancer. Int J Radiat Oncol Biol Phys 13:1327–1332, 1987.
27. Kurtz JM, Spitalier J-M, Amalric R: Results of salvage surgery for local recurrence following conservative therapy of operable breast cancer. Front Radiat Ther Oncol 17:84–90, 1983.
28. Kurtz JM, Spitalier J-M, Amalric R, Brandone H, Ayme Y, Bressac C, Hans D: Mammary recurrences in women younger than forty. Int J Radiat Oncol Biol Phys 15:271–276, 1988.
29. Larson D, Weinstein M, Goldberg I, Silver B, Recht A, Cady B, Wilen W, Harris JR: Edema of the arm as a function of the extent of axillary surgery in patients with stage I–II carcinoma of the breast treated with primary radiotherapy. Int J Radiat Oncol Biol Phys 12:1575–1582, 1986.
30. Leung S, Otmezguine Y, Calitchi E, Mazeron JJ, Le Bourgeois JP, Pierquin B: Locoregional recurrences following radical external-beam irradiation and interstitial implantation for operable breast cancer—a 23-year experience. Radiother Oncol 5:1–10, 1986.
31. van Limbergen E, van den Bogaert W, van der Schueren E, Rijnders A: Tumor excision and radiotherapy as primary treatment of breast cancer: analysis of patient and treatment parameters and local control. Radiother Oncol 8:1–9, 1987.
32. Loeffler JS, Goldberg ID, Risser TA, Come PC, Parker A, Rose C, Botnick L, Kurland G: Noninvasive cardiac evaluation after definitive radiation therapy for carcinoma of the breast. (Abstract 32) Int J Radiat Oncol Biol Phys 11(suppl 1):103, 1985.
33. Montague ED: Conservation surgery and radiation therapy in the treatment of operable breast cancer. Cancer 53:700–704, 1984.
34. Montague ED, Ames FC, Schell SR, Romsdahl MM: Conservation surgery and irradiation as an alternative to mastectomy in the treatment of clinically favorable breast cancer. Cancer 54:2668–2672, 1984.
35. Mustakallio S: Treatment of breast cancer by tumour extirpation and roentgen therapy instead of radical operation. J Fac Radiol 6:23–26, 1954.
36. Mustakallio S: Conservative treatment of breast carcinoma: review of 25 years follow up. Clin Radiol 23:110–116, 1972.
37. Osborne MP, Ormiston N, Harmer CL, McKinna JA, Baker J, Greening WP: Breast conservation in the treatment of early breast cancer: a 20-year follow-up. Cancer 53:349–355, 1984.

38. Peters MV: Cutting the "Gordian knot" in early breast cancer. Ann R Coll Phys Surg Canada 8:186–192, 1975.
39. Peters MV: The role of local excision and radiation in early breast cancer. *In* Breast Cancer: Early and Late. Proceedings of the 13th Annual Clinical Conference on Cancer, Houston, 1968. Chicago, 1970, pp 171–189.
40. Peters MV: Wedge resection and irradiation: an effective treatment in early breast cancer. JAMA 200:144–145, 1967.
41. Peters MV: Wedge resection with or without radiation in early breast cancer. Int J Radiat Oncol Biol Phys 2:1151–1156, 1977.
42. Pierquin B, Wilson J-F, Chassagne D: Modern Brachytherapy. New York, Masson Publishing USA, 1987.
43. Porritt A: Early carcinoma of the breast. Br J Surg 51:214–216, 1965.
44. Prosnitz LR, Weshler Z, Goldenberg IS, Lawrence R: Radiotherapy instead of mastectomy for breast cancer: the Yale experience. *In* Harris JR, Hellman S, Silen W (eds): Conservative Management of Breast Cancer. Philadelphia, JB Lippincott, 1983, pp 61–70.
45. Recht A, Connolly JL, Schnitt SJ, Silver B, Rose MA, Love S, Harris JR: The effect of young age on tumor recurrence in the treated breast after conservative surgery and radiotherapy. Int J Radiat Oncol Biol Phys 14:3–10, 1988.
46. Recht A, Silen W, Schnitt SJ, Connolly JL, Gelman RS, Rose MA, Silver B, Harris JR: Time-course of local recurrence following conservative surgery and radiotherapy for early stage breast cancer. Int J Radiat Oncol Biol Phys 15:255–261, 1988.
47. Rigby-Jones P: Carcinoma of the breast treated by excision of the lump and radiotherapy. (Abstract 969) 11th International Congress on Radiology, Rome, p 456.
48. Schnitt SJ, Connolly JL, Harris JR, Hellman S, Cohen RB: Pathologic predictors of early local recurrence in stage I and II breast cancer treated by primary radiation therapy. Cancer 53:1049–1057, 1984.
49. Solin LJ, Fowble B, Martz KL, Goodman RL: Definitive irradiation for early stage breast cancer: the University of Pennsylvania experience. Int J Radiat Oncol Biol Phys 14:235–242, 1988.
50. Solin LJ, Fowble B, Schultz DJ, Goodman RL: Age as a prognostic factor for patients treated with definitive irradiation for early stage breast cancer. Int J Radiat Oncol Biol Phys 16:373–381, 1989.
51. Veronesi U, Saccozzi R, Del Vecchio M, Banfi A, Clemente C, De Lena M, Gallus G, Greco M, Luini A, Marubini E, Muscolino G, Rile F, Salvadori B, Zecchini A, Zucali R: Comparing radical mastectomy with quadrantectomy, axillary dissection, and radiotherapy in patients with small cancers of the breast. N Engl J Med 305:6–11, 1981.
52. Veronesi U, Zucali R, Luini A: Local control and survival in early breast cancer: the Milan trial. Int J Radiat Oncol Biol Phys 12:717–720, 1986.
53. Zafrani B, Fourquet A, Vilcoq JR, Legal M, Calle R: Conservative management of intraductal breast carcinoma with tumorectomy and radiation therapy. Cancer 57:1299–1301, 1986.

Conservation Surgery and Radiation: The M. D. Anderson Cancer Center Experience

Frederick C. Ames, M.D., Anne T. Stotter, Ph.D., Mary Jane Oswald, B.S., Eleanor D. Montague, M.D., and Marsha D. McNeese, M.D.

Conservation surgery plus radiation therapy is generally accepted as an alternative to mastectomy for many patients with operable breast cancer based largely on the data from the prospective randomized trials carried out in Milan[6] and by the National Surgical Adjuvant Breast and Bowel Project[1] (reviewed in other chapters). Prior to the mid 1970s, however, patients were seldom considered for conservation surgery and radiation unless they refused mastectomy or were considered medically unable to undergo operation under general anesthesia. Only after data were accumulated and retrospectively analyzed was conservation surgery plus radiation used electively to treat operable breast cancer.[2] This chapter reviews the techniques, results, and complications of treatment of patients prospectively treated for invasive breast cancer at The University of Texas M. D. Anderson Cancer Center.

MATERIALS AND METHODS

From 1955 through 1987, a total of 577 patients were treated with conservation surgery and radiation for operable breast cancer at The University of Texas M. D. Anderson Cancer Center. Prior to 1976, however, few patients were offered tumor excision (segmental mastectomy) and radiation as an alternative to mastectomy. During that earlier period, some patients were treated with protracted high-dose radiation without excision or were treated with breast conservation and radiation for either noninvasive or more advanced disease. In many instances the biopsy carried out prior to referral served as the only tumor excision. Through 1975, therefore, only 71 patients with operable invasive breast cancer had been treated with excision and radiation comparable to current practice. Following a review of that earlier experience, we modified our treatment approach and increasingly considered patients for elective breast conservation and radiation as an alternative to mastectomy.[2-5] Results of treatment and complications in 419 patients with T1–T2, N0–N1 breast cancer prospectively treated with conservation surgery and radiation between 1976 and 1987 were reviewed.

Surgical Technique

Most patients underwent excision of all gross tumor with an attempt to achieve histologically proven clear surgical margins. More than one third of these patients, however, were referred after biopsy and removal of most or all of the tumor. In these patients, a reexcision was often done where feasible if diseased margins were involved or if they could not be assessed. Our previous review revealed an increased rate of local failure in such patients.[2] This was most often the case when the surgeon performed the biopsy as a diagnostic procedure with no intent to consider treatment by excision and radiation. Some patients refused reexcision, and in some others, it was not technically feasible for cosmetic reasons. Among patients who underwent reexcision under these circumstances, more than 50 percent had residual cancer at the biopsy site.[4] In addition, axillary dissection for staging was recommended to all patients, and most underwent a level I dissection through a separate incision.

Radiation Therapy

The breast was treated through medial and lateral tangential open and wedged fields using cobalt 60 without bolus to 4500 to 5000 cGy tumor dose in 5 weeks (25 fractions). The dose was calculated at a point approximately two thirds of the distance from the areola to the base of the breast in the quadrant of the primary tumor based on breast contours and computed tomographic (CT) treatment planning.[4] If there was tumor in a reexcision specimen, a boost of 1000 cGy in 5 days delivered through the reduced fields with electrons of appropriate energy was given. If margins were disease positive or unknown and reexcision was not done, an interstitial implant was used to deliver 1500 to 2000 cGy.

Patients with lateral T1, N0 tumors received radiation only to the breast. With central, medial, or node-positive tumors, the internal mammary and supraclavicular nodes were given a 4500 to 5000 cGy tumor dose in 5 weeks. A mixture of electrons and photons was used to treat the nodal areas in order to avoid heart and lung damage. A posterior axillary port using cobalt 60 was added for patients with large nodes (>3 cm) or extranodal extension to supplement the dose to the midaxilla.

Systemic Adjuvant Therapy

After 1976, many patients with histologically positive axillary nodes were considered for systemic adjuvant therapy using 5-fluorouracil, doxorubicin, and cyclophosphamide. For patients with four or more disease positive nodes, radiation was usually delayed until at least three cycles of the planned course of chemotherapy had been administered. Most other patients who received systemic therapy did so after the completion of the planned radiation therapy followed by a 3- to 6-week rest. A total of 70 of the 419 patients (17 percent) received systemic adjuvant therapy, including 62 of the 204 patients (30 percent) with stage II disease.

RESULTS

The 5-year overall and distant metastasis–free survival rates are 92 percent and 90 percent, respectively, for stage I disease patients and 82 percent and 81 percent for stage II patients.

With a median follow-up of 56 months, locoregional failures have occurred in 39 of the 419 patients (nine percent). This includes 15 of the 215 stage I disease patients (seven percent) and 24 of the 204 with stage II disease (12 percent). The actuarial 5-year survival rate for these patients after local failure is 67 percent, although the follow-up for some is short. In comparison the actuarial 5-year survival for patients with locoregional failures who were treated prior to 1976 is 44 percent.

COMPLICATIONS

The complications of conservation surgery and radiation therapy in this series are presented in Table 38–6. A concerted effort was made to register all probable treatment complications even though they were minor or produced no symptoms. Although 200 of these 419 patients (48 percent) had some type of complication, most were asymptomatic or had only minor symptoms. For example, 77 patients (18 percent) had evidence of pneumonitis or apical fibrosis on chest roentgenogram,

Table 38–6. COMPLICATIONS FROM CONSERVATION SURGERY AND RADIATION FOR OPERABLE BREAST CANCER, 1976–1987 (N = 419)

Complication	No. Patients, Any Degree Severity (%)		No. Patients, Moderate to Severe (%)	
Pneumonitis-Fibrosis	75	(18)	21	(5)
Breast-Skin Fibrosis	62	(15)	36	(9)
Axillary Fibrosis	5	(1)	2	(<1)
Rib Fracture	13	(3)	11	(3)
Loss of Motion	8	(2)	3	(<1)
Necrosis	3	(<1)	3	(<1)
Neuropathy	3	(<1)	2	(<1)
Arm Edema	36	(9)	17	(4)
Other*	67	(16)	24	(6)
Total Patients (%)	200†	(48)	94†	(22)

*Breast edema, fibrosis at field junction, etc.
†Some patients had more than one complication.

but only 21 (five percent) were symptomatic, and none of these was severe or permanent. Fibrosis in the breast, skin, or axilla or at field junctions was observed in a number of patients but has not resulted in significant morbidity. More recently these sequelae have been minimized by using a mixture of photons and electrons for irradiating the internal mammary or supraclavicular fields.[3]

One patient suffered tissue necrosis following radiation. She had systemic lupus and dermatomyositis. Two other patients had delayed healing in the axilla as a result of infected seromas. One of these patients was a chronic heavy smoker with severe chronic obstructive pulmonary disease, and the other had no identified associated disease. We have experienced breast necrosis after radiation in a patient with scleroderma and are currently reluctant to irradiate patients who have systemic collagen diseases. Brachial plexus neuropathy occurred in five patients but was mild and transient in three and only moderate in two.

Overall, although 94 patients (22 percent) had symptomatic complications of treatment, only 27 (six percent) had symptoms that were judged to be significant and were persistent. Of these 27 patients, six had arm edema, 13 had breast fibrosis, three had fibrosis and edema, and four had rib fractures. These complications could probably be minimized by altering the technique described previously and elsewhere.[2-5] At present, patients with clinical stage I or II disease undergo level I–II axillary dissection and do not receive irradiation to the axilla or internal mammary fields unless extensive nodal or extracapsular extension of disease is found. This has minimized arm edema and eliminated junctional fibrosis at the site of field overlap. The remaining patient developed tissue slough after she underwent a later breast augmentation in an outside hospital. Only five of these 27 patients with significant or persistent complications were treated after January 1982. Cosmesis was judged to be good or better in more than 80 percent of all patients.

References

1. Fisher B, et al: Five-year results of a randomized clinical trial comparing total mastectomy and segmental mastectomy with or without radiation in the treatment of breast cancer. N Engl J Med 312:665, 1985.
2. Montague ED, et al: Conservation surgery and irradiation for the treatment of favorable breast cancer. Cancer 43:1058, 1979.
3. Montague ED, et al: Conservation surgery and irradiation in clinically favorable breast cancer. In Harris JR, Hellman S, Silen W (eds): Conservative Management of Breast Cancer. New Surgical and Radiotherapeutic Techniques. Philadelphia, JB Lippincott, pp 53–60, 1983.
4. Montague ED: Conservation surgery and radiation therapy in the treatment of operable breast cancer. Cancer 53:700, 1984.
5. Montague ED, et al: Conservation surgery and irradiation as an alternative to mastectomy in the treatment of clinically favorable breast cancer. Cancer 54:2668, 1984.
6. Veronesi U, et al: Comparing radical mastectomy with quadrantectomy, axillary dissection and radiotherapy in patients with small cancers of the breast. N Engl J Med 305:6, 1981.

Retrospective Study of Small Breast Cancers Treated by Conservative Surgery and Radiotherapy at the Institut Gustave-Roussy

Danièle Sarrazin, M.D., Rodrigo Arriagada, M.D., John A. Dewar, M.D., Simone Benhamou, M.Sc., Ellen Benhamou, M.D., Philippe Lasser, M.D., Françoise Fontaine, M.D., Jean-Paul Travagli, M.D., Marc Spielmann, M.D., Thierry Le Chevalier, M.D., and Geneviève Contesso, M.D.

We undertook a prospective randomized trial comparing tumorectomy, axillary dissection, and breast irradiation with modified radical mastectomy.* There was no advantage in terms of overall or disease-free survival for mastectomy, and thus conservative treatment became our standard treatment. We and others (see references) now have a very substantial experience in conservative management of breast cancer; this section is an analysis of our overall results with this treatment for small breast cancers.

---

*See subsequent subsection of this chapter entitled, "Randomized Trial Comparing Conservative Treatment of Early Breast Cancers to Mastectomy at the Institut Gustave-Roussy."

PATIENTS AND METHODS

The series comprised 592 patients with unilateral invasive breast cancer treated at the Institut Gustave-Roussy (IGR) between June 1970 and April 1982. It includes three groups of patients: those treated in the conservative arm of the IGR trial; those treated conservatively at the time the trial was running but not included in the trial because they were either ineligible or refused mastectomy; and those treated conservatively after the trial closed (when conservation became the standard therapy).

The protocol followed is essentially that described for the conservative arm of the trial. Patients presented with T0, T1, T2, N0, N1a, and M0 tumors [Union Internationale Contre le Cancer (UICC) classification, 1979]. They were, however, treated conservatively only if the tumor, measured by the pathologist at the time of surgery, was less than or equal to 20 mm (1970–1979) or less than or equal to 25 mm (1980–1982). The exceptions were eight patients with tumors larger than 25 mm who were included because they were medically unfit for more extensive surgery or had declined mastectomy. In addition, there were 18 patients with multiple tumors (17 with two tumors, one with three tumors) who were treated conservatively for similar reasons.

Surgery

All patients underwent tumorectomy, and the adequacy of the margins was confirmed by the pathologist at the time of surgery. The primary surgery was performed at the Institut Gustave-Roussy in 84 percent of cases, and six percent had reexcision of the tumor bed after initial surgery elsewhere.

The policy for the axilla was to perform a lower axillary dissection and remove at least seven nodes. These were examined by the pathologist at the time of surgery, and if any were involved by tumor (N+), a complete axillary dissection was performed. Thirty-four patients (four percent) did not undergo axillary surgery because either they were unfit or their surgery had been performed elsewhere.

Radiotherapy

All patients received radiotherapy to the breast by the technique described in the last section of this chapter, entitled, "Randomized Trial Comparing Conservative Treatment of Early Breast Cancers to Mastectomy at the Institut Gustave-Roussy." Patients without evidence of nodal involvement (N−) had no further axillary treatment. After complete axillary dissection N+ patients proceeded to full nodal irradiation unless managed in the no radiotherapy arm of the second randomization of the trial (see last section of this chapter). It was found that the combination of axillary clearance and radiotherapy was associated with excessive morbidity,[8] so after 1981 N+ patients treated by axillary clearance had no axillary irradiation. The technique of nodal radiotherapy was the same as described in the last section of this chapter.

Systemic Treatment

Systemic treatment was used adjuvantly in 55 N+ patients, but in a nonsystematic manner. This form of therapy comprised, alone or in combination, ovarian irradiation in 23 patients, additive hormone therapy in 12 patients, immunotherapy [adjuvant treatment with polyadenylic-polyuridylic acid (Poly-A-Poly-U)] in 25 patients, and chemotherapy in four.

Statistical Analysis

Survival and the probabilities of relapse were calculated by the actuarial method. Comparisons were made by the log rank test.

RESULTS

The mean age of patients was 52 years (S. D., 11.7; range, 22–81). Mean length of follow-up was 78 months (S. D., 35 months), and only 8.3 percent of patients alive had not been reviewed within the past year. Clinically the tumors were small, being T0/T1 in 80 percent of cases and T2 in 19 percent. The macroscopic tumor diameter was less than or equal to 20 mm in 87 percent, and the mean macroscopic tumor diameter was 15.8 mm (S. D., 4.9; range, 2–30). The clinical UICC axillary nodal status was N0 in 64 percent, N1a in 26 percent, and N1b in ten percent. Thirty-six percent of patients were subsequently shown to be N+. There was no significant variation in the proportion of N+ patients according to tumor site (lateral, 37 percent; central, 33 percent; and medial, 34 percent).

Survival

Overall survival was 92 percent at 5 years and 80 percent at 10 years. The equivalent figures for disease-free survival were 78 percent and 61 percent, respectively. Both curves are shown in Figure 38–9.

Local/Regional Control

There were 36 local/regional relapses. Of these, 26 were in the breast (including two with associated ipsilateral supraclavicular nodal relapse), and the remaining ten were entirely outside the breast. In nine cases they were associated with a synchronous metastatic relapse. The 5-year actuarial rate of local/regional relapse was 6.5 percent, and the median time to local/regional relapse was 37 months (range, 11–125).

Considering the 26 relapses within the breast, the

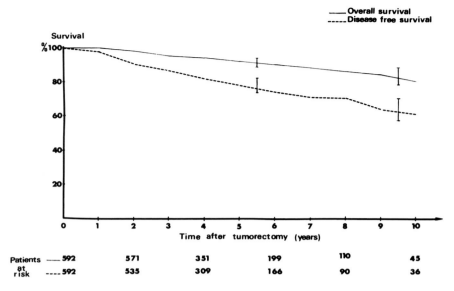

Figure 38–9. Actuarial overall and disease-free survival.

actuarial rate of relapse within the breast increased by approximately one percent per annum, being five percent at 5 years (Fig. 38–10). Following breast relapse, six patients were inoperable because of either an inflammatory relapse or the presence of distant metastases. One patient returned abroad and has been lost to follow-up. The remaining 19 patients underwent mastectomy, which was followed by systemic treatment in nine cases. All 19 patients remained locally controlled, although four have developed and died from distant metastases.

Ten patients relapsed in sites outside the breast. This group comprised, alone or in combination, five axillary relapses, five supraclavicular relapses, and three cutaneous relapses. Considering the axillary relapses, the mean time for axillary relapse was 31.4 months (S. D.,

17.5 months), and none were observed after 5 years. The probability of axillary relapse at 5 years was only 1.2 percent (95 percent confidence interval, 0.5 percent to 2.5 percent). It is of note that none of the N+ patients who underwent axillary clearance with or without axillary radiotherapy relapsed in the axilla.

Relapse outside the breast or an inoperable relapse within the breast was associated with a poor prognosis. Figure 38–11 depicts the actuarial survival after tumorectomy for patients (1) not relapsing locally or regionally, (2) who had had a mastectomy after breast relapse and (3) who had not had a mastectomy after breast or regional relapse. The survival of the last group is significantly inferior ($p<0.02$) to the other two groups, which do not differ significantly.

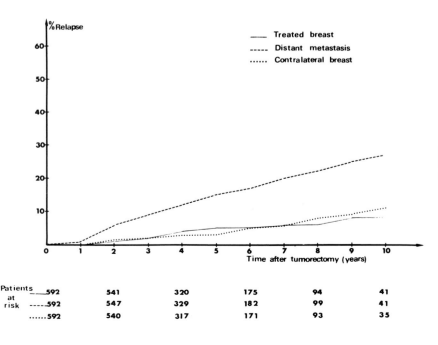

Figure 38–10. Actuarial curves of relapse within the breast compared with contralateral breast cancer and distant metastasis.

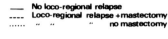

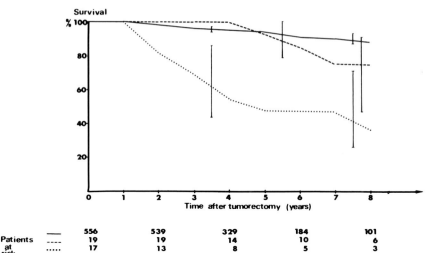

Figure 38–11. Actuarial survival after tumorectomy for patients with locoregional no relapse, relapse in the breast that had a mastectomy, and locoregional relapse without a mastectomy.

Distant Metastatic and Contralateral Breast Relapses

The actuarial rate of distant metastatic relapse was 15 percent at 5 years (Fig. 38–10). Ninety-five patients developed distant metastases, and of these, 44 have died of breast cancer.

The probability of relapse within the contralateral breast was three percent at 5 years (Fig. 38–10). A total of 26 patients developed contralateral breast cancer, an incidence (i.e., 1 percent per year) that was not significantly different from that of patients developing relapse within the treated breast.

CONCLUSIONS

The results of treatment of this larger series of patients confirm those previously obtained in the randomized trial. Essentially patients with small breast tumors (less than or equal to 25 mm) can be managed by tumorectomy, axillary dissection, and radiotherapy with an acceptable local control rate. In addition, it is important to note that relapse with an operable recurrence in the breast is not associated with a significantly impaired survival.

These results, however, have been obtained only in patients with relatively small tumors by using a meticulous surgical technique, adhering rigidly to a consistent radiotherapy protocol, and following the patients assiduously. Deviations from this treatment plan might well be associated with less favorable results. Further studies are necessary to define the upper limit of tumor size suitable for conservation therapy, to determine whether the tumorectomy must be macroscopically complete, and to ascertain whether variation of the radiotherapy protocol is associated with a decrease in local/regional control.

There was good local control within the axilla. Following axillary clearance in N+ patients, there were no axillary relapses regardless of whether the axilla was irradiated. This confirms the adequacy of axillary clearance as a therapeutic modality. Irradiation after axillary clearance is thus unnecessary and, in addition, is associated with excessive morbidity.

The rate of development of tumors in the contralateral breast was similar to that of relapse within the treated breast. This confirms the importance of careful long-term follow-up of these patients to detect relapse at both sites.

Overall survival, however, depends on the rate of distant metastatic relapse. The method of therapy (mastectomy or conservation treatment) has little effect on local control and hence survival. Thus the improvement in overall survival depends on the development of improved systemic therapy.

References

1. Amalric R, Santamaria F, Robert F, et al: Conservative therapy of operable breast cancer. Results at five, ten and fifteen years in 2216 consecutive cases. *In* Harris JR, Hellman S, Silen W (eds): Conservative Management of Breast Cancer. Philadelphia, JB Lippincott, 1983, pp 15–21.
2. Bedwinek JM, Lee J, Fineberg B, Ocwieza M. Prognostic indicators in patients with isolated local-regional recurrence of breast cancer. Cancer 47:2232–2235, 1981.
3. Berg JW: The significance of axillary node levels in the study of breast cancer. Cancer 8:776–778, 1955.
4. Bunting JS, Hemsted EH, Kremer JK: The pattern of spread and survival in 596 cases of breast cancer related to clinical staging and histological grade. Clin Radiol 27:9–15, 1976.
5. Bruce J, Carter DC, Fraser J: Patterns of recurrent disease in breast cancer. Lancet i:433–435, 1970.
6. Calle R, Vilcoq JR, Pilleron JP, Schlienger P, Durand JC: Conservative treatment of operable breast carcinoma by irradiation with or without limited surgery—ten year results. *In* Harris JR, Hellman S, Silen W (eds): Conservative Management of Breast Cancer. Philadelphia, JB Lippincott, 1983, pp 3–9.

7. Clark RM. Alternatives to mastectomy—the Princess Margaret Hospital experience. *In* Harris JR, Hellman S, Silen W (eds): Conservative Management of Breast Cancer. Philadelphia, JB Lippincott, 1983, pp 35–46.

8. Dewar JA, Sarrazin D, Benhamou E, Petit JY, Benhamou S, Arriagada R, Fontaine F, Castaigne D, Contesso G: Management of the axilla in conservatively treated breast cancer: 592 patients treated at Institut Gustave-Roussy. Int J Radiat Oncol Biol Phys 13:475–481, 1987.

9. Fisher B, Barrer M, Margolese T, et al: Five-year results of a randomized clinical trial comparing total mastectomy and segmental mastectomy with or without radiation in the treatment of breast cancer. N Engl J Med 312:665–673, 1985.

10. Harris JR, Recht A, Amalric R, et al: Time course and prognosis of local recurrence following primary radiation therapy for early breast cancer. J Clin Oncol 2:37–41, 1984.

11. Harris JR, Hellman S: The role of primary radiation therapy for early breast cancer at the Joint Centre for Radiation Therapy. *In* Harris JR, Hellman S, Silen W (eds): Conservative Management of Breast Cancer. Philadelphia, JB Lippincott, 1983, pp 47–52.

12. Hery M, Namer M, Verschoove J, Monticelli J, Boublil JL, Lalanne CM: Conservative treatment of breast cancer: a report on 108 patients. Int J Radiat Oncol Biol Phys 10:2185–2190, 1984.

13. Kaplan EL, Meier P: Non parametric estimation from incomplete observations. J Am Stat Assoc 53:457–481, 1958.

14. Kurtz JM, Spitalier JM, Amalric R: Late breast recurrence after lumpectomy and irradiation. Int J Radiat Oncol Biol Phys 9:1191–1194, 1983.

15. Lacour J, Lê M, Petit JY, Lasser P, Contesso G, Sarrazin D: Mastectomie radicale et modifiée dans le traitement du cancer du sein. Bull Cancer 64:593–602, 1977.

16. Lacour J, Lacour F, Spira A, et al: Adjuvant treatment with polyadenylic-polyuridylic acid in operable breast cancer: updated results of a randomised trial. Br Med J 288:589–592, 1984.

17. Montague ED, Schell SR, Romsdahl MM, Ames FC: Conservative surgery and irradiation in clinically favorable breast cancer—the MD Anderson experience. *In* Harris JR, Hellman S, Silen W (eds): Conservative Management of Breast Cancer. Philadelphia, JB Lippincott, 1983, pp 53–59.

18. Pierquin B: Conservative treatment for carcinoma of the breast: experience of Créteil—ten year results. *In* Harris JR, Hellman S, Silen W (eds): Conservative Management of Breast Cancer. Philadelphia, JB Lippincott, 1983, pp 11–14.

19. Recht A, Silver B, Schmitt S, Connolly J, Hellman S, Harris JR: Breast relapse following primary radiation therapy for early breast cancer. I. Classification, frequency and salvage. Int J Radiat Oncol Biol Phys 11:1211–1216, 1985.

20. Sarrazin D, Lê M, Rouëssé J, Contesso G, Petit JY, Lacour J, Viguier J, Hill C: Conservative treatment versus mastectomy in breast cancer tumors with macroscopic diameter of 20 millimeters or less. The experience of the Institut Gustave-Roussy. Cancer 53:1209–1213, 1984.

21. Schottenfeld D, Nash AG, Robbins GF, Beattie EJ: Ten-year results of the treatment of primary operable breast carcinoma. Cancer 38:1001–1007, 1976.

22. Vallagussa P, Bonadonna G, Veronesi U: Patterns of relapse and survival following radical mastectomy. Cancer 41:1170–1178, 1978.

23. Veronesi U, Saccozzi R, Del Vecchio M, et al: Comparing radical mastectomy with quadrantectomy, axillary dissection and radiotherapy in patients with small cancers of the breast. N Engl J Med 305:6–11, 1981.

Conservation Surgery and Irradiation in Stages I and II Disease at the Istituto Nazionale Tumori (Milan)

Umberto Veronesi, M.D.

The development of the new era in conservative treatment of breast cancer originates from many factors. The first is the change in the concept of the natural history of breast cancer, considered today a disease that spreads in the body fairly early, with the growth in distant organs being conditioned by biological and immunological factors; the extent of the removal of the primary carcinoma has little influence on its prognosis. The second is the change in the patient population as a result of the introduction on a large scale of information campaigns, screening programs, and new diagnostic tools such as mammography. Twenty years ago only a minority of cases presented with tumors less than 2 cm in diameter, whereas today this is the case in 30 percent to 50 percent of cases, at least in Western countries. The third factor is the observation of the failure of the aggressive surgical and radiotherapeutic procedures of the 1960s, with many trials showing that superradical operations and intense postoperative radiotherapy do not improve the prognosis of breast cancer patients. The fourth factor is the change in the attitude of women as to their participation in the decision process. Breast cancer patients today ask their surgeon for a complete description of the range of options available to treat their disease with the advantages and risks connected with each procedure.

FIRST MILAN TRIAL

In 1968 at the meeting of the World Health Organization (WHO) Committee of Investigators on Breast

Cancer Diagnosis and Treatment, a paper was presented by Veronesi, Banfi, and Saracci proposing a randomized international study comparing radical mastectomy with a conservative procedure consisting of a large breast resection (quadrantectomy) with a complete axillary dissection followed by radiotherapy (QUART) on the same breast.

The project was endorsed by the Committee by the end of 1969, but attempts to organize a coordinated international trial failed. At the Milan Institute the trial was implemented in 1973; the preliminary results were published in 1981,[2] and more consolidated results were made available in 1986.[1]

Only patients with clinical or mammographic evidence of a breast cancer smaller than 2 cm in diameter were selected for the trial. The absence of clinically metastatic nodes was another condition for eligibility. If the excisional biopsy and frozen section examination showed a carcinoma measuring up to 2 cm in diameter, the patients were randomized to one of two treatment groups: the first received the Halsted mastectomy, and the second received a conservative treatment (QUART). Patients with noninfiltrating carcinoma were excluded, as were patients older than 70 years or who had had previous malignant disease of any type. From 1973 to 1975, patients with histologically proven nodal metastases were further randomized to receive either radiotherapy to the supraclavicular and internal mammary nodes or no further treatment. From 1976 to 1980 the patients with histologically proven axillary metastases were all given adjuvant combination chemotherapy consisting of cyclophosphamide, methotrexate, and 5-fluorouracil (CMF) for 1 year.

Patients randomized to conservative treatment were treated with the quadrantectomy technique. The term "quadrantectomy" refers to an extensive breast resection that removes the entire quadrant of the breast containing the primary carcinoma, including the overlying skin and the fascia of the major pectoral muscle. This type of operation, although conservative, is considered a "locally radical" operation and not just a "debulking" operation, as many conservative procedures are.

When the primary cancer was located in the upper outer quadrants, the operation was performed en bloc, whereas when the primary site was in one of the other quadrants, the axillary dissection was performed through a separate incision. In all cases, to obtain a complete axillary dissection, the minor pectoralis muscle was resected, and all the axillary lymph nodes up to the apex of the axilla were removed. In more recent years, this technique has been substituted with one that preserves the minor pectoralis muscle.

Irradiation of the breast was an important part of the treatment. A dose of 50 Gy was delivered through two opposing tangential fields with high-energy photons (a cobalt unit or a 6 MeV linear accelerator), and another dose of 10 Gy was given with orthovoltage radiotherapy as a booster to the skin surrounding the scar.

Chemotherapy in node-positive patients was started 15 to 30 days after surgery; in the quadrantectomy

Table 38–7. MILAN I TRIAL: LOCAL RECURRENCES, SECOND PRIMARY BREAST CANCERS, AND DISTANT METASTASES, AS A FIRST EVENT

| | No. of Patients | | | |
| | Halsted | | Quart | |
	No.	%	No.	%
No. of patients	349		352	
Local recurrences	7	2.1	9	2.6
Second primary tumors				
Ipsilateral breast	—	—	8	2.3
Contralateral breast	18	5.2	18	5.1

group, it was begun simultaneously with radiotherapy in most cases. The average quantity of drugs administered was similar in the two treatment groups.

From 1973 to early 1980, 701 evaluable patients were entered into the trial; 349 were treated with the Halsted mastectomy and 352 with QUART. No significant differences between the two groups were present in any of the characteristics of the patients considered (i.e., age, menopausal status, tumor site by quadrant, dimensions of the primary cancer, incidence of axillary metastases, and previous biopsy). The two series therefore were strictly comparable.

Nine patients in the QUART group and seven in the Halsted group had local recurrences (Table 38–7 and Fig. 38–12). The nine patients with local recurrence in the QUART group underwent mastectomy; seven out of the nine are alive and well, and two died from distant metastases. Out of the seven patients with local recurrences in the Halsted group, five died from the disease. Eight patients treated with the conservative technique had a second cancer in the ipsilateral breast 4 to 10 years after the operation. The diagnosis of a second primary tumor in the ipsilateral breast was recorded after careful clinicopathological evaluation by surgeons, radiologists, and pathologists. Contralateral primary breast cancers were observed in 18 of the QUART patients and in 18 of the Halsted patients. By July 1988, there had been 55 deaths from breast cancer in the quadrantectomy group (15.6 percent) and 64 in the Halsted group (18.3 percent).

The data on overall survival and disease-free survival are shown in Figures 38–13 and 38–14. No differences between the two groups were recorded after 15 years of

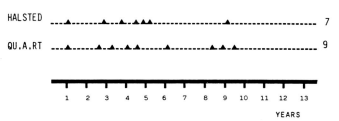

Figure 38–12. Milan Trial I. Local recurrences were observed for nine patients in the QUART group and seven patients in the Halsted group.

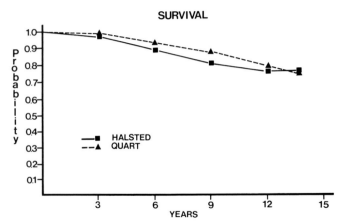

Figure 38–13. Survival curves according to type of treatment (Milan Trial I).

follow-up. Evaluation of disease-free survival by subgroups according to the presence or absence of axillary metastases showed a higher survival in the patients treated with the conservative procedure in the subgroup of patients with positive axillary nodes (Fig. 38–15).

In conclusion, the results of the first Milan trial showed that a less mutilating procedure can be substituted for mastectomy without alteration of the long-term survival rate and with a similar rate of local recurrence.

SECOND MILAN TRIAL

The Milan trial was the first controlled study proving the equal efficacy of a conservative treatment compared with that of the Halsted mastectomy. After publication of the results, the quadrantectomy and other nonmutilating operations were extensively introduced into sur-

gical practice in most Western countries. At the Milan Cancer Institute, by the end of 1987, more than 4000 breast cancer patients had been treated with conservative procedures. However, the main question remaining after the favorable conclusion of the trial was related to the real need for a combination of a "radical" local surgical procedure (quadrantectomy) with a "radical" local radiotherapy. Therefore a new trial was designed to compare the classic QUART procedure with a procedure consisting mainly of intensive radiotherapy preceded by a very limited resection (lumpectomy) that was a "debulking" rather than a "radical" procedure.

Thus the new procedure to be compared with QUART consisted of a lumpectomy (or tumorectomy) with axillary dissection followed by radiotherapy (TART) administered both by external irradiation with high energy (45 Gy) and by implantation of wires of iridium 192 (Fig. 38–16). The radioactive implantation was performed after the external irradiation was terminated, and therefore generally occurred some 2 months after the operation.

The study has enrolled 713 evaluable patients. The two series of patients are comparable as to site and size of the primary tumor, age, menopausal status, and rate of axillary dissection. The margins of resection were examined by pathologists and were found to be positive in 13 percent of the lumpectomy specimens and in two percent of the quadrantectomy specimens. These findings, however, according to the protocol, did not modify the therapeutic plan.

The preliminary results of the second Milan trial will be available in another 2 years.

THIRD MILAN TRIAL

A third trial was planned and initiated in 1987, the objective of which was to determine whether radiotherapy is needed after quadrantectomy or can be delivered

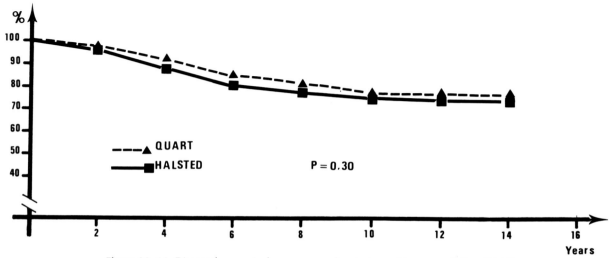

Figure 38–14. Disease-free survival curves according to type of treatment (Milan Trial I).

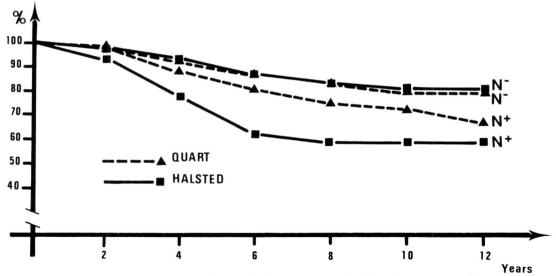

Figure 38–15. Disease-free survival curves of patients treated with Halsted mastectomy and with quadrantectomy, axillary dissection, and radiotherapy (QUART), according to absence (N−) or presence (N+) of axillary node metastases (Milan Trial I).

at the appearance of a local recurrence. The new trial compares the classic QUART technique with quadrantectomy and axillary dissection without radiotherapy (QUAD). The advantages of the latter procedure are not only that the treatment is easier, simpler, and less expensive, but also that it is better tolerated by the patient, and the follow-up of the operated breast is much easier, as it is deprived of the postirradiation fibrotic component that often makes the discovery of a recurrence difficult. Moreover, the late toxic effects of radiotherapy on the chest wall and on the cardiac muscle are avoided (Fig. 38–17).

Radiotherapy, according to the design of the trial, is administered only in the case of a local recurrence. The trial will therefore test whether delaying the radiotherapeutic treatment from the immediate postoperative period (when the hypothetical residual cancer cells are occult) to a later time (when overt recurrences appear)

reduces the efficacy of radiotherapy in controlling the disease locally.

Patient enrollment was initiated in December, 1987, and concluded by the end of 1989.

FUTURE DEVELOPMENTS

The experience in conservative treatments accumulated during recent years and the results of controlled therapeutic trials have made it possible to reach two important conclusions. The first is that certain treatments that preserve the breast, such as QUART, are definitely safe. The second is that patients treated with inadequate local/regional surgery or inadequate radiotherapy may be exposed to an excess of local/regional recurrences, which in turn may produce a lower overall survival. Therefore an effort should be made in the next

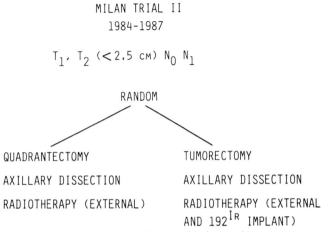

Figure 38–16. Design of Milan Trial II.

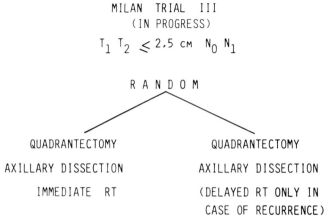

Figure 38–17. Design of Milan Trial III.

few years to identify the point at which an additional reduction of treatment may become dangerous.

Although the future trend is definitely in favor of increasingly reduced surgery, the adequacy of the new techniques must be carefully tested and evaluated. The problems to be faced by future trials will be the extent of the surgical act (limited excision vs. extensive resection, axillary dissection vs. no dissection, and total axillary dissection vs. axillary sampling), the type of radiotherapy (immediate vs. delayed, whole breast vs. limited direct field, boost vs. no boost, and regional node irradiation vs. no nodal irradiation), the comparison with other forms of surgery providing good cosmetic results (conservative treatments vs. total mastectomy plus immediate reconstruction), the size of primary to be submitted to conservative procedures, the pathological patterns requiring differentiated conservative tech-

niques (lobular carcinoma *in situ*, intraductal noninfiltrating carcinoma, Paget's disease, and minimal carcinomas).

The advent of conservative procedures in early breast cancer has created not only an atmosphere of confidence on the part of women toward the surgeons and radiotherapists involved in the treatment of breast cancer but also a high degree of expectancy for further progress, which clinical scientists should try not to disappoint.

References

1. Veronesi U, Banfi A, Del Vecchio M, et al: Comparison of Halsted mastectomy with quadrantectomy, axillary dissection, and radiotherapy in early breast cancer: long-term results. Eur J Cancer Clin Oncol 22:1085–1089, 1986.
2. Veronesi U, Saccozzi R, Del Vecchio M, et al: Comparing radical mastectomy with quadrantectomy, axillary dissection, and radiotherapy in patients with small cancers of the breast. New Engl J Med 305:6–11, 1981.

Randomized Trial Comparing Conservative Treatment of Early Breast Cancers to Mastectomy at the Institut Gustave-Roussy

Danièle Sarrazin, M.D., Monique G. Lê, M.D., R. Arriagada, M.D., Geneviève Contesso, M.D., Françoise Fontaine, M.D., Marc Spielmann, M.D., France Rochard, M.D., Thierry Le Chevalier, M.D., Jean Chavaudra, D.Sc., and Jean LaCour, M.D.

During the past two decades, the aim of research in early breast cancer treatment has been not only to increase long-term survival but also to improve the quality of survival by obtaining better aesthetic results and lower morbidity. To obtain such goals, two alternatives were possible: reducing surgery and reducing radiotherapy. Some authors have reported their experience of conservative surgical treatment in patients with small tumors, but these studies have not been controlled.* In addition, four randomized trials have been published[11, 14, 23–25, 30] comparing limited surgery and radiotherapy with mastectomy. Hayward[14] was the first to carry out a comparative trial of conservative therapy and mastectomy. He found no difference in 10-year survival rates but observed an increased local recurrence rate in the conservatively treated group, probably because the trial was initiated in the 1960s, and the patients could not have benefited from the most recent advances

in radiotherapy. In addition, a number of excessively large tumors were included.

A recent study of patients with tumors smaller than 2 cm, performed in Milan by Veronesi, showed no difference in favor of radical surgery: however, the conservative treatment studied was quandrantectomy with axillary dissection.[30] The role of even more limited surgery therefore remains to be analyzed.

Several studies of reduced nodal radiotherapy have been carried out, but none of them included only patients with tumors of less than 2 cm treated by conservative surgery. Moreover, the results of these studies are contradictory. Some show that radiotherapy decreases recurrence without modifying survival, while others report that radiotherapy can also decrease metastases and mortality.[3, 10, 16, 19, 22, 31]

The problems raised by reducing classic types of treatment have therefore not yet been solved. As early as 1971, the World Health Organization proposed a multicenter study aimed at comparing a conservative procedure (tumorectomy, axillary dissection, and radio-

---

*References 1, 6, 7, 12, 13, 15, 17, 18, 21, and 26.

therapy) to a modified radical mastectomy (Patey). This study was undertaken by the Institut Gustave-Roussy.

TRIAL TECHNIQUES AT THE INSTITUT GUSTAVE-ROUSSY

Eligibility of Patients

Between October 1972 and September 1979, patients with unilateral infiltrating breast cancer of 20 mm or less at mammography, i.e., T1a, N0, N1a or b, M0 [Union International Contre le Cancer (UICC) classification],[29] were considered for entry into the trial. Patients were orally informed of the possibilities of surgical treatment (tumorectomy, axillary dissection, and radiotherapy vs. modified radical mastectomy) according to the tumor size. Some patients refused mastectomy and were not included in the trial. The definitive criterion for inclusion was the tumor size measured macroscopically at the time of surgery: when the size before fixation was 20 mm or less and the tumor completely removed, the patient was included in the trial.

Patients older than 70 years, pregnant women, those unable to receive anesthesia and extended surgery, those refusing mastectomy, those with multifocal tumors, and those who could not be followed up for geographic reasons were excluded.

Patients included in this trial did not receive any systemic adjuvant treatment such as chemotherapy or hormonal therapy.

Surgical Techniques and First Randomization

All patients underwent local excision of the tumor, which was examined at the time of surgery by the pathologist. When it measured 20 mm or less at the macroscopic examination, the treatment was randomly allocated. The modified radical mastectomy did not include excision of the pectoral muscles. Tumorectomy consisted of the removal of the tumor with a margin of 2 cm of glandular tissue. According to Berg data[4] for all the patients, a lower axillary dissection and histological examination of a minimum of seven lymph nodes at the time of surgery were performed; if one or more positive nodes were detected, complete axillary dissection was undertaken. After October 1979, the first randomization was closed, and all eligible patients were treated by a conservative approach for previously reported reasons.[24] The design of the trial is summarized in Table 38–8.

Radiotherapy Modalities and Second Randomization

For patients with positive axillary nodes, a second randomization was performed in order to compare postoperative nodal irradiation with no further treatment.

Table 38–8. DESIGN OF THE TRIAL (OCTOBER 1972–OCTOBER 1979)*

First Randomization for All Eligible Patients†	N = 179	Second Randomization for N+ Patients‡	N = 58
Mastectomy	91		
N–	62		
N+	29 →	No further treatment	14
		→ Nodal irradiation	15
Tumorectomy + breast irradiation	88		
N–	59		
N+	29 →	No further treatment	11
		→ Nodal irradiation	18

*Between October 1979 and December 1980, 14 N+ patients systematically treated by tumorectomy were included in the second randomization. They are excluded from the current study (see text).

†All the patients had a lower axillary dissection.

‡All the N+ patients had a complete axillary dissection at the time of initial surgery, after histological examination of at least seven nodes from the lower axillary dissection.

After October 1979, the second randomization was continued for another year, and 14 N+ patients systematically treated by conservative procedure were included. This second part of the trial included only 72 patients, with a mean follow-up of fewer than 10 years. Because the power of statistical tests was very low, the 10-year results of this second part of the study are not reported here.

Irradiation Technique

The irradiation technique had been planned in such a way that a dose of 45 Gy (18 sessions—4½ weeks) could be delivered at the regional level (breast and lymph node areas) and a booster dose of 15 Gy (six sessions—10 days) on the tumor bed. The detailed prescription actually applied to patients in the different categories is given below.

Target Volumes

Target volumes included the breast, the chest wall, and (according to treatment modalities) the supraclavicular, axillary, and internal mammary nodes. The treatment plan was also supposed to allow a reasonable radiation dose to organs at risk such as the lung, the heart (left side localizations), the brachial plexus, the cervical spine, and the larynx.

Main Features of the Treatment Plan

The treatment was performed with cobalt 60 radiation and, for boost of some medial tumors, 8 or 10 MeV electron beams of a linear accelerator.

The fields were planned according to the following

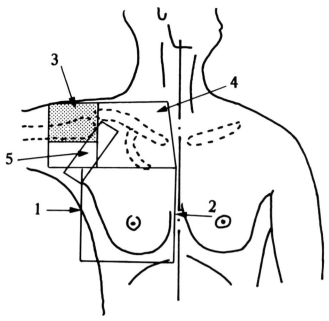

Figure 38–18. *Beam arrangement: 1 and 2,* Tangential fields (including the internal mammary chain). *3,* Anterior axillary and supraclavicular field. *4,* Reduced anterior supraclavicular field. *5,* Posterior axillary field.

principles for patients receiving a complete local/regional radiotherapy (Fig. 38–18):

1. One anterior supraclavicular and axillary field. This large field was used three times per week (three fractions of 2.5 Gy).

2. One anterior supraclavicular field and one posterior axillary field, both used once a week when the previous large field was not treated.

3. Two sets of two mammary fields, using tangential beams with wedge filters. The first set allowed the internal mammary chain and the whole mammary gland to be irradiated at a dose of 45 Gy. The second set involved smaller fields and was devoted to the booster irradiation of the tumor bed, performed in a second step.[2]

For both sets of mammary fields, the irradiation was performed four times per week.

Treatment Conditions and Treatment Planning

The patients were treated lying on the back. On the stretcher top, patients were adapted in a decline plane to allow the anterior part of the chest wall to be as horizontal as possible (better field matching between mammary and supraclavicular beams and decrease of the radiation dose to the lung), and an arm holder was utilized to allow the patient's arm to be kept at a right angle to the body.

The anatomical data were recorded using a mechanical device for the external outlines; a transverse tomograph was used for supine patients to provide the lung outlines and the chest wall thickness.

Treatment planning considered the dose distributions

in several transverse planes, allowing a good evaluation of the dose delivered to the axillary and internal mammary chain lymph nodes and of the dose distributions in the planes containing the tangential beam axis, the tumor bed, and the submammary region (Fig. 38–19).

It is indeed very important when performing the treatment planning to consider the dose distributions in several planes as a result of the anatomical situation and the difficulties of the tangential beam setting. The use of two different outlining devices requires a careful matching of the external and internal data. To improve the technique, evaluations were made using comprehensive computed tomography (CT) data; however, this method was unfortunately not available for routine treatments. Examples of dose distributions are presented in Figure 38–20.

Prescription Modalities

When performed, radiotherapy used cobalt 60 photon beams. For all patients treated by tumorectomy, the breast was irradiated to a dose of 45 Gy in 18 fractions (four fractions of 2.5 Gy per week) during 1 month. A booster dose of 15 Gy in six fractions during 10 days was given to the tumor bed, usually with cobalt 60 photon beams, but some medial tumors were boosted with an electron beam of adequate energy. Patients with histologically negative axillary nodes did not receive irradiation to nodal areas.

For patients with histologically positive axillary nodes randomly allocated to receive nodal irradiation (Table 38–8), a total dose of 45 Gy in 18 fractions during 1 month was given to the axillary, supraclavicular, and internal mammary areas. The supraclavicular and axillary nodes were treated three times per week by an anterior supraclavicular and axillary field delivering 2.5 Gy per fraction and once per week by anterior supraclavicular and posterior axillary fields, each delivering 2.5 Gy. The two latter fields overlapped to a variable extent

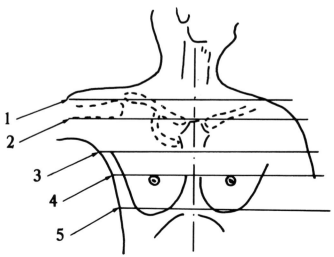

Figure 38–19. *Scheme of three transverse planes: 1,* Supraclavicular; *2,* sternal notch; *3,* second interspace; *4,* tangential beam axis; *5,* inframammary fold.

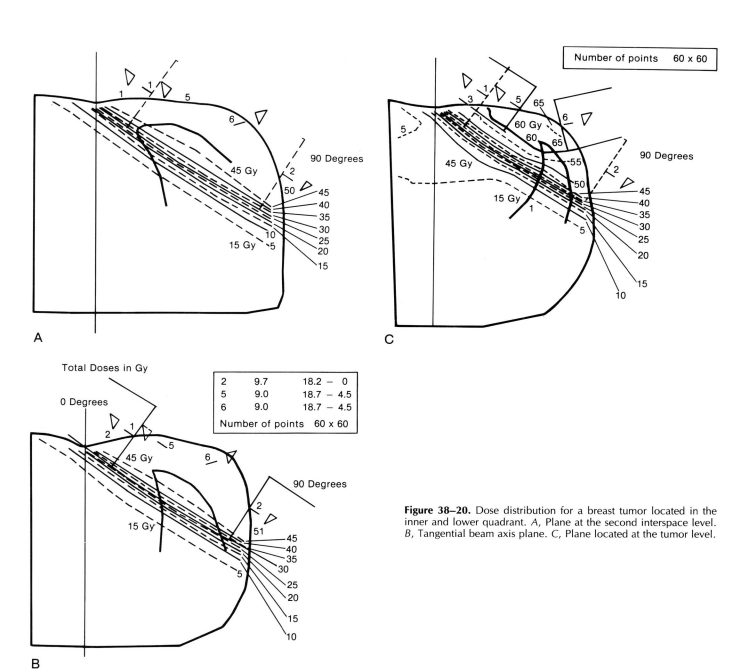

2	9.7	18.2 — 0
5	9.0	18.7 — 4.5
6	9.0	18.7 — 4.5
Number of points	60 x 60	

Figure 38–20. Dose distribution for a breast tumor located in the inner and lower quadrant. *A*, Plane at the second interspace level. *B*, Tangential beam axis plane. *C*, Plane located at the tumor level.

for each patient. The breast in the conservative group, or the chest wall in the mastectomy group, and the internal mammary chain were irradiated four times per week by two tangential fields delivering 2.5 Gy per fraction. The beam arrangements used have been previously described.[23, 24]

Statistical Analysis

Comparisons between the two treatment groups was based on the multifactorial Cox's model,[9] taking into account five major prognostic factors in order to decrease their possible confounding effects and to increase the test power. Thus relative risks of death, distant metastasis, contralateral breast cancer, and local/regional recurrence were estimated after adjustment for age, clinical tumor size, site of the tumor, histoprognostic grading of Scarff and Bloom,[5] and the number of histologically involved axillary nodes. Stratification for nodal irradiation was also performed. The survival rates were computed by the life table method.

Description of the Population

The number of patients included was 179; 91 had a mastectomy, and 88 had a conservative treatment. The two treatment groups were comparable in terms of age, clinical and histological tumor size, tumor site, histoprognostic grading, and number of histologically involved axillary nodes (Table 38–9). Among the 58 patients having positive axillary nodes who were included in the first randomization, 33 were randomized to nodal irradiation (15 from the mastectomy group and 18 from the conservative group, as shown in Table 38–8). For the total population, the mean follow-up was 10 years (S.D., 2 years).

Table 38–9. CHARACTERISTICS OF PATIENTS (FIRST RANDOMIZATION)

Characteristic	Tumorectomy (N = 88)	Mastectomy (N = 91)
Age, mean ± SD (yr)	51.4 ± 9.8	51.8 ± 9.1
Clinical dimension of tumor, mean ± SD (mm)	17.0 ± 5.5	17.4 ± 6.3
Histological dimension of tumor, mean ± SD (mm)	15.7 ± 3.8	15.6 ± 4.1
Percent of cases by no. of positive axillary nodes		
None	66	65
One to three	26	24
Four or more	8	11
Percent of cases with pathological grading		
1	33	30
2	45	43
3	22	27

Table 38–10. TEN-YEAR RATES OF DEATH, METASTASIS, CONTRALATERAL BREAST TUMOR, AND LOCAL/REGIONAL RECURRENCE ACCORDING TO THE ALLOCATED TREATMENT

	Mastectomy		Tumorectomy + RT*		
	No. of Events	10-Year Rate (%)	No. of Events	10-Year Rate (%)	Relative Risk†
Death	18	20	17	21	0.9
Relapse	35	42	28	34	0.8
Metastases	22	27	19	26	0.9
Contralateral breast tumor	6	9	5	9	0.9
Local/regional recurrence‡					
All sites	11	10	6	5	0.5
Chest wall/breast	9	9	5	7	i
Regional lymph nodes	4	5	1	1	i

*RT = Breast and tumor bed postoperative irradiation (45 Gy/18 fractions/30 days and 60 Gy/24 fractions/40 days, respectively).

†Compared with the mastectomy group and adjusted for age, clinical tumor size, tumor site, histoprognostic grading, and number of histologically involved axillary nodes.

‡The addition of the number of local and regional recurrences is greater than the total of local/regional recurrences, because two patients had both chest wall and nodal recurrences.

i = Irrelevant (small number of events in each stratum).

RESULTS

No difference between the two treatment groups was observed for the risks of death, distant metastasis, contralateral breast tumor, and local/regional recurrence (Table 38–10).

Survival and relapse-free survival curves are plotted in Figures 38–21 and 38–22. Similar results were observed in the two treatment groups. The relative risks of death and relapse were slightly lower for the conservative group than for the mastectomy group (0.9 and 0.8, respectively, vs. 1).

Contralateral breast cancer and distant metastasis rates are plotted in Figures 38–23 and 38–24. The number of events was similar in the two treatment groups. The relative risk of both contralateral breast cancer and distant metastases was slightly lower for the conservatively treated group than for the other group (Table 38–10).

Six local/regional recurrences occurred after conservative treatment and 13 after mastectomy (Fig. 38–25 and Table 38–10). Most of them were observed either in the breast or in the chest wall, as shown in Table 38–10. The relative risk of local/regional recurrence was twofold lower for the conservatively treated group than for the other group, but this difference was not significant. In our experience, tumorectomy produced a good cosmetic result in 92 percent of the cases (Fig. 38–26), according to definitions previously published.[10]

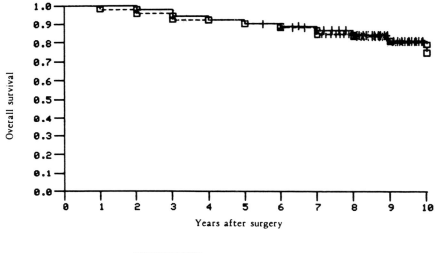

Figure 38–21. Overall survival rates (Kaplan Meier method).

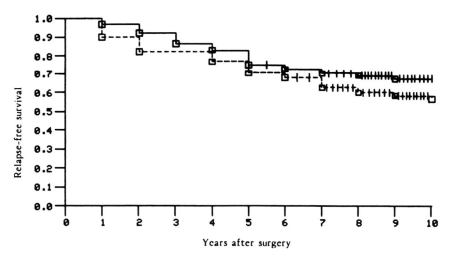

Figure 38–22. Relapse-free survival rate (Kaplan Meier method).

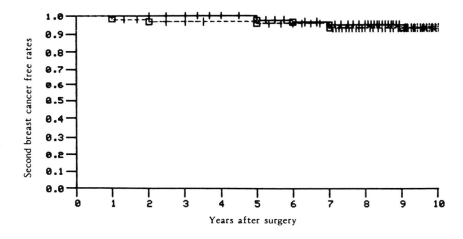

Figure 38–23. Second opposite breast cancer–free rate.

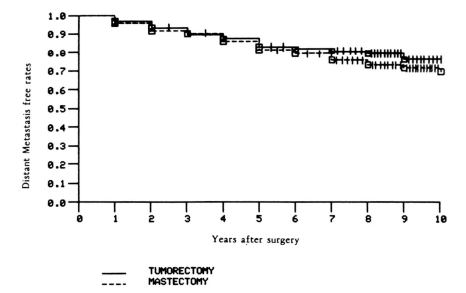

Figure 38–24. Distant metastasis–free rate.

DISCUSSION

Ten years after the initial treatment of early breast cancers, no detrimental effect in terms of overall survival, relapse-free survival, distant metastasis, contralateral breast cancer, or local/regional relapse rates was observed in patients treated by conservative management compared with those treated by classic mastectomy. In fact, the relapse-free survival rates were higher, although not significantly, in the conservatively treated group than in the mastectomy group. This trend may be because systematic irradiation of the breast in the conservatively treated group prevented local recurrences.

These results were obtained from a small series of 179 patients. With this number, the power to detect a difference of ten percent in 10-year survival rates between the two groups of treatment (70 percent versus 80 percent) was only 50 percent, with a type I error equal to 0.05. However, our results support the hypothesis that a conservative procedure does not decrease the chance of survival for patients with a small breast tumor. These results are consistent with those previously published in other randomized trials.[11, 30]

The two older trials[14] generally show worse results for the conservative treatment group than for the control group for both stage I and II patients. However, these trials essentially differed from others because the conservative therapy group had no axillary dissection, but did have irradiation of the axilla. Moreover, a low dose was delivered to both the breast and the axilla. These trials also included T2a and T3a tumors, and it is possible that, for large tumors, a conservative treatment may be inadequate to ensure long-term control.

Conversely, the Milan trial selected the smallest tumors, and included only T1 and N0 patients; 45 percent of them had a tumor measuring less than 1 cm. Our

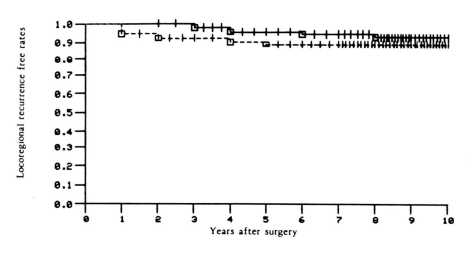

Figure 38–25. Locoregional recurrence–free rate.

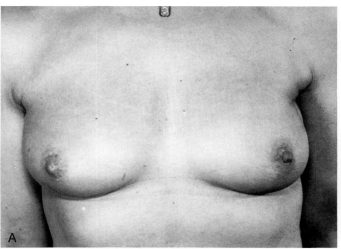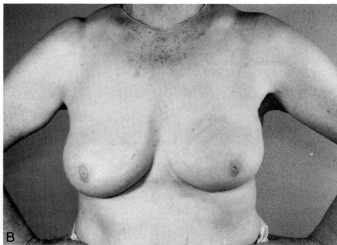

Figure 38–26. Cosmetic results. *A,* Excellent: no perceptible defect. *B,* Good: minor defect and asymmetry.

series included patients with larger tumors (only four percent of them had a tumor smaller than 1 cm), and more N1a–N1b patients (38 percent and five percent, respectively). The surgery performed as part of the Milan trial was more extensive than that for the Gustave-Roussy one (quadrantectomy vs. tumorectomy; Halsted vs. modified radical mastectomy). The radiotherapy technique was similar in the two series. However, 2 years after the start of the Milan trial, N+ patients received 12 cycles of combined chemotherapy using cyclophosphamide, methotrexate, and 5-fluorouracil (CMF) instead of lymph node radiotherapy. In spite of these differences between the Milan and Gustave-Roussy trials, the 5-year survival rates were similar for both conservative therapy groups (92 percent).

Finally, the National Surgical Adjuvant Breast and Bowel Project (NSABP) trial provides some evidence that conservative management might be extended to patients with tumors ranging in size from 2 to 4 cm. In this trial, the conservative treatment group was randomized in two arms (with and without breast irradiation). Although 27 percent of nonirradiated patients underwent mastectomy for local recurrence within 5 years of the initial treatment, these procedures do not decrease the chance of survival up to 5 years.

In summary, most of the results of randomized trials tend to support conservative treatment as a safe procedure to manage small breast cancers in terms of long-term local control and overall survival. This is well demonstrated for T1, small T2, N0–N1a, or N1b breast cancer.

Cosmetic results in the conservative group of this trial can be considered as satisfactory (Fig. 38–26), but better results can be obtained by improvement in the quality of surgery, decrease of the skin dose per fraction,[9] avoidance of treatment beam overlapping, and dose heterogenity using a three-dimensional computerized dosimetry.

The next step of our research will be to define more accurately the indications of conservative management according to the following guidelines:

1. To determine the extent to which conservative treatment can be applied to operable breast cancers as large as 4 or 5 cm, taking into account the tumor/breast size ratio.

2. To use histopathological criteria (tumor size, quality of surgical resection, histoprognostic grading, axillary nodal status, and extent of intraductal component) to identify the optimal predictors for a conservative treatment.

3. To use preoperative treatment with chemotherapy or radiotherapy to decrease the tumor size and allow breast conservation in large T2/T3 breast cancers.

4. Based on the good survival results observed in the NSABP trial[11] and the Princess Margaret Hospital experience,[7] to select according to good local prognostic criteria a small group of patients to be treated only by limited breast surgery and axillary dissection without irradiation. If these patients relapse, it will probably be possible to cure them with a second conservative surgery and irradiation.

Of course, all these guidelines should be studied in well-planned phase III trials to correctly evaluate the impact of these trends in breast cancer management.

ACKNOWLEDGMENT

We gratefully acknowledge the editorial advice of Dr. J. A. Dewar, Ninewells General Hospital, Dundee, Scotland.

References

1. Amalric R, Santamaria F, Robert F, Seigle J, Altshuler C, Pietra JC, Amalric F, Kurtz JM, Spitalier JM, Brandone H, Ayme Y, Pollet JL, Bressac C, Fondarai J: Conservation therapy of operable breast cancer. Results at five, ten and fifteen years in 2216 consecutive cases. *In* Harris JR, Hellman S, Silen W (eds): Conservative Management of Breast Cancer, Philadelphia, JB Lippincott, 1983, pp 15–21.
2. Arriagada R, Mouriesse H, Sarrazin D, Clark RM, Deboer G: Radiotherapy alone in breast cancer. I. Analyses of tumor

parameters, tumor dose, and local control: the experience of the Gustave-Roussy Institute and the Princess Margaret Hospital. Int J Radiat Oncol Biol Phys 11:1751–1757, 1985.
3. Bedwinek JM, Lee J, Fineberg B, Ocwieza M: Prognostic indicators in patients with isolated local-regional recurrence of breast cancer. Cancer 47:2232–2235, 1981.
4. Berg JW: The significance of axillary node levels in the study of breast cancer. Cancer 8:776–778, 1955.
5. Bloom HJG, Richardson WW: Histological grading and prognosis in breast cancer. Br J Cancer 11:359–377, 1957.
6. Calle R, Vilcoq JR, Pilleron JP, Schlienger P, Durand JC: Conservative treatment of operable breast carcinoma by irradiation with or without limited surgery—ten year results. In Harris JR, Hellman S, Silen W (eds): Conservative Management of Breast Cancer. Philadelphia, JB Lippincott, 1983, pp 3–9.
7. Clark RM: Alternatives to mastectomy—the Princess Margaret Hospital experience. In Harris JR, Hellman S, Silen W (eds): Conservative Management of Breast Cancer. Philadelphia, JB Lippincott, 1983, pp 35–46.
8. Cox DR: Regression models and life tables. J R Statist Soc 34:197–220, 1972.
9. Dewar JA, Benhamou S, Benhamou E, Arriagada R, Petit JY, Fontaine F, Sarrazin D: Cosmetic results following lumpectomy axillary dissection and radiotherapy for small breast cancer. Radiother Oncol 12:273–280, 1988.
10. Fisher B, Slack NH, Cavanaugh PJ, et al: Post-operative radiotherapy in the treatment of breast cancer. Ann Surg 172:711, 1970.
11. Fisher B, Bauer M, Margolese R, Poisson R, Pilch Y, Redmond C, Fisher E, Wolmark N, Deutsch M, Montague E, Saffer E, Wickerham L, Lerner H, Glass A, Shibata H, Deckers P, Ketcham A, Oishi R, Russel I: Five-year results of a randomized clinical trial comparing total mastectomy and segmental mastectomy with or without radiation in the treatment of breast cancer. N Engl J Med 312:665–73, 1985.
12. Harris JR, Hellman S: The results of primary radiation therapy for early breast cancer at the Joint Centre for Radiation Therapy. In Harris JR, Hellman S, Silen W (eds): Conservative Management of Breast Cancer. Philadelphia, JB Lippincott, 1983, pp 47–52.
13. Harris JR, Recht A, Amalric R, et al: Time course and prognosis of local recurrence following primary radiation therapy for early breast cancer. J Clin Oncol 2:37–41, 1984.
14. Hayward JL: The Guy's Hospital trials on breast conservation. In Harris JR, Hellman S, Silen W (eds): Conservative Management of Breast Cancer. Philadelphia, JB Lippincott, 1983, pp 78–90.
15. Hery M, Namer M, Verschoore J, Monticelli J, Boublil JL, Lalanne CM: Conservative treatment of breast cancer: a report on 108 patients. Int J Radiat Oncol Biol Phys 10:2185–2190, 1984.
16. Host H, Brenhovd IO: The effect of post-operative radiotherapy in breast cancer. Int J Radiol Oncol Biol Phys 2:1061, 1977.
17. Kurtz JM, Spitalier JM, Amalric R: Late breast recurrence after lumpectomy and irradiation. Int J Radiat Oncol Biol Phys 9:1191–1194, 1983.
18. Montague ED, Schell SR, Romsdahl MM, Ames FC: Conservative surgery and irradiation in clinically favorable breast cancer—the M.D. Anderson experience. In Harris JR, Hellman S, Silen W (eds): Conservative Management of Breast Cancer. Philadelphia, JB Lippincott, 1983, pp 53–59.
19. Paterson R, Russell MH: Clinical trials in malignant disease. Part III. Breast cancer—evaluation of post-operative radiotherapy. Fac Radiol 10:175–180, 1959.
20. Peto R, Pike MC, Armitage PV: Design and analysis of randomized clinical trials requiring prolonged observation of each patient. I. Introduction and design. II. Analysis and examples. Br J Cancer 34:585–612, 1976; 35:1–39, 1977.
21. Pierquin B: Conservative treatment for carcinoma of the breast: experience of Créteil—ten year results. In Harris JR, Hellman S, Silen W (eds): Conservative Management of Breast Cancer. Philadelphia, JB Lippincott, 1983, pp 11–14.
22. Recht A, Silver B, Schmitt S, Connolly J, Hellman S, Harris JR: Breast relapse following primary radiation therapy for early breast cancer. I. Classification, frequency and salvage. Int J Radiat Oncol Biol Phys 11:1211–1216, 1985.
23. Sarrazin D, Lê M, Fontaine MF, Arriagada R: Conservative treatment versus mastectomy in T1 or small T2 breast cancer. A randomized clinical trial. In Harris JR, Hellman S, Silen W (eds): Conservative Management of Breast Cancer. Philadelphia, JB Lippincott, 1983, pp 101–111.
24. Sarrazin D, Lê M, Rouëssé J, Contesso G, Petit JY, Lacour J, Viguier J, Hill C: Conservative treatment versus mastectomy in breast cancer tumors with macroscopic diameter of 20 millimeters or less. Cancer 53:1209–1213, 1984.
25. Sarrazin D, Pieddeloup C, Rouëssé J, Contesso C, Petit JY, Arriagada R, Fontaine F, Lê M: Essai thérapeutique de l'Institut Gustave-Roussy: traitement conservateur versus mastectomie dans les cancers du sein, d'un diamètre égal ou inférieur à 20 mm. In Pujol H, Dubois JB (eds): Les Traitements Conservateurs du Cancer du Sein. Montpellier, France, Sauramps Medical, 1984, pp 85–88.
26. Sarrazin D, Dewar JA, Arriagada R, Benhamou S, Benhamou E, Lasser P, Fontaine F, Travagli JP, Spielman M, Le Chevalier T, Contesso G: Conservative management of breast cancer. Br J Surg 73:604–606, 1986.
27. Sarrazin D, Lé MG, Arriagada R, Contesso G, Fontaine F, Spielmann M, Rochard F, Le Chevalier Th, Lacour J: Ten-year results of a randomized trial comparing a conservative treatment to mastectomy in early breast cancer. Radiother Oncol 14:177–184, 1989.
28. The Cancer Research Campaign: Management of early cancer of the breast. Report on an international multicentre trial. Br Med J 1:1035–1038, 1976.
29. TNM Classification des Tumeurs Malignes. Harmer MH (ed). UICC 3ème Edition, Genève, 1979, pp 47–56.
30. Veronesi U, Saccozzi R, Del Vecchio M, Banfi A, Clementi C, De Lenan M, Gallus G, Greco M, Luini A, Marubini, E, Muscolino G, Rilke F, Salvadori B, Zecchni A, Zucali R: Comparing radical mastectomy with quadrantectomy, axillary dissection and radiotherapy in patients with small cancers of the breast. N Engl J Med 305:6–11, 1981.
31. Wallgren A: A controlled study—pre-operative versus post-operative irradiation. Int J Radiol Oncol Biol Phys 2:1167, 1977.

Chapter 39

ADJUVANT SYSTEMIC THERAPY FOR EARLY STAGE BREAST CANCER

Michael J. Anderson, M.D. and Barnett S. Kramer, M.D.

HISTORICAL ASPECTS AND THEORY

During the past two decades, a major effort in cancer research has been applied to the development and evaluation of adjuvant therapy for breast cancer. The idea for this therapy is not new, but a great deal of information has been collected that has changed dramatically the oncologist's concept of strategy.

Nearly 100 years ago, the first approach to adjuvant therapy in treatment of breast cancer was oophorectomy as adjuvant endocrine therapy to involute the breast before or at the time of mastectomy.[166] About 50 years ago, others applied these same concepts using radiation-induced castration.[177] The introduction of adjuvant cytotoxic chemotherapy to the management of breast cancer occurred in the late 1950s. Early clinical observations and preclinical animal models provided a theoretical basis for subsequent work in this area. With the developing awareness of the relative plateau in cure rates of breast cancer,[8, 48] clinicians realized that the Halsted radical mastectomy,[94] based on anatomical principles of tumor confinement, was inadequate for cure in many patients, even when all clinically apparent disease could be surgically extirpated. The realization that "curative cancer surgery" resulted in a recurrence rate at 5 years of 20 percent in patients with negative nodes and approximately 70 percent in patients with positive nodes underscored the shortcoming of even the most aggressive local therapy.[65] This led to the important realization that the outcome of therapy for breast cancer patients could be improved only by control of subclinical distant disease for a substantial proportion of "early stage" patients. Finally, the curative effect of adjuvant chemotherapy as observed in animal models[59, 164] gave the foundation and hope with which to proceed with its application in human breast cancer.

Early Theoretic Constructs and Resulting Trials

The scientific background for the use of chemotherapy shortly after "curative" surgery began with the observation by Ashworth in 1869 of blood-borne tumor cells post mortem.[4] There were scattered similar observations by others, but the medical community showed no significant interest in this phenomenon until the observation in 1955 of tumor cells in the mesenteric venous blood in patients with colorectal carcinoma.[81] This piqued the interest of a number of investigators,[60] and in the ensuing few years, cancer cells in the peripheral blood were demonstrated in a number of clinical circumstances. When tumor cells were observed in the peripheral blood after procedures such as pelvic[159] and rectal[114] examination, surgical scrubbing of a tumor prior to surgery,[114] and cancer surgery,[51] the notion developed that blood-borne metastases were spawned by manipulation of the tumor at the time of surgery. Because Halsted's theory of anatomical tumor confinement still prevailed, it was believed that in spite of impeccable surgical technique, neoplastic cells dislodged during the mastectomy procedure and caused metastatic disease. Researchers set out to test whether the administration of chemotherapy during the perioperative period destroyed these circulating cells and prolonged survival in experimental animals. There were reports of successful destruction of peripherally disseminated cells with the administration of chemotherapeutic agents in experimental animals.[46, 124, 125] The prolongation of survival of animals transplanted with mammary adenocarcinoma and then treated with a combination of surgery and 6-mercaptopurine provided supportive experimental evidence.[60, 170, 72]

The first randomized adjuvant chemotherapy trial in breast cancer was begun in 1958.[79] It was performed under the auspices of the National Institutes of Health Cancer Chemotherapy National Service Center and was known as the National Surgical Adjuvant Breast Project (NSABP). It was designed to determine the efficacy of chemotherapy added to the Halsted radical mastectomy for improvement in survival and freedom from relapse for patients with breast cancer. This trial (NSABP B-01) evaluated the hypothesis that chemotherapy administered in the perioperative period could destroy tumor cells disseminated at the time of surgery and thus affect disease-free survival and overall survival of certain patients with breast cancer. After definitive surgery, patients were randomly assigned to receive adjuvant thiotepa or placebo. Initially 105 patients received thiotepa at a dosage of 0.8 mg/kg of body weight, with 0.4 mg/kg given at the time of the operation and 0.2 mg/kg given on each of two consecutive postoperative days. As a result of reported complications at this dose, the next 636 patients received 0.2 mg/kg at the time of surgery followed by 0.2 mg/kg on each of the first two postoperative days.[65] The first patient was entered onto NSABP B-01 on April 4, 1958, and patient entry was terminated after accrual of 826 acceptable patients on October 7, 1961.[65] Patients were considered eligible for inclusion if the following conditions were met:

1. The tumor was clinically confined to the breast and axilla.

2. The tumor did not have extensive skin involvement or ulceration and was moveable relative to the chest wall.

3. Axillary nodes were not fixed to the chest wall and there was no evidence of arm edema.

4. Histological evidence of malignancy was present.

5. A Halsted radical mastectomy had been performed en bloc.

6. The patient was between 30 and 70 years of age.

Analysis of the data did not reveal an overall difference in recurrence rate at 5 years in patients receiving thiotepa vs. placebo. Distribution of recurrence rates, however, suggested a beneficial effect of thiotepa in premenopausal women with four or more positive nodes. There was also a difference in survival in the same patient subset at 5 and 10 years after surgery favoring the treatment group (Table 39–1). The importance of this study was minimized at the time of evaluation because of the disappointment that all patients were not cured with the administration of chemotherapy. In retrospect, however, this was the first demonstration that the natural history of breast cancer could be altered by systemic chemotherapy at the time of surgery. Moreover, the study uncovered the importance of patient subsets in breast cancer therapy.[60]

A similar trial of a short course of adjuvant chemotherapy performed by the Scandinavian Adjuvant Chemotherapy Study Group[140] began in 1965 and ended in

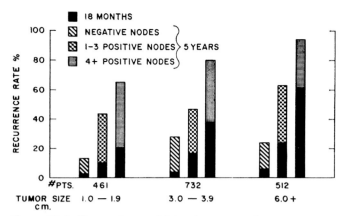

Figure 39–1. Tumor size, nodal involvement, and recurrence rate. (From Fisher B, et al: Cancer 24:1071, 1969. Reprinted by permission.)

1975. As in the NSABP study, the hypothesis was to eradicate the single tumor cells or clusters of cells that disseminated during surgery and resulted in metastatic disease years later. The treated group consisted of 507 patients who received cyclophosphamide 5 mg/kg/d I.V. for 6 days beginning on the day of surgery and were compared with 519 patients in a control group. Recent results showed a continued disease-free survival advantage for the treated group that became evident after 4 years.[140] Beneficial effect on crude survival was not as apparent but was significant up to 6 years after surgery.[140]

Current Theory

In parallel with these first adjuvant chemotherapy trials, a number of principles were being developed that related directly to the administration of surgical adjuvant chemotherapy. Among these principles was a better understanding of micrometastases, population cell kinetics, drug kill of tumor cells, and prognostic features of breast cancer. As previously noted, the origin of metastatic disease was explained at this time by the theory of tumor cells showering as a result of the manipulation of the primary cancer. Although criticized,[60] investigators produced evidence that seemed to indicate that this theory was not of primary importance in the natural history of the disease.[51, 163] Evidence of the natural progression of breast cancer indicated that preexisting micrometastases at the time of surgery had a greater bearing on disease outcome than did tumor cells disseminated as a result of surgery (Fig. 39–1).[77, 172] The presence and number of positive axillary nodes was an indicator of subclinical body burden of disease and of the presence of micrometastases at the time of diagnosis. Such data cast doubt on the view of regional nodes as protective "barriers" to tumor spread.

Clinical evidence now supports the concept that preexisting micrometastases are predominantly responsible for the eventual appearance of detectable metastatic disease. The Ludwig Breast Cancer Study Group reported on the timing and duration of adjuvant chemo-

Table 39–1. SURVIVAL RATES AT 5 AND 10 YEARS FOLLOWING RADICAL MASTECTOMY

Premenopausal Patients	Effect of TSPA			
	% at 5 Yr		% at 10 Yr	
	Placebo	TSPA	Placebo	TSPA
All	60	73*	49	58
Negative nodes	83	82	76	73
Positive nodes	41	61	28	41
1–3	67	67	50	48
≥4	24	57†	14	35

*$p < 0.01$.
†$p < 0.05$.
TSPA = thiotepa.
From Fisher B, et al: NCI Monogr 1:35–43, 1986. Reprinted with permission.

therapy for patients with node-positive breast cancer.[116] The study randomized 1229 pre- and postmenopausal patients with positive axillary lymph nodes into three treatment groups. The chemotherapy regimen was cyclophosphamide, methotrexate, and fluorouracil (CMF). One group received a single course of CMF beginning 36 hours after surgery, a second group received six courses of conventionally administered CMF beginning 25 to 32 days after surgery, and a third group received both chemotherapy regimens. At 42 months of follow-up, disease-free survival and overall survival significantly favored the longer treatments. The authors concluded that the single perioperative treatment was not as effective as longer courses and that starting the treatment perioperatively was no more effective than beginning 4 weeks after mastectomy. Preexistent micrometastases, rather than showering of tumor cells during surgery, appeared to be the major clinical problem.

There is also the current notion of sensitivity of tumor cells in relation to their proliferative state. The theory of growth fraction of tumor cell populations holds that tumors are composed of three cellular compartments.[172, 123] There is a compartment of proliferating cells (A) that has clonogenic potential and is responsible for tumor growth when cellular proliferation exceeds cell loss. There is a second compartment (B) that is nonproliferative but retains the potential for proliferation. This compartment is in equilibrium with compartment (A) and is recruited to replace a depleted clonogenic proliferating compartment. A third compartment (C) is composed of permanently nonproliferative, nonclonogenic cells that contribute only to tumor volume. A tumor's growth fraction is defined as the ratio A:B + C. The greater the value of the growth fraction, the more rapidly the tumor increases in size. Furthermore, tumor growth approximates the Gompertz equation,[164, 172] that is, an exponentially increasing doubling time with increase in tumor mass. This also reflects a decreasing growth fraction or a decrease in clonogenic proliferating cell number with tumor growth. Because chemotherapeutic agents interfere primarily with mitotically active cells, there is more potential for cell kill in smaller tumor masses with their associated larger growth fractions. This was shown in laboratory experiments[92] with the B16 transplantable mouse melanoma that revealed a direct relationship between cell numbers in the range of 10^3 to 10^9 and a cure rate achievable with chemotherapy. According to the concept of first-order kinetics of cell kill,[164, 195] a constant percentage of cell kill theoretically occurs, regardless of population size, as long as the tumor cell population is metabolically homogeneous relative to the chemotherapeutic agent applied. This theory further defines a small mitotically active cell population as most vulnerable to total cell kill.

The combination of evidence and theory gave credence to the potential for surgical adjuvant chemotherapy in curing small metastatic foci of tumor with a high growth fraction. Experiments in mouse tumor models in administering chemotherapy after surgical excision of the primary tumor yielded evidence in favor of adjuvant chemotherapy in four different tumor types:[165, 173] C3H mammary carcinoma, B16 melanoma, Lewis lung carcinoma, and line 26 colon carcinoma.

More recent theory has bolstered the appropriateness of administering chemotherapy when the tumor cell burden is at a minimum. A mathematical model was described by Goldie and Coldman relating drug sensitivity of tumors to spontaneous mutation rates.[88, 89] In the model, a given tumor maintains a constant mutation rate during its growth history. The theory states that, like microbial populations, drug-resistant phenotypes occur spontaneously and with a definite frequency. With the passage of time, the total population of resistant cells increases in mass, making chemotherapeutic cure less likely. This theory also predicts, however, that there is a period early in the growth of the tumor during which cure is possible with chemotherapeutic agents that are ineffective in the later stages of the tumor's development. Within each tumor, there are various other forms of tumor cell heterogeneity, including factors such as growth rate, karyotype, cell surface properties, antigenicity, and metastatic potential.[58] The cellular heterogeneity is a consequence of the emergence of new clonal subpopulations, the outcome of which is to render the cells less responsive to the host's (and the clinician's) attempts at control. Some known mechanisms of drug resistance, such as gene amplification and pleotropic drug resistance, also increase in likelihood with tumor growth.[90] This body of theoretical and laboratory evidence argues for adjuvant chemotherapy directed at a small population of subclinical metastatic cells present at the time of diagnosis in an attempt to destroy a relatively uniform cell population early in its exponential phase of growth.

In a retrospective look at NSABP B-01, it is perhaps more surprising that any benefit was found in survival in any subgroup from the short course of thiotepa therapy than that there was a lack of universal cure, which was the desired result. By current standards, thiotepa is not considered a particularly useful agent for breast cancer. The choice of thiotepa was a result of its modest effectiveness in palliation of breast cancer,[65] but at the time there was not a long list of drugs from which to choose. In addition, prognostic factors of breast cancer were less well defined at the time.[63]

After the demonstration of the prognostic importance of nodal groups, studies were stratified with an awareness of this most important indicator. In a review of the prognostic factors contributing to adjuvant chemotherapy in breast cancer, the main discriminants to be considered for patients receiving adjuvant chemotherapy[20] are axillary nodal metastases (1–3 vs. >4 vs. >10), micro- vs. macrometastases, receptor status, histological grade, tumor necrosis, vascular invasion, labeling index, and primary tumor size. Although theoretically all of these indicators should be considered in studies of adjuvant chemotherapy for breast cancer, in practice nodal status is the predominant indicator.[20]

Armed with a more refined understanding of the biology of early breast cancer and better antineoplastic agents, investigators were able to enter the next phase of adjuvant therapy trials.

ADJUVANT CHEMOTHERAPY TRIALS

Since the first adjuvant chemotherapy trial, NSABP B-01, a number of trials have been initiated. The largest studies with the longest follow-up data are those by the NSABP and the National Cancer Institute in Milan, Italy.[193]

NSABP

Since 1958, 12 randomized studies have been initiated by the NSABP to evaluate the efficacy of various adjuvant therapy regimens. A total of 9256 women with stages I and II breast cancer have been entered into these trials.[72] These studies, as initially designed, were aimed at comparing treatments and defining the basic biology of breast cancer. They proceeded with sequential protocols in which the design of each subsequent study was influenced by the results of its predecessor. The population of patients was similar among all of the studies.[72] Specifically, patients were included on study who had had a radical mastectomy (Halstead or modified) and were found to have one or more nodes positive for tumor with no other evidence of metastatic disease. The tumor must not have been fixed to the underlying muscle or chest wall, axillary nodes must have been movable relative to the chest wall and neurovascular bundle, and there could be no arm edema. Patients were excluded who were more than 75 years of age. Detailed descriptions of each study that include other criteria of patient selection, randomization, drug administration and modification, host and tumor characteristics, and statistical procedures have been reported.[61, 62, 64, 67, 68, 70, 71, 74, 78]

The investigators of NSABP adjuvant chemotherapy trials have published recent reviews of their findings.[62, 66, 72] The first protocol (B-01) compared women treated with Halsted radical mastectomy and thiotepa with those treated with the same surgical procedure and placebo. The doses and duration of thiotepa administration were either 0.2 or 0.4 mg/kg I.V. at the time of operation and 0.2 mg/kg on each of the first two postoperative days. Since results of the two different dose schedules did not reveal a difference in outcome, results were combined.[78] Increased disease-free survival and overall survival at 5 and 10 years after surgery in premenopausal patients with >4 positive nodes led to the next series of protocols.

NSABP B-01 was based on the theory that tumor cells shed from the primary tumor at surgery were responsible for metastatic disease that appeared years later. With the realization of the micrometastatic nature of breast cancer even at diagnosis, brief administration of drugs as in B-01 was deemed inadequate. Thus in NSABP B-05, melphalan given at a dosage of 0.15 mg/kg orally daily for 5 days every 6 weeks for 17 courses (2 years of therapy) was compared with a placebo.[72] The study randomized pre- and postmenopausal women younger than 75 years with one or more nodes positive for tumor. At 10 years of follow-up, there

was a statistically significant improvement for women ≤49 years of age in disease-free survival and overall survival in the melphalan treated group. The advantage was greatest in the 1–3 positive node subgroup but was also apparent for women with ≥4 positive nodes. Similar to the results of B-01, no advantage was seen in women ≥50 years of age. A significant improvement in overall survival, however, was shown in melphalan treated patients with poorly differentiated tumors, regardless of patient age.

The outcome of NSABP-05 led to the sequential addition of other agents to melphalan in future protocols. NSABP B-07 compared melphalan 6 mg/m² orally for 5 consecutive days every 6 weeks with melphalan 4 mg/m² orally and 5-fluorouracil (5-FU) 300 mg/m² intravenously for 5 consecutive days every 6 weeks.[64] The addition of 5-FU to melphalan resulted in a statistically insignificant trend toward improvement in disease-free survival in both the younger (≤49 years) and older (≥50 years) patient groups. Whereas the beneficial effect was noted in the younger women with 1–3 positive nodes, among the older women it was most pronounced in women with ≥4 positive nodes.

The third protocol in this series, NSABP B-08, compared the effects of melphalan and 5-FU in the same doses as in NSABP B-07 with melphalan and 5-FU with methotrexate 25 mg/m² added on days 1 and 5 of each 6-week cycle. The addition of methotrexate failed to show an advantage in any subset of patients over the two-drug regimen.[6, 72] NSABP B-11 added to melphalan and 5-FU adriamycin 30 mg/m² on days 1 and 21 of each 6-week cycle to a cumulative dose of 300 mg/m². Preliminary analysis indicates the three-drug regimen prolongs disease-free survival beyond the results of melphalan and 5-FU alone.[72] It should be noted that only in the first two trials, B-01 and B-05, was there an untreated control group. Although criticized for this, NSABP states that patients in a group demonstrating no benefit or detriment from therapy can justifiably serve as surrogates for untreated patients.[72]

From these NSABP studies, the following conclusions can be made:[72, 18]

1. The natural history of breast cancer can be altered by adjuvant chemotherapy prolonging disease-free survival and overall survival in node-positive premenopausal women.

2. There is an aspect of heterogeneity inherent in breast cancer that causes a nonuniform response to adjuvant chemotherapy.

3. Postmenopausal women after treatment with melphalan and 5-FU showed a statistically insignificant improvement in disease-free survival and overall survival.

4. Regardless of age and number of positive nodes, there was a significant overall survival advantage in women with poorly differentiated tumors treated with adjuvant chemotherapy.

Milan Trial

The Milan Cancer Institute began in 1973 to study a combination chemotherapy regimen in treatment of women with breast cancer and positive axillary lymph nodes.[13] The primary tumor of patients included on study could be clinically classified as a T1 (2 cm or less in its greatest dimension), T2 (>2, <5 cm), or T3 (>5 cm but with no fixation to the underlying pectoral facia or muscle). Surgery consisted of a conventional Halstead radical mastectomy or an extended radical mastectomy. The CMF drug combination was chosen because of its activity in patients with advanced breast cancer.[16] Cyclophosphamide (100 mg/m^2 p.o. q.d. days 1 through 14), methotrexate (40 mg/m^2 I.V. day 1 and 8), and 5-FU (600 mg/m^2 I.V. days 1 and 8) were administered on a 28-day schedule.

This prospective randomized study included 207 patients who were treated with CMF and 179 controls. The 10-year follow-up reports[14, 15, 23] indicate a persistent disease-free survival advantage in the CMF treated group (p <0.001) and a favorable overall survival trend (p = 0.10). The advantage in disease-free survival and overall survival, although suggestive in postmenopausal women, was statistically significant only in the premenopausal subset.

Furthermore, the number of histologically positive axillary lymph nodes continued to be prognostically important at the 10-year analysis, with the greatest benefit in disease-free and overall survival seen in the 1–3 positive node group. The investigators concluded that although the CMF regimen demonstrated a prolonged therapeutic advantage in a percentage of women with micrometastic disease regardless of menopausal status, the treatment outcome favored the premenopausal women.[18] Subsequent Milan Cancer Institute studies of adjuvant breast cancer chemotherapy included 12 vs. six cycles of CMF, sequential non–cross-resistant chemotherapy combinations, and negative axillary node patients.

Additional Controlled Trials

In addition to the NSABP and Milan controlled trials, there have been other studies that have evaluated this problem. Tables 39–2 and 39–3 summarize the larger adjuvant chemotherapy studies in node-positive women that included a local/regional treatment control group. With certain exceptions, results from these studies are similar. Although both the NSABP and Milan trials reported a disease-free and overall survival advantage in premenopausal women, advantages in postmenopausal women were marginal. Possible exceptions to this include the OSAKO trial,[168] which showed a significant disease-free survival advantage in postmenopausal women but not in premenopausal patients, and the Guy's/Manchester melphalan study, which failed to show a significant advantage in either disease-free survival or overall survival in premenopausal women given chemotherapy.[162] The largest of the trials, which evaluated only premenopausal women, was that performed by the Danish Breast Cancer Cooperative Group.[27, 28, 135] Total mastectomy with partial axillary dissection followed by local radiation therapy was performed prior to

randomization to one of the following: no further treatment, 12 monthly courses of cyclophosphamide (130 mg/m^2 p.o. days 1–14), or CMF (cyclophosphamide 80 mg/m^2 p.o. days 1–14, methotrexate 30 mg/m^2 I.V. days 1 and 8, and 5-fluorouracil 500 mg/m^2 I.V. days 1 and 8). Both total survival and disease-free survival at 7 years were statistically significantly increased for the cyclophosphamide and CMF treated groups compared to controls.

Tables 39–2 and 39–3 summarize the data related to menopausal status from trials that included a local/regional treatment control group. In each study in which disease-free survival was evaluated in premenopausal women, results favored the chemotherapy treated group and were often statistically significant. Overall survival was affected significantly only in premenopausal women in the NSABP, Milan, and Danish trials. In postmenopausal women, although there was a trend in improvement in disease-free survival in some studies, this was less pronounced than that in the premenopausal group. The findings of these studies support the theses that there is a definite and statistically significant disease-free survival advantage in premenopausal women with positive axillary nodes given chemotherapy, and that a statistically significant overall survival advantage has been shown for premenopausal women given chemotherapy in the NSABP, Milan, and Danish trials, but that only a statistically insignificant trend in disease-free survival has been demonstrated in postmenopausal women.

Heterogeneous Results of Clinical Trials

Even if the biological effects of adjuvant chemotherapy on tumor cells were uniform irrespective of patient age, the efficacy of adjuvant chemotherapy on overall survival is not likely to be uniform over the entire age spectrum because of competing causes of death. With advancing age, larger numbers of women will die as a result of causes other than breast cancer. Using the examples of Zelen and Gelman,[198] white women 50 to 54 years old experience a 10-year death rate of 5.3 percent from all causes other than breast cancer. Node-positive breast cancer has a 10-year death rate of about 70 percent. Therefore there will be approximately 13.2 breast cancer deaths relative to each death from other causes (70/5.3) in the 10-year period. This ratio will fall with increasing patient age at diagnosis of breast cancer and will alter the statistical efficiency of the study for any given number of patients included.

The issue of competing causes of death becomes more problematic in studies in which a larger proportion of older postmenopausal women are included in the study. The result of including such a population of women in a study is to decrease the statistical efficiency of the trials for the postmenopausal population. The actual sample size of postmenopausal women would have to be larger than the premenopausal group to result in an equivalent statistical efficiency. A Southwestern Oncology Group (SWOG) study is illustrative of the phenom-

Table 39–2. ADJUVANT CHEMOTHERAPY STUDIES WITH A LOCAL/REGIONAL TREATMENT CONTROL GROUP IN PREMENOPAUSAL NODE-POSITIVE PATIENTS

Author	Study Population	No. of Patients	Chemotherapy	Treatment Duration	Follow-up	Disease-free Survival (%)		Overall Survival (%)	
						Control	Chemotherapy	Control	Chemotherapy
Fisher et al[72] (NSABP B-05)	≤49 yr old	120	L-PAM	2 yr	10 yr	30*	46*	38*	61*
Bonadonna et al[14, 23] (Milan)	≤49 yr old	189	C,M,F	1 yr	10 yr	31‡	48‡	45	59
Senn et al[168] (Osako)	Pre- and perimenopausal	118	Ch,M,F,P,BCG	6 mo	8 yr	Not significant		Not significant	
Wheeler[194] (English Multi-center)	Pre- and perimenopausal	130	C,M,F,V	6 mo	1 yr	62 Not significant	86	No data	
Rubens et al[162] (Guy's/Manchester)	Premenopausal	156	L-PAM	96 wks	5–7.5 yr	52 Not significant	62	Not significant	
Padmanabhan et al[145] (Guy's/Manchester)	Premenopausal	211	C,M,F	1 yr	5 yr	52†	70†	68 Not significant	74
Morrison et al[133] (West Midlands)	Premenopausal	228	A,V,C,M,F,L	24 wk	54 mo	53	65*	Not significant	
Brinckner et al[28] (Danish Cancer Group)	Premenopausal	1032§	C	1 yr	68 mo	42‡	62‡	55 Not significant	70
			C,M,F	1 yr	68 mo	42‡	62‡	55*	70*
Smith et al[175] (Glasgow)	Premenopausal	322‖	C,M,F	13 mo	42 mo	Significant		Not significant	

*$p < 0.05$ for chemotherapy vs. control.
†$p < 0.005$ for chemotherapy vs. control.
‡$p < 0.0005$ for chemotherapy vs. control.
§Randomization to observation, C, or CMF.
‖Both pre- and postmenopausal patients.
Abbreviations: A, doxorubicin; C, cyclophosphamide; Ch, chlorambucil; F, 5-fluorouracil; L, leucovorin; L-PAM, L-PAM; M, methotrexate; V, vincristine.

enon.[144] Premenopausal and postmenopausal women with primary breast cancer and positive axillary nodes were randomized after stratification according to menopausal status and nodal involvement (1–3 nodes and ≥4 nodes) to receive CMF plus vincristine and prednisone (CMFVP) for 1 year or melphalan for 2 years. After 8 years median follow-up, overall disease-free survival was superior in all subsets but was not statistically significant in postmenopausal women. When deaths from other causes prior to recurrence are taken into account, a significant benefit for CMFVP is found in postmenopausal women as well.

If adjuvant chemotherapy is indeed effective treatment for only premenopausal women, then the next question is why? Tumor cell heterogeneity, medical oophorectomy, and dose intensity have been offered as

Table 39–3. ADJUVANT CHEMOTHERAPY STUDIES WITH A LOCAL/REGIONAL TREATMENT CONTROL GROUP IN POSTMENOPAUSAL NODE-POSITIVE PATIENTS

Author	Study Population	No. of Patients	Chemotherapy	Treatment Duration	Follow-up	Disease-free Survival (%)		Overall Survival (%)	
						Control	Chemotherapy	Control	Chemotherapy
Fisher, et al[72] (NSABP B-05)	≥50 yr old	229	L-PAM	2 yr	10 yr	29*	32*	44*	41*
Bonadonna et al[14, 23, 50] (Milan)	≥50 yr old	202	C,M,F	1 yr	10 yr	32*	38*	50*	52*
Senn et al[168] (Osako)	Postmenopausal	114	Ch,M,F,P,BCG	6 mo	8 yr	42†	56†	53*	65*
Wheeler[194] (English Multicenter)	Postmenopausal	120	C,M,F,V	6 mo	3 yr	74†	89†	No data	
Rubens et al[162] (Guy's/Manchester)	Postmenopausal	214	L-PAM	96 wk	5–7.5 yr	45*	51*	Not significant	
Padmanabhan et al[145] (Guy's/Manchester)	Postmenopausal	228	C,M,F	1 yr	5 yr	55*	59*	65*	70*
Morrison et al[133] (West Midlands)	Postmenopausal	234	A,V,C,M,F,L	24 wk	54 mo	Not significant		Not significant	
Smith et al[175] (Glasgow)	Postmenopausal	322‡	C,M,F	13 mo	42 mo	No data		Not significant	
Wallgren et al[191] (Stockholm-Gotland)	Postmenopausal	163	Ch or C,M,F	1 yr	49 mo	55†	48†	Not significant	
Tormey et al[62, 180, 183] (ECOG)	Postmenopausal	155	C,M,F,P	1 yr	5 yr	57*	60*	Not significant	

*Not significant
†$p < 0.5$ for chemotherapy vs. control.
‡Both pre- and postmenopausal patients.
Abbreviations: A, doxorubicin; C, cyclophosphamide; Ch, chlorambucil; F, 5-fluorouracil; L, leucovorin; L-PAM, L-PAM; M, methotrexate; P, prednisone; V, vincristine.

potential explanations. Tumor cell heterogeneity both within individual tumors and between pre- and postmenopausal groups of women may be contributing in an as-yet-undefined manner to the results of adjuvant trials. Major discriminants of histological variability other than nodal metastases have yet to be fully considered in adjuvant trials. There are some data to suggest that histological grade affects patient response to adjuvant chemotherapy regardless of menopausal status. The NSABP B-05 study revealed a significant disease-free survival and overall survival advantage for women ≤49 years and ≥50 years with high nuclear grade tumor histologies treated with melphalan.[62] At 10 years' follow-up, no advantage from melphalan was seen in all patients ≥50 years of age, but a significant overall survival advantage was observed in the same age group of patients with poorly differentiated tumors. There was no survival benefit in either age group with good nuclear grade.

Other studies support the results of NSABP. In the Danish Cancer Group Study,[135] premenopausal women with aggressive disease (≥4 nodes, tumor > 5 cm, and anaplasia grade 3 of 3) showed a statistically significant improvement in disease-free survival when treated with CMF vs. control. The Vienna Study[107] reported an overall survival difference in favor of women with undifferentiated and estrogen receptor (ER)–negative tumors given chemotherapy (79 percent vs. 41 percent, p <0.001; and 84 percent vs. 37 percent, p <0.05, respectively). No effect was seen in survival in patients with well or moderately differentiated tumors or in patients with ER-positive tumors. Data were not presented correlated to menopausal status. It is reported, however, that the ER-positive rate and median ER concentration increase with postmenopausal status and age.[37] Furthermore, ER-negative tumors are frequently poorly differentiated.[73] The data may support the thesis that premenopausal women respond favorably as a group of adjuvant chemotherapy because of an increased incidence of ER-negative, poorly differentiated tumors.

Certain studies exist that suggest that prophylactic surgical castration may increase disease-free survival and overall survival in premenopausal women with breast cancer (vide infra).[129] This prompts the hypothesis that adjuvant chemotherapy acts in premenopausal women by causing a temporary, if not permanent, amenorrhea.[148] Several studies have determined that amenorrhea occurring in premenopausal women during the administration of cytotoxic chemotherapy is caused by primary ovarian failure and not by alteration of pituitary or adrenal function.[53] There are no significant pituitary, ovarian, or adrenal hormonal profile alterations caused by chemotherapy in postmenopausal women.[53] Amenorrhea is permanent in the majority of the approximately 80 percent of premenopausal women who have disruption of menses during chemotherapy.[53, 145] There is, however, an inverse relationship between age and duration of treatment required to induce cessation of menses, with some younger women showing no evidence of ovarian suppression.

There are studies that support the concept that chemotherapy given to premenopausal women with breast cancer is effective, at least in part, because of induction of amenorrhea. In the Guy's/Manchester study, which randomized pre- and postmenopausal women to local control vs. CMF adjuvant chemotherapy,[145] only premenopausal women benefited from treatment with a statistically significant disease-free survival. Menstrual history was recorded in the premenopausal patients in 87 of 102 treated with CMF and in 89 of 109 controls. Of these women, 53 of 87 patients (61 percent) treated with CMF became permanently amenorrheic, as did ten of 89 controls (11 percent). Among premenopausal women with CMF-induced amenorrhea, there was a significant increase in disease-free survival and overall survival compared with controls (p = 0.0001 and 0.01, respectively) and with CMF treated women without amenorrhea (p = 0.02 and 0.01, respectively). There was no significant difference in either parameter between CMF treated women without amenorrhea and controls.

An Eastern Cooperative Oncology Group (ECOG) trial[184] that randomized pre- and postmenopausal women to 12 monthly cycles of intermittent CMF, CMF plus prednisone (CMFP), or CMFP plus continuous tamoxifen also determined a statistically significant disease-free survival and overall survival for patients who developed amenorrhea during therapy. A study of pre- and postmenopausal patients with one to three axillary lymph nodes involved randomized 491 patients to receive CMF or CMFP for 12 4-week cycles in Ludwig I.[118, 119] Of the 399 women who had menses during the 6 months prior to trial entry, 85 percent experienced amenorrhea for at least 3 months during treatment. Disease-free survival at 6 years for the amenorrhea-induced group was 75 percent, compared with 62 percent for the group that continued menses (p = 0.006). Reestablishment of menstrual function occurred in 20 percent of the patients who had experienced amenorrhea during treatment. Disease-free survival for these patients was 75 percent, compared with 78 percent for patients who did not resume menses.

Finally, in a retrospective analysis of the trial of 1032 pre- and perimenstrual women randomized to observation or adjuvant chemotherapy with cyclophosphamide or CMF, the Danish Breast Cancer Cooperative Group[28] determined that CMF and cyclophosphamide were equally effective in improving disease-free survival when compared with the local-treatment-only control groups. A statistically significant survival advantage was evident in the treated groups and was slightly more pronounced in the patients who received CMF. Amenorrhea occurred in 70 percent of patients who received cyclophosphamide, 63 percent of patients who received CMF, and 13 percent of the control group. When comparing the amenorrheic women with the women who continued menses within each group of patients, only in the cyclophosphamide treated women was there a statistical advantage to disease-free survival for the women who ceased to menstruate. In both the control and CMF groups, there was no statistical difference between women who continued or ceased menstruation. The authors believe that these data support the hypothesis that the results of adjuvant chemotherapy occur in part because of chemical castration (the cyclophosphamide group) and in part through a purely cytotoxic effect that is additive to the effect of chemical castration (the CMF group).

Not every review supports the hypothesis that adjuvant chemotherapy acts preferentially in premenopausal patients via the mechanism of induction of amenorrhea. A report of the initial CMF trial in Milan at 10 years' follow-up did not confirm a positive effect on disease-free survival in premenopausal women with amenorrhea.[14, 15] The 9-year disease-free survival has been reported related to amenorrhea and nodal status in premenopausal women ≤40 years of age.[17] Of 32 patients who received CMF, the survival of the 19 patients who did not experience drug-induced amenorrhea was identical to the 13 who experienced amenorrhea regardless of nodal status. The analysis was limited to women ≤40 years of age, since only two patients older than 40 years were evaluable in the subgroup that maintained menstrual function. Results of NSABP study B-05 agreed with the findings of the Milan trial regarding a lack of association of disease-free survival with depression of ovarian function.[76] The NSABP report divided the premenopausal group into those ≤39 years of age and those 40 to 49 years of age. The treated women in the younger group demonstrated a greater improvement in disease-free survival at 4 years relative to controls (69 percent vs. 32 percent; $p = 0.01$) than did those in the older age group (61 percent vs. 48 percent; $p = 0.09$). Amenorrhea, however, occurred in 73 percent of patients in the 40- to 49-year age group and in only 22 percent of women ≤39 years of age ($p < 0.001$). The dichotomy of results of ovarian suppression and disease-free survival benefit is used as evidence by NSABP to support the conclusion that although chemical castration may account for some of the effectiveness of adjuvant chemotherapy in premenopausal women, other factors are primarily responsible.

A dose-response effect, as suggested by the Milan group, is another possible explanation for the disparity of results between pre- and postmenopausal women. In a retrospective analysis of 901 women,[19] all of whom had received CMF in previous prospective Milan studies, the authors determined a dose-response effect indicating that CMF was effective only when given in a full or nearly full dose. Women receiving ≥85 percent of the planned dose had a 5-year disease-free survival of 77 percent compared with a 5-year disease-free survival of 45 percent in those receiving ≤65 percent of the planned dose (45 percent disease-free survival in the control population). The Milan update of this information at 9 years confirmed these initial findings.[17] Furthermore, this relationship was true in both of the subgroups of premenopausal and postmenopausal women. The analysis of the Milan data indicated that a higher proportion of women in the premenopausal group received ≥85 percent of the planned dose than did those in the postmenopausal group. When similar groups of women were compared (i.e., similar dose and similar number of involved axillary lymph nodes), the disease-free survival was the same in a statistically significant comparison regardless of menopausal satus. The Milan investigators used this information to suggest that "menopausal status should probably no longer be regarded as an important prognostic factor."[19] It must be borne in mind, however, that any retrospective dose-response analysis may be misleading, since it cannot establish a cause-and-effect relationship between dose and outcome. Factors that decrease the ability to give chemotherapy at full dose may also be associated with more aggressive disease and poorer outcome. No other investigating group has correlated a beneficial dose-response effect with menopausal status.

Other groups did not find conclusive evidence of a dose-survival relationship in general in breast adjuvant chemotherapy.[93, 168] In a Swiss adjuvant study, there was a suggestion that patients who received greater than 90 percent of full dose had better overall survival at 8 years ($p = 0.07$).[168] In a follow-up study comparing CMF administration for 6 months with CMF administration for 18 months, no clear-cut correlation between the administered drug dose and disease-free or overall survival was documented.[168] In a study at Memorial Sloan Kettering Cancer Center,[93] results of the dose-survival relationship were dependent on the method of calculation.

A number of other studies have shown no advantage in the dose-survival relationship.[100, 117, 118, 162, 188, 191] In the Guy's/Manchester CMF study, although the average doses represented 20 percent less CMF than was used in the Milan study, a dose-response relationship was not shown.[100] This was also true for the Guy's/Manchester melphalan study.[162] The Ludwig Breast Cancer Study Group evaluated dosage and disease-free survival in both studies involving pre- and postmenopausal women. Both studies involved the use of CMF with prednisone or tamoxifen or both (CMFP + T) and have been criticized for interpreting results as a function of CMF dose levels.[17] In the Ludwig III study of CMFP + T vs. P + T vs. control patients for postmenopausal women, differences in disease-free survival among three dose levels of CMF were not significant.[117] In the Ludwig I study of CMF vs. CMFP for pre- and perimenopausal women, significantly higher doses of CMF were administered with the addition of prednisone ($p ≤ 0.0001$).[118] In spite of this, there was no improvement in disease-free survival or overall survival for patients who received lower doses of CMF. In the Stockholm-Gotland study, although patients receiving greater than 86 percent of the ideal dose had a rate of recurrence approximately 70 percent of that for patients receiving lower doses, this difference was not statistically significant.[191] Finally, in a study analyzed similarly to that of the Milan group, the Southeastern Cancer Study Group randomized pre- and postmenopausal women to CMF for 6 to 12 months or to local/regional radiation therapy followed by 6 months of CMF. No significant differences in relapse rates regardless of number of nodes involved or menopausal status were detected.[188]

Hryniuk et al. reported an analysis of dose intensity

for chemotherapy in stage II breast cancer.[102] The analysis was retrospective and combined the results of a number of clinical trials. The inclusion of several trials that utilized different drugs required that the following assumptions be made:

1. Each of the drugs in a regimen was of equivalent activity.

2. Differences in drug scheduling could be ignored.

3. A dose intensity of zero could be assigned to missing drugs in partial CMF combinations.

4. Vincristine and prednisone did not contribute to the outcome of therapy in breast cancer.

5. For purposes of calculation of equivalent activity of dose, cyclophosphamide equaled 40 times the milligrams of melphalan.

The conclusion was that dose intensity correlates with disease-free survival rate for all four of the evaluated prognostic groups (i.e., women <50 years with 1–3 and >3 positive nodes, and those ≥50 years with 1–3 and >3 positive nodes). The authors distinguished between intended and actual dose intensity and acknowledged methodological difficulties in dose calculation and retrospective analysis of clinical trials.

These methodological difficulties are in part illustrated by the NSABP report that in the studies comparing melphalan to control and melphalan + 5FU to control, women receiving ≥85 percent of the dose of placebo had a significantly better disease-free survival than women receiving <65 percent of placebo.[152] An even more striking example is that of the report of the Coronary Drug Project Research Group, which sought to evaluate the efficacy of several lipid-influencing drugs on the long-term treatment of coronary artery disease.[44] Patients who took more than 80 percent of placebo had a highly statistically significant ($p < 10^{12}$) lower 5-year mortality than those who took <80 percent of placebo. There are, however, no available results from a randomized adjuvant chemotherapy trial in treatment of stage II breast cancer prospectively evaluating dose intensity as it correlates with disease-free survival or overall survival.

Optimal Adjuvant Chemotherapy Regimen

In 1958 the NSABP initiated sequential randomized clinical trials to assess the efficacy of various adjuvant chemotherapy regimens.[72] After protocol B-05 demonstrated a statistically significant disease-free survival and overall survival in premenopausal women, the next study, B-07, compared women treated with melphalan with those treated with melphalan and 5-FU. The addition of 5-FU to melphalan resulted in a statistically insignificant improvement in disease-free survival in both pre- and postmenopausal women and prompted a comparison of melphalan and 5-FU with melphalan, 5-FU, and methotrexate. The addition of methotrexate failed to show any advantage. This NSABP experience and the Milan CMF report[13] established the precedent for clinical trials comparing single-agent and multi-agent adjuvant chemotherapy.

There have been few studies similar to the NSABP clinical trials that have compared a single agent with a combination of drugs that included the single agent.[95] Two of these studies showed no statistical difference in disease-free survival or overall survival in women treated with monotherapy versus combination therapy.[36, 91] The Danish Breast Cancer Cooperative Group Study comparing cyclophosphamide with CMF therapy in pre- and perimenopausal women also found no statistically significant difference in outcome between groups of women according to treatment.[28] Noteworthy facts of this study are that the intended ideal CMF dose is 20 percent to 25 percent less than the Milan CMF dose and that the hematological toxicity of cyclophosphamide was slightly greater than that of CMF. This indicates that the two regimens were not equitoxic, making a comparison difficult.

Several studies have compared melphalan with CMF or a regimen similar to CMF (Table 39–4). The studies are heterogeneous, and none included a no-treatment control arm. Four of six comparisons defined a subgroup that benefited by receiving the combination chemotherapy;[1, 45, 49, 144] two of the studies demonstrated an overall survival advantage in premenopausal women receiving combination chemotherapy;[1, 144] one study showed a disease-free survival advantage in patients ≥50 years receiving combination chemotherapy.[49] Two of the six studies showed no difference in outcome between melphalan and combination chemotherapy.[34, 39] The entire body of evidence, however, indicates that the CMF combination is a superior regimen to melphalan alone.

Clinical investigators have compared the CMF combination to CMF plus additional agents in three studies. In Ludwig I, CMF was compared with CMFP in premenopausal women with one to three positive nodes.[87] At 4 years, the disease-free survival and overall survival were virtually identical in the two arms of therapy. Although there was less hematological toxicity with CMFP, more severe infections (eight of ten patients), greater weight gain (8 percent vs. 4 percent), and cushingoid appearance (17 percent) occurred in the CMFP regimen.

The Eastern Cooperative Oncology Group initiated a study comparing 12 monthly cycles of CMF with CMFP in premenopausal women. There was no significant overall or disease-free survival difference between the two regimens. Moreover, as in the Ludwig I study, toxicity was significantly increased by the addition of prednisone to the adjuvant regiment. Finally, CALGB performed a study comparing CMF with CMF + methanol extraction residue (MER) of Calmette-Guerin bacillus, and with CMFVP in pre- and perimenopausal women.[182] The CMF + MER arm was discontinued prior to the end of the trial. The comparison of CMFVP with CMF revealed no significant difference in disease-free survival or overall survival. Separate analysis demonstrated that CMFVP was superior to CMF in those patients with ≥4 involved nodes (median disease–free survival, 55.3 percent vs. 35.3 percent; $p = 0.010$). Among patients with 4–9 involved nodes, this difference was not observed, but it was demonstrated in both pre-

Table 39–4. RANDOMIZED TRIALS COMPARING MELPHALAN AND REGIMENS SIMILAR TO CMF IN NODE-POSITIVE PATIENTS

Author	Study Population	No. of Patients	Chemotherapy	Treatment Duration	Follow-up (yr)	Disease-free Survival (%)		Overall Survival (%)	
						Melphalan	*CMF*	*Melphalan*	*CMF*
Davis et al[49]	Pre- and postmenopausal	254	L-PAM vs. CMFV	1 yr	4.5	54†	66†	No significant difference	
Creech et al[45] (Fox Chase)	Pre- and postmenopausal	279	L-PAM vs. CMF	2 yr vs. 1 yr	NA	No significant difference		No data	
Osborne et al[144] (SWOG)	Pre- and postmenopausal	366	L-PAM vs. CMFVP	2 yr vs. 1 yr	8	41†	53†	54*	65*
Ahmann[1]	Pre- and postmenopausal	293	L-PAM vs. CFP	60 wk	2	31*‡	44*	40*‡	70*
Cohen et al[33, 39]	Pre- and postmenopausal	194	L-PAM vs. CFP vs. CFP + BCG	1 yr	2	No significant difference		No data	
Carpenter et al[34]	Pre- and postmenopausal	171	L-PAM vs. CMF	56 wk vs. 48 wk	3	No significant difference		90*	74*

*$p < 0.05$
†$p < 0.005$
‡Results pertain to premenopausal patients only. Results for postmenopausal patients were not statistically significant.
Abbreviations: BCG, Calmette-Guerin bacillus; C, cyclophosphamide; F, 5-fluorouracil; L-PAM, L-PAM; M, methotrexate; P, prednisone; V, vincristine.

and postmenopausal groups with ≥10 positive nodes. The disease-free survival advantage was not translated into a survival benefit. Both regimens were well tolerated.[185] The suggestion of these three studies is that there is no definite advantage in disease-free or overall survival by the addition of prednisone or vincristine and prednisone to the CMF regimen. Toxicity may be greater with the CMFP and CMFVP regimens.

Several studies have been conducted evaluating the use of doxorubicin in adjuvant chemotherapy regimens (Table 39–5). One trial, the West Midlands Oncology Association Study, has incorporated doxorubicin in multi-agent schedules and compared results with those in control populations.[133] The clinical trial evaluated node-positive patients randomized after surgery to no further therapy or to therapy using vincristine, doxorubicin, cyclophosphamide, methotrexate, and 5-FU with leucovorin every 21 days for eight cycles. Median follow-up was 54 months for 462 patients, with the recurrence rate significantly reduced in treated patients vs. controls. However, this effect was confined to premenopausal patients. There was no benefit in overall survival conferred by treatment of any subgroup of patients.

Three additional studies have compared a doxorubicin-containing regimen to another adjuvant chemotherapeutic protocol. The Central Pennsylvania Oncology Group studied 5-FU, doxorubicin, and cyclophosphamide versus melphalan alone administered to 52 post-

Table 39–5. RANDOMIZED TRIALS OF DOXORUBICIN-CONTAINING ADJUVANT REGIMENS IN NODE-POSITIVE PATIENTS

Author	Study Population	No. of Patients	Chemotherapy	Treatment Duration	Follow-up (yr)	Disease-free Survival (%)		Overall Survival (%)	
						Doxorubicin	*Other*	*Doxorubicin*	*Other*
Simmonds et al[171] (Central Pennsylvania Oncology Group)	Postmenopausal	52	L-PAM vs. CAF‡	2 yr	1.5	Not significant		Not significant	
Misset et al[132]	Pre- and postmenopausal	249	CMF vs. CAFV	2 yr	3	65*	52*	Not significant	
Morrison et al[133] (West Midlands Oncology association)	Pre- and postmenopausal	462	AVCMFL vs. control	6 mo	4.5	60*	54*†	Not significant	

*$p < 0.05$
†Significance confined to premenopausal patients.
‡Methotrexate substituted for doxorubicin when total doxorubicin dose = 320 mg/m².
Abbreviations: A, doxorubicin; C, cyclophosphamide; F, 5-fluorouracil; L, leucovorin; L-PAM, L-PAM; melphalan; M, methotrexate; V, vincristine.

menopausal patients with stage II breast cancer after surgery.[171] Chemotherapy was administered for 2 years, and methotrexate was substituted when the total dose of doxorubicin reached 320 mg/m^2. With a mean follow-up of 19.8 months, there was no difference in disease-free survival or overall survival between either group. The published 5-year results of the French Adjuvant Trial for Breast Cancer compared CMF therapy with therapy using a combination of doxorubicin, vincristine, cyclophosphamide, and 5-FU in a randomized group of 249 node-positive pre- and postmenopausal women.[132] Both the CMF and the doxorubicin-containing regimens were administered for 12 months. The difference in disease-free survival, but not overall survival, was statistically superior in premenopausal patients treated with the doxorubicin-containing regimen. Although not statistically significant, an improvement in disease-free survival in postmenopausal patients was also seen in the doxorubicin-treated group. Finally the NSABP is evaluating the addition of doxorubicin to two regimens.[72] In NSABP B-09, pre- and postmenopausal node-positive patients were randomized after surgery to melphalan plus 5-FU (PF) versus melphalan, 5-FU, and tamoxifen (PFT). In two later trials, NSABP randomized the subset of patients responsive to PFT between PFT and PFT plus doxorubicin (PAFT); those patients who showed no difference in their responses to PF and PFT in B-09 were randomized between PF and PF plus doxorubicin (PAF). Preliminary results indicate that the addition of doxorubicin to PF and PFT increases the disease-free survival resulting from either regimen alone; furthermore, patients ≥50 years of age achieved a statistically significant increase in overall survival with PAFT versus PFT. The conclusion of the evaluation of the available data concerning the addition of doxorubicin to adjuvant regimens is encouraging but preliminary. Further study of this strategy must be made prior to the inclusion of doxorubicin in treatment of stage II breast cancer patients in routine practice.

Optimal Duration of Adjuvant Therapy

A practical and clinically relevant problem in adjuvant chemotherapy administration is the optimal duration of therapy. Shorter courses diminish short-term toxicity of treatment and possibly decrease the chance of any long-term toxicities. Patient compliance is also enhanced. There are at least five studies that evaluate the question of outcome related to duration of therapy.

Two studies have evaluated short vs. long courses of CMF in this clinical setting.[176, 188] The Milan trial entered a total of 466 patients in a prospective randomized study from 1975 to 1978.[176] Within 4 weeks of surgery, patients younger than 70 years of age with T1–T3a breast cancer and histologically positive nodes were randomized to receive either six or 12 cycles of CMF. Patients were stratified according to the number of nodes involved (1–3 or >3), and both pre- and postmenopausal women were entered on study. No disease-free or overall survival advantage was seen between the two treatment groups. The authors concluded that the results of the study were sufficiently mature to say that six cycles of CMF are equivalent to 12 cycles with regard to overall and disease-free survival. They speculated that the maximum therapeutic effect may also be achieved with fewer than six cycles of CMF.

A second study of duration of adjuvant CMF administration was performed by the Southeastern Cancer Study Group.[188] Patients were entered on study as in the Milan protocol with similar stratification according to number of involved nodes (1–3 and >3). CMF was administered as originally described by Bonadonna et al.[13] There were 620 patients entered on study. At analysis at 42 months, the one group with an improved disease-free survival was the premenopausal group with 1–3 positive nodes who received 12 months of CMF. The authors of this study concluded that there was an improvement in disease-free survival with the longer course of CMF administered to this subset of patients.

Three other studies have evaluated drug regimens other than CMF differing only in duration. The Dana-Farber Cancer Institute initiated a study in 1974 and closed to entry in 1985 that evaluated 286 patients given cyclophosphamide 500 mg/m^2 I.V. and doxorubicin 45 mg/m^2 I.V. on day 1 of a 3-week cycle for 5 vs. 10 courses.[96] No significant differences were observed in either overall survival or disease-free survival among the patients randomized to the two arms of the study. The Southwest Oncology Group randomized 312 patients with positive axillary nodes and ER-negative tumors to 1 vs. 2 years of CMFVP.[158] There was no benefit to patients given the longer course of chemotherapy at a median follow-up of approximately 3 years. Finally, the Swiss Group (SAKK) has reported 351 evaluable patients who received six monthly 14-day cycles of oral chlorambucil, methotrexate, and 5-FU (LMF) or 12 monthly courses of LMF followed by one course every other month for a total of 18 courses during a period of 24 months.[109] After a mean observation time of 6 years, there was no difference in overall survival or disease-free survival between the two groups. It is noteworthy that the overall recurrence rate of 62.1 percent raises the issue of whether this regimen had any activity at all. Because the study lacked an untreated control group, this question cannot be answered. There is no evidence from any of these five studies that the longer course of chemotherapy benefited overall survival. Only one study showed an advantage in disease-free survival in a subgroup of patients receiving the longer course of chemotherapy (premenopausal with 1–3 positive nodes).[188] In a later analysis, this finding remains consistent but is felt by the authors not to be a valid conclusion from the study.[189] Therefore the available studies evaluating the duration of adjuvant chemotherapy seem consistent in their findings of no benefit seen from the longer courses of treatment.

Combinations of Non–cross-resistant Regimens

There is a continuing effort to improve the result of adjuvant therapy for breast cancer. A possibility for improvement is the addition of non–cross-resistant chemotherapy to an established regimen such as CMF. There is a theoretical foundation for this in a previously described mathematical tumor model. The Goldie-Coldman hypothesis relates drug sensitivity of tumors to spontaneous mutation rates, stating that a given tumor maintains a mutation rate during its growth history.[88, 89] According to this theory, truly non–cross-resistant combinations would afford a broader spectrum of cytolytic activity. The Norton-Simon hypothesis, which defends more intense schedules and higher doses in the use of adjuvant chemotherapy, also supports the use of non–cross-resistant regimens.[143]

A study from Milan evaluated the concept of non–cross-resistant combinations in advanced breast cancer.[25] This prospective study of 110 patients randomized initial therapy between CMF and adriamycin plus vincristine (AV) and found no significant difference between the treatment groups in the response rate, median duration of response, or median survival. Effective secondary treatment after crossover for progressive or relapsed disease occurred in 35 percent of those in the AV group and in 20 percent of those in the CMF group. The authors concluded that there is no cross-resistance between CMF and AV.

Similar regimens were used in a Milan study of adjuvant chemotherapy in postmenopausal women.[26] Six-year results of patients treated with CMFP for six cycles followed by AV for four cycles were reported. In an attempt to clinically evaluate the Norton-Simon hypothesis, patients were randomized to receive a standard dose regimen or progressive dose intensification. Although no difference in outcome was seen between the two randomized groups, there was a better-than-expected disease-free survival and overall survival when the results were retrospectively compared with adjuvant CMF therapy in previous Milan studies of postmenopausal patients. The authors' tentative conclusion of the positive effect of the sequential use of these regimens warrants further evaluation.

Finally, the Cancer and Leukemia Group B evaluated 89 node-positive stage II patients randomized to receive initial treatment with CMFVP followed by further randomization to additional CMFVP vs. vinblastine, adriamycin, thiotepa, and halotestin (VATH).[147] Disease-free survival was significantly superior in patients who received VATH. Furthermore, the disease-free survival advantage for patients who received VATH was present in patients at highest risk for relapse, including postmenopausal patients with ≥4 positive nodes, patients with ≥10 positive nodes, and ER-negative patients. Further study of this issue and of whether a difference in overall survival can be achieved is warranted.

NODE-NEGATIVE PATIENTS

With evidence that the biology of the natural history of stage II breast cancer can be altered with chemotherapy and hormonal therapy, investigators have concentrated efforts to improve the outcome of patients with stage I disease. Although these patients have a relatively good prognosis, the relapse rate is still significant. Moreover, women with stage I disease account for 40 percent to 50 percent of the total of newly diagnosed breast cancer patients.[83] In a study including 512 patients with breast cancer but with negative lymph nodes (both axillary and internal mammary), the 10-year disease-free survival was 72.8 percent, while the overall survival was 80.4 percent.[190]

It would be optimal to restrict the use of any adjuvant therapy in this subset of patients to those destined to relapse with disease. In this regard there is an attempt to evaluate for prognostic features that would indicate a high probability of recurrent breast cancer. In many studies, although not all, estrogen receptor–negative tumor status confers a higher likelihood of relapse and a poorer survival.[7, 126] Tumor size, anaplastic tumor morphology, diffuse hyperplasia of regional lymph nodes or a pattern of germinal center predominance in lymph nodes, extensive tumor necrosis, measurement of aneuploidy by flow cytometry, young age, and family history of breast cancer have all been claimed to have prognostic significance for early relapse in stage I breast cancer.[7, 80, 104, 126] The thymidine labeling index has been found to have predictive value independent of stage and estrogen receptor content and to select a subgroup of stage I patients with a relapse expectancy of approximately 50 percent at 4 years.[130, 131] Similarly, DNA flow cytometry measurements of both S-phase analysis and ploidy status have been shown to be predictors of relapse in node-negative patients.[54] Finally, although not evaluated in stage 1 breast cancer, amplification of the HER2/*neu* oncogene has been reported to be a predictor of overall survival and time to relapse.[174] However, other investigators have not been able to confirm this.[187] Elevation of *ras* oncogene expression has been shown to be associated with increased lymph node metastases.[174]

The NIH Consensus Conference of 1985 in Adjuvant Chemotherapy and Endocrine Therapy for breast cancer commented on patients with negative nodes. For both pre- and postmenopausal women with stage I disease, there was no therapy routinely recommended, but treatment could be considered for certain high-risk patients in each menopausal category.[136] Studies on which to base firm recommendations were unavailable at the time. More data have become available since the consensus conference.

Of the nine studies listed in Table 39–6, seven have described a disease-free survival benefit for node-negative women given adjuvant therapy. In the majority of these, the benefit is statistically significant in all or a subset of patients treated. All of the studies included both pre- and postmenopausal women in the study group. In three of the studies, an overall survival benefit was observed in the treated population. Jakesz et al.[108] and Bonadonna et al.[24] administered CMF in differing schedules to pre- and postmenopausal patients. Both studies realized an overall survival benefit in the treated group in a small number of patients. The control group in the Bonadonna et al. study exhibited high-risk char-

Table 39–6. RANDOMIZED TRIALS COMPARING LOCAL THERAPY WITH AND WITHOUT ADJUVANT CHEMOTHERAPY IN NODE-NEGATIVE PATIENTS

Author or Study	Study Population	No. of Patients	Chemo-therapy	Treatment Duration	Median Follow-up (yr)	Disease-free Survival (%)		Overall Survival (%)	
						Chemo-therapy	Control	Chemo-therapy	Control
Nissen-Meyer et al[139]	Pre- and postmenopausal	609	C	6 d	20	64*	55*	Not analyzed	
Senn et al[168] (Osako)	Pre- and postmenopausal	122	Ch,M,F,BCG	6 mo	9	68*	62*	82*	67*
Morrison et al[133]	Pre- and postmenopausal	467	Ch,M,F	6 mo	4.5	No significant difference		Not analyzed	
Jakesze et al[108]	Pre- and postmenopausal	128	C,M,F,Vbl	3 yr	6	No significant difference		74†	90†
Bonadonna et al[24] (Milan)	Pre- and postmenopausal	90	C,M,F	1 yr	4	91‡	53‡	93*	73*
Williams et al[196]	Pre- and postmenopausal; ER (−) tumors	52	CAV	18 wk	6	95§	68%	No significant difference	
NSABP-13[69]	Pre- and postmenopausal ER (−) tumors	679	M,F	1 yr	4	80‡	71‡	No significant difference	
Intergroup Study[155]	Pre- and postmenopausal ER (−) tumors; ER (+) tumors ≥3 cm	406	C,M,F,P	6 mo	3	84‡	69‡	Longer follow-up needed	
Ludwig V[121]	Pre- and postmenopausal	1275	C,M,F,L	Day 1 and 8, 36 hr after surgery	4	77 ± 2†*	73 ± 2†	90 ± 1*	86 ± 2*

*No significant difference.
†$p < 0.05$ for chemotherapy vs. control.
‡$p < 0.005$ for chemotherapy vs. control.
§Seven patients who were randomized to treatment arm referred chemotherapy and were included in the control group. Results were "statistically significant" when analyzed for treatment delivered.
Abbreviations: A, doxorubicin; BCG, Calmette-Guerin bacillus. C, cyclophosphamide; Ch, chlorambucil; F, 5-fluorouracil; L, leucovorin; M, methotrexate; P, prednisone, Vbl, vinblastine; V, vincristine.

acteristics with a disease-free survival of less than 50 percent at 5 years and an overall survival of approximately 65 percent at almost 5 years. These results are significantly worse than those for the majority of studies of stage I breast cancer patients. The disparity in survival between the treated patients and the control group and the statistical significance, however, are impressive.

Three recent studies may have a profound impact on the clinician's decision to treat node-negative breast cancer patients with chemotherapy. NSABP B-13 is a study of pre- and postmenopausal node-negative, ER-negative women in which 339 women were randomized to receive sequential methotrexate and 5-FU for 12 courses and 340 to receive surgical therapy alone.[69] At 4 years of follow-up, 80 percent of the treated women were disease-free, whereas 71 percent of the control population were disease-free ($p = 0.003$); there was no difference in survival outcome between pre- and postmenopausal women. The Ludwig Breast Cancer Study Group reported the Ludwig V study in which 848 pre- and postmenopausal women who received one course of CMF with leucovorin on days 1 and 8 begun within 36 hours after surgery were compared with 427 control patients.[121] At 4 years median follow-up, disease-free

survival was statistically superior at 77 percent (±2 percent) for the treated group compared with 73 percent (±2 percent) for the control group. A trend in overall survival favored the treated group. The largest benefit in disease-free survival was realized by the ER-negative group. Both pre- and postmenopausal women benefited in disease-free survival by receiving chemotherapy as compared to the control group.

Finally, the Intergroup Study (INT 0011), which included ECOG, CALGB, and SWOG, randomized ER-negative and ER-positive patients with tumors ≥3 cm to CMFP for six cycles or to no adjuvant therapy.[122] A disease-free survival independent of ER and menopausal status was realized, with 84 percent of 196 treated patients and 67 percent of 210 control patients disease free at a median follow-up of 3 years ($p = 0.0001$). None of these three trials has yet shown an overall survival benefit for adjuvant chemotherapy in node-negative women.

Further improvement in disease-free and overall survival may occur with better utilization of prognostic variables in node-negative breast cancer patients. This would allow rational treatment selection according to patients at highest risk for recurrence.

TOXICITY OF ADJUVANT THERAPY

The disease-free and overall survival benefits of adjuvant therapy must be balanced with acute, delayed, and psychological toxicities caused by treatment. Acute toxicity secondary to CMF-based regimens has been reported.[18, 183] In the ECOG report,[183] CMF, CMFP, or CMFPT was administered to 533 premenopausal women, CMFP or CMFPT was administered to 223 postmenopausal women, and toxicities were summarized. The report from Milan summarized toxicity data of CMF.[18] Acute toxicities included weight gain (3–4 kg) in almost 50 percent of women treated, alopecia requiring a wig in less than ten percent, nausea and vomiting in more than 90 percent, leukopenia less than 2500/mm^3 in ten percent, thrombocytopenia less than 75,000/mm^3 in less than ten percent, and hemorrhagic cystitis in less than 15 percent. Systemic infection was reported by ECOG as occurring in one percent of patients receiving CMF. The Milan report emphasized that none of the women treated with CMF required intensive supportive therapy for life-threatening toxicity. The addition of prednisone added toxicities of edema, cushingoid appearance, and increased weight gain. An increased incidence of thromboembolic disease during the months patients received CMF has also been reported in pre- and postmenopausal women.[112] Persistent amenorrhea has been reported in 40 percent of women younger than 40 years and in 95 percent of women older than 40 years who receive CMF.[18]

The primary concern with delayed toxicity is secondary malignancy. The risk of leukemia following adjuvant therapy with melphalan has been reported by the NSABP.[75] In this report of 8493 women entered on NSABP trials since 1971, the cumulative risk of leukemia for surgical controls was 0.06 percent after 10 years in patients free of metastases (three of 2068 patients). For 5299 women treated with a 2-year course of melphalan, however, the cumulative risk for leukemia for patients free of metastases or a second primary was 1.11 ± 0.30 percent at 10 years; when combined with the incidence of myeloproliferative syndrome, the risk was 1.54 ± 0.36 percent. There were 26 cases of acute myelogenous leukemia and seven cases of myeloproliferative syndrome in the treated women. The results indicated an increased risk of hematological malignancy following treatment in this setting with melphalan for 2 years.

The Milan trial reported the incidence of all second malignancies after adjuvant therapy with CMF.[186] From 1973 to 1978, 845 pre- and postmenopausal women were entered on two studies evaluating CMF as adjuvant chemotherapy. Of 666 women who received either 6 months or 12 months of CMF, there were no cases of leukemia. Furthermore, the incidence of second malignancies in general, including breast cancer, was equivalent to that in the 179 patients who did not receive chemotherapy. Median follow-up for the group was more than 10 years.

There have been four cases of leukemia following CMF therapy reported in the literature.[186] Three of these four patients received postoperative radiation and CMF for 12 or 24 to 36 months, whereas one received CMF alone for 12 months. Henderson cautioned that the population sample of the Milan study is too small to conclude that there is absolutely no danger in developing second malignancies after CMF.[97]

Recent attention has been given to the quality of life patients experience during the course of adjuvant chemotherapy. A recent analysis of the Ludwig Breast Cancer Study III evaluated time without symptoms and toxicity (TWiST).[85] The Ludwig III Study randomized 463 postmenopausal women 65 years old or younger to no therapy, therapy with 12 months of prednisone plus tamoxifen (P + T), or CMFP + T. Periods during which the patient experienced side effects from therapy were subtracted from overall survival and compared with the control group. It was determined that the CMFP + T group had a significantly longer TWiST than did controls, with values at 72 months of follow-up of 37.9 months for controls, 42.4 months for P + T, and 44.3 months for CMFP + T. The TWiST after relapse was not calculated. This was a symptom-related evaluation that did not include psychological or stress-related phenomena. Additional studies may soon evaluate this problem.[113]

META-ANALYSIS OF ADJUVANT CHEMOTHERAPY FOR BREAST CANCER

In spite of three decades of clinical effort and more than 80 randomized trials of theapy in early breast cancer,[155] the subset of the population of women with early breast cancer benefited by treatment and the degree to which overall survival and disease-free survival are improved are not definitive and are debated. Reasons for this may be a lack of statistical power because of inadequacy of sample size, length of follow-up necessary for demonstration of beneficial effect, and an inhomogeneous treatment effect. Small sample sizes are adequate for definitive results of clinical trials only with those therapies that, when compared to no therapy, show a large clinical benefit. The effect, however, of even a small percentage increase in overall survival in treated patients with early breast cancer would not be trivial, given the number of patients diagnosed annually with this disease.

Meta-analysis (or overview analysis) is a statistical methodology that has been used to evaluate issues in medicine that remain unresolved in spite of extensive evaluation. Previously used in the field of psychology and in the analysis of cardiovascular studies,[56] it is now being applied to analyze adjuvant therapies of breast cancer. This approach to research analysis is a structured review of medical literature. A number of review articles on the subject have appeared.[56, 84, 153] The analysis must be of adequate sample size relative to the degree of expected treatment benefit, and systematic bias must be minimized. Prior to selection of individual clinical trials, study criteria must be strictly established. The question to be answered by the meta-analysis must be specific. Variability of trials must be minimal to diminish the possibility of effective therapies being cancelled by ineffective therapies in the results of the overview analysis. Although debated, it has been stated that all eligible trials, not just all published trials, should be included, and that the quality of individual trials should meet minimal criteria. Objective end points of analysis should be selected. For example, overall survival is a more objective outcome parameter than disease-specific survival or disease-free survival. An objective of the overall analysis is to minimize the effects of minor, random variations by increasing the sample size. Statistical issues and techniques are discussed in review articles of the subject.[56, 84, 153]

Few overview analyses have been performed to evaluate adjuvant therapy for early breast cancer. Himel et al. applied a quantitative method for combining data of 31 published randomized controlled trials of adjuvant chemotherapy for breast cancer through 1984.[98] The treatment group differed from the control group as to the chemotherapy received, and patients were evaluated with regard to treatment effects on disease-free survival and overall survival. Fourteen studies compared regimens of chemotherapy (both multi-agent and single agent) greater than 6 months' duration with untreated controls, three studies compared a short course of chemotherapy with untreated controls, 11 studies compared groups treated with differing regimens, and three studies compared chemotherapy regimens differing in the duration of administration. Of the studies comparing longer treatment with an untreated control group, disease-free and overall survival were improved significantly in the patients treated with multiple agents but not in those treated with single agents. Of 626 patients evaluated in multiple agent trials at 5 years' follow-up, relapse-free survival was improved 9 ± 7 percent, and overall survival was increased 7 ± 6.5 percent. Restricting the analysis of relapse-free survival to premenopausal women in single agent and multiple agent trials, 400 women on study experienced a 17 ± 10 percent advantage for treated women at 5-year follow-up, whereas 633 postmenopausal women studied in the same category did not show a relapse-free survival advantage for the treated group. In studies comparing multiple and single agent chemotherapy, multiple agent regimens seemed to yield better relapse-free and overall survival rates, but results were not statistically significant. The same can be said for studies comparing patients treated with short-term chemotherapeutic regimens with untreated controls.

Richard Peto and colleagues from the Clinical Trials Unit, Oxford University, reported findings of a meta-analysis of adjuvant chemotherapy at the National Institutes of Health Consensus Development Conference on Adjuvant Chemotherapy and Endocrine Therapy for Breast Cancer in 1985. This report remains unpublished to date but has been included in the analysis for the recommendations for therapy from the NIH Concensus Conference[150] and has been qualitatively discussed.[41, 155] A brief quantitative overview is contained in Henderson's monograph.[95] Peto's overview analysis evaluated published and unpublished randomized clinical trials in

which chemotherapy was included in only one arm of the study.[95] There were nearly 15,000 women included in the trials, 25 percent of whom died within the first 5 years of follow-up. In the analysis of all trials evaluating patients receiving chemotherapy, odds of death decreased 14 ± 3 percent in the group receiving chemotherapy. All age groups benefited, but women younger than 50 years benefited by an odds-of-death reduction of 24 ± 5 percent vs. 8 ± 4 percent for women older than 50 years. If the analysis were restricted to CMF, women younger than 50 years realized an odds-of-death reduction of 34 ± 6 percent vs. 17 ± 6 percent for women older than 50 years. The absolute effect of all chemotherapy was to increase the overall survival by 9 percent at 5 years for women younger than 50 years and by three percent for women older than 50 years.

The largest overview analysis of the subject was performed by the Early Breast Cancer Trialists Collaborative Group, which analyzed 61 randomized trials of 28,896 women.[55] This study evaluated outcome by mortality in trials that began randomization of patients prior to January 1, 1985, to tamoxifen or cytotoxic chemotherapy for early breast cancer. Data was collected on age, nodal status, date of entry, and date of death. Four comparison groups of patients were evaluated: tamoxifen vs. controls, all chemotherapy vs. controls, multiple agent chemotherapy vs. single agent chemotherapy, and short-term chemotherapy vs. longer administration of the same chemotherapy. Each group is different from its comparison in the treatment of interest. Death at 1, 2, 3, 4, and 5 years was evaluated; little useful data were available beyond 5 years.

In 31 trials of chemotherapy versus no chemotherapy, 9069 women were entered, and 2872 were dead at the time of the analysis. The treated group exhibited an overall 14 ± 4 percent reduction in odds of death with an even greater effect in younger women. Women younger than 50 years at entry demonstrated a 22 ± 6 percent reduction in annual odds of death, whereas there was no definite advantage for women older than 50 years at entry. Ten trials examined the issue of multiagent vs. single agent chemotherapy with 3005 women entered. Multi-agent chemotherapy conferred a 21 ± 9 percent reduction in annual odds of death compared with single agent chemotherapy. When evaluating regimens of multi-agent chemotherapy, there was a suggestion that CMF was better than other regimens, but this was not statistically significant. Adding tamoxifen to chemotherapy did not improve survival. There was no improvement in survival with the more prolonged (6–24 mo) versus shorter (3–6 mo) regimens. For women with no nodal involvement (1589 women in the chemotherapy trials), although the proportional reduction in mortality was similar to that for women with positive nodes, the amount of information was limited and not statistically significant.

ADJUVANT HORMONAL THERAPIES

Rationale

For a variety of reasons, there has been a recent resurgence of interest in adjuvant hormonal manipulations for early stage breast carcinoma. With the initial hope in the early 1970s that a large percentage of women with early stage breast cancer would be cured with adjuvant chemotherapy, enthusiasm for hormonal therapies waned. In part, this was a result of the paradigm that hormonal therapy was "cytostatic" and would not be as effective as "cytolytic" chemotherapy. However, it is by no means clear, given the results presented earlier in this chapter, that chemotherapy is significantly increasing the number of women actually being cured; in most trials, the survival curves do not become completely flat at any point. Furthermore, the stigma of the term "cytostatic," which has been attached to hormonal agents based on in vitro studies, is not consistent with the observation of complete tumor regressions and dramatic partial remissions that occur in many trials of hormonal agents in metastatic breast cancer.

The possibility has even been raised that some of the benefits of adjuvant chemotherapy in premenopausal women with breast cancer are mediated through a "chemically induced castration." A recently reported study from the Danish Breast Cancer Cooperative Group supports this hypothesis.[28] More than 1000 women with breast cancer and axillary node involvement who had undergone total mastectomy with axillary sampling were randomly assigned to receive either radiation alone (RT), RT plus single agent oral cyclophosphamide, or RT plus CMF. Adjuvant chemotherapy was given in the latter two groups for 12 months. Both of these groups had a significant improvement in disease-free and overall survival compared with controls but were not significantly different when compared with each other. In a retrospective analysis of the RT + cyclophosphamide arm of the study, it was found that disease-free survival was not improved in the subset of women who did not undergo chemotherapy-induced amenorrhea. By contrast, disease-free survival was virtually identical for women who did vs. those who did not undergo treatment-induced amenorrhea in the adjuvant CMF arm.

Similar results were reported by Howell et al.[100] in a randomized study of CMF vs. no adjuvant therapy in 327 women who had undergone total mastectomy and axillary dissection. In that study, disease-free survival was better in patients who had chemotherapy-induced amenorrhea than in control patients; disease-free survival was intermediate in treated patients who had no amenorrhea. There were no significant differences in overall survival in the study. In an Eastern Cooperative Oncology Group study in premenopausal women comparing CMF vs. CMF plus prednisone vs. CMF plus prednisone and tamoxifen, patients who developed amenorrhea had improved disease-free survival as well as overall survival when compared with those who did not have cessation of menses.[182]

Not all observations have been consistent with the hypothesis that the effects of adjuvant chemotherapy are mediated through a "chemical castration." Neither the Milan trial of adjuvant CMF vs. no adjuvant therapy in node-positive women[22] nor the NSABP trial of adjuvant melphalan vs. placebo[76] in node-positive women

revealed significant differences in the benefits to treated women when analyzed for cessation of menses in premenopausal women. It therefore seems clear that not all of the effects of adjuvant chemotherapy are mediated through a chemical castration. It is possible, nevertheless, that hormonal effects of chemotherapy play some role in the benefits in premenopausal women.

The ability to routinely assay tumor tissue from primary resections for estrogen and progesterone receptor content may heighten the ability to identify those women most likely to benefit from adjuvant hormonal therapy. Because the receptor content could not be measured at the time of many of the early trials, it was not known whether there were subsets of patients who benefited more than others. The presumption underlying the belief that a receptor assay can be used to predict response to adjuvant hormonal manipulations is that the receptor content of the primary tumor correlates with the receptor status of the subclinical metastases that are already present at the time of diagnosis and that the receptor status of the multiple subclinical metastases are concordant among themselves. The presumption is not proven. Allegra et al. found an 85 percent concordance rate in ER status in 23 cases in which multiple metastases were assayed simultaneously.[2] In another study, receptor status was compared between primary breast tumors and metastatic or contralateral breast tumors that subsequently developed.[99] The concordance rate was only 46 percent. Of nine patients with ER-positive primary tumors, six subsequently had ER-negative metastases; of 19 patients with ER-negative primary tumors, nine developed ER-positive metastases. Four of six patients in the latter category responded to hormonal therapy for their metastatic disease. It is true that some of the assays may have been false negatives. Nevertheless, it is possible that such results may in part account for recent observations in some adjuvant trials (discussed in following sections) that adjuvant tamoxifen carries some benefit even in ER-negative women.

Trials of Adjuvant Ovarian Ablation

Oophorectomy was first proposed as an adjuvant therapy for primary breast cancer in 1889.[166] Remission of advanced breast cancer after bilateral oophorectomy was first reported in 1896,[11] and the first therapeutic radiation-induced castration was reported in 1905.[50] The first clinical trial of prophylactic radiation castration was reported in 1939.[178] However, early clinical trials of the concept in the 1940s and 1950s gave no definitive information, since they were not internally controlled.[5, 52] There have been six "randomized" studies of adjuvant ovarian ablation vs. no therapy (Table 39-7). In one of the trials, allocation to treatment vs. control was by month of birth.[40] In three of these studies, the method of ovarian ablation was external beam radiation,[28, 40, 138] and in the other three, surgical oophorectomy was performed.[30, 137, 151] The two modalities of castration are not necessarily equivalent, since in one of the trials of adjuvant ovarian radiation in premenopausal women,

Table 39-7. CONTROLLED TRIALS OF ADJUVANT CASTRATION FOR EARLY STAGE BREAST CANCER

Authors	Study Population	No. of Patients	Follow-up (yr)	Relapse-Free Survival (%)		Overall Survival (%)	
				Castration	Controls	Castration	Controls
Surgical Oophorectomy Studies							
Nevinny et al[137]	Pre- or postmenopause, node negative or positive	143	63 pts. followed >5 years	68	54	78	74
Ravdin et al[155] (NSABP)	Premenopause, node negative or positive	236	Up to 5	44	45 (Placebo grp.)	71	79 (Placebo grp.)
Bryant and Weir[30]	Premenopause, stage I or II	359	10	69*	53	71*	60
Ovarian Radiation Studies							
Nissen-Meyer[138]	Premenopause (stage I); postmenopause (stage I, II)	336	Up to 8	No significant overall differences found (significant in postmenopause)			
Cole[40]	Pre- and perimenopause, node negative or positive (pts. allocated by birth month)	598	Up to 15	Not significantly different overall		45	40
Meakin[129]	Age <45 (ovarian RT vs. none)	137	Up to 15	No significant differences found			
	Premenopause, age ≥45 (none vs. ovarian RT ± prednisone)	208		Significantly better survival and DFS for RT + prednisone vs. no adjuvant*			
	Postmenopause (none vs. ovarian RT ± prednisone	360		No significant differences found			

*Statistically significant difference between treated group and controls.
Abbreviations: RT, radiotherapy.

12.7 percent of the irradiated patients subsequently had return of menses.[40] However, prophylactic surgical castration has been compared to ovarian radiation in a randomized trial of 117 premenopausal women with breast cancer; disease-free survival was very similar with 7 years of follow-up, and crude survival was virtually identical.[138]

Of the three randomized trials of adjuvant oophorectomy in operable breast carcinoma, one showed a statistically significant improvement in disease-free survival and overall survival.[30] In that trial, reported by Bryant and Wier, premenopausal women with clinicopathological stages I and II invasive breast cancer were randomly assigned after mastectomy to no therapy vs. prophylactic bilateral oophorectomy. Analysis was performed on 359 patients. Disease-free survival at 5 and 10 years of follow-up was 73 percent and 69 percent, respectively, in the oophorectomy group, compared with 65 percent and 53 percent, respectively, in the controls. Crude survival at 5 and 10 years was 81 percent and 71 percent in the adjuvant therapy group vs. 77 percent and 60 percent in the controls. These differences were statistically significant. Survival differences at 10 years favoring the oophorectomy group occurred in both stage I and II patients, though not in women with four or more involved axillary nodes. It should be noted that there was a design flaw in this study. Patients were randomized prior to obtaining consent for oophorectomy. If a patient assigned to the operation refused (or if her physician refused on her behalf), her randomization card was replaced in the randomization deck, and she was not analyzed with the other patients who underwent castration. This could have led to unintentional bias.[35] The

authors do not state how many women fell into this category.

The remaining two randomized trials of prophylactic surgical castration show no differences in either disease-free or overall survival.[137, 151] However, it may be important that follow-up in both of these trials was only 5 years. In the positive trial discussed previously, survival differences did not become apparent for 5 years.[30]

There have been two randomized trials[128, 138] of prophylactic radiation-induced castration and one trial in which patients were allocated by month of birth[40] (Table 39-7). One of them, conducted at the Princess Margaret Hospital, has been reported after up to 15 years of follow-up and suggests improved disease-free survival as well as overall survival in certain subgroups.[128] A total of 779 pre- and postmenopausal women with clinical stage I, II, or III operable breast cancer were entered onto study. After surgery and local radiation, women younger than 45 years were randomized to receive no further treatment vs. ovarian radiation (2000 rad in five fractions). Women aged 45 years or older were randomized to no further treatment vs. ovarian radiation plus prednisone 7.5 mg per day for up to 5 years. No differences were observed in either disease-free survival or overall survival in postmenopausal women. In premenopausal women younger than 45, disease-free and overall survival were superior in the castrated women, but differences were not statistically significant. In premenopausal women ≥45 years of age, disease-free survival and overall survival were significantly better ($p = 0.04$ and 0.02, respectively) for the castrated women who received prednisone compared with the controls. Differences did not become significant until after 3 to 5 years. Women who received ovarian radiation alone had intermediate outcome. Unfortunately, a statistical test for heterogeneity was not reported for all three treatment arms in this subgroup of women, and no test was reported for overall results in all premenopausal women. Interpretation of these results must therefore be tempered by the fact that retrospective subgroup analyses are not "protected" by the randomization process and are therefore subject to error.[133] Moreover, a potential source of bias was present in the study, since 51 eligible randomized patients did not receive the treatment to which they were assigned and were not analyzed. The authors did not report an analysis with all randomized eligible study subjects.

A second randomized trial showed similar results favoring ovarian radiation.[138] Nissen-Meyer, reporting from the Norwegian Radium Hospital, conducted a study comparing prophylactic to therapeutic ovarian radiation. A total of 175 postmenopausal women (stage I and II) and 161 premenopausal women ("good risk" only patients) were entered. With up to 8 years' follow-up, disease-free survival was improved in both groups but was statistically significant only in postmenopausal women, and crude survival was significantly improved in the postmenopausal patients. Finally, a third large study of ovarian radiation in 598 pre- and perimenopausal women with stages I and II cancer showed no significant advantages for the radiation arm after 15 years of follow-up.[40]

Adjuvant Tamoxifen Trials

The rationale for the use of the antiestrogen tamoxifen as adjuvant therapy in both pre- and postmenopausal women comes from two recent randomized trials of tamoxifen vs. oophorectomy that suggest that the two modalities have similar efficacy in premenopausal women with metastatic breast cancer. A crossover-designed trial in 54 premenopausal women with advanced carcinoma (ER-positive or ER-unknown) showed response rates that were not statistically different between the two treatments—37 percent for oophorectomy vs. 27 percent for tamoxifen.[106] Time to progression and survival were virtually identical, though survival comparisons are difficult with a crossover design. The statistical power of the study was low, but a large advantage for the oophorectomy group was felt to be unlikely. A preliminary report from Buchanan et al. appears confirmatory.[31] In a randomized trial of 107 patients, the response rate to oophorectomy was 21 percent compared with 24 percent for tamoxifen, with no difference in overall survival.

In elderly women, tamoxifen appears to have activity that is roughly equivalent to combination chemotherapy. Taylor et al.[179] reported a trial in 181 women aged 65 or older with advanced breast cancer who were randomly assigned to treatment with tamoxifen or to a regimen of CMF. Response rates to tamoxifen were 45 percent vs. 38 percent for CMF. Survival favored the tamoxifen treatment group but was not statistically sig-

nificant. Moreover, tamoxifen appeared to show efficacy equal to that of CMF in ER-positive as well as ER-negative patients.

In North America, adjuvant trials have tended to concentrate on the use of chemotherapy in premenopausal women, reserving tamoxifen as a single agent for postmenopausal women. This may be because of the belief that premenopausal women may have enough circulating endogenous estrogens to overcome the effects of tamoxifen. As will be discussed, however, two European trials give reason to believe that tamoxifen may have an impact on survival irrespective of menopausal status. It is hopeful that tamoxifen will remain an area of investigative interest in the treatment of premenopausal women. If effective, it may have a therapeutic index superior to that of chemotherapy, at least in certain subsets of women.

There have been 11 randomized trials comparing adjuvant tamoxifen to either no adjuvant therapy or to placebo (Table 39–8).* Two of them show a statistically significant improvement in survival with tamoxifen therapy,[6, 9] and one additional trial shows improved survival of borderline statistical significance ($p = 0.06$).[167] Virtually all of the remaining published trials show either statistically significant improvement in disease-free survival or a trend in that direction. Importantly, several of the trials showing improvement in disease-free survival were placebo controlled.[38, 47, 145] Because the ultimate goal of adjuvant therapy is to extend survival, the trials showing significant survival advantages will be discussed in more detail. Disease-free survival is a more subjective end point and is not an adequate surrogate for survival. Nevertheless, some of the studies that do not show survival advantages have relatively brief follow-up and may eventually demonstrate prolongation of overall survival.

In the Nolvadex Adjuvant Trial Organization (NATO) study, reported in 1985[9] and updated in 1987,[10] 1285 premenopausal women with positive axillary nodes and postmenopausal women with positive or negative axillary nodes were randomized either to tamoxifen 10 mg orally twice daily or to no adjuvant therapy after mastectomy and axillary dissection. Overall survival was superior in the treated group ($p = 0.0062$), representing a 0.86 observed:expected mortality ratio in the tamoxifen group. Only 524 of the primary tumors (46 percent) were assayed for ER content. Interestingly, the hazard ratios for disease-free survival and overall survival were similar for patients with ER-positive and ER-negative tumors. Regression analysis also showed no interaction between treatment effect and either menopausal or nodal status. Results were virtually identical at the 6- and 8-year updates of the trial, though significant differences in survival did not emerge until the third and fourth years.

In a Scottish trial begun in 1978, node-negative premenopausal and node-negative or -positive postmenopausal women who had undergone definitive local ther-

---

*References 6, 9, 10, 38, 47, 117, 127, 146, 149, 156, 160, 161, 167, and 192.

Table 39–8. RANDOMIZED TRIALS COMPARING LOCAL THERAPY WITH AND WITHOUT ADJUVANT TAMOXIFEN

Author or Study	Study Population	No. of Patients	Duration of Tamoxifen (yrs)	Follow-Up (yrs)	Relapse-Free Survival (%)		Overall Survival (%)	
					Tamoxifen	*Control*	*Tamoxifen*	*Control*
Bartlett et al[6] (Scottish Trial)	Node negative, premenopause; node positive and negative, postmenopause	1312	5	2.5–8	60†	40†	60†	45†
Baum et al[9, 10] (NATO Trial)	Node negative, premenopause; node positive and negative, postmenopause	1285	2	Up to 8	Observed: expected ratio 0.81 in favor of tam†		Observed: expected ratio 0.86 in favor of tam†	
Senanayake[167] (IATO Trial)	"Poor risk patients with early breast cancer"	197	2	Up to 5 (median 2)	81* (crude)	68* (crude)	89‡ (crude)	82‡ (crude)
Palshoff et al[145]	Pre- and postmenopause; node positive and negative	343	2	44 mo (median)	79 (pre-) 76 (post-)*	65 (pre-) 64 (post-)*	NR	NR
Ribeiro[157] (Christie Hosp.)	Postmenopause, stages I–III	588	1	Up to 7	71*	65*	~60	~60
Pritchard et al[148]	Node positive, postmenopause	400	2	Median 5.8	~43†	~27†	No significant difference	
NSABP[38, 127]	Node negative, ER positive, age ≤70	2644	At least 5§	Up to 4	83†	77†	93	92
Wallgren et al[191]	Node negative, postmenopause (primary ≤3 cm)	656	2	Mean 49 mo (range 12–86)	No significant difference		No significant difference	
Rose et al[160, 161] (Denmark)	Postmenopausal high risk (node positive, tumor >5 cm, or skin or fascia invasion)	1650	1	Up to 6	44†	40†	51	51
Ludwig Study Group[117]	Node-positive, postmenopause	681	1	Up to 5	58†	44†	75	80
Cummings et al[47] (ECOG)	Node positive, age >65	170	2	41 mo (median)	76†	52†	80	72

*p < 0.05 for tamoxifen vs. control.
†p < 0.005 for tamoxifen vs. control.
‡p = 0.06 for tamoxifen vs. control.
§Patients receiving tamoxifen were randomized after 5 years to continue or to receive placebo.
Abbreviations: NATO, Nolvadex Adjuvant Trial Organisation; IATO, International Adjuvant Trial Organisation; pre-, premenopausal women; post-, postmenopausal women; tam, tamoxifen.

apy were randomized to receive prophylactic tamoxifen 20 mg daily for 5 years vs. therapeutic tamoxifen at first relapse.[6] A total of 1312 eligible patients younger than 80 years were randomized, and follow-up was reported up to 8 years. ER status was available in 57 percent of patients. As in the NATO trial, there was a statistically significant improvement in survival for the adjuvant tamoxifen arm (p = 0.002; hazard ratio = 0.71). Again as in the NATO trial, there was a consistent benefit regardless of ER, nodal, or menopausal status.

Preliminary results have been reported from a trial performed by the International Adjuvant Trial Organization (IATO) in node-positive patients with early breast cancer. After "definitive" local therapy, 399 patients were randomized to one of four arms: no adjuvant therapy, tamoxifen 40 mg orally per day for 2 years, CMF, and CMF plus tamoxifen. After a median follow-up of 2 years (range, 3 months to about 5 years), the tamoxifen arm showed an improved survival (p = 0.06) and disease-free survival (p = 0.02) compared with the control arm. The remaining two study arms gave very similar results to the tamoxifen alone arm but

were associated with more toxicity. No information was given on the effects of treatments in subgroups.

Duration of Treatment with Adjuvant Tamoxifen

If adjuvant tamoxifen is to be used, how long should it be administered? The answer is not yet known, but studies are currently in progress that address the issue. There are hints that tamoxifen should be continued for a prolonged period after treatment of the primary tumor.[6] The only two randomized trials that currently show an overall survival advantage for adjuvant tamoxifen[6, 9] employed tamoxifen for 2 and 5 years, respectively. A third trial showing improved survival (p = 0.06) employed tamoxifen for 2 years.[167] There is an NSABP trial in which women with node-negative, ER-positive primary tumors were randomized to receive tamoxifen vs. placebo.[38, 129] After 5 years, women on tamoxifen are then randomized to continue tamoxifen indefinitely or to placebo. Results from this study and from one by the Intergroup Trial[179] of similar design are still pending but may provide a definitive answer to the question. In the interim, it is probably appropriate to continue tamoxifen for at least 5 years.

Tamoxifen Toxicity

Tamoxifen in the adjuvant setting is a very well tolerated medication. The most frequent toxicity is mild, self-limited nausea that rarely requires discontinuation and may be decreased by taking the drug after meals. Hot flashes are also common, though more so in pre- than in postmenopausal patients. Atrophic vaginitis or vaginal discharge (rarely bloody) occurs infrequently. A randomized NSABP trial of tamoxifen in node-negative women was placebo controlled and allowed the comparison of toxicities of tamoxifen to a placebo; interestingly, hot flashes and vaginal discharge symptoms occurred in both groups.[127] Weight gain may also occur. Rare toxicities include leukopenia, thrombocytopenia, and possibly thrombophlebitis. The phenomenon of tamoxifen "flare" (increase in bone pain or hypercalcemia shortly after starting therapy) only occurs in the setting of widespread bony metastases and has not been reported in the adjuvant setting. Retinopathy has been reported with long-term (>1 year) use of tamoxifen,[110] but only at doses in the range of 60–100 mg/m², far above those used in the adjuvant setting.[12] Theoretical long-term toxicities of prolonged use of tamoxifen include osteoporosis and adverse effects on serum lipoproteins. Preliminary data suggest that these are not problems.[197]

One study does suggest a potentially serious late toxicity associated with the use of adjuvant tamoxifen. Fornander et al. have recently reported on the occurrence of new primary cancers in their adjuvant study.[82] A total of 1846 postmenopausal patients with early breast cancer were randomly assigned to receive tamoxifen 20 mg b.i.d. for 2 years or no therapy. At a median follow-up of 4.5 years (range, 0.5–10.5 years), there were 13 cases of uterine endometrial carcinoma in the tamoxifen group vs. two in the control group ($p < 0.01$). However, there were only 18 new primary breast cancers in the tamoxifen group vs. 32 in the control group ($p = 0.05$). All other second malignancies were evenly distributed between the study groups. The proposed explanation for the increased incidence of endometrial carcinoma is the partial estrogen agonist effect of tamoxifen. It may also be important that tamoxifen was given at twice the conventional dose.

Overall it is clear that if adjuvant tamoxifen improves overall survival of patients with breast cancer, it has an extraordinarily favorable therapeutic index, at least in the short term.

Other Adjuvant Hormonal Therapies

There have been few trials of other forms of adjuvant hormonal therapy for breast cancer, and even fewer have been randomized. A 2-year course of aminoglu-

tethimide plus hydrocortisone has been tested by the Collaborative Breast Cancer Project in a randomized placebo-controlled study of 189 node-positive postmenopausal women.[42, 43] The aminoglutethimide successfully suppressed circulating levels of dehydroepiandrosterone over the 2-year period that patients were treated. Comparison of efficacy (overall and disease-free survival) has not yet been presented, as the planned accrual to the trial is 400 patients. Toxicities were more common in the treated group (83 percent) than in the placebo group (24 percent) but were generally manageable, consisting primarily of lethargy, ataxia, skin rashes, and dyspepsia. A Copenhagen Breast Cancer Trial performed a study of diethylstilbesterol vs. tamoxifen vs. controls in postmenopausal women with operable breast cancer.[146] There were no significant differences in disease-free survival or overall survival, and more than 40 percent of the women receiving diethylstilbesterol discontinued therapy because of toxicity.

It is not likely that these alternate forms of hormonal therapy will be pursued extensively in the adjuvant setting, as they appear to be more toxic than tamoxifen, and it is improbable that they would be more effective when used alone compared with castration or tamoxifen.

Trials Evaluating the Addition of Hormonal Therapy to Chemotherapy

A somewhat separate issue is whether hormonal manipulations can improve the therapeutic efficacy of adjuvant chemotherapy. There are theoretical arguments both for and against this hypothesis. Hormonal therapy may act on a different subpopulation of malignant cells than those affected by "cytolytic" agents. On the other hand, endocrine treatments may decrease the overall cell turnover rate, rendering the micrometastases less sensitive to chemotherapy. There are in vitro data to support both possibilities, and it is fair to say that none of the information resolves the issue. A number of randomized trials have been performed comparing chemotherapy to chemohormonal therapy.* None show statistically improved survival with the addition of hormonal therapy to chemotherapy. Some show a trend toward enhanced survival in the hormonal treatment arm,[167, 192] whereas others show a trend toward worsened survival.[103] The NSABP trial of melphalan and 5-fluorouracil with and without tamoxifen showed opposite trends in survival for patients ≤age 49 vs. those >49.[66] Thus, the issue of the impact of hormonal therapy on concomitant chemotherapy remains unresolved.

Overview

In 1985, the recommendation made at the National Institutes of Health Consensus Development Conference on Adjuvant Chemotherapy and Endocrine Therapy for Breast Cancer[136] was that adjuvant tamoxifen

---

*References 66, 103, 105, 119, 158, 167, 181, 182, and 192.

should be considered standard therapy for postmenopausal women with hormone receptor–positive tumors and axillary node involvement. Because adjuvant hormonal therapy was not felt to clearly benefit any other subset of patients with early stage breast cancer, its use was felt to be investigational in those settings. There are now four large trials that suggest that adjuvant hormonal therapy (oophorectomy in one trial, radiation castration in one trial, and tamoxifen in two trials) prolongs survival in early stage breast cancer.[6, 9, 28, 30] Perhaps as important, two trials suggest that the benefits of tamoxifen extend to women regardless of menopausal, nodal, or hormonal receptor status.[6, 9] Moreover, the increments in survival are comparable to those achieved in the randomized adjuvant chemotherapy trials that have shown overall survival advantages (vide supra).

Can we then go beyond the recommendations of the National Institutes of Health Consensus Development Conferences in view of recent data? Probably not at this point. On the other hand, it may be reasonable to consider the use of adjuvant hormonal therapy in three additional subsets of women: node-negative postmenopausal patients, perhaps irrespective of hormone receptor status; node-positive, receptor-negative postmenopausal patients; and premenopausal women. It now seems reasonable to directly compare adjuvant hormonal therapy to chemotherapy. In fact, there is an ongoing Scottish trial comparing ovarian ablation to chemotherapy as adjuvant treatment in node-positive premenopausal women[6] and a trial in the Gynecological Adjuvant Breast Cancer Group comparing adjuvant tamoxifen to chemotherapy in receptor-positive women with 1–3 involved axillary lymph nodes.[111] Preliminary analysis of the latter study shows no significant differences between tamoxifen and chemotherapy in either disease-free or overall survival.

SUMMARY AND RECOMMENDATIONS

Given the proliferation of studies during recent years on the management of early stage breast cancer, what recommendations can be made to the physician faced with a patient who does not want to participate in a clinical trial? A number of algorithms would be reasonable. We have therefore chosen to list them in three categories: (1) treatment that should be considered standard in current therapeutics; (2) treatment that is reasonable but whose application depends on interpretation of current results; and (3) adjuvant therapy that is currently under study and may change soon.

Standard Practice

Node-Positive Premenopausal Women. A course of adjuvant chemotherapy using one of the standard regimens such as CMF should be recommended and should be given for about 6 months.

Node-Positive Postmenopausal Women (ER-Positive). A course of adjuvant tamoxifen should be administered for at least 5 years. Studies are under way to determine whether the period of treatment should be extended beyond 5 years.

Treatment Depending on Personal Interpretation

Node-Negative, ER-Negative (Pre- or Postmenopausal) Women. It is reasonable to prescribe a course of adjuvant chemotherapy, as there is strong evidence that chemotherapy will improve the disease-free survival. Although no one would deny that it is good to be alive and free of cancer, current debate concerns whether disease-free survival is an adequate surrogate for absolute survival. Disease-free survival is a more subjective end point than overall survival. At this point, most studies that show an improved disease-free survival do not show an improved overall survival. If the disease-free survival does not translate into overall survival, then one is left with the decision whether disease-free survival is objective and important enough to stand alone as an end point. The cost in terms of toxicity is moderate but in terms of dollars is considerable. Another reasonable option would be to use adjuvant tamoxifen. This choice is based on the two European studies that show a strong trend for improved overall survival even in ER-negative women. Toxicity is minimal, although the financial cost is considerable. Until the results of the studies are fully matured and the debate has abated, it is reasonable to follow these patients off of therapy.

Node-Negative, ER-Positive (Pre- or Postmenopausal) Women. Here there is similar debate, but the choices may be simpler: adjuvant tamoxifen or observation are both probably acceptable.

Node-Positive, ER-Negative, Postmenopausal Women. The choice of therapy is difficult. There is the suggestion of a modest improvement in disease-free and overall survival that is not statistically significant in the majority of trials that evaluate chemotherapy in this population of patients. There are also two trials of adjuvant tamoxifen that demonstrate a statistical improvement in disease-free survival (regardless of ER and menopausal status) with the administration of tamoxifen. Either therapy could be justified in this subgroup of women, but there has been no standard of practice established.

Adjuvant Therapy Currently Under Study

As mentioned in the section on adjuvant hormonal therapy, both the Scottish and NATO studies suggest a benefit with tamoxifen therapy to node-negative women irrespective of ER status and to node-positive postmenopausal women. There is a current Scottish study directly comparing adjuvant chemotherapy to ovarian ablation in node-positive premenopausal women. Results of that study may simplify decision making.

References

1. Ahmann DL, O'Fallon JR, Scanlon PW, Payne WS, Bisel HF, Edmonson JH, Frytak S, Hahn RG, Ingle JN, Rubin J, Creagan ET: A preliminary assessment of factors associated with recurrent disease in a surgical adjuvant clinical trial for patients with breast cancer with special emphasis on the aggressiveness of therapy. Am J Clin Oncol 5:371–381, 1982.
2. Allegra JA, Barlock A, Huff KK, Lippman ME: Changes in multiple or sequential estrogen receptor determinations in breast cancer. Cancer 45:792–794, 1980.
3. Allen H, Brook R, Jones SE, et al: Adjuvant treatment for stage II (node positive) breast cancer with adriamycin-cyclophosphamide (AC) ± radiotherapy. In Salmon SE, Jones SE (eds): Adjuvant Therapy of Cancer, III. Orlando, FL, Grune and Stratton, 1981, pp 453–462.
4. Ashworth TR: A case of cancer in which cells similar to those in the tumors were seen in the blood after death. Aust Med J 14:146, 1869.
5. Bailar JC III, Louis TA, Lavori PW, Polansky M: Studies without internal controls. N Engl J Med 311:156–162, 1984.
6. Bartlett K, Eremin O, Hutcheon A, Preece P, Scott JS, Forrest P, Chetty U, Prescott J, Rodger A, Smyth J, Habeshaw T, Kaye SB, McArdle CS, McCallum M, Smith DC, McMillan B, Robinson SM, Stewart HJ, White GK, Giles GR: Adjuvant tamoxifen in the management of operable breast cancer: the Scottish trial. Lancet 2:171–175, 1987.
7. Bauer T, O'Ceallaigh D, Eggleston J, Moore G, Baker R: Prognostic factors in patients with Stage I, estrogen receptor–negative carcinoma of the breast. Cancer 52:1423–1431, 1983.
8. Baum M: The curability of breast cancer. Br Med J 1:439, 1976.
9. Baum M, Brinkley DM, Dossett JA, McPherson K, Patterson JS, Rubens RD, Smiddy FG, Stoll BA, Wilson A, Richards D, Ellis SH: Controlled trial of tamoxifen as single adjuvant agent in management of early breast cancer: analysis at six years by Nolvadex Adjuvant Trial Organization. Lancet 1:836–840, 1985.
10. Baum M, Wilson AJ, Ebbs SR: The role of adjuvant endocrine therapy in primary breast cancer. In SE Salmon (ed): Adjuvant Therapy of Cancer, V. Orlando, FL, Grune and Stratton, 1987, pp 377–390.
11. Beatson GT: On the treatment of inoperable cases of carcinoma of the mamma: suggestions for a new method of treatment with illustrative cases. Lancet 2:104–107, 1896.
12. Beck M, Mills PV: Ocular assessment of patients treated with tamoxifen. Cancer Treat Rep 63:1833–1834, 1979.
13. Bonadonna G, Brusamolino E, Valagussa P, Rossi A, Brugnatelli L, Brambilla C, DeLena M, Tancini G, Bajetta E, Musumeci R, Veronesi U: Combination chemotherapy as an adjuvant treatment in operable breast cancer. N Engl J Med 294:405, 1976.
14. Bonadonna G, Rossi A, Valagussa P: Adjuvant CMF chemotherapy in operable breast cancer. Ten years later. World J Surg 9:707–713, 1985.
15. Bonadonna G, Rossi A, Valagussa P: Adjuvant CMF chemotherapy in operable breast cancer. Ten years later. Lancet 1:976–977, 1985.
16. Bonadonna G, Rossi A, Valagussa P, Banfi A, Veronesi U: The CMF program for operable breast cancer with positive axillary nodes. Cancer 39:2904–2915, 1977.
17. Bonadonna G, Valagussa P: Adjuvant systemic therapy for resectable breast cancer. J Clin Oncol 3:259–275, 1985.
18. Bonadonna G, Valagussa P: Current status of adjuvant chemotherapy for breast cancer. Semin Oncol 14:8–22, 1987.
19. Bonadonna G, Valagussa P: Dose-response effect of adjuvant chemotherapy in breast cancer. NEJM 304:10–15, 1981.
20. Bonadonna G, Valagussa P: Contribution of prognostic factors to adjuvant chemotherapy in breast cancer. Recent Results Cancer Res 96:34–45, 1984.
21. Bonadonna G, Valagussa P: Comment on "The methodologic dilemma in retrospectively correlating the amount of chemotherapy received in adjuvant therapy protocols with disease-free survival." Cancer Treat Rep 67:527–529, 1983.
22. Bonadonna G, Valagussa P, Rossi A, et al: Ten-year experience with CMF-based adjuvant chemotherapy in resectable breast cancer. Breast Cancer Res Treat 5:95–115, 1985.
23. Bonadonna G, Valagussa P, Tancini G, Rossi A, Brambilla C, Zambetti M, Bignami P, DiFronzo G, Silvestrini R: Current status of Milan adjuvant chemotherapy trials for node-positive and node-negative breast cancer. NCI Monog 1:45–49, 1986.
24. Bonadonna G, Valagussa P, Zambetti M, Buzzoni R, et al: Milan adjuvant trials for stage I-II breast cancer. In Salmon S (ed): Adjuvant Therapy of Cancer, V. Orlando, FL, Grune and Stratton, 1987, pp 211–222.
25. Brambilla C, Delena M, Rossi A, Valagussa P, Bonadonna G: Response and survival in advanced breast cancer after two noncross-resistant combinations. Br Med J 1:801–804, 1976.
26. Brambilla C, Rossi A, Valagussa BS, Bonadonna G: Adjuvant chemotherapy in postmenopausal women: results of sequential noncross-resistant regimens. World J Surg 9:728–737, 1985.
27. Brinker H, Mouvidsen H, Rank F, Rose C, Andersen KW: Evidence of a castration-mediated effect of adjuvant chemotherapy in a randomized trial of cyclophosphamide monotherapy versus CMF in premenopausal stage II breast cancer. Proc Am Soc Clin Oncol 4:56, 1985.
28. Brincker H, Rose C, Rank F, Mouridsen HT, Jakobsen A, Dombernowsky P, Panduro J, Andersen KW, on behalf of the Danish Breast Cancer Cooperative Group: Evidence of a castration-mediated effect of adjuvant cytotoxic chemotherapy in premenopausal breast cancer. J Clin Oncol 5:1771–1778, 1987.
29. Brooks R, Jones S, Salmon S, Chase E, Davis S, Moon T, Giordano G, Ketchel S, Jackson R: Adjuvant chemotherapy of axillary node-negative carcinoma of the breast using doxorubicin and cyclophosphamide. NCI Monogr 1:135–137, 1986.
30. Bryant AJS, Weir JA: Prophylactic oophorectomy in operable instances of carcinoma of the breast. Surg Gynecol Obstet 153:660–664, 1981.
31. Buchanan RB, Williams CJ, Hall V, Blamey RW, Webster DJ, Nolvadex Oophorectomy Study Group: Tamoxifen versus surgical oophorectomy in premenopausal women with advanced breast cancer. Proc Am Soc Clin Oncol 4:59, 1985.
32. Buzdar AU, Hortobogi GN, Marcus CE, Smith TL, Martin R, Gehan E: Results of adjuvant chemotherapy trials in breast cancer at MD Anderson Hospital and Tumor Institute. NCI Monogr 1:81–85, 1986.
33. Caprini JA, Oviedo MA, Cunningham MP, Cohen E, Trueneart R, Khandekar J, Scanlon E: Adjuvant chemotherapy in stage II and III carcinoma of the breast. JAMA 244:243–246, 1981.
34. Carpenter JT, Maddox WA, Laws HL, Wirtschefter D, Soong JS: Favorable factors in the adjuvant therapy of breast cancer. Cancer 50:18–23, 1982.
35. Chalmers TC, Celano P, Sacks HS, Smith H Jr: Bias in treatment assignment in controlled clinical trials. N Engl J Med 309:1358–1361, 1983.
36. Chlebowski RT, Weiner JM, Reynolds R, Luce J, Bulcavage L, Bateman JR: Long term survival following relapse after 5-FU but not CMF adjuvant breast cancer therapy. Breast Cancer Res Treat 7:23–29, 1986.
37. Clark GM, Osborne CK, McGuire WL: Correlations between estrogen receptor, progesterone receptor, and patient characteristics in human breast cancer. J Clin Oncol 2:1102–1109, 1984.
38. Clinical alert from the National Cancer Institute (May 18, 1988).
39. Cohen E, Scanlon EF, Caprini JA, Cunningham MP, Oviedo MH, Robinson B, Knox KL: Follow-up adjuvant chemotherapy and ehcmoimmunotherapy for stage II and III carcinoma of the breast. Cancer 49:1754–1761, 1982.
40. Cole MP: A clinical trial of an artificial menopause in carcinoma of the breast. In Namer M, Lalanne CM (eds): Hormones and Breast Cancer, 55. Paris, INSERM, 1975, pp 143–150.
41. Consensus Conference: Adjuvant chemotherapy for breast cancer. JAMA 254:3461–3463, 1985.
42. Coombes RC, Chilvers C, Powles TJ: Adjuvant aminoglutethimide therapy for postmenopausal patients with primary breast cancer. In Jones SE, Salmon SE (eds): Adjuvant Therapy of Cancer, IV. Orlando, FL, Grune and Stratton, 1984, pp 349–357.
43. Coombes RC, Chilvers C, Dowsett M, Gazet J-C, Ford HT,

Bettelheim R, Gordon C, Smith IE, Zava D, Powles TJ: Adjuvant aminoglutethimide therapy for postmenopausal patients with primary breast cancer: progress report. Cancer Res 42(suppl):3415s–3419s, 1982.

44. Coronary Drug Project Research Group: Infuence of adherence to treatment and response of cholesterol on mortality in the Coronary Drug Project. N Engl J Med 303:1038–1041, 1980.

45. Creech RH, Dayal H, Alberts R, Catalano RB, Shah MK, Grotzinger PJ: A comparison of L-PAM and low dose CMF as adjuvant therapy for breast cancer patients with nodal metastases. Proc AACR 24:148, 1983.

46. Cruz EP, McDonald GO, Cole WH: Prophylactic treatment of cancer: the use of chemotherapeutic agents to prevent tumor metastasis. Surgery 40:291–296, 1986.

47. Cummings FJ, Gray R, Davis TE, Tormey DC, Harris JE, Falkson G, Arseneau J: Adjuvant tamoxifen treatment of elderly women with stage II breast cancer: a double-blind comparison with placebo. Ann Int Med 103:324–329, 1985.

48. Cutler SJ, Myers H, Green SB: Trends in survival rates in patients with cancer. N Engl J Med 293:122, 1975.

49. Davis HL, Metter GE, Romirez G, et al: An adjuvant trial of L-phenylalanine (L-PAM) vs cyclophosphamide (C), methotrexate (M), 5-fluorouracil (F) and vincristine (V) (CMF-V) following mastectomy for operable breast cancer. (Abstract) Proc Am Soc Clin Oncol 22:426, 1981.

50. DeCourmelles F: Action atrophique glandulaire des rayons. CR Acad Sci (D) (Paris) 140:606, 1905.

51. Delarue NC: The free cancer cell. Can Med Assoc J 82:1175–1182, 1960.

52. Diehl LF, Perry DJ: A comparison of randomized concurrent control groups with matched historical control groups: are historical controls valid? J Clin Oncol 4:1114–1120, 1986.

53. Dnistrian AM, Schwartz MK, Fracchia AA, Kaufman RJ, Hakes T, Currie V: Endocrine consequences of CMF adjuvant therapy in premenopausal and postmenopausal breast cancer patients. Cancer 51:803–807, 1983.

54. Dressler L, Clark G, Owens M, Pounds DG, Oldaker T, McGuire T: DNA flow cytometry predicts for relapse in node negative breast cancer patients. Proc Am Soc Clin Oncol 6:57, 1987.

55. Early Breast Cancer Trialists' Collaborative Group: Effects of adjuvant tamoxifen and of cytotoxic therapy on mortality in early breast cancer: an overview of 61 randomized trials among 28,896 women. N Engl J Med 319:1681–1692, 1988.

56. Ellenberg SS: Meta-analysis: the quantitative approach to research review. Semin Oncol 15:472–481, 1988.

57. Engell HC: Cancer cells in the blood: a five to nine year follow-up study. Ann Surg 147:457–461, 1959.

58. Fidler IJ, Poste G: The cellular heterogeneity of malignant neoplasms: implications for adjuvant chemotherapy. Semin Oncol 12:207–221, 1985.

59. Fisher B: Biological and clinical considerations regarding the use of surgery and chemotherapy in the treatment of primary breast cancer. Cancer 40:574, 1977.

60. Fisher B: The clinical scientific basis of adjuvant chemotherapy in breast cancer. Recent Results Cancer Res 96:8–17, 1984.

61. Fisher B, Carbone P, Economou SG, Frelick R, Glass A, Lerner H, Redmond C, Zelen M, Band P, Katrych D, Wolmark N, Fisher E: L-phenylalanine mustard (L-PAM) in the management of primary breast cancer: a report of early findings. N Engl J Med 292:117–122, 1975.

62. Fisher B, Fisher ER, Redmond C: Ten year results from the NSABP clinical trial evaluating the use of L-phenylalanine mustard (L-PAM) in the management of primary breast cancer. J Clin Oncol 4:929–941, 1986.

63. Fisher B, Bauer M, Wickerham L, Redmond CK, Fisher E, Cruz A, Foster R, Gardner B, Lerner H, Margolese R, Poisson R, Shibata H, Volk H: Relation of number of positive axillary nodes to the prognosis of patients with primary breast cancer. An NSABP update. Cancer 52:1551–1557, 1983.

64. Fisher B, Glass A, Redmond C, Fisher E, Barton B, Such E, Carbone P, Economou S, Foster R, Frelick R, Lerner H, Levitt M, Margolese R, MacFarlane J, Plotkin D, Shibata H, Volk H: L-phenylalanine mustard (L-PAM) in the management of primary breast cancer: an update of earlier findings

and a comparison with those utilizing L-PAM plus 5-fluorouracil (5-FU). Cancer 39:2883–2903, 1977.

65. Fisher B, Ravdin RG, Ausman RK, Slack NH, More GE, Rudolf JN: Surgical adjuvant chemotherapy in cancer of the breast: results of a decade of cooperative investigation. Ann Surg 168:337–356, 1968.

66. Fisher B, Redmond C, Brown A, Fisher ER, Wolmark N, Bowman D, Wolter J, Bornstein R, Legault-Poisson S, Saffer EA, and other NSABP investigators: Adjuvant chemotherapy with and without tamoxifen in the treatment of primary breast cancer: 5-year results from the National Surgical Adjuvant Breast and Bowel Project Trial. J Clin Oncol 4:459–471, 1986.

67. Fisher B, Redmond C, Brown A, Wolmark N, Wittliff J, Fisher ER, Plotkin D, Bowman D, Sachs S, Wolter J, Frelick R, Desser R, LiCalzi N, Geggie P, Campbell T, Elias G, Prager D, Koontz P, Volk H, Dimitrov N, Gardner B, Lerner H, Shibata H: Treatment of primary breast cancer with chemotherapy and tamoxifen. N Engl J Med 305:1–6, 1981.

68. Fisher B, Redmond C, Brown A, Wickerham D, Wolmark N, Allegra J, Escher G, Lippman M, Savlov E, Wittliff J, Fisher E, Plotkin D, Bowman D, Wolter J, Bornstein R, Desser R, Frelick R: Influence of tumor estrogen and progesterone receptor levels on the response to tamoxifen and chemotherapy in primary breast cancer. J Clin Oncol 1:227–241, 1983.

69. Fisher B, Redmond C, Dimitrov N, Bowman D, Legault-Poisson S, Wickerham D, Wolmark N, Fisher E, Margolese R, Sutherland C, Glass A, Foster R, Caplan R: A randomized clinical trial evaluating sequential methotrexate and 5-fluorouracil for the treatment of node negative breast cancer patients with estrogen receptor negative tumors. N Engl J Med 320:473–478, 1989.

70. Fisher B, Redmond C, Fisher ER, and participating NSABP Investigators: The contribution of recent NSABP clinical trials of primary breast cancer therapy to an understanding of tumor biology—an overview of findings. Cancer 46:1009–1025, 1980.

71. Fisher B, Redmond C, Fisher ER, et al: A summary of findings from NSABP trials of adjuvant therapy. In Jones SE, Salmon SE (eds): Adjuvant Therapy of Cancer, IV. Orlando, FL, Grune and Stratton, 1983, pp 185–194.

72. Fisher B, Redmond C, Fisher ER, Wolmark N: Systemic adjuvant therapy in treatment of primary operable breast cancer: National Surgical Adjuvant Breast and Bowel Project Experience. NCI Monogr 1:35–43, 1986.

73. Fisher ER, Redmond CK, Liu H, Rockette H, Fisher B: Correlation of estrogen receptor and pathologic characteristics of invasive breast cancer. Cancer 45:349–353, 1980.

74. Fisher B, Redmond C, Wolmark N, et al: Breast cancer studies of the NSABP: an editorialized overview. In Salmon SE, Jones SE (eds): Adjuvant Therapy of Cancer, III. New York, Grune and Stratton, 1981, pp 359–369.

75. Fisher B, Rockette H, Fisher ER, Wickerham DL, Redmond C, Brown A: Leukemia in breast cancer patients following adjuvant chemotherapy or postoperative radiation: the NSABP experience. J Clin Oncol 3:1640–1658, 1985.

76. Fisher B, Sherman B, Rockette H, Redmond C, Margolese R, Fisher ER: L-phenylalanine mustard (L-PAM) in the management of premenopausal patients with primary breast cancer. Cancer 44:847–857, 1979.

77. Fisher B, Slack N, Bross IDJ, and cooperating investigators: Cancer of the breast: size of neoplasm and prognosis. Cancer 24:1071–1080, 1969.

78. Fisher B, Slack N, Katrych D, Wolmark N: Ten year follow-up results of patients with carcinoma of the breast in a cooperative clinical trial evaluating surgical adjuvant chemotherapy. Surg Gynecol Obstet 140:528–534, 1975.

79. Fisher B, Wickerham DL, Beazley R, Bornstein R, et al: The use of adjuvant therapy for primary breast cancer: an overview. In Margolese R (ed): Contemporary Issues in Clinical Oncology. New York, Churchill Livingstone, 1983, pp 93–121.

80. Fisher E: Prognostic and therapeutic significance of pathologic features of breast cancer. NCI Monogr 1:29–34, 1986.

81. Fisher ER, Turnbull RB Jr: Cytologic demonstration and significance of tumor cells in the mesenteric venous blood in patients with colorectal carcinoma. Surg Gynecol Obstet 100:102–108, 1955.

82. Fornander T, Rutqvist LE, Cedermark B, Glas U, Mattson A, Silfversward C, Skoog L, Somell A, Theve T, Wilking N, Askergren J, Hjalmar M-L: Adjuvant tamoxifen in early breast cancer: occurrence of new primary cancers. Lancet 1:117–120, 1989.
83. Friedman M, Dorr F, Perloff M: Adjuvant therapy for breast cancer patients with negative lymph nodes. NCI Monogr 1:139–144, 1986.
84. Gelber RD, Goldhirsch A: The concept of an overview of cancer clinical trials with special emphasis on early breast cancer. J Clin Oncol 4:1696–1703, 1986.
85. Gelber RD, Goldhirsch A: A new endpoint for the assessment of adjuvant therapy on postmenopausal women with operable breast cancer. J Clin Oncol 4:1772–1779, 1986.
86. Glick J: Commentary. Meeting highlights: adjuvant therapy for breast cancer. J Natl Cancer Inst 80:471–475, 1988.
87. Goldhirsch A, Gelber R: Adjuvant treatment for early breast cancer: The Ludwig breast cancer studies. NCI Monogr 1:55–70, 1986.
88. Goldie JH, Coldman AJ: A mathematic model for relating the drug sensitivity of tumors to their spontaneous mutation rate. Cancer Treat Rep 63:1727–1731, 1979.
89. Goldie JH, Coldman AJ: Quantitative model for multiple levels of drug resistance in clinical tumors. Cancer Treat Rep 67:923–931, 1983.
90. Goldie JH, Coldman AJ: Genetic instability in the development of drug resistance. Semin Oncol 12:222–230, 1985.
91. Gough MH, Durrant KR, Girard-Saunders AM, Paine C, McPherson K, Vessey M: A randomized controlled trial of prophylactic cytotoxic chemotherapy in potentially curable breast cancer. Br J Surg 72:182–185, 1985.
92. Griswold DP Jr: The potential for murine tumor models in surgical adjuvant chemotherapy. Cancer Chemother Rep 5(part 2):187–204, 1975.
93. Hakes T, Geller N, Petroni G, Currie V, Kaufman R: Confirmation of dose-survival relationship in breast adjuvant chemotherapy. Proc Am Soc Clin Oncol 3:122, 1984.
94. Halsted WS: Results of operations for the cure of cancer of the breast performed at Johns Hopkins Hospital from June, 1889–January, 1894. Ann Surg 20:497, 1894.
95. Henderson IC: Adjuvant chemotherapy and endocrine therapy in patients with operable cancer. In DeVita VT Jr, Hellman S, Rosenberg SA (eds): Cancer: Principles and Practice of Oncology, ed 2. Philadelphia, JB Lippincott, 1985: update, March 1987.
96. Henderson IC, Gelman RS, Harris JR, Cannellos GP: Duration of therapy in adjuvant chemotherapy trials. NCI Monogr 1:95–98, 1986.
97. Henderson IC: Second malignancies from adjuvant chemotherapy? Too soon to tell. J Clin Oncol 5:1135–1137, 1987.
98. Himel HN, Liberati A, Gelber RD, Chalmer TC: Adjuvant chemotherapy for breast cancer: a pooled estimate based on published randomized control trials. JAMA 256:1148–1159, 1986.
99. Holdaway IM, Bowditch JV: Variation in receptor status between primary and metastatic breast cancer. Cancer 52:479–485, 1983.
100. Howell A, George WD, Crowther D, Rubens RD, Bulbrook RD, Bush H, Howat JMT, Sellwood RA, Hayward JL, Fentiman IS: Controlled trial of adjuvant chemotherapy with cyclophosphamide, methotrexate, and fluorouracil for breast cancer. Lancet 2:307–311, 1984.
101. Howell A, Rubens RD, Bush H, George W, Howat J, Crowther D, Sellwood R, Hayward J, Knight R, Bulbrook R, Fentiman I, Chaudary M: A controlled trial of adjuvant chemotherapy with melphalan versus cyclophosphamide, methotrexate, and 5-fluorouracil in breast cancer. Recent Results Cancer Res 96:74–89, 1986.
102. Hryniuk WM, Levine MN, Levin N: Analysis of dose intensity for chemotherapy in early (stage II) and advanced breast cancer. NCI Mongr 1:87–94, 1986.
103. Hubay CA, Gordon NH, Pearson OH, Marshall JS, McGuire WL, and participating investigators: Eight-year follow-up of adjuvant therapy for stage II breast cancer. World J Sug 9:738–749, 1985.
104. Huseby R, Ownby H, Frederick J, Brooks S, Russo J, Brennan M: Node-negative breast cancer treated by modified radical mastectomy without adjuvant therapies: variables associated with disease recurrence and survivorship. J Clin Oncol 6:83–88, 1988.
105. Ingle JN, Everson LK, Wieand HS, Martin JK, Wold LE, Krook JE, Ahmann DL, Cullinan SA, Paulsen JK: Randomized trial of adjuvant therapy with cyclophosphamide (C), 5-fluorouracil (F), prednisone (P) with or without tamoxifen (T) vs. observation following mastectomy in postmenopausal women with node positive breast cancer: a collaborative trial of the North Central Cancer Treatment Group and Mayo Clinic. Proc Am Soc Clin Oncol 5:70, 1986.
106. Ingle JN, Krook JE, Green SJ, Kubista TP, Everson LK, Ahmann DL, Chang MN, Bisel HF, Windschitl HE, Twito DI, Pfeifle DM: Randomized trial of bilateral oophorectomy versus tamoxifen in premenopausal women with metastatic breast cancer. J Clin Oncol 4:178–185, 1986.
107. Jakesz R, Kolb R, Reiner G, Rainer R, Schemper M, Moser K: Effect of adjuvant chemotherapy in stage I and II breast cancer is dependent on tumor differentiation and estrogen status. Proc Am Soc Clin Oncol 4:69, 1985.
108. Jakesz R, Kolb R, Reiner G, Schemper M, et al: Adjuvant chemotherapy in node-negative breast cancer patients. In Salmon S (ed): Adjuvant Therapy of Cancer, V. Orlando, FL, Grune and Stratton, 1987, pp 223–233.
109. Jung WF, Alberto P, Brunner KW, Mermillod B, Barrelet L, Cavalli F: Short or long term chemotherapy for node-positive breast cancer: LMF 6 versus 18 cycles. SAKK study 27/76. Recent Results Cancer Res 96:175–177, 1984.
110. Kaiser-Kupfer MI, Lippman ME: Tamoxifen retinopathy. Cancer Treat Rep 62:315–320, 1978.
111. Kaufmann M, Maass H, Kubli F, Jonat W, Caffier H, Melchert F, Hilfrich J, Mahlke M, Stosiek U, Brunnett K, Kleine W, Schorscher H, Hohlweg-Majert P, Stiglmayer R, Wander HF: Risk adapted adjuvant chemo-hormonotherapy in operable nodal positive breast cancer. In SE Jones, SE Salmon (eds): Adjuvant Therapy of Cancer, IV. Orlando, FL, Grune and Stratton, 1984, pp 369–378.
112. Levine MN, Gent M, Hirsh J, Arnold A, Goodyear M, Hryniuk W, DePauw S: The thrombogenic effect of anti-cancer drug therapy in women with stage II breast cancer. N Engl J Med 318:404–407, 1988.
113. Levine MN, Guyatt GH, Gent M, DePauw S, Goodyear M, Hryniuk W, Arnold A, Findlay B, Skillings J, Bramwell V, Levin L, Bush H, Abu-Zahra H, Kotalik J: Quality of life in stage II breast cancer: an instrument for clinical trials. J Clin Oncol 6:1798–1810, 1988.
114. Long L, Jonasson O, Roberts S, McGrath R, McGrew E, Cole W: Cancer cells in the blood; results of simplified isolation technique. Arch Surg 80:910–919, 1960.
115. Lundy J, Grimson R, Mishriki Y, Chaos Oravez S, Fromowitz F, Viola M: Elevated ras oncogene expression correlates with lymph node metastasis in breast cancer patients. J Clin Oncol 4:1321–1325, 1986.
116. Ludwig Breast Cancer Study Group: Combination adjuvant chemotherapy for node-positive breast cancer: inadequacy of a single perioperative cycle. N Engl J Med 319:677–684, 1988.
117. Ludwig Breast Cancer Study Group: Randomized trial of chemo-endocrine therapy, endocrine therapy, and mastectomy alone in postmenopausal patients with operable breast cancer and axillary node metastasis. Lancet 1:1256–1260, 1984.
118. Ludwig Breast Cancer Study Group: Adjuvant combination chemotherapy with or without prednisone in premenopausal breast cancer patients with metastases in 1 to 3 axillary lymph nodes: a randomized trial. Cancer Res 45:4454–4459, 1985.
119. Ludwig Breast Cancer Study Group: Adjuvant chemotherapy (CMF) with or without low-dose prednisone (P) in pre-menopausal patients with metastases in 1 to 3 axillary lymph nodes: Ludwig Trial I (LBCS I). Proc Am Soc Clin Oncol 4:53, 1985.
120. Ludwig Breast Cancer Study Group: Chemotherapy with or without oophorectomy in high-risk patients with operable breast cancer. J Clin Oncol 3:1059–1067, 1985.
121. Ludwig Breast Cancer Study Group: Prolonged disease-free survival after one course of perioperative adjuvant chemother-

apy for node-negative breast cancer patients. N Engl J Med 320:491–496, 1989.

122. Mansour EG, Gray R, Shatila AH, Osborne CK, Tormey D, Gilchrist K, Cooper M, Falkson G: Efficiency of adjuvant chemotherapy in high risk node negative breast cancer: an intergroup study (INT 0011) N Engl J Med 320:485–490, 1989.

123. Mendelsohn ML: The growth fraction. A new concept applied to tumors. Science 132:1486, 1960.

124. McDonald GO, Long EP, Cruz WH: The effect of cancer inhibitor drugs on the "take" of Walker carcinosarcoma 256 in rats. Surg Forum 7:486–489, 1956.

125. McDonald GO, Livingston C, Boyles CF, Cole W: The prophylactic treatment of malignant disease with nitrogen mustard and triethylenethiophosphoramide (Thio-TEPA). Ann Surg 145:624–629, 1957.

126. McGuire W, Clark G, Dressler L, Owens M: Role of steroid hormone receptors as prognostic factors in primary breast cancer. NCI Monogr 1:19–23, 1986.

127. McGuire WL, Glick JH, Abeloff MD, Henderson IC, Fisher B, Osborne CK: Oncology Viewpoints: Adjuvant Therapy in Node-Negative Breast Cancer. New York, LP Communications, 1988.

128. Meakin JW, Allt WC, Beale FA, et al: Ovarian irradiation and prednisone following surgery and radiotherapy for carcinoma of the breast. Breast Cancer Res Treat 3(suppl):45–48, 1983.

129. Meakin JW: Review of Canadian trials of adjuvant endocrine therapy for breast cancer. NCI Monogr 1:111–113, 1986.

130. Meyer J: Cell kinetics in selection and stratification of patients for adjuvant therapy of breast carcinoma. NCI Monogr 1:25–28, 1986.

131. Meyer J, Friedman E, McCrate M, Bauer W: Prediction of early course of breast carcinoma by thymidine labeling. Cancer 51:1879–1886, 1983.

132. Misset JL, Delgado M, Plagne R, et al: Five year results of the French adjuvant trial for breast cancer comparing CMF to a combination of adriamycin, vincristine, cyclophosphamide and 5-fluorouracil. In Jones SE, Salmon SE (eds): Adjuvant Therapy of Cancer, IV. Orlando, FL, Grune and Stratton, 1984, pp 243–251.

133. Morrison JM, Howell A, Grieve RJ, Monpenny IJ, Kelly KA, Marson A, Waterhouse JA: The West Midlands Oncology Association trials of adjuvant chemotherapy for operable breast cancer. In Jones SE, Salmon SE (eds): Adjuvant Therapy of Cancer, IV. New York, Grune and Stratton, 1984, pp 253–261.

134. Moses LE: The series of consecutive cases as a device for assessing outcomes of intervention. N Engl J Med 311:705–710, 1984.

135. Mouridsen HT, Rose C, Brincker H, Thorpe SM, Rank F, Fischerman K, Andersen KW: Adjuvant systemic therapy in high-risk breast cancer: the Danish Breast Cancer Cooperative Group's trials of cyclophosphamide or CMF in premenopausal and tamoxifen in post-menopausal patients. In Senn H (ed): Recent Results in Cancer Research: Adjuvant Chemotherapy in Breast Cancer. New York, Springer-Verlag, 1984, pp 117–127.

136. National Institutes of Health Consensus Development Panel on Adjuvant Chemotherapy and Endocrine Therapy for Breast Cancer: Introduction and conclusions. NCI Monogr 1:1–4, 1986.

137. Nevinny HB, Nevinny D, Rosoff CB, Hall TC, Muench H: Prophylactic oophorectomy in breast cancer therapy: a preliminary report. Am J Surg 117:531–536, 1969.

138. Nissen-Meyer R: The role of prophylactic castration in the therapy of human mammary cancer. Eur J Cancer 3:395–403, 1967.

139. Nissen-Meyer R, Host H, Kjellgren K, Mansson B, Norin T: Treatment of node-negative breast cancer patients with short course of chemotherapy immediately after surgery. NCI Monogr 1:125–128, 1986.

140. Nissen-Meyer R, Host H, Kjellgren K, Mansson B, Norin T: Neoadjuvant chemotherapy in breast cancer: as single perioperative treatment and with supplementary long-term chemotherapy. In Salmon S (ed): Adjuvant Therapy of Cancer, V. Orlando, FL, 1987, pp 253–261.

141. Nissen-Meyer R, Kjellgren K, Malmiok K, Mansson B, Norin T: Surgical adjuvant chemotherapy: results with one short course with cyclophosphamide after mastectomy for breast cancer. Cancer 41:2088–2098, 1978.

142. Nolvadex Adjuvant Trial Organisation controlled trial of tamoxifen as single adjuvant agent in management of early breast cancer. Lancet 1:836–839, 1985.

143. Norton L, Simon R: Tumor size, sensitivity to therapy, and design of treatment schedules. Cancer Treat Rep 61:1307–1317, 1977.

144. Osborne CK, Rivkin SE, McDivitt RW, Greer S, Stephens R, Costanzi J, O'Bryan R: Adjuvant therapy of breast cancer: Southwest Oncology Group studies. NCI Monogr 1:71–74, 1986.

145. Padmanabhan N, Howell A, Rubens RD: Mechanism of action of adjuvant chemotherapy in early breast cancer. Lancet 2:411–414, 1986.

146. Palshoff T, Mouridsen HT, Daehnfeldt JL: Adjuvant endocrine therapy of primary operable breast cancer: report on the Copenhagen breast cancer trials. Eur J Cancer 2(suppl):183–187, 1980.

147. Perloff M, Norton L, Korzun A, Wood W, Carey R, Weinberg V, Holland J: Advantage of an adriamycin combination plus halotestin after initial cyclophosphamide, methotrexate, 5-fluorouracil, vincristine and prednisone (CMFVP) for adjuvant therapy of node-positive stage II breast cancer. Proc Am Soc Clin Oncol 5:70, 1986.

148. Pourquier H: The results of adjuvant chemotherapy are predominantly caused by the hormonal changes such therapy induces. In Favor. In VanScoy-Mosher MB (ed): Medical Oncology: Controversies in Cancer Treatment. Boston, GK Hall, 1981, pp 83–99.

149. Pritchard KI, Meakin JW, Boyd NF, DeBoer G, Paterson AHG, Ambus U, Dembo AJ, Sutherland DJA, Wilkinson RH, Bassett AA, Evans WK, Beale FA, Clark RM, Keane TJ: Adjuvant tamoxifen in postmenopausal women with axillary node positive breast cancer: an update. In SE Salmon (ed): Adjuvant Therapy of Cancer, V. Orlando, FL, Grune and Stratton, 1987, pp 391–400.

150. Proceedings of the NIH Consensus Development Conference on Adjuvant Chemotherapy and Endocrine Therapy for Breast Cancer. NCI Monogr 1:1, 1986.

151. Ravdin RG, Lewison EF, Slack NH, Dao TL, Gardner B, State D, Fisher B: Results of a clinical trial concerning the worth of prophylactic oophorectomy for breast cancer. Surg Gynecol Obstet 131:1055–1064, 1970.

152. Redmond C, Fisher B, Wieand HS: The methodologic dilemma in retrospectively correlating the amount of chemotherapy received in adjuvant therapy protocols with disease-free survival. Cancer Treat Rep 67:519–526, 1983.

153. Redmond CK, Rockett HE: Meta-analysis: considerations of its worth and its limitations. In Salmon SE (ed): Adjuvant Therapy of Cancer, V. Orlando, FL, Grune and Stratton, 1987, pp 467–475.

154. Report from the Breast Cancer Trials Committee, Scottish Cancer Trials Office (MRC), Edinburgh: Adjuvant tamoxifen in the management of operable breast cancer: the Scottish Trial. Lancet 2:171–175, 1987.

155. Review of mortality results in randomized trials in early breast cancer. Lancet 2:1205, 1984.

156. Ribeiro G, Swindell R: The Christie Hospital tamoxifen (Nolvadex) adjuvant trial for operable breast cancer—7 year results. Eur J Cancer Clin Oncol 21:897–900, 1985.

157. Rivkin SE, Knight WA III, McDivitt R, Cruz T, Foulkes M, Osborne CK, Fabian CJ, Costanzi JJ: Adjuvant therapy for breast cancer with positive axillary nodes designed according to estrogen receptor status. World J Surg 9:723–727, 1985.

158. Rivkin SE, Knight WA, Cruz A, Foulhes M, McDivitt R: Adjuvant chemotherapy and hormonal therapy for operable breast cancer with positive axillary nodes. Proc Am Assoc Cancer Res 25:181, 1984.

159. Roberts S, Watne A, McGrath R, McGrew E, Cole WH: Technique and results of isolation of cancer cells from the circulating blood. Arch Surg 76:334–336, 1958.

160. Rose C, Mouridsen HT, Thorpe SM, Andersen J, Blichert-Toft

M, Andersen KW: Anti-oestrogen treatment of postmenopausal breast cancer patients with high risk of recurrence: 72 months of life-table analysis and steroid hormone receptor status. World J Surg 9:765–774, 1985.

161. Rose C, Thorpe SM, Andersen KW, Pedersen BV, Mouridsen HT, Blichert-Toft M, Ramussen BB: Beneficial effect of adjuvant tamoxifen therapy in primary breast cancer patients with high oestrogen receptor values. Lancet 1:16–19, 1985.

162. Rubens RD, Knight RK, Fentiman IS, Howell A, Crowther D, George WD, Hayward JL, Bulbrook RD, Chaudary M, Bush H, Sellwood RA, Howart JM: Controlled trial of adjuvant chemotherapy with melphalan for breast cancer. Lancet 1:839–843, 1983.

163. Salsbury HJ: The significance of the circulating cancer cell. Cancer Treat Rev 2:55–72, 1975.

164. Schabel FM: Concepts for systemic treatment of micrometastases. Cancer 35:15, 1975.

165. Schabel FM: Surgical adjuvant chemotherapy of metastatic murine tumors. Cancer 40:558–568, 1977.

166. Schinzinger A: Ueber carcinoma mammae. Verh Dtsch Ges Chir 18:28–29, 1889.

167. Senanayake F: Adjuvant hormonal chemotherapy in early breast cancer: early results from a controlled trial. Lancet 2:1148–1149, 1984.

168. Senn HJ, Jungi WF: Swiss adjuvant trials with LMF (+BCG) in N− and N+ breast cancer patients. In Jones SE, Salmon SE (eds): Adjuvant Therapy of Cancer, IV. Orlando, FL, Grune and Stratton, 1984, pp 261–270.

169. Senn HJ, Mahler-Barett R, for the Osako and SAKK Groups: Update of Swiss adjuvant trials with LMF and CMF in operable breast cancer. In Salmon SE (ed): Adjuvant Therapy of Cancer, V. Orlando, FL, Grune and Stratton, 1987, pp 243–253.

170. Shapiro DM, Fugmann RA: A role for chemotherapy as an adjunct to surgery. Cancer Res 17:1098–1101, 1957.

171. Simmonds MA, Lipton A, Harvey HA, White D, et al: FAC vs L-PAM chemotherapy for adjuvant treatment of breast cancer in postmenopausal women. Proc Am Soc Clin Oncol 22:438, 1981.

172. Skipper HE: Kinetics of mammary tumor cell growth and implication for therapy. Cancer 28:1479–1499, 1971.

173. Skipper HE: Adjuvant chemotherapy. Cancer 41:936–940, 1978.

174. Slamon D, Clark G, Wong S, Levin W, et al: Human breast cancer: correlation of relapse and survival with amplification of the HER-2/neu oncogene. Science 235:177–182, 1987.

175. Smith DC, Crawford D, Dykes EH, Calman KC, Russell AR, McArdle CS: Adjuvant radiotherapy and chemotherapy in breast cancer. In Jones SE, Salmon SE (eds): Adjuvant Therapy of Cancer, IV. Orlando, FL, Grune and Stratton, 1984, pp 283–289.

176. Tancini G, Bonadonno G, Valagussa P, Mandrini S, Veronesi U: Adjuvant CMF in breast cancer: comparative 5-year results of 12 versus 6 cycles. J Clin Oncol 1:2–10, 1983.

177. Taylor GW: Artificial menopause in carcinoma of the breast. N Engl J Med 211:1138–1140, 1934.

178. Taylor GW: Evaluation of ovarian sterilization for breast cancer. Surg Gynecol Obstet 68:452–456, 1939.

179. Taylor SG IV, Gelman RS, Falkson G, Cummings FJ: Combination chemotherapy compared to tamoxifen as initial therapy for stage IV breast cancer in elderly women. Ann Int Med 104:455–461, 1986.

180. Taylor SG IV, Olsen JE, Cummings FJ, Knuiman M: Observation compared to adjuvant chemo-hormonal therapy in postmenopausal breast cancer: the ECOG trial. Proc Am Soc Clin Oncol 4:61, 1985.

181. Taylor SG, Kalish LA, Olson JE, Cummings F, Bennett J, Falkson G, Tormey D, Carbone P: Adjuvant CMFP versus CMFP plus tamoxifen versus observation alone in postmenopausal, node-positive breast cancer patients: three-year results of an Eastern Cooperative Oncology Group study. J Clin Oncol 3:144–154, 1985.

182. Tormey DC: Clinical results III: experience of randomized trials without surgical controls. In Senn JH (ed): Recent results in Cancer Research. Adjuvant Chemotherapy of Breast Cancer. New York, Springer-Verlag, 1984, pp 155–165.

183. Tormey DC, Gray R, Taylor SG IV, Knuiman M, Olson J, Cummings F: Postoperative chemotherapy and chemohormonal therapy in women with node-positive breast cancer. NCI Monogr 1:75–80, 1986.

184. Tormey DC, Taylor SG IV, Kalish LA, Olsen JE, Grage T, Gray R: Adjuvant systemic therapy in premenopausal (CMF, CMFP, CMFPT) and post-menopausal (observation, CMFP, CMFPT) women with node positive breast cancer. In Jones SE, Salmon SE (eds): Adjuvant Therapy of Cancer, IV. Orlando, FL, Grune and Stratton, 1984, pp 359–368.

185. Tormey DC, Weinberg VE, Hollan JF, Weiss RB, Glidewell OJ, Perloff M, Falkson G, Falkson H, Henry P, Leone LA, Rafla S, Ginsberg S, Silver R, Blom J, Carey RW, Schein PS, Lesnick G: A randomized trial of five and three drug chemotherapy and chemoimmunotherapy in women with operable node positive breast cancer. J Clin Oncol 1:138–145, 1983.

186. Valagussa P, Tancini G, Bonadonna G: Second malignancies after CMF for resectable breast cancer. J Clin Oncol 5:1138–1142, 1987.

187. Vande Vijver MJ, Peterse JL, Moo WJ, Wisman P, Lomans J, Dalesio O, Nusse R: Neuprotein over expression in breast cancer: association with comedo-type ductal carcinoma in sites and limited prognostic value in stage II breast cancer. N Engl J Med 319:1239–1245, 1988.

188. Velez-Garcia E, Moore M, Vogel CL, Marcial V, Keatcham A, Raney M, Smalley R: Post surgical adjuvant chemotherapy with or without radiation therapy in women with breast cancer and positive axillary nodes: the Southeastern Cancer Study Group (SECSG) experience. In Jones SE, Salmon SE (eds): Adjuvant Therapy of Cancer, IV. Orlando, FL, Grune and Stratton, 1984, pp 273–283.

189. Velez-Garcia E, Carpenter JT, Moore M, Vogel CL, et al: Post surgical adjuvant chemotherapy with or without radiotherapy in women with breast cancer and positive axillary nodes: progress report of a Southeastern Cancer Study Group (SEG) trial. In Salmon SE (ed): Adjuvant Therapy of Cancer, V. Orlando, FL, Grune and Stratton, 1987, pp 347–356.

190. Veronesi U, Cascinelli N, Greco M, Bufalino R, Morabito A, Galluzzo D, Conti R, DeLellis R, Delle Donne V, Piotti P, Sacchini V, Clemente C, Salvadori B: Prognosis of breast cancer patients after mastectomy and dissection of internal mammary nodes. Ann Surg 6:702–707, 1985.

191. Wallgren A, Baral E, Beling U, Carstensen J, et al: Tamoxifen and combination chemotherapy as adjuvant treatment in postmenopausal women with breast cancer. In Senn HJ (ed): Recent Results in Cancer Research. Adjuvant Chemotherapy of Breast Cancer. New York, Springer-Verlag, 1984, pp 197–203.

192. Wallgren A, Baral E, Carstensen J, Friberg S, Glas U, Hjalmar M-L, Kaigas M, Nordenskjold B, Skoog L, Theve N-O, Wilking N: Should adjuvant tamoxifen be given for several years in breast cancer? In Jones SE, Salmon SE (eds): Adjuvant Therapy of Cancer, IV. Orlando, FL, Grune and Stratton, 1984, pp 331–337.

193. Weiss RB, DeVita VT: Multimodal primary cancer treatment (adjuvant chemotherapy): current results and future prospects. Ann Int Med 91:251–260, 1979.

194. Wheeler TK: Four drug combination chemotherapy following surgery for breast cancer. In Jones SE, Salmon SE (eds): Adjuvant Therapy for Cancer, II, Orlando, FL, Grune and Stratton, 1979, pp 269–276.

195. Wilcox WS: The last surviving cancer cell. The chance of killing it. Cancer Chemother Rep 50:541–542, 1966.

196. Williams C, Buchanan R, Hall V, Taylor I, et al: Adjuvant chemotherapy for T1–2, N0, M0 estrogen receptor negative breast cancer: preliminary results of a randomized trial. In Salmon S (ed): Adjuvant Therapy of Cancer, V. Orlando, FL, Grune and Stratton, 1987, pp 233–242.

197. Wolter J, Ryan WG, Subbaiah PV, Bagdage JD: Apparent beneficial effects of tamoxifen on serum lipoprotein subfractions and bone mineral content in patients with breast cancer. Proc Am Soc Clin Oncol 7:10, 1988.

198. Zelen M, Gelman R: Assessment of adjuvant trials in breast cancer. NCI Monogr 1:11–17, 1986.

Chapter 40

LOCALLY ADVANCED BREAST CANCER

Sandra M. Swain, M.D. and Marc E. Lippman, M.D.

The term "locally advanced breast cancer" (LABC) can be applied to a heterogeneous group of patients with varying prognoses. In this chapter the definition will include all patients with stage III breast carcinoma according to the combined Union Internationale Contre le Cancer-American Joint Committee on Cancer (UICC-AJCC) recommendations of 1983 (Table 40-1).[15] The revised UICC staging published in 1987,[63] soon to be published by the AJCC, is similar, with one exception: patients with clinical T3 N0 disease will be considered stage IIB in the new classification.

LABC is still diagnosed at presentation in a substantial proportion of women, reported to be 11.6 percent to 29 percent of women with breast cancer.[56, 83] Therefore there are a considerable number of patients annually diagnosed with this stage of disease. The prognosis for most patients in this group is very poor with local therapy alone, suggesting that micrometastases are present at diagnosis. The emphasis of this chapter will

be the treatment of this stage of breast cancer as a systemic disease; local treatment will be briefly reviewed. For more information on local control by radiation therapy see section XIV, chapter 37 and section XVI, chapter 41. Treatment with combination chemotherapy will be discussed, followed by a review of inflammatory breast carcinoma. Next the National Cancer Institute experience with locally advanced breast cancer will be presented. Finally, future directions in the treatment of breast carcinoma will be considered.

NONINFLAMMATORY LOCALLY ADVANCED DISEASE

Historical Background

Haagensen and Stout were responsible for identifying the poor prognostic features of breast cancer that made it what they termed "categorically inoperable."[61] They reviewed the experience at Columbia Presbyterian Hospital in New York during the period from 1915 to 1942 and analyzed the experience with radical mastectomy in 1135 cases of breast cancer during that time. They were able to identify clinical features of breast cancer that were associated with a zero percent 5-year cure and a greater than 50 percent chance of local recurrence. These features included extensive edema of the skin of the breast (greater than one third of the breast), satellite tumor nodules in the skin, inflammatory carcinoma (defined by involvement of greater than one third of the breast with edema or erythema), intercostal or parasternal nodules, supraclavicular nodal metastases, edema of the arm, or distant metastases. If these findings were present, patients were included in the Columbia Clinical Class D or inoperable classification. Haagensen and

Table 40-1. AMERICAN JOINT COMMITTEE BREAST CANCER STAGING: STAGE III (1983)[15]

Stage IIIA	T0, T1, T2, T3	N2	MO
	T3	N0, N1, N2	MO
Stage IIIB	Any T	N3	MO
	Any T4	Any N	MO

N0 = Axillary nodes not considered to contain growth.
N1 = Axillary nodes considered to contain growth.
N2 = Axillary nodes fixed.
N3 = Supraclavicular or infraclavicular nodes or arm edema.
T1 = Tumors ≤2 cm.
T2 = Tumors >2 cm and ≤5 cm.
T3 = Tumors >5 cm.
T4 = Tumor of any size with direct extension to chest wall or skin, edema of skin (peau d'orange), ulceration, or satellite skin nodules.
MO = No distant metastases.

Stout also reported that patients who developed carcinoma during pregnancy or lactation had a poor survival. Only one of 20 patients survived 5 years, and this patient then developed a recurrence at 6 years.

Haagensen and Stout also identified other features they called the "grave signs" of breast cancer. These included ulceration, fixation of the tumor to the chest wall, axillary lymph nodes greater than 2.5 cm in diameter, edema of less than one third of the skin of the breast, and fixed axillary lymph nodes. They felt that any of these signs alone did not make the patient inoperable. There was evidence of 5-year clinical cure in five percent to 38 percent of these patients treated by radical mastectomy. Also, the local recurrence rate ranged from 13 percent to 40 percent. Any one of these signs placed a patient in Stage C of the Columbia Clinical Classification. If two of these signs were present, patients were placed into Stage D. The basis for this was that in their series, only one patient who had two grave signs present was disease free at 5 years.

Because of the poor survival with radical mastectomy in the treatment of locally advanced breast cancer, physicians began treating these patients with primary radiation therapy. Baclesse published his 5-year results of the treatment of 431 breast carcinomas treated with classical 200 kilovoltage (kV) roentgen rays as the sole modality of therapy.[9] He treated 95 patients who were classified as stage C, with a survival rate of 41 percent. This was comparable to Haagensen's survival rate with radical mastectomy as treatment in Stage C (42.9 percent). Baclesse also treated 200 Stage D patients with radiation therapy, with a 13 percent survival at 5 years. Six of the 27 5-year survivors in this group were not disease free.

These results and the experience of others, discussed in the next section, suggest that patients with locally advanced disease have systemic micrometastases at diagnosis. Therefore local therapy alone is not sufficient to cure most patients with this disease.

Classification

The AJCC classification for 1983 divides stage III disease into stage IIIA and stage IIIB.[1] Stage IIIA includes patients with tumors greater than 5 cm in diameter, which by definition are T3 tumors. These patients can have no evidence of clinical node involvement on physical examination (N0), axillary nodes that are felt to be clinically positive (N1), or matted and fixed nodes (N2). Patients with tumors that are less than 5 cm in diameter are also stage IIIA if they have N2 nodes. Stage IIIB includes patients with any size tumor and infraclavicular and supraclavicular node involvement or arm edema (N3). Also, a T4 tumor with any nodal stage is IIIB. T4 tumors include those with inflammatory carcinoma, peau d'orange, satellite skin nodules, ulceration, or direct extension to the chest wall.

The prognosis for stage IIIA patients is felt to be better than that for IIIB patients, with much better local control and overall survival. However, the survival de-

pends, as will be discussed, on the extent of metastases in axillary lymph nodes.

Size of Primary Carcinoma and Axillary Nodal Metastases

The likelihood of axillary nodal metastases corresponds directly to the size of the primary tumor at diagnosis: the extent of axillary involvement increases with increasing tumor size.

Fisher et al. presented data from two earlier studies that included tumor size and extent of axillary nodal involvement in 2578 patients.[46] Patients with tumors 6 cm or larger had a 63 percent incidence of axillary nodal involvement, compared with 38 percent in patients with 1.0–1.9 cm tumors. Of the 63 percent, 35 percent had one to three nodes involved, and 65 percent had four or more nodes involved, which was the reverse of the smaller tumors. Fisher et al. also analyzed survival and recurrence data according to the presence of nodal metastases and tumor size in 1048 patients. Patients with ≥6-cm tumors and one to three nodes involved had a recurrence rate of 63 percent, and those with four or greater axillary nodes had a 94 percent recurrence rate. Also, the patients with larger tumors (≥6 cm) had a higher overall mortality rate (55 percent compared with 22 percent in patients in the smaller tumor group). This analysis concluded that larger tumor size correlated with a higher incidence of axillary nodal metastases, a higher incidence of four or more positive nodes, a higher tumor recurrence rate, and greater breast cancer mortality.

Haagensen also reported an increasing incidence of axillary nodal involvement with increasing tumor size.[57] His patients with ≥5-cm tumors had a 52 percent incidence of nodal involvement compared with 28 percent for tumors less than 1 cm. Nemoto et al. also confirmed this finding.[92] Sixty-five percent of his patients with tumors greater than 5 cm had axillary nodal metastases. This translated into greater breast cancer mortality.

The report of Ariel of 1178 patients treated by radical mastectomy according to size of primary tumor also supports the observation that survival decreases with increasing tumor size.[6] Patients with tumors 1 cm or smaller had a 10-year survival of 68 percent, compared with 53 percent for 3-cm tumors and 11 percent for tumors 9 cm or greater.

Conclusions from the studies in the literature reveal a poorer prognosis with increasing tumor size and a direct relationship of primary tumor size to the extent of axillary nodal metastases.

Prognosis for Patients With Negative Axillary Nodes

Fracchia et al. reviewed their experience with stage III carcinoma and addressed the prognosis for patients with this stage of breast cancer and with pathologically negative axillary nodes.[50] In 488 patients with stage III disease, all treated by mastectomy, 58 (11.8 percent) had no nodal metastases. These patients had a 10-year survival of 75.3 percent. Thus a small group of stage III patients do have a favorable prognosis, and attempts should be made to identify these patients.

Another report also revealed a better prognosis for stage III patients with pathologically negative axillary nodes. Toonkel analyzed the survival of 58 patients with T3 tumors and negative axillary nodes at mastectomy.[125] The 5-year survival was 72 percent, and 10-year survival was 57 percent in these patients.

Fisher et al.'s patients with tumors ≥6 cm and negative axillary nodes had a recurrence rate of 24 percent, with a 5-year survival of 75 percent.[46] This compares to a 5-year survival rate of 15 percent in patients with the same tumor size but four or more involved nodes. Though the recurrence rate is low for patients with large tumors and negative nodes, it is higher than that for patients with smaller tumors. In Fisher et al.'s series, women with tumors 1.0–1.9 cm and negative nodes, the 5-year survival was 85 percent.

Nemoto et al. reported a 25 percent 5-year relapse rate in patients with tumors >5 cm and negative nodes.[92] This compares with a 13 percent recurrence in patients with tumors <2 cm in the same series. Valagussa reported a 19 percent 5-year recurrence rate in women with tumors >5 cm and negative nodes compared with eight percent in those with tumors <2 cm.[129]

Thus the small subset of patients with pathologically negative axillary nodes appears to have a much better prognosis than other patients with stage III disease. However, there is still a relapse rate at 5 years of 19 percent to 27 percent.[92, 129]

Other Predictors of Prognosis

The determination of axillary nodal metastases by physical examination alone is associated with a high false-negative rate. Several series in the literature report that even if axillary nodes are not palpable, 27 percent to 32 percent of patients will have histological involvement at nodal dissection.[24, 26, 60, 109] Therefore it is essential to use other methods to predict prognosis in patients with stage III disease if nodes are not palpable.

Stewart et al. analyzed estrogen receptor content in 124 patients with stage III breast cancer.[118] There was a significantly increased median disease-free and overall survival in patients with operable disease (T3a N0–N1) and pathologically negative nodes who had positive estrogen receptors vs. comparable patients with negative receptors ($p < 0.05$). This was not the case in patients with inoperable (T3b–T4 N0–N1 M0 or TX N2–N3 M0) breast carcinoma; in these patients estrogen receptor status had no effect on prognosis.

Silvestrini et al. have evaluated the utility of cell kinetics determined by thymidine labeling index (TLI) to predict which patients have a higher risk of recurrence in locally advanced breast cancer.[113] They evaluated the pretreatment labeling index (LI) in 52 patients and found that a high LI significantly predicted a higher recurrence rate, shorter time to disease progression, and a shorter 4-year survival when compared with a low LI. The 4-year survival of patients with a low LI was 68

percent vs. 37 percent for a high LI. The relapse-free survival, however, was comparable in the two groups; 24 percent for low LI and 19 percent for high LI. This study suggests that evaluation of tumor cell kinetics may predict which patients with large tumors will need very aggressive therapy because of the higher probability of relapse. This method could help identify women with clinical T3 N0 disease who have a poorer prognosis and need systemic treatment.

Treatment of Locally Advanced Breast Cancer

Surgery

The poor results following treatment of locally advanced disease with surgery alone have been discussed in the previous sections. Haagensen and Stout reported a zero percent 5-year cure rate in patients who met the criteria for inoperability listed previously.[61] Fracchia reported a 27 percent 10-year survival in a retrospective review of patients with stage III breast cancers treated by mastectomy alone.[50] However, in retrospective analyses, patients treated by mastectomy are usually in a better prognosis category. Another series analyzing results of surgical treatment of stage III breast cancer, by Arnold and Lesnick,[7] retrospectively reviewed records of 228 patients treated with surgery. Fifty patients were treated by mastectomy alone and had a median survival of 54 months and disease-free survival of 54 months. They compared this with results in patients treated with postoperative radiation therapy and found the latter's median survival to be 36 months and disease-free survival to be 24 months. Patients who received preoperative radiation therapy had a median overall survival of 30 months and disease-free survival of 20 months. Finally, patients who received preoperative chemotherapy and radiation therapy had a median survival of 29 months and disease-free survival of 17 months. These results again are subject to a selection bias. The results of the group of patients treated with pre- or postoperative radiation or preoperative chemotherapy did not differ significantly but were much worse than those for patients treated by mastectomy alone.

In summary, treatment of inoperable (as categorized by Haagensen and Stout[61]) locally advanced disease with surgery alone results in a poor survival rate. This suggests that these patients have systemic disease at diagnosis.

Radiation Therapy

The use of primary radiation therapy in the treatment of advanced breast cancer is discussed in more detail in chapter 37. The survival rates reported for radiation therapy alone are comparable to those for surgical treatment. Sheldon et al. reported the Joint Center for Radiation Therapy experience in 1987.[112] The survival of a group of 192 patients treated with radiation therapy was 23 percent at 10 years, with a relapse-free survival rate of 19 percent. Other series report 5-year survivals ranging from 11 percent to 60 percent (Table 40–2).* Guttman reported a 60 percent 5-year survival rate, which is much higher than most other investigators report.[54] All of her patients had multiple biopsy samples taken from regional lymph nodes, internal mammary nodes, and axillary nodes prior to treatment. They were included in her series if their biopsy results were positive. Many of these patients may have been classified as stage I or II by other physicians, as most do not do such extensive biopsies.

Zucali et al. retrospectively evaluated 454 consecutive patients with stage III disease treated with radiation therapy.[136] Radical mastectomy was performed in 133 of these patients after radiation therapy. This was not a randomized study, and therefore there was a selection bias in that patients receiving a subsequent mastectomy had a better prognosis. All had achieved complete clinical remission. Patients treated by radiation therapy alone had a median survival of 25 months, compared with 45 months in those patients who also had surgical treatment. Patients with clinical N0 disease had a median survival of 48 months, compared with 27 months in patients with evidence of any clinical nodal involvement ($p < 0.01$). Patients with supraclavicular nodal involvement had a very poor median survival (16 months), as did those with inflammatory cancer (14 months). A very interesting analysis was done of the histological findings after radiation therapy and mastectomy. A total of 131 patients had mastectomy specimens available for analysis. Twenty-five percent of these patients had no residual tumor in the breast, 32 percent had histologically negative axillary nodes, and only ten percent had neither residual tumor in the breast nor axillary nodal involvement. This suggests poor local control with radiation therapy alone in stage III patients.

Toonkel et al. treated 509 stage III and localized stage IV breast cancer patients (AJCC 1978 staging) with surgical procedures ranging from incisional biopsy to

Table 40–2. FIVE-YEAR SURVIVAL OF LOCALLY ADVANCED BREAST CANCER PATIENTS TREATED BY PRIMARY RADIATION THERAPY

Author	% 5-yr Survival
Zucali (1976)[136]	21
Vilcoq (1984)[131]	39
Fodor (1987)[48]	35
Atkins and Horrigan (1961)[8]	11
Treurniet-Donker (1980)[126]	11
Zaharia (1987)[135]	22
Golding (1976)[51]	35
Bouchard (1965)[17]	14
Strickland (1973)[120]	36
Fletcher and Montague (1965)[47]	36
Langlands (1976)[76]	14
Delarue (1965)[36]	28
Guttman (1967)[54]	60
Sheldon (1987)[112]	38

*References 8, 17, 36, 47, 48, 51, 54, 76, 112, 120, 126, 130, 131, and 135.

radical mastectomy followed by radiation therapy.[125] There were 381 patients who had removal of all gross carcinoma prior to radiation. The 5-year survival and disease-free survival rates were 50 percent and 38 percent, respectively. The local recurrence rate was 55 percent.

The survival results with radiation alone are not dissimilar from those with surgery alone. This suggests that the addition of systemic treatment is needed to optimize outcome.

Combination Chemotherapy

The prognosis for patients with locally advanced breast cancer is poor, with most patients developing distant metastases early in their illness. This suggests that micrometastases are present at the time of the initial diagnosis and that treatment should include systemic therapy. Physicians began treating these patients with chemotherapy either before or after local therapy in attempts to improve survival.

Randomized Studies. The results of several randomized studies are shown in Table 40–3.* Schaake-Koning et al. reported a randomized study of 118 LABC patients with the TNM classification of T3b–T4, any N, M0, or T1–T3 with a positive axillary apex biopsy result.[107] They excluded patients with supraclavicular or infraclavicular nodal involvement or inflammatory disease that could not be confined to standard radiation fields. The randomization was to radiation therapy alone (arm I) or to radiation followed by 12 cycles of cyclophosphamide, methotrexate, and 5-fluorouracil (CMF) and tamoxifen (arm II) or to induction chemotherapy with doxorubicin and vincristine (AV) for two cycles alternating with two cycles of CMF, followed by radiation, then four cycles of AV alternating with four cycles of CMF with tamoxifen given for the entire treatment period (arm III). The median follow-up was 66 months. There were 45 patients in arm I, 34 in arm II, and 39 in arm III. The actuarial 5-year survival was 37 percent for all three threatment arms. The relapse-free survival (RFS) was 14 months for arm I, 26 months for arm II, and 20 months for arm III ($p = 0.11$). Patients with a dose reduction of 30 percent or greater in more than four cycles had a better RFS than did those with less dose reduction ($p = 0.04$). Thus adjuvant chemohormonal therapy did not improve survival compared with radiation therapy alone in this group of LABC patients. However, caution must be taken in this interpretation. First, the number of randomized patients is small, and second, it may be that the chemotherapy given was not aggressive enough in this poor prognosis group of patients.

The only other randomized study with a radiation therapy alone treatment arm was presented in an abstract by Caceres et al.[28] Stage III patients were treated in this study with exclusions not stated. The details of radiation and chemotherapy are not given. The randomization was to radiation (RT) (34 patients) or to RT and

*References 3, 28, 38, 39, 53, 71, 95, 101, 107, and 116.

Table 40–3. COMBINATION CHEMOTHERAPY TREATMENT OF LOCALLY ADVANCED BREAST CANCER: RANDOMIZED STUDIES

Investigator (year)	Treatment	Number of Patients	Stage	Follow-up (median)	Median Time to Progression (months)	Median Survival (months)
Schaake-Koning (1985)[107]	RT	45	T3BT4NXM0 or		14	48*
	RT + CMF Tam	34	T3 + axillary	66	26	42*
	AV + CMF → RT → AVCMF Tam	39	biopsy		20	50*
Caceres (1980)[28]	RT	34			11	19.9
	RT + S	27	III (AJCC)	NA	8.9	17.8
	RT + CMF	26			14.6	24.6
DeLena (1978)[39]	AVx4 → RT → Ob	44	T3b–T4NXM0		11	
	+OX or estrogen (110 pts) → AV or CMF	37		NA	19	36 (all)
DeLena (1981)[38]	3 AV → RT → 7AV (132 pts) → S	67 (57 rec'd RT) — 65 (51 rec'd S)	III (excludes IBC + SCN)	NA	22 15	51.7 49.1
Perloff (1988)[101]	CAFVP → S → 2 years / RT → CAFVP (113 pts)	43 44	T3N1 T3N2 T4N0–N2	37	29.2 24.4	39.3 39.0
Spangenberg (1986)[116]					**5-Year RFS (%)**	**5-Year Survival (%)**
	A. RT + hormones → C × 2 year → C × 2 mo + CMFVel × 3 year	26	III inoperable	NA	NA NA	20 20
	B. S + hormones → RT + C → CMFVel	131	III operable	38.3 (mean)	40.4 26.8	62.5 56.3
					Crude Recurrence Rate (%)	
Papaioannou (1983)[95]	CAVMF ± Tam ± OX → S → RT → CAVMFTam / NoRT (205 patients)	48 57	III	NA	21 27	NA
					Crude 3-Year (%)	
					RFS	**OS**
Gröhn (1984)[53]	S → RT ± levamisole / VAC ± levamisole / RT + VAC ± levamisole	40 40 39	T3N0–N2	NA	32 47 87	57 72 90
					Crude 5-Year RFS (%)	
Klefström (1987)[71] (update Gröhn)	Same	Same	Same	At least 5 years	22 30 67	NA
Alagaratnam and Wong (1986)[3]	S + RT → TAM / CAF	40 31	III	33	35* 28*	NA

*Median determined approximately by survival curves in papers.

Abbreviations: A, doxorubicin; AJCC, American Joint Committee on Cancer (all III refer to 1983 staging); C, cyclophosphamide; F, 5-fluorouracil; IBC, inflammatory breast cancer; M, methotrexate; MRM, modified radical mastectomy; NA, not available; Ob, observation; OS, overall survival; OX, oophorectomy; P, prednisone; RFS, relapse-free survival; RT, radiation therapy; S, surgery; SCN, supraclavicular nodes; Tam, tamoxifen; V, vincristine; Vel, vinblastine.

total mastectomy (RT + TM) (27 patients) or to RT and CMF (RT + CMF) (26 patients). Median survival was prolonged with RT and CMF (24.6 months) compared with RT (19.9 months) and RT + TM (17.8 months). Local control was best in patients receiving RT + TM.

These studies have differing results, but it is still apparent that treatment with radiation alone is not optimal. The median survivals of 14 to 20 months with radiation alone in these two studies are inadequate. More aggressive and effective chemotherapeutic regimens may improve results.

Rubens et al. reported a feasibility study testing the ability to combine radiation and chemotherapy in the treatment of LABC.[105] Patients with T1 N2–N3 M0 or T3–T4 N1 M0 disease were eligible, and T3 N0 M0 patients were excluded. Patients were allocated alternately, not randomly, to either four cycles of AV followed by radiation and then eight cycles of CMF (group A) or radiation followed by four cycles of AV and then eight cycles of CMF (group B). There were 24 patients allocated. Four patients were 60 years of age or older and had dose reductions of drugs (one group A patient, three group B patients). Group B received less total dose of all drugs, but this was only significant for doxorubicin. The crude recurrence rate at 40 months follow-up was 50 percent in group A and 58 percent in group B. The median survival of the combined groups A and B was 36 months. Rubens et al. compared this result historically with patients treated at their institution with radiation alone. The historical control had a median survival of 25 months (difference not significant). The conclusions were that toxicity was acceptable when combining radiation with chemotherapy.

DeLena and colleagues reported a randomized study in LABC with a combined treatment modality approach.[39] They treated 110 patients with locally advanced disease with AV for four cycles followed in responders by radiation therapy. The dose of doxorubicin was 75 mg/m^2 intravenously (I.V.) on day 1 and vincristine 1.4 mg/m^2 I.V. on days 1 and 8, every 3 weeks. Patients who were off study at any time for progressive disease or no response received CMF. It should be noted that patients older than 60 years of age were given a lower dose of drugs (doxorubicin 60 mg/m^2; methotrexate 30 mg/m^2; 5-fluorouracil 400 mg/m^2). After radiation therapy was complete, patients who had no evidence of disease were randomized to maintenance chemotherapy with six more cycles of chemotherapy or to observation only. The regimen consisted of AV for patients achieving a complete response (CR) or partial response (PR) during induction and CMF for patients achieving less than a PR. The objective response rate to induction chemotherapy was 70 percent, with 15.5 percent CR and 54.5 percent PR. The median disease-free survival of all patients was 19 months for those who received maintenance and 11 months for those who did not ($p = 0.02$). The three-year survival was 52 percent for all patients. This was a significant improvement in survival compared historically to treatment with local therapy alone. Zucali et al. had reported a 3-year survival of 40.7 percent with radiation alone ($p = 0.02$).[136] This study concluded that the additional chemotherapy increased overall survival, and maintenance chemotherapy increased the disease-free survival.

DeLena et al. followed this study with another in an attempt to determine the optimal local therapy regimen for locally advanced patients after induction chemotherapy.[38] The objective of the study was to determine whether surgery combined with chemotherapy could improve local control and survival compared with radiation and chemotherapy. A total of 132 women with LABC (excluding those with inflammatory disease or supraclavicular nodal involvement) were treated with three cycles of induction chemotherapy. This consisted of doxorubicin 60 mg/m^2 I.V. on day 1 and vincristine 1.2 mg/m^2 I.V. on days 1 and 8 repeated every 3 weeks. Doxorubicin was decreased to 50 mg/m^2 after local therapy for a total of seven more cycles. Patients who had no objective response or who experienced progression of disease during induction received CMF. Prior to induction chemotherapy patients were randomized to radiotherapy (group A, 57 patients) or to mastectomy (group B, 51 patients). Fifty percent of patients in group A had an objective response to induction therapy (one percent CR, 49 percent PR), whereas 54 percent of those in group B had objective responses (six percent CR, 48 percent PR). The median duration of remission was 22 months for group A and 15 months for group B ($p = 0.58$). The median survival was 48 months for both groups. The locoregional recurrence rate was

equivalent in the two groups: 31 percent in group A vs. 30 percent for group B. This study concluded that the modality of local therapy affected neither survival nor local control.

Perloff et al. reported the results of a randomized study in 113 evaluable patients with stage III breast carcinoma.[101] Patients with clinical T3 N0 disease were excluded. All patients were treated with three monthly cycles of cyclophosphamide (100 mg/m^2 orally, days 1–14), doxorubicin (25 mg/m^2 I.V., days 1 and 8), 5-fluorouracil (500 mg/m^2 I.V., days 1 and 8), vincristine (1.4 mg/m^2 I.V., days 1 and 8), and prednisone (P) (40 mg/m^2 orally, days 1–14). If patients were operable they were randomized to either surgery or radiation therapy followed in either case with 2 years of CAFVP (with methotrexate substituted for doxorubicin after a total dose of 550 mg/m^2).

The objective of this study was to determine the modality of therapy for optimal local control. After induction therapy, there was a 69 percent objective response rate in the 113 patients. Eighty-one percent (91 patients) were eligible for randomization, but four refused. There were 43 patients randomized to surgery and 44 to radiation therapy. The duration of disease control was similar in either arm, with a median relapse-free survival of 29.2 months for surgically treated patients and 24.4 months for those receiving radiation ($p = 0.50$). The median survival was 39.3 months for surgery vs. 39 months for radiation. The doses of drugs given did not vary significantly by treatment arm. The local recurrence rate was 19 percent after surgical treatment and 27 percent after radiation therapy. Conclusions from this study agree with those of DeLena et al.,[38] though the prognosis of patients in the Perloff et al. study as a whole was poorer (DeLena et al. excluded inflammatory patients and included T3 N0 patients). However, these studies both point out that the modality of local therapy does not affect survival, and future directions should include systemic treatments that will affect drug-resistant tumor cells.

Several studies have attempted to determine optimal therapy for operable stage III breast cancer. These studies evaluated the use of adjuvant chemotherapy, radiation, or a combination of both in this group of patients.

Spangenberg et al. randomized 131 operable stage III patients to either radiation therapy followed by mono-chemotherapy for 2 years (B1) or polychemotherapy alone for 2 years (B2).[116] Patients with N2 nodes, N3 nodes, peau d'orange, or thoracic wall fixation were excluded. The B1 arm received cyclophosphamide 1500 mg I.V. postoperatively, 1000–1500 mg I.V. 1 week later, 500 mg orally 1 week for 6 weeks, then 250–500 mg orally weekly for 2 years. The B2 arm consisted of cyclophosphamide 900 mg/m^2, 5-fluorouracil 1000 mg I.V., vinblastine 8 mg/m^2 I.V., and methotrexate 2.5 mg orally every 6 hours, for 2 days postoperatively, followed by cyclophosphamide 500 mg/m^2 I.V. 1 week later and then 500 mg/week orally, methotrexate 2.5 mg orally every 6 hr for 1 day a week or month, 5-fluorouracil 1000 mg I.V. every 6 weeks, and vinblastine 10 mg I.V.

every 6 weeks (all for 2 years). All patients also received either additive or ablative hormonal therapy. The 5-year survival of the B1 group was 62.5 percent vs. 56.3 percent for B2. The 5-year DFS was 40.4 percent for B1 and 22.5 percent for B2 [not significant (NS)]. The 5-year local recurrence rate was 11.7 percent for B1 and 22.5 percent for B2 (NS). The conclusions were that polychemotherapy did not increase survival in operable patients. The doses actually received by patients are not presented in this paper. Problems with this study are that most of the chemotherapy is oral, and the issue of compliance is not addressed. Also, both of the regimens given have a very low dose intensity.

Papaioannou et al. designed a study to determine optimal local treatment for patients with LABC after induction chemotherapy.[95] Patients were randomized to receive either postoperative radiation therapy or no therapy. Patients with inflammatory cancer, satellite skin nodules, arm edema, or extensive (more than one third of the breast) peau d'orange, erythema, or ulceration were excluded. There were 205 patients entered, with 78 patients (38 percent) excluded entirely from analysis and 22 others with <6 months follow-up, which seriously affects the validity of the study. Forty-two patients assigned to the radiation and mastectomy arm were excluded, with 14 patients refusing radiation. Thirty-six patients assigned to mastectomy alone were excluded. Also, more patients in the radiation arm had negative nodes and fewer patients had four or more positive nodes. The planned treatment was two cycles of preoperative chemotherapy with CAVMF plus hormonal manipulation, and mastectomy, with one group to then receive RT and the other no RT. After local therapy, ten additional cycles of chemotherapy were given along with tamoxifen in all patients. The crude recurrence rates were similar: 21 percent for no RT and 27 percent for RT (NS). Local recurrence was also similar, with 10.5 percent for no RT and 8.3 percent for RT. The results of this study as a randomized comparison should be seriously questioned because of the large number of exclusions, and no firm conclusions should be drawn.

Gröhn et al.[53] and Klefström et al.[71] have reported the results of a randomized study in patients with operable stage III disease (T3 N0–N2). Patients were randomized to receive postoperative RT (40 patients), chemotherapy (CT) (40 patients), or a combination (RT + CT) (39 patients). Chemotherapy consisted of six cycles of VAC with or without levamisole. Half of the radiation alone patients received levamisole as immunotherapy. The doses of chemotherapy were vincristine 1.2 mg/m² I.V. day 1, doxorubicin 45 mg/m² I.V. day 1, and cyclophosphamide 200 mg/m² orally for 5 days, all every 4 weeks. The 5-year results as reported by Klefström follow. The crude 5-year DFS was 20 percent for RT, 30 percent for CT, and 67 percent for RT + CT. There was a significant DFS (p <0.001) and overall survival benefit (p <0.001) in those patients who received a combination of RT and CT compared with groups receiving either CT or RT alone. Also the 5-year analysis revealed a significant DFS benefit in those patients allocated to levamisole (60 patients received

levamisole and 59 patients did not; p = 0.035), but there was not a significant benefit in survival. The investigators stated that the numbers were too small to make absolute conclusions, but there was a trend toward increased DFS in the RT + CT + immunotherapy arm, suggesting benefit from the combination.

A prospective randomized adjuvant study was reported in operable stage III breast carcinoma by Alagaratnam and Wong.[3] All patients had a total mastectomy followed by radiation therapy. Three weeks after patients completed radiation therapy, they were randomized to receive either tamoxifen 40 mg/d until relapse or cyclophosphamide (500 mg/m² day 1), doxorubicin (50 mg/m² day 1), and 5-fluorouracil (500 mg/m² day 1 and 8) repeated every 3 weeks for nine or ten cycles. There was no significant DFS difference between treatment arms. The median disease-free survivals determined from graphs shown in the paper was about 35 months for patients receiving tamoxifen and 28 months for patients receiving FAC. The problem with this study is that the patients included may not have been consecutive patients. It is not stated in the paper how patients were chosen for randomization and how many refused. To assure more reliable results, randomization should occur prior to any treatment or in all treated patients to avoid selection bias.

Results of these randomized studies reveal a modest increase in survival with the use of combination chemotherapy regimens used in conjunction with local therapy. Clearly, the modality of local therapy does not affect overall survival but may affect local control as shown by the studies of DeLena et al.[38] and Perloff et al.[101] The use of more aggressive and intensive chemotherapeutic regimens or novel modalities of therapy are necessary to make a major advancement in this disease.

Nonrandomized Studies. There are many other studies in the literature that treated patients with various subsets of LABC with combination chemotherapy regimens. They are summarized in Table 40–4.* The median time to progression varies from 20.9 to 30 months, with 5-year DFS ranging from 28 to 78 percent depending on stage subset. The overall survival ranges from 38 to 50 months, with 5-year survivals ranging from 38 percent to 80 percent, again depending on the stage subset.

Sheldon et al. presented data suggesting that the addition of chemotherapy to radiation therapy as the primary local treatment resulted in a better RFS.[112] The 5-year RFS of patients treated with chemotherapy was 40 percent vs. 26 percent for those not treated. This study was not prospective or randomized, and patients received a spectrum of chemotherapeutic regimens varying from a single agent to multiple agents. Many patients also received hormonal manipulations.

Conte et al. treated 39 LABC patients with FAC chemotherapy and estrogenic recruitment with diethylstilbesterol (DES) prior to mastectomy.[34] Patients with clinical T3 N0 and T4 N0 disease (except those with inflammatory disease) were excluded. Patients were

---

*References 1, 10, 16, 18, 34, 64–66, 74, 81, 84, 89, 90, 99, 100, 110, 111, 117, and 124.

Table 40–4. COMBINATION CHEMOTHERAPY TREATMENT OF LOCALLY ADVANCED BREAST CANCER: NONRANDOMIZED STUDIES

Investigator (year)	Treatment	Number of Patients	Stage	Follow-up (median)	Median Time to Progression (months)	Median Survival (months)
Loprinzi (1984)[81]	S → CMF ± P ± Tam → RT → CMF(P) + AV	32	III (AJCC)	NA	29.5	>32 3-yr survival, 65%
Hu (1987)[66]	C + CAF/CMF → RT → S → CMF	14	T2N3M0 T3N1–2 T4AN1–2 T4dN1	42	Crude RFS, 43%	Crude OS, 86%

					Projected 5-Year	
					RFS	**OS**
Schwartz (1987)[110]	CMF ± Tam ± A → ± S → ± R → CMF ± Tam ± A	100	T2N2 T3N0–2 T4N0–2	27	responders, 67% nonresponders, 28%	87% 43%
Meek (1983)[84]	CMFP/CMF + RT → ± S → chemo ± A	12	LABC	17	NA	NA
Thalmo (1984)[124]	CAF → S → CAF + RT	16	III	10 (mean)	NA	NA
Morris (1983)[89]	CAF ± V ± P → ± S	12	LABC	>33 months	NA	26.6 (mean)
Aisner (1982)[1]						
Perez (1979)[99]	FAC → RT + FAC → FAC	10	T3N2–3 T4N2–3	14	NA	Crude OS, 50%
Sponzo (1979)[117]	RT → CFP → ± S	6	T3b	NA	NA	NA
	RT → CFP → CFP → ± S	7	T4			
Bitran (1983)[16]	S → RT → CMF	34	LABC (excludes N0–1)	>48	21.4%	NA
Morrow (1986)[90]	CAFTam → S → CAFTam + RT	31	III	24.3	20.9%	42%

Conte (1987)[34]	FAC + Des → S → CMF/FAC + Des	39	T3b–4N1–3	NA	**Actuarial 3-Year**	
					RFS	**OS**
					53.5%	60%
Shanta (1985)[111]	RT + MF endoxan ± OX → S → MEFV	109	III	NA	5-year RFS, 64%	NA

					5-Year	
					RFS	**OS**
					36%	56%
Hery (1986)[64]	AVCF → RT → AVCF ± EMmcM	22	III	>48	36%	ID
Boyages (1988)[18]	A. CA → RT → CMFP ± Tam	35	III and II with	24	36%	38%
	B. S → CA → RT → CMFP ± Tam	34	>10+ nodes	23	29%	>40%
Perloff (1982)[100]	Chem ± RT ± BCG → M RT	17	T3N1–2T4	NA	**5-Year**	
Hortobagyi (1987)[65]						
					RFS	**OS**
	FAC ± BCG or FAC → CMF	48	IIIA	60	78%	80%
	S + RT	126	IIIB		28%	48%
Balawajder (1983)[10]	±TtM/CMF → RT → ±S	108	III		**Actuarial 10-Year**	
					RFS	**OS**
				34 (mean)	14%	14%
					Actuarial 5-Year	
					27%	40%
					Actuarial 5-Year	
	Chem → R → S	30			36%	38%
	Chem → R	23			41%	46%
	R → S	17			21%	44%
	R	38			14%	38%
Koyama (1985)[74]	IA ITA Mmc F or A] S + OX or → IA SCA Mmc F or A] Adrenalectomy C or C Teg Tam or A Teg Tam	55	III (2 stage II)	78	NA	5 year OS, 57%
Swain and Lippman (present series)	CAMFTam Pre → ±S → RT + CAMFTam Pre → CAMFTam Pre	107	III	32	all 30 IIIA 33 IIIB 28	50 ID 43

Abbreviations: A, doxorubicin; AJCC, American Joint Committee on Cancer (all III refer to 1983 staging); BCG, Calmette-Guerin bacillus; C, cyclophosphamide; chemo, various chemotherapy regimens; Des, diethylstilbesterol; E, VP-16; F, 5-fluorouracil; IA, intraarterial; ID, indeterminate; ITA, internal thoracic artery; LABC, locally advanced breast cancer; M, methotrexate; Mmc; mitomycin C; NA, not available; OS, overall survival; OX, oophorectomy; P, prednisone; RFS, relapse-free survival; RT, radiation therapy; S, surgery with mastectomy; SCA, subclavian artery; Tam, tamoxifen; Teg, tegafur; Tt, thiotepa; V, vincristine.

treated with three cycles of DES (1 mg orally days 1–3), followed by 5-fluorouracil (600 mg/m² I.V. day 4), doxorubicin (50 mg/m² I.V. day 4), cyclophosphamide (600 mg/m² I.V. day 4). Patients then underwent radical mastectomy followed by three cycles of DES-FAC alternated with DES-CMF for three cycles. The objective response rate to preoperative chemotherapy was 71.8 percent, with 15.4 percent CR and 56.4 percent PR. The 3-year RFS was 53.5 percent, and survival was 60 percent. The investigators obtained serial Tru-cut biopsy samples prior to the first cycle, on day 4 prior to FAC, and 24 hours after the first FAC cycle in 25 patients to evaluate tumor cell kinetics. The median basal thymidine labeling index (TLI) was 2.8 percent and primer-dependent alpha DNA polymerase (PDP-LI) was 5.6 percent. There was a significant increase in TLI in 39 percent of patients and in PDP-LI in 70 percent of patients after DES, which did not depend on the presence of estrogen receptor. This study suggested that breast cancer cells in vivo were stimulated by estrogen regardless of estrogen receptor status and may be useful in recruiting cells into the cycle, facilitating the effectiveness of cytotoxic therapy.

Hortobagyi et al. reported the results in the treatment of 191 patients with LABC, excluding inflammatory breast carcinoma (174 evaluable patients).[65] These patients were treated between 1974 and 1985. Several changes in the treatment regimen took place during these years. Patients received induction chemotherapy with 5-fluorouracil (500 mg/m² I.V. days 1 and 8), doxorubicin (50 mg/m² I.V. day 1), and cyclophosphamide (500 mg/m² I.V. day 1) every 3 weeks for three to six cycles. Bacillus Calmette-Guerin (BCG) immunotherapy was given to the first 52 patients. Patients with objective responses or nonresponders who were inoperable received radiation therapy alone as the local therapy. The remaining patients received a combination of surgery and radiation. Chemotherapy was given for a total treatment duration of 2 years from 1974 to 1981 (after a total dose of 450 mg/m² doxorubicin, methotrexate was substituted). The maintenance treatment was changed to 1 year after 1981. Of the 174 patients included in the report, 48 had stage IIIA disease and 126 had stage IIIB. The overall objective response rate was 88 percent, with ten percent CR and 78 percent PR. The median follow-up was 60 months (72 months for stage IIIB and 36 months for IIIA). The median RFS for both groups was 29 months, and median survival was 66 months. The actuarial 5-year DFS for stage IIIA patients was 78 percent and for stage IIIB was 28 percent (p <0.002). The actuarial 5-year survival for stage IIIA was 80 percent and for stage IIIB was 48 percent (p = 0.005). The authors concluded that aggressive combination chemotherapy increased the disease-free and overall survival in both stage IIIA and stage IIIB patients compared with historical controls at the same institution treated with local therapy alone.

Two studies have used tamoxifen therapy in LABC. Veronesi et al. treated 46 postmenopausal women with inoperable T3–T4 breast carcinoma (about half had metastatic disease) with tamoxifen 10–20 mg daily for at least 6 weeks.[130] Eight patients (17 percent) had an objective response after the first 6-week evaluation, and a total of 14 (30 percent) had a response noted at subsequent evaluations. There were five patients with inflammatory disease; none had a response. The median survival for the series was 10 months.

Campbell et al. treated 51 postmenopausal women with LABC with tamoxifen 10–20 mg twice a day.[29] Estrogen receptor (ER) values were assessed in 40 patients. There was an objective response rate of 45 percent with seven clinical complete responses (14 percent) and 16 partial responses (31 percent). Sixty-three percent of ER-positive patients responded, whereas 33 percent of ER-negative and 36 percent of ER-unknown patients responded. The median survivals were not given but can be determined from the graphs presented in the paper. The median overall survival of the tamoxifen responders was 48 months and for the nonresponders was 18 months.

These studies report a low overall response rate (17 percent to 31 percent) with tamoxifen alone. This is much lower than that for combination chemotherapy, in which objective responses are seen in up to 98 percent of patients. Also the overall survival with tamoxifen alone is poor in these two studies. Tamoxifen may add to survival, but only after aggressive combination chemotherapy has been given to reduce tumor size.

The use of either radiation therapy or surgical methods alone is clearly inadequate for the treatment of locally advanced breast cancer. The results of these nonrandomized studies again suggest a very small increase in survival with the use of combination chemotherapy compared historically to treatment with local modalities alone.

Recommendations

It is recommended that patients with locally advanced breast cancer be treated aggressively with combination chemotherapy prior to local therapy. A doxorubicin-containing regimen should be used, as response rates are higher in studies using this drug. This should be followed by local therapy with radiation, surgery, or a combination of both. Local therapy should be individualized according to patient response to chemotherapy to obtain the best local control for that patient.

INFLAMMATORY BREAST CARCINOMA

The term "inflammatory breast cancer" was given to this condition of the breast by Lee and Tannenbaum in 1924.[77] They felt that a clear description was necessary so that the condition would be better recognized by all physicians. The following passage is from their description of this disease:[77]

". . . the breast of the affected side usually increases in size. . . . This enlargement is more often diffuse. . . . As the disease progresses the skin becomes deep red or reddish-purple and to the touch is brawny and infiltrated. The inflamed areas present a distinct raised periphery after the fashion of erysipelas."

In their paper, Lee and Tannenbaum described 28 cases of inflammatory breast carcinoma. They concluded that this was a distinct entity that was frequently mistaken for other diseases of the breast. In addition to the characteristic clinical signs, the pathology of the tumor varied and was not of any specific histology, and the distinct pathological feature was dermal lymphatic invasion.

Since this report, various investigators have also described this disease and confirmed these findings. Haagensen described one of the largest earlier series of patients with this disease.[55] His clinical findings are used by many as the classic criteria for the diagnosis and will be described in the following section.

Inflammatory carcinoma is uncommon and comprises one percent to four percent of most individual series.* The age at which inflammatory breast cancer is diagnosed is similar to that for the more common invasive breast carcinoma, with mean ages ranging from 45 to 54 years. This disease has also been reported in a 12-year-old child[30] and in males[127] but is extremely rare in these groups. The incidence of inflammatory breast cancer, which also includes "occult" inflammatory cancer, in the black population was 10.1 percent in the Surveillance, Epidemiology, and End Results (SEER) data.[78] This is substantially higher than that for white and other non-white patients.

Clinical Features

The breast is reddened and edematous, especially in the dependent part or inferior aspect. The color changes vary from reddish-purple to reddish-brown to faint pink, which may be mottled. These changes can occur beyond the normal extent of the breast. The breast is enlarged and frequently does not have an associated mass. At times the breast may feel warm and tender to the touch. Nipple retraction may be present later in the course of the disease.

Haagensen described the clinical features of this disease in his series of 89 patients.[55] The diagnosis was not made unless at least one third of the breast had redness or edema. A tumor mass was present in 57 percent of patients, erythema in 57 percent, breast enlargement in 48 percent, edema of the skin in 13 percent, warmth of the skin in eight percent, nipple retraction in 13 percent, and pain in 29 percent.

Other reports describe two types of inflammatory carcinoma: primary and secondary. Taylor and Meltzer described the primary type, with features matching Haagensen's description.[123] The secondary type, also reported by Taylor and Meltzer, occurred in a breast with a localized tumor present for some time with the eventual occurrence of inflammatory signs late in the course of the disease.

---

*References 11, 42, 43, 55, 62, 77, 82, 87, 93, 103, 119, and 123.

Pathology

There is no consistent histological type of breast carcinoma associated with inflammatory breast disease. The histology ranges from infiltrating ductal to medullary. Haagensen's series of 40 patients included 19 (47 percent) with the large cell undifferentiated type.[58]

In 1887 Bryant made the initial observation that dermal lymphatic invasion by tumor was present in inflammatory carcinoma.[23] This was also reported by other investigators making it an integral part of the diagnosis. Some have found involvement of subepidermal capillaries or venules, but most authors agree that the disease is primarily of the lymphatic vessels. Lymphatic blockage with subsequent capillary congestion is thought to be responsible for the edema and erythema seen clinically.

A controversy exists in the literature as to whether inflammatory carcinoma is a clinical or pathological diagnosis. Several investigators have attempted to define the disease more specifically. Ellis and Teitelbaum in 1974 proposed the name "dermal lymphatic carcinomatosis of the breast" and suggested making the presence of dermal lymphatic invasion mandatory for the diagnosis.[44] They reviewed the literature of all patients diagnosed with inflammatory cancer who were disease free at 5 years. They found eight such patients, seven of whom had pathological material available for review at the Mayo Clinic. Four of these seven had lymphatic invasion in the breast tumor, and six had axillary nodal involvement. The skin of the breast of four patients was found not to contain carcinoma in the dermal lymphatics. Slides of skin were not available from three patients, two of whom were still disease free. Therefore six patients were disease free, and four of these patients had negative skin biopsy results. Two other patients were described, one for whom no pathological material was available, and one who had no evidence of dermal lymphatic invasion. Ellis and Teitelbaum concluded that an improved disease-free survival was seen if no dermal lymphatic invasion was present.

Saltzstein in 1974[106] described four patients who had no clinical evidence of inflammatory carcinoma but had dermal lymphatic invasion histologically. These patients all died rapidly. He suggested the term "clinically occult inflammatory carcinoma" and concluded that inflammatory carcinoma was a histological rather than clinical diagnosis.

Lucas and Perez-Mesa attempted to clarify this controversy in a retrospective review of inflammatory carcinoma.[82] They found 79 patients and excluded 21 because of inadequate material, leaving 58 patients with clinical inflammatory disease and an additional 15 with "occult" disease. They also included patients with secondary inflammatory carcinoma if they had had an acute onset of inflammation in a breast with a long-standing tumor. Thirty-nine patients with clinical and pathological evidence of inflammatory carcinoma had a median survival of about 16 months; 19 with clinical signs alone had a median survival of about 14 months; and 15 with pathological evidence alone had a better median survival of about 40 months. These patients were not treated homogeneously but with different modalities of therapy, both local and systemic. These investigators concluded that patients with clinical evidence of inflammation regardless of pathological findings had an equally poor prognosis and therefore were justifiably included in the diagnosis of inflammatory carcinoma.

Finally, Levine et al. presented the SEER data in an attempt to make the criteria for the diagnosis more uniform.[78] There were 153 patients with both clinical and pathological diagnoses, with a 3-year relative survival rate of 34 percent; 2937 patients with clinical features alone had a 3-year survival rate of 60 percent; and 81 patients with pathological features alone had a 3-year survival of 52 percent. This suggests that the prognosis is better for those patients with a clinical diagnosis alone. The shortcomings of this analysis include the fact that it was a retrospective review, the data are from many different investigators, many clinical characteristics may not have been noted, skin biopsies were not routinely done, and patients were treated with many different modalities of therapy.

Classification

Inflammatory breast carcinoma is a T4 tumor by the standard TNM staging classification of the UICC and AJCC.[15, 63] This is considered stage IIIB breast carcinoma (see Table 40–1). The Columbia Clinical Classification of Haagensen classifies inflammatory breast carcinoma as Stage D.[59]

Investigators at the Institut Gustave-Roussy (Villejuif, France) have created a classification with the name of "poussee evolutirie" (PEV) for breast cancer that differs from the TNM staging.[75] This classification is descriptive and takes recent tumor growth and inflammatory signs into consideration. The PEV categories are defined as follows: PEV0, a tumor without recent increase in volume and without inflammatory signs; PEV1, a tumor showing marked increase in volume during the past 2 months but without inflammatory signs; PEV2, a tumor whose overlying breast tissue, skin in particular, is affected by subacute inflammation and edema involving less than one half of the breast surface; and PEV3, a tumor with acute or subacute inflammation and edema involving more than one half of the breast surface.

Prognostic Factors

The most important factor in breast cancer is the presence and extent of axillary nodal involvement with carcinoma; nodal disease is indicative of systemic microscopic metastatic disease. An overwhelming majority of inflammatory breast cancer patients not only have nodal involvement microscopically but also have clinically involved nodes. Haagensen described axillary nodal involvement in 100 percent of his 30 patients treated by radical mastectomy.[55] In his larger series, 81 of 89 patients had clinically involved nodes, with 50 percent

of these having massive nodes or nodes greater than 2.5 cm.[55] Taylor and Meltzer's 25 patients with primary inflammatory cancer included ten with supraclavicular nodal involvement.[123] Other reports also substantiate the high incidence of axillary nodal involvement in this disease.[43, 55, 77, 87, 103, 123]

The number of patients with inflammatory cancer who also have distant metastatic disease evident at diagnosis is higher than for the more common breast carcinomas.[19, 37, 55, 78, 123] Taylor and Meltzer found visceral or bone metastases in nine (36 percent) of their primary inflammatory patients.[123] Haagensen reported that 15 of his 89 patients (17 percent) had distant metastases at presentation (nine lung, five bone, and one brain metastases).[55] The most extensive report is the SEER report, revealing metastatic disease at diagnosis in 24 percent of 3171 white patients with inflammatory carcinoma diagnosed from 1975 to 1981.[78] The range of 17 percent to 36 percent for metastatic disease at diagnosis far exceeds that for other presentations of apparently localized breast cancer at diagnosis (about five percent).[78]

Treatment

Surgery

Taylor and Meltzer in 1938 treated six patients with primary inflammatory breast carcinoma with radical mastectomy.[123] These patients all developed either local, regional, or contralateral breast recurrences fairly rapidly. The average survival was 21 months, with a range of 11 to 34 months. Haagensen's 30 patients treated by radical mastectomy had a mean survival of 19 months. The only 5-year survivor experienced recurrence and died 68 months after surgery. Haagensen became convinced that radical mastectomy should not be performed in any patients with inflammatory disease and abandoned this method of treatment.

Several other physicians treating inflammatory carcinoma patients with radical mastectomy report equally poor results.[19, 33, 87, 119] Treves stated in 1959 that radical mastectomy was contraindicated in this disease based on the results of six reports in the literature.[128] In his review of 114 patients in whom radical mastectomy was performed, four patients (3.5 percent) were alive at 5 years.

Radiation Therapy

Many physicians in the late 1800s and early 1900s noted that when inflammatory breast cancer presented, it was frequently at a point that precluded surgical treatment alone. Therefore many patients were treated by radiation therapy alone.

Wang and Griscom treated a series of 33 patients with inflammatory breast cancer with radiation alone from 1944 to 1959.[133] Six of these had metastatic disease. Twenty-three of the patients were treated with orthovoltage radiation and ten with supervoltage radiation. Radiation therapy with orthovoltage treatment resulted in a mean survival of 14.3 months, and supervoltage treatment resulted in a mean survival of 30 months.

Chu et al. treated 62 inflammatory breast cancer patients with radical radiotherapy.[32] Fourteen patients also received hormonal manipulation, and 20 received adjuvant chemotherapy (four single agent, 16 CMFVP or CMF). The mean survival for the 28 patients who were treated by radiation therapy alone was 28 months and for the whole group was 24 months (median, 18 months).

Mean survivals in patients with LABC treated with radiation as the primary modality of therapy (some series also included hormonal manipulation) ranged from 4 to 28.5 months.* It can be seen that radiation therapy alone has little impact on survival.

Surgery and Radiation Therapy

The combination of surgery and radiation therapy has been used in inflammatory breast cancer in an effort to improve local control. Perez and Fields treated 12 patients with radiation and mastectomy.[99] The median DFS was 24 months, and median overall survival was 42 months. The mean survival from several other series ranged from 7 to 29.0 months.† Thus overall survival is still very low with the combination of radiation therapy and mastectomy. These survival rates are not significantly different from those for patients treated with either surgery or radiation therapy alone.

Combination Chemotherapy

It is clear that inflammatory breast carcinoma is a systemic disease at diagnosis, and local therapy alone is inadequate for treatment. Several investigators have treated this disease with a combination of different modalities of therapy such as hormonal manipulation or chemotherapy. However, these were not tested systematically until the early 1970s. The results of studies in the literature treating inflammatory breast cancer patients with combination chemotherapy regimens are seen in Table 40–5.

DeLena et al. began a randomized trial in LABC at the National Cancer Institute in Milan in 1973,[39] treating patients with AV prior to local therapy (the chemotherapy regimen is described in the combination chemotherapy section under "Noninflammatory Locally Advanced Disease"). There were 36 patients with inflammatory disease who achieved a 67 percent objective response to induction chemotherapy. There were seven complete responses (20 percent) and 17 partial responses (47 percent). The median survival for the inflammatory group was 25 months and 3-year survival was 25 percent; this includes patients who did and who did not receive maintenance chemotherapy. These results were not significantly different from those with radiation alone (3-year survival of 28 percent). Though this study did not

show a benefit for inflammatory carcinoma patients treated with chemotherapy compared with historical controls treated with radiation alone, it did suggest that maintenance chemotherapy increased disease-free survival in LABC overall. As noted previously, 16 of the inflammatory carcinoma patients were postmenopausal and had a substantial dose reduction. Also, not all inflammatory carcinoma patients received maintenance therapy. Therefore these data are not conclusive for inflammatory carcinoma patients but did stimulate other investigators to take a more aggressive approach with chemotherapy in treating this disease.

Buzdar et al. reported the results of combination chemotherapy treatment in 32 patients with inflammatory breast cancer at M. D. Anderson between 1973 and 1977.[27] The results were compared with an historical control group of 32 patients treated with radiation alone at the same institution. The treatment regimen consisted of 5-fluorouracil (500 mg/m^2 I.V. day 1 and 8, doxorubicin (50 mg/m^2 I.V. day 1), cyclophosphamide (500 mg/m^2 I.V. day 1) plus BCG (6 × 10^8 organisms by scarification days 9, 13, and 17) every 3 weeks for three or four cycles. Patients then received radiation therapy with twice-daily fractionation. The radiation consisted of 5100 rad to the breast and to the supraclavicular and internal mammary nodes, with a boost to the entire breast and skin. Patients then received 2 years of maintenance chemotherapy. The median follow-up was 62 months. The median disease-free interval was 22.8 months for the chemotherapy treated group compared with 9 months for the historical controls. The median survival was 30.1 months for those patients receiving chemotherapy and 18 months for the controls. There were locoregional failures in 26 percent of chemotherapy treated patients who received twice-daily fractionation, compared with 43 percent in the patients treated historically with once-daily fractionation radiation. The difference in local control was believed to be a result of the twice-daily fractionation.

Fastenberg et al. updated this series to include 63 patients treated from 1973 to 1981 at M. D. Anderson.[45] Fifty patients received 5-fluorouracil, doxorubicin, and cyclophosphamide (FAC) and immunotherapy, 12 received other doxorubicin-containing regimens, and one received CMF. Most patients were also treated with radiation therapy. In addition, 21 had a simple mastectomy during their primary treatment, and seven of these did not receive consolidative radiation therapy. The median follow-up was 60 months. Patients received a median of three cycles of chemotherapy. After demonstrating no further improvement on physical examination, patients treated after the initial report were treated by mastectomy. Fifty patients (87 percent) received maintenance chemotherapy first with FAC and then with CMF for 2 years. The objective response to induction therapy was 68 percent, with 14 percent CR and 54 percent PR. The median DFS was 24 months, with a median survival of 43 months. Evaluation of patients according to dermal lymphatic invasion on skin biopsy revealed a median DFS of 31 months for patients with positive biopsy samples (16 patients) and 46 months for

---

*References 12, 21, 32, 33, 35, 43, 58, 62, 77, 87, 94, 98, 102–104, 119, 123, 128, 133, and 136.
†References 11, 13, 19, 33, 43, 58, 77, 94, 98, 102, 103, and 131.

Table 40–5. COMBINATION CHEMOTHERAPY TREATMENT OF INFLAMMATORY BREAST CARCINOMA

Investigator (year)		Chemotherapy Regimen	Number of Patients	Median Time to Progression (months)	Median Survival (months)
Fastenberg (1985)[45]		FAC	63	24	43
DeLena (1978)[39]		AV	36	NA	25
Schäfer (1987)[108]		Chlorambucil + MAF	21 (15 primary, 6 secondary)	NA	43
Loprinzi (1984)[81]		CMF P ± Tam alt. AV ± Tam	9 (32 total)	29.5 (all)	>25
Burton (1987)[25]		CAFV	22	16.4	23.6
Pawlicki (1983)[97]		CMVF	72 (Total 87 LABC)	3-year RFS, 10%	3 year OS, 28%
Zylberberg (1982)[137]		CAVF + Mel + BCG	15	66% crude RFS	ID >56
Israël (1986)[68]		High-dose C + F	25	33	ID
Keiling (1985)[70]		CAVF + Mel	41	58 mo, RFS 54%	58 mo, OS 63%
				3-Year RFS	**3-Year OS**
	A. B.	CEpiVF ⎤ CEpiVF ⎦ + VindMTt	18 19	A. 86% B. 58%	A. 86% B. 77%
Schwartz (1987)[110]		CMF ± Tam ± A	17	NA	5-year OS, >85%
Knight (1986)[73]		CF + P	18	NA	23
Fowble (1986)[49]		CMFPTam or CAF	16 (19 total)	3-year RFS, 65%	3-year OS, 84%
Hagelberg (1984)[62]		CMF 8 CAVF 6 Misc (4)	18 (5 M1)	NA	38
Jacquillat (1987)[69]		Vel Tt + MFA + Tam	66 (+29 T3N1b)	**Observed 4-Year** RFS, 73%	OS, 62%
Perloff (1988)[101]		CAFVP	14	17.5	26.9
Conte (1987)[34]		Des + FAC	14	15	NA
Noguchi (1988)[93]	IA a)	ITA FMmc ⎤ -C SCA FMmc ⎦	14	**RFS** 5-year, 59%	**OS** 5-year, 63%
	IA b)	ITA A ⎤ -CTam Teg (9) SCA A ⎦ ATam Teg (5) (premenopausal OX) (postmenopausal adrenalectomy) in 2 patients	14	10-year, 53%	10-year, 47%
Perez (1987)[98]	a) b)	FAC + RT FAC + S + RT	23 32	18 41	25 46
Chevallier (1987)[31]		CMF → AVCF	64	19	32
Brun (1988)[22]		AVCF	26	12	31
				4-Year RFS	**4-Year OS**
Rouësse (1986)[104]	a) b)	AVM + VCF AVCMF + AVM + VCF	91 79	28% 46%	44% 66%
Swain and Lippman (present series)		CAMF + Tam Pre	45	23	36

Abbreviations: A, doxorubicin; Alt, alternately; BCG, Calmette-Guerin bacillus; C, cyclophosphamide; Des, diethylstilbesterol; Epi, epidoxorubicin; F, 5-fluorouracil; IA, intraarterial; ID, indeterminate; ITA, internal thoracic artery; LABC, locally advanced breast cancer; M, methotrexate; M1, metastases; Mmc, mitomycin C; Mel, melphalan; NA, not available; OS, overall survival; OX, oophorectomy; P, prednisone; Pre, premarin; RFS, relapse-free survival; RT, radiation therapy; S, surgery; SCA, subclavian artery; Tam, tamoxifen; Teg, tegafur; Tt, thiotepa; V, vincristine; Vel, vinblastine; Vind, vindesine.

patients with negative biopsy samples (ten patients) (*p* = 0.45). Evaluation of patients according to response to induction therapy revealed a DFS of 31 months for responders, which was significantly better than for non-responders (*p* = 0.01). This study concluded that disease-free and overall survival were improved with the use of combination chemotherapy when compared with local modalities alone. Also, since there was no difference in DFS according to the presence or absence of

dermal lymphatic invasion on skin biopsy, it was concluded that a clinical diagnosis of inflammatory breast cancer in itself portended a poor patient prognosis.

Another large nonrandomized series of patients treated for inflammatory breast cancer was reported by Perez and Fields in 1987.[99] The authors compared the treatment outcomes of different combined modality approaches in 95 patients treated at a single institution. A significant benefit in DFS and overall survival (OS) was found in patients receiving chemotherapy in their treatment regimens. The details of the chemotherapy were not given, but it was stated that patients received two or three cycles of FAC prior to mastectomy. The median DFS for patients receiving radiation alone (28 patients) was 8 months, compared with 41 months for patients receiving chemotherapy, surgery, radiation, and more chemotherapy (CSRC) (32 patients, p <0.0001). The median overall survival for radiation alone was 18 months vs. 47 months for the CSRC group (p = 0.0002). There was also a significant increase in survival in patients who received CSRC vs. those who received radiation and chemotherapy alone (23 patients, p = 0.02). Another interesting finding in this series of patients was a decrease in local recurrences in patients treated with a combination of the three modalities of therapy. The local recurrence rate was 16 percent for the CSRC group, 57 percent for the radiation and chemotherapy group, 33 percent for radiation and mastectomy, and 68 percent for radiation alone. However, firm conclusions cannot be drawn from this report, since patients were selected for treatment and not randomized.

The largest series of patients with inflammatory breast carcinoma was reported by Rouessé in 1986 from the Institut Gustave-Roussy in Villejuif, France.[104] This report presented results of treatment of 230 patients with inflammatory breast carcinoma. The difficulty in comparing these findings with those in the North American literature is the different classification system. These physicians used the PEV classification but stated that all patients would have been classified as T4b in the TNM classification. Three different protocols were used. Radiation alone was the treatment from 1973 to 1975 (group C). Group A, treated between 1976 and 1980, received three cycles of doxorubicin (40 mg/m² I.V. day 1), vincristine (1 mg/m² I.V. day 2), and methotrexate (3 mg/m² subcutaneously for six doses every 12 hours beginning day 3) (AVM), all repeated every 3 to 4 weeks prior to radiation for three courses, then one cycle during radiation, and five cycles postirradiation. Group B, treated between 1980 and 1982, received three cycles of doxorubicin (50 mg/m² I.V. day 1), vincristine (0.6 mg/m² I.V. day 2), cyclophosphamide (200 mg/m² intramuscularly (IM) days 3–5, methotrexate (10 mg/m² IM days 3–5), and 5-fluorouracil (300 mg/m² IM day 3–5) every 4 weeks for three courses, followed by radiation with one cycle of the AVM combination, and then five more cycles of AVM. Groups A and B both received maintenance with vincristine (1 mg/m² I.V. day 1), cyclophosphamide (200 mg/m² IM day 2–4), and 5-fluorouracil (300 mg/m² IM day 2–4) every 4 weeks for four to 12 cycles. The median number of maintenance cycles given to group A patients was nine and to group B was ten. Radiation therapy treatment was the same in all three groups. This included 4500 rad to the breast and drainage of lymph nodes with a 2000–3000 rad boost to the tumor. All patients had hormonal manipulation, which consisted of radiocastration for pre- or perimenopausal women and tamoxifen 20 mg daily for 1 year (after 1973) for postmenopausal women.

Patient characteristics were equal in all three groups. There were 60 patients in group C, 91 in group A, and 79 in group B. Patients classified as PEV2 and PEV3 were equally distributed, with 68 percent and 32 percent, respectively, in the control group, 69 percent and 31 percent in group A, and 73 percent and 27 percent in group B.

The objective response rate to induction chemotherapy was 14 percent in group A and 27 percent in group B (p = 0.04). The 4-year DFS and OS, respectively, were 16 percent and 28 percent for group C, 28 percent and 44 percent for group A, and 46 percent and 66 percent for group B, with p < 0.005 in groups C vs. A, p < 0.00001 in groups C vs. B, and p < 0.01 in groups A vs. B. There is a survival difference between groups C vs. A (p = 0.03) and between groups A vs. B (p < 0.001) and groups C vs. B (p = 0.0001). The authors also analyzed DFS and OS in 91 patients who did not relapse either during maintenance chemotherapy or within 3 months of the termination of treatment. They looked at length of administration of maintenance, since patients received differing numbers of cycles. They stated that there was no difference in DFS or OS seen with length of administration of chemotherapy. The data are not shown and are not analyzed by group A vs. group B. The DFS at 4 years for patients classified as PEV2 and PEV3, respectively, for each group were: group C, 8 percent and 0 percent (p = 0.0001); group A, 35 percent and 11 percent (p = 0.005); and group B, 52 percent and 30 percent (p = 0.11). There was an improvement in DFS in the PEV3 group who received more intensive chemotherapy (groups B vs. A, p = 0.03). There was no difference in DFS in the N2–N3 group receiving more intensive chemotherapy: group C, six percent; group A, 18 percent; and group B, 15 percent (NS). However, there was a benefit seen in those patients with N0–N1 disease. The 4-year DFS in group C was six percent, in group A 30 percent, and in group B 53 percent (all p = 0.00001). The majority of patients actually fall into the N0–N1 category: group C, 42 patients (70 percent); group A, 69 patients (76 percent); and group B, 65 patients (82 percent).

The conclusions from the study of Rouessé are that the more aggressive chemotherapy prolonged DFS in patients with PEV3 disease, which is similar to inflammatory carcinoma by TNM classification. Also patients with N0–N1 disease benefited from more dose-intensive chemotherapy. However, patients with a larger disease burden (N2–N3 disease) did not benefit from the more aggressive regimen used in this study. A more intensive induction may be needed for this group.

A different approach was used by Noguchi et al.[93] Patients with inflammatory breast cancer all received intraarterial (IA) infusional chemotherapy, surgical ablation, extended radical mastectomy, and adjuvant chemotherapy (Table 40–5). There were 28 patients treated, with complete histological necrosis of the tumor at mastectomy in 13 patients (46 percent). The median follow-up was 111 months. The local recurrence rate was 32 percent, which was not much different than that seen with radiation therapy and surgery. Leukopenia with WBC < 3000/mm³ occurred in 75 percent of patients treated with IA therapy alone, indicating that there was systemic distribution of the drugs. The median 10-year DFS was 53 percent, and OS was 47 percent.

The issue of whether the presence of dermal lymphatic invasion influences disease-free survival was addressed in two other small studies. Burton et al. treated patients with CAFV chemotherapy and found that the median DFS of patients with carcinoma in dermal lymphatics was 17 months (12 patients) compared with 15 months for those without dermal lymphatic invasion (five patients).[25] In Schafer et al.'s series of 21 patients treated with chlorambucil, methotrexate, 5-fluorouracil, and doxorubicin, the median distant disease–free survival was 22.5 months for patients with dermal lymphatic invasion and 12 months for patients without invasion (NS).[108] Therefore from the evidence presented, it seems that when clinical inflammatory signs are present, dermal lymphatic invasion is not necessary to make the diagnosis.

Table 40–5 includes most series in the literature treating inflammatory carcinoma patients with some combination chemotherapy regimen accompanied by radiation or surgery as local therapy. Response rates varied from 14 percent to 98 percent. Median disease-free survival ranged from 15 to 41 months, with median overall survival ranging from 23 to 46 months. These studies suggest a modest benefit with the addition of systemic therapy, but clearly innovative approaches are warranted.

NATIONAL CANCER INSTITUTE EXPERIENCE

The National Cancer Institute report analyzed 107 patients with locally advanced breast cancer treated at the National Cancer Institute from April 1980 to February 1988 with primary induction chemotherapy, including an attempted hormonal synchronization in 101 patients. Results of this study have been published previously.[115, 121]

The combination regimen of chemotherapy with hormonal synchronization was chosen based on prior studies from our laboratory demonstrating that antiestrogen-induced inhibition of breast cancer cell growth could be reversed by estrogen rescue.[41, 79, 91] Weichselbaum et al.[134] found that this antiestrogen treatment followed by estrogen rescue could increase the sensitivity of breast cancer cells to cytotoxic drug treatment.[134] Green et al. demonstrated by flow cytometry that tamoxifen caused a G_1 arrest in MCF-7 human breast cancer cells in culture.[52] Our laboratory has shown that subsequent estrogen treatment could induce a synchronous wave of DNA synthesis in human breast cancer cells.[2] This strategy was used in the present study prior to the administration of the cell cycle–specific agents methotrexate and 5-fluorouracil, with the hypothesis that tumor cells were synchronized by tamoxifen and recruited by estrogen, therefore making them more susceptible to these cytotoxic drugs. Allegra et al. treated a group of

metastatic breast cancer patients with antiestrogen therapy followed by estrogen rescue plus methotrexate and 5-fluorouracil and reported a complete remission rate of 56 percent.[4] A randomized study from the NCI used CAMF chemotherapy with and without hormonal synchronization in patients with metastatic and inflammatory breast cancer.[80] In this study, 13 of 14 patients with inflammatory breast cancer had an objective response rate of 93 percent, with all of these patients having local decrease only. Four of seven patients with inflammatory nonmetastatic disease treated in the hormonal synchronization arm had clinical complete responses compared with only one of six who did not receive hormonal synchronization. For this reason, hormonal synchronization was chosen for the present study.

Patients were eligible if they had locally advanced breast cancer or stage III disease according to the 1983 American Joint Committee staging classification.[15] The initial 13 patients with inflammatory breast cancer were part of the randomized study in advanced breast cancer comparing chemotherapy with and without attempted hormonal synchronization.[80] Therefore no hormonal synchronization was given to six patients. These initial patients also received different drug doses as described previously.[121] This protocol was closed as a randomized study in June 1983. Subsequent patients were accrued to the hormonal arm of this study. The drug regimen consisted of cyclophosphamide (500 mg/m² I.V. day 1), doxorubicin (30 mg/m² I.V. day 1), tamoxifen (40 mg orally days 2–6), premarin (0.625 mg orally every 12 hours in three doses day 7), methotrexate (300 mg/m² I.V. day 8 followed in 1 hour by 5-fluorouracil, 500 mg/m² I.V. day 8), and leucovorin (10 mg/m² orally every 6 hours in six doses day 9). A 25 percent dose escalation of either methotrexate or 5-fluorouracil in alternate cycles was used to achieve maximum doses of these drugs.

All patients were treated with induction therapy to the point of maximum objective response. If a patient was considered a clinical complete responder, an incisional biopsy was performed at the site of the original lesion. If a negative biopsy sample was obtained, the patient received a course of radical radiotherapy. Patients with residual disease in their biopsy sample or patients achieving a partial response or no change to induction chemotherapy received a total mastectomy with removal of any gross axillary disease followed by a course of radical radiotherapy. All patients continued to receive chemotherapy, with the exclusion of doxorubicin, while radiotherapy was administered. All other patients received chemotherapy for 6 months after local therapy was completed, with doxorubicin included in every cycle. In all cases, total dose of doxorubicin did not exceed 525 mg/m².

At the time of the current analysis, 107 patients have been entered into the study with 102 evaluable patients and a median follow-up of 32 months. There were 47 patients with stage IIIA disease, 56 with stage IIIB disease (45 inflammatory stage IIIB and 11 noninflammatory stage IIIB), and four with stage IV disease.

An overall objective response (CR + PR) occurred

in 97 of 102 patients (95 percent), with 50 CRs (49 percent) and 47 PRs (46 percent); there were five patients with no change (5 percent). No patients progressed while on induction therapy. The median number of cycles to achieve best response was five (range, 2–11) or 3.3 months (range, 6–33 weeks). Response by stage group is shown in Table 40–6.

There are 105 patients evaluable for relapse, with two patients lost to follow-up (one in October 1982 and the other in October 1985). These two patients are excluded from the relapse data but not from disease-free or overall survival data. There have been 42 of 105 patients (40 percent) who have relapsed. Thirteen of 47 (28 percent) stage IIIA patients have relapsed compared with 26 of 54 (48 percent) stage IIIB patients. There have been relapses in 21 of 44 (48 percent) of stage IIIB inflammatory carcinoma patients and in five of ten (50 percent) of IIIB noninflammatory carcinoma patients. Also, three of four stage IV patients (75 percent) have relapsed. The median time to progression for all patients was 30 months (33 months for stage IIIA; 28 months for all IIIB, $p = 0.08$ for IIIA vs. IIIB; 23 months for IIIB inflammatory carcinoma patients; and indeterminate for IIIB noninflammatory). The median survival for all patients was 50 months. The median survival for stage IIIA patients was indeterminate at this time, 43 months for stage IIIB, 39 months for IIIB inflammatory and indeterminate for IIIB noninflammatory ($p > 0.15$).

CONCLUSIONS

Patients with stage IIIA disease and negative lymph nodes have a prognosis that approaches that for patients with stage I or II disease. It is important to investigate novel methods to evaluate these tumors to determine which patients have a higher recurrence rate and therefore also need systemic therapy. One method available at the current time is a measurement of cell kinetics by the thymidine labeling index.[88] Other approaches include the use of DNA flow cytometry to measure cellular DNA content abnormalities[85] or HER2/*neu* oncogene amplication[114] in tumors, both of which have been associated with a poor patient prognosis.

Other patients with stage IIIA disease, such as those with N2 or matted axillary nodes, have a prognosis that is similar to that for patients with stage IIIB disease. Most of these patients will not live for 5 years with the use of local modalities of therapy alone. Patients with inflammatory disease clearly have a grave prognosis also. These patients must be treated with more intensive or altogether different modalities of therapy if there is to be any hope for cure.

Treatment of patients with locally advanced breast carcinoma should consist of an attempt at aggressive systemic eradication of micrometastases along with an optimal local therapy regimen. Radiation therapy and surgical treatment may both be necessary to decrease local recurrence rates, but clearly neither will influence survival. At the present time it is recommended that an intensive combination chemotherapy regimen be used prior to local therapy. This will reduce local tumor burden and thereby optimize local control, eradicate systemic micrometastases, and increase the probability of survival.

FUTURE DIRECTIONS

Future directions in the treatment of locally advanced breast cancer, especially inflammatory breast cancer, include the use of very high dose chemotherapy and autologous marrow transplant, which we have incorporated into our regimen at the National Cancer Institute. Patients with locally advanced disease are ideal candidates for this modality of therapy at the time of best response after induction chemotherapy.

A recent excellent review of all clinical trials using high-dose chemotherapy and autologous marrow transplant has been published by Antman and Gale.[5] They evaluated 27 trials in 172 previously treated and untreated stage IV breast cancer patients. There were 73 patients (previously treated) given high-dose single agent chemotherapy with various drugs, with a complete response rate of five percent and partial response rate of 26 percent. There were 40 patients treated with high-dose combination chemotherapy or single agent chemotherapy combined with radiation, with a 25 percent CR rate and 48 percent PR rate. The median duration of response ranged from 2 to more than 16 months. Six studies were evaluated that included 59 previously untreated patients with inflammatory or stage IV disease to whom high-dose single agent or combination chemotherapy was given with autologous bone marrow transplant. Three studies used high-dose therapy only, and the other three administered an induction regimen prior to high-dose therapy. The objective response rate was 81 percent, with 64 percent CR and 17 percent PR. The median duration of response ranged from 3 to 8 months, which does not differ significantly from that seen in stage IV patients treated with conventional chemotherapy. There were also six early deaths (ten percent) resulting from toxicity. The authors' conclusions were that single or multiple agent high-dose chemotherapy with or without radiation produced responses in a substantial number of patients resistent to more conventional doses. The use of high-dose therapy with autologous bone marrow support may best be used earlier in the disease rather than at a point at which there are

Table 40–6. CLINICAL RESPONSE BY STAGE TO INDUCTION CHEMOTHERAPY

Stage	Number of Patients (%)		
	CR	PR	CR + PR
IIIA	23 (52)	18 (41)	41 (93)
IIIB	27 (50)	25 (46)	52 (96)
Inflammatory	24 (55)	19 (43)	43 (98)
Noninflammatory	3 (30)	6 (60)	9 (90)
IV	0	4 (100)	4 (100)

Abbreviations: CR, complete response; PR, partial response.

widespread metastases and a large tumor burden. If used at this time, disease-free and overall survival may be prolonged.

One problem with high-dose chemotherapy is severe and prolonged myelosuppression with resultant infections and treatment-related deaths. There has been interest recently in using granulocyte-macrophage colony-stimulating factor (GM-CSF) to accelerate hematopoietic recovery in the setting of high-dose therapy to reduce treatment-related toxicity. Recombinant human GM-CSF has been shown to promote proliferation of granulocyte-macrophage progenitor cells.[86]

Brandt et al. have published a phase I study using recombinant human GM-CSF after high-dose chemotherapy with cyclophosphamide, carmustine, and cisplatin in 19 patients with breast cancer and melanoma.[20] The mean granulocyte count at day 15 (the end of GM-CSF) was significantly higher in these patients than in controls (1160 ± 1030 vs. 318 ± 314; $p = 0.0035$). Though these results are very preliminary, the study suggests that GM-CSF may be helpful in accelerating myeloid recovery, thereby decreasing treatment-related toxicity. This promising therapy is receiving much more evaluation in well-designed prospective studies at the present time.

Other future directions in the treatment of breast cancer are in the use of techniques to block the action of growth factors such as transforming growth factor α (TGFα). TGFα is stimulated by estrogen treatment in vitro in breast cancer cell lines[14] and may be an important autostimulatory component in the growth regulation of breast cancer. New therapies may be designed to interrupt TGFα by antibodies to the growth factor or its receptor.

Another growth factor important in the biology and regulation of breast cancer is insulin-like growth factor I (IGF-I), which is stimulated by estrogen treatment.[67] Future chemotherapeutic approaches could utilize anti–growth factor receptor molecules conjugated with toxins to tumor-specific agents. These approaches have produced encouraging results in animal model systems.[96, 132]

Transforming growth factor β (TGFβ) inhibits the growth of many normal and transformed cells. It is increased by the antiestrogen tamoxifen and may be responsible for the inhibition of growth of breast cancer that is seen clinically with the use of tamoxifen.[72] TGFβ also inhibits estrogen-independent cell lines in vitro and may have effects on stromal proliferation[40] and bone resorption.[122] It is possible that this growth factor may be utilized in the future in breast cancer treatment.

References

1. Aisner J, Morris D, Elias EG, Wiernik PH: Mastectomy as an adjuvant to chemotherapy for locally advanced or metastatic breast cancer. Arch Surg 117:882–886, 1982.
2. Aitken SC, Lippman ME: Hormonal regulation of net DNA synthesis in MCF-7 human breast cancer cells in tissue culture. Cancer Res 42:1727–1735, 1982.
3. Alagaratnam TT, Wong J: Tamoxifen versus chemotherapy as adjuvant treatment in stage III breast cancer. Aust N Z J Surg 56:39–41, 1986.
4. Allegra JC, Woodcock TM, Richman SP, et al: A phase II trial of tamoxifen, premarin, methotrexate and 5-fluorouracil in metastatic breast cancer. Breast Cancer Res Treat 2:93–100, 1982.
5. Antman K, Gale RP: Advanced breast cancer: high-dose chemotherapy and bone marrow autotransplant. Ann Int Med 108:570–574, 1988.
6. Ariel IM: Results of 1178 patients with breast cancer treated by radical mastectomy and postoperative irradiation where metastases to axillary lymph nodes occurred. J Surg Oncol 12:137, 1979.
7. Arnold DJ, Lesnick GJ: Survival following mastectomy for stage III breast cancer. Am J Surg 137:362–366, 1979.
8. Atkins HL, Horrigan WD: Treatment of locally advanced carcinoma of the breast with roentgen therapy and simple mastectomy. Cancer 85:860–864, 1961.
9. Baclesse F: Five-year results in 431 breast cancers treated solely by roentgen rays. Ann Surg 161:103–104, 1965.
10. Balawajder I, Antich PP, Boland J: An analysis of the role of radiotherapy alone and in combination with chemotherapy and surgery in the management of advanced breast carcinoma. Cancer 15:574–580, 1983.
11. Barber KW, Dockerty MB, Clagett OT: Inflammatory carcinoma of the breast. Surg Gynecol Obstet 112:406–410, 1961.
12. Barker JL, Montague ED, Peters LJ: Clinical experience of irradiation of inflammatory carcinoma of the breast with and without elective chemotherapy. Cancer 45:625–629, 1980.
13. Barker JL, Nelson AJ, Montague ED: Inflammatory carcinoma of the breast. Radiology 121:173–176, 1976.
14. Bates S, McManaway ME, Lippman ME, Dickson RB: Characterization of estrogen responsive transforming activity in human breast cancer cell lines. Cancer Res 46:1707–1713, 1986.
15. Beahrs OH, Myers MH (eds): Manual for Staging of Cancer, ed 2. Philadelphia, JB Lippincott, 1983, pp 127–135.
16. Bitran JD, Desser RK, Schifeling D, et al: Multimodality therapy of stage III adenocarcinoma of the breast. J Surg Oncol 22:5–8, 1983.
17. Bouchard J: Advanced cancer of the breast treated primarily with irradiation. Radiology 84:823–842, 1965.
18. Boyages J, Langlands AO: The efficacy of combined chemotherapy and radiotherapy in advanced non-metastatic breast cancer. Int J Radiat Oncol Biol Phys 14:71–78, 1988.
19. Bozzetti F, Saccozzi R, DeLena M, Salvadori B: Inflammatory cancer of the breast: analysis of 114 cases. J Surg Oncol 18:355–361, 1981.
20. Brandt SJ, Peters WP, Atwater SK, et al: Effect of recombinant human granulocyte-macrophage colony-stimulating factor on hematopoietic reconstitution after high-dose chemotherapy and autologous bone marrow transplantation. New Engl J Med 318:869–876, 1988.
21. Bruckman JE, Harris JR, Levene MB, et al: Results of treating stage III carcinoma of the breast by primary radiation therapy. Cancer 43:985–993, 1979.
22. Brun B, Otmezguine Y, Feuilhade F, et al: Treatment of inflammatory breast cancer with combination chemotherapy and mastectomy versus breast conservation. Cancer 61:1096–1103, 1988.
23. Bryant T: Diseases of the Breast. London, Cassell and Co Ltd, 1887, pp 171–194.
24. Bucalossi P, Veronesi V, Zingo L, et al: Enlarged mastectomy for breast cancer: review of 1213 cases. Am J Roentgenol Radium Ther Nucl Med 111:119–122, 1971.
25. Burton GV, Cox EB, Leight GS, et al: Inflammatory breast carcinoma, effective multimodal approach. Arch Surg 122:1329–1332, 1987.
26. Butcher HR: Radical mastectomy for mammary carcinoma. Ann Surg 170:833–884, 1969.
27. Buzdar AU, Montague ED, Barker JL, et al: Management of inflammatory carcinoma of breast with combined modality approach—an update. Cancer 47:2537–2542, 1981.
28. Caceres B, Zaharia M, Lingan M, et al: Combined therapy of stage III adenocarcinoma of the breast. Proc Am Acad Cancer Res 798:199, 1980.
29. Campbell FC, Morgan DAL, Bishop HM, et al: The management of locally advanced carcinoma of the breast by Nolvadex (tamoxifen): a pilot study. J Clin Oncol 10:111–115, 1984.

30. Chamadol W, Pesie M, Puapairoj A: Inflammatory carcinoma of the breast in a 12-year-old Thai girl. J Med Assoc Thailand 70:543–548, 1987.
31. Chevallier B, Asselain B, Kunlin A, et al: Inflammatory breast cancer—determination of prognostic factors by univariate and multivariate analysis. Cancer 60:897–902, 1987.
32. Chu AM, Wood WC, Doucette JA: Inflammatory breast carcinoma treated by radical radiotherapy. Cancer 45:2730–2737, 1980.
33. Chris SM: Inflammatory carcinoma of the breast: a report of 20 cases and a review of the literature. Br J Surg 38:163–174, 1950.
34. Conte PF, Alama A, Bertelli G, et al: Chemotherapy with estrogenic recruitment and surgery in locally advanced breast cancer: clinical and cytokinetic results. Int J Cancer 40:490–494, 1987.
35. Dao TL, MacCarthy JD: Treatment of inflammatory carcinoma of the breast. Surg Gynecol Obstet 105:289–294, 1957.
36. Delarue NC, Ash CL, Petras V, Fielden R: Preoperative irradiation in management of locally advanced breast cancer. Arch Surg 91:136–154, 1965.
37. DeLarue JC, Levin F, Mouriesse H, et al: Oestrogen and progesterone cytosolic receptors in clinically inflammatory tumors of the human breast. Br J Cancer 44:911–916, 1981.
38. DeLena M, Varini M, Zucali R, et al: Multimodal treatment for locally advanced breast cancer: results of chemotherapy-radiotherapy versus chemotherapy-surgery. Cancer Clin Trials 4:229–236, 1981.
39. DeLena M, Zucali R, Viganotti G, et al: Combined chemotherapy-radiotherapy approach in locally advanced (T_{3b}–T_4) breast cancer. Cancer Chemother Pharmacol 1:53–59, 1978.
40. Derynck R, Goeddel DV, Ullrich A, et al: Synthesis of messenger RNAs for transforming growth factors α and β and the epidermal growth factor receptor by human tumors. Cancer Res 47:707–712, 1987.
41. Donehower R, Allegra JC, Lippman ME, Chabner B: Combined effects of methotrexate and 5-fluoropyrimidine on human breast cancer cells in serum-free culture. Eur J Cancer 16:655–661, 1980.
42. Donnelly BA: Primary "inflammatory" carcinoma of the breast: a report of five cases and a review of the literature. Ann Surg 128:918–930, 1948.
43. Droulias CA, Sewell CW, McSweeney MB, Powell RW: Inflammatory carcinoma of the breast: a correlation of clinical, radiologic and pathologic findings. Ann Surg 184:217–222, 1976.
44. Ellis DL, Teitelbaum SL: Inflammatory carcinoma of the breast: a pathologic definition. Cancer 33:1045–1047, 1974.
45. Fastenberg NA, Buzdar AU, Montague ED, et al: Management of inflammatory carcinoma of the breast. A combined modality approach. Am J Clin Oncol 8:134–141, 1985.
46. Fisher B, Slack NH, Bross IDJ: Cancer of the breast: size of the neoplasm and prognosis. Cancer 24:1071–1081, 1969.
47. Fletcher GH, Montague ED: Radical irradiation of advanced breast cancer. J Roentgen 93:573–584, 1965.
48. Fodor J, Tóth J, Szentirmay Z, Gyenes G: Prognostic significance of residual disease after radiation therapy of stage III breast cancer. Radiother Oncol 10:17–22, 1987.
49. Fowble BF, Glover D, Rosato EF, Goodman RL: Combined modality treatment of inflammatory breast cancer. Proceedings of the American Society for Therapeutic Radiology and Oncology; Volume 12, Supplement 1:151–152, 1986.
50. Fracchia AA, Evans JF, Eisenberg BL: Stage III carcinoma of the breast: a detailed analysis. Ann Surg 19:705–710, 1980.
51. Golding P: The treatment of inoperable carcinoma of the breast in Portsmouth 1960–69. Proc Royal Soc Med 69:701–703, 1976.
52. Green MD, Whybourne AM, Taylor IW, Sutherland RL: Effects of antiestrogens on the growth and cell cycle kinetics of cultured human mammary carcinoma cells. In Sutherland RL, Jordan VC (eds): Nonsteroidal Antiestrogens. New York, Academic Press, 1981, pp 397–413.
53. Gröhn P, Heinonen E, Klefström P, Tarkkanen J: Adjuvant postoperative radiotherapy, chemotherapy, and immunotherapy in stage III breast cancer. Cancer 54:670–674, 1984.
54. Guttman R: Radiotherapy in locally advanced cancer of the breast: adjunct to standard therapy. Cancer 20:1046–1050, 1967.
55. Haagensen CD: Diseases of the Breast, ed 2. Philadelphia, WB Saunders, 1971, pp 576–584.
56. Haagensen CD: Diseases of the Breast, ed 2. Philadelphia, WB Saunders, 1971, p 629.
57. Haagensen CD: Diseases of the Breast, ed 3. Philadelphia, WB Saunders, 1986, p 656.
58. Haagensen CD: Diseases of the Breast, ed 3. Philadelphia, WB Saunders, 1986, pp 808–814.
59. Haagensen CD: Diseases of the Breast, ed 3. Philadelphia, WB Saunders, 1986, p 858.
60. Haagensen CD: Diseases of the Breast, ed 3. Philadelphia, WB Saunders, 1986, p 860.
61. Haagensen CD, Stout AP: Carcinoma of the breast: II. Criteria of operability. Ann Surg 118:859–870; 1032–1051, 1943.
62. Hagelberg RS, Jolly PC, Anderson RP: Role of surgery in the treatment of inflammatory breast carcinoma. Am J Surg 148:125–131, 1984.
63. Hermanek P, Sobin LH (eds): TNM Classification of Malignant Tumors: UICC International Union Against Cancer, ed 4. Berlin, Springer-Verlag, 1987, pp 93–99.
64. Hery M, Namer M, Moro M, et al: Conservative treatment (chemotherapy/radiotherapy) of locally advanced breast cancer. Cancer 57:1744–1749, 1986.
65. Hortobagyi GN, Kau SW, Buzdar AV, et al: Induction chemotherapy for stage III primary breast cancer. In Salmon S (ed): Adjuvant Therapy of Cancer, V. Orlando, FL, Grune and Stratton, 1987, pp 419–428.
66. Hu E, Stockdale FE, Turner B, et al: Combined modality therapy of locally advanced breast cancer: one institution's experience and a review of the literature. Anticancer Res 7:733–736, 1987.
67. Huff KK, Knabbe C, Lindsey R, et al: Multihormonal regulation of insulin-like growth factor-1-related protein in MCF-7 human breast cancer cells. Molec Endocrinol 2:200–208, 1988.
68. Israël L, Breau J-L, Morere J-F: Two years of high-dose cyclophosphamide and 5-fluorouracil followed by surgery after 3 months for acute inflammatory breast carcinomas: a phase II study of 25 cases with a median follow-up of 35 months. Cancer 57:24–28, 1986.
69. Jacquillat C, Weil M, Auclerc G, et al: Neo-adjuvant chemotherapy in the conservative management of breast cancer: a study of 205 patients. In Salmon S (ed): Adjuvant Therapy of Cancer, V. Orlando, FL, Grune and Stratton, 1987, pp 403–409.
70. Keiling R, Guiochet N, Calderoli H, et al: Preoperative chemotherapy in the treatment of inflammatory breast cancer. In Primary Chemotherapy in Cancer Medicine. New York, Alan R Liss, 1985, pp 95–104.
71. Klefström P, Gröhn P, Heinonen E, Holsti L, Holsti P: Adjuvant radiotherapy, chemotherapy, and immunotherapy in stage III breast cancer. Cancer 60:936–942, 1987.
72. Knabbe C, Lippman ME, Wakefield L, et al: Evidence that TGFβ is a hormonally regulated negative growth factor in human breast cancer. Cell 48:417–428, 1987.
73. Knight CD, Martin JK, Welch JS: Surgical considerations after chemotherapy and radiation therapy for inflammatory breast cancer. Surgery 99:385–391, 1986.
74. Koyama H, Nishizawa Y, Wada T, et al: Intra-arterial infusion chemotherapy as an induction therapy in multidisciplinary treatment for locally advanced breast cancer. A long-term follow-up study. Cancer 56:725–729, 1985.
75. Lacour J, Hourtoule FG: La place de la chirurgie dans le traitement des formes evolutives du cancer du sein. Mem Acad Chir 93:635–643, 1967.
76. Langlands AO, Kerr GR, Shaw S: The management of locally advanced breast cancer by x-ray therapy. Clin Oncol 2:365–371, 1976.
77. Lee BJ, Tannenbaum NE: Inflammatory carcinoma of the breast: a report of twenty-eight cases from the breast clinic of the Memorial Hospital. Surg Gynecol Obstet 39:580–595, 1924.
78. Levine PH, Steinhorn SC, Ries LG, Aaron JL: Inflammatory breast cancer: the experience of the Surveillance, Epidemiology, and End Results (SEER) Program. J Natl Cancer Inst 74:291–297, 1985.

79. Lippman ME, Bolan G, Huff K: The effects of estrogens and antiestrogens on hormone-responsive human breast cancer in long-term tissue culture. Cancer Res 36:4595–4601, 1976.
80. Lippman ME, Cassidy J, Wesley M, Young RC: A randomized attempt to increase the efficacy of cytotoxic chemotherapy in metastatic breast cancer by hormonal synchronization. J Clin Oncol 2:28–36, 1984.
81. Loprinzi CL, Carbone PP, Tormey DC, et al: Aggressive combined modality therapy for advanced local-regional breast carcinoma. J Clin Oncol 2:157–163, 1984.
82. Lucas FV, Perez-Mesa C: Inflammatory carcinoma of the breast. Cancer 41:1595–1605, 1978.
83. McWhirter R: Simple mastectomy and radiotherapy in the treatment of breast cancer. Br J Radiol 28:128, 1955.
84. Meek AG, Order SE, Abeloff D, et al: Concurrent radiochemotherapy in advanced breast cancer. Cancer 51:1001–1006, 1983.
85. Merkel DE, Dressler LG, McGuire WL: Flow cytometry, cellular DNA content, and prognosis in human malignancy. J Clin Oncol 5:1690–1703, 1987.
86. Metcalf D, Begley CG, Johnson CR, et al: Biologic properties in vitro of a recombinant human granulocyte-macrophage colony-stimulating factor. Blood 67:37–45, 1986.
87. Meyer AC, Dockerty MB, Harrington SW: Inflammatory carcinoma of the breast. Surg Gynecol Obstet 87:417–424, 1948.
88. Meyer JS, McDivitt RW, Stone KR, et al: Practical breast carcinoma cell kinetics: review and update. Breast Cancer Res Treat 4:79–88, 1984.
89. Morris D, Poplin E, Aisner J: Long term follow-up of patients treated with mastectomy as an adjuvant to chemotherapy for locally advanced or metastatic breast cancer. Proc Am Soc Clin Oncol 396:102, 1983.
90. Morrow M, Braverman A, Thalmo W, et al: Multimodal therapy for locally advanced breast cancer. Arch Surg 121:1291–1296, 1986.
91. Nawata H, Chong M, Bronzert D, Lippman M: Estradiol in dependent growth of a subline of MCF-7 human breast cancer cell line in culture. J Biol Chem 256:6895–6902, 1981.
92. Nemoto T, Vana J, Bedwani RN, et al: Management and survival of female breast cancer: results of a national survey by the American College of Surgeons. Cancer 45:2917–2924, 1980.
93. Noguchi S, Miyauchi K, Nishizawa Y, et al: Management of inflammatory carcinoma of the breast with combined modality therapy including intraarterial infusion chemotherapy as induction therapy. Cancer 61:1483–1491, 1988.
94. Nussbaum H, Kagan AR, Gilbert H, et al: Management of inflammatory breast carcinoma. Breast 3:25–29, 1977.
95. Papaioannou A, Lissaios B, Vasilaros S, et al: Pre- and postoperative chemoendocrine treatment with or without postoperative radiotherapy for locally advanced breast cancer. Cancer 51:1284–1290, 1983.
96. Pastan I, Willingham MC, Fitzgerald DP: Immunotoxins. Cell 47:641–648, 1986.
97. Pawlicki M, Skolyszewski J, Brandys A: Results of combined treatment of patients with locally advanced breast cancer. Tumori 69:249–253, 1983.
98. Perez C, Presant C, Philpott G, Ratkin G: Phase II study of concurrent irradiation and multi-drug chemotherapy in advanced carcinoma of the breast: a pilot study by the Southeastern Cancer Study Group. Int Radiat Oncol Biol Phys 5:1329–1333, 1979.
99. Perez CA, Fields JN: Role of radiation therapy for locally advanced and inflammatory carcinoma of the breast. Oncology 1:81–93, 1987.
100. Perloff M, Lesnick GJ: Chemotherapy before and after mastectomy in stage III breast cancer. Arch Surg 117:879–881, 1982.
101. Perloff M, Lesnick GJ, Korzun A, et al: Chemotherapy with mastectomy or radiotherapy for stage III breast carcinoma: a Cancer and Leukemia Group B study. J Clin Oncol 6:261–269, 1988.
102. Rao DV, Bedwinek J, Perez C, et al: Prognostic indicators in stage III and localized stage IV breast cancer. Cancer 50:2037–2043, 1982.
103. Rogers CS, Fitts WT: Inflammatory carcinoma of the breast: a critique of therapy. Surgery 39:367–370, 1956.
104. Rouëssé S, Sarrazin D, Mouriesse H, et al: Primary chemotherapy in the treatment of inflammatory breast carcinoma: a study of 230 cases from the Institut Gustave-Roussy. J Clin Oncol 4:1765–1771, 1986.
105. Rubens RD, Sexton S, Tong D, et al: Combined chemotherapy and radiotherapy for locally advanced breast cancer. Eur J Cancer 16:351–356, 1980.
106. Saltzstein SI: Clinically occult inflammatory carcinoma of the breast. Cancer 34:382–388, 1974.
107. Schaake-Koning C, Van Der Linden EH, Hart G, Engelsman E: Adjuvant chemo- and hormonal therapy in locally advanced breast cancer: a randomized clinical study. Int J Radiat Oncol Biol Phys 11:1759–1763, 1985.
108. Schäfer P, Alberto P, Forni M, et al: Surgery as part of a combined modality approach for inflammatory breast carcinoma. Cancer 59:1063–1067, 1987.
109. Schottenfeld D, Nash AG, Robbins GF, et al: Ten-year results of the treatment of primary operable breast carcinoma. Cancer 38:1001–1007, 1976.
110. Schwartz GF, Cantor RI, Biermann WA: Neoadjuvant chemotherapy before definitive treatment for stage III carcinoma of the breast. Arch Surg 122:1430–1434, 1987.
111. Shanta V, Krishnamurthi S, Sastry DVLN, Menon R: Multimodal approach in the therapy of stage III female breast cancers. J Surg Oncol 28:134–136, 1985.
112. Sheldon T, Hayes DF, Cady B, et al: Primary radiation therapy for locally advanced breast cancer. Cancer 60:1219–1225, 1987.
113. Silvestrini R, Daidone MG, Valagussa P, et al: Cell kinetics as a prognostic marker in locally advanced breast cancer. Cancer Treat Rep 71:375–379, 1987.
114. Slamon DJ, Clark GM, Wong SG, et al: Human breast cancer correlation of relapse and survival with amplification of the HER-2/neu oncogene. Science 235:177–182, 1987.
115. Sorace RA, Bagley CS, Lichter AS, et al: The management of nonmetastatic locally advanced breast cancer using primary induction chemotherapy with hormonal synchronization followed by radiation therapy with or without debulking surgery. World J Surg 9:775–785, 1985.
116. Spangenberg JP, Nel CJC, Anderson JD, Doman MJ: A prospective study of the treatment of stage III breast cancer. South Afr J Surg 24:57–60, 1986.
117. Sponzo RW, Cunningham TJ, Caradonna RR: Management of non-resectable (stage III) breast cancer. Int J Radiat Oncol Biol Phys 5:1475–1478, 1979.
118. Stewart JF, King RJB, Winter PJ, et al: Oestrogen receptors: clinical features and prognosis in stage III breast cancer. Eur J Cancer Clin Oncol 18:1315–1320, 1982.
119. Stocks LH, Patterson FMS: Inflammatory carcinoma of the breast. Surg Gynecol Obstet 143:885–889, 1976.
120. Strickland P: The management of carcinoma of the breast by radical supervoltage radiation. Br J Surg 60:569–573, 1965.
121. Swain SM, Sorace RA, Bagley CA, et al: Neoadjuvant chemotherapy in the combined modality approach of locally advanced nonmetastatic breast cancer. Cancer Res 47:3889–3894, 1987.
122. Tasjian AH, Voelkel EF, Lazzaro M, et al: α and β human transforming growth factors stimulate prostaglandin and bone resorption in cultured mouse calvaria. Proc Natl Acad Sci (USA) 82:4535–4538, 1985.
123. Taylor GW, Meltzer A: Inflammatory carcinoma of the breast. Ann Surg 33:33–49, 1938.
124. Thalmo W, Sand J, Marti J, et al: Clinical and pathological (Path) findings in locally advanced breast cancer (LABC) treated with cyclophosphamide-adriamycin-5-FU (CAF). Proc Am Soc Clin Oncol 498:127, 1984.
125. Toonkel LM, Fix I, Jacobson LH, et al: Locally advanced breast carcinoma: results with combined regional therapy. Int J Radiat Oncol Biol Phys 12:1583–1587, 1986.
126. Treurniet-Donker AD, Hop WCJ, Hoed-Sijtsema SD: Radiation treatment of stage III mammary carcinoma: a review of 129 patients. Int J Radiat Oncol Biol Phys 6:1477–1482, 1980.
127. Treves N: Inflammatory carcinoma of the breast in the male patient. Surgery 34:810–820, 1953.
128. Treves N: The inoperability of inflammatory carcinoma of the breast. Surg Gynecol Obstet 109:240–242, 1959.
129. Valagussa P, Bonadonna G, Veronesi V: Patterns of relapse and

survival following radical mastectomy. Cancer 41:1170–1178, 1978.

130. Veronesi A, Frustaci S, Tirelli U, et al: Tamoxifen therapy in postmenopausal advanced breast cancer: efficacy at the primary tumor site in 46 evaluable patients. Tumori 67:235–238, 1981.

131. Vilcoq JR, Fourquet A, Jullien D, et al: Prognostic significance of clinical nodal involvement in patients treated by radical radiotherapy for a locally advanced breast cancer. Am J Clin Oncol (Cancer Clin Trials) 7:625–628, 1984.

132. Vitella ES, Uhu JW: Immunotoxins: redirecting nature's poisons. Cell 41:653–665, 1985.

133. Wang CC, Griscom NT: Inflammatory carcinoma of the breast: results following orthovoltage and supervoltage radiation therapy. Clin Radiol 15:168–174, 1964.

134. Weichselbaum RR, Hellman S, Piro AJ, et al: Proliferation kinetics of a human breast cancer cell line *in vitro* following treatment with 17β-estradiol and 1-β-D-arabinofuranosylcytosine. Cancer Res 38:2339–2345, 1978.

135. Zaharia M, Caceres E, Valdivia S, et al: Radiotherapy in the management of locally advanced breast cancer. Int J Radiat Oncol Biol Phys 13:1179–1182, 1987.

136. Zucali R, Uslenghi C, Kenda R, Bonadonna G: Natural history and survival of inoperable breast cancer treated with radiotherapy and radiotherapy followed by radical mastectomy. Cancer 37:1422–1431, 1976.

137. Zylberberg B, Salat-Baroux J, Ravina JH, et al: Initial chemo-immunotherapy in inflammatory carcinoma of the breast. Cancer 49:1537–1543, 1982.

Chapter 41

MANAGEMENT OF LOCAL/REGIONAL RECURRENCE

Nancy Price Mendenhall, M.D., Gilbert H. Fletcher, M.D., and Rodney R. Million, M.D.

Local/regional recurrence (LRR) refers to a second clinical manifestation of breast cancer in either the primary site (breast, chest wall incision, or skin flaps) or regional lymphatics, including first echelon (axillary, internal mammary, Rotter's) or second echelon (supraclavicular) lymph nodes. LRR occurs in at least ten percent to 30 percent of patients undergoing radical or modified radical mastectomy.[6, 12, 19, 24, 28, 34, 35] The actual risk is greater, as physicians may not document LRR after distant metastases develop.

PRESENTATION

LRR is frequently not diagnosed clinically[26] or is diagnosed only after the disease has become extensive because of the subtlety of early clinical signs of recurrence, inexperience or inattentiveness of the physicians responsible for posttreatment follow-up,[7] and patient denial. The extent of disease at presentation is often greater than is apparent on physical exam.[22, 25] The time to local recurrence or initial disease-free interval varies inversely with initial stage of disease; in a study by Gilliland and coworkers,[16] the median time to local recurrence was 6.2 years, 4.3 years, and 2.1 years for patients with stage I, II, and III disease, respectively. Some of the more common clinical presentations are described in the sections that follow and shown in Figures 41–1 through 41–11.

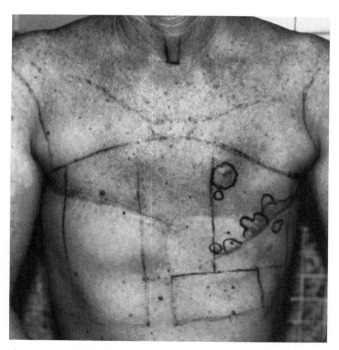

Figure 41–1. Multiple nodules of recurrent breast carcinoma ranging from 0.25 cm to 1 cm in diameter were palpable in the chest wall flap along the mastectomy incision in this 44-year-old woman six months following diagnosis of inflammatory carcinoma (T4 N2) treated with three courses of preoperative chemotherapy, simple extended mastectomy, and an additional four months of postoperative chemotherapy.

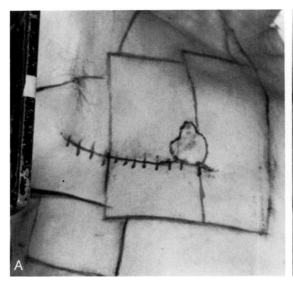
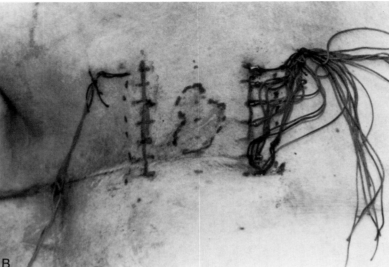

Figure 41–2. This 64-year-old woman underwent a right modified radical mastectomy in March 1984 and six months of postoperative chemotherapy for an estrogen and progesterone receptor–negative, 3-cm breast carcinoma with metastatic involvement of 15 of 18 nodes retrieved. In June 1985 a small nodule was noted in the superior chest wall flap, just above the mastectomy incision. Bone scan demonstrated multiple asymptomatic bone metastases. The nodule was excised, and the patient was placed on tamoxifen. In July 1986, the tumor progressed to a 2.5-cm area of tender multiple confluent nodules. *A,* External-beam treatment portals are shown with the tumor nodules encircled. Because distant metastases were present, a short course of therapy was indicated. A dose of 3000 cGy in ten fractions over 15 days was delivered to the chest wall with 8 MeV electrons with bolus, to the supraclavicular fossa with 8 mV x-rays, and to the internal mammary chain nodes with 14 MeV electrons. *B,* The chest wall recurrence was given an additional 2000 cGy over 50 hours with an interstitial radium needle implant. Complete regression of the chest wall tumor was obtained. The chest wall and regional lymphatics remained free of tumor until the patient's death from progression of distant metastases in March 1987.

Chest Wall Recurrence

Chest wall recurrence most commonly appears as tiny (1–2 mm), single or multiple, painless cutaneous nodules usually in close proximity to the scar (Figs. 41–1 and 41–2).[21] Initially these nodules may be diagnosed only by meticulous palpation of the skin flaps, but eventually they progress to distort, infiltrate, or ulcerate the skin of the operative flap. Erythema or purplish discoloration of the skin without palpable nodularity or with only minimal skin thickening (Fig. 41–3) may be the only sign of recurrence. Advanced signs of recurrence include skin induration or nodularity, pruritic or nonpruritic erythematous macules or papules (Fig. 41–4), obvious inflammatory skin changes, ridging, and carcinoma en cuirasse (Fig. 41–5). As the disease progresses, tumor

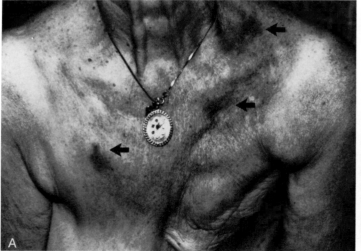
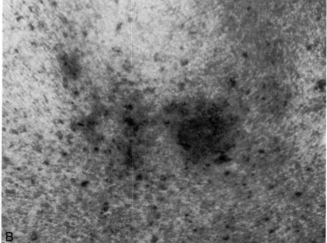

Figure 41–3. This 72-year-old woman initially presented with left axillary adenopathy of unknown origin. Mammogram and physical examination did not confirm any obvious primary tumor in the breast. She was treated with preoperative irradiation to the left breast and regional lymphatics followed by modified radical mastectomy. *A,* One and a half years after the initial treatment, multiple nonpalpable areas *(arrows)* of purplish skin discoloration were observed and were proved by biopsy to be recurrent breast carcinoma. *B,* Detail of recurrent disease involving the skin.

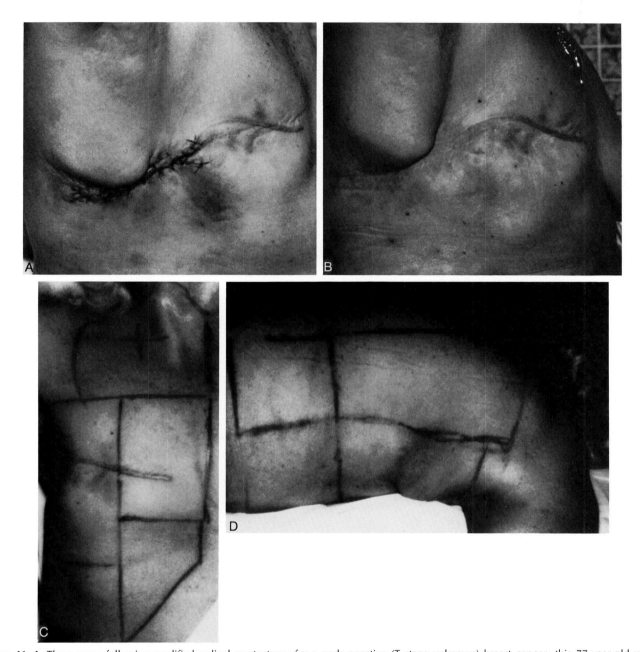

Figure 41–4. Three years following modified radical mastectomy for a node-negative (T stage unknown) breast cancer, this 77-year-old woman presented with an extensive chest wall recurrence. For six months prior to biopsy of the chest wall, the patient had repeatedly complained of skin erythema, thickening, and tenderness to her physician, who noted these findings but attributed them to irritation from her brassiere. *A,* Photograph obtained after biopsy shows marked leathery induration and erythema of skin along the lateral portion of the mastectomy incision and multiple satellite nodules in the inferior chest wall flap and along the medial portion of the mastectomy incision.

The estrogen receptor level in the recurrent tumor was 301 fmol per mg of protein and the progesterone receptor level was <1 fmol per mg. Because of the extent of the recurrence, radiotherapy was not thought to be feasible, so the patient was placed on tamoxifen. Regression of erythema and nodularity was judged to be 75 percent at three months *(B)* following administration of tamoxifen. Tattoos indicate sites of previous satellite nodules.

Following the response to tamoxifen, the chest wall was treated with radiation using cobalt 60 and 14 MeV electrons for the supraclavicular fossa, 8 MeV electrons with bolus for the chest wall fields, and 14 MeV electrons for the internal mammary chain field with the patient supine *(C)*. Because of the posterior extent of the recurrence, posterior lateral chest wall fields were also treated, with the patient in a prone position *(D)*. The initial treatment plan was 5000 cGy to the peripheral lymphatic areas and 6000 cGy to the entire chest wall, followed by an interstitial implant to the mastectomy scar and tattooed satellite nodules.

Moist desquamation of the chest wall precluded delivery of more than 5600 cGy. The peripheral lymphatic areas received 5000 cGy. The patient is alive without evidence of recurrent disease or other sequelae of treatment 2.5 years after beginning tamoxifen.

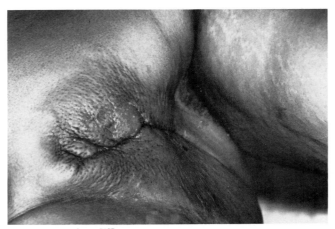

Figure 41–5. This 48-year-old woman presented with a 10-cm left breast mass in December 1987. Needle aspiration showed infiltrating ductal carcinoma. The patient was staged as IIIA and treated with three courses of CAF chemotherapy. A residual 7-cm mass was present in the breast at the time of simple mastectomy with dissection of the lower (level 1) axillary contents in March 1988. Pathology revealed residual infiltrating ductal carcinoma with a poorly differentiated histologic and nuclear grade, endothelial space invasion, and perineural invasion. The margins of resection were negative, and there was no dermal lymphatic invasion. Eight of 16 lymph nodes contained metastatic carcinoma that did not extend beyond the capsule of the lymph nodes. Postoperative chemotherapy was recommended but not given. Two weeks after a normal physical examination in June 1988, the patient presented to the emergency room with the sudden onset of massive arm edema and a tender reddened area on the chest wall. She admitted to pain in the upper aspect of the left arm. Physical examination revealed extensive carcinoma en cuirasse involving the left anterior chest wall with scattered nodules of tumor on the inferior chest wall flap and posterior to the mastectomy incision on the lateral portion of the back. There was massive edema of the arm with palpable tumor filling the infraclavicular axillary apical area.

CT scan of the chest confirmed tumor involving the axillary apex and surrounding the brachial plexus. Bone scan demonstrated diffuse metastatic disease. Chemotherapy was recommended for palliation.

may extend beyond the chest wall (Figs. 41–5 and 41–6).[21] Ipsilateral pleural effusion may signal chest wall recurrence in the intercostal musculature.[36]

Regional Lymphatic Recurrence

A painless mobile node detected in the supraclavicular fossa on physical examination is the most common presentation for regional recurrence (Fig. 41–7). Occasionally LRR is not discovered until the patient develops arm edema or brachial plexopathy (Figs. 41–8 and 41–9). LRR in the axillary apex presents as mobile nodes or a vague fullness palpable on the anterior chest wall in the infraclavicular area beneath the pectoralis major muscle, usually distinguishable from the coracoid process (Figs. 41–9 and 41–10).

Internal mammary node recurrence most often presents as a painless subcutaneous parasternal mass, with or without skin involvement (Figs. 41–10 and 41–11).[27] Occasionally an abnormality on chest roentgenogram is the first sign of an internal mammary node recurrence (Figs. 41–10 and 41–11). Patients with advanced disease may present with symptoms secondary to destruction of

the sternum or rib (Fig. 41–11), pleural effusion, or anterior mediastinal involvement with superior vena cava syndrome.[27]

In patients who have had a modified radical mastectomy for a large superior and central primary tumor, recurrence in Rotter's (interpectoral) nodes appears as a subcutaneous mass in the area beneath the pectoralis major muscle.[5, 29]

Axillary recurrence after complete axillary dissection is uncommon. Pain, arm edema, or a mass may be present on physical examination.

TREATMENT

Patient Selection

LRR is isolated (i.e., not associated with clinically apparent distant metastases at the time of diagnosis) in

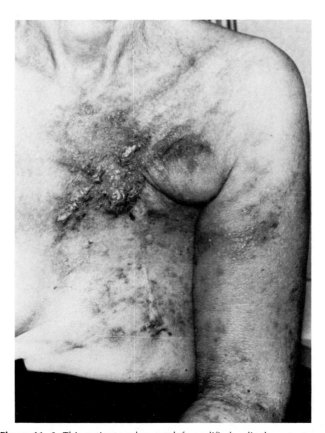

Figure 41–6. This patient underwent left modified radical mastectomy, three courses of adjuvant chemotherapy, and postoperative irradiation for clinically T3 N0 carcinoma with histological involvement of 23/23 nodes. Eight months after treatment, she developed progressive arm edema requiring aggressive management with a Jobst stocking and pump. At 16 months, she developed a pruritic rash involving the left chest wall flaps. The multiple flat and raised erythematous papules, confluent over the mastectomy incision, were confirmed on biopsy to be recurrent breast carcinoma. The tumor did not respond to CAF chemotherapy or mitomycin but progressed to involve the skin of the entire anterior chest wall and left upper extremity (as shown) as well as patchy areas of the skin of the back prior to her death as a result of pericardial and pleural effusions.

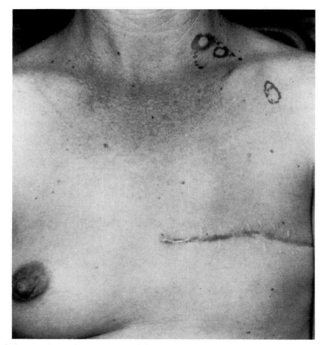

Figure 41–7. This 35-year-old woman had a left modified radical mastectomy in May 1985 for a Stage I (T1 N0) estrogen and progesterone receptor–negative adenocarcinoma of the breast with close surgical margins and lymphatic space invasion within the specimen. In August 1986 she had biopsy-proven recurrent disease in the left supraclavicular and infraclavicular nodes, as shown. The lymph nodes ranged from 0.5 cm to 1.5 cm in diameter and were located in the medial supraclavicular fossa, deep to the insertion of the sternocleidomastoid muscle and just beneath the clavicle in the midclavicular line. She received three courses of chemotherapy (CMF) with little response, radiation to the chest wall and lymphatic areas with complete regression of the tumor, and then another course of chemotherapy, during which she developed contralateral axillary nodal disease and distant metastases. She died of progressive disease in May 1987.

approximately two thirds of patients.[6, 37] However, it is regarded as a harbinger of distant metastases. In the series reported by Gilliland and coworkers,[16] all patients eventually developed distant metastases and died of breast cancer. Control of LRR, however, is associated with a better rate of freedom from distant metastases and survival.[5, 16, 20, 23] Uncontrolled local/regional disease can be painful and can present problems with hygiene and infection that alienate the patient from family and friends. As an obvious sign of treatment failure, it can be psychologically devastating to the patient. Radical treatment of early recurrences is therefore worthwhile.

A significant proportion of patients with isolated LRR will not be judged to be candidates for radical treatment.[5] For patients who are elderly, who are in poor medical condition, or who have extensive LRR, only palliative treatment may be justified. Palliation can often be obtained with hormonal manipulation, chemotherapy, or a brief course of irradiation; therapy in this setting should be relatively short and of low morbidity (Fig. 41–2). For patients who are young, are in good medical condition, and have limited disease in previously untreated sites, therapy should be aggressive and well

planned. These patients can survive 10 years or more and will be at risk for complications from treatment.

Initial studies should include chest roentgenogram, bone scan, and liver function tests. When the initial studies are equivocal, other tests such as chest CT scan, plain roentgenograms and magnetic resonance imaging of the bones, and technetium or CT scans of the liver may be useful. A CT scan of the brain should be performed if there are any neurological signs or symptoms present.

Biopsy

When planning the biopsy, it is important to take into consideration the overall management plan. To facilitate decisions regarding systemic therapy, tissue should be submitted for assay of estrogen and progesterone receptor levels (which may differ from those in the original tumor). When total excision of a gross tumor nodule can easily be accomplished, it may allow the radiation

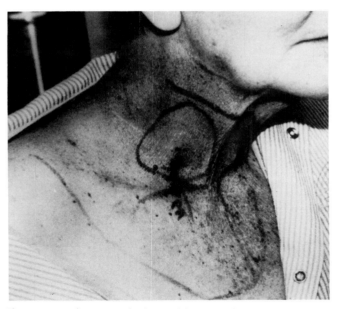

Figure 41–8. This patient had a modified radical mastectomy in 1974 for a T3 N1 M0 carcinoma of the left breast (three of the nine nodes retrieved were involved) followed by 2.5 years of adjuvant melphalan. In March 1980, she noted numbness and tingling in the right hand that did not respond to physical therapy. In October 1980 a biopsy-proven recurrence was found in the right supraclavicular fossa with an estrogen receptor level of 62 fmol per mg of protein. Her symptoms resolved with tamoxifen but recurred, together with weakness and pain in the right arm, in May 1983. In July 1983, she developed Horner's syndrome. She was treated for 1 year with chemotherapy (CMF). A 4 × 5 cm mass was noted in the medial right supraclavicular fossa and low neck, as shown; progression was suspected and she was referred for radiotherapy. On radiographic studies, the lesion extended from C3 to T2 with involvement of the bodies and transverse processes of C5 and C6 and grossly invaded the spinal canal. She had resolution of her paresthesias, improvement in the arm weakness, and regression of her tumor mass with 6000 cGy of radiation delivered in 120-cGy fractions twice a day. She developed pleural effusions 1 year after irradiation, however, and died in February 1986.

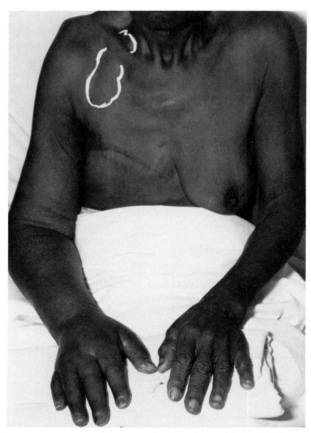

Figure 41–9. In 1967, this patient had a right modified radical mastectomy followed by 1 year of adjuvant chemotherapy for a breast carcinoma of unknown stage. She developed progressive arm edema in 1982, which was treated with pain medications. In 1984, she had surgery for presumed right carpal tunnel syndrome with progressive neurological loss in the right hand. In March 1987, she presented to the emergency room with a nonfunctioning right upper extremity with severe arm edema (despite a stocking), severe arm pain, and ulnar and radial nerve neuropathies. Recurrent carcinoma was confirmed with biopsy after a CT scan demonstrated a mass high in the right axilla, involving the pectoralis major muscle, with extension along the brachial plexus. Obvious disease was palpable in the right supraclavicular fossa. The patient did not respond to tamoxifen, megestrol acetate, or combination chemotherapy and was referred for irradiation in March 1988. She then had supraclavicular disease fixed to underlying tissues and infraclavicular disease fixed to the anterior chest wall (shown outlined in white). Bone scan was negative, and on CT scan of the chest the disease was localized to the supraclavicular and infraclavicular fossae with no evidence of other adenopathy or lung metastases.

therapist to use a lower dose or less penetrating radiation. An unnecessarily large or aggressive surgical procedure may require prolonged healing time before definitive treatment with radiation can be started. An ill-planned incision that potentially contaminates additional tissue can necessitate extension of radiation portals and place the patient at increased risk for complications. Close coordination with the radiation therapist is necessary. In selected cases, chest wall resection may be considered (Fig. 41–11).[30]

Radiation Therapy

No Prior Irradiation

Irradiation is the mainstay of management if the initial treatment did not include irradiation. Examples are shown in Figures 41–2, 41–4, 41–10, and 41–11.

Treatment Volume. If the recurrence is limited to the chest wall, irradiation fields should include the entire chest wall flap with generous margins and the peripheral lymphatics (i.e., ipsilateral internal mammary nodes and apical axillary and supraclavicular nodes). If the axilla is clinically involved at LRR or if, at initial presentation, indications for postoperative irradiation of the axilla existed (i.e., incomplete axillary dissection, nodes ≥2.5 cm in diameter, extranodal axillary disease[14]), then the axilla should be treated as well. For an isolated supraclavicular recurrence, treatment may be limited to the nodal site involved (Fig. 41–8). Treatment of isolated first echelon nodal recurrences (internal mammary nodes or axilla) should include elective treatment of the supraclavicular nodes as well. Because of the high incidence of occult chest wall disease,[26] the chest wall is also electively irradiated in first echelon nodal recurrences. The design of standard treatment fields for subclinical disease in the chest wall flaps, the internal mammary and supraclavicular nodes, and the axilla is discussed in detail in chapter 37. Additional boost treatment for clinically evident disease is tailored to the site and volume of disease. Examples are shown in Figures 41–2, 41–4, 41–8, 41–10, and 41–11.

Time-Dose Factors. All areas at risk for subclinical involvement are given 5000 cGy in 5 weeks at 200 cGy per fraction. The dose to areas around surgical incisions is boosted to 6000 cGy in 6 weeks at 200 cGy per fraction. For areas of gross involvement, the dose is boosted with an additional 1500 cGy to 2000 cGy at 200 to 250 cGy per fraction or by implant, if technically suitable.

Prior Irradiation

Retreatment with irradiation is not likely to be successful, may result in severe complications, and is generally not advised.

Combining Irradiation With Systemic Therapy

Chemotherapy or hormonal therapy alone should be used only in patients who are not suitable for irradiation. Occasionally a patient not judged to be a candidate for radical irradiation has an excellent response to systemic therapy and may become a candidate for irradiation (Fig. 41–4).

In patients who have not previously received systemic therapy, it is rational to use adjuvant hormonal manipulation or chemotherapy for postmenopausal patients

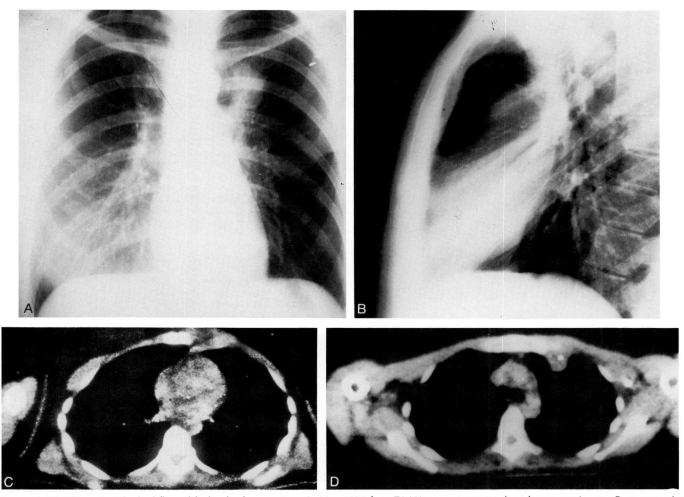

Figure 41–10. This patient had a left modified radical mastectomy in May 1977 for a T1 N0 upper outer quadrant breast carcinoma. Posteroanterior and lateral chest roentgenograms obtained on routine follow-up in 1978 were normal. She noted a rapidly growing parasternal nodule in July 1979. She also admitted to a several-month history of mild upper extremity pain and paresthesias relieved by arm elevation. Physical examination showed a 7.5 × 8.5 cm left parasternal nodule in the second interspace, a 1 × 2 cm subcutaneous nodule in the first interspace, and a tethered 5 × 5 cm node high in the left axilla. Biopsy confirmed recurrent breast carcinoma. *A* and *B,* PA and lateral chest roentgenograms in August 1979 demonstrated an anterior mediastinal mass at the level of the first and second intercostal spaces. *C* and *D,* CT scan sections from August 1979 showed destruction of the sternum by a mass consistent with internal mammary adenopathy and also demonstrated the subpectoral (infraclavicular) mass that was palpable high in the axilla.

Illustration continued on following page

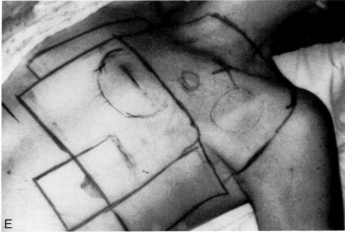

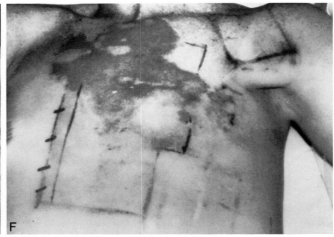

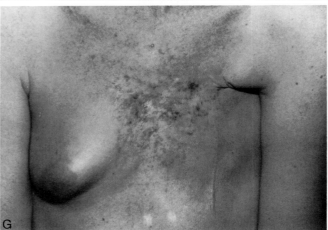

Figure 41–10 *Continued E,* Radiation treatment fields are shown; the three palpable recurrent nodules are circled. The patient received comprehensive chest wall and regional lymphatic irradiation and concomitant chemotherapy (CMF), which was continued for 1 year. Following 5000 cGy to the entire chest wall and supraclavicular fossa, the dose to the parasternal area was boosted through a shrinking-field technique with 14 MeV, 12 MeV, and 10 MeV electrons to 7500 cGy, and the dose to the left infraclavicular mass was boosted with 17 mV x-rays with a shrinking-field technique to 6500 cGy. *F,* A moist desquamation occurred at the end of treatment, most pronounced in areas of previous sun exposure. Her treatment was complicated by radiation pneumonitis, requiring prolonged steroid therapy, and symptomatic pericarditis, which was managed with aspirin. *G,* She is currently alive and well and has remained without evidence of disease 9 years after the LRR with only moderate telangiectasia and hyperpigmentation in the treatment field.

with estrogen receptor–positive tumors and to use chemotherapy for estrogen receptor–negative tumors or premenopausal patients. In our experience it has not been possible to use a doxorubicin-containing regimen concurrently with irradiation, and it has occasionally been difficult to complete the full course of irradiation, including the boost, with concomitant cyclophosphamide, methotrexate, and 5-fluorouracil (CMF). Chemotherapy is relatively ineffective in preventing LRR,[4, 9, 13, 15, 17, 32] and it is unlikely that chemotherapy alone will permanently eradicate recurrent local/regional disease (Fig. 41–1).[20] Therefore we do not recommend a lengthy delay in the start of irradiation to permit a prolonged course of chemotherapy. For patients with surgical resection of all gross tumor who require only modest doses of irradiation, radiation may be delivered concomitantly with CMF. For patients with gross residual disease after biopsy, chemotherapy may be delayed until completion of irradiation. Alternatively, two or three courses of chemotherapy may be given prior to irradiation so that information on the tumor's responsiveness to chemotherapy may be obtained (Fig. 41–7). The response achieved with 2 to 3 months of chemotherapy or hormonal therapy may significantly reduce gross tumor and facilitate subsequent irradiation (Fig. 41–11). Hormonal manipulation, if the tumor has high levels of estrogen

and progesterone receptors, can be started as soon as the diagnosis of LRR is made. It is critical, however, for the radiation therapist to evaluate the patient before any systemic therapy is given and, if possible, prior to surgical excision. Knowledge of the initial extent of LRR is imperative and may be impossible to obtain after the tumor responds to systemic treatment or the clinical picture is distorted by surgery.

The role of chemotherapy is unclear in patients who develop LRR following standard adjuvant chemotherapy [CMF or cyclophosphamide, doxorubicin HCl, and 5-fluorouracil (CAF)].

RESULTS OF TREATMENT AND PROGNOSTIC FACTORS

Results

Control of local/regional recurrences ranges from 35 percent to 60 percent.[1, 2, 5, 20, 23, 33] Five-year survival for series of patients treated primarily before 1960 with either surgery or irradiation ranged from 3.4 percent to 12 percent.[18, 31, 37] For patients treated primarily in the 1950s and 1960s with irradiation, 5-year survival ranged from 20 percent to 30 percent.[10, 11, 16] Five-year survival

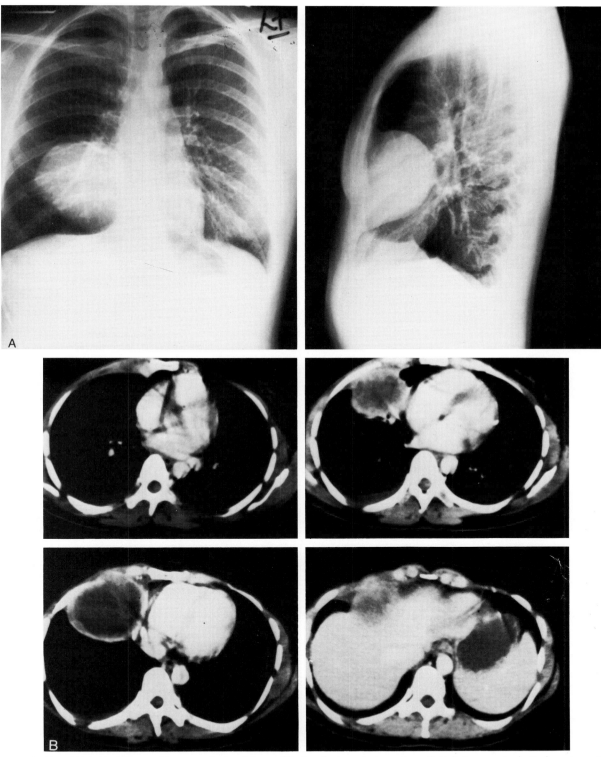

Figure 41–11. In May 1984 this 29-year-old woman had a right modified radical mastectomy for a 3 × 2.5 cm metaplastic breast carcinoma with squamous differentiation. Eight lymph nodes retrieved contained no tumor, and estrogen and progesterone receptor levels were negative. Chest roentgenogram was normal. *A,* In November 1984 she had right anterior chest wall pain, and chest roentgenogram demonstrated a 10-cm mass in the right lower chest. *B,* CT scan showed involvement of the anterior right fifth rib, as did bone scan. The mass was located in a parasternal position adherent to the right pericardium. Biopsy confirmed recurrent tumor. Metastatic evaluation was negative.

Illustration continued on following page

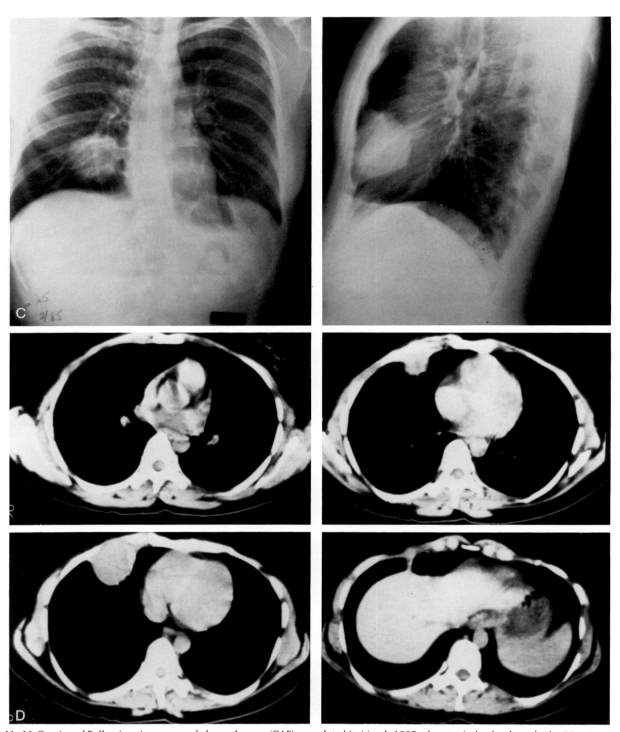

Figure 41–11 *Continued* Following six courses of chemotherapy (CAF) completed in March 1985, she was judged to have had a 50 percent reduction in the tumor as apparent on chest roentgenogram *(C)* and CT scan *(D)*, with stabilization of response after the third course of chemotherapy. In April 1985, she underwent resection of the residual mass, which grossly appeared to be a large, necrotic internal mammary lymph node that had grown into the anterior fifth rib and into the thoracic cavity, invading lung and adherent to pericardium. With the chest wall resection, a margin of lung was removed, which on histological examination was positive; tumor was also noted in the marrow of one of the resected ribs. Other margins were negative. A myocutaneous flap from the right latissimus dorsi was used to close the defect.

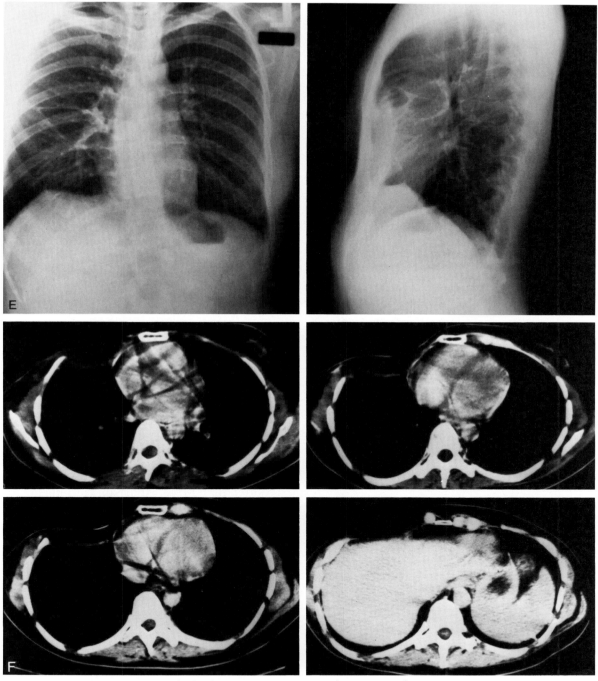

Figure 41–11 *Continued* Chest roentgenogram *(E)* and CT scan *(F)* after surgery are shown.

Illustration continued on following page

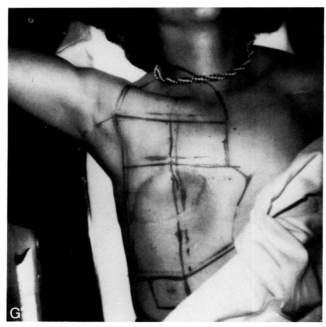

Figure 41–11 Continued G, External-beam treatment portals. From May through July 1985, the patient received 5000 cGy in 25 fractions over five weeks to the supraclavicular fossa (with 4000 cGy from cobalt 60 and 1000 cGy from 10 MeV electrons), the internal mammary nodes (with 12 MeV electrons), and the medial and lateral chest walls (6 MeV electrons). An additional 1000 cGy was delivered to the internal mammary nodes, myocutaneous flap, and incision (with 6 MeV and 12 MeV electrons) for a total dose of 6000 cGy. To spare the underlying heart, beeswax bolus was shaped to fit the chest wall defect during treatment of the portion of the medial chest wall that was included in the internal mammary chain portal. She received two courses of CMF chemotherapy concurrently and two more courses following irradiation, finishing treatment in August 1985. In November 1985, restaging studies (chest roentgenogram, bone scan, and CT scan of the chest) were negative. In December 1985, however, she developed a brain metastasis, which was treated aggressively with craniotomy and radiation. Thereafter she developed metastatic disease in the thyroid (March 1986), left supraclavicular area (May 1986), and lung (July 1986). She remained free of local/regional disease until her death in August 1986.

in selected subsets of patients treated primarily after 1970 with irradiation or irradiation and systemic therapy has ranged from 40 percent to 60 percent.[1, 2, 5, 20, 23, 33] Ten-year survival ranges from 20 percent to 30 percent in aggressively treated patients.[5, 23] It is unclear to what extent these improved results represent better patient selection, a delay of distant metastases and death as a result of systemic therapy, or the curability of some patients with LRR who are diagnosed with small tumor burdens.

Information on the benefits of adding systemic treatment to comprehensive irradiation of LRR is limited. In a retrospective review of all patients treated radically for LRR at the M. D. Anderson Hospital, Janjan and coworkers[20] compared the results of treatment in patients with irradiation alone, chemotherapy alone, or both modalities (Table 41–1). The groups were not comparable, but it was noted that the 5-year disease-free survival rate was better with chemotherapy alone than with radiotherapy alone, although there was no difference in 5-year overall survival. Chemotherapy used alone was less effective, however, than irradiation in achieving control of LRR.

Prognostic Factors

Long-term survivors after aggressive treatment for LRR include patients with single chest wall nodules,[5, 20] patients with parasternal recurrence,[18] and patients with axillary recurrence.[12, 23] Most factors thought to be significant for prognosis are related to tumor burden and tumor biology.

Tumor Burden

The size and number of recurrent lesions reflect tumor burden. Control rates[5, 20, 23] and survival rates[20] are better for patients with single chest wall nodules than for those with multiple chest wall nodules. Bedwinek and coworkers[3] also found higher local control and survival rates in patients with recurrences of smaller size.

Haagensen determined that patients with LRR after treatment of early breast cancer did better than those with LRR after treatment of an advanced tumor, although this has not been confirmed.[3, 5, 8, 18] Two series reported from M. D. Anderson Hospital did note higher local/regional control of LRR for patients who were histologically node-negative at mastectomy, compared with histologically node-positive patients.[5, 20] A higher survival rate in patients who were histologically node-negative at mastectomy has been noted in some series[10, 11, 16, 33] but not in others.[3, 8, 20, 23]

Table 41–1. PATTERNS OF TREATMENT FAILURE AND SURVIVAL IN PATIENTS TREATED FOR LOCAL/REGIONAL RECURRENCE FOLLOWING RADICAL OR MODIFIED RADICAL MASTECTOMY

Treatment of LRR	Incidence of Treatment Failure		5-Year Survival	
	Local/Regional	*Distant*	*Disease-Free*	*Overall*
Irradiation alone	20/57* (35%)	34/57 (60%)	22%†	60%
Chemotherapy alone	27/50* (54%)	24/50 (48%)	37%†	47%
Irradiation + chemotherapy	19/57 (33%)	36/57 (63%)	33%	45%

*$p = 0.049$.
†$p = 0.08$.
Modified from Janjan NA, et al: Cancer 58:1553, 1986.

Tumor Biology

The clinical parameter that best reflects tumor biology is initial disease-free interval (DFI), the time between initial treatment and first manifestation of recurrence or metastatic disease. Initial DFI has been correlated with prognosis; the shorter the initial DFI, the worse the prognosis.[3, 8, 18, 23, 33] Initial DFI may be affected by the tumor burden at initial presentation of disease[6, 11, 16, 18, 33] and by treatment (i.e., the use of adjuvant chemotherapy, hormonal manipulation, or postoperative irradiation).

References

 1. Aberizk WJ, Silver B, Henderson IC, Cady B, Harris JR: The use of radiotherapy for treatment of isolated locoregional recurrence of breast carcinoma after mastectomy. Cancer 58:1214–1218, 1986.
 2. Bedwinek JM, Fineberg B, Lee J, Ocwieza MA: Analysis of failures following local treatment of isolated local-regional recurrence of breast cancer. Int J Radiat Oncol Biol Phys 7:581–585, 1981.
 3. Bedwinek JM, Lee J, Fineberg B, Ocwieza MA: Prognostic indicators in patients with isolated local-regional recurrence of breast cancer. Cancer 47:2232–2235, 1981.
 4. Bonadonna G, Valagussa BS, Rossi A, Tancini G, Brambilla C, Zambetti M, Veronesi U: Ten-year experience with CMF-based adjuvant chemotherapy in resectable breast cancer. Breast Cancer Res Treat 5:95–115, 1985.
 5. Chen KK-Y, Montague ED, Oswald MJ: Results of irradiation in the treatment of locoregional breast cancer recurrence. Cancer 56:1269–1273, 1985.
 6. Ciatto S, Rosselli del Turco M, Pacini P, De Luca Cardillo C, Bastiani P, Bravetti P: Early detection of local recurrences in the follow-up of primary breast cancer. Tumori 70:179–183, 1984.
 7. Crile G Jr: The incidence of local recurrence of carcinoma of the breast. Surg Gynecol Obstet 156:497–498, 1983.
 8. Danoff BF, Coia LR, Cantor RI, Pajak TF, Kramer S: Locally recurrent breast carcinoma: the effect of adjuvant chemotherapy on prognosis. Radiology 147:849–852, 1983.
 9. DeLena M, Varini M, Zucali R, Rovini D, Viganotti G, Valagussa P, Veronesi U, Bonadonna G: Multimodal treatment for locally advanced breast cancer: results of chemotherapy-radiotherapy versus chemotherapy-surgery. Cancer Clin Trials 4:229–236, 1981.
10. Di Pietro S, Bertario L, Piva L: Prognosis and treatment of locoregional breast cancer recurrences: critical considerations on 120 cases. Tumori 66:331–338, 1980.
11. Fentiman IS, Matthews PN, Davison OW, Millis RR, Hayward JL: Survival following local skin recurrence after mastectomy. Br J Surg 72:14–16, 1985.
12. Fisher B, Redmond C, Fisher ER, Bauer M, Wolmark N, Wickerham OL, Deutsch M, Montague E, Margolese R, Foster R: Ten-year results of a randomized clinical trial comparing radical mastectomy and total mastectomy with or without radiation. New Engl J Med 312:674–681, 1985.
13. Fisher B, Bauer M, Margolese R, Poisson R, Pilch Y, Redmond C, Fisher E, Wolmark N, Deutsch M, Montague E, Saffer E, Wickerham L, Lerner H, Glass A, Shibata H, Deckers P, Ketcham A, Oishi R, Russell I: Five-year results of a randomized clinical trial comparing total mastectomy and segmental mastectomy with or without radiation in the treatment of breast cancer. New Engl J Med 312:665–673, 1985.
14. Fletcher GH: Textbook of Radiotherapy, ed 3. Philadelphia, Lea and Febiger, 1980.
15. Fowble B, Gray R, Gilchrist K, Goodman RL, Taylor S, Tormey DC: Identification of a subgroup of patients with breast cancer and histologically positive axillary nodes receiving adjuvant chemotherapy who may benefit from postoperative radiotherapy. J Clin Oncol 6:1107–1117, 1988.
16. Gilliland MD, Barton RM, Copeland EM III: The implications of local recurrence of breast cancer as the first site of therapeutic failure. Ann Surg 197:284–287, 1983.
17. Griem KL, Henderson IC, Gelman R, Ascoli D, Silver B, Recht A, Goodman RL, Hellman S, Harris JR: The 5-year results of a randomized trial of adjuvant radiation therapy after chemotherapy in breast cancer patients treated with mastectomy. J Clin Oncol 5:1546–1555, 1987.
18. Haagensen CD: Disease of the Breast, ed 2, revised reprint. Philadelphia, WB Saunders, 1971.
19. Host H, Brennhovd IO, Loeb M: Postoperative radiotherapy in breast cancer: long-term results from the Oslo study. Int J Radiat Oncol Biol Phys 12:727–732, 1986.
20. Janjan NA, McNeese MD, Buzdar AU, Montague ED, Oswald MJ: Management of locoregional recurrent breast cancer. Cancer 58:1552–1556, 1986.
21. Leggett CAC: Local recurrence of carcinoma of the breast. Aust NZ J Surg 50:298–300, 1980.
22. Lindfors KK, Meyer JE, Busse PM, Kopans DB, Munzenrider JE, Sawicka JM: CT evaluation of local and regional breast cancer recurrence. AJR 145:833–837, 1985.
23. Mendenhall NP, Devine JW, Mendenhall WM, Bland KI, Million RR, Copeland EM III: Isolated local-regional recurrence following mastectomy for adenocarcinoma of the breast treated with radiation therapy alone or combined with surgery and/or chemotherapy. Radiother Oncol 12:177–185, 1988.
24. A report of the Primary Therapy of Breast Cancer Study Group: Identification of breast cancer patients with high risk of early recurrences after radical mastectomy: II. Clinical and pathological correlations. Cancer 42:2809–2826, 1978.
25. Rosenman J, Churchill CA, Mauro MA, Parker LA, Newsome J: The role of computed tomography in the evaluation of postmastectomy locally recurrent breast cancer. Int J Radiat Oncol Biol Phys 14:57–62, 1988.
26. Roth D, Bayat H: The role of residual tumor in the chest wall in the late dissemination of mammary cancer. Ann Surg 168:887–890, 1968.
27. Rubin P, Bunyagidj S, Poulter C: Internal mammary lymph node metastases in breast cancer: detection and management. Am J Roentgenol Radium Ther Nucl Med 111:588–598, 1971.
28. Sarrazin D, Le M, Rouesse J, Contesso G, Petit J-Y, Lacour J, Viguier J, Hill C: Conservative treatment versus mastectomy in breast cancer tumors with macroscopic diameter of 20 millimeters or less: the experience of the Institut Gustave-Roussy. Cancer 53:1209–1213, 1984.
29. Scanlon EF: Local recurrence in the pectoralis muscles following modified radical mastectomy for carcinoma. J Surg Oncol 30:149–151, 1985.
30. Shah JP, Urban JA: Full thickness chest wall resection for recurrent breast carcinoma involving the bony chest wall. Cancer 35:567–573, 1975.
31. Spratt JS: Locally recurrent cancer after radical mastectomy. Cancer 20:1051–1053, 1967.
32. Stefanik D, Goldberg R, Byrne P, Smith F, Ueno W, Smith L, Harter K, Bachenheimer L, Beiser C, Dritschilo A: Local-regional failure in patients treated with adjuvant chemotherapy for breast cancer. J Clin Oncol 3:660–665, 1985.
33. Toonkel LM, Fix I, Jacobson LH, Wallach CB: The significance of local recurrence of carcinoma of the breast. Int J Radiat Oncol Biol Phys 9:33–39, 1983.
34. Veronesi U, Zucali R, Luini A: Local control and survival in early breast cancer: the Milan trial. Int J Radiat Oncol Biol Phys 12:717–720, 1986.
35. Wallgren A, Arner O, Bergstrom J, Blomstedt B, Granberg P-O, Raf L, Silfversward C, Einhorn J: Radiation therapy in operable breast cancer: results from the Stockholm trial on adjuvant radiotherapy. Int J Radiat Oncol Biol Phys 12:533–537, 1986.
36. Weichselbaum R, Marck A, Hellman S: Pathogenesis of pleural effusion in carcinoma of the breast. Int J Radiat Oncol Biol Phys 2:963–965, 1977.
37. Zimmerman KW, Montague ED, Fletcher GH: Frequency, anatomical distribution and management of local recurrences after definitive therapy for breast cancer. Cancer 19:67–74, 1966.

Chapter 42

MANAGEMENT OF SYSTEMIC METASTASES AND SEQUENTIAL THERAPY FOR ADVANCED DISEASE

William S. Dalton, M.D., Ph.D.

PROGNOSTIC FACTORS DETERMINING RESPONSE TO THERAPY

When diagnosed in its early stages, breast cancer is highly curable with available treatment strategies including surgery, radiotherapy, and adjuvant chemotherapy. That chemotherapy is effective in eradicating micrometastases and prolonging survival in premenopausal patients with early breast cancer is indisputable.[59] The efficiency with which combined chemotherapy is able to eliminate occult microscopic disease is related to the stage or tumor burden at the time of diagnosis.[53] Generally as the tumor burden increases (as measured by the number of axillary nodes containing malignant cells), the effectiveness of chemotherapy in eradicating systemic micrometastases declines. Once distant metastases become clinically apparent and are no longer microscopic, the disease is no longer curable by conventional means. This ability to develop distant metastases is the most devastating property of breast cancer and, unless the patient dies of other causes, will result in the patient's ultimate demise.

Although it is generally agreed that metastatic breast cancer is incurable, responses to therapy and survival duration after the first recurrence are highly variable.[2, 28, 55, 141, 144] This variability in response to therapy and survival duration demonstrates the biological heterogeneity of breast cancer.[25, 126] In some patients, the tumor burden is significantly reduced after hormone therapy or chemotherapy, with responses lasting for years after the first recurrence.[103] Yet in other patients, the tumor may recur very soon after treatment of the primary tumor; response to therapy is minimal, with the patient rapidly succumbing to the disease. Clinically, there are a number of characteristics that appear to be associated with the aggressiveness of the disease. These include the time interval between diagnosis of the primary tumor and development of overt metastatic disease, organ sites involved, and rate of tumor growth.[25, 57, 69, 103] More recently, biological characteristics have been associated with response to therapy and prognosis; these include the proliferative activity of the tumor, the hormone receptor status of the primary tumor, and perhaps the amplification or overexpression of certain proto-oncogenes.[39, 126, 177, 180] Drug resistance genes, such as the multidrug resistance gene 1 (MDR1), as described in in vitro systems, may also play a role in response to chemotherapy.[70, 139] In addition to the inherent biological characteristics of the tumor, certain host characteristics such as patient race, age, performance status, and disease-free interval may also influence the response to therapy of metastatic breast cancer.[69, 92, 133] Knowledge of the biological characteristics of the tumor and clinical characteristics of the patient may help in the selection of appropriate treatments for patients with metastatic disease. Identifying factors that influence the response and survival of patients also permits comparison of results between different clinical trials and indicates where new treatment strategies are needed for better treatment outcome.

Clinical Host Characteristics

A number of host factors have been analyzed to determine their prognostic importance in predicting survival and response to therapy following relapse. These variables predominantly have been related to either extent of tumor burden (such as number of metastatic sites and specific organ sites involved) or the rate of tumor progression (such as disease-free interval from time of initial diagnosis to time of relapse).[69, 92, 166] The most significant host characteristics that appeared to be related to response to chemotherapy and survival were actually an indication of tumor burden.[77] Some of these prognostic factors included poor performance status, abnormal biochemical and hematological values, organ sites involved, and number of metastatic sites. Other potential factors that have been studied for prognostic significance include age of patient at time of relapse, patient race, menopausal status, use of prior adjuvant chemotherapy, and psychosocial factors (Table 42–1).

In a study reported by Swenerton and colleagues,[166] 619 patients with metastatic breast cancer treated with a combination of 5-fluorouracil, adriamycin, and cyclophosphamide were analyzed retrospectively to identify host characteristics that might predict response to chemotherapy. Primary tumor characteristics such as size of primary, number of axillary metastases, and stage of diagnosis were not found to be of prognostic significance for response to therapy once metastatic disease developed. Patient age and menstrual status were also unrelated to outcome. Noncaucasian patients had a lower response rate and shorter survival than did caucasian patients. Factors that estimated the extent of disease or tumor burden such as poor performance status and abnormal biochemical and hematological values predicted a lower response rate to chemotherapy and shorter survival duration. Actual sites of metastatic disease were less important than factors that predicted the total tumor burden or extent of disease. There was a trend, however, for patients with bone involvement alone to have a longer survival than patients with metastases to other organ sites. A multivariate analysis of these same patients confirmed that an estimation of overall tumor burden was more important in predicting chemotherapeutic response than were the specific sites of organ involvement.[92] These investigators recommended treatment of metastatic disease at a time when the relative tumor burden was low to achieve the best possible results.

The presence of liver metastases is generally consid-

ered to be a poor prognostic factor in patients with breast cancer. However, very few patients with liver metastases as their sole metastatic site have been studied regarding response to therapy and survival. Zinser and colleagues[192] from M. D. Anderson Hospital reported a retrospective analysis of 233 patients with liver metastases. Patients with liver metastases alone or liver plus skeletal lesions survive longer than patients who had liver metastases and more than three other sites of metastatic disease. The investigators thus concluded that the extent of disease was a much better predictor of survival than the presence of liver metastases alone. Objective response rate to chemotherapy containing doxorubicin was approximately 60 percent in patients with hepatic metastases. Those patients who had normal albumin levels and good performance status had the best response rate and longest survival compared with patients with abnormal liver function tests and ascites. These studies showed that presence of liver metastases by itself was not an ominous factor but was generally a predictor of overall tumor burden. More than 80 percent of patients with hepatic metastases had lesions outside the liver.

In contrast to the poorer survival usually associated with visceral metastases, metastatic breast cancer confined to the skeletal system has been shown to have a favorable prognosis.[43, 151, 152] In a study of 86 patients with metastatic breast cancer confined to the skeletal system, the median survival was 48 months compared with a median survival of 17 months in patients with breast cancer metastatic to other disease sites.[152] In addition, these patients responded to both hormone therapy and chemotherapy. Sequential responses to hormonal therapy were frequent in this patient group.

The hormone receptor status, tumor characteristics, survival, and complications after first relapse were reported in 498 patients with first skeletal metastases and compared with 80 patients with liver metastases.[43] These investigators found that the patients with bony metastases had tumors that were better differentiated and more likely to have hormone receptors than those in patients with liver metastases. In addition, patients who presented with skeletal metastases as the first evidence of metastatic disease had a median survival of 24 months compared with 3 months after first relapse in the liver. Scheid and colleagues from M. D. Anderson reported a median survival of 28 months for patients with skeletal metastases only.[151] Objective response to chemotherapy was observed in 59 percent of patients.

Several studies have indicated that both age and menopausal status are unrelated to response to therapy or survival in patients with metastatic breast cancer.[69, 92, 166] However, a study by Nash et al.[133] using a multivariant regression model showed that patients younger than 40 years had a significantly shorter survival duration. A second study reported by Falkson investigated the effect of age at the time of first recurrence on survival in patients with metastatic breast cancer.[56] Patients with better performance status, fewer than three sites of metastases, and without visceral or nodal metastases had a better survival time. Patients who were

Table 42–1. POTENTIAL PROGNOSTIC FACTORS IN PREDICTING RESPONSE TO CHEMOTHERAPY

Factors related to tumor burden
   Performance status
   Number of metastatic sites
   Specific organ sites involved
   Abnormal hematological and biochemical values
   Disease-free interval
Other potential factors
   Age
   Menopausal status
   Use of prior adjuvant chemotherapy
   Psychosocial factors

younger, regardless of menopausal status, had shorter survival times. These investigators showed that patients younger than 35 years had a median survival of 491 days, compared with patients older than 45 years who had a median survival of 700 days.

The use of adjuvant cytotoxic chemotherapy to treat women with primary breast cancer has become a common practice during the past decade. Although adjuvant chemotherapy is effective in eliminating micrometastases in certain subgroups of women, relapse after adjuvant chemotherapy is a common problem.[59] The question of the emergence of drug resistance and shorter survival duration following relapse after the use of adjuvant chemotherapy has been studied by a number of investigators.[3, 27, 71, 104, 105] Valagussa et al.[178] reported equivalent response rates and response durations to salvage chemotherapy between patients who had received adjuvant CMF and patients who had not received any form of adjuvant chemotherapy. These investigators also noted that patients who received adjuvant cyclophosphamide, methotrexate, and 5-fluorouracil (CMF) responded to the same combination chemotherapy for the treatment of metastatic disease if the relapse-free survival was greater than 12 months. Kardinal and colleagues[104] found no difference in response rates, response duration, time to treatment failure, or survival between patients who had received prior adjuvant chemotherapy and those who had not. If patients relapsed 6 months or later following the completion of adjuvant chemotherapy, their responses to standard doses of cyclophosphamide, doxorubicin, and 5-fluorouracil were the same as those in patients untreated previously with adjuvant chemotherapy.

In a contrasting study, Ahmann et al.[3] found that patients who relapsed after receiving adjuvant chemotherapy consisting of doxorubicin and cyclophosphamide had a shorter median survival from the date of onset of recurrent disease (18 months vs. 28 months), a lower response rate to initial combination chemotherapy (38 percent vs. 69 percent), and a high incidence of central nervous system involvement at the time of relapse (11 percent). These investigators concluded that patients who failed adjuvant chemotherapy had a shorter survival time following relapse and a lower response to chemotherapy. In a similar retrospective review of patients who received a doxorubicin-containing regimen, Kau et al.[105] from M. D. Anderson observed that patients who relapsed after receiving adjuvant chemotherapy had a shorter survival from the time of first relapse, but that the survival from mastectomy was similar to that in patients who had never received adjuvant chemotherapy. These investigators concluded that although survival following the development of metastatic disease was shorter in patients who received adjuvant chemotherapy, it had no detrimental effect on overall survival.

It has long been speculated that certain psychological factors such as depression, emotional stress, and lack of social support could contribute to a shorter survival duration in patients with cancer.[167] Weisman and Worden[185] showed evidence that increased emotional stress contributes to a shorter survival. Similar obser-vations were noted by Greer and colleagues[76] as well as by Bloom,[18] who examined the relationship between stress and the lack of social support and the outcome of patients with breast cancer. Derogatis et al.[52] showed that patients who expressed their feelings about the disease and its treatment tended to live longer. In contrast, the study by Cassileth et al.[33] of 154 cancer patients revealed no significant relationship between psychosocial factors and length of survival. Similar results were described by Jamison et al.,[100] who analyzed psychosocial variables of 49 women with metastatic breast carcinoma. It was concluded that in this group of seriously ill patients, survival was not significantly influenced by psychosocial factors. It is generally concluded that although psychosocial factors are not a major determinant of survival at the time of development of metastatic disease, these factors undoubtedly influence the quality of life during treatment of metastatic disease.

Tumor Biology

Hormone Receptor Status and Response to Endocrine Therapy

Once a patient develops symptomatic recurrent breast cancer, the most common question is whether to treat the patient with hormone therapy or chemotherapy. The most important biological factor in determining response to hormone therapy is the presence of estrogen and progesterone receptors on the tumor specimen.[116, 126, 137] If the tumor does not contain these receptors, it is unlikely that the patient will respond to any hormonal treatment. In contrast, approximately 75 percent of patients with metastatic disease will respond if both receptors are present. The concentration of the receptor proteins in the tumor specimens also shows a direct relationship to likelihood of response. Tumors with high levels of receptor proteins (>100 Fmol/mg of cytosolic protein) are more likely to respond to hormonal treatments.[116, 137] In addition, the presence of both receptors and metastatic tissue also predicts a higher response rate compared with tumors that are positive for only estrogen or only progesterone receptors. It is generally recommended when the patient develops metastatic disease that a biopsy be obtained for determination of hormone receptor status. If a biopsy of the metastatic tumor is not feasible (i.e., the quantity of tissue is insufficient for determination of receptor status), then other characteristics may be used to predict response to hormone therapy. If the primary tumor was receptor positive, then it is reasonable to assume that the metastatic tumor will also be receptor positive, especially if no hormonal therapy has been administered in the interim.[8] Similarly, if the primary tumor was receptor negative, it is extremely unlikely that the metastatic tissue will be receptor positive. Sequential biopsies of metastatic tumor have also shown that the loss of the progesterone receptor is an adverse prognostic sign. A study by Osborne et al.[137] has demonstrated that intervening endocrine therapy may eliminate hormone-sensitive tumor cells and allow the emergence of tumor cells lacking the progesterone receptor. The survival duration of patients whose tumor cells became progesterone receptor negative was significantly shorter than that for those whose tumor cells remained progesterone receptor positive.

Other patient characteristics that appear to be related to hormonal responsiveness and may be used as a guide in administering hormonal therapy (especially when the receptor content of the tumor is unknown) include advanced age, postmenopausal status, prolonged disease-free interval after treatment of the primary tumor, and tumor sites primarily involving soft tissue and bones.[103] These clinical characteristics are usually indicative of a more indolent tumor that is likely to be hormone receptor positive.

Hormone Receptor Status and Response to Chemotherapy

A number of studies have investigated the relationship of cell kinetics to the presence of estrogen receptors in breast cancer. This relationship is based on the fact that estrogen receptor content is a biochemical marker of tumor differentiation; generally, the more well differentiated the tumor, the higher the estrogen receptor content.[78, 125] It has also been demonstrated that more well differentiated tumors tend to have a lower proliferative capacity.[111] Based on these two correlations, it is reasonable to speculate that tumors high in estrogen receptor content should have a low proliferative capacity. These correlations were observed by Meyer and others[127, 128] for breast carcinoma in relapse. These studies showed that a low labeling index was associated with minimal nuclear anaplasia, estrogen receptor positivity, and prolonged patient survival. Later Silvestrini et al. confirmed the observations of Meyer using tumor labeling index as a measure of proliferative activity.[153] Since estrogen receptor–negative tumors tend to have high proliferative activity, it has been speculated that they would respond better to chemotherapy. Most of the studies that have examined this question have been retrospective analyses. Lippman and coworkers[117] in 1978 reported in a retrospective study the relationship between estrogen receptors and the response rate to chemotherapy in 70 patients with metastatic breast cancer. These investigators found that those patients with low or absent estrogen receptor values had a higher response rate to chemotherapy than did those patients whose tumors were estrogen receptor positive. They concluded that the estrogen receptor values of tumors were important predictors of response to chemotherapy in metastatic breast cancer.

In contrast, Kiang et al.[106] analyzed the clinical data of 143 patients with advanced breast cancer and found that the response rate to chemotherapy was significantly higher in receptor-positive tumors than in receptor-negative tumors. In addition, response to hormonal therapy was unrelated to a subsequent response to chemotherapy. These investigators concluded that tumors high in estrogen receptor values respond better to

cytotoxic chemotherapy as well as hormonal therapy than do tumors that are low in estrogen receptors. Subsequent studies examining this controversy between the presence or absence of estrogen receptors and response to chemotherapy have generally shown no correlation between the presence of hormone receptors and response to chemotherapy.[146, 190] Those studies reporting a correlation between presence of hormone receptors and response to chemotherapy may be a result of biased patient selection. In a prospective study recently reported by Rosner et al.,[147] the predictive value of estrogen receptor status for response to chemotherapy was studied in 173 patients with metastatic breast cancer. In this study, there was no significant difference in overall responses between estrogen receptor–positive patients and estrogen receptor–negative patients. There was also no difference in overall survival between these two patient groups; however, those patients with estrogen receptor–positive tumors tended to have a longer duration of response than those patients with estrogen receptor–negative tumors.

Overall, unlike the case with hormonal therapy, the presence or absence of hormone receptors on breast cancer are unlikely to predict response to cytotoxic chemotherapy. As with using tumor cell kinetics as a predictive measure for response to chemotherapy, many factors are believed to influence response to cytotoxic chemotherapy, and no one particular factor is able to predict for response to chemotherapy.

Tumor Cell Kinetics

The relevance of tumor cell kinetics to disease-free survival and overall survival in early breast cancer is well established.[153, 162] Patients with tumors that have an abnormal DNA content and high percentage of cells in S phase have a worse prognosis than do those patients whose tumors have a normal DNA content and low proliferative capacity.[133] The influence of tumor cell kinetics on the response to chemotherapy or hormone therapy for advanced breast cancer has been studied less extensively.[172] Sulkes and coworkers[164] evaluated cell kinetics in patients with advanced breast cancer using an in vitro tritiated thymidine labeling index. Tumor cell uptake of tritiated thymidine was determined prior to treatment of 25 patients with disseminated breast cancer. All patients were subsequently treated with a doxorubicin-based combination chemotherapy. A tumor cell labeling index greater than nine percent predicted for a response to chemotherapy. None of the patients who had a labeling index of less than nine percent responded to treatment. In addition, those patients who responded to chemotherapy had a significantly longer survival as dated from the time of initiation of the combined chemotherapy. However, in those patients who were nonresponders, there was a higher frequency of prior chemotherapy, which may have decreased the likelihood of response to chemotherapy. In contrast, a study by Silvestrini et al.[154] measuring labeling index as a prognostic marker in locally advanced breast cancer found no relationship between pretreatment labeling index and response to chemotherapy. A high labeling index, however, did predict a higher progression rate at the end of the treatment regimen. Those patients with a higher labeling index had a shorter time to disease progression and a poorer probability of 4-year survival in comparison with patients with a low labeling index.

Zhang et al.[191] measured cytosolic thymidine kinase as an index of proliferative activity for 57 metastatic breast cancers and correlated this activity with the response or failure to subsequent hormonal therapy or chemotherapy. In this study, thymidine kinase did not predict response to hormone therapy; however, it was useful in predicting responses to chemotherapy. Those tumors with a high thymidine kinase activity indicative of a high proliferation rate were more likely to respond to chemotherapy than were those tumors with a low thymidine kinase activity. No statement could be made regarding duration of response and its relationship to proliferative activity based on this assay.

These studies indicate that the relationship between proliferative activity and response to chemotherapy is a complex one. The success of chemotherapy depends on a balance between the number of cells killed by chemotherapeutic drugs and the proliferation of cells surviving this chemotherapy. Thus the pretreatment measurements of proliferative activity using labeling index or other parameters such as flow cytometry are likely to be of limited prognostic value. These measurements may, however, prove useful in attempts to manipulate cell kinetics so that a greater number of cells may be recruited into the cell cycle, increasing the percentage of tumor cells susceptible to chemotherapy. Examples of this attempt to manipulate cell kinetics and using hormonal synchronization are discussed in chapters 40 and 44.

The relevance of tumor cell kinetics to hormonal response and its relationship to the presence of hormone receptors has also been studied in advanced breast cancer.[12, 128–130] The knowledge of hormone receptor status of tumor cells provides a rational biochemical basis for the treatment of patients with advanced breast cancer with endocrine therapy. Overall the response to hormonal therapy is approximately 60 percent in patients with estrogen receptor–positive tumors.[116] Studies have also demonstrated that the higher the estrogen receptor level in the tumor, the greater chance for response.[116, 137] Tumors that are positive for both the estrogen receptor as well as the progesterone receptor have a higher response rate to hormone therapy (70 percent) compared with tumors that are negative for both receptors (ten percent). The 30 percent to 40 percent failure rate of hormone therapy in hormone receptor–positive tumors demonstrates the biological heterogeneity of the tumor population.

One explanation for this heterogeneity may be a difference in cell kinetics. The relationship between cell kinetics and hormonal status and response to endocrine therapy was recently studied in 52 patients with advanced breast cancer.[138] Paradiso and colleagues[138] observed that tumors that grew slowly as determined by a low labeling index were mainly estrogen receptor positive, whereas fast proliferating tumors or those with a high labeling index were equally likely to be estrogen receptor positive or negative. Patients were more likely to receive a clinical benefit if their tumors were estrogen receptor positive and had a low labeling index (response rate of 88 percent) compared with those patients who had estrogen receptor–positive tumors and a high labeling index (response rate of 46 percent). However, the time to achieve maximum response was significantly longer for patients with slow proliferating, estrogen receptor–positive tumors than for those with fast proliferating, estrogen receptor–positive tumors. These investigators concluded that fast proliferating, estrogen receptor–positive tumors were able to escape hormonal control because of the presence of an autonomous subpopulation of tumor cells. A similar study was conducted by Baildam et al.[12] examining the relationship between DNA content of cancer cells and subsequent response to endocrine therapy in patients with advanced breast cancer. The highest proportion of estrogen receptor–positive tumors was found in the tetraploid tumors. Patients with diploid or tetraploid tumors survived longer and stayed in remission longer than did those patients with other aneuploid tumors. These studies demonstrate that cell kinetic analysis, in addition to the hormone receptor status of the tumor, may provide important information in identifying patients who are more likely to respond to endocrine therapy.

Cytogenetic and Molecular Biological Alterations: Correlations with Clinical Course of Disease

Based on the observations of hematological malignancies, cytogenetic and molecular analysis of breast tumors are currently being conducted to determine mechanisms of progression, patterns of metastases, response to therapy, duration of response, and survival. Cytogenetic studies of B cell neoplasms have demonstrated the correlation of specific sites of chromosomal alterations with loci of various cellular oncogenes. It is readily apparent from several lines of evidence that the aberrant expression of normal or mutated cellular oncogene sequences are involved in the malignant process. One of the most clearly documented mechanisms for inducing abnormal oncogene expression is some form of chromosomal alteration, such as chromosome translocation or gene amplification.[177] Preliminary cytogenetic studies of patients with metastatic breast cancer have demonstrated that alterations in chromosomes 3, 6, 7, and 11 predict for a poor response to either chemotherapy or hormone therapy. Also, survival duration from the time of diagnosis is short for these patients compared with those patients with no chromosomal abnormality.[49] Several proto-oncogene and oncogene abnormalities have been described in human breast cancer.[39, 180] The frequency of abnormalities appears to be related to the amount of tumor burden, and patients with metastatic disease appear to have the highest frequency of aberrancies in expression. Although this type of biological data is preliminary and the evidence is insufficient to clearly establish a causal relationship between aberrant oncogene expression and metastatic potential and response to therapy, the study of genetic phenomena and chromosome change in breast cancer will likely offer a biological explanation for these observations.

CHEMOTHERAPY FOR METASTATIC BREAST CANCER

Pharmacological Considerations

Of the many different types of cancers, metastatic breast carcinoma is considered to have a high response rate to cytotoxic chemotherapy. The response rate to a combination of cytotoxic drugs is approximately 70 percent, which is twice the response rate associated with other common metastatic tumors such as colon or lung. Despite this high response rate to chemotherapeutic drugs, the benefit in terms of survival is debatable.[2, 28, 144, 148] Undoubtedly, patients with life-threatening disease (such as those with metastases to the liver and lungs) do have a survival benefit when a durable response is achieved with combined chemotherapy. Other patients, however, who have more indolent disease (such as those with soft tissue or bone metastasis) are likely to gain little in terms of prolonged survival. In almost all patients, however, there is an improved quality of life, with decrease in pain and improved organ function associated with response to chemotherapy.[40] Thus the benefits associated with the use of cytotoxic drugs outweigh the risk of toxicity in patients who are truly symptomatic from their disease. Because treatment of metastatic breast cancer is primarily palliative, the choice of treatment must be individualized for each patient to maximize relief of symptoms with the lowest toxicity. For patients with more indolent non–life-threatening disease, hormone therapy or regional therapy such as radiation therapy may be the best treatment option. Other patients who have more rapidly progressing disease that may be life-threatening will require the use of cytotoxic drugs.

It is well recognized that a complete response to cytotoxic chemotherapy is not equivalent to cure in patients with metastatic breast carcinoma. Even patients who have long, durable remissions will eventually succumb to metastatic breast carcinoma if they do not die of other causes first. This is in obvious contrast to those patients who have prolonged survivals, if not cures, following the use of combination chemotherapy in the adjuvant treatment of primary breast cancer.[59] The development of drug resistance and the inability to cure metastatic breast cancer are likely caused by several factors. These factors include tumor growth kinetics (kinetic resistance), development of pharmacological sanctuaries (for example, loss of vascular supply and development of hypoxia in large tumors), and development of structural and metabolic changes in individual cells that confer drug resistance by spontaneous muta-

tion. The probability of developing any one of these factors is directly related to tumor mass.

The gompertzian function has been used to describe tumor growth rate in experimental systems.[77] According to this model, tumors initially grow rapidly, with a high percentage of cells involved in the cell cycle. Figure 42–1 demonstrates this type of growth curve in patients with breast carcinoma. As the tumor size increases, a plateau effect develops, and the apparent doubling time lengthens, with fewer cells actively proliferating. Figure 42–1 also demonstrates several chemotherapeutic principles and possible outcomes plotted against a gompertzian tumor growth curve. According to this model, the chance for cure is greatest when the tumor mass is smallest. As the tumor mass enlarges with time, the total number of cancer cells killed with chemotherapy is less, and the patient eventually dies of the disease.

A fundamental concept in cancer chemotherapy is the "cell-kill" hypothesis, derived from detailed studies in animal tumor systems. Basically, chemotherapy is thought to destroy cancer cells in a logarithmic fashion or by first-order kinetics. Simply stated, the proportion of tumor cells killed is a constant percentage of the total number of cells present and not a constant number of cells. For example, a log kill of 2 reduces a theoretical tumor burden of 10^9 cells to 10^7 cells, or a 99 percent reduction in tumor mass. The log cell kill for an individual or combination of drugs is dependent on the number of cells that are sensitive to these drugs. Most cytotoxic drugs kill cells by interfering with DNA synthesis or function. In general, cells are more sensitive to drugs when they are actively dividing and in the cell cycle as opposed to cells that are at rest.[24, 155, 169, 179] As demonstrated in Figure 42–1, by the time the tumor mass is detectable by standard methods (e.g., about 1 cm in diameter), tumor growth has reached a plateau and an increasing percentage of the cells are resting or not actively involved in cell division. The log cell kill is less for chemotherapeutic drugs during this phase of tumor growth. Presumably then, chemotherapeutic drugs could cure if the dose of drugs was sufficiently high to increase

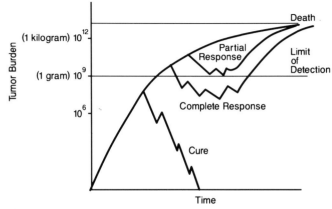

Figure 42–1. Growth curve of breast cancer demonstrating gompertzian kinetics.

the log cell kill or if the treatment was started early while the number of malignant cells present was small.

In addition to the kinetic resistance model for drug resistance, tumor cells may develop an intrinsic drug resistance to one or multiple drugs. Malignant cells, in contrast to normal cells, are generally considered to be more genetically unstable and prone to the generation of mutant clones.[74] Some of these mutations may allow for the development of drug resistance. Two mechanisms have been proposed for the emergence of drug resistance in cancer. One possibility is the drug itself induces mutations causing drug resistance; the other proposes that mutation to drug resistance occurs spontaneously and that drug exposure merely selects for resistant clones. Early work by Luria and Delbruck[122] and later work by Law[112] demonstrated that mutations to resistance occurred spontaneously and that resistant cells could exist prior to drug exposure. In 1979, Goldie and Coldman developed a mathematical model that related the curability of tumor to the appearance of drug-resistant mutants.[72–74] Two assumptions made in their mathematical model of drug resistance are: (1) drug-resistant cells arise spontaneously but at a measurable frequency (mutation rate), and (2) the number of resistant cells for a given tumor size depends on the mutation rate and the time at which the mutation developed during the tumor life span. Figure 42–2 demonstrates that as the tumor grows, it becomes more heterogeneous with the development of spontaneous mutations. Each of these spontaneous mutations may, in fact, confer resistance to a single drug or multiple drugs. The model predicts that the proportion of resistant cells increases as the tumor ages, and the likelihood of curing a given tumor with a single drug also decreases. Given the fact that most tumors have completed two thirds of their life span by the time they are detected, it is likely that a tumor has already developed multiple drug-resistant clones.

A great deal of research is now being conducted to investigate possible mechanisms of drug resistance as they occur in human cancers.[16, 70, 139] One noteworthy form of resistance has been termed "multidrug resistance" and is characterized by the simultaneous development of resistance to a wide variety of natural product agents, including doxorubicin and vincristine. This type of resistance is believed to be caused by the overexpression of an integral membrane protein called P glycoprotein or MDR1.[70, 139] This protein acts as an efflux pump that actively removes drug from the cell, resulting in a net decrease in intracellular drug accumulation. The P glycoprotein has been demonstrated in cancer cells from patients with metastatic breast cancer, but the significance of this finding remains to be determined.[149] It is likely that several mechanisms play a role in the development of drug resistance, including a decreased drug accumulation secondary to either reduced influx or enhanced efflux of drug from the cell; changes in subcellular distribution of drug that would alter drug concentrations at the target; alterations in the target (e.g., DNA); differences in DNA repair capacity; and changes in cellular metabolic systems that would facilitate detoxification of cytotoxic drugs. Such mechanisms are not likely to be mutually exclusive and may be operating in concert to contribute to the overall resistant phenotype in breast cancer cells.

Goldie and Coldman have recommended treatment strategies for cancers using currently available chemotherapeutic agents.[72] Their model predicts that the use of alternating non–cross-resistant treatments would be superior to the sequential use of these same treatments, because the latter approach would allow for the development and regrowth of doubly resistant cell lines. In order to achieve maximum cell kill with this strategy, it is important that each treatment be equally effective. In addition, it is assumed that the two treatments cannot be given simultaneously because of overlapping toxicity. This sort of approach has been used in certain cancers such as Hodgkin's disease, acute lymphocytic leukemia, and diffuse large cell lymphoma. Studies using a similar approach in the treatment of metastatic breast cancer, however, have not been as successful. These studies are preliminary, and studies using dose-intensive, alternating therapies are currently ongoing.

Efficacy of Individual Cytotoxic Drugs

As stated earlier, metastatic breast cancer has a high response rate to cytotoxic chemotherapy compared with other common cancers. Responses have occurred in a wide range of drugs, including alkylating agents, antitumor antibiotics, antimetabolites, plant alkaloids, and synthetic compounds (Table 42–2). Theoretically, this characteristic of responding to a wide variety of drugs should allow for an increased number of drug combinations that have unique mechanisms of action and are non–cross-resistant.

It is difficult to compare response rates for individual chemotherapeutic agents used in the treatment of breast cancer because of the heterogeneous patient populations studied for each individual drug. In the early development of effective chemotherapy, most patients had not received extensive prior therapy, and response rates in these relatively untreated patients might be expected to

Spontaneous Mutation to Drug Resistance with Tumor Progression in Breast Cancer

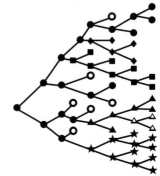

Figure 42–2. Heterogeneity of breast cancer caused by spontaneous mutations. Each symbol represents a new mutated clone.

be higher compared with those in patients who have been heavily pretreated. Early phase II trials in metastatic breast cancer evaluated primarily alkylating agents and antimetabolites. Phase II trials evaluating doxorubicin, generally considered the single most active agent for breast cancer, included patients who were either untreated or had received only one chemotherapeutic regimen. Most patients included in phase II trials of new agents for breast cancer have received a number of chemotherapeutic drugs, including doxorubicin. It is difficult, therefore, to compare the efficacy of individual chemotherapeutic agents because of the differences in patient populations studied. In addition, differences in criteria of response have varied from study to study, which makes it difficult to compare early trials with trials performed more recently. Table 42–2 shows the more commonly used agents and their approximate response rates in patients with metastatic breast cancer.

A number of alkylating agents have proven to be effective in the treatment of metastatic breast cancer. Cyclophosphamide is the most frequently used alkylating agent and has a response rate of approximately 26 percent. Cyclophosphamide may be given either orally or intravenously with equal efficacy. The dose-limiting factor is myelosuppression, with a nadir occurring at 8–14 days and recovery by 18–25 days. When compared with other alkylating agents, cyclophosphamide has been considered to be "platelet-sparing," but significant thrombocytopenia can also occur. Other toxicities such as hemorrhagic cystitis and cardiac toxicity are infrequent at the standard doses used.

Thiotepa and melphalan have also been used in the treatment of metastatic breast cancer and are considered to have less acute toxic effects, especially nausea and vomiting. Thiotepa was one of the first alkylating new agents used in the treatment of breast cancer but was replaced with cyclophosphamide.[75] Melphalan, although active in advanced breast cancer, has been primarily used in early breast cancer in the adjuvant setting because of its low acute toxicity.[151a] A significant drawback to the use of melphalan is the erratic bioavailability of the oral form.[6] Although the alkylating agents are

thought to share the same major mechanism of action, recent evidence has shown that many of the alkylating agents are non–cross-resistant and may even be synergistic.[171] Studies to evaluate the combination of high-dose alkylating agents with autologous marrow rescue are being performed.[9]

Doxorubicin is considered to be the single most active agent in the treatment of metastatic breast cancer.[173] As a single agent, the response rate varies between 28 percent and 43 percent for previously treated and untreated patients, respectively. The efficacy of doxorubicin is likely to be dose related. Using a combination of doxorubicin and cyclophosphamide, Jones and colleagues[102] observed that when the dose of doxorubicin was reduced from 40 mg/m^2 to 20 mg/m^2, the overall objective response rate went from 80 percent to 53 percent for this particular combination. Two more recent studies have confirmed the steep dose responsiveness to doxorubicin in metastatic breast cancer. Jones et al.[101] treated 26 patients with an intensive escalating dose of doxorubicin beginning at 25 mg/m^2/d for 3 days. The overall response rate of 85 percent and complete response rate of 38 percent were approximately double those previously reported with conventional doxorubicin doses. Toxicity was high, however, with 16 patients showing evidence of cardiotoxicity at a mean dose of 459 mg/m^2. Similarly, Carmo-Pereira and coworkers[32] treated 48 patients with metastatic breast cancer using either 35 or 70 mg/m^2 every 3 weeks. Both the percentage of objective responses and the median duration of response were significantly greater in the higher dose treatment group.

Cardiotoxicity is the dose-limiting factor for repeated administration. The incidence of congestive heart failure rises sharply after an accumulative dose of 450 mg/m^2. Based on the assumption that cardiotoxicity is related to peak concentrations of doxorubicin, attempts to reduce the incidence of cardiotoxicity have been made by giving the drug by either weekly or continuous infusion.[37, 176] There has been no evidence that the more frequent administration of lower doses of doxorubicin either increases or decreases its efficacy in comparison to bolus administration every 3 weeks.[186] Speyer et al.[159] reported the protective effect of the antioxidant bispiperazinedione (ICRF 187) against doxorubicin-induced cardiac toxicity in women with advanced breast cancer. Antitumor response was not changed by the use of ICRF 187, yet cardiac toxicity was significantly reduced. The use of antioxidants such as ICRF 187 may allow for further dose escalation of doxorubicin.

Mitomycin C is a second antitumor antibiotic used in the treatment of metastatic breast cancer.[17, 90] Activity as a single agent varies from 12 percent to 38 percent in patients who have been previously treated with CMF or doxorubicin.[90] This drug is most frequently combined with doxorubicin or vinblastine for second or third line chemotherapy, depending on the drug combination used in front line therapy. Thrombocytopenia and prolonged marrow suppression are associated with the use of mitomycin C.[140] Administration of the drug is usually limited to every 6 weeks because of prolonged myelo-

Table 42–2. ACTIVITY OF SINGLE AGENTS COMMONLY USED IN METASTATIC BREAST CANCER

Drug	Approximate Response Rate (percent)
Alkylating agents	
Cyclophosphamide	25
Melphalan	19
Thiotepa	17
Antitumor antibiotics	
Doxorubicin	35
Mitomycin C	20
Antimetabolites	
Methotrexate	23
5-Fluorouracil	21
Vinca alkaloids	
Vinblastine	21
Vincristine	10

suppression. Other serious toxicities associated with mitomycin C include pulmonary toxicity and cardiotoxicity.[90, 140] Renal toxicity may occur in association with microangiopathic hemolytic anemia. This latter toxicity is usually observed after a cumulative dose of 60 mg/m^2 and may occur long after the mitomycin C has been discontinued.[90]

Methotrexate and 5-fluorouracil (5-FU) represent the two most frequently used antimetabolites in the treatment of breast cancer. Both drugs as individual agents have a response rate of approximately 20 percent in patients with metastatic disease. Myelosuppression is generally considered to be the dose-limiting factor for both agents, with mucositis being a secondary concern. Methotrexate and 5-FU are frequently used in combination with cyclophosphamide as part of the CMF regimen, in which both drugs are administered on day 1 and day 8 of a 28-day cycle. Usually methotrexate precedes the administration of 5-FU. Both in vitro and in vivo studies have shown a possible synergism with this sequence.[14, 15] Conversely, if the drugs are given in the reverse sequence (5-FU preceding methotrexate) antagonism has been reported for experimental tumors. High-dose methotrexate (3 gm/m^2 or greater) with leucovorin rescue has been studied when given alone or in combination with other agents.[93, 189] No enhanced benefit regarding response rates or prolonged remissions can be attributed to the use of high-dose methotrexate alone. Leucovorin has also been combined with 5-FU to enhance the binding of 5-FU to thymidilate synthetase.[54, 123, 145] This regimen appears to be effective in drug-refractory patients, but with substantial gastrointestinal toxicity.

5-FU has been given as a single agent by long-term continuous infusion (200 to 300 mg/m^2/d) through a chronic indwelling venous catheter.[81] Patients were administered drug until toxicity but frequently received daily drug for 1–2 months. Overall response rate was 32 percent (8 of 25 patients) in this drug-refractory patient population, many of whom had received 5-FU as a bolus.

The *Vinca* alkaloids, vinblastine and vincristine, have both been used in combination chemotherapy for metastatic breast cancer.[1, 38] Until recently, vincristine was used more frequently than vinblastine because it was not myelosuppressive and could be combined with other drugs without compromising the dose of any of the other drugs in the combination. As a single agent, vincristine has a very low response rate compared with the other agents (see Table 42–2). In a study by Jackson et al.[98] using vincristine by continuous infusion at 0.5 mg/m^2/d for 5 days, the objective response rate was 13 percent. Thus whether vincristine is given as a bolus or by continuous infusion, it appears to be less active than the other agents commonly used in metastatic breast cancer. It is conceivable, however, that vincristine in combination with other cytotoxic agents may act synergistically. In vitro studies have shown that vincristine may increase the intracellular concentration of doxorubicin by inhibiting the efflux of doxorubicin.[187] Several clinical studies have suggested that the combination of vincristine and

doxorubicin may result in higher response rates than those obtained by doxorubicin alone.[21] In contrast, a prospective study by Steiner et al.[160] showed that the response rates and the duration of remissions were identical between patients treated with doxorubicin alone and those treated with doxorubicin plus vincristine. The group treated with the combination of doxorubicin plus vincristine did develop significantly more neurotoxicity. Similarly, other investigators have failed to demonstrate a therapeutic advantage in adding vincristine to various doxorubicin combinations, but toxicity has been increased.[38, 79] Reports by Ahmann et al.[1] and Segaloff et al.[150] also showed no therapeutic advantage in adding vincristine to various combinations of cyclophosphamide, methotrexate, 5-fluorouracil, and prednisone. Thus, the role of vincristine in the treatment of metastatic breast cancer is questionable.

The efficacy of vinblastine in the treatment of metastatic breast cancer appears to be more promising. However, the dose-limiting factor of vinblastine is myelosuppression, thereby limiting its usefulness in combination chemotherapy. Fraschini et al.[64] reported objective responses in 39 of 106 patients (37 percent) with metastatic refractory breast cancer treated with a 5-day continuous infusion of vinblastine at doses of 1.7–2.0 mg/m^2/d. Responses also occurred in patients who had become refractory to the bolus administration of *Vinca* alkaloids, indicating that steady-state concentration of the drug may be important.

Combination Chemotherapy

In patients with metastatic breast cancer, the use of combined chemotherapy has been associated with increased response rates compared with single agents.[29, 45, 75, 148] Greenspan was among the first to demonstrate that the objective response rates associated with the combination of thiotepa and methotrexate were more than double those produced by either of the agents used singly.[75] The therapeutic potential of combination chemotherapy was further reinforced when Cooper reported a response rate of 90 percent with cyclophosphamide, methotrexate, 5-fluorouracil, vincristine, and prednisone.[45] Although subsequent larger trials of this same five-drug combination have failed to reproduce this impressive response rate, the superiority of combination chemotherapy to single agents in terms of response rates has been confirmed.

The Eastern Cooperative Oncology Group compared single agent melphalan to the CMF regimen in patients with metastatic breast cancer.[29] The CMF combination was superior to melphalan alone in frequency of response, duration of response, and survival. This study therefore suggested that in addition to improving response rates, combined chemotherapy might also improve survival.[29]

Because of the relatively large number of drugs that are effective in the treatment of breast cancer, there are literally hundreds of possible combinations that may be empirically derived. It is obviously not possible to test and compare all the various combinations of drugs in a clinical setting. Therefore it is important to consider the following pharmacological principles in combining drugs to achieve potentially synergistic activity:

1. Each of the individual drugs should be effective against the tumor.

2. Toxicities should minimally overlap so that full doses of each drug may be used in combination.

3. Ideally, the drugs should have different mechanisms of action.

Over the years, a number of regimens have become "standard" in the treatment of metastatic breast cancer. Almost all the regimens use the alkylating agent cyclophosphamide, and one of the most commonly used regimens is the CMF combination.[29] Objective responses occur in approximately 50 percent to 60 percent of patients, and the complete response rate is usually less than 20 percent. Median survival ranges from 12 to 18 months when this regimen is used as the initial treatment program. The CMF regimen appears particularly well tolerated in elderly patients older than 65. Gelman and Taylor[68] showed that when doses were decreased according to pretreatment creatinine clearance ("modified" CMF), CMF could be administered safely to elderly patients.

The addition of prednisone to the CMF regimen adds approximately 15 percent to the response rate. Median duration of response may also be slightly increased, according to a study by the Eastern Cooperative Oncology Group.[173a] The increase in response frequency and response duration are modest and may be caused by the actual increase in dose of cyclophosphamide, methotrexate, and 5-FU in the CMFP regimen compared with that in the CMF regimen. The addition of prednisone decreases the incidence of vomiting, and nadir white counts are higher compared with those in the CMF regimen. On the other hand, the use of even moderate doses of prednisone for 14 days can be associated with cushingoid side effects, which the patient may find unacceptable.

Advantages of Doxorubicin Combinations

As mentioned earlier, doxorubicin is the most active single agent for the treatment of metastatic breast cancer.[173] Because of its high degree of activity and possible lack of cross-resistance between other agents used (especially the alkylating agents), doxorubicin has frequently been combined with various other agents (Table 42–3).

A comparison of reported results of trials comparing doxorubicin-containing regimens to methotrexate combinations is given in Table 42–4. Of the seven randomized controlled trials, two show a significant survival advantage using doxorubicin. Four of the trials demonstrate that the overall response rate is superior for the doxorubicin-containing regimens, indicating a greater degree of tumor cell kill by the doxorubicin-containing combinations. These trials demonstrate, therefore, the superiority of doxorubicin-containing regimens in terms

of response rates and response duration; however, the survival benefit appears to be modest.

Doxorubicin has been combined with a number of other active agents. Some of these combinations and approximate reported response rates are noted in Table 42–4. Doxorubicin has been combined with cyclophosphamide with and without 5-FU, producing overall response rates between 70 percent and 80 percent in previously untreated patients.[47] The *Vinca* alkaloids have also been combined with doxorubicin, but vinblastine appears to be more effective in combination chemotherapy than vincristine.[63, 121] Perloff and coworkers[142] and, later, Hart and colleagues[83] reported on the combination of vinblastine, doxorubicin, thiotepa, and fluoxymesterone in patients who had received prior chemotherapy for metastatic breast cancer. This particular regimen also appeared to be effective in patients who had been treated with prior doxorubicin chemotherapy. Tannir et al.[168] reported an overall response rate of 43 percent using a sequential continuous infusion of doxorubicin for 2 days, followed by vinblastine over a 4-day period. The combination of vinblastine plus doxorubicin appears to be an effective second line therapy for patients who have failed to respond to the combination of cyclophosphamide, methotrexate, and 5-fluorouracil.

Several factors must be taken into consideration when deciding whether to use a doxorubicin-containing regimen or other drug combinations when the patients is first diagnosed with metastatic disease. These considerations include whether the patient has received adjuvant chemotherapy, which drugs were used in the adjuvant therapy, whether the patient has underlying medical problems that would preclude the use of specific drugs, and the symptoms of the patient at time of presentation. When considering the best therapeutic approach for individual patients, it must be emphasized that the standard treatment modalities currently available do not cure metastatic disease, and the major goal is relief of symptoms. Therefore the benefit achieved with combination chemotherapy must be weighed against the risk of side effects and toxicity.

Salvage Regimens

Relapse following the initial treatment of metastatic breast cancer is inevitable. The four most commonly used drugs in the treatment of breast cancer are cyclophosphamide, doxorubicin, 5-fluorouracil, and methotrexate. Salvage chemotherapy must then make use of other agents that are active but non–cross-resistant to those agents used primarily after the diagnosis of metastatic disease. A common approach to a patient with newly diagnosed metastatic disease is to treat with a combination of 5-fluorouracil, doxorubicin, and cyclophosphamide (FAC). Objective remissions occur in 50 percent to 80 percent of patients, including 15 percent to 20 percent with a complete remission. In patients who achieve a durable remission, doxorubicin is discontinued after reaching a cumulative dose of 450 mg/m² because of the risk of cardiotoxicity.[182] Therapy is continued by replacing doxorubicin with methotrexate until

Table 42–3. MOST FREQUENTLY USED COMBINATION CHEMOTHERAPY REGIMENS

Regimen	Schedule	Cycle Length	Reference
Doxorubicin-Containing Regimens			
AC			
Doxorubicin	40 mg/m^2 I.V. d 1		
Cyclophosphamide	200 mg/m^2 p.o. d 3–6	3 weeks	102
CAF			
Cyclophosphamide	400–500 mg/m^2 I.V. d 1		
Doxorubicin	40–50 mg/m^2 I.V. d 1	3 weeks	26
5-Fluorouracil	400–500 mg/m^2 I.V. d 1 + 8		
VATH			
Vinblastine	4.5 mg/m^2 I.V. d 1		
Doxorubicin	45 mg/m^2 I.V. d 1		
Thiotepa	12 mg/m^2 I.V. d 1	3 weeks	142
Halotestin	10 mg p.o. TID daily		
Non-Doxorubicin–Containing Regimens			
CMF(P)			
Cyclophosphamide	100 mg/m^2 p.o. d 1–14		
Methotrexate	40–60 mg/m^2 I.V. d 1 + 8	4 weeks	29
5-Fluorouracil	600–700 mg/m^2 I.V. d 1 + 8		
Prednisone	40 mg/m^2 p.o. d 1–14		
Mitomycin-Vinblastine			
Mitomycin C	10 mg/m^2 I.V. d 1 and 28, then every 6–8 weeks		67
Vinblastine	5 mg/m^2 I.V. d 1, 14, 28, and 42, then every 3 weeks		

evidence of progressive disease. Using this approach, all four of the most active agents in the treatment of breast cancer are utilized in the initial treatment of metastatic disease.

Combination chemotherapy consisting of mitomycin C and vinblastine has been proposed for patients who progress on FAC or CMF regimens.[51, 67, 109, 121] As mentioned previously, these two drugs as individual agents produce response rates in 25 percent to 30 percent of patients. Konits and coworkers[109] reported their experience using mitomycin C (20 mg/m^2 I.V. every 6 weeks) in combination with vinblastine (0.15 mg/kg I.V. on

Table 42–4. COMPARISON OF DOXORUBICIN-CONTAINING REGIMENS WITH METHOTREXATE-CONTAINING REGIMENS IN METASTATIC BREAST CANCER: RESULTS OF RANDOMIZED TRIALS

Treatment	Evaluable Cases	Overall Response (%)	Median Duration Response (Months)	Median Survival (Months)	Reference
CMF	40	62	8	17	26
CAF	38	82	10	27	
p value		0.08	NS	0.13	
CMF	99	37	9.7	16	5
CAF	82	55	13.7	26.5	
p value		0.01	0.05	0.04	
CMFP	76	53	6.3	15.8	47
CAF	79	53	11.0	18.6	
p value		NS	NS	NS	
CMFVP	72	57	14	20	132
CAFVP	76	58	16	33	
p value		NS	NS	0.07	
CMFVP	130	40	7	14	157
CAF	135	54	7	17	
p value		0.01	NS	0.10	
CMFVP	86	50	9	16	175
CAFVP	107	71	14	19	
p value		0.003	0.07	0.24	
CMFVP	109	50	7	13	175
CAFVP	107	71	14	19	
p value		0.002	0.01	0.01	

Abbreviations: A, doxorubicin; C, cyclophosphamide; F, 5-fluorouracil; M, methotrexate; P, prednisone; V, vincristine.

days 1 and 21 of each cycle). Overall response rate in 31 patients was 40 percent, with a median duration of response of 127 days. Hematological toxicity, including thrombocytopenia, was significant, perhaps because of the relatively high dose of mitomycin C. Denefrio et al.[51] reported their results with a smaller but more frequent dosage schedule of mitomycin C at 6 mg/m² every 4 weeks combined with vinblastine at 5 mg/m² every 2 weeks. The hematological toxicity was less than that reported by Konits et al.,[109] but Denefrio and colleagues had only one response among 17 patients. In a study by Garewal et al.[67] using an intermediate dose of mitomycin C (10 mg/m²) in combination with 5 mg/m² of vinblastine, a response rate of 35 percent was reported in patients who had been heavily pretreated. These data suggest that there is a dose-response effect for mitomycin C, but that hematological toxicity must be taken into consideration.

In summary, the combination of mitomycin C and vinblastine appears to be an active regimen in refractory breast cancer. Response rates vary from 30 percent to 40 percent, with response durations lasting from 4 to 6 months when this combination is used as salvage chemotherapy.

Several studies have investigated the possibility of using various combinations of cytotoxic agents in an alternating fashion, as opposed to a sequential fashion.[4, 21, 46, 110] This approach is based on the Goldie-Coldman hypothesis and would ideally employ alternating combinations that are theoretically non–cross-resistant.[72, 73] Such an approach might preclude the emergence of drug-resistant cells and prolong response durations. In a study by Tormey et al.,[174] 23 patients were administered a combination of 11 different cytotoxic drugs and hormones during a 28-day period. This intensive regimen induced a complete response rate of 78 percent, but the response duration of 13 months was no greater than that seen for standard combinations. Other randomized trials comparing a single combination to alternating combinations have failed to improve response rates and durations of response.[58, 120, 181]

New Agents

Doxorubicin is the most active single agent in the treatment of breast cancer; however, its usefulness is limited by cumulative, dose-dependent, chronic cardiotoxicity. Retrospective studies by Von Hoff et al.[182] estimated the risk of cardiotoxicity at 3 percent to 4 percent after a cumulative dose of 450 mg/m², increasing to six percent to ten percent after 550 mg/m². The incidence of congestive heart failure rises rapidly with increasing doses. Because of the risk of cardiotoxicity, it is generally recommended that doses be limited to 450–550 mg/m² when doxorubicin is administered as a bolus infusion every 3 weeks.

One means of solving this problem is to develop new anthracycline analogues by altering the chemical structure and stereochemistry of doxorubicin and daunorubicin. Preclinical studies have shown that structure al-

terations of the anthracycline molecule may result in a better therapeutic index by lessening the potential for cardiac toxicity. Epirubicin (4'-epi-doxorubicin) was one of the first analogues to be studied.[22, 99] It is a stereoisomer of doxorubicin in which the hydroxl group at the 4 position of the aminosugar side chain is epimerized. Preclinical studies have shown that the antineoplastic activity of epirubicin was similar to that of doxorubicin, but acute and chronic toxicity, including cardiac toxicity, was less compared with doxorubicin.

Phase II studies comparing epirubicin with doxorubicin in the treatment of advanced breast cancer have now been reported.[22, 99] In a study by Jain et al.,[99] both epirubicin and doxorubicin produced an overall response rate of 25 percent in patients who had previously been treated with a non-anthracycline combination. The median duration of response to epirubicin was 11.9 months, compared with 7.1 months with doxorubicin. Cardiotoxicity occurred in both groups, but the median cumulative dose at which congestive heart failure occurred for epirubicin was 1134 mg/m², compared with 492 mg/m² for doxorubicin. In addition, fewer episodes of nausea and vomiting were observed in patients receiving epirubicin. In a similar phase II study by Brambilla et al.,[22] the overall response rates were 52 percent and 62 percent for doxorubicin and epirubicin, respectively. The median duration of response was 22 months for both agents. Acute toxicity comprised of vomiting, mucositis, and leukopenia occurred less frequently following administration of epirubicin when compared with doxorubicin. No specific comment could be made regarding cumulative cardiac toxicity because of the small number of patients. The authors concluded that epirubicin was as effective as doxorubicin but with less toxicity.

Epirubicin has also been compared with doxorubicin in phase III trials comparing combination chemotherapy with cyclophosphamide, 5-fluorouracil, and either doxorubicin or epirubicin. In a French study, 263 patients were randomized to treatment regimens consisting of fluorouracil, cyclophosphamide, and either epirubicin or doxorubicin.[10, 66] Overall response was produced in 50.4 percent of patients treated with the epirubicin combination compared with 52 percent for the doxorubicin treated group. There was no statistical difference between the two regimens in overall response rate or duration of response. In the patients treated with the doxorubicin regimen, three of 120 patients developed clinical congestive heart failure. In comparison, of the 124 evaluable patients treated with the epirubicin regimen, no episodes of congestive heart failure were observed. In addition, there was significantly less acute toxicity, including nausea and vomiting, alopecia, and neutropenia, for patients treated with epirubicin. The authors concluded that the epirubicin combination was as effective as the more commonly used doxorubicin regimen but was better tolerated.

Esorubicin (4'-deoxydoxorubicin) is another doxorubicin analogue that has also been evaluated because of the preclinical finding of decreased cardiac toxicity compared with doxorubicin. Two separate phase II studies have shown that this analogue, unlike epirubicin, is relatively inactive in advanced breast cancer.[30, 114]

A new daunorubicin analogue, 4-demethoxy-daunorubicin (4-DMDR), differs from daunorubicin in that it lacks the C-4 methoxyl group in the aglycone. Preclinical studies demonstrated more activity in solid tumors with less cardiotoxicity compared to either doxorubicin or daunorubicin. In addition, 4-DMDR could be administered orally and retain its activity.[50] Two phase II studies have evaluated oral 4-DMDR in patients with metastatic breast cancer.[108, 124] In both studies, the patients had progressed on front line chemotherapy but had not been previously treated with anthracyclines. Martoni and colleagues[124] reported an overall response rate of 30 percent and a median duration of 6 months. Kolaric et al.[108] reported an objective response rate of 23 percent with a median response duration of 4 months. Acute toxicity consisted of mild nausea and vomiting, leukopenia, and mild alopecia. There was no evidence of cardiac toxicity in either study.

The anthracenediones represent a new class of synthetic agents that have been recently evaluated for activity in breast cancer. Mitoxantrone is the most well characterized anthracenedione and has been frequently compared to doxorubicin because it is a planar, electron-rich chromophore possessing a dihydroxyquinone function.[183] Like doxorubicin, mitoxantrone binds DNA; however, it does not appear to be a classic intercalating agent, and the exact mechanism of action is unknown at this time.[20] In all animal tumors studied, the cytotoxicity of mitoxantrone was superior to that of doxorubicin.[183] In addition, cardiotoxicity as determined by a rat model was much less compared with that of doxorubicin.[36] Because of these promising preclinical results, mitoxantrone has been studied extensively in the treatment of breast cancer.[88, 158] A number of studies have shown that mitoxantrone as a single agent is effective in the primary treatment of metastatic breast cancer. A large multicenter phase II trial comparing mitoxantrone with doxorubicin in the treatment of metastatic breast cancer has been recently reported.[84] In this study, 165 patients were randomized to receive mitoxantrone, and 160 received doxorubicin. All patients had been treated with at least one prior regimen, but no patients had received prior doxorubicin. Both mitoxantrone and doxorubicin were administered intravenously on a 3-week schedule. The mitoxantrone dose was 14 mg/m^2, and the dose of doxorubicin was 75 mg/m^2. The overall response rate to mitoxantrone was 20 percent, compared with 29 percent for those who received doxorubicin. This difference was not significant at the $p < 0.05$ level. Median duration of response was similar (152 days for mitoxantrone and 124 days for doxorubicin). Median survival was also similar at 273 days for mitoxantrone and 268 days for doxorubicin.

The major toxicity for both treatment groups was myelosuppression, with the level of severity being identical. However, non-hematological toxicity was significantly less for the mitoxantrone treatment group, especially for nausea and vomiting and alopecia. Sixty-one percent of the patients treated with doxorubicin had severe alopecia, compared with only 5 percent of patients treated with mitoxantrone. Only one patient in the mitoxantrone treatment group developed congestive heart failure, compared with five patients who received doxorubicin. Using radionuclide angiography to evaluate left ventricular function demonstrated that mitoxantrone caused significantly less cardiac damage compared with doxorubicin.

This study concluded that mitoxantrone was slightly less active than doxorubicin. The duration of response for doxorubicin and mitoxantrone were identical, as was survival duration. Both acute and chronic toxicity appeared to be substantially less for mitoxantrone compared with doxorubicin.[80, 81, 84]

Because combined chemotherapy is generally considered to be more effective than treatment with a single agent, regimens containing mitoxantrone have been compared with similar regimens containing doxorubicin.[65, 89] In a study by Follezou et al.,[60] 142 patients were given cyclophosphamide plus 5-fluorouracil with either doxorubicin or mitoxantrone. The objective response rate in those patients receiving the doxorubicin combination was 42.8 percent, compared with 42.2 percent in the mitoxantrone treatment group. Median duration of response was 37 weeks for the doxorubicin group and 34 weeks for the mitoxantrone group. There was no significant cardiotoxicity in either group. Noncardiac toxicity was primarily myelosuppression and was similar for each group. Other acute toxicities, including nausea and vomiting and alopecia, were significantly less for the mitoxantrone-containing regimen. Similar results have been reported by Bennett et al.,[13] who studied 331 patients treated with either cyclophosphamide, mitoxantrone, and fluorouracil or cyclophosphamide, doxorubicin, and fluorouracil. In this study, however, the mitoxantrone regimen was slightly less effective in overall response, but the survival benefit was identical in the two treatment groups. Again, toxicity was significantly less in the mitoxantrone regimen compared with the doxorubicin regimen.

Leonard et al.[115] in comparing doxorubicin plus vincristine and prednisolone with mitoxantrone plus vincristine and prednisolone found that the doxorubicin-containing regimen was significantly more effective, with an overall response rate of 61 percent and an overall response rate of 35 percent compared with the mitoxantrone regimen. Median survival, however, was similar for both regimens. Toxicity, particularly alopecia and nausea and vomiting, was significantly lower for the mitoxantrone treated patients. The investigators cautioned, however, that subclinical cardiotoxicity was seen in both treatment groups and stated that cardiac toxicity was a potential hazard with either drug combination.

Although mitoxantrone and doxorubicin have frequently been compared because of their structural similarities, these two compounds do have distinct mechanisms of action and recently have been shown to have different mechanisms of resistance.[20, 48] Alberts et al.[7] reported that the combination of mitoxantrone plus doxorubicin was at least additive and potentially synergistic in vitro using the human breast cancer cell line

MCF-7. In a crossover design study comparing mitoxantrone with doxorubicin in advanced breast cancer, Neidhart and colleagues[134] demonstrated that ten percent of patients receiving doxorubicin and 21 percent of patients receiving mitoxantrone responded when these agents were administered after failure had occurred with the primary agent. These data suggested that the cross-resistance between the two agents was only partial. A recent Canadian study reported on the combination of mitoxantrone and doxorubicin in patients with advanced breast cancer.[62] Fifty percent of the patients responded to this regimen. As expected, myelotoxicity was the dose-limiting factor; however, symptoms of congestive heart failure occurred in three of 14 patients examined. Mitoxantrone in combination with doxorubicin, therefore, should be used with caution, given the possibility of increased cardiac toxicity.[62, 161]

Bisantrene, also an anthracene derivative, has also been studied in the treatment of metastatic breast cancer.[35, 61, 87] In comparison to mitoxantrone, bisantrene appears to be less active, with minimal activity in patients previously treated with doxorubicin. Hematological toxicity (leukopenia) is dose limiting, but nonhematological side effects are also significant. Phlebitic reactions are high, requiring that this drug be given via a central venous catheter, which further limits its usefulness.

Dose Response

As mentioned earlier, there are a number of factors that appear to predict for response rate and duration. Most of these factors are intrinsic to the tumor, including tumor mass and proliferative activity, and are generally beyond the control of the treating physician. One factor ·that may also play a role in determining treatment outcome and that is at least under partial control of the treating physician is the dose of drugs delivered to the patient. The efficacy and toxicity of drugs are generally related to dose. Intuitively, one would hypothesize that higher doses of drug would improve response and outcome. This principle of dose response holds true for many experimental tumors, and it has also been observed to apply to certain human tumors such as acute lymphocytic leukemia as well as certain solid tumors, including small lung carcinoma and testicular carcinoma. Extrapolating these results to the treatment of breast cancer has been more difficult.[85, 86]

Most studies analyzing the principle of dose response in the treatment of breast cancer have been largely retrospective. Hryniuk and Bush[94] emphasized dose intensity of various drugs in the treatment of metastatic breast carcinoma. In this retrospective analysis, dosages of the standard drugs cyclophosphamide, methotrexate, 5-fluorouracil, and doxorubicin were converted to the form of mg/m^2/wk. This was given the term "dose intensity" and allowed comparison among various drug regimens.[94, 95] The concept of dose intensity considers not only the absolute dose but the scheduling of drugs as well. A reduction in dose intensity may occur by either reducing the absolute dose or delaying treatment. Using this calculation, the investigators reported a direct relationship between response rate and average relative dose intensity. This relationship was seen for CMF as well as the doxorubicin-containing regimen CAF of Bull and Tormey.[26, 175]

Prospective studies evaluating the importance of dose have reported conflicting results. Studying doxorubicin as a single agent in the treatment of metastatic breast cancer, Carmo-Pereira et al.[32] found a clear benefit in terms of objective response and median duration of response in patients who received doxorubicin 70 mg/m^2 every 3 weeks compared with those patients who received a lower dose at 35 mg/m^2 every 3 weeks. In another prospectively randomized study, patients were randomized to either high-dose chemotherapy, receiving three cycles of high-dose FAC in a protected environment, with all subsequent cycles being administered at standard doses in the outpatient setting, or to chemotherapy using standard doses throughout treatment.[91] Therefore the only difference between the high-dose treatment group and the control group was in the first three cycles of treatment. During the first three cycles, the dose intensity for doxorubicin in the high-dose treatment group was 28.3 mg/m^2/wk, compared with 16.6 mg/m^2/wk for the standard dose group. There were no differences in overall, complete response, or partial response rates between the high-dose FAC and control groups. Median duration of response and survival were also similar. The investigators concluded that within the doses administered, there was no benefit for high-dose induction therapy.

Two prospective studies have tested the schedule, dose, and dose intensity of CMF-containing regimens in advanced breast cancer. In a study by Carmo-Pereira et al.,[31] 67 percent of patients in the intensive treatment group achieved an objective response vs. only 41 percent of patients in the standard dose treatment group. Median duration of response in the intensively treated group was 14 months vs. 11 months in the standard group. In a similar study by Tannock et al.,[169a] patients who received a higher dose of CMF had a response rate of 30 percent compared with the lower dose arm at 11 percent. Patients randomized to the higher dose treatment group survived longer than did those in the lower dose intensity arm; however, in this study, the two patient groups were imbalanced with respect to the interval from first relapse to randomization, and this imbalance may have accounted for the difference in survival.

Overall both retrospective and prospective studies would indicate that response rates are improved with higher doses of chemotherapy. The higher response rates may also translate into better palliation of disease-related complications. The trial of Tannock et al.[169a] suggested that better palliation was achieved by using higher dose chemotherapy. It would appear that lowering the dose in anticipation of reducing toxicity is not valid and that the reduction of doses may in fact reduce the probability of improved quality of life.

Treatment Duration

In addition to dose intensity, there are other pharmacological factors that may determine treatment results. These factors include drug scheduling, total dose of drug administered, and treatment duration. The studies of dose intensity would indicate that the greatest amount of drug given in the shortest amount of time may be the most effective; however, in order to achieve a significant amount of cell kill, the duration of therapy must also be considered. If effective drugs are administered below the minimum time necessary to eliminate drug-sensitive cancer cells, then the benefits of intensive therapy are lost. Conversely, prolonged therapy with cytotoxic agents may merely select for drug-resistant cells, and further therapy would only produce toxicity with no further cell kill. In a study by Coates et al.,[40] patients were prospectively randomized to receive either continuous chemotherapy administered until disease progression was evident, or intermittent therapy, whereby treatment was administered for only three cycles, then stopped and repeated for another three cycles only when there was evidence of disease progression. The same combinations of drugs were used in each treatment arm. Intermittent therapy resulted in significantly worse response rates and shorter times to treatment failure. In addition, the quality of life was significantly improved in those patients receiving continuous treatment compared with those receiving intermittent therapy. This was attributed to the fact that those in the continuous treatment group were more likely to have a response to therapy and, therefore, to experience palliation of symptoms. This study does not exclude the possibility that another type of intermittent therapy, such as discontinuing therapy after patients receive the maximum response, might not achieve a similar response rate and response duration compared with continuous therapy. Patients treated in this manner might also have improved quality of life with less toxicity than is experienced with continuous treatment. A reasonable approach might be to treat patients to maximum response plus an additional three courses and then discontinue treatment until there is evidence of progressive disease.

High-Dose Chemotherapy with Autologous Marrow Rescue

As discussed previously, there does appear to be a relationship between response to chemotherapy and doses of drugs employed. However, in the studies mentioned, the increase in dose of drugs has been modest, usually no greater than twofold, because of dose-limiting toxicity. For most chemotherapeutic drugs, the dose-limiting factor is myelosuppression. Recent studies have used transplantation of normal bone marrow cells to overcome this limitation. In this setting, the dose may be escalated as high as tenfold, depending on nonhematological toxicities encountered. Antman and Gale[9] recently reviewed 27 trials of high-dose therapy with autologous bone marrow transplantation in patients with

metastatic breast cancer. One hundred seventy-two patients received single or multiple agent chemotherapy, radiation, or both. Most of the patients treated in these trials had been heavily treated with multiple agents prior to receiving high-dose therapy. It appeared that multiple alkylating agents offered the best response rate (76 percent); however, no best regimen has yet been described. Although response rates were high, the durations of response were short, usually less than 6 months. These investigators felt that treatment with high-dose therapy earlier in the course of disease might produce more durable responses.

Peters et al.[143] reported a phase II trial using high-dose cyclophosphamide, cisplatin, and carmustine or melphalan and bone marrow support as initial therapy for metastatic breast cancer. Twelve of 22 patients treated obtained a complete response (55 percent), with an overall response rate of 73 percent. Median duration of response in the patients achieving a complete remission was 9 months. Studies using a single treatment of high-dose chemotherapy with autologous marrow rescue indicated that a large cell kill can be obtained by a single intensive treatment; however, this mode of therapy appears to be inadequate to eliminate enough cells to provide a long, durable remission. Other means are needed to eliminate the remaining surviving cells. Perhaps the use of hematopoietic growth factors, such as granulocyte-macrophage colony-stimulating factor (GM-CSF), will allow for multiple dose-intensive treatments to achieve a greater overall cell kill.[23]

Combined Chemohormonal Therapy

Great interest has recently developed regarding the possibility of combining chemotherapy and hormonal therapy. On first analysis, this combination would appear to be ideally suited for meeting the pharmacological precepts of combination therapy, (i.e., both treatments are effective in their own right, the mechanisms of action are very different for the two treatments, and the toxicities associated with the two treatments are non-overlapping, thereby allowing full doses of both treatments). One would anticipate, therefore, that the combination of chemotherapy and hormonal therapy would at least be additive if not synergistic. Further investigation, both in the laboratory and in the clinic, has demonstrated the interaction between these two treatment modalities to be very complex. Both synergism and antagonism have been observed in combination chemohormonal therapy, depending on which hormonal agent is used. This therapeutic approach has been analyzed in depth in chapters 40 and 44, and only a summary statement will be made regarding the use of combined chemohormonal therapy in the treatment of advanced breast cancer.

A large number of studies have tested the efficacy of combined chemohormonal therapy in the treatment of metastatic breast cancer.[11, 19, 35, 41, 57, 119] Many of the studies do not take into consideration the hormone receptor status of the tumor being treated, and this may explain some of the discrepant results observed in clinical trials. Some of these trials have shown an improvement in initial response rate with the addition of endocrine therapy to chemotherapy; however, this finding is not universal.[41, 57, 119, 131] The use of concurrent chemohormonal therapy has also been compared with the sequential use of both treatment modalities.[11, 25] Although initial treatment response is higher with the addition of chemotherapy compared with hormone therapy alone, the overall tumor response to the sequential use of hormone therapy and chemotherapy is similar.[11] Furthermore, overall survival is unaffected by the combination of chemohormonal therapy. These results would suggest that endocrine therapy as an initial treatment of patients with hormone receptor–positive disease is appropriate, followed by cytotoxic chemotherapy when hormone therapy fails. Most of these studies have been conducted using the antiestrogen tamoxifen. It is conceivable that using growth stimulatory hormones such as estrogens may produce a different outcome.

Hormone therapy in the treatment of breast cancer usually acts by one of two different mechanisms. Growth inhibitory hormones such as tamoxifen decrease tumor growth by blocking cells in the G_0/G_1 phase.[135] On the other hand, growth stimulatory hormones such as the estrogens actually increase tumor growth fraction by recruiting cells from the G_0 phase into the cell cycle.[136] This ability of hormones to modulate tumor growth fraction is likely to influence the cytotoxic potential of chemotherapeutic agents.[113] Studies by Weichselbaum and colleagues[184] have found that growth stimulatory hormones such as estradiol enhance cell proliferation, shorten overall cell cycle time, and increase the proportion of cells in the S phase. Subsequent use of cytotoxic agents such as doxorubicin results in increased cell kill compared with cells that are not exposed to estradiol.[97] In contrast, growth inhibitory hormones such as tamoxifen have been shown to inhibit the in vitro cytotoxicity of chemotherapeutic agents.[96] Sutherland et al.,[165] using the MCF-7 breast cancer cell line, found that tamoxifen inhibited cell growth in a dose-dependent manner. This inhibition in growth was accompanied by a dose-dependent decrease in the percentage of S phase cells with a concomitant increase in the percentage of cells in the G_0/G_1 phase of the cell cycle. This inhibitory effect of tamoxifen could be at least partially reversed by the use of estradiol. Thus in contrast to growth stimulatory agents such as estradiol, tamoxifen reduces the number of cells in the cell cycle, thereby reducing the number of cells vulnerable to cytotoxic agents. It is possible, therefore, that the simultaneous use of chemotherapy with antiestrogens could lead to reduced effectiveness of chemotherapy against rapidly growing tumors. This hypothesis is supported by the observations of Fisher et al.,[59] who reported poorer results from the adjuvant use of tamoxifen plus chemotherapy compared to chemotherapy alone in premenopausal, estrogen receptor–negative patients.

The capacity of estrogens to recruit resting breast cancer cells, and possibly enhance chemotherapeutic effects, has been tested in a number of clinical trials.

Kiang and coworkers[107] studied the use of estrogen with combination chemotherapy consisting of cyclophosphamide and 5-fluorouracil in postmenopausal women with advanced breast cancer whose tumors were either positive for estrogen receptors or of unknown estrogen status. The group given combined chemohormonal therapy survived significantly longer than those given sequential treatment of initial estrogen therapy followed by chemotherapy after failure or relapse. In patients whose tumors were estrogen receptor negative, survival was short regardless of the therapeutic method. Conte et al.[44] also reported a survival benefit for combined chemohormonal therapy in the subset of patients who experienced failure with adjuvant polychemotherapy.

Lippman et al.[118] reported a study attempting to increase the efficacy of cytotoxic chemotherapy in metastatic breast cancer by hormonal synchronization. Patients were randomized to receive either chemotherapy alone or tamoxifen followed by estrogen just prior to the administration of cytotoxic chemotherapy. Tamoxifen was used to theoretically synchronize the breast cancer cells, followed by estrogen to recruit cells into the cell cycle. Immediately following estrogen recruitment, patients were then given combined chemotherapy. Modest improvements in time to progression and survival were seen in a subset of patients given the chemohormonal therapy.

Future studies investigating combined chemohormonal therapy should take into consideration the hormone receptor status of the patient's tumor. Those patients with hormone receptor–positive tumors are more likely to benefit from this type of combination therapy. The type of hormone manipulation must also be considered when combining these agents with cytotoxic drugs. Growth inhibitory hormones such as tamoxifen may actually reduce the effectiveness of cytotoxic drugs. However, the use of growth stimulating agents such as estrogens or the combination of antiestrogens with estrogen rescue may enhance the efficacy of cytotoxic drugs and improve response rates. Further studies are necessary to confirm these observations.

An Approach to the Individual Patient

Despite the introduction of new therapeutic drugs and treatment modalities, metastatic breast cancer remains incurable by current standard treatments. Hormone therapy and chemotherapy offer substantial palliation for many patients. In order for these modalities to be effective, however, these treatments must be administered at optimal doses and schedule. Certain biological characteristics of the tumor, such as hormone receptor status, and clinical characteristics of the patient must also be considered in choosing the appropriate therapy. Other forms of treatment such as palliative radiation therapy, analgesics, antiemetics, and psychological support can also improve the quality of life for these patients.

In treating the individual patient, a number of factors must be considered. Some of these factors are outlined in the flow diagram in Figure 42–3. For most patients diagnosed with metastatic breast cancer, the goal of treatment will be palliation. Only in a well-controlled experimental setting should the primary goal become prolonged survival or cure. Treatments with the primary goal of cure, such as high-dose chemotherapy with autologous marrow rescue, may put the patient at considerable risk for toxicity or early death. This type of aggressive treatment should only be conducted after obtaining informed consent and in a setting where accurate and reliable data may be obtained to determine the efficacy of this type of treatment.

Figure 42–3 outlines an approach to the individual patient when the primary goal is palliation, as is the case for most patients with metastatic disease. The first item that must be determined for each individual patient is the presence of life-threatening disease. A patient who is symptomatic with visceral metastases or has rapidly progressing disease involving multiple sites generally should receive combination chemotherapy. If there is no contraindication to the use of doxorubicin, then the initial treatment used should contain this agent. Patients with heart disease or other possible contraindications to the use of doxorubicin may do better with the CMF regimen. Doses of these agents should be sufficient to produce an objective response, for only in those patients who achieve a response will palliation occur. As demonstrated by Gelman et al.,[68] doses may need to be adjusted according to physiological parameters such as creatinine clearance; however, a dosage reduction in an attempt to reduce toxicity on a purely empirical basis should be avoided.

If the patient responds to the chemotherapy, treatment should be continued until maximum response and for at least three courses thereafter. At that time, the cytotoxic chemotherapy may be discontinued and hormone therapy instituted if the patient's tumor is hormone receptor positive. If the patient's tumor is hormone receptor negative, then observation off chemotherapy may be warranted until there is evidence of disease progression. If the disease remains stable for more than 6 months, then reinstitution of the initially effective cytotoxic drugs may produce a significant objective response. If after two courses of this combination there is evidence of progressive disease, then second line chemotherapy using non–cross-resistant agents should be started.

For patients who do not respond to adequate doses of a doxorubicin-containing regimen, then salvage chemotherapy using mitomycin C or vinblastine may be considered. Another option would be to use experimental therapy such as dose intensification of standard agents, biological therapy, or therapy with a promising new phase II agent. Regional therapy such as radiation therapy or surgery may also be necessary for a life-threatening problem such as spinal cord compression.

If, on the other hand, it is determined that the newly diagnosed patient does not have life-threatening disease, then less toxic treatment such as hormone therapy should be instituted. If the patient is asymptomatic with

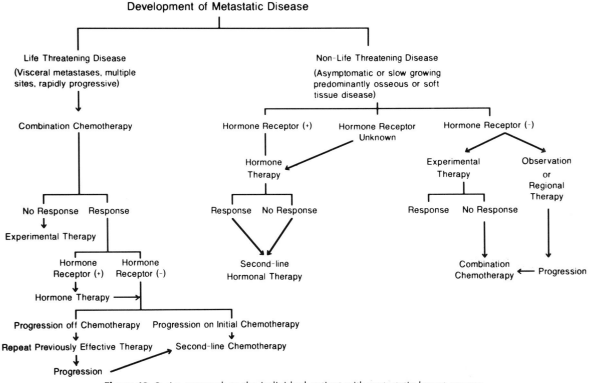

Figure 42–3. An approach to the individual patient with metastatic breast cancer.

non–life-threatening disease and the tumor is hormone receptor positive, then hormone therapy with tamoxifen is usually used. Objective responses may require prolonged administration of these agents, and discontinuation should not be premature if the patient remains asymptomatic. If the patient initially responds and then relapses or has no response to the initial hormone agent and remains asymptomatic, then second line hormonal therapy with a progestational agent or aminoglutethimide may be used. This same approach may be used in patients with newly diagnosed metastatic disease whose hormone receptor status is unknown.

For the patient with hormone receptor–negative disease but whose disease is non–life-threatening, then either observation or regional therapy alone may be warranted. Such regional therapy may include radiation therapy to bony metastases. On the other hand, patients with measurable disease who are asymptomatic may be considered for experimental therapy, e.g., with a new phase I or phase II agent. These patients will not have been heavily pretreated, and the likelihood of response to experimental therapy may be increased. If patients develop progressive disease after receiving regional therapy or experimental therapy, then the use of combination chemotherapy in these receptor-negative patients is indicated.

In conclusion, only through well-controlled clinical trials will advances be made in the treatment of metastatic disease. Although it is controversial whether combination chemotherapy can prolong survival of patients with metastatic disease, this is not an area for the therapeutic nihilist. It is unlikely that one therapeutic modality will produce significant survival benefit in these patients. Future studies may show that in order to control the disease, it will be necessary to use combined modalities such as high-dose intensive drugs and radiation in combination with hormones or growth factors to control or differentiate persistent malignant cells. The age of strictly empirically designed clinical trials in metastatic breast cancer must come to an end. Only by applying knowledge of tumor biology and logically intervening or manipulating these biological variables will substantial strides be made in the treatment of metastatic disease.

References

1. Ahmann DL, Bisel HF, Hahn RG, Eagan RT, Edmonson JH, Steinfeld JL, Tormey DC, Taylor WF: An analysis of a multiple-drug program in the treatment of patients with advanced breast cancer utilizing 5-fluorouracil, cyclophosphamide, and prednisone with or without vincristine. Cancer 36:1925–1935, 1975.
2. Ahmann DL, Schaid DJ, Bisel HF, Hahn RG, Edmonson JH, Ingle JN: The effect on survival of initial chemotherapy in advanced breast cancer: polychemotherapy versus single drug. J Clin Oncol 5(12):1928–1932, 1987.
3. Ahmann FR, Jones SE, Moon TE: The effect of prior adjuvant chemotherapy on survival in metastatic breast cancer. J Surg Oncol 37:116–122, 1988.
4. Ahmann FR, Pugh R: Short-term chemotherapy of poor-prognosis metastatic breast cancer with three non-cross resistant chemotherapy regimens. Cancer 59:239–244, 1987.
5. Aisner J, Weinberg V, Perloff M, Weiss R, Perry M, Korzun A, Ginsberg S, Holland JF: Chemotherapy versus chemoimmunotherapy (CAF V CAFVP V CMF each +/− Mer) for metastatic carcinoma of the breast: a CALGB study. Cancer and leukemia group B. J Clin Oncol 5(10):1523–1533, 1987.
6. Alberts DS, Chang SY, Chen G, Evans TL, Moon TE: Oral melphalan kinetics. Clin Pharmacol Ther 26(6):737–745, 1979.
7. Alberts DS, Einspahr J, Bregman MD: Additive activity of mitoxantrone and doxorubicin in vitro against human breast cancer. J Drug Dev 1(1):15–21, 1988.
8. Allegra JC, Barlock A, Huff KK, Lippman ME: Changes in multiple or sequential estrogen receptor determinations in breast cancer. Cancer 45:792–794, 1980.
9. Antman K, Gale RP: Advanced breast cancer: high-dose chemotherapy and bone marrow autotransplants. Ann Int Med 108:570–574, 1988.
10. Armand JP, Hurteloup P, Bastit P, Chevallier B, Bonneterre J, Monnier A, Chauvergne J, Vo Van ML, Hayat M, Mercier M, et al: Epirubicin in advanced breast cancer. Preliminary results. Proc Am Soc Clin Oncol 6:A254, 1987.
11. Australian and New Zealand Breast Cancer Trials Group, Clinical Oncological Society of Australia: A randomized trial in postmenopausal patients with advanced breast cancer comparing endocrine and cytotoxic therapy given sequentially or in combination. J Clin Oncol 4(2):186–193, 1986.
12. Baildam AD, Zaloudik J, Howell A, Barnes DM, Turnbull L, Swindell R, Moore M, Sellwood RA: DNA analysis by flow cytometry, response to endocrine treatment and prognosis in advanced carcinoma of the breast. Br J Cancer 55(5):553–559, 1987.
13. Bennett JM, Muss HB, Doroshow JM, Wolff S, Krementz ET, Cartwright K, Dukart G, Reisman A, Schoch I: A randomized multicenter trial comparing mitoxantrone, cyclophosphamide, and fluorouracil with doxorubicin, cyclophosphamide, and fluorouracil in the therapy of metastatic breast carcinoma. J Clin Oncol 6(10):1611–1620, 1988.
14. Benz C, Silverberg M, Cadman E: Use of high-dose oral methotrexate sequenced at 24 hours with 5-FU: a clinical toxicity study. Cancer Treat Rep 67(3):297–299, 1983.
15. Bertino JR, Mini E, Fernandes DJ: Sequential methotrexate and 5-fluorouracil: mechanisms of synergy. Semin Oncol 10(2):2–5, 1983.
16. Birkhead BG, Rankin EM, Gallivan S, Dones L, Rubens RD: A mathematical model of the development of drug resistance to cancer chemotherapy. Eur J Cancer Clin Oncol 23(9):1421–1427, 1987.
17. Bishop JF, Raghavan D, Woods R, Coates A, Burns I, Jeal PN, Hillcoat BL, Tattersall MNH: Mitomycin and mitoxantrone in previously treated patients with advanced breast cancer. Cancer Treat Rep 71:191–193, 1987.
18. Bloom JR: Social support, accommodation to stress and adjustment to breast cancer. Soc Science Med 16:1329–1338, 1982.
19. Boccardo F, Rubagotti A, Rosso R, Santi L: Chemotherapy with or without tamoxifen in postmenopausal patients with late breast cancer. A randomized study. J Steroid Biochem 23(6B):1123–1127, 1985.
20. Bowden GT, Roberts R, Alberts DS, Peng Y-M, Garcia D: Comparative molecular pharmacology in leukemic L1210 cells of the anthracene anticancer drugs mitoxantrone and bisantrene. Cancer Res 45:4915–4920, 1985.
21. Brambilla C, DeLena M, Rossi A, Valagussa P, Bonadonna G: Response and survival in advanced breast cancer after two non-cross-resistant combinations. Br Med J 1:801–804, 1976.
22. Brambilla C, Rossi A, Bonfante V, Ferrari L, Villani F, Crippa F, Bonadonna G: Phase II study of doxorubicin versus epirubicin in advanced breast cancer. Cancer Treat Rep 70(2):261–266, 1986.
23. Brandt SJ, Peters WP, Atwater SK, Kurtzberg J, Borowitz MJ, Jones RB, Shpall EJ, Bast RC, Gilbert CJ, Oette DH: Effect of recombinant human granulocyte-macrophage colony-stimulating factor on hematopoietic reconstitution after high-dose chemotherapy and autologous bone marrow transplantation. N Engl J Med 318(14):869–876, 1988.
24. Bruce WR, Merker BE, Valeriote FA: Comparison of the sensitivity of normal hematopoietic and lymphoma colony-forming cells exposed to vinblastine, vincristine, arabinosyl-

cytosine, and amethopterin. J Natl Cancer Inst 42:1015–1025, 1969.

25. Brufman G, Biran S: Prognostic factors affecting treatment results with combination chemotherapy in metastatic breast cancer. Anticancer Res 6:733–736, 1986.

26. Bull JM, Tormey DC, Li SH, Carbone PP, Falkson G, Blom J, Perline E, Simon R: A randomized comparative trial of adriamycin versus methotrexate in combination drug therapy. Cancer 41:1649–1657, 1978.

27. Buzdar AU, Legha SS, Hortobagyi GN, Yap H-Y, Wiseman CL, Distefano A, Schell FC, Barnes BC, Campos LT, Blumenschein GR: Management of breast cancer patients failing adjuvant chemotherapy with adriamycin-containing regimens. Cancer 47:2798–2801, 1981.

28. Canellos GP, DeVita VT, Gold GL, Chabner BA, Schein PS, Young RC: Combination chemotherapy for advanced breast cancer: response and effect on survival. Ann Intern Med 84(4):389–392, 1976.

29. Canellos GP, Pocock SJ, Taylor SG III, Sears ME, Klaasen DJ, Band PR: Combination chemotherapy for metastatic breast carcinoma. Prospective comparison of multiple drug therapy with L-phenylalanine mustard. Cancer 38:1882–1886, 1976.

30. Carlson RW, Billingham ME, Kohler M, Johnson FD, Doroshow JH, Torti FM: Esorubicin in refractory metastatic carcinoma of the breast: a northern California Oncology Group study. Cancer Treat Rep 71(4):427–428, 1987.

31. Carmo-Pereira J, Costa FO, Henriques E, and Carvalho V: A randomized trial of two regimens of cyclophosphamide, methotrexate, 5-fluorouracil, and prednisone in advanced breast cancer. Cancer Chemother Pharmacol 17:87–90, 1986.

32. Carmo-Pereira J, Costa FO, Henriques E, Godinho F, Cantinho-Lopes MG, Sales-Luis A, Rubens RD: A comparison of two doses of adriamycin in the primary chemotherapy of disseminated breast carcinoma. Br J Cancer 56(4):471–473, 1987.

33. Cassileth BR, Lusk EJ, Miller DS, Brown LL, Miller C: Psychosocial correlates of survival in advanced malignant disease. New Engl J Med 312:1551–1555, 1985.

34. Cavalli F, Gerard B, ten Bokkel Huinink W, Clavel M, Rozencweig M: Phase II evaluation of bisantrene in metastatic breast cancer. Cancer Treat Rep 69(3):337–338, 1985.

35. Cavalli F, Goldhirsch A, Joss R, Brunner KW: Hormonochemotherapy in the treatment of advanced breast cancer. J Steroid Biochem 23(6B):1129–1134, 1985.

36. Cheng CC, Zbinden G, Zee-Cheng RKY: Comparison of antineoplastic activity of aminoethylaminoanthraquinones and anthracycline antibiotics. J Pharm Sci 68:393–396, 1979.

37. Chlebowski RT, Paroly WS, Pugh RP, Hueser J, Jacobs EM, Pajak TF, Bateman JR: Adriamycin given as a weekly schedule without a loading course: clinically effective with reduced incidence of cardiotoxicity. Cancer Treat Rep 64:47–51, 1980.

38. Chlebowski RT, Pugh R, Weiner JM, Block JB, Bateman JR: Doxorubicin and CCNU with or without vincristine in patients with advanced refractory breast cancer. Cancer 52:606–609, 1983.

39. Cline MJ, Battifora H, Yokota J: Proto-oncogene abnormalities in human breast cancer: correlations with anatomic features and clinical course of disease. J Clin Oncol 5:999–1006, 1987.

40. Coates A, Gebski V, Stat M, Bishop JF, Jeal PN, Woods RL, Snyder R, Tattersall MHN, Byrne M, Harvey V, Gill G, Simpson J, Drummond R, Browne J, van Cooten R, Forbes JF: Improving the quality of life during chemotherapy for advanced breast cancer. N Engl J Med 31:1490–1495, 1987.

41. Cocconi G, De Lisi V, Boni C, Mori P, Malacarne P, Amadori D, Giovanelli E: Chemotherapy versus combination of chemotherapy and endocrine therapy in advanced breast cancer. A prospective randomized study. Cancer 51:581–588, 1983.

42. Coldman AJ, Goldie JH: Impact of dose-intense chemotherapy on the development of permanent drug resistance. Semin Oncol 14(4):29–33, 1987.

43. Coleman RE, Rubens RD: The clinical course of bone metastases from breast cancer. Br J Cancer 55:61–66, 1987.

44. Conte PF, Pronzato P, Rubagotti A, Alama A, Amadori D, Demicheli R, Gardin G, Gentilini P, Jacomuzzi A, Lionetto R, Monzeglio C, Nicolin A, Rosso R, Sismondi P, Sussio M, Santi L: Conventional versus cytokinetic polychemotherapy with estrogenic recruitment in metastatic breast cancer: results of a randomized cooperative trial. J Clin Oncol 5(3):339–347, 1987.

45. Cooper RG: Combination chemotherapy in hormone resistant breast cancer. Proc Am Assoc Cancer Res 10:15, 1969.

46. Cruciani G, Tienghi A, Molinari AL, Fiorentini G, Rosti G, Turci D, Marangolo M: Cyclophosphamide, methotrexate, 5-fluorouracil, alternating with adriamycin and mitomycin C in metastatic breast cancer: a pilot study. Tumori 73:303–307, 1987.

47. Cummings FJ, Gelman RS, Horton J: Comparison of CAF versus CMFP in metastatic breast cancer: analysis of prognostic factors. J Clin Oncol 3:932–940, 1985.

48. Dalton WS, Cress AE, Alberts DS, Trent JM: Cytogenetic and phenotypic analysis of a human colon carcinoma cell line resistant to mitoxantrone. Cancer Res 48:1882–1888, 1988.

49. Dalton WS, Yang JM, Leibovitz A, Villar H, Thompson FH, Trent JM: Chromosome analysis and clinical correlation of human breast carcinoma. Breast Cancer Res Treat 10(12):87, 1987.

50. De Lena M, Brandi M, Bozzi D, Calabrese P, Romito S: 4-demethoxydaunorubicin administered orally in advanced breast cancer. A phase II study. Tumori 74(1):65–70, 1988.

51. Denefrio JM, Est DR, Trover MB, Vogel CL: Phase II study of mitomycin C and vinblastine in women with advanced breast cancer refractory to standard cytotoxic therapy. Cancer Treat Rep 62:2113–2115, 1978.

52. Derogatis LR, Abeloff MD, Melisaratos N: Psychological coping mechanisms and survival time in metastatic breast cancer. JAMA 242:1504–1508, 1979.

53. DeVita VT: The relationship between tumor mass and resistance to chemotherapy. Cancer 51:1209–1220, 1983.

54. Doroshow J, Leong L, Margolin K, Flanagan B, Goldberg D, Bertrand M, Carr B, Akman S: Effective salvage therapy for refractory metastatic breast cancer with high dose continuous infusion folinic acid (HDFA) and intravenous bolus 5-fluorouracil (FURA). Proc Am Soc Clin Oncol 7:A129, 1988.

55. Falkson G, Gelman RS, Leone L, Rosoff AH, Falkson CI: Survival of premenopausal women with metastatic breast cancer. Proc Am Assoc Cancer Res 29:A782, 1988.

56. Falkson G, Gelman RS, Tormey DC, Cummings FJ, Carbone PP, Falkson HC: The Eastern Cooperative Oncology Group experience with cyclophosphamide, adriamycin, and 5-fluorouracil (CAF) in patients with metastatic breast cancer. Cancer 56:219–224, 1985.

57. Falkson G, Gelman RS, Tormey DC, Falkson CI, Wolter JM, Cummings FJ: Treatment of metastatic breast cancer in premenopausal women using CAF with or without oophorectomy: an Eastern Cooperative Oncology Group study. J Clin Oncol 5(6):881–889, 1987.

58. Ferrari L, Bajetta E, Gianni L, Verusio C, Bartoli C, Valagussa P, Bonadonna G: Four-drug sequential regimen in advanced breast cancer. Breast Cancer Res Treat 10:(2)151–157, 1987.

59. Fisher B, Redmond C, Brown A, Fisher ER, Wolmark N, Bowman D, Plotkin D, Wolter J, Bornstein R, Legault-Poisson S, Saffer EA, et al: Adjuvant chemotherapy with and without tamoxifen in the treatment of primary breast cancer: 5-year results from the National Surgical Adjuvant Breast and Bowel Project trial. J Clin Oncol 4:459–471, 1986.

60. Follezou JY, Palangie T, Feuilhade F: Randomized trial comparing mitoxantrone with adriamycin in advanced breast cancer. Presse Med 16(16):765–768, 1987.

61. Forastiere AA, Perry MC, Hughes AK, Wood WC: Bisantrene (NSC 337766) (CL 216,942) in advanced breast cancer. A cancer and leukemia group B study. Cancer Chemother Pharmacol 13:226–229, 1984.

62. Ford JM, Panasci L, Leclerc Y, Margolese R: Phase II trial of a combination of doxorubicin and mitoxantrone in metastatic breast cancer. Cancer Treat Rep 71(10):921–925, 1987.

63. Fraschini G, Esparza L, Tashima C, Jabboury K, Hortobagyi G: Simultaneous 5-day continuous infusion (CI) of vinblastine (V) and 5-fluorouracil (F) for the treatment of refractory metastatic breast cancer (MBC). Proc Am Assoc Cancer Res 28:196, 1987.

64. Fraschini G, Yap H-Y, Hortobagyi GN, Buzdar A, Blumen-

schein G: Five-day continuous infusion vinblastine in the treatment of breast cancer. Cancer 56:225–229, 1985.

65. Fraschini G, Yap H-Y, Mann G, Buzdar AU, Blumenschein GR, Hortobagyi GN: Chemotherapy with mitoxatrone in combination with continuous infusion vinblastine for metastatic breast cancer. Cancer 60(8):1724–1728, 1987.

66. French Epirubicin Study Group: A prospective randomized phase III trial comparing combination chemotherapy with cyclophosphamide, fluorouracil, and either doxorubicin or epirubicin. J Clin Oncol 6(4):679–688, 1988.

67. Garewal HS, Brooks RJ, Jones SE, Miller TP: Treatment of advanced breast cancer with mitomycin C combined with vinblastine or vindesine. J Clin Oncol 1(12):772–775, 1983.

68. Gelman RS, Taylor SG: Cyclophosphamide, methotrexate, and 5-fluorouracil chemotherapy in women more than 65 years old with advanced breast cancer: the elimination of age trends in toxicity by using doses based on creatinine clearance. J Clin Oncol 2:1404–1413, 1984.

69. George SL, Hoogstraten B: Prognostic factors in the initial response to therapy by patients with advanced breast cancer. J Natl Cancer Inst 60(4):731–736, 1978.

70. Gerlach JH, Kartner N, Bell DR, et al: Multidrug resistance. Cancer Surv 5:24–26, 1986.

71. Goldhirsch A, Gelber RD, Castiglione M: Relapse of breast cancer after adjuvant treatment in premenopausal and perimenopausal women: patterns and prognoses. J Clin Oncol 6(1):89–97, 1988.

72. Goldie JH: Drug resistance and cancer chemotherapy strategy in breast cancer. Breast Cancer Res Treat 3:129–136, 1983.

73. Goldie JH, Coldman AJ: The genetic origin of drug resistance in neoplasms: implications for systemic therapy. Cancer Res 44:3643–3653, 1984.

74. Goldie JH, Coldman AJ: Genetic instability in the development of drug resistance. Semin Oncol 12(3):222–230, 1985.

75. Greenspan E: Combination chemotherapy in advanced disseminated breast carcinoma. J Mt Sinai Hosp 33:1–27, 1966.

76. Greer S, Morris T, Pettingale KW: Psychological response to breast cancer: effect on outcome. Lancet 2:785–787, 1979.

77. Griswold DP: Body burden of cancer in relationship to therapeutic outcome: consideration of preclinical evidence. Cancer Treat Rep 70(1):81–86, 1986.

78. Guazzi A, Bozzetti C, Riva MI, Zaffe D, Cocconi G: Relationship between estrogen receptor concentration and cytomorphometry in breast cancer. Cancer 56:1972–1976, 1985.

79. Gundersen S, Kvinnsland S, Klepp O, Kvaly S, Lund E, Hst H: Weekly adriamycin versus VAC in advanced breast cancer. A randomized trial. Eur J Cancer Clin Oncol 22(12):1431–1434, 1986.

80. Hall VL, Buchanan RB, Williams CJ: Toxicity of mitoxantrone compared to doxorubicin in combination chemotherapy for advanced breast cancer. Proc Am Assoc Cancer Res 29:A790, 1988.

81. Hansen R, Quebbeman E, Beatty P, Ritch P, Anderson T, Jenkins D, Frick J, Ausman R: Continuous 5-fluorouracil infusion in refractory carcinoma of the breast. Breast Cancer Res Treat 10(2):145–149, 1987.

82. Harris AL, Cantwell BM, Ghani S, Dawes P, Evans RG, Lucraft H, Wilson R, Farndon J: A randomized trail of short course (9 weeks) mitoxantrone versus continuous chemotherapy in advanced breast cancer. Proc Am Soc Clin Oncol 6:A258, 1987.

83. Hart RD, Perloff M, Holland JF: One day VATH (vinblastine, adriamycin, thiotepa, and halotestin) therapy for advanced breast cancer refractory to chemotherapy. Cancer 48:1522–1527, 1981.

84. Henderson IC, Allegra JC, Woodcock T, et al: Randomized clinical trial comparing mitoxantrone with doxorubicin in previously treated patients with metastatic breast cancer. J Clin Oncol 7:560–571, 1989.

85. Henderson IC, Hayes DF, Gelman R: Dose-response in the treatment of breast cancer: a critical review. J Clin Oncol 6(9):1501–1515, 1988.

86. Hirshaut Y, Kesselheim H: Prolonged remissions of metastatic breast cancer achieved with a six-drug regimen of relatively low toxicity. Cancer 51:1998–2004, 1983.

87. Holmes FA, Esparza L, Yap H-Y, Buzdar AU, Blumenschein GR, Hortobagyi GN: A comparative study of bisantrene given by two dose schedules in patients with metastatic breast cancer. Cancer Chemother Pharmacol 18(2):157–161, 1986.

88. Holmes FA, Neidhart JA, Hortobagyi GN, Esparza L, Buzdar AU, Jabboury K: High dose mitoxantrone (M) in patients (PTS) with metastatic breast cancer (MCBC). Proc Am Soc Clin Oncol 6:A248, 1987.

89. Holmes FA, Yap H-Y, Esparza L, Buzdar AU, Blumenschein GR, Hug V, Hortobagyi GN: Mitoxantrone, cyclophosphamide, and fluorouracil in metastatic breast cancer unresponsive to hormonal therapy. Cancer 59(12):1992–1999, 1987.

90. Hortobagyi GN: Mitomycin-C in breast cancer. Semin Oncol 7(4):65–70, 1985.

91. Hortobagyi GN, Bodey GP, Buzdar AU, Frye D, Legha SS, Malik R, Smith TL, Blumenschein GR, Yap H-Y, Rodriguez V: Evaluation of high-dose versus standard FAC chemotherapy for advanced breast cancer in protected environment units: a prospective randomized study. J Clin Oncol 5(3):354–364, 1987.

92. Hortobagyi GN, Smith TL, Legha SS, Swenerton KD, Gehan EA, Yap H-Y, Buzdar AU, Blumenschein GR: Multivariate analysis of prognostic factors in metastatic breast cancer. J Clin Oncol 1(12):776–786, 1983.

93. Hortobagyi GN, Yap H-Y, Blumenschein GR, Buzdar AU, Barnes BC, Legha SS, Wiseman CL: Phase II evaluation of vinblastine, methotrexate, and calcium leukovorin rescue in patients with refractory metastatic breast cancer. Cancer 51:769–772, 1983.

94. Hryniuk W, Bush H: The importance of dose intensity in chemotherapy of metastatic breast cancer. J Clin Oncol 2(11):1281–1288, 1984.

95. Hryniuk WM, Pater JL: Implications of dose intensity for cancer chemotherapy. Semin Oncol 14(4):43–44, 1987.

96. Hug V, Hortobagyi GN, Drewinko B, Finders M: Tamoxifen-citrate counteracts the antitumor effects of cytotoxic drugs in vitro. J Clin Oncol 3(12):1672–1677, 1985.

97. Hug V, Johnston D, Finders M, Hortobagyi G: Use of growth-stimulatory hormones to improve the in vitro therapeutic index of doxorubicin for human breast tumors. Cancer Res 46:147–152, 1986.

98. Jackson DV, White DR, Spurr CL, Hire EA, Pavy MD, Robertson M, Legos HC, McMahan RA: Moderate-dose vincristine infusion in refractory breast cancer. Am J Clin Oncol 9(5):376–378, 1986.

99. Jain KK, Casper ES, Geller NL, Hakes TB, Kaufman RJ, Currie V, Schwartz W, Cassidy C, Petroni GR, Young CW, Wittes RE: A prospective randomized comparison of epirubicin and doxorubicin in patients with advanced breast cancer. J Clin Oncol 3(6):818–826, 1985.

100. Jamison RN, Burish TG, Wallston KA: Psychogenic factors in predicting survival of breast cancer patients. J Clin Oncol 5(5):768–772, 1987.

101. Jones RB, Holland JF, Bhardwaj S, Norton L, Wilfinger C, Strashun A: A phase I-II study of intensive-dose adriamycin for advanced breast cancer. J Clin Oncol 5:172–177, 1987.

102. Jones SE, Durie BGM, Salmon SE: Combination chemotherapy with adriamycin and cyclophosphamide for advanced breast cancer. Cancer 36:90–97, 1975.

103. Kamby C, Rose C: Metastatic pattern and response to endocrine therapy in human breast cancer. Breast Cancer Res Treat 8:197–204, 1986.

104. Kardinal CG, Perry MC, Korzun AH, Rice MA, Ginsberg S, Wood WC: Responses to chemotherapy or chemohormonal therapy in advanced breast cancer patients treated previously with adjuvant chemotherapy. A subset analysis of CALGB study 8081. Cancer 61(3):415–419, 1988.

105. Kau S, Buzdar A, Frye D, Fraschini G, Hortobagyi G: Survival experience of patients (PTS) failing adjuvant therapy in comparison to PTS with metastatic breast cancer. Proc Ann Meet Am Soc Clin Oncol 7:A32, 1988.

106. Kiang DT, Frenning DH, Goldman AI, Ascensao VF, Kennedy BJ: Estrogen receptors and responses to chemotherapy and hormonal therapy in advanced breast cancer. N Engl J Med 299:1330–1334, 1978.

107. Kiang DT, Gay J, Goldman A, Kennedy BJ: A randomized trial of chemotherapy and hormonal therapy in advanced breast cancer. N Engl J Med 313:1241–1246, 1985.
108. Kolaric K, Mechl Z, Potrebica V, Sopkova B: Phase II study of oral 4-demethoxydaunorubicin in previously treated (except anthracyclines) metastatic breast cancer patients. Oncology 44:82–86, 1987.
109. Konits PH, Aisner J, van Echo DA, et al: Mitomycin C and vinblastine chemotherapy for advanced breast cancer. Cancer 48:1295–1298, 1981.
110. Kosmidis P, Kondilis D, Lissaios B: Salvage chemotherapy (SC) for breast cancer patients treated with adjuvant adriamycin (A) containing regimen. Proc Am Soc Clin Oncol 6:A218, 1987.
111. Kute TE, Muss HB, Anderson D, Crumb K, Miller B, Burns D, Dube LA: Relationship of steroid receptor, cell kinetics, and clinical status in patients with breast cancer. Cancer Res 41:3524–3529, 1981.
112. Law LW: Origin of the resistance of leukaemic cells to folic acid antagonists. Nature 169:628–629, 1952.
113. Leclercq G, Devleeschouwer N, Danguy A, Verrijdt A, Heuson JC: In vitro synergism between estrogens and cytotoxic agents. J Steroid Biochem 23(6B):1111–1113, 1985.
114. Leitner SP, Casper ES, Hakes TB, Kaufman RJ, Winn RJ, Scoppetuolo M, Raymond V, Geller NL, Young CW: Phase II trial of 4'-deoxydoxorubicin in patients with advanced breast cancer. Cancer Treat Rep 69(11):1319–1320, 1985.
115. Leonard RCF, Cornbleet MA, Kaye SB, Soukop M, White G, Hutcheon AW, Robinson S, Kerr ME, Smyth JF: Mitoxantrone versus doxorubicin in combination chemotherapy for advanced carcinoma of the breast. J Clin Oncol 5:1056–1063, 1987.
116. Lippman ME, Allegra JC: Quantitative estrogen receptor analyses: the response to endocrine and cytotoxic chemotherapy in human breast cancer and the disease-free interval. Cancer 46:2829–2834, 1980.
117. Lippman ME, Allegra JC, Thompson EB, Simon R, Barlock A, Green L, Huff KK, Do HMT, Aitken SC, Warren R: The relation between estrogen receptors and response rate to cytotoxic chemotherapy in metastatic breast cancer. N Engl J Med 298:1223–1228, 1978.
118. Lippman ME, Cassidy J, Wesley M, Young RC: A randomized attempt to increase the efficacy of cytotoxic chemotherapy in metastatic breast cancer by hormonal synchronization. J Clin Oncol 2(1):28–36, 1984.
119. Lloyd RE, Jones SE, Salmon SE: Comparative trial of low dose adriamycin plus cyclophosphamide with or without additive hormonal therapy in advanced breast cancer. Cancer 43:60–65, 1979.
120. Loprinzi CL, Tormey DC, Rasmussen P, Falkson G, Davis TE, Falkson HC, Chang AYC: Prospective evaluation of carcinoembryonic antigen levels and alternating chemotherapeutic regimens in metastatic breast cancer. J Clin Oncol 4(1):46–56, 1986.
121. Luikart SD, Witman GB, Portlock CS: Adriamycin (doxorubicin), vinblastine, and mitomycin C combination chemotherapy in refractory breast carcinoma. Cancer 54:1252–1255, 1984.
122. Luria SE, Delbruck M: Mutations of bacteria from virus sensitivity to virus resistance. Genetics 28:491, 1943.
123. Marini G, Simoncini E, Zaniboni A, Gorni F, Marpicati P, Zambruni A: 5-Fluorouracil and high-dose folinic acid as salvage treatment of advanced breast cancer: an update. Oncology 44(6):336–340, 1987.
124. Martoni A, Pacciarini MA, Pannuti F: The new anthracycline 4-demethoxydaunorubicin by oral route in advanced pretreated breast cancer and melanoma. A pilot study. Drugs Exp Clin Res XI(2):127–131, 1985.
125. McCarty KS, Barton TK, Fetter BG, Woodard BH, Mossler JA, Reeves W, Daly J, Wilkinson WE, McCarty KS: Correlation of estrogen and progesterone receptors with histologic differentiation in mammary carcinoma. Cancer 46:2851–2858, 1980.
126. McGuire WL: Prognostic factors for recurrence and survival in human breast cancer. Breast Cancer Res Treat 10:5–9, 1987.
127. Meyer GS, Rao BR, Stevens SC: Low incidence of estrogen receptor in breast carcinomas with rapid rates of cellular replication. Cancer 40:2290–2298, 1977.
128. Meyer JS, Lee JY: Relationships of S-Phase fraction of breast carcinoma in relapse to duration of remission, estrogen receptor content, therapeutic responsiveness, and duration of survival. Cancer Res 40:1890–1896, 1980.
129. Meyer JS, Prey MU, Babcock DS, McDivitt RW: Breast carcinoma cell kinetics, morphology, stage, and host characteristics. Lab Invest 54(1):41–51, 1986.
130. Mitchell I, Deshpande N, Millis R, Rubens RD: Deoxyribonucleic acid (DNA) content of primary carcinoma and response to endocrine or cytotoxic drug therapies in patients with advanced breast cancer. Eur J Surg Oncol 11:251–256, 1985.
131. Mouridsen HT, Rose C, Engelsmann E, Sylvester R, Rotmensz N: Combined cytotoxic and endocrine therapy in postmenopausal patients with advanced breast cancer. J Steroid Biochem 23(6B):1141–1146, 1985.
132. Muss HB, White DR, Richards F II, Cooper MR, Stuart JJ, Jackson DV, Rhyne L, Spurr CL: Adriamycin versus methotrexate in five-drug combination chemotherapy for advanced breast cancer. Cancer 42:2141–2148, 1978.
133. Nash CH, Jones SE, Salmon SE, Davis SL, Moon TE: Prediction of outcome in metastatic breast cancer treated with adriamycin combination chemotherapy. Cancer 46:2380–2388, 1980.
134. Neidhart JA, Gochnour D, Roach R, Hoth D, Young D: A comparison of mitoxantrone and doxorubicin in breast cancer. J Clin Oncol 4(5):672–677, 1986.
135. Osborne CK, Boldt DH, Clark GM, Trent JM: Effects of tamoxifen on human breast cancer cell cycle kinetics: accumulation of cells in early G_1 phase. Cancer Res 43:3583–3585, 1983.
136. Osborne CK, Boldt DH, Estrada P: Human breast cancer cell cycle synchronization by estrogens and antiestrogens in culture. Cancer Res 44:1433–1439, 1984.
137. Osborne CK, Yochmowitz MG, Knight WA, McGuire WL: The value of estrogen and progesterone receptors in the treatment of breast cancer. Cancer 46:2884–2888, 1980.
138. Paradiso A, Lorusso V, Tommasi S, Schittulli F, Maiello E, De Lena M: Relevance of cell kinetics to hormonal response of receptor-positive advanced breast cancer. Breast Cancer Res Treat 11:31–36, 1988.
139. Pastan I, Gottesman M: Multiple-drug resistance in human cancer. N Engl J Med 316:1388–1393, 1987.
140. Pasterz RB, Buzdar AU, Hortobagyi GN, Blumenschein GR: Mitomycin in metastatic breast cancer refractory to hormonal and combination chemotherapy. Cancer 56:2381–2384, 1985.
141. Paterson AHG, Cyr M, Szafran O, Lees AW, Hanson J: Response to treatment and its influence on survival in metastatic breast cancer. Am J Clin Oncol 8:283–292, 1985.
142. Perloff M, Hart RD, Holland JF: Vinblastine, adriamycin, thiotepa, and halotestin (VATH). Therapy for advanced breast cancer refractory to prior chemotherapy. Cancer 42:2534–2537, 1978.
143. Peters WP, Shpall EJ, Jones RB, Olsen GA, Bast RC, Gockerman JP, Moore JO: High-dose combination alkylating agents with bone marrow support as initial treatment for metastatic breast cancer. J Clin Oncol 6(9):1368–1376, 1988.
144. Petru E, Schmahl D: No relevant influence on overall survival time in patients with metastatic breast cancer undergoing combination chemotherapy. J Cancer Res Clin Oncol 114:183–185, 1988.
145. Pronzato P, Amoroso D, Ardizzoni A, Bertelli G, Canobbio L, Conte PF, Cusimano MP, Fusco V, Gulisano M, Lionetto R, et al: Sequential administration of cyclophosphamide, methotrexate, 5-fluorouracil, and folinic acid as salvage treatment in metastatic breast cancer. Am J Clin Oncol 10(5):404–406, 1987.
146. Rosenbaum C, Marsland TA, Stolbach LL, Raam S, Cohen JL: Estrogen receptor status and response to chemotherapy in advanced breast cancer: the Tufts-Shattuck-Pondville experience. Cancer 46:2919–2921, 1980.
147. Rosner D, Nemoto T, Lane WW: Response to chemotherapy in metastatic breast cancer in relation to estrogen receptor status. Proc Am Assoc Cancer Res 29:A781, 1988.
148. Ross MB, Buzdar AU, Smith TL, Eckles N, Hortobagyi GN, Blumenschein GR, Freireich EJ, Gehan EA: Improved survival of patients with metastatic breast cancer receiving combination chemotherapy. Cancer 55:341–346, 1985.

149. Salmon SE, Grogan TM, Miller T, Scheper R, Dalton WS: P-glycoprotein staining predicts in vitro doxorubicin resistance in myeloma, lymphoma and breast cancer. J Natl Cancer Inst 81(9):4542–4549, 1989.

150. Segaloff A, Hankey BF, Carter AC, Escher GC, Ansfield FJ, Talley RW: An evaluation of the effect of vincristine added to cyclophosphamide, 5-fluorouracil, methotrexate, and prednisone in advanced breast cancer. Breast Cancer Res Treat 5:311–319, 1985.

151. Scheid V, Buzdar AU, Smith TL, Hortobagyi GN: Clinical course of breast cancer patients with osseous metastasis treated with combination chemotherapy. Cancer 58:2589–2593, 1986.

151a. Sears ME, Haut A, Eckles N: Melphalan (NSC-8806) in advanced breast cancer. Cancer Chemother Rep 50:271–279, 1966.

152. Sherry MM, Greco FA, Johnson DH, Hainsworth JD: Metastatic breast cancer confined to the skeletal system. An indolent disease. Am J Med 81:381–386, 1986.

153. Silvestrini R, Daidone MG, Gasparini G: Cell kinetics as a prognostic marker in node-negative breast cancer. Cancer 56:1982–1987, 1985.

154. Silvestrini R, Daidone MG, Valagussa P, Salvadori B, Rovini D, Bonadonna G: Cell kinetics as a prognostic marker in locally advanced breast cancer. Cancer Treat Rep 17(4):375–379, 1987.

155. Skipper HE, Schabel FM, Wilcox WS: Experimental evaluation of potential anticancer agents. XIII. On the criteria and kinetics associated with "curability" of experimental leukemia. Cancer Chemother Rep 35:1–111, 1964.

156. Smalley RV, Carpenter J, Bartolucci A, Vogel C, Krauss S: A comparison of cyclophosphamide, adriamycin, 5-fluorouracil (CAF) and cyclophosphamide, methotrexate, 5-fluorouracil, vincristine, prednisone (CMFVP) in patients with metastatic breast cancer. Cancer 40:625–632, 1977.

157. Smalley RV, Lefante J, Bartolucci A, Carpenter J, Vogel C, Krauss S: A comparison of cyclophosphamide, adriamycin, and 5-fluorouracil (CAF) and cyclophosphamide, methotrexate, 5-fluorouracil, vincristine, and prednisone (CMFVP) in patients with advanced breast cancer. Breast Cancer Res Treat 3:209–220, 1983.

158. Smyth JF, Cornbleet MA, Stuart-Harris RC, Smith IE, Coleman RE, Rubens RD, McDonald M, Mouridsen HT, Rainer H, van Oosterom AT: Mitoxantrone as first-line chemotherapy for advanced breast cancer: results of a European collaborative study. Semin Oncol 11(3):15–18, 1984.

159. Speyer JL, Green MD, Kramer E, Rey M, Sanger J, Ward C, Dubin N, Ferrans V, Stecy P, Zeleniuch-Jacquotte A, Wernz J, Feit F, Slater W, Blum R, Muggia F: Protective effect of the bispiperazinedione ICRF-187 against doxorubicin-induced cardiac toxicity in women with advanced breast cancer. N Engl J Med 319:745–752, 1988.

160. Steiner R, Stewart JF, Cantwell BMJ, Minton MJ, Knight RK, Rubens RD: Adriamycin alone or combined with vincristine in the treatment of advanced breast cancer. Eur J Cancer Clin Oncol 19(11):1553–1557, 1983.

161. Stewart DJ, Perrault DJ, Maroun JA, Lefebvre BM: Combined mitoxantrone plus doxorubicin in the treatment of breast cancer. Am J Clin Oncol 10(4):335–340, 1987.

162. Straus MJ, Moran RE: The cell cycle kinetics of human breast cancer. Cancer 46:2634–2639, 1980.

163. Stuart-Harris RC, Bozek T, Pavlidis NA, Smith IE: Mitoxantrone: an active new agent in the treatment of advanced breast cancer. Cancer Chemother Pharmacol 12:1–4, 1984.

164. Sulkes A, Livingston RB, Murphy WK: Tritiated thymidine labeling index and response in human breast cancer. J Natl Cancer Inst 62(3):513–515, 1979.

165. Sutherland RL, Green MD, Hall RE, Reddel RR, Taylor IW: Tamoxifen induces accumulation of MCF7 human mammary carcinoma cells in the G_0/G_1 phase of the cell cycle. Eur J Cancer Clin Oncol 19(5):615–621, 1983.

166. Swenerton KD, Legha SS, Smith T, Hortobagyi GN, Gehan EA, Hwee-Yura Y, Gutterman JU, Blumenschein GR: Prognostic factors in metastatic breast cancer treated with combination chemotherapy. Cancer Res 39:1552–1562, 1979.

167. Talmadge JE: Stress factors and breast cancer outcome. J Clin Oncol 5(3):333–334, 1987.

168. Tannir N, Yap H-Y, Hortobagyi GH, Hug V, Buzdar AU, Blumenschein GR: Sequential continuous infusion with doxorubicin and vinblastine: an effective chemotherapy combination for patients with advanced breast cancer previously treated with cyclophosphamide, methotrexate, 5-FU, vincristine, and prednisone. Cancer Treat Rep 68:1039–1041, 1984.

169. Tannock I: Cell kinetics and chemotherapy: a critical review. Cancer Treat Rep 62(8):1117–1133, 1978.

169a. Tannock IF, Boyd NF, De Boer G, Erlichmann C, Fine S, Larocque G, Mayers C, Perrault D, Sutherland H: A randomized trial of two dose levels of cyclophosphamide, methotrexate, and fluorouracil chemotherapy for patients with metastatic breast cancer. J Clin Oncol 6:1377–1387, 1988.

170. Taylor SG, Gelman RS, Falkson G, Cummings FJ: Combination chemotherapy compared to tamoxifen as initial therapy for stage IV breast cancer in elderly women. Ann Int Med 104:455–461, 1986.

171. Teicher BA, Cucchi CA, Lee JB, Flatow JL, Rosowky A, Frei E, III: Alkylating agents: in vitro studies of cross-resistance patterns in human cell lines. Cancer Res 46:4379–4383, 1986.

172. Thirlwell MP, Livingston RB, Murphy WK, Hart JS: A rapid in vitro labeling index method for predicting response of human solid tumors to chemotherapy. Cancer Res 36:3279–3283, 1976.

173. Tormey DC: Adriamycin (NSC-123127) in breast cancer: an overview of studies. Cancer Chemother Rep 6:319–327, 1975.

173a. Tormey DC, Gelman R, Bond PR: Comparison of induction chemotherapies for metastatic breast cancer. Cancer 50:1235–1244, 1982.

174. Tormey DC, Kline JC, Palta M, Davis TE, Love RR, Carone PP: Short term high density systemic therapy for metastatic breast cancer. Breast Cancer Res Treat 5:177–188, 1985.

175. Tormey DC, Weinberg VE, Leone LA, Glidewell OJ, Perloff M, Kennedy BJ, Cortes E, Silver RT, Weiss RB, Aisner J, Holland JF: A comparison of intermittent vs. continuous and of adriamycin vs. methotrexate 5-drug chemotherapy for advanced breast cancer. A cancer and leukemia group B study. Am J Clin Oncol 7:231–239, 1984.

176. Torti FM, Bristow MR, Howes AE, Aston D, Stockdale FE, Carter SK, Kohler M, Brown BW, Billingham ME: Reduced cardiotoxicity of doxorubicin delivered on a weekly schedule. Ann Int Med 99:745–749, 1983.

177. Trent JM: Cytogenetic and molecular biologic alterations in human breast cancer: a review. Breast Cancer Res Treat 5:221–229, 1985.

178. Valagussa P, Tancini G, Bonadonna G: Salvage treatment of patients suffering relapse after adjuvant CMF chemotherapy. Cancer 58:1411–1417, 1986.

179. Valeriote FA, Edelstein MB: The role of cell kinetics in cancer chemotherapy. Semin Oncol 4(2):217–226, 1977.

180. Venter DJ, Kumar S, Tuzi NL, Gullick WJ: Overexpression of the c-erbB-2 oncoprotein in human breast carcinomas: immunohistological assessment correlates with gene amplification. Lancet 2:69–71, 1987.

181. Vogel CL, Smalley RV, Raney M, Krauss S, Carpenter J, Velez-Garcia E, Fishkin E, Raab S, Moore MR, Stagg M: Randomized trial of cyclophosphamide, doxorubicin, and 5-fluorouracil alone or alternating with a "cycle active" non-cross-resistant combination in women with visceral metastatic breast cancer: a Southeastern Cancer Study Group project. J Clin Oncol 2(6):643–651, 1984.

182. Von Hoff DD, Layard MW, Basa P, Davis HL, Von Hoff AL, Rozencweig M, Muggia FM: Risk factors for doxorubicin-induced congestive heart failure. Ann Int Med 91:710–717, 1979.

183. Wallace RE, Murdock KC, Angier RB, Durr FE: Activity of a novel anthracenedione, 1,4-dihydroxy-5,8-bis{{{[(2-hydroxyethyl)amino]ethyl} amino]}}-9,10- anthracenedione dihydrochloride, against experimental tumors in mice. Cancer Res 39:1570–1574, 1979.

184. Weichselbaum RR, Hellman S, Piro AJ, Nove JJ, Little JB: Proliferation kinetics of a human breast cancer line in vitro following treatment with 17β-estradiol and 1-β-D-arabinofuranosylcytosine. Cancer Res 38:2339–2342, 1978.

185. Weisman AD, Worden JW: Psychosocial analysis of cancer deaths. Omega 6:61–75, 1979.

186. Weiss AJ, Metter GE, Fletcher WS, Wilson WL, Grage TB, Ramirez G: Studies on adriamycin using a weekly regimen demonstrating its clinical effectiveness and lack of cardiac toxicity. Cancer Treat Rep 60(7):813–822, 1976.

187. Willingham MC, Cornwell MM, Cardarelli CO, Gottesman MM, Pastan I: Single cell analysis of daunomycin uptake and efflux in multidrug-resistant and sensitive cells: effects of verapamil and other drugs. Cancer Res 46:5941–5946, 1986.

188. Yap H-Y, Blumenschein GR, Schell F, Buzdar AU, Valdivieso M, Bodey GP: Dihydroxyanthracenedione: a promising new drug in the treatment of metastatic breast cancer. Ann Inter Med 95:694–697, 1981.

189. Yap H-Y, Blumenschein GR, Yap B-S, Hortobagyi GN, Tash-ima CK, Wang A-Y, Benjamin RS, Bodey GP: High-dose methotrexate for advanced breast cancer. Cancer Treat Rep 63:757–761, 1979.

190. Young PCM, Ehrlich CE, Einhorn LH: Relationship between steroid receptors and response to endocrine therapy and cytotoxic chemotherapy in metastatic breast cancer. Cancer 46:2961–2963, 1980.

191. Zhang H-J, Kennedy BJ, Kiang DT: Thymidine kinase as a predictor of response to chemotherapy in advanced breast cancer. Breast Cancer Res Treat 4:221–225, 1984.

192. Zinser JW, Hortobagyi GN, Buzdar AU, Smith TL, Fraschini G: Clinical course of breast cancer patients with liver metastases. J Clin Oncol 5(5):773–782, 1987.

Chapter 43

STEROID AND PEPTIDE HORMONE RECEPTORS IDENTIFIED IN BREAST TISSUE

James L. Wittliff, Ph.D., Resad Pasic, M.D., Ph.D., and Kirby I. Bland, M.D.

INTRODUCTION

More than 200 years ago, Percival Pott observed that breast development was influenced by removal of the ovaries. In 1889, Schinzinger[170] gave a brief communication suggesting breast cancer exhibited hormone responsiveness. Sir George Beatson's report,[13] in 1896, described remissions in two women given bilateral oophorectomy as a treatment for breast cancer providing further evidence of hormonal dependency. Following these clinical observations, a throng of investigators has defined many of the elements of the hormone responsive mechanisms operating in normal and neoplastic breast.

These early studies of ovarian influence led to efforts to study estrogen localization in tissues and its excretion using ^{14}C-labeled hormones.[183] However, the specific radioactivities were too low to detect specific tissue association. Pioneering work by Glascock and Hoekstra[55] demonstrated that [^{3}H]hexestrol, a synthetic estrogenic substance, was selectively distributed in physiological target organs such as the uterus, vagina, mammary glands, and pituitary glands of young sheep and goats. Across the Atlantic, Jensen and Jacobson[81] confirmed that [6,7-^{3}H] estradiol-17β of high specific radioactivity was taken up and retained by organs of the rat, which responded to estrogen treatment in vivo. The three ensuing decades in the evolution of steroid and peptide research contained monumental scientific achievements.

Because the literature on the field of sex hormone–binding proteins and receptors is comprehensive, it is impractical to review even representative examples of each laboratory's contributions. The newer aspects of peptide hormone and growth factor receptors as prognostic factors in breast cancer are described. This is complemented by exciting investigations revealing that certain oncogenes are amplified and their protein products are overexpressed in breast cancer; elevated levels of these molecules are correlated with decreased relapse-free survival and overall survival. Because a detailed review is inappropriate, we apologize to any investigator whose noteworthy contributions have been deleted. Instead we have attempted to provide an overview of salient aspects of receptor biochemistry and their clinical application. This review includes receptor methods, quality control, and a description of each step from the time of biopsy until the delivery of the result by report. Values from receptor and oncogene analyses should be added to other clinical parameters such as axillary nodal involvement, menopausal status, location of the dominant metastatic lesion, proliferative rate, and DNA ploidy in selecting a treatment design for the patient with breast cancer.[33]

HORMONES INFLUENCING NORMAL BREAST DEVELOPMENT AND FUNCTION

Both peptide and steroid hormones influence many of the molecular processes involved in proliferation, differentiation, and secretion in normal breast tissue. Estrogen, progesterone, and certain glucocorticoids are known to influence differentiation of both parenchymatous and mesenchymal components, although the specific role of each of the hormones is unknown.[197] Androgen exerts a negative control on the proliferation of breast epithelium during early development. The actions of the steroid horomones are complemented by those of insulin, prolactin, and possibly growth hormone as well as by certain growth factors during pregnancy and lactation. These promote the orderly progression of resting breast cells of the female to a structurally and, finally, functionally differentiated state (Fig. 43–1). The functionally differentiated state is characterized histologically by an alveolar secretory appearance and by an increased rate of synthesis of milk proteins, lipids, and lactose.

Prior to the onset of lactation, breast tissue is composed predominantly of adipose cells surrounding a branched system of ducts of epithelial cells with connective tissue elements. Tissue composition shifts toward a

---

This chapter is dedicated to Dr. Condict Moore, a distinguished surgeon who has been teacher, academic colleague, and friend to generations of clinical scientists.

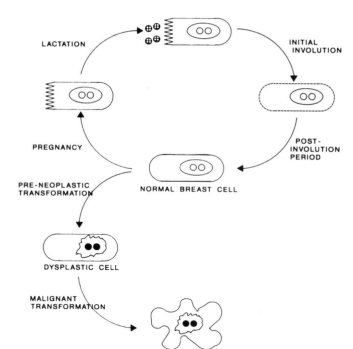

Figure 43–1. Stages in the differentiation of normal breast and malignant transformation.

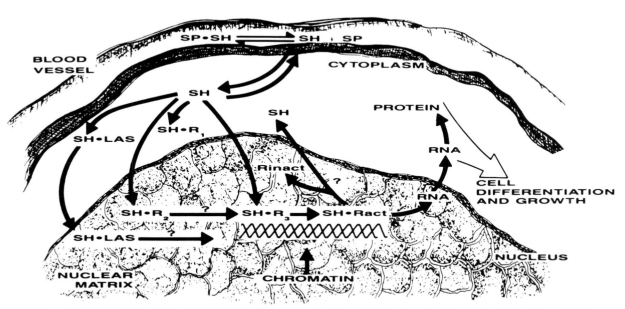

Figure 43–2. Schematic representation of hypothetical intracellular cascade of events following steroid receptor interaction with its receptor in a target cell. Steroid hormones (SH) normally circulate in the blood bound to albumin and certain specific serum proteins (SP) such as TeBG and CBG. As lipid molecules, steroids move across the cell membrane into the cytoplasm in a passive fashion and interact with their intracellular receptor proteins (R) in a reaction exhibiting high affinity and specificity. The exact location of the true receptor protein is unknown, but possibilities include association with the nuclear membrane (R_1), nuclear matrix (R_2), and chromatin (R_3). After association with the steroid, an apparent activation takes place that may involve phosphorylation. The activated steroid-receptor complex (SHR_{act}) associates with acceptor sites in chromatin and stimulates synthesis of nucleic acids and, subsequently, proteins characteristic of the biologic response (differentiation and growth) to the specific steroid hormone. In addition, steroid hormones may associate with low affinity sites (LAS) whose subsequent pathway is uncertain. The details of these intranuclear events are presently unclear. However, the presence of the receptor protein in a cell appears to be a prerequisite for response to a steroid hormone stimulus. (From Wittliff JL: In Donegan WL, Spratt JS (eds): Cancer of the Breast. Philadelphia, WB Saunders, 1988, pp 303–335. Reprinted with permission.)

higher concentration of lobuloalveolar cells that are responsible principally for the synthesis of milk constituents as the gland differentiates during pregnancy and lactation (see chapter 3, "Normal, Lactating, and Diseased States"). The mammary epithelium undergoes involution at the culmination of lactation. These events appear to be regulated by a host of factors, of which hormone receptors are central to organized differentiation and development.

The original "two-step mechanism" suggested independently by Gorski and coworkers[57] at the University of Illinois and by Jensen and colleagues[80b, 82] at the University of Chicago has evolved to the sequence of events shown in Figure 43–2 as the steroid hormone interacts with a target cell. These early studies used uterine tissues from rodents. Investigators from many laboratories using rodent and human tissues suggest that a similar cascade of events exists in normal and neoplastic mammary cells. Plasma proteins such as albumin, testosterone-estradiol–binding globulin (TeBG; formerly sex steroid–binding globulin), and corticosteroid-binding globulin (CBG) transport steroid hormones with a characteristic affinity and capacity for each. Albumin binds estradiol-17β (Fig. 43–2), the native female sex hormone, reversibly with a K_d value of 10^{-5} mol/L, whereas TeBG associates with the hormone exhibiting a K_d value of 10^{-7}–10^{-8} mol/L.

Steroid hormones enter target cells by passive diffusion and combine with specific receptor proteins in a reaction characterized by a high degree of ligand affinity and specificity (Fig. 43–2). For example, the estrogen receptor molecule is composed of numerous domains (Fig. 43–3), and a large part of the sequence near the carboxy-terminus (E domain) is responsible for steroid hormone binding.[62] The exact locations of receptor proteins in normal or neoplastic target cells are not clearly understood, although recent immunocytochemical and enzyme studies suggest a nuclear location.[86, 194] The steroid-receptor complex must undergo an activation step that may involve phosphorylation and other post-translational modifications of the receptor[121] prior

to high affinity association with the nuclear matrix and chromatin. Certain associated molecules such as the heat shock proteins[12] may be involved in this step. Then the activated (transformed?) steroid hormone–receptor complex associates with the chromatin in an event called retention. Specific regions of the receptor molecule known as the C domain are formed into two DNA binding fingers[61] that presumably have zinc ions coordinated within each structure. This sequence dictates association of the receptor molecule with the hormone response element of a specific gene regulated by the steroid hormone. Thereafter, RNA synthesis is stimulated in a yet undetermined manner, resulting in the formation of certain breast cell proteins.

Thus the steroid receptor appears to be a biological prerequisite for responsiveness to hormonal perturbations; in its absence, alterations in macromolecular synthesis do not occur at physiological hormone concentrations. Normal breast cells contain specific binding proteins for estrogen, progestin, glucocorticoid, and androgen of variable quantities depending on the stage of mammary gland differentiation.[120, 197] These receptors are also found in many breast cancers.[4]

Recent studies by a number of laboratories have established that the amino acid sequences of the steroid hormone receptors exhibit considerable homologies, especially in steroid- and DNA-binding domains.[171] Even more interesting is the finding that diverse receptor proteins such as those for vitamin D_3, retinoic acid, aryl hydrocarbons, and thyroid hormones show similar sequence homologies. The receptor for T_3 and T_4 hormones was discovered to be essentially identical to the *erb-a* oncogene protein product.

TISSUE PROCUREMENT, SPECIMEN HANDLING, AND PREPARATION

Breast biopsy specimens should be excised expeditiously and without trauma from the surgical technique.[23, 44, 45, 156] The specimens, well trimmed of normal

APORECEPTOR (65 Kd)

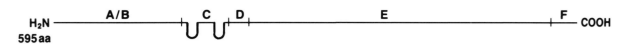

TRUNCATED RECEPTOR (50 Kd)

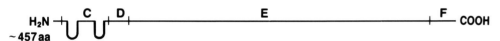

Figure 43–3. Proposed binding domains of the estrogen receptor protein. From gene cloning experiments,[61, 62] a 65- to 66-kDa protein was predicted that possessed the following domains: A/B, related to regulatory function such as by the DNA-dependent RNA polymerase; C, association of Zn^{2+}-binding fingers with hormone response element of the DNA; D, hinge region; E, high affinity association with steroid ligand; and F, unknown function. A truncated estrogen receptor of 50 kDa has been detected in several normal and neoplastic estrogen target organs. (From Wittliff JL, et al: *In* Kerlavage AR (ed): The Use of HPLC in Receptor Biochemistry. New York, Alan R Liss, 1989, pp 155–199. Reprinted with permission.)

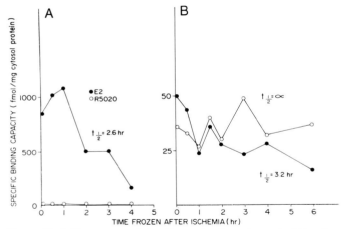

Figure 43–4. Time course of steroid receptor decay in surgical biopsies of breast cancer. The half-life of each receptor (● for estrogen and ○ for progestin) is highly tissue dependent. (From an unpublished study by Wittliff JL and Olson J.)

and necrotic tissue, must be transported from surgery and pathology to the clinical chemistry laboratory either in the frozen state or chilled in a petri dish or plastic bag immersed in ice. It is preferable to freeze the specimen immediately following excision at the time of frozen section diagnosis. However, an increasing number of specimens are transported directly to pathology for permanent section and may remain unfrozen for a considerable time. Specimens must be maintained on ice to retard both steroid and peptide hormone receptor degradation. Recent studies indicate the half-lives of estrogen and progestin receptors are highly variable in intact tumor biopsy specimens (Fig. 43–4), ranging from a half-life of as little as 30 minutes to no change in 6 hours at room temperature.[21, 200, 201] In general, the tissue should be frozen at -70°C within 30 to 45 minutes after removal and preferably maintained on ice or in a refrigerator in the interim. Optimum cutting temperature (OCT) compound does not influence receptor levels significantly if it is removed while frozen.[136] If a specimen is to be shipped to a distant laboratory for analyses, the snap-cap vials used for grid storage by electron microscopists are superb for freezing in liquid nitrogen or on dry ice.

Preservation of the biologic integrity of the tumor biopsy prior to arrival in the biochemistry laboratory is the shared responsibility of the pathologist and surgeon. The biopsy sent for receptor analyses must be representative of the tissue procured, and the specimen must be of sufficient volume (weight) for receptor analysis. Usually no less than 200 mg and preferably 400 to 500 mg of tumor are required to determine both estrogen and progestin receptors as well as the new prognostic factors. Intratumoral regional differences in steroid receptor status have been observed,[99, 113] emphasizing the need for submission of a representative sample. These results and others[110, 210] suggest a clonal heterogeneity relative to receptor status.

We examined the relationship between estrogen-binding capacity and the proportion of tumor epithelium in

a breast biopsy,[202] as human breast tumors are heterogeneous with regard to cell type. No correlation between the quantity of estrogen receptors in a breast biopsy specimen and the proportion of tumor epithelium was observed (Fig. 43–5). It was noted that numerous specimens containing less than 25 percent tumor epithelium exhibited very high estrogen-binding capacities (fmol/mg cytosol protein). Secondly, specific estrogen-binding capacities of individual tumor specimens containing the same quantity of tumor epithelium were highly variable. Estrogen receptor levels in these tumors varied from undetectable to more than several hundred fmol/mg cytosol protein. Although the estrogen-binding capacity of normal mammary gland might be expected to increase with increasing cellularity,[196, 197] this is not true of breast tumors. Quantitative differences in estrogen-binding capacity do not appear to be simply the result of the number of tumor cells in a sample; rather, this variation in activity reflects differences in the number of binding sites per breast tumor cell. We routinely recommend that small samples of the biopsy be forwarded for receptor analyses and fixed and stained to confirm the presence of tumor epithelium.[202, 207]

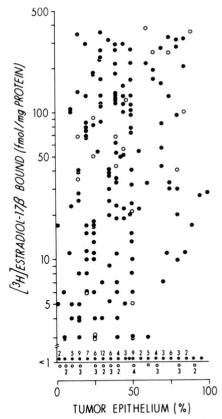

Figure 43–5. Relationship between specific estrogen-binding capacity and proportion of tumor epithelium in human breast carcinomas. At the time of estrogen receptor analysis, a representative sample of the breast biopsy was fixed in neutral formalin and processed for histologic examination. Relative concentration of tumor epithelium was estimated in specimens of primary (●) and metastatic (○) breast carcinomas and compared with estrogen-binding capacity. (From Wittliff JL, et al: In St Arneault, G, et al (eds): Recent Results in Cancer Research. New York, Springer-Verlag, 1976, pp 59–77. Reprinted with permission.)

An extract is made of the tumor biopsy by homogenization in an appropriate buffer soon after arrival in the laboratory. The thermostability of steroid receptors in tumor biopsies has been difficult to assess, partially because of the heterogeneous nature of the tissue and the quantity of steroid receptors. However, from studies in vitro, steroid receptors are labile proteins that undergo degradation or ligand dissociation in a temperature-dependent manner.[197] Rapid association of ligand with receptor aids in stabilization, suggesting that the time between cytosol preparation and introduction of the ligand should be as short as possible. Addition of sodium molybdate to homogenization buffer also aids in the stabilization of receptors released during cellular extraction.[147]

A comparison of receptor levels in fresh mastectomy specimens with those in biopsy specimens[112] suggests that there is only a small reduction in the proportion of estrogen receptor–positive mastectomy specimens compared with the biopsy specimens. This differential in quantitative measurements infers that each specimen, regardless of source, is clinically useful if maintained properly. However, we cannot emphasize enough the importance of selecting representative tissues from the biopsy specimen, since breast cancer exhibits intratumoral variation.[113]

QUALITY CONTROL MEASURES

Quality Assurance Programs for Cooperative Clinical Trials.

An increasing number of treatment protocols under investigation by cooperative trial groups in North America utilize defined levels of estrogen and progestin receptors to randomize therapy for breast and endometrial cancer patients.[49, 49a] To ensure that analyses for the sex steroid hormone receptors were performed in an accurate and uniform manner, the laboratory at the University of Louisville established a national reference facility under the sponsorship of the National Cancer Institute and the American Cancer Society initially. Since 1977 we have assisted in cancer treatment trials[206, 212a] with the National Surgical Adjuvant Breast and Bowel Project (NSABP), Cancer and Leukemia Group B (CALGB), Eastern Cooperative Oncology Group (ECOG), North Central Cancer Treatment Group (NCCTG), Southeastern Cancer Study Group (SECSG), Southwest Oncology Group (SWOG), as well as with the College of American Pathologists (CAP) (Fig. 43–6).

Currently, both female sex steroid receptors are being analyzed annually in tens of thousands of breast tumor specimens in the United States alone. As a means of examining how these data correlate with responses to specific therapeutic regimens, certain clinical cooperative groups, particularly the NSABP and SECSG, initiated experimental therapeutic protocols in the late 1970s requiring steroid receptor analyses of breast tumors. The establishment of assay uniformity and quality control was imperative to ensure meaningful correlations between laboratory results and clinical response.

LABORATORIES PARTICIPATING IN QUALITY ASSURANCE PROGRAMS TO ESTABLISH UNIFORMITY OF STEROID HORMONE RECEPTOR DETERMINATIONS IN THE CLINICAL LABORATORY

	NUMBER
Cancer and Leukemia Group B (CALGB)	39
College of American Pathologists (CAP)	65
Eastern Cooperative Oncology Group (ECOG)	50
Volunteer Survey (NP)	142
National Surgical Adjuvant Breast & Bowel Project (NSABP)	204
North Central Cancer Treatment Group (NCCTG)	18
Southeastern Cancer Study Group (SECSG)	45
Southwest Oncology Group (SWOG)	69

Figure 43–6. Laboratories participating in quality assurance programs to establish uniformity of steroid hormone receptor determinations in the clinical laboratory. (From Wittliff JL, Wittliff TH: J Clin Immunoassay 1990, in press. Reprinted with permission.)

Because the procedures and various programs for establishing uniformity of steroid receptors have been described in detail elsewhere[198, 204, 212a] they are mentioned here only briefly. Reports presented at the First International Workshop on Estrogen Receptors in Breast Cancer indicated that greater efforts must be made to establish uniformity and quality control of receptor methods.[107] In fact, one of the conclusions drawn from the 1979 NIH Consensus Development Conference was that "there is a need for quality control of steroid receptor assays."[6] Since 1977, the Hormone Receptor Laboratory at the University of Louisville has established a reference facility for monitoring quality assurance of steroid receptors in biopsy specimens of breast and endometrial carcinomas (Fig. 43–7).

Each shipment of reference powders is designed according to the specific need of the cooperative trial group and shipped on dry ice to the participating laboratories. Thus far, our laboratory has cooperated with the groups listed in Figure 43–6. We also collaborate with the College of American Pathologists in providing annual surveys. Currently we have assisted more than 400 laboratories in North America and have worked with various laboratories in Europe, South America, Asia, Australia, and Africa to establish quality assurance measures.

Tissue reference powders are composed of various quantities of frozen, pulverized organs such as uterus, breast, muscle, and liver as well as certain types of sera (of pregnancy) and are prepared using tissue grinders and liquid nitrogen. Often breast tumors were added to certain powders. Each of these reference powders is formulated in such a manner as to contain different combinations of estrogen receptors (ER) and progestin receptors (PR) (e.g., ER positive/PR negative; ER positive/PR positive) at different test levels. Return shipments are included in each survey. More recently we have developed lyophilized tissue reference powders

Information Sequence for Quality Assurance Program

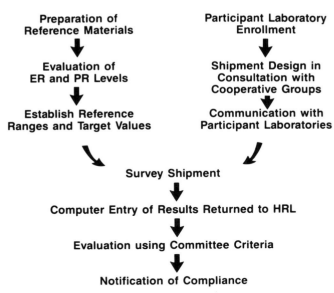

Preparation of Reference Materials

↓

Evaluation of ER and PR Levels

↓

Establish Reference Ranges and Target Values

Participant Laboratory Enrollment

↓

Shipment Design in Consultation with Cooperative Groups

↓

Communication with Participant Laboratories

↘   ↙

Survey Shipment

↓

Computer Entry of Results Returned to HRL

↓

Evaluation using Committee Criteria

↓

Notification of Compliance

Figure 43–7. Information sequence for quality assurance programs. This mechanism is utilized by laboratories participating in cooperative clinical trial groups in North America and by those participating in the survey program of the College of American Pathologists. (From Wittliff JL, Wittliff TH: J Clin Immunoassay 1990, in press. Reprinted with permission.)

for both the steroid hormone receptors and the epidermal growth factor (EGF) receptor that will greatly reduce the expense and time required to ship frozen powders. The exact composition is also based on the specific need of each clinical cooperative trial group.

To demonstrate the affinity and concentration of steroid receptors in a cytosol preparation, aliquots are incubated with increasing concentrations of various labeled steroids for 12 to 16 hr at 0°–3°C. Routinely, 2,4,6,7-[^{3}H]estradiol-17β and 17β-methyl-[^{3}H]promegestone (R 5020) are used as labeled ligands to measure estrogen and progestin receptors. Recently [^{125}I]iodoestradiol (Fig. 43–8), which is an excellent ligand for estrogen receptors, was synthesized.[72] A new ligand for the progestin receptor, [^{125}I]iodovinyl-nortestosterone (Figs. 43–8, 43–9), allows the detection of small quantities of these receptors in biopsy specimens weighing less than 200 mg. Binding observed in the presence of an excess of unlabeled inhibitor is related to nonreceptor or nonspecific (low affinity, high capacity) association of the ligand (see Fig. 43–9). Specific binding is estimated as the difference between total and nonspecific binding. The use of a double-label procedure also increases sensitivity.[65] Using Scatchard analysis[165] with software such as Accufit One-Site or Two-Site, the dissociation constant (K_d) or the association constant (K_a) may be determined from the slope of the plot (Fig. 43–9A).

The binding capacity is estimated from the intercept on the abscissa. The Accufit Competition software is

excellent for measuring the binding characteristics of the EGF receptor.[209] By definition, the higher the affinity of the binding site, the lower the dissociation constant, which is a measure of the tendency of the steroid-receptor complex to dissociate. The rate of this first order process is highly dependent on both the type of ligand used in the assay and the kind of receptor being measured. K_d values of 10^{-10} to 10^{-11} mol/L for estrogen and progestin receptors are good indicators that the biopsy specimen contains high affinity components. Similar affinities should be exhibited by the EGF receptor.[48] Usually specific binding capacity is expressed in femtomoles (10^{-15} mol) of labeled steroid bound per mg cytosol protein.[200]

It is generally accepted that an estrogen-binding capacity of less than 3 fmol/mg cytosol protein usually correlates with a lack of response to endocrine therapy of either the ablative or additive type.[201] Although there is a "borderline" range of values from 3 to 10 or 20 fmol/mg cytosol protein, estrogen and progestin receptor levels of >10 fmol/mg appear to represent a clinically significant level.[49, 49a] The equivalent cutoff values for the luteinizing hormone releasing hormone (LH-RH) and EGF receptor levels have not been determined.

Sucrose gradient centrifugation (Fig. 43–10), which separates the various forms of the steroid receptors, assesses certain molecular properties of these proteins in tumor extracts. We have used this method to ensure that the quality assurance for materials we distribute are representative of human tissue specimens.[202, 207, 208] Using this method, it has been determined that the sedimentation profiles of both estrogen and progestin receptors in human breast carcinomas fall into one of the following categories: tumors that contain specific steroid-binding components migrating at 8 S (Svedberg units) only, 4 S only, or both 8 S and 4 S (see Fig. 43–10); and those in which receptors are undetectable. The sedimentation coefficients of 8 S and 4 S are only approximate and are used operationally. Clinical significance of receptor polymorphism has been addressed.[92, 204, 210]

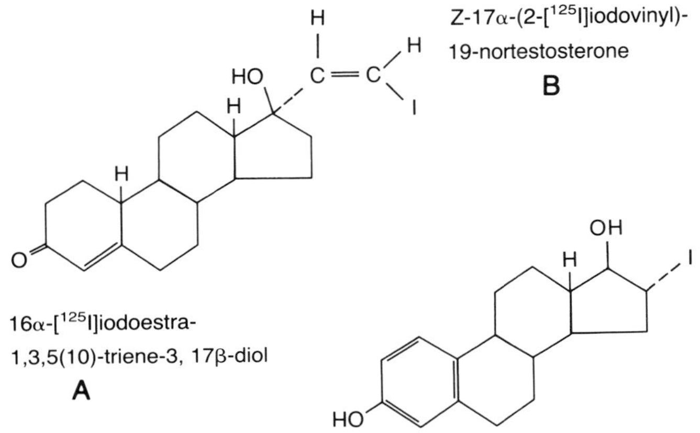

Z-17α-(2-[^{125}I]iodovinyl)-19-nortestosterone

B

16α-[^{125}I]iodoestra-1,3,5(10)-triene-3, 17β-diol

A

Figure 43–8. [^{125}I]-labeled ligands used in the determination of estrogen receptors (A) and progestin receptors (B). The specific radioactivity of [^{125}I] iodoestradiol ranges from 500 to 2200 Ci/mmol, while that of [^{125}I] IVNT is usually 400 to 500 Ci/mmol.

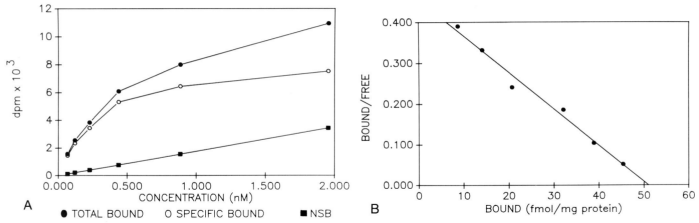

Figure 43–9. Titration analysis of progestin receptors in human breast carcinoma. A, Aliquots (0.1 ml) of cytosol prepared from frozen human breast tumors were incubated in triplicate with 0.1 ml [^{125}I]IVNT solutions in an homogenization buffer containing increasing amounts of radioactive ligand either in the absence (●) or presence (■) of a 200-fold excess of unlabeled R 5020. Specific binding (○) was estimated as the difference between total binding (●) and binding in the presence of the competitor (■). B, The titration data from A were plotted according to the method of Scatchard. This dissociation constant (K_d) determined from the slope of the curve was 5.2×10^{-11} mol/L for this preparation. The specific binding capacity of the progestin receptor complexes was estimated from the intercept on the x-axis and given a value of 81 fmol/mg for cytosol protein.

The Quality Control Analysis program is a set of menu-driven macros running on Lotus 1-2-3 version 2.01 spreadsheet software. The menu system provides easy access to the various data entry areas and has instructions included in key areas, avoiding the need for hard-copy documentation. After the data are entered, the program performs calculations on the data "ranges." Following the calculations, the data are output in two ways. The first is the Internal Report, which contains the raw data (for accuracy verification) and criteria

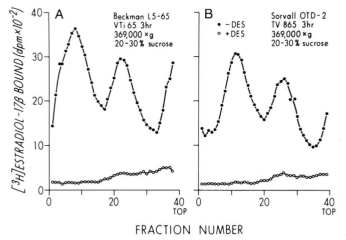

FRACTION NUMBER

Figure 43–10. Sucrose density gradient separation of the isoforms of estrogen receptors in human breast carcinoma. Cytosol prepared from two samples of human breast cancer was reacted with [^{3}H]estradiol-17β for 4 hours at 3°C in the presence (○) or absence (●) of a 200-fold excess of an unlabeled competitor. Separation was accomplished using vertical tube rotors in an ultracentrifuge cooled to 3°C. Note the presence of both 8 S and 4 S forms of these steroid receptors in each breast carcinoma sample analyzed.

ranges (for reference use). The program then produces the Quality Control Report, which is distributed to the participating members (see Figs. 43–6, 43–7).

A laboratory at an institution participating in a treatment trial of one of the cooperative groups is sent a set of two to four different tissue powders either frozen in dry ice or lyophilized and forwarded at ambient temperature. Often three vials of each powder are included to evaluate the intra-assay variability of each receptor measurement. A vial of unknown protein concentration is included to assess the influence of variation in this important determination. The laboratory analyzes these tissues using "in-house" methods and returns the results to the headquarters of the cooperative group for comparison with data generated by participant laboratories and by the Reference Laboratory at the University of Louisville (see Fig. 43–7). Criteria for evaluating agreement of the results are established by a committee in consultation with the Reference Laboratory that contacts each laboratory in writing regarding its performance relative to that of the other laboratories participating in the clinical trial. This important information is available to the physician treating the patient either by contacting the headquarters of the clinical trial group or by contacting the Reference Laboratory. It is required that receptor assays on breast tumor biopsy tissue be conducted by laboratories meeting the compliance criteria of one or more of the quality assurance programs of the cooperative groups (see Fig. 43–6).

It is essential that a laboratory utilize a daily quality control material and periodically participate in an extramural quality assurance program such as those established by the clinical cooperative groups. In this way, meaningful relationships between biochemical markers such as the steroid hormone receptors and clinical response to experimental therapies can be realized.

Sources of Variability in Assay Procedures

The lack of uniformity in the methods of receptor analyses in the clinical laboratory and in the expression of receptor results has been an extensive problem in the past.[93, 162, 203, 204] Some common sources of variability in receptor analyses we have noted by laboratories participating in our quality assurance survey during the past 13 years include the following:

1. Type and source of ligand and range of concentrations
2. Concentration and type of competitive inhibitor
3. Incubation time and temperature of reaction
4. Concentration of protein and type of assay selected
5. Method of calculation and outlier selection

The following additional parameters may complicate receptor analyses if not properly controlled:

1. Contribution of nonspecific (low affinity, high capacity) binding
2. Metabolism of the ligand
3. Ligand-receptor dissociation
4. Ligand association with specific serum proteins such as sex steroid–binding globulin and corticosteroid-binding globulin (steroid receptors)
5. Thermal lability, both in the biopsy specimen and in cell-free preparations
6. Ionic strength lability
7. Occupancy of binding sites by endogenous hormone
8. Proteolysis of the receptor
9. Receptor "inhibiting" substances

To verify precise quantification of the number of binding sites in a biopsy using a titration procedure (see Fig. 43–9) and provide some method to remove unbound ligand, it is necessary to use a broad range of labeled ligand concentrations approaching saturation. These must include a sufficient number of points below the saturation level so that an interpretable Scatchard plot is generated [Fig. 43–9(B)]. Some laboratories participating in cooperative clinical trials used too many saturating concentrations of ligand so that the points were "grouped" near the abscissa of the Scatchard plot, making it difficult to accurately estimate the dissociation constant as well as the number of specific binding sites.

The concentration and type of competitive inhibitor used to estimate the contribution of nonspecific (low affinity, high capacity) binding is another source of variation. This type of binding is largely a result of necrotic materials and blood in biopsy specimens which may contain albumin and other proteins such as TeBG and CGB known to associate specifically with steroid hormones. Diethylstilbestrol is a potent synthetic estrogen that does not bind to plasma proteins with high affinity. Thus it is a useful inhibitor in estrogen receptor analyses (see Fig. 43–10), since it only associates with intracellular binding components. We routinely use a 200-fold excess of unlabeled diethylstilbestrol in a titration assay. A similar quantity (200-fold excess) of unlabeled R 5020, a synthetic progestin, is utilized with [³H]R 5020 to estimate low affinity, high capacity binding. Because R 5020 and certain glucocorticoids may

associate with the same binding sites,[108] it is advisable to use low nanomolar concentrations of [³H]R 5020 to avoid measurement of glucocorticoid receptors.[197] The principal advantage of utilizing [³H]R 5020 as a ligand for the progestin receptor is that it does not associate to any great extent with CBG, which is known to bind the natural progestin (progesterone). Furthermore, dissociation from the progestin receptor and metabolism are reduced.

The sucrose gradient procedure (see Fig. 43–10) requires the use of a saturating concentration of labeled ligand, usually 3 to 5 nmol/L for either estradiol-17β or R 5020 as suggested from titration analyses (see Fig. 43–9). It is essential to use a competitive inhibitor of ligand binding to clearly estimate the receptor proteins. Albumin and other nonreceptor proteins often produce sediment in the 4 S to 5 S region of the sucrose gradient, where certain receptor species migrate as well, so ligand specificity should be evaluated. Using the newer techniques of high performance liquid chromatography (HPLC) for receptor isoform separation, unlabeled inhibitors are also employed to ensure specificity.[199]

Enzyme immunoassay (EIA) of steroid receptors is being used more frequently for small biopsy specimens from which limited amounts of cytosol are available (Fig. 43–11). As with ligand binding, it is essential that the performance of all instruments employed be checked routinely. This is particularly important in the EIA because the Quantum spectrophotometer supplied by

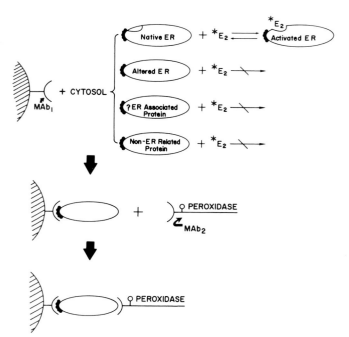

Figure 43–11. Schematic representation of enzyme-linked immunoassay for estrogen receptors using monoclonal antibodies. As shown it is predicted that liganded and unliganded receptors as well as those with defective ligand-binding sites would interact with monoclonal antibodies specific to the receptor. It is unclear to what extent estrogen receptor–associated proteins may also be identified with this procedure. (From Sato N, et al: J Chromatogr 359:475–487, 1986. Reprinted with permission.)

Abbott Laboratories provides the only data generated in the procedure. Because of the small volumes, the precision of pipetting cytosol should be well established using an intralaboratory comparison. Other sources of variation include (1) the quality and composition of pipette tips, (2) the source of reaction plates, (3) the time and temperature of reactions (antigen-antibody complex stability usually has a narrow limit), (4) the specificity of enzyme-labeled antibody and its clarity (diluted conjugates may aggregate after prolonged storage), (5) the humidity of the cluster plate environment, (6) the uniformity and precision of the washing procedure, and (7) the concentration of protein and type of assay selected. When our laboratory first establishes an EIA procedure for a new type of marker in tumor biopsy specimens, the linearity of the reaction is determined as a function of protein concentration. These reactions appear to provide a straightforward, rapid,

and accurate measurement of steroid receptors, which appear to have a concordance of 80 percent to 90 percent with steroid ligand-binding assays.[138, 182] Their sensitivity appears to be in the range of 1 to 3 fmol/mg cytosol protein.

The immunocytochemical assay (ICA) provides a semi-quantitative evaluation of receptors in tumor biopsy specimens (Fig. 43–12) that have been either frozen and fixed or fixed and embedded with paraffin.[104a] The kits provided by Abbott Laboratories for ER-ICA and PR-ICA are recommended only for use with frozen tissue. The reagents in these kits are used to ascertain the proportion and distribution of cells containing receptor protein. Various procedures have been recommended for assessing the intensity of staining and the percentage of positive tumor cells in a biopsy. These include a scale developed by McCarty et al.[105] Another means of semi-quantitation is the method of Remele et

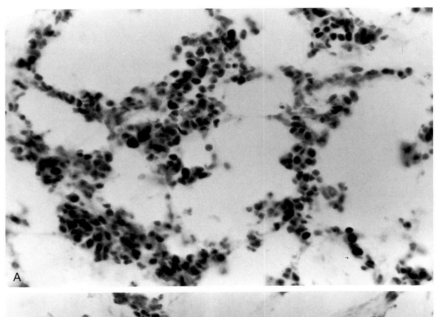

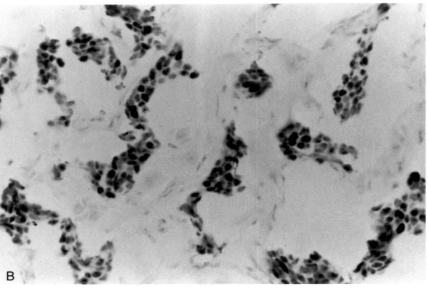

Figure 43–12. Immunohistochemical detection of estrogen and progestin receptors in human breast carcinomas. Using the ICA procedure with specific monoclonal antibodies, cells containing either estrogen receptors (A) or progestin receptors (B) are readily identified by peroxidase staining.

al.,[153] in which a score is determined between 0 and 12. A new method of assessing steroid receptors in tissue slices is the CAS Image Analysis System, which utilizes commercially available monoclonal antibodies and immunoperoxidase techniques.

Each of these methods has a particular set of variables that must be assessed before the method is clinically applied. It is essential that receptor assays of breast tumor biopsy specimens be conducted only by laboratories meeting the compliance criteria of one or more of the quality assurance programs. Wet laboratory workshops are conducted periodically, and quality control materials for setting up receptor assays for estrogen, progestin, glucocorticoid, androgen, epidermal growth factor, and LH-RH are available.[212a]

PHYSIOLOGICAL AND CLINICAL FACTORS INFLUENCING RECEPTOR LEVELS

Clinical and physiological factors must be considered when assessing the significance of the hormone receptor level (Table 43–1). Most of the data generated thus far were derived from studies of *steroid receptors* but appear to apply in most cases when considering *peptide hormone receptors*.

Biopsy specimens of infiltrating ductal carcinoma examined in our laboratory show a broad range of concentration values for steroid receptor, ranging from zero to almost 6000 fmol/mg cytosol protein. Thus far, no single histological feature has been determined that might explain the variation in the levels of estrogen receptors in human breast tumors.[22, 23, 96] However, some studies suggest that tumor cellularity and receptor levels are related to prognosis for operable breast cancer.[19] Prognosis was actually better for patients with low cellularity. Chua et al.[32] reported a strong correlation between estrogen receptor level, age, and histological grade of breast tumors from women in Singapore; Silfversward et al.[173] reported a positive correlation between receptor content and degree of differentiation in ductal carcinoma. Godolphin et al.[56] showed that receptors and staging were complementary indicators in breast cancer; lymphoid infiltration generally was correlated with low estrogen receptor values. Other studies investigated the relationship of pathologic features and receptor status.[30, 33, 76, 111, 113, 116, 146, 155, 202] At this time there is considerable variability in the results reported, and a well-controlled inter-laboratory study should be conducted to assess the relationship of parameters such as histological classification, nuclear grade, DNA content and ploidy, and lymphocytic infiltration to receptor status.

In general, the presence of both sex hormone receptors (and receptors for androgens and glucocorticoids) implies retention of regulatory mechanisms operating in the normal breast epithelium. Thus a loss in receptor content may be used with other neoplastic features as a means of identifying patients at increased risk of tumor recurrence or mortality.[134]

The proportion of tumor cells relative to surrounding connective tissue and adipose cells (see Fig. 43–5) does not appear to correlate with a variation in estrogen-binding capacity, although the former elements appear to contribute to the quantity of progestin receptors estimated in a biopsy sample.[202] Because fibroblasts may contain significant levels of specific progestin-binding components, it is imperative to utilize a biopsy specimen that incorporates as much of the malignant lesion as is technically possible. Adipose cells of normal breast do not contain specific estrogen receptors, although they may contain considerable concentrations of the steroid hormones, presumably because of their lipid solubility.[197] Using immunocytochemical assays (Fig. 43–12), the level of steroid receptors in a tumor biopsy sample reflects a heterogeneous cell population in which tumor cells may exhibit different degrees of hormone sensitivity (i.e., variable numbers of receptor molecules).[85, 94, 105]

Receptor level does not appear to correlate with size or location of the tumor in the breast, axillary node status, or clinical stage of the disease. Although larger tumors were reported to contain lower quantities of estrogen receptors, presumably because of increased necrosis,[107] this was not supported by more thorough investigations presented at the NIH Consensus Development Conference.[6]

Endocrine status and the concentrations of circulating estrogen and progesterone influence the number of specific binding sites on receptor proteins occupied in vivo by the steroid hormones (Tables 43–2 and 43–3).[21a] For example, estrogen-binding capacity in target organs varies during the menstrual cycle; binding capacity is low in mid cycle and is reduced further in the second phase.[29, 102, 104, 183] Pollow et al.[145] reported that there is insignificant binding of [³H]estradiol to receptors in breast tumors from patients with plasma estradiol-17β levels exceeding 300 pg/ml.

Both the incidence and concentration of steroid receptors in breast tumors were confirmed by Bland et al[21A] to be lower in premenopausal than in postmenopausal women (see Tables 43–2 and 43–3). Patient age also influences the level of receptors, with higher concentrations being exhibited in tumors from elderly patients.[1, 46, 106, 196] The elevated levels of endogenous estrogen in plasma of premenopausal women may mask receptor-binding sites. However, because estrogen stimulates the formation of its own receptor as well as progesterone receptor synthesis, the level of circulating estrogen may not be the only factor.[74, 75] In premenopausal patients with breast cancer, elevated circulating

Table 43–1. PHYSIOLOGICAL AND CLINICAL FACTORS INFLUENCING HORMONE RECEPTOR LEVELS IN BREAST CANCER

Race	Menopausal status
Sex	Day of cycle (premenopausal)
Age	Pregnancy and lactation
Organ site	Drug administration
Tumor cellularity and histological differentiation	Surgical technique of resection

Table 43–2. SPECIFIC BINDING CAPACITIES OF STEROID RECEPTORS IN BREAST TUMOR BIOPSY SPECIMENS ACCORDING TO PATIENT ENDOCRINE STATUS

Steroid-Binding Capacity (fmol/mg cytosol protein)*		Patient Endocrine Status	Tumor Receptor Status
Estrogen	*Progestin*		
90 ± 9 (10–1335)	237 ± 22 (10–3038)	Premenopausal	ER +, PR +
83 ± 16 (10–568)	—	Premenopausal	ER +, PR −
—	84 ± 18 (10–1151)	Premenopausal	ER −, PR +
286 ± 18 (10–5693)	337 ± 28 (10–5923)	Postmenopausal	ER +, PR +
176 ± 29 (10–2807)	—	Postmenopausal	ER +, PR −
—	75 ± 26 (10–977)	Postmenopausal	ER −, PR +

*Measured by multipoint titration analyses using Scatchard plots. Mean ± standard error of the mean of number of determinations shown in Table 43–4. Range shown in parentheses. A level of >10 fmol/mg cytosol protein was taken as an arbitrary cutoff point for the presence of receptors as utilized by the NSABP.[49]

Adapted from Bland KI, et al: Surg Forum XXXII:410–412, 1981.

progesterone may reduce the formation of estrogen receptors in comparison with quantities occurring in postmenopausal women when progesterone levels are lower.[6] We suggest that it is prudent to consider the menstrual status of a breast cancer patient when evaluating the significance of the specific steroid-binding capacity in the selection of a therapeutic regimen.

In general, levels of receptors in biopsy samples of metastatic breast carcinomas were similar to those observed in primary tumors.[6, 77, 203] However, the incidence of estrogen and progestin receptors is somewhat elevated in biopsy specimens from postmenopausal patients compared with those from premenopausal patients (see Table 43–3). Often metastatic lesions are less differentiated than primary breast tumors. Loss of expression of steroid hormone receptors during malignant transformation may reflect a more endocrine-independent growth pattern. For example, Meyer et al.[111] showed that a low incidence of estrogen receptor correlated with rapid rates of cellular replication. Recent studies expanded this observation.[113] Studies reported at the Consensus Development Conference with analyses of multiple sequential biopsies suggest there may be a progressive loss of estrogen receptors in breast tumors as the course of the disease advances.[6, 67, 77, 214] In 80 percent of tumors, estrogen receptor status of the asynchronous secondary tumor was similar to that of the primary lesion, even though variations in receptor levels

were observed in approximately half of the tumors.[2, 3] There was no consistent influence of breast site or time interval between primary and secondary cancer appearance on receptor variation.

We suggest that steroid receptors be reevaluated in the metastatic lesion whenever feasible and that every primary breast tumor be analyzed for steroid receptors, even if the patient does not have metastatic disease. Later in the course of disease progression, receptor levels may become even more useful if the metastatic lesions have disseminated to organs such as bone and brain that are not easily accessible to biopsy. We recommend the ICA (see Fig. 43–12) for measuring receptors in brain lesions.[104a]

Therapies using cytotoxic drugs or antihormones may eliminate receptor-containing cells or alter levels of receptors in tumor biopsies.[190, 191] For example, tamoxifen (Fig. 43–13) treatment of postmenopausal women with breast cancer causes an early increase in uterine progestin receptor and a decrease in levels of luteinizing hormone (LH) and follicle-stimulating hormone (FSH) as well as prolactin.[66, 83] Estrogen receptor levels were not altered by radiation of human breast cancer cells and in fact returned to normal after removal of antiestrogen inhibition.[27] Because of the half-life of tamoxifen-receptor complexes in vivo, it is recommended that tamoxifen administration be discontinued at least 3 weeks prior to biopsy for steroid receptor analyses.

Table 43–3. REPRESENTATIVE DISTRIBUTION OF STEROID RECEPTORS IN TUMOR BIOPSY SPECIMENS ACCORDING TO PATIENT ENDOCRINE STATUS*

Receptor Status of Tumor Biopsy Specimens	Endocrine Status of Patient			
	Premenopausal		Postmenopausal	
	No.	*%*	*No.*	*%*
ER +, PR +	222	45	520	63
ER +, PR −	58	12	128	15
ER −, PR −	136	28	137	17
ER −, PR +	72	15	41	5
Total	488		826	

*Fifty-five years of age was chosen as an age at which virtually every woman may be considered postmenopausal.

Adapted from Bland KI, et al: Surg Forum XXXII:410–412, 1981.

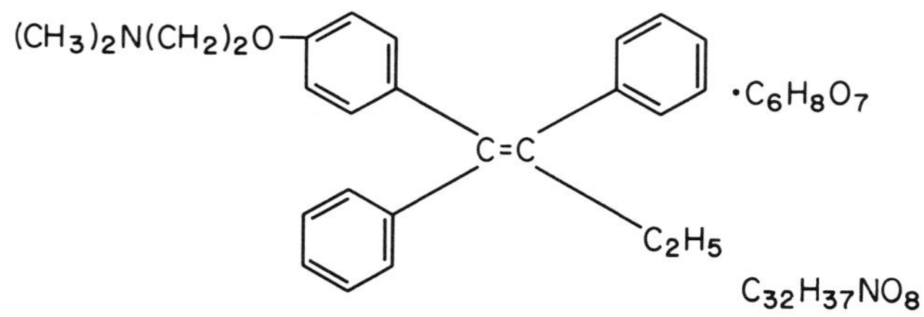

Z-2-[4-(I,2-dipheny-I-butenyl)phenoxy]-N,N-dimethylethanamine 2-hydroxy-I,2,3- propanetricarboxylate (1:1)

Figure 43–13. Structure of tamoxifen. Tamoxifen (Nolvadex) represents a potent inhibitor of [³H] estradiol binding by estrogen receptors and is itself an excellent ligand for this receptor, exhibiting a K_d value of 10^{-9} to 10^{-10} mol/L. The presence of estrogen receptor in a breast biopsy appears essential for a breast cancer patient to respond to this drug.

Table 43–4. METHODS OF DETERMINING THE PRESENCE OF STEROID HORMONE RECEPTORS

Method	Principle	Usage	Comments
Ligand titration	Sample incubated with increasing amounts of labeled ligand, with and without the presence of unlabeled inhibitor. Amount of specific binding is plotted by Scatchard plot, and the total number of binding sites and dissociation constant (K_d) are calculated.	Most frequently used	Requires 100–500 mg tissue dependent on ligand used. ^{125}I-labeled ligand allows assay of 100–200 mg biopsy.
Sucrose density gradient centrifugation	Molecular forms of receptors of different sizes are separated on sucrose gradient following centrifugation. Location and number of sites present are determined by labeled ligand binding (with and without inhibitor).	Infrequently used	Cannot calculate ligand affinity by this method.
High-performance liquid chromatography (HPLC) methods	Different receptor isoforms are separated as a result of specific molecular property of receptor proteins.	Research of molecular properties	Sensitive, rapid means of separation with high recovery. Calculation of K_d values approximate by these methods.
Size exclusion	Following binding with labeled ligand, receptors are separated on basis of molecular size and shape.		
Ion exchange	Following binding with labeled ligand, receptors are separated on basis of their surface charge properties.		
Chromatofocusing	Following binding with labeled ligand, receptors are separated on basis of their isoelectric points.		
Hydrophobic interaction	Following binding with labeled ligand, receptors are separated on basis of different surface hydrophobicity.		
Enzyme-linked immunoassay	Sandwich assay with immobilized monoclonal antibody to receptor. Following binding of specific receptor, second monoclonal antibody to another receptor epitope, labeled with horseradish peroxidase, is bound. Quantification using appropriate substrate is performed.	Frequency of use increasing	Provides estimate of receptor mass relative to ligand-binding capacity.
Immunohistochemical	Monoclonal antibody, specific for a steroid receptor, binds to tissue steroid receptor. Second antibody, labeled with peroxidase, is used to localize first antibody binding. Visualization of receptor in tissue with substrates for peroxidase stain.	Investigational, but shows promise for clinical applications as qualitative tests.	Used for qualitative identification on small tissue samples; fine needle aspirations.
Immunofluorescence	Fluorescein-labeled steroid is bound to tissue steroid receptors. Amount of bound steroid is visualized by fluorescence microscopy.	Rare, experimental	Used for qualitative identification on small tissue biopsy specimens.

Adapted from Wittliff JL: *In* Pesce AJ, Kaplan LA (eds): Methods in Clinical Chemistry. St. Louis, CV Mosby, 1987, pp 767–795.

Patients treated with toremifene should be handled in the same manner. Literature from studies on cells in culture[3] and in patients[29] suggest that tamoxifen may work as either an estrogen agonist or antagonist depending on its concentration. Furthermore, it may be used therapeutically to induce progestin receptors in human tumors.[29, 119]

Organ site of breast carcinoma metastases is a criterion used in the selection of therapy for the breast cancer patient. Estrogen and progestin receptors have been detected in biopsies obtained from breast carcinoma metastases from the adrenal gland, bone, colon, contralateral breast, kidney, liver, lung, lymph nodes, muscle, omentum, ovary, skin, stomach, and thyroid gland by our laboratory and others.[6, 198] The incidence and specific binding capacities of these metastatic lesions varied considerably; however, the ligand affinities and specificities of the receptors were characteristic of those in normal tissues. No correlation was observed between the presence of steroid receptors and the organ site of metastatic lesions in breast cancer.

Race apparently also has an influence on clinical prognosis[126, 189, 213] as well as on steroid receptor status.[118, 130, 131, 139, 141, 164] The relationship between receptor status and level with survival data in patients of different races suggests that black women with receptor-negative breast cancer have a decreased disease-free interval and overall survival. The development of reference ranges of sex steroid receptors in various racial groups and their clinical significance appears relevant.

METHODS OF STEROID HORMONE RECEPTOR ANALYSIS

Wittliff[198-201] has reviewed the details of many clinical and experimental methods in several recent publications, so these procedures will be discussed only briefly here. Table 43–4 outlines various methods used in steroid receptor determinations with comments regarding their utility.

Radioligand-Binding Procedures

The exact location of steroid receptors in a cell is currently debated, but increasing evidence suggests a nuclear association.[86, 194] These receptors are regulatory proteins found in cytosolic extracts of target cells. Cytosol is used operationally to define the soluble portion of the cell, both nuclear and cytoplasmic. Most steroid receptors exist in the presence of other binding components, thus complicating measurements of their binding properties. Receptors associate with their particular steroid hormone in a reversible fashion and with high affinity and ligand specificity.

Equations Describing Ligand-Receptor Interaction

Receptors are specific cellular proteins that communicate regulatory stimuli. A cellular response to a specific hormone will only be elicited when the characteristic hormone associates with the ligand recognition sites of the receptor protein (see Fig. 43–3). Receptor proteins vary widely in their characteristics and, in general, the *steroid receptors* are located in the *nucleoplasm* and *cytoplasm* (Fig. 43–2), whereas the *peptide hormone receptors* are associated with *cell membranes*.

These types of receptor assays are contingent on the binding of some ligand (Table 43–5) to a recognition site on the protein. Knowledge of the nature of the interaction between a steroid hormone and its binding site is thus important for an understanding of receptor measurements. This interaction is thought to be bimolecular in nature, and may be described by the equation

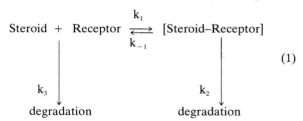

(1)

The rates of association and dissociation of steroid hormones with specific receptor binding sites are dependent on both incubation time and temperature. For example, the binding of [3H]estradiol to its receptor is usually maximal in 4 to 6 hours at 0°–3°C and remains unchanged for 20 additional hours of incubation.[200] At 25°C, apparent equilibrium is reached in 30 to 90 minutes and is maintained for 30 additional minutes before a gradual loss of binding activity is observed. Presumably this loss is caused by degradation of the receptor or by irreversible dissociation of the steroid-receptor com-

Table 43–5. STEROID HORMONES AND ANALOGUES USED AS LIGANDS FOR STEROID HORMONE RECEPTORS

Estrogen Receptors	Progestin Receptors	Androgen Receptors	Glucocorticoid Receptors
3H-estradiol-17β*	3H-progesterone	3H-testosterone	3H-hydrocortisone
3H-estrone	3H-R 5020* (promegestone)	3H-5α-dihydrotestosterone	3H-corticosterone
3H-estriol	3H-R 27987	3H-R 1881* (methyltrienolone)	3H-dexamethasone*
125I-iodoestradiol-17β*	3H-Org 2058	3H-cyproterone acetate	3H-dexamethasone mesylate
3H-R 2858 (moxestrol)	3H-medroxyprogesterone acetate	3H-mibolerone*	3H-triamcinolone acetonide*
3H-tamoxifen	3H-RU 486		
3H-tamoxifen-40H			
3H-tamoxifen aziridine			

*Most often employed in clinical assays.
Adapted from Wittliff JL: In Pesce AJ, Kaplan LA (eds): Methods in Clinical Chemistry. St Louis, CV Mosby, 1987, pp 767–795.

plexes. As a result of the temperature sensitivity of the estrogen-receptor complex at 25°C, the majority of binding reactions are performed overnight at 0°–3°C.

In the absence of any other binding components, an expression for the concentration of steroid hormone bound to the receptor can be derived from the equation for the law of mass action,

$$[R][S]/[RS] = K_d \qquad (2)$$

where [R] and [S] are the concentrations of unbound receptor and steroid hormone, respectively, and [RS] is the concentration of steroid-receptor complexes. The total receptor concentration is given by

$$[R]_t = [R] + [RS]. \qquad (3)$$

If B equals the concentration of receptor bound steroid and F equals the concentration of unbound (free) steroid, then

$$K_d = ([R]_t - B)F/B \qquad (4)$$

$$B = F[R]_t (F + K_d). \qquad (5)$$

Estimation of $[R]_t$ and K_d (or $K_a = 1/K_d$) can be facilitated by the rearrangement of eq. (4), and B can then be calculated using various forms of linear plots. The most commonly employed is the Scatchard[165] plot (see Fig. 43–9B), which will be discussed shortly. These equations can only be utilized after correction for nonreceptor binding, since all tissues contain steroid-binding components other than receptors.

Selection of Labeled Ligand and Inhibitor

A summary of many of the naturally occurring steroid hormones and their analogues used as ligands for steroid hormone receptors is given in Table 43–5. The principal physiological estrogen employed is [³H]estradiol-17β, since it exhibits a high affinity ($K_d = 10^{-10}$ mol/L) and specificity for its receptor.[197] The most commonly used commercially prepared radioactive steroid that is highly purified and reasonably stable is the [2,4,6,7-³H] estradiol-17β. The hexatritium-labeled steroid has a higher specific radioactivity but requires greater care to retard degradation. Labeled estrone and estriol are used primarily for research.

One of the most useful new estrogenic ligands is [16α-¹²⁵I]iodoestradiol-17β (see Fig. 43–8), an estrogen agonist that exhibits binding characteristics similar to native estradiol.[72] Because of its high radiospecific activity (1500–2000 Ci/mmol), it is being used in many studies of the molecular properties of the estrogen receptor[199, 211, 212] and may be employed in the new double-isotope methods for simultaneous measurements of both estrogen and progestin receptors.[65]

Increasing interest is being directed toward synthetic estrogens and antagonists such as moxestrol and triphenylethylene type compounds, including tamoxifen (see Fig. 43–13) and 4-hydroxy-tamoxifen (see Table

43–5). More recently, a tamoxifen aziridine analogue that has agonist, affinity labeling properties has been synthesized. Most of the ligands mentioned in this group would appear to be useful in a future generation of the current receptor method.

As shown in Table 43–5, the main naturally occurring progestin used as a receptor ligand is progesterone. Currently it is infrequently used because it rapidly associates with and dissociates from its binding sites in clinical specimens. The ligand employed most widely because of its high affinity ($K_d = 10^{-10}$ mol/L) for the progestin receptor and its ability to form the stable ligand-receptor complexes necessary for clinical assays is promegestone, also referred to as R 5020.[200] A new analogue of this steroid, R 27987, appears to be an even better ligand for both clinical and research analyses. An important chemical property for both of these compounds is their covalent association with the specific progestin-binding site when photoactivated. Thus affinity-labeled receptors can be prepared for structural studies. Other synthetic progestins employed infrequently are Organon-2058, RU-486, and medroxyprogesterone acetate (Fig. 43–14). The latter compound may assist in the development of a new type of assay, since it is a hormonal type drug used in the treatment of breast and endometrial cancer. We have recently developed the use of [¹²⁵I]iodovinyl-nortestosterone (see Figs. 43–8 and 43–9) for measurements of progestin receptors.

Although testosterone was used in early research on androgen receptors (Table 43–5), the affinity and spec-

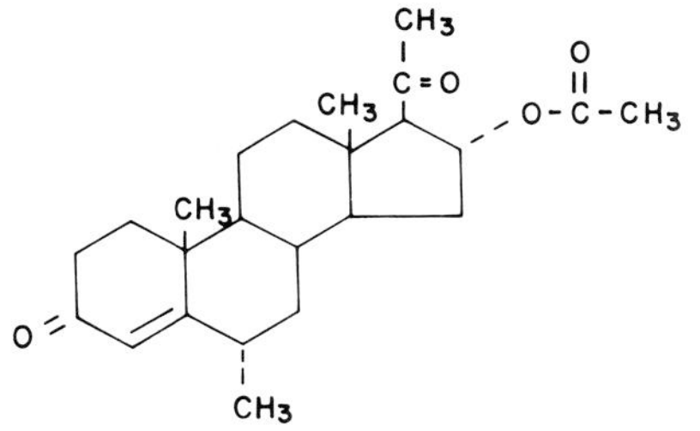

Medroxyprogesterone Acetate
(6α-methyl-17α-acetoxy-progesterone)

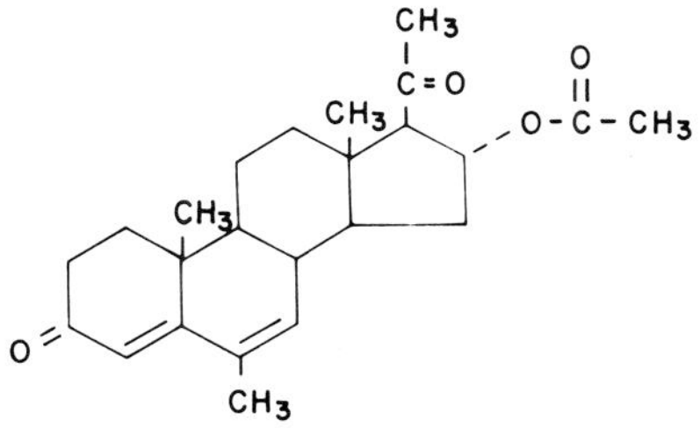

Megestrol Acetate
(17α-acetoxy-6-methylpregna-4,6-diene-3,20-dione acetate)

Figure 43–14. Therapeutic progestational agents known to associate with progestin receptors in breast carcinoma. Both medroxyprogesterone acetate (Provera) and megestrol acetate (Megace) bind to progestin receptors with K_d values ranging from 10^{-9} to 10^{-10} mol/L. Presence of progestin receptor in a tumor appears to be essential to elicit a therapeutic response to these agents.

ificity of the reaction between 5α-dihydrotestosterone and its binding site make it a widely used ligand for clinical determinations of androgen receptors. Because of the occasional problems with association-dissociation kinetics with receptors from certain androgen target organs, the synthetic agonist methyltrienolone (R 1881) is the ligand of choice for many procedures. Binding constants such as a K_d value of 10^{-9} mol/L and high specificity coupled with low metabolic alteration permit effective determination of androgen receptors in many solid tumors. Cyproterone acetate, an antagonist, is used primarily for research purposes. The most promising new ligand for androgen receptors is mibolerone (see Table 43–5), which does not associate with the glucocorticoid receptor and has a low affinity for the progestin receptor in our experience.

One of the most ubiquitous steroid receptors in humans is the glucocorticoid receptor.[12] Interestingly, glucocorticoids may be catabolic in one organ (such as in lymphocytes) and anabolic in others (such as in the liver). Again, there appears to be difficulty in using physiological glucocorticoids such as hydrocortisone or corticosterone (see Table 43–5) in routine clinical assays because of the rapid association-dissociation reactions that occur with their receptors. Most investigators in the clinical chemistry field utilize the agonists dexamethasone for glucocorticoid receptor determinations in lymphomas and leukemias[179] and triamcinolone acetonide for receptors in solid tumors.[197] More recently, an affinity ligand, dexamethasone mesylate, has been developed primarily as a research tool.

Ligand Saturation Analysis

To determine the affinity (K_d value) and concentration (N value) of receptors in a preparation, cytosol aliquots are incubated with increasing concentrations of various labeled ligands for 12 to 18 hours at 0°–3°C (Fig. 43–9A). Routinely, either [2,4,6,7-^{3}H]estradiol-17β or [16α-^{125}I]iodoestradiol-17β and 17α-methyl-^{3}H-promegestone (R 5020) are used as labeled ligands to measure estrogen and progestin receptors, respectively. Briefly, a series of test tubes are prepared with the various concentrations of labeled ligand, and the reactions are initiated by the addition of the receptor preparation. These assays are termed "total binding reactions," since they measure receptor and nonreceptor binding. The binding curve (Fig. 43–9A) will show a point of inflection suggesting saturable binding under the conditions usually employed. Simultaneously, a second series of test tubes are prepared containing the various concentrations of the labeled steroid and a 150- to 200-fold excess of an unlabeled inhibitor. These reactions are also initiated by the addition of the receptor preparation being analyzed. This latter series is termed "nonspecific binding," since it should measure all low affinity, high capacity association of ligand with nonreceptor components in the cytosol. This is also termed "nonsaturable binding."

One of the principal proteins contaminating cytosols is serum albumin, which often is present because of tumor necrosis. The K_d value for estrogen-albumin association is 10^{-5} to 10^{-6} mol/L, which is the lower affinity type of association. Thus at the labeled ligand concentration used in most receptor determinations, that is, 1–10 nmol/L, low affinity association of steroid with albumin-like proteins should be linear, indicating nonsaturability (Fig. 43–9A). Likewise, the upper slope of the total binding curve after saturation has been achieved should be similar to that of the nonspecific binding curve. This is a visual test that the titration has been conducted in a satisfactory manner reflecting a competent measurement of receptor binding. In practice, it is recommended that the binding curves be visually evaluated before proceeding with the actual Scatchard plot (Fig. 43–9B). Specific binding is estimated as the arithmetic difference between the total and nonspecific binding curves (Fig. 43–9A). Furthermore, the curve describing specific binding should exhibit saturability permitting measurement of a finite number of binding sites after data transformation.

Using Scatchard analysis, the apparent dissociation constant (K_d) or the association constant (K_a) may be determined from the slope of the plot according to the equation.

$$\text{Slope} = 1/K_d \text{ where } K_d = 1/K_a = k_{-1}/k_1 \qquad (6)$$

As shown in Figure 43–9B, the binding capacity is estimated from the intercept on the abscissa. By definition, the *higher* the affinity of the binding site, the *lower* the dissociation constant, which is a measure of the tendency of the steroid-receptor complex to dissociate. The rate of this first order process is highly dependent on both the type of ligand used in the assay and the kind of receptor being measured (see Table 43–5).

Sucrose Density Gradient Centrifugation

Sucrose gradient centrifugation separates forms of the steroid receptors based on their size (expressed as Svedberg units, or S) and shape (Fig. 43–10). Sedimentation profiles of both estrogen and progestin receptors in human breast carcinomas exhibit components migrating at 8 S only, 4 S only, or both 8 S and 4 S, whereas others do not exhibit receptors. The sedimentation coefficients given, that is, 8 S and 4 S, are only approximated for the sake of discussion. With two kinds of steroid receptors, each with four different types of profiles, there are at least 16 possible combinations.

Incorporation of standard (known) proteins permits more exact determination of the sedimentation coefficients of the steroid receptors in the biopsy. This method requires a relatively small tissue sample (200 mg). Briefly, a receptor preparation is incubated with a saturating concentration of the radioactive steroid similar to that used in the titration assay. Usually, cytosol prepared in either TRIS or phosphate buffers, pH 7.4 to 7.8, is incubated overnight at 1°–3°C with 2–3 nmol/L [^{3}H]estradiol-17β or 3–4 nmol/L [^{3}H]R-5020 in the presence and absence of a 150- to 200-fold excess of unlabeled competitor for sufficient time to reach reaction equilibrium. The reactions are terminated by the addition of small pellets of dextran-coated charcoal that have been prepared by centrifuging an aliquot of this reagent (as in the titration assay). This permits removal of the unbound steroid without dilution of the reaction mixture. After the labeled steroid-receptor complexes have formed and unbound steroid has been removed, usually 100–200 μl of the labeled complexes are carefully layered onto the linear gradient of sucrose that was prepared earlier. The gradient tube with receptor may then be centrifuged at 1°–3°C at high speed using an ultracentrifuge. Separation can be accomplished by centrifugation overnight using a swinging bucket rotor of the type supplied by Beckman (SW-60 Ti). If dissociation of labeled ligand during separation is suspected, as is often the case with progestin receptors, vertical tube rotors such as those supplied by Beckman and Sorvall Instruments can be employed (see Fig. 43–10). Swinging bucket type rotors usually require overnight centrifugation at 60,000 rpm (485,000 g), whereas good separation can be achieved within 3 to 4 hours at 60,000 rpm using vertical tube rotors (see Fig. 43–10). The desktop ultracentrifuge (Beckman Model TL-100) using the TLS-55 rotor with four buckets gave good preliminary results with estrogen and progestin receptors in a single biopsy specimen.[185] After centrifugation, the gradients are fractionated either from the top of the tube with a commercial pump or from the bottom of the tube by puncturing a hole and collecting fractions. Fractions are mixed with ligand scintillation fluor if a tritium-labeled ligand was used and are counted, correcting for the efficiency of the measurement. If an ^{125}I-labeled ligand is utilized (see Fig. 43–8), fractions may be counted directly in a gamma counter. In both cases, conversion of the measured radioactivity (cpm) to concentration of steroid bound is essential so that specific binding capacities can be calculated.

Programs developed in our laboratory are utilized to compute the specific binding capacities of the individual receptor species, such as 8 S and 4 S, expressing the data as total specific binding capacity and binding capacity of the individual isoforms. The quantity of specific steroid binding also can be estimated manually by summing the radioactivity under the individual peaks in the sedimentation profile (i.e., total binding) (Fig. 43–10) and subtracting these from the radioactivity in the profiles of the reaction performed in the presence of the radioactive ligand and an excess of unlabeled competitive inhibitors (nonspecific binding). The sucrose density gradient assay, as usually performed, represents a single point method of analysis that provides definitive evidence of the presence of steroid receptors. The presence of the 8 S species of the estrogen and progestin receptor has been suggested as a marker of an endocrine-responsive tumor.[208, 210]

Chromatographic Separation

Dynamic proteins such as the steroid receptors exhibit different properties of size, shape, surface charge, and hydrophobicity depending on the conditions of their environment. These properties may be exploited using various types of chromatography to separate various species of the receptors. Early chromatographic methods utilized conventional gel filtration and ionic exchange chromatography.[197] Many of the receptor species reported earlier may have been products of interactions with the packing matrices or the result of long incubation times.

We circumvented the problem of prolonged manipulation in receptor preparations with high-performance liquid chromatography (HPLC) in size exclusion, ion-exchange, chromatofocusing, and hydrophobic interaction modes, since they provide rapid, effective separation of receptor isoforms.[199, 211, 212] Because of the sensitivity of this technique coupled with radiochemically labeled ligands (see Fig. 43–8) of high specific activities (1500–2200 Ci/mmol) and superior protein recovery, the HPLC columns may be thought of as the biochemist's microscope (see Fig. 43–15). Receptor species and levels of association never identified previously may be explored. HPLC separation indicated these receptors exhibit polymorphism, suggesting their composition is far more complicated than originally assumed. The use of the term "fractionated receptors" was suggested to designate the pattern of the various steroid hormone–binding components (isoforms) displayed by a single receptor type.[200]

The configuration of the HPLC setup with in-line technology (Fig. 43–16) is typical of a multi-modality

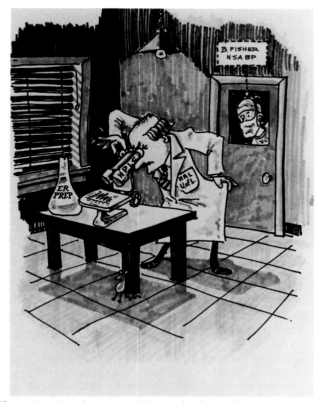

Figure 43–15. Advances in HPLC technology allow investigators to discern receptor polymorphism and levels of organization never revealed previously.

Instrumentation for High Performance Liquid Chromatography

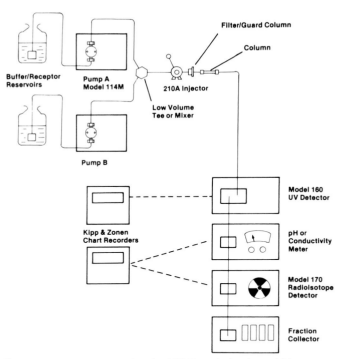

Figure 43–16. Instrumentation for HPLC analysis of steroid hormone receptors. (*From* Wittliff, JL: LC-GC Magazine 4:1092–1106, 1986. Reprinted with permission.)

approach. Briefly, a two-pump system is used for high-performance ion-exchange chromatography (HPIEC), high-performance chromatofocusing (HPCF), and high-performance hydrophobic interaction chromatography (HPHIC) with an ultraviolet detector, pH meter (Pharmacia), conductivity meter (Bio-Rad), and gamma or beta radioactivity detectors (Beckman) in-line before fraction collection. All chromatography is performed in a Puffer-Hubbard cold box at 3°–4°C. High-performance size exclusion chromatography (HPSEC) is conducted isocratically. Pre- and postcolumn derivatization and fluorescence may also be employed with this arrangement.

High-Performance Size Exclusion Chromatography

HPSEC separates soluble receptor isoforms based on characteristics of size and shape using either silica- or polymer-based stationary phases. The labeled receptor preparation is loaded on the column and separated with an aqueous mobile phase usually containing low ionic strength to minimize the effects of the hydrophobic surface and slightly catatonic character of the columns. Inclusion of polar organic solvents such as propanol may improve recovery and sharpen elution profiles. A representative example of estrogen receptor isoforms separated by HPSEC is shown in Figure 43–17.

High-Performance Ion-Exchange Chromatography

Polymorphism of steroid hormone receptors also may be detected by using HPIEC, which separates isoforms based on surface charge properties. The principle of this method is that receptor proteins are associated with either anion or cation exchangers associated with the

stationary phase by eluting them with a mobile phase containing a gradient of increasing ionic strength. Since this method results in recoveries of 85 percent to 100 percent, the molecular heterogeneity of receptors in a small tumor biopsy is easily detected within hours (Fig. 43–18). We have used this procedure to study receptor-antibody interaction[26] as a prelude to affinity chromatography.

High-Performance Chromatofocusing

HPCF represents another means of ascertaining receptor polymorphism, utilizing the surface charge properties of soluble proteins. Briefly, a stationary phase consisting of an ion exchanger is charged with a mobile phase at a pH sufficient to bind the receptor molecules, and the column is loaded with liganded receptor. This starting pH is usually in the mildly alkaline range, 8.6, and is reduced as a gradient by percolating a second mobile phase containing polyampholytes such as those supplied by Pharmacia at a lower pH (e.g., 4.5). Receptor isoforms are eluted at or near their pH values (Fig. 43–19). This is an extremely sensitive means of discerning small differences in receptor surface charge properties.[205]

High-Performance Hydrophobic Interaction Chromatography

HPHIC separates proteins on the basis of interactions between hydrophobic residues or patches on the protein surface and hydrophobic groups on the stationary phase.

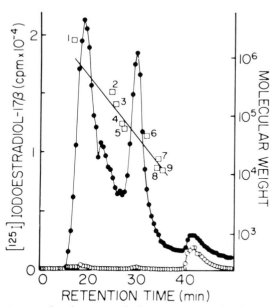

Figure 43–17. Identification and characterization of isoforms of the estrogen receptor from human breast cancer by HPSEC. Cytosol was prepared from a sample of human breast cancer and incubated with 3 to 4 nmol/L of [^{125}I]iodoestradiol-17β in the presence (○) and absence (●) of excess DES. A 200-μl aliquot of incubate was cleared of free steroid with dextran-coated charcoal and applied to a TSK3000 SW column. Hemoglobin was added to all samples before analysis or reanalysis as an internal marker. In addition, the HPSEC system was calibrated using a series of pure proteins (thyroglobulin, catalase, aldolase, bovine serum albumin, hemoglobin, ovalbumin, lysozyme, myoglobin, and cytochrome). (From Wittliff JL, Wiehle RD: *In* Hollander VP (ed): Hormonally Responsive Tumors. New York, Academic Press, 1985, pp 383–428. Reprinted with permission.)

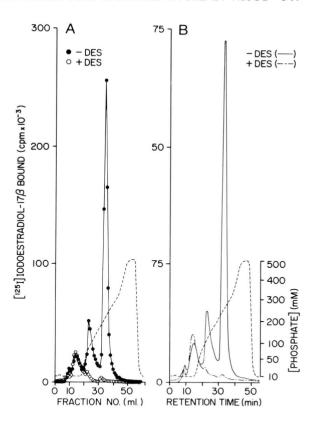

Figure 43–18. HPIEC separation of ionic isoforms of estrogen receptors from human breast cancer. Cytosol was prepared and incubated with 5 nmol/L [^{125}I] iodoestradiol-17β as described previously. Elution of the AX-1000 ion exchange column was performed on 200 μl of cytosol cleared of unbound ligand at 1.0 ml/min using a gradient of potassium phosphate at pH 7.4 (---). *A*, 1 ml fractions were collected and radioactivity measured manually with a gamma counter; *B*, radioactivity was recorded continuously using the Beckman Model 170 Radioisotope Detector in-line with a conductivity flow cell. Total binding is indicated by (●) in *A* and by (---) in *B*, and nonspecific binding is indicated by (○) in *A* and by (−·−·−·) in *B*. Recovery of radioactivity from the column was 97%. Specific binding was 167 fmol receptor/mg cytosol protein determined by multipoint titration analysis. (From Boyle DM, et al: J Chromatogr 327:369–376, 1985. Reprinted with permission.)

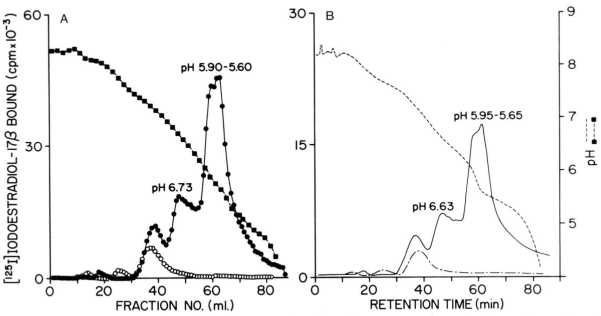

Figure 43–19. HPCF separation of ionic isoforms of estrogen receptors from human breast cancer. The sample of breast tissue and conditions used in this experiment were the same as described for Figure 43–18. The curves of [^{125}I]iodoestradiol-17β bound are the results of receptors separated protein determined by multipoint titration analysis. (From Boyle DM, et al) performed isocratically on 200 μl of cleared cytosol at 1.0 ml/min. The pH gradient is indicated as (■) in *A* and as (---) in *B*. *A*, 1-ml fractions were collected and radioactivity or pH measured manually; *B*, radioactivity and pH were recorded continuously using on-line Model 170 Radioisotope Detector with flow-through electrode. Recovery of radioactivity from the column was 97%. Specific binding was 167 fmol receptor/mg cytosol protein determined by multipoint titration analysis. (From Boyle DM, et al: J Chromatogr 327:369–376, 1985. Reprinted with permission.)

Briefly, the receptor preparation is made by combining 1–2 mol/L with a salt such as ammonium sulfate and quickly added to a column designed for HPHIC. The initial high salt conditions enhance hydrophobic interactions by removing water molecules from the protein surface. Receptor isoforms are eluted by a descending salt gradient, which allows the proteins to rehydrate, leading to their selective elution with retention of their biologic activity (Fig. 43–20). Receptor isoforms are collected and analyzed as indicated earlier. This procedure, which appears harsh, is actually one of the most useful for separating receptors that retain both their immuno-recognition and ligand-binding properties.

Affinity Chromatography

Two types of affinity chromatography have been employed for the study of the structural properties of steroid hormone receptors.[171, 197, 200] Ligand affinity chromatography employs the covalent association of an appropriate steroid or analogue with a stationary matrix such as Sepharose. Once bound, receptors may be eluted with increasing concentrations of a radiochemically labeled ligand characteristic of the receptor (see Table 43–5). A useful column employing diethylstilbestrol ligand was synthesized by Van Oosbree et al.[186] Antibody affinity chromatography utilizes either a polyclonal or monoclonal antibody against the receptor bound to a stationary phase such as Sepharose.[63, 64] In this case, the receptor is eluted by increasing concentrations of antibody or by altering the chemical environment (e.g., altering ionic strength). We have used the D547 mono-

clonal antibody against the estrogen receptor for its purification from human breast tumors.[26] Both of these procedures represent experimental methods that will be rarely encountered in the clinical laboratory.

Enzyme Immunoassay

Enzyme immunoassay is based on a sandwich technique that involves two monoclonal antibodies prepared against either the partially purified estrogen receptor from MCF-7 cells or progestin receptor from T47D human breast cancer cells (Abbott Laboratories, Inc.).[63, 64] The first antibody is immobilized on a polystyrene bead (see Fig. 43–11). Cytosol prepared in either TRIS or phosphate buffer containing 5 to 10 mmol/L sodium molybdate is incubated with the polystyrene bead for 18 hours at 3°C. After incubation, the immobilized receptor is incubated with a second monoclonal antibody that has been conjugated with horseradish peroxidase. The bead is washed to remove unbound conjugate and incubated with hydrogen peroxide and the enzyme substrate, ortho-phenylenediamine, to develop a color that is a measure of the quantity of estrogen receptor. The intensity of the color developed is read in a Quantum spectrophotometer set at 492 nm and incorporating software permitting automated calculation. A standard curve must be run separately for each receptor type using controls included in the kit, and the protein concentration of the cytosol preparation

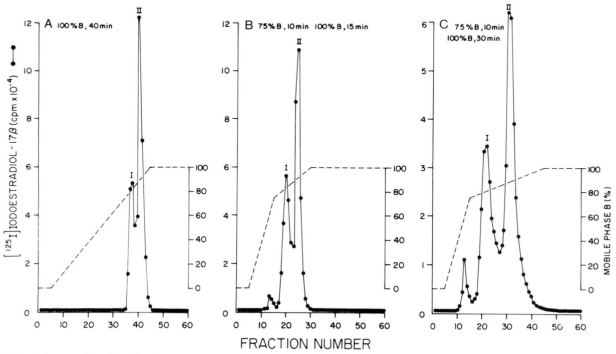

Figure 43–20. Influence of gradient development time on HPHIC separation of estrogen receptor isoforms from human breast cancer. Human breast cancer cytosol was separated on a HPHIC column and separated with gradient times reaching *(A)* 100% elution buffer in 40 min., *(B)* 75% elution buffer in 10 min followed by 100% elution buffer in the next 15 min, and *(C)* 75% elution buffer in 10 min, followed by 100% elution buffer in 30 min. All samples were adjusted to 1.5 mol/L ammonium sulfate and eluted with mobile phase buffer that did not contain the salt. (From Hyder SM, Wittliff JL: J Chromatogr 476:455–466, 1989. Reprinted with permission.)

must be measured. This procedure measures that mass of the receptor (in contrast to radioligand-binding techniques, which measure the steroid-binding capacity). However, most investigators relate the enzyme immunoassay results to specific steroid-binding capacity expressed as femtomoles per milligram (fmol/mg) of cytosol protein.

There appears to be considerable variation in the estrogen and progestin receptor levels measured by the multipoint titration assay compared with those observed with the enzyme immunoassay, with a greater receptor level observed by the EIA method.[7, 69, 84, 117, 125, 148, 182] The molecular basis of this observation is unclear and may be related to differences in the affinities of receptor isoforms for the monoclonal antibodies.[80, 163] In general, the results of these assays agree well,[182] and we[137] suggest that a cutoff value of 15 fmol/mg cytosol protein by EIA is equivalent to the accepted cutoff of 10 fmol/mg cytosol protein established for the ligand-binding assay by studies such as protocol B-09 of the NSABP (Fig. 43–21).[49] We recommend that this procedure be used as a companion to the ligand-binding method, particularly for small breast biopsy specimens (less than 200 mg) as well as for those from premenopausal patients with suspected breast cancer.

Immunocytochemical Assay

The ICA procedure was originally designed for use with frozen tissue sections.[105] Two specimens from the same tumor biopsy are mounted on separate microscope slides, fixed in formalin, methanol, and acetone, and treated with a blocking reagent to prevent nonspecific association of reagents added subsequently. One of the mounted specimens is incubated with a monoclonal antibody directed against either the estrogen or progestin receptor (see Fig. 43–12), whereas the other is incubated with a control antibody such as normal rat immunoglobulin (IgG) that allows evaluation of nonspecific binding. Each of the mounted tissues is then incubated with a bridging antibody such as goat antirat IgG that associates with the primary rat antibody made against human estrogen receptor and with normal rat IgG bound to the specimen incubated with control antibody. Next, a rat peroxidase/antiperoxidase complex is added to each of the mounted tissues, where it binds to the bridging antibody. Finally, the reaction is developed with a solution containing hydrogen peroxide and diaminobenzidine 4 HCl, which is converted to an insoluble reddish-brown product (see Fig. 43–12). Cells containing receptors are visualized with a light microscope. Control slides containing receptor-positive breast cancer cells are carried through the same procedure to ensure performance of the reactions.

Evaluation of the immunocytochemical analysis is largely qualitative,[138] utilizing both the intensity of staining and the percentage of positively reacting cells.[104a, 105] This procedure also may be used for fine needle aspiration biopsy samples.[51, 102a] More recently several investigators have shown that these antibodies react with receptors in paraffin-embedded sections, indicating that

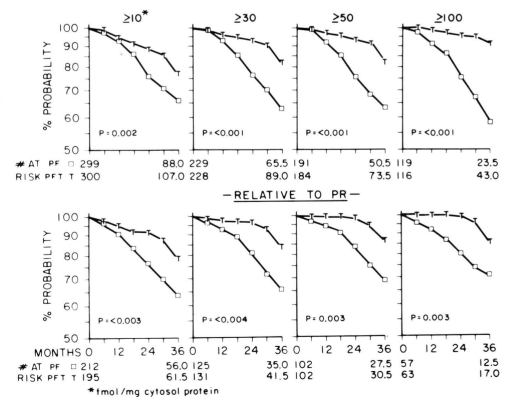

Figure 43–21. Disease-free survival of patients 50 years of age or older entered into protocol B-09 of the NSABP. The top four panels describe the disease-free survival relative to the estrogen receptor levels in breast tumor biopsy specimens, whereas the lower four panels describe those relative to progestin receptor levels. Patients receiving L-phenylalanine mustard and 5-fluorouracil alone (PF) or in combination with tamoxifen (PFT) are represented by the open squares and by the letter T, respectively. (From Fisher B, et al: J Clin Oncol 1:227–241, 1983. Reprinted with permission.)

stored tissue blocks may be evaluated.[5, 104a, 172] This procedure will be useful in microscopic breast cancer lesions in which insufficient tissue is present for ligand-binding analysis or EIA. It should also be useful in correlation studies with proposed new prognostic factors such as EGF and LH-RH receptors[48] as well as with the protein products from oncogene expression.[177]

Fluorescein-Linked Steroid Ligands

Often breast carcinomas are discovered that contain an insufficient amount of tissue for titration analyses of estrogen and progestin receptors to be performed. Another approach to estimate the level of receptors in small biopsy specimens has been the use of fluorescein-linked steroid hormones.[31] This provides a nonradiochemical means of detecting receptors in histologic preparations of breast and endometrial cancer. The method involves the incubation of tissue slices with a fluorescein-linked estrogen and visualization of the "receptor-bound" steroid under a fluorescence microscope.

Although the use of a fluorescein-linked steroid as a ligand for steroid hormone receptors would be desirable, especially for tissue biopsy sections of tumors, this procedure has been employed with very little success.[100] Thus far, the use of these compounds has two major disadvantages: (1) derivitization of estradiol in the 17β position reduces the affinity of the ligand for the specific binding sites on the receptor, and (2) bonds between the fluorescent steroid ligand and the spacer are labile, making assessment of the affinity constant difficult because of the presence of contaminating free estradiol. The unequivocal determination of estrogen receptors in tissue preparations has not been possible because of these and other complicating factors such as tissue autofluorescence and low affinity association.[17]

REFERENCE RANGES OF STEROID HORMONE RECEPTORS

Specific binding capacity is expressed as femtomoles (10^{-15} mol) of labeled steroid bound per mg cytosol protein. Since menopausal status influences receptor level (see Table 43–2) and distribution (see Table 43–3), reference ranges are considered in terms of this factor. The cutoff point for the presence of receptors is generally accepted to be 10 fmol/mg of receptor cytosol protein.[49, 49a, 198] This threshold value is utilized by the NSABP. The sensitivity of the assay and the biological data suggest that less than 3 fmol/mg cytosol protein is a clinically insignificant quantity of receptors in human breast tumors. K_d values of 1 to 9×10^{-10} mol/L to 1 to 9×10^{-11} mol/L are indicative of high affinity estrogen receptors, while 1 to 9×10^{-9} mol/L to 1 to 9×10^{-10} mol/L are indicative of the presence of high affinity progestin-binding components.[198, 200] Some tumors exhibit both estrogen and progestin receptors (see Table 43–3), whereas others exhibit either only the estrogen or only the progestin receptor.[6] Others do not exhibit either

steroid hormone receptor. In general, the progestin receptor level is high in tumors from premenopausal patients in the presence of the estrogen receptor but considerably lower and rarely observed in tumors that do not exhibit the estrogen receptor (see Table 43–2). Steroid hormone receptors are seen more often and at higher concentrations in breast tumors in postmenopausal patients than in those of premenopausal patients. The curious distribution in which the estrogen receptor is lacking and the progestin receptor is present is seen three times more often in biopsy specimens of premenopausal patients than in biopsy specimens of postmenopausal patients (see Table 43–3). This appears to result from the presence of circulating estrogens in the plasma of premenopausal patients that mask the steroid hormone receptors in a tumor biopsy specimen.

Evaluation of a similar set of patients by EIA would be useful in determining the influence of endogenous native ligand or hormonal type drugs such as tamoxifen (see Fig. 43–13) when associated with steroid hormone receptors. Receptor-ligand complexes appear to bind more tightly with the nuclear components (matrix and chromatin); thus radioligand-binding procedures may provide an underestimate of the number of receptors. The new monoclonal antibody–based EIA procedures should provide a means of estimating both ligand-associated and nonassociated forms of the receptor in biopsy samples if the validation data are sufficient.[7, 83, 163, 182] Because numerous physiological and clinical factors influence receptor levels (see Table 43–1), it is essential that the relevant information be indicated on the assay request form prior to analysis.

We recommend that a laboratory develop its own distribution profiles of steroid hormone receptors such as the ones described earlier[198, 200] and include the levels found in the various patient populations such as those presented in Tables 43–2 and 43–3. These should be compared with studies published in the literature to ensure that the laboratory is generating comparable information, thus indicating a valid procedure.

CLINICAL RELEVANCE OF STEROID RECEPTOR RESULTS

Steroid Receptors in Female Breast Cancer

It has been demonstrated conclusively that the presence of estrogen receptors provides a molecular basis for the distinction between human breast carcinomas that are responsive to hormonal therapy or organ ablative surgery and those that are not. From studies of these steroid-binding proteins in hormonally responsive tumors of rodents, Jensen and coworkers[82] originally suggested that the ability of a breast carcinoma to bind estrogen may be predictive of a patient's response to endocrine therapy. This was supported by their findings in which the presence of estrogen receptors in tumor biopsy specimens correlated with a favorable response to adrenalectomy.[81]

Since the original report of Folca and coworkers in

Table 43–6. RELATIONSHIP BETWEEN ESTROGEN-BINDING CAPACITY OF BREAST TUMOR BIOPSY SPECIMENS AND OBJECTIVE REMISSION AFTER ENDOCRINE MANIPULATION

	Specific Estrogen-Binding Capacity			
	Positive		Negative	
Therapeutic Manipulation	*No.*	*%*	*No.*	*%*
Additive hormone treatment	59/105	56	12/109	11
Ablative endocrine therapy	59/107	55	8/94	8
Total	118/212	56	20/203	10

Adapted from McGuire WL, et al (eds): Estrogen Receptors in Human Breast Cancer. New York, Raven, 1975.

1961,[52] numerous studies have shown that approximately half of all biopsy samples of malignant breast tumors contain estrogen receptors (Tables 43–6 and 43–7).[6, 107] Our personal experience during the past two decades from the analyses of more than 10,000 breast tumor biopsy specimens indicates that 60 percent to 65 percent of primary lesions and 45 percent to 55 percent of metastatic breast tumors exhibit more than 10 fmol/mg cytosol protein of estrogen receptor using ligand-binding procedures.

The collective results of investigators participating in the NIH Consensus Development Conference in 1979 are given in Tables 43–7 and 43–8. These results represent the level of response (50 percent to 60 percent) that might be expected of a breast cancer patient given hormonal manipulation when only estrogen receptor status is considered. These results also are in excellent agreement with the data presented in 1974 at the first International Workshop on estrogen receptors in human breast cancer (Table 43–6). Unfortunately, the field has not progressed sufficiently to determine the particular therapeutic modality that should be administered.

Numerous investigations support the thesis that the number of objective remissions in breast cancer patients given hormone therapy may be expected to increase with an elevation in specific estrogen-binding capacity of the tumor. In summarizing the collective reports from the NIH Consensus Development Conference,[6] there appears to be a spectrum of responses ranging from less than 6 percent objective remissions at estrogen receptor levels below 10 fmol/mg cytosol protein to more than 80 percent objective remissions at estrogen receptor levels of several hundred or more fmol/mg cytosol protein. Recent results suggest that only analyses providing quantification of the estrogen (and progestin) receptor should be used in the clinical laboratory.[6, 7, 34, 49, 56, 137]

Analyses of estrogen receptors in primary lesions indicate that patients with breast cancer containing these regulatory proteins exhibit an increased disease-free survival when compared with patients whose tumors did not contain estrogen receptors.[91] The disease-free interval of stage II patients appeared to be independent of the patient's menopausal status and the presence of metastases in the axillary lymph nodes. These data, which now have been supported by a number of studies,[18, 20, 53, 68, 133, 181] clearly indicate that the estrogen receptor is useful as a predictive index of response to endocrine manipulation and as a prognostic index of the course of the disease. Thus quantitative results from estrogen receptor analyses assume a major role in the management of the patient with carcinoma of the breast (see Fig. 43–21), as was suggested by the adjuvant trial conducted by the NSABP.[49, 49a]

The relationship between estrogen receptor content of a tumor and ability to predict either disease-free survival or overall survival appears to be related to the breast cancer stage and patient race. Crowe et al.[36] reported that estrogen receptor status and race, while individually acting as important variables, actually interact when survival data are considered. They conclude that black patients with estrogen receptor–negative tumors, particularly postmenopausal patients, are at very high risk of recurrence and death. The endocrine therapy of breast cancer is reviewed in detail in section XVII, chapter 44.

Not all women with breast tumors containing estrogen receptors respond to hormone therapy. One possibility for this binding may be that there is a defect in the intracellular cascade of events that normally control biological responsiveness to an endocrine stimulus. One of the approaches taken to assess the intactness of the estrogen response mechanism in breast tumors has been the determination of progestin receptors.[75] The assump-

Table 43–7. RELATIONSHIP BETWEEN ESTROGEN RECEPTOR STATUS OF BREAST TUMOR AND PATIENT'S OBJECTIVE RESPONSE TO ENDOCRINE THERAPY

	Estrogen Receptor Status	
Investigator	*Responses/ ER+ Tumors*	*Responses/ ER− Tumors*
Blamey et al	13/30	5/27
Dao and Nemoto	64/119	4/56
DeSombre and Jensen	39/62	4/108
Maass et al	64/93	3/76
Manni et al	68/105	0/12
McCarty et al	32/58	3/20
Nomura et al	29/45	0/36
Osborne et al	70/145	5/53
Paridaens et al	14/38	0/11
Rubens and Hayward	46/146	5/55
Singhakowinta et al	20/30	2/25
Skinner et al	17/30	5/44
Wittliff	46/76	0/44
Total	522/977 (53%)	36/567 (6%)

Adapted from the collective papers presented at the NIH Consensus Development Conference on Steroid Receptors in Breast Cancer. Cancer 46:2759–2963, 1980.

Table 43–8. RELATIONSHIP BETWEEN STEROID RECEPTOR STATUS OF BREAST TUMOR AND PATIENT'S OBJECTIVE RESPONSE TO ENDOCRINE THERAPY

Investigator	Steroid Receptor Status*			
	ER + /PR +	*ER + /PR −*	*ER − /PR −*	*ER − /PR +*
Brooks et al	4/6	2/7	—	—
Dao and Nemoto	10/13	18/31	2/28	—
Degenshein et al	26/33	3/14	0/14	1/1
King	10/11	3/15	2/9	0/2
McCarty et al	33/40	2/20	3/35	1/3
Nomura et al	7/10	8/12	2/20	0/1
Osborne et al	16/20	14/45	3/20	—
Skinner et al	9/12	2/6	3/30	2/3
Young et al	20/29	3/14	2/9	1/1
Total	135/174 (78%)	55/164 (34%)	17/165 (10%)	5/11 (45%)

*Number of patients responding to treatment/number of women with receptor status designated.

Adapted from the collective papers presented at the NIH Consensus Development Conference on Steroid Receptors in Breast Cancer. Cancer 46:2759–2963, 1980.

tion is that progestin receptor formation in breast carcinomas is regulated by estrogen receptors in a fashion similar to the mechanism in rodent uterine tissues as first described by Rao and Meyer.[150] Thus simultaneous determinations of the progestin receptor with the estrogen receptor (as shown in Table 43–8) should increase the accuracy for selecting the breast cancer patient most likely to respond to hormone therapy.

Table 43–8 provides a summary of results presented at the Consensus Development Conference.[6] From studies of the steroid receptor status of tumor biopsy samples, it was found that 78 percent of patients with breast tumors containing *both* receptors responded objectively to hormone therapy. If only the estrogen receptor was present, a 34 percent response rate was observed, whereas only ten percent of patients responded to endocrine manipulation if neither receptor was present in the breast tumor. Surprisingly, a few patients responded objectively to hormone therapy, although each had breast tumors containing only the progestin receptor. This appears puzzling if there is a relationship between estrogen and progestin receptors in responsive tumors and may be related to endocrine status of the patient as discussed earlier (see Tables 43–1 and 43–2).[1, 106] These latter data further suggest that the progestin receptor may be particularly important in the selection of premenopausal patients for endocrine manipulation.[21A]

Results of the recent adjuvant trial comparing cytotoxic chemotherapy with and without tamoxifen (Fig. 43–21) suggest that the progestin receptor may have particular significance in predicting hormonal responsiveness.[49] Patients with increased levels of progestin receptors who received both cytotoxic chemotherapy and tamoxifen exhibited an increased disease-free survival. Clark et al.[34] also concluded that progestin receptor level was of equal or greater value than estrogen receptor level for predicting disease-free survival of patients with breast cancer.

Steroid Receptors in Male Breast Cancer

Approximately 65 percent of male patients with advanced breast cancer respond to orchiectomy or adrenalectomy, indicating that the lesion is hormone dependent in many patients. The physiological and psychological impact of orchiectomy and adrenalectomy often compound the problem of correlating endocrine manipulation with the presence of estrogen receptors in these tumors. Relatively few receptor analyses have been reported, because these tumors are encountered infrequently.[47, 140]

An unusual example of estrogen receptor isoforms identified by sucrose gradient centrifugation is shown in Figure 43–22. Note that both primary and metastatic biopsy specimens contained 8 S and 4 S isoforms of estrogen receptor, whereas normal breast tissue did not exhibit either.[202] In addition to the similarity in molecular properties, the ranges of binding capacities and affinities of these receptors in male breast cancer were virtually identical to those in female breast cancer.[47] The principal difference between receptors in breast cancer in males and females is their incidence of appearance.[47, 140]

The collective results reported by Everson and colleagues[47] indicated that estrogen receptors were present in 29 of 34 tumor biopsy samples of male breast cancer. Estrogen receptor concentration was negatively correlated with patient age. Although the quantity of estrogen receptor appeared to be related to the level of progesterone receptor, the disease-free interval, and the duration of response, these were not statistically significant. An even higher percentage of estrogen and progestin receptors was reported by Pegoraro et al,[140] who employed both cytosolic and nuclear analyses of receptor proteins. Curiously, the presence of nuclear progestin receptor was not correlated with this receptor in cytosol preparations; estrogen receptors were detected

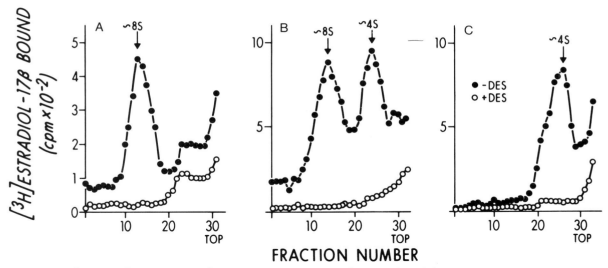

Figure 43–22. Sucrose density gradient separation of estrogen receptors in tissues from a male with breast cancer. The primary tumor is shown in A, and a metastatic lymph node containing both 8 S and 4 S isoforms of the estrogen receptor is shown in B. Normal breast (C) did not show either isoform. (From Wittliff JL, et al: In St Arneault G, et al (eds): Recent Results in Cancer Research. New York, Springer-Verlag, 1977, pp 59–77. Reprinted with permission.)

in both compartments in approximately 90 percent of the biopsy specimens examined.

Nine of 14 breast cancer biopsy samples from male patients had significant levels of progestin receptor, and several exhibited androgen and glucocorticoid receptors.[47] It has been our experience and that of others that gynecomastia seldom exhibits estrogen receptors, and usually these are limited to the 4 S species as detected by sucrose gradient centrifugation. However, we have observed low levels of progestin receptors, suggesting that a proportion of these molecules arise from connective tissue elements.

As in female breast cancer, clinical results from these reports do not sufficiently justify a specific therapeutic modality based on steroid receptor status of a biopsy sample. This is primarily because of the paucity of results. Pegoraro et al.[140] suggested that more detailed analyses of both cytoplasmic and nuclear values of these receptors may be useful to predict therapeutic responses.

The presence of sex hormone receptors in male breast cancer suggests that some patients may be candidates for an endocrine manipulation other than orchiectomy or medical adrenalectomy. During the past two decades, we have observed elevated concentrations (>100 fmol/ mg cytosol protein) of these receptors in a number of patients. In addition, recent analyses have detected the presence of EGF receptors and even overexpression of *HER-2/neu* protein. This suggests that therapeutic agents such as tamoxifen or toremifene, which inhibit estrogen binding, and medroxyprogesterone acetate or megestrol acetate, which inhibit progestin binding, may be useful in the management of this disease. Obviously the participation of widely distributed patients in an intergroup protocol would be necessary to conduct a meaningful clinical trial.

RECEPTOR-ASSOCIATED MOLECULES

Sex steroid hormone receptors function as regulatory proteins within responsive cells such as those of the breast and uterus. These receptors are now believed to undergo phosphorylation/dephosphorylation covalent modifications in the modulation of their activity.[8, 35] The mechanisms of phosphorylation/dephosphorylation of steroid receptors have been linked to both their ligand-binding activity and receptor activation,[161] and thus they may be considered as phosphoproteins. Additionally, estradiol and glucocorticoid receptors have been proposed either to be closely associated with or to actually exhibit protein kinase activity.[9, 174]

Bell and Munck[14] confirmed that initial binding of glucocorticoid to receptor in thymus cells may be regulated by a phosphorylation event that depended on adenosine triphosphate (ATP) supply. Others have shown that when crude preparations of receptors were incubated with phosphatases, both the steroid-binding capacity and activation/transformation process were affected.[11] Wiegel et al.[192, 193] reported that both A and B subunits of the progestin receptor from chick oviduct co-purified with a protein kinase which was even more effective than the cyclic adenosine monophosphate–dependent (cAMP-dependent) kinase in phosphorylating these receptor proteins. In contrast to our findings with estrogen receptors,[9] the kinase could be dissociated from both progestin receptor subunits by further chromatography,[192] indicating that neither receptor in itself possessed the kinase activity. Garcia et al.[55] also reported a Ca^{2+}-dependent kinase activity in highly purified progesterone receptor preparations from chick oviduct. Similar to Weigel's study, the Ca^{2+}-dependent kinase activity was separated from progesterone receptor subunits on further purification.[54] Experiments in vivo showed that progesterone receptor was a phosphoprotein when [^{32}P]orthophosphate was injected into oviducts of chickens. Subsequent purification of progesterone receptor showed it was a phosphoprotein containing covalently labeled phosphoserine.[39]

Many studies have shown that glucocorticoid receptors are also phosphoproteins. Housley and Pratt[75] first reported the phosphorylation in vivo of glucocorticoid receptor in the intact L929 mouse fibroblast cells. Grandics et al.[60] have also shown that rat hepatic glucocorticoid receptor is phosphorylated in vivo after injection of [^{32}P]orthophosphate into these animals. Similar to progesterone receptor, the glucocorticoid receptor appears to be a good substrate for cAMP-dependent protein kinase.[175] The two steroid receptors studied less extensively in the context of receptor phosphorylation, the androgen and estrogen receptors, also appear to be phosphoproteins. The androgen receptor has been successfully phosphorylated in vitro by a cAMP-dependent protein kinase.[58] Uterine estradiol receptor is reported to be phosphorylated on tyrosine residues in vitro by a purified calmodulin-stimulated nuclear kinase.[114]

Employing a novel use of a monoclonal antibody raised against estrogen receptor from MCF-7 breast cancer cells,[63] as outlined in Figure 43–23, we demonstrated that immunopurified estrogen receptors contain protein kinase activity.[9] Figure 43–24 illustrates the presence of protein kinase activity associated with the immobilized antibody diagramed in Figure 43–11. Phosphoproteins with molecular weights of 43, 47, and 57 kDa were detected. We also demonstrated the presence of phospholipid kinase activity in estrogen receptors from MCF-7 cells. These activities were easily ascertained in vitro on femtomolar quantities of receptor by virtue of the fact that estrogen receptor–monoclonal antibody complexes were immobilized on a single polystyrene bead. The estrogen receptor directed phosphorylation reaction, as with the majority of protein kinases, required ATP rather than guanosine triphosphate (GTP) as the phosphoryl donor and was highly dependent on the presence of Mg^{2+} (Fig. 43–24). Later studies have shown that phosphorylation occurred on serine residues. The specificity of the reaction catalyzed by immunopu-

Assessment of Protein Kinase Activity

Tissue Extract

↧

Associate with Immobilized Monoclonal Antibody

↧

Incubate with Mg^{2+}/ATP-^{32}P

↧

Elute Phosphoproteins/Separate by SDS-PAGE

Figure 43–23. Sequence for assessing protein kinase activity in breast tumor cytosol using immobilized monoclonal antibodies.

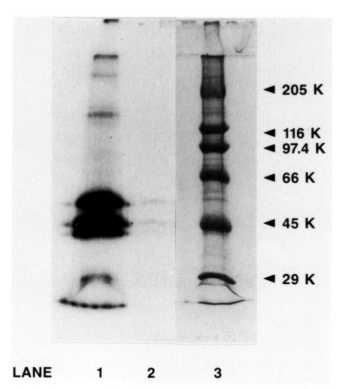

LANE   **1**   **2**   **3**

◄ **205 K**
◄ **116 K**
◄ **97.4 K**
◄ **66 K**
◄ **45 K**
◄ **29 K**

Figure 43–24. Nucleotide dependence of estrogen receptor phosphorylation activity from MCF-7 cells. ER was purified from MCF-7 cytosol using immobilized monoclonal antibody, and the immunocomplexes were washed extensively and incubated either with [γ-^{32}P]ATP or [γ-^{32}P]GTP. Reactions were terminated by removal of the reaction medium, and the [^{32}P]-labeled polypeptides were solubilized and separated by polyacrylamide-SDS gel electrophoresis. The slab gel was dried, and autoradiography was performed for 16 hrs at 25°C. Lane 1: MCF-7 MAb-receptor complex incubated with [γ-^{32}P]ATP as substrate showing the presence of phosphorylated proteins with molecular weights of 57, 47, and 43 kDa. Lane 2: same as Lane 1, but [γ-^{32}P]GTP was used as substrate. Note absence of phosphorylation activity. Lane 3 shows the corresponding molecular weight standards. Numbers on the right indicate the position of molecular weight standards in kilodaltons. (From Baldi A, et al: Biochem Biophys Res Commun 135:597–606, 1986. Reprinted with permission.)

rified estrogen receptor molecules from the estrogen receptor–positive cells (MCF-7) was shown when similar preparations from estrogen receptor–negative breast cancer cell lines (MDA and T-47D) showed minimal protein kinase activity. MCF-7 cytosol contains 90 to 100 fmol estrogen receptor/mg cytosol protein whereas MDA cytosol contains 1 to 5 fmol estrogen receptor/mg binding sites as determined by radioligand-binding analysis.

High-performance hydrophobic interaction chromatography (see Fig. 43–20) may be used to separate and characterize steroid hormone receptor isoforms with virtually complete retention of their biological activity.[79, 80, 201] Resolution may be achieved in the absence of organic solvents with virtually 100 percent recoveries of both the mass and the radioligand-binding activity associated with these labile regulatory proteins. It is intriguing that only one isoform of these receptors demonstrated the protein kinase activity.[79] This kinase activity does not appear to be an integral part of the receptor molecule itself but rather an associated protein, since biopsy specimens of some estrogen receptor–negative breast cancer exhibited the enzyme.[80] Our results suggest that the protein kinase activity of the estrogen receptor from rat uteri resides in the nonactivated isoform, although this has not been proven conclusively. The physiological significance of these observations remains to be resolved.

Our evidence regarding the phosphorylating activity of immuno-immobilized estrogen receptor led us to postulate a mechanism by which steroid hormone receptors may share similar properties with oncogene products, as discussed by Sluyser and Mester.[178] The kinase activity exhibited by estrogen receptor preparations from MCF-7 breast cancer cells is a serine kinase, in contrast to the tyrosine kinase mode exhibited by most of the oncogenic transforming products.[78] Further work is needed to establish the relationship between the metabolic capabilities of these receptors and those of oncogenic products.

A number of recent studies have shown that a non-steriod-binding protein, M_r-90,000 is associated with a number of steroid receptors[38, 152, 160] as well as with the aryl-hydrocarbon (Ah) receptor.[142] This protein, which has been termed the HSP-90 heat shock protein, appears to contribute a stabilizing effect on the protein with which it binds.[95] Although the specific functions have not been determined, it has been proposed that HSP-90 caps the DNA-binding domain of the glucocorticoid receptor, maintaining it in the inactive state.[12] Apparently, two molecules of HSP-90 associate with each molecule of the glucocorticoid receptor.[38] Dissociation of HSP-90 from the receptor may be significant in the activation of the regulatory component. HSP-90 also appears to be a phosphoprotein.

Utilizing the results of previous studies on the polymorphism of steroid receptors obtained with various modes of HPLC,[200, 201] and with immunopurified receptors exhibiting associated protein kinase activity, [9] we have developed a model for the composition of the estrogen receptor (Fig. 43–25). This model provides a possible explanation of the molecular heterogeneity of

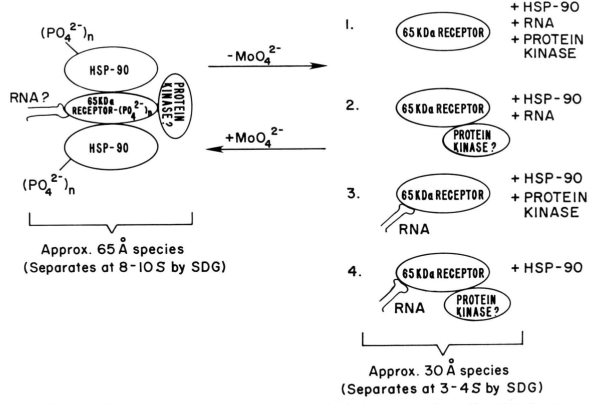

Figure 43–25. Possible composition of the estrogen receptor explaining the molecular heterogeneity observed by HPLC. The 65A receptor species separated by HPHIC appears to contain the 65-kDa estrogen receptor molecule complex with two molecules of the abundant protein HSP-90. Other cellular proteins, such as protein kinases, and small RNA molecules, have also been reported to be associated with this series. This complex is stabilized by the presence of molybdate ions and sediments at 9–10 S using sucrose density gradient centrifugation (SDG). In the absence of molybdate ions, as well as during prolonged manipulations, the large oligomeric complex appears to dissociate into smaller species (30 Å). The latter components sediment at 3–4 S using the sucrose density gradient centrifugation. Based on this model, heterogeneity exists in the composition of the 30 Å species, as shown on the right. The dissociation of the oligomeric complex during HPIEC in the absence of molybdate results in the exposure of highly charged species of estrogen receptors eluting at 180 mmol/L phosphate. In addition, other charged species are resolved at 50–100 mmol/L phosphate, which may be the result of association of the estrogen receptor with other molecules. The possibility exists that there are two or more distinct receptor molecules, which would imply that molecular heterogeneity is a reflection of different ionic forms. (From Hyder SM, Wittliff JL: J Chromatogr 476:455–466, 1989. Reprinted with permission.)

the estrogen receptor utilizing the 65-kDa molecule as the ligand-binding domain. The reader should keep in mind that this is only a model to be tested in human breast cancer, as earlier studies[208, 210] suggested that polymorphism was related to the clinical response to endocrine therapy.

METHODS OF PEPTIDE HORMONE RECEPTOR ANALYSIS

Saturation Analysis

Analyses of peptide hormone receptors by radioligand titration are conducted similarly to those described in detail for steroid hormone receptors (see Fig. 43–9, Table 43–4). Briefly, aliquots of membrane suspensions derived from the pellets obtained from the cytosol preparation (for estrogen and progestin receptor determinations) are incubated with increasing concentrations of [^{125}I]-labeled peptide hormone in the presence and absence of the unlabeled ligand. Software developed by Beckman Instruments in cooperation with Lundon Software (AccuFit Saturation One Site and Two-Site) provides an excellent means of transforming ligand-binding data using the method of Scatchard.[165] Both specific binding capacity expressed as fmol/mg membrane protein and the affinity constant, either K_a or K_d, are generated from a binding isotherm and Scatchard analysis.[101] In addition, a Klotz plot provides information relative to the selection of the range of labeled ligand concentrations.[90] Generally, we report both specific binding capacity and K_d value from clinical analyses of prolactin, somatostatin, LH-RH, and EGF receptors.[15, 16, 48]

Ligand Displacement

Ligand competition assays have been used widely in both clinical and basic research, particularly when the affinity constant of an unknown, unlabeled compound was to be explored.[97] In addition, we have used these to evaluate the ligand specificity of various receptor proteins as well as to identify receptor subtypes (isoforms).[48]

Briefly, a fixed concentration of radiolabeled ligand is incubated with a wide range of concentrations of the same unlabeled ligand using a membrane preparation of the tumor biopsy specimen being analyzed (Fig. 43–26). Generally, a sigmoid curve is developed that provides the I_{50} values indicating the molar concentration of unlabeled ligand required to reduce receptor binding with the labeled ligand by 50 percent.

The AccuFit Competition Software is excellent for data analysis. Association of either labeled or unlabeled ligand with receptor and nonreceptor proteins in a reaction is represented by a complex series of equations, particularly if more than one binding site is present. The program computes both the K_d value and specific binding capacity using equations that accurately describe the chemical equilibria. The data are then represented graphically as a logit-log transformation. This type of analysis appears to be better suited for clinical determinations of peptide hormone receptors in breast biopsy specimens.[209]

PEPTIDE HORMONE RECEPTORS IDENTIFIED IN BREAST CANCER

Prolactin Receptors

Only a sparse number of studies of the prolactin (PRL) receptor in breast cancer have been reported.[24, 25, 73, 135, 149] Although this pituitary hormone is known to be involved in breast development,[124] most laboratories have encountered methodological problems in assay of this steroid receptor.

A micro-method was developed for the determination and characterization of PRL receptors in human breast

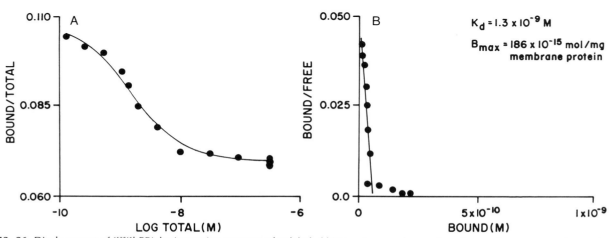

Figure 43–26. Displacement of [^{125}I]hPRL by increasing amounts of unlabeled hPRL using membranes from human breast cancer. Increasing amounts of unlabeled human prolactin were incubated with a constant quantity of [^{125}I]hPRL in the presence of a membrane fraction isolated from an infiltrating ductal carcinoma of the breast (A). Scatchard analysis (B) of the data indicated a single class of binding sites with a K_d value = 1.3 × 10^{-3} mol/L and a specific binding capacity of 186 fmol/mg membrane protein. (From Ben-David M, et al: Biomed Pharmacother 42:101–109, 327–334, 1988. Reprinted with permission.)

cancer specimens using either intact biopsy tissue or the pellet fraction remaining from biopsy specimens previously processed for steroid hormone receptors.[15] Labeled human PRL (hPRL) is used as the ligand. The specific [125I] PRL–binding of 307 human breast cancer specimens was evaluated by this micro-method (Fig. 43–26). A significant level of specific PRL-binding (3 to 25 fmol/mg membrane protein) was detected in 41 percent of American breast cancer patients and in 42 percent of Israeli patients.[16] Scatchard analyses, performed on pooled membrane fractions with the highest specific PRL binding, revealed one class of receptors having a dissociation constant, $K_d = 4.1 \times 10^{-9}$ mol/L, and specific binding capacity, $B_{max} = 1.3$ pmol/mg protein. When these preparations were exposed to 3 mol/L $MgCl_2$, which dissociates endogenously bound PRL from hormone-receptor complexes, the characterization of the "total" PRL receptors was possible. Two classes of receptors were then revealed. One class of receptors showed high affinity ($K_{d1} = 8.1 \times 10^{-10}$ mol/L) and low capacity ($B_{max} = 335$ fmol/mg protein) whereas the other possessed lower affinity ($K_{d2} = 8.2 \times 10^{-8}$ mol/L) but a higher capacity ($B_{max} = 34.4$ pmol/mg protein). No correlation was found with steroid receptor status (Fig. 43–27). Since PRL facilitates the growth of human breast cancer cell lines, these results suggest that many human breast cancers may be prolactin dependent. Routine determination of PRL receptors in biopsy samples of human breast cancer is now possible, allowing clinical correlations to proceed.

LH-RH Receptors

The hypothalamus produces a decapeptide called gonadotropin-releasing hormone (GnRH), also called luteinizing hormone–releasing hormone, which controls the release of leuteinizing hormone (LH) and follicle-stimulating hormone (FSH) from the anterior pituitary. The receptors for LH-RH are membrane associated at the surface of target cells such as those on a luteotrophic cell. Although the molecular composition of the receptor is unclear, it appears that there are two molecules of the binding protein in close proximity to each other and to a calcium channel.

A number of studies with clinical material as well as experimental systems suggest that analogues of LH-RH are useful for the treatment of hormone-dependent breast cancer.[28, 43, 71, 88, 89, 115, 151] Analogues that exhibit agonistic LH-RH activity, such as [D-Trp6]LH-RH, Zoladex, Buserelin, and Leuprolide, have produced objective responses in significant numbers of pre- and post-

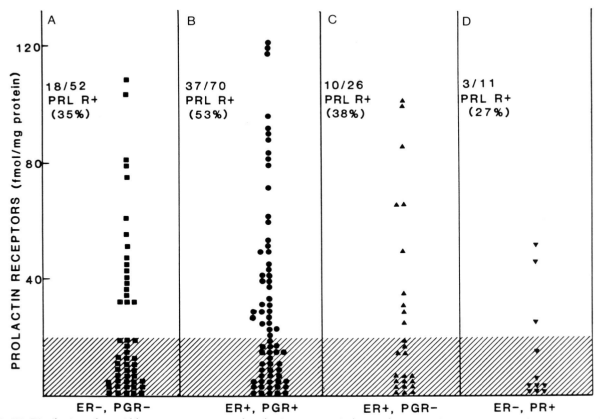

Figure 43–27. Distribution of steroid hormone receptors and prolactin receptors in human breast carcinoma. Receptors for estrogen and progestin were determined on cytosol, whereas those for hPRL receptors were determined on membrane fractions from 159 breast cancer biopsy specimens. The data were separated into the subgroups shown using a hPRL receptor level of 20 fmol/mg membrane protein or greater as positive. A cutoff value of 10 fmol/mg cytosol protein was used for estrogen and progestin receptors. (From Ben-David M, et al: Biomed Pharmacother 42:101–109, 327–334, 1988. Reprinted with permission.)

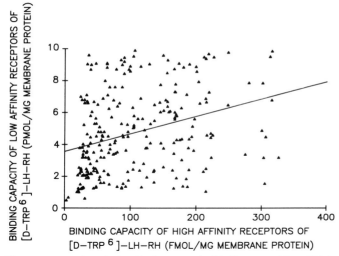

Figure 43–28. The relationship between the binding capacities of high affinity and low affinity receptors for [D-Trp⁶]LH-RH. Receptors for the LH-RH analog, [D-Trp⁶]LH-RH, were detected in 260 human breast cancer specimens using a radiolabeled ligand displacement assay. (From Fekete M, et al: J Clin Lab Anal 3:137–147, 1989. Reprinted with permission.)

menopausal women with breast cancer.[88, 89, 103] Although the antitumor effect of LH-RH analogues is thought to be primarily a result of estrogen deficiency, a detailed correlation of objective response by breast cancer patients treated with LH-RH analogues has not been conducted.[128, 143, 167]

Procedures for measuring LH-RH receptors in breast cancer biopsy specimens have been developed using the membranes remaining after the preparation of cytosol for steroid receptor analyses.[48] In 260 of 500 biopsy specimens (52%), two classes of [D-Trp⁶]-LH-RH receptors were detected (Fig. 43–28): one exhibited high affinity and low capacity (K_d = 8.2 x 10⁻¹¹ mol/L; B_{max} = 41 fmol/mg membrane protein), whereas the other had low affinity and high capacity (K_d = 1.3 x 10⁻⁷ mol/L; B_{max} = 7 pmol/mg membrane protein). LH-RH receptors have been reported in a number of human mammary tumor cell lines[42] as well as in breast cancer by other workers.[89, 103] Evaluation of LH-RH receptors in breast cancer patients treated with LH-RH agonists or antagonists is now possible. We recommend that this be conducted in a controlled setting such as that of a cooperative trial group.

Somatostatin Receptors

A well-characterized hypothalamic releasing hormone, somatostatin (a growth hormone release–inhibiting hormone, or GH-RIH) inhibits the secretion of growth hormone in the anterior pituitary and influences the release of pancreatic hormones. The mode of action of somatostatin has not been established physiologically and poses a particularly intriguing problem, since it has been found in a wide variety of organs, including the gut, median eminence sympathetic ganglia, and parafol-

licular region of the thyroid gland. Somatostatin receptors have been determined in experimental tumors[144, 166] and in small numbers of human breast cancers using autoradiography.[154]

Fekete et al.[48] developed a sensitive means for determination of the binding of a somatostatin analogue, [¹²⁵I]SS-14, to membrane preparations from human breast cancer biopsy specimens.[48] Approximately 36 percent of 178 biopsy specimens exhibited high affinity binding sites for this ligand. Of 45 samples that were negative for both estrogen and [D-Trp⁶]-LH-RH receptors, one third also showed high affinity binding sites for [¹²⁵I]SS-14. Only one class of receptor sites were detected with a K_d value = 1.4 x 10⁻⁹ mol/L. At least one specimen exhibited elevated membrane protein, indicating the utility of the competition inhibition assay. The clinical application of somatostatin analogues is in an embryonic stage, and the development of a sensitive receptor assay for SS-14 should allow study of the relationship between clinical response and receptor levels.

Epidermal Growth Factor Receptors

Epidermal growth factor is a single polypeptide chain with M_r = 6000 that is highly heat stable, partially because of three disulfide bridges. EGF is known to interact with a number of organs in the body, including the reproductive tissues. EGF receptor is a complicated molecule consisting of a large extracellular domain responsible for the association with EGF. The conformation of this domain is maintained by a large number of disulfide bridges and glycosylated residues. The transmembrane portion secures the receptor in the cytoplasmic membrane. The internal domain contains an ATP-binding site and exhibits tyrosine kinase.[40] Interestingly, the molecule can autophosphorylate itself on tyrosine residues located near the carboxy terminus.

EGF receptors have been reported in human breast cancer by several groups. An earlier study[50] suggested that there was an inverse relationship between EGF receptor levels and estrogen receptor concentrations. This was confirmed by Delarue et al.[37] and by our studies of a larger patient population (Figure 43–29).[48] Our recent investigations[48] and those of Sainsbury et al.[157–159] confirmed that there is an inverse relationship between EGF receptors and estrogen receptors in biopsy specimens of human breast cancer. Furthermore, Sainsbury et al. have shown that elevated EGF receptor is related to a shorter disease-free interval and diminished overall survival for breast cancer patients.[127, 129, 157] This appears reasonable based on the findings of Lippman et al.[98] that breast cancer growth is controlled by secretory growth factors.

A sensitive method for measuring EGF receptors in the membranes remaining after cytosol preparation for steroid receptor analyses is available (Fig. 43–30).[48, 209] Both commercially prepared [¹²⁵I]EGF and iodination of EGF using chloramine-T, iodogen beads, and lactoperoxidase in our laboratory provides a useful ligand

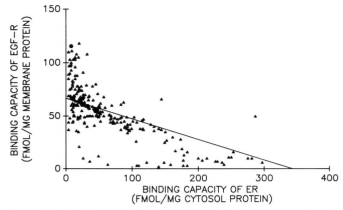

Figure 43–29. The relationship between the binding capacities of estrogen receptors (ER) and epidermal growth factor receptors (EGF-R). Using radioligand binding techniques, the levels of ER and EGF-R were determined in 253 human breast cancer specimens showing both receptor sites. (From Fekete M, et al: J Clin Lab Anal 3:137–147, 1989. Reprinted with permission.)

for these studies. Both titration and competition inhibition analyses (see Fig. 43–30) are performed routinely using the AccuFit Competition software. In an earlier study,[48] high affinity EGF receptors were present in 67 percent of 335 biopsy specimens of human breast cancer. Analysis of the ligand displacement curves as well as Scatchard analysis suggested [^{125}I]EGF bound to one class of receptor sites with a K_d = 1.5 x 10^{-9} mol/L. In more recent studies, we have detected EGF receptors with K_d values ranging from 10^{-10} to 10^{-11} mol/L, providing molecular evidence of receptor heterogeneity.[209] Currently we are correlating these with clinical parameters, including response to hormone therapy. Hanauske et al.[70] showed that EGF receptor levels were altered in patients following treatment with antineoplastic agents. Estrogen is known to regulate EGF receptors in model systems.[122] Even more interesting is the observation that progestin regulates the EGF receptor in breast tumors.[123] Growth factors and cancer are the focus of considerable research for signal transduction and its role in uncontrolled growth.[41, 59]

The *neu* oncogene, originally isolated from rat neuroblastomas, encodes a 185-kDa surface glycoprotein termed "p185 *neu*,"[169] which exhibits tyrosine kinase activity and is structurally similar to the EGF receptor.[10, 78] When various molecular properties and chromosomal localization studies were conducted, it was revealed that the EGF receptor was distinct from p185 *neu*.[168, 180] The native ligand for p185 *neu* is unknown but is the focus of research in many laboratories. The human homolog of *c-neu*, which is termed "*c-erb-B-2*," is reported to be amplified in human breast cancer.[176, 188] This amplification has been correlated with decreased disease-free survival and lower overall survival.[176, 184, 187] The oncogene has also been called *HER-2/neu*. More recently, it has been shown that the mRNA of *HER-2/neu* is overexpressed in some primary breast cancers.[87, 184] Finally, overexpression of the *HER-2/neu* protein product is correlated with amplification of

the oncogene and is related to decreased disease-free survival and overall survival for breast cancer patients.[109, 176, 177, 181a]

The role of EGF and other growth regulatory factors as well as oncogenes in breast cancer is discussed in section VII, chapters 19 and 20, and no extensive discussion will be provided here. To evaluate the relationship between expression of the *erb-B2* oncogene and its messenger RNA and protein product as a function of breast cancer natural history and therapeutic response, it is essential to have uniform methods of analyses. Procedures are evolving, and we are currently employing an ELISA procedure developed by DuPont for measuring the *erb-B-2* protein in homogenates of breast cancer. Furthermore, immunocytochemistry is being utilized to detect the protein's presence in frozen and paraffin-embedded sections. Other investigators

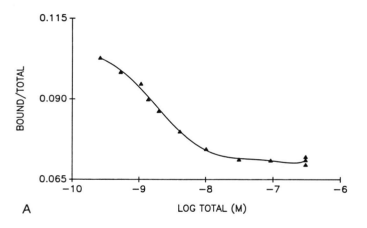

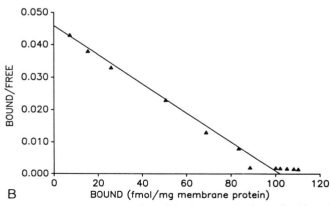

Figure 43–30. Representative ligand displacement analysis of epidermal growth factor receptors in human breast cancer. Displacement of [^{125}I]EGF was measured in the presence of increasing amounts of unlabeled EGF in the membrane of one specimen of human breast cancer *(A)*. Scatchard plot analysis was accomplished with the data from the displacement curve *(B)*. The individual data points are means of triplicate determination calculated and plotted by the LIGAND-PC computer program according to Rodbard et al.[154a] The coefficients of variations of parameters were six per cent and 11 per cent. (From Fekete M, et al: J Clin Lab Anal 3:137–147, 1989. Reprinted with permission.)

have indicated that immunohistochemical analysis of paraffin blocks is useful for correlative clinical studies.[132]

CONCLUSIONS AND RECOMMENDATIONS

Breast cancer patients most likely to respond to an additive or ablative endocrine manipulation (medical or surgical) may be identified from analyses of sex hormone receptors. Steroid hormone receptors should be considered along with clinical factors such as axillary nodal involvement, previous response to hormone therapy, disease-free interval, age, menopausal status, location of the dominant metastatic lesion, and other criteria for selecting therapeutic regimens for these women.

The most reliable methods of quantifying estrogen and progestin receptors are titration analysis using specific radiolabeled hormones or hormone analogues and enzyme immunoassay. Immunocytochemical methods should be used *only* as a confirmatory test of receptor presence and are appropriate for analyses of needle biopsies and fine needle aspirates. In general, when estrogen receptors are elevated in a tumor biopsy, a higher progestin-binding capacity is observed when considering both pre- and postmenopausal women. Usually a lower progestin receptor level is exhibited when estrogen receptors are absent, supporting the hypothesis that the formation of progestin receptor is dependent on estrogen activity. Levels of estrogen receptors that exceed 10 fmol/mg cytosol protein have been observed in 55 percent to 65 percent of primary breast tumors and in 45 percent to 55 percent of metastatic lesions. Breast tumors of postmenopausal women contain estrogen receptors more frequently than do tumors of premenopausal women. Benign breast lesions such as fibrocystic disease and fibroadenomas usually contain less than 10 fmol/mg cytosol protein of estrogen receptor but may exhibit progestin receptor. Almost 90 percent of male breast carcinomas contain estrogen receptors, and less than 50 percent contain progestin receptors. Approximately 55 percent of women with breast tumors containing estrogen receptors respond objectively to endocrine therapy, either additive or ablative, whereas less than

three percent of patients with tumors lacking these receptors respond objectively.

Progestin receptors are found in 45 percent to 60 percent of primary or metastatic breast tumors. The presence of significant quantities (>50 fmol/mg cytosol protein) of both female sex hormone receptors in a breast tumor is correlated with the observation that 75 percent to 80 percent of such patients will respond to endocrine manipulation, either additive or ablative. Furthermore, the quantity of both estrogen and progestin receptors in a breast tumor correlates with the patient's response to endocrine therapy. The incidence of response to hormone therapy increases with increasing receptor values.

The presence of 8 S isoforms of the estrogen and progestin receptors in a breast tumor (as detected by sucrose gradient centrifugation) appears to assist in selection of the patient likely to respond to endocrine therapy. This method is used primarily in the research setting. Using HPLC in various modes, it was demonstrated that both estrogen and progestin receptors exhibit polymorphism (presence of multiple isoforms) based on characteristics of size, shape, surface ionic charge, and hydrophobicity. Molecular heterogeneity appears to result from the various types of receptor modifications that occur from phosphorylation. This heterogeneity may also result from nonreceptor-associated activities such as protein kinase and HSP-90.

Preliminary reports have demonstrated that the levels of epidermal growth factor receptor associated with cytoplasmic membranes of breast cancers are inversely correlated with estrogen receptor concentrations. The presence of EGF receptor appears to be correlated with a decreased disease-free interval and overall survival. Furthermore, EGF receptor expression may be useful to ascertain prognosis in both node-negative and node-positive breast cancer.

Amplification of the *HER-2/neu* oncogene appears to correlate with decreased disease-free interval and overall survival by breast cancer patients. Overexpression of the protein p185 *neu* encoded by the *c-erb-B-2* oncogene, which is structurally similar to the EGF receptor, also appears to correlate with decreased time to relapse and to overall survival.

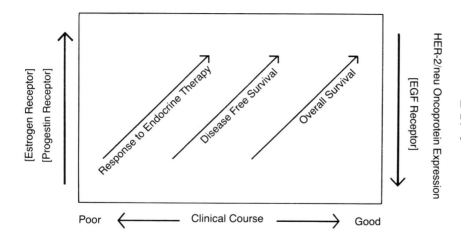

Figure 43–31. Prognostic factors employed in the management of breast cancer. (From Wittliff JL, Wittliff TH: J Clin Immunoassay, 1990, in press. Reprinted with permission.)

We recommend that both estrogen and progestin receptor analyses be performed on all tumor biopsy samples from patients with confirmed or suspected cases of breast cancer *prior to therapeutic manipulation.* Whenever possible the clinician should analyze EGF receptors and expression of *HER-2/neu* protein as well. One must be cognizant of laboratories complying with criteria assigned by quality assurance programs that establish uniformity of methods and data expression for these receptors and oncogene products.[212a] Collectively, these results are useful as predictive indicators of an endocrine-responsive tumor and as prognostic indices of a patient's clinical course (Fig. 43–31).

As suggested in previous published data, [201] a new generation of laboratory tests is evolving in which the analyses will be performed directly on the biopsy tissue. It is envisioned that tissue banks will be developed for long-term preservation of tumor biopsy samples so that biochemical parameters may be assessed as new clinical, chemical and molecular biological probes are developed.[212a] The tumor itself provides an enormous resource for the development of new markers of therapeutic response and for assessment of the physiological status of the patient with breast carcinoma.

ACKNOWLEDGMENTS

During the past decade, research in the Hormone Receptor Laboratory has been supported in part by grants from the American Cancer Society (BC-514B) and Phi Beta Psi sorority and by USPHS grants CA-19657, CA-34211, CA-32101, CA-37429, CA-25224, CA-42154, and CA-31946 from the National Cancer Institute and the College of American Pathologists.

References

1. Alghanem AA, Hussain S: The effect of age on estrogen and progesterone receptor in primary breast cancer. J Surg Oncol 30:29–32, 1985.
2. Allegra JC, Barlock A, Huff KK, Lippman ME: Changes in multiple or sequential estrogen receptor determinations in breast cancer. Cancer 45:792–794, 1980.
3. Allegra JC, Lippman ME: The effects of 17β estradiol to tamoxifen on the ZR-75-1 human breast cancer cell line in defined medium. Eur J Cancer 16:1007–1015, 1980.
4. Allegra JC, Lippman ME, Thompson B, et al: Distribution, frequency, and quantitative analysis of estrogen, progesterone, androgen and glucocorticoid receptors in human breast cancer. Cancer Res 39:1447–1454, 1979.
5. Andersen J, Poulsen HS: Immunohistochemical estrogen receptor determination in paraffin-embedded tissue. Cancer 64:1901–1908, 1989.
6. Anonymous: NIH Consensus Development Conference on Steroid Receptors in Breast Cancer. Cancer 46:2759–2963, 1980.
7. Anonymous: Symposium on Estrogen Receptor Determination With Monoclonal Antibodies. Cancer Res 46(suppl 1):4231–4314, 1986.
8. Auricchio F, Migliaccio A, Rotondi A: Inactivation of estrogen receptor *in vitro* by nuclear dephosphorylation. Biochem J 194:569–574, 1981.
9. Baldi A, Boyle DM, Wittliff JL: Estrogen receptors are associated with protein and phospholipid kinase activities. Biochem Biophys Res Commun 135:597–606, 1986.
10. Bargmann CI, Hung M-C, Weinberg RA: The neu oncogene encodes an epidermal growth factor receptor-related protein. Nature 319:226–230, 1986.
11. Barnett CA, Schmidt TJ, Litwack G: Effects of calf intestinal akaline phosphate, phosphatase inhibitors and phosphorylated compounds on the rate of activation of glucocorticoid-receptor complexes. Biochem 19:5446–5455, 1980.
12. Baulieu EE: Steroid hormone antagonists at the receptor level: A role for the heat-shock protein MW 90,000 (hsp 90). J Cell Biochem 35:161–174, 1987.
13. Beatson GT: On the treatment of inoperable cases of carcinoma of the mamma; suggestions for a new method of treatment with illustrative cases. Lancet II:104–107, 1896.
14. Bell PA, Munck A: Steroid-binding properties and stabilization of cytoplasmic glucocorticoid receptors from rat thymus cells. J Biol Chem 136:97, 1973.
15. Ben-David M, Kadar T, Wittliff JL, Biran S, Schally AB: Characterization of prolactin receptors and their distribution among American and Israeli women with breast cancer: implications for prediction of hormonal dependency and future treatment. Biomed Pharmacother 42:101–109, 1988.
16. Ben-David M, Wittliff JL, Fekete M, Kadar T, Biran S, Schally AV: Lack of relationship between the levels of prolactin receptors and steroid receptors in woman with breast cancer. Biomed Pharmacother 42:327–334, 1988.
17. Berns EMJ, Mulder E, Rommerts FFG, Blankenstein RA, de Graaf E, van der Molen HJ: Fluorescent ligands, used in histocytochemistry, do not discriminate between estrogen receptor-positive and receptor-negative human tumor cell lines. Breast Cancer Res Treat 4:195–204, 1984.
18. Bishop HM, Blamey RW, Elston CW, Haybittle JL: Relationship of oestrogen-receptor status to survival in breast cancer. Lancet II:283–284, 1979.
19. Black R, Prescott R, Bers K, Hawkins A, Stewart H, Forrest P: Tumour cellularity, oestrogen receptors and prognosis in breast cancer. Clin Oncol 9:311–318, 1983.
20. Blamey RW, Bishop HM, Blake JRS, et al: Relationship between primary breast tumor receptor status and patient survival. Cancer 46:2765–2769, 1980.
21. Bland KI, Freeman BE, Harris PL, He YJ, Wittliff JL: The effects of ischemia on estrogen and progesterone receptor profiles in the rodent uterus. J Surg Res 42:653–660, 1987.
21a. Bland KI, Fuchs A, Wittliff, JL: Menopausal status as a factor in the distribution of estrogen and progestin receptors in breast cancer. Surg Forum XXXII:410–412, 1981.
22. Blanco G, Alavaikko M, Ohala A, et al: Estrogen and progesterone receptors in breast cancer: relationships to tumor histopathology and survival of patients. Anticancer Res 4:383–390, 1984.
23. Bloom ND, Johnson F, Pertshuck L, Fishman J: Electrocautery: effects on steroid receptors in human breast cancer. J Surg Oncol 25:21–24, 1984.
24. Bonnetere J, Peyrat JPH, Beuscart R, Demaille A: Correlation between prolactin receptors, estradiol and progesterone receptors in human breast cancer. Eur J Cancer Clin Oncol 22:1331–1336, 1986.
25. Bonnetere J, Peyrat JPH, Beuscart R, Lefebvre J, Demaille A: Prognostic significance of prolactin receptors in human breast cancer. Cancer Res 47:4724–4628, 1987.
25a. Boyle DM, Wiehle RD, Shahabi NA, Wittliff JL: Rapid high-resolution procedure for assessment of estrogen receptor heterogeneity in clinical samples. J Chromatogr 327:369–376, 1985.
26. Brandt DW, Wittliff JL: Assessment of estrogen receptor-monoclonal antibody interaction by high-performance liquid chromatography. J Chromatogr 397:287–297, 1987.
27. Burke RE, Miva JG, Datta R, Zava DT, McGuire WL: Estrogen action following irradiation of human breast cancer cells. Cancer Res 38:2813–2817, 1978.
28. Butzow R, Huntaniemi I, Clayton R, Wahlstrom T, Andersson LC, Seppala M: Cultured mammary carcinoma cells contain gonadotropin-releasing hormone-like immunoreactivity, GnRH binding sites and chorionic gonadotropin. Int J Cancer 39:498–501, 1987.
29. Carlson JA, Allegra JC, Day TG Jr, Wittliff JL: Tamoxifen and

endometrial carcinoma alterations in estrogen and progesterone receptors in untreated patients and combination hormonal therapy in advanced neoplasia. Am J Obstet Gynecol 149:149–154, 1984.

30. Chambon AB, Goldberg JD, Venet L: Carcinoma of the breast inter-relationship among histopathologic features, estrogen receptor activity and age of the patient. Hum Pathol 14:368–372, 1982.
31. Chamness GC, Mercer WD, McGuire WL: Are histochemical methods for estrogen receptor valid? J Histochem Cytochem 28:792–798, 1980.
32. Chua DYF, Pang MWY, Rauff A, Aw S-E, Chan S-H: Correlation of steroid receptors with histologic differentiation in mammary carcinoma. Cancer 56:2228–2234, 1985.
33. Clark GM, McGuire WL: Prognostic factors in primary breast cancer. Breast Cancer Res Treat 3:69–72, 1983.
34. Clark GM, McGuire WL, Hubay CA, Pearson OH, Marshall JS: Progesterone receptors as a prognostic factor in stage II breast cancer. N Engl J Med 309:1343–1347, 1983.
35. Cohen P: The role of protein phosphorylation in normal hormonal control of cellular activity. Nature 296:613, 1982.
36. Crowe JP Jr, Gordon NH, Hubay CA, Pearson OH, Marshall JS, McGuire WL: The interaction of estrogen receptor status and race in predicting prognosis for stage I breast cancer patients. Surgery 100:599–605, 1986.
37. Delarue JC, Friedman S, Mouriesse H, May-Levin F, Sancho-Garnier H, Contesso G: Epidermal growth factor receptor in human breast cancers: Correlation with estrogen and progesterone receptors. Breast Cancer Res Treat 11:173–178, 1988.
38. Denis M, Gustafsson JA, Wikstrom AC: Interaction of the M_r-90,000 heat shock protein with the steroid-binding domain of the glucocorticoid receptor. J Biol Chem 263:18,520–18,523, 1988.
39. Dougherty JJ, Puri RK, Toft DO: Phosphorylation in vivo of chicken oviduct progesterone receptor. J Biol Chem 257:14,226–14,230, 1982.
40. Downward J, Parker P, Waterfield MD: Autophosphorylation sites on the EGF receptor. Nature 311:483–485, 1984.
41. Druker BJ, Mamon HJ, Roberts TM: Oncogenes, growth factors and signal transduction. Semin Med Beth Israel Hosp Boston 321:1383–1391, 1989.
42. Eidne KA, Flanagan CA, Harris NS, Millar RP: Gonadotropin-releasing hormone (GnRH)-binding sites in human breast cancer cell lines and inhibitory effects of GnRH antagonists. J Clin Endocrinol Metab 64:425–427, 1987.
43. Eidne KA, Flanagan CA, Miller RP: Gonadotropin-releasing hormone binding sites in human breast carcinoma. Science 229:989–991, 1985.
44. Ellis LM, Wittliff JL, Bryant MS, Sitren HS, Hogancamp WE, Souba WW, Bland KI: Effects of ischemia on breast tumor steroid hormone-receptor levels. Curr Surg 45:312–314, 1988.
45. Ellis LM, Wittliff JL, Bryant MS, Sitren HS, Hogancamp WE, Souba WW, Bland KI: Lability of steroid hormone receptors following devascularization of breast tumors. Arch Surg 124:39–42, 1989.
46. Elwood YN, Godolpin W: Oestrogen receptors in breast tumors: Association with age, menopausal status, epidemiological and clinical features in 735 patients. Br J Cancer 42:635–644, 1980.
47. Everson RB, Lippman ME, Thompson EB, McGuire WL, Wittliff JL, DeSombre ER, Jensen EV, Singhakowinta A, Brooks SC Jr, Neifeld JP: Clinical correlations of steroid receptors and male breast cancer. Cancer Res 40:991–997, 1980.
48. Fekete M, Wittliff JL, Schally AV: Characteristics and distribution of receptors for [D-TRP⁶]-luteinizing hormone-releasing hormone, somatostatin, epidermal growth factor, and sex steroids in 500 biopsy samples of human breast cancer. J Clin Lab Anal 3:137–147, 1989.
49. Fisher B, Redmond C, Brown A, Wickerham DL, Wolmark N, Allegra JC, Escher G, Lippman M, Savlov E, Wittliff JL, Fisher ER: Influence of tumor estrogen and progesterone receptor levels on the response to tamoxifen and chemotherapy in primary breast cancer. J Clin Oncol 1:227–241, 1983.
49a. Fisher B, Redmond C, Brown A, Womark N, Wittliff JL, et al: Treatment of primary breast cancer with chemotherapy and tamoxifen. New Engl J Med 305:1–6, 1981.
50. Fitzpatrick SL, Brightwell JJ, Wittliff JL, Barrows GH, Schultz GS: Epidermal growth factor binding by human breast tumor biopsies and relationship to estrogen receptor and progestin receptor levels. Cancer Res 44:3448–3453, 1984.
51. Flowers JL, Burton GV, Cox EB, Dent GA, Geisinger KR, McCarthy KS Jr: Use of monoclonal anti-estrogen receptor antibody to evaluate estrogen receptor content in fine needle aspiration biopsies. Ann Surg 203:250–254, 1986.
52. Folca PJ, Glascock RF, Irvine WT: Studies with tritium-labeled hexoestrol in advanced breast cancer. Lancet II: 796–798, 1961.
53. Gapinski PV, Donegan WL: Estrogen receptors and breast cancer: Prognostic and therapeutic implications. Surgery 88:386–393, 1980.
54. Garcia T, Buchou T, Renoir JM, Mester J, Baulieu EE: A protein kinase copurified with chick oviduct progesterone receptor. Biochem 25:7937, 1986.
55. Garcia T, Tuchima P, Mester J, Buchou T, Renoir JM, Baulieu EE: Protein kinase activity of purified components of the chicken oviduct progesterone receptor. Biochem Biophys Res Commun 113:960, 1983.
55a. Glascock RF, Hoekstra WG: Selective accumulation of tritium-labeled hexoestrol by the reproductive organs of immature female goats and sheep. Biochem J 72:673–682, 1959.
56. Godolphin W, Elwood JM, Spinelli JJ: Estrogen receptor quantitation and staging as complementary prognostic indicators in breast cancer. Study of 483 patients. Int J Cancer 28:677–683, 1981.
57. Gorski J, Toft D, Shyamala G, Smith D, Notides A: Hormone receptors: Studies on the interaction of estrogen with the uterus. Recent Prog Horm Res 24:45–80, 1968.
58. Goueli SA, Hottzman JL, Ahmed K: Phosphorylation of the androgen receptor by a nuclear cAMP-independent protein kinase. Biochem Biophys Res Commun 123:778–784, 1984.
59. Goustin AS, Leof EB, Shidley GD, Moses HL: Growth factors and cancer. Cancer Res 46:1015–1029, 1986.
60. Grandics P, Miller A, Schmidt TJ, Litwack G: Phosphorylation in vivo of the rat hepatic glucocorticoid receptor. Biochem Biophys Res Commun 120:59–65, 1984.
61. Green S, Kumar V, Theulaz I, Wahli W, Chambon P: The N-terminal DNA-binding 'zinc finger' of the oestrogen and glucocorticoid receptors determines target gene specificity. EMBO J 7:3037–3044, 1988.
62. Green S, Walter P, Kumar V, Krust A, Burnett JM, Argos P, Chambon P: Human oestrogen receptor cDNA sequence, expression and homology to v-erb-A. Nature 320:134, 1986.
63. Greene GL, Fitche FW, Jensen EV: Monoclonal antibodies to estrophilin: Probes for the study of estrogen receptors. Proc Natl Acad Sci USA 77:157–161, 1980.
64. Greene GL, Sobel NB, King WJ, Jensen EV: Immunochemical studies of estrogen receptors. J Steroid Biochem 20:51–56, 1984.
65. Grill H, Manz B, Belozsky O, Pollow K: Criteria for establishment of the double labeling assay for simultaneous determination of estrogen and progesterone receptors. Oncology 41:25–32, 1984.
66. Groom GV, Grifiths K: Effect of the anti-estrogen tamoxifen on plasma levels of luteinizing hormone, follicle-stimulating hormone, prolactin, oestradiol and progesterone in normal premenopausal women. J Endocrinol 70:421–428, 1976.
67. Hahnel R, Twaddle E: The relationship between estrogen receptors in primary and secondary breast carcinomas and in sequential primary breast carcinomas. Breast Cancer Res Treat 5:155–163, 1985.
68. Hahnel R, Woodings T, Vivian AB: Prognostic value of estrogen receptors in primary breast cancer. Cancer 44:671–675, 1979.
69. Hanna W, Mobbs BG: Comparative evaluation of ER-ICA and enzyme immunoassay for the quantitation of estrogen receptors in breast cancer. Am J Clin Pathol 91:182–186, 1989.
70. Hanauske AR, Osborne CK, Chamness GC, Clark GM, Forseth BJ, Buchok JB, Arteaga CL, Von Hoff DD: Alteration of

EGF-receptor binding in human breast cancer cells by antineoplastic agents. Eur J Cancer Clin Oncol 23:545–551, 1987.

71. Harvey HA, Lipton A, Max D: LH-RH analogs for human mammary carcinoma *In* Vickery GH, Nestor JJ Jr, Hafez ESE (eds): LH-RH and Its Analogs—Contraceptive and Therapeutic Applications. Lancaster, PA, MTP Press, 1983, pp 329–336.

72. Hockberg RB: Iodine-125-labeled estradiol: a gamma-emitting analog of estradiol that binds to the estrogen receptor. Science 205:1138–1140, 1979.

73. Holdaway IM, Friesen HG: Hormone binding by human mammary carcinoma. Cancer Res 37:1946–1952, 1977.

74. Horwitz KG, McGuire WL: Specific progesterone receptors in human breast cancer. Steroids 25:497–505, 1975.

75. Horwitz KG, McGuire WL, Pearson OH, Segaloff A: Predicting response to endocrine therapy in human breast cancer: a hypothesis. Science 189:726–727, 1975.

75a. Housley PR, Pratt WB: Direct demonstration of glucocorticoid receptor phosphorylation by intact L-cells. J Biol Chem 258:4630–4635, 1983.

76. Howat JMT, Barnes DM, Harris M, Swindell R: The association of cytosol oestrogen and progesterone receptors with histological features of breast cancer and early detection of disease. Br J Cancer 47:629–640, 1983.

77. Hull DF III, Clark GM, Osborne CK, Chamness GC, Knight WA III, McGuire WL: Multiple estrogen receptor assays in human breast cancer. Cancer Res 43:413–416, 1983.

78. Hunter T, Cooper JA: Protein-tyrosine kinases. Ann Rev Biochem 54:897, 1985.

79. Hyder MS, Sato N, Wittliff JL: Characterization of estrogen receptors and associated protein kinase activity by high-performance hydrophobic-interaction chromatography. J Chromatogr 397:251–267, 1987.

79a. Hyder SM, Shahabi NA, Wittliff JL: Microanalysis of estrogen receptors from human uteri by multidimensional HPLC. Biochromatography 3(5):216–224, 1988.

80. Hyder SM, Wittliff JL: High performance hydrophobic interaction chromatography as a means of identifying estrogen receptors expressing different binding domains. J Chromatogr 444:225–327, 1988.

80a. Hyder SM, Wittliff JL: Separation of two molecular forms of human estrogen receptor by hydrophobic interaction chromatography: gradient optimization and tissue-comparison. J Chromatogr 476:455–466, 1989.

80b. Jensen EV: Historical perspective. Cancer 46:2759–2761, 1980.

81. Jensen EV, Block GE, Smith S, Kyser K, DeSombre ER: Estrogen receptors and breast cancer response to adrenalectomy. Natl Cancer Inst Monogr 34:55–79, 1971.

81a. Jensen EV, Jacobson HI: Fate of steroid estrogens in target tissues. *In* Pincus G, Vollmer EP (eds): Biological Activities of Steroids in Relation to Cancer. New York, Academic Press, 1960, pp 161–178.

82. Jensen EV, Suzuku T, Kawashima T, Stumpf WE, Jungblut PW, DeSombre ER: A two-step mechanism for the interaction of estradiol with rat uterus. Proc Natl Acad Sci USA 59:632–639, 1968.

83. Jordan VC: Role of tamoxifen in the long-term treatment and prevention of breast cancer. Oncology 2:19–24, 1988.

84. Jordan VC, Jacobson HI, Keenan EJ: Determination of estrogen receptor in breast cancer using monoclonal antibody technology: results of a multicenter study in the United States. Cancer Res 46:4237–4240, 1986.

85. King WJ, DeSombre ER, Jensen E, Greene GL: Comparison of immunocytochemical and steroid-binding assays for estrogen receptor in human breast tumors. Cancer Res 45:293–304, 1985.

86. King WJ, Greene GL: Monoclonal antibodies localized oestrogen receptor in the nuclei of target cells. Nature 307:745–747, 1984.

87. King CR, Swain SM, Porter L, Steinberg SM, Lippman ME, Gelmann EP: Heterogenous expression of erbB-2 mRNA in human breast cancer. Cancer Res 49:4185–4191, 1989.

88. Klijn JGM, Dejong FH: Treatment with a lutenizing hormone-releasing hormone analogue (buserelin) in premenopausal patients with metastatic breast cancer. Lancet 1:1213–1216, 1982.

89. Klijn JGM, Dejong FH, Lamberts SWJ, Blankenstein MA: LH-RH agonist treatment in clinical and experimental human breast cancer. J Steroid Biochem 23:867–873, 1985.

90. Klotz IM: Numbers of receptor sites from Scatchard graphs: facts and fantasies. Science 217:1247–1249, 1982.

91. Knight WA, Livingston RB, Gregory EJ, McGuire WL: Estrogen receptor as an independent prognostic factor for early recurrence in breast cancer. Cancer Res 37:4669–4671, 1977.

92. Kute TE, Heidemann P, Wittliff JL: Molecular heterogeneity of cytosolic forms of estrogen receptors from human breast tumors. Cancer Res 38:4307–4313, 1978.

93. Leclerq G, Toma S, Paridenas R, Heuson JC (eds): Clinical Interest of Steroid Hormone Receptors in Breast Cancer. Berlin, Springer-Verlag, 1984, pp 186–191.

94. Lee SH: Cancer cell estrogen receptor of human mammary carcinoma. Cancer 44:1–12, 1979.

95. Lefebvre P, Danze PM, Sablonniere B, Richard C, Formstecher P, Dautrevaux M: Association of the glucocorticoid receptor binding subunit with the 90K nonsteroid-binding component is stabilized by both steroidal and nonsteroidal antiglucocorticoids in intact cells. Biochem 27:9186–9194, 1988.

96. Lesser ML, Rosen PP, Senei RT, et al: Estrogen and progesterone receptors in breast carcinoma: Correlation with epidemiology and pathology. Cancer 48:288–299, 1981.

97. Limbird L: Surface receptors: a short course on theory and methods. The Netherlands, Amsterdam, Martinus Nijhoff, 1986.

98. Lippman ME, Dickson B, Gelmann EP, Rosen N, Knabbe C, Bates S, Bronzert D, Huff K, Kasid A: Growth regulation of human breast carcinoma occurs through regulated growth factor secretion. J Cell Biochem 35:1–16, 1987.

99. Locher GW, Davis B, Zava DT, Goldhirsch A, Hartmann WH: Intratumoral regional differences in hormone receptor status of breast cancer. Geburtshilfe Fraunheilkd 44:304–306, 1984.

100. Lonsdorfer M, Clements NC Jr, Wittliff JL: Use of high performance liquid chromatography in the elevation of the synthesis and binding of fluorescein-linked steroids to estrogen receptors. J Chromatogr 266:129–139, 1983.

101. Lundeen JE, Gordon JH: Computer analysis of binding data. *In* O'Brien RA (ed): Receptor Binding in Drug Research. New York, Marcel Dekker, p 31–49, 1986.

102. Maass H, Engel B, Hohmeister H: Estrogen receptors in human breast cancer. Am J Obstet Gynecol 113:377–382, 1972.

102a. Magdelenat H, Merle S, Zajdela A: Enzyme immunoassay of estrogen receptors in fine needle aspirates of breast tumors. Cancer Res 46:4265–4267, 1986.

103. Manni A, Santen R, Harvey H, Lipton A, Max D: Treatment of breast cancer with gonadotrophin-releasing hormone. Endocr Rev 7:89–94, 1986.

104. Markopoulos C, Berger U, Wilson P, Gazet J, Coombes RC: Oestrogen receptor content of normal breast cells and breast carcinomas throughout the menstrual cycle. Br Med J 296:1349–1351, 1988.

104a. Martin AW, Wittliff JL: Immunohistochemical analysis of sex-hormone receptors in biopsies of human cancer. J Clin Lab Anal 1990 (in press).

105. McCarty KS Jr, Miller LS, Cox EB, Konrath J, McCarty KS Sr: Estrogen receptor analyses: correlation of biochemical and immunohistochemical methods using antireceptor antibodies. Arch Pathol Lab Med 109:716–721, 1985.

106. McCarty KS Jr, Silva JS, Cox EB, Leight GS, Wells SA, McCarty KS Sr: Relationship of age and menopausal status to estrogen receptor content in primary carcinoma of the breast. Ann Surg 197:123–127, 1983.

107. McGuire WL, Carbone PO, Vollmer EP (eds): Estrogen Receptors in Human Breast Cancer. New York, Raven Press, 1975.

108. McGuire WL, Raynaud JP, Baulieu E-E (eds.): Progesterone Receptors in Normal and Neoplastic Tissues. New York, Raven Press, 1977.

109. McKenzie SJ, Marks PJ, Lam T, Morgan J, Panicali DL, Trimpe KL, Carney WP: Generation and characterization of monoclonal antibodies specific for the human neu oncogene product. Oncogene 4:543–548, 1989.

110. Meyer JS: Hormone receptors in human malignancy of unknown origin: potential utility in clinical management. *In* Fer MF,

Oldham D, Greceo A (eds): Tumors of Unknown Origin and Poorly Differentiated Neoplasms. Orlando, Grune and Stratton, pp 519–539, 1986.

111. Meyer JS, Rao BR, Stevens SC, White WL: Low incidence of estrogen receptor in breast carcinomas with rapid rates of cellular replication. Cancer 40:2290–2298, 1977.

112. Meyer JS, Schechtman K, Valdes R Jr: Estrogen and progesterone receptor assays on breast carcinoma from mastectomy specimens. Cancer 52:2139–2149, 1983.

113. Meyer JS, Wittliff JL: Regional heterogeneity in breast carcinoma: thymidine labeling index, steroid hormone receptors, DNA ploidy. 1990, Intl J Cancer (in press).

114. Migliaccio A, Rotundi A, Auricchio F: Calmodulin-stimulated phosphorylation of 17β-estradiol receptor on tyrosine. Proc Natl Acad Sci USA 81:5921, 1984.

115. Miller WR, Scott WN, Morris R, Fraser HM, Sharpe RM: Growth of human breast cancer cells inhibited by a luteinizing hormone-releasing hormone agonist. Nature 313:231–233, 1985.

116. Mills RR: Correlation of hormone receptors with pathological features in human breast cancer. Cancer 46:2869–2871, 1980.

117. Mirecki DM, Jordan VC: Steroid and hormone receptors and human breast cancer. Lab Med 16(5):287–294, 1985.

118. Mohla S, Sampson CC, Kahn T, Enterline JP, Leffal L, White JE, Gabriel BW, Hunter JB: Estrogen and progesterone receptors in breast cancer in black Americans. Cancer 50:552–559, 1982.

119. Mortel R, Levy C, Wolff J-P, Nicolas J-C, Robel P, Baulieu EE: Female sex steroid receptors in postmenopausal endometrial carcinoma and biochemical response to an antiestrogen. Cancer Res 41:1140, 1981.

120. Moudgil VK (ed.): Molecular Mechanisms of Steroid Hormone Action. Berlin, Walter de Gruyter and Co, 1985, p 376.

121. Moudgil VK (ed.): Receptor Phosphorylation. Boca Raton, FL, CRC Press, 1989, p 384.

122. Mukku VR, Stancel GM: Regulation of epidermal growth factor receptor by estrogen. J Biol Chem 260:9820–9824, 1985.

123. Murphy LJ, Sutherland RL, Stead B, Murphy LC, Lazarus L: Progestin regulation of epidermal growth factor receptor in human mammary carcinoma cells. Cancer Res 46:728–734, 1987.

124. Nagasawa H: Prolactin and human breast cancer: a review. Eur J Cancer 15:267–279, 1979.

125. Nakao M, Sato B, Koga M, et al: Identification of immunoassayable estrogen receptor lacking hormone binding ability in tamoxifen-treated rat uterus. Biochem Biophys Res Commun 132:336–342, 1985.

126. Nemoto T, Vana J, Bedwani RN, Bakder HW, McGregor FH, Murphy GP: Management and survival of female breast cancer: results of a national survey by the American College of Surgeons. Cancer 45:2917–2924, 1980.

127. Nicholson S, Halcrow P, Sainsbury JRC, Angus B, Chambers P, Farndon JR, Harris AL: Epidermal growth factor receptor (EGFR) status associated with failure of primary endocrine therapy in elderly postmenopausal patients with breast cancer. Br J Cancer 58:810–814, 1988.

128. Nicholson JGM, Maynard PV: Anti-tumor activity of ICI 118630, a new potent luteinizing hormone-releasing hormone agonist. Br J Can 39:268–273, 1979.

129. Nicholson S, Sainsbury JRC, Needham GK, Chambers P, Farndon JR, Harris AL: Quantitative assays of epidermal growth factor receptor in human breast cancer: cut-off points of clinical relevance. Int J Cancer 42:36–41, 1988.

130. Nomura Y, Kobayashi S, Takatani O, Sugano H, Matsumoto K, McGuire WL: Estrogen receptor and endocrine responsiveness in Japanese versus American breast cancer patients. Cancer Res 37:106–110, 1977.

131. Normura Y, Tashiro H, Hamada Y, Shigemateu T: Relationship between estrogen receptors and risk factors of breast cancer in Japanese pre- and postmenopausal patients. Breast Cancer Res Treat 4:37–43, 1984.

132. Paik S, Hazan R, Fisher ER, Sass RE, Fisher B, Redmond C, Schlessinger J, Lippman ME, King CR: Pathologic findings from the national surgical adjuvant breast and bowel project:

133. Palshof T, Mouridsen HT, Daehnfeldt JL: Adjuvant endocrine therapy of primary operable breast cancer. Report on the Copenhagen Breast Cancer Trials. Eur J Cancer 16(suppl 1):183–187, 1980.

134. Parl F, Schmidt BP, Dupont WD, Wagner RK: Prognostic significance of estrogen receptor status in breast cancer in relation to tumor stage, axillary node metastasis, and histopathologic grading. Cancer 54:2237–2242, 1984.

135. Partridge RK, Hähnel R: Prolactin receptors in human breast carcinoma. Cancer 43:643–646, 1979.

136. Pasic R, Djulbegovic B, Wittliff JL: Influence of O.C.T. embedding compound on determinations of estrogen and progestin receptors in breast cancer. Clin Chem 35:2317–2319, 1989.

137. Pasic R, Djulbegovic B, Wittliff JL: Comparison of enzyme immunoassay with the multipoint titration procedure for the determination of estrogen and progestin receptors. 1990, (Submitted J Clin Lab Anal).

138. Pasic R, Sewell CL, Wittliff JL: Establishment of equivalency of sex steroid receptor levels in human breast cancer determined by radioligand binding, enzyme immunoassay and immunohistochemical analysis. 1990, to be submitted.

139. Pegoraro RJ, Karnan V, Nirmul D, Joubert SM: Estrogen and progesterone receptors in breast cancer among women of different racial groups. Cancer Res 46:2117–2120, 1986.

140. Pegoraro RJ, Nirmul D, Joubert SM: Cytoplasmic and nuclear estrogen and progesterone receptors in male breast cancer. Cancer Res 42:4812–4814, 1982.

141. Pegoraro RJ, Nirmul D, Reinach SG, Jordaan JP, Joubert SM: Breast cancer prognosis in three different racial groups in relation to the steroid hormone receptor status. Breast Cancer Res Treat 7:111–118, 1986.

142. Perdew GH: Association of the Ah receptor with the 90-kDa heat shock protein. J Biol Chem 263(27):13,802–13,805, 1988.

143. Plowman PN, Nicholson RI, Walker KJ: Remission of postmenopausal breast cancer during treatment with the luteinizing hormone releasing hormone agonist ICI 118630. Br J Cancer 54:903–909, 1986.

144. Pollak NM, Perdue JF, Margolese RG, Baer K, Richard M: Presence of somatomedin receptors on primary human breast and colon carcinoma. Cancer 38:223–230, 1987.

145. Pollow K, Schmidt-Gollwitzer M, Pollow B: Progesterone- and estradiol-binding proteins from normal human endometrium and endometrial carcinoma: a comparative study. *In* Wittliff JL, Dapunt O (eds): Steroid Receptors and Hormone-Dependent Neoplasia. New York, Masson Publishing, 1984, pp 69–94.

146. Ponsky JL, Gliga L, Reynolds S: Medullary carcinoma of the breast: an association with negative hormonal receptors. J Surg Oncol 25:76–78, 1984.

147. Raam S, Teixeira T: Effect of sodium molybdate on protein measurements: quality control aspects of steroid hormone receptor assays. Eur J Cancer Clin Oncol 21:1219–1223, 1985.

148. Raam S, Vrabel DM: Evaluation of an enzyme immunoassay kit for estrogen receptor measurements. Clin Chem 32:1496–1502, 1986.

149. Rae-Venter B, Nemoto K, Schneider SL, Dao LT: Prolactin binding by human mammary carcinoma: relationship to estrogen receptor protein concentration and patient age. Breast Cancer Res Treat 1:233–243, 1981.

150. Rao BR, Meyer JS: Estrogen and progestin receptors in normal and cancer tissue. *In* McGuire WL, Raynaud JP, Baulieu EE (eds): Progesterone Receptors in Normal and Neoplastic Tissues. New York, Raven Press, 1977, pp 155–169.

151. Redding TW, Schally AV: Inhibition of mammary tumor growth in rats and mice by administration of agonistic and antagonistic analogs of luteinizing hormone-releasing hormone. Proc Natl Acad Sci USA 80:1459–1462, 1983.

152. Redevilh G, Moncharmont B, Secco C, Baulieu E-E: Subunit composition of the molybdate stabilized "8-9s" nontransformed estradiol receptor purified from calf uterus. J Biol Chem 262:6969–6975, 1987.

153. Remele W, Bettendorf U: Mammakarzinon: Prognostisch wich-

tige rezeptorbestimmungen. Dtsch Arztebl 83:3359–3364, 1986.

154. Reubi JC, Maurer R, Von Werder K, Torhorst J, Klijn JGM, Lamberts SWJ: Somatostatin receptors in human endocrine tumors. Cancer Res 47:551–558, 1987.

154a. Rodbard D, Munson PJ, Thakur AK: Quantitative characterization of hormone receptors. Cancer 46:2907–2918, 1980.

155. Rosen PP, Menendez-Botet C, Nisselbaum JS, et al: Pathological review of breast lesions analyzed for estrogen receptor protein. Cancer Res 35:3187–3194, 1975.

156. Rosenthal LJ: Discrepant estrogen receptor protein levels according to surgical technique. Am J Surg 138:680–681, 1979.

157. Sainsbury JRC, Farndon JR, Needham GK, Malcolm AJ, Harris AL: Epidermal-growth-factor receptor status as a predictor of early relapse and death from breast cancer. Lancet I:1398–1402, 1987.

158. Sainsbury JRC, Farndon JR, Sherbet GV, Harris AL: Epidermal-growth-factor receptors and oestrogen receptors in human breast cancer. Lancet I:364–366, 1985.

159. Sainsbury JRC, Malcolm AJ, Appleton DR, Farndon JR, Harris AL: Presence of epidermal growth factor receptor as an indicator of poor prognosis in human breast cancer. J Clin Pathol 38:1225–1228, 1985.

160. Sanchez ER, Toft DO, Schlesinger MJ, Pratt WB: Evidence that the 90 kDa phosphoprotein associated with the untransformed L-cell glucocorticoid receptor is a murine heat shock protein. J Biol Chem 260:12398–12401, 1985.

161. Sando JJ, Hammond ND, Stratford CC, Pratt WB: Activation of thymocyte glucocorticoreceptors to the steroid binding form. The roles of reducing agents, ATP, and heat-stable factors. J Biol Chem 254:4779, 1979.

162. Sarfaty GA, Nash AR, Keightley DD (eds): Estrogen Receptor Assays in Breast Cancer: Laboratory Discrepancies and Quality Assurance. New York, Masson Publishing, 1981, pp 43–56.

163. Sato N, Hyder SM, Chang L, Thais A, Wittliff JL: Interaction of estrogen receptor isoforms with immobilized monoclonal antibodies. J Chromatogr 359:475–487, 1986.

164. Savage N, Levin J, De Moor NG, Lange M: Cytosolic oestrogen receptor content of breast cancer tissue in blacks and whites. S Afr Med J 59:623–624, 1981.

165. Scatchard G: The attraction of proteins for small molecules and ions. Ann NY Acad Sci 51:660–672, 1949.

166. Schally AV, Redding TW, Cai RZ, Paz JI, Ben-David M, Comaru-Schally M: Somatostatin analogs in the treatment of various experimental tumors. *In* On Hormonal Manipulations of Cancer: Peptides, Growth Factors and New (Anti) Steroidal Agents. New York, Raven Press, 1987, pp 431–440.

167. Schally AV, Redding TW, Comaru-Schally AM: Potential use of luteinizing hormone-releasing hormones in the treatment of hormone-sensitive neoplasms. Cancer Treat Res 68:281–289, 1984.

168. Schechter AL, Humg M-C, Vaidyanathan L, Weinberg RA, Yang-Feng TL, Franke U, Ulrich A, Coussens L: The *neu* gene: An *erbB*-homologous gene distinct from and unlinked to the gene encoding the EGF receptor. Science 229:976–978, 1985.

169. Schechter AL, Stern DF, Vaidyanathan L, Decker SJ, Drebin JA, Greene MI, Weinberg RA: The neu oncogene: an erb-b-related gene encoding a 185,000-Mr tumor antigen. Nature 312:513–516, 1984.

170. Schinzinger A: Uber carcinoma mammae. Bericht uber die Verhandlungen der Deutschen Gesellschaft fur Chirurgie, 18. Kongreßals Beilage zum Centralblatt fur Chir 29:55, 1889.

171. Shepel LA, Gorski J: Steroid hormone receptors and oncogenes. Biofactors 1:71–83, 1988.

172. Shintaku IP, Said JW: Detection of estrogen receptors with monoclonal antibodies in routinely processed formalin-fixed paraffin sections of breast carcinomas. Use of DNase pretreatment to enhance sensitivity of the reaction. Am J Clin Pathol 87:161–167, 1987.

173. Silfversward C, Gustafsson J-A, Gustafsson SA, Humla S, Nordenskjold TB, Wallgren A, Wrange O: Estrogen receptor concentrations in 269 cases of histologically classified human breast cancer. Cancer 45:2001–2005, 1980.

174. Singh VB, Moudgil VK: Protein kinase activity of purified rat liver glucocorticoid receptor. Biochem Biophys Res Commun 125:1067–1073, 1984.

175. Singh VB, Moudgil VK: Phosphorylation of rat liver glucocorticoid receptor. J Biol Chem 260:3684–3690, 1985.

176. Slamon DJ, Clark GM, Wong SG, Levin WJ, Ullrich A, McGuire WL: Human breast cancer: correlation of relapse and survival with amplification of the HER-2/neu oncogene. Science 235:177–182, 1987.

177. Slamon DJ, Godolphin W, Jones LA, Holt JA, Wong SG, Keith DE, Levin WJ, Stuart SG, Udove J, Ullrich A, Press MF: Studies of the HER-2/neu proto-oncogene in human breast and ovarian cancer. Science 244:707, 1989.

178. Sluyser M, Mester J: Oncogenes homologous to steroid receptors. Nature 315:546, 1985.

179. Steiner AE, Wittliff JL: Glucocorticoid receptors in normal human lymphocytes and human leukemia and lymphoma cells. J Clin Lab Anal 2:39–43, 1988.

180. Stern DF, Heffernau PA, Weinberg RA: A product of the neu proto-oncogene, is a receptor-like protein associated with tyrosine kinase activity. Mol Cell Biol 6:1729–1740, 1986.

181. Stewart JF, Rubens RD, Millis RR, King RJ, Hayward JL: Steroid receptors and prognosis in operable (stage I and II) breast cancer. Eur J Cancer Clin Oncol 19:1381–1387, 1983.

181a. Tandon AK, Clark GM, Chamness GC, Ullrich A, McGuire WL: HER-2/neu oncogene protein and prognosis in breast cancer. J Clin Oncol 7:1120–1128, 1989.

182. Thorpe SM: Monoclonal antibody technique for detection of estrogen receptors in human breast cancer: greater sensitivity and more accurate classification of receptor status than the dextran-coated charcoal method. Cancer Res 47:6572–6575, 1987.

183. Trams G, Maass H: Specific binding of estradiol and dihydrotestosterone receptors in human mammary cancers. Cancer Res 37:258–261, 1976.

183a. Twombly GH, Schoenewaldt EF: Tissue localization and excretion routes of radioactive diethylstilbestrol. Cancer 4:296–302, 1951.

184. van de Vijver M, Van de Bersselaar R, Deville P, Cornelisse C, Peterse J, Nusse R: Amplication of the neu (c-erb-B-2) oncogene in human mammary tumors is relatively frequent and is often accompanied by amplification of the linked c-erbA oncogene. Mol Cell Biol 7:2019–2023, 1987.

185. van der Walt LA, Wittliff JL: Assessment of progestin receptor polymorphism using HPLC. J Steroid Biochem 24:377–382, 1986.

186. Van Oosbree TR, Kim UH, Mueller GC: Affinity chromatography of estrogen receptors on diethylstilbestrol-agarose. Anal Biochem 136:321–327, 1984.

187. Varley JM, Swallon JE, Brammar WJ, Whittaker JL, Walker RA: Alterations to either c-erbB-2 (neu) or c-myc protooncogenes in breast carcinomas correlate with poor short-term prognosis. Oncogene 1:423–430, 1987.

188. Venter DJ, Tuzi NL, Kumar S, Gullick WJ: Overexpression of the c-erb-2 oncoprotein in human breast carcinomas: immunohistological assessment correlates with gene amplification. Lancet ii:69–72, 1987.

189. Walker ARP, Walter BF, Tshyabalala EN, Isaacson C, Segal I: Low survival of South African urban black women with breast cancer. Br J Cancer 49:241–244, 1984.

190. Wander HE, Blossey HC, Nagel GA, Kobberling J: The influence of various hormone therapies on steroid hormone receptor determinations in metastatic breast cancer. Aktuelle Onkologie 14:18–21, 1984.

191. Waseda N, Kato Y, Imura H, Kurata M: Effects of tamoxifen on estrogen and progesterone receptors in human breast cancer. Cancer Res 41:1984–1988, 1981.

192. Weigel NL: Isolation of protein kinases from chicken oviduct which phosphorylate the progesterone receptor *in vitro*. Abstract 2710, 1984. *Excerpta Medica* Abstracts of the 7th International Congress of Endocrinology. New York, Elsevier, 1984.

193. Weigel NL, Tash JS, Means AR, Schrader WT, O'Malley BW: Phosphorylation of hen progesterone receptor by cAMP de-

pendent protein kinase. Biochem Biophys Res Commun 102:513–517, 1981.
194. Welshons WV, Lieberman ME, Gorski J: Nuclear localization of unoccupied oestrogen receptors. Nature 307:747–749, 1984.
195. Williams MR, Walker KJ, Turkes A, Blamey RW, Nicholson RI: The use of an LH-RH agonist (ICI 118630, Zoladex) in advanced premenopausal breast cancer. Br J Cancer 53:629–636, 1986.
196. Wittliff JL: Specific receptors of the steroid hormones in breast cancer. Semin Oncol 1:109–118, 1974.
197. Wittliff JL: Steroid binding proteins in normal and neoplastic mammary cells. *In* Busch H (ed): Methods in Cancer Research, vol XI. New York, Academic Press, 1975, pp 293–354.
198. Wittliff JL: Steroid hormone receptors in breast cancer. Cancer 53:630–643, 1984.
199. Wittliff JL: HPLC of steroid-hormone receptors. Liquid Chromatogr-Gas Chromatogr 4(11):1092–1106, 1986.
200. Wittliff JL: Steroid hormone receptors. *In* Pesce AJ, Kaplan LA (eds): Methods in Clinical Chemistry. St. Louis, CV Mosby, 1987, pp 767–795.
201. Wittliff JL: Steroid receptors analyses, quality control and clinical significance. *In* Donegan WL, Spratt JS (eds): Cancer of the Breast. Philadelphia, WB Saunders, 1988, pp 303–335.
202. Wittliff JL, Beatty BW, Savlov ED, Patterson WB, Cooper RA Jr: Estrogen receptors and hormone dependency in human breast cancer. *In* St Arneault G, Ban P, Israel L (eds): Recent Results in Cancer Research. New York, Springer-Verlag, 1976, pp 59–77.
203. Wittliff JL, Daput O (eds): Steroid Receptors and Hormone-Dependent Neoplasia. New York, Masson Publishing, 1980.
204. Wittliff JL, Durant JR, Fisher B: Methods of steroid receptor analyses and their quality control in the clinical laboratory. *In* Soto R, DeNicola AF, Blaquier JA (eds): Physiopathology of Endocrine Diseases and Mechanisms of Hormone Action. New York, Alan R Liss, 1981, pp 397–411.
205. Wittliff JL, Feldhoff PA, Fuchs A, Wiehle RD: Polymorphism of estrogen receptors in human breast cancer. *In* Soto R, DeNicola AF, Blaquier JA (eds): Physiopathology of Endocrine Diseases and Mechanisms of Hormone Action. New York, Alan R Liss, 1981, pp 375–396.
206. Wittliff JL, Fisher B, Durant JR: Establishment of uniformity in steroid receptor analyses used in cooperative clinical trials of breast cancer treatment. *In* Henningsen B, Linder F, Steichele C (eds): Recent Results in Cancer Research, vol 71. Heidelberg, Spring-Verlag, 1980, pp 198–206.
207. Wittliff JL, Hilf R, Brooks WF Jr, Savlov ED, Hall TC, Orlando RA: Specific estrogen-binding capacity of the cytoplasmic receptor in normal and neoplastic tissues of humans. Cancer Res 32:1983–1992, 1972.
208. Wittliff JL, Lewko WM, Park DC, Kute TE, Baker DT JR, Kane LN: Steroid binding proteins of mammary tissues and their clinical significance in breast cancer. *In* McGuire WL (ed): Hormones, Receptors, and Breast Cancer, New York, Raven Press, 1978, pp 325–359.
209. Wittliff JL, Lin MT, van Aswegen C, Johnson WT, Wiehle RD: An improved assay for epidermal growth factor receptors in biopsies of endocrine responsive neoplasia. 1990, (sumbitted J Clin Lab Anal).
210. Wittliff JL, Savlov ED: Estrogen-binding capacity of cytoplasmic forms of the estrogen receptors in human breast cancer. *In* McGuire WL, Carbone PP, Vollmer EP (eds): Estrogen Receptors in Human Breast Cancer. New York, Raven Press, 1975, pp 73–91.
211. Wittliff JL, Wiehle RD: Analytical methods for steroid hormone receptors and their quality assurance. *In* Hollander VP (ed): Hormonally Responsive Tumors. New York, Academic Press, 1985, pp 383–428.
212. Wittliff JL, Wiehle RD, Hyder SM: HPLC as a means of characterizing the polymorphism of steroid hormone receptors. *In* Kerlavage AR (ed): The Use of HPLC in Receptor Biochemistry. New York, Alan R Liss, 1989, pp 155–199.
212a. Wittliff JL, Wittliff TH: Quality assurance programs for prognostic factors used in the management of endocrine responsive cancer. J Clin Immunoassay, 1990, in press.
213. Wynder EL, Kajitani T, Kuno J, Lucas JC, De Palo A, Farrow JA: Comparison of survival rates between American and Japanese patients with breast cancer. Surg Gynecol Obstet 117:196–200, 1963.
214. Young SC, Burkett RJ, Stewart C: Discrepancy in ER levels of breast carcinoma in biopsy vs mastectomy specimens. J Surg Oncol 29:54–56, 1985.

Chapter 44

ENDOCRINE THERAPY OF BREAST CANCER

S. P. Sheth, M.D. and Joseph C. Allegra, M.D.

Therapeutic hormonal manipulation for the management of systemic breast cancer has undergone a remarkable transition in the past two decades. In the early and middle parts of this century, surgical castration was the mainstay of therapy. In fact, most physicians believed that breast cancer in general was a surgical disease, and drugs were rarely mentioned. Since the 1950s there has been a resurgence of interest in drug therapy, and the pendulum has swung in the opposite direction, with the role of surgery limited to management of the primary tumor, infrequent local recurrence, and a rare oophorectomy. With the advent of new and exciting oral agents that are capable of perturbing the hormonal milieu, interest in surgical castration for the management of early and advanced breast cancer is waning.

SURGICAL APPROACH

Oophorectomy

In 1889, Schinzinger[133] postulated that because breast cancer seemed to be worse in young women, those women should be made older by removal of their ovaries, leading to atrophy of the breast and encapsulation of the breast cancer in the atrophying tissue. This method of treatment was first employed by Beatson[13] in 1896. He reported dramatic improvement following castration in three patients with inoperable breast cancer.

In the ensuing decade there were several reports by different investigators clearly showing regression of metastatic disease in approximately one third to two fifths of patients, with the median survival of the improved patients being two to three times that of the nonresponders (Table 44–1).[20, 85, 143]

In 1922 DeCourmelles[33] introduced radiation therapy to induce an artificial menopause. Dresser[35] in 1936 reported an improvement in a third of patients with osseous metastases treated with ovarian radiation. Thayssen[142] in 1948 reported improvement in 35 percent of patients treated by radiotherapeutic castration and also recorded a significantly longer 5-year survival in the castrated patients. Subsequently there were several reports dealing primarily with the rate of regression following therapeutic castration and the greater efficacy of oophorectomy compared with radiation therapy to the

ovaries. Now, however, on critical evaluation of those two modalities, it seems that both give similar results. The only major drawback to irradiation is the 8- to 10-week delay before the effect is evident.

With the recent availability of accurate reproducible methods of measuring receptor content of breast cancers and an effective oral triphenylethylene antiestrogen (tamoxifen), there have been several reports comparing oophorectomy to tamoxifen therapy.[24, 64, 120, 132] From these studies it can be concluded that tamoxifen is effective in approximately 30 percent of estrogen receptor (ER) unselected patients. The response rate is better in patients with estrogen receptor positive (ER +) and progesterone receptor positive (PR +) tumors. The data concerning oophorectomy following tamoxifen response or failure are less clear, but it may be reasonable to attempt this in patients with ER + tumors. (The value of tamoxifen in premenopausal women with node-negative breast cancer will be discussed later in this chapter.)

With this modest but clear improvement in survival following therapeutic castration, some investigators advocated prophylactic castration, hoping to prevent recurrence and thereby improve overall survival. This resulted in two decades of conflicting reports, with proponents of prophylactic castration presenting data justifying their theory.[55–58, 135] Most of those studies had a very small number of patients and lacked any randomization among prophylactic castration, therapeutic castration, and no castration. In reviewing the literature it does not appear that prophylactic castration following mastectomy decreases the potential relapse rate, nor

Table 44–1. RATES OF OBJECTIVE RESPONSE TO ABLATIVE THERAPY

Therapy	No. of Patients	Response Rate (%)	Range of Responses (%)
Ablation			
Oophorectomy	1674	33	21–41
Adrenalectomy	3739	32	23–46
Hypophysectomy	1174	36	22–58

Modified from Henderson IC, Canellos GP: N Engl J Med 302:1730, 1980.

does it prolong survival. This concept will be discussed in more detail in section XIV, chapter 39, dealing with adjuvant therapy.

In conclusion, bilateral oophorectomy still has a role in the management of premenopausal patients with metastatic breast disease, especially those with receptor positive tumors. Of those who show a response, the possibility of subsequent response to another hormonal modality is in the range of 40 percent to 50 percent.[71] Historically, patients who respond to sequential hormonal therapies survive longer than nonresponders.

Adrenalectomy

Hayward, in a book titled *Hormones and Breast Cancer*,[49] attributed failure of response to oophorectomy in some patients to the continued secretion of estrogens by the adrenal gland. Atkins[6] reported the removal of all but a small part of one adrenal gland in a series of six patients with advanced breast cancer. Two patients showed some improvement, but he abandoned the procedures because of a high complication rate.

It was after the discovery of synthetic cortisone in the early 1950s that total bilateral adrenalectomy became feasible. The earliest reports were from Huggins and Bergenstal.[59-61] In 1951, they reported six patients with advanced mammary cancer who underwent the procedure. Two patients were improved, one patient was moderately benefited, and there was no demonstrable evidence of regression in three patients.

In the following years this procedure gained wide acceptance in the therapy of metastatic breast carcinoma. It produced objective remissions in approximately 30 percent to 40 percent of the patients (Table 44-1). The mortality rate ranged from four percent to ten percent.[26, 32, 42, 46] This high morbidity and mortality and the fact that medical adrenalectomy showed comparable results (discussed in the next section) and was not an irreversible procedure like the surgical removal of glands led to a steep decline in utilization of surgical adrenalectomy.

There are a few reports of adrenalectomy-oophorectomy performed as a single combined procedure. Even though the response rate to the combined procedure higher, it did not result in an improved overall survival[62, 109] Replacement therapy for adrenalectomized patients is 50 to 70 mg cortisone per day orally with 0.1 mg of fluorohydrocortisone.

Hypophysectomy

The earliest reports regarding hypophysectomy are from Luft and Olivecrona.[94, 95] Of 50 patients with metastatic breast cancer, 20 demonstrated subjective or objective improvement for periods lasting from 3 to 27 months. Since then, numerous studies have been published.[66, 72, 73, 81, 94, 96, 115, 116, 119, 121] Most of these studies show a response rate of approximately 40 percent if patients are unselected by ER, which increases to 60 to 70 percent in receptor-positive patients. The highest response is seen in postmenopausal patients who are receptor positive and are 10 years or more from menopause.[98]

The two main approaches for hypophysectomy have been transfrontal and transsphenoidal; both have shown equal antitumor effect, although the transfrontal hypophysectomy appears to offer a more complete hormonal ablation.[12] The hormonal profile useful in predicting the completeness of the hypophysectomy contains basal and stimulated blood levels of the pituitary-derived polypeptide hormones, namely follicle-stimulating hormone (FSH), luteinizing hormone (LH), thyroid stimulating hormone (TSH), prolactin, and adrenocorticotrophic hormone (ACTH). The fact that complete ablation does not result in a greater antitumor effect makes meticulous testing unwarranted, except in situations where the extent of the replacement therapy is in question.

Replacement therapy generally consists of 40 to 50 mg of cortisone (10 mg in A.M., 10 mg 5:00 P.M., and 20 mg h.s.) with 0.1 to 0.3 mg of levothyroxine. Most patients develop transient diabetes insipidus postoperatively, which requires adequate fluid and electrolyte replacement, and a few patients who develop permanent diabetes insipidus require replacement therapy with posterior pituitary hormone.[12, 69, 80]

Harvey et al.[48] reported a comparative trial of transsphenoidal hypophysectomy and estrogen suppression with aminoglutethimide in advanced breast cancer. Three of 14 patients experienced partial objective tumor regression with a median duration of 4.6 months following hypophysectomy, whereas 10 of 21 patients who received aminoglutethimide responded with a median duration of 11.5 months.

Although several studies have reported minimal morbidity and mortality with the surgical approach, the advent of new therapeutic agents such as aminoglutethimide and tamoxifen (which will be discussed later in this chapter) that yield the same degree of response with minimal toxicity has led to a steep decline in the utilization of hypophysectomy.

NONSURGICAL APPROACH

In the 1960s, Jensen and Jacobson[65] and others[41, 141] demonstrated radiolabeled estradiol bound to some breast cancer specimens and correlated this with response to therapy. During the next 15 years, we have witnessed the standardization and increased use of reliable hormone receptor assays, which have simplified the selection of therapy in many patients. The steroid hormone receptor assay is performed on tissue cytosol (for a detailed account of hormonal assay techniques, see chapter 43). Only 100 to 200 mg of tissue is required. Cytoplasmic levels of estrogen receptor protein (ERP) and progesterone receptor protein (PRP) are usually reported as femtomoles (fmol) per mg of cytosol protein. A tumor with a level greater than 10 fmol/mg is usually considered positive, with 3–10 fmol/mg being borderline, and 0–3 fmol/mg being receptor negative. Although considerable effort is being made toward standardization of these values, there still is some variation in this cutoff for positivity among different laboratories.

The correlation between the presence of receptors and clinical response to all types of endocrine therapy has been well established. Approximately 50 percent to 60 percent of patients with receptor-positive tumors respond to hormonal therapy, whereas less than ten percent of receptor-negative tumors show any response to endocrine manipulations. Thus by using receptor status to select patients for hormonal therapy, the response rate is increased while patients with little chance of responding are spared exposure to ineffective treatment.

Estrogen, Androgen, and Progestin Therapy

Haddow et al.[7, 45] reported favorable effects of estrogenic hormones on advanced breast cancer in the early 1940s. Since then numerous studies have been published.[30, 53, 74, 86, 107, 108, 117, 118, 134, 139, 140] Approximately 30 percent to 35 percent of unselected postmenopausal patients demonstrate an objective response, while those with receptor-positive tumors exhibit up to a 50 percent overall response lasting up to 12–14 months. The most commonly used drug was diethylstilbestrol 15 mg p.o. daily in divided doses. Anorexia, nausea, and vomiting are the most distressing side effects. These can be minimized by using other preparations like conjugated estrogens (i.e., Premarin) 10 mg p.o. t.i.d. or synthetic estrogen (ethinyl estradiol; i.e., Estinyl) 3 mg daily. Prolonged use of all those preparations leads to fluid retention, increased libido, and withdrawal bleeding, but the most undesirable side effect is stress incontinence, especially in the elderly. The mechanism of action of high-dose estrogens is still not understood. It is felt that high pharmacological doses of estrogen are necessary for the effect, since some animal models demonstrate estrogen stimulation at a low dose and suppression at higher dosages.[88]

The other unexplained phenomenon is the uncommon flare of disease presenting as increased bone pain and hypercalcemia in patients with extensive bone metastasis who are started on estrogen therapy. If possible, the estrogen therapy should be continued, because this flare reaction may actually be the first sign of subsequent antitumor response. (For comparison of response rates of different sex steroid hormones, see Table 44–2.)

Androgens have also been studied extensively in postmenopausal patients and are considered less effective than estrogens.[74] However, some investigators believe that androgens show equal or superior results in patients with osseous metastases.[69]

Kennedy and Brown[70] reported a study that compared androgens, estrogens, or a combination of estrogen and androgen in 66 postmenopausal patients with advanced disease. Of the 22 patients receiving testosterone, three (13.6 percent) had objective improvement; ten of 22 patients (45.5 percent) on estrogen responded, and nine of 22 (40.9 percent) on the combined arm responded.

Table 44–2. OBJECTIVE RESPONSE RATE TO ADDITIVE FORMS OF ENDOCRINE THERAPY

Therapy	No. of Patients	Response Rate (%)	Range of Responses (%)
Hormones			
Estrogens	1683	26	15–38
Androgens	2250	21	10–38
Progestins	508	25	9–43
Corticosteroids	589	23	0–43
Antiestrogens			
Tamoxifen	504	35	22–49
Nafoxidine	283	31	28–38
Clomiphene	167	28	16–39

Modified from Henderson IC, Canellos GP: N Engl J Med 302:1730, 1980.

The duration of response and survival was similar in the responding patients in each therapy group.

The preparations available include testosterone propionate 100 mg intramuscularly (I.M.) three times a week or fluoxymesterone 10 mg p.o. twice a day. Side effects include fluid retention, nausea, vomiting, virilization, increased libido, erythrocytosis, hepatotoxicity, and hypercalcemia.

Since the first demonstration of responsiveness of breast cancer to progestational therapy by Escher and White in 1951,[37] there have been several studies showing response rates in the range of 20 percent to 40 percent.[4, 5, 34, 106, 123] Duration of response lasted 3–19 months, with a mean duration of approximately 12 months. There are several preparations available, but the most widely used is megestrol acetate (Megace). The usual dose is 40 mg orally four times a day. This drug is tolerated very well by most patients. There is no serious or life threatening toxicity reported, although there are some rare instances of deep vein thrombosis and carpal tunnel syndrome. Many of the patients do gain weight, but the increase is usually in the 2–5 lb range.

Morgan[103] reported a study comparing megestrol acetate and tamoxifen in postmenopausal patients with advanced breast cancer. One hundred and six patients participated. Forty-eight tamoxifen patients and 46 megestrol patients were evaluable. Patients characteristics were well balanced. Both treatments were well tolerated, and side effects were minimal, with weight gain being the most common side effect. Response rates were similar, with no organ site preference noted for either agent. The median duration of remission was not significantly different, and survival was also comparable in the responding patients.

Twenty-four patients who failed on tamoxifen were subsequently treated with megestrol acetate. A partial response was achieved in three of six patients who had demonstrated a prior response to tamoxifen. Twelve patients who failed on megestrol acetate were treated with tamoxifen, but none achieved an objective response.

Ross et al.[123] reported a study in which 49 advanced breast cancer patients who were treated with tamoxifen and either did not respond or subsequently relapsed were treated with megestrol acetate. Fifteen patients (31 percent) had partial remission, 16 (33 percent) had stable disease, and 17 (36 percent) had progressive disease, concluding that megestrol acetate is an effective agent for palliation of advanced breast cancer relapsing following a mixed response to tamoxifen therapy.

Medical Adrenalectomy

An aromatase inhibitor, aminoglutethimide (AG), developed as an anticonvulsant in the 1950s, was introduced for general use in the United States in 1960.[63] Documented adrenal insufficiency in patients receiving AG led to its restriction to investigational drug status in 1966. Further work showed that AG was capable of suppressing synthesis of all adrenal steroid hormones by blocking cholesterol side chain cleavage via inhibition of the enzymes 11β-hydroxylase and aromatase, thereby causing a "medical adrenalectomy." This led to several studies evaluating AG in metastatic breast cancer in postmenopausal patients.[44, 63, 125, 128] One thousand milligrams of AG and 40 mg of hydrocortisone (HC) as a replacement were administered orally daily. An objective response rate of 30 percent to 35 percent was observed in unselected patients, with a 50 percent response in women with estrogen-positive tumors.[127]

In 1981, Santen et al.[130] performed a randomized trial comparing bilateral surgical adrenalectomy and AG in postmenopausal women with metastatic breast cancer. Fifty-three percent of AG-HC treated patients and 43 percent of the surgical group responded objectively. An additional five percent in the adrenalectomy category experienced disease stabilization. No particular site of metastasis responded more favorably to one therapy when compared with the other. The duration of response and overall survival were similar. Santen et al. concluded that based on their experience, surgical adrenalectomy can logically be replaced by use of AG-HC.

Aminoglutethimide (Cytadren) inhibits the enzymatic conversion of cholesterol to pregneninolone, resulting in decreased production of adrenal glucocorticoids. It also blocks several other steps in the steroid synthesis, including the C-11, C-18, and C-21 hydroxylations and the hydroxylations required for the aromatization of androgens to estrogens. This blockade is not limited to the adrenal gland, as AG also inhibits aromatase in the adipose tissue, thereby limiting the peripheral conversion of androgens to estrogens. It is this latter effect that probably accounts for AG's antineoplastic effect; this inhibition required less administration of AG than necessary to inhibit normal steroidogenesis. AG is available in 250 mg tablets, is rapidly and completely absorbed after oral administration, and has a half-life of approximately 12 hours.

Side effects of aminoglutethimide are mainly dose dependent, with approximately 40 percent of the patients developing lethargy, ataxia, and dizziness at 1000 mg of AG per day,[129] while nearly all the patients developing these symptoms at dosages above 1500 mg/d.[91] A transient drug rash is reported in 30 percent to 35 percent of patients and consists of morbilliform macular lesions, often accompanied by fever, generally appearing within 7 to 14 days of therapy, and resolving spontaneously within 4 to 5 days without cessation of the drug.

Hypothyroidism may occur as a result of inhibition of thyroxine synthesis, so periodic thyroid function tests are recommended, with institution of replacement therapy when clinically indicated. Postural hypotension, leukopenia, neutropenia, and pancytopenia have been reported, especially with concurrent administration of chemotherapeutic agents. The current recommended dosage for AG is 250 mg orally four times a day together with 40 mg of hydrocortisone in divided doses (10 mg in the morning, 10 mg at 5:00 P.M., and 20 mg at bedtime). Dexamethasone should not be used as a replacement therapy, as AG induces rapid metabolism of dexamethasone.[91]

A new potent aromatase inhibitor, 4-hydroxyandrostene-3,17-dione (4-OHA), was evaluated in reports by Brodie et al,[21, 22] who treated 75 postmenopausal patients with 4-OHA. Effective suppression of estradiol levels were achieved. Fourteen of 52 patients (27 percent) responded in a group treated intramuscularly; of the patients treated orally, eight of 23 (35 percent) responded. Side effects included sterile abscess in six patients given I.M. injections, two allergic type reactions, and lethargy in four patients. Further testing will be required, but the preliminary data show 4-OHA to be as effective as AG without the problems of complete adrenal blockade and with potentially fewer side effects.

Antiestrogens

There is now convincing evidence supporting the hypothesis that estrogens play a major role in the growth of mammary cancer. Also, there is no question that depriving a tumor of estrogen by an ablative procedure (discussed in the first part of this chapter) leads to a response in approximately a third of patients.

Some clinical and laboratory data showed persistence of low levels of estrogen production and excretion.[25, 31, 43, 102, 137] This led to refining the approach to hormonal therapy of breast cancer by utilizing a new class of chemical compounds: the antiestrogens, nonsteroidal compounds that antagonize estrogen effects. Many of them are amino-ether derivatives of polycyclic phenols. Their main characteristic is blocking the uptake of estradiol in both experimental and human tumors.[10, 97] A number of nonsteroidal antiestrogens were synthesized, but most of them were abandoned because of poor activity, toxicity, or lack of overall superiority over tamoxifen.[15, 67, 77, 79, 150] We will discuss a few of them briefly and also look at the new compounds currently undergoing clinical trials.

Clomiphene citrate (Clomid)[149] is related to other triarylethylene compounds such as estrogen chlorotrianisene. This was the first antiestrogen to show activity in breast cancer.[50, 52] It has not been extensively studied, and it is not currently approved for treatment of breast cancer. Hecker and associates[50] published a study showing a 39 percent overall response with minimal side effects (nausea) and a mean duration of response of approximately 1 year.

Nafoxidine is a diphenyldihydronaphthalene-derived, synthetic nonsteroidal antiestrogen[82] extensively studied in Europe, with a few studies from the United States.[16, 17, 38, 131] The response rate varied between 20 percent and 35 percent (mean, 30 percent), with higher response in receptor-positive patients and virtually no response in receptor-negative patients. The usual dose is 60 mg orally three times a day. Nafoxidine was better tolerated than estrogens, but the side effects were not infrequent. Skin toxicity included dryness, icthyosis, and photosensitivity on prolonged usage (more than 3 months). Those effects were not life threatening but did result in interrupted therapy.

Trioxifen mesylate[146] was studied by Lee and coworkers.[83] They reported an overall response of 52 percent, with ten percent complete responders. The median time to progression was 12 months. Toxicity was mild and mainly consisted of nausea, vomiting, hot flashes, increased bone pain, fluid retention, and drug rash. Approximately three percent of patients developed hypercalcemia. Their overall impression was that trioxifen mesylate is an active agent with similar therapeutic efficacy and toxicity to tamoxifen.

Witte et al.[150] treated 36 patients with graded doses of trioxifen. The low-dose group had a 21 percent response rate in 24 patients, and the high-dose group had a 33 percent response rate in 12 patients. Toxicities were non–dose-dependent and consisted of nausea (31 percent) and leukopenia (41 percent). They concluded that trioxifen is no more efficacious than tamoxifen and has more toxicity.

Tamoxifen is a triphenylethylene antiestrogen active in the treatment of breast cancer. It has been studied extensively and currently enjoys wide clinical usage.[9, 28, 76, 84, 99, 104, 111, 136, 145, 148] The response rate is 30 percent in unselected patients, 50 percent in ER-positive patients, and 60 percent to 75 percent in ER-positive and PR-positive patients. Tamoxifen is a nonsteroidal agent that has demonstrated potent antiestrogenic properties in animal models. In dimethylbenzanthracene (DMBA)-induced rat mammary carcinoma, tamoxifen caused regression of tumors and also inhibited induction of tumors. In a major clinical study conducted by the National Surgical Adjuvant Breast and Bowel Project (NSABP, protocol B-09),[40] major benefit was seen when tamoxifen was added to the adjuvant chemotherapy regimen in postmenopausal patients with four or more positive axillary lymph nodes and receptor levels greater than 10 fmol/mg. In another randomized clinical trial (NSABP B-14),[39] tamoxifen was evaluated in the treatment of node-negative patients who had receptor-positive tumors. There were 2644 patients randomized in this double-blind placebo-controlled trial. There was no survival advantage during 4 years of follow-up, but there was a significant prolongation of disease-free survival among both the premenopausal and the postmenopausal

patients. Treatment failure was significantly reduced, not only locally but also with respect to distant metastases, in patients treated with tamoxifen. There were fewer new primary tumors in the opposite breast, and those women also had a decreased incidence of local recurrence after lumpectomy and primary breast irradiation.

Tamoxifen is available only in 10-mg tablets. The usual dose is 10 mg orally twice a day, and there is no dose-related difference in response rate.[148] The initial half-life is 7 to 14 hours, with secondary peaks 4 or more days later. This is believed to be a result of enterohepatic circulation. The prolonged half-life and relative lack of serious toxicity are the major attractions of tamoxifen therapy.

The side effects reported most frequently are hot flashes (15 percent), nausea (ten percent), and vomiting, but they are rarely severe enough to require discontinuation of therapy. Thrombocytopenia and leukopenia are seen in five to ten percent of patients and especially in those patients with preexisting bone marrow compromise; thus a periodic complete blood count is recommended.

Increased bone and tumor pain and local flare of disease have been reported. These are sometimes associated with good tumor response. Some patients with bone metastasis develop hypercalcemia after a few weeks of tamoxifen therapy; calcium levels should be checked in those patients and, if elevated, should be treated appropriately. Less common side effects include vaginal bleeding (less than five percent), vaginal discharge, menstrual irregularities, erythematous skin rash, and rarely, thromboembolic events.

New Antiestrogens

There are several new antiestrogens undergoing clinical trials, and a few of them show promising preliminary results. Toremifene[68] is a triphenylethylene antiestrogen with a high affinity to estrogen receptors. Tamoxifen 4-OH is a metabolite of tamoxifen and mifepristone[11] (Ru 486), an antiprogestin and antiglucocorticoid. Further studies are under way to define the usefulness of those agents.

Other New Agents Under Investigation

Luteinizing hormone releasing hormone (LH-RH), or gonadotrophin releasing hormone (Gn-RH), when released from the hypothalamus in a pulsatile manner stimulates the pituitary to secrete luteinizing hormone (LH) and follicle-stimulating hormone (FSH). This stimulates the ovaries to increase estrogen production. This led to the production of several LH-RH analogues that were initially tested in animals. When injected, they were found to paradoxically inhibit LH and FSH production and, therefore, estrogen production. It appears that in vivo LH-RH is released in a pulsatile manner, which is stimulating, but chronic release is inhibitory. Thus if the ovaries are exposed to chronic exogenous administration of those analogues, it could result in a "medical castration." In males, the inhibition of FSH and LH leads to castration levels of testosterone. LH-RH agonists have been extensively studied in males with prostatic cancer and found to be as effective as orchiectomy.[36]

The agonists currently available include leuprolide (D-LEU-6-Gn-RH proethylamide), nafarelin, and buserelin (Zoladex). Leuprolide has been approved for use in prostate cancer, but the others are still undergoing trials. We will briefly review a few of the recent studies (see Table 44–3).

Harvey et al.[47] reported on the Abbott study group trial of leuprolide in advanced breast carcinoma. Twenty-five premenopausal patients were treated with an escalating dosage schedule (1 mg, 5 mg, and 10 mg). There were no complete remissions; 11 of 25 (44 percent) had a partial response with a median duration of response of 39 weeks. Dose escalation did not result in improved response; six of 14 ER-positive patients responded, and four of ten ER-negative patients responded. Toxicity was minimal, and most frequently consisted of hot flashes, nausea, vomiting, headache, and amenorrhea. In another study,[48] 32 postmenopausal patients with advanced disease were treated with an escalating dosage of leuprolide; two of 20 (ten percent) responded at 1 mg, and one of 20 (five percent) responded at 10 mg/d. Thus it appears that low-dose leuprolide is effective only in premenopausal patients, confirming that its primary action is blocking ovarian estrogen production and not a direct tumoricidal effect.

Buserelin was tried by Klijn and DeJong[78] in 32 premenopausal patients with metastatic breast cancer. The initial treatment was intravenous, but was subsequently randomized between intranasal and subcutaneous routes. Overall, nine of 23 patients (39 percent) responded. In the intranasal group, four of 12 responded, and in the subcutaneous, five of 11. Buserelin was also tried in combination with tamoxifen (three of five patients responding) and with megestrol acetate (two of four responding).

Nicholson et al.[110] reported on the use of buserelin in premenopausal patients. The overall response was 31 percent. ER-negative patients did not respond, whereas ER-positive patients showed a 55 percent response, and ER unknown, 40 percent. Nine postmenopausal women were treated with buserelin, and two responded, ages 58 and 54 years. Pretreatment estrogen levels were not reported. Mathé et al[100] studied D Trp 6 LH-RH in 23

heavily pretreated women with metastatic breast cancer. Three of 11 premenopausal patients responded, and three of 15 postmenopausal patients responded.

A phase II study of buserelin was recently reported by Hoffken et al.[54] The overall response was 42 percent in 19 premenopausal patients with advanced breast cancer; five of 19 (26 percent) achieved a complete response, and three of 19 (16 percent) had a partial response. None of the four ER-negative patients responded, six of 11 ER-positive patients (55 percent) responded, and two of four ER-unknown (50 percent) showed response.

On analyzing those studies it appears that LH-RH agonists are active against breast cancer. Their mechanism of action is by suppressing FSH and LH secretion, which leads to decreased estrogen production. Although most of those studies had a small number of patients and only a few evaluated response by ER status, there was a strong correlation between ER status and response. This preliminary data is very encouraging. If safe and easy methods of administration become available, then LH-RH agonists may become the first line of therapy, replacing oophorectomy in premenopausal patients with advanced breast cancer.

ROLE OF CHEMOHORMONAL THERAPY IN BREAST CANCER

As discussed in previous sections, hormonal therapy used in an additive or ablative mode plays a major role in the treatment of advanced breast cancer. The new group of antiestrogens has added yet another tool to the armamentarium against breast cancer. The availability of receptor studies has enhanced the ability to choose appropriate therapy for pre- and postmenopausal patients. The pioneering work on single-agent and combination chemotherapy (discussed in chapter 42) has enhanced the ability to treat receptor-negative patients and those who have progressive disease on hormonal therapy.

There is no question that both hormonal therapy and cytotoxic chemotherapy have taken great strides in trying to alter the natural history of metastatic breast cancer. Unfortunately, these therapies are palliative, and all patients with metastatic breast cancer eventually die from the disease. The combination of cytotoxic chemotherapy and endocrine manipulation in chemohormonal therapy has been an attempt to move from a

Table 44–3. LHRH AGONISTS IN PREMENOPAUSAL PATIENTS

Study Group/Author(s)	ER +	ER −	Agent	No.	CR	CR + PR	
Abbott Study Group	6/14	4/10	Leuprolide	25	—	11/25	(44%)
Klijn JGM, DeJong FH[78]			Buserelin	32	—	9/23	(39%)
Nicholson RI, et al[110]	11/20	0/18	Buserelin	45	—	14/45	(35%)
Mathé G, et al[100]			D-Trp 6 LH-RH	11	—	3/11	(27%)
Hoffken K, et al[54]	6/11	0/4	Buserelin	19	5/19	8/19	(42%)
TOTAL	23/45	4/32				45/123	(37%)

From Hamm JT, Allegra JC: New Hormonal Therapy. In press. Reprinted by permission.

palliative mode to a curative mode as the combination of these two different approaches attempts to take advantage of the well-described heterogeneity in breast cancer. The hypothesis is based on the efficacy of hormones against the well-differentiated ER+ cells in the tumor, while cytotoxic chemotherapy is utilized to kill the more rapidly dividing cellular components.

With these facts in mind, it was postulated that the two therapies combined together as chemohormonal therapy might have either an additive or synergistic effect leading to higher complete remission rates and possible cure. Various trials were undertaken using different well-proven combination chemotherapy regimens added to hormonal agents (ablative or additive). In the late 1970s and early 1980s, these regimens were used in both metastatic breast cancer and also in the adjuvant setting.

The results of those trials unfortunately did not demonstrate the expected results and yielded many surprises. This section will present a brief review of representative studies.

During the past two decades, numerous trials were conducted whereby the value of hormonal agents added to cytotoxic chemotherapy was evaluated in advanced disease.[1-3, 14, 19, 75, 89, 112, 138, 147] Although the majority of trials have a simple design, analysis of the trials is difficult. The first difficulty encountered is sample size, with most of the studies having fewer than a hundred patients. Potential selection bias is also an issue, with each study having different inclusion and exclusion criteria. Third, the majority of trials have a group of patients with unknown receptor status, and the response rate for that subset of patients cannot be fully evaluated. Finally, different hormonal agents were utilized, making valid comparisons among different studies nearly impossible.

Cocconi et al.[27] tested cyclophosphamide, methotrexate, and 5-fluorouracil (CMF) against CMF + tamoxifen. They reported a 74 percent overall response rate in the chemohormonal arm, and a 51 percent response rate with chemotherapy alone. Despite the higher response rate, there was no statistically significant improvement in survival. Tormey et al.[144] studied dibromodulcitol (DI) and doxorubicin (DO), with and without tamoxifen. The overall response in the DIDO + TAM arm was 55 percent vs. 36 percent in the DIDO alone. This also did not result in any improvement in survival, although the overall response rate was higher. In an excellent review done by Lippman,[90] most of the studies showed a higher initial response rate, with complete and partial responses ranging from 30 percent to 70 percent. This was statistically significant, but additional follow-up demonstrated no difference in median duration of response or in overall survival (Table 44–4).

It is important to note that the responses achieved were at a cost of considerable toxicity and therefore altered quality of life. It does not appear appropriate at this point to recommend the routine combination of cytotoxic chemotherapy with endocrine therapy in the management of metastatic breast cancer.

Various theories have been suggested to explain why the combination of chemohormonal therapy did not yield the anticipated benefits. Perhaps breast cancer does not consist of only two clones of cells (i.e., chemosensitive and hormone resistant or hormone sensitive and chemoresistant). There is some experimental evidence that clones of cells exist that are hormone resistant and chemosensitive, but the evidence of the converse is not well established. There may also be cells that are resistant to both modalities. Also, if hormones are cytostatic and not cytotoxic and lead to an arrest of growth in G_0 or early G_1, then this effect may make cytotoxic chemotherapy less effective, with the chemohormonal combination leading to an antagonistic result. Finally, there could be drug interactions between the two therapies (e.g., the modulation of certain enzymes by a hormone), which would effect the metabolism of the cytotoxic drugs, leading to their decreased effectiveness.

These findings led to a phase II clinical trial at the University of Louisville designed to test a variation of standard combination chemohormonal therapy: synchronization-stimulation of tumor cells in order to potentially increase the chemoresponsiveness of breast cancer. In this trial, endocrine therapy was used to synchronize tumor cells, and these cells were then rescued by a second hormonal manipulation. The rescue aspect of this schema was an attempt to increase the number of cells in the S phase of the cell cycle. The cells were then subsequently treated with S phase–specific cytotoxic chemotherapy in an attempt to further enhance cell kill. This clinical trial schema was based on laboratory observations. Lippman et al.[88] have studied the effects of estrogens and antiestrogens on growth of human breast cancer cells in great detail. In a human breast cancer cell model in long-term tissue culture, they showed that estrogen stimulates the growth of human mammary carcinoma, whereas the antiestrogen tamoxifen inhibits growth. The tamoxifen growth inhibition can be "rescued" by physiological concentrations of an estrogen. They observed a marked rise in thymidine incorporation in the rescued cells to levels exceeding both control and estrogen-stimulated cells. These data suggest that cells were arrested by antiestrogen in a uniform stage of cell cycle. They postulated that when estradiol addition reversed the tamoxifen inhibition, a larger proportion of the cells entered the DNA synthetic phase of the cell cycle, and the nucleoside incorporation increased dramatically.

Combination chemohormonal therapy is therefore based on the observations that breast cancers exhibit cellular heterogeneity with regard to estrogen receptor status, that hormonal therapy and chemotherapy have different mechanisms of action and of toxicity, and further, that cell cycle–specific agents are most effective against rapidly dividing cells. It was our hypothesis that utilizing hormone therapy and chemotherapy in this manner would result in a better response than that resulting from either therapy alone.

Fifty-seven patients with histologically documented measurable advanced breast cancer were entered into this clinical trial between July 1980 and July 1984. Thirty

Table 44–4. RESULTS OF RANDOMIZED TRIALS OF CHEMOTHERAPY AND ENDOCRINE THERAPY VS. CHEMOTHERAPY IN PRE- AND POSTMENOPAUSAL WOMEN WITH ADVANCED DISEASE

Investigators	No. of Patients	Receptor Status	Therapy	Complete & Partial Response Rates (%)	Survival Months	p value
Cocconi G, et al[27]	62	NA	CMF + TAM	74	18	NS
	71		CMF	51	27	
Tormey DC, et al[144]	67	NA	DIDO + TAM	55	11.2	NS
	55		DIDO	36	8.9	
Mouridsen HT, et al[105]	115	NA	CMF + TAM	74		0.066
	105		CMF	49		
Brunner KW,	48	NA	CMFVP + DES	63	26.7	NS
Sonntag RW[23]	48		CMFVP	54	19.2	
Boccardo F, et al[18]	32	NA	CMFV-DOC + TAM	75		NS
	36		CMFV-DOC	42		
Rubens RD, et al[124]	36 +	NA	DOV + Prog	53	8	NS
	33		DOV	61	15	

Abbreviations: C, cyclophosphamide; DES, diethylstilbestrol; DI, dibromodulcitol; DO, doxorubicin; F, 5-fluorouracil; M, methotrexate; NS, not significant; P, prednisone; Prog, progesterone; TAM, tamoxifen; V, vincristine.
Modified from Lippman ME: Breast Cancer Res Treat 3:117–127, 1983.

of the patients, or 53 percent, had tumors that were estrogen receptor positive. Twenty were estrogen receptor negative, and seven had tumors of unknown estrogen receptor status. Patients received tamoxifen 10 mg orally twice a day for 10 days. The tamoxifen was then discontinued, and the patients received premarin, a conjugated estrogen, in a dosage of 0.625 mg orally twice a day for 4 days. On the fourth day of premarin therapy, the patients received methotrexate 200 mg/m^2 intravenously, followed in 1 hour by 5-fluorouracil 600 mg/m^2 intravenously. Twenty-four hours later, the patients were rescued with leucovorin orally at 10 mg/m^2 every 6 hours for six doses. The treatment cycle was repeated every 18 days.

Overall response rate was 62 percent, with 37 percent complete remissions and 25 percent partial remissions. Stable disease was achieved in 21 percent of patients, and only 17 percent of the patients exhibited progressive disease. There were no significant differences in response as a function of ER status, menopausal status, dominant site of disease, or prior therapy. The median duration of remission was 14 months. The median survival for the group overall was 24 months, with responders showing a twofold increase in their median survival. This was statistically significant.

A prior attempt to test this synchronization-stimulation concept was also undertaken at the National Cancer Institute, Medicine Branch. Patients were randomized between cyclophosphamide, methotrexate, 5-fluorouracil, and doxorubicin with or without tamoxifen and premarin. The group receiving the antihormone hormone combination had a significantly longer median duration of remission. Although complete remission rates in that trial did not approach our 37 percent complete remission rate, the overall treatment regimens were very different, and our patient population was more favorable. In the European Organization for Research on the Treatment of Cancer (EORTC)[126] study, aminoglutethimidethinylestradiol was followed by 5-fluorouracil-doxorubicin-cyclophosphamide chemotherapy. The overall response in 41 patients was 74 percent, with 37 percent of the patients achieving a complete remission. Median duration of remission and survival and ER status were not recorded. As in our clinical trial, these investigators found no difference in response rates as a function of dominant metastatic site, menopausal status, or ER status.

There are several other studies utilizing the same concept of sequential hormone priming followed by chemotherapy.[14, 19, 29, 92, 112, 113, 138] The response ranged from as low as six percent overall response in the study published by Bowman[19] to as high as 75 percent in the study published by Paridaens et al.[112] Overall, the median response ranged from 40 percent to 60 percent. Clearly, with multiple groups reporting promising and similar results, additional large-scale trials to further test these concepts are warranted.

References

1. Allegra JC: Methotrexate and 5-fluorouracil following tamoxifen and premarin in advanced breast cancer. Semin Oncol 10(suppl 2):23–28, 1983.
2. Allegra JC, Woodcock TM, et al: A phase II trial of tamoxifen, premarin, methotrexate, and 5-fu in metastatic breast cancer. Breast Cancer Res Treat 2:93–99, 1982.
3. Allegra JC, Woodcock TM, Seeger J, Stevens D: A phase II trial of tamoxifen, premarin, methotrexate, and 5-fluorouracil in metastatic breast cancer. *In* Klign JG (ed): Hormonal Manipulation of Cancer: Peptides, Growth Factors, and New Antisteroidal Agents. New York, Raven Press, 1987, pp 459–501.
4. Ansfield FJ, Davis HL, Ellerby RA, Ramirez G: A clinical trial of megestrol acetate in advanced breast cancer. Cancer 33:907–910, 1974.
5. Ansfield FJ, Davis HL Jr, Ramire G, Davis TE, Borden EC, Johnson RO, Bryan GT: Further clinical studies with megestrol acetate in advanced breast cancer. Cancer 38:53–55, 1976.
6. Atkins HJB: Carcinoma of the breast. Ann R Coll Surg (Engl) 38:133, 1966.
7. Badger GM, Elson LA, Haddow A, Hewett CL, Robinson AM: Inhibition of growth by chemical compounds. Proc R Soc London 130:255–299, 1942.
8. Baker WH, Kelly RM, Sohier WD: Hormonal treatment of

metastatic carcinoma of the breast. Am J Surg 99:538–543, 1960.

9. Band P, Israel L: Treatment of advanced breast cancer with tamoxifen—10 mg b.i.d.: preliminary report. (Abstract) Proceedings of the American Society of Clinical Oncology. Proc Am Assoc Cancer Res 17:237, 1976.

10. Barbosa J, Seal US, Doe RP: Antiestrogens and plasma proteins. J Clin Endocrinol Metab 36:666–678, 1973.

11. Barden S, Vignon F, Chalbos D, Rochefort H: RU486, a progestin and glucocorticoid antagonist inhibits the growth of breast cancer cells via the progesterone receptor. J Clin Endocrin Metab 60:692–697, 1985.

12. Bates T, Rubens RD, Bulbrook RD, Goodwin PR, Wang DY, Knight RK, Hayward JL: Comparison of pituitary function and clinical response after transphenoidal and transfrontal hypophysectomy for advanced breast cancer. Eur J Cancer 12:775–782, 1976.

13. Beatson GT: On the treatment of inoperable cases of carcinoma of the mamma. Lancet 2:104–107, 1896.

14. Benz C, Candara D, Miller B, Drakes T, Monroe S, Wilbur B, DeGregorio M: Chemoendocrine pharmacokinetics and toxicity. Cancer Treat Rep 71:283–289, 1987.

15. Black LJ, Goode RL: Uterine bioassay of tamoxifen, trioxifene and a new estrogen antagonist (LY 117018) in mice and rats. Life Sci 26:1453–1458, 1980.

16. Bloom HJC, Boesen E: Antioestrogens in treatment of breast cancer: value of nafoxidine in 52 advanced cases. Br Med J 2:7–10, 1974.

17. Bloom HJC, Roe FJC, Mitchley BCV: Sex hormones and renal neoplasia. Cancer 20:2118–2124, 1967.

18. Boccardo F, Robagotti A, Rosso R, Santi L: Chemotherapy with or without tamoxifen in advanced breast cancer, 5 year results of a randomized trial. (Abstract) J Steroid Biochem 19(suppl):2125, 1983.

19. Bowman D: A phase II evaluation of sequential tamoxifen, premarin, methotrexate, and 5-fluorouracil in refractory stage IV breast cancer. Proc ASCO C413, 1983.

20. Boyd S: On oophorectomy in the cancer of the breast. Br Med J 2:1161, 1900.

21. Brodie AMH, Dewsett M, Coombs RE: Aromatase inhibitors and control of breast cancer. Proc AACR, 25:472–473, 1987.

22. Brodie AMH, Garrett W, Hendrickson JR, Tsai-Morris Ch, Williams JG: Aromatase inhibitors, their pharmacology and application. J Steroid Biochem 19:53–58, 1983.

23. Brunner KW, Sonntag RW: Combined chemo and hormonal therapy in advanced breast cancer. Cancer 39:2923–2933, 1977.

24. Buchanan RN, Blamey RT, Durrant KR, Howell A, Paterson AG, Preece PE, Smith DC, Williams CJ, Wilson RG: A randomized comparison of tamoxifen with surgical oophorectomy in premenopausal patients with advanced breast cancer. J Clin Oncol 4:1326–1330, 1986.

25. Bulbrook RD, Greenwood FC: Persistence of urinary oestrogen excretion after oophorectomy and adrenalectomy. Br Med J 1:662–666, 1957.

26. Cade S: Adrenalectomy for breast cancer. Br Med J 1:1–5, 1955.

27. Cocconi G, DeLisi V, Boni C, Mori P, Malacarne P, Amadori D, Giovanelli E: Chemotherapy versus combination of chemotherapy and endocrine therapy in advanced breast cancer. Cancer 51:581–588, 1983.

28. Cole MP, Todd IDH: Tamoxifen (ICI 46474). Clinical experience in 129 patients with advanced breast cancer. In Namer M, Lalane CM (eds): Hormones and Breast Cancer. Paris, INSERM, 1976, p 245.

29. Conte PF, Pronzato P, Rubagotti A, Alama A, Amadori D, Demicheli R, Gardin G, Gentilini P, Jacomuzzi A, Lionetto R, Monzeglio C, Nicolin A, Rosso R, Sismondi P, Sussio M, Santi L: Conventional versus cytokinetic polychemotherapy with estrogenic recruitment in metastatic breast cancer: results of a randomized cooperative trial. J Clin Oncol 5:339–347, 1987.

30. Council on Drugs, Subcommittee on Breast and Genital Cancer, Committee on Research, AMA: Androgens and estrogens in the treatment of disseminated mammary carcinoma-retrospective study of 944 patients. JAMA 172:1271–1283, 1960.

31. Dao TL-Y: Estrogen excretion in women with mammary cancer before and after adrenalectomy. Science 118:21–22, 1953.

32. Dao TL, Huggins CB: Metastatic cancer of breast treated by adrenalectomy. JAMA 165:1793–1797, 1957.

33. DeCourmelles FV: La radiotherapie indirecte ou dirigee par les correlation organiques. Arch Elect Med 32:264, 1922.

34. DeLena M, Brambilla C, Valagussa P, Bonadonna G: High dose medroxyprogesterone acetate in breast cancer resistant to endocrine and cytoxic therapy. Cancer Chemother Pharmacol 2:175–180, 1979.

35. Dresser R: The effect of ovarian irradiation on the bone metastases of the cancer of the breast. AJR 35:384, 1936.

36. Eisenberger MA, O'Dwyer PJ, Friedman MA: Gonadotropin hormone-releasing hormone analogues: a new approach for prostatic carcinoma. J Clin Oncol 4:414–424, 1986.

37. Escher GC, White A (eds): Symposium on Steroids in Experimental and Clinical Practice. Philadelphia, P Blukiston & Son, 1951, pp 402–448.

38. European Breast Cancer Group, EORTC: Clinical trial of nafoxidine, an oestrogen antagonist in advanced breast cancer. Eur J Cancer 8:387–389, 1972.

39. Fisher B, Constantino J, Redmond C, Poisson R, Bowman D, Couture J, Dimitrov NV, Wolmark N, Wickerham DL, Fisher ER, Margolese R, Robidoux A, Shibata H, Terz J, Paterson AHG, Feldman MI, Farrar W, Evans J, Lickley HL, Ketner M: A randomized clinical trial evaluating tamoxifen in the treatment of patients with node-negative breast cancer who have estrogen receptor positive tumors. N Engl J Med 320:479–484, 1989.

40. Fisher B, Redmond C, Brown A, Fisher ER, Wolmark N, Bowman D, Plotkin D, Wolter J, Bornstein R, Legault-Poisson S, Saffer EA, and other NSABP investigators: Adjuvant chemotherapy with and without tamoxifen in the treatment of primary breast cancer: 5-year results from the national surgical adjuvant breast and bowel project trial. J Clin Oncol 4(4):459–471, 1986.

41. Folca PJ, Glascock RF, Irvine WT: Studies with tritium-labelled hexoestrol in advanced breast cancer. Lancet 2:796–798, 1961.

42. Galante M, Fournier DJ: Adrenalectomy for metastatic breast cancer. JAMA 163:1011–1016, 1957.

43. Greenwood FC, Bulbrook RD: Effect of hypophysectomy on urinary oestrogen in breast cancer. Br Med J 1:666–668, 1957.

44. Griffiths CT, Hall TG, Saba Z, Barlow J, Nevinny H: Preliminary trial of aminoglutethimide in breast cancer. Cancer 32:31–37, 1973.

45. Haddow A, Watkinson JM, Paterson E, Koller PC: Influence of synthetic oestrogens upon advanced malignant disease. Br Med J 2:393–398, 1944.

46. Harris HS, Spratt JS: Bilateral adrenalectomy in metastatic mammary cancer. Cancer 23:145–151, 1969.

47. Harvey HA, Lipton A, Max DT, Perlman HG, Diaz-Perches R, de la Garza J: Medical castration produced by the GnRH analogue leuprolide to treat metastatic breast cancer. J Clin Oncol 3:1068–1072, 1985.

48. Harvey HA, Santen RJ, Osterman J, Samojlik E, White D, Lipton A: A comparative trial of transsphenoidal hypophysectomy and estrogen suppression with aminoglutethimide in advanced breast cancer. Cancer 43:2207–2214, 1979.

49. Hayward J: Hormones and Cancer. London, Wm Heinemann, 1979, pp 638–670.

50. Hecker E, Begh I, Levy CM, Magnin CA, Martinez JC, Loureiro J, Garola RE: Clinical trial of clomiphene in advanced breast cancer. Eur J Cancer 10:747–749, 1974.

51. Henderson IC, Canellos GP: Cancer of the breast, the past decade. N Engl J Med 302:1730, 1980.

52. Herbst AL, Griffiths CT, Kistner RW: Clomiphene citrate (NSC-35770) in disseminated mammary carcinoma. Cancer Chemother Rep 43:39–41, 1964.

53. Herman JB, Adair FE, Woodward HQ: Effect of estrogenic hormone on advanced carcinoma of the female breast. Arch Surg 54:1–9, 1947.

54. Hoffken K, Becher R, Kurschel E, Doberauer C, Anders CU, Callies R, Miller B, Miller AA, Schmidt CG: LHRH analogue (buserelin) treatment in premenopausal patients with advanced breast cancer. Proc ASCO 204, 1987.

55. Horsely GW: Treatment of cancer of the breast in premenopausal patients with radical amputation and bilateral oophorectomy. Ann Surg 125:703–717, 1947.

56. Horsely GW, et al: Carcinoma of the breast. Va Med 87:62, 1957.

57. Horsley JS III: Twenty years experience with prophylactic bilateral oophorectomy in the treatment of carcinoma of the breast. Ann Surg 155:935, 1962.

58. Huck P: Artificial menopause as an adjuct to radical treatment of breast cancer. NZ Med J 51:364, 1952.

59. Huggins CB: Control of cancers of man by endocrinologic methods: review. Cancer Res 16:825–830, 1956.

60. Huggins CB, Bergenstal DM: Surgery of adrenals. JAMA 147:101–106, 1951.

61. Huggins C, Bergenstal DM: Inhibition of human mammary and prostatic cancers by adrenalectomy. Cancer Res 12:134–141, 1952.

62. Huggins C, Thomas LY: Adrenalectomy and oophorectomy in treatment of advanced carcinoma of the breast. JAMA 16:1388–1394, 1953.

63. Hughes SWM, Burley DM: Aminoglutethimide a "side effect" turned to therapeutic advantage. Postgrad Med J 46:409–416, 1970.

64. Ingle JN, Krook JE, Green SJ, Kubista T, Everson L, Ahmann D, Change M, Bisel H, Windschitl H, Twito D, Pfeifle D: Randomized trial of bilateral oophorectomy versus tamoxifen in premenopausal women with metastatic breast cancer. J Clin Oncol 4:178–185, 1986.

65. Jensen EV, Jacobson HI: Bais guides to the mechanism of estrogen action. Recent Prog Horm Res 18:387, 1962.

66. Jessiman AG, Matson DD, Moore FD: Hypophysectomy in the treatment of breast cancer. N Engl J Med 261:1199–1207, 1959.

67. Jones CD, Suarez T, Massey EH, Black LJ, Tinely FC: Synthesis and antiestrogenic activity of [3,4-dihydro-2-(4-methoxyphenyl)-1-naphthalene] 4-(1-pyrolidinyl) ethoxyphenyl methanone, methanesulfonic acid. J Med Chem 22:962–966, 1979.

68. Kangas L, Niemin AL, Blanco G, Gronroos M, Kallio S, Karjalainen A, Perila M, Sodervall M, Toivola R: A new triphenylethylene compound, FC-1157a. Cancer Chemother Pharmacol 17:109–113, 1986.

69. Kennedy BJ: Hormonal therapies in breast cancer. Semin Oncol 1:119–130, 1974.

70. Kennedy BJ, Brown JH: Combined estrogenic and androgenic hormone therapy in advanced breast cancer. Cancer 18:431–435, 1965.

71. Kennedy BJ, Fortuny IE: Therapeutic castration in the treatment of advanced breast cancer. Cancer 17:1197–1202, 1964.

72. Kennedy BJ, French LA, Peyton WT: Hypophysectomy in advanced breast cancer. N Engl J Med 255:1165–1172, 1956.

73. Kennedy BJ, Peyton WT, Frenich LA: Total hypophysectomy in advanced breast cancer. Bull Univ Minn Hosp 26:528–551, 1955.

74. Kennedy BJ, Theologides A, Fortuny I, Foley J, Brown J: Diethylstilbestrol and testosterone propionate therapy in advanced breast cancer. A comparison. Cancer Chemother Rep 41:11–14, 1964.

75. Kiang DT, Frenning DE, Juliette G, et al: Combination therapy of hormone and cytotoxic agents in advanced breast cancer. Cancer 47:452–456, 1981.

76. Kiang DT, Kennedy BJ: Tamoxifen (antiestrogen) therapy in advanced breast cancer. Ann Int Med 87:687–690, 1977.

77. Kistner RW, Smith W: Observations on the use of a nonsteroidal estrogen antagonist: MER-25. Surg Forum 10:725–729, 1959.

78. Klijn JGM, DeJong FH: Long-term LHRH-agonist (buserelin) treatment in metastatic premenopausal breast cancer. In Klijn JGM (ed): Hormonal manipulation of cancer: peptides, growth factors, and new anti-steroidal agents. New York, Raven Press, 1987, pp 343–352.

79. Kraft RO: Triparanol in the treatment of disseminated mammary carcinoma. Cancer Chemother Rep 25:1113–1115, 1962.

80. LaRossa JT, Strong MS, Melby JC: Endocrinologically incomplete transethmoidal trans-sphenoidal hypophysectomy with relief of bone pain in breast cancer. N Engl J Med 1:1332–1335, 1978.

81. Le Beau J, Perrault M: A propos de l'hypophysectomie totale dans le traitement du cancer. Semaine d hop de Paris 29:1095, 1953.

82. Lednicer D, Babcock JC, Lyster SC, Duncan GW: Derivatives of 1, 2-dihydronaphthalene as antifertility agents. Chem In, 9 March 1963, pp 408–409.

83. Lee WR, Buzdar AV, Blumenschien GR, Hortobagyi GN: Trioxifene mesylate in the treatment of advanced breast cancer. Cancer 57:40–43, 1986.

84. Lerner H, Band P, Israel L, Leung B: Correlation of estrogen receptor sites to response: report of 11 patients with breast cancer treated with tamoxifen. (Abstract) Proc Am Assoc Cancer Res 17:2, 1976.

85. Lett H: An analysis of 99 cases of inoperable carcinoma of the breast treated by oophorectomy. Lancet 1:227, 1905.

86. Lewison EF, Trimble FH, Ganelin RS: Advanced cancer treated with sex hormones. JAMA 162:1429–1437, 1956.

87. Lippman ME: Hormone stimulation and chemotherapy for breast cancer. (Editorial) J Clin Oncol 5:331–332, 1987.

88. Lippman M, Bolan G, Huff KK: The effects of estrogens and anti-estrogens in hormone-responsive human breast cancer in long term tissue culture. Cancer Res 36:4595–4691, 1976.

89. Lippman ME, Cassidy J, Wesley M, Young RC: A randomized attempt to increase the efficacy of cytotoxic chemotherapy in metastatic breast cancer by hormonal synchronization. J Clin Oncol 2:28–36, 1984.

90. Lippman ME: Efforts to combine endocrine chemotherapy in the management of breast cancer: do two and two equal three? Breast Cancer Res Treat 3:117–127, 1983.

91. Lipton A, Santen JR: Medical adrenalectomy using aminoglutethimide and dexamethasone in advanced breast cancer. Cancer 33:503–512, 1974.

92. Lipton A, Santen RJ, Harvey HA, Manni A, Simmonds M, White-Hershey D, Bartholomew MA, Walker BK, Dixon RH, Valdevia DE, Gordon RA: A randomized trial of aminoglutethimide ± estrogen before chemotherapy in advanced breast cancer. Am J Clin Oncol 10:65–70, 1987.

93. Ludwig Breast Cancer Study Group: Randomized trial of chemoendocrine therapy, endocrine therapy and mastectomy alone in postmenopausal patients with operable breast cancer and axillary node metastases. Lancet 1:1253–1256, 1984.

94. Luft R, Olivecrona H: Hypophysectomy in man: experiences in metastatic cancer of breast. Cancer 8:261–270, 1955.

95. Luft R, Olivecrona H: Erfahrungen uber Hypophysektomie bei mammakrebs und bei diabetes mit Kimmelstiel-Wilson syndrom. Schweiz Med Wchnschr 86:113–117, 1956.

96. Luft R, Olivecrona H, Sjogren B: Hypophysectomy in man. Nord Med 47:351–354, 1952.

97. Lunan CB, Klopper A: Antioestrogens. A review. Clin Endocrinol 4:551–572, 1975.

98. Manni A, Pearson OH, Bordkey J, Marshall JS: Transsphenoidal hypophysectomy in breast cancer. Evidence for an individual role of pituitary and gonadal hormones in support tumor growth. Cancer 44(6):2330–2337, 1979.

99. Manni A, Trujillo J, Pearson OH: Antiestrogen-induced remissions in stage IV breast cancer. (Abstract) Proc Am Assoc Cancer Res 17:279, 1976.

100. Mathé G, Keiling R, Prevot G, VoVan ML, Gastiaburu J, Vannetzel JM, Despax R, Jasmin C, Levi F, Musset M, Machover D, Ribaud P, Misset JL: LHRH agonist: breast and prostate cancer. In Klijn JGM (ed): Hormonal Manipulation of Cancer: Peptides, Growth Factors, and New Anti-steroidal Agents. New York, Raven Press, 1987, pp 315–319.

101. Maudelonde T, Romieu G, Ulmann A, Pujol H, Grenier J, Khalaf S, Cavalie G, Rochefort H: First clinical trial of the use of the antiprogestin RU 486 in advanced breast cancer. In Klijn JGM (ed): Hormonal Manipulation of Cancer: Peptides, Growth Factors, and New Anti-steroidal Agents. New York, Raven Press, 1987, pp 55–59.

102. Miller WR, Forrest APM: Oestradiol synthesis by a human breast carcinoma. Lancet 2:866–868, 1974.

103. Morgan LR: Megestrol acetate and tamoxifen in advanced breast cancer in postmenopausal patients. Semin Oncol 12(suppl 1):43–47, 1985.

104. Morgan LR, Schein PS, Hoth D, McDonald J, Posey LE, Beazley RW, Trench L: Therapeutic use of tamoxifen in advanced breast cancer: a correlation with biochemical parameters. (Abstract) Proc Am Assoc Cancer Res 17:126, 1976.

105. Mouridsen HT, Rose C, Englesman E, Sylvester R: CMF versus CMF + tamoxifen in advanced breast cancer, final analysis of a randomized EORTC study. (Abstract) J Steroid Biochem 19(suppl):2085, 1983.

106. Muggia FM, Cassileth PA, Ochoa M Jr, Flatlow FA, Gellhorn A, Hyman GA: Treatment of breast cancer with medroxyprogesterone acetate. Ann Int Med 68:328–337, 1978.

107. Nathanson IT: Sex hormones and castration in advanced breast cancer. Radiology 56:535–552, 1985.

108. Nathanson IT: Clinical investigative experience with steroid hormones in breast cancer. Cancer 5:754–762, 1952.

109. Nelsen TS, Dragstedt LR: Adrenalectomy and oophorectomy for breast cancer. JAMA 175:379–383, 1961.

110. Nicholson RI, Walker KJ, Turkes A, Dyas J, Gotting KE, Plowman PN, Williams M, Elston CW, Blamey RW: The British experience with the LHRH agonist Zoladex in the treatment of breast cancer. In Klijn JGM (ed): Hormonal Manipulation of Cancer: Peptides, Growth Factors, and New Anti-steroidal Agents. New York, Raven Press, 1987, pp 331–341.

111. O'Halloran MJ, Maddock PG: I.C.I. 46, 474 in breast cancer. J Irish Med Assoc 67:38–39, 1974.

112. Paridaens R, Blonk van der Wijst J, Julien JP, et al: Chemotherapy with estrogenic recruitment in advanced breast cancer. Thirteenth International Congress of Chemotherapy, 1983.

113. Paridaens R, Kiss R, deLauncit Y, Atassi G, Paridaens RJ, Klijn JGM, Clarysse A, Rotmentz N, Sylvester RJ. Chemotherapy with estrogenic recruitment in breast cancer. In Klijn JGM (ed): Hormonal Manipulation in Cancer: Peptides, Growth Factors, and New Anti-steroidal Agents. New York, Raven Press, 1987, pp 447–486.

114. Pearson OH, Hubay CA: Adjuvant treatment, stage II breast cancer. Breast Cancer Res Treat 1:77–82, 1981.

115. Pearson OH, Ray BS, Harrold CC, West CD, Li MC, Maclean JP: Hypophysectomy in treatment of advanced cancer. Trans Assoc Am Physicians 68:101–111, 1955.

116. Pearson OH, Ray BS, Harrold CC, West CD, Li MC, Maclean JP: Hypophysectomy in treatment of advanced cancer. JAMA 161:17–21, 1956.

117. Pearson OH, West CD, McLean JP, Li MC, Lipsett MB: Endocrine treatment of metastatic breast cancer. Am Surg 11:1075–1083, 1955.

118. Peters MV: Influence of hormone (androgen + estrogen) therapy of metastatic carcinoma. Surg Gynecol Obstet 102:545–552, 1956.

119. Picaza JA, Marrinello Z, Schultte JA, Marquez JF: Hypofisecromia y cancer humano: reporte preliminar. Arch Soc Estud Clin Habana 47:89–94, 1954.

120. Planting AST, Alexieva-Figusch J, Blonk VD, Wijst J, Van Putten WLJ: Tamoxifen therapy in premenopausal women with metastatic breast cancer. Cancer Treat Rep 69:363–367, 1985.

121. Ray BS, Pearson OH: Hypophysectomy in treatment of advanced cancer of breast. Ann Surg 144:394–403, 1956.

122. Rivkin SE, Glucksberg H, Rasmussen S: Adjuvant chemotherapy for operable breast cancer with positive axillary nodes. In Salmon NE, Jones SE (eds): Adjuvant Therapy of Cancer, III. New York, Grune and Stratton, 1982, pp 236–282.

123. Ross MB, Buzdar AV, Blumenschien GR: Treatment of advanced breast cancer with megestrol acetate after therapy with tamoxifen. Cancer 49:413–417, 1982.

124. Rubens RD, Begent MB, Knight RR, Sexton SA, Hayward JL: Combined cytotoxic and progesterone therapy for advanced breast cancer. Cancer 42:1680–1686, 1978.

125. Santen R, Wells SA Jr: The use of aminoglutethimide in the treatment of patients with metastatic carcinoma of the breast. Cancer 46:1066–1074, 1980.

126. Santen RJ (ed): Aminoglutethimide and estrogenic recruitment for the chemotherapy of breast cancer. Proc. 13th International Congr Chemotherapy—Vienna, symposium 96, part 218, 1983.

127. Santen RJ: Suppression of estrogens with aminoglutethimide and hydrocortisone as treatment of advanced breast carcinoma: a review. Breast Cancer Res Treat 1:183–202, 1981.

128. Santen RJ, Samojlik E: Medical adrenalectomy for treatment of metastatic breast carcinoma. In McGuire W (ed): Breast Cancer, vol 3. New York, Plenum, 1979, pp 79–114.

129. Santen JR, Samojlik E, Upton A, Harvey H, Ruby EB, Wells SA, Kendall J: Kinetic, hormonal and clinical studies with aminoglutethimide in breast cancer. Cancer 39:2948–2958, 1977.

130. Santen RJ, Worgul TJ, Samojlik E, Interrante A, Boucher A, Lipton A, Harvey H, White D, Smart E, Cox C, Wells S: Randomized trial comparing surgical adrenalectomy with aminoglutethimide plus hydrocortisone in women with advanced breast carcinoma. N Engl J Med 305:545–551, 1981.

131. Sasaki SH, Leung BS, Ed: Fletcher WS: Therapeutic use of nafoxidine in advanced breast cancer: a correlation with endocrine ablation and tumor estrogen receptor. (Abstract) Proc Am Assoc Cancer Res 16:271, 1975.

132. Sawka CA, Pritchard KI, Patterson AHG, Sutherland DJA, Thomson DB, Shelley WE, Myers RE, Mobbs BG, Malkin A, Meakin JW: The role and mechanism of action of tamoxifen in premenopausal women with metastatic breast cancer. Cancer Res 46:3152–3156, 1986.

133. Schinzinger U: Carcinoma mammee. (Abstract) Centralblatt Fur Chir 16:55, 1889.

134. Segaloff A: Progress report results of studies by the Co-operative Breast Cancer Group 1956–60. Cancer Chemother Rep 11:109–141, 1961.

135. Siegert AN: Kastration and mamma. Ca Strahlenther 87:62, 1952.

136. Sponzo RW, Barkley JM, Horton J, Cunningham TJ: Tamoxiphen (NSC 180,973) in the management of advanced breast cancer. (Abstract) Proc Am Assoc Cancer Res 17:68, 1976.

137. Stonesifier GL, Lowe RH, Cameron JL, Ganis FM: Conversion of hydrocortisone to estrogen in carcinoma of the breast after oophorectomy and adrenalectomy. Ann Surg 178:563–564, 1973.

138. Swain S, Lippman ME, Bagley C, Bader J, Danforth D, Steinberg S: Treatment of locally advanced breast cancer using primary induction chemotherapy with hormonal synchronization followed by radiation therapy with or without debulking surgery. Proc ASCO 6:192, 1987.

139. Symposium-discussion on advanced cases of carcinoma of the breast treated by stilbestrol. Proc R Soc Med 37:371–376, 1944.

140. Taylor SG III, Slaugheter DP, Smejkal W, Fowler EF, Preston FW: Effect of sex hormones on advanced carcinoma of the breast. Cancer 1:604–617, 1948.

141. Terenius L: Selective retention of estrogen isomers in estrogen-dependent breast tumors of rats demonstrated by in vitro methods. Cancer Res 28:328–337, 1968.

142. Thayssen VF: The influence of castration by roentgen on carcinoma of the breast. Acta Radiol (Stockh) 29:189, 1948.

143. Thomson A: Analysis of cases in which oophorectomy was performed for inoperable carcinoma of the breast. Br Med J 2:1538, 1902.

144. Tormey DC, Falkson G, Crowley J, Falkson HC, Voelkel J, Davis TE, et al: Dibromodulcitol and adriamycin + tamoxifen in advanced breast cancer. Am J Clin Oncol 5:33–39, 1982.

145. Tormey D, Lippman M, Bull J, Myers C: Evaluation of tamoxifen dose in advanced breast cancer. (Abstract) Proc Am Assoc Cancer Res 17:276, 1976.

146. Trioxifene mesylate, an investigational new drug. Clinical Investigators' Manual, Indianapolis, IN, Eli Lilly & Company.

147. Viladu P, Alonso MC, Avella A, Beltran M, Borras J, Ojeda B, Bosch X: Chemotherapy versus chemotherapy plus hormonotherapy in postmenopausal advanced breast cancer patients. Cancer 56:2745–2750, 1985.

148. Ward HWC: Antioestrogen therapy for breast cancer: a trial of tamoxifen at two dose levels. Br Med J 1:113–114, 1973.

149. William S Merrell Company: Clomiphene citrate (Climid). Clin Pharmacol Ther 8:891–897, 1967.

150. Witte RS, Pruitt B, Tormey DC, Moss S, Rose DP, Falkson G, Carbone PP, Ramirez G, Falkson H, Pretorius FJ: A phase I/II investigation of trioxifene mesylate in advanced breast cancer. Cancer 57:34–38, 1986.

Chapter 45

PALLIATIVE PROCEDURES FOR SPECIFIC PROBLEMS

Surgical Procedures for Advanced Local and Regional Malignancies of the Breast

Raphael E. Pollock, M.D., Ph.D., Stephen S. Kroll, M.D., and Charles M. Balch, M.D.

Surgery has an important role in the palliative treatment of local and advanced malignancy of the breast. It is the quickest and most effective way to establish a durable complete response for local disease control. There are some significant limitations, however. Surgical treatment of stage III breast cancer fails to treat distant micrometastases that are present in virtually all such patients and even fails locally in ten percent to 20 percent of patients who live 2 years or longer. On the other hand, improvements in palliation and even cure have resulted from the integration of surgery, chemotherapy, and radiotherapy in the treatment of these advanced problems. In order to understand the remarkable successes of current multimodality therapy for advanced breast disease, it is critical to examine the rationale and evolution of this therapeutic approach.

Locally advanced breast cancer encompasses four distinct clinical entities occurring in patients without clinically evident distant metastases. These include (1) locally recurrent (persistent) breast carcinoma, (2) inflammatory breast carcinoma, (3) stage IIIa breast cancer, and (4) stage IIIb breast carcinoma. Inflammatory and locally recurrent carcinoma are discussed elsewhere in this textbook. Stage IIIa disease includes any tumor with metastases to homolateral axillary lymph nodes that are fixed to each other or to other structures.[12] It also includes any tumor ≥5 cm with metastasis to non-fixed ipsilateral axillary nodes.[12] Stage IIIb disease includes any tumor with direct extension to the chest wall or skin with any form of axillary or internal mammary node involvement, or any tumor with internal mammary node involvement.[12] The most recent staging schema proposed by the American Joint Committee for Cancer (AJCC) has designated ipsilateral infra- or supraclavicular node involvement as M1 instead of N3 and designates this clinical presentation as stage IV disease. Likewise, a primary tumor ≥5 cm without lymph node involvement is now considered stage II rather than stage IIIa disease (Fig. 45–1).[12]

These staging changes have important ramifications, because most clinical research studies to date have been based on earlier staging schemes. Any clinical series prior to 1987 will therefore possibly include some patients who would currently be considered either stage II or IV rather than stage III. Because it is not feasible to retrospectively restage these studies, our discussion will be based on these earlier staging categories, except where otherwise indicated. Historically, stage IIIa lesions have been considered operable, whereas stage IIIb tumors have not been considered for surgical resection.

HISTORICAL CONSIDERATIONS: UNIMODALITY APPROACHES

The awareness of differences in natural biology (and therefore therapy) for locally advanced breast cancer stems from Haagensen and Stout's pioneering insights that derived from nearly 30 years of cumulative experience in breast cancer management. Based on a review of 1135 breast cancer patients treated with radical mastectomy at Presbyterian Hospital in New York (1915–1942), it was recognized that patients with certain features of locally advanced breast cancer were beyond cure, even by radical surgery.[7] Haagensen's "grave signs" included edema of the skin of the breast, skin ulceration, chest wall fixation, an axillary lymph node >2.5 cm diameter, and fixed axillary nodes. Patients with two or more signs had a 42 percent local recurrence rate and a two percent 5-year disease-free survival, hence their recommendation that these patients be treated with palliative radiotherapy alone.[7]

In 1949, Baclesse used radiotherapy alone to achieve local tumor control for selected patients with advanced breast cancer.[1] In 1965, Fletcher and Montague from the M. D. Anderson Cancer Center reported a 70 percent local control rate of advanced breast cancer using radiotherapy alone.[6] Distant metastasis occurred an average of 18 months later, with a 5-year overall survival rate of 25 percent. Other retrospective reviews of the 1960s–1970s included Harris et al.'s report of the Joint Center for Radiation Therapy experience, where 54 percent 5-year local tumor control and 30 percent 5-year overall survival were achieved using radical radiation therapy alone.[8] The National Cancer Institute, Milan, Italy, published their retrospective experience in 1973.[21] An encouraging 50 percent control rate was initially observed. However, 45 percent of these "controlled" patients relapsed within 18 months of beginning radiotherapy. Of these relapses, 82 percent were at a distant site. An overall 21 percent 5-year survival was achieved. It should be kept in mind that supervoltage radiotherapy as then administered was not benign. Fibrosis and skin ulceration, pathological fractures, and severe lymphedema of the ipsilateral arm were common and debilitating occurrences.

More recently, the Alabama Breast Project examined the efficacy of modified radical mastectomy versus radical mastectomy as unimodality therapy of stage III breast carcinoma in patients with a minimum of 10 years follow-up.[15] In this study, stage III patients treated by modified radical mastectomy represented only six percent of the total study population, yet accounted for 20 percent of the total local recurrences. In contrast, the stage III radical mastectomy patients were five percent of the total study population but incurred only six percent of the total local recurrences. Radical mastectomy significantly decreased the rate of local recurrence and improved survival when compared with modified mastectomy, albeit with greater morbidity. Observations such as those in the Alabama experience led to the realization that multimodality therapy might yield comparable survival but without the associated severe morbidities of unimodal radical interventions.

MULTIMODALITY APPROACHES

The unimodality experiences all demonstrated that good local control rates by surgery or radiotherapy alone did not correlate with good prognosis and ultimate survival. Clearly, hematogenous metastasis was not being controlled with either radical surgery or radical radiotherapy alone.[4] Consequently, in the early 1970s a change in treatment strategies occurred that incorporated systemic chemotherapy as an integral part of the primary management of locally advanced breast cancer.[14] Several major prospective multimodality trials were initiated, including the National Cancer Institute, Milan, Italy, trial begun in 1973 and the M. D. Anderson Cancer Center trial begun in 1974.

In the Milan trial, patients with IIIa or IIIb breast cancer were given four cycles of doxorubicin and vincristine, followed by 60 Gy to the breast and a 10 Gy boost to the area of residual tumor. Patients with complete response were randomized to no further treatment or to six more courses of chemotherapy. An 89 percent objective response rate occurred with this preoperative chemotherapy regimen. This included a 15.5

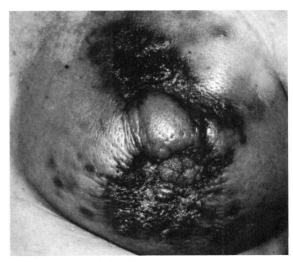

Figure 45–1. Patient with locally advanced breast cancer. Note prominent skin retraction and nipple distortion caused by large underlying primary tumor.

percent complete response, a 54.5 percent major response (>50 percent tumor size reduction), and a 19 percent minor response rate (<50 percent tumor size reduction). Of the patients responding to induction chemotherapy, 83 percent had a complete response after the addition of radiotherapy. This multimodality approach resulted in an overall 53 percent 3-year survival rate in these patients.[14]

In 1975, the National Cancer Institute, Milan, Italy, group began a second trial that ultimately enrolled 277 consecutive stage IIIa and IIIb patients.[20] In this trial, patients received three courses of doxorubicin and vincristine preoperatively. They were then randomized to radiotherapy or surgery (radical or modified radical mastectomy). After these treatments, the patients then received six additional courses of chemotherapy. The best local control was achieved when surgery was interposed between chemotherapy, where an 82.3 percent complete local control rate was achieved. These results were much better than when chemotherapy and radiotherapy were employed (without surgery), where there was a significantly smaller 63.9 percent local control rate. Freedom from disease progression was continuous for 5 years or longer in 25 percent of the chemotherapy/surgery/chemotherapy patients, which was significantly better than the 4.9 percent disease-free survival at 5 years achieved with a chemotherapy/radiotherapy regimen. Likewise, overall 5-year survival was 49.4 percent for chemotherapy/surgery/chemotherapy compared to a 19.7 percent 5-year overall survival rate achieved with chemotherapy/radiotherapy.

In 1974, a multimodality treatment protocol for locally advanced breast cancer was initiated at the M. D. Anderson Cancer Center.[11] It was postulated that the combined use of all three modalities (chemotherapy, surgery, and radiotherapy) would result in control of micrometastases and reduce local tumor bulk, thereby avoiding the need for either radical radiotherapy or radical mastectomy.

Between 1974 and 1985, 174 patients with noninflammatory stage III (operable and inoperable) breast cancer were treated with combination chemotherapy consisting of fluorouracil, doxorubicin (Adriamycin), and cyclophosphamide (FAC) as their initial form of therapy. After three cycles of induction chemotherapy, patients were assessed for clinical response and classified as (1) complete response; (2) major response; (3) minor response; (4) nonresponse, resectable; or (5) nonresponse, unresectable. Complete responders and unresectable nonresponders next received radiotherapy, followed by 6–12 courses of postradiotherapy chemotherapy. Major responders, minor responders, and resectable nonresponders were treated with mastectomy (total or partial) and level I/II axillary dissection, followed next by chemotherapy and lastly by radiotherapy. The specific chemotherapy and radiotherapy protocols (as currently used) are discussed in the text that follows. The median follow-up was 95 months. A complete remission was achieved in 16.7 percent of the patients, and 70.7 percent achieved a major partial response after the initial three FAC cycles. All but six of the 174 patients treated were eventually rendered disease-free after induction chemotherapy and local treatment. The stage IIIa patients had a 19 percent complete response and 73 percent partial response after induction chemotherapy. The complete response rate was 100 percent after induction chemotherapy followed by local therapies. At 5 years, an 84 percent survival and 78 percent disease-free survival had been achieved. In the 122 stage IIIb patients, induction chemotherapy yielded a seven percent complete response, an 80 percent partial response, and a 96 percent complete response after induction chemotherapy plus local therapy. Only three of 174 stage III patients (1.7 percent) suffered disease progression while receiving FAC induction chemotherapy. These initial responses translated into a 5-year 33 percent disease-free survival and a 56 percent overall survival (Fig. 45–2).

CURRENT PATIENT MANAGEMENT

The recent revision of the AJCC staging system for breast cancer will undoubtedly influence the manner in which certain subsets of patients are managed. Because ipsilateral supraclavicular or infraclavicular adenopathy is now categorized as stage IV disease,[12] the tendency will be to treat these individuals by chemotherapy alone. Because the multimodality experience suggests that some of these patients are potentially curable, it is hoped that the astute clinician will use multimodality programs for patients if the presence of ipsilateral periclavicular nodes is the only reason the patient is classified as stage IV.

Staging work-up includes a thorough physical examination, a complete blood count (CBC) with differential and platelet counts, a biochemical survey (SMA-12), chest roentgenogram, bilateral xeromammogram, bone scan, and liver imaging (liver ultrasound or computerized tomography). Patients with pain, an abnormal bone

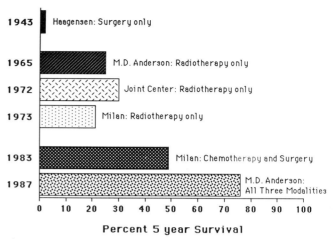

Figure 45–2. Comparison of 5-year survival rates for selected series of patients with locally advanced breast cancer.

scan, or elevated alkaline phosphatase levels have pertinent bone radiographs to rule out distant disease. Incisional biopsy or needle core biopsy is performed for both histopathological and hormone receptor examination.

There is a biological rationale for the sequence of modalities as currently used in the treatment of locally advanced breast cancer at the University of Texas M. D. Anderson Cancer Center (Fig. 45–3). Two to three courses of FAC induction chemotherapy are used first in a desire to achieve early control of distant micrometastasis (Table 45–1). Even though distant disease may be undetectable by current clinical diagnostic procedures, its presence is suggested by the high percentage

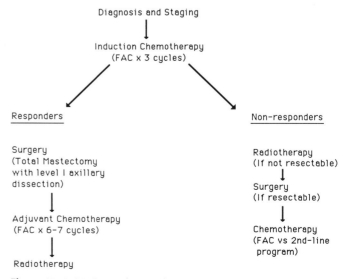

Figure 45–3. M. D. Anderson algorithm for the treatment of stage III breast carcinoma.

Table 45–1. M. D. ANDERSON CHEMOTHERAPY PROTOCOL FOR STAGE III BREAST CANCER

1. 5-fluorouracil 500 mg/m² I.V. on days 1 and 8.
2. Doxorubicin (Adriamycin) 50 mg/m² on day 1–2 as a 48-hr continuous infusion.
3. Cyclophosphamide 500 mg/m² I.V. on day 1.
4. Chemotherapy repeated at 21-day intervals.
5. Dose modification based on hematological toxicity as defined by weekly CBC with differential and platelet counts. If the lowest granulocyte count is <1000/mm³ or the lowest platelet count is <50,000/mm³, the doses of all drugs are reduced 20 percent.
6. Adjuvant chemotherapy is initiated after surgical treatment has been completed.
7. Adjuvant chemotherapy is continued as above until a total dose of 450–500 mg/m² doxorubicin has been administered.

of distant failures even when good local control was achieved with radiotherapy/surgery in the prechemotherapy era, as discussed previously. In addition, the use of induction chemotherapy may decrease primary tumor bulk sufficiently to convert some inoperable patients into candidates for mastectomy. The third reason for using induction chemotherapy is that patient responsiveness has been shown to correlate with overall survival, as will be discussed later. Consequently, patient responsiveness to induction chemotherapy may serve as an in vivo chemosensitivity assay to indicate the potential effectiveness of postoperative adjuvant chemotherapy.

If the patient has progressed after three courses of induction chemotherapy, surgical resection is attempted if feasible. Otherwise, radiotherapy is used, followed by surgical resection. If the patient has responded to induction chemotherapy, surgery is then generally used as the second modality. The issue of response versus progression of the primary is assessed by physical examination and repeat xeromammograms (Fig. 45–4). Criteria used for grading tumor regression are those of the Union Internationale Contre le Cancer (UICC).[10]

The surgical procedure is usually a total mastectomy with level I/II axillary dissection, defined as the nodal tissues lying between the thoracodorsal and long thoracic nerves (level I) as well as the nodal tissues underlying the pectoralis minor muscle (level II). This resection is generally performed 3 weeks after the last chemotherapy treatment in order to avoid granulocyte and platelet nadir effects commonly observed about 2 weeks after myelosuppressive chemotherapy. In the event of prolonged myelosuppression, the CBC with differential is followed until the granulocyte count is ≥1000/mm³, at which time surgical resection is performed. The technique of mastectomy is discussed elsewhere in this textbook. Occasionally, an en bloc chest wall resection is required for some stage IIIb lesions. The surgical goal is to achieve the best possible local control on the chest wall and the axilla so as to avoid the complex and difficult problems of chest wall recurrence (Fig. 45–5).

The mastectomy performed includes a level I and II axillary dissection for pathological node assessment. Because of the documented low incidence of "skip

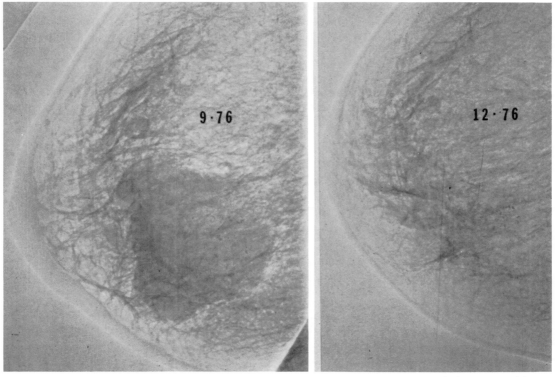

Figure 45–4. Mammography before and after three courses of FAC induction chemotherapy. Note the marked response of the primary tumor.

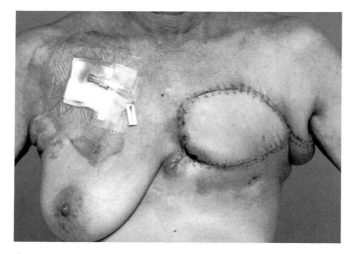

Figure 45–5. The same patient as in Figure 45–1 after preoperative induction chemotherapy. Full-thickness chest wall resection and mastectomy site have been reconstructed using a pedicle flap. Note the presence of a percutaneous subclavian chemotherapy catheter to be used for postoperative adjuvant chemotherapy.

metastasis" (metastatic deposits in level III without level I/II disease)[2] and because the patient will be receiving axillary radiotherapy, the possibility of uncontrolled axillary disease is minimal. In addition, the level I/II axillary dissection avoids the functional and cosmetic difficulties that can result from axillary radiotherapy in an already completely dissected axilla.[18] Surgery is used before radiotherapy because, having already debulked the tumor surgically, better radiotherapeutic local control can be achieved in the adjuvant setting.[16] There have been no inordinate infection or wound healing problems in postoperative patients treated by this multimodality approach (M. Edwards; personal communication).

The last reason for using surgery after induction chemotherapy but before radiotherapy is that it provides the opportunity for pathological assessment of primary tumor response at a point in the clinical course where operability has been achieved. The importance of this pathological assessment was suggested by Feldman et al., who examined 90 patients with locally advanced breast cancer treated from 1974–1981 at the M. D. Anderson Cancer Center.[5] All patients had at least 5 years of posttreatment follow-up. Group A consisted of patients without macroscopic cancer in their mastectomy specimen on gross pathological examination (15/90); group B had residual pathological macroscopic disease (75/90).

Relapse after 5-year follow-up was significantly higher in group B, as was death from recurrent breast cancer at 6 or more years (group A: 93 percent 5-year survival vs. group B: 30 percent 5-year survival; $p < 0.01$). The median disease-free survival was greater than 5 years in group A and only 22 months in group B. At the M. D. Anderson Cancer Center, pathological assessment of response to induction chemotherapy is used as an indicator of whether to continue "first line" FAC chemo-

therapy as a postoperative adjuvant or consider "second line" agents.

After total mastectomy with level I/II axillary dissection, adjuvant chemotherapy is given. Initially 12 courses were used, but no significant improvement in survival was noted when compared with six courses.[11] Therefore six courses of adjuvant chemotherapy are now standard (see Table 45–1). At the completion of chemotherapy, radiotherapy is then used (Table 45–2). The underlying rationale for this sequence is based on the awareness that radiotherapy and doxorubicin are poorly tolerated if given simultaneously.[11] In addition, local control is equally good with early or late radiotherapy; however, more distant failures have been observed with postoperative radiotherapy given before adjuvant chemotherapy. The use of systemic hormonal therapy has not yet been evaluated in the context of prospective multimodality trials of locally advanced breast disease. In the future, immunotherapy may also have an important and yet-to-be-defined role. An accurate understanding of the natural biology of locally advanced breast carcinoma, coupled with the ability to integrate extirpative and reconstructive surgery with the other available modalities, has radically improved our capacities to treat and even cure these formerly lethal problems.

RECONSTRUCTION OF DEFECTS FOLLOWING MASTECTOMY

The success of chemotherapy in controlling distant disease places an important new emphasis on local control of stage III breast cancer. Although in many patients local control can be achieved with a standard mastectomy, at times skin invasion or chest wall fixation may mandate the use of more radical ablative procedures. Such procedures are possible only if closure of the wound can be achieved. Fortunately, if wound closure by primary approximation of the wound edges is impossible, reconstructive techniques can be used to bring additional tissues into the wound and allow healing to occur. The surgeon performing the ablative procedure is then free to excise whatever is required to achieve local control of the tumor.

Table 45–2. M. D. ANDERSON RADIOTHERAPY PROTOCOL FOR STAGE III BREAST CARCINOMA

1. 50 Gy to the chest wall.
2. 10 Gy boost to the mastectomy scar.
3. 50 Gy to the interval mammary lymph node chain.
4. 50 Gy to the supraclavicular lymph node chain.
5. Electron beam is used when possible to treat internal mammary nodes in order to lessen risk of cardiotoxicity.
6. In patients with bulky residual disease after induction chemotherapy:
   a. 55 Gy in twice-daily fractionation delivered to the breast
   b. 10 Gy boost to areas of residual disease
   c. Lymph node chains treated as above

The choice of reconstructive method depends on the size and type of the defect that will be presented to the reconstructive surgical team. Such defects are best considered by dividing them into two groups: those in which the chest wall is intact and those in which it is not.

Intact Chest Wall

If the defect involves only skin and subcutaneous tissue, in some cases it can be handled with a skin graft. This rather simple maneuver will provide coverage that is reasonably functional and will stand up to postoperative radiotherapy once it has fully healed (Fig. 45–6). Unfortunately, it is also rather unattractive and less durable than a myocutaneous flap. In addition, skin grafts require an extended period of time for recipient site healing and healing of the donor site. For these reasons, and because of advances that have occurred in the ability to cover wounds with flaps, skin grafts are rarely used at the M. D. Anderson Cancer Center.

Most larger defects are best reconstructed with myocutaneous flaps.[3] Flaps provide durable skin coverage of normal quality and thickness and heal in a manner similar to a primarily closed wound. While use of a flap requires sacrifice of muscle function, that loss is generally well tolerated and may even go unnoticed by the patient. Because of these advantages, flaps have grown in popularity in recent years and have become the cornerstone of chest wall and breast reconstruction at the M. D. Anderson Cancer Center. Although many flaps are available for the reconstruction of mastectomy defects, the latissimus dorsi and the rectus abdominis myocutaneous flaps are exemplary because of their suitability and reliability.

Latissimus Dorsi Myocutaneous Flap

The latissimus dorsi myocutaneous flap was first described in 1897 by the Italian surgeon Tansini.[19] This

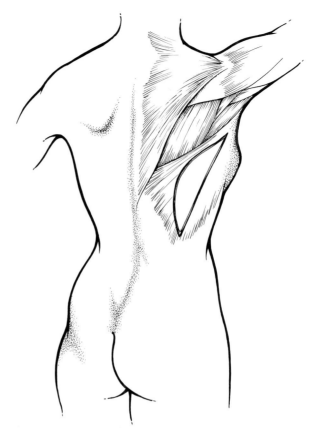

Figure 45–7. Drawing of the plan at the latissimus dorsi myocutaneous flap. Note underlying latissimus muscle. The shape of the skin paddle can be altered to fit the defect.

flap, which consists of a skin paddle based on the underlying latissimus dorsi muscle, is supplied with blood by both the thoracodorsal artery and by branches of the posterior intercostal arteries close to the spine (Fig. 45–7). The flap can survive on either of these two blood supplies; for chest wall and breast reconstruction the larger and dominant thoracodorsal pedicle is best used. The flap is isolated on its thoracodorsal vascular leash and rotated around its attachment point in the axilla. From there it will easily reach to the sternum and will generally fill a defect 8 cm in width and up to 20 cm in length (Fig. 45–8).

The two chief advantages of the latissimus dorsi flap are its lack of donor site morbidity and its reliable blood supply. Perhaps because of similar actions by the teres major and minor, patients notice little morbidity from use of the latissimus dorsi muscle in a flap. This flap is rarely lost perioperatively unless the thoracodorsal vessels have been damaged during the mastectomy. Even in that event, the flap will often survive on collateral flow between the thoracodorsal vessel and its serratus branch.

The chief disadvantage of the latissimus flap is its limited size. Although the muscular portion of the flap can be quite wide, the skin of the donor site in the back does not stretch well. If more than 8–10 cm of skin is

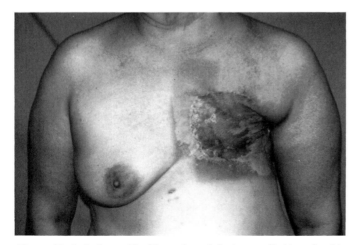

Figure 45–6. Patient with skin graft on left chest wall. Note the thin cover and poor cosmetic appearance.

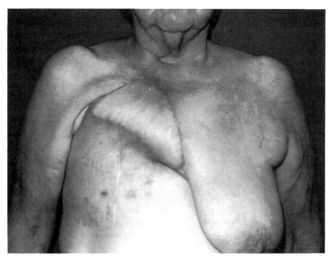

Figure 45–8. Patient with healed latissimus dorsi myocutaneous flap reconstruction of full-thickness chest wall defect.

mobilized in flap development, donor site primary closure can no longer be achieved. Although larger donor defects can be skin grafted, the use of skin grafts will compromise the ultimate cosmetic result.

Rectus Abdominis Flaps

The rectus abdominis myocutaneous flaps are large flaps of great usefulness. There are three versions of the flap that can be used for chest wall reconstruction: the vertical rectus flap, the single pedicle TRAM flap, and the double-pedicle TRAM flap.

The vertical rectus abdominis flap was the earliest of the rectus flaps to be described and is the easiest to perform.[17] The skin paddle is positioned vertically over the contralateral rectus abdominis muscle, where it is abundantly supplied with blood from the underlying muscle via perforating vessels (Fig. 45–9). Fortuitously, in most females the abdominal skin is lax or redundant. Consequently, large amounts of skin can be mobilized, and the donor site can still be closed primarily. The width of the skin paddle can frequently be greater than 15 cm.

The single pedicle transverse rectus abdominis myocutaneous (TRAM) flap[9] has become justifiably popular for postmastectomy breast reconstruction (Fig. 45–10). Adaptation of this technique, which uses a transversely oriented skin paddle, has been hindered by the less robust nature of its blood supply. Because a large part of the skin paddle does not lie directly over the muscle, the flap is dependent on the integrity of a small number

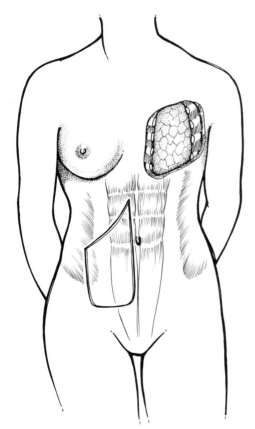

Figure 45–9. Drawing of plan for a vertical rectus abdominis myocutaneous flap for chest wall reconstruction.

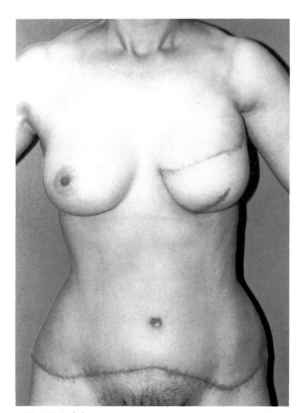

Figure 45–10. Left breast reconstruction with a single-pedicle TRAM flap. This patient did not have a chest wall defect.

Despite its decreased reliability, the single pedicle TRAM flap is useful in nonsmoking patients with an intact chest wall. Situated low on the rectus muscle, this flap has a long leash and a long axis of rotation, allowing it to rotate quite far laterally or high into the axilla. If the chest wall is intact, the viability of the flap is less critical, and a slightly higher risk of flap loss can therefore be tolerated.

The double pedicle TRAM flap is a variation on the single pedicle TRAM in which the blood supply is doubled by basing the flap on both rectus abdominis muscles (Fig. 45–11).[13] This overcomes the blood supply problems of the single pedicle TRAM flap and combines the reliability of the vertical rectus with the mobility and improved postoperative appearance of the TRAM concept. The decreased abdominal strength from the loss of two rectus muscles has been well tolerated. Because the blood supply is better, the flap can often be made quite large. In some cases, reconstruction of not only the chest wall cover but also an approximation of the missing breast can be accomplished (Figs. 45–12 and 45–13).

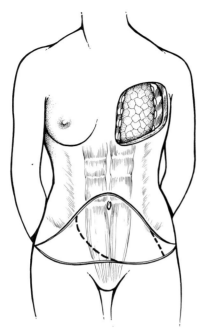

Figure 45–11. Drawing of plan for a double-pedicle TRAM flap to be used for chest wall reconstruction.

of perforating vessels that exist where the skin and the muscle overlap. In most healthy patients, this blood supply is adequate, and a large flap may be obtained. In smoking patients, diabetic patients, and patients in poor general health, this circulation may be inadequate and may limit the size and viability of the flap.

Chest Wall Not Intact

When the chest wall is not intact, the reconstruction problems are not different from those when the chest wall is intact, except that flap reliability becomes more

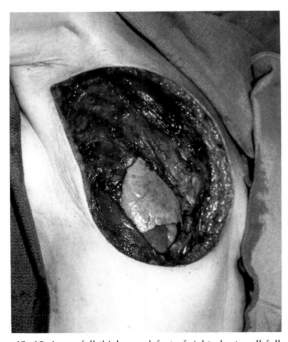

Figure 45–12. Large full-thickness defect of right chest wall following mastectomy and chest wall resection.

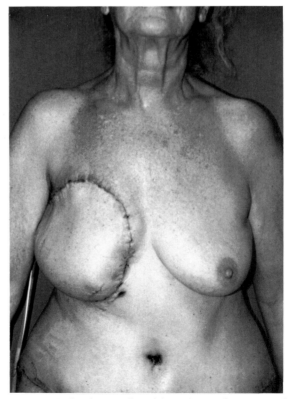

Figure 45–13. Right chest wall and breast mound reconstruction of patient shown in Figure 45–12.

critical. Reconstruction of the rib cage may not be necessary even after resection of up to five ribs or the entire sternum. If good flap coverage and respirator support is provided, sufficient scar tissue will form to stabilize the chest wall, usually after 4 to 7 days. This avoids implantation of synthetic materials such as Marlex mesh or acrylic that can lead to chronic pain or infection.

Because a fistula into the pleural cavity is poorly tolerated, flap reliability is of utmost importance when the chest wall is not intact. Consequently, the latissimus dorsi myocutaneous flap is a good choice for small defects that are within the arc of rotation. The flap is very reliable, and the underlying muscle can be sutured to the edges of the rib cage defect to help stabilize the chest. This creates a two-layer closure; even if some skin loss occurs, the underlying muscle can survive and protect the chest cavity.

For defects lower on the chest wall that would be difficult to reach with the latissimus or for very large defects that the latissimus flap would not cover, the vertical rectus abdominis flap and the double pedicle TRAM flap are good options. Both of these flaps are quite reliable; although there is only one layer of closure, the flaps are thick. This bulkiness helps to stabilize the chest wall and compensate for the loss of ribs.

Other methods and techniques that can be used in chest wall reconstruction include random and axial skin flaps, omental flaps, other myocutaneous flaps, and microvascular free flaps. However, the methods discussed have been so successful and versatile that these other approaches are rarely needed. Because variation is inherent in both human anatomy and the biological behavior of tumors, there will always be exceptional situations requiring alternative strategies. Nevertheless, appropriate use of the latissimus dorsi flap and the various rectus abdominis flaps will allow successful reconstruction of almost all defects that will be encountered in the treatment of locally advanced breast cancer.

References

1. Baclesse F: Roentgen therapy alone as the method of treatment of cancer of the breast. AJR 62:311–319, 1949.
2. Boova RS, Bonanni R, Rosata FE: Patterns of axillary nodal involvement in breast cancer. Ann Surg 196:642–644, 1982.
3. Bostwick J, Vasconez LO, Jurkiewicz MD: Breast reconstruction after a radical mastectomy. Plast Reconstr Surg 61:682, 1978.
4. Davila E, Vogel CL: Management of locally advanced breast cancer (stage III): a review. Int Adv Surg Oncol 7:297–327, 1984.
5. Feldman LD, Hortobagyi GN, Buzdar AU, Ames FC, Blumenschein GR: Pathological assessment of response to induction chemotherapy in breast cancer. Cancer Res 46:2578–2581, 1986.
6. Fletcher GH, Montague ED: Radical irradiation of advanced breast cancer. AJR 93:573–584, 1965.
7. Haagensen CD, Stout AP: Carcinoma of the breast: II. Criteria of operability. Ann Surg 118:859–870; 1032–1051, 1943.
8. Harris JR, Sawicka J, Gelman R, Hellman S: Management of locally advanced carcinoma of the breast by primary radiation therapy. Int J Radiat Oncol Biol Phys 9:345–349, 1983.
9. Hartrampf CR, Scheflan M, Black PW: Breast reconstruction with a transverse abdominal island flap. Plast Reconstr Surg 69:216, 1982.
10. Hayward JL, Carbone PP, Henson JC, et al: Assessment of response to therapy in advanced breast cancer. A project of the program on clinical oncology of the International Union Against Cancer. Cancer 39:1289–1294, 1977.
11. Hortobagyi GN, Ames FC, Buzdar AU, Kau SW, McNeese MD, Paulus D, Hug V, Holmes FA, Romsdahl MD, Fraschini G, McBride CM, Martin RG, Montague E: Management of stage III primary breast cancer with primary chemotherapy, surgery and radiation therapy. Cancer 62:2507–2516, 1988.
12. Hutter RVP: At last—worldwide agreement on the staging of cancer. Arch Surg 122:1235–1239, 1987.
13. Ishii CH, Bostwick J, Raine TJ, Coleman JJ, Hester TR: Double-pedicle transverse rectus abdominis myocutaneous flap for unilateral breast and chest wall reconstruction. Plast Reconstr Surg 76:901, 1985.
14. Lena MD, Zucali R, Viganotti G, Valagussa P, Bonadonna G: Combined chemotherapy-radiotherapy approach in locally advanced (T_{3b}–T_4) breast cancer. Cancer Chemother Pharmacol 1:53–59, 1978.
15. Maddox WA, Carpenter JT, Laws HT, Soong SS, Cloud G, Balch CM, Urist MM: Does radical mastectomy still have a place in the treatment of primary operable breast cancer? Arch Surg 122:1317–1319, 1987.
16. Montague E, Fletcher G: Local regional effectiveness of surgery and radiation therapy in the treatment of breast cancer. Cancer 55:2266–2272, 1985.
17. Robbins TH: Rectus abdominis myocutaneous flap for breast reconstruction. Aust NZ J Surg 49:527, 1979.
18. Spanos WJ, Montague ED, Fletcher GH: Late complications of radiation only for advanced breast cancer. Int J Radiat Oncol Biol Phys 6:1473–1476, 1980.
19. Tansini I: Sopra il mio nuovo processo di amputazione della mammella. Gazetta Medica Italiana 57:141, 1906.
20. Valagussa P, Zambetti M, Bignami P, Lena MD, Varini M, Zucali R, Rovini D, Bonadonna G: T_{3b}–T_4 breast cancer: factors affecting results in combined modality treatments. Clin Exp Metastasis 1:191–202, 1983.
21. Zucali R, Uslenghi C, Kenda R, Bonnadonna G: Natural history and survival of inoperable breast cancer treated with radiotherapy and radiotherapy followed by radical mastectomy. Cancer 37:1422–1431, 1976.

Palliative Radiation Therapy for Disseminated Breast Cancer

Nancy Price Mendenhall, M.D.

Radiation is an extremely useful tool in the management of localized problems in patients with disseminated breast cancer. Because the goal of treatment is palliative, only symptomatic patients or those likely to develop irreversible symptoms are treated. Once distant metastases are present, survival is limited. In planning treatment, an assessment of the patient's overall prognosis must be made based on the site and extent of metastases, the disease-free interval, the estrogen and progesterone receptor status of the tumor, the age and general medical condition of the patient, prior therapy, and the potential responsiveness of the tumor to other modalities. After assessing the patient's overall prognosis, a treatment regimen is selected based on the likelihood of response, expected time to response, expected duration of response, and likelihood of morbidity. Most patients with disseminated breast cancer will have multiple problems during the course of their disease that require palliative irradiation. As each treatment field is planned, it must be assumed that therapy may later be required to adjacent areas. The junction between adjacent fields potentially may be underdosed or overdosed. If feasible, potential field junctions should be placed over areas at low risk for tumor and normal tissue damage. Treatment of the more common presentations of disseminated breast cancer is discussed below; treatment of local/regional recurrence, with or without disseminated disease, is discussed in chapter 41.

BONE METASTASES

The most common problem for which irradiation is used in disseminated breast cancer is bone metastases. Breast cancer is the primary malignancy accounting for 40 percent to 60 percent of bone metastases in most series.[49, 59, 86, 96, 111]

The survival of patients with bone metastases from breast cancer is somewhat longer than survival of patients with bone metastases from other cancers. In the Radiation Therapy Oncology Group (RTOG) study of single-dose hemibody irradiation for multiple bone metastases, in which more than 80 percent of the patients had severe and constant pain and many patients were considered terminal, two of 129 patients were still alive more than 5 years after treatment.[93] The median survival for patients with metastatic breast cancer ranges from 4 months to 15 months in most series,[6, 31, 37, 39, 59, 93, 110, 114] with 2-year survival rates of only 15 percent to 20 percent. Gilbert and coworkers[39] reported a median survival of 15 months from treatment of first bony metastasis from breast cancer but found that 15 percent of patients with metastatic breast cancer died within less than 3 months of treatment.

Mechanism of Pain Relief

The mechanism by which irradiation relieves pain is unknown. Pain secondary to bone metastasis is thought to be caused by stretching of the periosteum, through which nerve fibers conducting pain sensation are known to pass. The rapidity of response to low doses of irradiation given to large fields and the effectiveness of many different dose regimens have led some researchers[17, 113, 125] to hypothesize that palliation from irradiation may depend on an effect on humoral factors such as prostaglandins through which pain may be mediated rather than on tumor shrinkage and relief of periosteal tension.

Response Rates

Various treatment regimens are favored at different institutions, and all produce excellent palliation, with complete response rates in the range of 50 percent to 60 percent and total response rates in the range of 70 percent to 90 percent (Table 45–3).[2, 13, 37, 39, 59, 82, 87, 96, 108, 111, 114]

Dose

Trodella and associates[111] noted no significant differences in overall response rates with various total or daily doses but concluded that 300-cGy daily fractions produced the best ratio of complete responses to partial responses (Fig. 45–14). The results of four prospective studies[51b, 69, 86, 110] from Odense University Hospital in Denmark, the Royal Marsden Hospital, the RTOG, and Rush Medical Center of various dose-fractionation schemes for palliation of bone metastases are summarized in Table 45–4. In the trials from Odense University, the Royal Marsden, and the RTOG, treatment regimens were prospectively randomized. Doses tested included extremely hypofractioned regimens of large

Table 45–3. NONCONTROLLED TRIALS OF VARIOUS RADIATION REGIMENS FOR PALLIATION OF BONE METASTASES

Author, Institution, Year	No. Patients (No. Treated Areas)	Dose/No. Fractions/ Duration	CR Rate* (%)	TR Rate* (%)	Percent Requiring Retreatment	Median Overall Survival	Percent Pts. in Study with Breast Cancer
Vargha et al[114] Mt. Sinai Hosp., New York 1969	119 (132)	4–18Gy/1f/1d	59	96 (98)	2	4 mo	39
Thomas[108] Univ. Hosp., Leiden 1976	65	n.d.	n.d.	71	n.d.	n.d.	100
Jensen and Roesdahl[59] Radiumcenter, Copenhagen 1976	64 (104)	3–7Gy/1f/1d	62	85	6	4 mo	84
Qasim[87] Weston Park Radiotherapy Hosp., Sheffield 1977	315	8–10Gy/1f/1d 20Gy/5f/5d	55 56	83 84	10 15	n.d. n.d.	38
Penn[82] London Hosp., Exeter 1976	144 (223)	8–15Gy/1f/1d 30Gy/10f/2wk	53 50	89 94	5 4	16%† 20%†	100
Allen et al[2] Swedish Hosp., Seattle 1976	110 (152)	10Gy/2f/2d 20Gy/8f/12d 20Gy/5f/7d	n.d.	77 (85)	15	n.d.	60
		40Gy/20f/45d 20Gy/4f/4d 40Gy/16f/25d	n.d.	78 (82)	18	n.d.	
		32Gy/8f/10d 30Gy/5f/7d 40Gy/10f/12d	n.d.	80 (86)	14	n.d.	
Gilbert et al[39] Kaiser Permanente, Los Angeles 1977	158	30–40Gy/3–4wk 20Gy/5f 13Gy/2f	n.d.	73	n.d.	12 mo	43
Garmatis and Chu[37] Memorial Sloan-Kettering, NY 1978	75 (158)	20–25Gy/8–10f/ 2wk	20	76	n.d.	15 mo	100
Schocker and Brady[96] Hahnemann Med. Coll., Philadelphia 1982	(384)	20–50Gy/1– 4.5wk	72	86	17	n.d.	53
Trodella et al[111] Univ. Cattolica del Sacro Cuore, Rome 1984	79	20–40Gy at 2– 4Gy/f	52 (67)	89 (95)	n.d.	n.d.	54

*Figures in parentheses represent results for only the patients with breast cancer.
†2-year survival rate.
Abbreviations: CR, complete response; f, fraction; Gy, 100 cGy; n.d. = no data; TR, total response.

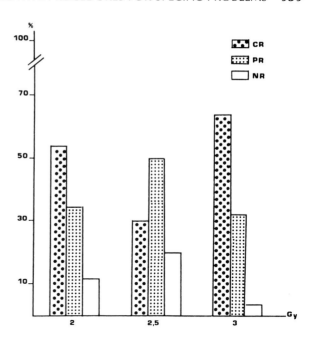

Figure 45–14. Relationship of therapeutic response and daily dose in Gy for bone metastases (3 Gy = 300 cGy). The graph shows the percentage of complete, partial, and no responses obtained with various fraction (daily dose) sizes in a retrospective study of the effectiveness of various treatment regimens for palliation of bone metastases conducted at the Universita Cattolica del Sacro Cuore. CR = complete response, PR = partial response, NR = no response. (From Trodella L, Ausili-Cefaro G, Turriziani A, Marmiroli L, Cellini N, Nardone L: Pain in osseous metastases: Results of radiotherapy. Pain 18:387–396, 1984. Reprinted by permission.)

doses delivered in one or two fractions (800 cGy × 1, 1000 cGy × 2), moderately hypofractionated regimens delivering a daily dose of 300 cGy, 400 cGy, or 500 cGy for 1 week, an intermediate regimen of 3000 cGy in 10 fractions over 2 weeks, and one relatively high-dose regimen of 4050 cGy delivered in 15 270-cGy fractions over 3 weeks. The conclusion from these reports was that there was no demonstrable benefit for long, protracted courses of treatment in the overall population of

patients with bone metastases. However, reanalysis of the RTOG data by Blitzer[8] (Table 45–5) with different statistical techniques and an emphasis on the parameters of complete pain relief prior to retreatment and complete relief from pain without narcotics has shown a benefit for the two more protracted, higher dose treatment regimens (3000 cGy in 10 fractions and 4050 cGy in 15 fractions) over the lower dose, hypofractioned regimens (1500 cGy, 2000 cGy, or 2500 cGy in five

Table 45–4. PROSPECTIVE RANDOMIZED TRIALS OF VARIOUS RADIATION THERAPY REGIMENS FOR PALLIATION OF BONE METASTASES

Author, Institution, Year	No. Patients	Type of Lesion	Dose/No. Fractions/ Duration	CR Rate (%)	TR Rate (%)	TR Rate in Breast Cancer Patients
Price et al[86] Royal Marsden 1986	288	n.d.	8Gy/1f/1d 30Gy/10f/2wk	45 28	72 64	88%
Tong et al[110] RTOG 1982	1016	Solitary	40.5Gy/15f/3wk 20Gy/5f/1wk	61 53	92 90	*
		Multiple	30Gy/10f/2wk 15Gy/5f/1wk 20Gy/5f/1wk 25Gy/5f/1wk	57 49 56 49	92 89 89 87	
Madsen[69] Odense Univ. Hosp. 1983	157	n.d.	24Gy/6f/3wk 20Gy/2f/1wk	n.d. n.d.	47 48	4/10 6/10
Hendrickson et al[51a] Rush Medical Center 1976	86	n.d.	9Gy/1f/1d 12Gy/2f 15Gy/5f 20Gy/10f	n.d. n.d. n.d. n.d.	86	82%
			20Gy/5f 30Gy/10f	n.d. n.d.	70	

*For all dose-fractionation schedules, breast and lung cancer metastases responded significantly better than did other histological types.
Abbreviations: CR, complete response; f, fraction; n.d., no data; TR, total response.

Table 45–5. RESULTS OF RADIATION TREATMENT OF BONE METASTASES

	Complete Pain Relief (Pain Score Only)		Pre-retreatment Complete Pain Relief (Pain Score Only)		Retreated		Complete Combined (Pain + Narcotic)	
	%	No.	%	No.	%	No.	%	No.
Solitary group								
270 cGy × 15 fractions	61	45/74	61	45/74	11	8/74	55	38/69
400 cGy × 5 fractions	53	38/72	49	35/72	24	17/72	37	25/68
Multiple group								
300 cGy × 10 fractions	57	96/167	55	92/167	12	20/167	46	72/158
300 cGy × 5 fractions	49	70/143	47	67/143	23	33/143	36	48/135
400 cGy × 5 fractions	56	87/155	52	81/155	15	24/155	40	59/147
500 cGy × 5 fractions	49	72/148	46	68/148	16	23/148	28	39/137
B_1 = coefficient for number of fractions								
Estimate	0.0409		0.0511		0.0790		0.0834	
p value	0.07		0.02		0.02		0.0003	

From Blitzer PH: Cancer 55:1469, 1985. Reprinted by permission.

fractions). The complete pain relief parameter in this RTOG study was based on subjective reports by the patient, and the combined pain relief parameter was based not only on the patient's subjective response but also on narcotic intake.

Time to Response

The time to response is usually rapid. Trodella and coworkers[111] reported that 60 percent of all patients treated respond within 5 to 7 days after beginning treatment. Tong et al.[110] reported that 96 percent of all patients getting at least a minimal response to irradiation did so within 4 weeks of treatment and that 50 percent of all patients getting a complete response did so within 4 weeks.

Duration of Response

Duration of response is difficult to assess, but one study[110] found that more than 70 percent of patients who responded did not relapse in the treated site before death. In an attempt to assess the durability of response, several studies have documented the percentage of patients responding to treatment who require retreatment of the same lesion. Retreatment rates range from two percent to 18 percent.[2, 59, 82, 87, 114] Retreatment rates underestimate the relapse rate, which ranges from 8.6 percent to 25 percent when documented.[2, 82] Two prospective randomized trials comparing different dose schedules have addressed the issue of duration of response.[69, 110] Madsen,[69] reporting on a trial conducted at the Royal Marsden Hospital of 800 cGy in one fraction vs. 3000 cGy in ten fractions over 2 weeks, found no difference in durability of response between the two regimens. Tong et al.,[110] reporting on an RTOG trial of various dose regimens stratified by whether the patient had solitary or multiple metastases, found no difference

in duration of response between short, hypofractioned regimens and more protracted regimens delivering higher doses. Schocker and Brady,[96] in discussing the same RTOG data, noted that retreatment rates appeared to be higher in the shorter, more hypofractioned regimens. In a reanalysis of the RTOG data with multivariate techniques and an emphasis on parameters of complete pain relief prior to retreatment as measured by both the patient's assessment of response and the pattern of narcotic usage, Blitzer[8] concluded that there was a significantly increased rate of retreatment following the shorter, hypofractionated regimens as well as a significant improvement in the rate of complete pain relief with the higher dose, more protracted regimens (Table 45–5). The rate of retreatment after the more protracted regimens was 11 percent and 12 percent for 40.5 Gy and 30 Gy, respectively, compared with 23 percent, 24 percent, 15 percent, and 16 percent for 15 Gy, 20 Gy, 20 Gy, and 25 Gy, respectively.

Pathological Fractures and Bone Healing after Irradiation

In the RTOG study of various dose-fractionation regimens for the treatment of bone metastases, the rate of pathological fracture after irradiation was eight percent when all sites were studied, 13 percent when only long bones were considered, and six percent when only spinal sites were considered.[110] In this study, the rate of pathological fracture in patients with a solitary metastasis was significantly higher after 4050 cGy than after 2000 cGy (18 percent vs. four percent, $p = 0.02$). Other studies have not found a correlation between the risk of pathological fracture and the dose of irradiation.[82, 87] Pathological fracture is a complication of malignancy that can frequently be avoided by attention to risk factors and prophylactic surgical intervention. Roentgenographic and clinical features that indicate a high risk of fracture include a lytic lesion greater than 2 cm in diameter on either anteroposterior or lateral view of the proximal femur, an avulsion fracture of the lesser trochanter, destruction of more than 50 percent of the cortex at any level, and persisting stress pain despite irradiation. A full discussion of the management of a patient at risk for pathological fracture follows in the next subchapter entitled, "Management of Osseous Metastases and Impending Pathological Fractures."

The initial response of bone to irradiation is focal hyperemia, leading to localized osteoporosis and structural weakening. In a patient receiving irradiation for a bone metastasis, the period at highest risk for fracture is 10 to 18 days after beginning irradiation. Bonarigo and Rubin[10] demonstrated interference by irradiation with the chondrogenetic phase of osteoblastic proliferation required for fracture healing. Once a fracture has occurred, irradiation may interfere with the normal healing mechanism, resulting in nonunion.[10, 49] In patients at risk for a pathological fracture, therefore, surgical intervention is best performed prophylactically prior to irradiation. If fracture does not occur, there is frequently bone healing after irradiation through a mechanism different from that required for fracture healing, not requiring a chondrogenetic phase.[49] Several researchers[13, 18, 37, 49] have reported healing on roentgenograms of bone metastases from breast cancer and other malignancies after irradiation in 25 percent to 85 percent of cases. Bouchard[13] noted that there is no roentgenographic evidence of bone repair for at least 2 months after beginning irradiation and that optimum healing usually requires 6 to 12 months.

Side Effects and Complications

Side effects and complications of treatment are related to the site, treatment volume, and dose-fractionation regimen. Transient acute reactions of incidentally irradiated mucosa occur, causing sore throat with treatment of the cervical spine; dysphagia with treatment of the thoracic spine; and nausea, vomiting, and occasionally diarrhea with treatment of the lumbar spine. Transient erythematous skin reactions are most pronounced with orthovoltage treatment, moderate with cobalt, and insignificant with higher energy photon irradiation from accelerators. Several researchers reported severe but transient nausea and vomiting lasting from a few hours up to 2 days associated with large single doses of irradiation to either the lumbar spine or pelvis.[69, 82, 87, 114] Additionally, Penn[82] reported a transient myelitis and Madsen[69] reported a permanent myelitis after a large single dose (10 Gy or 12 Gy) of irradiation to the lumbar spine.

Single-Dose Hemibody Irradiation

Many reports[6, 31, 93, 97] have documented the effect of single-dose hemibody irradiation on patients with widespread metastases. Treatment is delivered to either the upper hemibody or the lower hemibody through equally weighted anterior and posterior fields. Doses of 400 cGy to 800 cGy have been given to the upper hemibody and 800 cGy to 1000 cGy to the lower hemibody. The responses achieved with this approach are summarized in Table 45–6. Complete response rates have ranged from 20 percent to 65 percent and total response rates from 60 percent to 100 percent. The time to response has been very short. Salazar[93] reported that 50 percent of responses occurred within 48 hours and 80 percent within 1 week. Bartelink and coworkers[6] also noted that most responses occurred within 48 hours. In the study by Schorcht and associates,[97] the duration of response

Table 45–6. SINGLE-FRACTION HEMIBODY IRRADIATION FOR MULTIPLE BONE METASTASES

Author, Institution, Year	No. Patients, Dose	CR Rate (%)	TR Rate (%)	Time to Response (hr)	Median Duration of Response (mo)	Median Survival
Bartelink et al[6] Antoni van Leeuwenhoek Hosp., Amsterdam 1980	21 pts 8 Gy lower, 6 Gy upper	57	100	<48	3	n.d.
Fitzpatrick and Garrett[31] Princess Margaret Hosp., Toronto 1981	34 pts 8–10 Gy lower	65	82	n.d.	17 (CR) 2 (PR)	58 wk
Schorcht et al[97] Medical Academy Carl Gustav Carus, Dresden 1984	23 pts 8 Gy lower, 4–8 Gy upper	n.d.	60	n.d.	5–7* 0–1† 7–8‡ 2–5§	7.7 mo
Salazar et al[93] RTOG 1986	168 pts 8–10 Gy lower, 6–7 Gy upper	20	73	48	4	7.5 mo

*In patients with involvement of one or two systems.
†In patients with involvement of three or four systems.
‡In patients with disease-free interval >2 yr.
§In patients with disease-free interval ≤2 yr.
Abbreviations: CR, complete response; Gy, 100 cGy; PR, partial response; TR, total response.

Table 45–7. OVERALL TOXICITY OF MIDBODY IRRADIATION AND LOWER HALF-BODY IRRADIATION

| Scale | Acute (%) | | Subacute (%) |
	Nausea and Vomiting	Diarrhea	Hematological
0 None	51	80	62
1 Mild	18	7	7
2 Moderate	22	10	21
3 Severe	7	1	3
4 Life-threatening	2	2	7
5 Fatal	0	0	0

From Salazar OM, et al: Cancer 58:33, 1986. Reprinted by permission.

varied in different subsets of patients from 0 to 7.8 months; patients with long disease-free intervals prior to diagnosis of disseminated disease and a limited number of systems involved did best. In the study by Bartelink et al.[6] the median duration of either complete or partial response was approximately 3 months. Salazar and coworkers,[93] analyzing data from the RTOG trial of hemibody irradiation, defined the parameter of *net pain relief* as the proportion of remaining life with pain relief. As the mean survival time for patients obtaining some pain relief was 30 weeks and the mean duration of pain relief was 15 weeks, the net pain relief was 50 percent. In the same RTOG study, 50 percent of patients did not require retreatment.[93] The duration of response reported by Fitzpatrick and Garrett[31] was substantially longer, as was patient survival, possibly because all patients had had little or no prior therapy and all were premenopausal or perimenopausal and may have benefited from ovarian ablation. In fact, 41 percent of premenopausal patients in this study showed indirect effects of the lower hemibody irradiation (i.e., tumor response in areas not treated). The morbidity of this approach includes transient nausea, vomiting, diarrhea, bone marrow suppression, and occasional pneumonitis (Tables 45–7 and 45–8). When doses higher than 600 cGy to 700 cGy are delivered to the upper hemibody, pneumonitis is more common and may be fatal.[35, 85, 94]

Treatment Recommendations

Because response rates are good with a variety of dose-fractionation regimens, high-dose, protracted treatment regimens that may occupy a significant proportion of most patients' lives are not indicated in the majority of cases. Because of the risk of severe late complications with large-dose, hypofractionated regimens[48, 103] and the possibility of more durable responses with higher dose, protracted regimens,[8] the majority of patients at the University of Florida are treated with an intermediate regimen of 3000 cGy in ten fractions over 2 weeks.

In patients with a favorable presentation (i.e., a solitary bone metastasis in a patient in good health with a high estrogen receptor level or a long disease-free interval), treatment is more aggressive because survival may be prolonged. A dose of 4500 cGy to 5000 cGy over 5 to 5½ weeks is delivered (Fig. 45–15). When an extremity lesion is treated, attention is given to sparing a strip of skin the entire length of the affected limb to reduce the risk of subsequent edema (Fig. 45–15).

For patients with a very poor prognosis and multiple metastases, hemibody or sequential hemibody irradiation is the best choice. This approach saves the very ill patient many difficult trips to the department and offers excellent and rapid pain relief. The dose delivered to the upper hemibody is 600 cGy and to the lower hemibody is 800 cGy. Most patients are observed overnight in the hospital and managed aggressively for transient but often significant nausea and vomiting. When sequential treatment is given, a period of 4 to 6 weeks is usually required for marrow recovery before the second part of treatment. In a patient with a very poor prognosis who has a localized symptomatic area, 800 cGy or 1000 cGy may be given in a single fraction.

BRAIN METASTASES

One of the more common indications for palliative radiation therapy is brain metastasis. In most series[19, 27, 32, 40, 54, 77, 79, 101, 118] reporting results of palliative radiation for brain metastases, breast cancer is the primary malignancy in 20 percent to 40 percent of cases (Table 45–9).

Table 45–8. OVERALL TOXICITY OF UPPER HALF-BODY IRRADIATION

| Scale | Acute (%) | | | Subacute (%) | |
	Nausea and Vomiting	Fever	Diarrhea	Hematological	Pneumonitis
0 None	45	87	94	37	97
1 Mild	13	5	3	5	3*
2 Moderate	26	8	3	26	0
3 Severe	16	3	0	21	0
4 Life-threatening	0	0	0	11	0
5 Fatal	0	0	0	0	0

*One patient, not fatal, lasted 1 week, treated symptomatically.
From Salazar OM, et al: Cancer 58:34, 1986. Reprinted by permission.

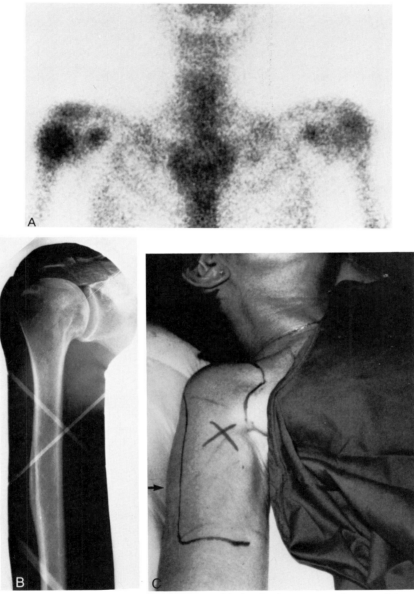

Figure 45–15. In August 1984, a 57-year-old woman underwent a right modified radical mastectomy for a medial central T1N0 estrogen receptor–positive breast carcinoma. In May 1988 the patient presented with vague discomfort in the left shoulder after playing tennis. Roentgenographic evaluation demonstrated a lytic lesion and fracture of the left proximal humerus. Bone scan showed increased uptake in the left proximal humerus and no other evidence of abnormality. On biopsy, recurrent estrogen receptor–positive breast carcinoma was found. The left proximal humerus was internally fixed and then irradiated to a dose of 5000 cGy in 25 fractions over five weeks. The patient resumed normal activities, including tennis. In May 1989 she presented with vague discomfort in the right shoulder. *A,* Bone scan demonstrated increased uptake in the proximal right humerus and no other areas of abnormality. *B,* The lytic lesion was easily seen on the simulation film. Because of the patient's high functional level, the demonstrated indolent biology of her tumor, the limited amount of metastastic disease, and the probability of prolonged survival, she was again treated aggressively. A customized block was made of Lipowitz's metal to treat the proximal humerus. A dose of 5000 cGy was delivered in 25 fractions over five weeks to the treatment volume. *C,* A strip of skin (arrow) was spared along the lateral aspect of the arm in an effort to decrease the risk of edema.

Table 45–9. NONCONTROLLED STUDIES OF PALLIATION OF BRAIN METASTASES WITH IRRADIATION

Author, Institution, Year	No. Pts.	Percentage with Breast Cancer (%)	Response Rate (%)	Median Duration of Survival
Chu and Hilaris[19] Memorial Hospital 1961	218	39	86‡	6.7 mo*, 2.2 mo†
Order et al[79] Yale 1968	108	14	60	6.3 mo
Hindo et al[54] Presbyterian- St. Luke's 1970	54	21	65	5.6 mo
Nisce et al[77] Memorial Hospital 1971	560	39	80‡	6 mo‡
Gilbert et al[40] So. California Permanente 1978	90	23	48(10/21)	3–7 mo
West and Maor[118] M. D. Anderson Hospital 1980	350	42	75	5.7 mo
Snee et al[101] Western General Hosp., Edinburgh 1985	90	100	81	4 mo
Egawa et al[27] Tokyo 1986	254	11	44§	4.6 mo

*In responders.
†In nonresponders.
‡Of breast cancer patients who completed prescribed treatment.
§Breast cancer only.

Response Rates

Most researchers report response rates of approximately 60 percent (see Table 45–9). The median duration of survival after irradiation for brain metastases is approximately 5 months. Response rates for palliation of common symptoms of brain metastases obtained in two RTOG studies are shown in Table 45–10.[12] The duration of response is difficult to assess. In one study, control of symptoms was documented at last follow-up in only 55 of the 242 patients for whom information was available.[118] In the RTOG trials, it was estimated that patients' symptoms remained palliated for 75 percent of their remaining life span.[12]

Dose

The Princess Margaret Hospital conducted a prospective randomized trial of various dose-fractionation

Table 45–10. SPECIFIC NEUROLOGICAL SYMPTOM RELIEF WITH BRAIN IRRADIATION

Symptom	First Study			Second Study		
	No. Pts.	Complete Response (%)	Overall Response (%)	No. Pts.	Complete Response (%)	Overall Response (%)
Headache	500	52	82	482	69	82
Motor loss	454	32	74	456	37	61
Impaired mentation	355	34	71	425	52	69
Cerebellar dysfunction	218	39	75	259	50	64
Cranial nerve	215	40	71	244	44	59
Increased intracranial pressure	165	57	83	No data	No data	No data
Convulsions, general	108	66	86	134	87	90
Convulsions, focal	85	58	76			
Sensory loss	175	41	77	No data	No data	No data
Lethargy	237	39	69	No data	No data	No data

From Borgelt BB, et al: Int J Radiat Oncol Biol Phys 6:6, 1980. Reprinted by permission.

schemes in patients irradiated for brain metastases.[32] The two regimens tested were 1000 cGy delivered in a single fraction and 3000 cGy delivered in ten fractions over 2 weeks. There was no difference in response rates, with responses obtained in 57 percent of the patients receiving 1000 cGy and 64 percent of the patients receiving 3000 cGy. The RTOG conducted two prospective randomized trials evaluating the efficacy of various dose-fractionation schemes.[12] In the first study, patients were randomized to receive 3000 cGy in either 2 weeks or 3 weeks or 4000 cGy in either 3 weeks or 4 weeks. In the second trial, patients received 2000 cGy in 1 week, 3000 cGy in 2 weeks, or 4000 cGy in 3 weeks. No benefit was demonstrated for any regimen. A subset analysis performed on favorable subgroups of patients, including ambulatory breast cancer patients with no soft tissue metastases, also showed no advantage with any of the dose-fractionation regimens tested.[38] A third trial compared conventional fractionation with an accelerated hyperfractionation scheme employing multiple daily treatments. Patients received either 3000 cGy delivered in ten fractions over 2 weeks or 3000 cGy delivered in 15 fractions, three fractions a day, over 1 week.[24] No difference was found between conventional treatment and multiple daily fractions in terms of response rate, neurological improvement, survival, or morbidity.

Corticosteroids

The primary role of steroids is to rapidly improve or stabilize neurological deficits until definitive treatment is under way. Steroids are also useful in managing patients with steroid-reversible neurological deficits following completion of definitive therapy and at the time of tumor progression. It is not clear whether steroids are beneficial for neurologically intact patients.

Borgelt and coworkers[12] suggested that patients treated with steroids and radiation may obtain a more rapid response than patients treated with radiation only. Horton et al.[55] have reported that the duration of response achieved with corticosteroids appears to be prolonged by the addition of radiation therapy. In a comprehensive review of the role of glucocorticoid treatment for brain metastases and epidural spinal cord compression, Weissman[117] found that steroids decrease or prevent peritumoral edema. He recommends a starting dose of 16 mg per day of dexamethasone with tapering of the dosage started as soon as definitive treatment is under way. The overall steroid course should last no longer than 14 to 21 days in most patients. The dose may be escalated to 100 mg per day in patients with progressive neurological deficits; after a 7-day trial, the dose should be tapered in these patients to the lowest dose that will maintain stable neurological function. The indication for long-term steroid treatment is the presence of a steroid-reversible deficit, not a fixed neurological deficit. Toxicity from prolonged steroid therapy includes not only weight gain, change in facial appearance, striae, acne, sleep disturbance, hiccough, and genital burning, but also life-threatening problems such as diabetes, proximal muscle weakness, suscepti-

bility to infections, peripheral edema, gastrointestinal perforation, and psychosis.

Side Effects and Complications

In most series, side effects are minimal. Transient alopecia may occur. High-dose single-fraction or hypofractionated regimens appear to result in more acute and late complications than do conventional fractionation regimens. In the prospective randomized trial from Princess Margaret Hospital comparing two dose-fractionation schemes, acute complications consisting of headache, nausea, vomiting, increased neurological deficit, and a decrease in the level of consciousness occurred in 47 percent of patients receiving 1000 cGy and 27 percent of patients receiving 3000 cGy.[32] In a study of patients treated with 1000 cGy in a single fraction, Hindo and associates[54] reported death within 48 hours of treatment in three of 54 patients, all of whom had severe neurological deficits. Sundaresan et al.[105] reported three cases of radiation necrosis resulting in severe debility or death after treatment regimens employing high doses per fraction and high overall doses (3900 cGy in 11 fractions to the whole brain).

Solitary Brain Metastasis

There is no prospective randomized trial evaluating the relative roles of surgical resection and postoperative whole-brain irradiation for a solitary brain metastasis.[76] Long-term survivors with aggressive treatment of a solitary metastasis from breast cancer as well as renal carcinoma have been reported.[26] Several reports[26, 36, 115] have suggested a benefit to surgical resection with or without postoperative whole-brain irradiation. The postoperative mortality, when reported, approximates 15 percent.[90, 115] Smalley et al.[100] demonstrated that whole-brain irradiation following surgical resection results in a decrease in the subsequent incidence of brain relapse and may prolong survival. Within the group of 1895 patients treated in the two RTOG trials of various dose-fractionation schemes discussed previously, there were 218 patients who had undergone prior surgery—either biopsy or surgical resection of a solitary metastasis.[12, 51] When the group was stratified by initial neurological function, there was no difference in improvement of neurological function with or without surgery. However, the overall rates of symptom relief for headache and motor loss were higher in patients who had undergone surgical resection of the metastasis prior to irradiation. In patients with no extracerebral disease, it appeared that the time to tumor progression was greater in patients who had undergone resection of the metastasis prior to irradiation. The conclusion of the study was that surgical intervention is indicated when (1) an intracranial lesion suspected to be malignant is present with no known primary cancer, and (2) an apparently solitary metastasis is located in an accessible, noncritical location.

Brachytherapy and Radiosurgery

There is limited experience with interstitial implantation of brain metastases with stereotactic placement of catheters that are loaded afterward with iridium.[53, 83] Limited experience has also been reported with high doses (2000–3000 cGy) of radiation delivered in a single fraction with very small fields and a stereotactic technique.[104] Both approaches offer the advantage of high-dose irradiation to the tumor and only a small volume of normal tissue. Further experience and follow-up will be needed to define the optimal role of these approaches.

Retreatment

Several studies[32, 63, 77, 79] have reported responses in one third to one half of patients given a second course of irradiation for recurrent brain metastases. Responses lasting an average of 1.5 months to 2.6 months were obtained in 50 percent to 69 percent of patients undergoing second and third courses of irradiation at Rush-Presbyterian.[98] In a study from the University of Colorado, however, Hazuka and Kinzie[50] found neurological improvement in only 27 percent of the 44 patients undergoing retreatment. The median survival after a second course of irradiation was only 8 weeks. Three brain necroses occurred, two of which were fatal. The authors concluded that retreatment was seldom worthwhile.[50]

Treatment Recommendations

All symptomatic patients are started on a course of steroid therapy to achieve as rapid a response as possible. The steroid dosage is tapered after the course of

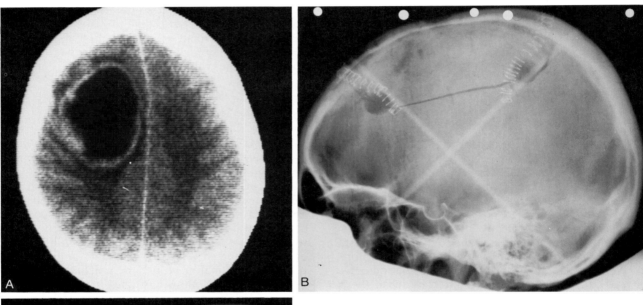

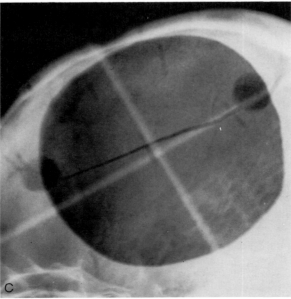

Figure 45–16. This 27-year-old woman underwent right modified radical mastectomy in 1983 for a medial T1N0 estrogen receptor–negative carcinoma of the breast. In November 1984, she had right chest wall pain and was found to have a large right internal mammary node recurrence. She was treated with cyclophosphamide, doxorubicin HC1, and 5-fluorouracil for six courses, obtaining an excellent response. The residual mass was resected, and postoperative irradiation was delivered to the chest wall and peripheral lymphatics. She presented in January 1986 with left hand weakness, headaches, and ataxia. *A,* Computerized tomography showed a large but solitary lesion in the right frontal area with moderate mass effect. Craniotomy was performed with gross resection of the fluid-filled cystic mass, which was consistent histologically with her primary breast cancer. After surgery all neurological signs and symptoms resolved. *B,* Postoperatively she received 4500 cGy to the whole brain in 25 fractions over five weeks followed by *(C)* a 500 cGy boost dose to the tumor bed delivered in three fractions through reduced lateral and anterior portals with wedge filters. Although other sites of distant disease developed, there was no further evidence of disease in the brain at the time of her death in August 1986.

Sign/Symptom	First Symptom		Symptoms at Diagnosis	
	No. Pts.	%	No. Pts.	%
Pain	125	96	125	96
Weakness	2	2	99	76
Autonomic dysfunction	0	0	74	57
Sensory loss	0	0	66	51
Ataxia	2	2	4	3
Herpes zoster	0	0	3	2
Flexor spasms	0	0	2	1

From Gilbert RW, et al: Ann Neurol 3:42, 1978. Reprinted by permission.

irradiation is started. The majority of patients receive 3000 cGy in ten fractions of 300 cGy over 2 weeks. For patients with solitary lesions judged to have a favorable prognosis (i.e., a long disease-free interval, control of the primary disease, and no evident extracerebral metastases), surgical resection is performed if feasible, followed by postoperative irradiation. After surgical resection, 4500 cGy is delivered to the whole brain in 25 fractions at 180 cGy a day; the dose to the tumor bed is boosted with an additional 500 cGy to 1000 cGy (Fig. 45–16). If surgical resection is incomplete or not feasible, consideration may be given to a brachytherapy boost after whole-brain irradiation.

SPINAL CORD METASTASES

Spinal cord compression complicates the course of disseminated cancer in five percent of cases and represents a true oncological emergency.[91] Breast cancer accounts for the primary malignancy in 15 percent to 25 percent of spinal cord compressions secondary to metastatic cancer.[23, 41, 60, 120, 124] The first symptom of epidural cord compression is pain in 80 percent to 95 percent of cases (Table 45–11).[5, 41] At the time of diagnosis, however, sensory and motor symptoms are common; sphincter dysfunction is less common and indicates an advanced lesion and a poor prognosis.[121] A high index of suspicion is imperative, as the outcome of treatment depends on early diagnosis and early treatment.[15]

Cord compression from metastatic disease may result from direct tumor extension through intervertebral foramina from mediastinal or retroperitoneal lymph nodes, soft tissue extension from metastatic disease in vertebral bodies, vertebral collapse from tumor destruction, or intramedullary metastases. The vast majority of cord compressions in metastatic breast cancer are complications of vertebral metastases, with occasional intramedullary metastases.[123]

Spinal cord compression traditionally has been treated with laminectomy, with or without postoperative irradiation,[120] or with irradiation alone.[41, 75, 81] Studies that retrospectively compare results in patients treated with

these three approaches have failed to conclusively demonstrate a better result with the addition of laminectomy.[21, 41, 121] Two studies specifically addressing the role of radiation therapy after laminectomy have shown better motor recovery with laminectomy plus postoperative irradiation than with laminectomy alone.[121, 124] White and coworkers[120] noted that a substantial number of patients who recovered the ability to ambulate after surgery alone subsequently lost it because of local recurrence. The only prospective randomized trial comparing laminectomy plus postoperative irradiation with irradiation alone demonstrated no advantage with either regimen for pain relief, improved ambulation, or sphincter function.[126]

A number of studies have shown that prognosis for ambulation is related to the initial functional status. The results of several studies of recovery of ambulation as a function of initial functional status are presented in Table 45–12.[120, 121, 124] Recovery of ambulation is rare in patients who are paraplegic at presentation.[5, 47, 102, 109, 120, 121, 124] It is likely that the only paraplegic patients with a reasonable chance of recovery are those in whom the paralysis is of very short duration.[70] A second factor very important for prognosis is the degree of blockage of cerebrospinal flow demonstrated at myelography. In the trial of irradiation with or without preceding laminectomy reported by Young et al.,[126] the proportion of patients who were ambulatory either immediately after treatment or 4 months after treatment relative to their initial functional status and degree of blockage demonstrated on pretherapy myelography is shown in Table 45–13. In patients who were not paraplegic at the time of treatment, six of seven patients without complete block were ambulatory after treatment vs. eight of 19 patients with complete block. Four months after treatment, four of seven patients without complete block remained ambulatory vs. only six of 19 patients with complete block. Other factors indicating a poor prognosis are rapid progression of symptoms, vertebral collapse, elevated protein in the cerebrospinal fluid, and complete sensory loss.[74]

Table 45–12. RESULTS OF TREATMENT OF SPINAL CORD COMPRESSION

Pretherapy Function	Posttherapy Function (% Patients Treated)		
	Ambulatory	Nonambulatory	Paraplegic
Ambulatory			
Memorial Hospital[120]	64	22	14
Massachusetts General Hospital[124]	53	37	10
Long Beach VA Hospital[121]	1/3	—	2/3
Nonambulatory			
Memorial Hospital[120]	34	47	19
Massachusetts General Hospital[124]	37	30	33
Long Beach VA Hospital[121]	71	14	14
Paraplegic			
Memorial Hospital[120]	10	14	76
Massachusetts General Hospital[124]	0	11	89
Long Beach VA Hospital[121]	31	26	43

Table 45–13. EFFECT OF MYELOGRAPHIC BLOCK ON 29 PATIENTS WITH SPINAL EPIDURAL METASTASES: MOTOR PERFORMANCE

Results	No Block			Block		
	No. Pts.	*No. Ambulatory*	*%*	*No. Pts.*	*No. Ambulatory*	*%*
Immediate results						
Ambulatory	4	4	100	7	4	57
Not ambulatory	3	2	67	12	4	33
Paraplegic	0	0	0	3	0	0
At 4 months						
Ambulatory	4	3	75	7	2	29
Not ambulatory	3	1	33	12	4	33
Paraplegic	0	0	0	3	0	0

From Young RF, et al: J Neurosurg 53:744, 1980. Reprinted by permission.

Side Effects and Complications

Early series reported laminectomy mortality rates of eight percent,[124] but more recent series show few non-tumor-related deaths with surgery or irradiation.[126] Side effects and complications of irradiation are similar to those observed after palliative irradiation for bone metastases.

Treatment Recommendations

Patients suspected of having cord compression should undergo immediate myelography. A new method for identifying cord compression is magnetic resonance imaging. The relative effectiveness of the two diagnostic regimens has not been proven in a prospective study, but satisfactory results may be obtained with either method. Decompressive laminectomy should be considered for previously irradiated areas of compression, progression of symptoms during the course of irradiation, complete blockage on myelogram, known or suspected radioresistant tumors, rapid onset of symptoms, compression secondary to vertebral collapse, and diagnosis when the primary tumor is not known. Most patients do not require laminectomy but begin treatment on corticosteroids and irradiation immediately after myelography. A dose of 3000 cGy delivered in ten fractions of 300 cGy over 2 weeks is given. In patients who are paraplegic or have severe weakness, 400 cGy to 500 cGy may be given once or twice, followed by smaller fractions (250 cGy to 275 cGy) for the remainder of the course, as experimental and clinical data suggest that higher initial daily doses are safe and may result in better responses.[92] It is important to base the extent of the treatment portal on the findings at myelogram or magnetic resonance imaging. The sensory level is often two to three vertebral levels below the lesion. It has been shown that a high proportion of the recurrences after irradiation are in lesions outside the treatment field that were present at the time of diagnosis but were missed by the treatment portal.[66] Another study[16] demonstrated that 75 percent of portals planned on the basis of clinical findings and plain roentgenograms were inadequate to cover the disease apparent on myelography. Treatment portals should include two vertebral bodies above and below the lesion defined at magnetic resonance imaging or myelography and any adjacent asymptomatic lesions. An occasional patient whose neurological defect progresses during the course of radiation therapy may be rendered ambulatory by decompressive laminectomy, so it is imperative that patients have close follow-up while under treatment.[21]

CHOROID METASTASES

The most common intraocular malignancy is metastatic tumor.[9, 30] The choroid is the intraocular structure most often affected by metastases.[9, 30] The most common site of metastatic involvement within the choroid is the posterior pole on the temporal side of the macula.[20, 89, 95] Breast cancer is the primary malignancy accounting for 60 percent to 70 percent of all metastatic choroid lesions.[9, 25, 30, 33, 42, 57, 80, 88, 122] Choroid metastases usually occur in conjunction with widespread metastases in other sites but are the first sign of distant metastases in 20 percent to 30 percent of cases.[20, 72, 107] In a large series[73] from the M. D. Anderson Cancer Center in Houston, 152 patients presented with ocular complaints and a history of breast cancer; 38 percent were found to have choroid metastases. Choroid metastases were also diagnosed on screening examination in nine percent of an additional 98 asymptomatic patients with a history of breast cancer. All patients found to have incidental choroid metastases had known stage IV disease, for a 14 percent rate of choroid involvement in asymptomatic stage IV disease. Bilateral involvement occurs in 25 percent to 40 percent of cases.[20, 25, 57, 72, 73, 88, 107] Choroid metastasis is a significant clinical problem because of the potential for uncontrolled choroid disease to produce the debilitating complications of blindness or glaucoma. Blindness results from elevation and detachment of the retina. Glaucoma may result from increased intraocular pressure secondary to rapid tumor growth, venous congestion from pressure on choroid vessels, or blockage of the iris angle by exfoliated tumor cells or anterior motion of the lens.[78] Patients usually present with blurred vision, scotomata, pain, and photophobia.[20] Choroid metastases may exhibit rapid growth, leading to blindness within days or weeks of initial presentation, and thus prompt management is indicated.

Results of Treatment

One third to one half of patients will have a marked response or complete resolution of symptoms after irradiation.[20, 25, 80, 88, 107] Another one third will obtain a partial response or stabilization of disease.[20, 25, 80, 88] A few patients continue to deteriorate after irradiation.[20, 80] Chu and coworkers[20] noted that 100 percent of patients with lesions occupying less than half of a quadrant of the eye ground obtained a response to irradiation, 77 percent of patients with more than half of a quadrant involved but minimal or no retinal detachment responded, and only 37 percent of patients with moderate to massive retinal detachment showed improvement. Most responses occur within 3 to 4 weeks of irradiation.[107] When there is retinal detachment, responses may occur later as subretinal fluid is resorbed.

Treatment

Conventional external-beam irradiation with photons is the standard treatment for choroid metastasis. Doses of 3000 cGy in ten fractions over 2 weeks or 4000 cGy in 20 fractions over 4 weeks are effective. Lesions in the posterior pole are adequately treated with a single lateral 4 cm × 4 cm field. The anterior field edge is placed just behind the lens, which is the most radiosensitive structure in the eye. The field is angled 5° posteriorly to avoid irradiation of the contralateral lens. For patients with bilateral involvement, opposed lateral fields may be used with either a 5° posterior tilt on both fields or half-beam blocks placed in the anterior half of the beams to eliminate divergence. Electron beam[20] and proton beam[46] therapy have been used in an attempt to limit normal tissue irradiation. Side effects and complications of standard photon beam therapy are rare, however, because of the doses delivered and techniques employed.[20, 68, 73, 80] Electron beam therapy does produce a significant skin reaction, which is not seen with high-energy photon irradiation, and proton beam is both expensive and inaccessible to the majority of patients. Responses to both chemotherapy[14, 65] and hormonal therapy[22, 28, 61] have been reported, so patients diagnosed incidentally with asymptomatic choroid metastases who are undergoing systemic therapy should be observed closely. Radiation therapy should be instituted at the first sign of progression, however, as results may depend on the extent of tumor.[20]

LIVER METASTASES

The prognosis for patients with hepatic metastases is quite poor. The median survival in 390 patients with untreated liver metastases was 75 days, with only seven percent of patients surviving more than a year.[58] The signs and symptoms most often associated with liver metastases are abdominal pain, nausea and vomiting, fevers and night sweats, ascites, anorexia, abdominal distention, jaundice, weakness, and fatigue.

Conventional Irradiation

In an excellent discussion of the role of radiation therapy in the treatment of liver metastases, Kinsella[62] noted that a major consideration is the radiation tolerance of the normal liver parenchyma. The clinical syndrome indicating acute radiation damage is radiation hepatitis, which usually occurs within 2 to 6 weeks of treatment and can be fatal.[56] This syndrome and its relation to radiation parameters of treatment volume, dose, and fraction size (daily dose) have been studied by Ingold and colleagues[56] from Stanford. The syndrome occurs uncommonly with doses to the whole liver of less than 3000 cGy to 3500 cGy delivered in fractions of 200 cGy or less per day. Other data suggest that the threshold for radiation hepatitis may be as low as 2500 cGy when the daily dose is greater than 200 cGy.[119] When smaller volumes of liver are treated, doses as high as 5500 cGy are tolerated.[56] Treatment regimens employing dose-fractionation schemes unlikely to produce radiation hepatitis have generally been regarded as unlikely to be effective in arresting the growth of metastatic carcinoma. However, several recent series have documented excellent palliative results with radiation therapy.[84, 99, 112] Total response rates ranged from 70 percent to 90 percent, with up to 44 percent obtaining complete pain relief.[84, 99] Improvement in jaundice and ascites was occasionally noted as well.[84] Sherman et al.[99] noted that pain relief usually persisted for most of the remainder of the patient's life. The RTOG conducted a prospective nonrandomized, noncontrolled study of optimal doses for patients with either solitary or multiple liver metastases.[11] For patients with solitary liver metastases, participating investigators were allowed a choice of 2040 cGy in 19 fractions or 3000 cGy in 15 fractions to the entire liver, each with an optional 2000-cGy boost dose to the metastasis. For patients with multiple liver metastases, the options were 3000 cGy in 15 fractions, 2560 cGy in 16 fractions, 2000 cGy in ten fractions, or 2100 cGy in seven fractions. The median survival for the patient population was 11 weeks. Twenty-two percent of patients died less than 4 weeks after treatment, and 20 percent lived more than 6 months after treatment. No differences in outcome were noted among the various regimens. A higher proportion of patients (17/18) with multiple metastases treated with 2100 cGy in seven fractions completed the treatment regimen than did those treated with a more protracted regimen. Complete and total response rates for various signs and symptoms of hepatic metastases are shown in Table 45–14. It was noted that patients with mild symptoms prior to treatment spent 80 percent of their remaining life with mild or no pain; patients with moderate or severe pain spent 63 percent of their remaining life with mild or no pain.

Table 45–14. THERAPEUTIC BENEFIT OF HEPATIC IRRADIATION (FOURTH WEEK ASSESSMENT)

Sign/Symptom	No. responding*/ No. evaluable†	%	Improvement (%)
Abdominal pain	43/78	55	24
Nausea/vomiting	17/35	49	34
Fever/night sweats	10/22	45	27
Ascites	7/21	33	29
Anorexia	18/65	28	9
Abdominal distension	13/49	27	10
Jaundice	8/30	27	17
Weakness/fatigue	15/81	19	7

*Patients dying within 4 weeks were considered to be nonresponders.

†Includes all patients with symptom initially present.

From Borgelt BB, et al: Int J Radiat Oncol Biol Phys. 7:589, 1981. Reprinted by permission.

New Radiotherapy Methods

In an effort to increase the effectiveness of irradiation in the treatment of hepatic metastases, approaches combining irradiation with intraarterial chemotherapy or misonidazole or using infusion of radioactive microspheres or radioactive isotope–labeled immunoglobulin have been investigated.

Irradiation in Combination with Intraarterial Chemotherapy

Kinsella[62] compiled the results (Table 45–15) of several recent trials of conventional radiation therapy in combination with infusional chemotherapy.[4, 34, 52, 62, 67, 116] Response rates ranged from 50 percent to 70 percent. Morbidity was tolerable, with no treatment-related deaths and only mild myelosuppression, mild nausea and vomiting, and occasional gastroenteritis. It is unclear whether combined modality therapy is better than conventional irradiation alone.

Irradiation in Combination with Misonidazole

The RTOG has tested the benefit of misonidazole, a hypoxic cell sensitizer, in conjunction with conventional radiation.[64] Patients were allocated in a prospective randomized fashion to receive 2100 cGy in seven fractions to the entire liver for metastatic disease, with or without misonidazole. The dose of misonidazole was 1.5 gm/m^2 given 4 hours before each dose of radiation. Patients were stratified by primary site, extent of metastatic disease, and Karnofsky performance rating. The end points of the study were relief of hepatic pain, improvement of Karnofsky status, decrease in alkaline phosphatase level, decrease in liver and tumor size, and survival. The addition of misonidazole did *not* significantly improve the therapeutic response to irradiation in any of the parameters studied. Abdominal pain was relieved in 80 percent of symptomatic patients; 54 percent of patients had complete pain relief. Palliation of pain occurred at a median time of 1.7 weeks after beginning treatment. The median duration of response was 13 weeks in symptomatic patients.

Infusion of Radioactive Microspheres

Microscopic liver metastases derive their blood supply from the portal system, whereas large, established hepatic metastases derive their blood supply from the hepatic arteries.[1, 7] It is reasonable, therefore, to assume that large, solitary hepatic metastases could be selectively treated by infusing a cytotoxic agent into the appropriate hepatic artery. Extensive work has been done with intraarterial infusion of 5-fluorouracil, both with portal vein infusion in the adjuvant setting in patients with colorectal carcinoma[106] and with hepatic arterial infusion for known hepatic metastases.[3, 45] In a similar fashion the radioactive isotope phosphorus-32 has been injected into both the superior mesenteric and the celiac arteries in an attempt to prevent liver metastases in patients with colorectal carcinoma.[43, 71] Addi-

Table 45–15. CLINICAL STUDIES OF COMBINED RADIATION AND INTRAARTERIAL CHEMOTHERAPY FOR HEPATIC METASTASES

Author	No. of Patients	Radiation Schedule	Chemotherapy Schedule	Response No.	Response %	Median Survival of Responders
Webber et al[116]	25	2500 cGy/2 wk, 250 cGy per f	FUDR, 25 mg/d to a total dose of 300–500 mg	13/25	52	11 mo
Herbsman et al[52]	13	2500–3000 cGy/3 wk, 150–200 cGy per f	FUDR, 0.25–0.5 mg/kg/d during and after hepatic irradiation	9/13	69	16 mo
Barone et al[4]	10	3000 cGy/2 wk, 300 cGy per f	5-FU, 6–10 mg/kg/d during and after hepatic irradiation	7/10	70	No data
Friedman et al[34]	21	1500–2100 cGy/1–2 wk, 300 cGy per f	5-FU, 10 mg/kg/d to a total dose of 2700–8000 mg and doxorubicin, 2.5–10 mg/kg/d to a total dose of 21–85 mg	10/21	48	No data
Lokich et al[67]	16	2500–3000 cGy/2 wk, 250–300 cGy per f	5-FU, 1 g/d or FUDR, 0.5 mg/kg/d only during irradiation	10/16	62	No data
Total	85			49/85	58	

Abbreviations: f, fraction; 5-FU, 5-fluorouracil; FUDR, Floxuridine.

Modified from Kinsella TJ: Semin Oncol 10:219, 1983.

tionally, radioactive yttrium-90–labeled microspheres have been injected in the hepatic arteries of patients with known liver metastases.[43, 71] Yttrium-90, with a half-life of only 64 hours, is attached to inert glass microspheres with a diameter of 15 μm. The size of the microspheres enables them to be trapped within a tumor capillary bed. This allows selective delivery of high doses (5000 cGy) of irradiation to the tumor with little irradiation of the surrounding liver parenchyma. Grady and coworkers[44] have also treated patients with metastatic liver disease with yttrium-90–labeled microspheres and hyperthermia. Most of the patients treated in this manner have had colorectal carcinoma. Response rates of 65 percent have been reported, but treatment-related morbidity is high, with some treatment-related deaths.[43] This unconventional approach is not applicable to the typical patient who has bilobar liver metastases.

Radioactive Isotope–Labeled Immunoglobulin

Treatment of primary liver cancer with radiolabeled antibody is being investigated.[29] If tumor-associated antigens can be identified for metastases from breast cancer and highly specific antibodies developed, this approach may be useful in the future for patients with metastatic breast cancer.

Treatment Recommendations

For patients expected to have a very short survival, single fractions of 600 cGy to 800 cGy can be delivered to the liver with good responses. It is not necessary to treat the entire liver in this setting. If the response is good, treatment can be repeated in 1 to 2 weeks. For the majority of patients, however, conventional treatment with 2100 cGy to 3000 cGy in 300-cGy fractions is recommended. The whole liver is treated with equally weighted anterior and posterior portals. The left kidney is blocked from the posterior portal after 1800 cGy when it is in the field.

References

1. Ackerman NB, Lien WM, Kondi ES, Silverman NA: The blood supply of experimental liver metastases. I. The distribution of hepatic artery and portal vein blood to "small" and "large" tumors. Surgery 66:1067–1072, 1969.
2. Allen KL, Johnson TW, Hibbs GG: Effective bone palliation as related to various treatment regimens. Cancer 37:984–987, 1976.
3. Ansfield FJ, Ramirez G, Davis HL Jr, Wirtanen GW, Johnson RO, Bryan GT, Manalo FB, Borden EC, Davis TE, Esmaili M: Further clinical studies with intrahepatic arterial infusion with 5-fluorouracil. Cancer 36:2413–2417, 1975.
4. Barone RM, Byfield JE, Frankel S: Combination infusional 5-fluorouracil and radiation therapy for the treatment of metastatic carcinoma of the colon to the liver. Dis Colon Rectum 22:376–382, 1979.
5. Barron KD, Hirano A, Araki S, Terry RD: Experiences with metastatic neoplasms involving the spinal cord. Neurology 9:91–106, 1959.
6. Bartelink H, Battermann J, Hart G: Half body irradiation. Int J Radiat Oncol Biol Phys 6:87–90, 1980.
7. Blanchard RJW, Grotenhuis I, LaFave JW, Perry JF Jr: Blood supply to hepatic V2 carcinoma implants as measured by radioactive microspheres. Proc Soc Exp Biol Med 118:465–468, 1965.
8. Blitzer PH: Reanalysis of the RTOG study of the palliation of symptomatic osseous metastasis. Cancer 55:1468–1472, 1985.
9. Bloch RS, Gartner S: The incidence of ocular metastatic carcinoma. Arch Opthalmol 85:673–677, 1971.
10. Bonarigo BC, Rubin P: Nonunion of pathologic fracture after radiation therapy. Radiology 88:889–898, 1967.
11. Borgelt BB, Gelber R, Brady LW, Griffin T, Hendrickson FR: The palliation of hepatic metastases: results of the Radiation Therapy Oncology Group pilot study. Int J Radiat Oncol Biol Phys 7:587–591, 1981.
12. Borgelt BB, Gelber R, Kramer S, Brady LW, Chang CH, Davis LW, Perez CA, Hendrickson FR: The palliation of brain metastases: final results of the first two studies by the Radiation Therapy Oncology Group. Int J Radiat Oncol Biol Phys 6:1–9, 1980.
13. Bouchard J: Skeletal metastases in cancer of the breast. Study of the character, incidence, and response to roentgen therapy. AJR 54:156–171, 1945.
14. Brinkley JR Jr: Response of a choroidal metastasis to multiple-drug chemotherapy. Cancer 45:1538–1539, 1980.
15. Bruckman JE, Bloomer WD: Management of spinal cord compression. Semin Oncol 5:135–140, 1978.
16. Calkins AR, Olson MA, Ellis JH: Impact of myelography on the radiotherapeutic management of malignant spinal cord compression. Neurosurgery 19:614–616, 1986.
17. Carr DB, Carr JM: Role of brain opiates in pain relief. In Stoll BA, Parbhoo S (eds): Bone Metastasis: Monitoring and Treatment. New York, Raven Press, 1983, pp 375–393.
18. Cheng DS, Seitz CB, Eyre HJ: Nonoperative management of femoral, humeral, and acetabular metastases in patients with breast carcinoma. Cancer 45:1533–1537, 1980.
19. Chu FCH, Hilaris BB: Value of radiation therapy in the management of intracranial metastases. Cancer 14:577–581, 1961.
20. Chu FCH, Huh SH, Nisce LZ, Simpson LD: Radiation therapy of choroid metastasis from breast cancer. Int J Radiat Oncol Biol Phys 2:273–279, 1977.
21. Cobb CA III, Leavens ME, Eckles N: Indications for nonoperative treatment of spinal cord compression due to breast cancer. J Neurosurg 47:653–658, 1977.
22. Cogan DG, Kuwabara T: Metastatic carcinoma to eye from breast. Effect of endocrine therapy. Arch Ophthalmol 52:240–249, 1954.
23. Constans JP, de Divitiis E, Donzelli R, Spaziante R, Meder JF, Haye C: Spinal metastases with neurological manifestations. Review of 600 cases. J Neurosurg 59:111–118, 1983.
24. D'Elia F, Bonucci I, Biti GP, Pirtoli L: Different fractionation schedules in radiation treatment of cerebral metastases. Acta Radiol (Oncol) 25:181–184, 1986.
25. Dobrowsky W: Treatment of choroid metastases. Br J Radiol 61:140–142, 1988.
26. Dosoretz DE, Blitzer PH, Russell AH, Wang CC: Management of solitary metastasis to the brain: the role of elective brain irradiation following complete surgical resection. Int J Radiat Oncol Biol Phys 6:1727–1730, 1980.
27. Egawa S, Tukiyama I, Akine Y, Kajiura Y, Yanagawa S, Watai K, Nomura K: Radiotherapy of brain metastases. Int J Radiat Oncol Biol Phys 12:1621–1625, 1986.
28. Ellis RA, Scheie HG: Regression of metastatic lesions of breast carcinoma following sterilization. Arch Ophthalmol 48:455–459, 1952.
29. Ettinger DS, Order SE, Wharam MD, Parker MK, Klein JL, Leichner PK: Phase I–II study of isotopic immunoglobulin therapy for primary liver cancer. Cancer Treat Rep 66:289–297, 1982.
30. Ferry AP, Font RL: Carcinoma metastatic to the eye and orbit. Arch Ophthalmol 92:276–286, 1974.
31. Fitzpatrick PJ, Garrett PG: Metastatic breast cancer: ovarian ablation with lower half-body irradiation. Int J Radiat Oncol Biol Phys 7:1523–1526, 1981.
32. Fitzpatrick PJ, Keen CW: The Princess Margaret and Ontario Cancer Foundation experience. In Weiss L, Gilbert HA,

Posner JB (eds): Brain Metastasis. Proceedings of the Workshop on Brain Metastasis, New York, 1978. Boston, GK Hall, 1978, pp 286–302.

33. Freedman MI, Folk JC: Metastatic tumors to the eye and orbit. Patient survival and clinical characteristics. Arch Ophthalmol 105:1215–1219, 1987.

34. Friedman M, Cassidy M, Levine M, Phillips T, Spivack S, Resser KJ: Combined modality therapy of hepatic metastasis. Cancer 44:906–913, 1979.

35. Fryer CJH, Fitzpatrick PJ, Rider WD, Poon P: Radiation pneumonitis: experience following a large single dose of radiation. Int J Radiat Oncol Biol Phys 4:931–936, 1978.

36. Galicich JH, Sundaresan N, Thaler HT: Surgical treatment of single brain metastasis. Evaluation of results by computerized tomography scanning. J Neurosurg 53:63–67, 1980.

37. Garmatis CJ, Chu FCH: The effectiveness of radiation therapy in the treatment of bone metastases from breast cancer. Radiology 126:235–237, 1978.

38. Gelber RD, Larson M, Borgelt BB, Kramer S: Equivalence of radiation schedules for the palliative treatment of brain metastases in patients with favorable prognosis. Cancer 48:1749–1753, 1981.

39. Gilbert HA, Kagan AR, Nussbaum H, Rao AR, Satzman J, Chan P, Allen B, Forsythe A: Evaluation of radiation therapy for bone metastases: Pain relief and quality of life. AJR 129:1095–1096, 1977.

40. Gilbert H, Kagan AR, Wagner J, Fuchs K, Nussbaum H, Rao AR: The Southern California Permanente Medical Group experience: functional results. In Weiss L, Gilbert HA, Posner JB (eds): Brain Metastasis. Proceedings of the Workshop on Brain Metastasis, New York, 1978. Boston, GK Hall, 1978, pp 303–313.

41. Gilbert RW, Kim J-H, Posner JB: Epidural spinal cord compression from metastatic tumor: diagnosis and treatment. Ann Neurol 3:40–51, 1978.

42. Giri DV: Metastatic carcinoma of the choroid secondary to mammary carcinoma in a man. Schweiz Med Wochenschr 69:1069–1072, 1939.

43. Grady ED: Internal radiation therapy of hepatic cancer. Dis Colon Rectum 22:371–375, 1979.

44. Grady ED, McLaren J, Auda SP, McGinley PH: Combination of internal radiation therapy and hyperthermia to treat liver cancer. South Med J 76:1101–1105, 1983.

45. Grage TB, Vassilopoulos PP, Shingleton WW, Jubert AV, Elias EG, Aust JB, Moss SE: Results of a prospective randomized study of hepatic artery infusion with 5-fluorouracil versus intravenous 5-fluorouracil in patients with hepatic metastases from colorectal cancer: a Central Oncology Group study. Surgery 86:550–555, 1979.

46. Gragoudas ES: Current treatment of metastatic choroidal tumors. Oncology 3(6):103–110, 1989.

47. Hall AJ, Mackay NNS: The results of laminectomy for compression of the cord or cauda equina by extradural malignant tumour. J Bone Joint Surg 55B:497–505, 1973.

48. Halle JS, Rosenman JG, Varia MA, Fowler WC, Walton LA, Currie JL: 1000 cGy single dose palliation for advanced carcinoma of the cervix or endometrium. Int J Radiat Oncol Biol Phys 12:1947–1950, 1986.

49. Harrington KD: Impending pathologic fractures from metastatic malignancy: evaluation and management. Instr Course Lect 35:357–381, 1986.

50. Hazuka MB, Kinzie JJ: Brain metastases: results and effects of re-irradiation. Int J Radiat Oncol Biol Phys 15:433–437, 1988.

51. Hendrickson FR, Lee M-S, Larson M, Gelber RD: The influence of surgery and radiation therapy on patients with brain metastases. Int J Radiat Oncol Biol Phys 9:623–627, 1983.

51a. Hendrickson FR, Shehata WM, Kirchner AB: Radiation therapy for osseous metastasis. Int J Radiat Oncol Biol Phys 1:275–278, 1976.

52. Herbsman H, Hassan A, Gardner B, Harshaw D, Bohorquez J, Alfonso A, Newman J: Treatment of hepatic metastases with a combination of hepatic artery infusion chemotherapy and external radiotherapy. Surg Gynecol Obstet 147:13–17, 1978.

53. Heros DO, Kasdon DL, Chun M: Brachytherapy in the treatment of recurrent solitary brain metastases. Neurosurgery 23:733–737, 1988.

54. Hindo WA, DeTrana FA III, Lee M-S, Hendrickson FR: Large dose increment irradiation in treatment of cerebral metastases. Cancer 26:138–141, 1970.

55. Horton J, Baxter DH, Olson KB, and the Eastern Cooperative Oncology Group: The management of metastases to the brain by irradiation and corticosteroids. Am J Roentgenol Radium Ther Nucl Med 111:334–336, 1971.

56. Ingold JA, Reed GB, Kaplan HS, Bagshaw MA: Radiation hepatitis. Am J Roentgenol Radium Ther Nucl Med 93:200–208, 1965.

57. Jaeger EA, Frayer WC, Southard ME, Kramer S: Effect of radiation therapy on metastatic choroidal tumors. Trans Am Acad Ophthalmol Otolaryngol 75:94–101, 1971.

58. Jaffe BM, Donegan WL, Watson F, Spratt JS Jr: Factors influencing survival in patients with untreated hepatic metastases. Surg Gynecol Obstet 127:1–11, 1968.

59. Jensen N-H, Roesdahl K: Single-dose irradiation of bone metastases. Acta Radiol Ther Phys Biol 15:337–339, 1976.

60. Khan FR, Glicksman AS, Chu FCH, Nickson JJ: Treatment by radiotherapy of spinal cord compression due to extradural metastases. Radiology 89:495–500, 1967.

61. King EF: Two cases of secondary carcinoma of choroid. Trans Ophthalmol Soc UK 74:229–234, 1954.

62. Kinsella TJ: The role of radiation therapy alone and combined with infusion chemotherapy for treating liver metastases. Semin Oncol 10:215–222, 1983.

63. Kurup P, Reddy S, Hendrickson FR: Results of re-irradiation for cerebral metastases. Cancer 46:2587–2589, 1980.

64. Leibel SA, Pajak TF, Massullo V, Order SE, Komaki RU, Chang CH, Wasserman TH, Phillips TL, Lipshutz J, Durbin LM: A comparison of misonidazole sensitized radiation therapy to radiation therapy alone for the palliation of hepatic metastases: results of a Radiation Therapy Oncology Group randomized prospective trial. Int J Radiat Oncol Biol Phys 13:1057–1064, 1987.

65. Letson AD, Davidorf FH, Bruce RA Jr: Chemotherapy for treatment of choroidal metastases from breast carcinoma. Am J Ophthalmol 93:102–106, 1982.

66. Loeffler JS, Glicksman AS, Tefft M, Gelch M: Treatment of spinal cord compression: a retrospective analysis. Med Pediatr Oncol 11:347–351, 1983.

67. Lokich J, Kinsella T, Perri J, Malcolm A, Clouse M: Concomitant hepatic radiation and intraarterial fluorinated pyrimidine therapy: correlation of liver scan, liver function tests, and plasma CEA with tumor response. Cancer 48:2569–2574, 1981.

68. Macmichael IM: Management of choroidal metastases from breast carcinoma. Br J Ophthalmol 53:782–785, 1969.

69. Madsen EL: Painful bone metastasis: efficacy of radiotherapy assessed by the patients: a randomized trial comparing 4 Gy × 6 versus 10 Gy × 2. Int J Radiat Oncol Biol Phys 9:1775–1779, 1983.

70. Makin WP: Treatment of spinal cord compression due to malignant disease. (Abstract) Br J Radiol 61:715, 1988.

71. Mantravadi RVP, Spigos DG, Grady ED, Tan WS, Karesh SG, Capek V: Treatment of hepatic malignancies by intravascular administration of radioisotopes. In Winkler C (ed): Nuclear Medicine in Clinical Oncology: Current Status and Future Aspects. Berlin, Springer-Verlag, 1986, pp 365–371.

72. Maor M, Chan RC, Young SE: Radiotherapy of choroidal metastases. Breast cancer as primary site. Cancer 40:2081–2086, 1977.

73. Mewis L, Young SE: Breast carcinoma metastatic to the choroid. Analysis of 67 patients. Ophthalmology 89:147–151, 1982.

74. Millburn L, Hibbs GG, Hendrickson FR: Treatment of spinal cord compression from metastatic carcinoma. Review of the literature and presentation of a new method of treatment. Cancer 21:447–452, 1968.

75. Mones RJ, Dozier D, Berrett A: Analysis of medical treatment of malignant extradural spinal cord tumors. Cancer 19:1842–1853, 1966.

76. Moser RP, Johnson ML: Surgical management of brain metastases: how aggressive should we be? Oncology 3(6):123–127, 1989.

77. Nisce LZ, Hilaris BS, Chu FCH: A review of experience with irradiation of brain metastasis. Am J Roentgenol Radium Ther Nucl Med 111:329–333, 1971.

78. de Ocampo G, Espiritu R: Bronchogenic metastatic carcinoma of the choroid. Am J Ophthalmol 52:107–110, 1961.

79. Order SE, Hellman S, von Essen CF, Kligerman MM: Improvement in quality of survival following whole-brain irradiation for brain metastasis. Radiology 91:149–153, 1968.

80. Orenstein MM, Anderson DP, Stein JJ: Choroid metastasis. Cancer 29:1101–1107, 1972.

81. Patterson RH Jr: Metastatic disease of the spine: surgical risk *versus* radiation therapy. Clin Neurosurg 27:641–644, 1980.

82. Penn CRH: Single dose and fractionated palliative irradiation for osseous metastases. Clin Radiol 27:405–408, 1976.

83. Prados M, Leibel S, Barnett CM, Gutin P: Interstitial brachytherapy for metastatic brain tumors. Cancer 63:657–660, 1989.

84. Prasad B, Lee M-S, Hendrickson FR: Irradiation of hepatic metastases. Int J Radiat Oncol Biol Phys 2:129–132, 1977.

85. Prato FS, Kurdyak R, Saibil EA, Carruthers JS, Rider WD, Aspin N: The incidence of radiation pneumonitis as a result of single fraction upper half body irradiation. Cancer 39:71–78, 1976.

86. Price P, Hoskin PJ, Easton D, Austin D, Palmer SG, Yarnold JR: Prospective randomised trial of single and multifraction radiotherapy schedules in the treatment of painful bony metastases. Radiother Oncol 6:247–255, 1986.

87. Qasim MM: Single dose palliative irradiation for bony metastasis. Strahlentherapie 153:531–532, 1977.

88. Reddy S, Saxena VS, Hendrickson F, Deutsch W: Malignant metastatic disease of the eye: management of an uncommon complication. Cancer 47:810–812, 1981.

89. Reese AB: Tumors of the Eye, ed 3. Hagerstown, MD, Harper & Row, 1976, pp 424–428.

90. Richards P, McKissock W: Intracranial metastases. Br Med J 1:15–18, 1963.

91. Richter MP, Coia LR: Palliative radiation therapy. Semin Oncol 12:375–383, 1985.

92. Rubin P, Miller G: Extradural spinal cord compression by tumor. Part I: experimental production and treatment trials. Radiology 93:1243–1260, 1969.

93. Salazar OM, Rubin P, Hendrickson FR, Komaki R, Poulter C, Newall J, Asbell SO, Mohiuddin M, van Ess J: Single-dose half-body irradiation for palliation of multiple bone metastases from solid tumors. Final Radiation Therapy Oncology Group report. Cancer 58:29–36, 1986.

94. Salazar OM, Rubin P, Keller B, Scarantino C: Systemic (half-body) radiation therapy: response and toxicity. Int J Radiat Oncol Biol Phys 4:937–950, 1978.

95. Sanders TE: Metastatic carcinoma of the iris. Am J Ophthalmol 21:646–651, 1938.

96. Schocker JD, Brady LW: Radiation therapy for bone metastasis. Clin Orthop 169:38–43, 1982.

97. Schorcht J, Herrmann T, Friedrich S, Jochem I, Winkler C: Single exposure of high-dose half-body irradiation in cases of carcinoma of the breast. Radiobiol Radiother 25:531–535, 1984.

98. Shehata WM, Hendrickson FR, Hindo WA: Rapid fractionation technique and re-treatment of cerebral metastases by irradiation. Cancer 34:257–261, 1974.

99. Sherman DM, Weichselbaum R, Order SE, Cloud L, Trey C, Piro AJ: Palliation of hepatic metastasis. Cancer 41:2013–2017, 1978.

100. Smalley SR, Schray MF, Laws ER Jr, O'Fallon JR: Adjuvant radiation therapy after surgical resection of solitary brain metastasis: association with pattern of failure and survival. Int J Radiat Oncol Biol Phys 13:1611–1616, 1987.

101. Snee MP, Rodger A, Kerr GR: Brain metastases from carcinoma of breast: a review of 90 cases. Clin Radiol 36:365–367, 1985.

102. Solisio EO, Akbiyik N, Alexander LL: Spinal cord compression from metastatic breast carcinoma: treatment by radiation therapy alone. J Natl Med Assoc 71:229–230, 1979.

103. Spanos WJ Jr, Wasserman T, Meoz R, Sala J, Kong J, Stetz J: Palliation of advanced pelvic malignant disease with large fraction pelvic radiation and misonidazole: final report of RTOG phase I/II study. Int J Radiat Oncol Biol Phys 13:1479–1482, 1987.

104. Sturm V, Kober B, Höver K-H, Schlegel W, Boesecke R, Pastyr O, Hartmann GH, Schabbert S, zum Winkel K, Kunze S, Lorenz WJ: Stereotactic percutaneous single dose irradiation of brain metastases with a linear accelerator. Int J Radiat Oncol Biol Phys 13:279–282, 1987.

105. Sundaresan N, Galicich JH, Deck MDF, Tomita T: Radiation necrosis after treatment of solitary intracranial metastases. Neurosurgery 8:329–333, 1981.

106. Taylor I, Brooman P, Rowling JT: Adjuvant liver perfusion in colorectal cancer: initial results of a clinical trial. Br Med J 2:1320–1322, 1977.

107. Thatcher N, Thomas PRM: Choroidal metastases from breast carcinoma: a survey of 42 patients and the use of radiation therapy. Clin Radiol 26:549–553, 1975.

108. Thomas P: Radiotherapy of metastases of mammary carcinoma. Radiol Clin 45:306–313, 1976.

109. Tomita T, Galicich JH, Sundaresan N: Radiation therapy for spinal epidural metastases with complete block. Acta Radiol Oncol 22:135–143, 1983.

110. Tong D, Gillick L, Hendrickson FR: The palliation of symptomatic osseous metastases. Final results of the study by the Radiation Therapy Oncology Group. Cancer 50:893–899, 1982.

111. Trodella L, Ausili-Cefaro G, Turriziani A, Marmiroli L, Cellini N, Nardone L: Pain in osseous metastases: results of radiotherapy. Pain 18:387–396, 1984.

112. Turek-Maischeider M, Kazem I: Palliative irradiation for liver metastases. JAMA 232:625–628, 1975.

113. Twycross RG: Analgesics and relief of bone pain. *In* Stoll BA, Parbhoo S (eds): Bone Metastasis. Monitoring and Treatment. New York, Raven Press, 1983, pp 289–310.

114. Vargha ZO, Glicksman AS, Boland J: Single-dose radiation therapy in the palliation of metastatic disease. Radiology 93:1181–1184, 1969.

115. Vieth RG, Odom GL: Intracranial metastases and their neurosurgical treatment. J Neurosurg 23:375–383, 1965.

116. Webber BM, Soderberg CH Jr, Leone LA, Rege VB, Glicksman AS: A combined treatment approach to management of hepatic metastases. Cancer 42:1087–1095, 1978.

117. Weissman DE: Glucocorticoid treatment for brain metastases and epidural spinal cord compression: a review. J Clin Oncol 6:543–551, 1988.

118. West J, Maor M: Intracranial metastases: behavioral patterns related to primary site and results of treatment by whole brain irradiation. Int J Radiat Oncol Biol Phys 6:11–15, 1980.

119. Wharton JT, Delclos L, Gallager S, Smith JP: Radiation hepatitis induced by abdominal irradiation with the cobalt 60 moving strip technique. Am J Roentgenol Radium Ther Nucl Med 117:73–80, 1973.

120. White WA, Patterson RH Jr, Bergland RM: Role of surgery in the treatment of spinal cord compression by metastatic neoplasm. Cancer 27:558–561, 1971.

121. Wild WO, Porter RW: Metastatic epidural tumor of the spine. A study of 45 cases. Arch Surg 87:825–830, 1963.

122. Willis RA: The Spread of Tumours in the Human Body. St. Louis, CV Mosby, 1952, pp 296–298.

123. Winkelman MD, Adelstein DJ, Karlins NL: Intramedullary spinal cord metastasis. Diagnostic and therapeutic considerations. Arch Neurol 44:526–531, 1987.

124. Wright RL: Malignant tumors in the spinal extradural space: results of surgical treatment. Ann Surg 157:227–231, 1963.

125. Yarnold JR: Role of radiotherapy in the management of bone metastases from breast cancer. J R Soc Med 78(suppl 9):23–25, 1985.

126. Young RF, Post EM, King GA: Treatment of spinal epidural metastases. Randomized prospective comparison of laminectomy and radiotherapy. J Neurosurg 53:741–748, 1980.

Management of Osseous Metastases and Impending Pathological Fractures

Dempsey S. Springfield, M.D.

Carcinoma of the breast has an affinity for the skeleton. Of the patients who succumb to this disease, the incidence of skeletal involvement has been reported to be as great as 73 percent.[1] Clinically, breast metastases are not uncommon, but less than half of patients with metastatic breast carcinoma will have clinically symptomatic skeletal lesions. These lesions should be treated when recognized and can usually be successfully managed with irradiation alone.[39] Delay in the recognition of bone metastasis may necessitate surgical stabilization in addition to irradiation to adequately treat impending pathological fractures. It is therefore important for the physician managing a patient with breast carcinoma to be aware of the significant percentage of patients who develop bone metastasis and the advantages of early diagnosis and therapy. The clinician should be cognizant of the possibility for the development of metastatic disease and should not be complacent in its recognition. It is discouraging to see a patient with bone metastasis that has been ignored until the fracture is clinically evident or the pathological progression of the osseous lesion is extensive and symptomatic (impending fracture). It is equally important for the patient to be aware of the significance of pain in an extremity, and all patients should be encouraged to report such symptoms to their physician, who should then obtain high-quality roentgenograms.

A plain film radiograph does not identify a metastatic lesion, but it does suggest whether the patient is at risk for sustaining a pathological fracture. The technetium 99m bone scan is very sensitive and will often reveal occult metastatic foci in bone. However, it is not absolutely essential to obtain bone scans, as repeat roentgenographs can be taken at monthly intervals. Should a metastatic lesion be present, it will in time become obvious on the plain radiograph and can usually be managed with irradiation. The physician must be cognizant of musculoskeletal pain in the patient with breast carcinoma, as the pain often is secondary to metastatic spread of disease.

Any bone can be involved with metastatic breast carcinoma; however, the spine, pelvis, skull, ribs, and femur, in decreasing order, are the most common sites affected.[39] The lumbar spine is the single most commonly involved osseous metastatic site, as approximately 20 percent of the osseous metastases involve this area. Metastatic frequencies for the ribs, pelvis, thoracic spine, skull, and femur are 15 percent, 14 percent, 13 percent, 12 percent and 11 percent, respectively. The humerus is not a common site for metastatic deposits (5.5 percent). However, when a pathological fracture occurs in this bone, the patient loses significant function, experiences pain, and the fracture usually does not heal spontaneously. Therefore the humerus should be included in the bones that must be evaluated closely for the possibility of metastatic deposits.

Skull and rib lesions can be irradiated whenever metastases are discovered, and early diagnosis has less importance than in long bone lesions. The early discovery of lumbar or thoracic spine lesions permits the metastatic foci to be best managed with irradiation as a solitary modality with little or negligible risk of neurological compromise. If treatment is delayed, lower extremity paralysis may develop, and recovery is less frequently obtained even with aggressive decompression. Lesions of the pelvis, femur, or humerus are important to identify and treat as early as possible to eliminate the pathological fracture that may occur should the metastatic foci be left untreated.

Patients with metastatic breast carcinoma to osseous sites often survive for considerable periods with established disease. For this reason, the physician should not withhold therapy for palliative purposes. This is of particular significance for patients with metastatic disease confined to the skeleton, as they frequently have a more indolent course than patients with bone and other organ system metastasis. Sherry and coinvestigators[33] observed a median survival of 48 months for 86 patients with metastatic breast carcinoma confined to the skeleton; however, median survival was only 17 months for patients with disease metastatic to other sites. With a response rate of 87 per cent, the group with only bone metastases responded better to hormonal and chemotherapy than those with metastases to other sites.

Metastatic tumor in the skeleton results in bone destruction with secondary bone formation. Usually bone destruction exceeds bone formation, and the net effect of the metastatic lesion is bone loss. On occasion bone formation will predominate, and the lesion will be seen on the radiograph as an osteoblastic abnormality. Metastases from breast carcinoma only rarely produce sufficient stroma for membranous bone formation, as is common with metastatic prostatic carcinoma, and the osteoblastic activity seen with metastatic breast carcinoma is reactive bone from adjacent periosteal and endosteal osteoblasts.

There are two mechanisms that initiate bone destruction in metastatic carcinoma.[10] First, in the presence of the metastatic foci, there is stimulation of local osteoclasts as the result of the secretion of a variety of osteoclast stimulating factors. Thereafter the stimulated osteoclast resorbs the contiguous local bone, initiating net loss of bone matrix. The second mechanism of destruction is resorption of local bone by the carcinoma. This event occurs in the later phases of metastatic destruction. Both mechanisms of bone loss are probably mediated through prostaglandin E_2 production, and the administration of prostaglandin inhibitors can diminish the degree of bone resorption and the subsequent net total loss of bone integrity.

Galasko[10] has completed a series of in vitro experiments with tissue cultures of breast carcinoma incubated with mouse calvarium to determine the osteolytic effect of the breast carcinoma cells. These experiments revealed that two thirds of breast tumors are osteolytic, while one third do not produce osteolysis in the cultured osseous cells. In the predominant cell lines that were osteolytic, the addition to the cell media of prostaglandin inhibitors or diphosphonates reduced the amount of lysis of the calvarium. The addition of these two inhibitors of bony lysis was more than additive. This work suggests that patients with osteolytic breast carcinoma may best be treated with nonsteroidal antiinflammatory agents that have prostaglandin inhibitor activity; however, this therapeutic treatment has only been infrequently initiated, and clinical experience is limited.

The strength of the bone matrix can be rapidly diminished by the osteolytic process of the metastatic lesion and subsequent destruction. Biomechanical studies provide data that the orthopedic surgeon uses to determine bone stability when a destructive lesion is confirmed.[9, 28] The strength and integrity of the bone matrix is best predicted by the extent of the defect in the bone cortex (e.g., partial- vs. full-thickness) and, if present, the size of the defect in relation to the diameter of the affected bone. Osteolytic defects that do not penetrate the cortex do not significantly reduce the strength of the bone; however, when the cortex is completely eroded, the bone strength is dramatically reduced. Fortunately the "extra" strength in the unaffected, normal bone is significant; thus structural weakening from full-thickness defects is not always clinically evident. A defect is considered clinically significant only when the bone is at risk for pathological fracture. Spontaneous breakage suggests that the bone fractures following minimal stress, such as occurs with torque of the skeleton (twisting) in bed with the foot in a stationary position.

With spontaneous fractures, the bone fails in tension, and because torsion initiates significant tension, pathological fractures are most commonly seen with torsional stresses of the axial skeleton and long bones. Metastatic lesions that, on measurement, are smaller than the diameter of the bone are called *stress-risers*. These neoplastic lesions reduce the strength of the bone to 40 percent or less of its inherent strength.[28] Whether this defect is a small drill-type hole or a pathological defect just less than the diameter of the bone, the percentage weakening of the bone matrix is essentially identical. Holes from osteolytic metastases with diameters that are measurably greater than the diameter of the affected bone are called *open-section defects* and reduce the inherent strength of the bone as much as 90 percent.

Often a bone can tolerate a stress-riser without becoming excessively weak, and should the underlying process be arrested, the involved segment will regain its original strength within 4 to 6 weeks. If the metastatic foci can be controlled with irradiation, the involved bony area can compensate for the osteolytic defect without filling the defect with bone. Thus a small defect can be successfully treated with irradiation alone, even if the bone does not remodel on the radiogram, it is uncommon for the bone to fracture. We recommend prophylactic internal fixation for defects with a measured diameter that is less than 50 percent of the diameter of the bone for patients who continue to have local pain 1 month after completion of their irradiation. Those lesions that are osteolytic, painful, and are equal to or greater than 50 percent of bone diameter have such a high risk for fracture that they are considered to be impending fractures, and immediate operative stabilization is recommended. Those bones with metastatic lesions producing a diffuse, permeative destruction are at significant risk for pathological fracture and should be internally stabilized prophylactically. Irradiation is given postoperatively.

The orthopedist should be more aggressive surgically with any lesion in the periacetabulum, proximal femur, and distal femur than with a lesion in the wing of the ilium, pubis, and scapula[3, 18] because of the added risk of fracture in the weight-bearing bones and the difficulty of treatment after such fractures occur compared with treatment before fracture. As a rule, if the patient undergoes surgery prior to the fracture, the technical procedure is considerably simplified for the surgeon, and morbidity and mortality for the patient are minimized. Furthermore, the patient does not suffer the intense pain associated with the fracture or experience the complications inherent with the restrictions of immobilization with bed rest. On occasion the orthopedist may be more aggressive than is absolutely essential, but the advantages of prophylactic fixation cannot be overemphasized. Some radiotherapists suggest that the majority of patients with metastatic foci, even those with large destructive lesions, are best managed with irradiation alone.[7, 35] Cheng et al.'s[7] results suggest that only patients with diffusely mottled destruction of the femoral neck require internal stabilization prior to irradiation; these management principles are disputed by the orthopedic community.

Although orthopedists and radiotherapists disagree as to the necessity for operative intervention in patients with impending fractures, they do agree with respect to the role of surgery in patients with a pathological fracture secondary to metastatic disease. Pathological fractures should have open reduction and internal fixation as soon as medically feasible, provided the operative procedure will result in sufficient stabilization to allow the patient pain-free movement. Early operative stabilization of the pathological fracture will permit the patient to be out of bed quickly and decrease the risk of superimposed illness that occurs with the immobilization of bed rest and pain medications. Irradiation is given postoperatively.

Prior to surgery in the patient with a metastatic breast lesion, a thorough physical examination is essential. It is incumbent on the surgeon to be certain of the necessity of the procedure as determined by a risk-benefit determination with operative planning. Patients with metastatic breast carcinoma not uncommonly have elevated serum calcium levels, prolongation of clotting parameters, myeloplastic anemia, and pulmonary compromise as a consequence of this systemic illness. These parameters must be evaluated in addition to the routine preoperative parameters prior to anesthetic induction. Additional metastatic bone lesions that require surgery can often be confirmed by palpating the entire skeleton, including the spine. Radiographs of the potentially involved bones (humerus, pelvis, and femur) are recommended, and if possible, a preoperative technetium 99m bone scan should be done. The technetium scan is an excellent method to evaluate the entire skeleton for metastatic deposits, as it is uncommon for a patient with a breast carcinoma metastasis to bone to have a normal bone scan.

No consensus exists as to the expected duration of a patient's survival prior to internal fixation of a pathological or impending pathological fracture, but estimates suggest a range of 6 weeks to 6 months. When the patient's expected survival is longer than the interval expected for recovery from the operation, surgery is indicated. Pathological fractures often do not have complete union, and frequently the patient is in constant pain, bedridden, and on large doses of narcotics until the fracture is operatively stabilized. Expected recovery is 3 to 4 days, assuming the physical therapist can initiate mobility that will reduce the amount of medication required for pain control. For patients with impending fractures, recovery is expeditious, and unless there are specific contraindications to surgery, operative stabilization is recommended, especially for osseous lesions of the lower extremity.

Operative stabilization of pathological fractures has become an accepted axiom in orthopedic management during the past decade, and results have dramatically improved, principally as a consequence of the availability and use of polymethylmethacrylate (PMMA).[8, 11, 17, 20, 26, 31, 37] PMMA is used primarily to enhance the fixation of metal devices placed in fractures that otherwise would not be of adequate strength to secure fixation screws; it is also used to replace a segment of the bone, improving the stability of the reconstruction.[2, 16, 18, 36] Prior to the availability of PMMA, it was not often possible to sufficiently stabilize a pathological fracture to allow the patient unrestricted activity, and the failure rate of internal fixation in these patients was unacceptably high.

Fractures of long bones are best treated with internal fixation devices either without or, more commonly, with PMMA. Intramedullary rods or plates and fixation screws can be operatively placed depending on the bone

that is fractured. Preferably, the fracture is reduced using closed techniques; thereafter an intramedullary rod is positioned for fixation without exposing the fracture site. When the fracture site must be exposed, either for reduction or to augment fixation with PMMA, the site of the gross (metastatic) tumor should be excised and rigid fixation applied. The first goal of the operation is to relieve pain and permit ambulation of the patient in the immediate postoperative period. The second goal of the operation is to provide sufficient stability and bone apposition so that a union will be achieved. If osseous union is not achieved, often the internal fixation device will fail before the patient succumbs to metastatic breast cancer. The patient should not defer activity for the bone to heal; however, fixation devices have limited stability, and should the patient live long enough and the fracture achieve complete union, the fixation device will fail. Therefore the surgeon should aim for osseous fixation that is immediately adequate for ambulation and sufficient to allow bone repair. Patients with insufficient bone matrix for primary healing should have bone grafting at the time of internal fixation. Also, metastatic breast carcinoma can be dangerously vascular. Although metastatic breast lesions are not extensively vascularized, it is important to consider preoperative angiography with therapeutic embolization to reduce the blood loss expected at the time of the stabilization of the fracture.[6]

All patients with metastatic carcinoma to bone that initiates an impending or pathological fracture should have irradiation following operative stabilizations.[5, 30] The usual recommended dose of irradiation varies between 2000 cGy/5 fractions/5 days and 3500 cGy/10 fractions/14 days. This therapeutic dose will usually control progression of the metastasis but will not inhibit osseous repair and fracture union. Because bone pain is the usual indication for irradiation of metastatic lesions and patients are asymptomatic after successful stabilization, radiotherapists are aware of the importance of this modality in the control of metastatic disease. If the lesion is not irradiated, further destruction of the bone matrix may occur, and the fixation will be lost.

SPECIFIC ANATOMICAL SITES FOR METASTASES

Spine

Metastatic involvement of the vertebrae by breast carcinoma is common, usually asymptomatic, and therefore not recognized except at autopsy. When symptomatic, however, as a consequence of a pathological fracture, it is difficult to determine whether the vertebral body is simply osteoporotic or a metastasis is present. If the patient has other metastases, it should be assumed that the spinal lesion represents an additional metastatic deposit, and the patient should be treated with irradiation. When metastatic disease has not been confirmed radiologically or histologically, a biopsy is required. A prebiopsy CT scan is of value to localize abnormalities of the vertebral body and increase the probability that diagnostic material can be obtained at the time of the biopsy. The biopsy can be successfully completed with a needle using CT guidance; however, when an open biopsy is the preferred approach, we recommend posterior exposure of the metastatic site with the biopsy done through the pedicle of the area with maximal involvement.

On occasion, the patient with metastatic breast carcinoma will develop progressive neurological compromise following anterior compression of the cord by the tumor. These neurological events may result after irradiation either from latent growth of the neoplasm or, more commonly, following collapse of the vertebral body with resultant sharp kyphosis. With these neurological symptoms, an anterior decompression and fusion is recommended.[14, 15] The anterior decompression should be radical, with removal of as much tumor as is technically possible. This will reduce the late risk of progressive neurological compromise. Cortical allografts are advised to replace the resected vertebral body.

Periacetabulum

The periacetabular metastasis is a difficult orthopedic problem to treat successfully, especially if the patient's femoral head begins to advance and protrude into the pelvis. When sufficient acetabular bone exists, irradiation is the treatment of choice after a limited curettage and packing with PMMA (Fig. 45–17).[7] More extensive

disease requires reconstruction of the hip joint with replacement of the acetabulum and femoral head (Fig. 45–18).[13, 19]

Femur

The proximal femur is the most common metastatic location that requires surgical intervention.[12, 22, 25, 27, 29] The combination of frequent involvement, large stress and torque forces placed on the bone, the consequences of a fracture, and the numerous devices available to stabilize the bone explain the frequency of surgical intervention. When the femoral head is damaged, it is best to replace it with a prosthesis.[21] The operation is a routine orthopedic procedure and can be done with minimal blood loss and without excess morbidity to the patient. It is important for the surgeon to have available a comprehensive set of bone prostheses in the event there is greater destruction of bone than was indicated on the preoperative radiographs. Both calcar femorale replacement and long-stem prosthetic devices should be available as well. If involvement of the calcar femorale is established, it should be resected, and when metastases in the femoral shaft are evident radiographically or at surgery, the stem of the prosthesis should extend beyond them.

Habermann et al.[12] reported that 19 of 23 patients with metastatic breast carcinoma and fractures of the femoral neck had acetabular involvement; however, even if this constellation of radiographical and clinical

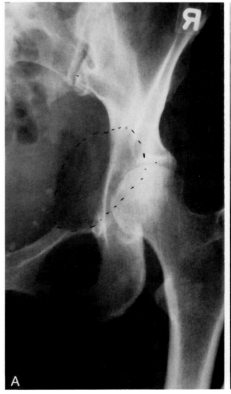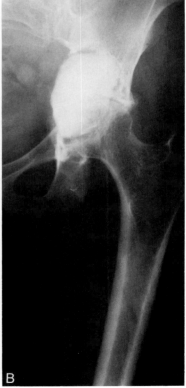

Figure 45–17. *A*, Radiograph of the hip with outline of the acetabular metastatic lesion. The patient had mild groin pain. The radiograph changes are subtle, and the clinician reviewing these films must carefully scrutinize for details of bony destruction. A technetium bone scan will often indicate areas of greatest concern, as almost all metastatic breast lesions have increased uptake. *B*, Plain x-ray film of the patient following curettage and polymethylmethacrylate (PMMA) packing of the cavity. The patient became asymptomatic after curettage and packing and was treated with 3000 rads postoperatively.

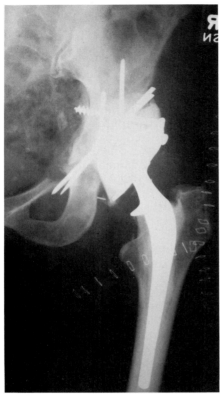

Figure 45–18. This woman had extensive acetabular destruction secondary to metastatic breast carcinoma and required an acetabular reconstruction. The lesion and involved bone were curetted. Following removal of gross tumor, the defect was replaced by PMMA reinforced with metal pins, and a prosthetic hip was used for the reconstruction. She also received postoperative irradiation. Thereafter, the patient could ambulate asymptomatically with the aid of a cane. The metal acetabular component is a protrusio ring and is applied to enhance stability of the acetabular components.

disease is not apparent on the plain roentgenogram, the effectiveness of the hemiarthroplasty will not be altered. If acetabular disease is apparent on the roentgenogram and the patient has a fractured femoral head or neck, a total hip replacement is recommended. Often the acetabular component may require augmentation with a protrusion ring.

Metastatic deposits of the femoral neck can be managed with either a proximal femoral replacement or internal fixation with or without PMMA. When the femoral head is uninvolved and the hip joint is normal, the neck fracture should be treated with reduction and internal fixation. If reduction cannot be obtained, hemiarthroplasty should be performed.

Involvement of the proximal femur, either the intratrochanteric or subtrochanteric area, is especially dangerous. The normal forces of torque and stress experienced by the bone with walking are as great as three times body weight.[9] When the metastatic lesion is discovered prior to fracture, an internal fixation device can be placed with little difficulty; this practice is recommended in the majority of patients. The Zickel nail is the only device designed specifically for subtrochanteric

fractures and is recommended when the patient has a subtrochanteric fracture of the femur (Fig. 45–19).[23, 29, 32, 38] This device is best used without PMMA. Avulsion fractures of the lesser trochanter have recently been reported as indicative of a metastasis, and with the presentation of this unusual injury, metastatic carcinoma should be suspected.[4]

Femoral shaft metastases are best treated with an intramedullary rod. PMMA is indicated when the rod is not able to provide sufficient stabilization and permit early ambulation. When numerous metastatic lesions are present within the femur or when the femur is diffusely involved with disease, PMMA augmentation of the intramedullary rod is indicated. A technique has been developed for the introduction of an intramedullary rod and PMMA into the femur from either the greater trochanteric approach or the knee (Fig. 45–20).[24] This method allows the stabilization of the entire femur with a limited surgical exposure.

Carcinoma metastatic to the distal femur is less common than to more proximal areas and, when seen, the more proximal sites should be examined carefully; as a rule, metastatic disease involves the bone from proximal to distal. Internal fixation of the fractured distal femur is best accomplished with a supracondylar blade plate (Fig. 45–21). PMMA is used to replace completely destroyed bone or to improve the fixation of screws.

Humerus

Disease metastatic to the humerus is better tolerated than carcinomatous foci in the lower extremity, unless the patient needs crutches for ambulation. When the patient has bone pain in the absence of a fracture, irradiation is recommended. If the patient has a humeral fracture, it is best treated with internal fixation and postoperative irradiation. With internal fixation, the bone is exposed, the gross disease curetted, and plate fixation completed (Fig. 45–22). Intramedullary fixation is an alternative, but it usually does not provide sufficiently rigid stabilization.

POSTOPERATIVE CARE

Postoperatively, the patient should be encouraged to use the extremity as soon as possible. An active rehabilitation program is important to maximize the patient's recovery. Patients with skeletal metastases are at greater risk of developing the complications of osteoporosis, kidney stones, and pulmonary emboli (the most dangerous) with bed rest. The generalized weakness and loss of will associated with pain and prolonged bed rest can be devastating to a patient with metastatic breast carcinoma. An aggressive program that allows early stabilization of fractures with a return to activity will improve the quality of life. Finally, the patient who has had a bone metastasis is at significantly increased risk for a second focus to develop; close follow-up will reduce the

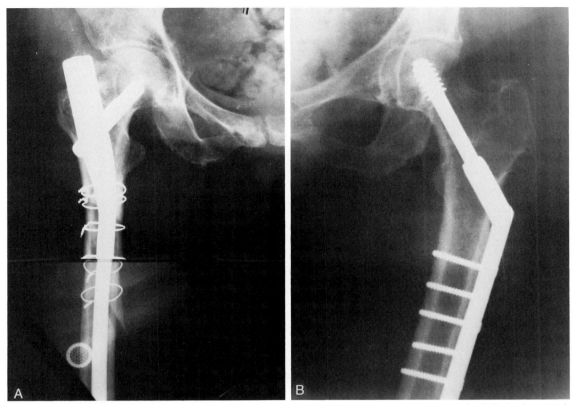

Figure 45–19. This patient with metastatic breast carcinoma had acute pain in her proximal thigh and sustained a fall. On her initial radiograph, a subtrochanteric femur fracture was diagnosed and she had internal fixation with a Zickel nail and five circulage wires. The Zickel nail was designed specifically for subtrochanteric femoral fractures and has been frequently placed for internal fixation of pathological subtrochanteric fractures. *B,* Radiograph of the same patient, who was evaluated and diagnosed with an "impending fracture" of the opposite femur. Thereafter, the patient had prophylactic internal fixation with a sliding hip screw and side plate. Both proximal femurs were irradiated postoperatively.

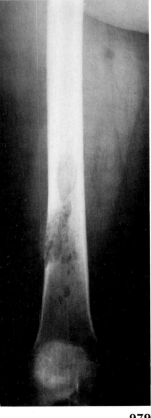

Figure 45–20. This woman had extensive destruction of the distal femur in the absence of a demonstrable fracture. She was considered to have an "impending fracture" and underwent prophylactic internal fixation. The method of bone fixation necessitated the introduction of an intramedullary rod through the intracondylar notch exposed with an arthrotomy of the knee. PMMA was injected into the medullary canal to enhance the strength of fixation. Thereafter, the patient was asymptomatic and received postoperative irradiation.

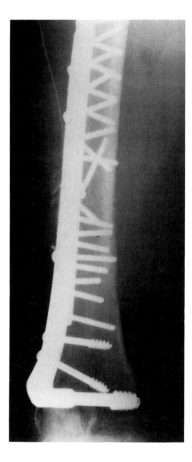

Figure 45–21. The method of internal fixation of a distal femoral lesion using a supracondylar plate and screws. This fixation technique requires extensive exposure of the bone for placement of the device and is indicated when the metastatic lesion requires curettage or biopsy.

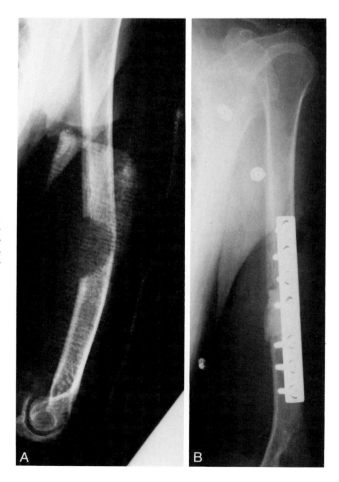

Figure 45–22. This woman's arm was painful for two months prior to x-ray. The breast metastasis has destroyed the majority of the bone in the mid-diaphysis of the humerus. B, The lesion was exposed and curetted and the bone replaced with PMMA. The entire construct was secured with a large bone plate and screws. A bone graft was placed to assist in osseous repair and union.

possibility of yet another pathological fracture if the lesion is identified early.

References

1. Abrams HL, Spiro R, Goldstein N: Metastasis in carcinoma. Cancer 3:74–85, 1950.
2. Anderson JJ, Erickson JM, Thompson RC, Chao LY: Pathologic femoral shaft fractures comparing fixation techniques using cement. Clin Orthop 131:273–278, 1978.
3. Beals RK, Lawton GD, Snell WE: Prophylactic internal fixation of the femur in metastatic breast cancer. Cancer 28:1350–1354, 1971.
4. Bertin KC, Horstman J, Coleman SS: Isolated fracture of the lesser trochanter in adults. An initial manifestation of metastatic disease. J Bone Joint Surg 66A:770–773, 1984.
5. Blake DD: Radiation treatment of metastatic bone disease. Clin Orthop 73:89–100, 1970.
6. Carpenter PR, Ewing JW, Cook AJ, Kuster A: Angiographic assessment and control of potential operative hemorrhage with pathologic fractures secondary to metastasis. Clin Orthop 123:6–8, 1977.
7. Cheng DS, Seitz CB, Eyre HJ: Nonoperative management of femoral, humeral and acetabular metastases in patients with breast carcinoma. Cancer 45:1533–1537, 1980.
8. Coran AG, Banks HH, Aliapoulios MA, Wilson RE: The management of pathologic fractures in patients with metastatic carcinoma of the breast. Surg Gynecol Obstet 127:1225–1230, 1968.
9. Fielding JW, Cochran GVB, Zickel RE: Biomechanical characteristics and surgical management of subtrochanteric fracture. Orthop Clin North Am 5:629–650, 1974.
10. Galasko CSB: Mechanism of lytic and blastic metastatic disease of bone. Clin Orthop 169:20–27, 1982.
11. Gristina AG, Adair DM, Spurr CL: Intraosseous metastatic breast cancer treatment with internal fixation and study of survivors. Ann Surg 197:128–134, 1983.
12. Habermann ET, Sachs R, Stern RE, Hirsh DM, Anderson WJ: The pathology and treatment of metastatic disease of the femur. Clin Orthop 169:70–82, 1982.
13. Harrington KD: The management of acetabular insufficiency secondary to metastatic malignant disease. J Bone Joint Surg 63A:653–664, 1981.
14. Harrington KD: Metastatic disease of the spine. J Bone Joint Surg 68A:1110–1115, 1986.
15. Harrington KD: The use of methylmethacrylate for vertebral body replacement and anterior stabilization of pathological fracture-dislocations of the spine due to metastatic malignant disease. J Bone Joint Surg 63A:36–46, 1981.
16. Harrington KD, Sim FH, Eric JE, Johnston JO, Dick HW, Gristina AG: Methylmethacrylate as an adjuvant in internal fixation of pathological fractures. Experience with three hundred and seventy-five cases. J Bone Joint Surg 58A:1047–1055, 1976.
17. Heisterberg L, Johansen TS: Treatment of pathological fractures. Acta Orthop Scand 50:787–790, 1979.
18. Jensen TM, Dillon WL, Reckling FW: Changing concepts in the management of pathological and impending pathological fractures. J Trauma 16:496–502, 1976.
19. Johnson JTH: Reconstruction of the pelvic ring following tumor resection. J Bone Joint Surg 60A:747–751, 1978.
20. Krebs H: Management of pathologic fractures of long bones in malignant disease. Arch Orthop Trauma Surg 92:133–137, 1978.
21. Lane JM, Sculco TP, Zolan S: Treatment of pathologic fractures of the hip by endoprosthetic replacement. J Bone Joint Surg 62A:954–959, 1980.
22. Levy RN, Sherry HS, Siffert RS: Surgical management of metastatic disease of bone at the hip. Clin Orthop 169:62–69, 1982.
23. Mickelson MR, Bonfiglio M: Pathologic fractures in the proximal part of the femur treated by Zickel nail fixation. J Bone Joint Surg 58A:1067–1070, 1976.
24. Miller GJ, Vander Griend RA, Blake P, Springfield DS: Performance evaluation of a cement augmented intramedullary fixation system for pathologic lesions of the femoral shaft. Clin Orthop 221:246–254, 1987.
25. Murray JA, Parrish FF: Surgical management of secondary neoplastic fractures about the hip. Orthop Clin North Am 5:887–901, 1974.
26. Perez CA, Bradfield JS, Morgan HC: Management of pathologic fractures. Cancer 29:684–693, 1972.
27. Poigenfurst J, Marcove RC, Miller TR: Surgical treatment of fractures through metastasis in the proximal femur. J Bone Joint Surg 50B:743–756, 1968.
28. Pugh J, Sherry HS, Futterman B, Frankel VH: Biomechanics of pathologic fractures. Clin Orthop 169:109–114, 1982.
29. Sangeorzan BJ, Ryan JR, Saleiccioli GG: Prophylactic femoral stabilization with the Zickel nail by closed technique. J Bone Joint Surg 68A:991–999, 1986.
30. Schocker JD, Brady LW: Radiation therapy for bone metastasis. Clin Orthop 169:38–43, 1982.
31. Schurman DJ, Amstutz HC: Orthopaedic management of patients with metastatic carcinoma of the breast. Surg Gynecol Obstet 137:831–836, 1973.
32. Schurman DJ, Amstutz HC: Treatment of neoplastic subtrochanteric fractures. Clin Orthop 97:108–113, 1973.
33. Sherry MM, Greco FA, Johnson DH, Hainsworth SD: Metastatic breast cancer confined to the skeletal system. An indolent disease. Am J Med 81:381–386, 1986.
34. Snell WM, Beals RK: Femoral metastases and fractures from breast cancer. Surg Gynecol Obstet 119:22–25, 1964.
35. Tong D, Gillick L, Hendrickson FR: The palliation of symptomatic osseous metastasis. Cancer 50:893–899, 1982.
36. Wang GJ, Reger SI, Maffeo C, McLaughlin RE, Stemp WG: The strength of metal reinforced methylmethacrylate fixation of pathologic fractures. Clin Orthop 135:287–290, 1978.
37. Welch CE: Pathologic fracture due to malignant disease. Surg Gynecol Obstet 62:735–744, 1936.
38. Zickel RE, Mouradian WH: Intramedullary fixation of pathologic fractures and lesions of the subtrochanteric region of the femur. J Bone Joint Surg 58A:1061–1066, 1976.
39. Zimskind PD, Surver JM: Metastasis to bone from carcinoma of the breast. Clin Orthop 11:202–215, 1958.

Management of Pleural Metastases in Breast Cancer

Jeffrey M. Crane, M.D. and Barnett S. Kramer, M.D.

Pleural effusions and metastatic pleural disease are frequent problems in patients with breast cancer. In Abrams et al.'s 1950 series of 1000 consecutive autopsies in cancer patients, pleural metastases were found in 65 percent of the 167 patients with breast cancer.[1] Perhaps because of both the frequency of breast cancer and the relative frequency of this metastatic site, the most common cause of a malignant pleural effusion in American women is carcinoma of the breast, occurring in 37 percent of 472 patients with malignant effusions at Duke Medical Center.[29]

Pleural metastases in breast cancer occur with approximate equal frequency in pre- and postmenopausal patients. In a retrospective series of 105 breast cancer patients, the mean age at diagnosis of pleural disease was 53 years (range, 25–83 years), with 60 percent of patients being postmenopausal.[3] The interval from initial diagnosis to recognized pleural metastases ranges from 0 to >20 years (mean, 41 months). Malignant pleural effusions from breast cancer are nearly always a result of hematogenous metastases to the pleura[1, 13, 17, 24] as opposed to the occasional local extension from the primary tumor through the chest wall.[13, 18, 34] For this reason, malignant effusions may be bilateral in five percent to 15 percent of cases.[13, 18, 37, 47] About 57 percent of pleural metastases (190/334 cases) are ipsilateral to the primary site of breast cancer.[17, 18, 34] Only four of these 334 cases had direct chest wall extension to the parietal pleura.[34] Moreover, pleural metastases usually occur in the setting of hematogenous metastases to other sites.[17, 34] Fentiman et al. reported that 60 of 105 patients (57 percent) had distant metastases preceding or concomitant with the demonstration of pleural metastases.[17] Forty-five of these had pleural effusions as the first manifestation of recurrent disease. Documenting the first site of systemic spread is a useful determinant of prognosis in patients with breast cancer.[15]

PATHOPHYSIOLOGY

The pleural cavity is a potential space, normally containing less than 5 ml of low protein fluid (approximately 2 gm/dl). The formation of this fluid is the result of a net hydrostatic-oncotic pressure of the capillaries of the parietal pleura moving fluid into the pleural space. In the normal state, 80 percent to 90 percent of this fluid is reabsorbed by the pulmonary venous capillaries

of the visceral pleura. The remaining ten percent to 20 percent is reabsorbed through the pulmonary lymphatics. In a 24-hour period, 5–10 l are exchanged across the pleural space from parietal to visceral pleura.[6, 55]

Accumulation of pleural fluid may result when any one of several pathophysiological events occur. These fall into the following categories:

1. Increased capillary permeability, usually related to inflammatory processes.

2. Increased hydrostatic pressure, as in congestive heart failure.

3. Increased negative intrapleural pressure, as in atelectasis.

4. Decreased oncotic pressure, as in any hypoalbuminemic state.

5. Increased oncotic pressure of pleural fluid, usually related to an inflammatory process or malignancy.

6. Impaired visceral lymphatic drainage, such as found in tumor infiltration of hilar or mediastinal lymph nodes or lymphatic interstitial spread.

Obviously, some of the causes of disturbed physiology of the pleura are not malignant. Hence it is important to document the cause of an effusion in any patient with breast cancer before attributing it to metastatic disease.

Certain types of pleural disease are related to malignancy, but without direct malignant spread. These have been called "para-malignant effusions" (Table 45–16). Causes include mediastinal lymphatic obstruction, postobstructive pneumonia or atelectasis, pulmonary embolism, superior vena cava syndrome, low oncotic pressure, and chylothorax from disruption of the lymphatics

Table 45–16. CAUSES OF PARAMALIGNANT EFFUSIONS

Mediastinal lymph node obstruction
Bronchial obstruction with pneumonia
Bronchial obstruction with atelectasis
Pulmonary embolism
Superior vena cava syndrome
Chylothorax
Mediastinal radiation
Drug reactions
    Methotrexate
    Procarbazine
    Cyclophosphamide

Adapted from Sahn SA: Clin Chest Med 6:113–125, 1985.

or following radiation therapy to the mediastinum.[41] The precise incidence of these "para-malignant" conditions is unknown in patients presenting with pleural effusions, since most are described in case reports. However, the medical history, physical examination, and supporting laboratory data should aid in differentiating these conditions from metastatic involvement of the pleura.

Attempts to define the causes of a pleural effusion begin with a characterization of the nature of the fluid as either transudative or exudative. There are only three circumstances in which tests of pleural fluid are diagnostic: (1) the presence of malignant cells, (2) bacteria on stain or culture, and (3) the presence of lupus erythematosus cells.[14, 27] Most of the remaining tests of pleural fluid lack sensitivity, specificity, or predictive accuracy. Therefore the history, physical examination, and ancillary laboratory investigations will guide the clinician in selecting the most appropriate algorithm for diagnosis and management.

SIGNS AND SYMPTOMS

Metastatic breast cancer involving the pleura rarely presents as adenocarcinoma of occult primary site, since at presentation most patients are known to have breast cancer.[1, 11, 13, 17, 24, 41, 44] Although as many as 25 percent of patients are asymptomatic, cough is the most common symptom. Dyspnea on exertion may be noted by 50 percent of patients.[41, 44] The accumulated fluid may be as much as 1 l in up to 60 percent of patients.[13] Approximately ten percent of patients will have a massive effusion, opacifying the entire hemithorax. In such cases, shift of the mediastinum into the contralateral hemithorax helps distinguish bronchial obstruction with lung collapse from a massive effusion.

DIAGNOSTIC TESTS

The initial diagnostic maneuver is thoracentesis. The gross appearance of the pleural fluid may be suggestive of the cause. Typically, malignant processes produce bloody fluid. However, although serous fluid may suggest a nonmalignant etiology, this is not always the case. Malignant effusions are serous in approximately ten percent to 20 percent of cases.[13, 14] Turbid, nonbloody fluid suggests a parapneumonic etiology, possibly secondary to bronchial obstruction with a postobstructive pneumonia present.[44, 48] Typically, a malignant effusion has fewer than 4000 leukocytes per μl and lymphocytes predominate (>50 percent).[41]

It is helpful to determine whether the pleural fluid is a transudative or an exudative,[31] since malignant effusions are usually exudative.[13, 14, 41, 48] A transudate is typically caused by diseases that alter hydrostatic or osmotic forces, with normal pleural surfaces.[14] As such, further evaluation of a transudative effusion by pleural

biopsy is usually not helpful.[14] There are exceptions, however, since ten percent to 20 percent of malignant effusions are transudative.[31, 41, 48] Hence if a nonmalignant cause for the effusion cannot be determined, a pleural biopsy or thoracoscopy is sometimes indicated.[45, 56] Exudates are caused by diseases that influence the permeability of the pleural tissues to protein, decrease the lymphatic flow from the pleural surface, or decrease pressure in the pleural space. In these instances, further characterization of the pleural exudate usually will provide additional discriminating information about the etiology of the exudate. A simple, two-stage evaluation of pleural fluid is a sensitive, specific, and cost-effective laboratory approach.[31, 36] First, pleural fluid:serum protein and pleural fluid:serum lactate dehydrogenase (LDH) ratios are determined. Light et al.[31] have demonstrated that a pleural fluid to serum protein ratio greater than 0.5 predicts an exudate with 97 percent accuracy. If the ratio is less than or equal to 0.5, a transudate is predicted with 83 percent accuracy. Similarly, a ratio of pleural fluid to serum LDH greater than 0.6 indicates an exudate with an accuracy of 98 percent; if the ratio is less than or equal to 0.6, a transudate is predicted with an accuracy of 77 percent.[31] Pleural fluid glucose concentration has been found to be decreased in approximately one third of nonmesothelioma malignant effusions.[16, 20]

In the patient with known metastatic breast cancer, a pleural fluid cytology specimen often will be positive. Cytology findings in different malignant effusions are of variable diagnostic accuracy, ranging from 42 percent to 92 percent in published series.[16, 21, 27, 29, 46, 48, 56] False-positive results in pleural fluid cytology specimens for metastatic carcinoma of various types are infrequent; Grunze reported a false-positive rate of only two percent.[21] The number and volume of samples available for cytologic review influence the diagnostic accuracy of the procedure. It is recommended that the sample volume be at least 250 ml (though not more than 1500 ml taken at one procedure). In the series reported by Salyer et al.[43] and Winklemann and Pfitzer,[56] a single sample of fluid had a diagnostic yield of approximately 53 percent; the second sample, 64 percent; and a third sample increased the cumulative accuracy to 69 percent.[43, 56] Automated flow cytometry analysis for aneuploidy may also enhance the accuracy of cytological examination of pleural fluid.[53] Pleural fluid carcinoembryonic antigen, though a poor screening test, may be helpful in the diagnostically difficult effusion.[33, 39] If cytology specimens from three thoracenteses are negative but malignancy is still suspected, then biopsy of the pleura, with diagnostic thoracoscopy, if available, has been proposed.[11, 24, 41, 43, 45, 56]

THERAPY

Therapy for breast cancer metastatic to the pleura or leading to pleural effusions may be broadly divided into three categories: local, systemic, and a combination of the two. The decision to treat the patient is contingent on the physician's knowledge of the growth rate of the patient's cancer, the patient's performance status, and prior exposure to chemotherapeutic agents.

A variety of cytotoxic and cytostatic therapies are currently available for advanced metastatic breast cancer. The appearance of a malignant pleural effusion is indicative of widespread systemic metastases in all patients. Although no presently available therapy for systemic disease is curative, there is effective palliative systemic treatment that may improve the pleural disease. Breast cancer is a chemo-, hormone-, and relatively radioresponsive neoplasm. The treatment given to the patient with a malignant effusion is directed at symptomatic control of the local process as well as, in many cases, the systemic spread of tumor. Systemic therapy in advanced breast cancer is addressed elsewhere in this text (chapters 42 and 44) and will not be further covered in this section.

Local therapy for the malignant pleural effusion may be useful when systemic therapy is ineffective. However, not all malignant effusions in breast cancer require local therapy. Local treatment is aimed solely at palliation and should be reserved for relief of the symptoms of the effusion. Choice of treatment will often depend on the life expectancy and performance status of the patient.[20, 43]

Therapeutic and diagnostic thoracentesis is best used initially, not only for diagnosis but also to relieve the patient's distressing pulmonary symptoms. After initial thoracentesis with removal of the pleural fluid, the rate of reaccumulation may be determined (typically 2–3 weeks in malignant effusions). However, repeated attempts at thoracentesis are rarely effective in the long-term control of malignant pleural effusions, and several investigators have found a 97 percent to 100 percent frequency of fluid reaccumulation within 1 month.[5, 30, 44] Furthermore, repeated thoracentesis can lead to a number of complications, including hypoxemia, reexpansion pulmonary edema, severe bradycardia or hypotension, and traumatic pneumothorax or hemothorax, as well as hypoproteinemia and loculation of the fluid remaining in the affected hemithorax, making later attempts at pleurodesis difficult. Sclerosis of the pleural space should be considered if there is rapid symptomatic fluid accumulation and the patient's life expectancy is at least several months.

Most studies of pleurodesis in malignant pleural effusions use tube thoracostomy as a means of delivering the therapy and draining reaccumulated fluid. Most of these studies focus on a variety of tumor types. Nevertheless, a large percentage of patients in most series have breast cancer. The data presented here will attempt to highlight information related specifically to breast cancer. Tube thoracostomy alone has been advanced as an effective means of controlling recurrent malignant pleural effusions. However, the support for this is derived from a study with incomplete data on response rates. If a strict definition of success (i.e., no fluid reaccumulation for at least 1 month) is applied, then only a minority of patients (11 percent to 43 percent) respond to tube thoracostomy alone.[5, 19, 25, 57]

Sclerosing agents are usually necessary in conjunction with tube thoracostomy and drainage. This allows the apposition of pleural surfaces and facilitates the action of the instilled sclerosing agent. Several studies have compared thoracentesis with instillation of a sclerosing agent (mechlorethamine, a nitrogen mustard) to tube drainage and sclerosing agent instillation.[5, 19] These studies support the importance of pleural surface apposition. Treatment with mechlorethamine using tube thoracostomy for drainage successfully sclerosed the pleural space for greater than 1 month in 66 percent of patients, whereas instillation via thoracentesis needle was successful in only 27 percent of patients. In these studies, it was felt that prior to the instillation of the sclerosing agent, pleural fluid drainage should be less than 50–100 cc per day. The less pleural fluid present before therapy, the better is the apposition of the surfaces and the more even the distribution of the sclerosing agent instilled.

Sahn[41] has indicated that sclerosing therapy is unlikely to be effective when either the pleural effusion or the sclerosing solution pH is less than 7.3. He therefore recommends that patients with pleural fluid pH <7.3, and especially those patients in whom survival is expected to be less than a few weeks, should undergo repeated thoracentesis instead of pleurodesis.[20, 42]

Those patients who fail to reexpand collapsed lobes following 24 hours of tube thoracostomy drainage and prior to sclerosing therapy should undergo bronchoscopy or thoracoscopy. Many of these patients will have collapse secondary to bronchial obstruction or to a trapped, tumor-encased lung. The use of a sclerosing agent in these cases is to be discouraged, as the results are uniformly poor.

Sclerosing agents affect the pleural surface by direct reaction, causing an inflammatory response in the pleural tissues leading to fibrotic sclerosis.[20] There is little apparent antitumor effect of the various agents used, and many are not antineoplastic agents. An excellent review of the subject is presented by Hausheer and Yarbro, summarizing the trials published using the various agents and addressing the relative merits and disadvantages of each agent.[24]

Tetracycline (15–20 mg/kg or 1 gm) administered via tube thoracostomy is considered by many to be the initial agent of choice for pleurodesis of malignant pleural effusions.[6, 40, 51] Its use yields a 70 percent to 100 percent response rate in several studies where patient follow-up was available for more than 1 month.[7, 41, 54, 57] Side effects of fever or pain are seen in approximately 50 percent of patients. Pain may be diminished by pretreatment of the pleural space with instilled lidocaine (15 ml of one percent solution in 50 ml of normal saline) via the chest tube and administration of narcotic premedication. When the tube thoracostomy has an output of less than 100 ml/d, a solution of tetracycline in 50 ml of normal saline is instilled via the chest tube. The tube is then clamped, and the patient is rotated, including Trendelenberg's position, to evenly distribute the solution over the pleural spaces. After 10 minutes, the chest tube is unclamped and reconnected to suction (-20 cm H_2O). Some prefer to allow the solution to remain in the pleural space for up to 8 hours before the tube is unclamped.

The use of bleomycin as a sclerosing agent in malignant pleural effusions is effective in 65 percent to 85 percent of patients.[8, 35] There is evidence that bleomycin may be successfully used as a sclerosing agent in patients failing pleurodesis with tetracycline.[26] Bleomycin is instilled in the same fashion as tetracycline, and the usual dose of 1.25 U/kg in 50 ml of normal saline is used in younger patients. Because of two episodes of possible drug-related deaths in elderly patients receiving more than 40 U/m^2 of bleomycin solution into the pleural space, this should be considered the maximum dose in the elderly.[52] The solution is evenly dispersed into the pleural cavity in the same fashion as tetracycline. The toxicity of bleomycin is actually less than tetracycline; several investigators used no pretreatment and reported pain in only four percent of patients and fever in 16 percent.[24] When tetracycline and bleomycin were compared, their efficacy was found to be equivalent, though no strict response criteria were applied.[22] However, bleomycin is much more expensive than tetracycline.

Hausheer and Yarbro[24] have extensively reviewed the use of other sclerosing agents, including mechlorethamine,[5, 6, 19] quinacrine,[9, 10, 44, 54] thiotepa,[4] fluorouracil,[50] and talc.[2, 3, 12, 23] Expense, toxicity, or unacceptable therapeutic yields render these agents as less desirable alternatives to tetracycline or bleomycin as initial therapy. Patients who fail tetracycline and bleomycin, however, may be candidates for talc pleurodesis.

Talc (1–2 gm in a 50 cc suspension) is likely the most effective sclerosing agent available.[2, 3, 12, 23, 38] However, its use often requires general anesthesia, perhaps because it is often used as an agent of last resort. Failure of the other agents to provide durable and effective pleurodesis is often a result of inherent anatomical restrictions to reinflation (i.e., tumor- or fibrosis-encased lung or obstruction of a main stem bronchus). In the few patients without such restrictions who fail tetracycline or bleomycin, talc may be administered without general anesthesia. Those patients who require pleurectomy for effective pleurodesis obviously will be served best by general anesthesia and talc pleurodesis.

Pleurectomy is rarely indicated and should be used only in those patients who fail other methods of controlling pleural effusions, who can tolerate major surgery, and whose life expectancy is reasonably long.[32] Pleurectomy, in competent hands, is nearly 100 percent effective in controlling malignant effusions, but perioperative mortality is approximately ten percent, and the rate of complications postoperatively is approximately 20 percent and includes air leaks, bleeding, respiratory insufficiency, and pulmonary embolism.[28]

External-beam radiotherapy is not effective as a sole treatment modality because of the large surface area, radiosensitivity of the underlying lung relative to the metastatic breast cancer cells, and complex dosimetry associated with treating these curved surfaces.[49]

PROGNOSIS

In the series we have reviewed, a variety of treatment modalities were used, both local and systemic. Median survival of patients with metastatic breast cancer with pleural involvement ranged from 6.5 months to 15.7 months, with a median survival from diagnosis of the pleural effusion of approximately 10 months.

Utilizing tetracycline or bleomycin by the methods previously described will control 70 percent to 85 percent of malignant effusions for greater than 1 month. Slightly less than half of these patients will succumb to breast cancer as a direct result of pleuropulmonary metastases, and the remainder will die as a result of distant metastases to other sites.

The opinions or assertions contained herein are the private views of the authors and are not to be construed as official or as reflecting the views of the Department of the Navy or the Department of Defense.

References

1. Abrams HC, Spiro R, Goldstein N: Metastases in carcinoma; Analysis of 1000 autopsied cases. Cancer 3:74–85, 1950.
2. Adler RH, Rappole BW: Recurrent malignant pleural effusions and talc powder aerosol treatment. Surgery 62:1000–1006, 1967.
3. Adler RH, Sayek I: Treatment of malignant pleural effusion: a method using tube thoracostomy and talc. Ann Thorac Surg 22:8–15, 1976.
4. Andersen AP, Brinker H: Intracavitary thiotepa in malignant pleural and peritoneal effusions. Acta Radiol 7:369–378, 1969.
5. Anderson CB, Philpott GW, Ferguson TB: The treatment of malignant pleural effusions. Cancer 33:916–922, 1974.
6. Austin EH, Flye MW: The treatment of recurrent malignant pleural effusions. Ann Thorac Surg 28:190–203, 1979.
7. Bayly TC, Kisner DL, Sybert A, McDonald JS, Tsou E, Schein PS: Tetracycline and quinacrine in the control of malignant pleural effusions: a randomized trial. Cancer 41:1188–1192, 1978.
8. Bitran JD, Brown C, Desser RK, Kozloff MF, Shapiro C, Billings AA: Intracavitary bleomycin for the control of malignant effusions. J Surg Oncol 16:273–277, 1981.
9. Borda I, Krant M: Convulsions following intrapleural administration of quinacrine hydrochloride. JAMA 201:1049–1050, 1967.
10. Borja ER, Pugh RP: Single dose quinacrine and thoracostomy in the control of pleural effusion in patients with neoplastic diseases. Cancer 31:899–902, 1973.
11. Canto A, Rivas J, Saumench J, et al: Points to consider when choosing a biopsy method in cases of pleurisy of unknown origin. Chest 84:176–179, 1983.
12. Chambers JS: Palliative treatment of neoplastic pleural effusion with intercostal intubation and talc instillation. West J Surg Obstet Gynecol 66:26, 1958.
13. Chernow B, Sahn SA: Carcinomatous involvement of the pleura: An analysis of 96 patients. Am J Med 63:695–702, 1977.
14. Chetty KG: Transudative pleural effusions: In Symposium on Pleural Diseases. Clin Chest Med 6:49–54, 1985.
15. Clark GM, Sledge GW, Osborne CK, McGuire WL: Survival from first recurrence: relative importance of prognostic factors in 1,015 breast cancer patients. J Clin Oncol 5:55–61, 1987.
16. Clarkson B: Relationship between cell type, glucose concentration, and response to treatment in neoplastic effusions. Cancer 17:914–928, 1964.
17. Fentiman IS, Millis R, Sexton S, Hayward JL: Pleural effusion in breast cancer: a review of 105 cases. Cancer 47:2087–2092, 1981.

18. Fentiman IS, Rubens RD, Hayward JL: The pattern of metastatic disease in patients with pleural effusions secondary to breast cancer. Br J Surg 69:193–194, 1982.

19. Fracchia AA, Knapper WH, Carey JT, et al: Intrapleural chemotherapy for effusion from metastatic breast carcinoma. Cancer 26:626–629, 1970.

20. Good JT Jr, Taryle DA, Sahn SA: Pleural fluid pH in malignant effusions: pathophysiology and prognostic implications. Chest 74:338, 1978.

21. Grunze H: The comparative diagnostic accuracy, efficiency, and specificity of cytologic techniques used in the diagnosis of malignant neoplasms in serous effusions of the pleural and pericardial cavities. *In* Symposium on Diagnostic Accuracy of Cytologic Technics, vol 8. 1984, pp 150–163.

22. Gupta N, Opfell RW, Padova J, et al: Intrapleural bleomycin vs. tetracycline for control of malignant pleural effusions: a randomized study. (Abstract) ASCO 189:366, 1980.

23. Harley HRS: Malignant pleural effusions and their treatment by intercostal talc pleurodesis. Br J Dis Chest 73:173–177, 1979.

24. Hausheer FH, Yarbro JW: Diagnosis and treatment of malignant pleural effusion. Semin Oncol 12:54–75, 1985.

25. Izbicki R, Weyhing BT III, Baker L, et al: Pleural effusions in cancer patients; a prospective randomized study of pleural drainage with the addition of radiophosphorous to pleural space vs. drainage alone. Cancer 36:1511–1518, 1975.

26. Jarvi OH, Kunnas RJ, Laitio MT, Tyrrko JES: The accuracy and significance of cytologic cancer diagnosis of pleural effusions. Acta Cytol 16:152–158, 1972.

27. Jay SJ: Diagnostic procedures for pleural disease. Clin Chest Med 6:33–48, 1985.

28. Jensik R, Cagle JE, Milloy F, et al: Pleurectomy in the treatment of pleural effusion due to metastatic malignancy. J Thorac Cardiovasc Surg 46:322–330, 1963.

29. Johnston WW: The malignant pleural effusion: a review of cytopathologic diagnoses of 584 specimens from 472 consecutive patients. Cancer 56:905–909, 1985.

30. Lambert CJ, Shah HH, Urschel HC Jr, et al: The treatment of malignant pleural effusion by closed trocartube drainage. Ann Thorac Surg 3:1–5, 1967.

31. Light RW, MacGregor MI, Luchsinger PC, et al: Pleural effusions: the diagnostic separation of transudates and exudates. Ann Int Med 77:507–513, 1972.

32. Martini N, Bains MS, Beattie EJ Jr: Indications for pleurectomy in malignant effusion. Cancer 35:734–738, 1975.

33. McKenna JM, Chandrasekhar AJ, Henkins RE: Diagnostic value of carcino-embryonic antigen in exudative pleural effusions. Chest 78:587–590, 1980.

34. Meyer PC: Metastatic carcinoma of the pleura. Thorax 21:437–443, 1966.

35. Paladine W, Cunningham TJ, Sponzo R, Donavan M, et al: Intracavitary bleomycin in the management of malignant effusions. Cancer 38:1903–1908, 1976.

36. Peterman TA, Speichler CE: Evaluating pleural effusions: a two stage laboratory approach. JAMA 25:1051–1053, 1984.

37. Porter EH: Pleural effusion and breast cancer. (Letter) Br Med J 1:251, 1965.

38. Prorok J, Nealon TF: Pleural symphysis by talc poudrage in the treatment of malignant pleural effusion. Bull Soc Chir 27:630, 1968.

39. Rittgers RA, Lowenstein MS, Feinerman AE, et al: Carcinoembryonic antigen levels in benign and malignant pleural effusions. Ann Int Med 88:631, 1978.

40. Rubinson RM, Bolooki H: Intrapleural tetracycline for control of malignant pleural effusion. A preliminary report. South Med J 65:847, 1972.

41. Sahn SA: Malignant pleural effusions. *In* Symposium on Pleural Diseases. Clin Chest Med 6:113–125, 1985.

42. Sahn SA, Good JT, Potts DE: The pH of sclerosing agents: a determinant of pleural symphysis. Chest 76:198–200, 1979.

43. Salyer WR, Eggleston JC, Erozan YS: Efficacy of pleural needle biopsy and pleural fluid cytopathology in the diagnosis of malignant neoplasm involving the pleura. Chest 67:536–539, 1975.

44. Sarma PR, Moore MR: Approach to the management of pleural effusion in malignancy. South Med J 71:133–136, 1978.

45. Scerbo J, Keltz H, Stone DJ: A prospective study of closed pleural biopsies. JAMA 218:377–380, 1971.

46. Stiksa G, Korsgaard R, Simonsson BG: Treatment of recurrent pleural effusion by pleurodesis with quinacrine. Scand J Resp Dis 60:197, 1979.

47. Stoll BA: Pleural effusion and breast cancer. (Letter) Br Med J 1:658, 1965.

48. Storey DD, Dines DE, Coles DT: Pleural effusion: a diagnostic dilemma JAMA 236:2183–2186, 1976.

49. Strober SJ, Klotz E, Kuperman A, et al: Malignant pleural disease—a radiotherapeutic approach to the problem. JAMA 226:296–299, 1973.

50. Suhrland LG, Weisberger AS: Intracavitary 5-fluorouracil in malignant effusions. Arch Int Med 116:431, 1965.

51. The treatment of malignant pleural and pericardial effusions. Med Lett Drugs Ther 23:59, 1981.

52. Trotter JM, Stuart JFB, McBeth JG, et al: The management of malignant effusions with bleomycin. Br J Cancer 40:310, 1979.

53. Unger KM, Raber M, Bedrosian CWM, Stein DA, Barlogie B: Analysis of pleural effusions using automated flow cytometry. Cancer 52:873–877, 1983.

54. Wallach HW: Intrapleural tetracycline for malignant pleural effusions. Chest 68:510–512, 1975.

55. Wang NS: Anatomy and physiology of the pleural space. *In* Symposium on Pleural Diseases. Clin Chest Med 6:3–16, 1985.

56. Winkelmann M, Pfitzer P: Blind pleural biopsy in combination with cytology of pleural effusions. Acta Cytol 25:373–376, 1981.

57. Zaloznik AJ, Oswald SJ, Langin M: Intrapleural tetracycline in pleural effusions: a randomized study. Cancer 51:752–755, 1983.

Management of Central Nervous System Metastases in Breast Cancer

Jeffrey M. Crane, M.D. and Barnett S. Kramer, M.D.

As a cause of central nervous system (CNS) metastases, carcinoma of the breast is second only to lung cancer. In autopsy series, CNS metastases (primarily brain, dura, and meninges) occur in 30 percent of breast cancer patients.[1, 42, 44] Of these, approximately 65 percent to 70 percent had been asymptomatic.[43] CNS metastases nearly always occur in the setting of widespread disease.[13, 43] In Tsukada et al.'s autopsy series, only three percent of CNS metastases were the sole site of metastatic spread, and 70 percent of patients with CNS disease died of either extra-CNS disease or a combination of both CNS and systemic disease.[43]

The CNS may be conveniently divided into three categories of metastatic disease. The major site of metastatic disease is the intracranial portion of the CNS. This site includes the extradural and subdural sites of metastases as well as the cerebrum, cerebellum, midbrain, and choroid plexus. The second anatomical category is the leptomeninges, an area of involvement that many investigators believe is increasing in frequency as more patients survive for longer periods with cancer.[5, 27, 35, 48] The third site of CNS metastases is the spinal cord. Extramedullary metastases account for 97 percent of cases in this category.[35]

The time to development of CNS metastases in breast cancer is extremely variable. CNS disease is occasionally symptomatic at the time of diagnosis, and metastases have been found as late as 19 years after the primary diagnosis.[16, 33] The disease-free interval as well as the underlying rate of growth of the primary disease are very important prognostic factors. Metastases to one site in the CNS predict an increased likelihood of metastatic involvement to other sites in the CNS.[35, 43] Although a combination of therapeutic modalities may secure symptomatic relief in CNS metastases, survival is usually short after the occurence of symptomatic CNS metastases.[43] Equally important, however, is the fact that once signs or symptoms of CNS metastases are detected, prompt and appropriate therapeutic palliation can usually prevent unfortunate neurological sequelae.

ANATOMICAL SITES OF SPREAD

Intracranial Disease

Intracranial disease accounts for the majority of CNS metastases from breast cancer (62 percent according to Tsukada et al.'s investigation[43]). Only one third of these are clinically suspected ante mortem. Presenting symptoms may be focal or global, in the case of increased intracranial pressure. The cranial dura are involved in approximately 54 percent of patients with CNS metastases. In Tsukada et al.'s series of 1044 autopsies of breast cancer patients, 16 percent of all patients had dural metastases. Half of all symptomatic patients had dural metastases as a component of their CNS disease. The incidence of cranial dura involvement was increased threefold when vertebral body metastases were present.[43]

Solitary metastases to the CNS occurred in 81 of 193 patients with intracranial metastases (42 percent) or 7.8 percent of all breast cancer patients autopsied. After the cranial dura, the cerebellum is the next most frequent site of both asymptomatic and symptomatic metastases in this series, accounting for 20 percent of all CNS metastases and approximately two thirds of solitary sites of CNS metastases.

Diagnosis

As noted previously, the majority of CNS metastases in breast cancer are asymptomatic, largely because of the preponderance of asymptomatic intracranial and cranial dura metastases. One review of 101 breast cancer patients with metastatic CNS disease indicated that 70 percent were receiving systemic chemotherapy at the time of their CNS metastases.[13] Despite attempts to presymptomatically diagnose various carcinomas metastatic to the brain, including breast cancer, overall survival has not been lengthened.[26] The likely explanation for this negative result lies in the fact that the majority of patients have concomitant extra-CNS metastases, and the majority of these, approximately 70 percent, die as a result of that extra-CNS disease. Also, very few breast cancer patients have disease sufficiently anatomically limited that they may be considered candidates for curative surgical or radiotherapeutic measures. Although most therapeutic interventions are termed "palliative," it is to be emphasized that the interventions frequently improve the quality and, occasionally, the quantity of life. Appropriate and prompt treatment may prevent the potentially crippling sequela of progressive CNS metastases.

Headache is a presenting complaint in approximately 50 percent of patients with intracranial (including dural) metastases.[10, 35] Many of these patients describe the headache in terms that strongly indicate the presence of elevated intracranial pressure. Classically, the headache is worse on awakening in the morning and abates within 30 minutes of arising, returning again the next morning. Papilledema is reported by Posner to be present in only 25 percent of patients with symptomatic metastatic intracranial disease.[35] Its absence, therefore, is not helpful. Posner also stresses that a careful examination of patients with systemic cancer will often disclose other signs of CNS disease not noted by the patient. As an example, he notes that although only 40 percent of patients with documented intracranial metastases complain of focal weakness, two thirds of them have focal weakness on careful physical examination. Similarly, impaired cognitive function could be found by careful mental status exam in three fourths of patients, but barely a third complained of behavioral or mental changes. Focal or generalized seizures were a presenting complaint in 15 percent of patients and were somewhat more frequent in patients with leptomeningeal metastases.[10, 35]

The best single test for the diagnosis of metastatic intracranial metastases remains computerized axial tomography (CAT), capable of defining mass lesions as well as peritumor edema as small as 5 mm. There is no current "gold standard" with which to determine negative predictive accuracy or sensitivity of CAT scanning except at necropsy. Necropsy studies performed in patients dying of small cell lung cancer, however, indicate that in symptomatic patients, CAT scanning of the brain has positive and negative predictive accuracies of 98 percent and 99 percent, respectively.[12] Furthermore, in symptomatic patients with suspected spinal cord compression by metastases, the frequency of concomitant intracranial metastases encourages prompt CAT scanning of the brain.[43] Radionuclide brain scanning has been generally replaced by CAT brain scanning, as have cerebral arteriography and pneumonencephalography. Lumbar puncture is generally indicated after CAT scan confirms normal intracranial pressure in patients with CNS metastases because of the common incidence of leptomeningeal or spinal cord metastases associated with intracranial metastases.[24, 43] The cerebrospinal fluid (CSF) of patients with isolated intracerebral metastases is commonly normal, but it may be abnormal in those patients with concomitant leptomeningeal metastases.[35] Plain skull roentgenograms play little or no role in the diagnosis of intracranial CNS metastases.[4, 43]

In the patient with breast cancer who has signs and symptoms of CNS metastases, the CAT scan finding of a solitary intracranial mass is usually indicative of metastasis. However, other causes of a solitary lesion should be considered such as brain abscess, primary brain tumors (such as gliomas or meningiomas), cerebral infarcts of either thrombotic or embolic arterial occlusion, and chronic subdural hematomas or effusions. These can often be excluded on the basis of CAT scan appearance. Multiple intracranial lesions seen on CAT scan in a patient with breast cancer are nearly always secondary to metastatic disease. If no intracranial mass lesion is seen in the symptomatic patient with breast cancer, diagnoses that should be considered include leptomeningeal metastases, endocrine-related paraneoplastic encephalopathy, carcinomatous neuromyopathy (such as subacute cerebellar degeneration), and rarely, sensorimotor neuropathy syndrome or progressive multifocal leukoencephalopathy.

Management

Although cure of intracranial metastases is rarely possible, palliation is often possible. Untreated, median survival is approximately 6 weeks.[13, 24, 29] Nevertheless, with aggressive combined modality therapy, including surgery, radiation therapy, and systemic chemotherapy in selected patients, a 1-year survival of 40 percent to 50 percent may be achieved.[5, 10, 13, 18, 24, 29, 42] Critical appraisal of the various treatment modalities is difficult, because none of the numerous studies are adequately controlled for critical variables such as age, rate of growth of underlying disease, number and site of brain metastases, and cell type and radiosensitivity of the primary lesion. However, it does appear that it is possible to define certain patient characteristics that predict for response to therapy, such as disease-free interval, number of brain metastases, and performance status.[13]

Corticosteroids are the most commonly used treatment for intracranial metastases. Corticosteroids, by themselves, improve symptoms of brain metastases in 60 percent to 75 percent of patients, often within 24 hours.[35] Used alone, however, their effect is only temporary, as their action is directed primarily at reduction of peritumor edema. They have no proven oncolytic effect on brain metastases. Glucocorticoids are favored, but no particular type is proven to be more efficacious than another. Nevertheless, a recent study suggests that the CNS pharmacokinetics of systemically administered dexamethasone is more favorable than prednisone.[2] Dexamethasone is usually begun with a loading dose of 10–25 mg followed by 16 mg/d in three or four daily oral or parenteral doses. This dose may be increased to as much as 100 mg daily if symptomatic improvement is not apparent within 24 hours. After several days the dose may be tapered to the minimum dose effective. There is no evidence that steroids are of any benefit in patients without CNS symptoms.[24] Used alone, the glucocorticoids exert their effect for an average of 1 to 2 months. If no other treatment is given, extension in survival is only approximately 1 month over that of untreated patients.[5] The side effects of steroids are numerous; the most bothersome are steroid-associated myopathy and insomnia. There is a possibility of an enhanced tendency to develop peptic ulcer disease with perforation. Glucose intolerance may also occur and may improve at a lowered dose of steroid.[5, 35]

Radiation therapy is the second most commonly used therapeutic modality in the treatment of cerebral metastases. The optimum radiation schedule, dose, and fractionation are not clearly established.[24] Doses vary from 2500 to 5000 rads given over a 1- to 5-week course of whole brain therapy, depending on estimated patient survival. The whole brain is treated because of the frequency of patients with multiple brain sites (60 percent of patients with brain metastases). However, in patients with solitary brain metastases, an additional boost of 500–1000 rads may be given to the lesion.[5, 18, 24]

In the mid 1970s, a National Cooperative Study sponsored by the Radiation Therapy Oncology Group (RTOG) evaluated more than 1000 patients with a variety of metastatic intracerebral metastases with regard to different schedules and doses of radiation therapy, the influence of steroids and chemotherapy, and primary tumor site and status.[24] Hendrickson's review of the results concluded that 3000 rads delivered to the whole brain given in ten or 15 fractions was equal to 4000 rads given in 15 or 20 fractions. There were no differences in median survival or in the proportion of patients with symptomatic improvement. Headache or convulsions were completely resolved in 55 percent and 67 percent, respectively, while fewer than 15 percent experienced either no change or worsening of these symptoms. Impaired mentation and motor loss were completely resolved in approximately a third of the patients, with partial resolution in 40 percent.

The concomitant use of systemic chemotherapy is advocated for those patients with brain metastases and evidence of extra-CNS systemic disease. As outlined in other chapters of this text, effective chemotherapy exists that can yield a 40 percent to 70 percent response rate in previously untreated metastatic breast cancer. However, since chemotherapy does not cross the blood-brain barrier in therapeutic levels, it does not affect CNS relapse.[13]

The routine use of phenytoin to prevent seizures is probably not necessary in all patients with brain metastases. Approximately 15 percent of patients will experience seizures at some point. Nevertheless, the toxicities of prophylactic phenytoins in the 85 percent of patients who don't need anticonvulsant therapy probably outweigh the benefits in the 15 percent who do. Anticonvulsants will usually ameliorate these patients.[5, 24, 35] It is our opinion that patients with documented brain metastases should not drive or operate heavy machinery.

Occasionally patients with brain metastases develop rapid neurological decompensation, suggesting tentorial or cerebellar herniation. In these situations the prompt use of osmotically active agents may stabilize and often improve the patient's symptoms.[5] Mannitol (20 percent in distilled water, 1–2 gm/kg body weight) or urea (30 percent solution, 1.5 gm/kg body weight) given intravenously are used in combination with intravenous glucocorticoids. Once the patient is stabilized, more definitive therapy with radiation, with or without surgery, can be undertaken.

Recurrence of symptomatic metastases after radiation of the brain is not uncommon, being five percent in the RTOG national study and as high as 83 percent in other studies.[13, 24] Retreatment may still be possible. However, CNS metastases were the primary cause of death in 60 percent of the patients who had recurrence.[13, 41]

The role of surgery in brain metastases is confined to those few patients (less than five percent) with breast cancer in whom the metastases are solitary, surgically approachable, and with no apparent metastatic sites outside the CNS.[5, 36] There is occasionally a need for surgical placement of a ventricular shunt if obstructive hydrocephalus is present in a candidate for surgical reversal of the obstruction.[42] Also, if meningeal carcinomatosis is evident, the placement of an Ommaya reservoir may be indicated for delivery of chemotherapy.[37] Three series have examined the role of surgery alone in the treatment of metastatic cancer to the brain, with 1-year postoperative survival varying from 22 percent to 31 percent of patients.[5, 36, 42] These results are better than the 14 percent to 21 percent 1-year survival of three series compiled one decade earlier and somewhat better than those results obtained utilizing radiotherapy alone.[24] However, the apparent improvement could well be a result of patient selection.

Because other microscopic CNS metastases are likely, whole brain radiation is usually given after surgical removal of a solitary metastasis.[5, 10, 24] In one series of patients undergoing resection of brain metastases from a variety of tumor types, those with breast cancer did better in general than the group as a whole.[10] Using a combined modality approach in patients with metastatic breast cancer with solitary metastases, three separate neurosurgical groups have reported a median survival of 9 to 12 months, with 13 percent to 25 percent of patients surviving 2 years.[10, 36, 42] Perioperative mortality was 10 percent to 21 percent. Although 66 percent to 90 percent of patients symptomatically improved after combined surgery and postoperative whole brain irradiation, many authors have noted a high risk of recurrence in the brain. Sundaresan and Galicich noted that of eight breast cancer patients who underwent surgery, six had solitary metastases at surgery; of these, five relapsed in the CNS within 2 years after craniotomy.[42] Postcraniotomy autopsy series have shown the continued presence of tumor at the margins of resection in 25 percent to 42 percent of cases in which death occurred within 30 days of supposed complete surgical resection.[5, 10]

Leptomeninges

Metastatic involvement of the leptomeninges is found in approximately six percent of breast cancer patients at autopsy.[44] Solitary leptomeningeal metastases are rare; Tsukada et al. found only three cases in 309 patients with CNS metastases (1,044 total breast cancer patients).[43] Of 59 patients found at autopsy to have leptomeningeal involvement, 32 had been symptomatic. None of the three patients with solitary meningeal spread had been symptomatic. As is the case with both childhood and some adult leukemias, leptomeningeal involvement appears to be increasing in frequency in breast cancer patients.[5, 27, 35, 48] Perhaps equally disturbing is the finding of concomitant leptomeningeal metastases in one third of breast cancer patients with symptomatic intracranial metastases.[17, 43, 48]

Diagnosis

Leptomeningeal carcinomatosis is the wide, multifocal spread of cancer in the subarachnoid space.[19, 27, 33] Since this spread may occur microscopically, asymptomatic patients may be found at necropsy.[43] The lag time from initial diagnosis of breast cancer to diagnosis of leptomeningeal metastases ranges in the literature from 1 to 120 months, with a median time of 25 months.[33, 48] There appears to be no difference in frequency between pre- and post-menopausal patients; hormone receptor status in these patients has not been reported.

Leptomeningeal spread of breast cancer usually presents with signs and symptoms similar to those of intracranial metastases, though the additional symptoms and signs of cranial neuropathies and of spinal root compression dominate the clinical picture.[27, 33, 48] Although headache is the most common presenting complaint, it occurs in only about a third of patients at diagnosis and in only about 50 percent at any time during the course of the illness. Global symptoms of hydrocephalus can occur as a result of tumor obstruction of CSF circulation.[43] Meningeal carcinomatosis may also extend to involve the parenchyma of the brain, nerve roots within the spinal cord, or the parenchyma of the spinal cord.[17] In this way, neurological symptoms throughout the neuroaxis may be produced through a variety of mechanisms. Cranial neuropathies or lower motor neuron signs (i.e., facial paralysis or urinary incontinence) may be caused by invasion of the nerves in the subarachnoid space. Focal neurological defects may arise from direct invasion of the brain parenchyma, resulting in focal or generalized seizures and hemiplegia. Central hypoventilation has also been described as a consequence of meningeal spread of breast cancer.[28]

Posner, in a review of patients with various types of primary cancer, states that "the diagnosis of meningeal carcinomatosis is suggested by the fact that patients have neurological symptoms or signs of either widespread or multifocal invasion of the neuroaxis rather than a single focal lesion."[35] The physician should be especially aware of the potential for leptomeningeal spread in the breast cancer patient with other CNS metastases or vertebral body metastases who presents with multifocal symptoms such as confusion, a change in affect or headache, or the spinal root symptoms of pain in the back or neck or radiculopathy. Nuchal rigidity, decreased deep tendon reflexes, or other spinal root signs are commonly present, and as many as 55 percent of the patients will demonstrate extensor plantar response, poor attention span, diplopia, or papilledema. The most frequently involved cranial nerves are the constellation of III, IV, VI (78 percent at presentation, 94 percent during the course of illness), followed by VII (42 percent and 70 percent) and VIII (30 percent and 38 percent), although involvement of each of the cranial nerves has been reported. Dysarthria and gait abnormalities are occasionally seen in these patients.[27, 33, 45]

The diagnosis of leptomeningeal carcinomatosis is confirmed by the finding of malignant cells in CSF but is not excluded by their absence.[17] Multiple lumbar punctures may be necessary to detect malignant cells. In one series, the diagnosis was established in 82 of 90 patients by the third lumbar puncture.[45] However, in most instances there is at least one of the following abnormalities: elevated CSF pressure (>150 mm H_2O in 98/137 patients); an increased number of white blood cells (64 of 90 patients, >5 cells/mm^3, predominantly lymphocytes); or elevated CSF protein levels (>50 mg/dl in 80/90 patients).[45] In two separate series, only one of 137 different CSF samples was completely normal (including chemistry analysis, cell count, and cytologic analysis), in patients ultimately proven to have leptomeningeal carcinomatosis.[28, 40] The measurement of CSF concentration of carcinoembryonic antigen (CEA) may also be helpful in both diagnosis and management of meningeal carcinomatosis of metastatic breast cancer.[45, 46]

In Tsukada et al.'s autopsy series of 1044 breast cancer patients, 17 of 59 patients with leptomeningeal metastases were not clinically suspected ante mortem.[43] Intracerebral metastases frequently are found on CAT brain scan in patients with leptomeningeal metastases. Thirty of 90 patients with leptomeningeal disease had other parenchymal CNS spread (16 brain, 14 to epidural cord) in one series,[45] and in only 18 of 90 patients was breast cancer spread confined solely to the leptomeninges. The CAT findings of hydrocephalus or of contrast enhancement of the basal cisterns or cerebral sulci suggest leptomeningeal spread.[45] However, CAT is not capable of detecting microscopic spread of metastases into the leptomeninges.

Myelography may occasionally indicate concomitant extradural spinal cord spread. In one series of various types of carcinomatous meningitis, seven of 18 patients had multiple nodular defects noted on nerve roots later confirmed at laminectomy as metastases.[45] The electroencephalogram has been performed in a series of patients with leptomeningeal carcinomatosis from varying primary cancers, and although not diagnostic, 75 percent were abnormal, primarily manifesting nonspecific diffuse slow waves.[43, 45]

Management

The treatment of leptomeningeal carcinomatosis is directed at prevention of further neurological deterioration and possible reversal of evolving signs and symptoms. As in most neurological deficits, once metastatic disease has caused a deficit, complete reversal with therapy is rare.[35] Indeed, even in the occasional patient with carcinomatous meningitis who survives more than 2.5 years following intensive therapy, post mortem examination frequently discloses persistent metastatic leptomeningeal involvement. Untreated patients usually succumb within 6 weeks of diagnosis.[27, 33, 45]

A variety of treatments for leptomeningeal carcinomatosis have been reported; none have been compared in controlled trials. The entire neuroaxis must be treated to effect long-term control of symptomatic disease.[45] Because myelosuppression results from irradiation of the entire craniospinal axis, it is recommended that only the site of primary neurological symptoms receive radiation therapy in patients receiving systemic chemotherapy (e.g., whole brain ports for cranial neuropathies). The usual dose of radiation is 3000–4000 rads. The remainder of the neuroaxis is then treated with intrathecal or intraventricular (via Ommaya reservoir) administration of methotrexate: 12 mg twice weekly via lumbar intrathecal route or 6.5 mg/m² (12 mg maximum) if given via Ommaya in preservative-free 0.9 percent saline.[30, 33, 35, 40, 45, 48]

The decision to place an Ommaya reservoir is usually contingent on an acceptable prognosis and functional status of the individual patient.[37, 48] The Ommaya reservoir permits more thorough exposure of the meningeal surfaces to methotrexate and allows intermittent therapeutic drug monitoring to ensure adequate therapeutic levels of methotrexate and avoidance of toxic CNS levels as well as weekly cytologic assessment of CSF.[6, 7, 37, 40] Once the CSF normalizes, the interval between doses lengthens until maintenance methotrexate is given once monthly.[35, 48] Should evidence of progressive leptomeningeal disease occur during the therapeutic course, despite confirmation of adequate methotrexate levels at the site of meningeal disease, a change to cytosine arabinoside (50 mg/m² given twice weekly)[6, 7] or thiotepa (10 mg total)[22] may be substituted for methotrexate. In addition, dexamethasone 16 mg/d in four divided doses is useful in moderate to severely symptomatic patients.[35, 48] There is no evidence that glucocorticoids, given for their edema-reducing effects, exert a direct cytotoxic effect.

Administration of methotrexate via repetitive lumbar punctures will fail to deliver drug to the subarachnoid space in five percent to ten percent of treatments, reaching instead the sub- or epidural space.[40] Furthermore, it has been noted that neoplastic meningitis results in disordered CSF circulation,[21, 32] even in the absence of extradural block, and the physician may be delivering a subtherapeutic ($<10^{-6}$ mg/L) dose of methotrexate to the focus of neoplastic meningitis. For these reasons, in those patients with leptomeningeal carcinomatosis with potentially good prognoses, the administration of methotrexate should be via Ommaya reservoir.

The response to treatment as outlined previously depends on the status of the patient's extra-CNS disease and the level or degree of neurological function or deficits prior to therapy.[47] Clearly, successful, durable results are most easily attained in patients who are diagnosed early in the course of their meningeal disease and who can tolerate combined therapy. It is uncommon for leptomeningeal metastases to be the sole site of metastatic disease, and effective systemic treatment of the patient's breast cancer is usually necessary. In two series of breast cancer patients, treated as outlined previously, the overall response rate was approximately 65 percent, with a median survival of responding patients of 4.5 to 7.2 months (range, 1–29 mo). Nonresponding patients succumb (median survival of 1 month), generally, to CNS disease, whereas approximately half of responding patients die as a result of extra-CNS dis-

ease.[33, 45] The overall survival at 1 year in treated patients is only about ten percent to 15 percent.[33, 45, 47]

Several toxicities can be associated with treatment. The use of combined whole brain irradiation and intraventricular methotrexate may rarely result in brain necrosis or multifocal leukoencephalopathy. Also, occasional marrow suppression is reported with these dosages of methotrexate but is reversible with folinic acid. More commonly, intrathecal (via lumbar puncture) or intraventricular (via Ommaya reservoir) methotrexate results in aseptic meningitis or arachnoiditis. Except in accomplished and experienced hospitals, the rate of complications with insertion and maintenance of the Ommaya device is approximately 20 percent. Though usually mild, these may include infections resulting from poor catheter placement in the subarachnoid space and the development of new neurological signs.[45]

Spinal Cord

Next to lung cancer, breast cancer is the second most common cause of symptomatic spinal cord compression.[1, 4, 9, 11, 16] The true incidence of spinal cord metastases in breast cancer is unknown, as no studies have systematically studied post mortem spinal cords in a large cohort of breast cancer patients. Thus, information is not available on the frequency of asymptomatic breast cancer patients with spinal cord metastases. Some authors, however, have estimated a frequency of approximately five percent to ten percent in patients with breast cancer.[1, 43] In Tsukada et al.'s series, the cord was examined only in those cases with clinical symptoms referrable to that site; 32 cases of spinal cord metastases were found among 96 examined cords; eight were found to be the sole site of CNS involvement.[43] Seventy-five percent of spinal cord metastases were associated with other sites of CNS metastases. In Barron et al.'s analysis of 127 necropsied cases of symptomatic involvement of the spinal cord and cauda equina by a variety of metastatic neoplasms, there were 20 cases of metastatic breast cancer.[4] Their review of all cases of breast cancer at autopsy at Montefiore Hospital indicated an incidence of 6.5 percent of metastatic spinal cord involvement. Compiling several series has shown up to a 12 percent incidence of cord metastases in breast cancer.[1, 4, 43]

Posner has reported that more than 97 percent of metastatic disease in the cord is extramedullary.[35] Edelson et al.'s series further substantiates the rarity of metastatic intramedullary disease.[15] Batson described the important role of the plexus of veins around the vertebral bodies with their anastomosis to the dural sinuses in metastasis to the CNS, concomitant with vertebral body disease. In Barron et al.'s 20 cases of breast cancer metastatic to the spinal cord, he noted the following four characteristics:[4]

1. Carcinoma of the breast was always an established diagnosis at the time of spinal cord disease.

2. The median duration of pain was often longer than for other metastatic carcinomas to the cord. However,

once neurological signs were present, progression to hemiparesis or hemiplegia was rapid.

3. The onset of spinal cord metastases in breast cancer was typically late in the course of the disease.

4. In patients with back pain, myelographic abnormalities, and breast cancer, the plain x-ray films of the spine were usually (94 percent) abnormal.

Diagnosis

Early diagnosis of extradural metastatic tumor tests the skills of every physician treating these patients. Although breast cancer patients may have pain secondary to a benign musculoskeletal problem, back pain may also be the first indication of metastasis to a vertebral body or spinal epidural space.[4, 9, 11, 35, 38, 42] Extremely variable in onset, spinal cord compression has been reported to occur up to 19 years from original diagnosis.[16] Despite advances in other aspects of oncology, the prognosis of patients with neurological impairment from extradural spinal cord compression has remained static over the past several decades.[11, 31] Irreversible hemiparalysis occurs in approximately one third of cancer patients with spinal cord compression.[16] Patients who cannot walk before treatment rarely walk again.[4, 9, 11, 16] Knowing this, the physician must diagnose compressive metastatic tumor in the early stage of back pain and with minimal or no neurological deficit. Once suspected, the diagnosis of spinal cord compression must be pursued until it is either confirmed or excluded. An algorithmic approach is outlined as follows.[34]

Metastatic breast cancer reaches the epidural space, leading to compression of the spinal cord either through invasion of the vertebral body and direct growth of the tumor into the spinal cord or through growth from the paravertebral gutter through the intravertebral foramina.[11, 35] Also, tumor deposits in the subarachnoid space may occur via hematogenous spread or seeding of the CSF via leptomeningeal metastases (as noted previously). All mechanisms are important, and in the latter two instances, it should be noted that plain roentgenograms and radionuclide scans will likely be normal. Fewer than three percent of cord compression syndromes in cancer patients will result from intramedullary metastases.[22] Intervertebral discs are rarely involved unless extension from adjacent osseous metastases are present.[20]

Localized back pain is by far the most common early symptom, lasting weeks to months and present in 90 percent to 95 percent of patients who are ultimately found to have epidural spinal cord compression (ESCC).[4, 11, 16, 34, 35] The pain may be radicular and is commonly exacerbated by recumbency, movement, coughing, or Valsalva maneuver. Once neurological signs other than local pain begin, development of other deficits often follows quickly. In one series, 30 percent of patients with radicular pain progressed to maximal neurological deficit within 1 week.[35]

The cord level of disease affects the presentation. In Barron et al.'s series of 127 patients with various types of cancer metastatic to the cord (of which breast cancer

was the second most predominant type), 14 of 14 patients with cervical spine ESCC presented with pain. Thoracic cord involvement, when painful, is usually bilateral. However, in thoracic spine ESCC, 37 percent of patients presented without back pain.[4] This latter group often presented with hemiparesis or paralysis. Patients with cauda equina or conus medullaris metastases commonly presented with severe pain radiating into the legs; sphincter disturbances presented early in the course of pain.[4] A benign condition such as Herpes zoster or herniated nucleus pulposus may mimic malignant cord compression. In those instances in which myelography discloses ESCC at the level of an intervertebral disc without neighboring vertebral body disease, more confirmatory evidence of metastatic ESCC may be needed. Metastases to the intervertebral disc space are rare, and such patients are also at risk for benign processes such as extradural abscess or herniation of the nucleus pulposus.[20] Radiation therapy is clearly not the best treatment for these processes.

Plain films of the area of pain should always be performed in a patient with breast cancer and focal or radicular back pain. A routine roentgenogram of the spine correctly predicts for the presence or absence of epidural solid tumor in more than 80 percent of cases[34, 38] and is more specific than a bone scan. Moreover, a negative plain film in a patient with a normal neurological exam virtually eliminates (0 of 20 patients in Rodichok et al.'s series) spinal epidural metastases as the cause of back pain in a patient with a solid tumor.[34, 38, 41]

The diagnosis of cord compression is made definitively by myelography.[4, 9, 16, 34, 35, 38] A myelogram is essential not only for diagnosis but also to delineate the extent of cord compression and therapeutic approach best utilized.[16, 35, 38, 41] The degree of myelographic block (i.e., greater than vs. less than 80 percent) also alters the prognosis and influences the urgency of therapy.[38] Furthermore, ten percent of examinations disclose unsuspected sites of tumor around the cord.[41] If a complete block prevents passage of the contrast material from a lumbar myelogram, then the cephalad limits of the defect should be imaged from above by cisternal puncture. This allows accurate port placement by the radiation oncologist or neurosurgical planning. Following the myelogram, the contrast should be left in the thecal sac in order to assess the response to therapy.

CAT scanning with metrizamide contrast has not replaced myelography for definitive diagnosis. CAT scanning with metrizamide contrast is very accurate in revealing the presence of epidural masses as well as their relationship to surrounding vertebral bodies, paravertebral gutter, and intervertebral discs. CAT scanning should be performed in all instances of plexopathy, since paravertebral gutter soft tissue metastases occur frequently in these patients.[34] Magnetic resonance imaging (MRI) is also very accurate and may eventually supersede myelography as the state of the art if MRI imaging quality improves.[8] However, in the only study thus far comparing MRI with myelography in the diagnosis of malignant ESCC from a variety of metastatic tumors, myelography was reportedly superior to MRI.[23]

In that study, MRI and myelography were equally accurate in detecting large lesions that caused complete subarachnoid block, but myelography was superior in detecting smaller but clinically significant extradural lesions; 18 of 19 cases were detected by myelography vs. 10 of 19 with MRI.

The appropriate treatment for any spinal cord compression depends on the type of primary tumor, the level of the block, the rapidity of onset, and the degree of block. Patients present with symptoms ranging from localized back pain to full blown myelopathy, and a method of determining urgency is helpful. A useful system has been outlined by Portenoy et al.[34] Three groups of differing degrees of myelopathy are described, with differing levels of urgency. The initial evaluation and the three algorithms are illustrated in Figures 45–23 through 45–26.

Patients with signs of stable and minor ESCC and most patients with radiculopathy or plexopathy and no evidence of ESCC are in category I (see Fig. 45–24). This evaluation would be considered less urgent, but investigations should be performed within 24 hours. If delay occurs, high-dose dexamethasone should be instituted.

In the presence of bony lesions on plain film and if the myelogram is negative and the CSF examination is incompatible with subarachnoid spinal cord involvement, local radiotherapy to the bony lesion or systemic therapy and analgesics would be appropriate.

Patients with evidence of radiculopathy (radicular pain, weakness, or reflex changes or sensory losses in one myo- or dermatome) require prompt evaluation (category II). Brachial or lumbosacral plexopathy also falls into category II. When signs or symptoms of ESCC are not evident, consideration must be given to tumor extension from the paravertebral gutter into the epidural space (Fig. 45–25), since a coincident plexopathy may obscure the diagnosis of myelopathy.

CAT scan is the study of choice in patients with plexopathy but may ultimately be replaced by magnetic

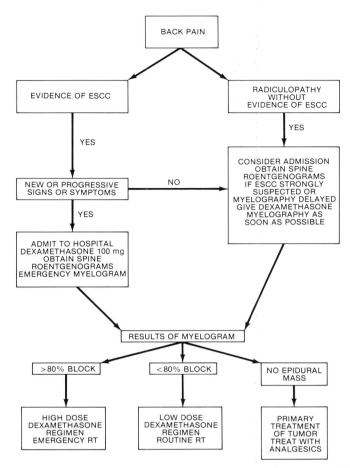

Figure 45–24. Management of cancer patient with back pain and evidence of ESCC or radiculopathy. (From Protenoy RK, et al: Neurology 37:135, 1987. Reprinted with permission.)

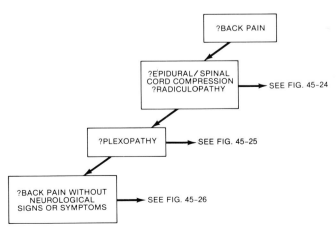

Figure 45–23. Initial evaluation of back pain in the cancer patient. (From Protenoy RK, et al: Neurology 37:135, 1987. Reprinted with permission.)

resonance imaging. Both provide excellent imaging of both osseous and soft tissue structures.[8, 39] Myelography and CSF examination is indicated only if the CAT scan is entirely normal but there is still strong suspicion of cord compression. Also, because Portenoy et al. have reported finding that 36 percent of patients with paraspinal tumor had epidural metastases on myelography, myelography should be performed in patients with CAT scan evidence of paravertebral masses.[34] Depending on the degree of block, the therapy should be given as outlined in Figure 45–25.

Patients presenting with back pain and no evidence of neurological deficit (category III) may undergo nonemergent evaluation as an outpatient. The approach to these patients, however, must be prompt and directed at the exclusion of the diagnosis of ESCC. Plain roentgenograms of the painful vertebral areas, including oblique areas, should be obtained initially (Fig. 45–26). In breast cancer, bony abnormalities corresponding to symptomatic site on plain films carry a high probability of epidural disease. If suspicion remains high, despite a normal plain film, based on historical characteristics of the patient's pain, then radionuclide bone scanning of the suspected area is indicated.[34, 38]

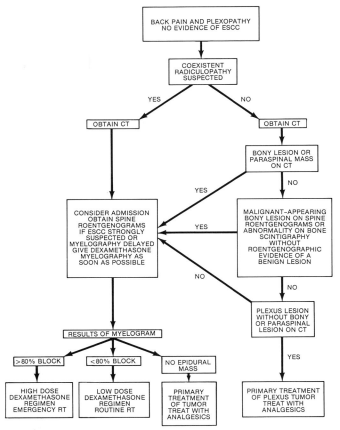

Figure 45–25. Management of cancer patient with suspected plexopathy. (From Portenoy RK, et al: Neurology 37:136, 1987. Reprinted with permission.)

Management

The patient presenting with a history of new or progressing signs or symptoms of ESCC has the minimum criteria for inclusion in category I (Fig. 45–24). As outlined, treatment would begin immediately using dexamethasone (100 mg I.V.). If an epidural lesion is identified, dexamethasone is then given orally and tapered over the course of the radiation therapy. Radiation therapy and dexamethasone are the standard therapeutic measures in most breast cancer patients with metastatic ESCC.[16, 35, 41] Breast cancer is a moderately radiosensitive tumor. A commonly recommended regimen is 400 rads/d for 3 days followed by 200 rads daily to a total dose of 3000–4000 rads.[25, 35] However, with the antiedema effects of corticosteroids, others report that it is not necessary to give the first few doses at higher fractionation.[9, 25] Using radiotherapy and dexamethasone alone in breast cancer ESCC, approximately 50 percent of patients will respond (as defined by preservation or restoration of neurological function for at least 4 weeks).[3, 16, 25, 41] Prognosis is determined primarily by severity and rapidity of onset of motor dysfunction, again emphasizing the need for prompt diagnosis and therapy.[3, 9, 25, 41] In one series, the response to high-dose dexamethasone was seen to have prognostic value.

Among patients with various primary tumors who had an objective response to steroids, 67 percent improved with radiotherapy.[3]

Current indications for surgical decompression include lesions located posteriorly in the cord, progression of signs during or after radiation therapy, recurrence in an area previously radiated heavily, or severe vertebral body instability.[3, 9, 11, 14, 16, 41] After surgical decompression, radiation should be given to any patient who has not previously received radiation to the area, as complete resection of tumor is virtually never possible. Added radiation is intended to decrease the risk of local recurrence.[11, 14, 16, 31, 41]

Prognosis

There are few situations in oncology in which rapid diagnosis and treatment enhance therapeutic benefits as much as in spinal cord compression. Undiagnosed and untreated, the consequences are devastating. Although there are no randomized prospective trials comparing surgical decompression and radiation therapy with radiation therapy alone, retrospective analysis indicates that both short- and long-term outcomes of the two approaches are very similar.[3, 4, 11, 14, 16, 41] As outlined previously, however, there are specific indications in which surgical decompression followed by radiation therapy is advocated.

In the two largest trials to date involving a variety of primary tumors subclassified as to radiosensitivity, patients with tumors (such as breast cancer, comprising 181 of 730 cases) considered to be radiosensitive had a favorable response (ability to ambulate) in 47 percent to 67 percent of cases.[11, 16] This corresponds closely with

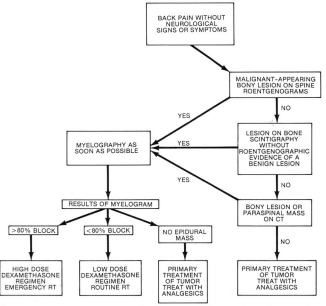

Figure 45–26. Management of cancer patient with back pain and no neurological signs or symptoms. (From Portenoy RK, et al: Neurology 37:137, 1987. Reprinted with permission.)

other authors' conclusions, with favorable results in 34 percent to 47 percent of patients with who were given radiation therapy alone. Pretreatment neurological grade (I = ambulatory, II = paraparetic, and III = paraplegic) had a profound influence on outcome. Those pretreatment grade I patients remained ambulatory in 79 percent of cases, those with grade II dysfunction remained or regained complete ambulatory ability in 34 percent of cases, and patients with grade III deficits had no full recovery of ambulation.[3, 4, 9, 14, 25, 41]

As with other metastatic tumors, overall survival is not significantly affected by local therapy. In retrospective analyses of series comprising heterogeneous types of metastatic carcinomas, only 30 percent of patients survived 1 year, and very few patients survived 5 years.[3, 4, 9, 25, 41] However, relieving the signs and symptoms of this complication and promptly preventing or reversing paraplegia are important goals for the physician.

The opinions or assertions contained herein are the private views of the authors and are not to be construed as official or as reflecting the views of the Department of the Navy or the Department of Defense.

References

1. Abrams HL, Spiro R, Goldstein N: Metastases in carcinoma; analysis of 1000 autopsied cases. Cancer 3:74–85, 1950.
2. Balis FM, Lester CM, Chrousos GP, et al: Differences in cerebrospinal fluid penetration of corticosteroids: possible relationship to the prevention of meningeal leukemia. J Clin Oncol 5:202–207, 1987.
3. Barcena A, Lobato RD, Rivas JJ, et al: Spinal metastatic disease: analysis of factors determining functional prognosis and the choice of treatment. Neurosurgery 15:820–827, 1984.
4. Barron KD, Hirano A, Araki S, Terry AD: Experiences with metastatic neoplasms involving the spinal cord. Neurology 9:91–106, 1959.
5. Black P: Brain metastasis: current status and recommended guidelines for management. Neurosurgery 5:617–631, 1979.
6. Blasberg RG: Methotrexate cytosine arabinoside, and BCNU concentration in brain after ventriculocisternal perfusion. Cancer Treat Rep 61:625–631, 1977.
7. Blasberg RG, Patlak CS, Shapiro WR: Distribution of methotrexate in the cerebrospinal fluid and brain after intraventricular administration. Cancer Treat Rep 61:633–641, 1977.
8. Bosley TM, Cohen DA, Schatz NJ, et al: Comparison of metrizamide computed tomography and magnetic resonance imaging in the evaluation of lesions at the cervicomedullary junction. Neurology 35:485–492, 1985.
9. Bruckman JE, Bloomer WD: Management of spinal cord compression. Semin Oncol 5:135–140, 1978.
10. Chan RC, Steinbok P: Solitary cerebral metastasis: the effect of craniotomy on the quality and duration of survival. Neurosurgery 11:254–257, 1982.
11. Constans JP, DeDiviths E, Donzelli R, et al: Spinal metastases with neurological manifestations. J Neurosurg 59:111–118, 1983.
12. Crane JM, Nelson MJ, Ihde DC, et al: A comparison of computed tomography and radionuclide scanning for detection of brain metastases in small cell lung cancer. J Clin Oncol 2:1017–1024, 1984.
13. Distefano A, Yong Yap Y, Hortobagyi GN, Blumenschein GR: The natural history of breast cancer patients with brain metastases. Cancer 44:1913–1918, 1979.
14. Dunn RC, Kelly WA, Wohns RNW, et al: Spinal epidural neoplasia; a 15 year review of the results of surgical therapy. J Neurosurg 52:47–51, 1980.
15. Edelson RN, Deck MDF, Posner JB: Intramedullary spinal cord metastases: clinical and radiographic findings in 9 cases. Neurology 22:1222–1231, 1972.
16. Gilbert RW, Jae-Ho K, Posner JB: Epidural spinal cord compression from metastatic tumor: diagnosis and treatment. Ann Neurology 3:40–51, 1978.
17. Glass JP, Melamed M, Chernik NL, et al: Malignant cells in cerebrospinal fluid (CSF): the meaning of a positive CSF cytology. Neurology 29:1369–1375, 1979.
18. Goldson AL, Streeter OE Jr, Ashayen E, Collier-Manning J, Barber JB, Fan KJ: Intraoperative radiotherapy for intracranial malignancies. Cancer 54:2807–2813, 1984.
19. Gonzalez-Vitale JC, Garcia-Bunuel R: Meningeal carcinomatosis. Cancer 37:2906–2911, 1976.
20. Goodkin R, Carr BI, Perrin RG: Herniated lumbar disc disease in patients with malignancy. J Clin Oncol 5:667–671, 1987.
21. Grossman SA, Trump DL, Chen DCP, et al: Cerebrospinal fluid flow abnormalities in patients with neoplastic meningitis. Am J Med 73:641–647, 1982.
22. Gutin PH, Levi JA, Wiernik PH, Walker MD: Treatment of malignant meningeal disease with intrathecal thiotepa: a phase II study. Cancer Treat Rep 61:885–887, 1977.
23. Hagenau C, Grosh Currie M, Wiley RG: Comparison of spinal magnetic resonance imaging and myelography in cancer patients. J Clin Oncol 5:1663–1669, 1987.
24. Hendrickson FR: Radiation therapy of metastatic tumors. Semin Oncol 2:43–46, 1975.
25. Khan FR, Glicksman AS, Chu FCH, et al: Treatment by radiotherapy of spinal cord compression due to extradural metastases. Radiology 89:495–500, 1967.
26. Lewi HJ, Roberts MM, Donaldson AA, Forrest APM: The use of cerebral computed assisted tomography as a staging investigation of patients with carcinoma of the breast and malignant melanoma. Surg Gynecol Obstet 151:385–386, 1980.
27. Little JR, Dale AJD, Okazaki H, et al: Meningeal carcinomatosis: clinical manifestations. Arch Neurol 30:138–143, 1974.
28. Marcus FS, Dandolos EM, Friedman MA: Meningeal carcinomatosis in breast cancer presenting as central hypoventilation: a case report with a brief review of the literature. Cancer 47:982–984, 1981.
29. Markesbery WR, Brooks WH, Gupta GD, Young AB: Treatment for patients with cerebral metastases. Arch Neurol 35:754–756, 1978.
30. McKelvey EM: Meningeal involvement with metastatic carcinoma of the breast treated with intrathecal methotrexate. Cancer 22:576–580, 1968.
31. Millburn L, Hibbs GB, Hendrickson FR: Treatment of spinal cord compression from metastatic carcinoma. Cancer 21:447–452, 1968.
32. Murray JJ, Greco FA, Wolff SN, et al: Neoplastic meningitis: marked variations of cerebrospinal fluid composition in the absence of extradural block. Am J Med 75:289–294, 1983.
33. Olson ME, Chernik NL, Posner JB: Infiltration of the leptomeninges by systemic cancer: a clinical and pathologic study. Arch Neurol 30:122–137, 1974.
34. Portenoy RK, Lipton RB, Foley KM: Back pain in the cancer patient: an algorithm for evaluation and management. Neurology 37:134–138, 1987.
35. Posner JB: Management of central nervous system metastases. Semin Oncol 4:81–91, 1977.
36. Ransohoff J: Surgical management of metastatic tumors. Semin Oncol 2:21–27, 1975.
37. Ratcheson RA, Ommaya AB: Experience with the subcutaneous cerebrospinal fluid reservoir; preliminary report of 60 cases. N Engl J Med 279:1025–1031, 1968.
38. Rodichok LD, Harper GR, Ruckdeschel JC, et al: Early diagnosis of spinal epidural metastases. Am J Med 70:1181–1188, 1981.
39. Sarpel S, Sarpel G, Yu E, et al: Early diagnosis of spinal-epidural metastasis by magnetic resonance imaging. Cancer 59:1112–1116, 1987.
40. Shapiro WR, Young DF, Mehta BM: Methotrexate distribution in cerebrospinal fluid after intravenous ventricular and lumbar injections. N Engl J Med 293:161–166, 1975.
41. Stark RJ, Henson RA, Evans SJW: Spinal metastases; a retro-

spective survey from a general hospital. Brain 105:189–213, 1982.
42. Sundaresan N, Galicich JH: Surgical treatment of brain metastases; clinical and computerized tomography evaluation of the results of treatment. Cancer 55:1382–1388, 1985.
43. Tsukada Y, Fouad A, Pickren JW, et al: Central nervous system metastasis from breast carcinoma; autopsy study. Cancer 52:2349–2354, 1983.
44. Viadana E, Cotter R, Pickren JW, et al: An autopsy study of metastatic sites of breast cancer. Cancer Res 33:179–181, 1973.

45. Wasserstrom WR, Glass JP, Posner JB: Diagnosis and treatment of leptomeningeal metastases from solid tumors. Cancer 49:759–772, 1982.
46. Yap BS, Yap HY, Fritsche HA, Blumenschein G, Bodey GP: CSF carcinoembryonic antigen in meningeal carcinomatosis from breast cancer. JAMA 244:1601–1603, 1980.
47. Yap HY, Yap BS, Rasmussen S, et al: Treatment for meningeal carcinomatosis in breast cancer. Cancer 50:219–222, 1982.
48. Yap HY, Yap BS, Tashima CK, et al: Meningeal carcinomatosis in breast cancer. Cancer 42:283–286, 1978.

Management of Pericardial Metastases In Breast Cancer

Jeffrey M. Crane, M.D. and Barnett S. Kramer, M.D.

Pericardial effusion has been reported in as many as 53 percent of breast cancer patients, though most are asymptomatic, and less than 25 percent are proven to be malignant.[4] Because the increasing use of echocardiography will increase the number of breast cancer patients with known effusions, it should be stressed that these patients only infrequently develop malignant effusions in the absence of other sites of metastatic disease. Buck et al. found no instances of proven malignant pericardial effusion in any patient with effusions without evidence of other metastases (lung, 63 percent; bone, 58 percent; soft tissue, 87 percent; and liver, 11 percent).[4]

Cardiac tamponade refers to any degree of cardiac compression secondary to increased intrapericardial pressure that results in a functional decompensation of the heart. Neoplastic cardiac tamponade results from either an accumulation of fluid containing malignant cells within the pericardium or a constriction of the pericardium by tumor, with or without fluid. The incidence of cardiac tamponade in breast cancer patients is unknown. Autopsy series of breast cancer patients reveal pericardial metastases in 12 percent to 35 percent of necropsied patients.[1, 11, 15] It is very uncommon for breast cancer to present initially with pericardial metastases; malignant pericardial effusions usually present insidiously in patients with a known history of breast cancer. Autopsy series do not report the frequency of cardiac tamponade as a result of pericardial metastases, and unless specifically searched for, pericardial effusion may not be apparent to the clinician. Most effusions are asymptomatic. Buck et al. found that 53 percent (20/38) of serially screened patients with advanced metastatic breast cancer had pericardial effusions by echocardiogram, and 85 percent of these were judged "small" by echocardiographic criteria.[4] Only one was ultimately diagnosed as malignant. The other 19 patients had no

progression of their effusions on follow-up. In a second group of breast cancer patients studied by the same authors, 32 patients without any evidence of metastatic disease were found on echocardiogram to have pericardial effusions.[4] Thirty of these were clinically or histologically benign; the remaining two had known predisposing heart disease and had no progression after 10 to 12 months of follow-up. Thurber et al.[25] noted that of patients with a variety of tumors metastatic to the pericardium, only 29 percent had cardiac symptoms prior to death and only 16 percent had pericardial effusions when autopsied. An ante mortem diagnosis of cardiac metastases is made in less than ten percent of autopsy-proven cases.[6, 25]

PATHOPHYSIOLOGY

As mentioned previously, many pericardial effusions in breast cancer patients are not malignant. Breast cancer patients may develop nonmalignant pericardial effusions secondary to infectious or metabolic diseases or secondary to treatment of the tumor. Both cyclophosphamide and radiation can induce pericardial injury. In 117 patients with breast cancer who underwent postoperative radiation therapy in Stewart et al.'s 1976 series, four developed radiation-induced heart disease.[23] In Buck et al.'s series of patients, one third had received cardiac irradiation; radiation pericarditis was implicated in a third of these and histologically proven in a third of those suspected.[4]

In patients with malignant pericardial effusion, the major route of metastatic spread of breast cancer to the heart and pericardium is via retrograde lymphatic permeation from involved mediastinal lymph nodes.[15] It is thought that the flow of lymph from the endocardium and interstitium of the myocardium is via the epicardial lymphatics to the mediastinal collecting system.[16] Kline[15] was able to find only one of 61 patients with various malignancies metastatic to the pericardium in whom there was no evidence of mediastinal node involvement. This was the only example he could find of pure hematogenous spread of metastases to the pericardium. Six of his 61 cases were thought to be a result of direct extension to the pericardium from involved mediastinal lymphatics.

The severity of cardiac tamponade is related to the rate of pericardial fluid accumulation, its volume, and the underlying functional status of the patient's myocardium. Gradual accumulation of fluid allows the pericardium to stretch to accommodate the pressure; the myocardium can also adapt to a gradual increase in pericardial pressure. Thus the pericardium may accommodate several liters of fluid when fluid accumulation is insidious. The critical point occurs when the reflex tachycardia and peripheral vasoconstriction are no longer adequate to compensate for the falling stroke volume. Venous return diminishes as pressures within the vena cava, the pulmonary venous and arterial systems, and the atria rise to the level of ventricular diastolic filling pressures and cardiac output precipitously falls. When the pericardium is thickened by tumor infiltration or radiation fibrosis, compensatory stretching is impossible, and the critical point is reached early. Occasionally, therefore, neoplastic and postirradiation constrictive pericarditis progress rapidly or present as cardiac tamponade. Spodick provides a detailed review of these events.[21]

CLINICAL MANIFESTATIONS

A variety of symptoms can occur in patients with cardiac tamponade resulting from various causes. These include apprehension or extreme anxiety, precordial pressure or retrosternal pain, dyspnea, orthopnea, cough, hoarseness, singultus (hiccups), and various gastrointestinal symptoms, including dysphagia, nausea, vomiting, and abdominal pain. At the extreme, cardiovascular collapse can occur.

The physical signs of pericardial effusion or cardiac tamponade are primarily related to the effects of decreased cardiac output and compensatory peripheral vasoconstriction. Common signs include diaphoresis, confusion (including coma), tachypnea, and pallor with or without peripheral cyanosis. Peripheral pulses are weak, and jugulovenous distention is evident. The presence of diminished systolic blood pressure as well as decreased pulse pressure should suggest the diagnosis of tamponade. Also useful is the physical finding of pulsus paradoxus. Moreover, a change in the magnitude of pulsus paradoxus may accurately reflect the clinical response to therapy of the effusion. Chest examination may disclose pleural effusions, absence of the apical cardiac impulse, and faint heart sounds. The pericardial knock commonly heard in constrictive pericarditis is usually not a component of pericardial effusion with tamponade. The presence of ascites, hepatomegaly, or hepatojugular reflex may be additional clues to pericardial effusion with tamponade in the cancer patient.

Electrocardiographic (EKG) findings may include low-voltage sinus tachycardia and other arrythmias, elevation of ST segments diffusely, and variable T wave abnormalities. Electrical alternans (both P and QRS-T complexes), termed "total electrical alternans," is unusual but is quite specific for pericardial effusions.[21] In fact, this EKG finding in the patient with metastatic breast cancer should immediately prompt investigation for suspected neoplastic pericardial effusion with incipient tamponade.[17] Partial electrical alternans (QRS complex only) is less specific, being present commonly in other nonmalignant or nontamponade conditions.[4]

The roentgenographic signs of pericardial effusion in metastatic malignancies are variable. A normal chest roentgenogram does not rule out the possibility of neoplastic pericarditis.[18] However, a globose "water bottle heart" shadow is frequently seen in neoplastic pericardial effusions. Even more commonly, simple enlargement of the cardiac silhouette is seen on serial chest x-ray films.[2] Of Thurber et al.'s 55 patients with pericardial metastases, only four had a normal chest x-ray film.[25]

The echocardiogram is a simple, relatively inexpensive, safe, rapid, and noninvasive test that is very sensitive for the diagnosis of pericardial effusion.[4, 8, 18, 21] Furthermore, abnormalities in anterior mitral valve leaflet motion suggest cardiac tamponade.[8] Right heart catheterization, with pressure-wave tracings of the vena cava, right atrium, right ventricle, and pulmonary artery along with pulmonary capillary wedge pressure measurement, is a sensitive and specific test for cardiac tamponade. However, the invasive test is rarely necessary to make a diagnosis.

Once a clinical diagnosis of cardiac tamponade has been made, the pericardial fluid must be removed as quickly as possible. There are few medical oncology emergencies in which as rapid an alleviation of the patient's discomfort may occur. However, cytologic reviews of the fluid may not provide pathological confirmation of the clinical diagnosis of a neoplastic pericardial effusion. The fluid is nearly always exudative. Approximately one third of pericardial effusions are serous; the remainder are serosanguinous or grossly bloody. Approximately 80 percent of specimens are positive for tumor.[5–7, 13, 19, 25, 26] False-positive results are rare.

TREATMENT

Sudden cardiovascular collapse and death are always possible in cardiac tamponade, whether of neoplastic or benign etiology.[4] Supportive care should be immediately instituted as emergency pericardiocentesis is prepared. Intravascular volume should be expanded with intravenous fluids. Normal saline will usually suffice, but five percent serum albumin or its synthetic analogues may be more effective in intravascular volume expansion in tamponade.[22] Blood and other volume expanders may also be used, and if needed, pressor agents may be initiated. In cases of dyspnea or tachypnea, the administration of oxygen will help to partially alleviate some of the patient's distressing symptoms. Positive end-expiratory pressure by mechanical ventilation reduces cardiac output via reduction in central venous return and thus should not be used.[21]

The only immediately effective treatment for pericardial effusion with tamponade is removal of the fluid. To save the patient's life, pericardiocentesis should be performed as soon as possible.[14] Pericardiocentesis is generally indicated when there is (1) cyanosis, dyspnea, a shock-like syndrome, or impairment of consciousness; (2) rising peripheral venous pressure above 130 mm H_2O; or (3) measured pulsus paradoxus exceeding 50 percent of the pulse pressure or falling pulse pressure below 20 mm Hg.[21] Cardiac arrythmias, bleeding, and myocardial trauma are potentially fatal complications of pericardiocentesis, and attempts to diminish these risks by EKG, blood pressure, and even fluoroscopic monitoring are recommended. Removal of the first 50–100 ml of fluid usually results in an impressive improvement in the patient's symptoms and signs of tamponade, but it is recommended that as much fluid as possible be removed.

Reaccumulation of the pericardial fluid is the rule, usually within 48 to 72 hours of the initial pericardiocentesis. Long-term control of the effusion may be accomplished by sclerosis of the pericardial sac with tetracycline. Other agents, including talc, bleomycin, nitrogen mustard, or thiotepa, have been used, but the efficacy, low cost and toxicity, and ease of administration of intrapericardial tetracycline (500–1000 mg dissolved in 20 ml of sterile saline) encourage its use initially.[7, 19, 20] The irritative, sclerosing action of tetracycline is best accomplished after the pericardial sac has been drained completely to allow apposition of the pericardial surfaces. Although some have noted diminished reaccumulation of fluid using only short-term catheter drainage of the pericardium,[9] the duration of the response to this limited approach is generally shorter (2 to 12 weeks) than that achieved with tetracycline (1 to 66 weeks). In two reported series, 21 of 26 patients with various solid tumors metastatic to the pericardium treated with tetracycline had complete resolution of the effusion for more than 30 days. Toxicity was generally mild, consisting of pain, fever, or (rarely) supraventricular tachycardia; these occurred in fewer than 20 percent of reported cases.[7, 22] Repeated instillation of tetracycline was necessary in some patients. The addition of lidocaine (100 mg) into the pericardial sac immediately before sclerosis diminished pain and did not impede successful sclerosis. Postsclerosis administration of a narcotic successfully alleviated painful pericardial irritation symptoms.

The value of radiation therapy delivered to the pericardium either alone or in conjunction with a pleuropericardial window following failed repetitive attempts at sclerosing therapy is well described.[3, 5, 11, 20, 21, 25] External beam irradiation has replaced instillational therapy with radioactive phosphorous (^{32}P), yttrium (^{90}Y) or gold (^{198}Au). External beam irradiation, 2500–3500 rads delivered in 3 to 4 weeks by anterior and posterior ports after pericardiocentesis to tap the effusion dry, controlled pericardial effusion in 11 of 16 breast cancer patients for a period ranging from 2 to 36 months.[5] All of these patients had cytologically confirmed malignant pericardial effusions.

If the patient has the potential for long-term survival and sclerosis or radiation fails, the creation of a pleuropericardial window has been reported to provide effective control of pericardial effusions in patients with tamponade resulting from cancer.[10, 12] In Hill and Cohen's small series, all patients achieved effective and durable palliation of their tamponade symptoms. The neoplastic diagnosis may also be confirmed with this procedure, if in doubt. Postoperative radiation therapy was given to some patients, and survival following surgery ranged from 3.5 to >21 months. In the series by Buck et al., ten of 19 patients with histological proof of neoplastic pericarditis were treated either with pericardiectomy or window procedure, and none had recurrence.[4] Median survival was 18.3 months from diagnosis. Postoperative complications from neoplastic pericardial disease are probably less frequent than those described for pleuropericardial windows performed for infectious etiologies.[10] Nevertheless, these complications, as well as the inherent problems of submitting a cancer patient to thoracotomy, must be weighed against the good results reported for sclerosis therapy. Most authors recommend sclerosis as first line therapy.[24] As second line therapy and in patients failing local sclerosing therapy and whose pericardium is not encased with tumor, pleuropericardial windows offer excellent long-term control of the symptoms of neoplastic pericardial effusion. Finally, pericardiectomy is the treatment of choice for radiation-induced pericardial effusion.[24]

Concomitant with local therapy directed toward the malignant effusion, systemic therapy with cytotoxic drugs or hormonal manipulation should be initiated in those patients who are candidates for aggressive management. Given the durable response rates to tetracycline sclerosis or pericardiectomy in some patients with neoplastic pericardial effusion and the frequency of extrapericardial disease, these patients should be considered for systemic chemotherapy.

PROGNOSIS

Untreated, neoplastic cardiac tamponade is rapidly fatal. Nevertheless, even if the acute episode is successfully managed, other systemic metastases are nearly always present, and long-term survival is unusual.

In those patients presenting with neoplastic tamponade as the first sign of pericardial metastases (from breast and other carcinoma primaries), the prognosis is grave. An exceptionally grave sign is total electrical alternans, and most patients have died within a few days despite removal of pericardial fluid.[17] Those patients without frank malignant tamponade have a much better prognosis, with a median survival of 12.8 months and

15 to 16 months for patients with complete response to local therapy.[20]

In Buck et al.'s series of breast cancer patients, of the 19 patients with histological proof of pericardial metastases treated with either pericardiectomy or a window procedure, survival ranged from 1 to 69 months (median, 18.3 months).[4] Of the three patients treated with a pericardiocentesis, all relapsed, requiring a surgical procedure. Survival in these three patients was between 20 and 40 months.

The opinions or assertions contained herein are the private views of the authors and are not to be construed as official or as reflecting the views of the Department of the Navy or the Department of Defense.

References

1. Abrams HL, Spiro R, Goldstein N: Metastases in carcinoma; analysis of 1000 autopsied cases. Cancer 3:74–85, 1950.
2. Abrams HL, Adam DF, Grant HA: The radiology of tumors of the heart. Radiol Clin North Am 9:299–326, 1971.
3. Biran S, Brutman G, Klein E, Hichman A: The management of pericardial effusion in cancer patients. Chest 71(2):182–186, 1977.
4. Buck M, Ingle JN, Giuliani ER, et al: Pericardial effusion in women with breast cancer. Cancer 60:263–269, 1987.
5. Cham WC, Freiman AH, Carsteus PHB, Chu FCH: Radiation therapy of cardiac and pericardial metastases. Radiology 114:701–704, 1975.
6. Cohen GU, Peery TM, Evans JM: Neoplastic invasion of the heart and pericardium. Ann Int Med 42:1238–1245, 1955.
7. Davis SD, Sharma SM, Blumberg ED, Kim CS: Intra pericardial tetracycline for the management of cardiac tamponade secondary to malignant pericardial effusion. N Engl J Med 299:1113–1114, 1978.
8. D'Cruz IA, Cohen HC, Prabhu R, et al: Diagnosis of cardiac tamponade by echocardiography: changes in initial valve motion and ventricular dimensions with special reference to paradoxical pulse. Circulation 52:460–465, 1975.
9. Flannery EP, Gregoratos G, Corder MP: Pericardial effusions in patients with malignant diseases. Arch Int Med 135:976–977, 1975.
10. Fredriksen RT, Cohen LS, Mullins CB: Pericardial windows or pericardiocentesis for pericardial effusions. Am Heart J 82:158–162, 1971.
11. Hanfling SM: Metastatic cancer to the heart: review of the literature and report of 127 cases. Circulation 22:474–483, 1960.
12. Hill GJ II, Cohen BI: Pleural pericardial window for palliation of cardiac tamponade due to cancer. Cancer 26:81–93, 1970.
13. Johnson WD: The cytological diagnosis of cancer in serous effusions. Acta Cytol 10:161–172, 1966.
14. Kilpatrick ZM, Chapman CB: On pericardiocentesis. Am J Cardiol 16:722–728, 1965.
15. Kline IK: Cardiac lymphatic involvement by metastatic tumor. Cancer 29:799–808, 1972.
16. Lokich JJ: The management of malignant pericardial effusions. JAMA 224:1401–1404, 1973.
17. Niarchos AP: Electrical alternans in cardiac tamponade. Thorax 30:228–233, 1975.
18. Pories WJ, Guandiani VA: Cardiac tamponade. Surg Clin North Am 55:573–589, 1975.
19. Shepherd FA, Ginsberg JS, Evans WK, et al: Tetracycline sclerosis in the management of malignant pericardial effusion. J Clin Oncol 3:1678–1682, 1985.
20. Smith FE, Lane M, Hudgins PT: Conservative management of malignant pericardial effusion. Cancer 33:47–57, 1974.
21. Spodick DH: Acute cardiac tamponade: pathologic physiology, diagnosis and management. Prog Cardiovasc Dis 10:64, 1967.
22. Stein L, Shubin H, Weil MH: Recognition and management of pericardial tamponade. JAMA 225:503–506, 1973.
23. Stewart JR, Cohn KE, Fajardo LF, et al: Radiation induced heart disease: a study of twenty-five patients. Radiology 89:302–310, 1976.
24. Theologides A: Neoplastic cardiac tamponade. Semin Oncol 5:181–192, 1978.
25. Thurber DL, Edwards JE, Anchor RWP: Secondary malignant tumors of the pericardium. Circulation 26:228–241, 1962.
26. Zipf RE, Johnston WW: The role of cytology in the evaluation of pericardial effusions. Chest 62:593–596, 1972.

Chapter 46

GENERAL CONSIDERATIONS FOR FOLLOW-UP

Lee M. Ellis, M.D. and Kirby I. Bland, M.D.

Despite advances in the treatment of breast cancer, up to 70 percent of patients will suffer recurrence of their malignancy.[38] Early identification of recurrent cancer, whether it is local, regional, or disseminated, aids in controlling malignant growth, thus allowing a greater probability for palliation or improved survival. The patterns of recurrence and overall prognosis strongly correlate with the stage of disease at the time of initial treatment.[60] However, because of the diverse biologic nature of breast cancer, predicting the patterns of recurrence remains a diagnostic problem. Further compounding the difficulty in diagnosing recurrent cancer is the ability of this heterogeneous tumor to remain dormant for years, only to recur as late as 20 years following treatment of the primary.

Recurrences can be classified as local, regional, or disseminated. *Local recurrence* is defined as the reappearance of cancer in the remaining breast tissue, scar, skin, chest wall, soft tissues, or the underlying muscles. *Regional recurrence* is defined as the presence of tumor in the regional lymph node basins, including internal mammary, axillary, supraclavicular, and Rotter's nodes. *Disseminated disease* is defined as metastatic disease at distant sites, most commonly occurring in bone, lung, pleura, soft tissues, and liver.

It is the responsibility of the physician following the patient after treatment of the primary breast cancer to recognize patterns and sites of recurrence and to be able to detect these recurrences at an early (and treatable) stage. This chapter addresses the efficacy of follow-up for patients with breast cancer and offers suggestions for management of patients in follow-up.

CHARACTERISTICS OF RECURRENCE DISEASE

The vast majority of relapses are either local/regional or confined to the skeletal system or chest (Table 46–

1).[28] Local/regional recurrences are best detected clinically, whereas osseous or thoracic metastases are most easily detected radiologically with symptomatology dictating radiological evaluation. However, as will be demonstrated later in this chapter, routine radiological surveillance does not significantly affect the natural history of the patient with recurrent breast cancer. Several factors contribute to the incidence of recurrent disease; this is addressed in detail in other chapters in this text. Overall, large, node-positive tumors that are poorly differentiated and estrogen receptor negative are more likely to recur than tumors without those characteristics. Kamby et al.[32] demonstrated the importance of initial stage of disease as a predictor for the site of recurrence. These investigators showed the relative increased incidence of local/regional recurrence in stage I disease vs. the relative predominance of distant metastasis in stage II diseases (Fig. 46–1). However, these investigators clearly state that screening for recurrent disease should *not* be directed toward any specific site.

Table 46–1. SITE OF FIRST RELAPSE

Site	Number of Relapses	Percent
Bone	171	21
Chest wall	150	19
Lung	153	19
Homolateral axilla	131	16
Liver	75	9
Opposite breast	51	6
Homolateral supraclavicular fossa	26	3
Brain	19	2
Other	33	4
Total	809	~100

From Heitanen P, et al: Ann Clin Res 18:143, 1986. Reprinted by permission.

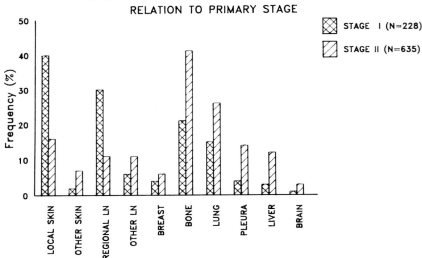

Figure 46–1. Distribution of patients according to primary stage and anatomical location of first recurrence. (From Kamby C, et al: Eur J Cancer Clin Oncol 23(12):1925–1934, 1987. Reprinted by permission.)

The most important prognostic indicator of recurrent disease and survival is the nodal status (Fig. 46–2).[60] Node-negative patients have a 20 percent to 25 percent incidence of relapse compared with node-positive patients, who have a 50 percent to 75 percent incidence of relapse (Tables 46–2 and 46–3). If more than 3 nodes are involved, then the incidence of recurrence is even higher. Node-positive patients also experience recurrence preferentially in distant organs and tissues. Should distant metastases be evident, the most common sites of disseminated disease include bone (49 to 60 percent), lung (15 to 22 percent), pleura (ten to 18 percent), soft tissue (seven to 15 percent) and liver (five to 15 percent).[38] Overall, ten to 30 percent of recurrences will be local, 60 to 70 percent will be manifested by distant metastases, and ten to 30 percent will be both local and distant.[28, 38, 60] In select patients, postoperative radiation therapy may decrease the local/regional recurrence rate

but has no effect on the overall relapse rate.[38] Systemic chemotherapy, however, has been shown to decrease total recurrence rates in sites that are inclusive of systemic metastases as well as local/regional disease.[4] Thus the overall frequency of metastatic relapse is significantly affected by adjuvant chemotherapy.

In order to determine frequency and duration (interval) of follow-up, it is necessary to be aware of the time period over which possible recurrence will appear. Although the majority of recurrences will occur within the first 36 months of treatment, breast cancer commonly remains occult and indolent for many years, necessitating prolonged follow-up. Romsdahl et al.[52] studied 177 patients with recurrent or metastatic breast cancer and found that 29 percent of these recurrences occurred during the first year, 30 percent the second year, 13 percent the third year, 27 percent the fourth through the eleventh year, and five percent after 12 years. Donegan determined that the peak incidence of local/regional recurrences were observed in the second

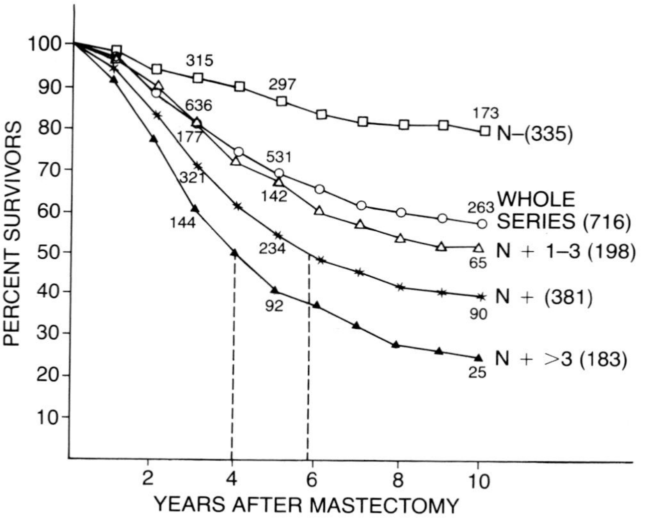

Figure 46–2. Breast cancer treated with radical mastectomy. Overall survival according to nodal status. (From Valagussa P, et al: Cancer 41:1170–1178, 1978. Reprinted by permission.)

Table 46–2. CUMULATIVE FAILURE PERCENT RELATED TO THE SITE OF FIRST RELAPSE IN AXILLARY NODE–POSITIVE PATIENTS (ACTUARIAL ANALYSIS)

Site of First Relapse	3 Yr	5 Yr	10 Yr
Local/regional* only	14.5	16.6	17.8
Distant	16.7	22.3	28.2
Bone	8.9	11.2	14.4
Viscera	6.8	8.8	10.9
Soft tissue	1.0	2.3	2.9
Multiple sites	17.3	19.6	23.3
Local/regional + distant	6.8	7.6	9.1
Multiple distant	10.5	12.0	14.2
Contralateral breast	3.2	5.1	6.2
Total	51.7	63.6	75.5

*Chest wall and/or ipsilateral supraclavicular region.
From Valagussa P, et al: Cancer 41:1170–1178, 1978. Reprinted by permission.

Table 46–3. CUMULATIVE FAILURE PERCENT RELATED TO THE SITE OF FIRST RELAPSE IN AXILLARY NODE–NEGATIVE PATIENTS (ACTUARIAL ANALYSIS)

Site of First Relapse	3 Yr	5 Yr	10 Yr
Local/regional* only	3.8	4.5	6.0
Distant	6.4	9.0	10.0
Bone	2.9	5.2	6.2
Viscera	2.6	2.6	2.6
Soft tissue	0.9	1.2	1.2
Multiple sites	3.0	4.4	7.2
Local/regional + distant	0.7	1.2	2.0
Multiple distant	2.3	3.2	5.2
Contralateral breast	1.8	3.1	4.7
Total	15.0	21.0	27.9

*Chest wall and/or ipsilateral supraclavicular region.
From Valagussa P, et al: Cancer 41:1170–1178, 1978. Reprinted by permission.

year following treatment.[20] Others[6, 58] observed similar recurrence patterns, with 75 percent to 80 percent of recurrences being detected within 3 years of treatment. It is important to note that as many as 20 percent of patients with breast cancer may suffer a recurrence more than 5 years after treatment of the primary cancer.

CLINICAL EVALUATION

The most important mode of detecting recurrent disease lies in the clinical evaluation and physical examination. In the study by Pandya et al. of 175 patients with node-positive breast cancer who relapsed, the first indicator of relapse was symptoms in 38 percent, physical findings at self-examination in 18.3 percent, physical examination by a clinician in 19.4 percent, abnormal blood chemistry findings in 12 percent, abnormal bone scans in eight percent, abnormal chest radiographs in 5.1 percent, and abnormal mammograms in 1.1 percent.[49] Therefore, 75 percent of cancers were detected clinically.

Similarly, Scanlon et al.[54] studied 194 patients with stage II and III breast cancer treated with chemoimmunotherapy. Patients were examined prior to each 6-week course of chemotherapy for the first year, and thereafter at 6-month intervals. Of the 38 patients (19.6 percent) who had recurrent disease, 29 were symptomatic and four were asymptomatic; all recurrences were detected on routine physical examination. Therefore, 33 of 38 patients (86.8 percent) had their recurrent disease detected by routine history and physical examination. A second group of 60 patients who developed recurrent breast cancer were evaluated off protocol. This group had postoperative follow-up monthly for the first 6 months, bimonthly for the next 6 months, quarterly for 6 months, and semiannually for life. Of the second group, 43 patients were symptomatic and 14 were discovered by routine history and physical examination, with three patients being asymptomatic. Combined, 90 of 98 recurrences (91.8 percent) were detected by routine history and physical examination. These authors concluded that history and physical examination, with careful monitoring of symptoms, will identify most recurrences at an early stage, diminishing the necessity for routine laboratory or radiological testing.

Valagussa et al.[61] reviewed the records of 278 patients with relapse after primary treatment for breast cancer following mastectomy or mastectomy and systemic chemotherapy. History and physical examination detected 78 percent of the recurrences in this series. The most frequently involved sites of recurrence were soft tissue in 38 percent, bone in 37 percent, and viscera in 34 percent. In symptomatic patients, occult sites of disease were detected in only eight percent of patients. Twenty-two percent of those who relapsed were asymptomatic and had recurrent cancer detected by routine radiographic examinations (67 percent by chest roentgenogram). Despite the latter observations, these investigators concluded that because the interval between the appearance of asymptomatic metastases and development of symptoms is probably short, early detection of recurrent disease probably does not dramatically affect prognostic outcome. Therefore they concluded that frequently repeated radiological or biochemical studies do not affect the natural history of recurrent breast cancer.

Others confirmed the overwhelming importance of the history and physical examination for the detection of recurrent breast cancer. Cantwell and associates[7] observed that 86.5 percent of patients with recurrent breast cancer had their recurrences detected by history and physical examination, whereas only 11.9 percent were detected by bone scans, and 2.3 percent by chest radiograph. Winchester et al.[68] studied 87 patients with recurrent breast cancer after mastectomy and confirmed that 79 recurrences (90.8 percent) were accompanied by clinical symptoms. Of those patients with recurrent disease, 38 percent developed osseous metastases, 16 percent recurred locally, ten percent had local and systemic disease, and ten percent had pulmonary metastasis. Only three of 87 recurrences (3.4 percent) were discovered by means other than history and physical examination.

Two major questions should be addressed. First, is routine screening for recurrent breast cancer efficacious (i.e., are recurrences detected earlier at routine, scheduled visits as compared with nonscheduled, interval visits)? Second, if a recurrence is detected in the asymptomatic stage, will early detection alter the natural course of this disease? The majority of the studies that address these issues have demonstrated that routine screening is *not* superior to interval evaluation of the patient with breast cancer and that early detection of recurrent disease does *not* affect survival, thus minimizing the importance of detecting asymptomatic recurrences. Holli and Hakama[30] demonstrated the ineffectiveness of routine follow-up in a Finland study of 551 breast cancer patients with 5-year follow-up. These investigators observed that recurrent disease was detected five times as often in patients who presented at spontaneous visits when compared with routine visits. However, false-positive clinical diagnosis of recurrent disease was more commonly observed at spontaneous visits. Marrazzo et al.[42] retrospectively reviewed 85 patients with breast cancer treated by radical mastectomy and evaluated follow-up parameters. Chemotherapy (cyclophosphamide, methotrexate, 5-fluorouracil; CMF) was given to 41 patients with positive axillary nodes. Thirty-two patients developed recurrent disease, with 28.1 percent of the recurrences being discovered in the asymptomatic state. Seventy-five percent of the recurrences were detected within 2 years of treatment. These authors acknowledge the lack of evidence demonstrating improved survival in the detection and treatment of asymptomatic recurrences. With compliance of follow-up protocols, these investigators concluded that asymptomatic patients need *not* undergo specific examinations at predetermined intervals. Brøyn and Frøyen[6] evaluated 81 women with recurrent breast cancer and determined that the majority of recurrences were diagnosed at nonroutine visits. Within the first 3 years, 75 percent of these recurrences were detected. These investigators concluded that commonly utilized parameters for follow-up were *not* of value in allowing early detection of recurrent cancer, and routine follow-up did *not* prolong survival. Thus these studies demonstrated no benefit for the early detection of recurrent breast cancer in the asymptomatic stage.

In contrast, others have found improved survival in patients with asymptomatic recurrences. Tomin and Donegan[58] studied 1230 women treated for breast cancer to evaluate patterns of recurrence and overall prognosis. Of the 248 cases analyzed for recurrent disease, 36 percent were diagnosed in asymptomatic patients, who enjoyed a greater survival when compared with those with symptomatic recurrences (Fig. 46–3). They concluded that few recurrences are detectable in asymptomatic patients; however, asymptomatic recurrences may influence "lead time" and thus enhance overall survival. Despite these findings, there was no difference in survival after recurrence between compliant (regular follow-up) or noncompliant (irregular follow-up) patients (Fig. 46–4). Others suggest that detection of recurrences in the asymptomatic state may afford an enhanced survival. Bedwinek et al.[3] found that when local/regional recurrences are detected when tumor volume is minimal, nearly 50 percent 5-year survival can be obtained. Specifically, the detection of asymptomatic local recurrences afforded a 5-year survival of 50 percent compared with 10.8 percent for symptomatic recurrences. The difference in survival for osseous metastases in symptomatic vs. asymptomatic patients approached statistical significance ($p = 0.06$). Dewar and Kerr[19] studied 546 patients treated for early breast cancer with or without radiation therapy. One hundred ninety-two relapses were detected; 93 were noted at routine visits vs. 99 found at unscheduled (interval) visits. Of those patients who suffered a relapse of their disease, routine evaluation was more likely to detect disease in the treated area or contralateral breast (74 percent) as opposed to disease at metastatic sites (26 percent). This study revealed that locally recurrent disease detected at a routine visit afforded a significantly better survival rate than for

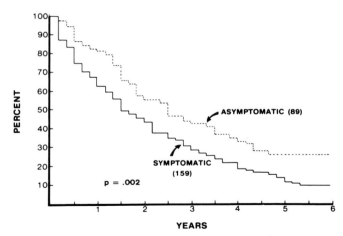

Figure 46–3. Survival after symptomatic vs. asymptomatic recurrences. Survival is significantly longer in patients with recurrent disease discovered in the asymptomatic state. (From Tomin R, Donegan WL: J Clin Oncol 5(1):62–67, 1987. Reprinted by permission.)

patients whose relapse was detected at an interval visit. Overall, however, a potentially curable relapse (local disease or disease in the contralateral breast) was detected in only one percent of routine visits, with only 0.39 percent of patients remaining free of disease at the completion of the study.

Controversy continues to exist regarding the value of routine follow-up for patients with breast cancer. This controversy has special significance in light of the necessity to establish cost-effective screening parameters in order to justify early detection. Routine interval visits may increase the "lead time" before overt recurrences are evident on physical, laboratory, or radiological examinations. With improvements in adjuvant therapy (radiation, chemotherapy, or immunotherapy) this "lead time" may be converted into improvement in survival rates and quality of life for the patient with recurrent breast cancer.

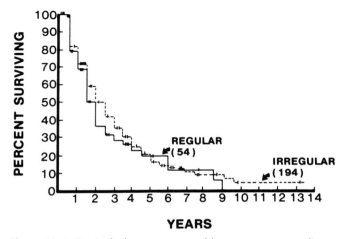

Figure 46–4. Survival after recurrence of breast cancer according to regular or irregular follow-up examinations. There is no difference in overall survival. (From Tomin R, Donegan WL: J Clin Oncol 5(1):62–67, 1987. Reprinted by permission.)

Bone Scans

Many clinical studies have documented the most common site of recurrent metastatic breast cancer to be osseous. Most of these lesions are osteolytic. The lesion must be greater than 1.5 cm in diameter with greater than 50 percent demineralization to allow adequate radiological visualization and detection.[22] Therefore routine skeletal surveys may not detect osseous metastases until advanced stages of growth. Lesions often remain asymptomatic until the periosteum is involved, initiating intense skeletal pain (see chapter 45, section entitled, "Management of Osseous Metastases and Impending Pathological Fractures").

Bone scan (technetium 99m–labeled phosphate) is more sensitive than skeletal roentgenograms and may increase the probability for detection of asymptomatic osseous metastases. Bone scans should be correlated with radiographs and clinical symptoms to rule out other abnormalities.[22] The incidence of positive bone scans (i.e., presumed osseous metastases) directly correlates with the stage of disease. With complaints of bone tenderness or pain, more than 35 percent of patients are observed to have an abnormal bone scan.[34] When these symptoms are associated with abnormal skeletal roentgenograms, then more than 80 percent will have an abnormal bone scan.[34] However, the value of routine bone scanning lies in the ability of the clinician to detect an asymptomatic recurrence. Bone scans may also aid in detecting unsuspected osseous disease in patients with documented recurrences at other sites. Kunkler and Merrick[34] found that for patients with documented local/regional recurrences, bone scans were positive in 37 percent of patients; when nonosseous metastases were present, bone scans were positive in 54 percent of patients.

The value of routine bone scanning in detecting asymptomatic recurrence in patients with breast cancer is minimal. Pedrazzini et al.[50] studied 1601 patients with node-positive breast cancer and determined that radionuclide scans would have detected first recurrences in only 2.4 percent of those studied. Thus this series suggests that bone scans were not indicated when the patient does not present with clinical evidence of osseous pathology (e.g., symptoms of bone pain or fractures).

Wickerham and colleagues[66] of the National Surgical Adjuvant Breast Project (NSABP) prospectively evaluated 2697 patients with stage II (node-positive) breast cancer in trial B-09. Bone scans were done every 6 months for the first 3 years and yearly thereafter. Only 0.6 percent of these scans were effective for detecting lesions in asymptomatic patients. In light of the lack of evidence suggesting that the early diagnosis and treatment of osseous metastasis improves survival, bone scans were suggested only for symptomatic patients. Pandya et al.[49] studied 175 patients with recurrent breast cancer in an Eastern Cooperative Oncology Group (ECOG) study. Bone scans were obtained every 3 months for the first year and every 6 months thereafter. These studies diagnosed asymptomatic osseous metastases in eight percent of patients studied; scans detected recurrences only in the first 2 years of follow-up. Chaudary et al.[11] studied 241 breast cancer patients with positive axillary nodes. Patients underwent modified radical mastectomy and adjuvant chemotherapy and were followed postoperatively for 2 years. A total of 832 bone scans in the 241 patients detected only 25 patients with bone metastases (10.4 percent), and only 13 of these patients (five percent) were asymptomatic. These investigators concur with others who suggest that routine serial bone scanning is not indicated in the follow-up of the asymptomatic breast cancer patient.

Other clinicians continue to advocate routine bone scanning with higher incidences for the detection of asymptomatic recurrence.[23] Citrin et al.[13] evaluated 75 patients with early breast cancer (stage I and II) who underwent routine preoperative bone scans and subsequent scanning at 6-month intervals. Eleven patients (14.7 percent) presented with abnormal bone scans, and 13 patients (17.3 percent) were determined to have an abnormal bone scan in subsequent follow-up (conversions). These conversions to positive scans in stage I and II disease seem to reiterate the propensity for patients to harbor occult (dormant) metastatic disease despite initial presentation as an early cancer. However, correlation with symptoms was not addressed in this study, and the number of patients discovered in an asymptomatic stage was not reported.

Selective bone scanning in patients at an increased risk for developing osseous metastases may prove more rewarding. McNeil et al.[43] have shown that the rate of conversion from negative bone scans to positive bone scans strongly correlates with stage of disease. These investigators found that the conversion rate for stage I disease was seven percent; for stage II, 45 percent; and for stage III, 58 percent. Most of these conversions occurred within the first 2 postoperative years. Coker et al.[14] likewise demonstrated that the conversion rates from negative to positive bone scans correlate with stage of disease, with conversion rates for stage I, II, and III disease being six percent, 26 percent, and 60 percent, respectively. It would seem likely that selective bone scanning in patients with stage II or III disease may be efficacious. However, many of these patients may be symptomatic, and the value of routine bone scan in the asymptomatic patient with even stage III disease has yet to be determined.

Biochemical Tumor Markers

Tumor markers are best utilized at present for the detection of metastases from colorectal cancer. Several biological markers specific for breast tumors are currently under investigation to study their effectiveness in detecting recurrent breast cancer in the asymptomatic stage (Table 46-4). For a tumor marker to be efficacious, it must fulfill the following criteria:

1. It must be produced by malignant tumor cell line.
2. It must be specific to the tumor cell line and not present in benign conditions.
3. It must be detected early in tumor growth.

Table 46–4. POTENTIAL SERUM BREAST CANCER TUMOR MARKERS

CA 15-3
CA 19-9
CA 549
CEA
MAM-6
Mammary Serum Antigen (MSA)
CA 50 (?)
CA 19-7 (?)

4. It must reflect changes in cell growth and correlate with therapy.
5. It must be easily accessible for analysis.
6. It must be cost effective.

Multiple Biochemical Markers

Biochemical analysis of serum is commonly used to follow patients with malignancy. Serum is easily obtained, and routine liver chemistry tests are relatively inexpensive. However, specificity and sensitivity are lost when individual parameters are assessed. Sensitivity increases with the number of parameters studied, but specificity is virtually unaffected. Alkaline phosphatase is the most sensitive serum marker for liver metastases, and levels are elevated in 58 percent of patients with hepatic metastases.[8] Although there are other causes of elevated alkaline phosphatase levels (i.e., osseous disease), an increase of this isoenzyme in patients with breast cancer will signify liver metastases 85 percent of the time.[8] Serum glutamate oxaloacetate transaminase (SGOT) is also a sensitive biochemical parameter to aid in the detection of liver metastases; levels are increased in 60 percent of patients with liver metastases.[8] Serum glutamate pyruvate transaminase (SGPT) is less sensitive than SGOT as an indicator of hepatic involvement.[8] Hypoproteinemia with a decrease in serum albumin levels may also be evident in patients with liver metastases; however, a significant number of breast cancer patients without liver metastases will also have decreased serum albumin levels that are related to other causes. Combining liver function studies with hepatic radionuclide imaging increases the diagnostic sensitivity for liver metastases but has not proved to be cost effective at this time.[67]

Tumor markers, along with physical and radiological examinations, may help detect a large percentage of patients with recurrent cancer in an early stage. Coombes et al.[15, 16] studied 141 patients with primary breast cancer with no evidence of metastases at initial evaluation. One third of these patients subsequently relapsed in follow-up.[15] Serial markers were obtained every 3 months; clinical examination, chest radiograph, bone scan, liver scan, bone marrow aspirate, and skeletal radiographs were performed every 6 months. Carcinoembryonic antigen, gamma glutamyl transpeptidase, and alkaline phosphatase were found to be the most useful chemical markers for detecting metastatic disease. These tests, in combination with the chest radiograph

and clinical examination, allowed the identification of 98 percent of patients with metastases, with only a 3.5 percent risk of false-positive tests. These authors found that the aforementioned studies provided a "lead time" of approximately 3 months prior to detection of overt metastasis.

Waalkes et al.[64, 65] studied multiple urine and serum markers in patients undergoing chemotherapy for breast cancer for node-positive disease. These investigators observed that overall, metastatic disease yielded a higher proportion of elevated values in multiple markers for patients diagnosed with recurrent disease than in patients without recurrent disease. This series evaluated biochemical markers to organ-specific sites and determined that gamma glutamyl transpeptidase and alkaline phosphatase were the best indicators of hepatic disease, and urinary hydroxyproline was the best biochemical marker for bone disease. Carcinoembryonic antigen was not site-specific, but levels were elevated in a high proportion of patients with hepatic or osseous involvement.

Lee[39] studied 500 patients who had undergone mastectomy for breast cancer. Blood was obtained for biochemical and hematological tests every 2 to 4 months in the first year and every 4 to 6 months thereafter. Patients with disseminated soft tissue or lung metastases had similar blood test results when compared with those without metastases. Patients with metastases to bone or other viscera were noted to have decreased albumin and total serum protein levels; gamma globulin and carcinoembryonic antigen levels were elevated when compared with those in patients without metastases.

Despite the common usage of routine determination of biochemical or hematological parameters, there is no objective evidence to support their use in the follow-up of the patient with breast cancer. However, if the clinician suspects recurrent disease, these tests may aid in supporting the clinical findings and even help to determine the organ system involved.

Carcinoembryonic Antigen

Carcinoembryonic antigen (CEA) is an oncofetal glycoprotein discovered by Gold and Friedman in 1965 in patients with adenocarcinoma of the colon. CEA is present on the cell surface membrane and is easily released into surrounding fluids. CEA is found normally in embryonic and fetal gut as well as certain malignant cells. This serum glycoprotein is commonly used as a tumor marker for colorectal cancer, but levels have also been found to be elevated in other malignancies. In addition, elevated serum CEA levels are found in patients with in various benign disease states such as colorectal polyps, pancreatitis, liver disease, and pulmonary infections. Heavy cigarette smokers may also have elevated serum CEA levels.

Several prospective studies have shown that serum CEA levels correlate with the stage of disease at the time of diagnosis.[40] Furthermore, serum CEA has been found to be an indicator of prognosis and may also predict response to therapy.[40] Many authors have examined the efficacy of monitoring serial serum CEA levels following potentially curative therapy for breast cancer in an attempt to identify patients with recurrent disease at an early stage. The spectrum of conclusions and recommendations ranges from those investigators who propose obtaining serial serum CEA levels every 3 months after treatment to others who adamantly insist that CEA monitoring has no role whatsoever in the follow-up of the patient with breast cancer.[1, 2, 10, 21, 25, 26, 33, 35, 36, 40, 41, 45]

Several studies have demonstrated that routine serial serum CEA determinations may help identify the patient with subclinical recurrent breast cancer. The importance of determination is that patients with recurrent disease can be identified while the malignancy is small and in its early stage of growth. Elevations of CEA prior to clinical evidence of disease may lead the clinician to obtain the appropriate studies in the search for recurrent disease. Thus the "lead time" obtained with an elevated CEA level prior to recognition of clinical disease may help identify the site of recurrence and afford earlier and more effective eradication of recurrent disease. Several investigators have reported "lead times" of 2 to 8 months prior to clinical manifestations of recurrent disease.[1, 10, 40] In a few studies, survival was improved by early discovery of recurrence, but in the majority of studies, survival was unaffected.

The empiric downfall in the reliability of monitoring serial serum CEA levels is the lack of sensitivity and specificity of the assay. As stated, other malignant and nonmalignant states are associated with elevated serum CEA levels. In one study of 2095 patients following mastectomy for breast cancer, 46 percent of patients *without* detectable metastases had a normal serum CEA level, and 41 percent of patients *with* verified metastases had a normal CEA level.[35] Thus false-negative results are obtained in greater than 40 percent of these cases. In another study, 67 percent of patients with an increased serum CEA level relapsed. However, there was no difference between the number of patients who suffered a recurrence without an increase in CEA levels and those who had an increased CEA level but without recurrence.[48]

In the majority of studies, 50 percent of patients with recurrent breast cancer have elevated serum CEA levels.[2, 10, 21, 30] Beard and Haskell reviewed several series studying the use of serial serum CEA monitoring in the early detection of recurrent breast cancer and found a 53 percent overall false-positive rate (patients with an elevated serum CEA without recurrent disease) (Table 46–5).[2] Furthermore, a subgroup of patients with con-

sistently low serum CEA levels develop metastatic disease.[33] Obviously, serum CEA is meaningless in this subset of patients.

Others have identified specific instances where serial monitoring of serum CEA may be useful.[21, 45, 48, 62] Van Der Linden et al.[62] found that serial serum CEA monitoring for the first 2 years after treatment may be helpful in screening for distant metastasis in patients with primary tumors ≥ 2 cm in diameter with positive axillary nodes and positive estrogen receptors. However, even these authors concluded that serial CEA determination is probably not cost effective.

An elevated serum CEA level (>5 ng/ml) is, in part, organ specific. Patients with an elevated serum CEA level are more likely to have visceral or osseous metastases than local or local/regional recurrent disease.[26, 36, 37, 41] If higher serum CEA levels (10 ng/ml) are used as the "cutoff point," then the only patients with elevated serum CEA levels and recurrent disease are those with disseminated metastases.[37]

Overall it does *not* appear that CEA monitoring is a useful or cost-effective test for determining recurrence of breast cancer.[24, 25] If levels are elevated, recurrence is more likely to be present in distant organs rather than present on the chest wall or in regional lymph node basins.

Miscellaneous Serum Tumor Markers

Other tumor-associated antigens have been studied in regard to their usefulness as tumor markers. Nearly all the studied markers have been found to be more sensitive and specific than serum CEA.

CA 15–3. CA 15–3 is a high-molecular-weight, carbohydrate breast cancer–associated antigen. Increases in serum CA 15–3 levels greater than 25 percent above baseline strongly correlate with disease progression.[27, 59] Higher levels are found in patients with multiple sites of metastases and osseous metastases.[31, 51] CA 15–3 has been found to be a sensitive and specific marker for breast cancer and is superior to serum CEA determinations in its sensitivity.[27, 51, 59] Increased serum CA 15–3 levels have been found to precede clinical evidence of recurrent breast cancer by up to 13 months ("lead time").[31] The high sensitivity and specificity of CA 15–3 makes this antigen a potentially highly efficacious marker for early recurrent breast cancer.

CA 549. CA 549 is a glycoprotein breast cancer–associated antigen. Elevated CA 549 serum levels correlate more closely with systemic disease than with local recurrence, and changes in serum CA 549 levels corre-

Table 46–5. CEA AND EARLY DETECTION OF RECURRENT BREAST CANCER

No. of Patients at Risk for Recurrence	Patients with Recurrence	No. of Patients with an Elevated CEA	Elevated or Rising CEA Level Preceding Documented Recurrence (True-Positive)	Elevated or Rising CEA Level *Without* Recurrence During Study (False-Positive)
1626	312 (19%)	227	107 (47%)	120 (53%)

From Beard DB, Haskell CM: Am J Med 80:241–245, 1986. Reprinted by permission.

late with clinical response to therapy.[9] However, results of prospective studies utilizing this serum antigen as a marker of early recurrent disease are not available at the present time.

MAM-6. MAM-6 is another tumor-associated glycoprotein found to be increased in the serum of patients with breast cancer. Serum MAM-6 levels correlate with the progression of metastatic disease and are more sensitive than serum CEA levels in detecting recurrent disease.[29] Rising levels may precede clinical evidence of metastases.

Mammary Serum Antigen. Mammary serum antigen (MSA) is a breast tumor–associated glycoprotein discovered in the early 1980s. Changes in MSA have been found to be correlated with the clinical course of patients with breast cancer in nearly 90 percent of cases. MSA monitoring is more sensitive than serum CEA in detecting recurrent disease but overall does not appear as promising as other previously mentioned tumor markers.[56, 57] False-positive results are a frequent occurrence.

The role of other potential antigens such as CA 50 and CA 19–7 as tumor markers has not yet been determined.

Chest Roentgenogram

Chest roentgenogram as a routine follow-up study may detect occult disease, but detection of occult disease by chest roentgenogram does not affect survival. Ciatto and Herd-Smith[12] studied 1697 breast cancer patients without evidence of distant metastases. Clinical examination and chest radiographs were obtained every 6 months for 3 years and then yearly thereafter. During a mean follow-up of 4.2 years, 523 patients (31 percent) relapsed. Total (both isolated and associated with other sites of metastases) and isolated intrathoracic metastases were 26 percent and 13 percent of total relapses, respectively. Pleural recurrences were the most symptomatic (89 percent), followed by multiple (35 percent) or single pulmonary nodules (five percent). The sensitivity of chest roentgenogram in detecting metastases was 86 percent. In this study, 50 percent of intrathoracic metastases were detected *with* concurrent disease. A trend toward prolonged survival was noted when intrathoracic metastases were detected in asymptomatic patients compared with symptomatic, but this trend did not reach statistical significance (20.2 months vs. 17 months). Thus this study does not support the use of routine chest roentgenograms in the follow-up of the patient with breast cancer. The previously noted study by Chaudary et al.[11] likewise supports the conclusion that routine chest radiographs are not indicated in the follow-up of the patient with breast cancer. In the latter study, only five percent of patients were found to have metastatic disease on chest radiograph; of those patients, 67 percent were asymptomatic. Thus only three percent of patients had intrathoracic metastases detected by chest radiograph during an asymptomatic stage.

Metastatic disease can be detected in the thorax in up to 40 percent of patients with recurrent disease.[38] Thus

chest roentgenogram should identify the patient with metastatic breast cancer in a significant number of cases. However, at the present time there is no evidence that early detection of intrathoracic metastases affects survival.

Diagnostic Studies for Liver Metastases

Routine liver scanning, computerized tomography, and radionuclide scanning have not been found to be efficacious in detecting hepatic metastases in the asymptomatic patient following treatment of primary breast cancer.[8, 55, 67] Routine hepatic echography is also not indicated and, with refinements in computerized tomography scanning, is rarely necessary. DeSouza and Shinde[18] reported a remarkably high incidence of asymptomatic liver metastases (up to 23 percent) in patients with breast cancer undergoing screening laparoscopic liver examination. However, others have not been as aggressive in searching for hepatic metastases, relying instead on noninvasive methods to detect asymptomatic hepatic involvement. Until further studies substantiate the efficacy of searching for asymptomatic hepatic metastases, hepatic imaging is not indicated as a routine screening modality.

Brain Scanning

Brain metastases following primary treatment of breast cancer are relatively rare. There is no role of brain scanning by either computerized tomography or radionuclide study in any patient with breast cancer *without* central nervous system symptoms. However, nearly half of patients with central nervous system symptoms will have demonstrable metastases by computerized tomography scan, providing important prognostic information. Computerized tomography scanning is superior to radionuclide scanning for investigation of central nervous system symptoms in patients with breast cancer.[17, 46]

Computerized Tomography Scan of the Chest

Current data do not support the use of routine computerized tomography (CT) scanning of the chest for the follow-up of asymptomatic breast cancer patients. However, patients with local/regional recurrence may harbor unsuspected disease in the upper abdomen or bone or soft tissues of the chest.[44, 63] Rosenman et al.[53] found that 22 of 33 patients (67 percent) with locally recurrent breast cancer had unsuspected disease noted by chest and upper abdominal computerized tomography scan that changed the treatment protocol in 30 percent. Others have also noted that CT scanning of the chest will detect unsuspected disease in a high percentage of patients with local/regional recurrences, prompting alterations in therapy.[44, 63] The most significant find-

Table 46–6. RECOMMENDED FOLLOW-UP OF THE PATIENT WITH BREAST CANCER FOLLOWING CURATIVE THERAPY

	Preoperative	Follow-up (Interval)
History and physical	Yes	q 3 months for 3 years, q 6 months for 2 years, yearly thereafter
Serum liver chemistry tests	Yes	As indicated
Chest roentgenogram	Yes	As indicated
Bone scan	Optional	As indicated (? with local recurrence)
Computerized tomography, abdomen and chest	No	As indicated (? with local recurrence)
Brain scan	No	As indicated

ing on CT scan that alters treatment planning is unrecognized disease in the internal mammary lymph node chain.

SUGGESTED GUIDELINES FOR FOLLOW-UP

Follow-up of the patient with breast cancer depends on facilities available to the clinician as well as patient compliance, personality, and stage of disease. Follow-up must be tailored to the individual patient and that patient's associated risk factors. Patients with multiple risk factors for recurrent disease, such as nodal disease and negative estrogen receptors or chest wall invasion, may need more frequent follow-up than patients with a small node-negative, hormone receptor–positive tumor.

Our recommendations (Table 46–6) for follow-up are based on the clinical studies previously referenced, clinical experience, and cost effectiveness. For reference, Table 46–7 outlines follow-up schedules utilized by other investigators. It should be noted that data are not available to support various time intervals of follow-up. With advances in the treatment of local/regional and systemic recurrences, more frequent follow-up may provide a longer "lead time" before clinical manifestations

of disease. The goal of the oncologist is to convert this "lead time" into an improvement in overall and disease-free survival. Based on these premises, our current recommendations are described as follows.

All patients should have routine serum liver chemistry tests, chest roentgenograms, mammograms, and bone scans completed *prior to* primary treatment. The patient should be evaluated clinically every 3 months for the first 3 years; thereafter, follow-up is every 6 months for the following 2 years. After 5 years in which there is no evidence of recurrent disease, the patient can be evaluated on an annual basis. The patient should be instructed in breast self-examination of the involved chest wall as well as the opposite breast. Chest roentgenogram and bone scan should be obtained only when physical examination or symptomatology warrants further investigation. Routine serum level or biological marker tests are not, at the present time, indicated in routine follow-up, unless examination or symptoms warrant the need for further investigation. Brain, liver, or computerized tomography scanning of the chest or abdomen are also not routinely indicated.

If local recurrence is detected, then ancillary studies unrelated to the site of local recurrence may be helpful in detecting asymptomatic metastases. Bone scan has been found to show evidence of metastatic disease in

Table 46–7. FOLLOW-UP SCHEDULES UTILIZED BY OTHER INVESTIGATORS

Authors	History and Physical Examination	Serum Chemistry Tests	Chest Roentgenogram	Bone Scan	Skeletal Survey	Liver Scan
Pandya et al.[49]	q 3 mo	q 3 mo	q 3 mo	q 3 mo x 1 yr; q 6 mo, x 1–5 yrs	q 3 mo	—
Valagussa et al.[61]	q 3 mo × 1 yr, q 4 mo after	q 6 mo × 3 yr, q yr after 3 yr	q 4 mo × 3 yr, q 6 mo after 3 yr	—	q 6 mo	Yearly
Tomin and Donegan[58]	q 3 mo × 2 yr q yr after 5 yr	q 6 mo for 5 yr	q 6 mo for 5 yr	—	As indicated	—
Winchester et al.[68]	q 6 mo, 3–5 yr, yearly after 5 yr	q 3–4 mo for 3 yr	Yearly	Yearly	As indicated	—
Marrazzo et al.[42]	q 3 mo	q 3 mo	q 3 mo	q 6 mo	Yearly	Yearly
Muss et al.[47]	q 6 mo	Yearly	Yearly	Yearly	—	—

one third of patients who harbor local/regional recurrent disease without symptoms of osseous metastases. Likewise, occult intrathoracic disease may be detected by computerized tomography scan of the chest in 67 percent of patients.[53] We recommend both bone scan and CT scan of the chest in patients who manifest local/regional recurrent disease.

It must be stressed that the vast majority of recurrences will be recognized by a detailed history and physical examination along with careful attention to symptomatology. Therefore the clinician should not rely solely on technological advances in order to detect recurrent or metastatic disease that is best recognized by a thorough medical evaluation.

As new tumor markers are developed and assessed, these diagnostic measures may play a more active role in detecting recurrent or metastatic breast cancer in follow-up. However, at the present time none of these modalities have sufficient specificity or sensitivity to recommend their use on a routine basis in follow-up. Furthermore, the cost of routine application of these tests cannot be justified at present.

Early detection of recurrent breast cancer does not significantly affect survival. However, recent advances in chemotherapy and immunotherapy suggest that the medical community has made meaningful progress in the control of systemic disease. The ultimate goal of enhancing disease-free and overall survival of breast cancer patients through early detection of relapses has not been realized by the clinician.

References

1. Ahlemann LM, Staab HJ, Anderer FA: Serial CEA determinations as an aid in postoperative therapy management of patients with early breast cancer. Biomedicine 32:194–199, 1980.
2. Beard D, Haskell CM: Carcinoembryonic antigen in breast cancer: Clinical review. Am J Med 80:241–245, 1986.
3. Bedwinek JM, Lee J, Fineberg B, et al: Prognostic medicators in patients with isolated local-regional recurrence of breast cancer. Cancer 47:2232–2235, 1981.
4. Bonadonna G, Brusamolino E, Valagussa P, et al: Combination chemotherapy as an adjuvant treatment in operable breast cancer. N Engl J Med 294:405–410, 1976.
5. Butzelaar RMJM, Van Dongen JA, De Graaf PW, Van Der Schoot JB: Bone scintigraphy in patients with operable breast cancer stages I and II. Final conclusion after five-year follow-up. Eur J Cancer Clin Oncol 20(7):877–880, 1984.
6. Brøyn T, Frøyen J: Evaluation of routine follow-up after surgery for breast carcinoma. Acta Chir Scand 148:401–404, 1982.
7. Cantwell B, Fennelly JJ, Jones M: Evaluation of follow-up methods to detect relapse after mastectomy in breast cancer patients. Ir J Med Sci 151:1–5, 1982.
8. Castagna J, Benfield JR, Yamada H, Johnson DE: The reliability of liver scans and function tests in detecting metastases. Surg Gynecol Obstet 134:463–466, 1972.
9. Chan DW, Beveridge RA, Bruzek DJ, Damron DJ, Bray KR, Gaur PK, Ettinger DS, Rock RC: Monitoring breast cancer with CA-549. Clin Chem 34(10):2000–2004, 1988.
10. Chatal JF, Chupin F, Ricolleau G, Tellier JL, Le Mevel A, Fumoleau P, Godin O, Le Mevel BP: Use of serial carcinoembryonic antigen assays in detecting relapses in breast cancer involving high risk of metastasis. Eur J Cancer 17:233–238, 1981.
11. Chaudary MM, Maisey MN, Shaw PJ, Rubens RD, Hayward JL: Sequential bone scans and chest radiographs in the postopera-

tive management of early breast cancer. Br J Surg 70(9):517–518, 1983.
12. Ciatto S, Herd-Smith A: The role of chest x-ray in the follow-up of primary breast cancer. Tumori 69:151–154, 1983.
13. Citrin DL, Furnival CM, Bessent RG, Greig WR, Bell G, Blumgart LH: Radioactive technetium phosphate bone scanning in preoperative assessment and follow-up study of patients with primary cancer of the breast. Surg Gynecol Obstet 143:360–364, 1976.
14. Coker DD, Lambrecht RW, Kehn BD: The value of initial and follow-up bone scans in patients with operable breast cancer. Milit Med 145(7):492–494, 1980.
15. Coombes RC, Gazet JC, Ford HT, Powles TJ, Nash AG, McKinna A: Treatment of malignant disease. Assessment of biochemical tests to screen for metastases in patients with breast cancer. Lancet 1(8163):296–298, 1980.
16. Coombes RC, Powles TJ, Gazet JC, Ford HT, McKinna A, Abbott M, Gehrke CW, Keyser JW, Mitchell PEG, Patel S, Stimson WH, Worwood M, Jones M, Neville AM: Screening for metastases in breast cancer: an assessment of biochemical and physical methods. Cancer 48:310–315, 1981.
17. Dearnaley DP, Kingsley DPE, Husband JE, Horwich A, Coombes RC: The role of computed tomography of the brain in the investigation of breast cancer patients with suspected intracranial metastases. Clin Radiol 32:375–382, 1981.
18. DeSouza LJ, Shinde SR: The value of laparoscopic liver examination in the management of breast cancer. J Surg Oncol 14:97–103, 1980.
19. Dewar JA, Kerr GR: Value of routine follow up of women treated for early carcinoma of the breast. Br Med J 291:1464–1467, 1985.
20. Donegan WL: Local and regional recurrence. In Donegan WL, Spratt JA (eds): Cancer of the Breast, ed 3. Philadelphia, WB Saunders, 1988, pp 648–663.
21. Falkson HC, Falson G, Portugal MA, Van Der Watt JJ, Schoeman HS: Carcinoembryonic antigen as a marker in patients with breast cancer receiving postsurgical adjuvant chemotherapy. Cancer 49:1859–1865, 1982.
22. Feig SA: The role of new imaging modalities in staging and follow-up of breast cancer. Semin Oncol 13(4):402–414, 1986.
23. Gerber FH, Goodreau JJ, Kirchner PT, Fouty WJ: Efficacy of preoperative and postoperative bone scanning in the management of breast carcinoma. New Engl J Med 297(6):300–303, 1977.
24. Gray BN: Value of CEA in breast cancer. Aust NZ J Surg 54:1–2, 1984.
25. Gray BN, Walker C, Barnard R: Value of serial carcinoembryonic antigen determinations for early detection of recurrent cancer. Med J Aust 1:177–178, 1981.
26. Haagensen DW, Kister SJ, Vandevoorde JP, Gates JB, Smart EK, Hansen HJ, Wells SA: Evaluation of carcinoembryonic antigen as a plasma monitor for human breast carcinoma. Cancer 42:1512–1519, 1978.
27. Hayes DF, Zurawski VR Jr, Kufe DW: Comparison of circulating CA 15–3 and carcinoembryonic antigen levels in patients with breast cancer. J Clin Oncol 4(10):1542–1550, 1986.
28. Hietanen P: Relapse pattern and follow-up of breast cancer. Ann Clin Res 18:134–143, 1986.
29. Hilkens J, Bonfrer JMG, Kroezen V, van Eykeren M, Nooyen W, de Jong-Baker M, Bruning PF: Comparison of circulating MAM-6 and CEA levels and correlation with the estrogen receptor in patients with breast cancer. Int J Cancer 39:431–435, 1987.
30. Holli K, Hakama M: Effectiveness of routine and spontaneous follow-up visits for breast cancer. Eur J Clin Oncol 25:251–254, 1989.
31. Kallioniemi O-P, Oksa H, Aaran R-K, Hietanen T, Lehtinen M, Koivula T: Serum CA 15–3 assay in the diagnosis and follow-up of breast cancer. Br J Cancer 58:213–215, 1988.
32. Kamby C, Rose C, Ejlertsen B, Andersen J, Birkler NE, Rytter L, Andersen KW, Zedeler K: Stage and pattern of metastases in patients with breast cancer. Eur J Cancer Clin Oncol 23(12):1925–1934, 1987.
33. Krieger G, Wander HE, Kneba M, Prangen M, Bandlow G, Nagel GA: Metastatic breast cancer with constantly low CEA blood levels. J Cancer Res Clin Oncol 108:341–344, 1984.

34. Kunkler IH, Merrick MV: The value of non-staging skeletal scintigraphy in breast cancer. Clin Radiol 37:561–562, 1986.
35. Lamert R, Leonhardt A, Ehrhart H, von Lieren H: Serial carcinoembryonic antigen (CEA) determinations in the management of metastatic breast cancer. Oncoder Biol Med 1(2):123–135, 1980.
36. Lee YTN: Carcinoembryonic antigen as a monitor of recurrent breast cancer. J Surg Oncol 20:109–114, 1982.
37. Lee YTN: Serial tests of carcinoembryonic antigen in patients with breast cancer. Am J Clin Oncol 6:287–293, 1983.
38. Lee YTN: Breast carcinoma: pattern of recurrence and metastasis after mastectomy. Am J Clin Oncol 7:443–449, 1984.
39. Lee YTN: Biochemical and hematological tests in patients with breast carcinoma: correlations with extent of disease, sites of relapse, and prognosis. J Surg Oncol 29:242–248, 1985.
40. Lokich JJ, Zamcheck N, Lowenstein M: Sequential carcinoembryonic antigen levels in the therapy of metastatic breast cancer. Ann Int Med 89:902–906, 1978.
41. Loprinzi CL, Tormey DC, Rasmussen P, Falkson G, Davis TE, Falkson HC, Chang AYC: Prospective evaluation of carcinoembryonic antigen levels and alternating chemotherapeutic regimens in metastatic breast cancer. J Clin Oncol 4(1):46–56, 1986.
42. Marrazzo A, Solina G, Pocosa V, Fiorentino E, Bazan P: Evaluation of routine follow-up after surgery for breast carcinoma. J Surg Oncol 32:179–181, 1986.
43. McNeil BJ, Pace PD, Gray EB, et al: Preoperative and follow-up bone scans in patients with primary carcinoma of the breast. Surg Gynecol Obstet 147:745–748, 1978.
44. Meyer JE, Munzenrider JE: Computed tomographic demonstration of internal mammary lymph-node metastasis in patients with locally recurrent breast carcinoma. Radiology 139:661–663, 1981.
45. Mughal AW, Hortobagyi GN, Fritsche HA, Buzdar AU, Yap HY, Blumenschein GR: Serial plasma carcinoembryonic antigen measurements during treatment of metastatic breast cancer. JAMA 249(14):1881–1886, 1983.
46. Muss HB, White DR, Cowan RJ: Brain scanning in patients with recurrent breast cancer. Cancer 38:1574–1576, 1976.
47. Muss HB, McNamara MCJ, Connelly RA: Follow-up after stage II breast cancer: a comparative study of relapsed versus nonrelapsed patients. Am J Clin Oncol (CCT) 11(4):451–455, 1988.
48. Pallazzo S, Ligvoni V, Molinari B, Greco LM, Mancini V: The role of carcinoembryonic antigen in the postmastectomy follow-up of primary breast cancer and in the prognostic evaluation of disseminated breast cancer. Tumor 70:57–59, 1984.
49. Pandya KJ, McFadden ET, Kalish LA, Tormey DC, Taylor SG IV, Falkson G: A retrospective study of earliest indicators of recurrence in patients on Eastern Cooperative Oncology Group adjuvant chemotherapy trials for breast cancer. Cancer 55:202–205, 1985.
50. Pedrazzini A, Gelber R, Isley M, Castiglione M, Goldhirsch A: First repeated bone scan in the observation of patients with operable breast cancer. J Clin Oncol 4(3)(March):389–394, 1986.
51. Pons-Anicet DMF, Krebs BP, Mira R, Namer R: Value of CA 15–3 in the follow-up of breast cancer patients. Br J Cancer 55:567–569, 1987.
52. Romsdahl MM, Sears ME, Eckles NE: Posttreatment evaluation of breast cancer. *In* Breast Cancer: Early and Late. Chicago, Year Book Medical, 1970, pp 291–299.
53. Rosenman J, Churchill CA, Mauro MA, Parker LA, Newsome J: The role of computed tomography in the evaluation of postmastectomy locally recurrent breast cancer. Int J Radiat Oncol Biol Phys 14(1):57–62, 1988.
54. Scanlon EF, Oviedo MA, Cunningham MP, Caprini JA, Khandekar JD, Cohen E, Robinson B, Stein E: Preoperative and follow-up procedures on patients with breast cancer. Cancer 46:977–979, 1980.
55. Sears HF, Gerber FH, Sturts DL, Fouty WJ: Liver scan and carcinoma of the breast. Surg Gynecol Obstet 140:409–411, 1975.
56. Stacker SA, Sacks NPM, Golder J, Tjandra JJ, Thompson CH, Smithyman A, McKenzie IFC: Evaluation of MSA as a serum marker in breast cancer: a comparison with CEA. Br J Cancer 57:298–303, 1988.
57. Tjandra JJ, Russell IS, Collins JP, Stacker SA, McKenzie IFC: Application of mammary serum antigen assay in the management of breast cancer: a preliminary report. Br J Surg 75:811–817, 1988.
58. Tomin R, Donegan WL: Screening for recurrent breast cancer—its effectiveness and prognostic value. J Clin Oncol 5(1):62–67, 1987.
59. Tondini C, Hayes DF, Gelman R, Henderson IC, Kufe DW: Comparison of CA15–3 and carcinoembryonic antigen in monitoring the clinical course of patients with metastatic breast cancer. Cancer Res 48:4107–4112, 1988.
60. Valagussa P, Bonadonna G, Veronesi U: Patterns of relapse and survival following radical mastectomy. Analysis of 716 consecutive patients. Cancer 41:1170–1178, 1978.
61. Valagussa P, Tess T, Rossi A, Tancini G, Banfi A, Bonadonna G: Adjuvant CMF effect on site of first recurrence, and appropriate follow-up intervals, in operable breast cancer with positive axillary nodes. Breast Cancer Res Treat 1:349–356, 1981.
62. Van Der Linden JC, Baak JPA, Postma T, Lindeman J, Meyer CJLM: Monitoring serum CEA in women with primary breast tumours positive for oestrogen receptor and with spread to lymph nodes. J Clin Pathol 38:1229–1234, 1985.
63. Villari N, Fargnoli R, Mungai R: CT evaluation of chest wall recurrences of breast cancer. Eur J Radiol 5:206–208, 1983.
64. Waalkes TP, Abeloff MD, Ettinger DS, Woo DB, Gehrke CW, Mrochek JE: Multiple biological markers and breast carcinoma: a preliminary study in the detection of recurrent disease after primary therapy. J Surg Oncol 18:9–19, 1981.
65. Waalkes TP, Enterline JP, Shaper JH, Abeloff MD, Ettinger DS: Biological markers for breast carcinoma. Cancer 53:644–651, 1984.
66. Wickerham L, Fisher B, Cronin W, Stolbach L, Abramson N, Bowman D, Deckers PJ, Eisenberg P, Foster R, Glass A, Kay S, Kyle A, Prager D, Pritchard K: The efficacy of bone scanning in the follow-up of patients with operable breast cancer. Breast Cancer Res Treat 4:303–307, 1984.
67. Wiener SN, Sachs SH: An assessment of routine liver scanning in patients with breast cancer. Arch Surg 113:126–127, 1978.
68. Winchester DP, Sener SF, Khandekar JD, Oviedo MA, Cunningham MP, Caprini JA, Burkett FE, Scanlon EF: Symptomatology as an indicator of recurrent or metastatic breast cancer. Cancer 43:956–960, 1979.
69. Zwaveling A, Albers GHR, Felthuis W, Hermans J: An evaluation of routine follow-up for detection of breast cancer recurrences. J Surg Oncol 34:194–197, 1987.

Chapter 47

SPECIAL PROBLEMS RELATED TO THE OPERATIVE SITE: LOCAL RECURRENCE, THE AUGMENTED BREAST, AND THE CONTRALATERAL BREAST

Edward M. Copeland III, M.D.

Breast screening and follow-up care is important for every woman, but especially for one who has had breast cancer. Throughout this book, follow-up care has been discussed relative to specific topics. There are certain circumstances, however, that deserve special attention.

RECURRENCE IN THE OPERATIVE SITE FOLLOWING MASTECTOMY

Although chest wall recurrences are related to initial stage of the primary disease, the operative site should be evaluated every 3 to 4 months for the first 2 postoperative years and every 6 months thereafter regardless of the stage of the primary disease. At the very least, the patient should understand the value of careful evaluation of the wound and be more aware of any changes that require a physician's attention.

Seven percent to 32 percent of patients will eventually develop a local recurrence of breast cancer.[65] Although related to extent of disease on the chest wall at the time of primary resection and to the aggressiveness of perioperative radiation therapy, chest wall recurrence does not appear to be related to the proximity of the primary to the pectoralis major muscle fascia, provided the areolar plane between the breast and the underlying fascia is not involved at the time of mastectomy.[2] Sixty percent to 80 percent of all chest wall recurrences will appear within the first 2 years after mastectomy, but they can occur throughout the lifetime of the patient.[16, 19, 69, 95] From 45 percent to 85 percent of patients who have local recurrence will have a previous or simultaneous distant metastasis.[6, 12, 20, 57] Adjuvant radiation therapy at the time of primary treatment has been shown to decrease the rate of local/regional recurrence after surgery, but any survival benefit from radiation therapy is unclear.[22, 25–27, 88] It has been difficult to prove that adjuvant chemotherapy given postoperatively to patients at high risk for local recurrence (advanced stage II and stage III disease) reduces local recurrence rates in the absence of adjuvant chest wall radiation therapy. Undoubtedly, chemotherapy given preoperatively to patients with advanced local disease reduces the risk of local recurrence in those patients who respond to treatment. These patients are, however, usually treated by appropriate mastectomy and chest wall radiation therapy as well, making the impact of chemotherapy on local recurrence difficult to evaluate. Delivery of chemotherapy postoperatively is no doubt impeded by the interruption of blood supply and scar in the healing wound where residual breast cancer is deposited.

Nevertheless, three recent studies using different cytotoxic chemotherapy protocols in a large number of node-negative patients who received no radiotherapy have been completed.[23, 24, 62] These patients were randomized to treatment with postoperative chemotherapy vs. observation only. The group receiving chemotherapy had a prolonged disease-free interval and a reduction in local and regional recurrences at a maximum follow-up of 4 years (Table 47–1). Survival advantages were not detected for either group. Possibly chemotherapy may only delay the inevitable recurrence and will not replace chest wall radiation therapy as the major deterrent to chest wall relapse following surgery. Future follow-up of these patient groups may be enlightening.

Classic teaching has been that local recurrence heralds the discovery of distant metastases and should be treated as such. Very few studies, however, have evaluated patients who have local recurrence as the first and only site of failure. Common sense would dictate that an occasional malignant nodule on the chest wall might represent a new primary in residual breast tissue left on the skin flaps at the time of mastectomy or a single cluster of cells in the scar deposited at the time of operation. In such instances, cure should be obtainable

Table 47–1. LOCAL/REGIONAL RECURRENCE AS FIRST SITE OF TREATMENT FAILURE IN LYMPH NODE-NEGATIVE PATIENTS

Type of Adjuvant Therapy	Surgery Alone (%)	Surgery + Adjuvant (%)
Methotrexate, 5-FU[24] ER negative	8.0	4.0*
Tamoxifen[23] ER positive	3.0	1.0*
Cyclophosphamide, methotrexate 5-FU, leucovorin[62]		
ER positive	3.9	0.9†
ER negative	8.1	1.1†

*p <0.05.
†Significance of values not started.

by appropriate local therapy. Gilliland et al.[32] reported 60 patients with ipsilateral chest wall recurrence of breast cancer and no detectable distant metastases. These authors made several interesting observations. More than 50 percent of the nodules were solitary and easily removed. Only ten percent of patients had more than five nodules. The majority of the recurrences were in the mastectomy scar or immediate vicinity. Mean disease-free interval between treatment of the primary cancer and discovery of the chest wall recurrence, and time interval between local recurrence and death, were directly related to stage of initial disease (Tables 47–2 and 47–3). All stage I patients had at least a 2-year disease-free interval, and this interval was as long as 21 years in some patients. Surgical resection resulted in the best local control. Even in the most favorable group of patients with no detectable distant metastases at the time of local recurrence, all 60 patients eventually died of metastatic breast cancer. Consequently, this report supports the concept that chest wall recurrence is a distant metastasis. Mendenhall et al.,[63] however, reported a small subset of patients who were aggressively treated for local recurrence and who had 5- and 10-year actuarial survival rates of 50 percent and 34 percent, respectively. These patients have not yet been followed as long as those studied by Gilliland et al.[32]

Certainly local recurrence should be treated aggressively. Short-term prognosis and patient comfort improve markedly if local control of the recurrence can be obtained. Those lesions amenable to surgical removal

Table 47–2. TIME INTERVAL BETWEEN TREATMENT OF PRIMARY TUMOR AND DISCOVERY OF CHEST WALL RECURRENCE

Stage	(No.)	Mean Disease-free Interval (yrs)	Range (yrs)
I	(11)	6.2	2.5–21.0
II	(9)	4.3	1.2–6.8
III	(31)	2.1	0.2–11.0

Stage I vs. II, p = 0.26; stage I vs. III, p = 0.01; stage II vs. III, p = 0.11.
Adapted from Gilliland MD, et al: Ann Surg 197:284–287, 1983.

Table 47–3. TIME INTERVAL BETWEEN LOCAL RECURRENCE AND DEATH

Stage (No.)	Average Time Interval (yrs)	Range (yrs)
I (11)	7.2	1.0–23.0
II (9)	6.0	2.1–13.0
III (31)	2.5	0.3–6.3

p <0.05, stage III vs. stage I or II.
Adapted from Gilliland MD, et al: Ann Surg 197:284–287, 1983.

(including major chest wall resections) should be treated surgically. Shah and Urban[82] reported a 43 percent 5-year survival rate utilizing full-thickness chest wall resection for isolated chest wall recurrences. The recent advent of free flaps, made possible by microsurgery, and better prosthetic materials have extended the limits of chest wall resection.

If not previously utilized, radiation therapy is indicated. Our current policy is to treat the chest wall and internal mammary nodes to 5000 cGy in 25 fractions with electron beam. The supraclavicular nodes are treated with a combination of photons and electrons to a dose of 5000 cGy in 25 fractions as well. This dose may be boosted through reduced fields to areas of gross disease.[63]

The role of chemotherapy in the setting of isolated local/regional recurrence is not clear; however, treatment philosophies developed for other high-risk patients dictate it be used based on the hormone receptor and menopausal status of the patient. Again, no data on sequencing of multimodality treatment exists, but it would be reasonable to deliver appropriate chemotherapy either before or after surgical resection and before radiation therapy.

RECURRENCE IN THE RECONSTRUCTED BREAST

There remains some controversy about immediate vs. delayed reconstruction after mastectomy. The advantages of immediate reconstruction are an immediate breast form on the chest wall and possible reduction in psychological trauma. Immediate reconstruction also eliminates another operation and anesthetic required for the delayed reconstructive procedure. Disadvantages are potential compromise of prompt delivery of adjuvant therapy, the magnitude of the prolonged surgical procedure, and the possible masking of chest wall recurrence. In fact, up until several years ago, an empirical interval of 2 years between mastectomy and reconstruction was recommended in order to not mask recurrent disease during this "critical" time interval. Studies by Gilliland et al.[33] and others[29, 31] demonstrated that almost no patients with stage I disease who experienced recurrence on the chest wall did so in the first 2 years postoperatively. Therefore waiting a designated time interval is of no practical value in patients with stage I disease.

In an occasional early report of chest wall recurrence as the first site of treatment failure in a reconstructed breast, the entire capsule surrounding the silicone implant was infiltrated with metastatic breast cancer.[94] Fortunately, subsequent reports of chest wall recurrence after reconstruction have not been of this form of en cuirass disease.[29, 31] For example, with the implant in place subpectorally, Georgiade et al.[31] had no problem with early detection of four local recurrences in 50 patients reported. Likewise in this series, five patients on final pathological evaluation of the initial specimen had unsuspected evidence of nipple-areolar involvement. Therefore these authors did not recommend use of autologous nipple-areolar complex for reconstruction.

If a reconstruction procedure were to mask a chest wall recurrence, the best candidate would be the transverse abdominal island flap (TAIF) method of reconstruction in which a composite graft of autologous muscle and fat from the abdominal wall is transported with its blood supply intact to the chest wall. A recurrence deep to this tissue potentially could go undetected for some period of time. In fact, of the five recurrences reported by Hartrampf and Bennett[39] in their series of 300 patients reconstructed by the TAIF method, only one recurrence was delayed in its discovery (for 3 months). Thus it would appear that the only two potential contraindications to immediate breast reconstruction are the increased length of the operation and the need for adjuvant postoperative radiotherapy or chemotherapy. From early reports, however, satisfactory cosmetic and oncological results are being obtained from radiation therapy or chemotherapy with a silicone- or saline-filled implant in place.[48, 84] It is really too early to tell, however, what the ultimate effects will be of having an implant in place during adjuvant therapy.

BREAST CANCER AFTER SUBCUTANEOUS MASTECTOMY

Brief mention should be made of the possibility of developing breast cancer after prophylactic subcutaneous simple mastectomy.[10] Since the nipple-areolar complex is left intact after this operation, breast tissue obviously remains on the chest wall in the nipple since the ducts pass through it to exit on the surface. Also, in an attempt to not devascularize the nipple-areolar complex, a pledget of breast parenchyma may be left beneath the nipple. Subcutaneous mastectomy is often done via an incision in the inframammary crease; consequently, breast tissue is not dissected from the skin flaps under direct vision. Likewise, the axillary tail of the breast may be inadequately excised, since it is at the most distant site from the inframammary incision and troublesome bleeding may be encountered in this area. Patients undergoing subcutaneous mastectomy should be made aware of the possibility of some breast tissue remaining on the chest wall, especially if the operation is being done as prophylaxis against breast cancer. Breast cancer is both a multicentric and multifocal disease, particularly in patients with atypical hyperpla-

sia, a strong family history of breast cancer, and *in situ* disease. Since these are the individuals who are often offered subcutaneous mastectomy as a prophylactic operation, the risk of developing breast cancer in residual ductal tissue after the operation is even higher.

Although no operation assures the removal of all breast tissue, the best[41, 43] chance for complete extirpation is by simple mastectomy in which the nipple-areolar complex is excised as part of the specimen and the breast tissue is removed from the skin flaps under direct vision.

RECURRENCE IN THE INTACT IRRADIATED BREAST

For the properly selected patient, segmental resection (lumpectomy), axillary dissection, and postoperative radiation therapy to the intact breast results in survival rates equal to those for modified radical mastectomy.[22, 78] One fear, however, has been that a recurrence in the breast may have the same grave prognostic implications as a chest wall recurrence following mastectomy.[32] The best way for any surgeon to settle this debate is to properly select patients for lumpectomy and to minimize or eliminate recurrences. Because the latter is not entirely possible, a review of current knowledge about recurrent disease is valuable.

Factors that favor recurrence after lumpectomy are positive surgical margins at the time of lumpectomy (inadequate incision),[22, 38, 71, 79] lymphatic invasion,[59] anaplasia,[15, 38, 79] associated *in situ* disease in both the primary cancer and surrounding parenchyma,[38, 71, 79] tumor necrosis,[59] invasive lobular carcinoma,[59] inadequate radiation dose,[15] and a delay of radiation therapy for longer than 7 weeks after lumpectomy.[15] Several of these factors are controversial. For example, not every investigator has found that positive margins,[15] associated *in situ* disease,[15] or histological subtype[15] result in a higher recurrence rate. Also, each of these unfavorable prognostic factors was derived from series of patients compiled from institutions with strict criteria for patient selection for lumpectomy. Predictably, patients with advanced stage II and stage III disease would have higher local recurrence rates; however, very few such patients are in the reported series.

An idea of the magnitude of risk for recurrence can be obtained from studies by Harris et al.[38] Patients who had a combination of the three risk factors of *in situ* disease in the tumor and adjacent tissue and anaplasia had a 37 percent local recurrence rate at 8 years compared to eight percent for all other patients. Local recurrence was reduced by a radiation boost to the lumpectomy site. Survival rate was 69 percent for patients with all three risk factors compared with 90 percent for the remainder of the patients. These authors have also noted a greater actuarial risk of local recurrence at 5 years for patients who have an incomplete excision (36 percent) compared with those patients in whom excision is complete (8 percent).

Kurtz and colleagues[51] have followed 276 patients with

T1 and T2 lesions treated by lumpectomy only for 10 to 21 years. No chemotherapy was employed, and radiation therapy was administered appropriately. The recurrence rate in the treated breast was 15.6 percent. Contralateral breast cancer developed in 7.2 percent of patients. Breast recurrence was rare in the first 2 years postoperatively (data similar to the infrequency of early chest wall recurrence after mastectomy for stage I disease).[32] Only 63 percent of all eventual failures occurred before 5 years, and 53 percent of failures in patients with T1 lesions occurred 5 or more years postoperatively. Thus the true recurrence rate in the intact irradiated breast may not be known for many years.

Somewhat contrary to this concept of late recurrence are recent data from the NSABP B-06 protocol, which identified the majority of failures following lumpectomy to occur in the first 39 months of the study.[22] Accrual of only a few additional patients with recurrence occurred during the next 4 years of the study. Salvage surgery has been most often by modified radical mastectomy. In the series by Kurtz et al.,[51] 49 percent of patients had positive axillary lymph nodes in the mastectomy specimen, a figure much higher than would have been predicted at the initial operation had axillary dissections been done. Five-year survival after salvage mastectomy was 62 percent, again a lower figure than is expected for patients with T1 or T2N0 lesions. Why then was the pathological situation and survival worse for the cohort of patients with recurrent disease? Probably those patients who had local recurrences also had more aggressive cancer. In fact, early recurrence after mastectomy had a distinctly unfavorable prognosis. The type of local failure affects survival as well. An isolated breast parenchymal recurrence without inflammation is much more amenable to cure by mastectomy than is nodal or dermal relapse.[15] The prognosis for dermal relapse appears to be as poor as that for relapse on the chest wall after mastectomy.[15, 32]

It is difficult to know whether an isolated recurrence in the irradiated breast is a true recurrence or a new primary cancer.[71] The ipsilateral mammary tissue is still available for malignant degeneration. Schnitt et al.,[80] for example, found evidence of multicentricity in 22 percent of patients undergoing salvage mastectomy for solitary mammary recurrences. In the experience of the Prince Margaret Hospital in Toronto,[14] however, multicentricity seldom became clinically apparent after radiation therapy. Nevertheless, a new primary malignancy is possible. Kurtz et al.[50] reported 52 patients who were treated for a mammary recurrence by a repeat lumpectomy and axillary dissection rather than by mastectomy. The 5- and 10-year actuarial survival rates calculated from the date of the second operation were 79 percent and 64 percent, respectively. Seventy-three percent of patients were disease-free at a mean of 6 years after salvage surgery. This data compares quite favorably to previous series reported by these authors[51] and others[14, 15, 64] in which salvage surgery was done by modified radical mastectomy. In fact, the physician teams at both the Prince Margaret Hospital[14] and the Institute Gustave-Roussy[15] have concluded that a relapse

in the breast alone, if appropriately treated, does not adversely affect survival.

It would appear that mammary parenchymal recurrences after lumpectomy[14, 15, 51, 64] are distinctly different entities from chest wall recurrences after mastectomy.[32, 63] Mammary recurrence does not necessarily herald a distant metastasis, although the biological behavior of these tumors is somewhat aggressive. Early detection will no doubt prove to be important. A posttreatment mammogram is required to establish a new baseline, since the lumpectomy scar will be visible and radiation fibrosis may distort the image. Otherwise, follow-up is the same after lumpectomy as after modified radical mastectomy. Any suspicious areas in the breast must be biopsied; therefore, areas of fibrotic tissue are commonly removed, particularly near the scar. After 5 to 7 years, radiation fibrosis will usually stabilize, and a previously firm breast should become compliant. An experienced examiner is required to follow the irradiated breast, and patients should request to be examined by the same individual at each physician visit.

PRIMARY BREAST CANCER IN THE AUGMENTED BREAST

Safe and effective methods for breast augmentation have been available now for more than 20 years, and estimates are that well over one million women have undergone augmentation,[17, 93] many of whom have reached the prevalent age for the development of breast cancer. Consequently, reports of breast cancer in augmented breasts are now beginning to appear[8, 17, 18, 34, 83] and are stimulating debate about the possibility of the implant material, usually silicone, being causative. Experimental data from subcutaneous implantation of silicone has not shown a causal relationship with malignancy.[11, 44, 55]

Several large retrospective studies in women who have undergone augmentation showed no increase in the risk of breast cancer.[18, 37, 61] Deapen et al.[17] reported 3111 women in whom frequency distribution epidemiological analysis would have predicted 15.7 breast cancers. Only nine breast cancers were actually detected. Of the subpopulation of 447 women in this series who had implants in place for 10 years or more, 3.5 cases of breast cancer were expected, and only three were detected. Breast cancers that were identified seemed no more virulent than those in the general population. The conclusion from this study was that breast implants do not appear to increase the risk of breast cancer. The study was done, however, by 35 plastic surgeons in the Los Angeles County area who submitted their augmentation mammaplasty patients' records for review. Those who developed breast cancer were identified through a population-based cancer registry (The Los Angeles County Cancer Surveillance Program). Although errors inherent to this method of patient accrual do not invalidate the study, certainly the discovery of the patients with breast cancer relied on accurate record keeping by a multitude of physicians in the Los Angeles County area.

Silverstein et al.[83] approached the question from a different perspective. Of the 753 patients treated for primary breast cancer during a 66-month period, 20 had previously undergone a subglandular augmentation mammoplasty with a silicone gel–filled prosthesis. The authors make the point that the augmented group had a worse prognosis than did the general population of nonaugmented patients with breast cancer. None of the cancers in the augmented patients were occult or *in situ*, and 13 patients (65 percent) had positive axillary lymph nodes. All had palpable masses, none of which were discovered mammographically. Although the authors do not suggest that silicone is a causative agent, they do agree with us that women with augmentation have several disadvantages relative to breast cancer detection. The implant, when placed in a retromammary position in a small-breasted woman, compresses the breast parenchyma against the skin and obscures the normal parenchymal pattern (Fig. 47–1). Detection of small clusters of microcalcifications is impaired. Regardless of the plane of the mammogram, the implant will obscure some portion of the breast parenchyma from visualization. When scar and capsule formation occur, stellate masses may occur in the area of the capsule, give a false-positive appearance on mammogram, and present as an indistinct mass on physical examination. If silicone gains access to the breast parenchyma (i.e., from a ruptured implant), granulomas develop that are palpably indistinguishable from carcinoma and may appear as a calcified mass on mammogram.[66] Distortion of the physical examination and the mammographic pattern is not as pronounced when the implant is retromammary in a large-breasted woman or is in the subpectoral position. However, some "blind areas" still exist on the mammogram.

Prior to augmentation, all women should have a mammogram and have their risk of breast cancer assessed. For those with a strong family history of breast cancer, small dense breasts, atypical hyperplasia on a previous biopsy, or a previous contralateral breast cancer, the disadvantages of losing mammography as a potential tool for early detection should be weighed carefully against the cosmetic advantages. Certainly the woman should be apprised of the problem so that she can actively participate in the decision for augmentation. Following augmentation, annual mammograms should be considered when the patient reaches 35 years of age, and all suspicious lesions require biopsy.

The implant does not appear to alter the growth characteristics of the malignancy, although compression of lymphatics and distortion of flow are possibilities, as is the potentiation of neovascularization of the tumor. An initial fear was that a primary breast cancer in an augmented patient might be first detected as an en cuirass mass surrounding the retromammary implant. To the contrary, in reports to date,[8, 17, 18, 61, 83] the breast cancers have been freely mobile and not attached to the implant capsule (Fig. 47–2). In fact, in large-breasted patients, the lesions are readily visible by mammography (Fig. 47–3).[8]

Treatment regimens for patients developing breast cancer in an augmented breast have not been established. Modified radical mastectomy should remain the standard treatment until experience with breast conservation techniques is established. In the rare published experience with radiation of an intact augmented breast, it would appear that the implant may remain in place and that appropriate radiation therapy will not necessarily result in distorted capsule formation.[48] To date, most of this experience is by personal communication and is anecdotal. There has been no long-term follow-up relative to eventual cosmetic result or local recurrence. Likewise, the effect of cytotoxic chemotherapeutic agents on capsule scar formation is unknown. Doxorubicin does alter wound healing in both human beings and experimental animals.[9] Lumpectomy in those patients who are otherwise candidates for the operation should be reserved for special circumstances, and modified radical mastectomy with appropriate adjuvant therapy should be utilized.

RISK OF THE CONTRALATERAL BREAST

Although the contralateral breast has been discussed in multiple chapters in this book relative to the risk of developing breast cancer, a brief summary is provided here. Environmental, genetic, morphological, and biochemical factors affect both breasts equally when both are at risk. From four percent to 15 percent of surviving breast cancer patients develop a contralateral primary breast cancer, a risk two to six times higher than that

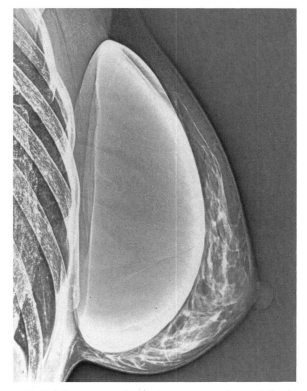

Figure 47–1. Retromammary implants compress and potentially obscure from view several areas of breast parenchyma.

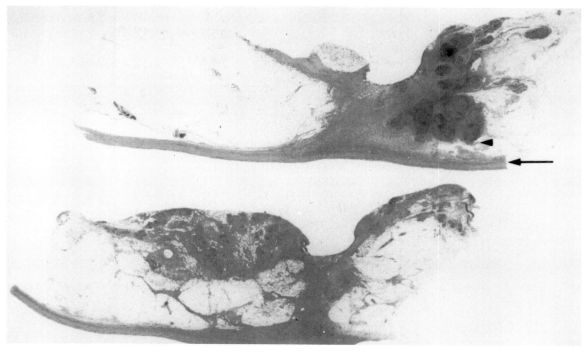

Figure 47–2. Photomicrograph of a breast cancer that developed in a patient with an augmented breast. Note the fibrous capsule around the silicone implant *(arrow)*. The arrowhead points to the advancing border of an adenocarcinoma and demonstrates no attachment to the capsule. (From Bingham H, et al: Ann Plast Surg 20:236–237, 1988. Reprinted by permission.)

for the general population.[13, 14, 70] This risk remains relatively constant throughout the lifetime of the patient.[40, 70, 73] The relationship between extent of disease in the initially affected breast and the development of contralateral breast cancer is equivocal and may be inverse.[1, 42, 46, 70] The use of radiation therapy to the intact breast or chest wall after mastectomy does not appear to further increase the risk of breast cancer in the contralateral breast.[45, 51, 71]

Horn and Thompson[45] reviewed 292 women with an incident contralateral breast cancer. Factors associated with an increased risk for the opposite breast were invasive lobular carcinoma, a positive progesterone assay in the initial primary cancer, and AB blood type.

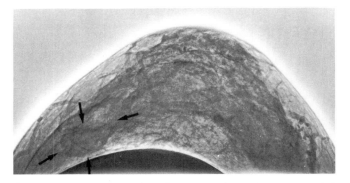

Figure 47–3. Mammogram from the patient whose photomicrograph is depicted in Figure 47–2. The breast cancer was freely mobile from the implant capsule by physical examination and not attached by mammogram. (From Bingham H, et al: Ann Plast Surg 20:236–237, 1988. Reprinted by permission.)

Interestingly, adjuvant chemotherapy significantly lowered the risk.

The need for contralateral breast biopsy in patients with invasive carcinoma is controversial. The work of Urban[85, 87] and Leis[52–54] indicates a potential for detecting a contralateral breast cancer at an early stage; Wanebo et al.[89] have adopted this approach because, in their opinion, the prognosis for patients who develop a contralateral breast cancer is unfavorable. Other investigators, however, have not been able to document any value of a contralateral biopsy in the absence of a detectable physical or radiographic abnormality of the contralateral breast.[3, 49, 58, 68, 73] Diligent lifelong surveillance of the opposite breast seems most appropriate and avoids unnecessary overtreatment from data obtained from contralateral "blind" breast biopsy.

A plan for follow-up management of a normal contralateral breast in patients with *in situ* breast cancer is difficult to obtain from reports in the literature. Data on bilaterality often include patients with a previous or synchronous breast cancer and greatly overestimate the actual risk of a normal contralateral breast. For example, in one of the earliest reports of a large series of patients with minimal breast cancer followed for up to 20 years, 59 percent of patients with lobular carcinoma *in situ* had bilateral breast cancer,[28] yet none of the patients with a normal contralateral breast at risk developed subsequent breast cancer. Seven percent of patients with intraductal carcinoma and the opposite breast at risk developed a subsequent breast cancer (Table 47–4). Likewise, in a recent report by Baker and Kuhajda,[7] six percent of patients who initially had in-

Table 47–4. BILATERALITY IN MINIMAL BREAST CANCER

Status of Opposite Breast	LIS	ICS	MIC
No contralateral disease	7	97	12
Contralateral disease			
Previous invasive carcinoma	3	16	8
Previous noninvasive carcinoma	0	1	0
Simultaneous invasive carcinoma	5	10	1
Simultaneous noninvasive carcinoma	2	4	—
Subsequent invasive carcinoma	0	5	0
Subsequent noninvasive carcinoma	0	3	0
No data	0	1	0
Metastasis from opposite breast	0	1	0
Total contralateral primary carcinoma	10 (59%)	39 (29%)	9 (42%)

Abbreviations: LIS, lobular carcinoma *in situ*; ICS, intraductal carcinoma; MIC, invasive ductal carcinoma less than 0.5 cm in size.
Adapted from Frazier TG, et al: Am J Surg 133:697–701, 1977.

vasive lobular carcinoma developed a subsequent cancer in the contralateral breast. Lobular carcinoma *in situ* was not a reliable marker for predicting the presence of either synchronous or metachronous invasive cancer in the opposite breast. The combination of both invasive and *in situ* lobular carcinoma, however, may portend to a significant increase in the expected incidence of contralateral breast cancer.[35] The actual incidence of invasive carcinoma occurring in either breast at the time of diagnosis of lobular carcinoma *in situ* is about five percent.[47, 75, 77]

Estimates of bilateral multicentricity of lobular carcinoma *in situ* range from 25 percent to 69 percent,[21, 67, 72, 90] and subsequent development of breast cancer in either breast ranges from four percent[92] to 67 percent.[60] A convincing report by Haagensen[36] places the incidence of subsequent invasive breast cancer in either breast at 15 percent. More than half of these invasive lesions develop more than 15 years after the lobular carcinoma *in situ* is diagnosed.[47, 76] Therefore, in those clinical series in which a large percent of patients have lobular carcinoma *in situ*, only a few breast cancers ever develop.

The treatment for the contralateral breast in a patient with lobular carcinoma *in situ* would seem to be careful surveillance throughout the remainder of the patient's life. In fact, most investigators now recommend only close follow-up for the ipsilateral breast if the *in situ* disease is adequately excised.[30] Since both breasts are at equal risk for the development of invasive cancer, the treatment for both breasts should be the same. Thus if total mastectomy is the selected surgical therapy, it should be applied bilaterally. However, treating lobular carcinoma *in situ*, a precursor lesion, with mastectomy when breast conservation is used routinely for selected patients with invasive cancer seems paradoxical.

Studies on the bilaterality of intraductal carcinoma are inconclusive. Reports from the Memorial Sloan-Kettering Institute indicate an incidence as high as 26 percent,[5, 74, 86] yet long term follow-up data on the opposite breast yields an actual breast cancer incidence of only four to seven percent.[28, 91] Consequently, most investigators recommend close follow-up by physical examination and mammography just as is done for invasive breast cancer.[56, 81]

Prophylactic simple mastectomy for the contralateral breast should probably be reserved for those patients who have multiple associated risk factors such as florid lobular carcinoma *in situ* and invasive lobular carcinoma in the ipsilateral breast, multiple first-degree relatives with breast cancer,[4] or a contralateral breast that is difficult to follow clinically because of the denseness and nodularity of the breast tissue.

References

1. Adami H-O, Hansen J, Jung B, Lindgren A, Rimsten A: Bilateral carcinoma of the breast: epidemiology and histopathology. Acta Radiol Oncol 20:305–309, 1981.
2. Ahlborn TN, Gump FE, Bodian C, Habif DV, Kister S: Tumor to fascia margin as a factor in local recurrence after modified radical mastectomy. Surg Gynecol Obstet 166:523–526, 1988.
3. Andersen LI, Muchardt O: Simultaneous bilateral cancer of the breast—evaluation of the use of a contralateral biopsy. Acta Chir Scand 146:407–409, 1980.
4. Anderson DE: Genetic considerations in breast cancer. *In* Breast Cancer: Early and Late. Chicago, Year Book Medical, 1969, pp 27–36.
5. Ashikari R, Hajdu SI, Robbins GF: Intraductal carcinoma of the breast (1960–1969). Cancer 28:1182–1187, 1971.
6. Auchincloss H: The nature of local recurrence following radical mastectomy. Cancer 11:611–619, 1958.
7. Baker RB, Kuhajda F: The incidence of synchronous and metachronous cancers in the contralateral breast of patients with lobular breast cancer. Ann Surg 210:444–448, 1989.
8. Bingham H, Copeland EM, Hackett R, Caffee HH: Breast cancer in a patient with silicone breast implants after 13 years. Ann Plast Surg 20:236–237, 1988.
9. Bland KI, Palin WE, von Fraunhofer JA, Morris RR, Adcock RA, Tobin GR: Experimental and clinical observations of the effects of cytotoxic chemotherapeutic drugs on wound healing. Ann Surg 199:782–790, 1984.
10. Bowers DG, Radlauer CB: Breast cancer after prophylactic subcutaneous mastectomies and reconstruction with silastic prostheses. Plast Reconstr Surg 44:541–544, 1969.
11. Brown JB, Fryer MP, Ohlwiler DA: Study and use of synthetic materials, such as silicons and Teflon, as subcutaneous prostheses. Plast Reconstr Surg 26:264–279, 1961.
12. Bruce J, Carter DC, Fraser J: Patterns of recurrent disease in breast cancer. Lancet 1:433–435, 1970.
13. Burns PE, Dabbs K, May C, Lees AW, Birkett LR, Jenkins HJ, Hanson J: Bilateral breast cancer in Northern Alberta: risk factors and survival patterns. Can Med Assoc J 130:881–886, 1984.
14. Clark RM, Wilkinson RH, Mahoney LJ, Reid JG, MacDonald WD: Breast cancer: a 21-year experience with conservative surgery and radiation. Int J Radiat Oncol Biol Phys 8:967–975, 1982.
15. Clarke DH, Le MG, Sarrazin D, Lacombe M-J, Fontaine F, Travagli J-P, May-Levin F, Contesso G, Arriagada R: Analysis of local-regional relapses in patients with early breast cancers

treated by excision and radiotherapy: experience of the Institut Gustave-Roussy. Int J Radiat Oncol Biol Phys 11:137–145, 1985.

16. Dao TL, Nemoto T: The clinical significance of skin recurrence after radical mastectomy in women with cancer of the breast. Surg Gynecol Obstet 117:447–453, 1963.

17. Deapen MD, Pike MC, Casagrande JT, Brody GS: The relationship between breast cancer and augmentation mammoplasty: an epidemiologic study. Plast Reconstr Surg 77:361–367, 1986.

18. DeCholnoky T: Augmentation mammoplasty: study of complications in 10,941 patients by 265 surgeons. Plast Reconstr Surg 45:573–577, 1970.

19. Demaree EW: Local recurrence following surgery for cancer of the breast. Ann Surg 134:863–867, 1951.

20. Donegan WL, Perez-Mesa CM, Watson RF: A biostatistical study of locally recurrent breast carcinoma. Surg Gynecol Obstet 122:529–540, 1966.

21. Fechner RE: Ductal carcinoma involving the lobule of the breast: a source of confusion with lobular carcinoma in situ. Cancer 28:274–281, 1971.

22. Fisher B, Bauer M, Margolese R, Poisson R, Pilch Y, Redmond C, Fisher E, Wolmark N, Deutsch M, Montague E, Saffer E, Wickerham L, Lerner H, Glass A, Shibata H, Deckers P, Ketcham A, Oishi R, Russell I: Five-year results of a randomized clinical trial comparing total mastectomy and segmental mastectomy with or without radiation in the treatment of breast cancer. N Engl J Med 312:665–673, 1985.

23. Fisher B, Costantino J, Redmond C, Poisson R, Bowman D, Couture J, Dimitrov NV, Wolmark N, Wickerham DL, Fisher ER, Margolese R, Robidoux A, Shibata H, Terz J, Paterson AHG, Feldman MI, Farrar W, Evans J, Lickley HL, Ketner M, et al: A randomized clinical trial evaluating tamoxifen in the treatment of patients with node-negative breast cancer who have estrogen-receptor-positive tumors. N Engl J Med 320:479–484, 1989.

24. Fisher B, Redmond C, Dimitrov NV, Bowman D, Legault-Poisson S, Wickerham L, Wolmark N, Fisher ER, Margolese R, Sutherland C, Glass A, Foster R, Caplan R, et al: A randomized clinical trial evaluating sequential methotrexate and fluorouracil in the treatment of patients with node-negative breast cancer who have estrogen-receptor-negative tumors. N Engl J Med 320:473–478, 1989.

25. Fisher B, Redmond C, Fisher ER, Bauer M, Wolmark N, Wickerham L, Deutsch M, Montague E, Margdese R, Foster R: Ten-year results of a randomized clinical trial comparing radical mastectomy and total mastectomy with or without radiation. N Engl J Med 312:674–681, 1985.

26. Fisher B, Slack NH, Cavanaugh PJ, Gardner B, Ravdin RG, and cooperating investigators: Postoperative radiotherapy in the treatment of breast cancer. Results of the NSABP clinical trial. Ann Surg 172:711–732, 1970.

27. Fletcher GH, Montague ED: Does adequate irradiation of the internal mammary chain and supraclavicular nodes improve survival rates? Int J Radiat Oncol Biol Phys 4:481–492, 1978.

28. Frazier TG, Copeland EM, Gallager HS, Paulus DD Jr, White EC: Prognosis and treatment in minimal breast cancer. Am J Surg 133:697–701, 1977.

29. Frazier TG, Noone RB: An objective analysis of immediate simultaneous reconstruction in the treatment of primary carcinoma of the breast. Cancer 55:1201–1205, 1985.

30. Frykberg ER, Santiago F, Betsill WL Jr, O'Brien PH: Lobular carcinoma in situ of the breast. Surg Gynecol Obstet 164:1–17, 1987.

31. Georgiade GS, Georgiade NG, McCarty KS, Ferguson BJ, Seigler HF: Modified radical mastectomy with immediate reconstruction for carcinoma of the breast. Trans South Surg Assoc 92:41–49, 1980.

32. Gilliland MD, Barton RM, Copeland EM: The implications of local recurrence of breast cancer as the first site of therapeutic failure. Ann Surg 197:284–287, 1983.

33. Gilliland MD, Larson DL, Copeland EM: Appropriate timing for breast reconstruction. Plast Reconstr Surg 72:335–337, 1983.

34. Gottlieb V, Muench AG, Rich JD, Pagadala S: Carcinoma in augmented breasts. Ann Plast Surg 12:67–69, 1984.

35. Gump FE: Personal communication in discussion of Baker RB,

36. Kuhajda F: The incidence of synchronous and metachronous cancer in the contralateral breast of patients with lobular breast cancer. American Surgical Association, Colorado Springs, Colorado, April, 1989. Ann Surg 210:444–448, 1989.

36. Haagensen CD: Lobular neoplasi (lobular carcinoma in situ). In Haagensen CD (ed): Diseases of the Breast. Philadelphia, WB Saunders, 1986, pp 192–241.

37. Harris HI: Survey of breast implants from the point of view of carcinogenesis. Plast Reconstr Surg 28:81–83, 1961.

38. Harris JR, Connolly JL, Schnitt SJ, Cady B, Love S, Osteen RT, Patterson WB, Shirley R, Hellman S, Cohen RB, Silen W: The use of pathologic features in selecting the extent of surgical resection necessary for breast cancer patients treated by primary radiation therapy. Ann Surg 201:164–169, 1985.

39. Hartrampf CR Jr, Bennett GK: Autogenous tissue reconstruction in the mastectomy patient: a critical review of 300 patients. Trans South Surg Assoc 98:70–81, 1986.

40. Harvey EB, Brinton LA: Second cancer following cancer of the breast in Connecticut, 1935–82. NCI Monogr 68:99–112, 1985.

41. Hicken NF: Mastectomy: clinical pathologic study demonstrating why most mastectomies result in incomplete removal of mammary gland. Arch Surg 40:6–14, 1940.

42. Hislop TG, Elwood JM, Coldman AJ, Spinelli JJ, Worth AJ, Ellison LG: Second primary cancers of the breast: incidence and risk factors. Br J Cancer 49:79–85, 1984.

43. Holleb AI, Montgomery R, Farrow JH: The hazard of incomplete simple mastectomy. Surg Gynecol Obstet 121:819–822, 1965.

44. Hoopes JE, Edgerton MT, Shelley W: Organic synthetics for augmentation mammoplasty: their relation to breast cancer. Plast Reconstr Surg 39:263–270, 1967.

45. Horn PL, Thompson WD: Risk of contralateral breast cancer: associations with histologic, clinical and therapeutic factors. Cancer 62:412–424, 1988.

46. Horn PL, Thompson WD, Schwartz SM: Factors associated with the risk of second primary breast cancer: an analysis of data from the Connecticut Tumor Registry. J Chron Dis 40:1003–1011, 1987.

47. Hutter RVP: The management of patients with lobular carcinoma in situ of the breast. Cancer 53:798–802, 1984.

48. Jacobson GM, Sause WT, Thomson JW, Plenk HP: Breast irradiation following silicone gel implants. Int J Radiat Oncol Biol Phys 12:835–838, 1986.

49. King RE, Terz JJ, Lawrence W Jr: Experience with opposite breast biopsy in patients with operable breast cancer. Cancer 37:43–45, 1976.

50. Kurtz JM, Amalric R, Brandone H, Ayme Y, Spitalier J-M: Results of wide excision for mammary recurrence after breast-conserving therapy. Cancer 61:1969–1972, 1988.

51. Kurtz JM, Spitalier J-M, Amalric R: Late recurrence after lumpectomy and irradiation. Int J Radiat Oncol Biol Phys 9:1191–1194, 1983.

52. Leis HP Jr: Bilateral breast cancer. Surg Clin North Am 58:833–841, 1978.

53. Leis HP Jr: Managing the remaining breast. Cancer 46:1026–1030, 1980.

54. Leis HP Jr, Urban JA: The other breast. In Gallager HS, Leis HP Jr, Snyderman RK, Urban JA (eds): The Breast. St Louis, CV Mosby, 1985, pp 487–496.

55. Lilla JA, Vistnes LM: Long-term study of reactions to various silicone breast implants in rabbits. Plast Reconstr Surg 57:637–649, 1976.

56. Lippman ME, Lichter AS, Danforth DN Jr: Diagnosis and Management of Breast Cancer. Philadelphia, WB Saunders, 1988, pp 312–325.

57. Marshall KA, Redfern A, Cady B: Local recurrence of carcinoma of the breast. Surg Gynecol Obstet 139:406–408, 1974.

58. Martin JK Jr, van Heerden JA, Gaffey TA: Synchronous and metachronous carcinoma of the breast. Surgery 91:12–16, 1982.

59. Mate TP, Carter D, Fischer DB, Hartman PV, McKhann C, Merino M, Prosnitz LR, Weissberg JB: A clinical and histopathologic analysis of the results of conservation surgery and radiation therapy in stage I and II breast cancer. Cancer 58:1995–2002, 1986.

60. McDivitt RW, Hutter RVP, Foote FW, Stewart FW: In situ lobular carcinoma: a prospective follow-up study indicating cumulative patient risks. JAMA 201:96–100, 1967.

61. McGrath MH, Burkhardt BR: The safety and efficacy of breast implants for augmentation mammoplasty. Plast Reconstr Surg 74:550–560, 1984.

62. Members of The Ludwig Breast Cancer Study Group: Prolonged disease-free survival after one course of perioperative adjuvant chemotherapy for node-negative breast cancer. N Engl J Med 320:491–496, 1989.

63. Mendenhall NP, Devine JW, Mendenhall WM, Bland KI, Million RR, Copeland EM: Isolated local-regional recurrence following mastectomy for adenocarcinoma of the breast treated with radiation therapy alone or combined with surgery and/or chemotherapy. Radiother Oncol 12:177–185, 1988.

64. Montague ED: Conservation surgery and radiation therapy in the treatment of operable breast cancer. Cancer 53:700–704, 1984.

65. Montague ED, Fletcher GH: Local regional effectiveness of surgery and radiation therapy in the treatment of breast cancer. Cancer 55:2266–2272, 1985.

66. Morgenstern L, Gleischman SH, Michel SL, Rosenberg JE, Knight I, Goodman D: Relation of free silicone to human breast cancer. Arch Surg 120:573–577, 1985.

67. Newman W: In situ lobular carcinoma of the breast: report of 26 women with 32 cancers. Ann Surg 157:591–599, 1963.

68. Nielsen M, Christensen L, Andersen JA: Contralateral cancerous breast lesions in women with clinical invasive breast carcinoma. Cancer 57:897–903, 1986.

69. Pawlias KT, Dockerty MB, Ellis FH: Late local recurrent carcinoma of the breast. Ann Surg 148:192–197, 1958.

70. Prior P, Waterhouse JAH: Incidence of bilateral tumours in a population-based series of breast cancer patients. I: Two approaches to an epidemiological analysis. Br J Cancer 37:620–634, 1978.

71. Recht A, Silver B, Schnitt S, Connolly J, Hellman S, Harris JR: Breast relapse following primary radiation therapy for early breast cancer. I. Classification, frequency and salvage. Int J Radiat Oncol Biol Phys 11:1271–1276, 1985.

72. Ringberg A, Palmer B, Linell F: The contralateral breast at reconstructive surgery after breast cancer operation—a histological study. Breast Cancer Res Treat 2:151–161, 1982.

73. Robbins GF, Berg JW: Bilateral primary breast cancers: a prospective clinicopathological study. Cancer 17:1501–1527, 1964.

74. Rosen PP: Lobular carcinoma in situ and intraductal carcinoma of the breast. In McDivitt RW, Oberman HA, Ozzello L, et al (eds): The Breast. Baltimore, Williams & Wilkins, 1984, pp 59–105.

75. Rosen PP, Braun DW, Lyngholm B, et al: Lobular carcinoma in situ of the breast: preliminary results of treatment by ipsilateral mastectomy and contralateral breast biopsy. Cancer 47:813–819, 1981.

76. Rosen PP, Lieberman PH, Braun DW, et al: Lobular carcinoma in situ of the breast: detailed analysis of 99 patients with average follow-up of 24 years. Am J Surg Pathol 3:225–251, 1978.

77. Rosen PP, Senie R, Schottenfeld D, Ashikari R: Noninvasive breast carcinoma: frequency of unsuspected invasion and implications for treatment. Ann Surg 189:377–382, 1979.

78. Sarrazin D, Monique LE, Rouesse J, Contesso G, Petit J-Y,

79. Schnitt SJ, Connolly JL, Harris JR, Hellman S, Cohen RB: Pathologic predictors of early local recurrence in stage I and II breast cancer treated by primary radiation therapy. Cancer 53:1049–1057, 1984.

80. Schnitt SJ, Connolly JL, Recht A, Silver B, Harris JR: Breast relapse following primary radiation therapy for early breast cancer: Detection, pathologic features and prognostic significance. Int J Radiat Oncol Biol Phys 11:1277–1284, 1985.

81. Schnitt SJ, Silen W, Sadowsky NL, Connolly JL, Harris JR: Current concepts: ductal carcinoma in situ (intraductal carcinoma) of the breast. N Engl J Med 318:898–903, 1988.

82. Shah JP, Urban JA: Full thickness chest wall resection for recurrent breast cancer involving the bony chest wall. Cancer 35:567–573, 1975.

83. Silverstein MJ, Handel N, Gamagami P, Waisman JR, Gierson ED, Rosser RJ, Steyskal R, Colburn W: Breast cancer in women after augmentation mammoplasty. Arch Surg 123:681–685, 1988.

84. Stabile RJ, Santoto E, Dispaltro F, San Filippo LJ: Reconstructive breast surgery following mastectomy and adjunctive radiation therapy. Cancer 45:2738–2743, 1980.

85. Urban JA: Bilaterality of cancer of the breast: biopsy of the opposite breast. Cancer 20:1867–1870, 1967.

86. Urban JA: Biopsy of the "normal" breast in treating breast cancer. Surg Clin North Am 49:291–301, 1969.

87. Urban JA, Papchristou D, Taylor J: Bilateral breast cancer: biopsy of the opposite breast. Cancer 40:1968–1973, 1977.

88. Wallgren A, Arner O, Bergstrom J, Blomstedt B, Granberg P-O, Raf L, Silfversward C, Einhorn J: Radiation therapy in operable breast cancer: results from the Stockholm trial on adjuvant radiotherapy. Int J Radiat Oncol Biol Phys 12:533–537, 1986.

89. Wanebo HJ, Senofsky GM, Fechner RE, Kaiser D, Lynn S, Paradies J: Bilateral breast cancer: risk reduction by contralateral biopsy. Trans South Surg Assoc 96:131–141, 1984.

90. Warner NE: Lobular carcinoma of the breast. Cancer 23:840–846, 1969.

91. Webber BL, Heise H, Neifeld JP, Costa J: Risk of subsequent contralateral breast carcinoma in a population of patients with in situ breast carcinoma. Cancer 47:2928–2932, 1981.

92. Wheeler E, Enterline JT, Roseman JM, Tomasulo JP, McIlvaine CH, Fitts WT Jr, Kirshenbaum J: Lobular carcinoma in situ of the breast: long-term follow-up. Cancer 34:544–563, 1974.

93. Whidden P: Augmentation mammoplasty. Transplant Implant Today 3:43–51, 1986.

94. Zaworski RE, DerHagopian RP: Locally recurrent carcinoma after breast reconstruction. Ann Plast Surg 3:326–329, 1979.

95. Zimmerman KW, Montague ED, Fletcher GH: Frequency, anatomical distribution and management of local recurrences after definitive therapy for breast cancer. Cancer 19:67–74, 1966.

Section XIX

Special Clinical Problems in Breast Cancer

Chapter 48

BILATERAL BREAST CARCINOMA

Arthur J. Donovan, M.D.

In 1800, Nisbett[20] reported a case of bilateral breast cancer. Kilgore[15] published a major study of the subject in 1921. Foote and Stewart,[9] in 1945, wrote an excellent review of the pathology of bilateral breast cancer. They are frequently quoted from that paper to the effect that "the most frequent antecedent of cancer of one breast is the history of having had cancer in the opposite breast." Robbins and Berg,[23] in 1964, published a detailed study of bilateral breast cancer. They estimated that, when compared with the risk in a patient without breast cancer, the diagnosis of cancer in one breast increased by a factor of five the risk of cancer in the opposite breast. The fact that cancer would affect both breasts is an obvious consequence of the fact that both breasts are presumably exposed to the same carcinogenic stimulus. Indeed, it is surprising that bilateral breast cancer is not more frequent.

The occurrence of bilateral breast cancer may be either synchronous or metachronous. Synchronous usually is defined as both cancers diagnosed at the same time. Admittedly, a second cancer detected shortly after the first was undoubtably present at the time of the initial diagnosis. In either synchronous or metachronous cancer, a distinction must be made between a second primary breast cancer and metastasis from one breast to the opposite breast. This distinction may not be easy. One could require that a diagnosis of bilateral primary breast cancer be accepted only if there is an arbitrarily defined disease-free interval between the detection of the tumor in the first and second breast. This is not a realistic requirement. Separate primary cancers of different histological types can occur synchronously. Conversely, soft tissue recurrence of breast cancer may only become manifest decades after the treatment of the initial tumor. A metastasis in the opposite breast can remain dormant for protracted periods. Furthermore, there are not absolute criteria to distinguish between a

second primary breast cancer and metastatic cancer. A different histological pattern in the tumors in the two breasts is extremely strong evidence for a double primary, but even this criterion is not absolute. Cancer of one breast may have differing pathological patterns in different areas of the same tumor mass or in multifocal areas of cancer in the same breast. The presence of *in situ* cancer within the cancer in the second breast is generally accepted as strong evidence of a second primary. Metastatic cancers are more likely to be in adipose tissue at the periphery of the breast or in the axillary tail. Metastatic tumors are less likely to be stellate and are irregularly infiltrative of breast tissue. All authorities would agree that direct presternal tracking of tumor from the first breast to the second breast establishes the tumor in the second breast to be an extension of the first. If metastases are present other than in the axillary nodes, the tumor in the second breast is usually arbitrarily considered metastatic rather than primary. Series of cases reported as bilateral primary breast cancer undoubtedly include instances of metastasis to the second breast, and cases excluded from series as metastatic are probably in some instances primary.

The criteria stated by Chaudary et al.[5] are generally consistent with these findings and include the following:

"1. The demonstration of *in situ* change in the contralateral tumour was considered absolute proof that the contralateral lesion was a primary tumour.

2. The tumour in the second breast was considered to be a new primary if it was histologically different in type from the cancer in the first breast.

3. The carcinoma in the second breast was considered to be a new primary if its degree of histological differentiation was distinctly greater than that of the lesion in the first breast.

4. In the absence of definite histological difference, a carcinoma in the breast was considered to be compatible

with an independent lesion provided there was no evidence of local, regional, or distant metastases from the cancer in the ipsilateral breast."

McSweeny and Egan[19] have noted that the mammographic patterns may be significantly different between a primary and a metastatic tumor of the breast. A metastatic tumor tends to be more diffuse, to be associated with edema of the breast, to lack the fine calcifications characteristic of primary cancer, and to be a more circumscribed mass. A metastatic tumor is radiologically less likely to have fingerlike projections into surrounding breast tissue than is a typical infiltrating cancer.

The patient is given the benefit of the doubt. The tumor in the second breast is assumed to be a second primary unless there is direct tracking from one breast to the other or distant metastases are present. The tumor in the second breast is treated on the assumption that the tumor may not only be controlled locally, but that long-term survival can occur. This is in contrast to the dismal long-term prognosis when mastectomy from breast cancer is followed by recurrence in the operative field.

In the discussions that follow, reference to bilateral breast cancer will refer to separate primary cancers. The diagnosis and treatment of metastatic cancer will not be considered, nor will recurrent cancer in the same breast following wide local excision with or without radiation therapy to the breast. Metastatic cancer in the opposite breast will be treated by the modalities available for soft tissue recurrence—primarily radiation therapy and chemotherapy. These therapies are thoroughly discussed elsewhere in this text.

RISK FACTORS

Several factors other than breast cancer itself increase the likelihood that a second primary cancer will occur in the opposite breast. Multifocal areas of cancer in one breast are believed by some to be predictive of an increased risk of cancer in the opposite breast.[17, 18, 23] Certainly, initial diagnosis at a favorable pathological stage and a premenopausal age[1] and long survival increase the risk.[23] Fisher and associates[7] from the National Surgical Breast Adjuvant Project, in a careful study of more than 1000 women with breast cancer followed for 10 years, reported an increased risk of bilateral disease with original cancers greater than 2 cm in diameter, invasive or in situ lobular cancer, or tubular cancer. None of these features obtained a relative risk of greater than two or occasionally three times that of other women with breast cancer. Two factors that warrant special consideration are lobular carcinoma in situ (lobular neoplasia) and a family history of breast cancer.

Lobular Carcinoma *In Situ*

Lobular carcinoma in situ (LCIS) in one breast is an established risk factor for bilateral breast cancer. The

process was described by Foote and Stewart[8] in 1941. Haagensen et al.[11] prefer the term "lobular neoplasia" as signifying that this lesion is a harbinger of cancer elsewhere in the breasts but is rather innocuous in itself. The term "lobular carcinoma in situ" is the one more widely employed. The pathology and treatment of LCIS are discussed in detail in chapters 8 and 35.

Lobular carcinoma in situ may be detected on biopsy of a palpable mass that is itself a benign process. A mass rarely consists solely of LCIS. LCIS may be present in tissue removed by a needle-directed excisional biopsy of a mammographically detected lesion, such as an area of stippled calcification, or may be present adjacent to an infiltrating ductal or lobular breast cancer. Multiple foci will be present in the same breast in more than half of the cases.[13, 28] Synchronous random biopsy of the other breast of women with a diagnosis of LCIS often documents the same process in the opposite breast. The frequency of synchronous bilateral LCIS varies in different studies. Cases detected prior to, synchronous with, and following the diagnosis of infiltrative or other in situ cancer are often combined as a percentage of incidence. Urban et al.[29] have had the greatest experience with random contralateral biopsy in women with breast cancer. They report on noninfiltrative cancer in the opposite breast but do not distinguish between intraductal cancer and LCIS. Wanebo et al.[30] reported that among seven cases of LCIS subject to synchronous random contralateral biopsy, three patients had bilateral LCIS. Rosen[24] has estimated that when the first breast shows only LCIS, the risk of concurrent LCIS in the opposite breast by random biopsy is approximately one in three, and whole organ sections might increase the yield to two of three cases.

Approximately 25 percent of patients with a diagnosis of LCIS will subsequently develop invasive cancer.[10, 11] Both the breast in which the diagnosis of LCIS is initially made and the opposite breast are at almost equal risk—ten to 15 percent each. Haagensen's data as to risk of cancer in the ipsilateral and contralateral breast of a cohort of women with LCIS are reproduced in Table 48–1. Interestingly, only about half of the overt cancers that develop in the opposite breast will be invasive lobular carcinoma.[6] The remainder will be other types, predominantly infiltrating ductal cancer. Although the diagnosis of lobular carcinoma in situ in one breast is a marker for high risk for development of invasive carcinoma in the same or the opposite breast, the interval between the original diagnosis and the development of overt cancer may be prolonged. The mean disease-free interval is probably ten to 15 years.

Family History

The significance of a family history of breast cancer can be considered in two ways relative to bilateral breast cancer. Does bilateral breast cancer increase the risk of breast cancer in relatives of such a patient, or is bilateral breast cancer more frequent in women with a family history of breast cancer? In published discussions, these

Table 48–1. THE INTERVAL AFTER THE DIAGNOSIS OF LOBULAR NEOPLASIA RELATED TO THE DEVELOPMENT OF AN INITIAL CARCINOMA* (Columbia-Presbyterian)

Interval in Years After Diagnosis of Lobular Neoplasia	Breasts with Lobular Neoplasia Not Amputated			Contralateral Breasts		
	Number of Breasts at Risk	*Numbers of Carcinomas Developing During Interval*	*Cumulative Probability of Carcinoma by End of Interval (%)*	*Number of Breasts at Risk*	*Number of Carcinomas Developing During Interval*	*Cumulative Probability of Carcinoma by End of Interval (%)*
0–1	280	0	0	276	3	1
1–2	272	2	1	268	1	1
2–3	269	2	1	267	3	3
3–4	266	5	3	263	1	3
4–5	261	1	4	262	7	6
6–10	253	9	8	246	4	7
11–15	173	6	12	183	1	8
16–20	10	6	18	122	4	12
21–25	59	1	19	66	1	14
26–35	32	0	19	32	2	23
36–47	8	0	—	8	0	—

*Twelve patients have been excluded. Two had no follow-up and ten had carcinoma in one breast prior to the diagnosis of lobular neoplasia in the other breast.

From Bodian C, Haagensen CD: *In* Haagensen CD (ed): Diseases of the Breast, ed 3. Philadelphia, WB Saunders, 1986. Reprinted by permission.

two questions often become confused. In the discussion that follows it must be remembered that the relationship of a family history of breast cancer to the overall risk of breast cancer is not the subject under consideration, but rather the relationship of a family history of breast cancer to bilateral breast cancer.

Anderson and Badzioch[3] report the lifetime risk of breast cancer by age 70 to be 28 percent if a women at age 30 has two sisters with breast cancer, one of whom has bilateral disease, and 14 percent if neither sister has bilateral disease. These observations support the belief that bilateral breast cancer may increase the risk of breast cancer in first degree relatives. Fisher and associates[7] found that a family history of breast cancer doubled the risk for bilateral cancer but was not statistically significant beyond 1.5 percent per year, as compared with an incidence of slightly less than one percent for women without a family history of breast cancer. Adami and colleagues[2] noted a six percent incidence of bilateral disease in "familial" cases and five percent in "nonfamilial" cases, which does not support family history as a risk factor for bilateral disease. Harris et al.[12] studied the risk of bilateral breast cancer in patients with familial disease defined as two first degree relatives with breast cancer. They state that the risk was three times greater than that in an unselected population. The cumulative risk at 20 years for a second primary is stated as 37.1 percent. They actually only report 21 second primaries among 198 patients at risk, or an 11 percent incidence of bilateral primary breast cancer.[12] Ottman et al.[21] reported that 26.8 percent of patients younger than 50 years with bilateral cancer had a family history of breast cancer, compared with 7.1 percent of patients with unilateral cancer. These findings are contrary to those of Fisher et al.[7] and Adami et al.[2] Additionally, Ottman et al. observed that sisters of patients diagnosed before age 50 with bilateral disease had a five times greater risk for development of breast cancer than did

sisters of patients with unilateral disease. A review of these sometimes conflicting reports leads to the conclusion that, most probably, a family history of breast cancer is not as important as bilateral breast cancer in predicting an increased risk of breast cancer in first degree relatives.

INCIDENCE

Reports on the incidence of bilateral breast cancer vary significantly, reflecting a number of factors. Mammography of the opposite breast at the time of diagnosis of breast cancer has increased the rate of early detection of synchronous cancer in the opposite breast, either invasive or noninvasive.[5] Varying age at initial diagnosis and varying lengths of follow-up in reported series have a major impact on the reported incidence of bilaterality.

A woman whose breast cancer is diagnosed at an early age and who has prolonged disease-free survival has a greater number of years of exposure to whatever factors are responsible for breast cancer. With increasing years of survival, there is an increasing risk of development of cancer in the opposite breast. Chaudary et al.[5] report a threefold increased risk of bilateral cancer for women whose first cancer was diagnosed before the age of 40 as compared with women diagnosed after age 40. Adami and associates[1] calculated the risk of bilateral breast cancer as 13.3 percent if the first cancer occurred before age 50 and 3.5 percent if the first tumor was detected after age 50. The data that are the basis for these calculations are summarized in Table 48–2. Bodian and Haagensen[4] summarized their own data along with those from studies by Hankey and associates and Prior and Waterhouse, all of which showed a similar effect of age at diagnosis of a first breast cancer on risk of a second breast cancer. Table 48–3 shows their results. Women whose first breast cancer is diagnosed post-

Table 48–2. CALCULATED CUMULATIVE RISK OF BILATERAL DISEASE BY AGE AT FIRST DIAGNOSIS

Age at First Diagnosis	Incidence Unilateral (a)	Incidence Bilateral (b)	Cumulative Risk: Percent b/a
<40	52	5	9.6
40–49	166	24	14.5
50–59	243	10	4.1
60–69	347	16	4.6
70–79	319	8	2.5
80+	158	3	1.9
Total	1285	66	5.1

From Adami HO, Bergstron R, Hansen J.: Cancer 55:643–647, 1985. Reprinted by permission.

menopausally have a lower incidence of bilateral breast cancer.

Robbins and Berg[23] estimated that the risk of development of clinically overt cancer in the opposite breast was approximately one percent per year. A risk of slightly less than one percent has been reported by Fisher and investigators of the NSABP.[7] The incidence was greatest in the first year after initial treatment. Currently, the absolute risk is approximately five to seven cases per 1000 women at risk per year.[5] The risk is quite constant for approximately 20 years of follow-up and then gradually falls. Bodian and Haagensen[4] summarized a number of published reports of absolute risk; their data are reproduced as Table 48–4. The generally reported incidence of synchronous bilateral primary breast cancer is in the range of one to two percent,[27] and the reported incidence of metachronous clinically overt cancer varies from one to 12 percent. This wide range reflects, at the least, variable age at first diagnosis, variable duration of follow-up, and variable criteria for the diagnosis of primary and metastatic cancer in the opposite breast. Wanebo et al.'s[30] report of a seven percent incidence of metachronous bilateral primary breast cancer is representative. They summarized the incidence of bilateral cancer in reported series that was 3.7 percent among 22,563 cases, with 29 percent synchronous and 71 percent metachronous. Data from this study are reproduced in Table 48–5. The incidence by years of follow-up as reported by Robbins and Berg[23] is depicted in Figure 48–1.

In 1969, Urban[28] reported a 14 percent incidence of bilateral breast cancer. among 488 cases, with 10 percent of these synchronous. Two thirds of the cases were noninfiltrating and included those detected by random biopsy of the opposite breast at the time of initial diagnosis of breast cancer. Urban[29] further reported in 1977 on 954 biopsies of the opposite breast at the time of initial treatment of 1204 patients with breast cancer. In 653 patients (68 percent), there were positive or suspicious findings on mammography or physical examination; the biopsy was not random. Infiltrating cancer was found in 50 cases and noninfiltrating cancer in 46 cases. Among 301 truly random biopsies, there were

five infiltrating and 18 noninfiltrating cancers. The combined incidence of infiltrating bilateral cancers detected by clinically indicated or synchronous random biopsy was six percent; the incidence for truly random biopsy was 1.6 percent.

The difference between the reported incidence of clinically overt synchronous bilateral breast cancer and that detected by random biopsy of the opposite breast or by serial sectioning of the breast is most notable and requires comment. The highest incidence of simultaneous bilateral breast cancer detected by random breast biopsy has been established by the studies of Urban.[28, 29] He adopted a policy of biopsy of the opposite breast when the diagnosis of breast cancer was made; these results have just been discussed. Wanebo et al.[30] reported a series of 62 synchronous contralateral biopsies. Seven cancers were diagnosed based on purely random biopsy without clinical or radiological indication and another six by indicated biopsy. Only three of the 13 were invasive lesions. King and colleagues[14] performed random biopsy of the opposite breast in 109 women without clinical indication. These investigators detected four noninvasive lesions and one invasive lesion; the latter had been suspected by mammography. They abandoned the practice of random biopsy as unrewarding.

Reports of a much higher incidence of cancer on pathological studies of random biopsy than are identified on the basis of mammography, physical examination, or during long-term follow-up raise the question as to whether a number of these histologically identified cancers are indeed nonthreatening in the biological sense and would not develop clinical significance in the patient's lifetime. Many are noninvasive. Indeed, there is no firm evidence as to how many patients in whom a

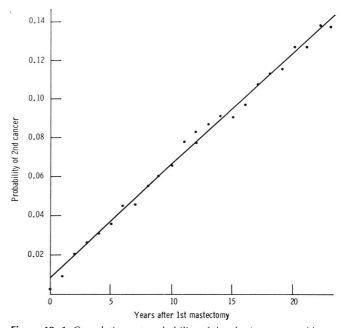

Figure 48–1. Cumulative net probability of developing a second breast cancer (other causes for removal from series have been corrected). (From Robbins GF, Berg JW: Cancer 17:1501–1527, 1964. Reprinted by permission.)

Table 48–3. NUMBER OF CASES AND RELATIVE RISK OF A PRIMARY CARCINOMA OF THE SECOND BREAST BY AGE AT INITIAL CARCINOMA OF THE BREAST

Age at Initial Carcinoma	Prior and Waterhouse (Birmingham, England, 1936–64)*			Hankey et al. (State of Conn't 1935–75)†			Columbia Presbyterian Medical Center, New York (Author's Case Series)					
	Number of Cases		Relative Risk	Number of Cases		Relative Risk	Private Patients (1936–79)			Clinic Patients (1935–66)		
							Number of Cases		Relative Risk	Number of Cases		Relative Risk
	Observed	Expected	Obs./Exp.	Observed	Expected	Obs./Exp.	Observed	Expected	Obs./Exp.	Observed	Expected	Obs./Exp.
Less than 40	42	5.13	8.2 } 5.3	430	75.1	5.7	19	2.53	7.5 } 5.9	4	1.04	3.9 } 5.6
40–44	47	11.70	4.0				26	5.15	5.0	11	1.64	6.7
45–49	66	18.36	3.6 } 3.4	454	127.6	3.6	24	7.44	3.2 } 3.2	2	1.35	1.5 } 0.9
50–54	52	16.37	3.2				24	7.46	3.2	1	2.01	0.5
55–59	37	16.51	2.2				15	6.46	2.3	0	1.08	—
60–64	18	17.83	1.1 } 1.3	660	277.9	2.4	9	4.17	2.2 } 2.3	2	1.30	1.5 } 1.3
65–69	25	16.90	1.5				11	3.77	2.9	1	1.81	0.6
70 and over	23	28.96	0.8				10	5.20	1.9	4	1.23	3.3
Total	310	131.76	2.4	1544	480.6	3.2	138	42.18	3.3	25	11.46	2.2

*Prior P, Waterhouse JAH: Br J Cancer 37:620, 1978.
†Hankey BF, et al.: J Natl Cancer Inst 70:797, 1983.
From Bodian C, Haagensen CD: *In* Haagensen CD (ed): Diseases of the Breast, 3rd ed. Philadelphia, WB Saunders, 1986. Reprinted by permission.

Table 48–4. BILATERAL CARCINOMA OF THE BREAST: PERCENT OF CASES WITH SIMULTANEOUS PRIMARY BILATERAL CARCINOMA AND AVERAGE ANNUAL RISK OF DEVELOPING SUBSEQUENT PRIMARY CARCINOMA OF THE SECOND BREAST (SUMMARY OF PUBLISHED REPORTS)

Author	Source of Data	Year of Initial Carcinoma	Total Number Primary Cases	Simultaneous Bilateral		Number Unilateral Cases with Follow-up	Maximum Years of Follow-up	Patient-Years at Risk	Number Bilateral Cases	Average Annual Risk per 1000	Trend over Period
				Number	Percent						
Hubbard (1955)	Minnesota University Hospitals	1932–39	267	3	1.1	264	9	1,540.5	9	5.8	Not stated
Robbins and Berg (1964)	New York Memorial Hospital	1940–43	1,458	4	0.3	1,454	24	12,818.0	87	6.8	Constant
Schottenfeld and Berg (1971)	New York Memorial and J. Ewing Hospitals	1949–62	9,792	58	0.6	9,734	13	Not stated	248	6.1	Not stated
Slack et al. (1973)	Various U.S. locations— Patients entered in NSABP	1961–68	—	—	—	2,734	6	12,217	52	4.3	Decline after 3 years
Veronesi et al. (1974)	Milan National Cancer Institute	1928–65	6,986	45	0.6	6,941	Not stated	43,612	189	4.3	Not stated
Schoenberg† (1977)	Connecticut—All primary cases	1935–64	18,010	101	0.6	17,909	30	96,934.9	596	6.1	Not stated
Sakamoto et al. (1978)	Tokyo—Cancer Institute Tokyo	1946–75	3,365	12	0.4	3,353	18	23,406	80	3.4	Constant
Donegan and Spratt (1979)	Missouri—Ellis Fischel State Cancer Hospital	1940–65 1940–58	2,620 711	52 7	2.0 1.0	704	7	2,727.5	14	5.1	Constant
Prior and Waterhouse (1978)	Birmingham, England Cancer Registry	1936–64	21,967	89	0.4	21,878	29	91,233	310	3.4	Constant
Hankey et al. (1983)	Connecticut Tumor Registry	1935–75	—	—	—	27,175	N.S.‡	217,200	1,544	7.1	Not stated

*Radical mastectomy patients only.
†These data presumably included in Hankey et al. (1983).
‡N.S. = not stated.
From Bodian C, Haagensen CD: *In* Haagensen CD (ed): Diseases of the Breast, ed 3. Philadelphia, WB Saunders, 1986. Reprinted by permission.

Table 48–5. OCCURRENCE OF BILATERAL BREAST CANCER (SYNCHRONOUS AND METACHRONOUS) AND INTERVAL BETWEEN THE PRIMARY AND SECOND CANCER

Author	Bilateral Cancer/ Total Patients	Synchronous Cancer Patients	Metachronous Patients	Interval Between First and Second Cancer
Al-Jurf (Univ. of Iowa,* 1981)	104/5608	26	78	123 months
P. Burns (Alberta, UK, 1981)	66/1351	3	63	10 years
S. Schell (M.D. Anderson, 1981)	106/2231	48	58	7 months to 10 years
Stage I/II Br Ca Bailey (St. George, England, 1980)	39/911	17	22	5 years, 8 months
J. Buls (Melbourne, 1976)	76/NS	21	55	Majority, 5 years
H. Kesseler (NYU/Columbia, 1976)	35/967	17	18	Unknown
E. Lewison (Johns Hopkins, 1971)	42/490	8	34	6 Years
C. McLaughlin (Univ. Nebraska)	38/475	NS	NS	Majority, 5 years
N. Slack (Nat. Surg. Adj.) Stage I/II Br Ca	52/2734	0	52	1 to 67 months
J. Hermann (NYMC, 1973)	31/418	3	28	6.3 years
J. Devitt (Ottawa, 1970)	28/1530	17	11	NS
J. Farrow (Memorial NY, 1957)	202/5576	21	18	5 to 10 years
T. Hubbard (Minnesota, 1952)	17/272	0	17	Majority, 5 years
Total	836/22563 (3.7%)	81 (29%)	454 (71%)	

NS = not stated.
From Wanebo HJ, et al: Ann Surg 201:667–677, 1985. Reprinted by permission.

microscopic focus of noninvasive cancer is detected in the opposite breast by random biopsy will, without further treatment, develop overt bilateral breast cancer.

DETECTION

Efforts at detection should include all women with proven breast cancer, with particular attention to those in a high-risk group, such as women with LCIS and a family history, particularly of bilateral breast cancer. Cancer in the second breast can be detected by physical examination, mammography, or random biopsy. The traditional technique for detection has been meticulous physical examination of the breast performed at regular intervals after the original detection of breast cancer and repeated for the remainder of the patient's life. The fact that survival for decades does not eliminate risk establishes that there is no reason for complacency, even after prolonged survival.

The development of mammography and its increased diagnostic sensitivity has provided another method for detection of bilateral breast cancer. When a cancer of one breast is suspected or proven, a mammogram is performed on the opposite breast to identify a covert synchronous cancer. The second cancer may be identified either in the form of a "gathering" or as an area of stippled calcification. The cancer may be either invasive or noninvasive. Periodic mammography, at least annually, should be performed in the follow-up of patients with a diagnosis of breast cancer. A metachronous tumor may be detected before it is apparent on physical examination.

McSweeny and Egan[19] previously reported that when mammography was employed, 27.2 percent of bilateral cancer was detected synchronously. Furthermore, there was a concurrent reduction in the incidence of metachronous cancer. Although mammography has not altered the reported incidence of bilateral breast cancer, the percent of the total that are synchronous and noninvasive has increased.[19]

Chaudary et al.[5] reported a fivefold increase in the incidence of synchronous bilateral cancer after introduction of routine mammography. Sears and associates[25] report a similar increase in incidence of synchronous diagnosis attributed to use of xeroradiography. These data would suggest that mammography has a significant role in the detection of minimal ($<$ 1 cm) cancer in the opposite breast, whether invasive or noninvasive, and at a time when the prognosis is highly favorable (i.e., at an earlier clinical and pathological stage).

Senofsky and colleagues[26] compared stage of disease and methods for detection of the second breast cancer in patients with a careful follow-up program that included physical examination and periodic mammography. These patients were compared to historical controls followed only by physical examination. Among 33 cases diagnosed before mammography, 15.2 percent were synchronous, as compared with 28.1 percent diagnosed with mammography. The very favorable impact of routine mammography on early stage of disease of the

second cancer is summarized in Table 48–6. Nevertheless, despite routine follow-up mammography, approximately one fourth of the tumors that developed in the opposite breast were identified by the patients on self-examination.

The subject of random biopsy in detection of cancer in the opposite breast has already been discussed. Such a policy has not been widely adopted in the majority of clinics because of the low yield of invasive cancer and the reasonably satisfactory results of treatment of a metachronous second cancer, which will be discussed in the next section.

TREATMENT

If the physician concludes after consultation with pathologists and consideration of all factors involved that the patient does indeed have a bilateral synchronous or metachronous primary breast cancer, both breast cancers should be treated with intent to "cure." This policy is pursued in the absence of metastases beyond the breasts and axillae or demonstrable presternal tracking.

Pack[22] concluded that the higher incidence of cancer in the opposite breast justified prophylactic removal of the second breast. Leis[16, 17] studied this problem over a number of years and recommended prophylactic mastectomy in patients with selected indications. These indications included a family history of breast cancer, multifocal cancer in the first breast, and age less than 50 years with favorable stage I breast cancer (i.e., a tumor less than 1 cm in diameter and histological types such as noninvasive cancer or colloid, medullary, tubular, or comedocarcinoma). There has not been a randomized study or, indeed, a convincing nonrandomized study that has established a benefit in survival for patients subjected to prophylactic mastectomy. Advantages in survival that are cited are based largely on probabilities. Leis,[16] in one report of 91 cases of prophylactic mastectomy, cited a 17 percent incidence of unsuspected cancer, of which two thirds were noninfiltrative.

The fact that more than 90 percent of women with cancer of one breast will not develop clinically overt

Table 48–6. FAVORABLE IMPACT OF MAMMOGRAPHY ON THE EARLY DETECTION OF BILATERAL BREAST CANCER (SYNCHRONOUS AND METACHRONOUS)

	Synchronous (%)	Metachronous (%)
I (BEM)	15.2	84.8
II (AEM)	28.1	71.9
	39.5*	60.5*

*Includes blind contralateral biopsy.

Abbreviations: AEM; after effective mammography; BEM; before effective mammography.

From Senofsky GM, et al: Cancer, 57:597–602, 1986. Reprinted by permission.

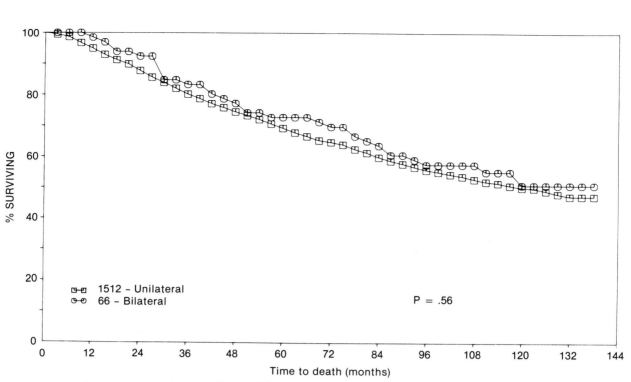

Figure 48–2. Survival of patients with unilateral and bilateral breast cancers. (From Fisher ER, et al: Cancer 54:3002–3011, 1984. Reprinted by permission.)

cancer of the opposite breast has led to reluctance on the part of surgeons to perform prophylactic mastectomy. One exception may be the case of a young woman with an early stage cancer in one breast and a family history of breast cancer in more than one first degree relative, particularly if one of these relatives had bilateral breast cancer (see section V, chapter 13). In such a patient, dense mammary dysplasia that would make both mammography and physical examination less reliable would be an additional consideration.

These are, in my opinion, two logical recommendations for treatment of LCIS. Based on the increased risk for subsequent invasive breast cancer that is almost equal in either breast, bilateral mastectomy can be advised or, conversely, careful follow-up with regular physical examination and mammography. Haagensen,[11] who certainly cannot be accused of antisurgical bias or a conservative surgical attitude in the treatment of breast cancer, favors the latter alternative for LCIS. This judgment is based on favorable prognosis when the cancer is detected and treated, the long interval that may occur before development of the cancer, and his conclusion that bilateral mastectomy is too radical an approach when a focus of LCIS is detected in the breast. Further discussion of treatment of LCIS is included in section XIII, chapter 35.

Invasive primary cancer of the opposite breast, whether synchronous or metachronous, should be treated by the methods discussed in section X, chapter 29. The treatment planned and magnitude of the operation will depend on the stage of disease.

Thus the treatment of the patient with a diagnosis of

cancer in one breast and who is at risk for bilateral breast cancer remains one of careful observation, with physical examination at intervals of at least every 3 months during the first 3 years following initial treatment. Thereafter, physician evaluation is continued every 6 months until 5 years have elapsed, and yearly thereafter. The patient should also have at least annual mammography and should be instructed in the techniques for self-examination of the breast. If a second primary cancer is detected, treatment should be as appropriate for stage of disease.

PROGNOSIS

The prognosis for the patient with bilateral breast cancer is quite favorable. That such would be true after appropriate treatment of bilateral noninvasive cancer would be expected. In a women with invasive cancer in one breast and *in situ* cancer in the other, the prognosis depends on the stage of the invasive cancer. Numerous studies have shown that survival after treatment of a second invasive breast cancer is dependent on the stage of the disease at the time of diagnosis of both cancers.[10] A graph depicting survival from the report by Fisher and associates[7] of the NSABP is shown in Figure 48–2. Although overall survival was the same for patients with bilateral and unilateral cancer, the survival in bilateral cases diagnosed within 2 years of the first cancer was less favorable—35 percent vs. 70 percent. Obviously, a patient whose disease-free interval is less than 2 years following treatment of the first cancer is at much greater risk of death from the first cancer than a patient who has survived the first cancer for greater than 5 or 10 years before developing a second cancer. Fracchia and associates,[10] from Memorial Sloan-Kettering, reported on survival after treatment in 403 patients with bilateral breast cancer. With bilateral noninvasive disease, there was no recurrence. With invasive disease in one breast and noninvasive disease in the other breast, cancer-free survival was dependent on the stage of the invasive cancer. The 5-year survival in patients with bilateral invasive disease was 60 percent for synchronous disease and 54 percent for metachronous disease.

References

1. Adami HO, Bergstron R, Hansen J: Age at first primary as a determinant of the incidence of bilateral breast cancer. Cancer 55:643–647, 1985.
2. Adami HO, Hansen J, Jung B, Rimsten A: Characteristics of familial breast cancer in Sweden: absence of relation to age and unilateral versus bilateral disease. Cancer 48:1688–1695, 1981.
3. Anderson DE, Badzioch MD: Risk of familial breast cancer. Cancer 56:383–387, 1985.
4. Bodian C, Haagensen CD: Bilateral carcinoma of the breast. *In* Haagensen CD (ed): Diseases of the Breast, ed 3. Philadelphia, WB Saunders, 1986.
5. Chaudary MA, Millis RR, Hoskins EOL, Halder M, Bulbrook RD, Cuzick J, Hayward J: Bilateral primary breast cancer: a prospective study of disease incidence. Br J Surg 71:711–714, 1984.
6. Davis N, Baird RM: Breast cancer in association with lobular carcinoma in situ. Clinicopathologic review and treatment recommendation. Am J Surg 147:641–645, 1984.
7. Fisher ER, Fisher B, Sass R, Wickerham L: Pathologic findings from the National Surgical Adjuvant Breast Project (protocol no. 4). XI. Bilateral breast cancer. Cancer 54:3002–3011, 1984.
8. Foote FW, Stewart FW: Lobular carcinoma in situ: a rare form of mammary cancer. Am J Pathol 17:491–495, 1941.
9. Foote FW Jr, Stewart FW: Comparative studies of cancerous versus noncancerous breasts. Ann Surg 121:197–222, 1945.
10. Fracchia A, Robinson D, Legaspi A, Greenall MJ, Kinne DW, Groshen S: Survival in bilateral breast cancer. Cancer 55:1414–1421, 1985.
11. Haagensen CD, Lane N, Lattes R, Bodian C: Lobular neoplasia (so-called lobular carcinoma in situ) of the breast. Cancer 42:737–769, 1978.
12. Harris RE, Lynch HT, Guirgis HA: Familial breast cancer: risk to the contralateral breast. J Natl Cancer Inst 60:955–960, 1978.
13. Hutter RVP: The management of patients with lobular carcinoma in situ of the breast. Cancer 53:798–802, 1984.
14. King RE, Terz JJ, Lawrence W Jr: Experience with opposite breast biopsy in patients with operable breast cancer. Cancer 37:43–45, 1976.
15. Kilgore AR: The incidence of cancer in the second breast. JAMA 7:454–457, 1921.
16. Leis HP Jr: Selective elective prophylactic contralateral mastectomy. Cancer 28:956–961, 1971.
17. Leis HP Jr, Mersheimer WL, Black MM, De Chabon A: The second breast. NY J Med 65:2460–2468, 1965.
18. Lesser ML, Rosen PP, Kinne DW: Multicentricity and bilaterality in invasive breast carcinoma. Surgery 91:234–240, 1982.
19. McSweeney MB, Egan RL: Bilateral breast carcinoma. Cancer Res 90:41–48, 1984.
20. Nisbett U: A case of the cause of cancer of both breasts, the one ulcerated the other schirrous. Med Phys J 4:296–298, 1800.
21. Ottman R, Pike MC, King MC, Casagrande JT, Henderson BE: Familial breast cancer in a population-based series. Am J Epidemiol 123:15–21, 1986.
22. Pack GT: Argument for bilateral mastectomy. (Editorial) Surgery 29:929–931, 1951.
23. Robbins GF, Berg JW: Bilateral primary breast cancers. A prospective clinicopathological study. Cancer 17:1501–1527, 1964.
24. Rosen PP: Lobular carcinoma in situ and intraductal carcinoma of the breast. Mongr Pathol 25:59–105, 1984.
25. Sears HF, Janus C, McDermott A, Grotzinger P: Bilateral breast carcinoma: prospective evaluation of factors assisting diagnosis. J Surg Oncol 32:203–207, 1986.
26. Senofsky GM, Wanebo HJ, Wilhelm MC, Pope TL Jr, Fechner RE, Broaddus W, Kaiser DL: Has monitoring of the contralateral breast improved the prognosis in patients treated for primary breast cancer? Cancer 57:597–602, 1986.
27. Slack NH, Bross IDJ, Nemoto T, Fisher B: Experiences with bilateral primary carcinoma of the breast. Surg Gynecol Obstet 136:433–440, 1973.
28. Urban JA: Bilateral breast cancer. Cancer 24:1310–1313, 1969.
29. Urban JA, Papachristou D, Taylor J: Bilateral breast cancer. Biopsy of the opposite breast. Cancer 40:1968–1973, 1977.
30. Wanebo HJ, Senofsky GM, Fechner RE, Kaiser D, Lynn S, Paradies J: Bilateral breast cancer. Risk reduction of contralateral biopsy. Ann Surg 201:667–677, 1985.

Chapter 49

CANCER OF THE MALE BREAST

Morton C. Wilhelm, M.D. and Harold J. Wanebo, M.D.

Cancer of the male breast is a rare disease, accounting for less than one percent of cancer in males as well as less than one percent of all breast cancer. Although the first description of male breast cancer was made by an English surgeon, John of Aderne, in 1307 and was followed subsequently by case reports by such notables as Ambroise Paré and Fabricius Hildanus in the sixteenth and seventeenth centuries,[31] large series were not reported until well into the twentieth century.

Male breast cancer occurred in approximately 0.7 percent of the cases of breast cancer in the United States in 1987.[27] This incidence has changed little over the past 20 years.[12] In Manchester, England, a 0.7 percent incidence was reported, unchanged from the previous report in 1977.[21a] Higher rates are reported in blacks, including 2.4 percent among West Africans in the report by Ajayi et al.[1] and a three percent incidence in black males by Nirmul et al.[19] An unusually high incidence is reported in Zambia, where 15 percent of all breast cancer is in males.[18] In Virginia, there is a disproportionately higher percentage of male breast cancer in black males (24 percent) in comparison with black females (16 percent).[33]

Male breast cancer presents at an older age than that found in females, with the average age at presentation being 63.6 years. It is quite rare in young males, with only seven cases reported in patients younger than 26 years.[24] A higher incidence of breast cancer has been reported among Jewish males and is suggested by a higher rate in Israel than in the United States.[29] Information regarding familial incidence is sparse.[4, 8, 23] Bilateral breast cancer in males occurs in about two percent of all cases.

Testicular hormonal factors appear to have a prominent role in male breast cancer.[2] There is a twentyfold increased incidence of Klinefelter's syndrome in male breast cancer patients, and recent information suggests a breast cancer risk of three percent among males with Klinefelter's syndrome.[10] The complication of mumps infection in males 20 years of age or older carries an increased risk of breast cancer, though other viral infections do not impart an increased risk.[18] A history of infectious orchitis was found in eight percent of 53 males with breast cancer, in contrast to only two percent with gynecomastia and none in colon cancer patients.[26] Although clinical gynecomastia has been observed in as-

sociation with male breast cancer in some series (these are largely uncontrolled data), microscopic gynecomastia was identified in 42 percent of male breast cancer cases by Heller et al.[13] and 27 percent by Scheike et al.[25b] There is no histological evidence of progression from gynecomastia to cancer, however, as gynecomastia is fairly common in normal adult males and little convincing evidence relates gynecomastia to male breast cancer.[3]

Occupational hazards may exert an effect. A review of the occupations of males with breast cancer show a higher frequency of chronic work exposure to heat in steel mills, blast furnaces, and rolling mills, which suggests that increased environmental temperatures may have a suppressive effect on testicular function, possibly potentiating the development of breast cancer.[18]

The significance of estrogens in male breast cancer has been considered. An increase urinary excretion of estrogen has been reported in male breast cancer patients by Dao et al.,[5] although this is denied by Ribeirio,[21a] who analyzed endogenous hormonal profiles in 31 male breast cancer patients and found no significant difference from controls. In his study, though there were modest but not significant increases in estradiol-17β and testosterone ($p = 0.11$), there were more distinctive increases in luteinizing hormone (LH) and follicle-stimulating hormone (FSH) ($p = 0.06$). More study is needed to provide a definitive answer to this question.

The development of breast cancer after radiation therapy for childhood cancer has been reported, and survivors of such treatment should be observed regularly.[16] The incidence of increased second primary cancer in males with breast cancer has been reported.[9] In a review of male breast cancer, the Virginia Tumor Registry has documented second malignancies in 11.2 percent of male patients with breast cancer.[33] The increased incidence of second malignancies may be related to age and environmental exposure (many of the lesions are cutaneous), as well as dietary factors (some series have increased frequencies of colorectal cancer).

Male breast cancer is commonly detected when it presents as a palpable mass. Public awareness of male breast cancer is leading to detection at an earlier stage. Other signs suggestive of male breast cancer include ulceration and nipple discharge, which should prompt immediate investigation. Diffuse unilateral or bilateral enlargement of the breast in the adolescent, though of concern for the individual and possibly suggestive of a systemic disorder, is rarely caused by breast cancer. Unilateral and bilateral enlargement in the young adult may be associated with a testicular tumor, and the testicles should be examined carefully in a male presenting with breast enlargement. In the elderly male, breast enlargement should also be evaluated carefully to rule out breast cancer. Previous or coexisting diseases, testicular tumors, or medications can also cause unilateral or bilateral breast enlargement in the male (Table 49–1).

Male breast cancer usually presents as a firm subareolar mass that is nontender. Tenderness is associated more commonly with gynecomastia. The distinction between a benign and malignant mass in the male breast is usually obvious. Although carcinoma is generally found in the elderly male, it has been reported in the young male.[24] Tissue evaluation is essential should the mass persist or if there is concern regarding possible malignancy.

Mammography is of limited use in the male because of the technical difficulty in obtaining the study. In obese males with large breasts and in some patients with gynecomastia, mammography has been a useful diag-

nostic procedure. The fatty breast is easy to penetrate, and the glandular pattern in gynecomastia is readily identified. Calcifications similar to those found in females have been identified in males with breast cancer. Evaluation of the opposite breast is essential in males with carcinoma of one breast. Ultrasonography has not been as beneficial as mammography in identifying male breast cancer.[14]

Galactograms performed on males with a nipple discharge have aided in localization of the abnormal ductal area when no mass is palpable.[7] Fine needle aspiration may help to distinguish between carcinoma and gynecomastia. In doubtful cases, however, a negative fine needle aspiration for cytology does not rule out carcinoma, and an open biopsy should be performed.

Estrogen and progesterone receptor studies should be performed on all males with breast cancer. Fresh tissue should be given to the pathologist at the time of biopsy, as additional tissue may not be available later. Male breast cancer receptor studies have revealed a high level of receptor activity in as many as 80 percent of the cases.[21a, 31]

PATHOLOGY

Male breast cancer is ductal in origin. Lobular carcinoma is extremely rare, although one case has been reported involving a patient with Klinefelter's syndrome.[25a] Infiltrating ductal carcinoma makes up 85 percent of cases, whereas intraductal carcinoma and papillary carcinoma are each found in approximately five percent of cases.[13] Tubular and colloid carcinoma are uncommon, and sarcoma is rarely reported.[30] Paget's disease does occur and is similar pathologically to that in females. Microscopic gynecomastia has been reported in up to 40 percent of cases, whereas clinical gynecomastia is rarely associated with male breast cancer.[13]

TREATMENT OF PRIMARY BREAST CANCER

The central location of the tumor and the proximity of the tumor to the pectoral muscles led to the radical mastectomy as the treatment of choice for male breast cancer.[12] In recent years, however, a modified radical mastectomy or a simple mastectomy with postoperative radiation therapy has been advocated. Simple mastectomy with postoperative radiation therapy has been the treatment of choice since 1961 at the Christie Hospital and Holt Radium Institute in Manchester, England.[21a] The M. D. Anderson Hospital advocates the same treatment approach.[22]

The survival after treatment for male breast cancer has been reported significantly worse than in female patients with breast cancer, especially if positive nodes are present (Table 49–2).[13, 21a, 28] Other studies found no difference in survival when patients were considered by stage.[9, 31]

The Virginia Tumor Registry contains 154 analytical

Table 49–1. MALE BREAST DISEASE: PREDISPOSING FACTORS

Benign breast enlargement (gynecomastia)*
  Etiology
    Disease
      Chronic renal disease
      Chronic hepatic disease
      Malnutrition
      Abnormal thyroid function
      Adrenal insufficiency
      Klinefelter's syndrome
      Testicular tumors
    Medications

Digitalis	LSD
Thiazides	Androgens
Spironolactone	Methyldopa
Diazepam	Cimetidine
Exogenous estrogens	Isoniazid
Cyclophosphamide	Amphetamine
Heroin	Reserpine
Methadone	Tricyclic antidepressants
Marijuana	

Male breast cancer
  Familial association
    Incidence of associated breast cancer in female relatives, 10–12 percent
  Ethnic—Racial
    Increased incidence in Jewish and black males
  Predisposing disease
    Mumps orchitis
    Testicular tumor
    Klinefelter's syndrome
  Other predisposing conditions
    Radiation of childhood cancer
    Occupational exposure to high environmental temperatures

*Although there are reports of gynecomastia in association with breast cancer, and there is a 27–42 percent frequency of microscopic gynecomastia in male breast cancer, there is no histological or statistical evidence to show gynecomastia as a premalignant lesion.

Table 49–2. SURVIVAL IN MALE BREAST CANCER

	Author				
	Heller et al [13]	*Spence et al* [28]	*Erlichman et al* [9]	*van Geel et al* [31]	*Ribeiro* [21a]
No. patients	97	81	89	104	292
Time period (yr)	5–10	5–10	5–10	5–10	5–10
Overall survival (%)	40–72	17–38	44 (1934–66)	54	38–53
			58 (1966–81)		
Node-negative (%)	79–90	60–82	50–77	52–70	70–82
Node-positive (%)	11–59	10–44	25–37	33–58	42–60
Stage (%)					
I	80–100	60–82	65–70	29–70	65–80
II	19–63	10–44	35–58	33–58	42–55
III	25–45	2–16	10	23–63	3–25
IV	—	0–8	—	13	0–4

cases of male breast cancer from 1970 to 1984. The overall 5-year survival was 37.8 percent for blacks compared with 70.78 percent for whites. At each stage, a decreased survival for black males was evident when compared with whites. Similar survival data were evident for black females in the Virginia Tumor Registry. More data are needed for an analysis of the significance of this finding. The overall 5- and 10-year survival for patients with male breast cancer was 78 percent and 59 percent, respectively with negative nodes and 59 percent and 27 percent with positive nodes. The majority of cases were treated with some form of mastectomy, with the trend away from the Halsted radical; some lumpectomies are recorded. The local recurrence rate after surgical treatment of male breast cancer has been reported to be as high as 20 percent to 26 percent,[9, 31] prompting increased use of postoperative radiation therapy. Although adjuvant radiation did not affect survival, the local recurrence rate was reduced.[9, 15, 21a] Possibly the high local and regional recurrence rates are related to the central location of the tumor and the intimate proximity of the tumor to the underlying muscle and chest wall in the male in comparison to the female breast.

Adjuvant Therapy

Reports of the use of adjuvant therapy for male breast cancer are infrequent. Ribeiro has reported the use of adjuvant tamoxifen therapy (20 mg of tamoxifen given for 12 months) in 23 patients with stage II (axillary nodal involvement) and stage III disease confined to the breast.[21a] Receptor studies were available in eight patients, seven of whom were positive for both estrogen and progesterone receptors.[11] One patient was negative for hormone receptors. Ribeiro reported a 5-year survival rate of 55 percent for this group, compared with 28 percent for a previously untreated, similar stage group. Erlichman has recommended adjuvant chemotherapy in males with stage II cancer in view of the benefits of its use in female breast cancer, but provided no treatment data.[9] The low occurrence rate of the disease has thus far precluded randomized studies.

Metastatic Disease

Metastatic disease in male breast cancer has been treated by hormonal manipulation for years. The detection of positive hormone receptors in 80 percent of male breast cancers has further stimulated and directed hormonal manipulation in the management of metastatic disease. In general, the achievement of an objective response (either partial or complete tumor regression) usually translates into a prolongation of survival. Such is the case in the M. D. Anderson series in which a response to hormonal therapy resulted in a statistically significant prolongation of survival in comparison to nonresponders. Mean survival for orchiectomy was 42 vs. 16 months for responders and nonresponders, respectively; for additive hormonal therapy, 27 vs. 16 months; and for hormonal therapy in general, 40 vs. 14 months.[15] Previous response to orchiectomy or hormonal therapy did not predict further hormonal response. The disease-free interval (DFI) appeared to best correlate with increased response rates; patients with a DFI of more than 12 months had superior survival to those with a DFI less than 12 months. Antiestrogens (tamoxifen) produced a 25 percent response rate in this series.[15] In the past, additive hormone (diethylstilbestrol) has produced objective regression of metastatic or recurrent disease. In Ribeiro's series, 38 percent of 55 male breast cancer patients had an objective response.[21b] The availability of tamoxifen has facilitated hormone therapy without the previous side effects of additive therapy; receptor activity generally enhances the likelihood of an objective remission. Ribeiro has reported a 37.5 percent response rate after tamoxifen therapy, with responses ranging from 8 to 60 months.[21a] Ablative therapy is also effective and was used more in the past. In a review of the Rosewell Park experience with orchiectomy, a 50 percent response rate was reported.[20] Adrenalectomy after orchiectomy was effective in 80 percent of the cases, and these investigators even demonstrated responses in a small subset of three patients who were orchiectomy nonresponders.

Hormonal therapy for metastatic male breast cancer is as effective as it is for female breast cancer and possibly may be more effective. The proper sequence of therapy with respect to tamoxifen, aminoglutethimide, and ablation needs to be studied further. The ready acceptance of medical therapy by the patient will certainly influence this decision. Fortunately the high rate of estrogen and progesterone receptor activity generally enhances the likelihood of an objective remission. The response is unknown, however, with respect to receptor-negative tumors.

The use of nasally administered buserelin in the treatment of lung metastases in male breast cancer has been reported.[32] Buserelin is a gonadotropin-releasing hormone analogue with minimal side effects that shows promise as another method of hormonal manipulation for metastatic breast cancer.

Chemotherapy for the treatment of male breast cancer has not been used as frequently as in females because of the generally good response of male breast cancer to hormonal manipulation. An overall response rate of 35 percent in male breast cancer patients treated by Cooper's regimen (cyclophosphamide, methotrexate, 5-fluorouracil, vincristine, and prednisone) or doxorubicin-containing combinations has been reported.[17] This response appears to be similar to that reported in female breast cancer series.

SUMMARY

Male breast cancer is an uncommon disease with an incidence that has remained fairly stable. An increased incidence seems to occur in Jewish males, individuals with Klinefelter's syndrome, and in males with mumps orchitis occurring after the age of 20. A slight increased incidence in blacks has been reported. The tumor presents as a mass and is of the ductal type pathologically. Treatment is by simple or modified mastectomy with the use of postoperative radiation therapy to reduce local recurrence in high-risk patients. There appears to be a higher local recurrence rate in males, possibly because of central location of the tumor and the closer proximity of the tumor to underlying muscle and chest wall. Overall survival rates for node-negative patients correspond favorably with those of females, but survival in node-positive male patients appears worse, suggesting a need for adjuvant therapy in that group. The role of adjuvant therapy has not been determined, but the use of tamoxifen may be beneficial in node-positive patients. Adjuvant chemotherapy in high-risk patients needs to be explored. Hormonal manipulation, either by medication or ablation, gives a good response in the management of metastatic disease. The effectiveness of chemotherapy is less known, but early studies suggest a response similar to that in female breast cancer patients.

References

1. Ajayi DO, Oseghe DN, Ademiluyi SA: Carcinoma of the male breast in West Africans and a review of world literature. Cancer 50:1664–1667, 1982.
2. Brown P, Terez J: Breast cancer associated with Klinefelter's syndrome. J Surg Oncol 10:413–415, 1978.
3. Cole FM, Qizilbosh AA: Carcinoma in situ of the male breast. J Clin Pathol 32:1128–1134, 1979.
4. Crichlow RW: Carcinoma of the male breast. Surg Gynecol Obstet 134:1011–1019, 1972.
5. Dao TL, Morreal C, Nemoto T: Urinary estrogen excretion in men with breast cancer. N Engl J Med 289:138–140, 1973.
6. Dershaw D: Male mammography. AJR 146:127–131, 1986.
7. Detraux P, Benmussa M, Tristant H, Garel L: Breast disease in the male: galactographic evaluation. Radiology 154:605–606, 1983.
8. Donegan WL, Perez-Mesa CM: Cancer of male breast. A 30-year review of 28 cases. Arch Surg 106:273–279, 1973.
9. Erlichman C, Murphy KC, Elhakim T: Male breast cancer: a 13 year review of 89 patients. J Clin Oncol 2:903–909, 1984.
10. Evans DB, Crichlow RW: Carcinoma of male breast and Klinefelter's syndrome—is there an association? CA 37:246–250, 1987.
11. Friedman MA, Hoffman PG, Dandolos EM, et al: Estrogen receptors in male breast cancer. Cancer 47:134–137, 1981.
12. Haagensen CD: Diseases of the Breast, ed 3. Philadelphia, WB Saunders, 1985.
13. Heller K, Rosen P, Schattenfeld D, Ashihari R, Kinne D: Male breast cancer. Ann Surg 188:60–65, 1978.
14. Jackson VP, Gilman RL: Male breast carcinoma and gynecomastia. Radiology 149:533–536, 1983.
15. Kantarjian H, Yap HY, Hortobagyi G, Buzder A, Blumenschein G: Hormonal therapy for metastatic male breast cancer. Ann Int Med 143:237–240, 1983.
16. Li FP, Corberg J, Vawter G, Frine W, et al: Breast carcinoma after cancer therapy in childhood. Cancer 51:521–523, 1983.
17. Lopez M, DiLauro L, Popaldo P, Lozzero B: Chemotherapy in metastatic male breast cancer. Oncology 42:205–209, 1985.
18. Mabuchi A, Bross D, Kessler I: Risk factors in male breast cancer. J Natl Cancer Inst 74:371–375, 1985.
19. Nirmul D, Pegoraro, RJ, Naidoo C, Joubert SM: The sex hormone profile of male patients with breast cancer. Br J Cancer 48:423–427, 1983.
20. Patel JK, Nemoto T, Dao T: Metastatic breast cancer in males: assessment of endocrine therapy. Cancer 53:1344–1346, 1984.
21a. Ribeiro G: Male breast cancer: review of 301 cases from Christie Hospital and Holt Radium Institute, Manchester. Br J Cancer 51:115–119, 1985.
21b. Ribeiro GG: The results of diethylstilbestrol therapy for recurrent and metastatic carcinoma of the male breast. Br J Med 33:465, 1976.
22. Robinson R, Montague E: Treatment results in males with breast cancer. Cancer 49:403–406, 1982.
23. Russ JE, Scanlon E: Identical cancers in husband and wife. Surg Gynecol Obstet 150:664–666, 1980.
24. Saltzstein EC, Tanof M, Latomoca R: Breast carcinoma of a young male. Arch Surg 113:880–881, 1978.
25a. Sanchez AG, Villanueva AG, Redondo C: Lobular carcinoma of breast in a patient with Klinefelter's syndrome. A case with bilateral synchronous histologically different breast tumors. Cancer 57:1181–1183, 1986.
25b. Scheike O, Visfeldt J: Male breast cancer, 4. Gynecomastia in patients with breast cancer. Acta Pathol Microbiol Scand 81:359, 1973.
26. Schattenfeld D, Lilenfield A, Diamond H: Some observations on the epidemiology of breast cancer among males. Am J Public Health 53:890–897, 1963.
27. Silverberg E, Lubero J: Cancer Statistics. CA 37:2–19, 1987.
28. Spence RA, MacKenzie G, Anderson JR, Lyons AR, Bell M: Long-term survival following cancer of the male breast in Northern Ireland. Cancer 55:648–652, 1985.
29. Steintz R, Katz L, Ben-Hur M: Male breast cancer in Israel: selected epidemiological aspects. Isr J Med Sci 17:816–821, 1981.
30. Tanino M, Tatsuzama T, Fenda T, Nakajiva H, Suquira H, Odoshimo S: Lymphosarcoma of the male breast. Dis Breast 10:13–15, 1989.
31. van Geel AN, van Slooten EA, Mavrunac M, Hart AA: A retrospective study of male breast cancer in Holland. Br J Surg 72:724–727, 1985.
32. Vorobiof DA, Falkson G: Nasally administered buserelin inducing complete remission of lung metastases in male breast cancer. Cancer 59:688–689, 1987.
33. Wilhelm MC, Wanebo HJ: Male breast cancer in Virginia: a review. Manuscript in preparation.

Chapter 50

CARCINOMA OF THE BREAST IN PREGNANCY AND LACTATION

Herbert C. Hoover, Jr., M.D.

Breast cancer, the most frequent cancer and cause of cancer deaths in women, is also the most likely cancer to be seen in pregnancy or lactation.[12] The occurrence of breast cancer during pregnancy and lactation presents a challenging clinical problem that is further compounded by its infrequent occurrence and the emotional issues involved. One of life's most joyous experiences can become a nightmare, often unnecessarily. Because most physicians deal with this clinical situation infrequently, anecdotal experiences of their own or their colleagues can easily lead to the propagation of misinformation. We will attempt to clarify the major questions related to the diagnosis, therapy, and prognosis of cancer of the breast in pregnancy and lactation.

HISTORICAL ASPECTS

From the time of Billroth[3] until Halsted's pioneering work, breast cancer diagnosed during pregnancy was considered incurable. Halsted, in 1896, performed a radical mastectomy on a lactating female who was reported to be alive and well more than 30 years later. This long-term follow-up was provided by Bloodgood as a part of a report by Kilgore[27] showing a 70 percent 5-year survival in lactating females with node-negative breast cancer and an 11.5 percent 5-year survival in patients with nodal involvement. These early writings also rejected the idea that milk fistulas would uniformly result from a breast biopsy during pregnancy or lactation. Bloodgood also mentioned that general anesthesia apparently had no harmful effect on the fetus and intimated that breast cancer occurring during pregnancy should, in fact, be treated in a manner similar to that in the nonpregnant women. However, an attitude of gloom was propagated by the 1943 article by Haagensen and Stout[15] stating that breast carcinoma developing during pregnancy and lactation was categorically inoperable. This was based on their experience with only 20 patients, 19 of whom had positive nodes, who had all died of their breast cancer. Haagensen[16] changed his view later after more extensive experience, but the pessimistic attitude was widely prevalent and continues often today.

However, studies in the past 30 years have convincingly demonstrated that the poor results are caused by delay in diagnosis and reluctance to treat patients aggressively during pregnancy.

EPIDEMIOLOGY

Because the incidence of breast cancer peaks between the ages of 50 and 55, the frequent coexistence of pregnancy and breast cancer would not be expected. White and White[45] reviewed 1296 such cases, including 60 of their own, in 45,881 breast carcinoma cases, for an incidence of approximately 2.8 percent. Of 300,860 pregnancies reviewed, there were only 93 cancers documented, or three breast cancers per 10,000 pregnancies. Wallack and associates,[44] in a large review of the literature, put the incidence figure even lower, with breast cancer associated with pregnancy or lactation in only one percent to two percent of breast cancers. In most series, the average age of patients has been 34 to 35 years. With the current trend toward postponing childbearing to the mid to late 30s, it is expected that the incidence of breast cancer diagnosed during pregnancy and lactation will increase.

ETIOLOGY

Even though pregnancy and cancer are the only two biological conditions in which antigenic tissue is tolerated by a seemingly intact immune system,[14] there is no evidence to implicate pregnancy or lactation in either the etiology or the progression of breast cancer. There is evidence for depressed cell-mediated immunity as evidenced by an abnormal lymphocyte response to phytohemagglutinin in vitro and by impairment of in vivo responses to common recall antigens used in testing for delayed cutaneous hypersensitivity.[37] Additionally, some of the pregnancy-induced hormonal changes such as the elevation of circulating corticosteroids could be immunosuppressive.[29] These changes could theoretically promote more rapid tumor growth but are unlikely to play any major etiological role. Based on our assumptions concerning the biology of breast cancer, we would assume that a cancer manifesting itself during pregnancy had its inception months or even years before conception. Of course, the etiology of breast cancer remains unknown, but there appears to be nothing unique about breast cancer in pregnancy.

CLINICAL PRESENTATION

Delay in diagnosis appears to be the primary and perhaps the only reason for the generally worse prognosis for all patients overall with breast cancer diagnosed during pregnancy and lactation.[1, 6, 7, 17, 23, 28, 32, 35, 38, 39] The duration of symptoms before diagnosis averaged 5 to 15 months in some series, which is considerably greater than in series of nonpregnant patients. This delay can be attributed to physician as well as to patient neglect. During pregnancy, the breasts become tense and often have a multinodular consistency. A discrete mass can be difficult to feel or can become obscure as the breasts hypertrophy. Because of the pregnancy, masses are often ignored even when noticed by patients or physicians, with the plan being to evaluate them further if they persist after delivery. Mammography is often not recommended during pregnancy because of the radiation exposure to the fetus and the poor imaging obtained in the tense, hyperplastic breast tissue. The latter is a significant problem, but the former need be of no major concern with proper abdominal and pelvic shielding and modern techniques.

As a consequence, virtually all series of patients with breast cancer during pregnancy report a more advanced cancer stage than in nonpregnancy series. Ribeiro and Palmer[39] reported on 88 patients with breast cancer concurrent with pregnancy. Nineteen had inoperable, advanced tumors. Of the 69 operable patients, 89 percent were found to have positive nodes in the ipsilateral axilla. Holleb and Farrow[23] reported 72 percent with positive nodes in 117 patients. These figures are far in excess of the 40 percent to 50 percent node-positive rate reported in most series of breast cancer in nonpregnant women.[20]

DIAGNOSIS

Primary care physicians, especially obstetricians and gynecologists, play a pivotal role in the diagnosis of breast cancer during pregnancy and lactation. It is especially important that a careful breast exam be performed at the initial obstetrical visit before the breasts become engorged and very difficult to examine carefully. As mentioned earlier, studies suggest that both patients and their physicians often fail to recognize the potentially serious nature of breast masses during pregnancy.

There should be nothing special about the diagnostic work-up of pregnant or lactating patients with breast masses, except that xeroradiography tends to not be as helpful as usual as a result of the parenchymal changes associated with gestation. Increased water density of the breasts reduces the discriminatory capacity of mammography.[22] Radiation exposure to the fetus should be negligible with proper shielding of the abdomen in modern techniques. In one series of 368 pregnant women undergoing mammography, there was no apparent damage to the fetus.[29] However, in a patient with a discrete palpable mass, a mammogram would rarely influence therapy and need not be obtained.

Any dominant mass should be evaluated promptly in pregnant or lactating patients. Evaluation should normally begin with a fine needle aspiration to distinguish cystic from solid lesions. Any solid mass requires a biopsy, which can almost always be performed under local anesthesia.

The breast masses sampled in patients during pregnancy show the same spectrum of histopathology found in nonpregnant patients. Additionally, the likelihood of finding a carcinoma appears to be similar to that in breast masses sampled in the nonpregnant population.[5] Byrd et al.[5] found that 22 percent of breast biopsy samples in pregnancy showed malignancy compared with 19 percent in all patients overall. Although the earlier literature[45] implied that inflammatory carcinoma was seen more frequently during pregnancy, modern series do not show this.

Steroid hormone receptors may be difficult to demonstrate in breast cancer tissue during pregnancy unless special methods are utilized.[13, 26, 40, 41] Pregnancy may depress levels of estrogen and progesterone receptor detectable in breast cancer cytosol fractions and cause false-negative results. High levels of estrogens circulating in pregnant patients cause receptor translocation into the nucleus and occupy all the cytoplasmic receptors, leaving none available for assay. During pregnancy, unbound estrogen should first be removed by treatment of cytosol with dextran charcoal. Exchange assays then can be performed to detect occupied estrogen receptors within cytosol and nuclei. To my knowledge, there are no data available on estrogen receptors in breast cancer during pregnancy that have any meaningful prognostic significance.

For biopsies done during lactation, some surgeons prefer to suppress lactation preoperatively using bromocriptine, although there is no evidence to support this practice. The risk of milk fistulas is very low for peripheral lesions but can occasionally cause a problem in deep, central lesions.

There is no evidence that a breast biopsy constitutes any significant risk to either the mother or the fetus even if general anesthesia is required, assuming that proper precautions are used. Byrd et al.[5] report only one fetal loss in 134 breast biopsies performed on pregnant patients under general anesthesia. The one loss was in an older patient not known to be pregnant at the time of the operation, and therefore the procedure was done without the usual precautions.

ANESTHETIC CONSIDERATIONS

Some anesthetic considerations should be mentioned for those patients who do require general anesthesia for a biopsy or for those patients who require partial or total mastectomy. There are some unique management considerations because of the physiological changes produced by pregnancy and the physical effects of an enlarged, gravid uterus. The special problems posed by general anesthesia in pregnant patients are discussed in several recent publications,[2, 8, 24, 30, 33, 34] which have been extensively reviewed by Wallack et al.[44] and will be briefly summarized here.

There are a number of cardiovascular and hematological alterations during pregnancy that require anesthetic adjustments. Blood volume increases by approximately 35 percent, but this is primarily in the plasma volume rather than red cell volume, giving a physiological dilutional anemia. By term, the heart rate increases 10 to 15 beats per minute. Along with the increase in blood volume and heart rate is a 30 percent to 50 percent increase in cardiac output. There is a slight decrease in the systemic vascular resistance as well. The lower hemoglobin content leads to a decrease in oxygen carrying capacity, and the task of maintaining oxygen saturation and cardiac output becomes critical. A high inspired oxygen concentration (at least 50 percent) and the avoidance of agents that depress cardiac output are advised.

Pregnancy also alters coagulation parameters. The platelet count increases nearly 50 percent, as does the fibrinogen level. The hypercoagulable state can lead to an increased risk of thromboembolism.

In the supine position, a gravid uterus may interfere with blood flow because of pressure on the distal aorta and inferior vena cava, making positioning during anesthesia of great importance. Tilting the operating table slightly to the left and putting a cushion under the patient's right hip can help to displace the uterus to the left and away from major vascular structures.

A large gravid uterus raises the level of the diaphragm significantly, thus compromising lung volumes. Decreased functional residual capacity along with a pregnancy-associated increase in respiratory rate can lead to a more rapid buildup of anesthetic vapor within the aveoli and thus a more rapid induction of anesthesia. Forced hyperventilation and maternal respiratory alkalosis can affect the fetus adversely by causing progressive fetal acidosis. The anesthetist must exercise great care in maintaining "normal for pregnancy" ventilatory balance. Also, serum cholinesterase activity is decreased by approximately 20 percent, causing a prolonged metabolism of succinylcholine.

Because of the decreased functional residual capacity and diminished ability to store oxygen coupled with the increased oxygen consumption in pregnancy, the pregnant patient is predisposed to hypoxemia during even brief apneic episodes. Preoxygenation for several minutes should always precede endotracheal intubation. Intubation itself should be carefully performed because of the hypervascularity that occurs in the respiratory tract mucosa in most pregnant women.

It is well known that gastric emptying time is prolonged in pregnancy, reaching as high as 60 percent above normal as the patient approaches term. The

pressure on the stomach makes reflux much more likely as well. Hypergastrinemia not uncommonly leads to more acidic gastric secretions. Therefore pregnant patients require special intubation techniques to avoid aspiration of this very damaging acidic material.

There are no published studies to confirm any deleterious effects of anesthetic agents on the developing fetus. There are many studies looking at the offspring of narcotic addicts that have shown no long-term effect of morphine, heroin, or methadone other than low birth weight.[4]

Fetal monitoring should be used whenever possible so that early fetal distress can be recognized and appropriate adjustments made. Otherwise, it is thought that general anesthesia poses no real hazard as long as careful attention is given to the unique requirements of the situation.

STAGING EVALUATION

Once the diagnosis of breast cancer is made, staging of the disease is critical before therapeutic decisions are made. Since all of the staging work-up, with the exception of blood studies, involve radiation exposure, there is more controversy concerning the extent of work-up that should be performed in breast cancer patients who are pregnant. Liver function tests, and calcium and CEA evaluation can give some useful information but do not give a definitive diagnosis or localization of metastatic disease.

A thorough understanding of the radiation risk to the fetus is helpful to the clinician deciding on the diagnostic tests to pursue. Hall[18] has published much useful information on this subject. Radiation delivered during the preimplantation phase from fertilization to embryonic implantation in the uterine wall (days 0 to 10) can result in the death of the embryo. As little as 10 rad can be lethal in the mouse. He did find that those embryos that survived irradiation during this period appeared to develop normally. Irradiation during organogenesis (days 11 to 56) can lead to major developmental malformations. In humans, the most frequently noted defect is microcephaly. Again, doses as low as 10 rad may be sufficient to produce a measurable increase in birth defects. Doses exceeding 100 rad are felt to produce congenital abnormalities in 100 percent of cases, based on the atomic bomb experience.[25, 31] After day 57, during the fetal stage when additional growth is occurring, larger doses of irradiation are required to give significant effects. After weeks 25 to 30, the fetus is far more resistant to damaging effects of radiation.[9] The majority of the reports on the effects of ionizing radiation on the developing organs are extrapolations from animals to man with doses involved that are much higher than are pertinent to our considerations in the radiological evaluation for metastasis in breast cancer but are more relevant in considering therapeutic breast irradiation. However, there are insufficient data in the literature to quantify the long-term risk to the fetus with the extremely low radiation doses involved in most scanning procedures. For example, the radiation dose to the fetus from a bone scan is approximately 0.1 rad.

Even though we conclude that any radiological staging procedure is probably safe in a pregnant patient, we cannot say this with certainty. Therefore bone scans are generally not recommended unless major therapeutic decisions are to be based on their outcome. This is similar to our policy in stages I and II nonpregnant patients with carcinoma of the breast, where the diagnostic yield in an asymptomatic patient is not felt to be high enough to justify the expense of a bone scan on a routine basis. Harbert[19] reviewed a large number of studies showing a three percent true-positive yield from bone scans in 533 patients with stage I breast cancer, seven percent in 696 patients with stage II disease, and 25 percent in 278 patients with stage III disease. When pregnant patients with stage I or II disease have skeletal pain, a bone scan is preferred to radiographic evaluation, as the radiation exposure from the scan would be considerably less than a skeletal survey. In clinical stage III disease where a significantly higher positive scan rate would be expected, we still prefer to defer a bone scan until the later stages of pregnancy or preferably after delivery unless we would decide to treat with systemic therapy at that stage of the pregnancy if bone metastases were demonstrated. This raises complex issues as to which patients should be considered for termination of pregnancy, a topic that will be discussed in the section on treatment.

Carcinogenesis from radiation exposure is another possible risk to the fetus. Although the association between fetal radiation exposure and cancer was not clearly shown in the atomic bomb experience, a recent study of twins showed that twins who developed cancer or leukemia were twice as likely to have been exposed to x-rays in utero as were control sets of twins.[21] Rather than take any chances, it is best to avoid any radiation exposure during pregnancy unless the data are critically important. This would not apply to routine chest roentgenograms, which can be done with essentially no risk to the fetus with proper abdominal and pelvic shielding. However, in stage I breast cancer, the chance of finding a positive chest radiograph is sufficiently low that the radiograph could be deferred until delivery of the fetus. There is no role for brain or liver scans in these patients. Any patient with central nervous system symptoms would be better served by a computed tomography scan, and the liver can be evaluated with ultrasound at no risk to the fetus.

TREATMENT

Although Haagensen and Stout concluded in 1943[15] that the prognosis was so poor that mastectomy was not justified in patients with breast cancer that developed during pregnancy or lactation, Haagensen did not persist with that point of view for long. He soon realized that his initial experience with 20 patients, who all died, was not representative of the prognosis.[16] Virtually all reports since then have stressed that surgical treatment

should be essentially the same as that of the nonpregnant patient in all stages of disease. A more controversial topic has been whether termination of pregnancy should be advised. Obviously the therapeutic decisions will be influenced by the stage of pregnancy and the stage of disease, so we must consider the treatment plan accordingly.

Because the risk of spontaneous abortion during mastectomy is extraordinarily low,[5] mastectomy or other breast procedures should be performed promptly on diagnosis at any stage of pregnancy. A mastectomy allows a normal pregnancy to continue with minimal risk to the mother or the fetus. This is especially true since no modern series suggest that abortion benefits the course of patients with breast cancer.[10, 11] Therefore any decision to terminate the pregnancy should be based on considerations other than abortion's influence on the progression of the disease. Termination of pregnancy has no role in the management of stage I and II breast cancer patients. Likewise, there is no substantial evidence that oophorectomy influences the course of breast cancer during pregnancy and lactation.

With the trend toward breast conservation and radiation for breast cancer, some pregnant women with early stages of breast cancer will want to consider that option. It should be strongly discouraged except in cases where radiation therapy could reasonably be withheld until after delivery. Using the standard technique of whole breast irradiation followed by a boost dose to the tumor bed, the dose scattered to the fetus would be unacceptably high.[29] There are two sources of radiation dosage outside the radiation beam: (1) internal scatter within the body, and (2) leakage radiation from the head of the machine. With proper lead blocks, the leakage rate can be reduced to a very low range of less than 2 rad. Internal scatter, however, is dependent on field size, photon energy, and proximity to the field edge. Shielding cannot modify this scatter. Early in pregnancy, when the distance between the breast and uterus is great, the internal scatter dose may be only 10 to 20 rad for a total course of treatment. However, when the top of the uterus approaches the xiphoid, doses up to 100 rad or more may be given.[29]

Obviously special treatment arrangements can be made for women who insist on breast conservation. This could involve primary excision using a small boost of irradiation to the area, with delivery of full breast irradiation after the patient gives birth. The patient would have to be aware of the potential risk, however, at even this low dose to the fetus. Every effort should be made to discourage such an approach. A more reasonable alternative would be simple surgical removal of the primary with observation until delivery, when further therapy could be given.

Adjuvant chemotherapy has become standard for node-positive, premenopausal women with breast cancer. It is thought that therapeutic delay may diminish the benefits of adjuvant therapy, and the decision to initiate chemotherapy during pregnancy is one that requires serious consideration.

Unfortunately the risks associated with chemotherapy

during pregnancy are not clear. Most of the hard data are from research in laboratory animals where the period of greatest risk is the initial portion of the pregnancy. Schapira and Chudley[42] found the incidence of teratogenicity of chemotherapeutic agents given to humans in the first trimester of pregnancy to be only 12.7 percent, whereas Sweet and Kinzie[43] reported an 11.5 percent incidence. Neither reported evidence for teratogenicity from the administration of chemotherapeutic agents in the second and third trimesters of pregnancy (Table 50–1). Most of the data involve single drug use only, and little is known about the combination regimens usually used in breast cancer patients.

Additionally, there are no good studies on the long-term consequences of fetal exposure to chemotherapeutic agents. In general, the use of chemotherapeutic agents during the first trimester of pregnancy should be discouraged, but their use during the second and third trimester probably induces very few fetal abnormalities.

Stages I and II (Operable) Breast Cancer

Modified radical mastectomy is the treatment of choice for stage I or II patients. A second choice would be total tumor excision to be followed by whole breast irradiation after delivery. In patients with positive axillary lymph nodes, chemotherapy should be delayed until the second trimester of pregnancy. My personal recommendation is to delay all chemotherapy in node-positive patients until after delivery. With determination of fetal age and maturity, consideration should be given to an early cesarean section to minimize the delay in beginning chemotherapy.

Stages III (Locally Advanced) and IV (Distant Metastases) Breast Cancer

In patients with locally advanced or metastatic carcinoma diagnosed early in the pregnancy where both chemotherapy and radiation therapy would normally be recommended, serious consideration must be given to termination of the pregnancy. In the later stages of pregnancy, nonsurgical therapy could potentially be delayed until after delivery, but one must weigh the risks of observing an advanced breast cancer for a prolonged period of time. As mentioned earlier, chemotherapy can be used with little known risk during the second and third trimester, but, unfortunately, good data for standard breast chemotherapy combinations are lacking. If radiation therapy is imperative at any stage of pregnancy, termination of pregnancy may be the most reasonable alternative. The mother's life expectancy is often limited, and damage to the fetus is a significant possibility.

There are no "right" answers to many of the therapeutic dilemmas encountered in patients developing breast cancer during pregnancy. A thorough discussion of all the risk factors involved with any approach must be presented to the patient and her family, who must be a part of these often difficult decisions.

Table 50–1. EFFECT OF ANTINEOPLASTIC AGENTS DURING PREGNANCY

	First Trimester		Second and Third Trimesters	
Drug	No. of Women Treated	No. of Cases of Fetal Malformations Observed	No. of Women Treated	No. of Cases of Fetal Malformations Observed
Alkylating agents				
Mechlorethamine hydrochloride	6	0	5	0
Cyclophosphamide	6	3	2	0
Chlorambucil	2	1	4	0
Busulfan	22	2	10	0
Triethylene melamine	3	0	5	0
Thiotepa	0	0	1	0
Antimetabolites				
Aminopterin	52	10	3	0
Methotrexate	0	0	5	0
Mercaptopurine	20	1	28	0
Azathioprine	35	0	1	0
Azaserine	1	0	0	0
Antimitotics				
Colchicine	10	0	3	0
Urethane	3	1	5	0
Dactinomycin	0	0	1	0
Vinblastine	2	0	2	0
Other				
MVP*	1	1	0	0
MOPP†	1	0	1	0
Total	164	19	76	0

*MVP, regimen of mechlorethamine hydrochloride, vinblastine sulfate, and procarbazine.
†MOPP, regimen of mechlorethamine hydrochloride, vincristine sulfate (Oncovin), procarbazine and prednisone.
Table modified from Sweet DL, Kinzie J: J Reprod Med 17:241, 1976.

Table 50–2. TREATMENT RESULTS IN OPERABLE BREAST CANCER IN PREGNANCY OR LACTATION

| Author-Year | No. of Patients | 5-Year Survival | | |
		Positive Nodes (%)	Negative Nodes (%)	Overall (%)
Peters,[35] 1962	60	23	62	37
Holleb and Farrow,[23] 1962	119	17	65	30
Rissanen,[39a] 1968	33	36	80	43
Donegan,[11] 1978	24	31	86	48
Ribeiro et al,[38] 1986	121	25	79	37
Total	357	26*	74*	39*

*Mean percentage.

PROGNOSIS

The rarity of breast cancer in pregnancy or lactation dictates that all reports of the entity are retrospective. Most report on only a few patients, making statistical analysis difficult or impossible. Nearly all have considered pregnancy and lactation together, assuming no differences between the two. With all of the shortcomings of small, retrospective studies, some general conclusions can be drawn. Table 50–2 lists several series chosen as those most likely to be representative based on their size and presentation of objective data. They clearly show that pregnant or lactating women who are diagnosed early with negative axillary lymph nodes have an expected outcome similar to that of nonpregnant females. Nugent and O'Connell[32] have shown this fact clearly in a small series comparing the distribution of stages of disease in pregnant patients with breast cancer with that in women younger than 40 years who were not pregnant (Table 50–3). The usual trend toward a higher stage of disease at diagnosis was found in pregnant patients, with 74 percent of patients having positive nodes compared with 37 percent node-positive nonpregnant women. When 5-year survival was compared in these groups both by stage and overall, no difference was noted (Table 50–4).

The challenge is clearly to affect this dread disease by making the diagnosis earlier. The bulk of evidence supports the opinion that pregnancy does not worsen the prognosis except by obscuring the disease for many months, allowing the metastatic process to progress. Hopefully, increased vigilance on the part of physicians seeing these patients early in pregnancy can reverse this trend.

OTHER CONSIDERATIONS

Metastatic Tumor to the Fetus

Some women with breast cancer diagnosed during pregnancy or lactation may fear that cancer cells have spread to their fetus and could grow there. This has been reported in melanoma and choriocarcinoma[36] but, to my knowledge, not in breast cancer.

Pregnancy Following Treatment of Breast Cancer

Many young women successfully treated for breast cancer desire additional children. Several studies[21, 35] have, in fact, shown an improved survival among breast cancer patients who later become pregnant. Some have argued that this phenomenon relates to patient selection in that only women without an early recurrence and with a good prognosis live to become pregnant. Peters[35] argues that improved survival among patients whose pregnancy occurred within a short interval after mastectomy is evidence against a selection process. She demonstrated an improvement in survival of 23 percent at 5 years and 28 percent at 10 years when 96 patients who became pregnant following breast cancer treatment were compared with 96 patients of similar age and clinical stage in whom pregnancy did not occur. In 41 patients treated for primary operable carcinoma of the breast, Harvey et al.[21] demonstrated no detrimental effect of subsequent pregnancy even among patients with positive axillary nodes or among those whose pregnancies occurred less than 2 years following mastectomy. Abortion gave no improvement in the survival rate. They con-

Table 50–3. STAGES OF BREAST CANCER AT DIAGNOSIS IN PATIENTS YOUNGER THAN 40 YEARS

| Stage | No. (%) | |
	Pregnant (N=19)	Nonpregnant (N=155)
I (negative nodes)	4 (21)	84 (54)
II (positive nodes)	14 (74)	57 (37)
III (distant disease)	1 (5)	14 (9)

Nugent P, O'Connell TX: Breast cancer in pregnancy. Arch Surg 120:1221–1224, 1985. Reprinted by permission.

Table 50–4. FIVE-YEAR SURVIVALS OF PREGNANT AND NONPREGNANT WOMEN YOUNGER THAN 40 YEARS

| Stage | Survival No. (%) | | |
	Pregnant	Nonpregnant	p Value
I	4/4 (100)	59/84 (70)	0.57
II	7/14 (50)	27/57 (48)	1.00
III	0/1 (0)	1/14 (7)	1.00
Overall	11/19 (57)	87/155 (56)	1.00

Nugent P, O'Connell TX: Breast cancer in pregnancy. Arch Surg 120:1221–1224, 1985. Reprinted by permission.

cluded, as have most other authors of recent series, that there are no therapeutic grounds for recommending avoidance or termination of pregnancy among patients without evidence of recurrent disease following treatment for breast cancer.

References

1. Anderson JM: Mammary cancers and pregnancy. Br Med J 1:1124–1127, 1979.
2. Attia RR, Ebeidan-Fischer JE: Gastrin: placental, maternal and plasma cord levels: its possible role in maternal residual gastric acidity. Abstr Am Soc Anesthesiolog 547, 1976.
3. Billroth TH: Die Krankheiten der Brustdrusen. *In* Hackley CE (ed): Surgical Pathology. Stuttgart, Enke, 1880.
4. Blinick G, Jerez E, Wallach RC: Methadone maintenance, pregnancy and progeny. JAMA 255:477, 1973.
5. Byrd BF, Bayer DS, Robertson JC, et al: Treatment of breast tumors associated with pregnancy and lactation. Ann Surg 155(6):940, 1962.
6. Canter JW, Oliver GC, Zaloudek CJ: Surgical diseases of the breast during pregnancy. Clin Obstet Gynecol 26:853–864, 1983.
7. Cheek JH: Cancer of the breast in pregnancy and lactation. Am J Surg 126:729–731, 1973.
8. Cohen SE: Why is the pregnant patient different? Semin Anesth 1:73, 1982.
9. Dekaban AS: Abnormalities in children exposed to X-radiation during various stages of gestation: tentative time table of irradiation injury to the human fetus, part I. J Nucl Med 9:471–477, 1968.
10. Donegan WL: Mammary carcinoma and pregnancy. *In* Dunphy JE (ed): Major Problems in Clinical Surgery. Philadelphia, WB Saunders, 1967, pp 170–178.
11. Donegan WL: Mammary carcinoma in pregnancy. *In* Hall EJ (ed): Radiobiology for the Radiologist. New York, Harper and Row, 1978, pp 397–410.
12. Donegan WL: Cancer and pregnancy. CA 33:194–214, 1983.
13. Garola RE, McGuire WL: An improved assay for nuclear estrogen receptor in experimental and human breast cancer. Cancer Res 37:333–337, 1977.
14. Gleichner N, Siegel I: Common denominators of pregnancy and malignancy. *In* Gleichner N (ed): Reproductive Immunology. New York, Alan R Liss, 1981, pp 339–353.
15. Haagensen CD, Stout AP: Carcinoma of breast; criteria of operability. Ann Surg 118:859–870, 1943.
16. Haagensen CD: The treatment and results in cancer of the breast at the Presbyterian Hospital, New York. Am J Roentgenol 62:328, 1949.
17. Haagensen CD: Cancer of the breast in pregnancy and lactation. Am J Obstet Gynecol 98:141–149, 1967.
18. Hall EJ: Effects on the embryo and fetus. *In* Hall EJ (ed): Radiobiology for the Radiologist. Hagerstown, MD, Harper and Row, 1973, pp 231–239.
19. Harbert JC: Efficacy of bone and liver scanning in malignant disease: facts and options. *In* Harbert JC (ed): Nuclear Medicine Annual, 1982. New York, Raven Press, 1982.
20. Harris JR, Hellman S, Canellos GP, Fisher B: Cancer of the breast. *In* DeVita VT, Hellman S, Rosenberg SA (eds): Cancer: Principles and Practice of Oncology, ed 2. Philadelphia, JB Lippincott, 1985, pp 1119–1177.
21. Harvey EB, Borce JD, Honeyman M, et al: Prenatal x-ray exposure and childhood cancer in twins. N Engl J Med 315:541, 1985.
22. Hoeffken W, Lanyi M: Mammography. Philadelphia, WB Saunders, 1977.
23. Holleb AI, Farrow JH: The relation of carcinoma of the breast in pregnancy in 283 patients. Surg Gynecol Obstet 115:65–71, 1962.
24. Huseymeyer RP, Davenport HT: Prophylaxis for Mendelson's syndrome before elective cesarean section: a comparison of cimetidine and magnesium trisilicate mixtures of regimens. Br J Obstet Gynecol 87:565, 1980.
25. Jablon S, Kato H: Childhood cancer in relation to pre-natal exposure to atomic bomb radiation. Lancet 2:1000, 1970.
26. Katzenellenbogen JA, Jonhson HJ, Carlson KE: Studies on the uterine, cytoplasmic estrogen binding protein. Thermal stability and ligand dissociation rate. An assay for empty and filled sites by exchange. Biochemistry 12:4092–4099, 1973.
27. Kilgore AR: Tumors and tumor-like lesions of breast in association with pregnancy and lactation (with a note by Bloodgood JC). The treatment of tumors of the breast during pregnancy and lactation. Arch Surg 18:2079–2098, 1929.
28. King RM, Welch JS, Marten JK, Coulam CB: Carcinoma of the breast associated with pregnancy. Surg Gynecol Obstet 160:228–232, 1985.
29. Lichter AS, Lippman ME: Special situations in the treatment of breast cancer. *In* Lippman ME, Lichter AS, Danforth DN (eds): Diagnosis and Management of Breast Cancer. Philadelphia, WB Saunders, 1988, pp 414–438.
30. Mendelson CL: Aspiration of stomach contents into the lungs during obstetric anesthesia. Am J Obstet Gynecol 53:191, 1946.
31. Miller R, Mulvihill S: Small head size after atomic irradiation. Teratology 14:355, 1976.
32. Nugent P, O'Connell TX: Breast cancer in pregnancy. Arch Surg 120:1221–1224, 1985.
33. Nunn JF: Applied Respiratory Physiology, ed 2. Boston, Butterworth, 1977, p 397.
34. Pedersen H, Finster M: Anesthetic risks in the pregnant surgical patient. Anesthesiology 51:439, 1979.
35. Peters MV: Carcinoma of the breast associated with pregnancy. Radiology 78:58–67, 1962.
36. Potter JF, Schoeneman M: Metastasis of maternal cancer to the placenta and fetus. Cancer 25:380–388, 1970.
37. Purtilo DT, Halgren HM, Yunis EJ: Depressed maternal lymphocyte response to phytohemagglutinin in human pregnancy. Lancet 1:769, 1972.
38. Ribeiro G, Jones DA, Jones M: Carcinoma of the breast associated with pregnancy. Br J Surg 73:607–609, 1986.
39. Ribeiro GG, Palmer MK: Breast carcinoma associated with pregnancy: a clinician's dilemma. Br Med J 2:1524–1527, 1977.
39a. Rissanen PM: Carcinoma of the breast during pregnancy and lactation. Br J Cancer 22:663–668, 1968.
40. Sakai F, Saez S: Existence of receptors bound to endogenous estradiol in breast cancers in premenopausal and postmenopausal women. Steroids 27:99–110, 1976.
41. Sarrif WM, Durant JR: Evidence that estrogen-receptor–negative progesterone-receptor–positive breast cancer and ovarian cancer contain estrogen receptor. Cancer 48:1215–1220, 1981.
42. Schapira DV, Chudley AE: Successful pregnancy following continuous treatment with combination chemotherapy before conception and throughout pregnancy. Cancer 54:800–803, 1984.
43. Sweet DL, Kinzie J: Consequences of radiotherapy and antineoplastic therapy for the fetus. J Reprod Med 17:241, 1976.
44. Wallack MK, Wolf JA, Bedwinek J, et al: Gestational carcinoma of the female breast. Curr Prob Cancer 7(9):1–58, 1983.
45. White TT, White WC: Breast cancer and pregnancy, a report of 49 cases followed 5 years. Ann Surg 144:384–393, 1956.

Chapter 51

THE UNKNOWN PRIMARY PRESENTING WITH AXILLARY LYMPHADENOPATHY

Daniel W. Tench, M.D. and David L. Page, M.D.

Carcinoma presenting as metastatic disease in lymph nodes is not uncommon. Location of the lymph nodes and histologic features of the metastatic tumor guide the search for the primary lesion. The rare presentation of adenocarcinoma compatible with breast primary in an axillary lymph node without an identifiable primary lesion poses special considerations in diagnosis and therapeutic decision making. This problem and its natural history was first outlined by Halsted[9] in 1907:

"I have twice seen extensive carcinomatous involvement of the axilla due to mammary cancer, which later in neither instance became palpable or demonstrable for a considerable period after the axillary glands had attained conspicuous dimensions. In each case the 'axillary tumors' had been removed, in one of them a year before, and in the other perhaps two years prior to my first examination which, though made in the most careful manner, failed to find the slightest evidence of cancer of either breast. In the course of a few months thereafter the mammary disease manifested itself in both patients.

"A third patient was operated upon for enlarged glands about two and a half years before she consulted me concerning the local axillary recurrence of the disease, and more especially to be relieved of severe neuralgic pains in the arms and legs. In this woman I found a large mass of axillary glands, which proved to be cancerous; but I found nothing in the breast except a quite definite parchment-like induration at the base of the nipple, which was retracted not at all, or merely to a barely appreciable degree."

In 1909 Cameron[3] recommended ipsilateral mastectomy in the face of axillary adenocarcinoma and a clinically benign breast. This course of action has been the usual mode of therapy in reported series and is predicated on the assumption that a solitary axillary metastasis of adenocarcinoma is likely to represent breast carcinoma in female patients with no other obvious malignancy after a limited workup in search of another primary tumor. Despite the introduction of sensitive modern mammographic modalities, which have redefined the "occult primary," there remain cases in which the breast fails to reveal its tumor, and therapy must be undertaken on the basis of relative certainty.

INCIDENCE AND NATURAL HISTORY

The three largest reported series of patients in the premammographic era had a range of 0.3 percent to 1 percent of breast carcinomas presenting as axillary metastases. Interestingly, Vilcoq et al.[17] report a similar incidence of 0.9 percent from the Institute Curie in Paris in mammographically benign breasts. Thus the addition of mammography has not allowed a marked decrease in the number of clinically undetected primary tumors (Table 51–1). It is likely that these numbers are slightly magnified as a result of the practice of referring patients with unusual manifestations of disease to the larger centers from which these reports arise. The median age and age range of these patients do not differ significantly from those of breast carcinoma patients in general.

In the majority of these cases an axillary swelling had been present for several months or less. Ashikari et al.[1] report that 64 percent of their cases were noted for less than 1 month, and almost 90 percent of those of Owen et al.[13] were present for less than 6 months. Also of note is the fact that some malignant neoplasms presenting in the axilla may be of other than breast origin. Melanoma is an evident possibility, and sweat gland tumors need also to be considered (section IV, chapters 9 and 11). The carcinomas most likely to present at any distant site should also be considered as possible sources for metastases to the axillae: thyroid, kidney, lung, stomach, and liver. In the series of Feuerman et al.[5] these were patients with carcinoma of the lung, stomach, colon, and pancreas who developed axillary metastases. All of these patients in the latter series had an evident symptomatic primary neoplasm.

Table 51–1. PRESENTATION OF BREAST CARCINOMA AS AXILLARY ADENOPATHY

Investigator	Year	Number	%
Fitts et al.[6]	1963	13 of 1300	1.00
Haagensen et al.[8]	1971	18 of 6000	0.30
Owen et al.[13]	1954	25 of 5451	0.45
Vilcoq et al.[17]	1982	11 of 1250	0.90

GROSS AND MICROSCOPIC ANATOMY

The size of the axillary node on clinical examination has varied widely from 0.9 cm to 5 cm, with most nodes between 2 and 5 cm. Among those patients who underwent formal axillary node dissection (usually at the time of mastectomy), one third had only the presenting solitary metastasis, whereas the remainder had additional nodes involved.

The histologic features of carcinoma in the involved lymph node have received relatively little attention despite the crucial role these studies have in predicting whether in fact the primary tumor is likely to have arisen from the breast. Most of the large studies simply report that the node contained carcinoma compatible with the breast primary. Haupt et al.[10] studied 43 cases of breast cancer presenting with axillary nodes and found a distinctive histologic pattern consisting of diffuse sheets of large apocrine-like cells without well-formed glands (Fig. 51–1). This pattern alone was present in 65 percent of their cases, while glandular structures more typical of carcinomas in the breast predominated in 23 percent. In 13 percent a mixture of these apocrine and glandular elements was present.

Owen et al.[13] report a high incidence of medullary carcinomas. These cases may well represent typical carcinomas with a heavy lymphocytic infiltrate, high grade nuclear features, and apocrine histology rather than pure medullary carcinomas, since the required gross circumscription of medullary carcinoma is not reported in these cases. Occasionally only in situ carcinoma is found in the specimen.[1, 2, 12, 19] In these series lobular carcinoma in situ (LCIS) accounts for only slightly fewer cases than ductal carcinoma in situ (DCIS). Together LCIS and DCIS make up 8 percent to 10 percent of the tumors found in clinically benign breasts with axillary metastases.[15] It is likely that the failure to demonstrate invasive tumor in this situation is largely a sampling problem.

It is mandatory to consider the possibility that the axillary tumor is actually a primary tumor. Careful analysis to determine that lymph nodal tissue is actually present should be done, because breast tissue extends into the axilla.

Of the 201 cases reported in which the results of mastectomy or biopsy are available, 68 percent contained tumor in resected breast tissue (Table 51–2). Slightly more than half were located in the upper outer quadrant. As the mode of presentation and the difficulty in finding tumor in surgically removed tissue suggest, these are small carcinomas. Ten of 16 cases of Patel et al.[14] were microscopic. In most series the majority of cases are 1 to 2 cm or less. However, in at least three instances, the primary lesion was 5 cm or greater and had a diffuse pattern of growth accounting for its nonpalpable nature.[6, 12, 14]

WORKUP

Obviously most unilateral lymphadenopathy does not represent metastatic carcinoma. The rationale involved in the decision to perform a biopsy on an enlarged lymph node is commonplace yet so complex that it need not be discussed in detail here. However, we wish to emphasize that the usual main concern is to exclude metastatic carcinoma, and fine needle aspiration of a superficial node should be considered. This procedure is simple, is accurate, requires no special equipment, and is associated with essentially no morbidity (see section VIII, chapter 26). If the aspiration yields carcinoma, lymph node biopsy can be planned in light of the results of a limited workup and with reference to the need for estrogen receptor analysis or other special studies. The extent of the workup of a woman with axillary carcinoma and benign breasts has been addressed,[12, 14] with the consensus of opinion being that studies need not be exhaustive. Physical examination should include careful thyroid, pelvic, and rectal exams as well as a search for other palpable lymph nodes and pigmented skin lesions. Other mandatory studies include chest radiographs, measurement of liver enzymes, and, of course, mammography. Bone scans are recommended by some and may be performed to establish a baseline. The efficacy of mammography in identifying or suggesting a mammary carcinoma in the setting of a solitary axillary metastasis has varied widely in reported series, ranging from 5 percent to 59 percent and averaging 25 percent (Table 51–2). This variation probably is a reflection of differences in methodology and interpretation as well as case definition.

In any case, the major determinant of further workup after detection of palpable axillary lymph nodes is the mammogram. In the event that a suspicious mammographic lesion is detected, the immediate course of action is evident. If the axillary lymph node is not greatly enlarged, the breast biopsy may be performed first, in the routine manner. When this breast biopsy evidences invasive carcinoma, then the usual pathways of clinical practice will be followed. These patients will be properly regarded as having preoperative axillary palpable adenopathy.

When the surgical biopsy of a mammographically detected lesion is negative in the presence of a palpable axillary node, then one returns to the clinical setting of this chapter and the clinical algorithm as outlined in Figure 51–2.

If the axillary tumor shows solid sheets of malignant cells, mucin stains demonstrating intracellular positivity can be helpful in determining that the tumor is an adenocarcinoma rather than other types of tumor such as melanoma and lymphoma, which may share this pattern of growth. Immunoperoxidase studies performed on paraffin-embedded tissue are quite reliable in classifying a poorly differentiated malignant neoplasm as epithelial, melanocytic, or lymphoid but are of limited help in pointing toward breast as the primary once it has been determined that the tumor is an adenocarcinoma. Electron microscopy demonstration of intracellular canaliculi, apical desmosomes, and secretory vesicles has been shown to be helpful in cases that appear undifferentiated by light microscopy.[11] Estrogen and progesterone receptor positivity is only suggestive of a

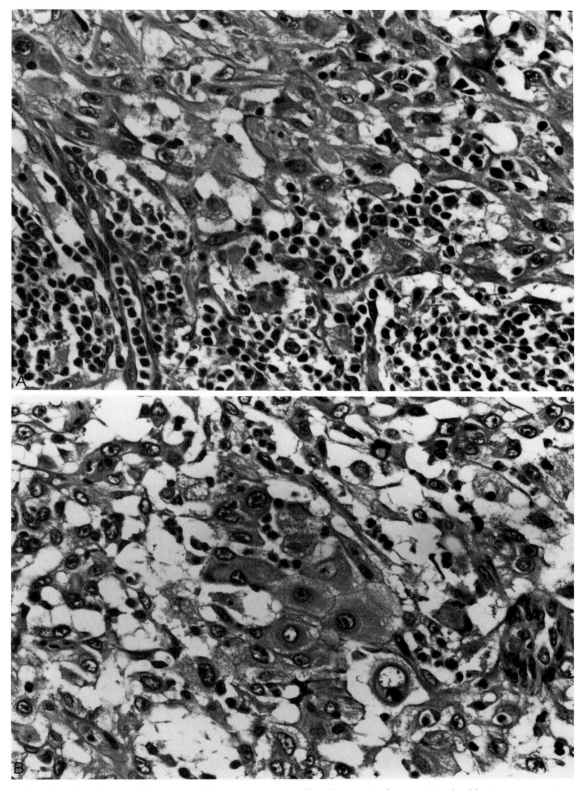

Figure 51–1. Axillary lymph node containing metastatic breast carcinoma cells with apocrine features. No gland lumina are seen. Large tumor cells have abundant granular, eosinophilic-to-clear cytoplasm and large single nucleoli. ×650

Table 51–2. RESULTS OF TISSUE EXAMINATION AND MAMMOGRAPHY

Investigator	No.	% Tumor in Breast*	Quadrant, if known (%) Upper Outer	Other	Abnormal Mammogram
Ashikari et al.[1]	42	65	71	29	3/25
Feuerman et al.[5]	10	70			
Fitts et al.[6]	13	85	55	45	
Haagensen[7]	28	84	42		
Haupt et al.[10]	43	72			11/43
Kemeny et al[12]	20	45			1/20
Owen et al.[13]	25	60	42	58	
Patel et al.[14]	29	55	55	45	10/17
Weinberger and Stetten[18]	5	100	50	50	
Westbrook and Gallagher[19]	18	75			6/17
Total	233	68			

*Of those examined histologically, totalling 201 cases.

breast primary but must be considered at the time of lymph node biopsy for the purpose of determining therapy. Awareness of the need for estrogen receptor studies at the time of initial node biopsy is especially important, since this may be the only tumor-containing tissue that will be available for study.

MANAGEMENT

The majority of women reported in these studies have had ipsilateral mastectomies. However, Kemeny et al.[12] retrospectively reported 20 women with axillary pres-

entation of breast carcinoma, 11 of whom received mastectomies, whereas seven had only axillary dissection or biopsy alone or in combination with radiation or chemotherapy. They show no difference in survival between those treated by mastectomy and those treated without mastectomy and conclude that mastectomy is unnecessary. Vilcoq et al.[17] recommend removal of the axillary mass followed by radiotherapy to the breast and axilla. Eleven patients over a 13-year period were thus treated, with a 91 percent 5-year survival. Feigenberg et al.[4] recommend upper outer quadrant sector mastectomy based on the statistical likelihood that this quadrant harbors the tumor. Only three of the eight women in their series were treated in this fashion. These three demonstrated tumor in the upper outer quadrant.

As axillary presentation of breast carcinoma is rare, questions of appropriate therapy are not likely to be answered on the basis of randomized prospective trials. However, we can tell a woman who has an axillary metastasis "consistent with breast primary" and who has a negative "other primary" workup that there is a greater than 90 percent chance that the ipsilateral breast contains tumor. Even if that breast is removed and no tumor is demonstrated, still the odds are that the breast does contain tumor that has not been located.

The reported equivalent or somewhat better prognosis following mastectomy for this form of breast carcinoma as compared to historical controls argues in favor of this approach. Based on the pathological findings of mastectomy specimens from the largest series (see Table 51–2), the sector mastectomy approach would be expected

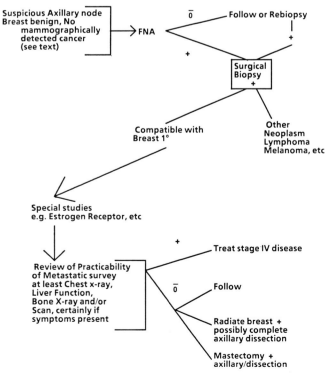

Figure 51–2. Flow chart outlining approach to female patient with suspected metastatic axillary carcinoma. FNA = fine needle aspiration.

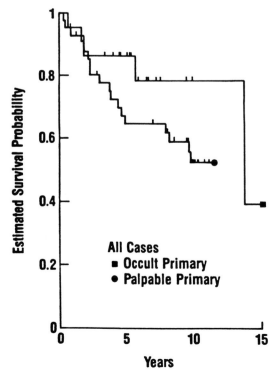

Figure 51–3. Survival of women (N = 22) with occult primary breast cancers of measurable size compared with similar patients presenting with palpable primary tumors. From Rosen PP, Kimmel M: Hum Pathol 21:518–523, 1990.

to leave as many as one half of the tumors behind in other quadrants. Upper outer quadrantectomy is an unproven approach but may be acceptable if the tumor is located within the resected tissue, is not multifocal, and does not have an extensive diffuse *in situ* component, and surgical margins are free. Should the tumor not be found in this quadrant, then consideration of further therapy may be appropriate. Axillary dissection should be performed in all surgically treated cases for adequate staging, prevention of axillary recurrence, and for further determining the need of adjuvant chemotherapy.

PROGNOSIS

The prognosis of women with axillary metastases from occult breast carcinomas has been shown to be no worse and perhaps slightly better than that of stage-matched patients with palpable breast cancer. The larger series of studies report "a better prognosis than is observed for the average carcinoma of the breast with nodal metastases,"[13] survival rates "higher than that for any group of our patients with carcinoma of the breast except for those without axillary metastases,"[6] and "prognosis is as good or better than it is for palpable breast cancer with axillary metastases."[19] The most recent study from Memorial Sloan-Kettering[16] compares 22 patients with occult breast carcinoma and axillary metastases whose mastectomy specimens contained measurable invasive tumor and matched them on the basis of tumor size, number of involved lymph nodes, tumor type, and age at diagnosis with patients presenting with palpable tumors (Fig. 51–3). Those with occult lesions demonstrated a more favorable, although not statistically different, prognosis.

References

1. Ashikari R, Rosen PP, Urban JA: Breast cancer presenting as an axillary mass. Ann Surg 183:415–417, 1976.
2. Breslow A: Occult carcinoma of second breast following mastectomy. JAMA 226:1000–1001, 1973.
3. Cameron HC: Some clinical facts regarding mammary cancer. Br Med J 1:577–582, 1909.
4. Feigenberg Z, Zer M, Dintsman M: Axillary metastases from an unknown primary source: A diagnostic and therapeutic approach. Isr J Med Sci 12:1153–1158, 1976.
5. Feuerman L, Attie JN, Rosenberg B: Carcinoma in axillary lymph nodes as an indicator of breast carcinoma. Surg Gynecol Obstet 114:5–8, 1962.
6. Fitts WT, Steiner GC, Enterline HT: Prognosis of occult carcinoma of the breast. Am J Surg 106:460–463, 1963.
7. Haagensen CD: Problems in differential diagnosis. Metastases of mammary carcinoma in axillary nodes without a palpable breast tumor. *In* Haagensen CD (ed): Diseases of the Breast, ed 3. Philadelphia, WB Saunders, 1986, p 548.
8. Haagensen CD, Bodian D, Haagensen DE: Breast carcinoma, risk and detection. *In* Haagensen CD (ed): Diseases of the Breast, Philadelphia, WB Saunders, 1971, p 441.
9. Halsted W: The results of radical operations for the cure of carcinoma of the breast. Ann Surg 46(1):1–19, 1907.
10. Haupt HM, Rosen PP, Kinne DW: Breast carcinoma presenting with axillary lymph node metastases: An analysis of specific histopathologic features. Am J Surg Pathol 9:165–175, 1985.
11. Iglehart JD, Ferguson BJ, Shingleton WW, et al: An ultrastructural analysis of breast carcinoma presenting as isolated axillary adenopathy. Ann Surg 196:8–13, 1982.
12. Kemeny MM, Rivera DE, Tarz JJ, Benfield JR: Occult primary adenocarcinoma with axillary metastases. Am J Surg 152:43–47, 1986.
13. Owen HW, Dockerty MB, Gray HK: Occult carcinoma of the breast. Surg Gynecol Obstet 98:302–308, 1954.
14. Patel J, Nemoto T, Rosner D, et al: Axillary node metastasis from an occult breast cancer. Cancer 47:2923–2927, 1981.
15. Rosen PP: Axillary lymph node metastases in patients with occult noninvasive breast carcinoma. Cancer 46:1298–1306, 1980.
16. Rosen PP, Kimmel M: Occult breast carcinomas presenting with axillary lymph node metastases: A follow-up of 48 patients. Hum Pathol 21:518–523, 1990.
17. Vilcoq JR, Calle R, Ferme F, et al: Conservative treatment of axillary adenopathy due to probable subclinical breast cancer. Arch Surg 117:1136–1138, 1982.
18. Weinberger HA, Stetten D: Extensive secondary axillary lymph node carcinoma without clinical evidence of primary breast lesion. Surgery 29:217–222, 1951.
19. Westbrook KC, Gallagher HS: Breast carcinoma presenting as an axillary mass. Am J Surg 122:607–611, 1971.

Chapter 52

MANAGEMENT OF THE PATIENT AT HIGH RISK

David L. Page, M.D. and William D. Dupont, Ph.D.

Patients are only considered at elevated risk for the development of carcinoma if the risk is reliably determined to approach double that of the general population. Note that use of the word "patients" rather than "women" in this operational definition denotes a clinical setting. Lesser degrees of risk may be important in nonclinical settings but are not considered here. Elevated risk is of unquestioned clinical importance when its magnitude approaches five times the general population. Note that comments on magnitude of relative risks (RR) are inherently confusing without an immediate reference group, because the term indicates a comparison. This reference group is usually a population of women without the risk factor or the general population. The age of a patient as well as the number of years at risk are of great import. Usually RR figures should be understood to have been derived while controlling the two comparison groups for age and number of years at risk. Application and derivation of risk statements are discussed in detail in the section entitled, "Slightly Increased Risk Lesions."

This chapter is primarily concerned with women identified to be at high risk because of histological determinants from breast biopsy. Nonanatomic factors such as familial associations are covered more completely elsewhere (see section V, chapter 13). Nulliparity, delayed parity, and other indicators of breast cancer risk are not discussed here but are acknowledged to be indicators of slight magnitude.

Symptomatic or painful breast disease has no known risk correlates or implications. Mammographic patterns may be associated with cancer risk[5, 12] but are not known to be sufficiently reliable to form the basis for clinical judgments. However, women with breasts that are dense on mammography should certainly be strongly encouraged to engage in yearly mammographic surveillance (see chapter 14).

By elevated risk, not otherwise specified, we mean any risk of breast cancer that is reliably identified and is of a magnitude that at least approaches twice that of the general population. When making more specific reference to the implications and magnitude of elevated risk, it is stratified as follows:

Slight or mild risk elevation:	1.5–2 times
Moderate elevation:	4–5 times
High elevation:	9–11 times

The levels are further discussed in chapter 14 and were the focus of a consensus conference organized by the College of American Pathologists and the American Cancer Society in 1985.[14]

This chapter will first summarize the relevant background material of chapters 6, 8, and 14 and then proceed with clinical management recommendations for women at heightened risk for breast cancer.

BACKGROUND

Between invasive carcinoma and nonproliferative breast tissue lies a group of lesions whose association with cancer and cancer risk varies. In this background section we will summarize information from chapters 6, 8, and 14, which deal with the pathology and epidemiology of these lesions. The extreme and clinically malignant example of this group is *palpable comedo carcinoma in situ*. It may be regarded as a true carcinoma because of poor prognosis following local excision.[17] About 50 percent of locally excised, palpable comedo carcinomas recur within 3 years. Many of these lesions may also have at least microscopic areas of invasion. Although regarded as a type of ductal carcinoma *in situ* (DCIS), the comedo lesions must be regarded separately from the others (see chapter 8).

The other *carcinomas in situ* (CIS) are discussed here as prototype examples of high-risk lesions. Indeed, they represent the highest risk against which the other elevated risk lesions may be best understood. The CIS lesions are discussed in detail elsewhere (see chapter 8), with only their risk associations highlighted here. Microscopic DCIS as well as lobular carcinomas *in situ* are associated with substantially less risk than palpable comedo *in situ* cancers and may be classified as high-risk, precancerous lesions.[14] It is against these high-risk lesions that the moderately elevated risk lesions of atypical hyperplasia should be compared and understood. These lesions do not necessarily progress to invasive cancer even when treated with biopsy only, although the risk of the patient developing cancer is substantial.

The vast majority of the *microscopic in situ ductal carcinomas* (micro DCIS) have a cribriform or papillary morphology and may be termed collectively as noncomedo carcinoma *in situ.* "Microscopic" may be taken loosely here, as it has been in other publications, to mean usually inapparent on gross examination of tissue but including mammographically detected lesions. These lesions are associated with a tenfold increase in risk of invasive cancer after treatment by surgical biopsy only. They were found in approximately 0.25 percent of biopsy specimens originally diagnosed as benign in the premammographic era[22] and are seen currently in greatly increased numbers because of their greater incidence in women undergoing open biopsy as a result of mammographically detected, nonpalpable lesions.[16, 24] We studied 28 consecutive patients with these lesions who were treated with biopsy only[9] and found that seven developed invasive cancer during an overall average follow-up period of 14 years. In this series the later carcinomas appeared an average of 7 years after biopsy. All seven of these cancers recurred in the same quadrant of the ipsilateral breast, indicating that micro DCIS is biologically monofocal. The recurrence rate at 15 years adjusted for withdrawals was 29 percent. Rosen et al.[28] found a similar incidence of microscopic, noncomedo DCIS, and eight of their 30 patients who were similarly treated had a subsequent and homolateral presentation of clinically evident carcinoma.

Lobular carcinoma in situ (LCIS) is associated with a magnitude of risk of invasive breast cancer similar to that of micro DCIS (see chapters 8 and 14). This risk is approximately ten times that of the general population.[29] The absolute risk of invasive breast cancer after LCIS is about 20 percent at 15 years (adjusted for withdrawals). Subsequent invasive cancer is equally likely to occur in either breast. This is roughly the same experience as reported by Haagensen et al.[13] However, the magnitude of risk was somewhat less in women in Haagensen et al.'s study, probably reflecting the inclusion of cases having less completely developed lesions that others would include in the atypical hyperplasia category.

Atypical hyperplasias (AH) occupy the borderland between unequivocally benign lesions and *in situ* carcinoma. These worrisome lesions are characterized by having some but not all of the features required for a diagnosis of *in situ* carcinoma.[23] It is important to realize that these lesions are relatively rare. Approximately four percent of benign biopsy samples contained atypical hyperplasia in the premammographic era.[7] During the 1950s and 1960s, women who underwent biopsies revealing these lesions presented with clinical lumps or lumpiness that prompted a surgical biopsy to diagnose or to rule out the presence of carcinoma.

The incidence of the atypical hyperplasias is undoubtedly different in different subgroups. The determination of this expected incidence is incomplete at this time. However, this incidence has been found to be somewhat less in a sample of women whose breasts were examined after unexpected death[3] than in women who presented with suspicious lumps. The incidence of atypical hyperplasias in a forensic autopsy series of women in an ethnically high-risk group for breast cancer (analogous to those women studied in the Nashville follow-up group)[7] was only 2.5 percent after the entire breast had

been examined.[3] However, the incidence of atypical hyperplasias in biopsy specimens obtained as a result of mammographic findings is in the range of ten percent.[30]

The age incidences of atypical hyperplasia also vary greatly as would be expected for a biological phenomenon linked to breast cancer.[23] Advancing age is also the strongest determinant of breast cancer risk other than female sex. In a large series of women undergoing surgical biopsy in the premammographic era, this age variation in atypical hyperplasias was noted to feature a peak incidence for hyperplasia in the immediate premenopausal age group. After menopause the incidence of atypical ductal hyperplasia continued to increase, whereas that of atypical lobular hyperplasia decreased (see chapter 14). There are two histologically distinct forms of atypical hyperplasia, named "lobular" (ALH) and "ductal" (ADH) because of their morphological similarities to lobular and ductal carcinoma *in situ*, respectively. Both of these lesions, however, probably originate within terminal ductal lobular units[33] and are associated with similar cancer risks. Women with atypical hyperplasia are at four to five times the breast cancer risk of women of similar age from the general population. The 15-year absolute risk of invasive cancer is about ten percent for these women.

In a cohort study,[23] 18 of 150 women with ADH subsequently developed breast cancer as compared with 16 of 126 women with ALH in an average follow-up of 17 years. Subsequent breast cancers occurred in the same breast as the original biopsy in 56 percent of these ADH patients and 69 percent of these ALH patients,[23] indicating that each breast should be considered at risk. A first degree family history of breast cancer (mother, daughter, or sister) doubles the cancer risk among women with atypical hyperplasia (see chapter 14). We estimated the 15-year absolute risk of breast cancer for these women to be 20 percent, which is comparable to the risk associated with microscopic *in situ* carcinoma as noted previously.

In contrast to atypical lesions, other benign breast lesions are associated with a modest or no increase in breast cancer risk. In our review of 10,366 consecutive benign biopsies in the premammographic era, 26 percent had *proliferative disease without atypia* (PDWA), and 70 percent lacked proliferative disease.[7] Women with PDWA had an almost twofold increase in breast cancer risk, whereas women without proliferative disease had no elevation in breast cancer risk. This latter result should be cause for considerable reassurance to women who have received this diagnosis. Note that this group includes a large majority of women undergoing breast biopsy on the indication of suspicion of cancer on clinical grounds. Thus it includes mostly women who have been identified because of lumps due to fibrous, adenotic, and cystic changes. Thus, these palpable abnormalities cannot be considered in themselves to be markers of increased cancer risk. We and many others[14, 19] prefer that the term "fibrocystic disease" be avoided and replaced with less negative or pejorative terms such as "fibrocystic change."

CLINICAL IMPLICATIONS OF HIGH RISK

The results of longitudinal studies providing outcome information on women with high-risk breast lesions do not lead to simple therapeutic decisions. Clinical management requires consideration of the degree of cancer risk, the level of anxiety of the patient, her willingness to participate in intensive long-term follow-up, and the importance of the patient's breasts to her self-image.

Translating these levels of risk into clinical management guidelines is not complete or at least has not achieved a concisely stated consensus. Indeed, some[4] are of the belief that such information is dangerous or potentially dangerous because it gives little guidance and produces anxiety. It may be little improved over the situation prior to these follow-up studies in which a "worrisome" histology was reported and this information relayed to the patient without even a glimpse at the implied level of risk. However, this risk information is available and, considering the level of concern about breast cancer already present in the community, should be used. Hopefully the information may actually aid in resolving anxieties about cancer. This may be done by focusing attention on the small proportion of women with substantial risk elevation and the corresponding large proportion at no or only slight elevation of risk.

CLINICAL MANAGEMENT

An approach toward clinical management predicated on this improved but still probabilistic knowledge of risk for breast cancer development is a new arena for most of us. We are steeped in the approach of having a definitive diagnosis that is linked to a specific therapy without having many intervening variables and certainly without having several generally acceptable clinical approaches in each situation.

The most frequent personal response to any indication of excess breast cancer risk probably will be greater than that merited by the facts themselves. Increased risk of cancer is relayed to patients in phrases that trigger some anxiety at the very least. We believe that both the anxiety and the medical implications should be addressed. Our suggested guidelines for clinical management of the different levels of risk follow.

In general, the acceptance of levels of risk from histopathological data have followed suggestions from a consensus conference held in 1985.[14] These levels of risk are as noted briefly in the introduction to this chapter as well as in chapter 6.

High-Risk Lesions

The high-risk lesions (some *in situ* carcinomas) are discussed here primarily to give a backdrop or template for the understanding of the moderate-risk lesions (the atypical hyperplasias). Both the magnitude of risk and variety of accepted approaches to clinical management should be considered. The high level of risk is under-

stood to approximate the magnitude of that associated with lobular carcinoma *in situ*. These women with LCIS are understood to have a risk of subsequent carcinoma development that in relative terms is approximately ten times that of the general population. There may be some differences associated with extensiveness of disease or age at presentation that are currently not well understood. This restriction derives largely from our lack of experience with women presenting in the younger and older age groups.[21] Thus the great majority of women who undergo biopsy for benign breast disease other than fibroadenoma are in the pre- and perimenopausal group from 35 to about 55 years of age. This uncertainty with younger and older women extends to those groups discussed in the sections that follow.

Clinical management of lobular carcinoma *in situ* as a practical matter involves a decision between extremes. The original diagnoses were made by only a few institutions in the 1940s and occasioned no action clinically.[11, 15, 20] As the diagnosis of LCIS was accepted in the 1960s and early 1970s, a simple mastectomy on the side involved with a large biopsy on the other side became a frequent clinical practice.[27] However, at other institutions this was not done, and these women were put under careful clinical surveillance as in the study of Haagensen et al.[13] The fact that the latter group was found on follow-up to have no deaths from metastatic carcinoma after treatment of the carcinomas that developed[13] has led many to believe that careful clinical follow-up is appropriate for this disease. It is important to note that this experience of Haagensen et al. was in the premammographic era. We can only assume that detection of smaller invasive carcinomas will be greatly facilitated by close surveillance with mammography.

Undoubtedly some physicians will continue to extirpate breast tissue, an option which must be conceded to be appropriate in some clinical settings. The historical and management perspectives are comprehensively reviewed in section XIII, chapter 35, as is the treatment of ductal carcinoma *in situ*.

No-Elevated-Risk Conditions

In this category may be placed approximately 70 percent of women who undergo biopsy on the basis of nodules or nodularity presenting to a surgeon in the era prior to mammography. With the different selectivity associated with mammographic evaluation, it is likely that this balance in the different histological findings will change somewhat. We have no reason to believe that the hyperplastic lesions themselves should have different indications but rather that their relative incidence and prevalence will be different. Recent evaluation of breast biopsies performed on the indication of mammography supports this contention and documents an increased prevalence of the atypical hyperplasias.[2, 30]

The microscopic patterns seen in virtually all breast biopsies involve irregularities in distribution of lobules, some variability and focal increase in fibrosis, and (particularly in the immediate period prior to menopause) the presence of cysts. This common complex has, of course, given rise to the term "fibrocystic disease" and may now be better relayed as "fibrocystic change," because there is no reason to believe a "disease" is present. Any other condition that is not associated with increased risk may also be accepted as a "no-elevated-risk" situation. Those conditions that are demonstrated to predict increased risk are discussed in the sections that follow.

Slightly-Increased-Risk Lesions

The term "slightly increased risk" is assigned to those conditions that have a statistically significant elevation in cancer risk of a magnitude that approaches twice that of the general population controlled for age and number of years at risk. We will consistently highlight the variable of years at risk. It is important not to extrapolate such risks to time intervals that are much longer than those documented in the literature. In particular we believe that projecting risk over the entire lifetime of an individual patient is misleading and usually overstates the magnitude of the patient's absolute risk.

The various methods of stating magnitude and relevance of increased risk should be understood by anyone counseling women thought to have increased risk. Most of our discussions are presented in terms of relative risk, which is a complex statement of a fraction divided by a fraction. Thus the statement that women with AH have a four times increased risk of cancer is derived as follows: Incidence of CA in women with AH ÷ Incidence of CA in general = RR, (incidence of CA in AH = women with AH developing cancer ÷ all women with AH) or Relative Risk equals

$$\frac{\text{Women with AH developing CA}}{\text{All women with AH}} \div \frac{\text{Women in ref. pop'n developing CA}}{\text{All women in ref. pop'n}}$$

Note that the choice of the reference population is a major influence on the credibility and magnitude of the end result. The variables of age at biopsy and number of years followed are critical and are carefully accounted for in credible studies, making the study and reference groups comparable. The RR is a construct designed for the comparison of groups to determine the credibility of the effect of one factor on another. By its nature it groups different sorts of persons in one statement. Thus it should only be used in application to a single patient after careful thought to comparability. This comparability is derived from a consideration of age and number of years at risk. These are just the factors amalgamated in the RR statement, which must be dissected out when a statement of risk is individualized. A clinically relevant statement is made in terms of absolute risk (AR). This states the percentage likelihood of an event occurring in a certain period of time. Absolute risk is stated as ten percent in 10 to 15 years. In general terms we do not feel that risk should be interpreted beyond that length of time. Moreover, we have also recently shown

that RR is not constant with time. Thus the all too common practice of taking presumed lifetime risk of breast cancer in North America (about ten percent) and multiplying it by an RR figure is incorrect. Such a prediction can be shown to be false even when the RR remains constant for the remainder of the patient's life. Studies have been performed that approach 20 years of follow-up but have observed few events after 15 years. Thus prediction should be confined to the next 10 to 15 or 20 years maximally; AR should be used preferentially in the clinical setting with an individual patient but should be carefully sculpted to the setting. AR may be derived from RR as seen in Fig. 52–1. However, the relative risk is assumed to be constant for the full 20 years, and for proliferative disease, RR falls when observed 10 years after biopsy (chapter 14). This latter observation emphasizes the tenuous nature of prediction beyond 10 to 15 years.

Conditions associated with slightly increased risk connote a risk of breast cancer similar to that associated with a weak (few or distant relatives only) family history of breast carcinoma (see chapter 13). These histological changes collectively termed "proliferative disease without atypia" (PDWA) (see chapter 6) are quite frequent and were long thought to be part of the spectrum of such broadly embracing terms as "mammary dysplasia" and "fibrocystic disease." The reported magnitude of risks are statistically significant, but whether they are medically significant is somewhat doubtful. Thus the risk for breast cancer of the general female population of North America is approximately 1.5 percent per year, or 15 per 1000 women between the ages of 40 and 50 years.[6] The average incidence in the decade between the ages of 40 and 50 years for women with a slight risk elevation would be about 25 per 1000.

We believe that the best way to relay this information to a patient is in terms of the next 10 to 15 years. The reliable knowledge of what will happen after that time is not available. Events separated by more than a decade in the future become clouded, particularly by the possibility of different associations with carcinoma development in different age groups, and greatly altered by competing causes of death, which go up very quickly following the age of 65.[6, 31]

The current suggestion followed by most practitioners at this time is that women falling in this slightly elevated risk group should merely be encouraged to follow the recommendation for a yearly mammogram commencing at approximately the age of 40. There seems to be no other indication to do anything else except to also encourage self-examination in these women. The greatest importance of this group is to delineate and define the majority of women who have had a breast biopsy and have no elevation of risk or the same breast cancer risk as that in the general population.

Despite the lack of certainty as to the cancer preventive effect of increased clinical surveillance on women with elevated risk, it is the only known alternative to denial. The approach to patients with these lesions should be made with humility, because we do not know if the anxiety we may cause could outweigh any thera-

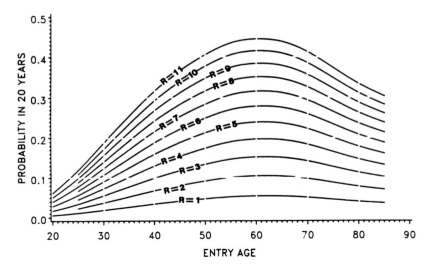

Figure 52–1. Breast cancer morbidity in U.S. women. "Probability in 20 Years" indicates the risk of developing breast cancer within 20 years of a patient's entry age. This is the age at which she is first known to have increased risk of developing cancer; she is assumed not to have developed breast cancer before this age. The lines labeled R = 1, 2, . . ., 11 denote her relative risk of breast cancer. These curves are based on the assumption that the relative risks remain constant over the 20-year interval; they use morbidity and mortality data from the SEER and NCHS data bases for American women in 1983. (From Dupont WD: Stat Med 8:641–651, 1989. Reprinted by permission of John Wiley & Sons, Ltd.)

peutic benefit that we may provide. We recommend little additional surveillance for women with slight risk elevation. This should include nothing more than a somewhat stronger encouragement of yearly mammography than might be done for the general population. This level of slight risk that approaches twice that of the general population is not a range that should occasion a great degree of concern. It is thought that encouraging mammography in women with slight risk elevation may increase detection.[1] Alexander et al.[1] are evaluating a screening program in which the general population is screened every 3 years, with more frequent screening for women with elevated risk.

Moderately-Increased-Risk Lesions

For women with a moderately elevated risk of subsequent carcinoma development, careful surveillance is mandatory. They should be told that this surveillance by mammography will, in all probability, reduce their risk of death from breast carcinoma to that experienced by the general population. This concept and promise is not made with the proof of specific experience but is certainly strongly supported by the experience of Haagensen et al.[13] Women with lobular neoplasia and related lesions who were followed by Haagensen using only clinical exams had no deaths from breast carcinoma, despite a moderate to high level of risk of developing carcinomas. Occasionally, particularly if they have a positive family history, women with moderate risk lesions will approach a relative risk of ten times. This risk is similar to that associated with lobular carcinoma *in situ*, a lesion long known to be associated with high risk of breast cancer (see previous discussion of LCIS).

In addition to women with *in situ* carcinomas, women treated for primary carcinoma in one breast may also be considered in this category. The subsequent risk for the contralateral breast is well accepted to be 0.7 percent to one percent per year, at least for the first 10 years (see chapters 12 and 48). Again, several clinical management possibilities are available, but breast removal

is only occasionally performed.[32] The magnitude of risk for these patients is comparable to that for women with AH at biopsy.

Of greatest concern here is the problem of the length of time at which this elevated risk persists. Although many prefer to be concerned with cumulative risk, which purports to deal with a lifetime risk, we are strongly in favor of the idea that clinical decision making should be based on knowledge of events in the ensuing 10 to 15 years and not beyond.[8] These are the limits of certainty that may be derived from follow-up studies. It is our experience (see chapter 14), particularly with older women, that these elevated risks will fall 10 to 15 years after detection.[8]

It is evident from the previous discussion that patient management decisions are difficult and no precise guidelines may be given. Probably the most important single factor is the individual woman's level of concern. It is overly dramatic to relay this variable as one of "cancerphobia," but that is the most familiar term. Our fervent belief is that once a high-risk lesion is determined, that no decision be rushed. It is not a medical emergency or an emergent situation of any type. Even the carcinomas *in situ* of greatest magnitude and extent have not been demonstrated to threaten life within several months following biopsy. Indeed, the "latent" period between detection of the microscopic ductal carcinomas *in situ* as well as lobular carcinoma *in situ* and the appearance of invasive carcinoma averages 10 years or more (chapters 8 and 35). Thus no harm is likely to result if several months pass between the detection of a high-risk or moderately high-risk lesion and formalizing a clinical decision; the decision should be made without the overlay of immediate drama and stress. It should also be made in the full knowledge of the impact of this diagnosis and risk assessment on the individual woman's quality of life. However difficult it might be to understand risk elevation in the sense of a group or defined population, it is certainly even more difficult to do so in the case of an individual. Thus if the individual's level of concern is extremely high (e.g., impairing sleep, etc.), the patient and her physicians should seriously consider the removal of breast tissue in the hope of reducing risk.[32]

As noted, mammographic surveillance is widely accepted as a clinical alternative over extirpative surgery for most women. The logic of this decision rests largely in the following knowledge:

1. Mastectomy would remove many more breasts than ever would develop cancer.

2. The patient's breast cancer risk will more closely approximate that of slightly elevated risk if she remains free of cancer for 10 years after biopsy indicating moderate risk.[8]

3. The current era of mammography should only improve the good prognosis after treatment of later developing breast cancer in women with moderate and high risk followed closely by palpation.[13]

There is no generally accepted program for clinical surveillance of women with moderate risk. However, yearly mammography with clinical examination once or twice yearly should be considered almost mandatory along with a recommendation for breast self-examination.[18] Whether more frequent mammographic examinations would have practical utility is questionable. The reason for this is based on the intrinsic rate of growth to detectability of many breast cancers. However, there is no specific reason to refuse twice yearly mammography for these women if it brings a calmer acceptance of the situation. A repeat mammogram at 5 to 6 months after initial diagnosis is useful for slightly different reasons (e.g., the possible effect of scarring at the biopsy site may be assessed and the early evaluation of a possible coexisting carcinoma may be accomplished). This suggestion is analogous to the guidelines made following radiation therapy (see section XIV, chapters 37 and 38).

There are a few differences between ductal and lobular pattern atypias, which are otherwise similar in many respects. The carcinomas developing after LCIS and ALH are much more likely to be infiltrating lobular carcinomas. This unusual (but not rare) carcinoma is often, but not always, diffusely infiltrating so that detection is difficult. Thus mammograms should be evaluated with care for subtle cues such as asymmetry between the breasts.

It is abundantly clear that many factors will impinge on the clinical management of the woman with moderate- and high-risk lesions. Although indications for biopsy (surgical or needle) will remain the same as for other women, it is also clear that biopsies will be performed more frequently in this group on less certain indications. When frequent biopsies are necessary, then preventive surgical strategies will become more seriously considered.[32] However, with the passage of time and the advance of age, the cancer risk for those women not developing carcinoma at 10 years after biopsy approximates that of women with lesions denoting slightly elevated risk[8] (see chapter 14).

Nonanatomic Risk Factors

Family history of breast cancer, mammographic patterns of increased density, nulliparity, delayed parity, and other nonanatomic indicators of elevated breast cancer risk are not further discussed here. However, we would like to highlight the interaction of positive family history (FH) with the moderate risk anatomic indicators of atypical hyperplasia. Not only are the risks of later carcinoma for women with AH and FH synergistically interactive (see chapter 14), but the emotional set of a woman with memories of suffering family members will have great impact on decisions made for clinical management. It is in these women that the strategies with greatest physical impact such as total glandular ("subcutaneous") mastectomy will be most likely considered. Even for these women, we believe that several months should pass before undertaking a final decision. We feel that it should be certain the woman knows that the anxiety and hindrance of life-style is and will be personally relentless.

Other interventional strategies are being tested, mostly those that affect diet or the endocrine milieu. Reduction of saturated fatty acids in the diet may lessen cancer risk, but that remains controversial. The same is true for agents such as tamoxifen and the luteinizing hormone-releasing hormone (LH-RH) agonists. The former acts as an antiestrogen in breast,[10, 26] and the latter reduces endogenous estrogens to low levels.[25] These clinical trials will take time but are promising.

References

1. Alexander FE, Roberts MM, Huggins A, Muir BB: Use of risk factors to allocate schedules for breast cancer screening. J Epidemiol Community Health 42:193–199, 1988.
2. Anderson TJ: Premalignant benign disease-fact or fiction? Br J Clin Practice 42:31–35, 1988.
3. Bartow SA, Pathak DR, Black WC, Key CR, Teaf SR: Prevalence of benign, atypical, and malignant breast lesions in populations at different risk for breast cancer. Cancer 60:2751–2760, 1987.
4. Baum M: Management of the "at risk" breast. Br J Clin Pract 42:41–46, 1988.
5. Boyd NF, O'Sullivan B, Fishell E, Simor I, Cooke G: Mammographic patterns and breast cancer risk: methodologic standards and contradictory results. J Natl Cancer Inst 72:1253–1259, 1984.
6. Dupont WD: Converting relative risks to absolute risks: a graphical approach. Stat Med 8:641–651, 1989.
7. Dupont WD, Page DL: Risk factors for breast cancer in women with proliferative breast disease. N Engl J Med 312:146–151, 1985.
8. Dupont WD, Page DL: Relative risk of breast cancer varies with time since diagnosis of atypical hyperplasia. Hum Pathol 20:723–725, 1989.
9. Eusebi V, Foschini MA, Cook MG, Berrino F, Azzopardi JG: Long-term follow-up of in situ carcinoma of the breast with special emphasis on clinging carcinoma. Semin Diagn Pathol 6:165–173, 1989.
10. Fentiman IS: The endocrine prevention of breast cancer. Br J Cancer 60:12–14, 1989.
11. Foote FW, Stewart FW: Lobular carcinoma in situ. Am J Pathol 17:491–495, 1941.
12. Goodwin PJ, Boyd NF: Mammographic parenchymal pattern and breast cancer risk: a critical appraisal of the evidence. Am J Epidemiol 127:1097–1108, 1988.
13. Haagensen CD, Lane N, Lattes R, Bodian C: Lobular neoplasia (so-called lobular carcinoma in situ) of the breast. Cancer 42:737–769, 1978.
14. Hutter RVP: Consensus meeting. Is "fibrocystic disease" of the breast precancerous? Arch Pathol Lab Med 110:171–173, 1986.

15. Hutter RVP, Foote FW: Lobular carcinoma in situ. Cancer 24:1081–1085, 1969.
16. Lagios MD, Margolin FR, Westdahl PR, Rose MR: Mammographically detected duct carcinoma in situ. Cancer 63:618–624, 1989.
17. Lewis D, Geschickter CF: Comedo carcinomas of the breast. Arch Surg 36:225–244, 1938.
18. Locker AP, Caseldine J, Mitchell AK, Blamey RW, Roebuck EJ, Elston CW: Results from a seven-year programme of breast self-examination in 89,010 women. Br J Cancer 60:401–405, 1989.
19. Love SM, Gelman RS, Silen W: Fibrocystic "disease" of the breast: a non-disease. N Engl J Med 307:1010–1014, 1982.
20. McDivitt RW, Hutter RVP, Foote FW, Stewart FW: In situ lobular carcinoma: a prospective follow-up study indicating cumulative patient risks. JAMA 201:96–100, 1967.
21. Page DL, Dupont WD: Histopathologic risk factors for breast cancer in women with benign breast disease. Semin Surg Oncol 4:213–217, 1988.
22. Page DL, Dupont WD, Rogers LW, Landenberger M: Intraductal carcinoma of the breast: follow-up after biopsy only. Cancer 49:751–758, 1982.
23. Page DL, Dupont WD, Rogers LW, Rados MS: Atypical hyperplastic lesions of the female breast. A long-term follow-up study. Cancer 55:2698–2708, 1985.
24. Patchefsky AS, Schwartz GF, Finkelstein SD, Prestipino A, Sohn SE, Singer JS, Feig SA: Heterogeneity of intraductal carcinoma of the breast. Cancer 63:731–741, 1989.
25. Pike MC, Ross RK, Lobo RA, Key TJA, Potts M, Henderson BE: LHRH agonists and the prevention of breast and ovarian cancer. Br J Cancer 60:142–148, 1989.
26. Powles TJ, Hardy JR, Ashley SE, Farrington GM, Cosgrove D, Davey JB, Dowsett M, McKinna JA, Nash AG, Sinnett HD, Tillyer CR, Treleaven JG: A pilot trial to evaluate the acute toxicity and feasibility of tamoxifen for prevention of breast cancer. Br J Cancer 60:126–131, 1989.
27. Rosen PP, Braun DW Jr, Lyngholm B, Urban JA, Kinne DW: Lobular carcinoma in situ of the breast: preliminary results of treatment by ipsilateral mastectomy and contralateral breast biopsy. Cancer 47:813–819, 1981.
28. Rosen PP, Braun DW Jr, Kinne DE: The clinical significance of pre-invasive breast carcinomas. Cancer 46:919–925, 1980.
29. Rosen PP, Lieberman PH, Braun DW Jr, Kosloff C, Adair F: Lobular carcinoma in situ of the breast: detailed analysis of 99 patients with average follow-up of 24 years. Am J Surg Pathol 2:225–251, 1978.
30. Rubin E, Alexander RW, Visscher DW, Urist MM, Maddox WA: Proliferative disease and atypia in biopsies performed for mammographically detected nonpalpable lesions. Cancer 61:2077–2082, 1988.
31. Seidman H, Mushinski MH, Gelb SK: Probabilities of eventually developing or dying of cancer—United States, 1985. Cancer 35:36–56, 1985.
32. Shack RB, Page DL: The patient at risk for breast cancer: pathologic and surgical considerations. Perspect Plast Surg 2:43–62, 1988.
33. Wellings SR, Jensen HM, Marcum RG: An atlas of subgross pathology of the human breast with special reference to possible precancerous lesions. J Natl Cancer Inst 55:231–273, 1975.

Section XX

Special Problems With Rehabilitation and Care of the Patient With Breast Cancer

Chapter 53

NURSING CARE FOR THE PATIENT WITH BREAST CANCER

Marilyn Brown, R.N., B.S.N., Holly Eyles, R.N., O.C.N., and Kirby I. Bland, M.D.

The opportunity for nursing interventions is multitudinal when caring for the patient with breast cancer. Depending on the setting this can begin with the challenge of teaching breast cancer prevention, screening, and identification of risk factors in the well-patient population. When a breast lesion that is suggestive of cancer is identified and diagnosed, the nurse offers emotional support to the patient and family and prepares the patient for tests and anticipated procedures. Interventions continue with postoperative nursing care and rehabilitative teaching and may include the patient receiving systemic therapy. This chapter will discuss nursing considerations for the patient with breast cancer and address the psychosocial, physiological, and educational aspects of care during each stage of diagnosis and treatment.

ROLE OF THE NURSE IN THE SCREENING AND DETECTION PROCESS

The number of women who die each year from breast cancer can be potentially reduced through screening and early detection.[8] The survival rates from this disease are directly linked to the stages in which the cancer is diagnosed. The nurse can have an impact on the screening and early detection process in a variety of settings by taking advantage of the opportunity to educate women, their families, and the general public about the benefits of early detection. The nurse must build awareness and understanding of the cancer risk, dispel myths and misconceptions about breast cancer, emphasize recognition of warning signs and symptoms, and establish the importance of periodic screening and early detection.

A lack of knowledge or confusion of the known risk factors for the disease may result in unnecessary anxiety in some women while offering false reassurance to others. Building awareness and understanding of the major risk factors and how they influence susceptibility can augment patient motivation to initiate beneficial health practices.[8] The presence or absence of risk factors is not used to determine which women should be screened but rather as a guide for the age at which to begin screening and the intervals at which the process is repeated. Numerous factors have been implicated to increase a woman's susceptibility to breast cancer, but very little is understood of the relationship of these factors to cause. Major risk factors include a positive family history of breast cancer (patients with mothers, daughters, or sisters with breast cancer have the highest risk), a history of previous breast cancer, or a suspicious or premalignant histology on a previous biopsy.[6, 10] For a detailed discussion of these risk factors, refer to section V, chapter 13 for considerations of pedigree analysis and family cancer syndromes. Section III, chapter 6 and section V, chapter 14 review the evaluation and treatment considerations for benign pathological lesions in high-risk patients.

There are several commonly held misconceptions by

the general public regarding breast cancer. Results from a recent survey conducted by Gross and Yarbro[8] revealed that more than half of women believed oral contraceptives and postmenopausal replacement hormones increased their risk of developing breast cancer. No evidence exists to support a causal relationship. Many people also erroneously believe that mild trauma or injury to the breast initiates breast cancer. The general public's knowledge with regard to breast cancer has greatly improved during the past decade, but the need for patient education remains great.

The vast majority of breast cancers diagnosed today are invasive ductal carcinomas, which most often present as a painless single, unilateral irregularly shaped mass that is sometimes associated with skin changes. The more advanced cancers (T3, T4) are usually associated with skin dimpling or nipple retraction, changes in size or shape of the breast, skin edema or discoloration, and a hard, fixed mass in the axilla. Nipple discharge is more commonly associated with benign breast disease but can also be associated with a malignancy (Chapter 3). Paget's disease, which is a more infrequent presentation of a subareolar breast cancer, presents with a crusting, oozing, or bleeding nipple surface.

The American Cancer Society recommends three methods of screening for breast cancer: breast self-exam (BSE), physical examination, and mammography. Monthly BSE should be performed by all women older than 20 years, and clinical exams should be obtained at least every 3 years from age 20 to age 40 and annually thereafter. Baseline mammography should be obtained between the ages of 35 and 40, every 1 to 2 years thereafter, and annually after age 50. For those women in the high-risk category, more frequent screening intervals may be recommended.[4]

If the patient is not familiar with BSE techniques, this can be demonstrated using either the patient's breasts or a breast model (e.g., Mammacare). Re-demonstration by the patient provides specific feedback to correct errors.[9] Pamphlets available from the American Cancer Society and National Cancer Institute are also helpful teaching aids. Figure 53–1 provides an illustrated example of the techniques used to perform a breast self-examination.

In many instances the nurse is involved in acquiring the patient's history during the screening process. The history should begin with an evaluation of the major risk factors. Other pertinent data to include are the age at menarche or menopause, number of pregnancies, age at pregnancies, and history of estrogen and/or steroid usage and smoking. It is also important to include any history of previous breast biopsy for benign breast disease (e.g., proliferative disease and fibroadenoma). If the patient reports a lump in her breast, a description should be included of the duration of the lesion, the changes in size or characteristics of its growth, and associated skin changes or nipple discharge.

ROLE OF THE NURSE IN DIAGNOSIS

A suspicious mammogram or physical examination most commonly initiates the confirmation of a breast cancer. Therefore one would anticipate the patient's anxiety level to be high. The primary goal of nursing intervention during the diagnostic period is the reduction of anxiety through support and education.

Nurses involved with patients during this period are often employed in outpatient settings such as a physician's office or clinic. This setting may place serious time constraints on nursing personnel for patient education, but the nurse must be cognizant of this crucial period for patient education and prioritize time accordingly. The recent study by Lierman[10] concludes that even in light of all the recent media attention given to the diagnosis and treatment of breast cancer, most patients have significant deficiencies or inaccurate knowledge regarding the potential diagnosis of this disease.

Patient teaching is most effective in a quiet, comfortable, and private setting. Basic terminology such as benign, malignant, and biopsy should be reviewed. The nurse should also assess patient concerns and possible misconceptions surrounding the word "cancer." The teaching must also include a basic description of the planned diagnostic technique such as fine needle aspiration, excisional, and needle-localized breast biopsy. (For a detailed description of the different biopsy procedures and their indications refer to section X, chapter 28.) Procedures should be explained emphasizing the safety and effectiveness of each, but education regarding the procedure alone may not be sufficient to reduce fear and anxiety. Education should reinforce the fact that the majority of breast masses are not malignant and that the presence of breast cancer may not necessitate breast removal. In addition to the underlying phobia of breast cancer, women undergoing any examination of the breast may experience apprehension and embarrassment, which are natural responses.[8] Nurses should be sensitive to a woman's reaction when performing or assisting with the exam.

Diagnosis of breast cancer must be made by the procurement of pathological tissues from the biopsy. This may be done either by fine needle aspiration in the physician's office or as an outpatient operative procedure. It is recommended that nurses who assist patients during this period should observe both an excisional and needle-localized breast biopsy, which are two commonly performed operative procedures used in the diagnosis of breast cancer. Procedures such as fine needle aspiration or Tru-cut biopsy may be performed in the physician's office, during which the nurse may be asked to assist in the procurement of diagnostic tissue.

Complications from any type of biopsy are rare, but patients should be instructed to notify the physician should they experience fever, chills, or malodorous wound drainage postoperatively. Patients should also be informed that bruising at the incision site is common and will gradually resolve over a 2- to 3-week period.

Biopsies are commonly performed under systemic sedation and/or local anesthesia in the outpatient setting and are therefore rarely uncomfortable. Should the administration of pain medication be necessary after the procedure, a mild analgesic is usually sufficient. Steri-

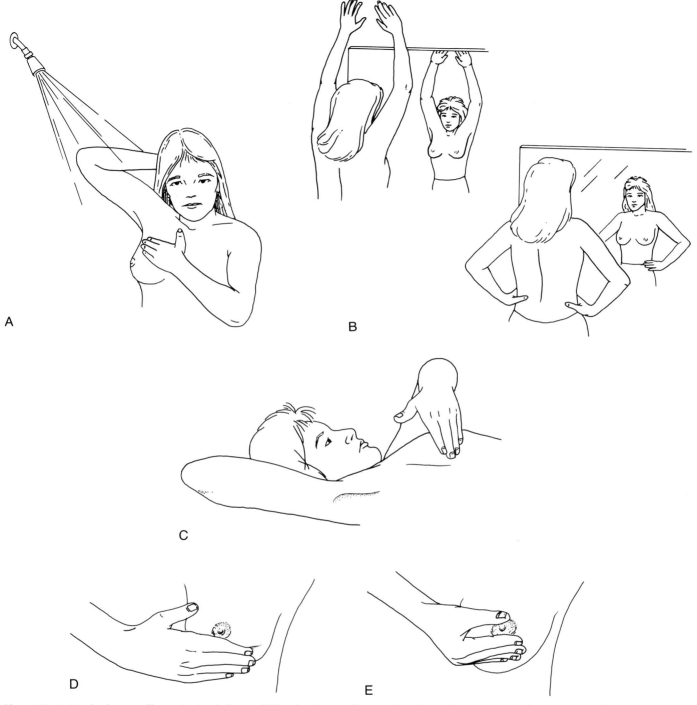

Figure 53–1. Regular breast self-examination helps establish what is normal breast tissue for each woman. Any skin or contour changes, masses, or lumps should be reported to the physician immediately. PERFORMING THE EXAMINATION. *A,* In the shower: Begin the examination in the shower or bath as hands glide more easily over wet skin. With fingers flat, move gently over every part of each breast. Use right hand to examine left breast, left hand for right breast. Check for lumps, knots, or thickening. *B,* In front of the mirror: Inspect breasts with arms at the side. Raise arms overhead, looking for any changes in the contour of each breast, dimpling of skin, or changes in the nipple. Rest palms on hips and press down firmly to flex the chest muscles. *C,* Lying down: To examine the right breast, place a pillow or folded towel under the right shoulder. Place the right hand behind the head—this distributes breast tissue more evenly. With the left hand, fingers flat, press gently in small circular motions. Begin at the superior margin of the breast and move in a clockwise motion, making a full circle. Move out approximately 1 inch and repeat. Keep circling until every part of breast, including nipple-areola, is covered. *D,* Repeat sequence for left breast, examining this breast with right hand. Positioning is mirror image of step *C*. *E,* Squeeze the nipple and areola of the breast between thumb and index finger. Any discharge, clear or bloody, should be reported to the doctor immediately. Now repeat on left breast, using right hand in a similar fashion.

strips are placed over the incision site at the time of surgery, and an occlusive sterile gauze is placed over the wound site. Patients should be instructed to keep the incision covered and dry until their postoperative visit. Patients can usually resume their normal daily activities 2 to 3 days following the biopsy. Many patients find it more comfortable to wear a bra continuously for the first 2 weeks postoperatively.

The preliminary pathology results of frozen section analysis are often given to the patient immediately following the biopsy; these results may be equivocal, and the results of the permanent section are needed to definitively determine treatment.[5] However, if the diagnosis of breast cancer is highly suspected clinically, the biopsy and definitive procedure may be performed as a one-stage procedure on the same day. These women present a special nursing challenge because of the uncertainty involved in the preoperative preparation. It is important to reassure any patient who expresses concern regarding this one-step approach and reiterate that a mastectomy will be employed only with definitive confirmation of pathology at the time of biopsy. Written (informed) consent for the procedure (biopsy and mastectomy) must be obtained *prior to* anesthetic induction.

If the diagnosis of cancer is established, the nurse must be prepared to interpret the serious nature of the illness, while at the same time emphasizing the optimistic aspects of appropriate therapy. Nurses must therefore be very familiar with diagnostic terminology, prognosis, and adjuvant therapy utilized in the treatment of breast cancer.

ROLE OF THE NURSE IN THE PREOPERATIVE OR EARLY DIAGNOSTIC PERIOD

Surgery is the standard treatment for the vast majority of breast cancers. The recent trends in operative approaches may present a special challenge for the nurse caring for the patient preoperatively. For the nurse working in the hospital setting, there may be no preoperative period, as cost-effective trends established in the past decade encourage (mandate) physicians to admit patients to specialty units *following* surgery. Therefore preoperative interventions often must be initiated in the outpatient setting. If a patient is admitted to the hospital preoperatively, it is usually on the afternoon prior to her surgery to evaluate coexisting medical illnesses that may increase morbidity and mortality with usage of general anesthesia. Either situation allows the nurse only a small period of time to work with these potentially complex nursing problems.

The focus of nursing intervention during this period is on the anticipation of the forthcoming stressful experience, enabling the patient to mobilize her own resources to begin recognizing her feelings and understanding her responses. The paramount issues in the early diagnostic, preoperative, and postoperative periods are psychosocial.[10] When formulating a care plan, patient individuality is a key factor to consider. No two patients will experience the same perceptions or have similar coping patterns; therefore the care plan must be tailored accordingly. A nonindividualized approach can be a "turn-off" for patients in this period, which is predictably laden with depression, and may undermine the development of an open and trusting nurse-patient relationship.

The sensual and physical presence of the breast to each individual woman comprises a complex interaction of cultural and psychological factors. Studies suggest that the emotional suffering following a mastectomy far outweighs the physical pain.[15] Any disturbance such as the loss or disfigurement of a breast affects self-esteem, which in turn may affect role function and interpersonal relationships.[10] A self-esteem inventory including to what extent the woman views her breasts as essential to her sense of worth and sexual gratification is an essential element in preoperative interventions. It is also essential that the physician and nursing staff make the patient aware of the impending stress with the forthcoming therapeutic and diagnostic events. The nurse can best prepare the patient to anticipate this stress and begin working through these depressive periods to allow establishment of effective coping mechanisms. Accurate expectations may increase the woman's perception of psychosocial control. A vague undefined threat is more often upsetting than known threats and anticipated stressful events.[10] This anticipatory guidance requires a concerned approach to patient teaching by employing good communication skills (e.g., the importance of listening and use of body language).

The patient may be scheduled for one of a variety of surgical procedures. The most common surgical procedure is the modified radical mastectomy or segmental mastectomy, also referred to as a tylectomy or lumpectomy. This latter procedure is usually accompanied with an ipsilateral axillary lymph node dissection. These procedures together with other variants of mastectomies are discussed in detail in chapter 29.

Preoperative patient education should include the expectations for the immediate postoperative period regarding pain, care of the wound site, and drainage catheters. The nurse should be mindful that high anxiety levels may interfere with information processing, especially when therapy and diagnostic studies may themselves enhance the anxiety level.[5] Therefore the information must be presented in such a way that patient comprehension is ensured. On occasion, denial and anxiety may require repetition for adequate comprehension. The uncertainties that emerge as the diagnostic and therapy processes continue only serve to enhance anxiety and the concerns for prognosis.

Sexual concerns can be extremely disturbing for many women undergoing breast surgery. The loss of femininity and sexual attractiveness are potential threats to the patient's identity, which may result in the fear of rejection or sexual withdrawal.[10] The woman having total breast removal is most affected by these factors. Sexual relations may also be affected by contributing factors such as physical discomfort, toxicity of treatments, or stress from the diagnosis. The patient's relationship with her partner also plays an important role. Patients with open, trusting, and supportive partners are better able to cope with their sexual concerns. Patients who are single, divorced, or separated are more profoundly threatened by a mastectomy and its psychosexual implications than are those women with an established relationship partner. These concerns may be difficult for patients to discuss and are more easily and effectively addressed in a trusting and supportive nurse-patient relationship. More complex psychological issues may require the perception of the nurse to identify the need for additional professional help.

When preparing patients for their recovery period, nurses should keep in mind that most women are able to resume *normal* lives following surgery, regardless of their need for further treatment. However, it is the more problematic aspect of psychosocial adjustment that requires the focus of many of these interventions preoperatively and throughout the recovery period.

NURSING CARE OF THE POSTMASTECTOMY PATIENT

Routine Postoperative Care

The patient usually returns from surgery with an occlusive, light-pressure dressing inclusive of a closed-suction drainage apparatus for the wound (i.e., Hemovac or Jackson-Pratt tubing), which is connected to continuous bulb suction at approximately 60 to 80 mm Hg pressure. The introduction of Silastic reservoirs makes mobility possible while ensuring continuous suction of the wound.

Fluids are given by mouth 2 to 4 hours postoperatively, and the patient may be allowed a light meal on the evening of the procedure. Early ambulation is encouraged, but mobility is limited in the ipsilateral arm or shoulder above the elbow. The use of an arm sling may be helpful in encouraging the desired immobility. It is important to keep the ipsilateral shoulder immobile to ensure flap adherence to the axillary space and chest wall. This important postoperative nursing instruction diminishes wound morbidity and hospital stay. A typical example of postoperative orders is depicted in Figure 53–2.

Immediately following the patient's arrival on the ward, a sign above the bed should be posted warning hospital personnel to avoid use of the ipsilateral arm for injections, intravenous fluid administration, phlebotomy, and the use of blood pressure cuffs.

Patients usually experience moderate pain in the axilla and chest wall that is controlled by oral or intramuscular analgesia. Hyperesthesias and paresthesias may also occur in the immediate postoperative period. These neurological manifestations occur with division of segments of the intercostobrachial nerve (1–3) that are sensory to the skin of the axilla and medial upper arms (see chapters 2, 29, and 31).[3] Patients should be instructed that these neurological manifestations are normal expectations following the mastectomy and should

subside in 3 to 6 weeks; however, insensate skin of these areas may persist for 8 to 10 months postoperatively. Prophylactic antibiotics are *not* routinely a part of postmastectomy care unless prevailing medical considerations necessitate such therapy. If erythema and cellulitis occur in the first week postoperatively, patients may benefit from topical antibacterial creams (e.g., Silvadene). Evidence of devascularization ischemia and necrotic tissues should prompt debridement to prevent progressive local and systemic infection.

Suction catheter drainage is usually maintained for 3 to 5 days postoperatively. The necessity for continual catheter drainage depends on the character and volume of the drainage. When serosanguineous drainage is less than 20 to 25 ml during a 24-hour period, the drains may be removed. At this time, if the flaps are firmly adherent, the physician may order active range-of-motion exercises to be initiated on the following day. It is important to emphasize that these exercises may be initially uncomfortable but will prevent future discomfort and will allow the preoperative range-of-motion to be restored. Figures 53–3 through 53–6 are illustrative of these recommended postoperative exercises. Exercises that may be initiated before the drains are removed include isometric exercises such as squeezing a rubber ball and wrist flexion. Isometric exercises increase blood flow but do not enhance lymphatic flow.

The patient undergoing lumpectomy will return with a dressing similar to that for the patient with an excisional biopsy. Usually these patients have undergone an axillary dissection. Their physiological recovery period is less complex and shorter than that of women undergoing total mastectomy, but the psychosocial issues are similar. Lumpectomy patients usually require irradiation of their remaining breast tissue. Radiation therapy is not without its side effects and complications.[15] For many women this may present serious concerns. For the nursing care of women undergoing radiation therapy for breast cancer, please refer to radiation oncology nursing texts.

Nursing Care of Complications

Lymphedema

Significant lymphedema is a complication occurring in less than five percent of all patients undergoing modified radical or radical mastectomy. Risk factors that enhance the probability for lymphedema include complete (Levels I–III) axillary node dissection, obesity, wound infection, poor nutritional status, and postoperative radiation therapy.[3] Lymphedema may occur days, weeks, and even years following extirpative surgery. The incidence is significantly higher if the patient undergoes a radical mastectomy.[7] Postoperative education with regard to the importance of range-of-motion exercise, protection against injury to the ipsilateral extremity, the avoidance of needles and blood pressure cuffs to the extremity, and the early recognition of symptoms is very important in the prevention of lymphedema (see chapter 32).

PHYSICIAN'S ORDERS
SHANDS HOSPITAL
at the
UNIVERSITY OF FLORIDA

*Generic equivalent permitted unless this square
initiated by physician.*

DATE/TIME	DOCTOR'S ORDERS	

8/5/90
10:15 am
	POSTOPERATIVE ORDERS FOLLOWING MASTECTOMY
	
	1. S/P right modified radical mastectomy.
	
	2. Vital signs every 2 hr × 4, then q 8 hr.
	
	3. Clear liquids PO when fully alert. Regular diet in A.M.
	
	4. Right upper extremity in sling.
	
	5. Sign at beside: "No BP/needle sticks, or blood draws in right arm."
	
	6. Record I and O every shift.
	
	7. Jackson-Pratt drains to continuous bulb suction—record drainage every shift. Notify patient to alert nursing staff if tubing is disconnected.
	
	8. D5 1/2 NS (*a* 80 cc/hr. D/C and heparin lock IV when tolerating PO liquids.
	
	9. Incentive spirometer q 4H.
	
	10. Ambulate with assistance this P.M. when alert; ambulate at least every shift.
	
	11. Elevate HOB 20 degrees.
	
	12. Medications: (A) Morphine sulfate 6–8 mg IM Q 4–6 hr p.r.n. for pain, *or*
	
	    (B) Tylenol 650 mg q 3–4 hr PO for pain.
	
	    (C) Dalmane 30 mg PO HS p.r.n. sleep.	

Figure 53–2. A typical example of postoperative orders following mastectomy.

The early recognition of severe lymphedema may require hospitalization for the mechanical expression of fluid with the use of an intermittent pneumatic tourniquet device such as the Jobst pump. (An Ace bandage or a compression elastic arm sleeve may be worn when the pump is not in use.) The patient may also be fitted for a custom-tailored sleeve that has a specific pressure (30 to 50 mm Hg) at its distal surface for continuous, long-term treatment.

Daily arm circumference measurements are very useful in determining the patient's progress. Proper measurement of the lymphedematous arm of the patient

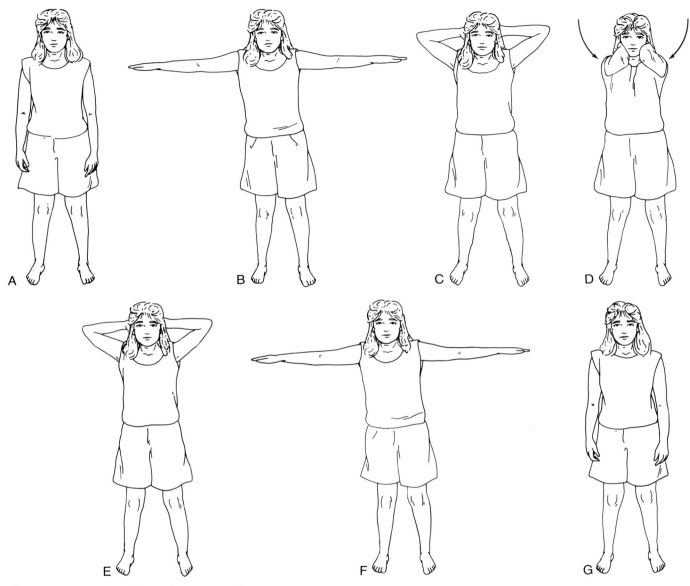

Figure 53–3. Exercise 1: Elbow pull-in. *A*, Stand facing straight ahead with feet 6 to 12 inches apart. *B*, Extend arms sideways to shoulder level. *C*, Bend elbows and clasp fingers at the back of neck. *D*, Pull elbows in toward each other until they touch. *E*, Return to position *(C)* with elbows bent. *F*, Unclasp fingers and extend arms sideways at shoulder level. *G*, Return to original position; rest and repeat.

involves obtaining precise tape measurement of both upper arms 6 cm above and below the olecranon process to evaluate therapeutic progress.

The patient may require systemic antibiotics if there is accompanying cellulitis. Diuretics and a low-salt diet may also be used to decrease lymphatic volume.

Wound Infection

Infection of the postmastectomy wound is rare, occurring in less than five percent of all patients.[3] Infection usually supervenes progressive tissue ischemia and necrosis and may be a serious and debilitating complication. It is important, therefore, that thorough wound assessment and documentation be performed. A subtle change in vital signs may also be indicative of early infection, and this observation should be communicated

to the patient's physician. Infection may precipitate cellulitis in the ipsilateral arm, and if this develops, intravenous antibiotic therapy is usually employed with good success. Topical irrigation of the wound may be ordered prophylactically to reduce bacterial flora.

Seromas

The use of closed-system wound drainage has greatly decreased the incidence of seromas, which are tumorlike collections of serum in the underlying tissue. They are almost always manifested during the first postoperative week and are usually treated by retaining the suction apparatus until drainage diminishes; if the catheter has already been removed, a pressure dressing may be applied.

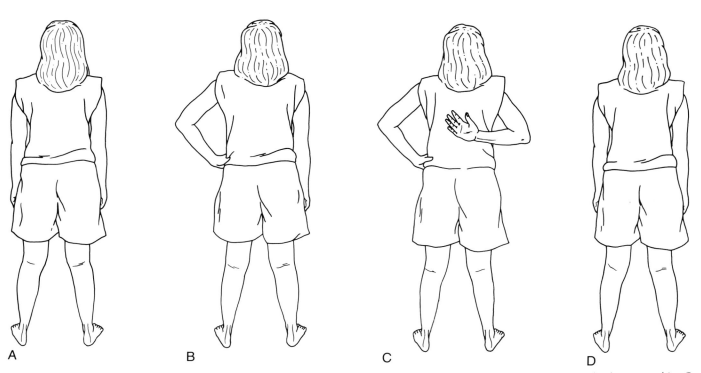

Figure 53–4. Exercise 2: Scratcher. *A,* Stand facing straight ahead with feet 6 to 12 inches apart. *B,* Place hand of unoperated side on your hip. *C,* Bend elbow at operated arm, placing back of hand in the middle of back. Gradually work the hand up your back until your fingers reach the opposite shoulder blade. *D,* Slowly lower your arm; rest and repeat.

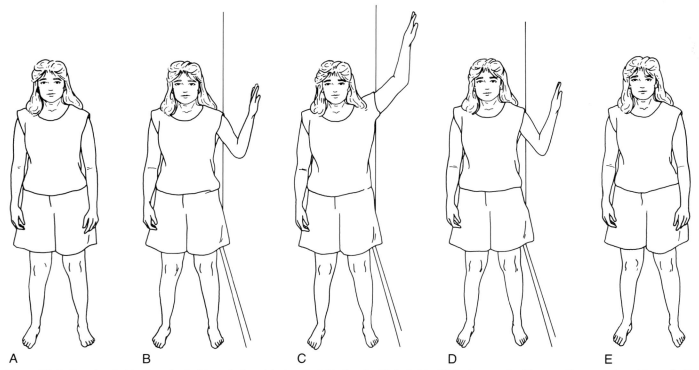

Figure 53–5. Exercise 3: Hand wall climbing. *A,* Stand facing straight ahead with feet 6 to 12 inches apart with operative arm closest to wall. *B,* Bend elbow and place palm against wall at shoulder level. *C,* Walk hand up wall until incisional pulling or pain occurs. Mark the level so progress can be checked. *D,* Slowly work hand down to shoulder level. *E,* Return to original position; rest and repeat.

of the pleural space and closed thoracostomy are necessary for therapy.

Hemorrhage

The use of closed-suction drainage allows the nurse the early recognition of this complication. In the first 24 hours, the character of the drainage should be monitored at least every 2 to 4 hours. If hemorrhage occurs in the postoperative period, the resulting liquid hematoma may be aspirated and a pressure dressing applied. Early recognition of this complication can prevent large blood loss and the need for blood transfusion. Continual bleeding beneath the flap may require reoperation to control the bleeding site.

As with all surgery requiring general anesthesia, there is a compromise in respiratory status with inhalation of anesthetic gases. This is especially important to keep in mind for the elderly patient or smoker. Coughing and deep breathing, early ambulation, and use of the incentive spirometer should be utilized routinely to prevent respiratory complications.

DISCHARGE TEACHING

At discharge, the nurse should provide instruction and advice for the immediate and long-term postoperative periods. The physician, patient, and family should recognize that providing a rationale increases patient compliance. It is therefore important to stress that following an axillary dissection, the affected extremity is much more susceptible to infection that could result in permanent lymphedema. Table 53–1 provides an example of discharge instructions for patients following mastectomy and axillary dissection. Patients should be instructed that compliance with these basic tenets will promote proper wound healing, which is important to overall recovery and to cosmesis.

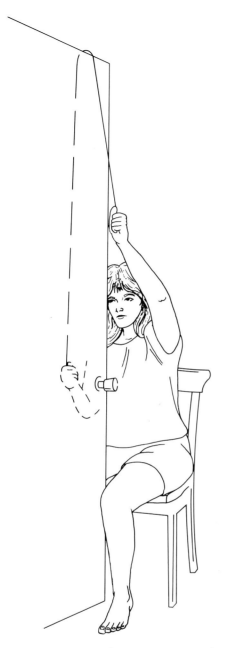

Figure 53–6. Exercise 4: Door pulley. *Equipment*: A 6-foot rope or 6 feet of bandage; a door and chair. *Procedure*: Place knots in the rope at each end and toss it over the door with the unaffected arm. Sit on armless chair with soles placed firmly on floor and door held closely between the legs. Hold the ends of the rope between the third and fourth fingers. Slowly pull the rope down with the unaffected arm, and raise the operative arm. Keep the raised arm close to the head and raise as far as is comfortable. Reverse the motion and raise the unaffected arm; rest and repeat.

Pneumothorax

Pneumothorax is a very rare complication resulting from entry of the parietal pleura during surgery and is seen most frequently in patients undergoing radical mastectomy.[3] Respiratory distress develops during the immediate postoperative period when occurrence is unrecognized in the operating room; immediate aspiration

Table 53–1. POSTMASTECTOMY DISCHARGE INSTRUCTIONS

1. Do not lift heavy objects (greater than 5 lbs) until wound has healed and the swelling has resolved.
2. No creams, powders, or deodorant should be applied to the axilla (armpit) until complete wound healing has occurred.
3. If you leave the hospital with a drain, record accurate daily measurements for your next physician's visit.
4. Do not take tub baths until wound has healed; showers only.
5. Do not drive an automobile for 2 weeks.
6. If you experience chills, fever, or an increase in pain or bleeding, call your physician immediately.
7. Avoid all unnecessary sun exposure while wound is healing. If you are in the sun, keep the affected area covered or wear a sun block agent (SPF 23 or greater).
8. Avoid constrictive clothing or jewelry on the affected arm and fingers.
9. *Always* protect the involved arm from injury (i.e., wear gloves while gardening, a thimble when sewing, and a mitt when cooking).
10. *Always* remind medical personnel to use the opposite arm for injections, blood draws, and blood pressure readings.

ROLE OF THE NURSE IN THE RECOVERY AND REHABILITATIVE PERIODS

The role of the nurse in the recovery and rehabilitative periods is to aid in the restoration of the patient's physical and emotional well-being. The interventions are thus aimed at promoting the patient's adaption to the far-reaching effects of breast cancer. The psychological impact of the diagnosis and treatment may result in a variety of effects on both the psyche and the interpersonal relationships of the patient. During this period the patient may experience feelings of inadequacy, fear, rejection, guilt, anger, and shame. Family members may feel resentful, ambivalent, and overburdened with the stress of the illness.[4] This is a period when the patient needs increased support from family and friends. Therefore the nurse may play a vital role in both identifying and working through these emotions in order to facilitate understanding by the patient and her family of these complex issues. The coping strategies identified earlier now play an important role in the patient's psychosocial recovery.

During this period, peer support groups such as The American Cancer Society's *Reach to Recovery* and *I Can Cope* provide the much needed support and sharing with other women who have experienced similar feelings and circumstances. By sharing knowledge and coping strategies, the goal of the volunteers, who often have had mastectomies themselves, is to help minimize the emotional problems that confront the patient. These programs are initiated by a volunteer who will visit the patient during her hospital stay. After discharge the patient may wish to attend local weekly meetings. Referral to these programs may require a physician's order; most professionals involved in the care of breast cancer patients welcome the participation of these support groups.

The recovery from breast cancer surgery depends greatly on many factors, including the type of surgery, stage of disease, and the patient's age and general state of health. However, the majority of patients should be able to dress, bathe, and groom themselves before their hospital discharge. Normal preoperative social and physical functions should be resumed 3 to 4 weeks after surgery.

Rehabilitative exercises are begun at the physician's discretion, which is often during the first week following surgery (see Figs. 53–3 to 53–6). Dissection of the axilla may result in limited shoulder range of motion and muscle contractures of the affected arm and shoulder. It must be emphasized that these exercises should be continued daily after discharge. If the patient develops muscle tightness or discomfort, she should be reassured that such is to be expected. Thereafter the patient should be advised to rest the involved shoulder extremity and continue the exercise. The patient should expect to see return of normal range of motion 2 to 3 months following surgery, and preoperative arm strength should be obtained within 6 months.[4]

Another major goal of rehabilitation is the restoration of a normal appearance. This may be achieved with a temporary prosthesis made from a soft preformed material. The prosthesis is commonly used at discharge until 4 to 6 weeks following surgery while the wound is healing. Permanent prostheses are available in a wide variety of shapes and sizes to help symmetrically duplicate the woman's original bustline. These devices are available in many different materials that feel much like the natural breast. Small prostheses, sometimes called equalizers, are available for women who have had lumpectomies. Breast prostheses are sold in surgical supply stores, lingerie shops, and department stores or may be custom-made at medical institutions. Most insurance policies cover the cost of the device, but a prescription written by the referring physician may be necessary to ensure payment by the third-party carrier.

Breast cancer follow-up usually requires a physician's office visit every 3 months for the first 2 years. If there is no evidence of recurrent disease, visits may only be required every 6 months from years 3 to 5 and annually thereafter. Mammograms are required on a yearly basis. Other tests such as chest radiographs, bone scans, and hemogram and liver function tests are required on a periodic basis. Should the patient require chemotherapy or radiation therapy, more frequent visits will be necessary for the first year and possibly thereafter. The recovery period provides the best opportunity to stress the importance of follow-up compliance as early detection of recurrence has a great impact on the probability of survival.

NURSING CARE OF THE PATIENT UNDERGOING RECONSTRUCTIVE SURGERY

Reconstructive surgery may be psychologically essential to restore self-esteem, which may have been diminished from the mastectomy.[4] This surgery may be completed synchronously with the mastectomy or months or years later. Immediate reconstruction has the obvious advantage of eliminating the need for a separate operative procedure and reducing the emotional trauma of the loss of a breast. However, the risks of wound complications may be increased. Reconstruction should be delayed when chemotherapy or radiation therapy is necessary postoperatively, when surgical margins are compromised, or when prognostically unfavorable findings are evident pathologically (e.g., vascular invasion or high mitotic rate).

There are several variants of breast reconstructive procedures, which are usually tailored to the individual needs of the patient and type of mastectomy performed. If the woman's remaining breast tissue can be utilized in the reconstruction, the prosthesis may be placed subpectorally. This usually requires a brief hospital stay and recovery period. If more extensive surgery is required or if the remaining skin is inadequate for proper restoration of volume, a donor area for transfer of autogenous tissue from the thorax (latissimus dorsi flap) or abdomen (transcutaneous rectus abdominis muscle, or TRAM flap) is used in the reconstruction. These operations require a lengthy hospitalization and recovery period. Should complications occur (e.g., infection or tissue necrosis) the implant may need to be removed or the transferred tissues may be compromised.

The formation of a fibrous capsule of scar tissue around the implant causing capsular contraction may occur at any time after reconstruction. This contracture may cause the implant to change its position, contour, or palpatory characteristics. Should this occur, surgical intervention may be necessary to excise the capsule of scar tissue and release the implant.

Because of the risk of cancer recurrence, the nipple and areola are removed during the total mastectomy. However, a variety of methods exist as reconstruction alternatives. Even with the best techniques available, the nipple and areola never assume the original contour, configuration, and color and are insensate to stimulation.

Presently, the majority of third-party carriers cover reimbursement for reconstruction, but each patient should contact her insurance company and determine the requirements and specific qualifications that may pertain to the planned constructive procedure.

Breast self-exam and mammography are most important following reconstruction. Both the residual ipsilateral tissues and the opposite breast are at risk for recurrence, which approximates 0.7 to 1 percent per annum. In addition, experts suggest that adherence to the recommended guidelines should also apply to the reconstructed breast.[4]

The decision of the patient to undergo the reconstruction process is a personal and private issue among the patient, the spouse, and the physician and should be made only after careful assessment of the risks, benefits, and economics of the procedure. The nurse is often called on to facilitate this decision process and should be aware and informed of such issues. (For a detailed discussion of reconstructive surgery, refer to section X, chapter 30.)

NURSING CARE OF THE PATIENT RECEIVING SYSTEMIC THERAPY

Systemic therapy for breast cancer is used both for the control of disseminated disease and as adjuvant therapy for the prevention of systemic spread. For those patients receiving chemotherapy for palliation, the goal of systemic therapy is to achieve the most effective "tumor-kill" with the drug combination using the least toxic therapies available. The goal of adjuvant therapy is to enhance breast cancer cure rates (e.g., disease-free and overall survival); it may require less toxic treatment regimens. Systemic therapy may also include hormonal therapy to manipulate estrogen levels, as estrogens are considered to be potential stimulatory agents of hormonally-sensitive breast cancer cells. This variant of hormonal therapy may be applied for both early (stage I or II) and metastatic disease if indicated by receptor assays.

For those patients with tumor pathologically con-

firmed in the lymph nodes (stage II), the chemotherapy treatments commonly used may produce undesirable side effects. These patients require continual education and support during their treatment.

Recent studies have indicated that systemic therapy may improve survival rates for those patients with tumor confined to the breast or node-negative tumors.[8] With the recommended systemic doses of chemotherapy in the treatment population, side effects may present a challenge for nurse management.

For the patient with widespread disease, systemic therapy may include both chemotherapy and hormonal therapy. For these patients, their quality of life is the most important consideration to further interventional therapy. Nurses play an important role in the evaluation of many of the side effects that may diminish the quality of life and in aiding the patient in the prevention of same. The breast cancer patient may present the ultimate nursing challenge, as many of the treatments may produce toxic side effects that may render the patient ill despite all efforts to avoid these complications of cytotoxic regimens.

Before initiating chemotherapy, the nurse should explain potential side effects and what steps to take with their occurrence. The most frequently observed side effects include alopecia, nausea and vomiting, leukopenia, stomatitis, and fatigue.

Alopecia. The amount of hair loss that occurs with systemic chemotherapy is directly related to the chemotherapeutic agent used in therapy. The nurse should be familiar with the drugs that are most apt to cause hair loss and adjust her teaching plan accordingly. However, it should be understood that some patients lose their hair even with mild dosage schedules, and therefore this side effect should be discussed with all patients. The nurse should suggest to the patient that she obtain a hair piece prior to receiving chemotherapy or shortly thereafter. This recommendation is made before initiating chemotherapy, as patients find it easier to match the hair piece to their own coloring and style while their own hair is still intact. Many insurance companies will reimburse the patient for a wig if it is written as a prescription for a "prosthetic hair piece." The use of scarves, turbans, and stylish hats can also be suggested to the patient. The American Cancer Society's "Look Good, Feel Better" program offers assistance to the patient in the application of cosmetics to enhance appearance while receiving chemotherapy. The patient should be advised that use of hair coloring dyes, permanents, and hot electric rollers may increase hair loss as a result of damage to fragile hair strands.

Nausea and Vomiting. Various medications are available to aid in the prevention of nausea and emesis in the patient receiving systemic chemotherapy. The nurse should become familiar with these drugs and collaborate with the physician as to the best regimen applicable for each patient. The patient should have prescriptions for both oral as well as suppository antiemetics to use after the chemotherapy in the event that orally administered medications may be difficult to administer in the nauseous state. Patients should be given emergency phone numbers that they may call should they experience nausea and vomiting of such severity as to cause dehydration. The nurse should also teach antiemetic preventive techniques such as encouraging the patient to eat smaller meals at more frequent intervals and to eat foods that are soft and bland and easy to digest. Carbohydrates are often the foods that are best tolerated, and this information should be relayed to the patient.

Leukopenia. The nurse should instruct the patient in the basic physiology and function of blood cellular components. The nurse should relate to the patient the mechanism of pancytopenia such that expectations related to the cytotoxic therapy are comprehended by the patient and her family. The patient should receive specific instructions about the steps to implement should she develop a fever during the nadir of leukocytes. The seriousness of the expectant pancytopenia should be emphasized to the patient and her family so that they understand the importance of obtaining medical assistance from their physician or local emergency room should fever and life-threatening blood counts develop. *This may be the most important teaching that a nurse can provide to the patient receiving systemic chemotherapy.* The nurse should instruct the patient to avoid crowds and visits with people who are ill with viral or bacterial infections while the leukopenia persists. The nurse should also stress to the patient that she is at risk for hemorrhage when her platelet count is low (< 60,000 cell/mm^3). These individuals should report any evidence of petechiae or other promontory symptoms of bleeding. Showing the patient a photograph of petechiae may be helpful to assist in the identification of this phenomenon.

Stomatitis. Inflammation of the mucous membranes of the oral cavity may produce tenderness, pain, and diminished taste sensation. This may result in speaking difficulty, fungal and bacterial infections, and anorexia. Oral hygiene measures should be encouraged with brushing and flossing after every meal. Instructions for thrombocytopenic patients should include the use of a soft bristle toothbrush for dental hygiene. Further, these patients should avoid aspirin-containing products. Soft, bland, high-protein foods should be recommended. Topical analgesics such as viscous xylocaine are especially helpful for symptomatic relief.

Fatigue. Some degree of fatigue and lethargy is experienced in essentially every patient undergoing chemotherapy. It is important for the nurse to stress that normal daily activities may be too strenuous, especially for the first few days following treatment. Accompanying emotional alterations may include sudden mood swings and depression.[4] Family discussions about lifestyle disruptions should be acknowledged before therapy, and alternatives should be encouraged prior to the initiation of treatment.

CYTOTOXIC CHEMOTHERAPEUTIC AND HORMONAL AGENTS USED IN THE TREATMENT OF BREAST CANCER

To apprise the nursing and paramedical personnel of the expectant toxic side effects evident with drug admin-

istration, a list of drugs commonly used for systemic chemotherapy in patients with breast cancer and a listing of some of the more frequent, specific side effects that occur with these drugs is included.

Cyclophosphamide (Cytoxan). Hemorrhagic cystitis may be a complication in patients receiving cyclophosphamide. The nurse should instruct the patient to report any blood in the urine and to drink 1 to 2 qts of fluid in the 24-hour period following administration of the drug. Patients should also be instructed to void frequently to ensure that toxic antimetabolites are not in contact with bladder mucosa. If the patient is taking cyclophosphamide by mouth, it is best administered in the morning followed by liberal hydration throughout the day. It is inadvisable to take the drug before retiring at night, as adequate hydration is difficult to ensure during these hours. Cyclophosphamide may also cause the syndrome of inappropriate antidiuretic hormone secretion (SIADH), and the nurse should continually assess the patient for the symptoms. When this drug is administered intravenously too rapidly, the patient may experience both burning in the oropharyngeal area and a metallic taste. Following administration of high-dose cyclophosphamide, the patient may experience cardiac toxicity, and therefore the nurse should evaluate for heart complications, especially ST depressions evident on electrocardiogram.[13]

Methotrexate (Mexate). Methotrexate can initiate severe mucositis, nausea, and leukopenia. Photosensitivity complications may be prevented by instructing the patient to avoid exposure to sunlight, to wear protective clothing, and to use sun block with a sun protection factor (SPF) of at least 15. When given as high-dose therapy, methotrexate can cause renal failure. This may be minimized by alkalinization of the urine and administration of large volumes of fluid orally or intravenously. Thereafter, the patient will receive folinic acid (Leucovorin) rescue after high-dose methotrexate therapy to diminish the toxicity from the resulting folic acid deficiency.[13]

5-Fluorouracil (Adrucil, Fluorouracil). 5-Fluorouracil administration may cause severe stomatitis, diarrhea, partial loss of nails (onchyatrophy), hyperpigmentation, and maculopapular rash. Again, patients should be instructed to avoid sunlight, wear protective clothing, and use sun block (SPF 15 minimum) lotion.

Doxorubicin (Adriamycin). Doxorubicin may cause cardiac toxicity abnormalities on the electrocardiogram. The nursing staff may note sinus tachycardia, T wave flattening, ST-T segment depression, voltage reduction, and arrhythmias. The patient may experience congestive heart failure. The nurse should be cognizant of the total cumulative dose of doxorubicin, which should not exceed 450 mg/m^2 for the patient with prior irradiation therapy, since the risk of congestive heart failure increases markedly with dosages above this level. For patients in whom irradiation was not utilized in therapy, the total cumulative dose should not exceed 550 mg/m^2.[13] The nurse should instruct the patient to expect orangered colored urine for one or two voidings following therapeutic administration of the drug. Doxorubicin is a potent vesicant and will cause tissue necrosis if it leaks into tissue following injection. The therapy for doxorubicin extravasation is difficult and ranges from early operative debridement, use of hydrocortisone intradermally, topical dimethyl sulfoxide (DMSO) and hydrocortisone, and the use of cold topical compresses. The nurse should be aware of the institutional policy and procedures regarding administration and extravasation of doxorubicin or other vesicants. Doxorubicin can also cause toxic chemosclerosis, with streaking along the course of the vein in which the drug is injected. The nurse should instruct the patient of the "recall" phenomena that may occur with patients receiving doxorubicin who have also received radiation therapy. This "recall" is a skin reaction in the area of the previous radiotherapy fields and produces a violaceous dermatitis with desquamation of the involved skin.[13]

Vincristine (Oncovin). Vincristine may produce profound neurotoxicity in patients receiving this drug. The peripheral neuropathy is manifested by numbness, pain, and tingling in the fingers and toes. The nurse should assess for wrist drop, foot drop, atrophy, cramps, ataxia, and difficulty with ambulation. As vincristine may cause constipation, the nurse should assess the bowel routine of the patient and make appropriate interventions such as exercise, hydration, increase of bulk and fiber in the diet, and possibly the use of laxatives to prevent this complication. Vincristine is also a vesicant, and the choice for extravasation is injection of hyaluronidase (Wydase) with application of heat compresses.[13]

Etoposide (VP-16). Etoposide can cause hypotension if infused too rapidly. The nurse should check the drug stability chart and infusion time on the product package insert for recommended time of each specific dose. During prolonged infusions the nurse should also inspect the fluid for clarity, as etoposide is often observed to precipitate.[13]

Vinblastine (Velban). Vinblastine produces a nadir of leukocytes in 4 to 10 days; thus the nurse should be cognizant of assessing the patient's white blood cell count at this time. Vinblastine may cause neurological toxicities similar to those caused by vincristine.[13]

Tamoxifen (Nolvadex). Tamoxifen is an oral medication having antiestrogen properties. The patient may experience hot flashes, nausea, vomiting, and a temporary increase in bone and tumor pain. Hypercalcemia may occur in patients with bone metastases. Patients may also experience menstrual irregularities (e.g., vaginal bleeding and discharge) and skin rash. The nurse should instruct the patient to receive regular ophthalmological examinations to access any visual change as tamoxifen, in some cases, has been reported to cause ocular damage. Patients receiving tamoxifen should be instructed to store the drug in a cool, dry place. These patients should also be admonished to avoid the use of estrogen therapy, such as the use of estrogen cream to counteract the vaginal dryness that may occur from tamoxifen therapy.[13] Recent studies have shown a slight increased risk of uterine cancer for patients receiving tamoxifen. The nurse should assess for abnormal uterine bleeding in patients' receiving this drug and ensure that adequate gynecological examinations are performed.[9a]

Megestrol Acetate (Megace). Megestrol acetate is an oral form of progesterone. The nurse should be aware of coexistent hypercalcemia, fluid retention, and liver function abnormalities.[13]

Prednisone (Deltacortisone). Many patients receive prednisone in conjunction with their cytotoxic therapy for breast cancer. Although the precise mode of action is unknown, steroids are believed to bind to the cytoplasmic receptor proteins of tumor cells to exert antitumor effects.[13] The nurse must assess for the various side effects evident with prednisone administration, which include gastrointestinal distress (including hemorrhagic gastritis) and immunosuppression. Patients should be instructed to take this medication with food or milk to decrease dyspepsia. Any steroid will augment sodium retention, which may initiate fluid retention and cause subsequent hypertension and/or heart failure. Steroids also promote the renal loss of potassium, which may produce muscle weakness. The expectant decrease in glucose tolerance may initiate adult-onset diabetes. Less commonly, changes in mental status such as psychoses, euphoria, and insomnia may occur.

Melphalan (L-PAM, phenylalanine mustard). Side effects of melphalan include hair loss, dermatitis, and pulmonary fibrosis.[13]

Mitomycin (Mutamycin, Mitomycin-C). Gastrointestinal disturbances with mitomycin are usually mild; however, bone marrow toxicity can be delayed but cumulative, and therefore the nurse should assess the patient accordingly. Renal toxicity has also been documented with mitomycin usage, and the nurse should evaluate for symptoms of compromised renal status. Mitomycin is a vesicant with no known antidote at this writing. Therefore, in patients with suspected extravasation, close monitoring is warranted with consultation from the surgeon. Debridement of the involved site of extravasation may be essential.[13]

Fluoxymesterone (Halotestine, Ora-Testryl). The nurse should instruct the patient receiving fluoxymesterone that virilization with increased facial hair, acne, clitoral hypertrophy, increased libido, and voice deepening may occur. Prolonged use of this exogenous androgen may physiologically induce serious liver damage and necessitates frequent monitoring of liver function.[13]

The nurse may, at this time, identify patients who are at risk for poor venous access and collaborate with the surgeon to obtain an implantable venous access device before initiation of chemotherapy. Breast cancer patients are at risk for developing venous complications of the upper extremities as they only have use of the arm contralateral to the primary neoplasms for venous access, and therefore access is limited. Many times the most feared aspect of chemotherapy for the patient is the venipuncture; placement of a venous access device may assist in alleviation of this phobia for the patient.

Systemic therapy places an additional stress on an already emotionally burdened patient and family. Through education, support, and the effort to promote realistic expectations from both the patient and her family, the nurse may alleviate much of the physical and psychosocial stress that is inevitable with the treatment of the breast cancer patient.

References

1. Anderson J: Coming to terms with mastectomy. Nurs Times 84:41–44, 1988.
2. Batehup L: Relieving pain for a patient with breast cancer. Nurs Times, Nov. 19, 1986, pp 36–39.
3. Bland KI, Heuser JS, Polk HC Jr, Spratt JS: The postmastectomy patient: wound care, complications and follow-up. *In* Rosato FE, Strombeck FE (eds): Surgery of the Breast. Stuttgart, Georg Thieme Verlag, 1986, pp 158–163.
4. The Breast Cancer Digest. Bethesda, MD, National Cancer Institute, 1984, pp 32–198.
5. Breast Lumps, A Guide to Understanding Breast Problems and Breast Surgery. Daly City, CA, Kramnes Communications, 1984, pp 1–15.
6. Casciato AC, Lowitz BB (eds): Manual of Bedside Oncology. Boston, MA, Little, Brown, 1983, pp 187–203.
7. Getz DH: The primary, secondary and tertiary nursing interventions of lymphedema. Cancer Nurs 8(3):177–184, 1985.
8. Gross J, Yarbro CH: Nursing Management of Breast Cancer. Seminars in Oncology, Nursing Series. Orlando, FL, Grune & Stratton, 1985, pp 155–223.
9. How to Examine your Breasts. A pamphlet by the American Cancer Society, Inc., New York, NY, 1977.
9a. Killackey MA, Hakes TB, Pierce VK: Endometrial adenocarcinoma in breast cancer patients receiving antiestrogens. Cancer Treat Rep 69:237–238, 1985.
10. Lierman L: Support for mastectomy: a clinical nursing research study. AORN 39(7):1150–1157, 1984.
11. Master Care Plan: The Patient with Breast Cancer. RN, Oct. 1986, p 31.
12. McNally JC, Campbell SJ, Somerville ET (eds): Guidelines for Cancer Nursing Practice. Kansas City, MO, Grune & Stratton, 1979, pp 6–11.
13. Physicians' Desk Reference. Oradell, NJ, Medical Economics Company, 1990.
14. Reach to Recovery: exercises after mastectomy/patient guide. A pamphlet by the American Cancer Society, Inc., New York, NY, 1983.
15. Rutherford DE: Assessing psychosexual needs of women experiencing lumpectomy cancer. Nursing 11(4):244–248, 1988.
16. Ziegfeld CR (ed): Core Curriculum for Oncology Nursing. Philadelphia, WB Saunders, 1987, pp 107–114.

Chapter 54

REHABILITATION

Thomas A. Gaskin, M.D., Marilyn C. Doss, M.A., Patricia Ann Kelly, P.T., and Jane McGee Colburn, M.A.

"The cancer patient who is cured of his malignancy but is left a physical or emotional cripple represents a sort of tawdry triumph of our therapeutic skills."[36] Rehabilitation is the process for minimizing physical, psychological, and vocational dysfunction that may result from the disease or its treatment. These disabilities or dysfunctions are not exclusively found in patients with breast cancer, although breast cancer is an appropriate model because of its prevalence, its demography, and the presence of essentially all categories of disability. The tragedy of curing a woman of breast cancer but having her life devastated by the physical or emotional effects of the cancer or its treatment occurs far too commonly. Our society has made the breast a focus of aesthetics and affection. Nevertheless, it is a fallacy that maladjustment to the cosmetic deformity of mastectomy constitutes the principal disability that a woman faces. The woman with breast cancer faces physical, sexual, psychosocial, and vocational disabilities.[36] The impact of these disabilities spreads far beyond the individual and involves her family, friends, and workplace.[10] This places an additional burden on the patient, her family, and those who treat her. Correction of these disabilities follows the same general principles and approaches as the treatment of the disease itself. The following items are essential:

1. Knowledge of the disabilities
2. Prospective action to prevent or minimize disabilities
3. An organized system of assessment
4. Interventions of varying complexity that may involve a variety of individuals with varying degrees and types of expertise (team approach) (Table 54–1)
5. Surveillance and reassessment to monitor effectiveness

PSYCHOSOCIAL REHABILITATION

Many cancer diagnoses are emotionally devastating, and breast cancer is one of these, affecting most, if not all, areas of a woman's life. Although major psychiatric illness is not common, serious anxiety and depression are, and this emotional suffering is far more intense than the physical: "I was fine until the day he came in and told me I had positive nodes. To me that meant, 'You've got cancer kid, and you're gonna die.' "[8, 50] For women who are less aware of the significance of the pathology report, the breast cancer diagnosis alone is enough to evoke the preceding response. The myths, fears, and understanding of breast cancer that each woman takes to the diagnosis determine not only her initial reaction but also her subsequent coping. For many, cancer is still the prototype for evil, a sinister force over which they have no control, one of mankind's most dreaded problems resulting in the worst of all deaths.

Existential concerns and religious questions surface even before diagnosis is confirmed. Thoughts about life and death, unanswerable questions, and ultimate concerns are common. What is happening? Must I die now? What did I do to deserve this? Am I a bad person? Helpless uncertainty, fear of isolation, feelings of worthlessness, anxiety, and depression result. Women may question the nature of God and their faith, wonder if they are being punished, or feel shame and guilt. The thoughts and fears are not rational. Self-esteem is affected as a woman judges herself; past regrets grow out of proportion. She fears a drastic change or end of her goals, dreams, duties, and roles, and the impact on her family is tremendous as loved ones are swept into the patient's devastation.[57] Psychosocial oncology helps patients and their families cope and adapt in order to relieve this distress and regain equilibrium. A person's perception of what has happened creates much of the suffering, which is related to the following themes:

1. The diagnosis—the worst thing that can happen
2. The loss of personal control
3. The uncertainty about the outcome and course of the disease
4. The ups and downs associated with hope for a cure and discordance between this hope and what has been read or observed
5. The debilitating nature of the disease[49]

From a psychosocial point of view, breast cancer has been given more attention than any other type of cancer, and there are few surprises in the literature. Regardless of prognosis, a significant number of women experience important changes, many of which are negative, in their lives for several years. Repressed anger and latent depression are common, becoming clinical problems in many women.[48] Anxiety, fear, and depression are documented among the majority of patients in most studies, with fear being one of the greatest disrupters of quality of life.[26, 51]

Table 54–1. REHABILITATION TEAM MEMBERS FOR INTERVENTIONAL APPROACH*

Rehabilitation Team Member	Cancer Center	500 Bed Hospital	200–300 Bed Hospital	Small Community Hospital	Physician's Office	Ambulatory Health Service
Physician (M.D.)	Psychiatrist or specially trained	Interested or specially trained	Interested and/or attending	Interested and/or attending	M.D.	M.D.
Nurse	Nurse coordinator	Nurse coorindator	Nurse	Nurse	Nurse	Nurse
Chaplain	Chaplain	Chaplain	Chaplain	Chaplain	Refer	Refer
Physical therapist (P.T.)	P.T.	P.T.	P.T. part-time	P.T. part-time	Refer P.T. center or visiting nurse (V.N.)	Refer P.T. center or V.N.
Occupational therapist (O.T.)	O.T.	O.T.	O.T. part-time or consultant	O.T. consultant or center	Refer O.T. center or V.N.	Refer O.T. center or V.N.
Social worker	Social worker	Social worker	Possible social worker or refer	Refer or V.N.	Refer community agency or V.N.	Refer community agency or V.N.
Psychiatrist or clinical psychologist	Psychiatrist	Psychiatrist or clinical psychologist	Consulting	Consulting	Refer	Refer
Speech and hearing specialist	Speech pathologist	Speech pathologist or consultant	Refer	Refer	Refer	Refer
Prosthodontist	Prosthodontist	Prosthodontist consultant	Consult	Refer	Refer	Refer
Prosthetist or orthotist	Prosthetist orthotist consultant	Prosthetist orthotist consultant	Consultant	Consultant or refer	Refer	Refer
Vocational counselor	Counselor on call	On call	Refer	Refer	Refer	Refer

*Adapted from Dietz, J. H., Rehabilitation Oncology. New York, John Wiley & Sons, 1981.

A careful history reveals those most vulnerable to acute distress and maladaptive coping. The meaning of the diagnosis is an important predictor of adjustment, along with the woman's age and menstrual status, the absence or presence of a social support system (including spouse, family, and friends), and her premorbid coping and psychological stability.[24, 26, 31] Patients who cope more positively have some commonalities. They confront the reality of what has happened and tend to focus on solutions to their distress. They take appropriate actions to relieve distress and are open to alternatives. They maintain communication with significant others, including their physicians. They seek emotional support but at the same time are quite self-reliant.[57] The percentage of patients who exhibit maladaptive coping varies depending on the study, but they, too, have some common characteristics. Those identified as poor copers avoid the reality of what has happened, and they feel powerless, pessimistic, and overwhelmed. They have few successful problem-solving skills and may have had many life failures prior to developing breast cancer, resulting in their feeling defeated at the outset and viewing their cancer as a final, crushing burden.[31, 57]

Positive coping strategies can be learned, and with education and counseling many women have discovered new ways to adapt to their disease.[13] Cancer can be demythologized, fear greatly reduced, and a patient's feeling of control restored. Many women today are asking for participation in and responsibility for their health care, viewing their physicians as partners. They need the physician's encouragement to change. We cannot assume that psychosocial needs will or should be met outside the health care system, just as we cannot take for granted that women will deal well with the psychosocial issues related to breast cancer. Psychosocial management is an integral part of good patient care. Information, education, and support have been shown to improve adjustment to breast cancer. Unfortunately, counseling and communication between physicians and patients does not always accompany good clinical care, and psychosocial support and referral may be nonexistent, resulting in compromised patient trust and ill will toward the physician, regardless of the quality of medical care practiced.[9, 12, 24]

Support in the health care setting begins with the physician during the first meeting prior to a definitive diagnosis and continues throughout treatment and follow-up. The physician's attitude toward psychosocial support programs may well determine whether the patient will use them. The physician's level of support and understanding is always conveyed to the patient. Although it may be very difficult to listen to the expression of powerful feelings and to encourage their expression, it is not difficult to be knowledgeable about available support programs and refer patients to them. Many patients need permission through referral from their physicians to participate in the support programs available in hospitals, outpatient offices and clinics, and the community. Peer visitation programs, education and counseling groups, and exercise programs for women with breast cancer have overlapping goals. They vary in format and structure, but they all have as a primary goal the reduction of the distress of cancer and cancer treatment and the promotion of positive coping. These programs usually encourage the expression of feelings and concerns associated with the disease, and they teach or model effective ways to deal with fear, anxiety, depression, and anger. In addition, education about breast cancer and breast cancer treatment may be offered as well as information about community resources. Participants are encouraged to be active and get involved in their care. The veteran patient who has adapted well is of tremendous help to those newly diagnosed or not coping well with their disease and treatment.

The reported benefits of participation in counseling, education, and other support programs are impressive. Almost all studies found reduction of fear, depression, anxiety, and maladaptive coping among the majority of women. Others reported improved relationships with family and friends, enhanced self-concept, and increased life satisfaction.[17, 22, 29, 38, 43, 52, 56, 57, 65] Being with women in a common predicament has other benefits. Women move out of self-absorption, and as they reach out and offer help or comfort to others, they discover they are also helped. They discover their own value and uniqueness. In addition, the experience of catharsis with those who understand helps women break through the very painful loneliness of having breast cancer.

Support and education programs are not a replacement for physician counseling and caring; they are an adjunct. In addition to good clinical treatment, the patient wants care and comfort. Conflicting expectations of physician and patient create many barriers and account for much of today's dissatisfaction with the health care system. A breast cancer patient focuses on many issues, and paramount is the uncertainty of survival; she will feel frustrated and cheated if her physician does not pay attention to her fears and concerns.[8] One woman eloquently describes this need for care and comfort:

"Please dare to be vulnerable. We all live in our own little world, wearing our masks of everyday. It is much easier to keep our masks on than to remove them and be open to others. Dare to find out about us by asking us relevant questions. Serious questions. Can you be open to asking us such things as, 'Are you able to understand the seriousness of your disease?' 'Are you afraid of the treatment you are receiving?' 'Are you managing okay with the medical bills?'

You may not really want to know all about us and carry our burdens on your shoulders, but if, by asking, you can let us unload occasionally, it helps so much. Please do not be afraid to be a friend.

"It is wonderful when physicians and other professionals are able to suggest other tools to help us cope with our disease. We are usually well aware of surgery, radiation, and chemotherapy. I am thinking of such things as learning how to relax, eating better, and the benefits of exercise. Our faith may be a very important tool in our getting well. These and other kinds of approaches may not help everyone, but they may help many. If we are encouraged and allowed to seek out appropriate alternative aids, it is nice. It is especially nice when our physicians are open to talking about it. If you offer the proper tools to us, we can feel more in control and know what types of treatments and new forms of self-help are credible for us to investigate.

"Most of all, I guess we just ask you to listen—not at the end of the bed, flipping through the chart or standing in the doorway, but look at us and listen. We may not be able to tell you what you really need to know. We may be grouchy or weepy. We may be trying to cope with a stiff upper lip and a thin smile and hope you can hear our faint and fearful words. But if you can listen with your eyes and ears and heart, we will know. It means so very much."[23]

PHYSICAL REHABILITATION

Occupational and physical therapy have important roles in helping women with breast cancer overcome their most obvious disability. The physical disabilities are related primarily to mastectomy but are also found in women who have had partial mastectomy and axillary dissection.[18] A variety of factors play a part in determining the type and extent of disabilities encountered, which include decreased range of motion in the shoulder on the operated side, lymphedema, scar tissue, decreased strength in the arm and shoulder girdle, changes in sensation, and pain. Contributing factors are preexisting problems, major and minor nerve injury, extent of lymphatic dissection, removal or denervation of muscles, postoperative wound problems including seroma and infection, type of incision, and even such details as type of surgical dressing.

Restricted range of motion of the shoulder on the operated side is a common sequela of operations on the breast and axilla.[1] Goniometric measurements may be used to document the extent of limitation and provide a baseline by which improvement can be measured, but for all practical purposes, limitation in flexion, abduction, adduction, and internal and external rotation is readily apparent to the patient and the treatment team (Table 54–2). Preoperative assessment is seldom practical but should be considered if there are preexisting problems with any of the areas that might be affected by the treatment of the breast cancer. Interventions to prevent, minimize, or correct range of motion limitations begin with the surgical dressing. Dietz, a prominent authority on rehabilitation of cancer patients, recommends that "postoperative dressings and positionings should keep the arm in abduction and slight elevation."[14] Degenshein has suggested more elaborate positioning

Table 54–2. ASSESSING RANGE OF MOTION*

Using the arm on your operated side are you able to
1. Brush and comb your hair?
2. Get a T-shirt, blouse that does not unbutton, or tight-necked sweater over your head?
3. Pull on a pair of pants or pantyhose and pull them up?
4. Close a back-fastening bra?
5. Completely zip up a dress with a back-fastening zipper?
6. Wash the upper part of your back, i.e., shoulder-blade area, on the same side as the operation?
7. Wash the upper part of your back, i.e., the shoulder-blade area, on the opposite side from the operation?
8. Reach into a cupboard over your head?
9. Make a double bed?
10. Carry a grocery bag containing three 1-pound cans, a 3-pound roast, a 3-pound bag of apples, and one or two other items so that the bag weighs approximately 10 pounds?

*Adapted from Wingate, L., Efficacy of physical therapy for patients who have undergone mastectomies. Physical Therapy, June, 1985.

and cautions, "There is no justification for burying the arm for several days into the dressing against the chest wall since this leads to a significant number of frozen shoulders."[11]

Postoperative shoulder movement is begun on different schedules by different surgeons based on a wide variety of indicators, including days after operation, status of drains, and presence of sutures.[1, 5, 20, 30, 42, 47, 60, 62] It is our practice to allow, but not insist on, shoulder motion immediately postoperatively as pain allows and to begin active range-of-motion exercises when the drains are removed. This practice admittedly is not based on documented evidence of superiority of this schedule over another. The brief length of postoperative hospital stay now common usually dictates that range-of-motion exercises are begun after discharge from the hospital. The range-of-motion exercises described in Reach to Recovery literature from the American Cancer Society are provided to the patient. Reinforcement of these exercises and monitoring of progress is a standard part of the first (and subsequent) postoperative visits. An exercise program such as STRETCH (see later discussion) can be invaluable in assisting in the preservation of range of motion. If, however, range of motion has not returned by the end of convalescence and normal wound healing, then individual occupational or physical therapy treatments should be begun.

Scar tissue (wound contracture) may contribute to range-of-motion limitations, physical deformity, and discomfort. Deep friction massage, use of moisturizers, and prolonged stretching of fibrous bands can help minimize the effects of wound contracture. Rarely, operative release may be necessary. Radiation therapy may worsen the restrictions and increase the need for continuing therapy.[45]

Muscle weakness may result from removal of muscle, prolonged immobilization, or nerve injury. A kinesiological study by Nikkanen et al. reports a 25 percent decrease in muscle strength on the operated side compared with the muscle strength on the control side.[41] While there are physical causes for much of the muscle weakness seen after breast surgery, it is not uncommon for women to become "one armed" after a mastectomy or axillary dissection. The resultant favoring of the affected extremity is a prominent cause of loss of muscle strength and reduced range of motion. The primary interventions are muscle strengthening and education to dispel the myth that muscular activity will reactivate the malignancy.[42, 46]

Lymphedema is the result of a number of factors: recurrent or persistent neoplasia, infection, cicatrix, and surgical removal of lymphatic channels. Continued dependent positioning of the arm and inadequate muscle contraction are also contributing factors, factors that can be minimized by physical and occupational therapy interventions.[33, 67] Assessment by volumetric measurement is accurate but cumbersome. Circumferential measurement is more practical and can be easily done in the occupational or physical therapy department, the physician's office, or at home with ease and with reproducible results. Dietz, again, is a valuable resource for instructions for preventing and controlling lymphedema (Table 54–3).[13] Reach to Recovery literature contains much of this practical information also. Positioning of the arm and restoration of muscular contraction are ways to improve mild lymphedema. Intermittent compression, centripetal massage, and the use of an elastic

Table 54–3. INSTRUCTIONS TO PATIENTS FOR PREVENTION AND CONTROL OF LYMPHEDEMA*

1. Protect the shoulder, arm, and hand on the affected side from burns.
   Hold cigarettes in the opposite hand.
   Wear padded noninflammable gauntlet gloves when reaching into the oven.
   Never get sunburned. Tan very gradually.
2. Avoid constriction of the arm on the affected side.
   Keep watchbands and jewelry loose.
   Keep dress sleeves and straps of underclothing loose.
   Carry heavy purses and packages on the opposite side.
   Have blood pressure taken using the unaffected arm.
3. Avoid injury and infection of the arm on the affected side.
   Never cut cuticles; leave them alone or use cuticle cream.
   Wear canvas gloves when gardening.
   Wear lined rubber gloves when using steel wool or cleaning.
   Have injections, finger pricks, and blood samples done on the opposite arm.
   Wear a thimble when sewing.
   Avoid pricking a finger with the needle.
   Use an electric shaver for underarms.
   Avoid scratches and nicks.
4. Care for minor injuries promptly.
   If there is the slightest break in the skin, wash it immediately with soap and water, and cover it with a bandage.
   Report any unusual soreness or swelling to your physician at once.
   Use a topical antibiotic ointment if prescribed by your physician.
5. Contact your physician immediately if the arm becomes painful, swollen, hot, or reddened.
6. Avoid using the arm for rapid movements in heavy work, especially when the movement is such that it would force blood and tissue fluids toward the hand.
7. Keep your regular appointments for follow-up examinations.
8. Continue your normal activities.

*Adapted from Dietz, J. H., Rehabilitation Oncology. New York, John Wiley & Sons, 1981.

compression garment are additional methods for more refractory lymphedema.[19, 28, 33, 54, 55, 62, 66, 67]

Posture is commonly affected in women following breast surgery. A subjective study of 114 women examined for physical disabilities following a variety of treatment for breast cancer revealed only 14 who were felt to have "normal" posture subjectively. Range-of-motion limitations, cicatrix, lymphedema, and pain may influence posture, but protective posturing may also result from the patient's increased self-consciousness of the loss and asymmetry. The postural deviations commonly seen are rounded shoulders, forward head, and asymmetry of shoulder level. Shoulder level asymmetry may be higher or lower on the affected side. Protective posturing may lead to increased tension, which is often found in the trigger-point areas of the upper trapezius.

The primary intervention for posture abnormalities is correction of any underlying cause (such as range-of-motion limitation) and, primarily, education and awareness. Relaxation techniques, acupressure, and exercises to improve mobility and strength are valuable adjuncts.[32]

Physical and occupational therapy provide education and techniques for minimizing a variety of physical disabilities that, if not corrected, could result in significant change in appearance and in modification of activities of daily living.[68] Physical and education techniques can promote a sense of control and wellness correlated with improved function and cosmesis. The value of this should not be underestimated as a factor in the overall recovery and adjustment of the woman with breast cancer.[61]

SEXUAL REHABILITATION

Sexuality is more than the union of an erect penis with a lubricated vagina. For a woman, it is the expression of her gender on her personality, her view of "self," and her relationship with others.[4] Changes in sexuality accompany many malignancies; breast cancer has no monopoly on this phenomenon.[44] Breast cancer, however, has an especially pronounced impact because of its commonness and because of the status of the breast in our sexual culture. The concept of breast removal as mutilation is not a twentieth century invention: Decius punished St. Agatha (the patron saint of breast cancer) in 251 A.D. by amputating her breasts.[25] The effect of breast removal has some almost universal effects on a woman's expression of her gender. The basic underlying factor is a change in self-image that manifests itself by difficulty in expressing intimacy and in selecting clothing and in avoidance of participation in many sports and activities that involve brief clothing.

Evaluation of sexual dysfunction is omitted in most clinical situations, perhaps because of reluctance (embarrassment?) by most physicians. However, detailed evaluation and treatment are probably beyond the scope of most clinical practices. The following factors should be included in detailed evaluations:

1. *Etiology.* Etiological factors including physical deformity, change in self-image, pharmacological disruptions of the hormone milieu, decrease in energy level resulting from chemotherapy, local discomfort from radiation, or psychological problems related to inadequate or mythical information are common in breast cancer.

2. *Demographic Factors.* Socioeconomic background and education are both related to expressions of sexuality, receptiveness to adjustment, and capacity to adapt.

3. *Sexual Background.* Sexual expression after breast cancer is largely affected by the quality of sexual expression before breast cancer, including existing self-esteem, quality of the relationship, and degree of sexual functioning.[34]

Therapy

The following PLISSIT therapeutic model of Annon has four levels:[2]

1. First Level: *Permission* to have sexual thoughts, feelings, and activities.

2. Second Level: *Limited information* to correct misinformation and myths.

3. Third Level: *Specific suggestions* of ways to overcome specific problems.

4. Fourth Level: *Intensive therapy* to overcome deep-seated and perhaps long-standing problems by either partner.

The simplest evaluation—"Are you having problems with your sex life?"—is often sufficient simply by raising the issue. Raising the issue and recognizing that there may be a problem infers that sexual desires and behavior are "OK." That inference will often suffice as therapy.

Restoration of sexual functioning carries benefits far beyond the private sexual behavior of a couple by enabling the woman's femininity to express itself in all of her relationships, including her very important relationship with herself.

Mildred Witkin has movingly and lucidly presented the following data[63, 64]:

1. Sexual self-concept superseded mortality as the primary concern of most recovering mastectomy patients.

2. The attitude of the partner—husband or lover—was crucial to that self-concept.

3. Most partners were eager to help.

4. Psychosexual counseling was welcomed and found to be appropriate.

VOCATIONAL REHABILITATION

Employment discrimination against people with a history of cancer has been well documented (Tables 54–4 and 54–5).[3, 16, 35] The cause of the discrimination, in some cases, may arise from myths regarding communicability but most commonly is based on economic prejudice.[21] Prejudice exists despite convincing evidence that "selective hiring of persons who have been treated for cancer, in positions for which they are physically qualified, is a sound industrial practice."[58] In recent years the problem of job discrimination has been magnified by two factors: the increasing number of women in the work force and the curability of certain malignancies

Table 54–4. SUMMARY OF STUDIES THAT MEASURE EMPLOYMENT FOLLOWING MASTECTOMY*

Year	Investigators	Number	Percentage of Nonworking Patients
1970	Schottenfeld and Robbins	316	16.0
1971	Torrie	1400	23.0
1974	Craig, et al	134	22.4
1976	Feldman	49	10.2
	Maguire	94	10.4
1977	Winick and Robbins	297	12.0
	Amberger, et al	55	30.8
1978	Feldman	56	14.0
1979	Greenleigh Associates (ACS-California)	237	24.5

*Adapted from Barofsky, I., Job Discrimination: A Measure of the Social Death of the Cancer Patient. Western States Conference on Cancer Rehabilitation, Bull Publishing Company, 1982.

(primarily lymphatic and hematological but also testicular cancer) that afflict young men.[53] These two factors have increased the number of able-bodied, previously employed individuals who can no longer secure employment and who are at a risk for becoming medically indigent.[27]

Our society increasingly places emphasis on what we do as a measure of who we are. Aside from a source of income, a job provides an identity and a sense of self-worth.[37]

Health insurance is a benefit of employment, and when a person loses employment, that often means loss of health insurance. Individual policies for a person with a history of cancer are either unavailable or carry extraordinary premiums beyond the reach of an unemployed person. Suitability for employment often means more than suitability for the position—it means insurability.[12, 15]

By and large employers are not obligated to provide employment for anyone and yet there are legal safeguards and remedies to protect certain classes of employees from discrimination.[59]

The Fifth and Fourteenth Amendments of the United

Table 54–5. SUMMARY OF EMPLOYMENT DISCRIMINATION STUDIES*

Investigators	Number	Discrimination Measure
Feldman (1976)	130	22 percent of sample reports at least one job rejection due to cancer
Smith, et al (1977)	95	13.7 percent of sample reports at least one job rejection due to cancer
Koocher and O'Malley (1981)	60	25 percent of sample reports employment discrimination

*Data consist of the percentage of patients who claim to be victims of frank job discrimination, but this is not considered a reflection of their current employment status. (Adapted from Barofsky, I.: Job Discrimination: A Measure of the Social Death of the Cancer Patient. Western States Conference on Cancer Rehabilitation, Bull Publishing Company, 1982.)

States Constitution provide some general protections against actions of government—and actions of government can be widely interpreted to include actions of those who do substantial business with the government. The Rehabilitation Act of 1973 is most often cited as the source of relief for cancer patients. This act, however, applies to "disabled" persons and several courts have ruled that recovered cancer patients are not disabled. The person with a history of cancer who faces job discrimination (most commonly a young person or a blue collar worker) may find little relief.

"The American Cancer Society saw the Rehab Act as inadequate, and the same applied to the state laws. Though 47 or 48 states have some kind of protection for the handicapped and disabled, only a few included cancer patients. The model is California's state law, which says pointblank, 'you will not discriminate against cancer patients.' There have been a number of cases where the courts have looked at a cancer patient, seen nothing physically wrong, and deemed the person not handicapped."[39]

In 1987, HR 1546 was introduced to prohibit employment discrimination against a person because of a history of cancer. Specifically, HR 1546 would allow relief against an employer who engaged in the following practices:

Failure or refusal to hire, deny a promotion to, or fire an individual because of cancer history.

Limiting, segregating, or classifying employees in any way because of cancer history.

Requiring that an individual meet medical standards unrelated to essential job requirements or reveal medical information unnecessary to job performance.

Giving and acting upon the results of an ability test if designed to or used to discriminate because of cancer history.

Retaliation against an employee if he or she participates in an investigation or hearing regarding the employer's practices.

Failure to provide reasonable accommodations for an employee to fulfill the essential job requirements.[39]

For the individual practitioner or other professional who may serve as the patient's advocate and advisor, there are two practical caveats to remember. A *leave of absence* to allow sufficient time to undergo treatment, recover, and resume employment may be preferable to attempting to work while ill. A person who tries to work while under the physical and emotional strains of noxious therapies will often not be able to perform satisfactorily and thereby risk dismissal. The frustrations of trying to work while sick can make the options of medical retirement seem attractive. Subsequent recovery, however, may result in termination of benefits leaving the person without a job and without health insurance or income.

The second caveat is to advise patients *never* to lie on the employment application form. A false answer "no" to the question of a history of cancer justifies termination and denial of benefits.[59]

THE TEAM APPROACH

Rehabilitation is important in the treatment of women with breast cancer and applicable to essentially all women who have it.[9] As in any treatment, accurate assessment of the problems and competent interventions are needed. Cancer care is a prototype of multidisciplinary care with the "team approach." Rehabilitation fits well into this concept.[62] The team composition will vary in different environments and must often be extended beyond the primary treatment group (see Table 54–1).[46, 47] The concept of an extended team is useful because it allows a treatment unit of any size to avail itself of community or regional resources or to use a specially organized group such as STRETCH to expand its expertise and effectiveness.[12]

A satisfactory assessment instrument is an astute and sensitive physician or nurse involved in treatment. A questionnaire (Appendix 1) is followed by an interview with a nurse clinician, counselor, or other trained professional as a thorough and efficient means, although not without bias, of identifying psychosocial problems.[7] Physical restrictions can be quantitated by physical and occupational therapists.

Interventions, in the same way, may require little more than the immediate treatment group, family, and friends. Beyond those there are many resources of professionals and volunteers, which can become part of the extended team (Appendix 2).

Professionals. These include those in physical therapy, occupational therapy, psychological care, pastoral care, sexual therapy, and vocational rehabilitation counseling.

Volunteer. The American Cancer Society has long been in the forefront of rehabilitation activities.[9] *Reach to Recovery* has been an extremely successful program. A specially trained volunteer who has had breast cancer visits the woman in the postoperative, or occasionally, the preoperative period to provide an information list, a temporary prosthesis, and firsthand experience with encouragement. The program has been expanded to include a group for husbands of married patients.

The American Cancer Society also has information and referral services, transportation services, loan and gift items, and financial assistance. Additionally it sponsors or supports community programs such as TOUCH, STRETCH, Bosom Buddies, and others, which provide a variety of services.

For the optimal functioning of the team—especially the extended team—the involvement, leadership, and direction of the physician is desirable if not essential.

STRETCH

STRETCH is an exercise-based rehabilitation program for women that began in February, 1985. Inspired by a number of women with breast cancer who left group exercise programs and requested private instruction, the exercise instructor broached the problem with the Lurleen B. Wallace Cancer Center, National Cancer Institute–designated comprehensive cancer center at the University of Alabama in Birmingham.

A pilot project was begun in collaboration with the community's surgeons, physical and occupational therapists, oncology counselors, and others. The women were studied for physical and psychosocial disabilities before, during, and after completion of an 8-week exercise program. Using that information, and help from the American Cancer Society, a standardized regimen of exercise and education was established.

Specifically designed for postsurgery patients, the exercise routines consist of five major segments:

1. *Warm-up* (10 to 15 minutes). Slow rhythmic head-neck exercises; gentle stretching and flexibility routines; arm-leg and arm-shoulder motions; all done slowly and deliberately.

2. *Floor Routine* (10 minutes). Abdominal exercises, including curls and sit-backs (no sit-ups); back, leg, and static stretches; all at a smooth rhythmic pace.

3. *Upper Body Concentration* (10 minutes). Mobility improvements; exercises require use of a dowel to position arm, hand, and shoulder correctly.

4. *Cool Down* (10 to 15 minutes). Relaxation routines.

5. *Group Discussion* (30 minutes). Speakers are periodically invited to address the group on educational, service, and social topics relating to the group's needs or requests.

What began as an exercise program may become a support group. Need for exercise is consistently reported as the reason for entering the program and physical improvement as the most important benefit, but emotional support—which is seldom listed as a reason for entering the program—is cited as the second most important benefit.

The physical benefits are improvement in flexibility and strength, reduction of arm swelling, endurance, becoming "two-handed" again, and the sense of well-being that comes with fitness. The exercises are designed for this purpose. The psychosocial benefits first come from seeing that other women don't look "funny" in exercise clothing. The education sessions are directed at basic information about the disease but also at reconstruction, clothing styles, sexual adjustment, assertiveness, and a number of optional topics. The reconstruction sessions evolved quickly into a personal demonstration of results by women who had undergone a variety of operations. The camaraderie that permeates the group fosters intense personal interaction monitored and directed by professionals. These shared experiences and discussions in a loosely controlled environment among women ostensibly brought together for the purpose of exercise has enabled the program to function as a support group. The support, however, is not crisis intervention but rather is directed at the common problems experienced by most women with breast cancer. The value of this program lies in its simplicity, reproducibility, its attention to both physical and psychosocial disabilities, and its applicability to most women with breast cancer.

References

1. Aitken DR, Minton JP: Complications associated with mastectomy. Surg Clin North Am 63:1131–1152, 1983.
2. Annon JS: A proposed conceptual scheme for the behavioral treatment of sexual problems. *In* Behavioral Treatment of Sexual Problems. Honolulu, HA, Enabling Systems, Inc., September, 1975.
3. Barofsky I: Job discrimination: a measure of the social death of the cancer patient. *In* Western States Conference on Cancer Rehabilitation. Palo Alto, CA, Bull Publishing, 1982.
4. Barton A: Sexual rehabilitation of the cancer patients. *In* Syllabus of Rehabilitation of the Cancer Patient in the Community Hospital. Princeton, AL, Baptist Medical Center, 1984.
5. Beeby J, Broeg PE: Treatment of patients with radical mastectomies. Phys Ther 50:40–43, 1970.
6. Bloom JR: Psychosocial measurement and specific hypotheses: a research note. J Consult Clin Psychol 47:637–639, 1979.
7. Bloom JR, Ross RD: Measurement of the psychosocial aspects of cancer: sources of bias. *In* Cohen J, Cullen JW, Martin LR (eds): Psychosocial Aspects of Cancer. New York, Raven Press, 1982.
8. Cassileth BR, Cohen I (eds): Interview with a mastectomy couple. *In* The Cancer Patient—Social and Medical Aspects of Care. Philadelphia, Lea and Febiger, 1979.
9. Cerra FB: A Manual for Practitioners. American Cancer Society, 1982.
10. Cohen MM: Psychosocial morbidity in cancer: a clinical perspective. *In* Cohen J, Cullen JW, Martin LR (eds): Psychosocial Aspects of Cancer. New York, Raven Press, 1982.
11. Degenshein GA: Mobility of the arm following radical mastectomy. Surg Gynecol Obstet. July, 145, 1977.
12. Dietz JH: Rehabilitation Oncology. New York, John Wiley and Sons, 1981.
13. Dietz JH: Rehabilitation and readaptation for the patient with breast cancer. The Breast. St Louis, CV Mosby, 1978.
14. Dietz JH: Rehabilitation of the cancer patient—cancer of the breast. Med Clin North Am 53: 1969.
15. Entmacher PS: Insurance for the cancer patient. Washington, DC, Georgetown University Medical Center Cancer Symposium, January, 1974.
16. Feldman FL: Employment issues, concerns and alternatives for cancer patients. *In* Western States Conference on Cancer Rehabilitation. Palo Alto, CA, Bull Publishing, 1982.
17. Ferlic M, Goldman A, Kennedy BJ: Group counseling in adults with advanced cancer. Cancer 43:760–766, 1979.
18. Gaskin TA, et al: STRETCH: a rehabilitation program for breast cancer. South Med J 82(4):467–469, 1989.
19. Getz DH: The primary, secondary and tertiary nursing interventions of lymphedema. Cancer Nurs 8:177–184, 1985.
20. Grabois M: Physical rehabilitation following mastectomy. Texas Med 78:53–55, 1982.
21. Halliday WR: Medicovocational rehabilitation of the cancer patient: obstacles and resources. A National Forum on Comprehensive Cancer Rehabilitation and its Vocational Implications. Richmond, Medical College of Virginia, November, 1980.
22. Herzoff N: A therapeutic group for cancer patients and their families. Cancer Nurs December, 1979.
23. Hill AF, Hamilton PK, Ringer L: I'm A Patient Too. New York, Nick Lyons Books, 1986.
24. Holland JC, Mastrovito R: Psychologic adaptation to breast cancer. Cancer (suppl). August, 1980.
25. Holneck FE: Biographical Dictionary of the Saints. Herden Book Company, 1924.
26. Jamison KR, Wellisch DK, Pasnau RO: Psychosocial aspects of mastectomy: 1. The woman's perspective. Am J Psychiat April, 135:432–436, 1978.
27. Koplin AN: The implications of cancer for the labor union. Georgetown University Medical Center Cancer Symposium. Washington, DC, January, 1974.
28. Lerner R, Requena R: Upper extremity lymphedema secondary to mammary cancer treatment. Am J Clin Oncol 9:181–187, 1986.
29. Linn M, Linn B, Harris R: Effects of counseling for late stage cancer patients. Cancer 49:1048–1053, 1982.
30. Lotze MT, Duncan MA, Gerber LH, Woltering EA, Rosenberg SA: Early versus delayed shoulder motion following axillary dissection. Ann Surg 193:288–295, 1981.
31. Mages N, Castro J, Fobair P, Hall J, Harrison I, Mendelsohn G, Wolfson A: Patterns of psychosocial response to cancer: can effective adaptation be predicted. Int J Radiat Oncol Biol Phys 7: 1981.
32. Marchant J: Rehabilitation of the mastectomy patient. Nurs Times. April 21, 73:564–566, 1977.
33. Markowski J, Wilcox JP, Helm PA: Lymphedema incidence after specific postmastectomy therapy. Arch Phys Med Rehab 62:449–452, 1981.
34. May HT: Psychosexual sequelae to mastectomy: implications for therapeutic and rehabilitative interventions. J Rehab January, February, March 1980.
35. Mayo Clinic Cancer Rehabilitation Program, Rochester, MN: A Study of Discrimination Toward Cancer Patients by Insurers and Vocational Rehabilitation Agencies. NCI Contract No. CN4-45120-F, 1977.
36. Mellete SJ: Comprehensive cancer rehabilitation. Syllabus of Rehabilitation of the Cancer Patient in the Community Hospital. Princeton, AL, Baptist Medical Center, 1984.
37. Mellete SJ: The problem of employability after cancer treatment. Proceedings of the American Cancer Society Fourth National Conference on Human Values and Cancer, 1984.
38. Miller C, Denner P, Richardson V: Assisting the psychosocial problems of the cancer patient: a review of current research. Int J Nurs Studies 13:161–166, 1976.
39. Miller J: Legislation protects cancer patients from employment discrimination. Oncology Times 9, Number 9(16):1, 41, 1987.
40. Miller MW, Nygren C: Living with cancer: coping behaviors. Cancer Nurs 1:297–302, 1978.
41. Nikkanen TAV, Vanharanta H, Helenius-Reunanen H: Swelling of the upper extremity, function and muscle strength of shoulder joint following mastectomy combined with radiotherapy. Ann Clin Res 10:273–279, 1978.
42. Pollard R, Callum KG, Altman DG, Bates T: Shoulder movement following mastectomy. Clin Oncol 2:343–349, 1976.
43. Ringler K, Whitman H, Gustafson J, Coleman F: Technical advances in leading a cancer patient group. Int J Group Psychother 31:329–344, 1981.
44. Rosenbaum EH, Rosenbaum IR, Bullard JS, Bullard D: How you can help cancer patients solve their sexual concerns. Your Patient and Cancer December, 1983.
45. Ryttov N, Blichert-Toft M, Madsen EL, Weber J: Influence of adjuvant irradiation on shoulder joint function after mastectomy for breast carcinoma. Acta Radiol Oncol 22:29–33, 1983.
46. Sachs SH, Davis JM, Reynolds SA, Spagnola M, Hall P, Bloch A: Postmastectomy rehabilitation in a community hospital. J Fam Pract 11:395–401, 1980.
47. Schmid WL, Kiss M, Hibert L: The team approach to rehabilitation after mastectomy. AORN J 19:821–836, 1974.
48. Scott DW, Eisendrath SJ: Dynamics of the recovery process following initial diagnosis of breast cancer. J Psychosoc Oncol 3: 1985/1986.
49. Silberfarb PM, Maurer LH, Crouthamel CS: Psychosocial aspects of neoplastic disease: 1. Functional status of breast cancer patients during different treatment regimens. Am J Psychiatr April, 137:450–455,1980.
50. Silberfarb PM: Psychiatric themes in the rehabilitation of mastectomy patients. Int J Psychiatr Med 8:159–167, 1978.
51. Sinsheimer LM, Holland JC: Psychological issues in breast cancer. Semin Oncol 14(1):75–82, 1987.
52. Spiegel D, Bloom J, Yalom I: Group support for patients with metastatic cancer. Arch Gen Psychiatr 38:527–533, 1981.
53. Stone RW: Employing the recovered cancer patient. Georgetown University Medical Center Cancer Symposium, Washington, DC, January, 1974.
54. Swedborg I: Effectiveness of combined methods of physiotherapy for post-mastectomy lymphoedema. Scand J Rehab Med 12:77–85, 1980.
55. Swedborg I: Effects of treatment with an elastic sleeve and intermittent pneumatic compression in post-mastectomy patients with lymphoedema of the arm. Scand J Rehab Med 16:35–41, 1984.

56. Vachon M, Lyall W: Applying psychiatric techniques patients with cancer. Hosp Comm Psychiatr 27:582–584, 1976.

57. Weisman A: Coping With Cancer. New York, McGraw-Hill, 1979.

58. Wheatley GM, Cumnick WR, Wright BP, Van Keuren D: The employment of persons with a history of treatment for cancer. Cancer 33:441–445, 1974.

59. Wheeler AP: Employment discriminations and the cancer patient: rights and remedies. Syllabus of Rehabilitation of the Cancer Patient in the Community Hospital. Princeton, AL, Baptist Medical Center, 1984.

60. Willhite OD: Pre and post operative rehabilitation exercises for the mastectomy patient. Home Healthcare Nurse Jan/Feb, 1984.

61. Wingate L: Efficacy of physical therapy for patients who have undergone mastectomies. Phys Ther 65:896–900, 1985.

62. Winick L, Robbins GF: The post-mastectomy rehabilitation group program. Am J Surg 132:599–602, 1976.

63. Witkin MH: Sex therapy and mastectomy. J Sex Marit Ther 4:290–304, 1975.

64. Witkin MH: Psychosexual counseling of the mastectomy patient. J Sex Marit Ther 4: 1978.

65. Worden W, Weisman A: Do cancer patients really want counseling? Gen Hosp Psychiatr 2: 1980.

66. Zanolla R, Monzeglio C, Balzarini A, Martino G: Evaluation of the results of three different methods of post-mastectomy lymphedema treatment. J Surg Oncol 26:210–213, 1984.

67. Zeissler RH, Rose GB, Nelson PA: Post-mastectomy lymphedema: late results in treatment in 385 patients. Arch Phys Med Rehab 53:159–166, 1972.

Appendix 1

PSYCHOSOCIAL SCREENING QUESTIONNAIRE
Summary

Counselor _____ Date _____

Name _____ DOB _____ Age _____ Sex _____ Race _____

Marital Status _____ Religion _____

Address: Street _____ City _____ State _____

         Zip Code _____

Phone # _____ Social Security # _____ Insurance _____

Occupation _____ Education Level _____

Date of Diagnosis _____ Diagnosis _____

Present Therapy: None _____ Surgery _____ Radiation _____ Chemotherapy _____ Other _____

Names of Family Members: Spouse _____ Children _____

         Parents _____ Other _____

Major Concerns: Health _____ Religious _____ Finance/Work _____ Family _____

         Friends _____ Self-esteem _____ Future _____

_____

Recommendations and Interventions: _____

_____
_____
_____
_____
_____
_____
_____
_____
_____
_____
_____
_____
_____
_____
_____
_____
_____
_____
_____
_____

TO OUR PATIENTS

During your visits to the Hematology/Oncology Outpatient Facility, the doctors, nurses, and oncology counselors will be concerned about how your illness may be interfering with various areas of your life. This form will help us to become aware of these concerns.

On the following forms are listed many of the concerns that have been expressed by other cancer patients. Please mark any item that represents a problem for you and for which you would like to receive some assistance. Your family members may be helpful in identifying particular concerns and may help you fill out this form.

When you have finished, please return this form to the reception desk. We will review your concerns with you either today during your visit or on subsequent visits. This information will also be made available to your doctor.

NAME _____DATE _____

Would you like more information about any of the following topics? (Please check all that apply)
_____ The Comprehensive Cancer Center
_____ The University of Alabama in Birmingham Hospitals and Clinics
_____ Resources within the Medical Center (such as physical therapy)
_____ Resources within your own community (such as Visiting Nurse Service)
_____ Your disease and side effects
_____ Your treatment (such as chemotherapy or radiation therapy) and side effects
_____ Your medications (such as high blood pressure medications and side effects)
_____ Where to get legal help
_____ Where to get financial help
_____ Where to make religious contacts in your community
_____ Other _____

How much does fatigue (or feeling tired) interfere with your normal activities?
_____ Always
_____ Sometimes
_____ Never

How much does pain interfere with your normal activities?
_____ Always
_____ Sometimes
_____ Never

Do you need any help with transportation getting to and from medical appointments?
_____ Yes
_____ No

Are you having difficulty with any of the following activities? (Please check all that apply)
_____ Moving your arms or legs normally
_____ Walking or going up and down stairs
_____ Getting in and out of the car, tub or shower, bed
_____ Getting on and off the toilet
_____ Other _____

Do you need additional help with any of the following activities? (Please check all that apply)
_____ Personal hygiene and getting dressed
_____ Child care
_____ Housekeeping
_____ Home maintenance
_____ Getting around easily in your home
_____ Living alone
_____ Other _____

Do you need any medical equipment, supplies or teaching for home care?
_____ Yes—what kind? _____
_____ No

Do you have any of the following concerns? (Please check all that apply)
_____ Inability to return to your regular work or school schedule
_____ A decrease in earnings
_____ A change in the way you do your regular work or school activities
_____ A decrease in the amount of time you can spend at work or school
_____ Other _____

Are you concerned about your ability to participate in any of the following? (Please check all that apply)
_____ Home activities and hobbies
_____ Sexual activity or interest
_____ Community activities
_____ Social relationships
_____ Exercise or sports
_____ Religious services
_____ Other _____

Are any of the following particularly troublesome for you? (Please check all that apply)
_____ Concern about your family
_____ Feeling sad
_____ Feeling angry or upset
_____ Difficulty sleeping
_____ Changes in your appearance
_____ Difficulty relaxing
_____ Worry about the future
_____ Concern about friends
_____ Other _____

Do you think your family needs help with any of the following? (Please check all that apply)
_____ More information about your illness or treatment
_____ Ways to improve communications among family members
_____ Being able to cope with your illness
_____ Being able to participate in your care
_____ Other _____

Has your illness or treatment interfered with your relationships with any of the following people? (Please check all that apply)
_____ Your spouse
_____ Your family
_____ Your friends
_____ Other people _____

Before your diagnosis, how discouraged or down did you usually get?

_____ Very
_____ A little
_____ Not at all

Have you ever seen anyone for emotional problems?

_____ Inpatient at a hospital
_____ Outpatient
_____ Never

In the past, have you expected things to turn out well or badly? _____

Are you:

_____ Very pessimistic
_____ More pessimistic than optimistic
_____ More optimistic than pessimistic
_____ Very optimistic

Looking back over the past few years, if you could do some things over, what would they be?

_____ Everything
_____ Specific things
_____ Nothing

If you are receiving chemotherapy, please describe any problems or side effects you are experiencing related to this treatment.

_____
_____
_____

Is there anything else you would like to comment about?

_____
_____
_____

Of all the concerns you have identified, which ones do you wish to have addressed by our staff, the hospital, or community resources?

_____
_____
_____

Appendix 2

Baptist Medical Center Princeton
REFERRAL TO CANCER PROGRAM SERVICES

Diagnosis _____

Date Diagnosed _____

This form should be completed for all diagnosed cancer patients who are experiencing difficulties accepting the diagnosis or recommended treatment.

I WOULD LIKE FOR THIS PATIENT TO BE EVALUATED FOR HELP IN THE FOLLOWING AREAS:

I. EDUCATION (Relative to) (Contact: Oncology Clinical Nurse Specialist)
 _____ Treatment Modalities: Chemotherapy/Radiotherapy/Surgery
 _____ Symptoms Management: Pain/Alopecia/Stomatitis
 _____ Hickman/Infusaid
 _____ Availability and focus of "Living with Cancer" series
 _____ Other _____

II. SUPPORT NETWORKS
 A. Social Work Services (Contact: Social Work Services)
 _____ Support counseling relative to dealing with the social, emotional, psychological obstacles preventing participation in the recommended treatment/management.
 Community Support Services:
 _____ Reach to Recovery
 _____ Lost Chord
 _____ Ostomy Association
 _____ Other _____

 B. Pastoral Care (Contact: Pastoral Care Department)
 _____ Counseling
 _____ T.O.U.C.H.

 C. Hospice (Contact: Hospice)
 _____ Home Care Support
 _____ Inpatient Follow Up
 _____ Bereavement and Survivors Group

Date _____Physician's Signature _____ M.D.

_____

EVALUATION COMMENTS:
Summary of Findings: _____

_____

_____

Recommendations: _____

_____

_____

Date _____Signature _____

PHYSICIAN'S RESPONSE TO EVALUATIVE REMARKS: _____

_____

_____

_____

Used and devised by the Division of Hematology and Oncology, The Medical Center of the University of Alabama, Birmingham.

Chapter 55

PSYCHOSOCIAL PROBLEMS ASSOCIATED WITH THE DIAGNOSIS AND TREATMENT OF BREAST CANCER

Lesley J. Fallowfield, D.Phil. and Michael Baum, Ch.M.

The diagnosis and treatment of cancer exerts a major impact on a patient's sense of well-being, creating a plethora of serious psychosocial as well as medical problems. Despite the impressive advances made in treating certain cancers, diagnosis is still perceived by many with a dread and fear akin to that of receiving a death sentence.[47] The considerable psychiatric morbidity associated with cancer is provoked by both knowledge of having a life-threatening disease and fear of the various toxic and sometimes mutilating treatments that patients know they will have to face. Table 55–1 illustrates the psychosocial problems that breast cancer patients must confront. They are multi-faceted and assume different levels of importance at different stages of the disease and its treatment. In this chapter we will look at the pre- and postoperative needs of women with breast cancer and review some of the research on the efforts of specialist oncology counselors and others to ameliorate this psychosocial distress. Wherever possible, we illustrate the points being made with quotations taken from taped interviews with breast cancer patients in England participating in our own research studies.[15b, 16, 17]

PSYCHOSOCIAL FACTORS: ETIOLOGY OF DISEASE

Personality Factors

The notion that certain personality traits are causally linked with the development of cancer is not new; Galen commented in the second century A.D. that "melancholic" women were more likely to develop breast cancer than "women of more sanguine" disposition. Empirical support for such an association between personality characteristics and cancer is limited, but there is some evidence to suggest that certain personality traits predispose one to the expression of cancer[1] and mediate the course and outcome of the disease. Emotional

inhibition, particularly the suppression of anger and hostility,[38] is often cited as an etiological factor in cancer-prone individuals, together with self-sacrifice[65] and negative mood states.[66]

One methodological difficulty with most of this work, however, is that of ascribing measurable personality differences between cancer patients and control groups to cause or effect. The mechanism of denial, for example, is an important coping strategy for a person adapting to the role of cancer patient[25] and can confound personality assessments. Much published work on the subject is from retrospective data, as obtaining reliable premorbid personality data from cancer patients is difficult.

In one methodologically sound work on breast cancer, Greer and Morris[22] interviewed women admitted for breast biopsies before they were given their diagnoses. They found a higher incidence of cancer in women with abnormal expression of emotion [i.e., those who never or rarely expressed anger or emotions (extreme suppressors) or those who frequently indulged in outbursts of temper or never concealed emotions (extreme expressors)]. However, there was no difference between groups using the Eysenck Personality Inventory (EPI).[15]

Schonfield[67] compared personality factors in Israeli women with either benign or cancerous breast lesions using the Minnesota Multi-phasic Personality Inventory (MMPI).[24] He found no real difference between the two groups using this rating scale. Likewise, a recent study by Priestman et al.[58] found no personality differences between 200 patients with benign or malignant breast lumps using the EPI.

Hormonal and Immunological Factors

Psychoimmunology is the study of the way in which the brain and the immune system interact to influence an individual's susceptibility to disease. An understanding of the biological mechanisms that might link the brain and immune system could provide a plausible

Table 55–1. PSYCHOSOCIAL PROBLEMS ASSOCIATED WITH THE DIAGNOSIS AND THERAPY OF BREAST CANCER

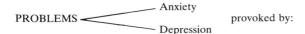

PROBLEMS

Anxiety

Depression

provoked by:

1. Knowledge of life-threatening disease
   — Uncertainty of prognosis
   — Inadequate information
   — Stigma of cancer
   — Fear of painful, undignified death
2. Coping with treatments: surgery, radiotherapy, or drugs
   — Loss of femininity, self-esteem
   — Rejection
   — Loss of libido
   — Toxicity of CMF, ulcers, nausea, alopecia
   — Hirsutism

explanation for the apparent impact that psychosocial variables such as personality exert on the development of cancer.

Exposure to stress undoubtedly affects immunosuppression in both animals and humans. Bereavement is a particularly noxious stressor, and there is plenty of evidence to show that recently bereaved people are more susceptible to disease and death themselves. An Australian study by Barthrop et al.[5] revealed that recently bereaved people had depressed lymphocyte function 6 weeks after the bereavement. In another rather different study of stress in humans, Kiecolt-Glaser, et al.[31] found that the natural killer cells of final-year medical students were significantly less active on examination day than they had been a month previously. Direct evidence that cell-mediated immunity influences cancer development is hard to obtain from humans because of ethical constraints and the difficulty of controlling potentially confounding variables; animal models therefore provide further clues. Laboratory rats subjected to tumor cell implants and then given uncontrollable electric shocks have depressed lymphocytes and mitogen response in comparison with animals who can control the shocks.[35]

Psychological stress can produce changes in the levels of circulating hormones, neurotransmitters, and neuromodulators (such as insulin, vasopressin, cortisol, testosterone, endorphins, and encephalins). There is evidence that cells of the immune system have surface receptors for many of these substances, and thus we have a plausible explanation of how psychological factors might influence the immune system. As far as breast cancer is concerned, Bulbrook and Hayward[9] conducted a prospective study on women at risk of developing breast cancer. They analyzed the hormone metabolites of urine and found that patients who subsequently developed breast cancer had significantly different levels of androgen and corticosteroid metabolites than did controls who were disease free.

Although much of this neuroendocrine and immunological work is still somewhat speculative, it could well

provide some interesting approaches to the treatment or prevention of cancer through behavior modification or other psychological interventions. We should at least remain open-minded to such ideas.

Stress and Life Events

There have been many anecdotal observations claiming that exposure to stressful life events is associated with an increased risk of breast cancer. In the nineteenth century the surgical pathologist, Sir James Paget, stated that " . . . deep anxiety, deferred hope and disappointment are quickly followed by the growth and increase of cancer."[53a] Le Shan's[37] historical review suggested that "the most consistently reported psychological factor has been the loss of a major emotional relationship prior to the first noted symptoms of the neoplasm."

Where is the sound scientific basis for such assertions? An epidemiological study by Parkes et al.[56] showed that cancer was the primary cause of death among people who died within 6 months after bereavement. The first attempt at a statistical study on breast cancer patients was by Herbert Snow in 1893.[71] He reported that in 156 of 250 women presenting with either breast or uterine cancers, "there had been immediately antecedent trouble, often in very poignant form as the loss of a near relative." Controlled studies conducted during the past two decades, however, provide little evidence to support such clinical observations. At least seven studies of women with breast cancer conducted in the U.S., Israel, and Europe report no significant relationship between loss of an important other and the development of cancer.[14, 22, 30, 51, 58, 67, 70]

Life events inventories that catalogue a variety of stressors encountered by patients provide a popular if not altogether sound method of measuring exposure to stress in the social milieu. They have proved useful in establishing associations between antecedent stress and various medical problems, such as cardiac disease and hypertension.[76] None of the three reported studies that have used a life events inventory with breast cancer patients have shown that women with malignant breast disease have experienced a greater number of stressful life events than have those with benign disease or healthy controls.[58, 67, 70] One of these studies (Schonfield[67]) found a significantly higher incidence of stressful life events in patients with benign disease and another (Priestman[58]) reported that stress exposure via life events was higher in controls than in breast disease patients.

In summary then, it appears that despite a vast literature of clinical observations suggesting the existence of a cancer-prone personality type and claims that emotional stress is related to the development of breast cancer, there is a dearth of well-controlled empirical support for such ideas. Much of the research is characterized by a plethora of methodological difficulties. Those studies that attempt to look at large numbers of unselected patients prospectively using standardized tests find little evidence that breast cancer patients have experienced more of life's stressors than noncancer patients or healthy controls. Evidence, however, from recent psychoimmunological research shows potential mechanisms supporting the notion that the experience of stress can produce an endocrine response that may impair the immune system, which can in turn increase tumor growth, but stress-associated pathologies such as breast cancer might only be observed if the host already has a predisposition to its development.

ADDRESSING THE PSYCHOLOGICAL NEEDS OF THE BREAST CANCER PATIENT

There have been consistent reports in the literature during the past 30 years showing that the diagnosis of breast cancer and its treatment, usually involving amputation of the breast, carries with it high levels of psychiatric morbidity.[4, 41, 49] The provision of satisfactory psychosocial support is therefore increasingly advocated. Evidence of the psychotherapeutic benefits of such things as counseling is equivocal and will be discussed later in this chapter, but assuming that adjuvant psychosocial therapy is necessary, what are the specific problems and stressors encountered by women during the different stages of the disease?

Preoperative Needs

On Finding the Lump

Several studies[16, 29, 40] report that women find the time between finding the lump and diagnosis the most psychologically stressful part of the whole experience, as the following quotation from a patient in one of our studies aptly demonstrates:[17]

"It was a living nightmare, that three weeks—knowing what it was, but not knowing for sure. Nothing that has happened since—the mastectomy or the treatment sessions were as bad as that time. Thinking it might be cancer and it was spreading everywhere was all I could do night and day."

This period was described by Bard and Sutherland[4] as the anticipatory phase, with women experiencing extreme anxiety about what is ahead of them. In Maguire's[40] 1976 study, only eight percent of his sample claimed not to have been at all concerned. Most women realize the significance of their symptoms immediately; in 1974, Knopf[32] found that at least 80 percent of the general public were aware that a breast lump could mean cancer. It is difficult these days to pick up a magazine or listen to a radio or television program that doesn't contain an item about breast cancer, so those figures are probably an underestimate of women who recognize that they could well have cancer if they have a breast lump. Lay populations in both the United States and Britain consistently overestimate the mortality figures for cancer and underestimate the cure rate;[33] thus many patients suffer extreme anxiety leading to considerable social and mental dysfunction. Scott[68] measured cognitive function and anxiety in 85 women while they were awaiting breast biopsy and then 6 weeks later when biopsy had been reported as negative. She found severe impairment in concentration and critical thinking together with high anxiety rates prior to biopsy. At 6 to 8 weeks post-biopsy, anxiety decreased and cognitive ability improved. Renneker and Cutler[60] suggested that fear of losing the breast was the primary focus of concern for the majority of women with a breast lump, although most other studies show fear of cancer rather than surgery as the main reason for anxiety.

Fear of Cancer and of Breast Loss Leading to Delay. Denial is a protective coping strategy employed by many of us in everyday life and a common feature among breast cancer patients. Although denial can be viewed as a psychologically protective mechanism, paradoxically it can be a biologically damaging strategy: some patients fail to report suspicious lumps, delaying medical attention until the unpleasant symptoms of advanced cancer are impossible to disregard and difficult to treat. An early study by Aiken-Swan and Paterson[2] identified two groups of patients with symptoms who had delayed consulting a doctor: one group was genuinely ignorant of the implications of their symptoms, and the other group was so overwhelmed by fear of doctors, hospitals, illness in general, and cancer in particular that they delayed reporting their symptoms.

Most studies report that "delayers" are older women of lower social class and education than "nondelayers,"[11, 21, 80] which to a certain extent accounts for their lack of awareness of the seriousness of symptoms. Frank denial, with patients ignoring or concealing their illness, is actually quite rare; rather than use denial, patients more often exhibit suppression in order to avoid upsetting themselves, their relatives, and their friends. Living as we do in a society that places so much emphasis on the breasts as symbols of femininity and sexuality, it is easy to see how the mere thought of breast loss could impose a major threat to self-esteem.

In summary, investigators have attributed delay to both fear of mastectomy[19, 21] and fear of cancer.[10, 21, 80] Delayers also differ from nondelayers in personality characteristics. Greer[21] reported that 62 percent of patients who had delayed presenting for treatment with breast lumps were "habitual deniers" in the face of stress in other life crises. Worden and Weisman[82] found that delayers avoided the word "cancer" and showed higher levels of manifest anxiety, tension, fatigue, and confusion.

On Hearing the Diagnosis

Women respond very differently to being given a diagnosis of breast cancer. By the time they reach the doctor's clinic, many women will have diagnosed breast cancer and given themselves a mutilating mastectomy and died a lonely, painful, and undignified death a hundred times over.

"I went through hell, back, and beyond that fortnight before I saw Mr. X. I imagined the worst—no chest, no hair, and dying anyway."

For some of these patients, diagnosis comes as a relief—at least some of the uncertainty has been diffused, and patients can start the adjustment and coping process.

"When he said, 'the tests show that it's cancer,' I was actually quite relieved. It might sound silly, but at last someone told me and I could stop worrying about what it might be. I couldn't wait to have the operation and start living again. I slept for the first time in 2 weeks that night."

For other patients the diagnosis comes as a complete shock, either because they genuinely had no idea that the lump might be serious or because they had successfully used denial to suppress their suspicions of the significance of their symptoms.

"It came as a total shock. I was absolutely stunned. All the time I'd thought that it was going to be a cyst. I didn't want to even think that it was malignant."

A seminal paper reported in the United Kingdom by Morris and colleagues[49] identified essentially five principal categories of response to diagnosis:

1. *Denial*, when patients rejected the seriousness of the evidence offered to them and seemed reluctant to engage in detailed discussion of the subject:

"They told me before that it was just mastitis, so I tried to think that was all it was again. I'm not the sort of person to ask a lot. I'd rather they didn't tell me."

2. *Fighting spirit*, where patients exhibited a positive, hopeful approach, soliciting as much information as possible:

"I am not giving in whatever happens. I'm going to fight this thing."

3. *Stoic acceptance*, with patients displaying quiet acknowledgement of the diagnosis and a phlegmatic approach to what lay ahead:

"I knew what he was going to say. I was quite prepared. I know that it's out of my hands—what will be will be. It's pointless worrying."

4. *Anxious/depressed acceptance*, with patients reacting with excessive anxiety or depression, viewing all results of their information gathering with pessimism but able nevertheless to carry on with usual activities:

"I don't know how I'd have got through that week if I hadn't been so busy with the children: but then they made it worse too—I kept thinking, 'God, they're going to be orphans.' "

5. *Helplessness/hopelessness*, when patients become so totally engulfed by the knowledge of their diagnosis that they view the future with extreme pessimism and suffer considerable social dysfunction. They are unable to view themselves as anything other than actively ill or dying:

"We're not lucky people in our family—my Dad died of cancer and my Mum. I know I'm going to go that way too. The only thing I like is my garden, but I haven't planted any bulbs even—what's the point? I won't see them will I?"

Doctor-Patient Information and Communication. The past 25 years have witnessed a vast change in doctors' attitudes about informing patients that they have cancer. In the U.S., Novak and colleagues[53] reported that the proportion of patients who had been explicitly told that their diagnosis was cancer rose from ten percent in 1961 to 90 percent in 1978. This change were probably a result of U.S. medicolegal constraints as well as social pressures that patients be fully informed.

In the U.K., many more people are made aware of their diagnosis,[34] but there is clearly room for improvement. A recent study by Newall et al.[52] comparing attitudes toward the presentation of information to cancer patients in the U.K. and U.S. revealed important differences: 98 percent of the U.S. patients claimed to have been told frankly that they had cancer, whereas one third of the British patients claimed that euphemisms such as "growth" or "tumor" were used.

A poorly informed breast cancer patient is more likely to be an anxious patient. In a study done by ourselves and Peter Maguire[17] in England, 101 patients who had been randomized to either mastectomy or breast conservation for early breast cancer were asked about the adequacy of the information that they received from their doctors. More than half the patients perceived that information as inadequate. Patients in this trial might have been expected to have more information about their illness and surgical options than is perhaps always possible in a busy outpatient department, as surgeons were required to obtain fully informed consent from patients prior to randomization. Affective disorders of anxiety or depression were found 12 months postoperatively in 46 percent of the poorly informed patients; in contrast, only 23 percent of the women who perceived their information as good were anxious or depressed a year later.

One of the obvious difficulties for both clinician and breast cancer patient is that there are several occasions during their interactions when diagnostic and prognostic information *is* inherently uncertain. This can be interpreted by the patient as unsatisfactory information, when in truth the surgeon actually has little clear information to impart. Superimpose on this the fact that patients will often see a different doctor at each outpatient visit who may well assume that certain important aspects of diagnosis and treatment have already been discussed, and the problem is further exacerbated. Many patients in our study comment that after hearing the word "cancer," they were too shocked to take in what was said thereafter:

"After he said 'cancer,' I just didn't know what he was going on about. I was all by myself and so shocked, I just couldn't believe it. I thought it was a bit callous. He might just as well have not bothered. It just went in one ear and out the other."

Allowing the anxious patient to invite a companion into the consulting room may ameliorate some of these problems.[16]

Postoperative Needs

During the Hospital Stay

Although anxious about the forthcoming operation, many hospitalized women experience some respite from the emotional traumas they have experienced since finding the lump and its diagnosis. It is not uncommon for women to exhibit postmastectomy euphoria as a result of being parted from their cancerous lump. Most women focus on the fact of their cancer and the somatic symptoms postoperatively and only really start to worry about other psychosocial issues later.

"I was so cheerful when I was in hospital, everyone said how great I was. I mean it felt so good to be rid of that awful thing at last. I didn't even care about the pain. It was only when she (the nurse) did the dressing that I started to think what a freak I was now. There was a travel program on the ward T.V. that night, and when I saw all those topless suntanned women on holiday I just cried and cried."

Unfortunately few nurses have been formally taught the skills necessary to deal with some of the emotional traumas breast cancer patients undergo. Much nurse training is concerned with attending to physical needs. Indeed, the staffing of wards is often too inadequate to permit nurses to utilize appropriate counseling skills even if they possess them.[74] Nurses often try to "jolly" patients along, and this form of reassurance only serves to neutralize or make light of a woman's concerns. This encourages patients to deny or suppress negative feelings rather than to help them cope with problems in a way that will not be maladaptive in the future.[23]

It is also vitally important that the breast prosthesis fitter contact any patient requiring a prosthesis before that patient leaves the hospital. Contact by a trained oncology counselor who can facilitate discussions between patients and their partners about the meaning breast cancer has for their relationship might well be useful at this time also.

At Home: Effects on Family and Friends

No woman gets breast cancer in a social vacuum; the effects of the diagnosis and treatment have important implications for family and friends, and their ability to provide a woman with general emotional and practical support can influence long-term adjustment enormously. Sound empirical work in this area is somewhat sparse, but two studies worthy of note emphasize the role of the male partner in helping a woman to achieve good adjustment.[7, 81] Reassurance of continued love and affection by the woman's partner after mastectomy can be a major source of positive support.

"You hear so much these days about men going off with younger women, I must admit I didn't really think about the cancer and losing my life. I was more worried about losing my husband when he saw what I looked like. He's never been much good at illness and things. It's funny you know, though, he was really great and told me that it wasn't breasts he'd married, but me, and he'd rather have me with one breast, one arm, one eye, one leg, than not at all. If anything, the physical side of things—you know, sex and that—is better than it's been for years."

Unfortunately, not all men react in this way. Pfefferbaum et al.[57] and Wellisch[79] describe the psychological trauma that men experience during the pre- and postoperative periods: along with their fears about confronting their wife's or partner's disfigurement, all have to come to terms with the fact of her cancer and the possibility that treatment might not be successful. Researchers such as Gyllenskold[23] have urged that psychological support be provided for the whole family on the grounds that unless a woman's family can come to terms with her illness, they will be unable to help or support her effectively.

Adjuvant Therapy

Radiotherapy. Several authors have highlighted the psychological and physical distress associated with radiotherapy.[26, 27, 69] Many patients become depressed, and most complain of an unremitting enervating fatigue that persists long after the course of treatment itself has finished.

A recent study in the United Kingdom, however, by Hughson et al.[28] compared psychosocial outcome in 47 breast cancer patients given postoperative radiotherapy with 38 patients receiving no further treatment postmastectomy. Approximately one third of all patients experienced anxiety and depression. At 3 and 6 months postoperatively, the radiotherapy-treated group had significantly more somatic symptoms and social dysfunction, but at 12 months postoperatively, there were no differences between groups. It is worth mentioning that the patients in this study received 15 fractions over 3 weeks—considerably less than is usual for breast conservation patients. There is some evidence that the radiotherapy given to patients treated with local excision is an important contributory factor in psychological morbidity.[16, 17]

Many factors contribute to psychological and somatic symptoms. Radiotherapy in the United Kingdom is usually provided in specialist centers dealing with predominantly cancer patients. Patients may have to be admitted for treatment for geographical reasons, leading to increased anxiety at being away from home; other patients may have to travel long distances daily for several weeks, thus increasing the fatigue and imposing a greater financial burden on the family. Long waiting periods, sometimes in inadequate departments, together with other seriously ill patients can make certain patients extremely fearful and depressed. Finally, lay people often harbor fears about radiation therapy because of the paradox that although radiation can cause cancer, it is also used to treat it.

Despite these problems for patients with early breast cancer, one cannot deny that radiotherapy often greatly enhances quality of life in patients with advanced disease. Locally advanced disease can be controlled, and radiotherapy provides considerable relief for painful bony secondaries.

An efficient appointments system, upgrading of the

radiotherapy department waiting areas, good information from well-trained staff, and provision of an oncology counseling service for patients and their families might well ameliorate much of the psychosocial distress associated with radiotherapy.

Chemotherapy. There is widespread debate and controversy over the benefits of giving cytotoxic chemotherapy to women with breast cancer. The toxicity associated with most chemotherapeutic regimens imposes a major disruption in the lives of both patients and their families, and in their enthusiasm to treat patients, oncologists show a marked tendency to underestimate the unpleasant side effects of their treatment.[55] Most American clinicians favor routine adjuvant chemotherapy for all breast cancer patients with involvement of axillary nodes. British clinicians are generally less enamored with the putative benefits and tend to support adjuvant endocrine therapy for its low toxicity and encouraging effects on survival.

In addition to the largely unavoidable pharmacological side effects of treatment, some patients experience conditioned physical responses of anxiety and nausea at the mere thought of coming for treatment.[50] These problems can be so aversive that patients refuse further treatments. The important role of the psychologist in helping such patients will be discussed later.

Despite the miseries of vomiting, nausea, hair loss, and other side effects, many patients are willing to put up with these if they are told that it will improve their chances of survival. Although they experience intense relief at the end of treatment and most somatic symptoms disappear, psychological and physical effects can persist. Meyerowitz et al.[48] found that more than 50 percent of breast cancer patients who had received adjuvant chemotherapy described problems linked to their therapy 2 years after treatment had ceased. In another study by McArdle et al.[46] comparing psychiatric morbidity in stage II breast cancer patients treated by mastectomy followed by either radiotherapy or chemotherapy, there was significant psychological morbidity 12 months postmastectomy in patients receiving chemotherapy. This trend persisted and was still evident 6 months after completion of the chemotherapy.

Two studies have shown that the greater the objective toxicity of different chemotherapy regimens, the greater the psychological morbidity. Palmer et al.[54] used self-rating questionnaires to compare psychosocial outcome of an aggressive cytotoxic combination of drugs with a low toxicity single-agent regimen. Maguire and his colleagues[42] used a semistructured psychiatric interview to assess the status of women receiving cyclophosphamide, methotrexate, and 5-fluorouracil (CMF); melphalan; or no chemotherapy postmastectomy. CMF significantly increased the risk of affective disorders. Anxiety and depression in this group of women were severe enough in some instances to merit psychiatric treatment.

In patients with advanced disease, Priestman and Baum[59] employed visual analogue self-rating scales to compare outcome in patients treated with either endocrine or cytotoxic therapy. The cytotoxic group reported far more treatment-related side effects but paradoxically described their sense of general well-being as better than the endocrine therapy group. This perverse result can probably be explained by the significant difference in objective response between the two treatment groups. The cytotoxic therapy group experienced greater symptomatic relief from objective tumor shrinkage than distress from the side effects of treatment.

For the patient with advanced disease, the relief at cessation of active treatment is often less than the intense psychological strain of assuming that no more can be done for them. These patients obviously require counseling about the limitations of cytotoxic therapy and need reassurance that they will continue to receive support and symptomatic relief. Other patients attain much psychological release by being given the option to participate in clinical trials that might help others.

"I don't want to just die for nothing. I'll try anything if it will help them (doctors) find a cure. My daughters or grandchildren might get it—I'd like to think I'd helped."

Reconstruction

Some women are helped to adjust more readily to mastectomy either by having immediate reconstructive surgery or by the offer of it at a later date. Surprisingly few patients (less than ten percent in both the United States and the United Kingdom) actively seek reconstruction. It is not clear whether this is a result of clinicians discouraging women by expressing disappointment with some of the implant techniques, lack of awareness that such options exist, financial considerations, or a reflection of the fact that many women do adjust to wearing a prosthesis. Wendy Schain and her colleagues[64] have suggested five primary factors that influence the seeking of reconstructive surgery: availability of information, economics, medical considerations, psychological factors, and interpersonal factors. The study by Rowland et al.[61] of 150 women who had breast reconstruction revealed that most were extremely satisfied with the cosmetic result and found that psychosocial and sexual functioning improved after reconstruction. One important benefit was that fears of recurrence diminished when the overt reminder (i.e., the flat chest wall and mastectomy scar) was removed. Insurance companies in the United States recognize the importance of reconstruction and reimburse the cost as a rehabilitative procedure. The general finding of most studies seems to be that reconstruction minimizes some of the psychological distress of mastectomy and that the earlier this is done, the better. Immediate reconstruction appears to protect women's self-esteem, minimize self-consciousness, and enhance sexuality more than if reconstructive surgery is delayed. The use of the permanent tissue expander facilitates immediate breast reconstruction, and because filling of the expander is controlled, earlier problems of skin flap necrosis and wound breakdown are eliminated.[6]

COMPARISON OF PSYCHOSOCIAL OUTCOME: MASTECTOMY VS. LUMPECTOMY

The psychological problems encountered by women treated for breast cancer by mastectomy have been well documented in both the academic literature and lay press. Much of this original work drew on uncontrolled series of patients or anecdotal reports. Two of the earliest methodologically sound studies conducted in the United Kingdom by Maguire et al.[41] and Morris et al.[49] compared the psychiatric status of women being treated for malignant breast lumps with women admitted for biopsy of benign breast lumps. Both studies found high levels of anxiety, depression, and sexual dysfunction among the mastectomy-treated women. For many, these problems were unremitting and severe enough to merit psychiatric intervention. Awareness of the psychological morbidity associated with mastectomy, together with abhorrence of the procedure by both surgeons and patients, has led to increased numbers of surgeons performing breast conservation surgery for its assumed cosmetic and psychological benefits. The advocates of breast conservation have been further encouraged by the results from various trials demonstrating no difference in relapse-free intervals or survival in patients treated by local excision and radiotherapy vs. those treated by mastectomy.[18]

Although there is a prima facie case that mastectomy produces high levels of anxiety and depression,[41, 49] there is to date no satisfactory published evidence supporting the intuitive assumption made by many that women undergoing local excision and radiotherapy for early breast cancer are protected from psychiatric morbidity.

There are at the time of this writing only six studies, shown in Table 55–2, comparing the psychological outcome of lumpectomy with that found in mastectomy. (For a more recent and comprehensive review see Hall and Fallowfield, 1989.)[23a] Sanger and Reznikoff[62] reported a study in the United States of 40 women, 20 of whom underwent mastectomy and 20 who underwent a breast conservation procedure. The surgeon made the treatment decision for the mastectomy group, whereas all those who had breast conservation made that decision themselves. The mastectomy patients volunteered for the psychological study by responding to advertisements in a store specializing in prosthesis fitting or via a cancer self-help group. The lumpectomy patients were referred by their radiotherapist or surgeon. Thus the two treatment groups are not comparable. This, together with the fact that psychological assessment was extremely limited, makes it difficult to accept the authors' conclusions that there is no difference in psychological adjustment. They themselves also comment that " . . . the physicians had refused to permit the testing of women they deemed to be having psychological difficulties."[62]

Another study from the United States by Wendy Schain[63] described questionnaire data from 38 patients randomized to receive either mastectomy (20 patients) or excision biopsy plus radiotherapy (18 patients).[63] She found similar psychological problems in both treatment groups, with the only significant difference being a less negative body image reaction among the conservatively treated women. Unfortunately, assessment via a nonstandardized postal questionnaire on such a small sample might not be a sensitive enough measure of the psychological variables in breast cancer.

Steinberg et al.[73] reported psychosocial data from United States breast cancer patients, 46 of whom underwent mastectomy and 21 of whom had local excision and radiotherapy. Half the breast conservation sample were given the choice of treatment, and half were referred for the breast saving procedure. Responsibility for decision making in the mastectomy patients could not be assessed. Their study shows no difference between groups on any standardized psychiatric scales, but

Table 55–2. PSYCHOSOCIAL OUTCOME OF MASTECTOMY VS. BREAST CONSERVATION (BC)

Authors	Patients	Assessments	Outcome
Sanger and Reznikoff[62]	40	Rorschach (ink-blot), Locke and Wallace Body Cathexis Scale, MMPI	No difference.
Schain[63]	38	Nonstandard questionnaire	Less negative body image in BC group.
Steinberg et al.[73]	67	SADS, POMS, BDI, Nonstandard questionnaire	No difference on standardized tests; BC group less self-conscious.
Ashcroft et al.[3]	40	Body satisfaction, LDS, STAI, Locke and Wallace, Holmes and Rahe, LES	Little or no difference on psychosocial measures but less concern with appearance in BC group.
Haes and Welvaart[13]	41	CPSC, Nonstandard tests of marital and body image and quality of life	Less negative body image in BC group; no other differences.
Fallowfield et al.[17]	101	PSE, RSCL, HAD	No difference, but more overt concern with cancer in BC group.

MMPI = Minnesota Multiphasic Personality Inventory; SADS = Shelfield Anxiety and Depression Scale; POMS = Profile of Mood States; BDI = Beck Depression Inventory; LDS = Leeds Depression Scale; STAI = Spielberger Trait Anxiety Inventory; LES = Holmes and Rahe Life Events Schedule; CPSC = Cancer Patients Symptom Checklist.

some small differences on self-rating scales of feelings of attractiveness and femininity. The authors then acknowledge that " . . . our emotionally distressed patients from both groups declined to participate."[73]

In Europe, de Haes and Welvaart[13] assessed psychosocial outcome in 41 women randomized to treatment. They report less negative body image problems in the local excision group but few other major differences.

In Britain, Ashcroft et al.[3] looked at 40 patients who were given a choice of treatment when possible. No actual figures are given anywhere in the paper, but the authors conclude that careful preoperative assessment and help with decision making ameliorates any development of psychiatric morbidity.

Fallowfield et al.[17] have reported retrospective data from a randomized study of 101 patients in the Cancer Research Campaign's Breast Conservation Trial. They showed that the psychological outcome was similar in both treatment groups. Details of the design of this multicenter study have been described elsewhere, but it should be remembered that the protocol invited participants to ascertain whether women had a treatment preference. Women with no apparent preference for a certain treatment were randomized to receive either mastectomy or lumpectomy. There is a possibility therefore that the psychological profile of women who have little expressed autonomy over their body might not be representative of breast cancer patients in general.

High levels of anxiety or depression comparable to those found in other empirical studies were experienced by women who underwent mastectomy, but Table 55–3 shows that the degree of psychiatric morbidity among the patients treated with local excision and radiotherapy was unfortunately just as high. Much has been written about the decline in self-esteem, self-image, and sexual functioning that follows mastectomy, the implication being that breast loss per se is the primary cause of psychosocial and sexual disturbance in breast cancer. The psychological data challenge this assumption, as does the finding that one third of the patients in the CRC study reported a loss of interest in love-making irrespective of their treatment group.

There are to date, therefore, no firm data demonstrating that breast conservation patients are protected from psychological morbidity, although less radical surgery clearly confers advantages in terms of body image for most women treated by local excision and avoids the nuisance value of the external prosthesis. The fear of cancer and disappointment with the cosmetic appearance of the treated breast expressed by some women must be addressed, as the following quote reveals:

"When he said they'd just remove a little lump, I felt relieved. I mean, no one really wants to lose a breast do they? But when I look at what's left I wonder if it was worth it. I mean, I'm still a freak aren't I? I don't like touching it or looking at it, and I'm scared to death it's going to come back again."

These data suggest that lumpectomy patients may require just as much psychological support as the mastectomy patients.

RECOGNITION AND REDUCTION OF PSYCHIATRIC MORBIDITY

Role of the Clinician: Treatment Choice

There is overwhelming evidence that a diagnosis of breast cancer and its treatment provoke considerable psychiatric morbidity. Despite this, many surgeons either fail to detect it or deal with it effectively only if it is recognized. An interesting study by Lee and Maguire[36] of patients attending a breast clinic found that when patients revealed their distress either verbally or nonverbally, these cues were in general not picked up or responded to by the surgeon. Other members of the hospital team, in particular the ward nurses, are not much better at recognizing the significant emotional difficulties being expressed by patients.[40, 42] Other researchers have shown that many women with breast cancer attempt to disguise their feelings of grief or anxiety,[16, 77] which makes recognition difficult unless clinicians make efforts to encourage women to reveal their concerns.

As there is still no consensus as to the most appro-

Table 55–3. PSYCHIATRIC MORBIDITY EXPERIENCED WITH MASTECTOMY VS. BREAST CONSERVATION (LUMPECTOMY AND RADIOTHERAPY) GROUPS

	Psychiatric Morbidity*			
	Anxiety state	*Depressive illness*	*Anxiety state and depressive illness*	*Either or both affective disorders*
Mastectomy group (n = 53)	14 (26)	11 (21)	8 (15)	17 (32)
Lumpectomy group (n = 48)	15 (31)	13 (27)	10 (21)	18 (38)

	Self Report on Rotterdam Symptom Checklist Assessing Lack of Sexual Interest*	
	"Not at all" to "a little"	*"Somewhat" to "very much"*
Mastectomy group (n = 48)†	30 (62)	18 (38)
Lumpectomy group (n = 39)†	24 (62)	15 (38)

*Figures are numbers (percentages) of patients.
†Fourteen elderly or single women in the two groups without sexual partners did not answer question.
From Fallowfield LJ, et al: Br Med J 293:1331–1334, 1986. Reprinted by permission.

priate treatment for breast cancer, surgeons have the option to tailor therapy to individual patients' needs. This requires extra time and counseling skills, but there is some evidence that certain patients given help with decision making actually adjust better to the treatment eventually given.[3] It is too simplistic an assessment of women to assume, however, that all women want to make that choice for themselves. Many prefer to leave the final decision to their surgeon, and they have that right. For these women, shouldering the burden of choosing among treatments on which the experts themselves disagree can only provoke needless further anxiety.

All women suffer uncertainty about their disease and fear recurrence or metastatic spread. It is not uncommon to find overt expression of these anxieties among women who have had breast conservation, given that it is still a relatively new treatment. Radiotherapy to "clear up any remaining cells" only amplifies these fears. False reassurance only destroys faith if things go badly, but there is much the surgeon can say about the survival statistics that can permit patients to maintain optimism, hope, and a positive attitude.

Role of the Specialist Nurse or Counselor

An increasingly important member of the breast care team is the specialist nurse. She can be trained to detect psychiatric morbidity and can then refer patients for appropriate therapy. Studies have shown that psychiatric morbidity declines in centers with a properly trained specialist nurse.[43] Not all patients require referral to a psychiatrist; nurses with counseling skills can ameliorate those borderline cases of psychosocial dysfunction not needing pharmacological or psychiatric intervention.

The evidence that counseling per se is beneficial for patients, however, is at best equivocal. Watson's[78] comprehensive and thoughtful review evaluating counseling studies concluded that a blanket service for all was probably unnecessary. Efforts must be made to improve the methods for identifying those women most at risk and likely to benefit. She also points out the dangers of assuming that all sorts of counseling may be therapeutic; some programs may well remove a patient's ability to utilize her own unique coping strategy.

Role of the Clinical Psychologist

The theoretical bases of behavioral and cognitive psychology have provided some powerful and effective treatment options for women crippled by depression and anxiety. These patients can derive considerable benefit from a psychologist skilled in anxiety management techniques or cognitive behavior therapy, as several studies have now shown.[20, 72]

Anxiety management training initially teaches patients how to identify their own internal cues for anxiety. They can then learn to induce anxiety through mental imagery and bring it back under control through muscular relaxation and imagery. This ability gives patients the confidence to exert self-control over symptoms of anxiety irrespective of the provoking stimulus. There is some evidence that relaxation therapy, together with cognitive therapy, can ameliorate fears of recurrent disease.[75] In cognitive behavior therapy, the patient is helped to shift perspective from a negative to a more positive viewpoint. The benefits of the psychological techniques of anxiety management and systematic desensitization have also been demonstrated in those patients receiving chemotherapy who experience anticipatory nausea and vomiting or become needle phobic.

Role of the Sex Therapist

There are sparse methodologically sound data about the impact that breast cancer has on sexual functioning, although Diana Bransfield has provided an excellent review.[8] Reports of the body image problems and loss of interest in sexual activity postmastectomy considered breast loss to be the major cause of this dysfunction. However, women who have conservative surgery suffer a deterioration in their sex lives comparable to that experienced by mastectomy patients.[17] Some patients and their partners therefore might be helped by referral to a sex therapist for Masters and Johnson type conjoint therapy,[45] but not all would necessarily welcome this. Lieber et al.[39] reported a study showing that although desire for sexual intercourse declined for 87.5 percent of their breast cancer patients, half of these women reported an increased desire for other affectionate behavior such as kissing and physical closeness. The surgeon can help by fostering open communication with the patient regarding sexuality.

Role of the Psychiatrist

Patients with unremitting depression or anxiety sometimes require psychiatric help. This may mean inpatient care and pharmaceutical intervention. There is often a surprising reluctance by physicians to refer patients for psychiatric help because of the assumption that affective disorders are natural reactions to a diagnosis of cancer and therefore not worthy of treatment. Mianserin, one of the new generation antidepressants with few side effects, has been shown to offer cancer patients effective relief.[12] Short courses of anxiolytics such as lorazepam help overly anxious patients, and the anxiety-related insomnia suffered by many breast cancer patients is often eased by an hypnotic such as Temazepam. With the acute symptoms of anxiety and depression under control, patients can profit from longer term psychotherapy and support. This might be offered by either the psychiatrist with a particular interest in the problems of cancer patients or a clinical psychologist or oncology counselor.

Role of Volunteer Groups

Some hospitals encourage volunteers from the Mastectomy Association (in the United Kingdom) or Reach to Recovery (in the United States) to provide advice or prosthesis fitting service. Many of these volunteers have had breast cancer themselves. There have been doubts raised about the potentially harmful effects of visits from a nonqualified person who might not have resolved all her own difficulties and could transmit these on to the patient.[44] The volunteer/counselor is not necessarily appropriate unless careful selection, training, and supervision are given.[15a] As more women are treated conservatively, they may not have contact with the mastectomy counselor if her primary role is one of prosthesis fitting. This might well leave a large number of breast cancer patients with no counseling or support service at all.

CONCLUSIONS

Psychology has mischievously been described as the subject that tells you what you already know in a language that you cannot understand. We hope this chapter has done something to allay the suspicions of clinical and nursing staff about the role that psychologists and allied professionals have to play in the management of patients with carcinoma of the breast. Clearly the psychological studies described do not tell us what we already know, as much of the data are counterintuitive. For example, methodologically sound studies have failed to corroborate the popular myth that stress is in some way connected with the development of breast cancer. Furthermore, studies on patients treated either by mastectomy or conservative techniques have indicated a high degree of psychological morbidity among those treated conservatively and hitherto judged to be protected from the emotional damage inflicted by mastectomy.

We wish to conclude this chapter with some simple practical advice by which the quality of a patient's life can be improved:

1. Before the "bad news" interview, identify whether the patient is happily married or has a close companion or other confidant. With her consent, try to involve the best individual identified by the patient in the initial interview so that you have a committed ally in your attempts to provide psychosocial support.

2. Identify the patient most at risk of developing serious psychological morbidity after the diagnosis and treatment of breast cancer. She is likely to be the one without a husband or powerful network of family support. Someone recently widowed or divorced or going through some other life crisis (e.g., moving, a husband's unemployment, or problems with her children) is also at risk. A previous history of depressive illness or chronic anxiety should alert the doctor to the likelihood of serious problems of adaptation.

3. Employ a professional, adequately trained counselor in the clinic. Ideally, this should be a mature nurse who has spent at least a year in a training program for counselors. Counseling skills do not necessarily exist among well-motivated paramedical staff, and they are not learned by "experience." These are professional skills that have to be respected. Very few doctors have the time or talent to fulfill this role adequately.

4. Open up lines of communication with a friendly neighborhood department of psychological medicine. It is best to work with an individual psychiatrist to deal with the serious problems identified by the professional counselor. Paradoxically, most psychiatrists are more interested in "madness" than the psychological problems generated by organic disease. Only pressure from interested clinicians will change this tendency.

5. Many patients are made unnecessarily miserable by prolonged outpatient waiting times in ugly or threatening hospital environments. Proper appointment systems must be made and adhered to, and the waiting areas should be brightened up with paintings, potted plants, and even tropical fish tanks. The role of music in the waiting area has yet to be researched.

6. Many women will inevitably suffer mastectomy in the future because the size or position of the tumor relative to the size of the breast makes breast conservation technically impossible. They will therefore need to be provided with an adequate prosthesis to compensate for their loss. Many women describe their feelings of disgust and humiliation by the deficiencies and inadequacies of the service provided. Prosthetic fitters should be adequately trained and should be female. A temporary prosthesis should be fitted before the patient leaves the hospital and an appointment made for 6 weeks thereafter for the fitting of the most aesthetically pleasing prosthesis. This is the patient's right and should not be hindered by artificial financial constraints and bureaucracy. The provision of the prosthesis should be treated with the same respect as the prescription of the cytotoxic drug.

7. Patients treated by local excision and postoperative radiotherapy are not automatically guaranteed a clean psychological bill of health. Their needs must be recognized and their anxieties dealt with. These women need the message continually reinforced that preserving the breast does not jeopardize their life. Constant obsessive reexamination and repeat mammographies do nothing to palliate this anxiety. Once a group of clinicians has embarked on this policy, they should have the courage of their convictions, recognizing that in the few cases where local control fails, delayed mastectomy can salvage the situation without having put the patient's life at risk.

8. The follow-up for patients having been treated for early carcinoma of the breast is often relegated to the most junior member of staff, and as a result there is little continuity of care. It has to be remembered that however trivial the visit in the eyes of the clinician, it is a momentous life event for the patient. She will be sleepless for nights beforehand, wondering whether this next visit will demonstrate the feared recurrence that will be the early signal of her impending death. Ideally, these patients should always be seen by the same responsible clinician.

9. When ultimately a patient's breast cancer does recur and she is under treatment for advanced disease, it should be recognized that treatment is only palliative; such patients are all condemned to die within 1 or 2 years. The exception to this general rule is the patient with local relapse in the breast after previous conservative surgery for the primary disease (see chapters 29, 38, 41, and 45). There is little evidence at present that any particular treatment strategy significantly prolongs survival when compared with any other policy. It is essential therefore to remember that the criterion of benefit should be quality of survival rather than length of survival. Ideally, some form of assessment of quality of life should be incorporated into treatment and research protocols.

10. Finally, when patients have exhausted the benefits of conventional active treatment, a good terminal care support group should be able to cope with all residual symptoms and the stress of dying felt both by the patient and her immediate family. Although active therapy should cease at this stage, many patients who wish that their death not be in vain may be happy to volunteer for phase I and II trials of promising new therapy.

This list should not be seen as a list of commandments, but as a list of admonitions, where with available knowledge and available resources we can do better in reducing suffering and increasing long-term well-being for the woman with carcinoma of the breast.

ACKNOWLEDGMENTS

The authors would like to thank Mrs. Ruth Sutton, secretary at the Cancer Research Campaign's Clinical Trials Centre, for her contributions to this chapter and the Cancer Research Campaign for their financial support.

References

1. Abse DW, Wilkins MM, van de Castle RL, Buxton WD, Demars JP, Brown RS, Kirschner LG: Personality and behavioural characteristics of lung cancer patients. J Psychosom Res 18:101–113, 1974.
2. Aiken-Swan J, Paterson R: The cancer patient's delay in seeking advice. Br Med J i:623–627, 1955.
3. Ashcroft JJ, Leinster SJ, Slade PD: Breast cancer—patient choice of treatment: preliminary communication. J Roy Soc Health 78:43–46, 1985.
4. Bard M, Sutherland AM: Psychological impact of cancer and its treatment. Cancer 8:656–672, 1955.
5. Barthrop RW, Lazarus L, Luckhurst E, Kiloh LG, Penny R: Depressed lymphocyte functioning after bereavement. Lancet i:834–836, 1977.
6. Becker H, Maraist F: Immediate breast reconstruction after mastectomy using a permanent tissue expander. South Med J 80(2):154–160, 1987.
7. Bloom JR: Social support, accommodation to stress and adjustment to breast cancer. Soc Sci Med 16:1329–1338, 1982.
8. Bransfield DD: Breast cancer and sexual functioning: a review of the literature and implications for future research. Int J Psychiatr Med 12(3):197–211, 1982–1983.
9. Bulbrook RD, Hayward JL: Abnormal urinary steroid secretion and subsequent breast cancer. Lancet i:512–519, 1967.
10. Buls JG, Jones IH, Bennett RC, Chan DPS: Women's attitudes to mastectomy for breast cancer. Med J Austr 2:236–338, 1976.
11. Cameron A, Hinton J: Delay in seeking treatment for mammary tumours. Cancer 21:1121–1126, 1968.
12. Costa D, Mogos I, Toma T: Efficacy and safety of mianserin in the treatment of depression of women with cancer. Acta Psychiatr Scand 72(suppl 320):85–92, 1985.
13. De Haes JCJM, Welvaart K: Quality of life after breast cancer surgery. J Surg Oncol 28:123–125, 1985.
14. Ewertz M: Bereavement and breast cancer. Br J Cancer 53:701–703, 1986.
15. Eysenck HJ, Eysenck SGB: Manual of the Eysenck Personality Inventory. London, University of London Press, 1964.
15a. Fallowfield LJ: Counselling for patients with cancer. Br Med J 297:727–728, 1988.
15b. Fallowfield LJ: Breast Cancer. The Experience of Illness Series. Tavistock/Routledge, London, 1990 (in press).
16. Fallowfield LJ, Baum M, Maguire GP: Addressing the psychological needs of the conservatively treated breast cancer patient. J Roy Soc Med 80(11):696–700, 1987.
17. Fallowfield LJ, Baum M, Maguire GP: Effects of breast conservation on psychological morbidity associated with diagnosis and treatment of early breast cancer. Br Med J 293:1331–1334, 1986.
18. Fisher B, Fisher ER, Redmond C: Ten year results of a randomized clinical trial comparing radical mastectomy and total mastectomy with or without radiation. N Engl J Med 312:674–681, 1985.
19. Gold MA: Causes of patient delay in disease of the breast. Cancer 17:564–577, 1964.
20. Gordon WA, Freidenbergs I, Diller L, Hibbard M, Wolf C, Levine L, Lipkins R, Ezrachi O, Lucido D: Efficacy of psychosocial intervention in cancer patients. J Consult Clin Psychol 48(6):743–759, 1980.
21. Greer HS: Psychological aspects. Delay in the treatment of breast cancer. Proc Roy Soc Med 67:470–473, 1974.
22. Greer HS, Morris T: Psychological attributes of women who develop breast cancer. A controlled study. J Psych Res 19:147–153, 1975.
23. Gyllenskold K: Breast cancer—the psychological effects of the disease and its treatment. London, Tavistock Publications, 1982.
23a. Hall A, Fallowfield LJ: Psychological outcome of treatment for early breast cancer: A review. Stress Med 5:167–175, 1989.
24. Hathaway SR, McKinley JC: Minnesota Multiphasic Personality Inventory. New York, Psychological Cooperation, 1951.
25. Hinton J: Dying, rev ed. NY, Penguin, 1967.
26. Holland JC, et al: Reactions to cancer treatment: assessment of emotional response to adjuvant radiotherapy as a guide to planned intervention. Psych Clin North Am 2(2):347–358, 1979.
27. Hughes J: Emotional reactions to the diagnosis and treatment of early breast cancer. J Psychosom Res 26(2):277–283, 1982.
28. Hughson AVM, Cooper AF, McArdie CS, Smith DC: Psychological effects of radiotherapy after mastectomy. Br Med J 294:1515–1518, 1987.
29. Jamison KR, Wellisch DK, Pasnau RO: Psychosocial aspects of mastectomy I: the woman's perspective. Am J Psychiatr 135(4):432–436, 1978.
30. Jones D, Goldblatt PO, Leon DA: Bereavement and cancer: some data on deaths of spouses from the longitudinal study of Office of Population Censuses and Surveys. Br Med J 289:461–464, 1984.
31. Kiecolt-Glaser JK, Glaser R, Strain EC, Stout JC, Tarr KL, Holliday JE, Speicher CE: Modulation of cellular immunity in medical students. J Behav Med 9:5–21, 1984.
32. Knopf A: Cancer: changes in opinion after 7 years of public education in Lancaster. Manchester, England, Manchester Regional Committee on Cancer, 1974.
33. Knopf A: Changes in women's opinions about cancer. Soc Sci Med 10:191–195, 1976.
34. Lancet Editorial. In cancer, honesty is here to stay. Lancet ii:245, 1980.
35. Laudenslager M, Ryan SM, Drugan RC, Hyson RL, Maier SF: Coping and immunosuppression: inescapable but not escapable shock suppresses lymphocyte proliferation. Science 221:568–570, 1983.
36. Lee ECG, Maguire GP: Emotional distress in patients attending a breast clinic. Br J Surg 62:162, 1975.

37. Le Shan L: Psychological states as factors in the development of malignant disease: a critical review. J Natl Cancer Inst 22:221–218, 1959.

38. Le Shan L, Worthington R: Personality as a factor in the pathogenesis of cancer. A review of the literature. Br J Med Psych 29:49–56, 1956.

39. Lieber L, Plumb MM, Gerstenzang ML, Holland JC: The communication of affection between cancer patients and their spouses. Psychosom Med 38(6):379–389, 1976.

40. Maguire GP: The psychological and social sequelae of mastectomy. *In* Howells JG (ed.): Modern Perspectives in the Psychiatric Aspects of Surgery. NY, Brunei Mayel, 1976, pp 390–421.

41. Maguire GP, Lee EG, Bevington DJ, Küchemann CS, Crabtree RJ, Corwell CE: Psychiatric problems in the first year after mastectomy. Br Med J 1:963–965, 1978.

42. Maguire GP, Tait A, Brooke M, Thomas C, Sellwood R: Effect of counselling on the psychiatric morbidity associated with mastectomy. Br Med J 281:1454–1456, 1980.

43. Maguire GP, Tait A, Brooke M, Thomas C, Howat JM, Sellwood R: Psychiatric morbidity and physical toxicity associated with adjuvant chemotherapy after mastectomy. Br Med J 2:1454–1456, 1980.

44. Mantell JE: Cancer patients' visitor programmes: a case for accountability. J Psychosoc Oncol 1:45–50, 1983.

45. Masters NH, Johnson VE: Human Sexual Inadequacy. Boston, Little, Brown, 1970.

46. McArdle CS, Calman KC, Cooper AF, Hughson AV, Russell AR, Smith DC: The social, emotional, and financial implications of adjuvant chemotherapy in breast cancer. Br J Surg 68:261–264, 1981.

47. McIntosh J: Processes of communication, information seeking and control associated with cancer. A selective review of the literature. Soc Sci Med 8:167–187, 1974.

48. Meyerowitz BE, Watkins IK, Sparks FC: Psychosocial implications of adjuvant chemotherapy. Cancer 52:1541–1545, 1983.

49. Morris T, Greer HS, White P: Psychological and social adjustment to mastectomy (a 2 year follow-up study). Cancer 40(5):2381–2387, 1977.

50. Morrow GR, Morell C: Behavioural treatment for the anticipatory nausea and vomiting induced by cancer chemotherapy. N Engl J Med 301:1476–1480, 1982.

51. Muslin HL, Gyarfus K, Pieper WJ: Separation experience and cancer of the breast. Ann NY Acad Sci 125, 1966, pp 802–806.

52. Newall D, Gadd EM, Priestman TJ: Presentation of information to cancer patients: a comparison of two centres in the UK and USA. Br J Med Psychol 60:127–131, 1987.

53. Novack BH, Plumer R, Smith RL, Ochitill H, Morrow GR, Bennett JM: Changes in physicians attitudes towards telling the cancer patient. JAMA 241(9):897–900, 1979.

53a. Paget J: Surgical Pathology. London, Longmans Green, 1870.

54. Palmer BV, Walsh GA, McKinna JA, Greening WP: Adjuvant chemotherapy for breast cancer: side effects and quality of life. Br Med J 281:1594–1597, 1980.

55. Parliament MB, Danjoux CE, Clayton T: Is cancer treatment toxicity accurately reported? Int J Radiat Oncol 11:603–608, 1985.

56. Parkes CM, Benjamin B, Fitzgerald RG: Broken heart: a statistical study of increased mortality among widowers. Br Med J 1:740–743, 1969.

57. Pfefferbaum B, Pasnau RO, Jamison K, Wellisch DK: A comprehensive program of psychosocial care for mastectomy patients. Int J Psych Med 8:63–71, 1978.

58. Priestman TJ, Priestman SG, Bradshaw C: Stress and breast cancer. Br J Cancer 51:493–498, 1985.

59. Priestman TJ, Baum M: Evaluation of quality of life in patients receiving treatment for advanced breast cancer. Lancet i:899–901, 1976.

60. Renneker R, Cutler M: Psychological problems of adjustment to cancer of the breast. JAMA 148:833–838, 1952.

61. Rowland J, et al: Psychological response to breast reconstruction. Syllab Sci Proc Am Psych Assoc, 1984, 39(suppl 142):301, 1984.

62. Sanger CK, Reznikoff M: A comparison of the psychological effects of breast-saving procedures with the modified radical mastectomy. Cancer 48:2341–2346, 1981.

63. Schain W: Psychosocial and physical outcomes of stage I breast cancer therapy: mastectomy v. excisional biopsy and irradiation. Br Cancer Res Treat 3:377–382, 1983.

64. Schain W, Wellisch DK, Pasnau RO, Landsverk J: The sooner the better: a study of psychological factors in women undergoing immediate versus delayed breast reconstruction. Am J Psychiatr 142(1):40–46, 1985.

65. Schmale AH, Iker HP: The effect of hopelessness and the development of cancer. Psychosom Med 28:716–721, 1966.

66. Schmale AH, Iker HP: Hopelessness as a predictor of cervical cancer. Soc Sci Med 5:95–100, 1971.

67. Schonfield J: Psychological and life-experience differences between Israeli women with benign and cancerous breast lesions. J Psych Res 19:225–234, 1975.

68. Scott DW: Anxiety, critical thinking and information processing during and after breast biopsy. Nursing Res 32:24–29, 1983.

69. Silberfarb PL, Maurer LH, Crouthamel CS: Psychosocial aspects of neoplastic disease I: functional status of breast cancer patients during different treatment regimens. Am J Psychiatr 137:450–455, 1980.

70. Snell L, Graham S: Social trauma as related to cancer of the breast. Br J Cancer 25:721–734, 1971.

71. Snow HL: Cancer and the Cancer Process. London, Churchill, 1893.

72. Sobel HJ, Worden JW: Helping cancer patients to cope: a problem solving intervention program for health care professionals. New York, BMA Audio Cassettes, Division of Guildford Publications, 1982.

73. Steinberg MD, Juliano MA, Wise L: Psychological outcome of lumpectomy versus mastectomy in the treatment of breast cancer. Am J Psychiatr 142(1):34–39, 1985.

74. Stockwell F: The Unpopular Patient. London, RCN, 1972.

75. Tarrier N, Maguire P, Kincey J: Locus of control and cognitive therapy in mastectomy patients. Br J Med Psychol 56:265–268, 1983.

76. Totman R: What makes "life-events" stressful? A retrospective study of patients who suffered a first myocardial infarction. J Psychosom Res 23:193, 1979.

77. Wabrek AJ, Wabrek CJ: Mastectomy: sexual implications. Primary Care 3:803–810, 1976.

78. Watson M: Psychosocial intervention with cancer patients: a review. Psychol Med 13:839–846, 1983.

79. Wellisch DK, Jamison KR, Pasnau RO: Psychosocial aspects of mastectomy II: the man's perspective. Am J Psychiatr 135(5):543–546, 1978.

80. Williams EM, et al: Delay in the presentation of women with breast disease. Clin Oncol 2:327–331, 1976.

81. Witkin MH: Psychosexual counselling of the mastectomy patient. J Sex Marit Ther 4:20–28, 1982.

82. Worden JW, Weisman AD: Psychosocial components of lagtime in cancer diagnosis. J Psychosom Res 19:69–79, 1975.

Index